Metabolic Drug Interactions

Metabolic Drug Interactions

Editors

René H. Levy, Ph.D.
*Professor
Department of Pharmaceutics
and Neurologic Surgery
University of Washington
Seattle, Washington*

Kenneth E. Thummel, Ph.D.
*Associate Professor
Department of Pharmaceutics
University of Washington
Seattle, Washington*

William F. Trager, Ph.D.
*Professor
Department of Medicinal Chemistry
University of Washington
Seattle, Washington*

Philip D. Hansten, Pharm. D.
*Professor
Department of Pharmacy
University of Washington
Seattle, Washington*

Michel Eichelbaum, M.D.
*Professor and Chairman
Department of Clinical Pharmacology
Eberhard-Karls-University
Tubingen, Germany
Director
Dr. Margarete Fischer-Bosch Institute
of Clinical Pharmacology
Stuttgart, Germany*

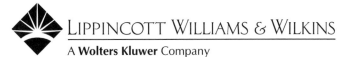

LIPPINCOTT WILLIAMS & WILKINS
A **Wolters Kluwer** Company
Philadelphia · Baltimore · New York · London
Buenos Aires · Hong Kong · Sydney · Tokyo

Acquisitions Editor: Anne M. Sydor
Developmental Editor: Pamela Sutton
Production Editor: Tony DeGeorge
Manufacturing Manager: Tim Reynolds
Cover Designer: David Levy
Compositor: Lippincott Williams & Wilkins Desktop Division
Printer: Maple Press

© 2000 by LIPPINCOTT WILLIAMS & WILKINS
530 Walnut Street
Philadelphia, PA 19106 USA
LWW.com

Printed in the USA

Library of Congress Cataloging-in-Publication Data
Metabolic drug interactions / René H. Levy...[et al.].
   p. ; cm.
   Includes bibliographical references and indexes.
   ISBN 0-7817-1441-9 (alk. paper)
   1. Drug interactions. 2. Drugs—Metabolism. I. Levy, René H.
   [DNLM: 1. Drug Interactions. 2. Metabolism—drug effects. QU 38 M587 2000]
   RM302.M48 2000
   615′.7045—dc21
                                                                99-056725

10 9 8 7 6 5 4 3 2 1

Contents

Section I: Prediction of Drug Interactions From *In Vitro* Studies: Basic Principles

Section II: Enzymes and Transporters

Section III: Drugs As Substrates of Metabolic Enzymes
Treatment of CNS Diseases

Treatment of Cardiovascular Diseases

Treatment of Microbial Diseases

Treatment of Inflammation

Treatment of Other Diseases

**Section IV: Drugs as Inhibitors of Metabolic Enzymes
Treatment of CNS Diseases**

Treatment of Cardiovascular Diseases

Contributing Authors

Susan M. Abel-Rahman, Pharm.D.
Assistant Professor
Departments of Pharmacy and Pediatrics
University of Missouri, Kansas City
2411 Holmes Street, M3-C19
Kansas City, Missouri 64108; and
Departments of Clinical Pharmacology and
  Experimental Therapeutics
Children's Mercy Hospital
2401 Gillham Road, HHC-600
Kansas City, Missouri 64108

Gail D. Anderson, Ph.D
Associate Professor
Department of Pharmacy
University of Washington
Box 357630, H375 Health Sciences Building
Seattle, Washington 98195-7630

J. Malcolm O. Arnold, M.D.
Departments of Medicine and Pharmacology
  and Toxicology
University of Western Ontario
London, Ontario; and
Research Scientist
Department of Medicine
London Health Sciences Centre
Victoria Campus
375 South Street
London, Ontario N6A 4G5 Canada

Janne T. Backman, M.D.
Research Associate
Department of Clinical Pharmacology
University of Helsinki
Haartmaninkatu 4
FIN-00290 Helsinki, Finland

David G. Bailey, B.Sc.Pharm., Ph.D.
Associate Professor
Departments of Medicine and Pharmacology
  and Toxicology
University of Western Ontario
London, Ontario; and
Research Scientist
Department of Medicine
London Health Sciences Centre
Victoria Campus
375 South Street
London, Ontario N6A 4G5 Canada

Theo K. Bammler, Ph.D
Research Scientist
Department of Environmental Health
University of Washington
4225 Roosevelt Way NE, Suite 100
Seattle, Washington 98195-7610

Christopher Banfield, MD
Department of Drug Metabolism and
  Pharmacokinetics
Schering-Plough Research Institute
2015 Galloping Hill Road
Kenilworth, New Jersey 07033

Donald J. Birkett, Ph.D.
Professor and Head
Department of Clinical Pharmacology
Flinders University
Adeleaid, South Australia 5000 Australia; and
Head
Flinders Medical Center
Bedford Park, South Australia 5042, Australia

William R. Brian, Ph.D.
Assistant Director
Departments of Clinical Metabolism and
*   Pharmokinetics*
Sanofi-Synthelabo Research
9 Great Valley Parkway
Malvern, Pennsylvania 19355

Kim Brøsen, M.D., Ph.D.
Professor
Institute of Public Health
Department.of Clinical Pharmacology
University of Southern Denmark
Odense University
Winslowparken 19
DK-5000 Odense; and
Consultant
Clinical Chemistry Department (KKA)
Odense University Hospital
Søndre Boulevard 29
DK-5000 Odense, Denmark

Dagmar Busse, M.D.
Clinical Pharmacologist
Dr. Margarete Fischer-Bosch Institute for
*   Clinical Pharmacology*
Auerbachstrasse 112
D-70376 Stuttgart, Germany

Susan P. Carpenter, Ph.D.
Postdoctoral Research Fellow
Puracyp
505 Coast Boulevard South
La Jolla, California 92037

Kan Chiba, Ph.D.
Professor
Department of Pharmaceutical Sciences
Chiba University
1-33 Yayoi-cho, Inage-Ku
Chiba-shi, Chiba 263-8522 Japan

Robert P. Clement, Ph.D.
Director
Department of Drug Metabolism and
*   Pharmacokinetics*
Schering-Plough Research Institute
2015 Galloping Hill Road
Kenilworth, New Jersey 07033-1300

Jerry M. Collins, Ph.D.
Director
Laboratory of Clinical Pharmacology
Food and Drug Administration
4 Research Court, Room 314
Rockville, Maryland 20850

Barry J. Cusack, M.D.
Associate Professor
Clinical Pharmacology and Gerontology
*   Research Unit*
Department of Veterans Affairs Medical Center
*   (111) and Mountain States Medical Research*
*   Institute*
500 W. Fort Street
Boise, Idaho 83702

C. Lindsay DeVane, Pharm.D.
Professor of Psychiatry and Behavioral
*   Sciences*
Medical University of South Carolina
67 President Street
Charleston, South Carolina 29425-0742

Tina M. deVries, Ph.D.
Senior Director
Department of Research and Development
Warner Chilcott Laboratories
100 Enterprise Drive, Suite 280
Rockaway, New Jersey 07866

David L. Eaton, Ph.D.
Professor
Department of Environmental Health
University of Washington
4225 Roosevelt Way NE, Suite 100
Seattle, Washington 98195-7610

David J. Edwards, Pharm.D.
Associate Professor
Pharmacy Practice
College of Pharmacy and Allied Health
*   Professions*
Wayne University
1400 Chrysler Drive
Detroit, Michigan 48202

Michel Eichelbaum, M.D.
Professor and Chairman
Department of Clinical Pharmacology
Eberhard-Karls-University
Tubingen, Germany; and
Director
Dr. Margarete Fischer-Bosch Institute of
*   Clinical Pharmacology*
Auerbachstrasse 12
D-70376 Stuttgart, Germany

Maurice G. Emery, Pharm.D., Ph.D.
Senior Research Pharmacologist
Department of Metabolism, Radiochemistry,
*   and Cellular Toxicity*
Abbott Laboratories
Building AP9-LL, 100 Abbott Park Road
Abbott Park, Illinois 60064

Volker Fischer, Ph.D.
Director
Department of Drug Metabolism and
*   Pharmacokineticcs*
Novartis Institute for Biomedical Research
59 Route 10
East Hanover, New Jersey 07936-1080

Martin F. Fromm, M.D.
Clinical Pharmacologist
Dr. Margarete Fischer-Bosch Institute of
*   Clinical Pharmacology*
Auerbachstrasse 112
D-70376 Stuttgart, Germany

S. Thomas Forgue, Ph.D
Research Scientist
Lilly Laboratory for Clinical Research
550 North University Boulevard
Indianapolis, Indiana 46202

Michael Goldberg, M.D., Ph.D.
Adjunct Research Professor of
*   Medicine*
Department of Clinical Pharmacology
Thomas Jefferson University School of
*   Medicine*
132 South 10th Street
Philadelphia, Pennsylvania 19107-5244; and
Senior Director, Scientific Staff
Department of Clinical
*   Pharmacology*
Merck Research Laboratories
10 Sentry Parkway
Blue Bell, Pennsylvania 19422

Mitchell D. Green, M.S.
Senior Research Assistant
Department of Pharmacology
University of Iowa
2-511 Bowen Science Building
Iowa City, Iowa 52242

David J. Greenblatt, M.D.
Professor and Chairman
Department of Pharmacology and Experimental
*   Therapeutics*
Tufts University School of Medicine
136 Harrison Avenue
Boston, Massachusetts 02111; and
Program Director
General Clinical Research Center
New England Medical Center
Boston, Massachusetts 02111

Robert L. Haining, Ph.D.
Research Assistant Professor
Department of Medical Chemistry
University of Washington
Box 357610
Seattle, Washington 98195

Stephen D. Hall, Ph.D.
Professor
Department of Medicine
Indiana University
Indianapolis, Indiana 46202; and
Co-director
Department of Clinical Pharmacology
Indiana University School of Medicine
Wishard Memorial Hospital
OPW 320, 1001 W. 10th Street
Indianapolis, Indiana 46202

Philip D. Hansten, Pharm. D.
Professor
Department of Pharmacy
University of Washington
1959 NE Pacific Street
Seattle, Washington 98195-7610

Mary F. Hebert, Pharm. D.
Associate Professor
Department of Pharmacy
University of Washington
Box 357630, H375 Health Sciences Building
Seattle, Washington 98195-7610

John R. Horn, Pharm. D.
Department of Pharmacy
University of Washington
Box 357630, H375 Health Sciences Building
Seattle, Washington 98195-7610

Yves Horsmans, M.D., Ph.D.
Professor
Department of Gastroenterology
Catholic University of Louvain; and
Associate
Department of Gastroenterology
Cliniques Universitaires St. Luc
10 Avenue Hippocrate
Brussels 1200 Belgium

Andra E. Ibrahim, M.D.
Assistant Professor
Department of Anesthesiology
University of Washington
1959 NE Pacific, Box 356540
Seattle, Washington 98195-6540

Graham R. Jang, Ph.D.
Research Investigator
Department of Metabolism and
  Pharmokinetics
Bristol-Meyers Squibb
Pharmaceutical Research Institute
P.O. Box 4000
Princeton, New Jersey 08543-4000

David R. Jones, Ph.D.
Assistant Scientist
Department of Medicine
Division of Clinical Pharmacology
Indiana University School of Medicine
Wishard Memorial Hospital
OPW 320, 1001 W. 10th Street
Indianapolis, Indiana 46220

Evan D. Kharasch, M.D., Ph.D.
Professor
Department of Anesthesiology
University of Washington
1959 N.E. Pacific Street, Box 356540
Seattle, Washington 98195-6540; and
Anesthesiology Service
Puget Sound Veterans Affairs Medical Center
Seattle, Washington 98108

Kari T. Kivistö, MD
Assistant Professor
Department of Clinical Pharmacology
University of Helsinki
Haartmaninkatu 4
FIN-00290 Helsinki, Finland

Kaoru Kobayashi, Ph.D
Research Associate
Laboratory of Biochemical Pharmacology and
  Toxicology
Department of Pharmaceutical Sciences
Chiba University
1-33 Yayoi-cho, Inage-ku
Chiba-shi, Chiba 263-8522 Japan

Dennis R. Koop, Ph.D.
Associate Professor
Department of Physiology and Pharmacology
Oregon Health Sciences University
3181 SW Sam Jackson Park Road
Portland, Oregon 97201

Kent L. Kunze, Ph.D.
Department of Medicinal Chemistry
University of Washington
Box 357610, H164 Health
  Sciences Building
Seattle, Washington 98195

Ronald M. Laethem, Ph.D.
Research Investigator
Department of Bioanalysis and Drug
  Metabolism
Glaxo Wellcome Inc.
3030 Cornwallis Road
Research Triangle Park, North Carolina 27709

J. Steven Leeder, Pharm.D., Ph.D.
Associate Professor
Department of Pediatrics
University of Missouri, Kansas City
Kansas City, Missouri 64108; and
Director, Clinical Pharmacology
  Laboratory
Department of Clinical Pharmacology and
  Toxicology
Children's Mercy Hospital
2401 Gilham Road
Kansas City, Missouri 64108-4698

Martin S. Lennard
Reader
Section of Molecular Pharmacology and
  Pharmacogenetics
Division of Clinical Sciences (CSUHT)
University of Sheffield
The Royal Hallamshire Hospital (L Floor)
Glossop Road
Sheffield S10 2JF United Kingdom

René H. Levy, Ph.D.
Chair and Professor
Department of Pharmaceutics
Professor
Department of Neurological Surgery
University of Washington
Box 357610, H272 Health
  Sciences Building
Seattle, Washington 98195-7610

Soraya Madani, Ph.D.
Pharmacokinetics Reviewer
Center for Drug Evaluation and
  Research
Food and Drug Administration
5600 Fishers Lane—HFD 870
Rockville, Maryland 20857

James B. Mangold, Ph.D.
Department of Drug Metabolism and
  Pharmacokinetics
Novartis Pharmaceuticals
59 Route 10
East Hanover, New Jersey 07936

John S. Markowitz, Pharm.D.
Assistant Professor
Department of Pharmaceutical Sciences
College of Pharmacy; and
Clinical Coordinator
Department of Pharmacy
Medical University of South Carolina
171 Ashley Avenue
Charleston, South Carolina 29425

Gary G. Mather
CEDRA Corporation
8609 Cross Park Drive
Austin, Texas 78754

Patrick J. P. Maurel, Ph.D.
Directeur de Recherche
INSERM U128
IFR24
1919 Route de Mende
34293 Montpellier, France

Ross A. McKinnon, B.Pharm., Ph.D.
Senior Lecturer
School of Pharmacy and
   Medical Sciences
University of South Australia
North Terrace
Adelaide, South Austrialia 5000 Australia

John O. Miners, Ph.D.
Professor
Department of Clinical Pharmacology
Flinders University School of Medicine and
   Flinders Medical Centre
Bedford Park
Adelaide, South Australia 5042 Australia

Michael Murray, Ph.D., D.Sc.
Head
Molecular Pharmacologic Unit
Heart Research Institute
Missenden Road
Campertown, New South Wales 2050 Australia

Sidney D. Nelson, Ph.D.
Professor
Department of Medicinal Chemistry
Dean
School of Pharmacy
University of Washington
Box 357631, H375 Health
   Sciences Building
Seattle, Washington 98195-7610

Pertti J. Neuvonen, M.D., Ph.D.
Professor and Chairman
Department of Clinical Pharmacology
University of Helsinki; and
Head Physician
Department of Clinical
   Pharmacology
Helsinki University Central Hospital
Haartmaninkatu 4
FIN-00290 Helsinki, Finland

Curtis J. Omiecinski, Ph.D.
Professor
Department of Environmental Health
University of Washington
4225 Roosevelt Way NE
Seattle, Washington 98105-6099

Mary F. Paine, Ph.D.
Research Assistant Professor
Division of Pharmacology
School of Pharmacy
University of North Carolina
CB #7360 Beard Hall
Chapel Hill, North Carolina 27599-7360; and
General Clinical Research Center
University of North Carolina Hospitals
101 Manning Drive
Chapel Hill, North Carolina 27599-7600

Ronald E. Polk, Pharm. D.
Professor of Pharmacy and Medicine
School of Pharmacy
Virginia Commonwealth University
410 North 12th Street, Smith Building
Richmond, Virginia 23298-0581

J. Robert Powell, Pharm. D.
Parke Davis
2800 Plymouth Road
Ann Arbor, Michigan 48105

Sheldon H. Preskorn, M.D.
Psychiatric Research Institute
Department of Psychiatry
University of Kansas
School of Medicine
1010 North Kansas
Wichita, Kansas 67214-2878

Michael P. Pritchard, Ph.D.
Biomedical Research Centre
University of Dundee
Level 5
Ninewells Hospital and Medical School
Dundee DD1 9SY United Kingdom

Rebecca B. Raftogianis, Ph.D.
Associate Member
Department of Pharmacology
Fox Chase Cancer Center
7701 Burholme Avenue
Philadelphia, Pennsylvania 19111

Judy Raucy, Ph.D.
Staff Scientist
La Jolla Institute for Experimental Medicine
505 Coast Boulevard South, Suite 412
La Jolla, California 92037

Allan E. Rettie, Ph.D.
Professor
Department of Medicinal Chemistry
Dean
School of Pharmacy
University of Washington
Box 357610, H172 Health Sciences Building
Seattle, Washington 98195

Barbara J. Ring, M.S.
Associate Senior Toxicologist
Department of Drug Disposition
Eli Lilly & Company
Lilly Corporate Center, Mail Drop 0825
Indianapolis, Indiana 46285

John B. Schenkman, Ph.D.
Professor
Department of Pharmacology
University of Connecticut Health Center
263 Farmington Avenue
Farmington, Connecticut 06070

Cosette J. Serabjit-Singh, Ph.D.
Director
Departments of Science Development,
  Bioanalysis and Drug Metabolism
Glaxo Wellcome Inc.
5 Moore Drive
Research Triangle Park, North Carolina 27709

Mujeeb U. Shad, M.D.
Senior Psychopharmacology Fellow
Departments of Psychiatry and Behavioral
  Sciences
University of Kansas School of Medicine
Wichita and Psychiatric Research Institute
1010 North Kansas
Wichita, Kansas 67214-2878

Danny D. Shen, Ph.D.
Professor
Departments of Pharmaceutics and Pharmacy
University of Washington
Box 357610, H272 Health Sciences Building
Seattle, Washington 98195-7610

Jeffrey A. Silverman, Ph.D.
Director
Department of Molecular and Cellular Biology
AvMax Inc.
385 Oysterpoint Boulevard, Building 9A
South San Francisco, California 94080

John T. Slattery, Ph.D.
Department of Pharmaceutics
University of Washington
Box 357610, H272 Health Sciences Building
Seattle, Washington 98195-7610

J. David Spence, M.D., F.R.C.P.C., M.B.A.
Professor
Clinical Neruological Sciences, Internal
  Medicine, and Pharmacology
University of Western Ontario; and
Director
Stroke Prevention and Artherosclerosis
  Research Centre
Siebens-Drake/Robarts Research Institute
1400 Western Road
London, Ontario N6G 2V2 Canada

Thomas R. Tephly, M.D., Ph.D.
Professor
Department of Pharmacology
University of Iowa
2-512 Bowen Science Building
Iowa City, Iowa 52242

Kenneth E. Thummel, Ph.D.
Associate Professor
Department of Pharmaceutics
University of Washington
Box 357610, H272 Health Sciences
  Building
Seattle, Washington 98195-7610

Timothy S. Tracy, Ph.D.
Associate Professor
Basic Pharmaceutical Sciences
West Virginia University
P.O. Box 9530
Morgantown, West Virginia 26506-9530

William F. Trager, Ph.D.
Professor
Department of Medicinal Chemistry
University of Washington
Box 357610, H172 Health Sciences Building
Seattle, Washington 98195-7610

Jashvant D. Unadkat, Ph.D.
Professor
Department of Pharmaceutics
University of Washington
Box 357610, H272 Health Sciences Building
Seattle, Washington 98195-7610

Robert E. Vestal, M.D.
Senior Medical Director
Early Clinical Development
Covance Incorporated
2121 N. California Boulevard, Suite 500
Walnut Creek, California 94596; and
Clinical Professor
Department of Medicine
University of Washington School of Medicine
Seattle, Washington 98195

Lisa L. von Moltke, M.D.
Research Assistant Professor
Department of Pharmacology and Experimental
  Therapeutics
Tufts University School of Medicine
136 Harrison Avenue
Boston, Massachusetts 02111; and
Associate Staff Physician
Department of Medicine
New England Medical Center
Boston, Massachusetts 02111

Jun-Sheng Wang, M.D.
Research Associate
Department of Clinical Pharmacology
University of Helsinki
Haartmaninkatu 4
FIN-00290 Helsinki, Finland

Yi Wang, Ph.D.
Senior Fellow
Department of Pharmaceutics
University of Washington
Box 357610, H272 Health Sciences
  Building
Seattle, Washington 98195-7610

Richard M. Weinshilboum, M.D.
Professor
Department of Pharmacology
Mayo Medical School
200 First Street, SW
Rochester, Minnesota 55905

C. Roland Wolf, Ph.D.
Professor/Director
Biomedical Research Centre
University of Dundee
Level 5
Ninewells Hospital and
  Medical School
Dundee DD1 9SY Scotland, United Kingdom

Steven A. Wrighton, Ph.D.
Research Advisor
Department of Drug Disposition
Eli Lilly & Company
Lilly Corporate Center,
  Mail Drop 0825
Indianapolis, Indiana 46285

Ulrich M. Zanger, Ph.D.
Staff Scientist
Dr. Margarete Fischer-Bosch
  Institute of Clinical
  Pharmacology
Auerbachstrasse 112
D-70376 Stuttgart, Germany

Foreword

Until about a decade ago, practicing physicians had little or no interest in understanding the enzyme systems responsible for the metabolism of the drugs they prescribed. The characterization of these enzymes and the interactions affecting them was considered an esoteric job of a small group of laboratory scientists, and the wealth of information that was being generated in these studies failed to produce any major impact on general prescribing. As is often the case in the history of medical progress, it took an epidemic of therapeutic disasters to alert physicians to the practical implications of knowledge considered up to that point to be largely of academic interest. The discovery in the early 1990s that inhibition of cytochrome CYP3A4 isoenzymes was involved in the appearance of serious cardiac toxicity in patients taking antihistamine or prokinetic drugs in combination with certain antibiotics or antifungals was instrumental in creating an unprecedented awareness of the value of *in vitro* studies for the prediction of clinically important metabolic drug interactions.

Interest in the variability of drug metabolizing enzymes was also stimulated by the explosion of studies on genetically determined drug oxidation polymorphisms, and by the development of refined methodological tools in molecular biology. Drug regulatory agencies and pharmaceutical companies were quick to realize the potential value of these studies in promoting a safer use of existing drugs, and in designing even better drugs for the future. More importantly, this awareness started to spread among medical practitioners and to be applied in routine clinical management. This initiated a gradual but irreversible shift in the approach to drug interactions, away from the "telephone directory" philosophy (i.e., the poorly digestible memorization of long lists of potentially dangerous drug combinations) to a new approach whereby interactions are predicted and understood on the basis of few, simple mechanistic concepts. In some specialties, such as psychiatry, treating physicians sometimes even surpass pharmacologists in their knowledge of substrates, inducers, and inhibitors of the isozymes involved in the biotransformation of the most commonly prescribed medications. In other specialties, this acquisition process has been slower, but it is occurring at an increasingly faster pace.

Exploitation of existing knowledge in this area has been hampered by the lack of an up-to-date publication collating the myriad data that accumulated over the years in a structured format. Dr. Levy and his co-editors should be praised for undertaking the daunting task of filling this deficiency. The results of their effort are superb. Thanks to the contribution of an impressive panel of leading experts from all over the world, *Metabolic Drug Interactions* provides a unique and rational approach to understanding the enzymes responsible for drug metabolism in humans, the factors involved in their expression and regulation, the medications which may affect their activity and the underlying mechanisms, and, most importantly, the implications of this knowledge from the academic, industrial, regulatory, and therapeutic viewpoints. The first part of the book deals with general aspects such as principles and mechanisms of metabolically-based drug interactions, the use of *in vitro* data to predict interactions *in vivo*, and the classification and characteristics of the different drug metabolizing enzyme systems. The central chapters deal with therapeutic classes of drugs and provide up-to-date reviews of the capacity of individual drugs within each class to act as substrates, inhibitors, or inducers of specific enzymes. The last section takes a critical look at the implications of these data regarding prediction and management of clinically important drug interactions. Comprehensive lists of references at the end of each chapter provide invaluable guidance to the reader seeking more specialized information. Because of its unique format, the book will be useful not only to scientists involved in research on drug metabolism and drug interactions, but also to clinical pharmacists and to clinicians striving for more rational drug prescribing. Filling the gap between basic science and clinical practice was surely a major objective in the planning of this book, and it has been accomplished admirably.

Emilio Perucca, M.D., Ph.D.

Preface

*Each year, large numbers of new drug-drug interactions are discovered, precluding the possibility that any prescriber could memorize them all.**

Since the early days of clinical pharmacology, caregivers could only rely on memorization of pairs of interacting drugs to identify patients at risk of receiving drug interactions. In the last decade, a paradigm shift has occurred in our understanding. Advances in the molecular biology of cytochromes P450 and other enzymes highlighted the usefulness of *in vitro* methodologies in the study of human drug metabolism. Based on such studies, it became possible to make valuable inferences on the likelihood of clinical drug interactions. Within a few years, scientists from academia, industry, and regulatory agencies developed prediction rules for any drug based on knowledge of isozymes involved in its metabolism and its inhibition/induction spectra.

In 1997 the Food and Drug Administration and the European Agency for the Evaluation of Medicinal Products issued new guidelines to stipulate the need for *in vitro* drug interaction studies and to define how results from such studies could be used for "class labeling." This type of information is now considered an intrinsic part of the safety assessment of any new drug and is included in reference texts for clinicians, such as the *Physicians' Desk Reference*.

Also within the last few years, the public has been sensitized by the popular media to the issue of drug interactions by a succession of events: several fatal interactions were reported, studies showed that dangerous drug combinations continue to be dispensed, and some drugs were withdrawn from the market based on drug interaction potential. The resulting increased expectations placed on practitioners, as well as the expansion of this body of knowledge, created the need for a reference text focused on the scientific basis of metabolic drug interactions. This volume represents an attempt to organize and synthesize the literature on metabolic drug interactions and to present it for use by clinicians and scientists. The information is organized as follows:

Section I presents the basic rules of interpretation of *in vitro* data from the academic, industrial, and regulatory perspectives.
Section II presents metabolic enzymes and transporters.
Section III discusses drugs as substrates of metabolic enzymes and is arranged by therapeutic class:
    Central nervous system diseases;
    Cardiovascular diseases;
    Microbial diseases;
    Inflammation;
    Other.
Section IV discusses drugs as inhibitors of metabolic enzymes and is arranged by therapeutic class:
    Central nervous system diseases;
    Cardiovascular diseases;
    Microbial diseases;
    Other.
Section V discusses drugs as inducers of metabolic enzymes.
Section VI is devoted to the identification of patients at special risk of drug interactions.

Sections III, IV, and V are the core of this book. Within these sections, the reader can find specific drug interactions by searching the contents by disease category and therapeutic drug class of interest.

---

*Guidance for Industry, USFDA, April 1997.

When a therapeutic class is not represented, the reader is referred to the Appendix, which includes recently approved drugs for which limited information on metabolism is available. Another approach finding specific interactions is to consult the Drug Interaction Index, which has been carefully constructed for this purpose.

This book was a "work in progress" for over one year in 1998 and 1999. During that period, the field continued to expand at an accelerating pace. We have made every effort to include the most current information. However, as the field continues to move ahead while we produce the book, it is not possible to include every recent advance. We plan to address this by updating the book frequently, and we welcome all comments and criticisms.

The Editors

Acknowledgments

We are greatly indebted to the eminent cast of authors for undertaking the challenge of synthesizing *in vitro* and *in vivo* data for each therapeutic class. We are even more thankful to them after seeing the result of their work as a composite product. We wish to express our gratitude to Mr. Brian Rasmussen for his excellent editorial skills and coordination throughout all phases of this endeavor. We also thank the staff of Lippincott Williams & Wilkins, and particularly Dr. Anne Sydor, who provided personal attention and superior leadership from concept to product.

SECTION I

Prediction of Drug Interactions from *In Vitro* Studies: Basic Principles

CHAPTER 1

Metabolically-Based Drug–Drug Interactions: Principles and Mechanisms

Kenneth E. Thummel, Kent L. Kunze, and Danny D. Shen

HISTORICAL CONTEXT

The characterization of drug–drug interactions has been a standard part of drug development programs for the past two decades. Before release to the general public, a new drug entity (NDE) must be tested for its ability to modulate the pharmacokinetic or pharmacodynamic effects of coprescribed medications, and for the reverse effects of these established medications on the NDE. Many clinically important drug–drug interactions involve the modulation of drug metabolism or transport processes. However, until recently, there has been only limited emphasis placed on understanding and predicting the scope and mechanism of metabolically or transport-based drug interactions during the period of new drug development. Decades ago, pharmacotherapy encompassed a limited number of drug products, and most had a relatively large therapeutic range. Clinically significant drug–drug interactions were uncommon and studies between the NDE and existing therapeutic agents were generally restricted to drugs, such as warfarin and theophylline, with a narrow therapeutic index and proven susceptibility to metabolic inhibition or induction. In general, interaction studies with an NDE were performed without much regard for the mechanistic basis for the interaction, resulting in much information on negative interactions and little specific guidance on the type of drugs that ought not be administered together with the NDE.

K. E. Thummel: Department of Pharmaceutics, University of Washington, Box 357610 H272 Health Sciences Building, Seattle, Washington 98195

K. L. Kunze: Department of Medicinal Chemistry, University of Washington, Box 357610 H164 Health Sciences Building, Seattle, Washington 98195

D. D. Shen: Departments of Pharmaceutics and Pharmacy, University of Washington, Box 357610 H272 Health Sciences Building, Seattle, Washington 98195

With the recent acceleration in drug development and the tremendous expansion in the number of potent and potentially toxic drugs, the need for rational design of interaction studies and a better understanding of interaction mechanisms has become essential. Much of this new emphasis occurred in response to the discovery of potentially fatal, metabolically based interactions between the first nonsedating antihistamine, terfenadine, and widely prescribed antifungal and antibiotic agents. Terfenadine undergoes extensive first pass metabolism to an active (H_1 antagonist) metabolite. The bioactivation reaction is catalyzed by the hepatic and intestinal enzyme CYP3A4 (1). It was discovered, after marketing, that profound inhibition of CYP3A4 by some azole antifungal agents (e.g., ketoconazole) and macrolide antibiotics (e.g., erythromycin) (2) resulted in the accumulation of terfenadine to plasma levels much higher than that seen under monotherapy, eliciting an undesired blockade of cardiac K^+ channels and a potentially life-threatening prolongation of the QTc interval (3–5). Although not every individual who received terfenadine along with ketoconazole or erythromycin experienced an adverse interaction, all were put at some level of risk, contributing to the eventual withdrawal of the drug from the US market.

It has been argued that a careful preclinical characterization of the enzymes catalyzing terfenadine metabolism and identification of the drugs that could modulate that process, would have allowed clinicians to anticipate and avoid adverse drug interactions. Certainly, the frequency of the interaction between terfenadine and potent CYP3A4 inhibitors in the population was greatly reduced by heightened awareness and a black box warning on the package labeling (6). However, without prior knowledge of the cardiovascular effects of terfenadine, it would have been difficult to appreciate the toxicologic importance of the inhibitory metabolic interaction. In addition, the interactions might never have been avoided entirely given human error with prescription practices.

What should be done with prospectively generated drug–drug interaction data? In every case, some level of cost-benefit analysis must be considered. In some circumstances, an interaction may be an unavoidable part of effective and indispensable therapy in the absence of alternative medications. This is currently the case for the human immunodeficiency virus (HIV)-1 protease inhibitors, which are potent inhibitors of CYP3A that can adversely alter the metabolic clearance of numerous drugs, including important comedicants (7) (see Chapter 31). In contrast, for mibefradil, a recently withdrawn calcium channel antagonist (8), serious adverse interactions were deemed unacceptable given the treatment population and the availability of therapeutic alternatives (9). Although it may never be possible to arrive at an unambiguous cost-benefit analysis before drug approval, a clear understanding of the potential frequency and magnitude of the problem should facilitate the drug development process and improve patient safety. This chapter presents basic principles and mechanisms of metabolically based drug–drug interactions and pharmacokinetic approaches for *in vivo* predictions based on *in vitro*–derived kinetic data.

MECHANISMS OF DRUG–DRUG INTERACTIONS

The ability to probe the mechanism of a metabolic drug–drug interaction has improved tremendously in recent years, primarily because of the availability of new molecular and analytic tools and a greatly expanded knowledge of the biochemistry of drug metabolism processes. Although metabolic drug interactions may occur with any one of the numerous drug-metabolizing enzymes, the majority are associated with the cytochrome P450 family of enzymes. Recent reviews on the biochemistry and molecular mechanisms of cytochrome P450–catalyzed biotransformations are available (10–12) and are also presented in Chapters 5 through 12.

For simplicity, it is assumed that the conversion of substrate to product is catalyzed by a single enzyme and can be described kinetically by the Michaelis-Menten equation (Equation 1-1), where v is the rate of product formation (or substrate disappearance if eliminated by a single enzyme), S is the substrate concentration, V_{max} is the maximal velocity of the reaction (also, $k_{cat} \cdot E_{total}$), and K_m is the Michaelis constant representing the concentration of substrate that results in half-maximal velocity.

$$S + E \underset{k_{-1}}{\overset{k_1}{\rightleftharpoons}} ES \xrightarrow{k_{cat}} E + P$$

$$v = \frac{V_{max} \cdot S}{K_m + S} \qquad [1\text{-}1]$$

More complex scenarios may influence the magnitude of a drug–drug interaction *in vivo* (discussed in more detail in later paragraphs). They include the formation of a major metabolite from more than one enzyme, formation of multiple products by one or more enzymes and nonenzymatic processes of drug elimination. Moreover, enzymatic reactions may exhibit nonhyperbolic kinetics *in vitro*, a phenomenon that has been associated with CYP3A4- and CYP2C9-catalyzed reactions (13,14). Mathematic treatment of nonhyperbolic drug metabolism kinetics and drug–drug interactions is complex and has been presented elsewhere (14). In this chapter, reversible, metabolically based drug interactions are represented as a modification of the hyperbolic relationship between v and S (15).

Enzyme Inhibition

Reversible Inhibition

Enzyme inhibition is the most frequently encountered form of metabolically based drug–drug interaction. It can occur by mechanisms that range from rapidly reversible, to slowly reversible, to irreversible. Competitive inhibition involves a mutually exclusive competition between the binding of substrate or inhibitor for the catalytic site of the enzyme of interest. As described by Equation 1-2 the reaction velocity, or $v_{(i)}$, is a function of the concentration of substrate (S) and inhibitor (I) at the enzyme active site and their respective affinities (K_m for substrate and K_i for inhibitor) for binding to the enzyme.

$$v_{(i)} = \frac{V_{max} \cdot S}{K_m(1 + I/K_i) + S} \qquad [1\text{-}2]$$

Conceptually, the competitive inhibitor increases the concentration of substrate necessary to reach half-maximal velocity, yielding an apparently higher K_m at any given concentration of inhibitor.

For reversible noncompetitive inhibition (Equation 1-3), substrate and inhibitor binding to the enzyme are not mutually exclusive.

$$v_{(i)} = \frac{\left(\dfrac{V_{max}}{1 + I/K_i}\right) \cdot S}{K_m + S} \qquad [1\text{-}3]$$

Thus, the effect of a noncompetitive inhibitor on the reaction velocity cannot be overcome by addition of excess substrate. Conceptually, the noncompetitive inhibitor reduces the maximal velocity that can be achieved at saturating substrate concentrations.

For uncompetitive inhibition (Equation 1-4), the inhibitor binds only to the substrate–enzyme complex.

$$v_{(i)} = \frac{\left(\dfrac{V_{max}}{1 + I/K_i}\right) \cdot S}{\dfrac{K_m}{(1 + I/K_i)} + S} \qquad [1\text{-}4]$$

Both the maximal velocity and apparent K_m terms are effectively reduced in the presence of inhibitor. However, the uncompetitive inhibitor has a negligible effect at concentrations of substrate that are well below the true K_m.

In clinical practice, uncompetitive inhibition is an uncommon event because substrate–enzyme saturation occurs rarely *in vivo*. Similarly, because substrate elimination *in vivo* usually conforms to first order kinetics (e.g., $S \ll K_m$), the ratio of the reaction velocity in the presence $[v_{(i)}]$ and absence (v) of a competitive or noncompetitive inhibitor will be independent of substrate concentration (Equation 1-5).

$$\frac{v_{(i)}}{v} = \frac{1}{1 + I/K_i} \qquad [1\text{-}5]$$

When more than one enzyme is involved in the metabolic elimination of a drug, the rate of substrate disappearance can be expressed as the sum of the individual processes. The effect of an inhibitor of one enzyme on the rate of substrate metabolism will be dependent on the fractional contribution of the affected pathway in the uninhibited state and the I/K_i ratio; Equation 1-6 illustrates the relationship for a selective competitive inhibitor of enzyme 2 in a two-enzyme elimination system.

$$v_{(i)} = \frac{V_{\max(1)} \cdot S}{K_{m(1)} + S} + \frac{V_{\max(2)} \cdot S}{K_{m(2)}(1 + I/K_i) + S} \qquad [1\text{-}6]$$

Slowly Reversible or Irreversible Inhibition

Many inhibitors of cytochrome P450s exert an effect that is only slowly reversible or irreversible. A common event is the formation of a stable complex between inhibitor and the one-electron–reduced ferrous heme of the enzyme. Heme ligands include parent drug molecules as well as products of P450-catalyzed metabolism, both of which contain unshared electrons that are available for heme coordination (16,17). A group of well-characterized inhibitory heme ligands are derived from substituted alkyl amines that undergo successive *N*-dealkylation to primary amines, followed by oxidation to yield a substituted nitroso metabolite that complexes with ferrous iron (18,19) (Fig. 1-1). One feature of metabolite inhibitor

complex (MI complex) formation is that it requires time for the accumulation of the complex before a full inhibitory effect emerges. *In vivo*, this may involve 1 to 3 days of inhibitor administration, as described for the inhibition of CYP3A4 by the macrolide antibiotic, erythromycin (20,21). However, for some MI complex inhibitors such as troleandomycin, inactivation of CYP3A4 appears to occur rapidly. This is illustrated by the inhibition of midazolam clearance after administration of a single 500-mg troleandomycin dose 2 hours before 1-mg intravenous midazolam dose (Fig. 1-2) (22).

The effect of a drug–metabolite pair that generates an MI complex differs from the reversible inhibitor in that inhibition may persist well after the elimination of the precursor to the inhibitor complex. Thus, general mathematic relationships between the inhibitor concentration and effect are complex. The extent of inhibition depends on the initial concentration of the precursor inhibitor, the efficiency of sequential catalysis to the ultimate inhibitor, and the stability of the MI complex. If it is assumed that the complex does not dissociate appreciably before normal proteolytic degradation, inhibition can be considered irreversible. Indeed, Wrighton and colleagues (23) described the chromatographic purification of a hepatic CYP3A–MI complex formed *in vivo* after administration of troleandomycin in the rat. CYP3A4 complexes with similar stability may be generated in humans.

In addition to MI complex formation, some drugs can inhibit cytochrome P450 by way of an irreversible or suicide mechanism. Classic examples include the 17α-acetylenic steroids such as ethinyl estradiol and gestodene (24), which are metabolized by CYP3A4 and bind irreversibly to the heme prosthetic group or to amino acid nucleophiles. Again, inhibition of the enzyme by compounds of this type is time- and inhibitor concentration–dependent. The kinetics of irreversible enzyme inhibition can be described with the following catalytic scheme (25):

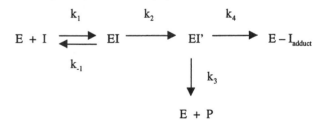

For *in vitro* systems in which there is no new enzyme synthesis, the observed initial rate constant for inactivation (k_{obs}) will be a function of the initial inhibitor concentration (I_0) and kinetic constants for the inactivation process (Equation 1-7):

$$k_{obs} = \frac{k_{inact} \cdot [I_0]}{K_{i,app} + [I_0]} \qquad [1\text{-}7]$$

where k_4 represents the maximal irreversible inactivation rate constant (also referred to as k_{inact}) for covalent binding of the reactive intermediate to enzyme, and $K_{i,app}$ is

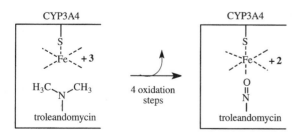

FIG. 1-1. Inhibition of CYP3A4 by troleandomycin through formation of a metabolite–inhibitor complex. A series of successive P450-catalyzed oxidations must occur to generate the stable complex.

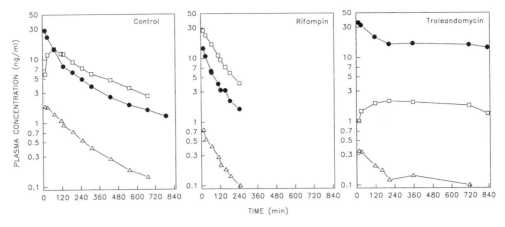

FIG. 1-2. Effect of rifampin and troleandomycin on intravenous midazolam disposition. Plasma concentrations of midazolam (*solid circles*), unconjugated 1'-OH-midazolam (*triangles*), and 1'-OH-mida-zolam-glucuronide (*squares*) are shown for a healthy volunteer after no pretreatment, rifampin (600 mg each morning for 5 days) pretreatment, and troleandomycin (500 mg given orally 2 hours before mida-zolam) pretreatment. (From Kharasch ED, Russell M, Mautz D, et al. The role of cytochrome P450 3A4 in alfentanil clearance. Implications for interindividual variability in disposition and perioperative drug interactions. *Anesthesiology* 1997;87:36–50.)

the inhibitor concentration that will produce an observed inactivation rate constant that is one-half k_{inact}. As seen in Fig. 1-3, which illustrates the inactivation of CYP1A2 by furafylline (26), the initial loss of catalytic activity proceeds at an apparent log-linear rate, with a slope that is a hyperbolic function of the initial inhibitor concentration (I_o). For experiments of this type, the inhibitor is incubated with active enzyme for varying lengths of time and at varying initial concentrations. At the end of this preincubation phase, the enzyme and inhibitor are diluted into

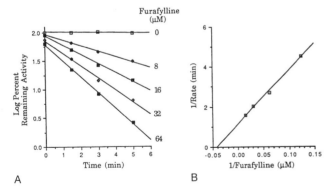

A   B

FIG. 1-3. (A) Time-dependent loss of human liver microsomal P450 1A2 activity by furafylline. P450 1A2 activity (R)-6-hydroxywarfarin formation was measured using (R)-warfarin at a concentration of 3.0 mM. **(B)** Double-reciprocal plot of the relationship between inactivation rate and furafylline concentration. The reversible binding constant K_i for the association of furafylline with P450 1A2 was found to be 22.6 (± 1.8) μM and the rate constant for inactivation k_{inact} was 0.87 (± 0.03) min^{-1}. (From Kunze KL, Trager WF. Isoform-selective mechanism-based inhibition of human cytochrome P450 1A2 by furafylline. *Chem Res Toxicol* 1993;6:649–656. Reproduced with permission of American Chemical Society.)

a larger volume of buffer containing substrate and remaining catalytic activity is measured. Parameter estimates are generated from a plot of the natural log percent activity remaining as a function of preincubation time with inhibitor.

From the aforementioned metabolic scheme, it should be noted that only a fraction of the activated enzyme inhibitor complex (EI') may be converted to the irreversibly inhibited enzyme adduct. Some may be converted to a parallel stable product (P), releasing enzyme for further catalysis. The partitioning of EI' into one pathway or the other (partition ratio) represents the ratio of the respective microrate constants for stable product (k_3) formation and inactivation (k_{inact}). It can be measured by quantitation of the two products at the end of the preincubation phase. For furafylline, a partition ratio of 5 was determined (27).

Although suicide inhibitors may also exert an effect *in vivo* through competitive or noncompetitive inhibition, clinical consequences are generally thought to be mediated through an irreversible mechanism. Under this condition, two factors must be considered to arrive at a quantitative prediction of *in vivo* effect: (a) the magnitude of the inhibitor dose and its fractional conversion to an enzyme adduct relative to the total enzyme pool and (b) the rate of inactivation relative to the natural half-life of the enzyme. For example, both ethinyl estradiol and gestodene are excellent and rapid inhibitors of CYP3A4 *in vitro*, but they are given at a clinical dose (100–200 nmol/day) that is low in comparison to the total average hepatic (5500 nmol) CYP3A4 pool (28), which appears to turn over with a half-life of approximately 24 hours. Thus, significant inhibition of hepatic CYP3A is unexpected unless an individual expressed very low levels of CYP3A.

A more plausible scenario for a significant drug interaction with oral gestodene administration is the inhibition of intestinal CYP3A and first pass gut wall metabolism. The total pool of CYP3A in human small intestine has been estimated at approximately 70 nmol (28). Given a reported partition ratio of 9 for gestodene, it is possible that the drug could inactivate a significant fraction of the intestinal pool after multiple dose administration and increase the bioavailability of high first pass substrates such as saquinavir, verapamil, and midazolam. Another example of covalent enzyme inactivation of CYP3A4 is with the antiprogestin agent mifepristone (RU486) (29), although this drug and others in its class, lilopristone and onapristone, may also inhibit CYP3A4 by an MI complex mechanism (30).

Enzyme Induction

Enzyme induction is less frequently encountered in clinical practice than enzyme inhibition, but it can have just as profound an effect on the pharmacokinetics of drugs metabolized by the susceptible enzyme. Increased levels of enzyme in an eliminating organ, such as the liver, generally results in an increase in the intrinsic metabolic clearance, increased extraction efficiency, and a reduced area under the concentration (AUC)-time profile. Depending on the drug, enzyme induction may also result in an increase in the systemic exposure and fraction metabolized to one or more metabolites. Both changes may alter the efficacy or safety profile of the therapeutic agent.

Enzyme induction can occur by way of a change in the rate of enzyme synthesis or the rate of enzyme degradation (Equation 1-8). Enzyme synthesis is generally considered to be a zero-order process, whereas enzyme degradation is first order. Either an increase in the synthesis rate (R_o) or decrease in the degradation rate constant (k_{degr}), or both, will result in an increased steady-state pool of enzyme (E_{ss}).

$$E_{ss} = \frac{R_o}{k_{degr}} \qquad [1\text{-}8]$$

Transcriptional Activation

Most enzyme induction phenomena proceed by way of a mechanism of increased protein synthesis. Although there are several ways in which this can occur, including increased mRNA translation efficiency, increased stability of mRNA, increased efficiency of mRNA processing, and increased DNA transcription, the latter mechanism is most commonly described for cytochrome P450 enzymes (31). Of the major drug-metabolizing P450 isoforms, the expression of CYP1A2, CYP2E1, and CYP3A4 in human liver is induced by the chronic administration of one or more xenobiotics. Evidence for the induction of other human hepatic P450 isozymes *in vivo* has been

described (see respective enzyme chapters), but is less well established.

In the case of CYP1A1/2 (32), the intracellular signals that mediate an induction response have been well characterized, involving the binding of an inducer to a cytosolic AH receptor, dissociation of heat-shock 90 proteins from the receptor, translocation of the receptor–ligand complex into the nucleus, binding to the Arnt protein, and binding of the Ah receptor–Arnt complex to response elements on the CYP1A genes, resulting in increased gene transcription. As discussed in Chapter 6, constituents in cigarette smoke and some drugs appear to induce hepatic CYP1A2 and extrahepatic 1A1 by this mechanism.

Similar schemes for the induction of other P450 isozymes have also been elucidated to varying degrees. Of major importance for drug metabolism is the induction of CYP3A4 by several structurally diverse drugs, which appears to be initiated, in part, by inducer binding to a nuclear receptor, hPXR (33) or hPAR (34), and binding of the receptor/9-cis retinoic acid heterodimer to CYP3A4 response elements, resulting in increased gene transcription. Discovery of the PXR receptor provides a molecular basis for the diversity of drugs that can upregulate CYP3A4 *in vitro* and *in vivo* and helps explain tissue localization of CYP3A4 and species differences in inducer potency and specificity (33,35). Multiple classes of drugs bind to the PXR receptor, and the human form is most highly expressed in liver and small intestine.

As implied from the mechanisms described, P450 induction by a transcriptional mechanism involves an increased rate of enzyme synthesis. The kinetic effect is represented by an increase in V_{max} (product of E_{ss} and k_{cat}). As discussed later, the time-course and magnitude of an inductive response will be complex and will depend on the dose and route of administration of inducer (i.e., concentration-time profile), the time-course of intracellular events leading to the production of new enzyme, and the rate of enzyme degradation.

Although induction of extrahepatic P450s may profoundly influence the toxic effects of xenobiotics, induction of P450s in the intestinal mucosa appears to be the only phenomenon of quantitative significance for drug clearance. CYP3A4 is the dominant P450 of the small intestine mucosa, and its expression and catalytic activity can be induced by rifampin (36,37). The effect of other known CYP3A4 inducers (i.e., phenytoin, phenobarbital, dexamethasone) has not been studied; however, expression of the PXR receptor in small intestinal tissues (33) suggests that induction of intestinal CYP3A4 is likely.

Protein Stabilization

Equation 1-8 shows that enzyme induction may also occur by a drug-mediated decrease in the rate of enzyme degradation. In theory, this could be accomplished with a change in the cellular machinery responsible for protein turnover. Alternatively, a drug might change the susceptibility of an enzyme to the degradation process. It is the second case, induction by protein stabilization, that has been described most extensively in the P450 literature. For example, several *N*-substituted imidazoles (38) and macrolide antibiotics (39,40) induce different rat liver P450 isozymes through protein stabilization with the parent drug or a metabolite (MI complex formation). Whether human P450s can be induced *in vivo* by a similar mechanism is unknown.

Induction of human and rodent CYP2E1 by a protein stabilization mechanism has been studied extensively and is presented in detail in Chapter 53. Briefly, experimental evidence indicates that hepatic CYP2E1 exists in two kinetically distinct pools, with half-lives of 7 hours and 37 hours, respectively (41,42). Ligands such as isoniazid and ethanol bind to CYP2E1 and convert enzyme from the fast pool to the slow degradation pool. This results in an accumulation of CYP2E1 to achieve a new steady-state based on the modified enzyme half-life. Evidence also indicates that ligand binding to the enzyme active site *in vivo*, while reducing the rate of enzyme degradation, also results in an inhibition of catalytic activity (43–45).

The biochemical nature of the two CYP2E1 pools has not been identified explicitly. However, investigators have proposed different mechanisms for enzyme degradation: an adenosine triphosphate (ATP)-dependent ubiquitin conjugation followed by proteasomal degradation (42,46) or Mg/ATP-dependent phosphorylation and subsequent proteolysis (47–50) that accounts for the respective rapid degradation phase, and an autophagosomal/autolysosomal process that produces the slow phase.

PHARMACOKINETIC CONSIDERATIONS

A systematic *in vitro* characterization of enzyme-catalyzed biotransformation processes controlling the *in vivo* clearance of an NDE and the modulation of enzyme function by the NDE can be used prospectively to make accurate qualitative, and sometimes quantitative, predictions of clinically relevant drug–drug interactions before widespread exposure in the treatment population. This includes interactions that involve induction through increased enzyme synthesis or decreased degradation, and enzyme inhibition through reversible, slowly reversible, and irreversible binding of the modulator to the enzyme.

Inhibition of Hepatic Metabolism

Theoretic Framework

General premises for *in vitro*–to–*in vivo* predictions of an inhibitory drug–enzyme interaction are that inhibition is reversible, that the extent of inhibition is determined by the unbound concentration of inhibitor at the enzyme active site and the enzyme inhibitory constant (K_i), and that substrate concentrations at the enzyme active site are well below the K_m (i.e., first order elimination kinetics). As discussed earlier, there are exceptions that involve formation of stable inhibitor–enzyme complexes or irreversible suicide complexes that are much less amenable to quantitative prediction.

The relationship between the concentration of inhibitor and the metabolic intrinsic clearance for a single enzyme-catalyzed reaction is relatively simple:

$$\frac{Cl_{int}}{Cl_{int(i)}} = 1 + \frac{[I]}{K_i} \qquad [1\text{-}9]$$

where the ratio of the intrinsic clearance (Cl_{int}) in the absence or presence of inhibitor (i) will be determined by the fraction of the total enzyme pool existing as an inhibitor–enzyme complex, as predicted by the relative magnitude of the inhibitor concentration [*I*] and the inhibition constant (K_i). There are additional assumptions implicit in Equation 1-9. It is stipulated that the inhibition constant determined *in vitro* is directly applicable to the *in vivo* interaction and that the *in vitro* inhibitory constant is determined relative to unbound inhibitor concentration. In addition, the unbound inhibitor concentration at the enzyme active site *in vivo* is assumed to be equivalent to the unbound concentration in plasma; inhibitor distribution in the liver is perfusion limited rather than diffusion limited, and there is no significant active uptake or efflux of inhibitor.

Extensive uptake of the inhibitor into the hepatocyte by a diffusional process, resulting in a liver/plasma partition ratio greater than unity, will not necessarily result in a disequilibrium between unbound concentrations at the enzyme active site ($I_{u,e}$) and plasma ($I_{u,p}$). If intracellular binding and debinding events are rapid, extensive intrahepatic tissue binding of inhibitor should be treated as just another distribution pool and does not directly affect unbound drug availability to the enzyme active site. In the absence of evidence to the contrary, it is assumed that the inhibitor gains access to the active site of the enzyme from the aqueous cytosol. However, it is possible that an inhibitor could move directly to the active site from the lipid membrane of the endoplasmic reticulum through a continuous hydrophobic domain (51). It is also conceivable that conditions that might increase the solubility of inhibitor in the cytosol (i.e., increased fatty acids and triglycerides associated with obesity or possibly a high-fat meal), could result in greater enzyme inhibition than would be predicted from the unbound plasma inhibitor concentration.

The relationship presented in Equation 1-9 assumes that the concentration of inhibitor is unchanging during the period of substrate elimination, but this is unlikely in clinical practice. The ratio of intrinsic clearances of substrate would be better described as a continuous function reflecting the time-dependent change in the inhibitor concentration (52,53). However, for predictive purposes, it is usually appropriate to substitute the average inhibitor concentration observed during the substrate dose interval. Alternatively, the peak inhibitor concentration can be used to obtain a conservative estimate of the expected interaction. However, for enzyme substrates with a high first pass, it is also important to consider the degree of overlap in the peak time for substrate and inhibitor.

Quantitative In Vitro–*to–*In Vivo *Comparisons*

Inhibition of the metabolism of a substrate will result in an increase in its AUC time curve and blood concentration at steady-state (C_{ss}). Mathematic relationships that describe the magnitude of expected change have been developed. Route of administration of the substrate, baseline intrinsic clearance for the affected pathway, fraction of dose metabolized through that pathway, and sites of metabolism and excretion are all important variables. Considering the simplest case in which drug is administered orally, reproducibly absorbed, and cleared exclusively by the liver by way of a single inhibitable pathway, the ratio of AUC and steady-state substrate concentration (C_{ss}) in the presence (i) and absence of unbound inhibitor (I_u) is as follows (54):

$$\frac{AUC_{(i)}}{AUC} = \frac{C_{ss(i)}}{C_{ss}} = 1 + \frac{I_u}{K_i} \qquad [1\text{-}10]$$

The equation reflects the inverse relationship between intrinsic clearance and systemic blood levels of the enzyme substrate.

Although few drugs conform exactly to all inherent assumptions described for the affected substrate in Equation 1-10, for some there is a good approximation. For example, tolbutamide is well absorbed and eliminated in humans primarily by a CYP2C9-catalyzed hydroxylation reaction, and its AUC after oral administration is altered significantly (approximately four-fold increase) and predictably by coadministration of the potent CYP2C9 inhibitor sulfaphenazole (55,56). Sulfaphenazole inhibits CYP2C9 *in vitro* with a K_i of approximately 0.2 to 0.6 μM (57,58). Because unbound concentrations of sulfaphenazole after oral administration appear to exceed the K_i several-fold (53), a large change in tolbutamide AUC is expected. Similarly, *S*-warfarin is eliminated predominantly by CYP2C9-catalyzed 7-hydroxylation (63% of dose) and 6-hydroxylation (16% of dose) (57,59). Chronic administration of fluconazole to steady-state (mean I_{ss} approximately 60 μM) caused a 2.8-fold increase in oral *S*-warfarin AUC (60). Again, because the K_i for inhibition of CYP2C9 in liver microsomes by fluconazole was found to be 7 to 8 μM (61), and because the plasma protein binding of fluconazole is negligible (13% bound), the observed 2.8-fold increase in *S*-warfarin AUC was entirely predictable.

When the metabolic elimination of a drug by way of a specific pathway represents only a fraction of the total body clearance, the relationship between the expected AUC change and inhibitor must also take into consideration the fraction metabolized (f_m) by way of the inhibitable pathway. Again, if metabolism is restricted to the liver, to first order, and to low intrinsic clearance, or high intrinsic clearance but with negligible extrahepatic metabolism, one can arrive at the following relationship (54,62–64):

$$\frac{AUC_{(i)}}{AUC} = \frac{1}{\dfrac{f_m}{1 + I/K_i} + (1 - f_m)} \qquad [1\text{-}11]$$

In this situation, there are parallel pathways of metabolism or excretion. As f_m varies from a value of $1 \rightarrow 0$, the effect of the inhibitor on the substrate AUC will be reduced. However, from a mechanistic perspective, it is still possible to quantitate the absolute magnitude of the enzyme-specific interaction if the fraction metabolized can be determined independently.

In some instances, mass balance analysis of urine and feces can provide reasonable estimates of the fraction metabolized. Such an approach was taken in the characterization of an interaction between quinidine and propranolol (65). Quinidine is a very potent inhibitor of CYP2D6 with a reported liver microsomal K_i of approximately 6 to 8 nM for inhibition of *R*- and *S*-propranolol 4-hydroxylation (66). Propranolol is eliminated *in vivo* by multiple metabolic pathways, including glucuronidation, *N*-deisopropylation, 5-hydroxylation, and 4-hydroxylation. CYP2D6 is the predominant catalyst of 4-hydroxy propranolol formation *in vitro* and *in vivo*. Coadministration of a single 50-mg quinidine dose with oral *R/S* propranolol resulted in only a 1.9-fold increase in *R/S* propranolol AUC, but a 92% reduction in the formation clearance ($f_m \times Cl$) to *R/S* 4-hydroxy propranolol. The profound inhibition of the CYP2D6 pathway reflects an expected peak unbound quinidine concentration to microsomal K_i ratio (I_u/K_i) of approximately 10, based on the known pharmacokinetic properties of the drug (67,68).

Alternative scenarios of drug administration (i.e., intravenous) or incomplete drug absorption require modification of the basic mathematic relationships presented earlier; these have been detailed elsewhere (53). In general, if a drug with a high intrinsic clearance is administered intravenously rather than orally, then one can expect a much diminished effect of an enzyme inhibitor on the systemic AUC of the substrate, regardless of the importance of the inhibitable metabolic pathway to the *in vivo* elimination of substrate. This scenario appears to explain the differing effects of chlorpromazine on systemic (no change) and oral (30% decrease) propranolol clearance (69). The systemic clearance of propranolol is 16 mL/min/kg (68), a value approaching hepatic blood flow (21.6 mL/min/kg) (70). Assuming a well-stirred model for hepatic clearance

(71), the intrinsic metabolic clearance of propranolol is approximately 2.8-fold higher than hepatic blood flow.

In situations in which the intrinsic hepatic metabolic clearance is no higher than hepatic blood flow (or plasma flow if the substrate is effectively excluded from red blood cells [RBCs]), significant inhibitory interactions are still expected. Examples include two selective CYP3A-catalyzed reactions: the inhibition of erythromycin demethylation by ketoconazole (72) and the inhibition of midazolam 1'-hydroxylation by fluconazole (73). In a complex study in cancer patients, Jamis-Dow and colleagues (72) were able to demonstrate reductions in an "instantaneous" measure of the erythromycin demethylation rate (erythromycin breath test) that were well correlated with circulating ketoconazole levels. Furthermore, a 50% reduction in the breath test measure was reasonably explained by consideration of measured plasma ketoconazole concentrations (IC_{50} approximately 2 μM), the plasma free fraction of ketoconazole (0.01), and an estimated K_i value of approximately 50 nM for liver microsomal CYP3A-catalyzed erythromycin demethylation (74). In the interaction study with intravenous midazolam, multiple-dose oral fluconazole administration reduced the systemic clearance of midazolam by 50%. Midazolam is cleared from the body almost exclusively by CYP3A-catalyzed 1'- and 4-hydroxylation (75,76). The mean fluconazole concentration measured 30 minutes after the intravenous midazolam dose was 29 μM, for a calculated unbound concentration of 25 μM, which was appreciably higher than the reported K_i (approximately 15 μM) for inhibition of human liver microsomal midazolam 1'-hydroxylation (77).

A mathematic expression for reversible inhibition of the hepatic metabolism of a drug with a high hepatic intrinsic clearance, and hence, high first pass, as well as significant renal elimination can also be derived (78). The relationship between the I/K_i ratio and predicted change in systemic AUC will be more complex than Equations 1-10 and 1-11, and will be be dependent on the fractional metabolic and renal clearances and the extent of hepatic first pass. Because renal clearance accounts for a greater fraction of the total systemic clearance, the effect of a hepatic enzyme inhibitor on the oral AUC will be partially masked, in comparison to a drug with an equivalent first pass effect but negligible renal clearance. In practice, however, it is difficult to imagine a drug that would be eliminated from the body in this prescribed manner, because highly efficient hepatic metabolism would likely be incongruous with a highly efficient renal elimination process.

In Vitro–to–In Vivo *Discrepancies: Reversible Inhibition*

Although the inhibitory effects of fluconazole on systemic midazolam clearance can be explained quantitatively based on unbound fluconazole concentrations in plasma and the *in vitro* fluconazole K_i, the same cannot be said for the effect of another systemic antimycotic agent, itraconazole, on the same systemic midazolam clearance process. In parallel study populations, Olkkola and colleagues (73) showed that oral itraconazole was even more effective than fluconazole at reducing systemic midazolam clearance (79% versus 50% decrease). However, the interaction with itraconazole is unexpected based on a liver microsomal K_i value of 270 nM (79), the mean plasma itraconazole concentration measured 30 minutes after the midazolam dose (499 nM) and a very low itraconazole plasma free fraction (0.002) (68). In this case, the calculated I_u/K_i ratio for this interaction is less than 0.01, for a prediction of no interaction.

Failures to accurately explain significant *in vivo* metabolically based interactions based on calculated I_u/K_i ratios abound in the literature. For example, the fluoroquinolone antibiotics enoxacin and ciprofloxacin inhibit CYP1A2-catalyzed theophylline metabolic clearance *in vivo* (80,81), with unbound plasma inhibitor concentrations that do not alter theophylline metabolism *in vitro* (82). Although the failure to adequately explain the *in vivo* interaction based on *in vitro* kinetic data is perplexing, the differential effect of the fluoroquinolones on the different pathways of theophylline elimination is still highly informative. In an inhibitor dose-effect study, Zhai and colleagues (83) demonstrated the selectivity of enoxacin and ciprofloxacin for inhibition of CYP1A2-catalyzed elimination pathways. As seen in Figure 1-4, a

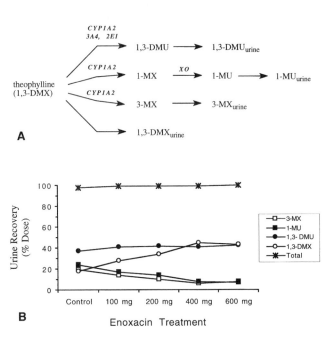

FIG. 1-4. Effect of enoxacin dose on the urinary excretion of theophylline and its metabolites. **(A)** Theophylline (1,3-DMX) is eliminated from the body by four parallel pathways, renal excretion of unchanged drug, CYP1A2-catalyzed formation of 1-methylxanthine (1-MX), 3-methylxanthine (3-MX), and formation of 1,3-dimethyluric acid (1,3-DMU) catalyzed by multiple enzymes including CYP1A2. **(B)** Increasing dose of enoxacin changes the fraction of dose excreted in urine through selective inhibition of CYP1A2.

mass balance of the theophylline dose revealed an enoxacin dose-dependent decrease in the urine recovery of 3-methyl xanthine and 1-methyl uric acid (secondary metabolite of 1-methyl xanthine), with a parallel increase in the recovery of unchanged theophylline (1,3-dimethyl xanthine). In contrast, recovery of 1,3-dimethyl uric acid (primary product of 8-oxidation) remained relatively unchanged with increasing enoxacin dose. From mass balance principles, when a major metabolic pathway is selectively inhibited, there should be an increase in the fraction of dose eliminated by unaffected parallel pathways. Total clearance of the drug will decrease because of a decrease in the formation clearance of the inhibited pathways, but the fractional clearances for the uninhibited pathways remain unchanged. Because the recovery of 1,3-dimethyl uric acid did not increase or decrease, it can be concluded that its formation was catalyzed to a similar extent by CYP1A2 and at least one noninhibitable enzyme.

A similar inability to accurately explain the effect of selective serotonin reuptake inhibitors (SSRIs) on CYP2D6-catalyzed metabolic processes has also been described. Various members of the class inhibit *in vivo* at circulating unbound concentrations that are significantly below the reported microsomal K_i (e.g., fluoxetine: K_i approximately 220 nM; I_u approximately 25 nM) (84,85). The presence of circulating metabolites with comparable inhibitory potency has been noted for some drugs (e.g., norfluoxetine and fluoxetine), but this still fails to adequately account for the *in vivo* effect. It is interesting to note that although there is a general failure to predict a significant *in vivo* interaction from the fluoroquinolones and SSRIs with the use of Equation 1-10 or 1-11, there is a good rank-order for the potency of inhibition *in vitro* and *in vivo* within each drug class (see Chapters 42 and 46). This suggests a common cause for the discrepancy, such as active or passive hepatic uptake of inhibitor that results in an inequality between the unbound concentration of inhibitor in plasma and the unbound concentration at the enzyme active site. Indeed, some investigators have suggested that, for the SSRIs, the "effective" inhibitor concentration at the enzyme active site should be adjusted upward from the total plasma concentration based on an *in vitro* determined liver/water partition ratio for the inhibitor (86). Although this provides an empiric explanation for these particular interactions, broader application to other inhibitors is risky without a clear mechanistic basis for the approach.

In some instances, significant *in vivo* drug–drug interactions can be better explained by consideration of the inhibitory effects of a metabolite rather than the parent molecule. For example, the calcium channel blocker diltiazem is an effective inhibitor of the oral clearance of a number of CYP3A4 substrates, including cyclosporine (87), midazolam (88), triazolam (89), and quinidine (90). Total (339 nM) and unbound (75 nM) steady-state plasma diltiazem concentrations following conventional dosing regimens (68,91) are well below the reported *in vitro* K_i (50–75 μM) for its inhibition of liver microsomal CYP3A4 (92). However, diltiazem is oxidized by CYP3A4 to primary and secondary metabolites, which have been shown to be much more potent inhibitors of CYP3A4 than the parent molecule. *N*-desmethyl and *N,N*-didesmethyl diltiazem exhibit a reversible K_i of 2 and 0.1 μM, respectively (93). Although total circulating concentrations of desmethyl diltiazem (155 nM) are still well below the respective K_i (93), it was argued that the *N,N*-didesmethyl metabolite, which has been detected in human urine (94,95), may be the ultimate inhibitor of CYP3A4 *in vivo*. A potentially alternative or complementary explanation for the *in vitro* and *in vivo* discrepancy with diltiazem considers its potential effect on the gut wall availability of orally administered CYP3A4 or P-glycoprotein substrates (see later discussion).

In Vitro–*to*–In Vivo *Discrepancies: Slow or Irreversible Inhibition*

As mentioned previously, some of the macrolide antibiotics can potentially inhibit CYP3A4 by multiple mechanisms. Although they all act as reversible inhibitors *in vitro*, time-dependent formation of an MI complex can sometimes be demonstrated, as is the case for erythromycin (19). *In vivo*, inhibition with erythromycin is not immediately apparent. Single-dose administration of the drug reportedly had no effect on the systemic clearance of alfentanil, a selective CYP3A4 substrate (22,96), whereas multiple-dose administration for 7 days resulted in a clinically significant (26%) reduction in total alfentanil clearance (20). Additional time-dependent inhibitory interactions with erythromycin and other CYP3A4 substrates can be deduced from the literature (3,21,87,97). Expected steady-state concentrations of erythromycin in plasma following a conventional oral dosing protocol are 2 to 7 μM for total drug and 0.3 to 1.1 μM for unbound drug (68), concentrations that are well below the range of K_i values (13–194 μM) reported for reversible inhibition of CYP3A4 (see Chapter 10). Similarly, plasma concentrations of clarithromycin (total = 2.7 to 4 μM and unbound = 1.4 to 2 μM) are much lower than its reported K_i (10–28 μM) for CYP3A4 (see Chapter 10), yet it is a good inhibitor of systemic and first pass midazolam metabolism *in vivo* (98).

Collectively, the data with erythromycin and clarithromycin suggest that these drugs inhibit CYP3A4 *in vivo* by MI complex formation. Thus, prediction of an interaction *in vivo* requires knowledge of the kinetics for formation of the complex as well as the stability of the MI complex and normal turnover of the enzyme. There may also be an additional complicating factor if total enzyme levels are induced by a protein stabilization mechanism, as suggested from animal data. However, the simplest pharmacokinetic scenario is to treat the complex as a pseudoirreversible adduct. In this case, the observed *in vivo* effect will depend on the K_i, k_{inact}, and inhibitor concentration for formation of the ultimate complex (as presented in Equation 1-7), as well as the dose and pharmacokinetics of the inhibitor, the partition ratio, the total enzyme pool, and the enzyme degradation half-life. None of these data, however, are known for the macrolide antibiotics and only a few of the suicide CYP3A4 inhibitors.

A theoretical treatment of the pharmacokinetic consequences of irreversible enzyme inactivation has been presented recently by Ito and colleagues (53). The authors have provided a series of simulations for the expected *in vivo* time-course of changes in hepatic enzyme content and intrinsic clearance based on a range of parameter estimates associated with cytochrome P450 inactivation and protein turnover. These efforts are highly instructional, confirming the complexity of these types of drug–drug interactions. For example, single-dose simulations illustrate the important relationship between the time of administration of the inhibitor relative to the substrate and the resulting effect on substrate blood concentrations (Fig. 1-5). As the authors noted, too short an interval can result in the complete elimination of substrate before significant inactivation of the enzyme pool has occurred. Too long an interval will allow the enzyme to recover before dosing of the substrate. This theoretic approach should be adaptable to multiple-dose administration of the inhibitor for clinical applications. However, it remains to be seen whether it will be amenable to quantitative *in vitro*–to–*in vivo* predictions.

Inhibition of Gut Wall First Pass Metabolism

Clinical Observations

CYP3A4 is the dominant P450 isozyme of the mucosal enterocytes of the human small intestine (see Chapter 10). Recent reports suggest that several low bioavailability substrates of CYP3A4 undergo some degree of first pass metabolism in the small intestine and the liver. These include cyclosporine (99), midazolam (100), verapamil (101), nifedipine (37), and tirilazad (102). If first pass gut wall metabolism is extensive, inhibitors of CYP3A4 could affect the systemic AUC of the substrate through the inhibition of first pass gut wall metabolism as well as hepatic metabolism. In this case, one would expect a much greater change in the blood AUC of an orally administered CYP3A substrate, in comparison to the change after intravenous dosing of substrate.

This hypothesis was tested directly for cyclosporine (103), midazolam (73), and tirilazad (102). Results indicate that ketoconazole, itraconazole, or fluconazole inhibit both hepatic and intestinal metabolism of one or more substrate (Table 1-1). The percent increase in substrate AUC with oral administration was 2.5- to 5.0-fold higher than the change observed with intravenous dosing. This route-specific difference could not be explained by consideration of an isolated hepatic interaction (i.e., a change in CL and F_H), suggesting a significant intestinal drug–drug interaction with oral substrate administration.

Inhibition of intestinal and hepatic first pass metabolism may also explain results from a recent itraconazole–felodipine interaction study (104). Multiple-dose itraconazole administration, with the last dose given 1 hour before felodipine, led to an increase in felodipine half-life of only 71% (for a computed 40% reduction in systemic clearance if the volume of distribution remained constant) in the face of a 536% increase in the oral felodipine AUC. Prediction of the change in hepatic (systemic) clearance and hepatic availability, based on a well-stirred model for hepatic metabolic extraction, does not

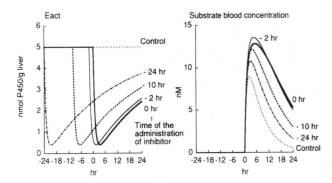

FIG. 1-5. Effects of administration interval of a suicide enzyme inhibitor and substrate on the active enzyme level in the liver and substrate concentration. Simulations were performed with parameter estimates and the model described by Ito and colleagues (53). (Reproduced with permission of the American Society for Pharmacology and Experimental Therapeutics.)

TABLE 1-1. *Inhibition of hepatic and intestinal drug metabolism*

Substrate	Inhibitor	Substrate—AUC (% increase from control)	
		Intravenous	Oral
Cyclosporine[a]	Ketoconazole	87	431
Tirilazad[b]	Ketoconazole	67	309
Midazolam[c]	Itraconazole	224	564
Midazolam[c]	Fluconazole	104	260

[a]Cyclosporine administered 10 hr after ketoconazole dose (200 mg qd)
[b]Tirilazad administered 2 hr after ketoconazole (200 mg qd)
[c]Midazolam administered 2 hr after itraconazole (200 mg qd) or fluconazole (400 mg, day 1; 200 mg qd)

fully explain the increase in felodipine oral bioavailability. Profound inhibition of intestinal first pass felodipine metabolism may be involved.

In theory, *in vivo* inhibition of intestinal CYP3A4 could substantially exceed that predicted from observed circulating inhibitor concentrations, especially if the inhibitor and substrate are administered simultaneously. The same argument can be made regarding the inhibition of hepatic first pass metabolism. However, portal blood concentrations of unbound inhibitor are likely to be only modestly higher than systemic concentrations. In a study of midazolam kinetics in liver transplant patients, portal concentrations were found to be approximately two-fold higher than arterial concentrations at the time of peak absorption (100). Even though this ratio will vary from drug to drug, our results with midazolam may represent an upper limit, in that midazolam was rapidly absorbed from the gut lumen after intraduodenal administration of a drug solution. Although there has been considerable speculation on the subject, the relative difference in inhibitor concentration between the mucosal compartment and in portal blood during the absorptive phase is unknown.

Persistent Inhibition of Intestinal CYP3A4

It has also been suggested, but not proven, that the profound and preferential inhibition of intestinal metabolism by high-affinity reversible CYP3A inhibitors, such as ketoconazole, persists well beyond the time window of inhibitor absorption. For example, the differential effects of ketoconazole on intravenous and oral cyclosporine clearance illustrated in Table 1-1, occurred even though the last dose of inhibitor was given a full 10 hours before the substrate, well after the intestinal absorption of the inhibitor was complete. Similarly, administration of itraconazole at 3, 12, or 24 hours before a single oral dose of triazolam resulted in a 183%, 193% and 157% increase in triazolam AUC, respectively, despite substantial elimination of itraconazole from the systemic circulation over the same time period (105); the highest itraconazole concentrations achieved during the triazolam elimination period were 175, 55, and 45 ng/mL, respectively. The mechanism for these phenomena is not clear. It could involve accumulation of uncharacterized metabolites (i.e., hydroxy metabolites of itraconazole and ketoconazole that inhibit CYP3A), but it may also involve a more general process of sequestration of high concentrations of the inhibitor within the enterocyte during first pass. Implicit in this hypothesis, however, is the assumption that the sequestered inhibitor slowly redistributes to the intracellular enzyme site in a direct fashion without first coming to equilibrium with inhibitor concentrations in the systemic circulation.

In a recent study of a quinidine–nifedipine interaction involving CYP3A4, Koley and colleagues (106) found

that quinidine behaved as a noncompetitive inhibitor of nifedipine oxidation by inducing a shift in CYP3A4 conformation that did not allow nifedipine oxidation. In addition, nifedipine binding to the quinidine–CYP3A4 complex was enhanced, yielding a ternary complex that was more stable than the nifedipine–CYP3A4 binary complex. Thus, under first pass conditions, high saturating concentrations of both inhibitor and substrate may substantially deplete the active enzyme pool via formation of a slowly dissociating inhibitor–substrate–enzyme complex.

Not all inhibitors of CYP3A act in this manner. Fluconazole is a much less potent inhibitor of CYP3A4 *in vitro* and *in vivo* (32,33), and it is more water soluble than other azole antifungals. It inhibits both systemic and first pass midazolam metabolism (73). In addition, oral fluconazole is only a slightly more effective inhibitor of oral midazolam clearance than intravenous fluconazole (107), suggesting that inhibition is not greater toward intestinal CYP3A.

Inhibition of intestinal first pass metabolism also appears to occur with the administration of some dialkylamine inhibitors that exhibit relatively low reversible affinity for CYP3A (see Chapter 10). For example, a retrospective analysis of the erythromycin–midazolam interaction suggests that midazolam systemic clearance decreased by 32%, whereas the oral clearance was reduced by 78% (108). Again, based on the well-stirred model of hepatic extraction, the change in the apparent hepatic clearance and hepatic availability of midazolam does not fully explain the change in oral clearance and strongly suggests inhibition of intestinal first pass midazolam metabolism.

Inhibition of CYP3A4 activity in the small intestine may occur through the formation of a slowly reversible metabolite–heme complex as discussed earlier. By this mechanism, inhibition of first pass metabolism with erythromycin could occur at systemic concentrations well below the reversible inhibition constant (K_i), because it depends on the fraction of the cumulative dose that is converted to the proximal inhibitory metabolite. If dissociation of the complex is slow relative to its rate of formation, it will accumulate over time. Based on the relatively low amount of CYP3A in the small intestine versus the liver (28) and an obligatory exposure of these enzymes to the entire inhibitor dose (i.e., transcellular absorption), this could lead to a preferential reduction in intestinal first pass extraction compared to hepatic first pass.

The assumption that there can be intestinal metabolism of erythromycin raises additional intriguing issues with regard to the dynamics of inhibition. In order to form an MI complex with CYP3A, the erythromycin must undergo four successive oxidations. Only the last step need be catalyzed by CYP3A, but it is likely that all are. However, if the primary or subsequent metabolites are released from the enzyme during the catalytic sequence, it is likely that the metabolite will not compete effectively for the enzyme-active site against potentially saturating concentrations of parent inhibitor found during the absorption phase. Thus, at a minimum, inhibition would be delayed until the parent inhibitor is cleared. If metabolites (of hepatic or intestinal origin) are re-presented to intestinal enzyme at a later time, metabolic steps toward MI complex formation could proceed unimpeded.

Interindividual Variability

A poorly appreciated but potentially clinically significant aspect of intestinal CYP3A-dependent drug interactions is the possibility that the magnitude of inhibition will vary with the individual level of CYP3A expression in the small intestine. We have reported that the level of CYP3A4 protein and intrinsic midazolam hydroxylation activity in microsomes from the small intestine mucosa can vary widely between individuals (28,109). This large variability is borne out *in vivo*, in that the predicted and directly measured first pass intestinal midazolam extraction ratio ranged between a negligible fraction to as high as 77% (110) and between 14% and 59% (100), respectively. For drugs in which intestinal first pass extraction is considerable, the change in oral bioavailability may also be quite variable in the presence of an inhibitor. For example, in a group of ten healthy subjects, multiple oral dosing of diltiazem increased the AUC of oral triazolam between 20% and 520% (89). Similarly, the selective intestinal CYP3A inhibitor grapefruit juice increased the oral AUC of felodipine (5% to 470%), midazolam (26% to 100%), and terfenadine (21% to 485%) to highly variable degrees (111–116). For felodipine, the percent increase in C_{max} and AUC were positively correlated with the baseline parameter (111,117). This relationship was confirmed in a later study by comparison of CYP3A4 content in duodenal biopsy specimens obtained from subjects before ingestion of grapefruit juice, with the increase in felodipine C_{max} observed over baseline after 16 glasses of grapefruit juice were taken over the course of 6 days (118). These findings may reflect the selectivity of grapefruit juice for gut CYP3A4 and the intersubject variation in first pass gut wall metabolism of felodipine.

Enzyme Induction

Time-Course and Magnitude of Induction: Transcriptional Activation

Although there is no theoretical limit to the extent of enzyme induction, studies with isolated human hepatocyte or precision-cut tissue slice systems indicate that microsomal cytochrome P450 inducers usually elicit a two- to eight-fold increase in enzyme levels or catalytic activity (e.g., CYP3A4 and rifampin) (119–123). If it is assumed that a change in enzyme synthesis in the presence of an inducer is relatively rapid and remains constant with maintained exposure to inducer, then enzyme content and V_{max} in the eliminating organ will increase to a new steady-state level as a function of the half-life for enzyme degradation, according to Equation 1-12 (124):

$$V_{max(t)} = V'_{max} - (V'_{max} - V_{max}) \cdot e^{-k'_{degr} t} \quad [1\text{-}12]$$

where $V_{max(t)}$ is the apparent maximum velocity at any time after introduction of the inducer, V'_{max} represents the maximum reaction velocity at steady-state with the inducer, and k'_{degr} is the enzyme degradation rate constant in the presence of inducer. V'_{max} can also be defined as $k_{cat} \cdot (R_o/k')$, where R_o is the enzyme synthesis rate and k_{cat} is the rate constant for dissociation of the enzyme–substrate complex to product and unbound enzyme.

As discussed, drugs may induce an enzyme by affecting either its synthesis rate or degradation rate. If it can be assumed that an inducer does not affect K_m (an important exception being an induction by protein stabilization; see Chapter 54), the following equation can be written for the intrinsic metabolic clearance (Cl_{int}):

$$Cl_{int(t)} = Cl'_{int} - (Cl'_{int} - Cl_{int}) \cdot e^{-k'_{degr} t} \quad [1\text{-}13]$$

Furthermore, the time-course of change in the steady-state blood concentration of a drug eliminated by the induced enzyme can be predicted by the time-course of change in drug clearance, because steady-state drug concentration and clearance are inversely related. Different routes of substrate administration have been considered (125). The blood concentration of the affected drug at any time after constant rate coadministration of an inducer will be a complex function of the baseline and maximally induced clearance of the affected drug, its volume of distribution, and the degradation half-life of the enzyme in the presence of inducer. Assuming the simple case of a constant-rate infusion of the affected drug, and where the half-life of the affected drug is shorter than the half-life of enzyme degradation, the decline in blood concentration from baseline to an induced state mirrors the change in enzyme content and intrinsic clearance (124) (Fig. 1-6). If the half-life of the affected drug is very long relative to the enzyme half-life, then the time to reach steady-state blood concentrations will be controlled primarily by the slower drug elimination process.

For most cases of enzyme induction, there will be some lag time for the absorption and accumulation of the inducer in the blood and liver to steady-state, and a maximal increase in gene transcription. If accumulation of the inducer is slow and if the change in synthesis or degradation is a function of the blood level of the inducer, then the time-course of change in enzyme level after initiation of inducer administration will take on added complexity. The mathematics for this scenario have also been considered (126). In general, there is a delay in the time to reach

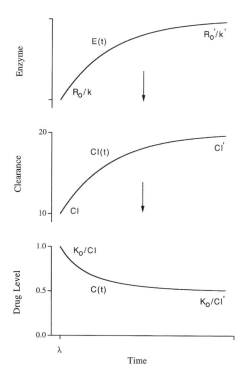

FIG. 1-6. Relationship between increase in enzyme level, E(t), and the corresponding increase in clearance, Cl(t), and decrease in blood concentration (K$_o$/Cl). The drug was administered by constant rate intravenous infusion (K$_o$) and the two-fold increase in the ratio of enzyme synthesis to degradation rate constant from baseline (R$_o$/k) to an induced state (R$_o$'/k') was assumed to occur instantaneously at time I. (Adapted from Levy RH, Lai AA, Dumain MS. Time-dependent kinetics. IV. pharmacokinetic theory of enzyme induction. *J Pharm Sci* 1979;68:398–399. With permission of the American Pharmaceutical Association.)

the new steady-state and a protracted de-induction phase, compared to the time-course that would result if the changes in synthesis or degradation were instantaneous.

It might also be expected that the level of enzyme would fluctuate to some degree in response to the kinetics of the inducer during repeated dosing. Indeed, as pointed out by Abramson (126), the contribution of the inducer kinetics to the time profile for substrate may completely obscure any relationship between the enzyme half-life and the time-course of systemic clearance and steady-state substrate blood levels. An extreme case is the phenomenon of autoinduction, wherein the enzyme inducer increases its own clearance. Perhaps the best known example of an autoinducer is the anticonvulsant drug carbamazepine. Carbamazepine is cleared from the body predominantly by CYP3A-catalyzed 10,11-epoxidation (127). Using stable-isotope–labeled carbamazepine to measure the apparent clearance at various times during chronic administration of unlabeled carbamazepine to children, Bertilsson and colleagues (128) found that carbamazepine clearance increased approximately two-fold between day 1 and day 146 to 162 of

therapy, and that a fully induced steady-state was not achieved until about day 21 to 36 of therapy.

Despite the clinical importance of the time-course of enzyme induction and de-induction, there has been remarkably little information published in the literature. Some of the best data have been generated with the use of an endogenous probe for CYP3A induction (129), 6β-hydroxylation of cortisol. Ohnhaus and colleagues (130), reported that 6β-hydroxy cortisol excretion increased steadily with daily rifampin administration but did not reach a maximum until day 11 to 14. De-induction of CYP3A occurred after discontinuation of rifampin, but was still incomplete after 7 days. Multiple-dose phenytoin administration caused a similar rapid increase in the urinary 6β-hydroxycorisol/cortisol ratio, with an apparent induction plateau achieved after approximately 4 days (131). Interestingly, the peak time for the inductive effect of phenytoin corresponded roughly to the time at which steady-state phenytoin concentrations were achieved. In contrast, the time-course for CYP3A induction with phenobarbital appears to occur more slowly; a significant increase in urinary 6β-hydroxycortisol excretion was detected only after 13 days of inducer administration (130). This delayed effect was similar to the protracted time-course for induction of warfarin clearance by phenobarbital (132). In this case, the time to reach a new steady-state of plasma warfarin concentration appeared to require 16 days of continuous inducer administration. De-induction required a similar period of time. Again, this may be related to the time required to reach steady-state phenobarbital levels in blood and the removal of inducer after discontinued administration (plasma phenobarbital half-life, approximately 99 hours), rather than a long half-life for P450 degradation.

There are only limited data available on the turnover of human P450s, and all of it is indirect. Urinary 6β-hydroxycortisol excretion data, mentioned previousely, suggests that the half-life of CYP3A is 24 to 48 hours. In a study of hepatic CYP2E1 kinetics, Emery and colleagues reported a mean enzyme degradation half-life of 50 hours, based on the time-course for the return of chlorzoxazone clearance following suicide inactivation of the enzyme pool with a single oral dose of disulfiram (133). Using these values as a benchmark, it should take 5 to 10 days of constant administration of an enzyme inducer to achieve a new steady-state in plasma concentrations of the affected drug, but this may take longer for some inducers or substrates that exhibit a longer blood elimination half-life than the enzyme half-life.

Although the magnitude of change in the steady-state blood concentration of a substrate affected by enzyme induction will depend on the predicted change in intrinsic metabolic clearance, there are other important pharmacokinetic considerations. If the substrate is dosed intravenously and hepatically cleared, then the magnitude of effect will depend on the baseline hepatic extraction ratio. For drugs with a high baseline intrinsic clearance or extraction ratio, the biochemical effect of an inducer should be partially or completely masked by a blood flow limitation. For example, the systemic clearance of three different CYP3A4 substrates—lidocaine, alfentanil, and midazolam—were increased 15%, 175%, and 164%, respectively, by multiple dose rifampin administration (22,134). The respective baseline plasma clearances of lidocaine, alfentanil, and midazolam in these studies were 7.5, 5.3, and 3.3 mL/min/kg and were inversely correlated with the percemnt change in clearance as predicted by pharmacokinetic theory. In a similar finding, Fleishaker and colleagues (135) reported a modest 92% increase in tirilazad clearance following multiple-dose phenytoin administration for individuals with a baseline clearance value of 6.0 mL/min/kg.

In theory, the effect of inducers on the AUC of a high intrinsic clearance substrate for the affected enzyme will be more profound when the substrate is given by the oral versus intravenous route, because the oral AUC is inversely proportional to the intrinsic clearance and is independent of hepatic blood flow. In a comparison of lidocaine elimination in healthy volunteers and patients receiving chronic phenytoin therapy, Perucca and colleagues (136) reported no significant difference in the systemic clearance of the drug (0.77 and 0.85 L/min for volunteers and patients, respectively), but a 61% lower AUC following an oral lidocaine dose in patients compared to volunteers. This prediction is also evident in the reported effects of rifampin on oral midazolam clearance. Multiple dosing of rifampin increased the apparent oral clearance (Cl/F) of midazolam 23-fold (137). However, the dramatic change in oral midazolam disposition following rifampin or phenytoin plus carbamazepine (138) administration may be due, in part, to an induction of gut wall CYP3A4 and increased gut wall first pass metabolism (136). Although there is no published model describing simultaneous liver and intestinal enzyme induction, one can deduce from first principles that the effect of a CYP3A inducer on the absolute bioavailability (F) and the oral clearance (Cl/F) would be multiplicative in nature and greater than what would occur if a single organ was involved.

Time-Course and Magnitude of Induction—Protein Stabilization

A kinetic model that relates the simultaneous inhibition and induction of CYP2E1-dependent drug clearance to the concentration of the inhibitor/inducer in blood and its enzyme dissociation constant (K_i) has recently been described (139). It appears to successfully predict the induction of human CYP2E1 by isoniazid and ethanol in humans (139). A detailed presentation of this type of interaction is described in Chapter 53. Briefly, the

inducer will elevate hepatic CYP2E1 enzyme levels when blood concentrations exceed the K_i. However, under first order elimination conditions for the substrate, the inducer will also simultaneously inhibit CYP2E1-dependent catalytic activity until blood levels fall below the inhibition constant. After that point, a brief period of increased catalytic activity may occur and last until baseline steady-state CYP2E1 levels are restored.

REFERENCES

1. Yun CH, Okerholm RA, Guengerich FP. Oxidation of the antihistiminic drug terfenadine in human liver microsomes. Role of cytochrome P-450 3A(4) in N-dealkylation and C-hydroxylation. *Drug Metab Dispos* 1993;21:403–409.
2. Jurima-Romet M, Crawford K, Cyr T, Inaba T. Terfenadine metabolism in human liver. In vitro inhibition by macrolide antibiotics and azole antifungals. *Drug Metab Dispos* 1994;22:849–857.
3. Honig P, Woosley R, Zamani K, Conner D Jr. LRC. Changes in the pharmacokinetics and electrocardiographic pharmacodynamics of terfenadine with concomitant administration of erythromycin. *Clin Pharmacol Ther* 1992;52:231–238.
4. Honig PK, Wortham DC, Zamani K, Conner DP, Cantilena LR. The terfenadine-ketoconazole interaction: pharmacokinetic and electrocardiographic consequences. *JAMA* 1993;269:1513–1518.
5. Honig PK, Wortham DC, Zamani K, Cantilena LR. Comparison of the effect of the macrolide antibiotics erythromycin, clarithromycin and azithromycin on terfenadine steady-state pharmacokinetics and electrocardiographic parameters. *Drug Invest* 1994;7:148–156.
6. Carlson AM, Morris LS. Coprescription of terfenadine and erythromycin or ketoconazole: an assessment of potential harm. *JAMA* 1996;NS36:263–269.
7. Barry M, Gibbons S, Back D, Mulcahy F. Protease inhibitors in patients with HIV disease. Clinically important pharmacokinetic considerations. *Clin Pharmacokinet* 1997;32:194–209.
8. Ernst ME, Kelly MW. Mibefridil, a pharmacologically distinct calcium antagonist. *Pharmacotherapy* 1998;18:463–485.
9. Gibaldi M. Drug recalls and warnings. In: Rasmussen B, ed. *Drug Therapy 1999*. New York: McGraw-Hill, 1999:369–371.
10. Guengerich FP. Human cytochrome P450 enzymes. In: De Montellano PR, ed. *Cytochrome P450*, 2nd ed. New York: Plenum Press, 1995:473–535.
11. Parkinson A. An overview of current cytochrome P450 technology for assessing the safety and efficacy of new materials. *Toxicol Pathol* 1996;24:45–57.
12. Guengerich FP. Role of cytochrome P450 enzymes in drug-drug interactions. *Adv Pharmacol* 1997;43:7–35.
13. Ueng Y-F, Kuwabara T, Chun Y-J, Guengerich FP. Cooperativity in oxidations catalyzed by cytochrome P450 3A4. *Biochemistry* 1997;36:370–381.
14. Korzekwa KR, Krishnamachary N, Shou M, et al. Evaluation of atypical cytochrome P450 kinetics with two-substrate-models: evidence that multiple substrates can simultaneously bind to cytochrome P450 active sites. *Biochemistry* 1998;37:4137–4147.
15. Segel IH. *Enzyme kinetics: behavior and analysis of rapid equilibrium and steady-state enzyme systems*. New York: John Wiley and Sons, 1975.
16. Franklin MR. A new class of inhibitory cytochrome P-450 complexes formed during metabolism: a comparison with amphetamine and SKF 525-A type complexes. *Chem Biol Interact* 1976;14:337–346.
17. Pershing LK, Franklin MR. Cytochrome P-450 metabolic-intermediate complex formation and induction by macrolide antibiotics; a new class of agents. *Xenobiotica* 1982;12:687–699.
18. Babany G, Larrey D, Pessayre D, eds. *Macrolide antibiotics as inducers and inhibitors of cytochrome P-450 in experimental animals and man*, vol 11. London: Taylor & Francis, 1988:61–98.
19. Lindstrom TD, Hanssen BR, Wrighton SA. Cytochrome P-450 complex formation by dirithromycin and other macrolides in rats and human livers. *Antimicrob Agents Chemother* 1993;37:265–269.
20. Bartkowski RR, Goldberg ME, Larijani GE, Boerner T. Inhibition of alfentanil metabolism by erythromycin. *Clin Pharmacol Ther* 1989;46:99–102.

21. Rosenstiel NV, Adam D. Macrolide antibacterials. Drug interactions of clinical significance. *Drug Safety* 1995;13:105–122.

22. Kharasch ED, Russell M, Mautz D, et al. The role of cytochrome P450 3A4 in alfentanil clearance. Implications for interindividual variability in disposition and perioperative drug interactions. *Anesthesiology* 1997;87:36–50.

23. Wrighton SA, Maurel P, Schuetz EG, Watkins PB, Young B, Guzelian PS. Identification of the cytochrome P-450 induced by macrolide antibiotics in rat liver as the glucocorticoid responsive cytochrome P-450p. *Biochemistry* 1985;24:2171–2178.

24. Guengerich FP. Mechanism-based inactivation of human liver cytochrome P450 IIIA4 by gestodene. *Chem Res Toxicol* 1990;3:363–371.

25. Waley SG. Kinetics of suicide substrates: practical procedures for determining parameters. *Biochem J* 1985;227:843–849.

26. Kunze KL, Trager WF. Isoform-selective mechanism-based inhibition of human cytochrome P450 1A2 by furafylline. *Chem Res Toxicol* 1993;6:649–656.

27. Racha JK, Rettie AE, Kunze KL. Mechanism-based inactivation of human cytochrome P450 1A2 by furafylline: detection of a 1:1 adduct to protein and evidence for the formation of a novel imidazomethide intermediate. *Biochemistry* 1998;37:7407–7419.

28. Paine MF, Khalighi M, Fisher JM, et al. Characterization of inter- and intra-intestinal differences in human CYP3A-dependent metabolism. *J Pharmacol Exp Ther* 1997;283:1552–1562.

29. He K, Woolf TF, Hollenberg PF. Mechanism-based inactivation of cytochrome P-450-3A4 by mifepristone (RU486). *J Pharmacol Exp Ther* 1999;288:791–797.

30. Jang G, Benet L. Antiprogestin-mediated inactivation of cytochrome P450 3A4. *Pharmacology* 1998;56:150–157.

31. Dogra S, Whitelaw ML, May BK. Transcriptional activation of cytochrome P450 genes by different classes of chemical inducers. *Clin Exp Pharmacol Physiol* 1998;25:1–9.

32. Sogawa K, Fujii-Kuriyama Y. Ah receptor, a novel ligand activated transcription factor. *J Biochem* 1997;122:1075–1079.

33. Lehmann JM, McKee DD, Watson MA, Willson TM, Moore JT, Kliewer SA. The human orphan nuclear receptor PXR is activated by compounds that regulate CYP3A4 gene expression and cause drug interactions. *J Clin Invest* 1998;102:1016–1023.

34. Bertilsson G, Heidrich J, Svensson K, et al. Identification of a human nuclear receptor defines a new signaling pathway for CYP3A induction. *Proc Natl Acad Sci USA* 1998;95:12208–12213.

35. Kliewer SA, Moore JT, Wade L, et al. An orphan nuclear receptor activated by pregnanes defines a novel steroid signaling pathway. *Cell* 1998;92:73–82.

36. Kolars JC, Schmiedlin-Ren P, Schuetz JD, Fang C, Watkins PB. Identification of rifampin-inducible P450IIIA4 (CYP3A4) in human small bowel enterocytes. *J Clin Invest* 1992;90:1871–1878.

37. Holtbecker N, Fromm M, Kroemer HK, Ohnhaus EE, Heidemann H. The nifedipine-rifampin interaction. Evidence for induction of gut wall metabolism. *Drug Metab Dispos* 1996;24:1121–1123.

38. Ritter JK, Franklin MR. Induction and inhibition of rat hepatic drug metabolism by N-substituted imidazole drugs. *Drug Metab Dispos* 1987;15:335–343.

39. Pessayre D, Descatoire V, Tinel M, Larrey D. Self-induction by oleandomycin of its own transformation into a metabolite forming an inactive complex with reduced cytochrome P-450. Comparison with troleandomycin. *J Pharmacol Exp Ther* 1982;221:215–221.

40. Delaforge M, Jaouen M, Mansuy D. Dual effects of macrolide antibiotics on rat liver cytochrome P-450. *Biochem Pharmacol* 1983;32:2309–2318.

41. Song BJ, Veech RL, Park SS, Gelboin HV, Gonzalez FJ. Induction of rat hepatic N-nitrosodimethylamine demethylase by acetone is due to protein stabilization. *J Biol Chem* 1989;264:3568–3572.

42. Roberts BJ, Song B-J, Soh Y, Park SS, Shoaf SE. Ethanol induces CYP2E1 by protein stabilization. Role of ubiquitin conjugation in the rapid degradation of CYP2E1. *J Biol Chem* 1995;270:29632–29635.

43. Pantuck EJ, Pantuck CB, Ryan DE, Conney AH. Inhibition and stimulation of enflurane metabolism in the rat following a single dose or chronic administration of ethanol. *Anesthesiology* 1985;62:255–262.

44. Zand R, Slattery SD, Thummel KE, Kalhorn TF, Adams SP, Wright JM. Inhibition and induction of CYP2E1-catalyzed oxidation by isoniazid in humans. *Clin Pharmacol Ther* 1993;54:142–149.

45. Chien JY, Peter RM, Nolan CM, Wartell C, Slattery JT, Nelson SD, Caruthers RL Jr., Thummel KE. Influence of NAT2 phenotype on the inhibition and induction of acetaminophen bioactivation with chronic isoniazid. *Clin Pharmacol Ther* 1996;61:24–34.

46. Tierney DJ, Haas AL, Koop DR. Degradation of cytochrome P450 2E1: selective loss after labilization of the enzyme. *Arch Biochem Biophys* 1992;293:9–16.

47. Johansson I, Eliassson E, Ingelman-Sundberg M. Hormone-controlled phosphorylation and degradation of CYP2B1 and CYP2E1 in isolated rat hepatocytes. *Biochem Biophys Res Comm* 1991;174:37–42.

48. Eliasson E, Johansson I, Ingelman-Sundberg M. Substrate-, hormone-, and cAMP-regulated cytochrome P450 (2E1) degradation. *Proc Natl Acad Sci USA* 1990;87:3225–3229.

49. Eliasson E, Mkrtchian S, Ingelman-Sundberg M. Hormone- and substrate-regulated intracellular degradation of cytochrome P450 (2E1) involving MgATP-activated rapid proteolysis in the endoplasmic reticulum membranes. *J Biol Chem* 1992;267:15765–15769.

50. Neve EPA, Eliasson E, Pronzato MA, Albano E, Marianari U, Ingelman-Sundberg M. Enzyme-specific transport of rat liver cytochrome P450 to the Golgi apparatus. *Arch Biochem Biophys* 1996;333:459–465.

51. Edwards RJ, Murray BP, Singleton AM, Boobis AR. Orientation of cytochromes P450 in the endoplasmic reticulum. *Biochemistry* 1991;30:71–76.

52. Shaw PN, Houston JB. Kinetics of drug metabolism inhibition: Use of metabolite concentration-time profiles. *J Pharmacokinet Biopharm* 1987;15:497–510.

53. Ito K, Iwatsubo T, Kanamitsu S, Ueda K, Suzuki H, Sugiyama Y. Prediction of pharmacokinetic alterations caused by drug-drug interactions: metabolic interaction in the liver. *Pharmacol Rev* 1998;50:387–411.

54. Rowland M, Matin SB. Kinetics of drug-drug interactions. *J Pharmacokinet Biopharm* 1973;1:553–567.

55. Pond SM, Birkett DJ, Wade DN. Mechanisms of inhibition of tolbutamide metabolism: phenylbutazone, oxyphenbutazone and sulfaphenazole. *Clin Pharmacol Ther* 1977;22:573–579.

56. Veronese ME, Miners JO, Randles D, Gregov D, Birkett DJ. Validation of the tolbutamide metabolic ratio for population screening with use of sulfaphenazole to produce model phenotypic metabolizers. *Clin Pharmacol Ther* 1990;47:403–411.

57. Rettie AE, Eddy AC, Heimark LD, Gibaldi M, Trager WF. Characteristics of warfarin hydroxylation catalyzed by human liver microsomes. *Drug Metab Dispos* 1989;17:265–270.

58. Doecke CJ, Veronese ME, Pond SM, et al. Relationship between phenytoin and tolbutamide hydroxylations in human liver microsomes. *Br J Clin Pharmacol* 1991;31:125–130.

59. Rettie AE, Korzekwa KR, Kunze KL, et al. Hydroxylation of warfarin by human cDNA-expressed cytochrome P-450: a role of P-4502C9 in the etiology of (S)-warfarin-drug interactions. *Chem Res Toxicol* 1992;5:54–59.

60. Black DJ, Kunze KL, Wienkers LC, et al. Warfarin-fluconazole II. A metabolically based drug interaction: in vivo studies. *Drug Metab Dispos* 1996;24:422–428.

61. Kunze K, Wienkers L, Thummel K, Trager W. Warfarin-fluconazole I. Inhibition of the human cytochrome P450-dependent metabolism of warfarin by fluconazole: in vitro studies. *Drug Metab Dispos* 1996;24:414–421.

62. Aarons L. Kinetics of drug-drug interactions. *Pharmacol Ther* 1981;14:321–344.

63. Tucker GT. The rational selection of drug interaction studies: implications of recent advances in drug metabolism. *Int J Clin Pharmacol Ther Toxicol* 1992;30:550–553.

64. Kunze KL, Trager WF. A rational approach to management of a metabolically based drug interaction. *Drug Metab Dispos* 1996;24:429–435.

65. Zhou HH, Anthony LB, Roden DM, Wood AJJ. Quinidine reduces clearance of (+) propranolol more than (−) propranolol through marked reduction in 4-hydroxylation. *Clin Pharmacol Ther* 1990;47:686–693.

66. Marathe PH, Shen DD, Nelson WL. Metabolic kinetics of pseudoracemic propranolol in human liver microsomes. Enantioselectivity and quinidine inhibition. *Drug Metab Dispos* 1994;22:237–247.

67. Ueda CT, Williamson BJ, Dzindzio BS. Absolute quinidine bioavailability. *Clin Pharmacol Ther* 1976;20:260–265.

68. Benet LZ. Pharmacokinetics. In: J.G. Hardman, Limbird LE, Molinoff

PB, Ruddon RW, Gilman AG, eds. *Goodman and Gilman's: The pharmacological basis of therapeutics,* 9th ed. New York: McGraw-Hill, 1996:14.

69. Vestal RE, Kornhause DM, Hollifield JW. Inhibition of propranolol metabolism by chlorpromazine. *Clin Pharmacol Ther* 1979;25:19–24.

70. Pirttiaho HI, Sotaniemi EA, Pelkonen RO, Pitkänen U. Hepatic blood flow and drug metabolism in patients on enzyme-inducing anticonvulsants. *Eur J Clin Pharmacol* 1982;22:441–445.

71. Wilkinson GR. Clearance approaches in pharmacology. *Pharmacol Rev* 1987;39:1–47.

72. Jamis-Dow CA, Pearl ML, Watkins PB, Blake DS, Klecker RW, Collins JM. Predicting drug interactions in vivo from experiments in vitro. Human studies with paclitaxel and ketoconazole. *Am J Clin Oncol* 1997;20:592–599.

73. Olkkola KT, Ahonen J, Neuvonen PJ. The effect of systemic antimycotics, itraconazole and fluconazole on the pharmacokinetics and pharmacodynamics of intravenous and oral midazolam. *Anesth Analg* 1996;82:511–516.

74. Riley RJ, Howbrook D. In vitro analysis of the activity of the major human hepatic CYP enzyme (CYP3A4) using [*N*-methyl-14C]-erythromycin. *J Pharmacol Toxicol Methods* 1998;38:189–193.

75. Kronbach T, Mathys D, Umeno M, Gonzalez FJ, Meyer UA. Oxidation of midazolam and triazolam by human liver cytochrome P450IIIA4. *Mol Pharmacol* 1989;36:89–96.

76. Thummel KE, Shen DD, Podoll TD, et al. Use of midazolam as a human cytochrome P450 3A probe: I. In vitro-in vivo correlations in liver transplant patients. *J Pharmacol Exp Ther* 1994;271: 549–556.

77. Gibbs MA, Thummel KE, Shen DD, Kunze KL. Inhibition of CYP3A in human intestinal and liver microsomes: comparison of Ki values and impact of CYP3A5 expression. *Drug Metab Dispos* 1999;27: 180–187.

78. Gillette JR, Pang KS. Theoretical aspects of pharmacokinetic drug interactions. *Clin Pharmacol Ther* 1977;22:623–639.

79. Moltke LLv, Greenblatt DJ, Schmider J, et al. Midazolam hydroxylation by liver microsomes in vitro: inhibition by fluoxetine, norfluoxetine, and by azole antifungal agents. *J Clin Pharmacol* 1996;36: 783–791.

80. Rogge MC, Solomon WR, Sedman AJ, Welling PG, Tothaker RD, Wagner JG. The theophylline-enoxacin interaction: I. Effect of enoxacin dose on theophylline disposition. *Clin Pharmacol Ther* 1988;44:579–587.

81. Schwartz J, Jauregui L, Letteri J, Bachmann K. Impact of ciprofloxacin on theophylline clearance and steady-state concentrations in serum. *Antimicrob Agents Chemother* 1988;1:75–79.

82. Sarkar M, Polk RE, Guzelian PS, Hunt C, Karnes HT. In vitro effect of fluoroquinolones on theophylline metabolism in human liver microsomes. *Antimicrob Agents Chemother* 1990;34:594–599.

83. Zhai S, Kunze KL, Loi C-M, Vestal RE. Evaluation of a model for the prediction of decreased theophylline clearance by individual and combined inhibitors of cytochrome P450 1A2 (*in press*).

84. Stevens JC, Wrighton SA. Interaction of the enantiomers of fluoxetine and norfluoxetine with human liver cytochromes P450. *J Pharmacol Exp Ther* 1993;266:964–971.

85. Bergstrom RF, Peyton AL, Lemberger L. Quantification and mechanism of the fluoxetine and tricyclic antidepressant interaction. *Clin Pharmacol Ther* 1992;51:239–248.

86. Moltke Lv, Greeblatt D, Cotreau-Bibbo M, Duan S, Harmatz J, Shader R. Inhibition of desipramine hydroxylation in vitro by serotonin-reuptake-inhibitor antidepressants, and by quinidine and ketoconazole: a model system to predict drug interactions in vivo. *J Pharmacol Exp Ther* 1994;268:1278–1283.

87. Yee GC, McGuire TR. Pharmacokinetic drug interactions with cyclosporine (Part II). *Clin Pharmacokinet* 1990;19:400–415.

88. Backman JT, Olkkola KT, Aranko K, Himberg J-J, Neuvonen PJ. Dose of midazolam should be reduced during diltiazem and verapamil treatments. *Br J Clin Pharmacol* 1994;37:221–225.

89. Varhe A, Olkkola KT, Neuvonen PJ. Diltiazem enhances the effects of triazolam by inhibiting its metabolism. *Clin Pharmacol Ther* 1996;59: 369–375.

90. Langaniere S, Davies RF, Carignan G, et al. Pharmacokinetic and pharmacodynamic interactions between diltiazem and quinidine. *Clin Pharmacol Ther* 1996;60:255–264.

91. Yeung PKF, Buckley SJ, Hung OR, et al. Steady-state plasma concen-

trations of diltiazem and its metabolites in patients and healthy volunteers. *Ther Drug Monit* 1996;18:40–45.

92. Pichard L, Fabre I, Fabre G, et al. Cyclosporin A drug interactions. Screening for inducers and inhibitors of cytochrome P-450 (cyclosporin A oxidase) in primary cultures of human hepatocytes and in liver microsomes. *Drug Metab Dispos* 1990;18:595–605.

93. Sutton D, Butler A, Nadin L, Murray M. Role of CYP3A4 in human hepatic diltiazem N-demthylation: inhibition of CYP3A4 activity by oxidized diltiazem metabolites. *J Pharmacol Exp Ther* 1997;282:294–300.

94. Sugawara Y, Ohashi M, Nakamura S, et al. Metabolism of diltiazem. I. Structures of new acidic and basic metabolites in rat, dog and man. *J Pharmacobio-Dynamics* 1988;11:211–223.

95. Sugawara Y, Nakamura S, Usuki S, et al. Metabolism of diltiazem II. Metabolic profile in rat, dog and man. *J Pharmacobio-Dynamics* 1988;11:224–233.

96. Kharasch ED, Thummel KE. Human alfentanil metabolism by cytochrome P450 3A3/4. An explanation for the interindividual variability in alfentanil clearance? *Anesth Analg* 1993;76:1033–1039.

97. Ludden TM. Pharmacokinetic interactions of the macrolide antibiotics. *Clin Pharmacokinet* 1985;10:63–79.

98. Gorski JC, Jones DR, Haehner-Daniels BD, Hamman MA, O'Mara EM, Hall SD. The contribution of intestinal and hepatic CYP3A to the interaction between midazolam and clarithromycin. *Clin Pharmacol Ther* 1998;64:133–143.

99. Kolars JC, Awni WM, Merionn RM, Watkins PB. First-pass metabolism of cyclosporin by the gut. *Lancet* 1991;338:1488–1490.

100. Paine MF, Shen DD, Kunze KL, et al. First-pass metabolism of midazolam by the human intestine. *Clin Pharmacol Ther* 1996;60:14–24.

101. Fromm MF, Busse D, Kroemer HK, Eichelbaum M. Differential induction of prehepatic and hepatic metabolism of verapamil by rifampin. *Hepatology* 1996;24:796–801.

102. Fleishaker JC, Pearson PG, Wienkers LC, Pearson LK, Graves GR. Biotransformation of tirilazad in humans: 2. Effect of ketoconazole on tirilazad clearance and oral bioavailability. *J Pharmacol Exp Ther* 1996;277:991–998.

103. Gomez DY, Wacher VJ, Tomlanovich SJ, Hebert MF, Benet LZ. The effects of ketoconazole on the intestinal metabolism and bioavailability of cyclosporine. *Clin Pharmacol Ther* 1995;58:15–19.

104. Javala KM, Olkkola KT, Neuvonen PJ. Itraconazole greatly increases plasma concentrations and effects of felodipine. *Clin Pharmacol Ther* 1997;61:410–415.

105. Neuvonen PJ, Varhe A, Olkkola KT. The effect of ingestion time interval on the interaction between itraconazole and triazolam. *Clin Pharmacol Ther* 1996;60:326–331.

106. Koley AP, Robinson RC, Markowitz A, Friedman FK. Drug-drug interactions: effect of quinidine on nifedipine binding to human cytochrome P450 3A4. *Biochem Pharmacol* 1997;53:455–460.

107. Ahonen J, Olkkola KT, Neuvonen PJ. Effect of route of administration of fluconazole on the interaction between fluconazole and midazolam. *Eur J Clin Pharmacol* 1997;51:415–419.

108. Olkkola KT, Aranko K, Luuila H, et al. A potentially hazardous interaction between erythromycin and midazolam. *Clin Pharmacol Ther* 1993;53:298–305.

109. Lown KS, Kolars JC, Thummel KE, et al. Interpatient heterogeneity in expression of CYP3A4 and CYP3A5 in small bowel: lack of prediction by the erythromycin breath test. *Drug Metab Dispos* 1994;22:947–955.

110. Thummel KE, O'Shea D, Paine MF, et al. Oral first-pass elimination of midazolam involves both gastrointestinal and hepatic CYP3A-mediated metabolism. *Clin Pharmacol Ther* 1996;59:491–502.

111. Bailey DG, Bend JR, Arnold JMO, Tran LT, Spence JD. Erythromycin-felodipine interaction: magnitude, mechanism, and comparison with grapefruit juice. *Clin Pharmacol Ther* 1996;60:25–33.

112. Kupferschmidt HHT, Ha HR, Ziegler WH, Meier PJ, Krähenbühl S. Interaction between grapefruit juice and midazolam in humans. *Clin Pharmacol Ther* 1995;58:20–28.

113. Edgar B, Bailey D, Bergstrand R, Johnsson G, Regardh CG. Acute effects of drinking grapefruit juice on the pharmacokinetics and dynamics of felodipine—and its potential clinical relevance. *Eur J Clin Pharmacol* 1992;42:313–317.

114. Bailey DG, Spence JD, Munoz C, Arnold JMO. Interaction of citrus juices with felodipine and nifedipine. *Lancet* 1991;377:268–269.

115. Benton RE, Honig PK, Zamani K, Cantalina LR, Woosley RL. Grapefruit juice alters terfenadine pharmacokinetics, resulting in prolonga-

115. tion of repolarization on the electrocardiogram. *Clin Pharmacol Ther* 1996;59:383–388.
116. Rau SE, Bend JR, Arnold MO, Tran LT, Spence JD, Bailey DG. Grapefruit juice—terfenadine single-dose interaction; magnitude, mechanism, and relevance. *Clin Pharmacol Ther* 1997;61:401–409.
117. Bailey DG, Arnold JMO, Spence JD. Grapefruit juice and drugs. How significant is the interaction? *Clin Pharmacokinet* 1994;26:91–98.
118. Lown KS, Bailey DG, Fontana RJ, et al. Grapefruit juice increases felodipine oral availability in humans by increasing intestinal CYP3A protein expression. *J Clin Invest* 1997;99:2545–2553.
119. Donato M, Castell J, Gomez-Lechon M. Effect of model inducers on cytochrome P450 activities of human hepatocytes in primary culture. *Drug Metab Dispos* 1995;23:553–558.
120. Schuetz EG, Beck WT, Schuetz JD. Modulators and substrates of p-glycoprotein and cytochrome P4503A coordinately up-regulate these proteins in human colon carcinoma cells. *Mol Pharmacol* 1996;49:311–318.
121. Li A, Rasmussen A, Xu L, Kaminski D. Rifampicin induction of lidocaine metabolism in cultured human hepatocytes. *J Pharmacol Exp Ther* 1995;274:673–677.
122. Lake BG, Ball SE, Renwick AB, et al. Induction of CYP3A isoforms in cultured precision-cut human liver slices. *Xenobiotica* 1997;27:1165–1173.
123. Curi-Pedrosa R, Daujat M, Pichard L, et al. Omeprazole and lansoprazole are mixed inducers of CYP1A and CYP3A in human hepatocytes in primary culture. *J Pharmacol Exp Ther* 1994;269:384–392.
124. Levy RH, Lai AA, Dumain MS. Time-dependent kinetics. IV. pharmacokinetic theory of enzyme induction. *J Pharm Sci* 1979;68:398–399.
125. Levy RH, Dumain MS, Cook JL. Time-dependent kinetics. V. Time course of drug levels during enzyme induction (one compartment model). *J Pharmacokinet Biopharm* 1979;7:557–578.
126. Abramson FP. Kinetic models of induction: I. Persistence of the inducing substance. *J Pharm Sci* 1986;75:223–232.
127. Kerr BM, Thummel KE, Wurden CJ, et al. Human liver carbamazepine metabolism. Role of CYP3A4 and CYP2C8 in 10, 11-epoxide formation. *Biochem Pharmacol* 1994;47:1969–1976.
128. Bertilsson L, Höjer B, Tybring G, Osterloh J, Rane A. Autoinduction of carbamazepine metabolism in children examined by a stable isotope technique. *Clin Pharmacol Ther* 1980;27:83–88.
129. Ged C, Rouillon JM, Pichard L, et al. The increase in urinary excretion of 6β-hydroxycortisol as a marker of human hepatic cytochrome P450IIIA induction. *Br J Clin Pharmacol* 1989;28:373–387.
130. Ohnhaus E, Breckenridge A, Park B. Urinary excretion of 6β-hydroxycortisol and the time course measurement of enzyme induction in man. *Eur J Clin Pharmacol* 1989;36:39–46.
131. Fleishaker JC, Pearson LK, Peters GR. Phenytoin causes a rapid increase in 6β-hydroxycortisol urinary excretion in humans—a putative measure of CYP3A induction. *J Pharm Sci* 1995;84:292–294.
132. Park BK, Breckenridge AM. Clinical implications of enzyme induction and enzyme inhibition. *Clin Pharmacokinet* 1981;6:1–24.
133. Emery MG, Jubert C, Thummel KE, Kharasch ED. Duration of cytochrome P4502E1 inhibition and estimation of functional CYP2E1 enzyme half-life following single dose disulfiram administration in humans. *Drug Metab Dispos* 1999;291:213–219.
134. Reichel C, Skodra T, Nacke A, Spengler U, Sauerbruch T. The lignocaine metabolite (MEGX) liver function test and P-450 induction in humans. *Br J Clin Pharmacol* 1998;46:535–539.
135. Fleishaker JC, Pearson LK, Peters GR. Induction of tirilazad by phenytoin. *Biopharm Drug Disp* 1998;19:91–96.
136. Perucca E, Richens A. Reduction of oral bioavailability of lignocaine by induction of first-pass metabolism in epileptic patients. *Br J Clin Pharmacol* 1979;8:21–31.
137. Backman JT, Olkkola KT, Neuovnen PJ. Rifampin drastically reduces plasma concentrations and effects of oral midazolam. *Clin Pharmacol Ther* 1996;59:7–13.
138. Backman JT, Olkkola KT, Ojala M, Laaksovirta H, Neuvonen PJ. Concentrations and effects of oral midazolam are greatly reduced in patients treated with carbamazepine or phenytoin. *Epilepsia* 1996;37:253–257.
139. Chien JY, Thummel KE, Slattery JT. Pharmacokinetic consequences of induction of CYP2E1 by ligand stabilization. *Drug Metab Dispos* 1997;25:1165–1175.

CHAPTER 2

From *In Vitro* to *In Vivo:* An Academic Perspective

René H. Levy and William F. Trager

The availability of human microsomes and specific cDNA-expressed enzymes has revolutionized the study of drug metabolism by melding the traditional approaches of medicinal chemists with those of pharmacokineticists, particularly in the unraveling of inhibition-based drug interactions (1–4). In drug development, new standards are rapidly evolving that make enzymology of the metabolism of a drug a critical element of its pharmacologic profile (5–7). As a result, a large body of *in vitro* data has been generated on various drugs with the aim of applying this knowledge to *in vivo* behavior. Even though the scientific return of such an approach is profound, practical guidelines to assess the validity of the extrapolations that can be made from *in vitro* data are not available. Variables that could obscure linear extrapolations are multiple and include differences among various *in vitro* systems, the role of drug concentration, the validity of enzyme "probes," the specificity of inhibitors, and time-dependent phenomena (1,8–11). This overview analyzes the variables that must be considered when attempting to project *in vitro* drug and enzyme behavior to drug disposition *in vivo* and proposes a set of principles that addresses the problem of inhibition-based drug interactions from a practical clinical perspective.

SUBSTRATE AND INHIBITOR CHARACTERISTICS ASSOCIATED WITH MAJOR VERSUS MINOR INTERACTIONS

In any inhibition-based clinical drug interaction, three critical entities are involved: the drug (substrate), the enzymes responsible for drug clearance, and the inhibitor

R. H. Levy: Department of Pharmaceutics and Neurologic Surgery, University of Washington, Box 357610, H272 Health Sciences Building, Seattle, Washington 98195
W. F. Trager: Department of Medicinal Chemistry, University of Washington, Box 357610, H172 Health Sciences Building, Seattle, Washington 98195.

(precipitant). A major interaction is defined as one that leads to a more than 50% increase in the plasma level of a substrate with a narrow therapeutic index. Such a drug has a ratio of toxic/minimum effective concentration of less than 3 (examples are found among antidepressants, anticoagulants, and anticonvulsants). A minor interaction is defined as one that leads to a less than 50% increase in plasma level of a substrate with a narrow therapeutic index. The occurrence of a major or minor interaction depends on the metabolic characteristics of the drug, the relative contributions of a given enzyme to the total clearance of the drug, and the selectivity, potency, and inhibition mechanism of the inhibitor.

Substrate Characteristics: Major Metabolite–Major Enzyme

The simplest metabolic model involves a drug that is cleared by one primary metabolite whose formation is catalyzed predominantly by one hepatic enzyme. In quantitative terms, it is assumed that the fraction metabolized (f_m) to the primary metabolite is larger than 0.7 and that the contribution of the major enzyme (E_c) is also larger than 0.7, where E_c is the fraction of the formation clearance of the primary metabolite (CL_f) catalyzed by this enzyme

$$E_c = CL_{fe}/CL_f \qquad [2\text{-}1]$$

E_c, like f_m, varies between 0 and 1 and is equal to 1 when the major enzyme is the sole catalyst in forming the primary metabolite. Even though the formation clearance of the primary metabolite could eventually approximate total body clearance (CL_t) of the drug in such a system, the focus should be on the fraction of total drug clearance catalyzed by a given enzyme. The concept of fraction metabolized thus evolves from the fraction of total clearance associated with formation of a given metabolite, f_m, to the fraction of total drug clearance catalyzed by a given enzyme, f_{me}, where

$$f_{me} = f_m \cdot E_c \qquad [2\text{-}2]$$

and

$$f_{me} = CL_f/CL_t \cdot CL_{fe}/CL_f = CL_{fe}/CL_t \qquad [2\text{-}3]$$

Under the aforementioned assumptions, $f_{me} > 0.49$. Inhibition of this major or dominant enzyme results in a decrease in CL_f and thus in CL. At a given inhibitor concentration, the larger f_m or E_c, the greater the effect of enzyme inhibition on total clearance and thus the greater potential for a major interaction.

Inhibitor Characteristics

When a drug exhibits the metabolic characteristics defined earlier (one primary metabolite formed mostly by one enzyme), the critical parameter in its potential to interact with other precipitants becomes the potency of the precipitant (inhibitor) to inhibit the major enzyme. If one assumes that the inhibitor freely associates and dissociates with the major enzyme (competitive inhibition), then potency is defined by the ratio of inhibitor unbound plasma concentration, I (which is assumed to reflect its concentration at the site of metabolism), to its *in vivo* inhibitory constant, K_{iiv}. In this situation, the selectivity of the inhibitor is not a factor as long as it inhibits the enzyme of interest. Quantitatively, the degree of interaction can be expressed by Equation 2-4:

$$C_i/C = CL/CL_i \sim CL_f/CL_{fi} = 1 + I/K_{iiv} \qquad [2\text{-}4]$$

where C_i and C equal the average steady-state (area under concentration [AUC]/τ) plasma concentrations of the drug in the presence and absence of inhibitor, respectively, and CL_i and CL_{fi} refer to the respective total and formation clearances in the presence of inhibitor. Under the aforementioned assumption that $f_{me} > 0.49$, $C_i/C > 1.5$ when $CL_i < 0.67$ CL. A major interaction is expected when I/K_{iiv} is larger than 0.5, whereas a minor interaction occurs if I/K_{iv} is less than 0.25.

One corollary of Equation 2-4 is that therapeutic agents that behave as potent inhibitors of specific cytochrome P450s must reach plasma levels well in excess of their K_{iiv}. Examples are quinidine inhibition of P450 2D6 ($K_{iv} = 20$–40 nM, I = 5–15 µM) and fluconazole inhibition of P450 2C19 ($K_{iv} = 10$–20 µM, I = 50–75 µM). A second and perhaps even more powerful corollary of this equation is that inhibition is substrate independent, that is, the same degree of inhibition expressed by I/K_{iiv} will be operative regardless of the drug metabolized by this enzyme. Examples of substrate independence are found among the interactions of warfarin, tolbutamide, and phenytoin with the P450 2C9 inhibitors sulfaphenazole, phenylbutazone, miconazole, and fluconazole (12) (see Chapters 17, 29, 41, and 47).

Substrate Characteristics: Multiple Metabolites–Multiple Enzymes

A more complex and perhaps more common model of metabolic behavior is one in which two or more enzymes generate one or more metabolites accounting for more than 90% of the dose. If such a drug is coadministered with a broad spectrum inhibitor with high potency toward all those enzymes, the total clearance of the drug will be affected appreciably, as in the previous case, and a major interaction will occur. If the inhibitor is selective (inhibits only one of the contributing enzymes), the interaction is expected to be minor even if the inhibitor has a high potency, because the fraction of drug clearance catalyzed by one enzyme, f_{me}, is likely to be small.

Substrate Characteristics: Multiple Metabolites–Major Enzyme

This substrate model encompasses both the simple and complex models described above. It considers the possibility of a single enzyme generating multiple metabolites from a drug. Although any one metabolite need not be major, the overall fraction of drug clearance catalyzed by this single enzyme could be large (larger than 0.7) when the contributions of all the metabolites formed by this enzyme are summed. Any inhibitor of this enzyme will simultaneously affect all the metabolites produced by the enzyme; this case then becomes equivalent to the major metabolite–major enzyme case in which the inhibitor can produce a major interaction if it is highly potent.

ROLE OF *IN VITRO* STUDIES IN INVESTIGATING THE MECHANISM OF AN INTERACTION

Assume that in the clinic a major inhibition interaction is encountered with a drug that is cleared predominantly by metabolism. What role do *in vitro* studies play in establishing the mechanism of this interaction?

Metabolic Fate of a Substrate

Knowledge of the metabolic fate of the drug must be obtained to determine whether it belongs to the simple or complex model, that is, if formation of a single metabolite accounts for at least 50% of the clearance or if multiple metabolites are formed with no single major pathway. This knowledge originates with *in vivo* human studies that account for the fate of the drug in terms of fractions of the total metabolic clearance associated with individual metabolites. Although it is not possible to determine from *in vitro* systems whether a drug is cleared predominantly by metabolism, it does appear that, in many instances, the relative fraction of metabolic clearance associated with a given metabolite *in vivo* is conserved in *in vitro* systems. Thus, it is not only reasonable but highly informative to conduct *in vitro* experiments to determine (a) whether a single enzyme catalyzes the formation of the dominant metabolite, (b) the identity of the enzyme, and (c) the properties of the inhibitor, because none of these parameters can be obtained easily from *in vivo* experimentation.

Identification of Enzymes Responsible for Substrate Clearance

Once the pathways of metabolism that lead to clearance of the substrate have been defined in terms of specific metabolites *in vitro* and *in vivo,* they must next be characterized in terms of the enzymes catalyzing their formation. The linkage between *in vitro* and *in vivo* data occurs by way of the enzyme responsible for formation of a given metabolite, that is, the information obtained *in vitro* is "projected" to the *in vivo* situation.

Progress in this area has been enhanced by the increased availability of human liver preparations and cDNA-expressed human cytochrome P450s. For example, incubation of the substrate of interest with a human liver microsomal preparation allows researchers to establish the identity and relative importance of primary oxidative metabolites. Then, the use of isoform-selective inhibitors and antibodies (coupled to several different human liver microsomal preparations of defined metabolic activity) allows preliminary identification of the enzymes catalyzing the metabolism of the substrate. Confirmation of the identified enzymes can be achieved by incubation of the substrate with the cDNA-expressed forms. To illustrate how these tools can be used to identify metabolic enzymes, two examples taken from our own work, carbamazepine and warfarin, are provided.

Example: Carbamazepine

Until recently, it was not possible to address the interactions associated with carbamazepine because there was no knowledge of the enzymes involved in its metabolism (13). Carbamazepine is biotransformed to three primary metabolites: carbamazepine-10,11-epoxide, and 2-hydroxycarbamazepine, and 3-hydroxycarbamazepine, of which carbamazepine-10,11-epoxide is the most significant (a 40%–60% fraction of dose based on urinary excretion measurements in epileptic patients) (14). The relative importance of these pathways *in vitro* was essentially the same as that found *in vivo*. The effects of a panel of cytochrome P450 isoform-selective chemical inhibitors on the formation of the 10,11-epoxide metabolite were assessed in a human liver microsomal preparation. Inhibitors of CYP1A2, CYP2C9/10, CYP2C19, CYP2D6, and CYP2E1 had no significant effect, whereas triacetyloleandomycin (TAO, a selective

CYP3A4 inhibitor) inhibited formation of the 10,11-epoxide metabolite by 70% (15). In the same incubation, formation of 2- and 3-hydroxycarbamazepine was not affected by TAO. Addition of a polyclonal antibody against CYP3A4 resulted in selective concentration-dependent inhibition of carbamazepine-10,11-epoxide formation with a maximum of 60% (and no effect on the production of the other two metabolites). A reasonable correlation ($r^2 = 0.57$, $p < 0.05$) between carbamazepine-10,11-epoxide formation rate and CYP3A4 content, as measured by Western blot analysis, was obtained in a panel of livers.

Purified reconstituted CYP3A4 catalyzed the 10,11-epoxidation of carbamazepine, but not the formation of the other two hydroxylated metabolites. This finding was confirmed by incubations of carbamazepine with cDNA-expressed CYP3A4 cell lysates and by the finding that plots of epoxide formation rate versus carbamazepine concentration obeyed Michaelis-Menten kinetics (13). The series of studies outlined earlier established with a high degree of certainty that CYP3A4 plays a dominant role in the metabolism of carbamazepine and made it possible to begin to rationalize the interactions of carbamazepine with numerous inhibitors, particularly erythromycin, troleandomycin, and other macrolide antibiotics (16) (see Chapter 17).

Example: Warfarin

It had long been known from *in vivo* drug interaction studies (17–19) that the major route of whole body clearance of (S)-warfarin, the pharmacologically potent enantiomer in the clinically available racemic form of the anticoagulant, was by way of formation of the pharmacologically inactive (S)-7-hydroxywarfarin metabolite. This single metabolite accounted for greater than 60% of (S)-warfarin clearance, but whether its formation was because of the action of a single or multiple enzymes was not known. When human liver became available, studies were conducted to compare the *in vitro* metabolic fate of the two enantiomers of the drug to their well-established *in vivo* metabolic profiles in an initial attempt to determine whether the fate of the drug in the two different environments could be correlated. The results of these studies (20) indicated that, *in vitro*, a high-affinity (low K_m) enzyme was responsible for the formation of both (S)-6- and (S)-7-hydroxywarfarin in a ratio of about 1:3. Together these two metabolites accounted for 80% to 85% of the *in vivo* clearance of (S)-warfarin. Subsequently, work with human cytochrome P450s expressed from cDNA clones indicated that, of the 11 isoforms examined, only a single cytochrome P450, CYP2C9, catalyzed formation of (S)-7-hydroxywarfarin (21). This particular enzyme also catalyzed formation of (S)-6-hydroxywarfarin in a ratio of 1:3.5 relative to the formation of (S)-7-hydroxywarfarin, as found earlier in the human liver microsomal preparations. Kinetic analysis indicated that the K_m for the formation of these two metabolites by expressed CYP2C9 was identical to that determined from microsomal preparations. In addition, the Ki values for sulfaphenazole inhibition of the formation of (S)-6- or (S)-7-hydroxywarfarin from (S)-warfarin by expressed CYP2C9 or human liver microsomes were identical. Also, drugs such as phenytoin (22,23), miconazole (18), amiodarone (19), and fluconazole (24,25), which inhibit the formation of (S)-7-hydroxywarfarin *in vivo,* also inhibit its formation *in vitro.* All of the evidence was consistent with a single enzyme, CYP2C9, being responsible for the majority of the clearance (85%) of the active enantiomer, (S)-warfarin, via the formation of two inactive hydroxylated metabolites (see Chapter 29).

FROM *IN VITRO* TO *IN VIVO*

In Vivo–In Vitro Assumption

It may be argued that the validity of *in vitro* studies rests on the assumption that the enzyme catalyzing the formation of a given metabolite *in vitro* must also be the same enzyme that catalyzes formation of the metabolite *in vivo.* For the majority of substrates studied to date, it appears that the relative contribution of a given metabolite to the *in vivo* metabolic clearance is largely conserved in microsomal preparations *in vitro.* In fact, the correspondence in fractional clearances between *in vitro* and *in vivo* experiments provides some of the primary evidence supporting the assumption that the same enzyme is operating both *in vitro* and *in vivo.*

Role of Concentration in Identification of Enzymes Responsible for Substrate Clearance

The importance of using therapeutic concentrations in the identification of enzymes involved in the formation of a particular metabolite cannot be overemphasized. An example of this point has been provided recently by Yasumori and colleagues (8) and Kato and Yamazoe (9) in the case of diazepam. Diazepam is metabolized by *N*-demethylation to nordiazepam and by 3-hydroxylation to temazepam. *In vivo,* formation of nordiazepam is a major pathway accounting for approximately 50% of the dose, whereas 3-hydroxylation accounts for approximately 30%. However, a number of early studies in human liver microsomal preparations suggested that 3-hydroxylation was the larger pathway (26–28). Yasumori and colleagues (8) showed that the discrepancy was because of the use of supratherapeutic concentrations. Yasumori and colleagues found that when diazepam concentrations decreased from 200 μM to 20 μM and finally 4 μM that the 3-hydroxylation/*N*-demethylation ratio also decreased from 4.55 to 1.27 and 0.73. They also observed that an

anti-2C antibody did not inhibit *N*-demethylation at 200 μM but exhibited an 80% to 90% inhibition at 20 μM. Because therapeutic concentrations are 1 to 2 μM, only data from incubation at a low substrate concentration has *in vivo* relevance.

If two enzymes are involved in the formation of a single metabolite, the relative contribution of each enzyme is determined by comparison of the intrinsic clearances (V_{max}/K_m values). This is why kinetic studies must be carried out both in microsomal and expressed systems to calculate the enzyme parameters, K_m, V_{max}, and intrinsic clearance. In the case of diazepam, Yasumori and coworkers and Kato and Yamazoe calculated the kinetic parameters for the two enzymes (presumably CYP2C19 and CYP3A) involved in the formation of nordiazepam (8,9). Results of their studies indicated that the low K_m enzyme (presumably CYP2C19) was absent in subjects who were poor metabolizers of (S)-mephenytoin.

In Vivo K_i (K_{iiv})

When the fraction of total drug clearance catalyzed by a given enzyme has been established *in vitro* and correlates to what is observed *in vivo,* approaches to resolving differences in inhibitor behavior in the two environments can be addressed. It becomes possible then to characterize inhibitor behavior *in vivo* using the same principles that operate *in vitro,* that is, the extent of inhibition *in vivo* will be dependent on the ratio of inhibitor unbound plasma concentration to the K_i actually operating *in vivo* (competitive inhibition). This type of K_i has been symbolized as K_{iiv} and is defined by Equation 2-4.

The concept of an *in vivo* K_i is particularly powerful because it describes the behavior of the inhibitor in the subject patient, without necessitating assumptions of correspondence between plasma and hepatocyte inhibitor concentrations or between K_i values operating *in vitro* and *in vivo* (29). Furthermore, the *in vivo* K_i allows a prediction of the extent of interaction in a given patient as a function of plasma concentration of the inhibitor (30,31). No other method presently available provides this type of prediction. In fact, inhibition studies have been typically carried out with a fixed dose of inhibitor and no allowance has been made for plasma concentration of inhibitor to explain intersubject variability in extent of interaction. Based on the concept of *in vivo* K_i, we propose that the design of inhibition-based interaction studies should include at least two doses of inhibitor and measurement of the steady-state plasma concentration of inhibitor. Such designs would allow the calculation of *in vivo* K_i values for each subject using Equation 2-4 (31). Also, the *in vivo* K_i determined for an enzyme–inhibitor pair should be generalizable because it is a constant that is independent of substrate. Thus, once determined, it should be applicable to any substrate of the enzyme and provide a basis for prediction of the degree of interaction.

Finally, the future availability of *in vivo* K_i values will provide a framework for comparison with their corresponding *in vitro* K_i values and thus allow an elucidation of the variables governing quantitative *in vitro–in vivo* correlations.

Role of Concentration in Determining Inhibitor Effectiveness *In Vivo*

When enzymes that contribute to the metabolic clearance of a drug have been identified (i.e., two enzymes), the role of the inhibitor can be assessed. If the observed interaction is major, then inhibition of either enzyme that accounts for greater than 50% of the clearance of the drug is most likely to be the cause. If the interaction is minor, inhibition of either enzyme could be the cause, depending on the relative potencies of the inhibitor toward the two enzymes. Of particular value is knowledge of the *in vitro* potency of the inhibitor, as measured by the K_i, for inhibiting the activity of each of the enzymes involved in the metabolism of the drug. To use *in vitro* K_i values for the purpose of quantitative *in vivo* predictions, the following guideline is generally used. The inhibitor will effectively decrease the catalytic function of a given enzyme *in vivo* if its K_i for that enzyme is lower than its unbound plasma concentration. If the K_i exceeds the unbound inhibitor concentration, inhibition will be unlikely. This interpretation assumes that the "effective" inhibitor concentration that is in equilibrium with the intracellular concentration of inhibitor–substrate complex is equal to the unbound plasma inhibitor concentration ("free drug" hypothesis) and that the *in vitro* K_i value is conserved *in vivo*. Potential problems associated with the determination of accurate *in vitro* K_i values are discussed in Chapter 1. Serious mispredictions of at least an order of magnitude are possible if care is not taken to avoid or correct for depletion of the inhibitor through metabolism and specific or nonspecific binding to the incubation matrix (32,33).

With regard to the *in vivo* hepatocellular concentration of inhibitor, the definition of "effective" is somewhat controversial. In the absence of any active uptake or efflux processes or any extracellular or intracellular diffusional barrier, the unbound concentration of inhibitor in the hepatocellular cytosol should be equivalent to the unbound concentration in plasma. This would be true even if there was extensive partitioning of the inhibitor into hepatic tissues, resulting in a much greater total concentration of inhibitor in hepatic tissue than that in plasma. If only the unbound cytosolic concentration of inhibitor drives the formation of an enzyme–inhibitor complex, nonspecific binding of inhibitor within the parenchymal cell becomes irrelevant. The limited number of cases examined to date suggest this assumption makes a reasonable starting point. Examples of reasonably accurate *in vitro*-to-*in vivo* prediction of an interaction include the inhibitory effect of ketoconazole on intravenous tirilazad clearance (34) and the effect of fluconazole on oral (S)-warfarin clearance (25).

Although the free drug hypothesis applies to some inhibitors, it is possible that, for others, simplifying assumptions about rapid distributional equilibrium and the inhibitor-enzyme binding equilibrium is inappropriate. An inhibitor may access the enzyme active site by way of the endoplasmic reticulum membrane rather than cytosol, such that the membrane concentration of inhibitor controls the extent of inhibitor–enzyme complex formation. It is also possible that active uptake of the inhibitor can increase the unbound intracellular concentration above that of the plasma unbound concentration, as has been described for cimetidine (35) and itraconazole (36) inhibition of midazolam hydroxylation in rat liver. When the "effective" hepatocyte concentration is much higher than plasma concentration, it is possible for significant inhibition *in vivo* to occur despite a plasma concentration that is less than the *in vitro* K_i.

In addition to unknowns pertaining to the disposition of the inhibitor *in vivo*, the K_i determined *in vitro* may not be conserved *in vivo* because of enzyme sensitivity to different physicochemical environments. In theory, the *in vivo* binding affinity of the inhibitor for enzyme may increase or decrease relative to the *in vitro* state. Additional factors that may complicate *in vitro*-to-*in vivo* predictions, particularly for CYP3A-dependent drug metabolism, include the possibility of a coadministered inhibitor affecting significant intestinal first pass metabolic extraction, the time-dependent formation of inhibitory metabolites from a "proinhibitory" parent molecule, or the formation of ternary inhibitor–enzyme–substrate complexes. These are discussed in greater detail in Chapters 1, 10, 24, and 46.

Because of the potential complications cited earlier, more conservative approaches using either total plasma or total liver inhibitor concentration for the *in vitro*-to-*in vivo* prediction have been considered. In these circumstances, it is essential to follow up the prediction with an *in vivo* interaction study before any change in pharmacotherapy is adopted. For example, itraconazole is a potent inhibitor of CYP3A4, with an estimated *in vitro* K_i of 270 nM (37). Steady-state itraconazole concentrations (200 mg twice daily) are 10-fold higher, 2.7 μM (38), but because of extensive binding to plasma proteins (39), the steady-state unbound concentration of itraconazole is estimated to be far lower (5.3 nM) than the *in vitro* K_i. Although no systemic interaction would be predicted, itraconazole has been shown to be a potent inhibitor of systemic midazolam clearance and causes even more profound effects when the CYP3A substrate is given orally (40,41). Although the poor *in vitro*-to-*in vivo* prediction with itraconazole may be due in part to the accumulation of an inhibitory metabolite, it may also reflect the failure of the unbound inhibitor hypothesis.

COROLLARIES

Drugs Metabolized by the Same Isoform Interact with the Same Inhibitors

All drugs for which clearance is controlled by the same enzyme should exhibit the same interaction profile, that is, they will interact with the same inhibitors. This is because the interaction between enzyme and inhibitor at the active site of the enzyme, as measured by the K_i, is a constant that is independent of the substrates of that enzyme. One enzyme for which the principle of isoform specificity and substrate independence has been illustrated is P450 2C9 (42). It was shown that three drugs—phenytoin, warfarin, and tolbutamide, for which P450 2C9 controls a significant fraction of the clearance—interact with the same set of inhibitors: sulfaphenazole, phenylbutazone, fluconazole, azapropazone, cotrimoxazole, propoxyphene, miconazole, amiodarone, disulfiram, metronidazole, and stiripentol (12).

Drugs Metabolized by the Same Isoform Do Not Automatically Interact

The ultimate determinant of whether the metabolism of one of a pair of drugs metabolized by the same enzyme will interfere with the metabolism of the other is the ratio of the concentration of each drug to its K_i. This principle is illustrated by the unidirectional interaction between phenytoin and warfarin. Although they have different kinetic origins, for the sake of simplicity, K_i and K_m are equated here. Even though phenytoin inhibits the metabolism of (S)-warfarin, (S)-warfarin has no apparent effect on the metabolism of phenytoin. This is because phenytoin reaches therapeutic concentrations equal to or higher than its K_m; it exhibits nonlinear kinetics with an *in vivo* Km (2–3 μM) close to the value measured *in vitro,* (approximately 10 μM), whereas the plasma concentration of (S)-warfarin is always below its *in vitro* K_m value (4 μM).

When a Substrate Becomes an Inhibitor

An inhibitor of an isoform may or may not be a substrate for that isoform. For example, omeprazole inhibits CYP2C19, the enzyme responsible for a significant portion of its clearance, whereas fluconazole, which inhibits CYP2C9 and interacts with phenytoin, (S)-warfarin, and tolbutamide, is eliminated mostly by renal excretion. Similarly, quinidine is a potent inhibitor of CYP2D6, yet its oxidative elimination appears to be catalyzed by CYP3A4. These considerations emphasize the importance of determining the isoform inhibitory profile of a drug and not just the profile of the isoforms for which it is a substrate.

REFERENCES

1. Birkett DJ, MacKenzie PI, Veronese ME, Miners JO. In vitro approaches can predict human drug metabolism. *Trends Pharmacol Sci* 1993;14:292–294.
2. Gonzalez FJ. In vitro systems for prediction of rates of drug clearance and drug interactions [editorial; comment]. *Anesthesiology* 1992;77:413–415.
3. Houston JB. Utility of in vitro drug metabolism data in predicting in vivo metabolic clearance. *Biochem Pharmacol* 1994;47:1469–1479.
4. Peck CC, Temple R, Collins JM. Understanding consequences of concurrent therapies [editorial; comment]. *JAMA* 1993;269:1550–1552.
5. Wrighton SA, Vandenbranden M, Stevens JC, et al. In vitro methods for assessing human hepatic drug metabolism: their use in drug development [published erratum appears in *Drug Metab Rev* 1994;26(1–2): 483]. Drug *Metab Rev* 1993;25:453–484.
6. Rodrigues AD. Use of in vitro human metabolism studies in drug development. An industrial perspective. *Biochem Pharmacol* 1994;48: 2147–2156.
7. Chiu SH. The use of in vitro metabolism studies in the understanding of new drugs. *J Pharmacol Toxicol Methods* 1993;29:77–83.
8. Yasumori T, Li QH, Yamazoe Y, Ueda M, Tsuzuki T, Kato R. Lack of low Km diazepam N-demethylase in livers of poor metabolizers for S-mephenytoin 4′-hydroxylation. *Pharmacogenetics* 1994;4:323–331.
9. Kato R, Yamazoe Y. The importance of substrate concentration in determining cytochromes P450 therapeutically relevant in vivo. *Pharmacogenetics* 1994;4:359–362.
10. Newton DJ, Wang RW, Lu AY. Cytochrome P450 inhibitors. Evaluation of specificities the in in vitro metabolism of therapeutic agents by human liver microsomes. *Drug Metab Dispos* 1995;23:154–158.
11. Houston JB, Carlile DJ. Prediction of hepatic clearance from microsomes, hepatocytes, and liver slices. *Drug Metab Rev* 1997;29:891–922.
12. Levy RH, Bajpai M. Phenytoin: interactions with other drugs: mechanistic aspects. In: Levy RH, Mattson RH, Melrum BS, eds. *Antiepileptic drugs,* 4th ed. New York: Raven, 1995:329–338.
13. Kerr BM, Thummel KE, Wurden CJ, et al. Human liver carbamazepine metabolism. Role of CYP3A4 and CYP2C8 in 10,11-epoxide formation. *Biochem Pharmacol* 1994;47:1969–1979.
14. Faigle JW, Feldmann KF. Carbamazepine: biotransformation. In: Levy RH, Mattson R, Melrum B, Penry JK, Dreifuss FE, eds. *Antiepileptic drugs,* 3rd ed. New York: Raven Press, 1989:491–504.
15. Faigle JW, Feldmann KF. Antiepileptic drugs. In: Levy RH, Mattson RH, Melrum BS, eds. *Antiepileptic drugs,* 4th ed. New York: Raven, 1995:499–513.
16. Levy RH, Wurden CJ. Carbamazepine: interactions with other drugs. In: Levy RH, Mattson RH, Melrum BS, eds. *Antiepileptic drugs,* 4th ed. New York: Raven, 1995:543–554.
17. Toon S, Low LK, Gibaldi M, et al. The warfarin-sulfinpyrazone interaction: stereochemical considerations. *Clin Pharmacol Ther* 1986;39: 15–24.
18. O'Reilly RA, Goulart DA, Kunze KL, et al. Mechanisms of the stereoselective interaction between miconazole and racemic warfarin in human subjects. *Clin Pharmacol Ther* 1992;51:656–667.
19. Heimark LD, Wienkers L, Kunze K, et al. The mechanism of the interaction between amiodarone and warfarin in humans. *Clin Pharmacol Ther* 1992;51:398–407.
20. Rettie AE, Eddy AC, Heimark LD, Gibaldi M, Trager WF. Characteristics of warfarin hydroxylation catalyzed by human liver microsomes. *Drug Metab Dispos* 1989;17:265–270.
21. Rettie AE, Korzekwa KR, Kunze KL, et al. Hydroxylation of warfarin by human cDNA-expressed cytochrome P-450: a role for P-4502C9 in the etiology of (S)-warfarin-drug interactions. *Chem Res Toxicol* 1992;5:54–59.
22. Panegyres PK, Rischbieth RH. Fatal phenytoin warfarin interaction [letter]. *Postgrad Med J* 1991;67:98.
23. Veronese ME, Mackenzie PI, Doecke CJ, McManus ME, Miners JO, Birkett DJ. Tolbutamide and phenytoin hydroxylations by cDNA-expressed human liver cytochrome P4502C9 [published erratum appears in *Biochem Biophys Res Comm* 1991 Nov 14;180(3);1527]. *Biochem Biophys Res Comm* 1991;175:1112–1118.
24. Kunze KL, Wienkers LC, Thummel KE, Trager WF. Warfarin-fluconazole. I. Inhibition of the human cytochrome P450-dependent metabolism of warfarin by fluconazole: in vitro studies. *Drug Metab Dispos* 1996;24:414–421.
25. Black DJ, Kunze KL, Wienkers LC, et al. Warfarin-fluconazole. II. A

metabolically based drug interaction: in vivo studies. *Drug Metab Dispos* 1996;24:422–428.

26. Inaba T, Tait A, Nakano M, Mahon WA, Kalow W. Metabolism of diazepam in vitro by human liver. Independent variability of N-demethylation and C3-hydroxylation. *Drug Metab Dispos* 1988;16:605–608.

27. Reilly PE, Thompson DA, Mason SR, Hooper WD. Cytochrome P450IIIA enzymes in rat liver microsomes: involvement in C3-hydroxylation of diazepam and nordazepam but not N-dealkylation of diazepam and temazepam. *Mol Pharmacol* 1990;37:767–774.

28. Beischlag TV, Kalow W, Mahon WA, Inaba T. Diazepam metabolism by rat and human liver in vitro: inhibition by mephenytoin. *Xenobiotica* 1992;22:559–567.

29. Kunze KL, Trager WF. Warfarin-fluconazole. III. A rational approach to management of a metabolically based drug interaction. *Drug Metab Dispos* 1996;24:429–435.

30. Tran A, Rey E, Pons G, et al. Influence of stiripentol on cytochrome P450-mediated metabolic pathways in humans: in vitro and in vivo comparison and calculation of in vivo inhibition constants. *Clin Pharmacol Ther* 1997;62:490–504.

31. Levy RH, Kerr BM, Farwell J, Trager WF, Kunze KL, Thummel KE. A novel method to quantify the extent of drug interactions in individual patients: application ot carbamazepine-stiripentol. *Epilepsia* 1993;34:69.

32. Obach RS. Nonspecific binding to microsomes: impact on scale-up of in vitro intrinsic clearance to hepatic clearance as assessed through examination of warfarin, imipramine, and propranolol. *Drug Metab Dispos* 1997;25:1359–1369.

33. Obach RS. The importance of nonspecific binding in in vitro matrices, its impact on enzyme kinetic studies of drug metabolism reactions, and implications for in vitro-in vivo correlations [letter]. *Drug Metab Dispos* 1996;24:1047–1049.

34. Fleishaker JC, Pearson PG, Wienkers LC, Pearson LK, Peters GR. Bio-transformation of tirilazad in human: 2. Effect of ketoconazole on tirilazad clearance and oral bioavailability. *J Pharmacol Exp Ther* 1996;277:991–998.

35. Takedomi S, Matsuo H, Yamano K, Yamamoto K, Iga T, Sawada Y. Quantitative prediction of the interaction of midazolam and histamine H2 receptor antagonists in rats. *Drug Metab Dispos* 1998;26:318–323.

36. Yamano K, Yamamoto K, Kotaki H, Sawada Y, Iga T. Quantitative prediction of metabolic inhibition of midazolam by itraconazole and ketoconazole in rats: implication of concentrative uptake of inhibitors into liver. *Drug Metab Dispos* 1999;27:395–402.

37. von Moltke LL, Greenblatt DJ, Schmider J, et al. Midazolam hydroxylation by human liver microsomes in vitro: inhibition by fluoxetine, norfluoxetine, and by azole antifungal agents. *J Clin Pharmacol* 1996;36:783–791.

38. Barone JA, Koh JG, Bierman RH, et al. Food interaction and steady-state pharmacokinetics of itraconazole capsules in healthy male volunteers. *Antimicrob Agents Chemother* 1993;37:778–784.

39. Benet LZ, Oie S, Schwartz JB. Design and optimization of dosage regimens; pharmacokinetic data. In: Hardman JG, Limbird LE, Molinoff PB, Ruddon RW, Gilman AG, eds. *Goodman and Gilman's the pharmacological basis of therapeutics,* 9th ed. New York: McGraw-Hill, 1996:1752.

40. Olkkola KT, Backman JT, Neuvonen PJ. Midazolam should be avoided in patients receiving the systemic antimycotics ketoconazole or itraconazole. *Clin Pharmacol Ther* 1994;55:481–485.

41. Olkkola KT, Ahonen J, Neuvonen PJ. The effects of the systemic antimycotics, itraconazole and fluconazole, on the pharmacokinetics and pharmacodynamics of intravenous and oral midazolam. *Anesth Analg* 1996;82:511–516.

42. Levy RH. Cytochrome P450 isozymes and antiepileptic drug interactions. *Epilepsia* 1995;36:S8–S13.

CHAPTER 3

Industrial Viewpoint: Application of *In Vitro* Drug Metabolism in Various Phases of Drug Development

Barbara J. Ring and Steven A. Wrighton

The effectiveness of a drug on the physiologic state of a patient depends on its concentration at the appropriate site of action in the body. Processes that control the circulating blood concentration of a drug may impact the effectiveness and safety of that drug. One of the major determinants of drug concentration in the body is its rate of biotransformation or metabolic clearance. Hence, natural or pharmacologically induced variability in the rate of biotransformation can potentially lead to deleterious results. Possible clinically significant outcomes of changes in the metabolism of a drug include toxicity caused by higher than acceptable concentrations of the drug as a result of decreased clearance of the drug or, alternatively, levels of compound that are not efficacious because of increased clearance. A major cause of alterations in the clearance of a drug is through the coadministration of additional drugs that affect the catalytic activities of enzymes involved in the biotransformation of the drug of interest.

A number of factors increase the potential clinical risks associated with alterations in the metabolism of a drug. For example, perturbation in the metabolism of a drug with a narrow therapeutic index has great potential to result in serious side effects. Drug–drug interactions that decrease only slightly the metabolism of a narrow therapeutic index drug result in elevated levels of the drug and may result in serious toxicity. Similarly, interactions that increase the metabolism of narrow therapeutic index drugs may result in decreased levels and effectiveness of

the drug. It is also important to have an understanding of the dependence of a particular route of metabolism on the overall clearance of the drug. If the clearance of the drug is less than 50% dependent on the particular route of metabolism being altered, the overall effect of altering this route of metabolism on total drug clearance would be in question regardless of the degree of change observed (1). Furthermore, there can be great interpatient variability in the level of the enzymes involved in drug metabolism. For example, a bank of human liver samples characterized for cytochrome P450 (CYP or P450) levels can exhibit CYP3A activities that vary by as much as 15-fold (2). In addition, the variable expression of several of the drug metabolizing enzymes have been shown to be under genetic control (3). These genetic polymorphisms result in a population of patients that are deficient in one or more of the drug-metabolizing enzymes and thus have reduced metabolic capabilities. These variabilities in enzyme levels among people lead to differences in the clearance of drugs in the general population. The timing of the administration of drugs can also play a role in interaction potential, particularly if gut metabolism and transport of the drug plays a role in the bioavailability of the compounds. Finally, the physician's or patient's lack of awareness of the potential for drug–drug interaction with concomitant medication may lead to changes in a biotransformation of the drugs with possible deleterious results.

One way in which the metabolism of a drug may be altered is through the coadministration of another drug that may affect, in some manner (e.g., inhibition or induction), the enzymes responsible for the metabolism of the agent in question. The overall clinical significance of

B. J. Ring and S. A. Wrighton: Department of Drug Disposition, Eli Lilly and Company, Lilly Corporate Center, Mail Drop 0825, Indianapolis, Indiana 46285

these types of interactions has been debated. However, a recent report indicates that the incidence of clinically significant drug–drug interactions occur in approximately 3% to 5% of patients taking a few drugs (4). Significant interactions increase dramatically in patients taking 10 to 20 drugs simultaneously (4). In a study of the geriatric population, it was shown that 60% of the patients examined took drugs that had a potential for drug interactions (5). Fourteen percent of those geriatric patients exhibited side effects caused by drug–drug interaction, which resulted in hospitalization in most cases (5). Therefore, the ability to predict the potential for drug interactions has important consequences in the management of drug therapy in many patients.

Biotransformation of lipophilic xenobiotic compounds into more hydrophilic metabolites occurs through reactions that are classified as either phase I or phase II. Phase I reactions, usually through oxidation or hydrolysis, introduce or expose polar functional groups on the compound, rendering the drug more hydrophilic. Phase II reactions involve conjugation with endogenous agents such as glucuronic acid, sulfate, glutathione, or amino acids onto a functional group on the compound or metabolite, resulting in excretion in the urine or feces. One of the most important and well-characterized enzyme systems responsible for phase I drug metabolism are the P450s. Because of their prominent role in drug metabolism, the P450s are often involved in drug interactions. Three families of P450s are primarily responsible for xenobiotic metabolism: CYP1, CYP2, and CYP3. These three families of P450s account for approximately 70% of total P450s in the human liver with approximately 50% being comprised of members of the CYP3A and CYP2C subfamilies (approximately 30% and 20%, respectively) (6). As for their role in drug metabolism, CYP3A participates in the metabolism of approximately 50% of all drugs with 2D6 contributing to approximately 25%, 2C9 to approximately 15%, and CYP1A2 to approximately 5% (7). Thus, these four P450s participate in the metabolism of 95% of all drugs. The flavin-containing monooxygenases (FMOs) are another phase I enzyme system that are able to oxidize compounds that contain nucleophilic heteroatoms.

The examination of drug–drug interactions in the pharmaceutical industry has traditionally been performed in an ad hoc fashion during the clinical investigation of the drug. The drug–drug interaction studies undertaken for inclusion in a new drug application (NDA) include studies with coadministered drugs with a low therapeutic index or those commonly prescribed with the new chemical entity (NCE). Recent studies by the Food and Drug Administration indicate that in an NDA, the most commonly reported drug–drug interaction studies include coadministration of the NCE with cimetidine (commonly prescribed), digoxin (low therapeutic index), warfarin (low therapeutic index), theophylline (low therapeutic

index), and propanolol (commonly prescribed) (8). In many cases, such studies lack the focus necessary to appropriately answer interaction questions that may be important for the NCE. For example, this ad hoc approach for examining potential drug–drug interactions failed to predict a potentially deadly interaction with terfenadine. Recent *in vitro* studies have demonstrated that CYP3A mediates the metabolism of terfenadine to its active metabolite (9). However, at the time that terfenadine was developed, the *in vitro* techniques used to determine the P450s responsible for metabolism and thereby predict drug–drug interactions were not available. Therefore, *in vivo* studies that focused on examining the effect of the inhibition of terfenadine metabolism by CYP3A were not performed. Following initial case reports and later through well-designed clinical drug–drug interaction studies, it was determined that the inhibition of CYP3A-mediated metabolism of terfenadine has the potential to result in terfenadine levels that are elevated enough to result in ventricular arrhythmias and, potentially, death (10,11). What stands out in the list of the aforementioned compounds that are normally examined *in vivo* for drug interactions is a lack of a drug that can be used as a model for CYP3A interactions. Therefore, this potentially fatal interaction with terfenadine treatment and coadministered compounds that interact with CYP3A would not have been identified in the most commonly used *in vivo* screen.

Recently, *in vitro* techniques have become widely used as a tool to help predict potential drug–drug interactions in humans. The utility of these studies is that *in vitro* data concerning the potential for drug–drug interactions can be obtained early enough in drug development to help focus *in vivo* interaction studies and predict pharmacokinetic variability (e.g., identify special populations). In fact, many pharmaceutical companies are performing these types of studies before *in vivo* efficacy and safety studies. Furthermore, regulatory agencies have issued guidances to the industry that indicates that these *in vitro* predictions are highly useful in guiding the *in vivo* studies and should be performed before the onset of large clinical trials (12–14). These techniques have also been used when questions concerning drug–drug interactions arise late in development or during the postmarketing of a compound.

Two *in vitro* approaches to questions concerning potential drug–drug interactions have been developed and are widely accepted. In the first approach, *in vitro* studies examine the potential of a new drug to inhibit the metabolism of drugs administered concurrently. A systematic approach, focusing on the ability of the NCE to interact with the known important drug-metabolizing enzymes, can be used to answer these questions. In the second *in vitro* approach to drug–drug interactions, the enzymes responsible for the metabolism of an NCE are determined. Information on how the catalytic activities of these drug-metabolizing enzymes are affected by other drugs can be used to predict the potential that these compounds may have on the metabolism of the NCE, if they are given concurrently. An additional *in vitro* technique used to predict drug–drug interactions is based on the ability of the NCE to induce or increase the drug-metabolizing enzymes in human hepatocytes. This approach is currently under development by numerous laboratories (15–17) and is gaining acceptance. The regulatory agencies in charge of ensuring efficacy and safety for marketed drugs in the United States, Australia, and Europe have responded to the availability of these techniques and have issued guidelines that outline for the pharmaceutical researcher their views as to the appropriate use of these tools to predict drug–drug interactions and pharmacokinetic variability (12–14).

IN VITRO TECHNIQUES

Many *in vitro* techniques are used by the pharmaceutical industry to model the human metabolism of drugs and thus predict potential drug interactions (2,18–20). These *in vitro* techniques can be placed in two broad categories that vary based on their complexity with respect to the number and types of drug-metabolizing enzymes present. The first type of *in vitro* metabolic study is the use of enzyme-based techniques. The second and more complex system is the use of cellular-based systems to study metabolism.

Enzyme-Based Techniques

The most reductionist approach to enzyme-based systems for examination of *in vitro* drug metabolism is through the use of purified enzymes. Initially, isolated enzymes were used to examine the metabolic capabilities of P450s purified from human liver tissue. However, the labor-intensive purification techniques necessary to isolate these enzymes and the necessity of adding lipid and enzymes (e.g., cytochrome b_5 and P450 reductase) to the incubation system have made their use arduous. Furthermore, the requirements for detergent, lipid, and enzymes in the incubation system, which are necessary for the enzyme to be metabolically competent but vary with the different forms of P450s, raise questions in relating results obtained with the purified enzyme systems to the *in vivo* situation.

Recent advances in molecular biology have allowed researchers to isolate cDNAs encoding the drug-metabolizing enzymes. In these systems, the cDNA encoding for the human metabolizing enzyme of interest is transfected into a host cell. These host cells have included human and other mammalian cell lines, *Escherichia coli*, yeast, and insect cells. These expressed enzyme systems are used as a source from which it is possible to isolate individual or defined mixtures of the drug-metabolizing enzymes. The

recent commercial availability of purified enzyme from cells expressing the drug-metabolizing enzymes, along with an easy-to-use incubation system containing the required lipid and cofactors, have made their use routine (21). However, many of the same questions concerning the relevance of the results obtained with purified enzymes to the *in vivo* situation remain with use of these enzymes isolated from cDNA expression systems.

Microsomes or other subcellular fractions prepared from cells expressing the cDNA for human metabolizing enzymes are commonly used to qualitatively determine whether a particular enzyme is capable of metabolizing an NCE. The utility of this approach is that the metabolism by a single enzyme can be examined in a membrane environment. In this fashion, the potential involvement of a specific enzyme in the metabolism of a compound can be examined, isolated from the influence of other drug metabolizing enzymes, but in a more physiologically relevant environment than can be obtained with the use of purified enzymes.

Quantitative conclusions regarding the relative abilities of different expressed enzymes to metabolize a compound of interest are limited. One problem is that transfection into nonhuman, nonhepatic cellular hosts may result in expressed enzymes that exhibit substrate affinity (K_m) and metabolic capacity (V_{max}), which is different than that observed for the native enzyme (21). Although the reason for this difference is often unknown, the differences in the lipid environment and concentrations and type of enzymes, such as P450 reductase and cytochrome b_5, in these cells appear to play a role in the catalytic activity of the expressed enzyme (22,23). Furthermore, the level of expression of enzyme and the ratio of P450 to coenzymes may be different from batch to batch. In addition, different drug-metabolizing enzymes may exhibit different levels of expression even within the same host cell. Therefore, interpretation of the *in vivo* relevance of a particular reaction studied in isolation can be difficult. With current understanding of the lipid, environmental, and coenzyme influences on P450 catalytic activity, the greatest utility of expressed enzymes is in determining which enzyme is capable of metabolizing the NCE.

As a next step in model complexity, subcellular fractions can be prepared from cells that naturally express the metabolizing enzymes. These subcellular fractions are isolated from cells using differential centrifugation (24). The fractions isolated include the cytosolic fraction of the cell (cellular homogenate with the major organelles removed), which contain many soluble phase II (conjugating) enzymes. The most commonly used subcellular fraction used is the microsomal fraction of cells (vesicles of endoplasmic reticulum) containing membrane-bound phase I (CYP and FMO) oxidative enzymes.

Because phase I metabolism is most often the rate-limiting step in the metabolism of drugs, microsomes prepared from human liver are a primary tool used for *in vitro* interaction studies. When properly harvested, human liver samples, snap-frozen and stored at approximately −80°C, show little loss of metabolic potential, even when stored over many years. Microsomes prepared from these samples have been found to retain their metabolic potential over a long period of time, even with multiple freeze and thaw cycles (25). As a result, these human liver microsomal samples are a ready source of the enzymes responsible for drug metabolism. It should also be noted that similar isolation techniques can be used to prepare microsomal fractions from extrahepatic sources of tissue for examination of drug metabolism.

The metabolism data obtained through the use of microsomes prepared from human liver appear to have a greater relevance to the *in vivo* situation than data obtained through the use of isolated enzyme systems. One reason for this increased relevance is that the native liver tissue contains a lipid environment, cytochrome b_5, and P450 reductase, which are similar to that seen *in vivo*. In addition, the phase I metabolism of an NCE can be examined in this microsomal system which contains a complete complement of CYPs and FMOs in their native environment. Therefore, the relative importance of different routes of metabolism obtained following liver microsomal incubations more closely approximates that observed *in vivo* rather than the information obtained examining multiple pathways by different isolated enzyme preparations.

Subcellular fractions may also be used to examine the ability of a drug to be metabolized by or interact with the phase II drug-metabolizing enzymes. To perform these *in vitro* interaction studies, the appropriate subcellular fraction containing the enzyme of interest must be used. Furthermore, the cofactors required for these reactions must be added. Often, as in the case of the uridine diphosphate glucuronosyltranferases (UDPGT) and glutathione transferases, a family of enzymes appear to have overlapping substrate specificities (26,27). Because of the lack of isoform-specific substrates, interaction studies *in vitro* can be performed with phase II enzymes by focusing on the interactions between the actual compounds of interest. For example, *in vitro* methods have been used to determine the UDPGTs responsible for the glucuronidation of propofol (28); it was determined that propofol was glucuronidated by both the I and II families of UDPGT. A variety of potential inhibitors of profolol glucuronidation were identified, including fentanyl, which has also been identified *in vivo* as an inhibitor of profolol clearance.

Cellular-Based Techniques

The two cellular-based systems commonly used to examine human xenobiotic metabolism are hepatocytes and liver slices. The use of an intact cell system to examine metabolism is, at least in theory, desirable because of its greater physiologic relevance to the intact organism.

These systems contain all the phase I and phase II enzyme systems along with their appropriate cofactors that are found in the liver *in vivo*.

Although liver slices and hepatocyte cultures are often used to determine the metabolism of a compound, there has been limited use of these models for drug–drug interaction studies (16,29–31). The current culture techniques for these cellular systems do not lead to the maintenance of constitutive expression of the P450s and phase II enzymes (32,33). Therefore, although these techniques may be useful for metabolite production and possibly induction studies, they are not useful models to examine the absolute rate of the metabolism of an NCE. As a result, their utility for inhibitory drug–drug interaction studies is limited.

The use of primary monolayer cultures of human hepatocytes shows utility as a system to model the induction of the drug-metabolizing enzymes. Currently, the examination of induction by an NCE is most often determined *in vivo* in animal models. However, it is well known that the P450s capable of xenobiotic metabolism show species differences in substrate specificity and regulation of expression (34); therefore, extrapolation of animal data to the human may lead to inaccurate predictions. The levels of P450s present in human hepatocytes are readily increased with known inducing compounds (15–17). Therefore, human hepatocytes appear to give the researcher an ability to examine the induction potential of an NCE in an *in vitro* system.

Primary hepatocytes have been proposed as useful *in vitro* models of drug inhibition (30,31). For example, the apparent K_i of inhibition obtained in studies with cultures of primary hepatocytes predicted the potent inhibition by ketoconazole or itraconazole on the CYP3A-mediated metabolism of terfenadine (30). Other inhibitors of CYP3A were also found to be inhibitors of terfenadine metabolism in these cultures of human hepatocytes. These studies suggest that, after further validation, it may be possible to use hepatocytes, with their full complement of phase I and phase II enzymes, to predict the inhibition of the metabolism of a compound in the presence of a second agent.

A major drawback with the use of primary hepatocyte cultures is the requirement for fresh human tissue. This is an important problem in that the freezing and thawing of hepatocytes results in problems with cellular viability. A number of researchers have been examining this problem in detail and may solve this storage problem.

DRUG INTERACTIONS—DETERMINING THE POTENTIAL OF A NEW CHEMICAL ENTITY TO INHIBIT THE CATALYTIC ACTIVITIES OF THE P450s

The identification of substrates that are selectively metabolized by an individual P450 (Table 3-1) have given

TABLE 3-1. *Form-selective catalytic activities of the human cytochromes P450*

Cytochrome P450	Form-selective catalytic activity
CYP1A2	Phenacetin *O*-deethylase
	Caffeine N3-demethylase
	Theophylline 8-hydroxylase
	Ethoxyresorufin *O*-deethylase
CYP2A6	Coumarin 7-hydroxylase
CYP2B6	*S*-Mephenytoin *N*-demethylase
CYP2C8	Taxol 6-hydroxylase
CYP2C9	Tolbutamide 4-hydroxylase
	Diclofenac 4′-hydroxylase
	S-Warfarin 4′-hydroxylase
CYP2C19	*S*-Mephenytoin 4′-hydroxylase
CYP2D6	Bufuralol 1′-hydroxylase
	Debrisoquine 4-hydroxylase
	Dextromethorphan *O*-demethylase
CYP2E1	*N*-Nitrosodimethylamine
	N-demethylase
	Chlorzoxazone 6-hydroxylase
CYP3A	Midazolam 1′-hydroxylase
	Testosterone 6β-hydroxylase
	Erythromycin *N*-demethylase
	Nifedipine oxidation

researchers tools to examine the inhibition of metabolism mediated by that CYP (2,35). In these studies, the NCE is examined for its ability to inhibit catalytic activities mediated by individual CYPs. The results from these studies, usually in the form of K_i or IC_{50} values, predict the potential that an NCE has to inhibit a specific CYP. This is invaluable information to the clinician who can design clinical interaction studies that are relevant for a particular NCE. Furthermore, the pharmaceutical company may report the results obtained in the *in vitro* drug interaction studies to the regulatory agencies and include them in the product insert, sometimes in lieu of clinical interaction studies. These options are particularly useful in an industry in which costs of developing drugs continue to escalate.

In vitro interaction studies can also be used when there is a specific question concerning the interaction between an NCE and a specific compound. In these studies, it is important to understand the biotransformation of the substrate being examined. For example, if a minor route of metabolism is inhibited, the overall significance of the inhibition of that route of metabolism on the clearance of the substrate would be minimal and likely not clinically significant (1). Again, when these *in vitro* studies are performed properly, it is possible that they may be used in place of *in vivo* interaction studies.

Studies examining the potential of an NCE as an inhibitor of metabolism mediated by a specific CYP are performed with an understanding of enzyme kinetics (36). In these studies, the metabolism of the form-selective substrate of a P450 (or specific substrate of interest) is determined over a wide range of concentrations of the substrate to determine K_m (the substrate concentration at half maximal velocity and a measure of the substrate

affinity for the enzyme of interest) and V_{max} (the maximal velocity of the reaction). To determine the effectiveness of a particular NCE as an inhibitor of the enzyme of interest, several concentrations of inhibitor (NCE) are added to the incubations at each substrate concentration and the rate of formation of the metabolite of interest is determined. The data are then used to determine the type of enzyme inhibition exhibited by the NCE, yielding an apparent K_i value (dissociation constant of the enzyme–inhibitor complex). To determine an accurate K_i value, data must be fit to the appropriate model of enzyme inhibition. These models of inhibition include competitive, noncompetitive, uncompetitive, and mixed competitive and noncompetitive (36).

When inhibition by an NCE of the metabolism of a form-selective substrate by a specific P450 is examined, the resulting K_i value determined is a constant for that enzyme–inhibitor complex and is independent of the substrate used in its determination. Therefore, the K_i value can be used to make predictions concerning the interaction potential of the NCE for all reactions that are mediated by the particular CYP being examined. Often, these studies are performed early in development of the drug and little is known about the anticipated therapeutic circulating concentration of the NCE. In these cases, the researcher can inform the clinician that, if circulating levels of the NCE approach the K_i value for the interaction, there is a potential for interaction to occur. Later in development, steady-state and maximal concentrations of the NCE are determined *in vivo*. At this time, predictions can be made concerning the inhibitory propensity of the NCE for the enzymes examined in the patient population. When making predictions concerning the inhibitory propensity of the NCE, a variety of factors must be understood. The dependence of a particular route of metabolism for a compound that may be inhibited needs to be known. If the inhibited route of metabolism accounts for less than 50% of the clearance of the compound, the overall effect of the inhibition of that pathway on total drug clearance would be in question (1). A consideration of the inhibitor concentration at the site of metabolism is also important. Because it is not possible to determine the concentration of inhibitor within the cell at the site of the drug-metabolizing enzymes, the circulating concentration of inhibitor is often used in these predictions. Furthermore, the binding of the inhibitor to protein will affect the total drug concentration able to interact with the enzyme. Pharmacokinetic theory indicates that only unbound drug would be available to the enzyme. However, the exact relationship between unbound plasma concentration of an NCE and its unbound concentration at the cellular site of metabolism is unknown. Thus, a number of assumptions are required to use the K_i value determined *in vitro* to predict *in vivo* inhibition.

When anticipated therapeutic concentrations of an NCE are known and the K_i value for a particular

TABLE 3-2. *Olanzapine inhibition of various CYP form-selective catalytic activities*

Enzyme	Catalytic activity	Type of inhibition	$K_i(\mu M)^a$
CYP3A	Midazolam 1'-hydroxylation	Noncompetitive	491 ± 33
CYP2D6	Bufuralol 1'-hydroxylation	Competitive	89 ± 5
CYP2C9	Tolbutamide 4-hydroxylation	Noncompetitive	715 ± 73
CYP1A2	Phenacetin O-deethylation	Competitive	37 ± 2
CYP2C19	S-Mephenytoin 4'-hydroxylation	Noncompetitive	920 ± 65

^{a}K_i ± standard error of the parameter estimate

drug–enzyme interaction has been determined, one can predict the *in vivo* inhibition by the NCE of metabolism mediated by that particular enzyme. In these determinations, the predicted percent inhibition, expressed in Equation 3-1 (36), is equal to:

$$1 - \frac{\text{inhibited velocity of the biotransformation}}{\text{uninhibited velocity}} \cdot 100 \quad [3\text{-}1]$$

The Michaelis-Menten formula is placed into Equation 3-1 to represent uninhibited velocity, and the formula for the particular type of inhibition observed for this enzyme–inhibitor complex is used for the inhibited velocity. In the case of competitive, noncompetitive, and mixed type inhibition, if the additional assumption is made that the K_m value of the inhibited reaction is substantially greater than the substrate concentration (which is the most conservative assumption to make), the relationship, expressed in Equation 3-2, reduces to:

$$\text{Percent inhibition} = \frac{(I)}{(I + K_i)} \cdot 100 \quad [3\text{-}2]$$

Where *I* is the inhibitor concentration.

Instead of determining K_i values, some researchers determine the concentration of inhibitor, which inhibits 50% (IC_{50}) of the turnover of a single concentration of a form-selective substrate. If an IC_{50} value calculated for the NCE is much higher than the expected circulating concentration for that inhibitor, it can be predicted with some assurance that an NCE would not be a clinically significant inhibitor of metabolism mediated by that CYP. However, there are problems in using this abbreviated approach for predicting the potential for a significant *in vivo* interaction. The major concern with this approach is the relationship between the IC_{50} and K_i values for the inhibition of an enzyme by a drug. Specifically, care should be taken in using an IC_{50} to predict drug interactions because IC_{50} equals the K_i value only in the case of noncompetitive inhibitors. With competitive (37) or mixed competitive and noncompetitive inhibition, the equality relationship between IC_{50} and K_i values does not necessarily hold true. For example, with competitive inhibition, the IC_{50} is equal to $K_i(1 + (S/K_m))$, where *S* is substrate concentration. Therefore, when $S = K_m$, the IC_{50} is $2K_i$, and if the single concentration of substrate used in the determination of IC_{50} exceeds the K_m value for the biotransformation, the IC_{50} value can be substantially

greater than the K_i value for the inhibitor. Because the type of inhibition is not discerned from studies determining only IC_{50}, the conservative assumption must be made that the IC_{50} may be greater than the actual K_i value for the inhibitor. Thus, when attempting to predict the *in vivo* significance of the inhibition of an enzyme by an NCE, if only IC_{50} values are used, an underestimation of the potential *in vivo* inhibition is possible.

An example of *in vitro* studies performed to determine the potential for inhibition of CYPs by an NCE has been reported for olanzapine (Zyprexa) (38), an antipsychotic marketed for the treatment of schizophrenia. Olanzapine was examined for its ability to inhibit form-selective catalytic activities for CYP2C9, CYP2D6, CYP3A, CYP1A2, and CYP2C19. For these studies, the rate of formation of the specific metabolite from each of the form-selective substrates was determined at five substrate concentrations, both without or in the presence of one of four different inhibitor (olanzapine) concentrations. Using these data, the enzyme kinetics of these biotransformations were modeled by nonlinear regression analysis to each of the four types of inhibitor models previously described. For each CYP selective biotransformation, the best fit model of inhibition by olanzapine was determined using a number of standard criteria (39). These analyses yielded apparent K_m and V_{max} values for each P450 selective biotransformation and a K_i value for olanzapine as the inhibitor. Olanzapine was found to exhibit competitive inhibition of CYP1A2- and CYP2D6-mediated metabolism, and noncompetitive inhibition of CYP3A-, CYP2C9-, and CYP2C19-mediated metabolism with a range of K_i values from 37 to 920 μM (Table 3-2) (38).

Having determined the K_i value and type of inhibition for each P450 for olanzapine, the *in vivo* potential of olanzapine to inhibit these P450s was predicted. Steady-state plasma concentrations of olanzapine reach approxi-

TABLE 3-3. *Predicted inhibition of in vivo catalytic activity of CYPs 3A, 2D6, 2C9, 1A2, and 2C19 by 0.2 µM Olanzapine*

Enzyme	Predicted inhibition (%)
CYP3A	0.04
CYP2D6	0.20
CYP2C9	0.03
CYP1A2	0.60
CYP2C19	0.02

TABLE 3-4. *Olanzapine inhibition of CYP-mediated reactions: comparison of* in vitro *prediction and* in vivo *drug interactions*

Drug	Enzyme	*In vitro* prediction	Result
Warfarin	2C9	No interaction	No change in pharmacokinetics
Imipramine	2D6	No interaction	No change in pharmacokinetics
Diazepam	3A and 2C19	No interaction	No change in pharmacokinetics
Theophylline	1A2	No interaction	No change in pharmacokinetics

mately 0.2 µM. Therefore, in the calculation of the predicted inhibition *in vivo* for each of the P450s by olanzapine, the value of 0.2 µM was entered for the concentration of the inhibitor along with the previously determined K_i values. Because, in all cases, olanzapine inhibition of the P450-examined modeled as competitive or noncompetitive inhibition, Equation 3-2 was used.

The predicted percent inhibition by olanzapine of metabolism mediated by all five of the CYPs examined was less than 1% (Table 3-3). Therefore, the *in vitro* data predict that olanzapine would be unlikely to cause clinically significant drug–drug interactions mediated by any of the five CYPs examined.

Clinical drug–drug interaction studies were performed coadministering olanzapine with drugs metabolized by the various P450s. As shown in Table 3-4, such studies *in vivo* were performed with substrates of each of the P450s examined *in vitro*. Therefore, the relationship between the *in vitro* prediction and clinical experience was directly determined. The *in vitro* results predicted in all cases that olanzapine coadministration would not alter the metabolic clearance of drugs metabolized by these P450s. These clinical results confirmed the *in vitro* predictions demonstrating the lack of pharmacokinetic interactions between olanzapine and the substrates of CYP1A2, CYP2C9, CYP2D6, and CYP3A examined (see Table 3-4). The results of these *in vitro* inhibition experiments are also summarized in the product insert for olanzapine (40). If the effect of an inhibitor is assumed to be substrate independent, the lack of interaction with other substrates for the same P450 isoforms is expected.

DRUG INTERACTIONS—IDENTIFICATION OF THE ENZYMES RESPONSIBLE FOR THE METABOLISM OF A NEW CHEMICAL ENTITY

Another approach to analyzing drug interactions *in vitro* with an NCE is through the identification of the enzymes responsible for the oxidative metabolism of the NCE. With the identification of the routes of metabolism, predictions can be made concerning the impact that perturbations (including genetic polymorphisms, inhibition, and induction) in a particular route of metabolism would have on the *in vivo* clearance of the NCE.

These studies begin with enzyme kinetic analyses of the *in vitro* formation of the metabolites of a compound by human liver microsomes. These analyses determine which oxidative metabolites of an NCE are formed and

the number of enzymes that may be able to form a particular metabolite. The formation of each of the metabolites of an NCE is determined over a wide range of substrate concentrations. The data are then examined through the use of an Eadie-Hofstee plot (36). A plot that yields a linear relationship is consistent with one enzyme forming the metabolite. A resultant curvilinear Eadie-Hofstee plot suggests the involvement of more than one enzyme in the formation of a particular metabolite. In either case, the apparent kinetic parameters of K_m and V_{max} can be determined for the enzymes responsible for the formation of that metabolite under the conditions examined. These results are used in two ways. First, if more than one oxidative metabolite is formed in human liver microsomal incubations, then predictions concerning the relative rank order *in vivo* of the rates of formation of these metabolites can be made. To make these predictions, the intrinsic clearance for a particular route of metabolism is calculated by dividing the V_{max} value by the K_m value of the reaction. Those routes of metabolism with large calculated intrinsic clearance values would be preferred over those routes with smaller intrinsic clearance values. Second, if more than one enzyme is capable of forming a metabolite, then substrate concentrations in subsequent incubations are determined that will examine metabolism mediated by the specific physiologically relevant enzyme.

To identify the enzymes responsible for the metabolism of an NCE, a three-pronged approach outlined in Figure 3-1 is often used. The first step is to determine the formation rate of the metabolites of interest by a bank of human liver samples, which has been characterized with respect to form-selective activities for various drug-metabolizing enzymes (i.e., P450s). The formation rate of the metabolites of the NCE is then correlated to the form-selective

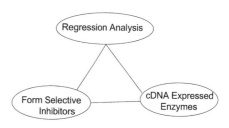

FIG. 3-1. A three-pronged approach often used to identify the enzymes responsible for the metabolism of a new chemical entity.

enzymatic activities determined for the livers. The correlation analyses yield information on whether the formation rates for the metabolites of the NCE regress or are significantly related to the catalytic activity of a specific drug-metabolizing enzyme. This gives the first suggestion as to the identity of enzymes responsible for the production of a particular metabolite. If more than one significant correlation is observed between the formation of the metabolite and the form-selective activities, then multivariate regression analysis is performed to determine whether several enzymes participate in the reaction.

The second step in identifying the enzymes responsible for NCE metabolite formation is to examine the ability of the specific drug-metabolizing enzymes to form the metabolites of the NCE. Microsomes prepared from cells that have been engineered to express the various cDNAs for the enzymes of interest are incubated with the NCE and those capable of forming the metabolite of interest are determined. If the resulting data correspond to the data obtained by correlation analysis, then no further work needs to be done. However, occasionally a variety of CYPs are found to be capable of forming a particular metabolite at similar rates. In these situations, the determination of which expressed enzymes are able to form the metabolite will not give a quantitative answer as to the relative importance of a particular enzyme in the formation of the metabolite *in vivo* and additional studies need to be performed.

Another approach to determine the role of the various drug-metabolizing enzymes in the formation of the metabolites of an NCE is through the use of enzyme-specific chemical inhibitors. A variety of inhibitor probes have been characterized as selectively inhibiting specific enzymes (Table 3-5). When used at the appropriate concentration, if significant inhibition of the formation of the metabolites of the NCE by the selective inhibitors is observed, the involvement of the enzyme being inhibited in this formation is indicated. However, care must be taken in the design of inhibitor studies because, at high concentrations, many inhibitors show nonspecific effects, often inhibiting several P450s. Furthermore, as indicated in Table 3-4, form-selective inhibitors of CYP2A6,

CYP2B6, and CYP2E1 have not been identified. Although the purported CYP2E1 inhibitor, DDC, was found in the study of Newton and colleagues (41) to be selective for CYP2E1, other laboratories have reported results that indicate that this inhibitor can also inhibit several other P450s (42–44). Furthermore, the reported CYP2B6 inhibitor, orphenadrine, was found to also inhibit CYP2E1- and CYP1A2-mediated metabolism (44,45).

A similar approach taken to confirm the role of specific enzymes in the biotransformation of an NCE is through the use of inhibitory antibodies (46). The increasingly commercial availability of antibodies that recognize and inhibit a specific P450 is making this technique more widely available. However, the major concern with antibody use is the potential for cross-reactivity with CYPs that are related to the CYP that the antibody is prepared against. Therefore, an understanding of the specificity of the antibody (potentially batch specific) must be known before conclusions can be reached with this technique (44).

Occasionally, aggregate results from these different approaches to enzyme identification suggest the involvement of multiple enzymes in the formation of a metabolite of an NCE or give conflicting results concerning which enzymes are involved in metabolite formation. In these cases, multivariate regression techniques can be used to determine which enzymes are significant regressors in the formation of a particular metabolite (39,47). This technique helps eliminate the problem associated with spurious coregression of unrelated catalytic activities observed in univariate regression techniques. In addition, the involvement of covert (hidden) enzymes in the metabolism of an NCE can be determined. In this case, if the y-intercept of the univariate regression analysis is significantly different from zero, additional enzymes may be participating in this biotransformation. Multivariate regression analysis can be used to attempt to identify this hidden regressor.

An example of the use of these techniques to identify the enzymes responsible for the metabolism of an NCE has been reported for olanzapine. These techniques were

TABLE 3-5. *Specific form selective inhibitors of the cytochromes P450*

Cytochrome P450	Inhibitor	Type of inhibition	Reference
CYP1A2	Furafylline	Mechanism based	58
	α-Naphthoflavone	Reversible	59
CYP2A6	8-Methoxypsoralen	Mechanism based	60
CYP2B6	None known		
CYP2C9	Sulfaphenazole	Reversible	41
CYP2D6	Quinidine	Reversible	41
CYP2E1	Diethyldithiocarbamate (DDC) (specificity in question—see text)	Mechanism based	41
CYP3A	Ketoconazole	Reversible	41
	Gestodene	Mechanism based	41
	Troleandomycin	Mechanism based	41

used in the identification of the enzymes responsible for the biotransformation of olanzapine to 2-hydroxy methyl-(2OH), 4′-N-oxide (NO)-, and N-desmethyl (NdM)-olanzapine (39). As indicated previously, the first step in these studies was to determine the kinetics of the formation of the various metabolites by human liver microsomes. Both 2OH-olanzapine and NdM-olanzapine exhibited biphasic formation kinetics. The K_m value for the high-affinity enzyme was found to be approximately 60 and 40 μM for the formation of 2OH- and NdM-olanzapine, respectively. Kinetic analysis of NO-olanzapine formation indicated that the enzyme generating this metabolite was not saturated over the concentration range of olanzapine examined. The intrinsic clearance values determined for all three routes of the oxidative metabolism of olanzapine indicated that, on average, the relative rate of formation of these metabolites would be NdM-olanzapine > NO-olanzapine >> 2OH-olanzapine. These results suggested that the formation of the N-demethylated and N-oxidized olanzapine metabolites would be the predominant oxidative routes of olanzapine metabolism, with the formation of 2OH-olanzapine being a minor route of metabolism.

Next, the formation rate of each metabolite at substrate concentrations assuring only the participation of the high-affinity, physiologically relevant enzyme was determined in a bank of 14 human livers characterized using form-selective catalytic activities for the P450s and FMO. The rates of formation of the metabolites of olanzapine were then correlated with the levels of the various characterized enzymes. Significant correlations were observed between CYP2D6 and CYP2C9 activities and the formation of 2OH-olanzapine. However, results from multivariate correlation analyses indicated that CYP2D6 activity was the only significant regressor in the formation of this metabolite. The formation of NO-olanzapine significantly correlated only with the FMO activity. NdM-olanzapine formation significantly correlated with CYP1A2 and CYP2C19 activities. Again, the use of multivariate regression techniques demonstrated that only activity for CYP1A2 was a significant regressor with the formation of NdM-olanzapine.

To confirm these results, different cDNA-expressed P450s were examined for their ability to form the metabolites of olanzapine. At substrate concentrations reflecting the low K_m enzymes, CYP2D6 produced 2OH-olanzapine and CYP1A2 produced NdM-olanzapine at rates significantly greater than the other P450s, confirming the results of the correlation analyses. Several of the CYPs examined were able to form NO-olanzapine, but at a low rate of turnover. Therefore, incubation conditions known to distinguish FMO-mediated reactions from those mediated by P450s (48) were examined because FMO activity in the bank of human liver samples was the only significant regressor for the formation of NdM-olanzapine. FMO involvement in the formation of the metabolite was confirmed due to the

observations that the formation of NO-olanzapine was enhanced at pH 8.5 as compared to formation rate at pH 7.4, and the activity was lost when the microsomes were heated at 55°C for 2 minutes in the absence of NADPH (reduced form of nicotinamide adenine dinucleotide phosphate). Furthermore, FMO inhibitors thiourea and thiobenzamide significantly inhibited the formation of NO-olanzapine.

Taken together, these results indicate that NdM-olanzapine formation is mediated by CYP1A2 and NO-olanzapine formation is mediated by FMO, and that these are the major oxidative routes of olanzapine metabolism. Furthermore, CYP2D6 is responsible for the formation of 2OH-olanzapine, which represents a minor route of olanzapine clearance. Therefore, the predictions made following these *in vitro* studies were that as the major metabolic pathway factors that affect CYP1A2-mediated metabolism should also affect olanzapine clearance. In addition, although 2OH-olanzapine is formed by the polymorphically expressed CYP2D6, clearance of olanzapine should be minimally affected by perturbations in this minor route of metabolism.

Clinical studies supporting these predictions were performed. In particular, cigarette smoking, which induces CYP1A2 activity, produced a 33% increase in oral clearance of olanzapine (49). Furthermore, coadministration of olanzapine and the potent CYP1A2 inhibitor fluvoxamine resulted in a 50% increase in the plasma concentration of olanzapine (50). The clinical data also indicated that men had a greater olanzapine clearance than women (49), confirming the reported gender difference in CYP1A2 catalytic activity (51). Furthermore, as predicted by the demonstration that CYP2D6 is involved in the formation of a minor metabolite, the pharmacokinetics of olanzapine in individuals known to be deficient in CYP2D6 catalytic activity were similar to those observed in normal patients (49).

CONCLUSION

The information presented herein, demonstrates the utility of using *in vitro* metabolism techniques to examine potential drug–drug interactions of an NCE and its pharmacokinetic variability before its exposure to large populations. With concurrent administration of an NCE and other drugs commonly used during clinical trials, these techniques can accurately predict the effect that the NCE may have on the metabolism of coadministered drugs. These techniques also can determine what effect a coadministered drug may have on the metabolism of the NCE. These *in vitro* techniques have given the pharmaceutical industry the ability to screen for potential drug–drug interactions and determine metabolic issues in special populations in a rapid, more efficient manner than traditional *in vivo* studies.

The strength of this *in vitro* model for predicting potential drug–drug interactions resides in the increasing understanding of the hepatic human P450s. Research is ongoing to further our understanding of the manner in which these enzymes function in drug metabolism, the factors that alter their catalytic activities, and move from qualitative to quantitative predictions. One of the many questions being pursued is how can *in vitro* data be better used to predict *in vivo* interactions. A greater understanding of how the major metabolizing enzymes function and are regulated is imperative to the attainment of this goal. An understanding is needed of the *in vivo* consequences, if any, of activation kinetics or the stimulation of enzyme activity by substrates themselves or other molecules that have been observed in *in vitro* incubations (52,53). In a related area, enzymes such as CYP3A behave as if they have multiple binding sites or conformers *in vitro* (54). Research needs to be performed examining the role that multiple binding sites or conformers play in *in vivo* metabolism.

According to Shimada and colleagues (6), approximately 70% of the enzymes involved in hepatic xenobiotic metabolism have been identified. Another important question to pursue is to determine the role that the "missing" enzymes play in metabolism. In addition, some of the known P450 enzymes, such as CYP2B6, CYP2C8, and CYP2C18, are not as well understood as many of the other P450 enzymes; therefore, their full role in metabolism and drug interactions may not be appreciated.

Current understanding of the other enzymes involved in the biotransformation of drugs, such as the FMOs and phase II enzyme systems, are not as advanced as current knowledge of the P450s. Specific substrates and inhibitors of these enzyme systems would help in the ability to examine metabolism through these pathways and thereby add to the ability to predict potential drug interactions. Furthermore, if maintenance and long-term storage techniques are perfected for liver slices or hepatocytes, an invaluable tool to examine integrated metabolism and enzyme regulation would be added to the current repertoire.

There is also a growing appreciation of extrahepatic sites of xenobiotic biotransformation. This is exemplified by the presence of CYP3A in the intestinal epithelium and the major role that it appears to play in the first pass metabolism of certain drugs. The integration of active transport systems with biotransformation systems makes the intestine potentially a very important site of metabolism for some compounds. Thus, it is important to consider intestinal metabolism and drug transport processes when examining drug interactions, particularly with orally dosed compounds (55). To effectively examine the role of the intestine in drug metabolism, both the drug metabolizing enzymes and the transporters present must be characterized and appropriate *in vitro* models must be determined to predict potential drug interactions.

Finally, many researchers are working on computational models in an attempt to understand the binding characteristics of substrates and inhibitors of drug-metabolizing enzymes. This is exemplified by the knowledge that, to bind to CYP2D6, a substrate must have a basic nitrogen that is 5 to 7 angstroms from the oxidation site (56,57). If such models for this and other enzymes can be validated, it may be possible to predict potential interactions with computer programs.

As discussed herein, *in vitro* models of drug metabolism are playing an increasingly important role in drug development. Through ongoing research, current knowledge is increasing, as is understanding of how substrates and inhibitors interact with the enzymes involved in drug metabolism. This information will improve the ability to predict potential drug–drug interactions and thereby ensure the safe use of drugs.

REFERENCES

1. Tucker GT. The rational selection of drug interaction studies: implications of recent advances in drug metabolism. *Int J Clin Pharmacol Ther Toxicol* 1992;30:550–553.
2. Wrighton SA, VandenBranden M, Stevens JC, Shipley LA, Ring BJ. In vitro methods for assessing human hepatic drug metabolism: their use in drug development. *Drug Metab Rev* 1993;25:453–484.
3. Guengerich FP. Human cytochrome P450 enzymes. In: Ortiz de Monellano PR, ed. *Cytochrome P450*, 2nd ed. New York: Plenum Press, 1995: 473–535.
4. Nies AS, Spielberg SP. Principles of therapeutics. In: Hardman JG, Limbird LE, Molinoff PB, Ruddon RW, Gilman AG, eds. *Goodman and Gilman's: The Pharmacological basis of therapeutics*, 9th ed. New York: McGraw-Hill, 1996:51.
5. Doucet J, Chassagne P, Trivalle C, et al. Drug-drug interactions related to hospital admissions in older adults: a prospective study of 1000 patients. *J Am Geriatr Soc* 1996;44:944–948.
6. Shimada T, Yamazaki H, Mimura M, Inui Y, Guengerich FP. Interindividual variations in human liver cytochrome P450 enzymes involved in the oxidation of drugs, carcinogens and toxic chemicals: studies with liver microsomes of 30 Japanese and 30 caucasians. *J Pharmacol Exp Ther* 1994;270:414–423.
7. Benet LZ. Pharmacokinetics. In: Hardman JG, Limbird LE, Molinoff PB, Ruddon RW, Gilman AG, eds. *Goodman and Gilman's: The pharmacological basis of therapeutics*, 9th ed. New York: McGraw-Hill, 1996:14.
8. Uppoor RS, Murroum P, Burnett A, et al. Most common interactant drugs in drug-drug interaction (DDI) studies. *Clin Pharmacol Ther* 1998;63:147.
9. Yun C-H, Okerholm RA, Guengerich FP. Oxidation of the antihistaminic drug terfenadine in human liver microsomes. *Drug Metab Dispos* 1993;21:403–409.
10. Honig PK, Woosley RL, Zamani K, Conner DP, Cantilena LR. Changes in the pharmacokinetics and electrocardiographic pharmacodynamics of terfenadine with concomitant administration of erythromycin. *Clin Pharmacol Ther* 1992;52:231–238.
11. Honig PK, Wortham DC, Zamani K, Conner DP, Mullin JC, Cantilena LR. Terfenadine-ketoconazole interaction. *JAMA* 1993;269: 1513–1518.
12. US Food and Drug Administration. *Guidance for industry—drug metabolism/drug interaction studies in the drug development process: studies* in vitro. US Food and Drug Administration, Rockville, MD, 1997.
13. European Agency for the Evaluation of Medicinal Products. *Note for guidance on the investigation of drug interactions*. European Agency for the Evaluation of Medicinal Products, London, 1997.
14. Australian Drug Evaluation Committee. *Draft TGA note for guidance—drugs metabolised by CYP450 isoforms*. Australian Drug Evaluation Committee, 1997.

15. Donato MT, Castell JV, Gomez-Lechon MJ. Effect of model inducers on cytochrome P450 activities of human hepatocytes in primary culture. *Drug Metab Dispos* 1995;23:553–558.
16. Lake BG, Charzat C, Tredger JM, Renwick AB, Beamand JA, Price RJ. Induction of cytochrome P450 isoenzymes in cultured precision-cut rat and human liver slices. *Xenobiotica* 1996;26:297–306.
17. Strom SC, Pisarov LA, Dorko K, Thompson MT, Scheutz JD, Scheutz EG. Use of human hepatocytes to study P450 gene induction. *Methods Enzymol* 1996;272:388–401.
18. Rodrigues AD. Use of in vitro human metabolism studies in drug development. *Biochem Pharmacol* 1994;48:2147–2156.
19. Lin JH, Lu AYH. Inhibition of cytochrome P-450 and implication in drug development. *Ann Rep Med Chem* 1997;32:295–304.
20. Fuhr U, Weiss M, Kroemer HK, et al. Systematic screening for pharmacokinetic interactions during drug development. *Int J Clin Pharmacol Ther* 1996;34:139–151.
21. Shaw PM, Hosea NA, Thompson DV, Lenius JM, Guengerich FP. Reconstitution premixes for assays using purified recombinant human cytochrome P450, NADPH-cytochrome P450 reductase, and cytochrome b$_5$. *Arch Biochem Biophys* 1997;348:107–115.
22. Guengerich FP, Martin MV, Guo Z, Chun Y-J. Purification of functional recombinant P450s from bacteria. *Methods Enzymol* 1996;272:35–44.
23. Gillam EM, Guo Z, Guengerich FP. Expression of modified cytochrome P450 2E1 in *Escherichia coli*, purification, and spectral and catalytic properties. *Arch Biochem Biophys* 1994;312:59–66.
24. van der Hoeven TA, Coon MJ. Preparation and properties of partially purified cytochrome P-450 and reduced nicotinamide adenine dinucleotide phosphate-cytochrome P-450 reductase from rabbit liver microsomes. *J Biol Chem* 1974;249:6302–6310.
25. Pearce RE, McIntyre CJ, Madan A, et al. Effect of freezing, thawing, and storing human liver microsomes on cytochrome P450 activity. *Arch Biochem Biophys* 1996;331:145–169.
26. Burchell B, Brierley CH, Rance D. Specificity of human UDP-glucuronosyltransferases and xenobiotic glucurondidation. *Life Sci* 1995; 57:1819–1831.
27. Seidegard J, Ekstrom G. The role of human glutathione transferases and epoxide hydrolases in the metabolism of xenobiotics. *Environ Health Persp* 1997;105:791–799.
28. Le Guellec C, Lacarelle B, Villard P-H, Point H, Catalin J, Durand A. Glucuronidation of propofol in microsomal fractions from various tissues and species including humans: effect of different drugs. *Anesth Analg* 1995;81:855–861.
29. Ekins S. Past, present, and future applications of precision-cut liver slices for in vitro xenobiotic metabolism. *Drug Metab Rev* 1996;28:591–623.
30. Li AP, Jurima-Romet M. Applications of primary human hepatocytes in the evaluation of pharmacokinetic drug-drug interactions: evaluation of model drugs terfenadine and rifampin. *Cell Biol Toxicol* 1997;13: 365–374.
31. Pichard L, Fabre I, Fabre G, et al. Cyclosporin A drug interactions. *Drug Metab Dispos* 1990;18:595–606.
32. Morel F, Beaune PH, Ratanasavanh D, et al. Expression of cytochrome P-450 enzymes in cultured human hepatocytes. *Eur J Biochem* 1990; 191:437–444.
33. Skett P, Bayliss M. Time for a consistent approach to preparing and culturing hepatocytes? *Xenobiotica* 1996;26:1–7.
34. Wrighton SA, Stevens JC. The human hepatic cytochromes P450 involved in drug metabolism. *Crit Rev Toxicol* 1992;22:1–21.
35. Parkinson A. An overview of current cytochrome P450 technology for assessing the safety and efficacy of new materials. *Toxicol Pathol* 1996; 24:45–57.
36. Segel IH. *Enzyme kinetics*. New York: John Wiley and Sons, 1975.
37. Cheng Y-C, Prusoff WH. Relationship between the inhibition constant (K_i) and the concentration of inhibitor which causes 50 per cent inhibition (I_{50}) of an enzymatic reaction. *Biochem Pharmacol* 1973;22: 3099–3108.
38. Ring BJ, Binkley SN, VandenBranden M, Wrighton SA. In vitro interaction of the antipsychotic agent olanzapine with human cytochromes P450 CYP2C9, CYP2C19, CYP2D6 and CYP3A. *Br J Clin Pharmacol* 1996;41:181–186.
39. Ring BJ, Catlow J, Lindsay TJ, et al. Identification of the human cytochromes P450 responsible for the in vitro formation of the major oxidative metabolites of the antipsychotic agent olanzapine. *J Pharmacol Exp Ther* 1996;276:658–666.
40. *Physicians' desk reference*, 52nd ed. Montvale, NJ: Medical Economics, 1998.
41. Newton DJ, Wang RW, Lu AYH. Cytochrome P450 inhibitors: evaluation of specificities in the in vitro metabolism of therapeutic agents by human liver microsomes. *Drug Metab Dispos* 1995;23:154–158.
42. Chang TKH, Gonzalez FJ, Waxman DJ. Evaluation of triacetyloleandomycin, α-naphthoflavone and diethyldithiocarbamate as selective chemical probes for inhibition of human cytochromes P450. *Arch Biochem Biophys* 1994;311:437–442.
43. Ono S, Hatanaka T, Hotta H, Satoh T, Gonzalez FJ, Tsutsui M. Specificity of substrate and inhibitor probes for cytochrome P450s: evaluation of in vitro metabolism using cDNA-expressed human P450s and human liver microsomes. *Xenobiotica* 1996;26:681–693.
44. Ekins S, VandenBranden M, Ring BJ, Wrighton SA. Examination of purported probes of human CYP2B6. *Pharmacogenetics* 1997;7: 165–179.
45. Guo Z, Raeissi S, White R, Stevens J. Orphenadrine and methimazole inhibit multiple cytochrome P450 enzymes in human liver microsomes. *Drug Metab Dispos* 1997;25:390–393.
46. Gelboin HV. Cytochrome P450 and monoclonal antibodies. *Pharmacol Rev* 1993;45:413–453.
47. Sharer JE, Wrighton SA. Identification of the human hepatic cytochromes P450 involved in the in vitro oxidation of antipyrine. *Drug Metab Dispos* 1996;24:487–494.
48. Cashman JR, Park SB, Yang S-C, Wrighton SA, Jacob P, Benowitz NL. Metabolism of nicotine by human liver microsomes: stero-selective formation of trans-nicotine N'-oxide. *Chem Res Toxicol* 1992;5: 639–646.
49. Ereshefsky L. Pharmacokinetics and drug interactions: update for new antipsychotics. *J Clin Psychiatry* 1996;57(suppl 11):12–25.
50. Maenpaa J, Wrighton SA, Bergstrom R, et al. Pharmacokinetic and pharmacodynamic interactions between fluvoxamine and olanzapine. *Clin Pharm Ther* 1997;61:225.
51. Jennings TS, Nafziger AN, Davidson L, Bertino JS. Gender differences in hepatic induction and inhibition of theophylline pharmacokinetics and metabolism. *J Lab Clin Med* 1993;122:208–216.
52. Korzekwa KR, Krishnamachary N, Shou M, et al. Evaluation of atypical cytochrome P450 kinetics with two-substrate models: evidence that multiple substrates can simultaneously bind to cytochrome P450 active sites. *Biochemistry* 1998;37:4137–4147.
53. Ueng Y-F, Kuwabara T, Chun Y-J, Guengerich FP. Cooperativity in oxidations catalyzed by cytochrome P450 3A4. *Biochemistry* 1997;36: 370–381.
54. Koley AP, Buters JTM, Robinson RC, Markowitz A, Friedman FK. CO binding kinetics of human cytochrome P450 3A4. *J Biol Chem* 1995; 270:5014–5018.
55. Wacher VJ, Wu C-Y, Benet LZ. Overlapping substrate specificities and tissue distribution of cytochrome P450 3A and P-glycoprotein: implications for drug delivery and activity in cancer chemotherapy. *Mol Carcinogen* 1995;13:129–134.
56. Koymans L, Donne-Op Den Kelder GM, Koppele Te JM, Vermeulen NPE. Cytochromes P450: their active-site structure and mechanism of oxidation. *Drug Metab Rev* 1993;25:325–387.
57. DeGrott MJ, Bijloo GJ, Van Acker FAA, Fonseca Guerra C, Snijders JG, Vermeulen NPE. Extension of a predictive substrate model for human cytochrome P4502D6. *Xenobiotica* 1997;27:357–368.
58. Sesardic D, Boobis AR, Murray BP, et al. Furafylline is a potent and selective inhibitor of cytochrome P4501A2 in man. *Br J Clin Pharmacol* 1990;29:651–663.
59. Tassaneeyakul W, Birkett DJ, Veronese ME, et al. Specificity of substrate and inhibitor probes for human cytochromes P450 1A1 and 1A2. *J Pharmacol Exp Ther* 1993;265:401–407.
60. Koenigs LL, Peter RM, Thompson SJ, Rettie AE, Trager WF. Mechanism-based inactivation of human liver cytochrome P450 2A6 by 8-methoxypsoralen. *Drug Metab Dispos* 1997;25:1407–1415.

CHAPTER 4

Regulatory Viewpoint: Prediction of Drug Interactions from *In Vitro* Studies

Jerry M. Collins

Clinical pharmacologists in academia, industry, and government have always had a strong interest in understanding and preventing adverse consequences of drug–drug metabolic interactions. In the past, clinical observations *in vivo* have been the source of essentially all information. Learning about drug interactions in the clinic, however, is inefficient and can be disastrous.

The study of drug metabolism *in vitro* presents an alternative approach to clinical studies and, although metabolic study *in vitro* is not new, much information from such studies has been gained recently.

From a regulatory viewpoint, the primary motivation for studies *in vitro* is a desire to learn something relevant to clinical use. Over the past 5 years, clinicians have become increasingly confident in their ability to predict clinical correlates from data obtained *in vitro*, but a complete understanding of the strengths and weaknesses of correlations *in vitro*-to-*in vivo* can only be determined through comparative clinical trials. Most pharmaceutical sponsors have one or more excellent studies that either validate the principles or challenge clinicians to further understand the situation. Slowly, at national and international conferences, these data are being presented. Even the largest pharmaceutical firms can benefit substantially from a pooling of experience and placement of these data into the public domain.

In the regulatory sector, there is an avalanche of data awaiting review. It is critically important to focus on the real opportunities for improved drug development and regulation. These opportunities are not going to arise in the future; they are already here. Qualitatively and quantitatively, the information available currently is different

from that available in the past. Reviewers need to be mindful of the relevant questions that can impact drug utilization, and then they must evaluate the tools that are available for seeking the answers.

There is a long list of relevant issues for drug development: Will the new drug inhibit the metabolism of other drugs or have its own metabolism inhibited by other drugs? Will this new drug induce metabolism of other drugs or be induced itself by other drugs? Are there intersubject variables that complicate interpretation of results, such as ethnic, racial, or genetic differences, or is there an impact of diet, age, or gender? An important frame of reference for considering these issues is that none of them are "problems invented by the technology"; rather, all of these issues existed before the maturing of this technology.

Bases for the New Paradigm

One advantage to the current approach for acquiring and using information on drug metabolism and interactions is that there is a better understanding of how contemporary tools can be applied, even though many of them have been available for at least two decades. One exception is that recombinant enzymes have replaced purification of enzymes, enabling the construction of a molecular framework. In turn, mapping of genes and their protein products has facilitated a generalization from compound-specific results to pathway-specific interpretations. This conceptual approach to data interpretation is perhaps the major critical shift that has driven recent advances in drug studies *in vitro*.

Because high-quality experimental metabolic data have been generated for decades as part of the drug development process, it is possible to overlook the revolutionary nature of changes that have occurred recently. Rather

J.M. Collins: Laboratory of Clinical Pharmacology, Food and Drug Administration, 4 Research Court, Room 314, Rockville, Maryland 20850

than thinking "maybe someone will figure out later how it will help," clinicians have moved on to an expectation that "we know how it will help if we have this information now."

The generation and interpretation of these data are no longer an occasional process restricted to "famous" molecules, but a process that is timely and consistent. Above all, researchers have changed from accepting predominantly idiosyncratic manifestations of interactions to systematically using prospective predictions and intervention.

There has also been a major shift from using animal-derived data to using human-based data. Except for comparative studies to assess interspecies differences, animal studies have declined in importance. Part of this shift is driven by an appreciation for the uncertainty in cross-species metabolic pathways. From the practical side, the well-organized, readily available supply of human tissue has fueled this shift.

The Old Paradigm: Zidovudine as an Example

The development of drugs for treatment of patients with human immunodeficiency virus (HIV) infection provides the clearest example of how far the field of drug interactions has developed. Ten years ago, zidovudine (AZT) was approved by the Food and Drug Administration as the first drug for use in this therapeutic area. At that time, my colleagues and I were involved in the first human studies of this agent (1). When the first subjects received treatment, we had no information on human metabolism from studies *in vitro*, and information from animals *in vivo* suggested that the drug was not metabolized. It became obvious, however, that "extra peaks" appeared in plasma and urine. Subsequently, it was shown that 70% to 80% of an AZT dose was glucuronidated (2). Several years later, when we wrote a review article on AZT kinetics (3), we still did not have any information on how to generalize the empirical observations. Later in this chapter, this experience for AZT is contrasted with the data-rich environment available for the HIV protease inhibitors as they have entered the market.

REGULATORY RESPONSE: LABORATORY RESEARCH

The FDA supported the clinical research that discovered and determined the mechanisms for the serious, and occasionally fatal, metabolic interactions between terfenadine and ketoconazole, and, more broadly, among several antihistamines and antiinfectives (4). This sequence of events underscored the need for capturing this type of information earlier in the development process (5). The FDA then established a focused program of regulatory research in the area of drug metabolism and drug interactions; a key element of this regulatory response was a laboratory-based research program.

The overall paradigm for focused regulatory research is to identify a specific need (in this case, metabolism and interactions) and assemble a research team to develop core expertise. As progress is made, internal research findings, external knowledge (e.g., peer-reviewed literature), and the accumulation of review experience combine to set the stage for establishing guidance to industry for drug development programs. The reviewers and researchers work together at the policy level on guidance development and then form the nucleus of a team that can provide training to other primary review staff, as well as serve as secondary reviewers (internal consultants) as Investigational New Drug Application (IND) and New Drug Application (NDA) submissions are evaluated.

Table 4-1 outlines the general pattern for research at the FDA, which focuses on those areas in which a need for hands-on experience has been determined. Initial hypotheses can be subjected to reality checks and refinement through collaboration with other federal agencies that include drug development as part of their mission (e.g., several institutes at National Institutes of Health and the US Army). Once the concepts are polished from these experiences, guidance can be written that addresses the state-of-the-art, without overlooking available tools or without overestimating validation capabilities.

Paclitaxel: Interspecies Metabolic Differences

The FDA first became involved in drug–drug metabolic interaction studies in a collaborative effort with the National Cancer Institute (NCI), just before the approval of the antitumor drug paclitaxel. Even when used as monotherapy for anticancer treatment, paclitaxel is coadministered with a variety of agents to minimize allergic reactions to the drug and its vehicle, Cremophor. The most common set of drugs includes two antihistamines (e.g., cimetidine plus diphenhydramine) and a corticosteroid (e.g., dexamethasone). The FDA had intended to undertake a series of studies in rats, but discovered a mismatch in CYP450 metabolism between rats and humans (6), as shown in Fig. 4-1.

For paclitaxel, the parent drug is the principal chemical species of biologic interest, both for toxicity and antitumor effects. Thus, the rat was still a relevant model for toxicity studies in general. Conversely, when collaborating on a phase 1 study of iododeoxydoxorubicin (7), the exposure to mice in toxicity studies was retrospectively found to be primarily to parent drug, whereas humans were primarily exposed to a metabolite. Because both the parent and the metabolite have biologic activity in this

TABLE 4-1. *Role of Food and Drug Administration Research*

Acquire hands-on experience
Reality check by way of federal collaborations
Credibility for regulatory policy

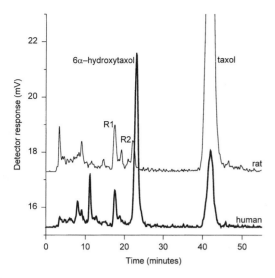

FIG. 4-1. Comparison of metabolic profile for paclitaxel in hepatic microsomes from humans (*lower tracing*) and rats (*upper tracing*). (From Jamis-Dow CA, Klecker RW, Katki AG, Collins JM. Metabolism of taxol by human and rat liver in vitro: a screen for drug interactions and interspecies differences. *Cancer Chemother Pharmacol* 1995;36:107–114.)

case, the investigators had inadvertently studied toxicity of the wrong chemical species before human trials.

Penclomedine: Develop the Metabolite?

The FDA's next experience was also with an investigational drug under development by NCI—the alkylating agent penclomedine (PEN). It can be demonstrated *in vitro* that PEN is oxidized to demethylpenclomedine (DMPEN), although it is difficult to maintain catalytic activity in the presence of reactive alkylating compounds. In collaboration with the phase 1 investigators at Johns Hopkins University, the FDA showed (8) rapid disappearance of parent drug from plasma, with rapid appearance and persistence of metabolite. Based on the data in Fig. 4-2, it was estimated that the area under concentration versus time curve (AUC) for DMPEN was 500-fold greater than for PEN but that their antitumor activities were similar. The parent molecule is a potent neurotoxin; all patients experienced symptoms at high doses. By inference, metabolite must not be very neurotoxic, because the patients had onset of neurotoxicity during the infusion, with decreasing intensity after the infusion period ended. Because the metabolite levels were sustained between doses and accumulated throughout the cycle, its timecourse was disconnected from the neurotoxicity.

This scenario with PEN and DMPEN is reminiscent of that for terfenadine. Parent terfenadine is highly cardiotoxic, whereas its metabolite fexofenadine is relatively noncardiotoxic. Both terfenadine and its metabolite have beneficial antihistaminic effects. Long after the initial

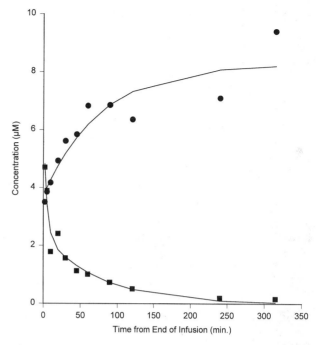

FIG. 4-2. Concentration-time profiles for penclomedine (■; PEN) and its metabolite, demethylpenclomedine (●; DMPEN), following a 1-hour intravenous infusion of penclomedine to patients on the first day of a 5-day treatment cycle. Only trace levels of PEN were detectable before the next day's infusion, but DMPEN accumulated throughout the cycle, reaching 50-μM levels. (From Hartman NR, O'Reilly S, Rowinsky EK, Collins JM, Strong JM. Murine and human in vivo penclomedine metabolism. *Clin Cancer Res* 1996;2:953–962.

introduction of terfenadine to the market, fexofenadine has replaced the parent compound.

What can be learned from the terfenadine experience in relation to PEN and DMPEN? In this case, a rapid determination that the parent molecule is the toxic species is helpful, because investigators may still have the energy and enthusiasm to pursue the metabolite before they grow weary of this class of molecules.

CAI: Which Metabolite Is Important?

When evaluating data from studies *in vitro*, interpretation of the significance of the metabolites and their pathways depends on the question being asked. CAI, which is another investigational anticancer drug under development by NCI, is an excellent example for demonstrating the different types of questions that can be answered. Microsomal studies at the FDA found a variety of metabolites (9), but 84% of the metabolism went to a compound designated as M3. This is the only microsomal pathway that would be important for modulating the circulating levels of CAI in patients; all other pathways are quantitatively unable to make a large difference in parent levels, even if completely inhibited. For example, the first metabolite eluting on an high-performance liquid chromatography (HPLC) analysis, M1, accounts for only 2% of the microsomal metabolism of CAI.

On the other hand, the relative importance of M1 and M3 is reversed when the focus is shifted to the body's exposure to circulating metabolites. Although most CAI does become transformed to M3, there is a rapid conversion of M3 by glucuronidation to a conjugate, which is efficiently excreted in urine. This sequential metabolism was found by using slices of human liver, in which the microsomal products were immediately available to secondary biotransformation, mimicking the situation *in vivo*. Thus, when plasma from patients taking CAI was examined, essentially no M3 was found circulating in the body.

Even though 40-fold lower amounts of M1 were formed compared with M3, there was not rapid secondary conversion of M1, and it was found to circulate in the body in concentrations similar to that of the parent drug. The focus of further studies of bioactivity, either toxicity or antitumor effect, ought to be M1, not M3, despite the 40-fold difference in primary formation rates.

Fenoldopam: Non-P450, Parallel Pathways, Stereospecific Metabolism

Fenoldopam, an antihypertensive agent recently approved by the FDA, illustrates several distinctive points. Upon examination of the metabolism of fenoldopam (a drug which originally was tested clinically in the late 1970s), it was found that cytochrome P450 had no role in fenoldopam metabolism (10). In fact, there were three major metabolites formed in parallel: methylation via catechol O-methyl transferase, glucuronidation, and sulfation. The presence of multiple parallel routes minimizes the chance that inhibition of any single pathway will substantially shift parent concentrations that circulate in the body.

In addition to the non-P450 pathways, another interesting facet of fenoldopam is that it is administered as a racemate, and differences in the stereospecificity of these metabolic pathways were found. As shown in Fig. 4-3, each stereoisomer has its own "fingerprint" of relative pathway importance.

Losigamone: Interactions Between Stereoisomers

Every racemate has inherent potential for metabolic drug–drug interactions, because one enantiomer can interact with the other. For the example of fenoldopam, although the stereoisomers have somewhat different metabolic profiles, they appear to be noninteracting. That is not always the case. The experimental anticonvulsant losigamone (LSG) is also administered as a racemate. Working with the Epilepsy Branch at NIH, McNeilly and Strong at the FDA showed (11) that not only does each enantiomer have its own metabolic profile but the patterns are also completely non-overlapping. Unlike the case for fenoldopam, there is a very strong interaction between the two enantiomers. As shown in Fig. 4-4,

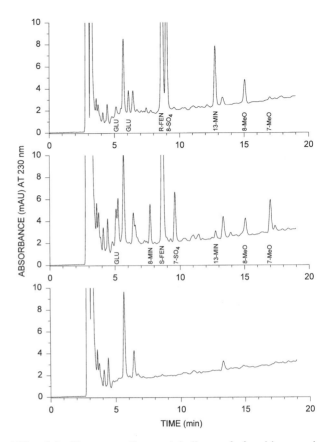

FIG. 4-3. Stereospecific metabolism of fenoldopam in human hepatic slices: R-FEN **(top panel)**; S-FEN **(middle panel)**; blank **(bottom panel)**. (From Klecker RW, Collins JM. Stereoselective metabolism of fenoldopam and its metabolites in human liver microsomes, cytosol, and slices. *J Cardiovasc Pharmacol* 1997;30:69–74).

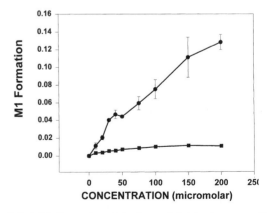

FIG. 4-4. Inhibition of metabolism of (+) losigamone in the presence of its (-)enaniomer. (Adapted from Torchin CD, McNeilly PJ, Kapetanovic IM, Strong JM, Kupferberg HJ. Stereoselective metabolism of a new anticonvulsant drug candidate, losigamone, by human liver microsomes. *Drug Metab Dispos* 1996;24:1002–1008.)

metabolism of +-LSG is completely inhibited by the -LSG. These findings do not preclude development of the racemate, but it is one of the factors that should be considered when making such decisions.

Saquinavir: Intestinal Metabolism

Returning to the area of anti-HIV drugs, in contrast to the nearly complete lack of metabolic information available for AZT at the time of its initial approval, the development and regulation of HIV protease inhibitors have benefited substantially from early attention to metabolism and drug interactions. Indeed, this class of molecules has a variety of major interactions with the other drugs typically used in the polypharmacy milieu of therapeutics for acquired immunodeficiency syndrome. However, their powerful activity against viral load in the body has provided a compelling motivation to understand these interactions, so that their power is not lost in a large set of adverse reactions.

Because of strong signals regarding low bioavailability and potential first pass metabolism, the FDA undertook some studies of saquinavir, the first molecule in its class to reach FDA review. The sponsor had already done metabolic work with human liver microsomes and found substantial involvement of P450 3A4, which increased the FDA's interest. Because the drug was being given orally, the FDA laboratory specifically sought to compare hepatic metabolism with intestinal metabolism, especially because the drug appeared to be transformed via the P450 3A pathways.

Saquinavir was incubated with samples from a bank of human intestinal microsomes, and a series of metabolites was found (12). The reaction rate was vigorous, so it was necessary to dilute the microsomal protein substantially to slow down the rate and avoid substrate depletion. The intestinal metabolic profile was identical with that of human liver microsomes. Incubation of saquinavir with recombinant human P450 3A4 also produced a similar profile (Fig. 4-5). Selective inhibitory concentrations of ketoconazole (K_i of 20 nM) also confirmed that 3A4 was the dominant enzyme. In addition to assisting the phenotyping of the enzymatic pathway, the ketoconazole information has practical clinical utility. If a patient's dose of saquinavir has been titrated to a stable dose, and then a fungal infection develops and concomitant therapy with ketoconazole is initiated, then the circulating levels of saquinavir would be expected to increase.

It is not sufficient to determine the effects of other drugs upon the metabolism of a new molecular entity (NME). The ability of the NME to impact upon the metabolism of other drugs is equally important. When the effect of saquinavir on the metabolism of terfenadine was examined, the K_i was 0.7 μM. Although not as impressive as the K_i for inhibition of saquinavir by ketoconazole, this concentration of saquinavir was neverthe-

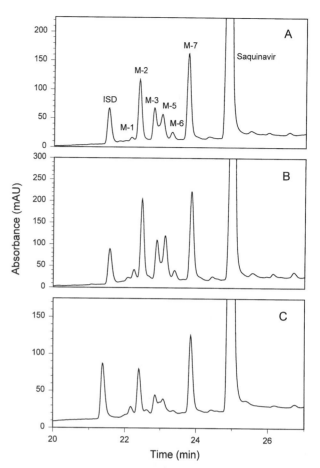

FIG. 4-5. Metabolism *in vitro* of the human immunodeficiency virus protease inhibitor saquinavir in microsomes prepared from **(A)** human liver, **(B)** human intestinal mucosa, and **(C)** recombinant human CYP450 3A4. (From Fitzsimmons ME, Collins JM. Selective biotransformation of the HIV protease inhibitor saquinavir by human small intestinal cytochrome P450 3A4: potential contribution to high first-pass metabolism. *Drug Metab Dispos* 1997;25:256–266.)

less in a range that was likely to be achievable and, thus, clinically relevant.

Intentional Strategy for Metabolic Inhibition

In general, drug–drug interactions are nuisances, because inhibition may produce safety issues and induction may produce loss of efficacy. However, in carefully selected cases, it can be desirable to intentionally exploit drug–drug interactions. The most common rationale is to increase the exposure of a scarce, expensive, or poorly bioavailable drug.

It is become increasingly clear that HIV protease inhibitors work best in combination with each other and with other anti-HIV drugs. The clinical study of the combination of saquinavir with ritonavir, a related protease inhibitor, was intentionally pursued to determine whether a metabolic interaction could provide potential advantages in terms of overcoming low patient exposures to saquinavir. Because ritonavir and yet another protease inhibitor, indinavir, were on-track for approval at about the same time, the FDA chose to gain some experience with this class of potential interactions and found that indinavir inhibited saquinavir metabolism in human intestinal microsomes in a potent fashion, with a K_i of 0.2 μM.

LABELING: TRANSLATING INFORMATION INTO PRACTICAL USE

The situation for the HIV protease inhibitors is much more data-rich than for AZT. The challenge rests in the translation of these data into "labeling," that is, instructions for use. What type of interaction is so serious that it leads the sponsor and FDA to contraindicate concomitant use? What level of interactions leads to warnings or precautions, that is, less serious signals about concomitant use?

How can the bench data and clinical observations be gathered into a package that does not overwhelm the prescriber and patient? How can the current state of knowledge be prioritized, and how is labeling updated as additional data are obtained? Predictably, some commentators have already found that "information overload" leads prescribers away from engaging in a serious consideration of the problem. Less commonly, for life-threatening diseases, but certainly to some degree, there is also a tendency to withhold otherwise useful therapy simply because the potential for drug–drug interactions looms ominously. HIV protease inhibitors have forced this issue to the forefront because they are so effective that they have changed the course of the disease. However, as a class, they have a high degree of drug–drug interaction, and they are never given as monotherapy.

The labeling for ritonavir is an extraordinary effort to cope with the avalanche of available information. More than a few critics have said that the ritonavir labeling is itself overwhelming, and not everyone is comfortable with the extrapolated scenarios for drugs never tested *in vitro* or in the clinic. Nonetheless, the systematic survey broke new ground. Table 2 of the ritonavir labeling (13) assessed the potential impact of ritonavir upon the metabolism of other drugs likely to be used in the target population. At one point, there were so many interactions being identified that one could assume everything is affected, but that is an overreaction, and one of the strengths of Table 2 is that it provides some reassurance about the *absence* of interactions in some cases. It is recommended that ritonavir always be taken in combination with at least one of the nucleoside analogues that are reverse transcriptase inhibitors. Thus, the reporting in Table 2 that ritonavir does not substantially impact upon AZT pharmacokinetics is highly relevant.

Whereas Table 2 broke new ground for the quantity of clinically derived data that were presented for drug interactions, Table 3 of the ritonavir label pushed into new territory by including a mixture of 80% extrapolation and 20% data. The 200 most commonly used drugs in the target population were assessed and classified in terms of small, medium, or large interaction potential. In addition to other challenges, these tables are reminders that interactions, like all pharmacologic responses, often need to be graded in severity of impact.

These approaches for ritonavir are not the final solution for user-friendly product labeling. All sectors of the community have learned a lot from this approach, and all are responsible for improving upon it. Every drug–drug interaction cannot be tested rigorously in the clinic. Thus, researchers need to determine their comfort zone for making clinical prescribing judgments on the basis of laboratory data. In particular, a type of "class labeling" that characterizes potential interactions based on metabolic pathways needs to be determined, rather than defining the therapeutic class or general similarity of molecular structure.

In addition to providing information that is user-friendly, there is a major challenge to ensure that the advice is not rapidly obsolete. This situation is rapidly getting more complicated. Since 1997, the FDA has approved more than 100 NMEs. Their interactions with the existing armamentarium is no small challenge considering that only two drugs are interacting, but in some therapeutic settings, and certainly in the elderly populations, it is rare that only two drugs are given at any one time.

REGULATORY GUIDANCE

Decisions regarding the approval of specific products, particularly high-profile or "priority" drugs, are the most widely visible actions of a regulatory agency. These decisions are the endpoint of negotiations among staff from the FDA and the sponsor of the drug, with additional input being given from advisory committees composed of academicians, practitioners, and consumer representatives. The science is always decided on a case-by-case basis, but general issues are cast within a scientific policy framework that is intended to provide guidance for common areas across all drugs, or for a class of drugs.

Consistent with the philosophy that product-specific research is the responsibility of the sponsor, regulatory research on specific products is only feasible in a small number of cases. Most regulatory research is geared to support scientific policy, which can guide the actions of review staff and the expectations of drug developers.

The FDA's first effort at regulatory policy in this area of drug–drug interactions was released in April 1997. It is available through the internet ("Guidance for Industry. Drug Metabolism/Drug Interaction Studies in the Drug Development Process: Studies *In Vitro*." Universal Reference Locator (URL) is http://www.fda.gov/cder/guidance/clin3.pdf). The regulatory science in the guidance was supported by many of the examples in this chapter and included input from the FDA, the clinical research conducted at universities under contract from FDA/Center for Drug Evaluation and Research (CDER), from consultation with reviewers at CDER who evaluate mountains of data every day, and from other groups who generate and analyze this type of data.

A follow-up document for clinical studies is in preparation ("Guidance for Industry. Metabolic Drug-Drug Interaction Studies *In Vivo:* Study Design, Data Analysis, and Impact on Dosing and Labeling"). The outline and goals have been presented at an advisory committee meeting, with an opportunity for input from industry, professional organizations, and the public.

After internal approval, it will also be posted on the world wide web for further comment.

REFERENCES

1. Klecker RW, Collins JM, Yarchoan R, et al. Plasma and cerebrospinal fluid pharmacokinetics of 3′-azido-3′-deoxythymidine: a novel pyrimidine analog with potential application for the treatment of patients with AIDS and related diseases. *Clin Pharmacol Ther* 1987;41:407–412.
2. Blum MR, Lao SHT, Good SS, deMiranda P. Pharmacokinetics and bioavailability of zidovudine in humans. *Am J Med* 1988;85(suppl 2A):189–194.
3. Collins JM, Unadkat J. Zidovudine pharmacokinetics. *Clin Pharmacokin* 1989;17:1–9.
4. Honig PK, Wortham DC, Zamani K, Conner DP, Mullin JC, Cantilena LR. Terfenadine-ketoconazole interaction. *JAMA* 1993;269:1513–1518.
5. Peck CC, Temple R, Collins JM. Understanding consequences of concurrent therapies. *JAMA* 1993;269:1550–1552.
6. Jamis-Dow CA, Klecker RW, Katki AG, Collins JM. Metabolism of taxol by human and rat liver in vitro: a screen for drug interactions and interspecies differences. *Cancer Chemother Pharmacol* 1995;36:107–114.
7. Gianni L, Vigano L, Surbone A, et al. Pharmacology and clinical toxicity of 4′-iodo-4′-deoxydoxorubicin: an example of successful application of pharmacokinetics to dose escalation in phase I trials. *J Natl Cancer Inst* 1990;82:469–477.
8. Hartman NR, O'Reilly S, Rowinsky EK, Collins JM, Strong JM. Murine and human in vivo penclomedine metabolism. *Clin Cancer Res* 1996;2:953–962.
9. Ludden LK, Strong JM, Kohn EC, Collins JM. Similarity of metabolism for CAI in human liver tissue in vitro and in humans in vivo. *Clin Cancer Res* 1995;1:399–405.
10. Klecker RW, Collins JM. Stereoselective metabolism of fenoldopam and its metabolites in human liver microsomes, cytosol, and slices. *J Cardiovasc Pharmacol* 1997;30:69–74.
11. Torchin CD, McNeilly PJ, Kapetanovic IM, Strong JM, Kupferberg HJ. Stereoselective metabolism of a new anticonvulsant drug candidate, losigamone, by human liver microsomes. *Drug Metab Dispos* 1996;24:1002–1008.
12. Fitzsimmons ME, Collins JM. Selective biotransformation of the HIV protease inhibitor saquinavir by human small intestinal cytochrome P450 3A4: potential contribution to high first-pass metabolism. *Drug Metab Dispos* 1997;25:256–266.
13. *Physicians' Desk Reference*, 52nd ed. Montvale, NJ: Medical Economics, 1998.

SECTION II

Enzymes and Transporters

CHAPTER 5

Cytochromes P450: Historical Overview

John B. Schenkman

RECOGNITION OF CYTOCHROME P450

Effect of Carbon Monoxide on Microsomal Metabolism

The story of cytochrome P450, like a tree, has many roots and branches. Its roots go back to many beginnings. There was a period when investigators such as B. B. Brodie were examining the metabolism of drugs and chemicals by liver microsomes (1–4) and the induction of such metabolism by drug substrates (5–7). At the same time, investigators such as Millers were studying liver microsomal metabolism of carcinogens and the induction of the metabolism by these substrates (8,9). Microsomal metabolism of steroids, too, was a subject of interest in this period. Ryan and Engel (10) noted that carbon monoxide would inhibit bovine adrenal microsomal steroid C21 hydroxylation and that the inhibition could be reversed by light. Although reduced and oxidized bovine adrenal microsomal spectra were recorded and cytochrome b5 was seen, spectra were not run under carbon monoxide. Ryan and Engel did note that "This light reversible carbon monoxide inhibition suggests the participation of the cytochrome in the hydroxylating system. No direct evidence for a cytochrome [b5] carbon monoxide complex is available...." Conney and coworkers (11) also noted inhibition of liver microsomal aminoazo dye metabolism by carbon monoxide.

The Carbon Monoxide–Binding Pigment and Role in Microsomal Monooxygenations

In that same period, Garfinkel and Klingenberg both reported that carbon monoxide addition to liver microsomes, in the presence of either NADH or dithionite, resulted in the appearance of a broad absorption peak

at 450 nm in ultraviolet (UV)/visible spectra (12,13). According to Omura (14), the original observation of the 450-nm carbon monoxide–binding peak was made (but never published) by G. R. Williams, whose stay at the Johnson Foundation of the University of Pennsylvania overlapped that of Klingenberg. The studies of Garfinkel were a continuation of the studies of Klingenberg. The nature of the carbon monoxide–binding pigment was not known at that time, but in the reports of Klingenberg and of Garfinkel, it was indicated that microsomal cytochrome b5 could only account for about half of the measured microsomal heme. It was not until 1962 that the carbon monoxide–binding pigment was identified as a hemoprotein by Omura and Sato (15), and was tentatively named cytochrome P450 after the position of the absorption peak. Total microsomal heme was seen to equal the amount of cytochrome b5 plus cytochrome P450. Sato, too, had been a visiting scientist at the Johnson Foundation, and his stay there overlapped that of Klingenberg. Another Johnson Foundation researcher, Estabrook, and his coworkers examined the carbon monoxide inhibition of the steroid C21 hydroxylase reaction in bovine adrenal cortex microsomes (16). They showed the presence of the 450-nm pigment in the adrenal microsomes and were able to reverse the inhibition maximally by light of 450 nm. The magnitude of the 450-nm peak was seen to depend on the carbon monoxide to oxygen ratio, and the extent of steroid 21-hydroxylation showed the same dependency on that ratio. From this, the researchers concluded that the cytochrome P450 was the terminal oxidase of the bovine adrenal microsomal steroid C21 hydroxylase (16) and the liver microsomal drug oxidase (17), and functions in oxygen activation. Microsomal cytochrome P450 was then shown to be the substrate-binding component of the monooxygenase system (18–22). A wide variety of substrates of the P450 monooxygenase system were identified, the vast majority of which caused one or another modification of the spectral properties of the hemoprotein (23). In the 1970s,

J.B. Schenkman: Department of Pharmacology, University of Connecticut Health Center, 263 Farmington Avenue, Farmington, Connecticut 06030

when it was recognized that a number of cytochrome P450 enzymes existed, attempts were made to determine substrate specificities of the different forms.

MULTIPLICITY OF CYTOCHROME P450

Early Indications of Multiple Forms

From these modest beginnings, a massive tree of studies on cytochrome P450 has grown. Branches extend to the role of cytochrome P450 in metabolism of drugs, to the role of cytochrome P450 in the activation of toxicants, mutagens, and carcinogens, to the molecular biology of cytochrome P450, and to the forms of cytochrome P450 in different species and phyla. By 1968, indications had begun to appear that suggested the presence of more than one form of cytochrome P450. Based on the differential sensitivities to inhibition by carbon monoxide of testosterone 16α-, 6β-, and 7α-hydroxylation products formed by liver microsomes, it was suggested that "one or more CO-binding cytochromes function in the hydroxylation of testosterone in liver microsomes" (24). That was not inconsistent with studies by early biochemical pharmacologists who had shown many drug-, steroid-, and chemical-metabolizing enzyme activities to be present in liver microsomes and were able to demonstrate differential induction of the different activities by some substrates (7,25,26). Other evidence for more than one P450 monooxygenase included multiple pH-sensitive peaks in the reduced ethylisocyanide-difference spectrum of liver microsomes (27,28) and the lack of linearity of Lineweaver-Burk plots of drug-metabolizing activities (29,30). The latter studies suggested multiple forms of cytochrome P450 with overlapping substrate specificities. Even so, as late as 1969, cytochrome P450 was thought of as being a single entity in liver microsomes. This was because the addition of carbon monoxide and reducing equivalents only produced a single peak, and because the metabolism of one substrate was competitively inhibited by the addition of another substrate. For example, the N-demethylation of ethylmorphine (31) and the N-dealkylation of 7-deoxycoumarin (32) were competitively inhibited by hexobarbital and a number of other drugs. Pretreatment of laboratory rodents with barbiturates, such as phenobarbital (33), or polycyclic hydrocarbons, such as benzo(a)pyrene or 3-methylcholanthrene (34,35), caused an increase in the microsomal content of cytochrome P450 (Fig. 5-1). Induction studies showed the carbon monoxide complex of polycyclic aromatic hydrocarbon–inducible cytochrome P450 to have an absorption peak shifted a few nanometers toward lower wavelengths and properties different from the constitutive and phenobarbital-induced enzymes in microsomes (28,35–38). Inhibitors of RNA synthesis and protein synthesis (e.g., actinomycin D and puromycin) blocked the

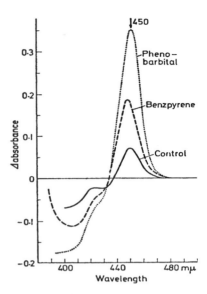

FIG. 5-1. Cytochrome P450 in liver microsomes of untreated, phenobarbital-treated, and benzo(a)pyrene-treated female weanling rats. Animals were injected with agents for 3 days at 80 mg phenobarbital/kg or 20 mg benzo(a)pyrene/kg and starved 48 hours before killing. Spectra were of the dithionite reduced plus carbon monoxide versus dithionite reduced microsomes at 2 mg per milliliter.

induction of the aryl hydrocarbon hydroxylase (9,39). Phenobarbital induction of cytochrome P450 and of drug metabolism by liver microsomes was also blocked by actinomycin D and by puromycin (40). These studies indicated a need for RNA synthesis and for protein synthesis in the induction process. Indeed, phenobarbital treatment of rats was shown to increase the levels of cytoplasmic mRNA coding for phenobarbital-inducible cytochrome P450 approximately 30-fold in liver (41). At this point, it was no longer possible to deny the presence of more than one species of cytochrome P450.

Induction and Characterization of Individual Forms of Cytochrome P450

The 1970s were a period of intense effort aimed at isolation and purification of cytochrome P450, and evidence for its existence in multiple forms accumulated rapidly. The response of the enzymes to inducing substrates greatly aided in these efforts, increasing levels of the hemoproteins in the liver microsomes. Barbiturates and polycyclic hydrocarbons were among the first agents shown to elevate the drug-metabolizing enzymes (6,7). Two different forms of cytochrome P450 were recognized after phenobarbital and polycyclic hydrocarbon pretreatment. These agents have come to be known as inducers of the CYP2 and CYP1 gene families, respectively. The two forms were shown to have different substrate specificities (36,42). Remmer (26) had noted that glucocorticoids, too, could elevate drug-metabolizing enzyme activity in liver microsomes of rats. Subsequently, steroids, such as pregnenolone 16α-carbonitrile and dexamethasone, were found to be a third category of inducer of drug metabolizing activities (43,44) and to induce the CYP3 family of genes. The different inducers caused a number of changes in kinetic constants that were indicative of multiple forms of cytochrome P450 (44). Such treatments were shown to increase the content of different specific protein bands containing heme at around 50,000 mass in sodium dodecylsulfate polyacrylamide electrophoresis (SDS-PAGE) (45–47).

In reconstitution studies, it was shown (42) that the selectivity of the cytochrome P450s for substrates lay with the hemoprotein, in that benzphetamine metabolism was selectively metabolized at a high rate with the phenobarbital-induced form of cytochrome P450 but poorly when the reaction was catalyzed by the 3-methylcholanthrene-induced form of cytochrome P450; the reverse was seen when the substrate chosen was benzo(a)pyrene. This would indicate a selectivity in metabolite formation by different forms of cytochrome P450 that might be used to identify different forms of the enzyme in microsomes and that would have to be considered in the kinetics of elimination of multiple drugs that share a common drug-metabolizing enzyme. The ability of different forms of cytochrome P450 to metabolize steroids and to produce different isomeric and epimeric products from testosterone (48–51), dichlorobiphenyls (52), and warfarin (53) with rat and rabbit enzymes was recognized, and attempts were made to use those agents as a means of identifying different forms of cytochrome P450 in different tissues based on the metabolite patterns. Similar studies were carried out with human forms of cytochrome P450 (54,55). As different forms of cytochrome P450 have been isolated and identified, attempts have been made to characterize them with respect to drug and toxicant metabolism. For example, a form of rat liver cytochrome P450 was isolated and characterized with respect to metabolism of a number of different substrates, including 4-hydroxylation of debrisoquine (56). This form (P450 UT-H, CYP2D6) was shown to be the only one of nine purified forms of rat P450 with appreciable activity and to be responsible for almost all of the debrisoquine 4-hydroxylase activity in rat liver microsomes (57).

Isolation and Purification of Different Forms of Cytochrome P450

A major breakthrough in the isolation of purified forms of cytochrome P450 was the observation that detergents made it possible to separate the hemoprotein from phenobarbital-induced rabbit liver microsomal membranes (58). Earlier, a number of microsomal proteins had been solubilized by proteases, including cytochrome b5 (59), NADH-cytochrome b5 reductase (60), and NADPH-

cytochrome P450 reductase (61). However, attempts to purify P450 hemoprotein with proteases were unsuccessful, and only yielded particles stripped of cytochrome b5 and NADPH-cytochrome P450 reductase (62), or converted the hemoprotein to cytochrome P420, a degradation form. Purification of cytochrome P450 was made possible by the recognition that addition of polyols, such as glycerol, to the solvent systems stabilized the hemoprotein (63,64) and that detergents were highly effective at solubilizing cytochrome P450 from the microsomal membranes (58,65–67). The success of Lu and Coon was followed by the purification of several differentially induced forms of cytochrome P450, mainly in the rat and rabbit (48,68–70), and subsequently of constitutive forms of cytochrome P450 (71–73).

Along with the purification of multiple forms of cytochrome P450 came multiple nomenclatures for the different cytochrome P450s, almost one nomenclature per laboratory carrying out purification. It was difficult in the 1980s to know whether the form studied in one laboratory was the same as or different from that studied in another laboratory (51,74–76). Many laboratories were involved in isolation and purification of forms of P450 from rodent microsomes (68–70,73,77–83), and each laboratory used its own nomenclature as well as its own preferred substrates and antibodies for characterization. The use of amino terminal amino acid sequencing of purified cytochrome P450 helped to identify and compare the different forms of cytochrome P450 isolated by the different laboratories. However, whereas amino terminal amino acid sequencing was a useful tool for comparison of most forms of cytochrome P450 initially, it soon became apparent that this alone would not suffice. The procedure is labor intensive and time consuming and requires a considerable amount of pure protein. A number of forms of cytochrome P450 are not inducible and are present in concentrations of less than 5% of the total P450 hemoprotein in the liver microsomes (56,57,84,85). The total P450 levels in some tissues are even less than that (86). Such forms are not readily purified from tissues in amounts sufficient for sequencing. Furthermore, amino terminal amino acid sequences can lead to confusion, in that a number of forms of cytochrome P450 exist with highly similar primary structures, such as phenobarbital-induced rat hepatic P450 (87), in which three forms differing in size but with the same amino-terminal amino acid sequence were seen. Two laboratories reported on the primary sequence of rabbit P450 isozyme 2 (CY2B4) with sequences differing by 14 residues (88,89). Subsequently, diethylaminoethyl (DEAE) cellulose and HPLC separations of the apparently pure rabbit cytochrome P450 isozyme 2 yielded three fractions (90). The use of molecular biology techniques to examine the problem provided an answer. Five different transcripts coding for isozyme 2 were found in rabbit liver cDNA clones from livers of phenobarbital-treated animals (70). Deduced sequences for the gene products revealed as few as six amino acid differences between one form (B1) and that reported for isozyme 2 (B0), and 11 amino acid differences between another form (B2) and isozyme 2 (90). A fifth form, Bx, was subsequently deduced that differed by only four residues (91). Subsequently, three of the deduced proteins—B0, B1, and Bx—were isolated from rabbit livers and identified by peptide mapping and sequencing (92).

FORMS OF CYTOCHROME 450

Nomenclature of Cytochrome P450

Rapid developments in the field of molecular biology greatly expanded the ability to detect, identify, and produce forms of cytochrome P450 that are expressed in extremely small amounts in tissues. Various inducers were shown to increase the rates of formation of P450 mRNA, from which many cDNA clones were prepared. These were used to detect, screen, and isolate new forms of cytochrome P450 found in different tissues of laboratory animals (93–98). This facilitated the identification and enumeration of forms of cytochrome P450 found in different tissues of the various species of organisms, as well as providing a unifying basis for naming of the different forms (99–102). Through the 1980s there were many reports of deduced sequences of newly detected microsomal forms of cytochrome P450. Currently, cytochrome P450 forms are named on the basis of evolutionary relationships in primary amino acid sequence alignments. Members in a gene family generally have more than 40% sequence identity with other members in the family and less than 40% sequence identity with another gene family. (There are a few exceptions to this rule.) Mammalian members of the same subfamily have a greater than 55% amino acid sequence identity and appear to lie within the same cluster on a chromosome. For example, P450 1A1 and P450 1A2 and P450 1B1 all have greater than 40% sequence identity and thus fit within the same CYP1 family and not, for example, in the CYP2 family. P450 1A1 and 1A2 both reside in the CYP1A subfamily by virtue of having greater than 55% amino acid sequence identity. Actually, the sequence identity between rabbit P450 1A1 and 1A2 is greater than 70%. In contrast, the sequence alignment identity between rabbit P450 2B5 and P450 1A1 is only 32%.

Mammalian Cytochrome P450 Gene Families

In the latter part of the 1980s, in part because of the low availability of some forms, the tools of molecular biology became of greater importance for the identification, expression, and study of the properties of additional forms of cytochrome P450, including those found in tissues other than the liver. The cDNA of many forms have been isolated, sequences deduced, proteins expressed, and catalytic activities determined in heterologous systems (103–107). Of the approximately 30 different families of cytochrome P450, only three have importance in drug, xenobiotic, and steroid metabolism in the vertebrate body, those in CYP 1, 2, and 3 families. Family 1 includes those forms that are involved in metabolism of polycyclic aromatic hydrocarbons, heterocyclic compounds, methylxanthines, and aromatic amines. Family 2 includes a large number of steroid- and drug-metabolizing enzymes, as well as forms capable of metabolism of a very wide range of organic chemicals. These enzymes are the most versatile of the xenobiotic metabolizing enzymes. Family 3 contains a smaller number of cytochrome P450 enzymes, but these forms, like those in family 2, metabolize a range of drugs and xenobiotics as well as being responsible for the 6β-hydroxylation of testosterone. There are two subfamilies in the CYP1 family: CYP1A and CYP1B. The former subfamily contains two members, 1A1 and 1A2 (Fig. 5-2), and based on sequence identities, orthologous to both genes appear to be present in most vertebrates. Orthologous genes are those that have counterparts in different species, that is, that have been derived from a common ancestral gene before the species diverged and often exhibit the same catalytic activities. These are given the same gene designation. For example, a human ortholog of rat CYP2E1 exists and has 78% amino acid sequence identity with the rat enzyme (103), hence it is also called CYP2E1. At least ten different mammalian CYP1A1 and seven CYP1A2 genes have been sequenced to date (http://drnelson. utmem.edu/genesperspecies.html). CYP1A2 was first isolated from human liver as phenacetin O-dealkylase (108), an activity it shares with the orthologous rat enzyme (109). Whereas the CYP1A1 protein has not

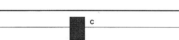

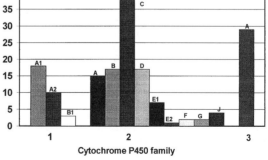

FIG. 5-2. Subfamilies of mammalian cytochrome P450 involved in xenobiotic metabolism. Genes for orthologous forms of cytochrome P450 in subfamilies 1A and 2E are also indicated. (Data from http://drnelson.utmem.edu/ nelsonhomepage.html#P450names.)

been isolated from the human liver, the CYP1A1 and CYP1A2 cDNAs have been isolated from human liver, and indications are that, as in rat liver, the former is expressed in barely detectable levels (109–111), if at all. In mouse liver, the constitutive levels of CYP1A2 mRNA is a bit higher than the level of 3-methylcholanthrene fully induced CYP1A1 mRNA (112). Three CYP1B1 genes have been identified: in rat, mouse, and human. Family 2 consists of eight subfamilies that contain mammalian genes 2A to 2G and 2J (see Fig. 5-2). Subfamily 2C is the largest, with 43 mammalian genes. A number of very similar genes are found in the 2A, 2B, and 2C subfamilies and, although assigned different subfamily numbers, have been suggested as being orthologous (76). Subfamily 2E consists of two members. There are eight orthologous CYP2E1 genes in the different species, and, to date, only one CYP2E2 gene has been reported; that was in rabbit. Family 3 has, at present, one subfamily, CYP3A, containing 27 mammalian genes.

From studies with rodent enzymes, it was recognized that the different forms of cytochrome P450 had overlapping substrate specificities, but that some forms have greater turnover of some substrates than others do. Attempts have been made to correlate microsomal metabolism of some substrates with certain forms. For example, benzo(a)pyrene is efficiently metabolized by a family 1 form of cytochrome P450. CYP1A1 exhibits high activity toward benzo(a)pyrene and for 7-ethoxycoumarin O-dealkylation, whereas CYP1A2 also metabolizes these substrates, but at a somewhat reduced rate (113,114). In contrast, in the metabolism of methylxanthines (e.g., caffeine and theophylline), CYP1A2 exhibits the higher activity (106). A similar broad spectrum of activity is exhibited by the CYP2C subfamily of enzymes toward drug substrates, with many enzymes able to metabolize the individual agents, but with one or another form exhibiting higher activity. For example, many forms of cytochrome P450 in rat liver microsomes metabolize mephenytoin, but CYP2D1 exhibits the greatest activity (57). From this it would appear that some forms of cytochrome P450 are more efficient at metabolism of certain substrates, and such specificity can result in unusual effects as a consequence of polymorphisms in certain forms.

Cytochrome P450 and Homeostasis

The large number of forms of cytochrome P450 in liver microsomes and tissues of animals suggests a need for the different forms and a role for at least some of them in the maintenance of homeostasis in the body. Earlier studies support this conclusion. Liver microsomes were shown to be capable of metabolism of a wide variety of drugs and substrates, and this metabolism was seen to be differentially altered by a number of physiologic and pathophysiologic conditions. For example, in rats made diabetic with alloxan, metabolism of aniline was doubled

but that of hexobarbital and a number of other drugs decreased by half or more (115,116). Similarly, starvation and adrenalectomy altered metabolism of drugs and chemicals by rat liver microsomes (117) and increased the level of certain SDS-PAGE–detectable forms of cytochrome P450 (118). In starved male rats or in rats made diabetic by the administration of streptozotocin, a number of changes were seen in levels of several forms of cytochrome P450. CYP2E1 increased more than eight-fold, CYP2C7 increased by 70%, and others (e.g., CYP2C11 and CYP2C13) decreased to barely detectable levels within a week in male rat liver microsomes (119–121). The orthologous CYP2E1 enzyme in humans responds similarly to diabetes, as determined in circulating lymphocytes of poorly controlled diabetic patients (122). Other forms of cytochrome P450 are also altered in diabetes, including CYP2A1 (elevated four-fold), CYP2A2 (decreased 80%), and CYP3A1/2 (decreased 50%) (123). Several forms of cytochrome P450 are also influenced by elevations in blood pressure. For example, in the spontaneously hypertensive rat, CYP2C11 and CYP3A1/2 were both increased several-fold, and CYP2A1 was decreased more than 50% in agreement with the similar homeostatic changes in microsomal 16α, 6β-, and 7α-hydroxylation of testosterone attributed to these forms, respectively (124). Although sex differences are seen in the individual liver microsomal forms and in total levels of cytochrome P450 in rats and some strains of mice, no such differences are seen in other species. However, developmental changes in rodent hepatic cytochrome P450 are seen (125), as is tissue-specific expression of a number of forms of cytochrome P450 (126–129), suggesting a role for these enzymes in maintaining the internal milieu.

Human Forms of Cytochrome P450

In the 1980s through the 1990s, a number of investigators began turning their interest to forms of human cytochrome P450. Early studies on human liver microsomes revealed the presence of low levels of both cytochrome b5 and cytochrome P450 in necropsy specimens. The cytochrome P450 levels decline with time after death and, in specimens older than 5 hours, the cytochrome P450 could not be detected (130). When cytochrome P450 was present, the microsomes had the ability to metabolize a number of drug substrates also metabolized by rat liver microsomes: aminopyrine, aniline, and benzo(a)pyrene. Similar levels were found in liver biopsy material (131). Much higher levels were, however, reported for necropsy material by one laboratory, which also demonstrated metabolism of codeine, hexobarbital, and aniline in the liver microsomes (132). Shortly thereafter, Kaschnitz and Coon (133) were able to separate cytochrome P450 from human liver microsomes, and several other laboratories were able to partially purify forms of human cytochrome P450 (134–136). Some of the first forms of human cytochrome P450 were isolated from human autopsy material (135) and from organ donor liver (137). In the latter study, six forms of cytochrome P450 were isolated and characterized with respect to substrate metabolism. One of these was primarily responsible for microsomal debrisoquine 4-hydroxylation (CYP2D6) and another for phenacetin O-dealkylation (CYP1A2) (108). Another form was identified as responsible for the nifedipine oxidase of microsomes (CYP3A3/4) (138). Subsequently, cDNA-derived heterologously expressed forms of cytochrome P450 have been used to determine catalytic activities of the enzymes (139–143).

At present, 39 functional human genes have been sequenced, of which 19 are in subfamilies 1, 2, and 3 (drnelson.utmem.edu/genesperspecies.html). Two are present in subfamily 1A and one is present in subfamily 1B (Fig. 5-3). Three are in 2A, one in 2B, four in 2C, and one each in 2D, 2E, 2F, and 2J subfamilies. Four active genes are found in subfamily 3A. CYP3A constitutes the major portion of cytochrome P450 forms expressed in the human liver and, as such, is of major importance in the clearance of drugs from the body. Human cytochrome P450 3A, like its rodent counterparts, metabolizes testosterone to the 6β-hydroxy metabolite. At least four 3A forms exist in human liver: 3A3, 3A4, 3A5, and 3A7; these are responsible for the greatest portion of testosterone β-hydroxylation, a major route in humans (144). Using cDNA expressed proteins, it was shown that the decreasing order of testosterone 6β-hydroxylase activity was 3A4 > 3A3 > 3A5 (55).

Polymorphism of Human Forms of Cytochrome P450

Once human forms of cytochrome P450 were available, it became possible to examine and explain the observed phenomenon of polymorphisms in oxidative metabolism of different drugs by humans. Polymorphisms have been observed in humans in the oxidative metabolism of debrisoquine (CYP2D6) (145), tolbutamide (CYP2C8-10) (146), and mephenytoin (CYP2C19) (147,148), as well as in forms of CYP2E1. In the latter gene, the polymorphism is in the transcription regulatory region and results in an increase in the rate of gene expression (149). A form of rat cytochrome P450 with high activity for 4-hydroxylation of debrisoquine (UT-H, CYP2D1) was shown to be the form responsible for the major metabolism of this drug by rat liver microsomes, using antibodies raised to the purified protein (56). Subsequently, the gene was cloned and used to explain the DA rat debrisoquine polymorphism (150). The human liver debrisoquine 4-hydroxylase, UT-DB (CYP2D6) was purified with the help of the antibody to rat UT-H (108) and was shown to be responsible for this activity in human liver microsomes. The 4-hydroxylation of mephenytoin in humans has recently been shown to use distinctly different forms of cytochrome P450 than are used for metabolism of tolbutamide (139,151). The latter is metabolized primarily by P450 2C9. This gene is associated with the metabolism of the anticoagulant warfarin, with dilantin, and with some nonsteroidal antiinflammatory agents (143). As more forms of cytochrome P450 are isolated and characterized with respect to drug substrates, other polymorphisms will be identified. Although no polymorphisms have as yet been associated with CYP2C9, a number of variants exist.

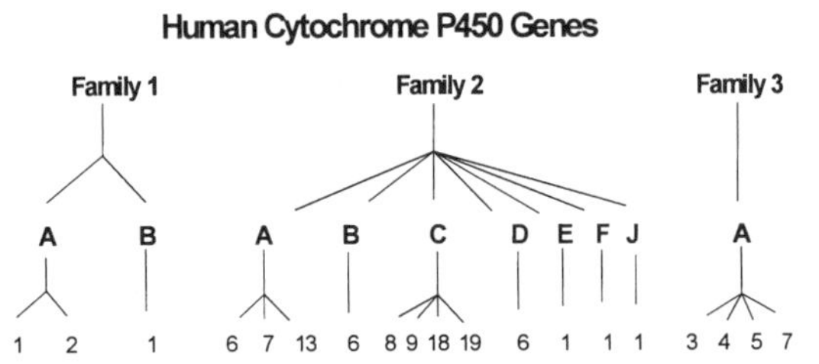

ACKNOWLEDGMENT

The author would like to gratefully acknowledge the many suggestions of Dr. Ingela Jansson and her help in critiquing and proofing this paper.

FIG. 5-3. Human cytochrome P450 genes in the xenobiotic-metabolizing CYP 1, 2, and 3 families. (Data from http://drnelson.utmem.edu/genesperspecies.html.)

REFERENCES

1. Brodie BB, Axelrod J, Cooper JR, et al. Detoxication of drugs and other foreign compounds by liver microsomes. *Science* 1955;121:603–604.
2. Axelrod J. The enzymatic demethylation of ephedrine. *J Pharmacol Exp Ther* 1955;114:430–438.
3. LaDu B, Gaudette L, Trousof N, Brodie BB. Enzymatic dealkylation of aminopyrine (pyramidon) and other alkylamines. *J Biol Chem* 1955;214:741–752.
4. Posner HS, Mitoma C, Udenfriend S. Enzymatic hydroxylation of aromatic compounds. II. Further studies of the properties of the microsomal hydroxylating system. *Arch Biochem Biophys* 1961;94:269–279.
5. Remmer H, Alsleben B. Die Aktivierung der Entgiftung in den Lebermikrosomen wahrend der Gewönung. *Klin Wschr* 1958;36:332–333.
6. Remmer H. Der beschleunigte Abbau von Pharmaka in den Lebermikrosomen unter dem Einfluss von Luminal. *Naunyn-Schmiedeberg's Arch Exp Pathol Pharmak* 1959;235:29–290.
7. Conney AH, Gillette JR, Inscoe JK, Trams ER, Posner HS. Induced synthesis of liver microsomal enzymes which metabolize foreign compounds. *Science* 1959;130:1478–1479.
8. Conney AH, Miller EC, Miller JA. The metabolism of methylated aminoazo dyes. V. Evidence for induction of enzyme synthesis in the rat by 3-methylcholanthrene. *Cancer Res* 1956;16:450–459.
9. Conney AH, Gilman AG. Puromycin inhibition of enzyme induction by 3-methylcholanthrene and phenobarbital. *J Biol Chem* 1963;238:3682–3685.
10. Ryan KJ, Engel LL. Hydroxylation of steroids at carbon 21. *J Biol Chem* 1957;225:103–114.
11. Conney AH, Brown RR, Miller JA, Miller EC. The metabolism of methylated aminoazo dyes. VI. Intracellular distribution and properties of the demethylase system. *Cancer Res* 1957;17:628–633.

12. Garfinkel D. Studies on pig liver microsomes. I. Enzymic and pigment composition of different microsomal fractions. *Arch Biochem Biophys* 1958;77:493–509.

13. Klingenberg M. Pigments of rat liver microsomes. *Arch Biochem Biophys* 1958;75:376–386.

14. Omura T. History of cytochrome P-450. In: Omura T, Ishimura Y, Fujii-Kuriyama Y, eds. *Cytochrome P-450.* Tokyo: Kodansha, 1993: 1–15.

15. Omura T, Sato R. A new cytochrome in liver microsomes. *J Biol Chem* 1962;237:1375–1376.

16. Estabrook RW, Cooper DY, Rosenthal O. The light reversible carbon monoxide inhibition of the steroid C21-hydroxylase system of the adrenal cortex. *Biochem Z* 1963;338:741–755.

17. Cooper DY, Levin S, Narasimhulu S, Rosenthal O, Estabrook RW. Photochemical action spectrum of the terminal oxidase of mixed function oxidase systems. *Science* 1965;147:400–402.

18. Narasimhulu S, Cooper DY, Rosenthal O. Spectrophotometric properties of a triton-clarified steroid 21-hydroxylase system of adrenocortical microsomes. *Life Sci* 1965;4:2101–2107.

19. Remmer H, Schenkman J, Estabrook RW, et al. Drug interaction with hepatic microsomal cytochrome. *Mol Pharmacol* 1966;2:187–190.

20. Imai Y, Sato R. Substrate interaction with hydroxylase system in liver microsomes. *Biochem Biophys Res Commun* 1966;88:489–503.

21. Cammer W, Schenkman JB, Estabrook RW. EPR measurements of substrate interaction with cytochrome P-450. *Biochem Biophys Res Commun* 1966;23:264–268.

22. Whysner JA, Ramseyer J, Kazmi GM, Harding BW. Substrate induced spin state changes in cytochrome P-450. *Biochem Biophys Res Commun* 1969;36:795–801.

23. Schenkman JB, Sligar SG, Cinti DL. Substrate interaction with cytochrome P-450. *Pharmacol Ther* 1981;12:43–71.

24. Conney AH, Levin W, Ikeda M, Kuntzman R, Cooper DY, Rosenthal O. Inhibitory effect of carbon monoxide on the hydroxylation of testosterone by rat liver microsomes. *J Biol Chem* 1968;243: 3912–3915.

25. Remmer H. Die Beschleunigung der Evipanoxidation und der Demethylierung von Methylaminoantipyrin durch Barbiturate. *Naunyn-Schmiedeberg's Arch Exp Pathol Pharmak* 1959;237: 296–307.

26. Remmer H. Die Verstärkung der Abbaugeschwindigkeit von Evipan durch Glykocorticoide. *Naunyn-Schmiedeberg's Arch Exp Pathol Pharmak* 1958;233;181–191.

27. Imai Y, Sato R. Evidence for two forms of P450 hemoprotein in microsomal membranes. *Biochem Biophys Res Commun* 1966;23: 5–11.

28. Sladek NE, Mannering GJ. Evidence for a new P-450 hemoprotein in hepatic microsomes from methylcholanthrene treated rats. *Biochem Biophys Res Commun* 1966;24:668–674.

29. Wada F, Shimakawa H, Takasugi M, Kotake T, Sakamoto Y. Effect of steroid hormones on drug-metabolizing enzyme systems in liver microsomes. *J Biochem* 1968;64:109–113.

30. Pederson TC, Aust SD. Aminopyrine demethylase. Kinetic evidence for multiple microsomal activities. *Biochem Pharmacol* 1970;19: 2221–2230.

31. Rubin A, Tephley TR, Mannering GJ. Kinetics of drug metabolism by hepatic microsomes. *Biochem Pharmacol* 1964;13:1007–1016.

32. Ullrich V, Weber P. The O-dealkylation of 7-ethoxycoumarin by liver microsomes. A direct fluorometric test. Hoppe-Seyler's *Z Physiol Chem* 1972;353:1171–1177.

33. Orrenius S, Ernster L. Phenobarbital-induced synthesis of the oxidative demethylating enzymes of rat liver microsomes. *Biochem Biophys Res Commun* 1964;16:60–65.

34. Remmer H, Estabrook RW, Schenkman J, Greim H. Reaction of drugs with microsomal liver hydroxylase: its influence on drug action. *Naunyn-Schmiedeberg's Arch Exp Pathol Pharmak* 1968;259:98–116.

35. Alvares AP, Schilling G, Levin W, Kuntzman R. Studies on the induction of co-binding pigments in liver microsomes by phenobarbital and 3-methylcholanthrene. *Biochem Biophys Res Commun* 1967;29: 521–526.

36. Sladek NE, Mannering GJ. Induction of drug metabolism II. Qualitative differences in the microsomal N-demethylating systems stimulated by polycyclic hydrocarbons and by phenobarbital. *Mol Pharmacol* 1969;5:186–195.

37. Bidelman K, Mannering GJ. Induction of drug metabolism. V. Independent formation of cytochrome P-450 and P1-450 in rats treated with phenobarbital and 3-methylcholanthrene simultaneously. *Mol Pharmacol* 1970;6:697–701.

38. Nebert DW. Microsomal cytochromes b5 and P450 during induction of aryl hydrocarbon hydroxylase activity in mammalian cell culture. *J Biol Chem* 1970;245:519–527.

39. Nebert DW, Gelboin HV. Substrate-inducible microsomal aryl hydroxylase in mammalian cell culture II. Cellular responses during enzyme induction. *J Biol Chem* 1968;243:6250–6261.

40. Orrenius S, Ericsson JLE, Ernster L. Phenobarbital-induced synthesis of the microsomal drug-metabolizing enzyme system and its relationship to the proliferation of endoplasmic membranes. *J Cell Biol* 1965;25:627–639.

41. Adesnik M, Bar-Nun S, Maschio F, Zunich M, Lippman A, Bard E. Mechanism of induction of cytochrome P-450 by phenobarbital. *J Biol Chem* 1981;256:10340–10345.

42. Lu AYH, Kuntzman R, West S, Conney AH. Reconstituted liver microsomal enzyme system that hydroxylates drugs, other foreign compounds and endogenous substrates. I. Determination of substrate specificity by the cytochrome P-450 and P-448 fractions. *Biochem Biophys Res Commun* 1971;42:1200–1206.

43. Lu AYH, Somogyi A, West S, Kuntzman R, Conney AH. Pregnenolone-16α-carbonitrile: a new type of inducer of drug-metabolizing enzymes. *Arch Biochem Biophys* 1972;152:457–462.

44. Powis G, Talcott RE, Schenkman JB. Kinetic and spectral evidence for multiple species of cytochrome P-450 in liver microsomes. In: Ullrich V, Roots I, Hildebrandt A, Estabrook R, Conney A, eds. *Microsomes and drug oxidation.* Oxford: Pergamon Press, 1977:127–135.

45. Alvares AP, Siekevitz P. Gel electrophoresis of partially purified cytochrome P-450 from liver microsomes of variously-treated rats. *Biochem Biophys Res Commun* 1973;54:923–929.

46. Welton AF, Aust SD. Multiplicity of cytochrome P450 hemoproteins in rat liver microsomes. *Biochem Biophys Res Commun* 1974;56: 898–906.

47. Van der Hoeven TT, Coon MJ. Preparation and properties of partially purified cytochrome P-450 and reduced nicotinamide adenine nucleotide phosphate-cytochrome P-450 reductase from rabbit liver microsomes. *J Biol Chem* 1974;249:6302–6310.

48. Haugen DA, van der Hoeven TA, Coon MJ. Purified liver microsomal cytochrome P450. *J Biol Chem* 1975;250:3567–3570.

49. Waxman DJ, Ko A, Walsh C. Regioselectivity and stereoselectivity of androgen hydroxylations catalyzed by cytochrome P-450 isozymes purified from phenobarbital induced rat liver. *J Biol Chem* 1983;258: 11937–11947.

50. Cheng K-C, Schenkman JB. Testosterone metabolism by cytochrome P-450 isozymes RLM3 and RLM5 and by microsomes. Metabolite identification. *J Biol Chem* 1983;258:11738–11744.

51. Waxman DJ. Interactions of hepatic cytochromes P-450 with steroid hormones. Regioselectivity and stereospecificity of steroid metabolism and hormonal regulation of rat P-450 enzyme expression. *Biochem Pharmacol* 1988;37:71–84.

52. Kaminsky LS, Kennedy MW, Adams SM, Guengerich FP. Metabolism of dichlorobiphenols by highly purified isozymes of rat liver cytochrome P-450. *Biochemistry* 1981;20:7379–7384.

53. Fasco MJ, Vatsis KP, Kaminsky LS, Coon MJ. Regioselective and stereoselective hydroxylation of R and S warfarin by different forms of purified cytochrome P-450 from rabbit liver. *J Biol Chem* 1978; 253:7813–7820.

54. Kaminsky LS, Dunbar DA, Wang PP, et al. Human hepatic cytochrome P-450 composition as probed by in vitro microsomal metabolism of warfarin. *Drug Metab Dispos* 1984;12:470–477.

55. Waxman DJ, Lapenson DP, Aoyama T, Gelboin HV, Gonzalez FJ, Korzekwa K. Steroid hormone hydroxylase specificities of eleven cDNA-expressed human cytochrome-P450s. *Arch Biochem Biophys* 1991;290:160–166.

56. Larrey D, Distlerath LM, Dannan GA, Wilkinson GR, Guengerich FP. Purification and characterization of the rat liver microsomal cytochrome P-450 involved in the 4-hydroxylation of debrisoquine, a prototype for genetic variation in oxidative drug metabolism. *Biochemistry* 1984;23:2787–2795.

57. Distlerath LM, Larrey D, Guengerich FP. Genetic polymorphism of debrisoquine 4-hydroxylation: identification of the defect at the level of a specific cytochrome P-450 in a rat model. In: Omenn G, Gelboin H, eds. *Banbury Report 16: Genetic variability in responses to chem-*

ical exposure. New York: Cold Spring Harbor Laboratory, 1984: 85–95.

58. Lu AYH, Coon MJ. Role of hemoprotein P-450 in fatty acid ω-hydroxylation in a soluble enzyme system from liver microsomes. *J Biol Chem* 1968;243:1331–1332.

59. Strittmatter P, Velick SF. The isolation and properties of microsomal cytochrome. *J Biol Chem* 1956;221:253–264.

60. Strittmatter P, Velick SF. A microsomal cytochrome reductase specific for diphosphopyridine nucleotide. *J Biol Chem* 1956;221:277–286.

61. Phillips AH, Langdon RG. Hepatic triphosphopyridine nucleotide-cytochrome c reductase: isolation, characterization, and kinetic studies. *J Biol Chem* 1962;237:2652–2660.

62. Nishibayashi H, Sato R. Preparation of hepatic microsomal particles containing P-450 as sole heme constituent and absolute spectra of P-450. *J Biochem* 1968;63:766–779.

63. Silverman DA, Talalay P. Studies on the enzymic hydroxlation of 3,4-benzpyrene. *Mol Pharmacol* 1967;3:90–101.

64. Ichikawa Y, Yamano T. Reconversion of detergent- and sulfhydryl reagent-produced P-420 to P-450 by polyols and glutathione. *Biochim Biophys Acta* 1967;131:490–497.

65. Miyake Y, Gaylor JL, Mason HS. Properties of a submicrosomal particle containing P-450 and flavoprotein. *J Biol Chem* 1968;243:5788–5797.

66. Lu AYH, Junk KW, Coon MJ. Resolution of the cytochrome P-450-containing ω-hydroxylation system of liver microsomes into three components. *J Biol Chem* 1969;244:3714–3721.

67. Sato R, Satake H, Imai Y. Partial purification and some spectral properties of hepatic microsomal cytochrome P450. *Drug Metab Dispos* 1973;1:6–12.

68. Guengerich FP. Separation and purification of multiple forms of microsomal cytochrome P450. *J Biol Chem* 1978;253:7931–7939.

69. Botelho LH, Ryan DE, Levin W. Amino acid compositions and partial amino acid sequences of three highly purified forms of liver microsomal cytochrome P-450 from rats treated with polychlorinated biphenyls, phenobarbital, or 3-methylcholanthrene. *J Biol Chem* 1979;254:5635–5640.

70. Imai Y, Hashimoto-Yutsudo C, Satake H, Girardin A, Sati R. Multiple forms of cytochrome P-450 purified from liver microsomes of phenobarbital and 3-methylcholanthrene pretreated rabbits. *J Biochem* 1980;88:489–503.

71. Koop DR, Coon MJ. Purification and properties of P-450 LM3b, a constitutive form of cytochrome P450 from rabbit liver microsomes. *Biochem Biophys Res Commun* 1979;91:1075–1081.

72. Agosin M, Morello A, White R, Repetto Y, Pedemonte J. Multiple forms of noninduced rat liver cytochrome P450: metabolism of 1-[4′-ethylphenoxy)-3,7-dimethyl-6,7-epoxy-trans-2-octene by reconstituted preparations. *J Biol Chem* 1979;254:9915–9920.

73. Cheng K-C, Schenkman JB. Purification and characterization of two constitutive forms of rat liver microsomal cytochrome P-450. *J Biol Chem* 1982;257:2378–2385.

74. Lu AYH, West SB. Multiplicity of mammalian microsomal cytochromes P-450. *Pharmacol Rev* 1980;31:277–295.

75. Schenkman JB, Favreau LV, Mole J, Kreutzer DL, Jansson I. Fingerprinting rat liver microsomal cytochromes P-450 as a means of delineating sexually distinctive forms. *Arch Toxicol* 1987;60:43–51.

76. Soucek P, Gut I. Cytochromes P-450 in rats: structures, functions, properties and relevant human forms. *Xenobiotica* 1992;22:83–103.

77. Coon MJ, Blake RC II, Oprian DD, Ballou DP. Mechanistic studies with purified components of the liver microsomal hydroxylation system: spectral intermediates in reaction of cytochrome P-450 with peroxy compounds. *Acta Biol Med Germ* 1979;38:449–458.

78. Guengerich FP, Dannan GA, Wright ST, Martin MV, Kaminsky LS. Purification and characterization of liver microsomal cytochromes P-450: electrophoretic, spectral, catalytic, and immunochemical properties and inducibility of eight isozymes isolated from rats treated with phenobarbital or β-naphthoflavone. *Biochemistry* 1982;21:6019–6030.

79. Johnson EF, Schwab GE. Constitutive forms of rabbit-liver microsomal cytochrome P-450: enzymatic diversity, polymorphism and allosteric regulation. *Xenobiotica* 1984;14:3–18.

80. Tamburini PP, Masson HA, Bains SK, Makowski RJ, Morris B, Gibson GG. Multiple forms of hepatic cytochrome P-450. Purification, characterisation and comparison of a novel clofibrate-induced isozyme with other major forms of cytochrome P-450. *Eur J Biochem* 1984;139:235–246.

81. Waxman DJ, Walsh C. Cytochrome P-450 isozyme 1 from phenobarbital-induced rat liver: purification characterization, and interactions with metyrapone and cytochrome b5. *Biochemistry* 1983;22:4846–4855.

82. Waxman DJ. Rat hepatic cytochrome P-450 isoenzyme 2c. Identification as a male-specific, developmentally induced steroid 16α-hydroxylase and comparison to a female-specific cytochrome P-450 isoenzyme. *J Biol Chem* 1984;259:15481–15490.

83. Jansson I, Mole J, Schenkman JB. Purification and characterization of a new form (RLM2) of liver microsomal cytochrome P-450 from untreated rat. *J Biol Chem* 1985;260:7084–7093.

84. Kamataki T, Maeda K, Yamazoe Y, Nagai T, Kato R. Sex difference of cytochrome P-450 in the rat: purification, characterization, and quantitation of constitutive forms of cytochrome P-450 from liver microsomes of male and female rats. *Arch Biochem Biophys* 1983;225:758–770.

85. Thomas PE, Bandiera S, Reik LM, Maines SL, Ryan DE, Levin W. Polyclonal and monoclonal antibodies as probes of rat hepatic cytochrome P-450 isozymes. *Fed Proc* 1987;46:2563–2566.

86. Orrenius S, Ellin Å, Jakobsson SV, et al. The cytochrome P-450-containing mono-oxygenase system of rat liver kidney cortex microsomes. *Drug Metab Dispos* 1973;1:350–356.

87. Backes WL, Jansson I, Mole JE, Gibson GG, Schenkman JB. Isolation and comparison of four cytochrome P-450 enzymes from phenobarbital-induced rat liver: three forms possessing identical NH2-terminal sequences. *Pharmacology* 1985;31:155–169.

88. Tarr GE, Black SD, Fujita VS, Coon MJ. Complete amino acid sequence and predicted membrane topology of phenobarbital-induced cytochrome P-450 (isozyme 2) from rabbit liver microsomes. *Proc Natl Acad Sci USA* 1983;80:6552–6556.

89. Ozols J, Heinemann FS, Johnson EF. The complete amino acid sequence of a constitutive form of liver microsomal cytochrome P-450. *J Biol Chem* 1985;260:5427–5434.

90. Gasser R, Negishi M, Philpot RM. Primary structures of multiple forms of cytochrome P-450 isozyme 2 derived from rabbit pulmonary and hepatic cDNAS. *Mol Pharmacol* 1988;32:22–30.

91. Ryan R, Grimm SW, Kedzie KM, Halpert JR, Philpot RM. Cloning, sequencing, and functional studies of phenobarbital-inducible forms of cytochrome P450 2B and 4B expressed in rabbit kidney. *Arch Biochem Biophys* 1993;304:454–463.

92. Jansson I, Mole JE, Schenkman JB. The isolation and comparison of multiple forms of CYP2B from untreated and phenobarbital-treated rabbit liver microsomes. *Arch Biochem Biophys* 1995;316:275–284.

93. Fujii-Kuriyama Y, Taniguchi T, Mizukami Y, Sakai M, Tashiro Y, Muramatsu M. Molecular cloning of a complementary DNA of phenobarbital-inducible cytochrome P-450 messenger RNA from the rat. *Proc Japan Acad* 1980;56:603–608.

94. Fujii-Kuriyama Y, Mizukami Y, Kawajiri K, Sogawa K, Muramatsu M. Primary structure of a cytochrome P-450: coding nucleotide sequence of phenobarbital-inducible cytochrome P-450 cDNA from rat liver. *Proc Natl Acad Sci U S A* 1982;79:2793–2797.

95. Hardwick JP, Gonzalez FJ, Kasper CB. Cloning of DNA complementary to cytochrome P-450 induced by pregnenolone-16α-carbonitrile. *J Biol Chem* 1983;258:10182–10186.

96. Kawajiri K, Gotoh O, Sogawa K, Tagashira Y, Muramatsu M, Fujii-Kuriyama Y. Coding nucleotide sequence of 3-methylcholanthrene-inducible cytochrome P-450d cDNA from rat liver. *Proc Natl Acad Sci USA* 1984;81:1649–1653.

97. Leighton JK, Kemper B. Differential induction and tissue-specific expression of closely related members of the phenobarbital-inducible rabbit cytochrome P-450 gene family. *J Biol Chem* 1984;259:11165–11168.

98. Yabusaki Y, Shimizu M, Murakami H, Nakamura K, Oeda K, Ohkawa H. Nucleotide sequence of a full-length cDNA coding for 3-methylcholanthrene-induced rat liver cytochrome P-450MC. *Nucl Acids Res* 1984;12:2929–2938.

99. Nebert DW, Adesnik M, Coon MJ, et al. The P450 gene superfamily: recommended nomenclature. *DNA* 1987;6:1–11.

100. Nebert DW, Nelson DR, Adesnik M, et al. The P450 superfamily: updated listing of all genes and recommended nomenclature for the chromosomal loci. *DNA* 1989;8:1–13.

101. Nelson DR, Kamataki T, Waxman DJ, et al. The P450 superfamily—update on new sequences, gene mapping, accession numbers, early trivial names of enzymes, and nomenclature. *DNA Cell Biol* 1993;12:1–51.

102. Nelson DR, Koymans L, Kamataki T, et al. P450 superfamily: update on new sequences, gene mapping, accession numbers and nomenclature. *Pharmacogenetics* 1996;6:1–42.

103. Song B-J, Gelboin HV, Park S-S, Yang CS, Gonzalez FJ. Complementary DNA and protein sequences of ethanol-inducible rat and human cytochrome P-450s. *J Biol Chem* 1986;261:16689–16697.

104. Crespi CL, Langenbach R, Kudo K, Chen YT, Davies RL. Transfection of a human cytochrome P-450 gene into the human lymphoblastoid cell line, AHH-1, and use of the recombinant cell line in gene mutation assays. *Carcinogenesis* 1989;10:295–301.

105. Umeno M, McBride OW, Yang CS, Gelboin HV, Gonzalez FJ. Human ethanol-inducible P450IIE1: complete gene sequence, promoter characterization, chromosome mapping, and cDNA-directed expression. *Biochemistry* 1988;27:9006–9013.

106. Fuhr U, Doehmer J, Battula N, et al. Biotransformation of caffeine and theophylline in mammalian cell lines genetically engineered for expression of single cytochrome P450 isoforms. *Biochem Pharmacol* 1992;43:225–235.

107. Fuhr U, Woodcock BG, Siewert M. Verapamil and drug metabolism by the cytochrome-P450 isoform CYP1A2. *Eur J Clin Pharmacol* 1992;42:463–464.

108. Distlerath LM, Reilly PEB, Martin MV, Davis GG, Wilkinson GR, Guengerich FP. Purification and characterization of the human liver cytochromes P-450 involved in debrisoquine 4-hydroxylation and phenacetin O-deethylation, two prototypes for genetic polymorphism in oxidative drug metabolism. *J Biol Chem* 1985;260:9057–9067.

109. Sesardic D, Edwards RJ, Davies DS, Thomas PE, Levin W, Boobis AR. High affinity phenacetin O-deethylase is catalysed specifically by cytochrome P450d (P450IA2) in the liver of the rat. *Biochem Pharmacol* 1990;39:489–498.

110. Thomas PE, Reik LM, Ryan DE, Levin W. Induction of two immunochemically related rat liver cytochrome P-450 isozymes, cytochromes P-450c and P-450d, by structurally diverse xenobiotics. *J Biol Chem* 1983;258:4590–4598.

111. Goldstein JA, Linko P. Differential induction of two 2,3,7,8-tetrachlorodibenzo-p-dioxin-inducible forms of cytochrome P-450 in extrahepatic versus hepatic tissues. *Mol Pharmacol* 1984;25:185–191.

112. Gonzalez FJ, Tukey RH, Nebert DW. Structuralgene products of the Ah locus. Transcriptional regulation of cytochrome P1-450 and P3-450 mRNA levels by 3-methylcholanthrene. *Mol Pharmacol* 1984;26:117–121.

113. Soucek P, Gut I. Cytochromes P-450 in rats: structures, functions, properties and relevant human forms—review. *Xenobiotica* 1992;22:83–103.

114. Funae Y, Imaoka S. Cytochrome P450 in rodents. In: Schenkman J, Greim H, eds. *Cytochrome P450.* Berlin: Springer-Verlag, 1993:221–238.

115. Dixon RL, Hart LG, Fouts JR. The metabolism of drugs by liver microsomes from alloxan-diabetic rats. *J Pharmacol Exp Ther* 1961;133:7–11.

116. Kato R, Gillette JR. Sex differences in the effects of abnormal physiological states on the metabolism of drugs by rat liver microsomes. *J Pharmacol Exp Ther* 1965;150:285–291.

117. Kato R, Takanaka A, Onoda K. Effect of adrenalectomy or alloxan diabetes on the substrate interaction with cytochrome P-450 in the oxidation of drugs by liver microsomes. *Biochem Pharmacol* 1971;20:447–458.

118. Past MR, Cook DE. Effect of diabetes on rat liver cytochrome P-450. *Biochem Pharmacol* 1982;31:3329–3334.

119. Favreau LV, Malchoff DM, Mole JE, Schenkman JB. Responses to insulin by two forms of rat hepatic microsomal cytochrome P-450 that undergo major (RLM6) and minor (RLM5b) elevations in diabetes. *J Biol Chem* 1987;262:14319–14326.

120. Favreau LV, Schenkman JB. Composition changes in hepatic microsomal cytochrome P-450 during onset of streptozocin-induced diabetes and during insulin treatment. *Diabetes* 1988;37:577–584.

121. Imaoka S, Terano Y, Funae Y. Changes in the amount of cytochrome P450s in rat hepatic microsomes with starvation. *Arch Biochem Biophys* 1990;278:168–178.

122. Song BJ, Veech RL, Saenger P. Cytochrome P450IIE1 is elevated in lymphocytes from poorly controlled insulin-dependent diabetics. *J Clin Endocrinol* 1990;71:1036–1040.

123. Thummel KE, Schenkman JB. Effects of testosterone and growth hormone treatment on hepatic microsomal P450 expression in the diabetic rat. *Mol Pharmacol* 1990;37:119–129.

124. Schenkman JB, Thummel KE, Favreau LV. Physiological and pathophysiological alterations in rat hepatic cytochrome P450. *Drug Metab Rev* 1989;20:557–584.

125. Kato R, Yamazoe Y. Sex-specific cytochrome P450 as a cause of sex-related and species-related differences in drug toxicity. *Toxicol Lett* 1992;6(5):661–667.

126. Warner M, Gustafsson J-Å. Extrahepatic microsomal forms: brain cytochrome P450. In: Schenkman J, Greim H, eds. *Cytochrome P450.* Berlin: Springer-Verlag, 1993:387–397.

127. Strobel HW, Stralka DJ, Hammond DK, White T. Extrahepatic microsomal forms: gastrointestinal cytochromes P450, assessment and evaluation. In: Schenkman J, Greim H, eds. *Cytochrome P450.* Berlin: Springer-Verlag, 1993:363–371.

128. Ding X, Coon MJ. Extrahepatic microsomal forms: olfactory cytochrome P450. In: Schenkman J, Greim H, eds. *Cytochrome P450.* Berlin: Springer-Verlag, 1993:351–361.

129. Arinç E. Extrahepatic microsomal forms: lung microsomal cytochrome P450 isozymes. In: Schenkman J, Greim H, eds. *Cytochrome P450.* Berlin: Springer-Verlag, 1993:373–386.

130. Schenkman JB, Gurtoo HL, Dondero T, Johns DG. Cytochrome P-450 of human liver microsomes. *J Clin Invest* 1969;48:483.

131. Alvarez AP, Schilling G, Levin W, Kuntzman R, Brand L, Mark CL. Cytochromes P-450 and b5 in human liver microsomes. *Clin Pharmacol Ther* 1969;10:655–659.

132. Darby FJ, Newnes W, Price-Evans DA. Human liver microsomal drug metabolism. *Biochem Pharmacol* 1970;19:1514–1517.

133. Kaschnitz RM, Coon MJ. Drug and fatty acid hydroxylation by solubilized human liver microsomal cytochrome P-450: phospholipid requirement. *Biochem Pharmacol* 1975;24:295–297.

134. Kitada M, Kamataki T, Itahashi K, Rikihisa T, Kato R, Kanakubo Y. Immunochemical examinations of cytochrome P-450 in various tissues of human fetuses using antibodies to human fetal cytochrome P-450, P450HFLa. *Biochem Biophys Res Commun* 1985;131:1154–1159.

135. Wang P, Mason PS, Guengerich FP. Purification of human liver cytochrome P450 and comparison to the enzyme isolated from rat liver. *Arch Biochem Biophys* 1980;199:206–219.

136. Beaune P, Dansette P, Flinois JP, Columelli S, Mansuy D, Leroux JP. Partial purification of human liver cytochrome P450. *Biochem Biophys Res Commun* 1979;88:826–832.

137. Wang PP, Beaune P, Kaminsky LS, et al. Purification and characterization of six cytochrome P-450 isozymes from human liver microsomes. *Biochemistry* 1983;22:5376–5383.

138. Beaune PH, Umbenhauer DR, Bork RW, Lloyd RS, Guengerich FP. Isolation and sequence determination of a cDNA clone related to human cytochrome P-450 nifedipine oxidase. *Proc Natl Acad Sci USA* 1986;83:8064–8068.

139. Brian WR, Srivastava PK, Umbenhauer DR, Lloyd RS, Guengerich FP. Expression of a human liver cytochrome P450 protein with tolbutamide hydroxylase activity in *Saccharomyces cerevisiae*. *Biochemistry* 1989;28:4993–4999.

140. Brian WR, Sari M-A, Iwasaki M, Shimada T, Kaminsky LS, Guengerich FP. Catalytic activities of human liver cytochrome P-450 IIIA4 expressed in *Saccharomyces cerevisiae*. *Biochemistry* 1990;29:11280–11292.

141. Gonzalez FJ, Crespi CL, Czerwinski M, Gelboin HV. Analysis of human cytochrome-P450 catalytic activities and expression. *Tohoku J Exp Med* 1992;168:67–72.

142. Gonzalez FJ, Gelboin HV. Human cytochromes P450: evolution, catalytic activities and interindividual variations in expression. In: Gledhill B, Mauro F, eds. *New horizons in biological dosimetry.* New York: Wiley-Liss, 1991;11–20.

143. Goldstein JA, Demorais SMF. Biochemistry and molecular biology of the human CYP2C subfamily. *Pharmacogenetics* 1994;4:285–299.

144. Kawano S, Kamataki T, Yasumori T, Yamazoe Y, Kato R. Purification of human liver cytochrome P-450 catalyzing testosterone 6β-hydroxylation. *J Biochem* 1987;102:493–501.

145. Mahgoub A, Dring LG, Idle JTR, Lancaster R, Smith RL. Polymorphic hydroxylation of debrisoquine in man. *Lancet* 1977;2:584–586.

146. Scott J, Poffenbarger PL. Pharmacogenetics of tolbutamide metabolism in humans. *Diabetes* 1979;28:41–51.

147. Wedlund PJ, Aslanian WS, McAllister CB, Wilkenson GR, Branch RA. Mephenytoin hydroxylation deficiency in caucasians: frequency of a new oxidative drug polymorphism. *Clin Pharmacol Ther* 1984;36:773–780.

148. Meier UT, Meyer UA. Genetic polymorphism of human cytochrome

P-450 (S)-mephenytoin 4-hydroxylase: studies with human autoanti-bodies suggest a functionally altered cytochrome P-450 isozyme as cause of the genetic deficiency. *Biochemistry* 1987;26:8466–8474.

149. Kato S, Shields PG, Caporaso NE, et al. Cytochrome-P450IIE1 genetic polymorphisms, racial variation, and lung cancer risk. *Cancer Res* 1992;52:6712–6715.

150. Gonzalez FJ, Matsunaga T, Nagata K, et al. Debrisoquine 4-hydroxy-lase: characterization of a new gene P450 gene subfamily, regulation, chromosome mapping, and molecular analysis of the DA rat poly-morphism. *DNA* 1987;6:149–161.

151. Srivastava PK, Yun C-H, Beaune PH, Ged C, Guengerich FP. Separa-tion of human liver microsomal tolbutamide hydroxylase and (S)-mephenytoin 4'-hydroxylase cytochrome P-450 enzymes. *Mol Phar-macol* 1991;40:69–79.

CHAPTER 6

CYP1A

John O. Miners and Ross A. McKinnon

INTRODUCTION

In humans, and indeed other mammalian species, the CYP1A subfamily comprises just two members, CYP1A1 and CYP1A2. The *CYP1A* genes each contain seven exons and have been localized to human chromosome 15 (15q22-qter) (1). Unlike other *CYP* genes, the first exon is noncoding. Human CYP1A1 and CYP1A2 share 68% amino acid sequence identity. Overall, there is marked sequence conservation among mammalian *CYP1A* genes, especially in exons 2, 4, 5, and 6, which has been postulated to be an evolutionary response to dietary and general environmental factors in higher species (1). CYP1A may also be essential for the development of key physiological functions because neonatal lethality has been reported in mice homozygous for a targeted mutation in the *CYP1A2* gene (2).

Considerable attention has focused on CYP1A, given the capacity of these enzymes to activate a range of procarcinogenic xenobiotics to mutagenic species. For example, CYP1A1 is able to activate polycyclic aromatic hydrocarbons such as benzo(a)pyrene, whereas CYP1A2 has been implicated in the activation of aflatoxin B1, 2-acetylaminofluorene, and a number of arylamines and food-derived aminoimidazoazarenes (3,4). This has stimulated considerable interest in possible relationships between CYP1A activity and chemical carcinogenesis. There is also increasing awareness of the importance of CYP1A2 in human hepatic drug metabolism. CYP1A2 contributes to the biotransformation of caffeine, clomipramine, clozapine, cyclobenzaprine, flutamide, imipramine, lisofylline, mianserin, olanzapine, ropinirole, tacrine, theophylline, and (R)-warfarin.

Despite their evolutionary relatedness, CYP1A1 and CYP1A2 display markedly different expression patterns. Whereas CYP1A2 is constitutively expressed in mammalian liver, constitutive CYP1A1 expression appears to be low and largely extrahepatic. Low-level CYP1A1 expression has been demonstrated in human liver at both the messenger RNA (mRNA) and protein levels, but this is unlikely to be significant in the hepatic metabolism of therapeutic agents (5,6). Similar to many drug-metabolizing P450s, both CYP1A1 and CYP1A2 display inducibility by xenobiotics. Although a diverse collection of xenobiotics have been identified as inducers of CYP1A, the prototypic inducers are the polycyclic aromatic hydrocarbons. The induction of CYP1A1 by these chemicals appears to be tissue independent, whereas CYP1A2 induction is primarily limited to liver.

CYP1A REGULATION

CYP1A Induction

CYP1A1 and *CYP1A2* were among the earliest P450 genes identified as responsive to xenobiotic exposure, and the molecular basis of this induction has subsequently been the focus of much attention. There is now compelling evidence that CYP1A1 induction is mediated solely by a ligand-activated transcription factor receptor termed the *a*ryl *h*ydrocarbon (Ah) receptor (AhR). Although always mediated by the AhR, the precise mechanism of CYP1A1 upregulation may vary according to the nature of the inducer. CYP1A2 induction also is generally AhR mediated, but recent evidence also suggests the existence of AhR-independent pathways.

CYP1A1 induction was originally demonstrated by using carcinogenic polycyclic aromatic hydrocarbons such as 3-methylcholanthrene (3-MC). Subsequently, halogenated aromatic hydrocarbons, including 2,3,7,8-

J. O. Miners: Department of Clinical Pharmacology, Flinders University School of Medicine and Flinders Medical Centre, Bedford Park, South Australia 5042, Australia

R. A. McKinnon: School of Pharmacy and Medical Sciences, University of South Australia, North Terrace, Adelaide, South Australia 5000, Australia

tetrachlorodibenzo-*p*-dioxin (abbreviated dioxin or TCDD), were shown to produce a more potent and sustained response, and TCDD is now considered the prototypic CYP1A inducer. In addition to polycyclic aromatic hydrocarbons, which are presumably involved in CYP1A induction in cigarette smokers and consumers of charcoal-broiled beef, a diverse array of compounds and factors have been identified as possible CYP1A inducers *in vitro* and/or *in vivo*, and these are listed in Table 6-1. The extent of induction of CYP1A activity *in vivo* by certain of these factors may be substantial. Although variable induction of CYP1A2 by cigarette smoking has been reported, metabolic clearances of substrates for this enzyme can be almost two-fold higher in smokers compared with nonsmokers (7,8). Similarly, therapeutic doses of rifampicin may almost double the plasma clearances of drugs metabolized by CYP1A2 *in vivo* (9).

CYP1A induction reported after exposure to substituted benzimidazoles, especially omeprazole, has generated considerable interest, given the widespread clinical use of these drugs and the substrate profile of human CYP1A2. Omeprazole-mediated induction of both CYP1A1 and CYP1A2 was initially observed in primary cultures of human hepatocytes from patients with hepatocellular carcinoma and also in liver biopsies from patients administered therapeutic doses of omeprazole (10). However, subsequent investigations have provided conflicting results concerning the extent and importance of this phenomenon. In particular, studies using methylxanthines as markers of CYP1A2 activity *in vivo* reported little or no induction, even in subjects deficient in CYP2C19 (the main enzyme involved in omeprazole metabolism: for example, ref. 11). It appears that the disparity between studies may be explained largely by dosage differences, especially considering the observation that omeprazole induction of human CYP1A2 is dose dependent (10,12). It would seem that very high doses of omeprazole may be capable of inducing CYP1A expression, but induction of CYP1A would appear to be of little significance with usual therapeutic regimens.

Mechanisms of CYP1A Induction

Ah Receptor (AhR)-mediated Induction

The induction of CYP1A enzymes is predominantly transcriptional, although posttranscriptional effects have been reported for CYP1A2 (13,14). As noted previously, transcriptional induction of CYP1A expression is mediated by xenobiotic binding to the Ah or dioxin receptor. The AhR is a unique transcription factor, belonging to a subfamily of basic helix–loop–helix proteins termed basic helix–loop–helix/PAS (bHLH/PAS). This subfamily derives its name from the presence within the protein of the PAS A and B domains, two regions of homology with Per (a circadian rhythm factor from *Drosophila*), Arnt (the AhR nuclear translocator protein), and Sim (a neurogenic factor from *Drosophila*). The Arnt protein is critical to the function of the AhR as a transcription factor (see later). Typical of most transcription factors, the AhR and Arnt are modular in nature with multiple functional domains. Ligand binding by AhR has been localized to the vicinity of the PAS B domain, whereas the HLH domains of both proteins form an interface for their dimerization. Dimerization of Arnt and liganded AhR is essential for binding to DNA. Both the AhR and Arnt interact with DNA via their basic amino terminus regions. Trans-activating domains have been localized to the C-terminus of both proteins. In the case of CYP1A1, it appears that the trans-activating domain of the AhR plays a pivotal role in induction, whereas the role of the Arnt trans-activation domain seems less important (15,16).

The molecular events after xenobiotic binding to the AhR have been the focus of extensive investigation (reviewed in refs. 17 and 18), and recently a consensus working model has emerged (reviewed in ref. 19) (Fig. 6-1). According to this model, the latent AhR resides in the cytoplasm of the cell in a complex with the molecular chaperone, heat-shock protein 90 (hsp90). Hsp90 is believed to mask a nuclear localization signal within the receptor. Ligand binding presumably alters the conforma-

TABLE 6-1. *Factors implicated in the induction of mammalian CYP1A1 and/or CYP1A2 activity*

Altitude	β-Naphthoflavone
Bilirubin	Omeprazole
Caffeine	Pan-fried meat (high levels of heterocyclic amines)
Charcoal-broiled beef	Polybrominated biphenyls
(high polycyclic aromatic hydrocarbon content)	Polychlorinated biphenyls
Cigarette smoke (source of polycyclic	2,3,7,8-Tetrachlorodibenzo-*p*-dioxin
aromatic hydrocarbons and other chemicals)	Rifampicin
Cruciferous vegetables	
Heavy exercise	
3-Methylcholanthrene (and other polycyclic aromatic hydrocarbons)	

Adapted with permission from Eaton DL, Gallagher EP, Bammler TK, Kunze KL. Role of cytochrome P4501A2 in chemical carcinogenesis: implications for human variability in expression and enzyme activity. *Pharmacogenetics* 1995;5:259–274.

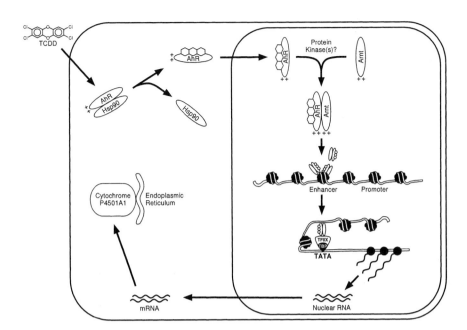

FIG. 6-1. Model for CYP1A1 induction. Reproduced with permission from Whitlock JP, Okino ST, Dong L, et al. Induction of cytochrome P4501A1: a model for analyzing mammalian gene transcription. *FASEB J* 1996;10: 809–817.

tion of the receptor, exposing a nuclear localization signal, with the resultant translocation of the receptor to the nucleus. Once located in the nucleus, the AhR dimerizes with its partner protein Arnt, probably after phosphorylation. The liganded dimer then binds to specific DNA target sequences variously designated "Ah-responsive elements" (AhREs), "xenobiotic-responsive elements" (XREs), or "dioxin-responsive elements" (DREs). Transfection experiments indicate that these sequences function as classic enhancers. AhREs are found in the upstream region of several genes known to be Ah responsive or polycyclic aromatic hydrocarbon inducible. This includes *CYP1A1* and *CYP1A2*, along with several genes that encode drug-metabolizing conjugating enzymes (e.g., *UGT1A6*). These coordinately regulated genes are frequently termed the Ah gene battery (reviewed in ref. 20).

The *CYP1A1* gene features six AhRE sequences, which lie approximately 1 kb upstream of the transcription start site. Although binding of the AhR/Arnt dimer to AhRE sequences in the *CYP1A1* gene is clearly responsible for elevated transcription levels, the precise mechanism still remains unclear. In addition to the AhRE enhancers, there are several other control elements, including a region that lies immediately upstream of the transcription start site. This element appears to act as a transcriptional promoter and also seems to be AhR and Arnt dependent, although no AhRE site is found within its sequence (21). Receptor complex binding to upstream AhREs probably facilitates the recruitment of several transcription factors (e.g., TATA-box binding protein) to the promoter (22,23). Thus a putative role for the AhR/ARNT heterodimer is to disrupt the chromatin structure of the *CYP1A1* promoter region, prob-

ably by transactivation, creating more favorable access for factors with direct roles in enhancing transcription. A further well-defined regulatory sequence of the *CYP1A1* gene is the negative regulatory element (NRE), located approximately 700 to 800 bases upstream of the transcriptional start site (24). A recent study has identified the Oct-1 transcription factor as a negative regulator of the rat *CYP1A1* gene through the NRE sequence (25).

Ligand-independent AhR-mediated Induction

In recent years it has become clear that many agents capable of inducing CYP1A enzymes, including omeprazole, have chemical structures that render them unlikely AhR ligands. Despite low receptor affinity, omeprazole is nevertheless able to induce the formation of a nuclear AhRE-binding complex in treated cell lines (26–28). Moreover, there is convincing evidence for Ah-dependent omeprazole CYP1A1 induction from studies using mutant forms of the human receptor to abrogate response (27). Collectively, these findings suggest ligand-independent activation of the AhR by omeprazole. Evidence for ligand independent Ah activation also is provided by experiments demonstrating induction of CYP1A1 after the release of human keratinocytes from cell substratum and in cell suspensions despite ligand absence (29,30). To explain the apparent paradoxic findings regarding omeprazole induction of CYP1A1, it has been suggested that omeprazole is a precursor of a novel class of AhR ligands (27), or alternatively, omeprazole triggers the activation of intracellular signal-transduction pathways that are different from those involved in induction by prototypic AhR ligands (28).

AhR-Independent CYP1A Induction

The recent availability of AhR null mouse lines has provided a valuable model for assessing the possibility of AhR-independent induction of CYP1A. In a recent study, piperonyl butoxide and acenaphthylene were shown to induce CYP1A2 and another AhR-regulated P450, CYP1B1, in a AhR null mouse line (31). In contrast, CYP1A1 induction was not observed. Phenobarbital also was capable of inducing CYP1A2 in the AhR null mice. These findings suggest the existence of a mechanism for increased CYP1A2 levels that is AhR independent. It is presently unclear if this reflects a novel induction pathway, or alternatively, enhanced constitutive expression.

Pharmacogenetics

AhR Polymorphism

A genetic polymorphism in the AhR was originally identified from studies of inducible benzo(a)pyrene metabolism among inbred mouse strains having genes for high- and low-affinity Ah receptors (reviewed in ref. 32). C57BL/6 (B6) and DBA/2 (D2) are the prototype mouse strains that display highest and lowest CYP1A1-inducibility/AhR-affinity phenotypes, respectively. There is convincing evidence from studies using these strains that allelic differences in the AhR locus are associated with profound differences in individual susceptibility to many toxicities affecting multiple organ systems (32). Notably, those with the low-affinity phenotype exhibit decreased tumor risk after exposure to carcinogenic polycyclic aromatic hydrocarbons. Cloning and sequencing of AhR cDNAs from several inbred mouse lines has allowed the molecular basis of the polymorphism to be studied (33–35). Among the various strains studied, 12 amino acid differences have been identified, only one of which (Ala375Val) is in the putative ligand-binding domain of the receptor. This polymorphism, together with a second, which determines the position of the translation stop codon, is critical in determining AhR affinity (34,35).

Similar to the inbred mouse lines, human populations display marked heterogeneity in CYP1A1 inducibility phenotypes, indicative of differences in the affinity of the AhR (reviewed in ref. 36). There is evidence to suggest a bimodal distribution of CYP1A1-inducibility/AhR-affinity phenotypes, with 10% of human subjects exhibiting the high-affinity phenotype, and 90%, the low. Despite efforts to identify the molecular basis of the human AhR polymorphism, the mechanism currently remains unknown. Both mouse and human studies are consistent with a polyallelic mode of inheritance in which one or two amino acids are responsible for differences in phenotype, but it is likely that several other amino acids act as modifiers for the trait. The human AhR cDNA has been cloned and encodes a protein of 848 amino acids, with the residue corresponding to the critical mouse site resid-

ing in exon 9 (37,38). A recent study has focused on this region by sequencing DNA from members within a single multigeneration family exhibiting the high- and low-affinity binding traits, but no differences in the encoded amino acids were observed (39).

Since its identification, interest in the human AhR polymorphism has been intense because of the possible relationship between genetic differences at the AhR locus and adverse human health. Accidental exposure of human populations to potent AhR ligands such as TCDD has led to manifestations of malignancies, early onset of menopause, immunosuppression, and chloracne, but no direct cause-and-effect relationship between the AhR genotype polymorphism and these toxicities has been demonstrated. A correlation between CYP1A1 inducibility in cigarette smokers and susceptibility to lung cancer was reported 25 years ago (40). Subsequent studies in a number of independent laboratories have also suggested that among cigarette smokers, the high-affinity AhR phenotype is at higher risk of bronchogenic carcinoma, presumably due to enhanced activation of procarcinogens present in cigarette smoke (41–43). A similar relationship has also been demonstrated between the high-affinity AhR phenotype and cancers of the oral cavity (44). Although collectively these studies support a link between malignancies of tissues in direct contact with cigarette smoke and AhR phenotype, others have found no such correlation (45,46). It has been proposed that the contradictory results may reflect difficulties associated with the technically demanding lymphocyte culture assay, which is typically used to determine the phenotype of individuals. This has recently prompted alternative approaches to phenotyping by using reverse transcription–polymerase chain reaction (RT-PCR) to quantitate CYP1A1 mRNA levels (47). There remains a need for a simple, reliable, and noninvasive biomarker for assessing AhR/CYP1A1-inducibility phenotype in large populations. Whereas DNA genotyping would be ideal, the inability to identify a molecular basis for the human AhR polymorphism currently prevents such an approach.

AhR Null Mouse Line

Based on a number of experimental findings, including developmental expression and conservation across mammalian species, it has long been proposed that the AhR protein is of physiological significance. To define accurately any role in mammalian development and/or survival, mouse lines bearing two null alleles of the AhR gene have been produced (48,49). As expected, administration of TCDD to homozygous *AhR* null mice does not result in CYP1A1 and CYP1A2 induction as seen in wild-type animals. Basal CYP1A2 expression also is reduced, indicating a previously unknown role for the AhR in constitutive P450 gene expression (discussed later). Interestingly, the two independent *AhR* null lines demonstrate divergent phenotypes. Analysis of the first *AhR* null line demonstrated immune system impairment and hepatic fibrosis in homozygous mutants (48). The other line also displayed abnormal liver development with a spectrum of hepatic defects, confirming a role for the AhR in liver growth and development, but mice were free of the immune impairment observed in the first *AhR* null line (49).

Constitutive and Tissue-specific CYP1A Expression

As noted previously, CYP1A2 is expressed in a constitutive manner in human liver, albeit at varying levels (4–6). Whereas CYP1A2 expression was thought to occur only in liver, low-level expression has been described more recently in brain and umbilical vein endothelium (4). Factors controlling the constitutive expression of CYP1A2 remain poorly understood. CYP1A2 expression is extinguished in cultured cells and greatly diminished in primary hepatocytes, indicative of a role for hepatocyte-enriched transcription factors in constitutive expression. Recent studies with the *AhR* null mouse line have implicated the receptor in constitutive expression of CYP1A2 because expression of this protein was substantially reduced in AhR-deficient animals (48). Constitutive expression of a second AhR-inducible gene (*UGT1A6*) also was significantly reduced in the null mouse line. It is thus possible that the AhR is involved in the regulation of hepatic transcription factors that influence the constitutive expression of CYP1A2, as well as liver growth and development.

Although low-level expression of CYP1A1 has been reported in human liver (5,6), CYP1A1 is considered to be primarily an extrahepatic enzyme in mammalian species (4,50–52). Low-level CYP1A1 expression has been reported in human placenta, lung, and pulmonary macrophages, lymphocytes, and cultured epidermal keratinocytes. Treatment of laboratory animals with polycyclic aromatic hydrocarbons induces CYP1A1 expression in liver and extrahepatic tissues, whereas CYP1A2 induction is limited to liver (52). A similar pattern of inducibility appears to occur in cigarette-smoking humans (50,51). As discussed previously, extrahepatic CYP1A1 induction may have implications for the development of chemical-induced malignancies in a number of tissues, particularly lung. Moreover, because some drug substrates for CYP1A2 also may be metabolized by CYP1A1 (53,54), hepatic and extrahepatic induction of both isoforms may contribute to the higher plasma clearance of CYP1A2 substrates observed in cigarette smokers.

CYP1A1 Polymorphism

In addition to the AhR polymorphism that influences CYP1A1 inducibility, several structural polymorphisms have been identified in the *CYP1A1* gene itself. There is a restriction fragment length polymorphism (*m1*) in the 3′-noncoding region of the *CYP1A1* gene affecting the size of *Msp* I fragments (55). In Japanese populations, this structural polymorphism has been suggested to be associated with an increased incidence of lung cancer (56), and with a mutation (*m2*; Ile462Val) in the heme-binding region of CYP1A1, which results in a 50% increase in enzyme activity (57). When this polymorphism is combined with the null mutation for glutathione-*S*-transferase μ (GSTM1), a nine-fold increased risk of lung cancer was observed in Japanese cigarette smokers (58). In contrast to the results in Japan, studies in other populations have failed to demonstrate any relationship between the *Msp* I restriction fragment length polymorphism, the heme-binding region mutation, and lung cancer (59–61). Contrasting findings between Japanese and other ethnic groups may be in part explained by different allelic frequencies; the frequency of the recessive phenotype is 7 times higher in Japanese populations than in whites. In addition, the *Msp* I polymorphism may be in linkage disequilibrium with another mutation important for CYP1A1 inducibility or another tumorigenic gene in Japanese.

Two other structural polymorphisms have been identified in the *CYP1A1* gene. The first of these (*m3*), located in intron 7 of the gene, was identified in African-Americans and appears to be restricted to this population group (62,63). An association between the African-American CYP1A1 polymorphism and cancers of the lung and breast has been suggested, but such an association remains controversial (64–66). The remaining polymorphism (*m4*) is a transversion occurring in exon 7 (resulting in a Thr461Asp substitution), which is directly adjacent to the codon affected by the *m2* polymorphism (67). The *m4* mutation appears not to represent a susceptibility factor for lung cancer.

CYP1A2 Polymorphism

Wide interindividual variability has been reported in the expression of CYP1A2 in humans. For example, CYP1A2 mRNA content varied 43-fold in 21 livers, whereas rates of caffeine *N*3-demethylation and 4-aminobiphenyl N-oxidation, both CYP1A2 catalyzed reactions, varied 57-fold and 130-fold, respectively, in 22 livers (6,68). The distribution of CYP1A2 has been investigated *in vivo* by using different caffeine-based urine and plasma metabolite ratios (see CYP1A Substrate Probes), but results are conflicting. Depending on the ratio used, log normal, bimodal, and trimodal distributions of CYP1A2 activities have resulted (69–75). It is almost certain that the different metabolic ratios used contributed to these disparate findings, because all are subject to a variable extent to confounding factors (see CYP1A Substrate Probes). Furthermore, the composition of the various populations studied varied (inclusion or exclusion of smokers), and inappropriate segregation analyses may have led to the misinterpretation of data (4,76). A more selective study of caffeine urine metabolite ratios in 68 nuclear families was not consistent with familial resemblance (75).

To date, no specific polymorphisms of the *CYP1A2* gene have been identified. Importantly, no differences in nucleotide sequence have been identified in the exons, exon–intron junctions, and 5′-flanking region of the *CYP1A2* gene from supposed "poor" and "extensive" metabolizers of caffeine (phenotyped by using a urine metabolite ratio) (74). Sequence analysis of a PCR-amplified CYP1A2 cDNA from a liver expressing low amounts of CYP1A2 mRNA and protein indicated loss of exon 4 in this clone (6). However, the abnormally and normally spliced mRNA were subsequently identified in all livers examined, with the normally spliced species being the more abundant.

Other Factors Influencing CYP1A Expression

Based on methylxanthine disposition data, age appears to be an important determinant of CYP1A2 expression in humans. Premature neonates have markedly diminished capacity to metabolize caffeine and theophylline (77,78), both CYP1A2 substrates (see later). For example, mean plasma caffeine clearance (0.009 L/h/kg) and elimination half-life (103 hours) are approximately 14-fold lower and 25-fold higher than the respective parameters in adults (77,79). Theophylline metabolism and plasma clearance correlate significantly with postconceptual age and reach adult values after 50 weeks (78), presumably reflecting CYP1A2 maturation. There is evidence suggesting that caffeine and theophylline plasma clearances are higher in children (1–12 years) than in adults (80,81), although it is not clear to what extent increased CYP1A2 expression contributes to this phenomenon. CYP1A2 activity appears not to decline significantly in old age (82).

Gender-related differences in methylxanthine elimination tend to be relatively minor (73,83). However, there is a progressive decline in caffeine plasma clearance during the second and third trimesters of pregnancy, with a return to nonpregnant values soon after parturition (84). It was speculated that this alteration in clearance arose from an effect of steroid hormones on the expression of the enzyme (i.e., CYP1A2) responsible for caffeine metabolism. Application of various caffeine urinary metabolic ratios has provided conflicting evidence concerning the distribution of CYP1A2 activities in different ethnic groups (69,71). Reported differences may, however, be due to experimental artifacts rather than to altered expression (see CYP1A Substrates: Caffeine). As noted previously, allele frequencies of polymorphisms in the *CYP1A1* gene may vary between ethnic groups (see CYP1A1 Polymorphism).

CYP1A SUBSTRATE AND INHIBITOR PROBES

The contribution of a given CYP isoform to the metabolism of a compound is most appropriately determined by using an intact system, such as the microsomal fraction, which contains a full complement of P450 enzymes and associated proteins. This may be achieved by using isoform-selective chemical (or antibody) inhibitors, a number of which have been developed for CYP1A. Furthermore, given the contribution of CYP1A2 to hepatic drug metabolism and the possible relationships between the susceptibility to certain chemical-induced cancers and phenotypic differences in the expression of both CYP1A isoforms, numerous substrates have been used to investigate CYP1A expression and regulation *in vitro* and *in vivo*. The selectivity of CYP1A substrate and inhibitor probes is discussed here.

CYP1A Substrates

Caffeine

There has been considerable interest in recent years in the development of caffeine (CA; 1,3,7-trimethylxanthine) as a substrate probe for CYP1A and other xenobiotic metabolizing enzymes in vitro and in vivo (71,85). The near-ubiquitous dietary consumption of CA, together with its relative safety and favorable pharmacokinetic characteristics (complete absorption, moderately high clearance, and relatively short half-life), potentially make this compound a highly useful metabolic probe for use in humans.

Pathways of CA biotransformation are shown in Fig. 6-2. Five primary metabolic pathways contribute to CA

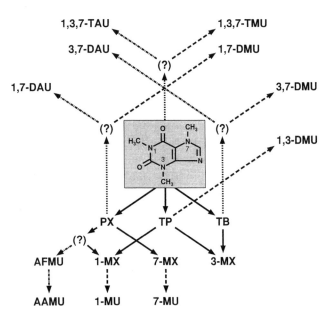

FIG. 6-2. Pathways of caffeine biotransformation in humans. See text for abbreviations.

clearance in humans (85). N1-Demethylation to form theobromine (TB; 3,7-dimethylxanthine), N3-demethylation to form paraxanthine (PX; 1,7-dimethylxanthine) and N7-demethylation to form theophylline (TP; 1,3-dimethylxanthine) account, on average, for 80%, 11%, and 4%, respectively, of CA metabolism in humans (86). Formation of the C8-hydroxylated metabolite 1,3,7-trimethyluric acid (TMU) and the C8–N9 bond scission product 6-amino-5-(N-formylmethylamino)-1,3-dimethyluracil (1,3,7-TAU), which are derived from a common intermediate, account for the remainder of CA metabolic clearance. A similar pattern of CA metabolism is observed *in vitro* at substrate concentrations comparable to CA plasma concentrations observed after normal dietary intake (less than 100 μM), but TMU formation dominates at higher concentrations (53,87).

Once formed, PX, TB, and TP are subject to extensive metabolism (see Fig. 6-2). Each of these dimethylxanthines can undergo two separate N-demethylation reactions to form the corresponding monomethylxanthine (1-, 3-, and 7-MX). The N7-demethylation of PX appears to proceed by way of an unstable ring-opened intermediate. Subsequent internal rearrangement or acetylation of this species results in the formation of 1-MX and 5-acetylamino-6-formylamino-3-methyluracil (AFMU). Deformylation of AFMU, which may occur spontaneously in urine, produces 5-acetyl-6-amino-3-methyluracil (AAMU). Further oxidation (*viz.*, 8-hydroxylation) of 1- and 7-MX, but not 3-MX, produces 1- and 7-methyluric acid (1- and 7-MU). PX, TB, and TP also undergo 8-hydroxylation, giving rise to a dimethyluric acid (1,3-, 1,7-, or 3,7-DMU). Dimethylaminouracil (DAU) formation, arising from C8–N9 bond scission, occurs only with those dimethylxanthines methylated at N7 (i.e., PX and TB).

The relative conversion of CA to each dimethylxanthine (i.e., PX, TB, TP) and the extent of secondary biotransfor-mation determines the proportions of the various CA metabolites excreted in urine *in vivo*. As would be expected, those compounds derived from PX, whose formation accounts for 80% of CA clearance, are the most abundant urinary metabolites. Indeed, the N7-demethylation products of PX (i.e., AFMU, 1-MX, 1-MU) account for almost 60% of all metabolites formed from CA in vivo.

Evidence supporting the involvement of hepatic CYP1A2 in the conversion of CA to PX, TB, and TP is overwhelming. Human liver CA N1-, N3-, and N7-demethylation all exhibit biphasic kinetics (Fig. 6-3), with high (K_m < 0.33 mM) and low (K_m > 19 mM) affinity components (53). Rates of each of the high-affinity reactions correlated highly with known CYP1A2 activities in microsomes from panels of human livers and were inhibited by compounds known to be alternate substrates or inhibitors of this enzyme. Moreover, the conversion of CA to PX, TB, and TP was catalyzed by recombinant or purified human CYP1A2, with K_m values matching those calculated for the high-affinity human liver activities (see Fig. 6-3) (53,68,87). CYP1A1 also has the capacity to convert CA to PX (53), but activity is lower than that for CYP1A2 and, as noted earlier, constitutive expression of this isoform in liver is low (or absent) in comparison to CYP1A2. Consistent with these *in vitro* data, plasma CA clearance is known to be increased by cigarette smoking and decreased by the CYP1A2 specific inhibitor furafylline (see later) in humans (8,71,88). Taken together, these data indicate that rates of hepatic CA N-demethylation generally reflect the activity of CYP1A2.

Because PX formation is the dominant CA metabolic pathway in humans, assessment of hepatic CYP1A2 activity *in vitro* is normally based on measurement of CA N3-demethylation. This approach is, however, valid only at appropriately low substrate concentrations. As the CA concentration of microsomal incubations increases above

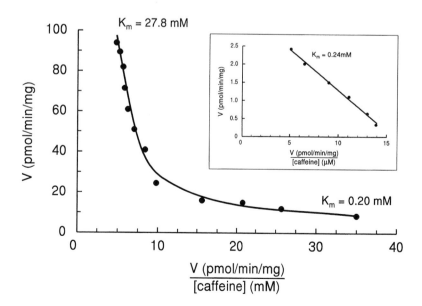

FIG. 6-3. Kinetics of caffeine N3-demethylation by human liver microsomes and complementary DNA (cDNA)-expressed CYP1A2 (inset). Data taken, with permission, from Tassaneeyakul W, Mohamed Z, Birkett DJ, et al. Caffeine as a probe for human cytochromes P450: validation using cDNA-expression, immuno-inhibition and microsomal kinetic techniques. *Pharmacogenetics* 1992;2:173–183; and Tassaneeyakul W, Birkett DJ, McManus ME, et al. Caffeine metabolism by human hepatic cytochromes P450: contributions of 1A2, 2E1 and 3A isoforms. *Biochem Pharmacol* 1994;47:1767–1773.

0.1 mM, there is an increasing contribution from the isoforms (probably CYP 2A6, 2E1, and 3A) responsible for the low-affinity component of CA N3-demethylation (53,87). CYP1A1 is also likely to contribute to PX formation in tissues that express this enzyme, particularly in individuals exposed to CYP1A inducers.

Theoretically, the most valid index of CYP1A2 activity *in vivo* is the intrinsic clearance for CA N3-demethylation. Plasma CA clearance is an acceptable alternative because N1-, N3-, and N3-demethylation, all of which are catalyzed by CYP1A2, account for more than 90% of CA elimination. Calculation of these parameters is, however, not feasible in population-screening studies because of the need for intensive blood and urine collection. Given these difficulties, attention has focused on the use of urinary CA metabolite ratios as indirect indices of CYP1A2 activity. Six different urinary ratios have been proposed as surrogate markers of CYP1A2 (76), and these are listed in Table 6-2. Most are based on CA N3-demethylation, that is, the conversion of CA to PX (see Fig. 6-2).

A comparison of ratios 1, 2, and 4 to 6 in 237 subjects administered CA found that most correlated with each other poorly, demonstrating that the various ratios do not reflect the same parameter (89). More recently, the validity of the six metabolic ratios listed in Table 6-2 was assessed by using computer simulations based on literature values of CA kinetic parameters (76). The results demonstrated that the sensitivity of the ratios to confounding variables was in many cases greater than their sensitivity to discriminate CYP1A2. In particular, ratios 1 to 5, which use the urinary excretion of CA or PX as the denominator, are sensitive to changes in urine flow rate, whereas ratios 1 and 2 are additionally influenced by sampling time. Metabolic ratio 6 was the most robust because it is least affected by changes in urine flow (76). Even so, wide variability has been observed in studies investigating the relationship between this ratio and plasma CA clearance (71,72,90). As noted earlier (CYP1A2 Pharmacogenetics), the application of urinary CA metabolic ratios has led to controversial and conflicting claims concerning the multimodality of CYP1A2 dis-

tribution and possible consequences for cancer susceptibility. It is now clear that the uncritical use of metabolic ratios may lead to erroneous conclusions.

In contrast to the urinary metabolic ratios, computer simulation showed the ratio of PX to CA in plasma or saliva measured 5 to 7 hours after CA ingestion was, at least theoretically, a valid marker of CYP1A2 activity (76). The ratio of PX to CA in plasma or saliva has been reported to correlate highly with plasma CA clearance (72,91). Another option worthy of attention is the use of salivary CA half-life based on a limited number of blood or saliva samples, because the volume of distribution of CA is relatively invariant (76).

Theophylline

The primary metabolic pathways of TP (1,3-dimethylxanthine) are N1- and N3-demethylation and 8-hydroxylation to form 3-MX, 1-MX, and 1,3-DMU, respectively (see Fig.˘ 6-2) (85). Once formed *in vivo*, 1-MX is converted almost entirely to 1-MU by xanthine oxidase. Unlike CA, the predominant route of metabolism of TP in humans is 8-hydroxylation. Both *in vivo* and *in vitro*, 50% to 60% of TP metabolism occurs by 8-hydroxylation, 20% to 25% by 1-demethylation, and 15% to 20% by 3-demethylation. Human liver microsomal inhibition studies and the use of recombinant CYP isoforms has demonstrated that CYP1A2 is responsible for the N1- and N3-demethylations of TP, although like CA, CYP1A1 also may contribute to these reactions in tissues in which it is expressed (92–94). CYP1A2 is also the major catalyst for 1,3-DMU formation, with an additional contribution from CYP2E1 and possibly CYP3A4.

A comparison of TP and CA metabolism in 12 subjects showed that the ratios of 1-MU and 3-MX to TP in plasma and in urine (12-hour collection) correlated highly with the respective partial metabolic clearances (95). However, only the TP plasma ratios correlated with the ratio of PX to CA in plasma, and neither the TP plasma nor urine ratios correlated with the "standard" CA urinary ratio (AFMU + 1-MU + 1-MX)/(1,7-DMU; ratio 6 of Table 6-2). These data highlight further the limitations of urine (and probably plasma) metabolic ratios. Although the N-demethylation pathways of TP may serve as surrogate measures of CYP1A2 activity *in vitro*, this drug has few advantages over CA *in vivo*. Despite its simpler metabolism, TP is less convenient to administer, has a narrower therapeutic index, and concentrations of the demethylated metabolites in blood are low.

TABLE 6-2. *Caffeine urinary metabolic ratios used as surrogate markers of CP1A2 activity*

Ratio	Components
1	PX/CA
2	1,7 – DMU + PX/CA
3	PX + TB + TP/CA
4	AFMU + 1 – MX + 1 – MU + PX/CA
5	AFMU + 1 – MX + 1 – MU/PX
6	AFMU + 1 – MX + 1 – MU/1,7 — DMU

Adapted with permission from Rostani-Hodjegen A, Nurminen S, Jackson PR, Tucker GT. Caffeine urinary metabolite ratios as markers of enzyme activity: a theoretical assessment. *Pharmacogenetics* 1996;6:121–149.

Phenacetin

Like the CA N-demethylations, the conversion of phenacetin to acetaminophen (paracetamol; Fig. 6-4) exhibits biphasic kinetics in human liver microsomes (54,96). Mean apparent K_m values of the high- (9 μM)

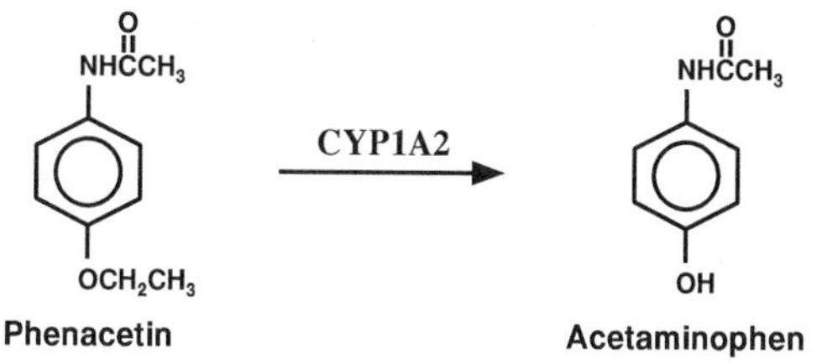

FIG. 6-4. Conversion of phenacetin to acetaminophen (paracetamol).

and low-affinity (322 μM) reactions differ more than 30-fold. The high-affinity component of phenacetin O-deethylation is inhibited by furafylline and other CYP1A inhibitors and was found to correlate highly with CA $N3$-demethylation activity in microsomes from a panel of human livers (51,54). Moreover, apparent K_m values for the high-affinity microsomal reaction and phenacetin O-deethylation by complementary DNA (cDNA)-expressed CYP1A2 were shown to be close in value (54). Whereas CYP1A1 additionally has the capacity to deethylate phenacetin, the intrinsic clearance for this enzyme is five-fold lower than that for CYP1A2 (54). Although the high-affinity component of phenacetin O-deethylation provides a valid and readily measurable marker of CYP1A2 activity in human liver microsomes, care is necessary in selecting a substrate concentration that differentiates the high- and low-affinity reactions (54). Phenacetin is no longer approved for use in humans *in vivo*.

7-Ethoxyresorufin

The O-dealkylations of a number of alkoxyresorufins, most notably 7-ethoxyresorufin, have been used widely as substrate probes for CYP1A and other isoforms (97). Kinetic analyses of cDNA-expressed human CYP1A1 and CYP1A2 demonstrated an element of selectivity in the O-deethylation of 7-ethoxyresorufin by these enzymes (98). The apparent K_m (87 vs. 240 μM) was lower, and the turnover number (7.6 vs. 1.9 per minute) was higher for CYP1A1 compared with CYP1A2. Apart from CYP1A1, recombinant CYP1A2 exhibited substantially higher 7-ethoxyresorufin O-deethylase activity than did other cDNA-expressed CYP isoforms, and this activity in human liver microsomes was inhibited by furafylline and anti-CYP1A antibodies (97,99). Thus it would appear that 7-ethoxyresorufin is a selective substrate for human liver CYP1A2, although clearly there will be a major contribution from CYP1A1 in tissues in which it is expressed. However, a need for caution with the use of 7-ethoxyresorufin as a CYP1A-specific probe has been noted (97). Furafylline, even at high concentrations, did not completely abolish hepatic 7-ethoxyresorufin O-deethylation, and there was some evidence from antibody inhibition of a variable contribution of CYP2C or CYP3A subfamily isoforms. The kinetics of

human liver microsomal 7-ethoxyresorufin O-deethylation appear not to have been characterized and hence the concentration dependence of the possible contribution of non-CYP1A isoforms to this pathway remains unclear.

(R)-Warfarin

Numerous CYP isoforms are known to contribute to the stereo- and regioselective oxidation of warfarin and the various metabolic pathways of racemic warfarin therefore potentially serve as markers for multiple isoform activities *in vivo* and *in vitro*. It has been demonstrated using recombinant enzymes that CYP1A1 and CYP1A2 catalyze the 6- and 8-hydroxylation of (R)-warfarin, with CYP1A2 showing high selectivity for 6-hydroxylation, and CYP1A1, weak selectivity for 8-hydroxylation (100,101). Confirmatory studies with human liver microsomes showed that furafylline was a potent, mechanism-based inhibitor of this pathway and that rates of (R)-warfarin 6-hydroxylation correlated significantly with immunoreactive CYP1A2 content and CA $N3$-demethylation activity (101,102). It has been suggested that, given the differing regioselectivities of CYP 1A1 and 1A2 for (R)-warfarin, the 6-hydroxylation to 8-hydroxylation ratio may additionally differentiate these isoform activities in different tissues (101). Although warfarin is a useful model substrate for CYP1A and other isoforms (notably CYP2C9), assay conditions are generally complex, and the narrow therapeutic index of the drug poses problems for its use *in vivo*.

Other Substrates

Although it has been known for some time that 7-ethoxycoumarin O-deethylation may exhibit biphasic kinetics in human liver microsomes (96), more recent studies have demonstrated that the kinetics of this reaction differ according to the relative CYP isoform content of human liver. Although biphasic kinetics occur in the majority of livers, Michaelis–Menten kinetics are apparent in livers in which the relative expression of CYP1A2 compared with CYP2E1 is high (103). Antibody inhibition and comparative kinetic studies with human CYP isoforms confirmed that CYP1A2 was responsible for the high-affinity component of 7-ethoxycoumarin O-deethylation, whereas CYP2E1 and possibly CYP2B6 are the low-affinity enzymes. The intrinsic clearance for 7-ethoxycoumarin O-deethylation by CYP1A1 is more than 30 times greater than that for CYP1A2 (103), indicating a likely major contribution of CYP1A1 to this reaction in tissues in which it is expressed.

Benzo(a)pyrene hydroxylation and acetanilide 4-hydroxylation, the latter forming acetaminophen, are other pathways used frequently to assess CYP1A activity *in vitro*, particularly in laboratory animals. CYP1A1 is the human isoform with highest benzo(a)pyrene hydroxylase activity, and it is almost certain that CYP1A1 is the major contributor to this reaction in tissues in which it is present (98,104,105). In liver, however, multiple enzymes, including CYP3A4, CYP1A2, and possibly CYP2C subfamily members, probably contribute to benzo(a)pyrene hydroxylation (104,105). The turnover number for acetanilide 4-hydroxylation is eight-fold higher for CYP1A2 compared with CYP1A1 (98). Furthermore, an anti-CYP1A antibody known to inhibit recombinant human CYP1A2 decreased human liver microsomal acetanilide 4-hydroxylation by 60% (106). Whereas CYP1A2 would appear to be a contributor to hepatic acetanilide 4-hydroxylation, the capacity of non-CYP1A isoforms to catalyze this reaction appears not to have been defined.

There is increasing evidence supporting the validity of the cognition activator tacrine as a selective human hepatic CYP1A2 substrate probe. The conversion of tacrine to stable ring-hydroxylated metabolites is almost abolished by furafylline, and formation of the major metabolite, 1-hydroxytacrine, was shown to correlate with immunoreactive CYP1A2 content and theophylline N1-demethylation in microsomes from a panel of human livers (107,108).

CYP1A Inhibitors

Furafylline

An investigation of the pharmacokinetics and tolerability of furafylline, a 1,3,8-trisubstituted xanthine (1,8-dimethyl-3-(2′-furfuryl)methylxanthine; Fig. 6-5), revealed that administration of this compound resulted in the accumulation of CA and the development of methylxanthine-like toxicity in subjects consuming CA-containing beverages (88). A single dose (90 mg) of furafylline was further shown to prolong plasma CA elimination half-life almost 10-fold and to decrease plasma concentrations of PX. Subsequent studies confirmed that furafylline was an inhibitor of both human liver microsomal CA N3-demethylation and the high-affinity component of phenacetin O-deethylation and that selectivity for CYP1A2 was high (102,109,110). Detailed kinetic analyses further demonstrated that furafylline was a potent mechanism-based inhibitor of CYP1A2 (102,

110,111), with reported K_i and k_{inact} values ranging from 3 to 23 μM and 0.07 to 0.87 per minute, respectively.

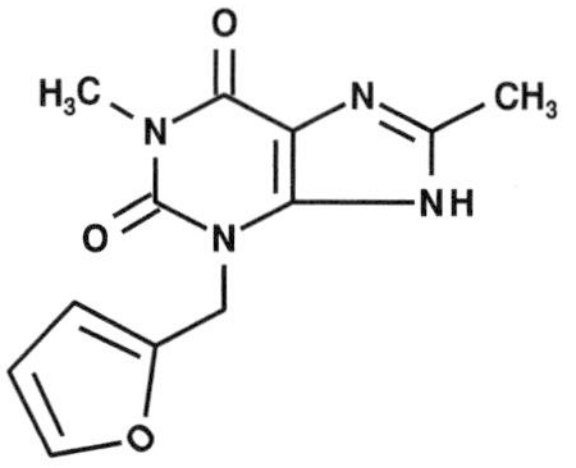

Whereas the majority of CYP1A2 inhibitors also affect CYP1A1 (54), initial findings suggested that furafylline interacted minimally with CYP1A1 because there was no inhibition of the aryl hydrocarbon hydroxylase activity of placental samples from women who were smokers (51). Marked selectivity for CYP1A2 over CYP1A1 was demonstrated unequivocally by using recombinant enzymes (110,111). Although the inactivation-rate constants for both isoforms were of a similar order, K_i values differed markedly (7 vs. 1,000 μM). Thus the affinity of furafylline for CYP1A2 is two orders of magnitude greater for CYP1A2 compared with CYP1A1. At appropriately low concentrations (e.g., 10 μM..) and under conditions that favor mechanism-based inhibition, furafylline is therefore a highly selective inhibitor of human CYP1A2 activity *in vitro* and the preferred chemical probe for inhibition of this isoform. Furafylline is not, however, available tor use in humans *in vivo*.

7,8-Benzoflavone (α-Naphthoflavone)

7,8-Benzoflavone (BF), also known as α-naphthoflavone, has found widespread use as a CYP1A inhibitor *in vitro*. BF has indeed been shown to be a potent inhibitor of both the CYP1A1- and CYP1A2-catalyzed O-deethylation of phenacetin (54). Moreover, median inhibitory concentration (IC_{50}) values for the two enzymes differed by an order of magnitude, and at low concentrations, BF may differentiate CYP1A2. However, there is evidence to suggest that BF may inhibit isoforms other than CYP1A. Notably, BF affects CYP2C8 and CYP2C9 activities at concentrations similar to those causing CYP1A inhibition (112). At higher concentrations, BF also may inhibit CYP2A6 and CYP2B6. Use of BF as a CYP1A-inhibitory probe is considered inappropriate.

Fluvoxamine

Because furafylline is not available for use in human subjects, attention has focused on the identification of alternative drugs that may be used as CYP1A inhibitor probes *in vivo*. The selective serotonin-reuptake inhibitor fluvoxamine causes inhibitory interactions with a number of drugs metabolized by CYP1A2, including caffeine, clomipramine, clozapine, imipramine, tacrine, and theophylline. For example, plasma CA clearance was reduced by 80% in subjects pretreated with fluvoxamine for 12 days (113). The potent inhibition of hepatic CYP1A2 by fluvoxamine has been confirmed *in vitro*. Fluvoxamine inhibited all pathways of TP metabolism in human liver microsomes, with an apparent K_i value of about 0.1 μM for both the N1- and N3-demethylation pathways (114). Little or no effect was observed on hepatic CYP2A6,

FIG. 6-5. Structure of furafylline.

CYP2E1, or CYP3A activities, or on placental ethoxyre-sorufin O-deethylation (CYP1A1). The selectivity of flu-voxamine for inhibition of CYP1A2 over CYP1A1 also has been demonstrated by using cDNA-expressed iso-forms (115).

On the basis of these data, fluvoxamine has been pro-posed as a selective inhibitor probe for CYP1A2 (114,115), but this is questionable. Fluvoxamine addi-tionally inhibits CYP2C19- and CYP2D6-catalyzed reac-tions *in vivo* (116,117). In particular, fluvoxamine pre-treatment inhibited the CYP2C19-catalyzed partial clearances of chloroguanide by about 60% in extensive metabolizers.

Other Inhibitors

A number of other compounds, including ellipticine and isosafrole, have been investigated for their ability to inhibit CYP1A. Comparative studies with recombinant enzymes demonstrated that the affinity of isosafrole for CYP1A2 is 14-fold higher than that for CYP1A1 (115). In contrast, ellipticine is a nonselective CYP1A inhibitor (54). It should be recognized, however, that the ability of these compounds to inhibit human CYP isoforms other than those of the 1A subfamily appears not to have been investigated in a systematic manner.

Apart from xenobiotic probes, *antibodies* have been used to identify, localize, quantify, and inhibit CYP1A. Antiprotein antibodies, both polyclonal and monoclonal, have been used, and certain of these are able to differenti-ate CYP1A1 and CYP1A2 (54). The recent development of three-dimensional models for CYP has allowed the identification of the regions of a number of isoforms involved in substrate binding, and this in turn has made it possible to produce antipeptide antibodies directed to regions of enzymes involved in catalytic activity. For example, an antibody raised against residues 291 to 302 of human CYP1A2 has been shown to bind specifically to CYP1A2, both as the recombinant enzyme and in human liver microsomes (118). Moreover, the antibody was able to abolish hepatic microsomal phenacetin O-deethylase activity. Although this and other inhibitory antibodies pro-vide a means for identifying the contribution of CYP1A2 to the metabolism of any given substrate, being complex to produce, they provide no advantage over the now readily available chemical inhibitor furafylline.

REFERENCES

1. Gonzalez FJ. The molecular biology of cytochrome P450s. *Pharma-col Rev* 1989;40:243–288.
2. Pineau T, Fernandez-Salguero P, Lee SST, et al. Neonatal lethality associated with respiratory distress in mice lacking cytochrome P4501A2. *Proc Natl Acad Sci USA* 1995;92:5134–5138.
3. Guengerich FP. Metabolic activation of carcinogens. *Pharmacol Ther* 1992;54:17–61.
4. Eaton DL, Gallagher EP, Bammler TK, Kunze KL. Role of cyto-chrome P4501A2 in chemical carcinogenesis: implications for human variability in expression and enzyme activity. Pharmacogenetics 1995; 5:259–274.
5. McKinnon RA, Hall PM, Quattrochi LC, Tukey RH, McManus ME. Localization of CYP1A1 and CYP1A2 mRNA in normal liver and hepatocellular carcinoma by in situ hybridization. *Hepatology* 1991; 14:848–856.
6. Schweikl H, Taylor JA, Kitareewan S, Linko P, Nagorney D, Goldstein JA. Expression of *CYP1A1* and *CYP1A2* genes in human liver. *Phar-macogenetics* 1993;3:239–249.
7. Grygiel JJ, Birkett DJ. Cigarette smoking and theophylline clearance and metabolism. *Clin Pharmacol Ther* 1981;30:491–496.
8. Kotake AN, Schoeller DA, Lambert GH, Baker AL, Schaffer DD, Josephs H. The caffeine CO_2 breath test: dose response and route of N-demethylation in smokers and non-smokers. *Clin Pharmacol Ther* 1982;32:261–269.
9. Robson RA, Miners JO, Wing LMH, Birkett DJ. Theophylline-rifampicin interaction: non-selective induction of theophylline meta-bolic pathways. *Br J Clin Pharmacol* 1984;18:445–448.
10. Diaz D, Fabre I, Daujat M, et al. Omeprazole is an aryl hydrocarbon-like inducer of human hepatic P-450. *Gastroenterology* 1990;99: 737–747.
11. Andersson T, Holmberg J, Walan A. Pharmacokinetics and effect on caffeine metabolism of the proton pump inhibiters omeprazole, lanso-prazole and pantoprazole. *Br J Clin Pharmacol* 1998;45:369–375.
12. Rost LK, Brosicke H, Heinemeyer G, Roots I. Specific and dose-dependent enzyme induction by omeprazole in human beings. *Hepa-tology* 1994;20:1204–1212.
13. Porter TD, Coon M. Cytochrome P-450: multiplicity of isoforms, sub-strates, and catalytic and regulatory mechanisms. *J Biol Chem* 1991; 266:10019–10022.
14. Savas U, Jefcoate CR. Dual regulation of cytochrome P450EF expres-sion via the aryl hydrocarbon receptor and protein stabilization in C3H/10T1/2 cells. *Mol Pharmacol* 1994;45:1153–1159.
15. Reisz-Porszasz S, Probst MR, Fukunaga BN, Hankinson O. Identifi-cation of functional domains of the aryl hydrocarbon receptor nuclear translocator protein (ARNT). *Mol Cell Biol* 1994;14:6075–6086.
16. Ko HP, Okino ST, Ma Q, Whitlock JP. Dioxin-induced *CYP1A1* tran-scription in vivo: the aromatic hydrocarbon receptor mediates trans-activation, enhancer-promoter communication, and changes in chro-matin structure. *Mol Cell Biol* 1996;16:430–436.
17. Swanson HI, Bradfield CA. The Ah receptor: genetics, structure and function. *Pharmacogenetics* 1993;3:213–230.
18. Hankinson O. The aryl hydrocarbon receptor complex. *Annu Rev Pharmacol Toxicol* 1995;35:307–340.
19. Whitlock JP, Okino ST, Dong L, et al. Induction of cytochrome P4501A1: a model for analyzing mammalian gene transcription. *FASEB J* 1996;10:809–817.
20. Nebert DW, Puga A, Vasiliou V. Role of the Ah receptor and the dioxin-inducible (Ah) gene battery in toxicity, cancer, and signal transduction. *Ann N Y Acad Sci* 1993;685:624–640.
21. Jones KW, Whitlock JP. Functional analysis of the transcriptional pro-moter of the CYP1A1 gene. *Mol Cell Biol* 1990;10:5098–5105.
22. Robertson RW, Zhang L, Pascoe DA, Fagan JB. Aryl hydrocarbon-induced interactions at multiple DNA elements of diverse sequence: a multicompartment mechanism for activation of cytochrome P4501A1 (CYP1A1) gene transcription. *Nucleic Acids Res* 1994;22:1741–1749.
23. Okino ST, Whitlock JP. Dioxin induces localized, graded changes in chromatin structure: implications for CYP1A1 transcription. *Mol Cell Biol* 1995;15:3714–3721.
24. Hines RN, Mathis JM, Jacob CS. Identification of multiple regulatory elements on the human P4501A1 gene. *Carcinogenesis* 1988;9: 599–605.
25. Sterling K, Bresnick E. Oct-1 transcription factor is a negative regu-lator of rat CYP1A1 expression via an octamer sequence in its nega-tive regulator element. *Mol Pharmacol* 1996;49:329–337.
26. Quattrochi LC, Tukey R. Nuclear uptake of the Ah (dioxin) receptor in response to omeprazole: transcriptional activation of the *CYP1A1* gene. *Mol Pharmacol* 1993;43:504–508.
27. Dzeletovic N, McGuire J, Daujat M, et al. Regulation of dioxin recep-tor function by omeprazole. *J Biol Chem* 1997;272:12705–12713.
28. Backlund M, Johansson I, Mkrtchian S, Ingelman-Sundberg M. Sig-nal transduction-mediated activation of the aryl hydrocarbon receptor in rat hepatoma H4IIE cells. *J Biol Chem* 1997;272:31755–31763.

29. Sadek CM, Allen-Hoffman BL. Cytochrome P450IA1 is rapidly induced in normal keratinocytes in the absence of xenobiotics. *J Biol Chem* 1994;269:16067–16074.

30. Sadek CM, Allen-Hoffman BL. Suspension mediated induction of Hepa1c1c7 CYP1A1 expression is dependent on the AH receptor signal transduction pathway. *J Biol Chem* 1994;269:31505–31509.

31. Ryu DY, Levi PE, Fernandez Salguero P, Gonzalez FJ, Hodgson E. Piperonyl butoxide and acenaphthylene induce cytochrome P450 1a2 and 1b1 mRNA in aromatic hydrocarbon-responsive receptor knockout mouse liver. *Mol Pharmacol* 1996;50:443–446.

32. Nebert DW. The Ah locus: genetic differences in toxicity, cancer, mutation and birth defect. *Crit Rev Toxicol* 1989;20:153–174.

33. Schmidt JV, Carver LA, Bradfield CA. Molecular characterisation of the murine AhR gene: organisation, promoter analysis and chromosomal assignment. *J Biol Chem* 1993;268:22203–22209.

34. Ema M, Sogawa K, Watanabe N, et al. cDNA cloning and structure of mouse putative Ah receptor. *Biochem Biophys Res Commun* 1992;184:246–253.

35. Poland A, Palen D, Glover E. Analysis of the four alleles of the murine aryl hydrocarbon receptor. *Mol Pharmacol* 1994;46:915–921.

36. Nebert DW, McKinnon RA, Puga A. Human drug metabolizing polymorphisms: effects on risk of toxicity and cancer. *DNA Cell Biol* 1996;15:273–280.

37. Dolwick KM, Schmidt JV, Carter LA, Swanson HI, Bradfield CA. Cloning and expression of human Ah receptor cDNA. *Mol Pharmacol* 1993;44:911–917.

38. Itoh S, Kamataki T. Human Ah receptor cDNA: analysis for highly conserved sequences. *Nucleic Acids Res* 1993;21:3578–3581.

39. Micka J, Milatovich A, Menon A, Grabowski GA, Puga A, Nebert DW. Human Ah receptor (AhR) gene: localization to 7p15 and suggestive correlation with CYP1A1 inducibility. *Pharmacogenetics* 1997;7:95–101.

40. Kellermann G, Shaw CR, Luyten-Kellermann M. Aryl hydrocarbon hydroxylase inducibility and bronchogenic carcinoma. *N Engl J Med* 1973;329:934–937.

41. Kouri RE, McKinney CE, Slomiany DJ, Snodgrass DR, Wray NP, McLemore TL. Positive correlation between high aryl hydrocarbon hydroxylase activity and primary lung cancer as analyzed in cryopreserved lymphocytes. *Cancer Res* 1982;42:5030–5037.

42. Guirgis HA, Lynch HT, Mate T, et al. Aryl hydrocarbon hydroxylase activity in lymphocytes from lung cancer patients and normal controls. *Oncology* 1976;33:105.

43. Korsgaard R, Trell E. Aryl hydrocarbon hydroxylase and bronchogenic carcinomas associated with smoking. *Lancet* 1978;1:1103.

44. Trell E, Korsgard R, Kitzing P, Lundgren K, Nattiasson I. Aryl hydrocarbon inducibility and carcinoma of the oral cavity. *Lancet* 1978;1:109–111.

45. Lieberman J. Aryl hydrocarbon hydroxylase in bronchogenic carcinoma. *N Engl J Med* 1978;298:686.

46. Paigen B, Gurtoo HL, Minowada J, et al. Questionable relation of aryl hydrocarbon hydroxylase to lung cancer risk. *N Engl J Med* 1977;297:346–350.

47. Landi MT, Bertazzi PA, Shields PG, et al. Association between CYP1A1 genotype, mRNA expression and enzymatic activity in humans. *Pharmacogenetics* 1994;4:242.

48. Fernandez-Salguero P, Pineau T, Hilbert DM, et al. Immune system impairment and hepatic fibrosis in mice lacking the aryl-hydrocarbon receptor. *Science* 1995;268:722–726.

49. Schmidt JV, Su GH-T, Reddy JK, Simon MC, Bradfield CA. Characterisation of murine AhR null allele: involvement of the receptor in hepatic growth and development. *Proc Natl Acad Sci USA* 1996;93:6731–6736.

50. Rannug A, Alexandric A-K, Persson I, Ingelman-Sundberg M. Genetic polymorphism of cytochromes P450 1A1, 2D6 and 2E1: regulation and toxicological significance. *J Environ Med* 1995;37:25–36.

51. Sesardic D, Pasanen M, Pelkonen O, Boobis AR. Differential expression and regulation of members of the cytochrome P4501A gene subfamily in human tissues. *Carcinogenesis* 1990;11:1183–1188.

52. Sesardic D, Cole KJ, Edwards RJ, et al. The inducibility and catalytic activity of cytochromes P450c(1A1) and P450d(1A2) in rat tissues. *Biochem Pharmacol* 1990;39:499–506.

53. Tassaneeyakul W, Mohamed Z, Birkett DJ, et al. Caffeine as a probe for human cytochromes P450: validation using cDNA-expression,

54. Tassaneeyakul W, Birkett DJ, Veronese ME, et al. Specificity of substrate and inhibitor probes for human cytochromes P450 1A1 and 1A2. *J Pharmacol Exp Ther* 1993;265:401–407.

55. Bale AE, Nebert DW, McBride OW. Subchromosomal localisation of the dioxin-inducible P_1450 locus (CYP1) and description of two RFLPs detected with a 3' P_1450 cDNA probe. *Cytogenet Cell Genet* 1987;46:574.

56. Kawajiri K, Nakachi K, Imai K, Yoshii A, Shinoda N, Watanabe J. Identification of genetically high risk individuals to lung cancer by DNA polymorphisms of the cytochrome P450IA1 gene. *FEBS Lett* 1990;263:131–133.

57. Hayashi S-I, Watanabe J, Nakachi K, Kawajiri K. Genetic linkage of lung cancer-associated MspI polymorphisms with amino acid replacement in the heme binding region of the human cytochrome P450IA1 gene. *J Biochem (Tokyo)* 1991;110:407–411.

58. Nakachi K, Imai K, Hayashi S, Kawajiri K. Polymorphisms of the CYP1A1 and glutathione S-transferase genes associated with susceptibility to lung cancer in relation to cigarette dose in a Japanese population. *Cancer Res* 1993;53:2994.

59. Shields PG, Bowman ED, Harrington AM, Doan VT, Weston A. Polycyclic aromatic hydrocarbon-DNA adducts in human lung and cancer susceptibility genes. *Cancer Res* 1993;53:3486.

60. Hirvonen A, Husgafvel-Pursiainen K, Karjalainen A, Antilla S, Vainio H. Metabolic P450 genotypes and assessment of individual susceptibility to lung cancer. *Pharmacogenetics* 1992;2:259–263.

61. Tefre T, Ryberg D, Haugen A, et al. Human CYP1A1 gene: lack of association between the *MspI* restriction fragment length polymorphism and incidence of lung cancer in a Norwegian population. *Pharmacogenetics* 1991;1:20–25.

62. Crofts F, Cosma GN, Currie D, Taioli E, Toniolo P, Garte SJ. A novel CYP1A1 gene polymorphism in African-Americans. *Carcinogenesis* 1993;14:1729–1731.

63. Mrozikiewicz PM, Cascorbi I, Brockmoller J, Roots I. *CYP1A1* mutations 4887A, 4889G, 5639C and 6235C in the Polish population and their allelic linkage, determined by peptide nucleic acid-mediated clamping. *Pharmacogenetics* 1997;7:303–307.

64. Taioli E, Trachman J, Chen X, Toniolo P, Garte SJ. A *CYP1A1* restriction fragment length polymorphism is associated with breast cancer in African-American women. *Cancer Res* 1995;55:3757.

65. London SJ, Daly AK, Fairbrother K, et al. Lung cancer risk in African-Americans in relation to a race-specific CYP1A1 polymorphism. *Cancer Res* 1995;55:6035.

66. Kelsey KT, Wiencke JK, Spitz MR. A race-specific genetic polymorphism in the *CYP1A1* gene is not associated with lung cancer in African Americans. *Carcinogenesis* 1994;15:1121–1124.

67. Cascorbi I, Brockmoller J, Roots IA. A C4887A polymorphism in exon 7 of human *CYP1A1*: population frequency, mutation linkages, and impact on lung cancer susceptibility. *Cancer Res* 1996;56:4965–4969.

68. Butler MA, Iwasaki M, Guengerich FP, Kadlubar FF. Human cytochrome P450PA (P4501A2), the phenacetin O-deethylase, is primarily responsible for the hepatic 3-demethylation of caffeine and N-oxidation of carcinogenic arylamines. *Proc Natl Acad Sci USA* 1989;86:7696–7700.

69. Butler MA, Lang NP, Young JP, et al. Determination of CYP1A2 and NAT2 phenotypes in human populations by analysis of caffeine urinary metabolites. *Pharmacogenetics* 1992;2:116–127.

70. Kalow W, Tang B-K. Use of caffeine metabolite ratios to explore CYP1A2 and xanthine oxidase activities. *Clin Pharmacol Ther* 1991;50:508–519.

71. Kalow W, Tang B-K. The use of caffeine for enzyme assays: a critical appraisal. *Clin Pharmacol Ther* 1993;53:503–514.

72. Fuhr U, Rost KL. Simple and reliable CYP1A2 phenotyping by the paraxanthine/caffeine ratio in plasma and saliva. *Pharmacogenetics* 1994;4:109–116.

73. Vistisen K, Poulson HE, Loft S. Foreign compound metabolism capacity in man measured from metabolites of dietary caffeine. *Carcinogenesis* 1992;13:1561–1568.

74. Yokoi T, Sawada M, Kamataki T. Polymorphic drug metabolism: studies with recombinant Chinese hamster cells and analyses in human populations. *Pharmacogenetics* 1995;5:S65–S69.

75. Catteau A, Bechtel YC, Poisson N, Bechtel PR, Bonaiti-Pellie C. A

population and family study of CYP1A2 using caffeine urinary metabolites. *Eur J Clin Pharmacol* 1995;47:423–430.

76. Rostami-Hodjegan A, Nurminen S, Jackson PR, Tucker GT. Caffeine urinary metabolite ratios as markers of enzyme activity: a theoretical assessment. *Pharmacogenetics* 1996;6:121–149.

77. Aranda JV, Cook CE, Gorman W, et al. Pharmacokinetic profile of caffeine in the premature newborn infant with apnea. *J Pediatr* 1979; 94:663–668.

78. Kraus DM, Fischer JH, Reitz SJ, et al. Alterations in theophylline metabolism during the first year of life. *Clin Pharmacol Ther* 1993; 54:351–359.

79. Lelo A, Birkett DJ, Robson RA, Miners JO. Comparative pharmacokinetics of caffeine and its primary demethylated metabolites paraxanthine, theobromine and theophylline in man. *Br J Clin Pharmacol* 1986;22:177–182.

80. Campbell ME, Spielberg SP, Kalow W. A urinary metabolite ratio that reflects systemic caffeine clearance. *Clin Pharmacol Ther* 1987;42: 157–165.

81. Grygiel JJ, Birkett DJ. Effect of age on patterns of theophylline metabolism. *Clin Pharmacol Ther* 1980;28:456–462.

82. Blanchard J, Sawers SJA. Comparative pharmacokinetics of caffeine in young and elderly men. *J Pharmacokinet Biopharm* 1983;11: 109–126.

83. Nafziger AN, Bertino JS. Sex-related differences in theophylline pharmacokinetics. *Eur J Clin Pharmacol* 1989;37:97–100.

84. Aldridge A, Bailey J, Neims AH. The disposition of caffeine before and after pregnancy. *Semin Perinatol* 1981;5:310–314.

85. Miners JO, Birkett DJ. The use of caffeine as a metabolic probe for human drug metabolising enzymes. *Gen Pharmacol* 1996;27: 245–249.

86. Lelo A, Miners JO, Robson RA, Birkett DJ. Quantitative assessment of caffeine partial clearances in man. *Br J Clin Pharmacol* 1986;22: 183–186.

87. Tassaneeyakul W, Birkett DJ, McManus ME, et al. Caffeine metabolism by human hepatic cytochromes P450: contributions of 1A2, 2E1 and 3A isoforms. *Biochem Pharmacol* 1994;47:1767–1773.

88. Tarrus E, Cami J, Roberts DJ, Spickett RGW, Celdran E, Segura J. Accumulation of caffeine in healthy volunteers treated with furafylline. *Br J Clin Pharmacol* 1987;23:9–18.

89. Notarianni LJ, Oliver SJ, Bennet PN, Silverman BW. Caffeine as a metabolic probe: a comparison of the metabolic ratios used to assess CYP1A2 activity. *Br J Clin Pharmacol* 1995;39:65–69.

90. Denaro CP, Wilson M, Jacob P, Benowitz NL. Validation of urine caffeine metabolite ratios with use of stable isotope labelled caffeine clearance. *Clin Pharmacol Ther* 1996;59:284–296.

91. Fuhr U, Rost KL, Engelhardt R, et al. Evaluation of caffeine as a test drug for CYP1A2, NAT 2 and CYP2E1 phenotyping in man by *in vivo* versus *in vitro* correlations. *Pharmacogenetics* 1996;6:159–176.

92. Robson RA, Miners JO, Matthew AP, et al. Characterisation of theophylline metabolism by human liver microsomes: inhibition and immunochemical studies. *Biochem Pharmacol* 1988;37:1651–1659.

93. Gu L, Gonzalez FJ, Kalow W, Tang BK. Biotransformation of caffeine, paraxanthine, theobromine and theophylline by cDNA-expressed human CYP1A2 and CYP2E1. *Pharmacogenetics* 1992;2: 73–77.

94. Ha HR, Chen J, Freiburghaus AU, Follath F. Metabolism of theophylline by cDNA-expressed human cytochromes P450. *Br J Clin Pharmacol* 1995;39:321–326.

95. Rasmussen BB, Brosen K. Theophylline has no advantages over caffeine as a putative model drug for assessing CYP1A2 activity in humans. *Br J Clin Pharmacol* 1997;43:253–258.

96. Boobis AR, Kahn GC, Whyte C, Brodie MJ, Davies DS. Biphasic *O*-deethylation of phenacetin and 7-ethoxycoumarin by human and rat liver microsomal fractions. *Biochem Pharmacol* 1981;30:2451–2456.

97. Burke MD, Thompson S, Weaver RJ, Wolf CR, Mayer RT. Cytochrome P450 specificities of alkoxyresorufin O-dealkylation in human and rat liver. *Biochem Pharmacol* 1994;48:923–936.

98. Penman BW, Chen L, Gelboin HV, Gonzalez FJ, Crespi CL. Development of a human lymphoblastoid cell line constitutively expressing

99. Lee QP, Fantel AG, Juchau MR. Human embryonic cytochrome P450s: phenoxazone ethers as probes for expression of functional isoforms during organogenesis. *Biochem Pharmacol* 1991;42:2377–2385.

100. Rettie AE, Korzekwa KR, Kunze KL, et al. Hydroxylation of warfarin by cDNA-expressed cytochrome P450: a role for P4502C9 in the etiology of *S*-warfarin drug interactions. *Chem Res Toxicol* 1992;5: 54–59.

101. Zhang Z, Fasco M, Huang Z, Guengerich FP, Kaminskey LS. Human cytochromes P450 1A1 and 1A2: *R*-warfarin as a probe. *Drug Metab Disp* 1994;23:1339–1345.

102. Kunze KL, Trager WF. Isoform-selective mechanism based inhibition of human cytochrome P4501A2 by furafylline. *Chem Res Toxicol* 1993;6:649–656.

103. Yamazaki H, Inoue K, Mimura M, Oda Y, Guengerich FP, Shimada T. 7-ethoxycoumarin *O*-deethylation catalyzed by cytochromes P450 1A2 and 2E1 in human liver microsomes. *Biochem Pharmacol* 1996; 51:313–319.

104. McManus ME, Burgess WM, Veronese ME, Huggett A, Quattrochi LC, Tukey RH. Metabolism of 2-acetylaminofluorene and benzo(a)pyrene and activation of food-derived heterocyclic amine mutagens by human cytochromes P450. *Cancer Res* 1990;50: 3367–3376.

105. Bauer E, Guo Z, Ueng YF, Bell C, Zeldin D, Guengerich FP. Oxidation of benzo(a)pyrene by recombinant human cytochrome P450 enzymes. *Chem Res Toxicol* 1995;8:136–142.

106. Liu G, Gelboin HV, Myers MJ. Role of cytochrome P450 1A2 in acetanilide 4-hydroxylation as determined with cDNA expression and monoclonal antibodies. *Arch Biochem Biophys* 1991;284:400–406.

107. Spaldin V, Madden S, Woolf TF, Pool WF, Park BK. The effect of enzyme inhibition on the metabolism and activation of tacrine by human liver microsomes. *Br J Clin Pharmacol* 1994;38:15–22.

108. Spaldin V, Madden S, Adams DA, Edwards RJ, Davies DS, Park BK. Determination of human hepatic cytochrome P4501A2 activity *in vitro*: use of tacrine as an isoenzyme-specific probe. *Drug Metab Disp* 1995;23:929–934.

109. Sesardic D, Boobis AR, Murray BP, et al. Furafylline is a potent and selective inhibitor of cytochrome P4501A2 in man. *Br J Clin Pharmacol* 1990;29:651–663.

110. Clarke SE, Ayrton AD, Chenery RJ. Characterization of the inhibition of CYP1A2 by furafylline. *Xenobiotica* 1994;24:517–526.

111. Tassaneeyakul W, Birkett DJ, Veronese ME, McManus ME, Tukey RH, Miners JO. Direct characterization of the selectivity of furafylline as an inhibitor of cytochromes P450 1A1 and 1A2. *Pharmacogenetics* 1994;4:281–284.

112. Chang THK, Gonzalez FJ, Waxman DJ. Evaluation of triacetyloleandomycin, α-naphthoflavone and diethyldithiocarbamate as selective chemical probes for inhibition of human cytochromes P450. *Arch Biochem Biophys* 1994;311:437–442.

113. Jeppesen U, Loft S, Poulson HE, Brosen K. A fluvoxamine-caffeine interaction study. *Pharmacogenetics* 1996;6:213–222.

114. Rasmussen BB, Maenpaa J, Pelkonen O, et al. Selective serotonin reuptake inhibitors and theophylline metabolism in human liver microsomes: potent inhibition by fluvoxamine. *Br J Clin Pharmacol* 1995;39:151–159.

115. Pastrakuljic A, Tang B-K, Roberts EA, Kalow W. Distinction of CYP1A1 and CYP1A2 activity by selective inhibition using fluvoxamine and isosafrole. *Biochem Pharmacol* 1997;53:531–538.

116. Jeppesen U, Gram LF, Vistisen K, Loft S, Poulsen HE, Brosen K. Dose-dependent inhibition of CYP1A2, CYP2C19 and CYP2D6 by citalopram, fluoxetine, fluvoxamine and paroxetine. *Eur J Clin Pharmacol* 1996;51:73–78.

117. Jeppesen U, Rasmussen BB, Brosen K. Fluvoxamine inhibits the CYP2C19 catalyzed bioactivation of chloroguanide. *Clin Pharmacol Ther* 1997;62:279–286.

118. Adams DA, Edwards RJ, Davies DS, Boobis AR. Specific inhibition of human CYP1A2 using a targeted antibody. *Biochem Pharmacol* 1997;54:189–197.

CHAPTER 7

CYP2C

Allan E. Rettie, Dennis R. Koop, and Robert L. Haining

INTRODUCTION

The cytochrome P450s are a superfamily of oxidative enzymes involved in the metabolism of endogenous compounds as well as the metabolic clearance of a variety of drugs and other xenobiotics (1). Oxidative metabolism of xenobiotics is carried out principally by members of the CYP1, CYP2, CYP3, and CYP4 families, of which the CYP2C subfamily is the most complex in mammalian species (2). The CYP2C subfamily is composed of at least four members, CYP2C8, CY2C9, CYP2C18, and CYP2C19, the genes for which are located together on chromosome 10 (3–5).

This review will deal with each of these four isoforms in terms of (a) their initial identification, tissue distribution, and physical properties; (b) substrate specificity; (c) pharmacogenetic variability; and (d) regulation of expression and catalytic function.

IDENTIFICATION, PHYSICAL PROPERTIES, AND TISSUE DISTRIBUTION

Purification and cDNA Cloning

The revolution in our understanding of the enzymes composing the CYP2C subfamily that has occurred over the last 10 years is due to a combination of knowledge derived from classic protein-purification procedures, complementary DNA (cDNA) cloning, and heterologous expression of the individual genes. The first isolation of these enzymes from human liver, which provided N-terminal sequence data consistent with their placement in the

A. E. Rettie and R. L. Haining: Department of Medicinal Chemistry, University of Washington, Box 357610 H172 Health Sciences Building, Seattle, Washington 98195

D. R. Koop: Department of Physiology and Pharmacology, Oregon Health Sciences University, 3181 SW Sam Jackson Park Road, Portland, Oregon 97201

CYP2C family, was reported in the middle to late 1980s for CYP2C8 (6,7) and CYP2C9 (7,8). N-terminal sequencing data were critical for matching the purified proteins to the sequences of cDNA clones that were being isolated at that time for CYP2C8 (9,10) and CYP2C9/10 (10,11). CYP2C10, which differs from wild-type CYP2C9 (Tyr358, Gly417) at only two amino acid positions (Cys358, Asp417), is now believed to be a cloning artifact, because extensive genotyping studies have not detected mutant alleles at either locus in either white or Asian populations (12,13). In the ensuing years, cDNAs for CYP2C18 and CYP2C19 also were described (14,15) and CYP2C19 purified eventually from human liver by Wrighton et al. (16). However, isolation of these enzymes from human tissues is not a trivial endeavor. This approach requires substantial quantities of nonpostmortem tissue, is laborious, and has yet to yield purified samples of CYP2C18, which is expressed at very low levels in human liver (17). Therefore, several laboratories have reported the heterologous expression of the human CYP2Cs in a variety of cell systems, notably yeast (18,19), *Escherichia coli* (20,21), and insect cells (22–24).

Physical Properties

The expression of recombinant CYP2C8, CYP2C9, CYP2C18, and CYP2C19 from heterologous systems yields proteins that exhibit Soret maxima at 451 nm, 450 nm, 450.5 nm, and 452 nm, respectively, for the reduced-carbon monoxide difference spectra (21,25). Despite very small differences in molecular weights calculated from protein sequences deduced from the individual cDNA sequences, the purified human CYP2C proteins migrate on sodium dodecylsulfate–polyacrylamide gel electrophoresis (SDS-PAGE) gels (Fig. 7-1) with apparent molecular masses of 55 kDa (CYP2C9), 53.5 kDa (CYP2C8), 52.5 kDa (CYP2C18), and 52 kDa (CYP2C19). This discrete migration behavior has facilitated the immunoquantitation of these isoforms in human tissues.

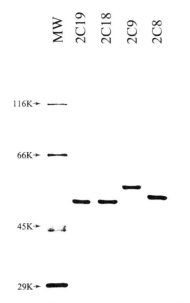

FIG. 7-1. Sodium dodecylsulfate–polyacrylamide gel electrophoresis (SDS-PAGE) of purified human CYP2C isoforms (10 pmol each) expressed and isolated from the baculovirus/*T. ni.* expression system according to procedures detailed in Haining RL, Hunter AP, Veronese ME, Trager WF, Rettie AE. Allelic variants of human cytochrome P450 2C9: baculovirus-mediated expression, purification, structural characterization, substrate stereoselectivity, and prochiral selectivity of the wild-type and I359L mutant forms. *Arch Biochem Biophys* 1996;333:447–458.

Tissue Expression

The absolute quantitation of the CYP2C isoforms present in human liver microsomes has been reported by several laboratories (17,26,27). CYP2C9 is clearly the most abundant CYP2C protein expressed among the various samples analyzed, with estimates ranging from 40 ± 10 pmol/mg, n = 6 (15) to 89 ± 9 pmol/mg, n = 17 (27). This isoform also exhibited the least variation in protein expression levels. Richardson et al. (17) found mean levels of CYP2C8 and CYP2C19 in most samples of 19 ± 9 pmol/mg (n = 5) and 27 ± 5 pmol/mg (n = 4), respectively, although some microsomal preparations showed CYP2C8 and CYP2C19 levels as high as 70 pmol/mg. Similar absolute levels and variability have also been reported by Lasker et al. (27). The CYP2C18 protein concentration was below detection limits, less than 2.5 pmol/mg, in the one study that examined this isoform, a finding that probably explains why this is the only member of the CYP2C subfamily that has not been isolated directly from human liver tissue.

Clearly, CYP2C9 is the dominant human CYP2C isoform, accounting for up to 30% of the total hepatic P450 content (27). A minimal CYP2C9 promoter is located between the translation start site and nucleotide −155 (28). This region contains an HPF-1 domain consensus sequence to which nuclear proteins have been shown to bind. Therefore, Ibeanu and Goldstein (28) have suggested that the HPF-1 site is an important *cis*-acting element that directs hepatic expression of CYP2C9.

Although messenger RNA (mRNA) for one or other of the CYP2C isoforms is detectable by sensitive reverse transcription–polymerase chain reaction (RT-PCR) procedures in a wide variety of tissues including human breast tissue (29), brain (30), bronchoalveolar macrophages (31), and placenta (32), convincing demonstrations of significant levels of CYP2C protein in human extrahepatic tissues is limited. It is notable that two members of the CYP2C family have been purified recently from rabbit intestine (33). In addition, it has been shown that immunoreactive CYP2C9 and CYP2C19 are readily detected in human intestinal microsomes (34).

Currently there is considerable interest in human gut P450 metabolism because of the potential for some drugs to undergo prehepatic first-pass extraction in the intestine, thereby limiting their oral bioavailability. However, it is not clear at present whether this in vivo phenomenon extends to substrates for isoforms other than CYP3A4 (see Chapter 10).

SUBSTRATE SPECIFICITY

Arachidonic Acid

Comparison of the cDNA sequences for the human CYP2Cs reveals that the four proteins share 89% to 96% amino acid homologies (25). Therefore, it is not surprising that several compounds are substrates for more than one of the isoforms. However, a relatively rare example of metabolic reactions that all four human CYP2C isoforms have in common is the epoxidation of arachidonic acid (AA). This endogenous substrate is epoxidized by CYP2C8, CYP2C9, and CYP2C19 to characteristic mixtures of the 8,9-, 11,12-, and 14,15-epoxides (35–37), and we have found recently that CYP2C18 is also an efficient AA epoxygenase. Comparative high-performance liquid chromatography (HPLC) radiochromatograms for each of the four purified human CYP2C isoforms are shown in Fig. 7-2. CYP2C9 and CYP2C18 exhibit almost identical profiles, with the AA 14,15-epoxide metabolite predominating. In contrast, CYP2C8 forms equivalent amounts of only the 11,12- and 14,15-epoxides. CYP2C19 generates all four isomers, but the 8,9- and 14,15-epoxides predominate.

The stereoselectivity of AA epoxide formation has been investigated for CYP2C8 and CYP2C9 (34,38). The chirality of AA epoxide metabolites generated by CYP2C8 matched that of the enantiomers present *in vivo* in human kidney cortex (39). As a consequence, it has been suggested that CYP2C8 is at least partly responsible for the metabolism of endogenous AA pools (38). How-

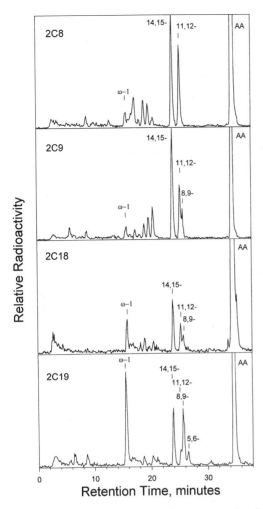

FIG. 7-2. High-performance liquid chromatography (HPLC) radiochromatograms depicting the ω-1-hydroxy, 14,15-, 11,12-, 8,9-, and 5,6-epoxide arachidonic acid metabolites formed by each purified human CYP2C according to methods described in Daikh BE, Lasker JM, Raucy JL, Koop DR. Regio- and stereoselective epoxidation of arachidonic acid by human cytochromes P450 2C8 and 2C9. *J Pharmacol Exp Ther* 1994;271:1427–1433.

ever, the vast majority of known substrates for the human CYP2C isoforms are not endogenous compounds. In the following section, each isoform's substrate specificity toward drugs and other xenobiotics is discussed on an individual basis.

Substrate Specificity of CYP2C8

The prototypic substrate for CYP2C8 is taxol (paclitaxel). The major metabolite of the drug formed in human is 6α-hydroxypaclitaxel, and *in vitro* studies have shown that this metabolite is formed selectively, and with relatively high affinity, only by CYP2C8 (21,40). In addition, several studies have demonstrated excellent correlations between immunoreactive levels of

CYP2C8 and the rate of formation of 6α-hydroxypaclitaxel in human liver microsomes (21,41); therefore taxol can be considered to be a diagnostic substrate probe for this isoform.

CYP2C8 also has the capacity to metabolize benzphetamine (6), retinoic acid (42), tolbutamide (43), benzo(a)pyrene (44), carbamazepine (45), and (R)-ibuprofen (41), although it may not be the dominant metabolic isoform for any of these substrates. Therefore, CYP2C8 appears to have the narrowest substrate specificity of the three CYP2C isoforms expressed at significant levels in human liver.

Xenobiotic Substrates for CYP2C9

The characteristic feature of CYP2C9 catalysis is the preference exhibited by this isoform for a wide range of weakly acidic drugs. Of special note is the CYP2C9-mediated metabolism of the low therapeutic index drugs, tolbutamide (43), (S)-warfarin (46), and phenytoin (47), because decreases in the clearance of these drugs, as a consequence of either genetic factors or concomitant administration of alternate substrates or inhibitors, can have profound clinical consequences.

Warfarin

The anticoagulant agent warfarin is administered as a racemic mixture, although the (S) enantiomer is responsible for the bulk of the therapeutic activity (48). In humans, (S)-warfarin is eliminated principally by hydroxylation on the coumarin nucleus at the 7-position (49). Early studies with human liver microsomes identified a high-affinity P450 enzyme component responsible for (S)-warfarin 7-hydroxylation (50). Subsequent kinetic studies with recombinant enzymes and the inhibitor sulfaphenazole identified CYP2C9 as the principal isoform involved in the conversion of (S)-warfarin to its inactive 6-hydroxy and 7-hydroxy metabolites (46).

CYP2C9 does not detectably metabolize (R)-warfarin [less than 5% of the rate of metabolism of (S)-warfarin]; however, the (R) enantiomer is an effective inhibitor of CYP2C9 with a K_i of approximately 7 μM (51). This K_i value is approximately equal to the K_m for (S)-warfarin, which indicates that both enantiomers have a similar affinity for the enzyme, but that the binding orientation of the (R) enantiomer is such that efficient oxygen transfer to this substrate is precluded.

Warfarin is a coumarin anticoagulant; however, coumarin itself is not a substrate for CYP2C9, instead being metabolized by CYP2A6 at the 7-position on the coumarin ring (52). Both CYP2C9 and CYP2A6 cosegregate in terms of the human isoform selectivity for metabolism of valproic acid (53). Therefore, it is possible that CYP2C9 and CYP2A6 share some common electrostatic determinants of substrate binding.

Phenytoin and Related Hydantoins

The anticonvulsant agent, phenytoin (diphenylhydantoin), is a prochiral molecule whose major primary pathway of metabolism in humans is aromatic hydroxylation on the pro-S phenyl group to form (S)-5-(4-hydroxyphenyl)-5-phenylhydantoin [(S)-p-HPPH) (54,55)]. CYP2C9 exhibits high affinity for phenytoin and catalyzes the hydroxylation reaction in vitro with the prochiral stereoselectivity observed in vivo (56).

Mephenytoin (3-methyl-5-ethyl-5-phenylhydantoin) is a chiral anticonvulsant compound, closely related in structure to phenytoin. (S)-mephenytoin is a substrate for CYP2C9, but unlike phenytoin, it is not detectably metabolized on the aromatic ring by CYP2C9. Instead, CYP2C9 directs metabolism to the hydantoin ring, forming nirvanol slowly by N-demethylation (57). In contrast, (S)-mephenytoin is rapidly p-hydroxylated by CYP2C19 (16,18). The structural features of these hydantoin ligands that dictate whether CYP2C9 or CYP2C19 dominates their metabolism have not been clearly delineated. However, limited in vivo data suggest that N-alkylation of the hydantoin ring may bias metabolism in favor of CYP2C9 (58).

Tolbutamide

The sulfonylurea hypoglycemic agent tolbutamide is metabolized in vivo in humans almost exclusively by CYP2C9-mediated benzylic hydroxylation (59). In vitro studies have shown that both CYP2C8 and CYP2C19 also have the capacity to generate this metabolite (21,43,60,61). However, the selectivity exhibited in vivo for CYP2C9 is likely a combination of higher K_m values and relatively lower expression levels of these two enzymes relative to CYP2C9. Torasemide, a loop diuretic agent related structurally to tolbutamide, also undergoes CYP2C9-mediated benzylic hydroxylation (62). As noted in a recent review by Miners and Birkett (63), it seems likely that CYP2C9 will also contribute to the metabolism of other chemically related oral hypoglycemic agents and diuretic agents.

Tienilic acid

Tienilic acid (TA) is a uricosuric diuretic agent that was withdrawn from the United States market in 1980 because of an unacceptable incidence (1:10,000) of immunoallergic hepatitis (64). TA-induced hepatitis has been associated with the appearance, in patient serum, of circulating anti-liver and anti-kidney microsomal type 2 autoantibodies (65), which are directed against a three-site conformational epitope on CYP2C9 (66). Oxidation of TA is catalyzed selectively by CYP2C9, which forms 5-hydroxy TA as the major stable metabolite (67). It has been proposed that CYP2C9 first generates an electrophilic thiophene sulfoxide, which reacts either with water to yield 5-hydroxy TA, or with a nucleophilic amino acid residue of CYP2C9 to form the covalent adduct, which serves as the starting point for the production of autoantibodies (68).

Other Carboxylate-containing Substrates

The arylacetic and arylpropionic acids represent an important class of nonsteroidal antiinflammatory drugs (NSAIDs). Several members of this therapeutic group, including diclofenac (69,70), flurbiprofen (71), and naproxen (72) are hydroxylated or O-demethylated selectively by CYP2C9. Ibuprofen (41) and piroxicam (T.S. Tracy, personal communication, 1998) also are good, but less selective, substrates for CYP2C9, because they are metabolized to a significant extent by other CYP2C isoforms, particularly at high substrate concentrations. In addition, valproic acid is hydroxylated and desaturated by CYP2C9 (53), although oxidation is a relatively minor clearance pathway for this anticonvulsant drug.

Molecular Modeling of CYP2C9 Active Site

The distinctive substrate specificity of CYP2C9 has prompted several efforts to model the active site of the enzyme. Because many of the substrates discussed earlier exist as anions at physiologic pH, Mancy et al. (73) have considered that a cationic site exists on the protein that interacts with the anionic site on the ligand. Early modeling studies, which focused largely on TA derivatives, generated a model for the substrate binding site of CYP2C9 in which the distance between the hydroxylation site and the putative anionic site was 7.8 ± 1.8 angstroms, and the angle between these loci was 82 ± 15 degrees (73). Alternatively, the substrate specificity has been rationalized in terms of a hydrogen bond donor/acceptor model in which the distance between the ligand's hydrogen bond donor heteroatom and the site of metabolism is 6.7 ± 1.0 angstroms, and the angle is 133 ± 21 degrees (74). Our group has generated a CoMFA model for CYP2C9 ligands by using more than 20 coumarin structures of defined stereochemistry (75). Because not all good ligands for the enzyme are obligate anions at physiologic pH, this view of the active site of CYP2C9 highlights areas of positive charge donation on the enzyme, as well as sites for π–π interaction between the enzyme and the nonmetabolized C-9 phenyl ring of the coumarin derivatives. Site-directed mutagenesis studies suggest that the latter interaction may occur with Phe114 on CYP2C9 (76). In addition, it has become clear that residues Lys241, Ser286, and Asn289 are critical determinants of the CYP2C9 selectivity for carboxylate-containing drugs (70,77).

Substrate Specificity of CYP2C18

Very few xenobiotic substrates have been identified for CYP2C18. The enzyme can function as a low K_m diazepam N-demethylase (78) and appears to have some minor capacity to hydroxylate omeprazole and lansoprazole (79,80), at least *in vitro*. Mansuy's group (81) demonstrated that CYP2C18 is as effective a catalyst of TA 5-hydroxylation as CYP2C9. However, at present there is no evidence that CYP2C18 contributes to the clearance of any of these drugs *in vivo*.

Substrate Specificity of CYP2C19

The prototypic substrate for this isoform is (*S*)-mephenytoin, which undergoes *p*-hydroxylation on its aromatic ring by CYP2C19 but not to any significant extent by CYP2C8, CYP2C9, or CYP2C18 (18). The exclusive participation of CYP2C19 in this metabolic pathway is the basis for the use of (*S*)-mephenytoin as an *in vivo* probe drug for phenotyping CYP2C19 status (82).

Omeprazole

The antiulcer drug omeprazole is also an effective probe drug for CYP2C19 status in humans when the 5-hydroxylation pathway is analyzed (83,84). The corresponding *in vitro* studies with recombinant CYP2C enzymes suggest slightly less CYP2C19 specificity than is observed for (*S*)-mephenytoin (80). Similar results have been reported for lansoprazole 5-hydroxylation (85).

Diazepam

CYP2C19 catalyzes both N-demethylation and C-3 ring hydroxylation of diazepam (78). Several other human P450 isoforms can catalyze diazepam metabolism (86); however, analysis of *in vitro* kinetic parameters and the effects of isoform-selective inhibitors suggests that CYP2C19 and CYP3A4 are the principal contributors to diazepam N-demethylation at low substrate concentration in human liver microsomes (78).

Proguanil

Metabolism of the antimalarial drug proguanil to its cyclized active metabolite, cycloguanil, exhibits widespread interindividual variability, which cosegregates with the (S)-mephenytoin polymorphism (87,88). However, in vitro studies with recombinant enzymes have not yet been reported.

Enzymatic Determinants of CYP2C19 Substrate Specificity

These examples illustrate a major difference in the substrate specificities of CYP2C19 and CYP2C9, in that

CYP2C19 readily accepts basic and neutral drugs that are not substrates for CYP2C9 (25). Site-directed mutagenesis studies have shown that replacement of amino acids 99, 220, and 221 of CYP2C9 with the corresponding residues from CYP2C19 is sufficient to convert CYP2C9 into a high-activity omeprazole 5-hydroxylase (89). Interestingly, the high omeprazole activity CYP2C9 mutant did not metabolize (S)-mephenytoin. This suggests that omeprazole and (S)-mephenytoin make contact with different subsets of amino acids within the active site of CYP2C19.

PHARMACOGENETIC VARIABILITY

Chromosome Localization

The CYP2C subfamily is clustered together on chromosome 10q1.24, from centromere to telomere in the order: 2C18, 2C19, 2C9, and 2C8 (3). Cursory examination of the data available on the genetically determined expression of these enzymes reveals the CYP2C subfamily to be a veritable lexicon on polymorphic variability. This encompasses traditional population pharmacogenetics, in which deviations from unimodality are evident from examination of a drug's pharmacokinetics in relatively small numbers of subjects [e.g., the CYP2C19-dependent (S)-mephenytoin polymorphism], and the current trend in "reverse pharmacogenetics," in which DNA sequence analysis can be the first indicator of polymorphism, and analysis of any metabolic consequences occurs secondary to identification of the molecular basis for the defect.

CYP2C19 Pharmacogenetics

Mephenytoin is an anticonvulsant hydantoin drug administered as a racemic mixture. In humans, the (S)-enantiomer is usually eliminated rapidly by aromatic hydroxylation (90). However, in whites, 2% to 5% of individuals exhibit an (S)-mephenytoin hydroxylation defect (91,92). Subsequent studies showed that this defect was more prevalent in Asians, where 13% to 23% of individuals were affected (93,94). The deficient pathway for these mephenytoin "poor metabolizers" (PMs) was one of aromatic hydroxylation, which implicated a P450 enzyme, but one which clinical pharmacology studies were quick to show was distinct from that responsible for the debrisoquine PM phenotype described in the late 1970s (91,95,96). As a consequence, much of the research on the CYP2C subfamily conducted throughout the 1980s was driven by the goal of elucidating the identity of this human liver (S)-mephenytoin hydroxylase. However, this proved to be a highly demanding task because of the close structural, immunochemical, and catalytic similarities between this isoform and other members of the CYP2C subfamily (97). Nevertheless, by 1991, Guengerich's group (98) were able to conclude that the protein involved in polymorphic (S)-mephenytoin 4'-hydroxylation was closely related to, but distinct from, CYP2C8, CYP2C9, and CYP2C10. In the same year, CYP2C18 was cloned from human liver (14,15), and for a brief period, this isoform attracted attention as the putative (S)-mephenytoin hydroxylase (15). However, this complex situation was finally resolved by the demonstration, using all of the cDNA-expressed human CYP2C isoforms, that stereoselective hydroxylation of (S)-mephenytoin was catalyzed only by CYP2C19 (18).

The major molecular genetic defect responsible for the (S)-mephenytoin polymorphism is as a single G→A mutation in exon 5 of CYP2C19 (CYP2C9*2), which creates an aberrant splice site (99). This shifts the reading frame, introduces a premature stop codon, and generates a truncated, inactive protein. Goldstein's group (100) have also characterized the CYP2C19*3 allele, a premature stop codon in exon 4, which occurs only in Asians. The CYP2C19*2 and CYP2C19*3 alleles account for more than 99% of Asian PM alleles, but only about 85% of white PM alleles (101). Two additional rare alleles, CYP2C19*4, a mutation in the initiation codon, and CYP2C19*5, an Arg433→Trp mutation in the heme-binding region that abolishes enzyme activity, have recently been described (102,103). Collectively, these five null alleles account for more than 90% of the mephenytoin PM alleles in whites and essentially all of the Asian PMs.

CYP2C9 Pharmacogenetics

Although several variant CYP2C9 cDNAs have been isolated from human liver libraries (5,10,11,15,47,104), extensive PCR-based analysis of human genomic DNA has provided convincing evidence only for expression of the R144C (CYP2C9*2) and I359L (CYP2C9*3) allelic variants (12,13). These two alleles exhibit ethnic differences in expression, and initial indications from genotyping experiments are that higher mutant allele frequencies occur in whites (about 10%) than in Chinese or African-American populations (fewer than 2%) (12,105).

Functional Consequences for Expression of CYP2C9 Alleles

Unlike the CYP2C19 defects described earlier, both CYP2C9*2 and CYP2C9*3 are non-null alleles, in that they code for functional protein, albeit with reduced levels of enzyme activity (22,61,105,106). This reduction in catalytic efficiency is most marked for CYP2C9*3 (22,105), because, in addition to significant decreases in

V_{max} for a given substrate, apparent K_m values increase markedly relative to the wild-type enzyme. Consequently, in vitro determinations of catalytic efficiency (V/K) suggest that in vivo clearances of a CYP2C9 substrate could be decreased by more than 10-fold if an individual carries two copies of the CYP2C9*3 gene (22).

There are several excellent in vivo correlates of the in vitro data for CYP2C9*3. At least one phenotypic tolbutamide PM has been shown to be homozygous for CYP2C9*3 (105). In addition, a patient who was found to be ultrasensitive to the anticoagulant effects of warfarin in the clinic was genotyped as homozygous for CYP2C9*3 (107).

This polymorphism has also caused complications during drug development. Losartan, a CYP2C9 substrate (108), was found to exhibit anomalous pharmacokinetics in two patients from a cohort of 200 who were given the investigational drug during late clinical trials. These two individuals did not metabolize the compound appreciably to its major acid metabolite, and subsequently both were genotyped as homozygous for CYP2C9*3 (109). One of these patients consented to further studies involving tolbutamide and phenytoin, and, as expected, the half-lives for both of these CY2C9 probe substrates were found to be substantially prolonged.

Even CYP2C9*1*3 heterozygotes may have pharmacogenetically determined alterations in drug response. Studies conducted recently in Japanese heart disease patients have shown that the oral clearance of (S)-warfarin is reduced in heterozygotes relative to a control wild-type population (110).

In contrast, the clinical significance of expression of the CYP2C9*2 allele is much less clear. Although in vitro studies with the recombinant variant consistently find K_m values to be unaltered (61,105), the effect on V_{max} has been reported to vary greatly. Crespi et al. (106) suggested that this variability could be expression-system dependent and reflective of different degrees of saturation of CYP2C9*2 with cytochrome P450 reductase, either coexpressed with the P450 or added exogenously. In vivo studies are sparse and have been conducted, to date, only with *1*2 heterozygotes. Furuya et al. (112) reported a small decrease in the median maintenance dose of warfarin in heterozygotes carrying the *2 allele. This is consistent with reduced warfarin metabolism catalyzed by the CYP2C9*2 gene product. However, because no *2*2 homozygotes were evaluated, and the patients were not genotyped for the *3 allele, the study remains inconclusive. Interestingly, one tolbutamide PM has been reported to be a mixed, *2*3 heterozygote (105). Therefore at present, the weight of available evidence suggests that expression of the CYP2C9*2 allele probably does cause a minor reduction in the metabolic clearance of at least some substrates, but the magnitude of this effect is small relative to that caused by the CYP2C9*3 allele.

CYP2C8 Variability

Although there are no clinical indicators of a CYP2C8 polymorphism in humans, several studies are suggestive of bimodality in the expression of immunoreactive CYP2C8 in human liver (6,15,42). Whereas the majority of microsomal preparations that have been analyzed vary by about fivefold, occasional samples have been identified in which little or no immunoreactive CYP2C8 is present (15,27). The factors underlying these extremes in expression of CYP2C8 are unknown.

Although the various cDNAs that have been cloned for CYP2C8 do display a degree of microheterogeneity (9,10,15,21), studies have not been conducted to determine whether these single nucleotide polymorphisms occur at any significant frequency in the human population, or whether these (putative) allelic variants possess altered catalytic properties.

CYP2C18 Polymorphisms

At least one allelic variant of the enzyme (Thr/Met385) has been cloned (15), and a nonfunctional allele detected in the Japanese population (113). In addition, polymorphic variability in the 5′-upstream regulatory region has been reported for the enzyme. This has attracted some (academic) interest because it appears to cosegregate with the CYP2C19*2 polymorphism (114). However, in the absence of convincing evidence for either expression of CYP2C18 protein or the existence of specific drug substrates for the enzyme, no case can be made for significant clinical consequences as a result of any CYP2C18 polymorphism(s).

REGULATION OF CYP2C EXPRESSION AND CATALYTIC FUNCTION

Developmental Regulation

Immunoreactive CYP2C proteins are not expressed at detectable levels in human fetal liver microsomes (115,116) but, like many hepatic P450 proteins, appear in the first few weeks after birth, reaching about 50% of the adult concentration by age 1 year (117). Interestingly, when the expression levels of various P450 isoforms were examined in postmortem liver samples from sudden infant death syndrome (SIDS) infants, immunoreactive CYP2C levels were increased markedly relative to controls (118). These authors speculated that the enhanced expression of CYP2C proteins in SIDS might be linked to an increase in levels of AA epoxide metabolites, which could conceivably relax pulmonary smooth muscle sufficiently to induce a fatal apnea.

Induction

At present, the effect that well-recognized P450 inducers such as rifampin and phenobarbital have on the induc-

tion of the individual human CYP2C isoforms can probably best be assessed by evaluating the available clinical literature, which is replete with studies describing inducer–drug interactions with CYP2C-selective substrates. This topic has been reviewed recently, at least for CYP2C9 (63), and so only a few additional salient points are discussed here.

As noted earlier, (S)-warfarin clearance to the major 7-hydroxy and 6-hydroxy metabolites is a CYP2C9-dependent process in humans. Trager and coworkers (119) have shown that rifampin increases the formation clearance of both of these metabolites approximately threefold. Rifampin effects of a similar magnitude have also been found for losartan, phenytoin, and tolbutamide (63), suggesting that commonly used rifampin dosing regimens (450 to 1,200 mg daily) are likely to cause clinically important interactions with other CYP2C9 substrates. Clinical data also suggest that rifampin significantly induces CYP2C19, because dosing patients with 600 mg rifampin for 22 days increased their urinary excretion of 4′-hydroxymephenytoin by 40% to 180% in mephenytoin extensive metabolizers (EMs), but not PMs (120).

The effect of barbiturates on CYP2C-dependent metabolism is less clear. Although total warfarin blood levels are decreased and anticoagulant effect diminished in patients receiving phenobarbital, amylobarbital, or secobarbital (121), studies examining the disposition of (S)-warfarin have not been performed to allow the conclusion that CYP2C9, specifically, is induced by barbiturates. Moreover, phenobarbital is reported to have little effect on the disposition of losartan (122) or phenytoin (123, 124). However, interpretation of these studies might be complicated by the fact that phenobarbital is known to alter liver mass and liver blood flow. Primary cultures of human hepatocytes may be a valuable tool for studying the response of specific human P450 isoforms to various xenobiotics, because the system lends itself to a more mechanistic, molecular approach to the question of isoform inducibility. However, the method is technically demanding and has been limited by the availability of suitable tissue preparations. Nonetheless, Li et al. (125) have been able to demonstrate a consistent induction of CYP3A proteins by the well-characterized inducer, rifampin, and so, with this important positive control in place, it should be possible soon to extend this method to other P450 enzymes, including the human CYP2Cs.

Purification and cDNA cloning studies indicate that at least two CYP2C isoforms are expressed in monkey liver, one more closely related to human CYP2C9 and the other to human CYP2C19 (126). Treatment of patas and cynomologus monkeys with phenobarbital in their drinking water for 14 days, to a final dosage of 15 mg/kg body weight, resulted in about a twofold induction of an immunoreactive CYP2C protein in these nonhuman primates (127). Unfortunately, the identity of the specific CYP2C isoform induced by phenobarbital was not elucidated. It is possible that nonhuman primates may represent a useful *in vivo* model for induction of the human CYP2C isoforms, although a clearer understanding of the relationship between orthologous human and monkey CYP2C isoforms is desirable. Both of these latter approaches offer the possibility of studying primate CYP2C induction events at the mRNA level, which may be particularly useful for CYP2C8 and CYP2C18, for which no induction data are currently available.

Finally, CYP2C9 enzyme activity has been demonstrated recently to be activated *in vitro* by dapsone and some related compounds (72). However, the *in vivo* significance of this finding remains to be established.

Inhibition

CYP2C8 and CYP2C18

No diagnostic inhibitors for these two isoforms are in general use. However, Mansuy (128) reported preliminary studies on the development of compounds related to TA, which interact selectively with CYP2C18. Further development of these analogues may ultimately provide useful *in vitro* tools for selectively inhibiting both CYP2C8 and CYP2C18.

CYP2C9

Sulfaphenazole is the prototypic inhibitor for CYP2C9. It acts in a competitive fashion with an apparent K_i for CYP2C9 of about 200 nM (46,129,130). In contrast, sulfaphenazole is at least a hundredfold less potent an inhibitor of the other human P450 isoforms, including CYP2C8, CYP2C18, and CYP2C19 (81). Consequently, sulfaphenazole is widely used to diagnose whether CYP2C9 is a contributor to *in vitro* metabolism catalyzed by human liver microsomes.

Inhibition of CYP2C9 activity *in vivo* can give rise to clinically significant interactions because several key drug substrates for the enzyme have low therapeutic indices. A notable example is the anticoagulant drug warfarin. Inhibition of the CYP2C9-dependent metabolic clearance of the more biologically potent (S)-enantiomer significantly increases the risk of serious hemorrhage. This phenomenon has been documented *in vivo* for sulfinpyrazone (49), phenylbutazone (131), fluconazole (132), amiodarone (133), and miconazole (134). Many of these compounds also predictably inhibit the metabolism of phenytoin, tolbutamide, and several other CYP2C9 substrates both *in vivo* and *in vitro* [see review article (63) for a full discussion of CYP2C9 inhibitors].

CYP2C19

No high-affinity, diagnostic inhibitors have been identified for CYP2C19. *In vitro* studies generally use the prototypic substrate, (S)-mephenytoin, at concentrations ranging from 50 to 250 μM when it is necessary to evaluate the participation of CYP2C19 in human liver microsomal catalysis. An alternative selective *in vitro* inhibitor of CYP2C19 may be the investigational antiepileptic drug, topiramate (135). An earlier suggestion that tranylcypromine could be used in this capacity (136) may not be valid because it is also a potent inhibitor of CYP2C9 (137).

In vivo observations demonstrate that fluvoxamine (138) and omeprazole (139) exert inhibitory effects on the bioactivation of proguanil and chloroguanide, although these two compounds are clearly not isoform-selective inhibitors of CYP2C19. Inhibition of CYP2C19-catalyzed metabolism *in vivo* has also been invoked to explain drug–drug interactions arising from coadministration of phenytoin with omeprazole, felbamate, fluoxetine, imipramine, diazepam, and cimetidine (140).

CONCLUDING REMARKS AND FUTURE DIRECTIONS

In terms of rationalizing the substrate specificity and potential for inhibitory drug interactions involving the human CYP2C isoforms, it is clear that the availability of high-resolution structures beyond those constructed by the iterative interplay of molecular modeling, site-directed mutagenesis, and nuclear magnetic resonance (NMR) ligand studies will have the greatest impact. Progress toward this goal is incremental but has been spurred recently by advances in the molecular engineering of the CYP2C enzymes such as the functional expression of soluble bacterial P450–CYP2C hybrids (141) and progress toward the preparation of truncated, soluble monomeric CYP2C isoforms (142). Ultimately these approaches can be expected to provide protein targets that may prove amenable to crystallization or to structural elucidation by NMR.

ACKNOWLEDGMENT

We thank Drs. F.J. Gonzalez, M.E. Veronese, and J.A. Goldstein for the provision of cDNAs for each of the human CYP2C isoforms. We also acknowledge Ms. Bethany Klopfenstein for assistance with the arachidonic assay metabolite assays. This work was supported in part by National Institutes of Health Grant GM32165 (A.E.R.) and AA08608 (D.R.K.).

REFERENCES

1. Nelson DR, Koymans L, Kamataki T, et al. P450 superfamily: update on new sequences, gene mapping, accession numbers and nomenclature. *Pharmacogenetics* 1996;6:1–42.
2. Gonzalez FJ, Nebert DW. Evolution of the P450 gene superfamily: animal-plant "warfare," molecular drive and human genetic differences in drug oxidation. *Trends Genet* 1990;6:182–186.

3. Gray IC, Nobile C, Muresu R, Ford S, Spurr NK. A 2.4-megabase physical map spanning the CYP2C gene cluster on chromosome 10q24. *Genomics* 1995;28:328–332.

4. Inoue K, Inazawa J, Suzuki Y, et al. Fluorescence in situ hybridization analysis of chromosomal localization of three human cytochrome P450 2C genes (CYP2C8, 2C9, and 2C10) at 10q24.1. *Jpn J Hum Genet* 1994;39:337–343.

5. Meehan RR, Gosden JR, Rout D, et al. Human cytochrome P-450 PB-1: a multigene family involved in mephenytoin and steroid oxidations that maps to chromosome 10. *Am J Hum Genet* 1988;42:26–37.

6. Wrighton SA, Thomas PE, Willis P, et al. Purification of a human liver cytochrome P-450 immunochemically related to several cytochromes P-450 purified from untreated rats. *J Clin Invest* 1987; 80:1017–1022.

7. Lasker JM, Raucy J, Kubota S, Bloswick BP, Black M, Lieber CS. Purification and characterization of human liver cytochrome P-450-ALC. *Biochem Biophys Res Commun* 1987;148:232–238.

8. Shimada T, Misono KS, Guengerich FP. Human liver microsomal cytochrome P-450 mephenytoin 4-hydroxylase, a prototype of genetic polymorphism in oxidative drug metabolism: purification and characterization of two similar forms involved in the reaction. *J Biol Chem* 1986;261:909–921.

9. Okino ST, Quattrochi LC, Pendurthi UR, McBride OW, Tukey RH. Characterization of multiple human cytochrome P-450 1 cDNAs: the chromosomal localization of the gene and evidence for alternate RNA splicing (published erratum appears in *J Biol Chem* 1988;263:2576). *J Biol Chem* 1987;262:16072–16079.

10. Kimura S, Pastewka J, Gelboin HV, Gonzalez FJ. cDNA and amino acid sequences of two members of the human P450IIC gene subfamily. *Nucleic Acids Res* 1987;15:10053–10054.

11. Umbenhauer DR, Martin MV, Lloyd RS, Guengerich FP. Cloning and sequence determination of a complementary DNA related to human liver microsomal cytochrome P-450 S-mephenytoin 4-hydroxylase. *Biochemistry* 1987;26:1094–1099.

12. Wang SL, Huang J, Lai MD, Tsai JJ. Detection of CYP2C9 polymorphism based on the polymerase chain reaction in Chinese. *Pharmacogenetics* 1995;5:37–42.

13. Stubbins MJ, Harries LW, Smith G, Tarbit MM, Wolf CR. Genetic analysis of the human cytochrome P450 CYP2C9 locus. *Pharmacogenetics* 1996;6:429–439.

14. Furuya H, Meyer UA, Gelboin HV, Gonzalez FJ. Polymerase chain reaction-directed identification, cloning, and quantification of human CYP2C18 mRNA. *Mol Pharmacol* 1991;40:375–382.

15. Romkes M, Faletto MB, Blaisdell JA, Raucy JL, Goldstein JA. Cloning and expression of complementary DNAs for multiple members of the human cytochrome P450IIC subfamily. *Biochemistry* 1991;30:3247–3255.

16. Wrighton SA, Stevens JC, Becker GW, VandenBranden M. Isolation and characterization of human liver cytochrome P450 2C19: correlation between 2C19 and S-mephenytoin 4′-hydroxylation. *Arch Biochem Biophys* 1993;306:240–245.

17. Richardson TH, Griffin KJ, Jung F, Raucy JL, Johnson EF. Targeted antipeptide antibodies to cytochrome P450 2C18 based on epitope mapping of an inhibitory monoclonal antibody to P450 2C51. *Arch Biochem Biophys* 1997;338:157–164.

18. Goldstein JA, Faletto MB, Romkes S-M, et al. Evidence that CYP2C19 is the major (S)-mephenytoin 4′-hydroxylase in humans. *Biochemistry* 1994;33:1743–1752.

19. Lecoeur S, Bonierbale E, Challine D, et al. Specificity of in vitro covalent binding of tienilic acid metabolites to human liver microsomes in relationship to the type of hepatotoxicity: comparison with two directly hepatotoxic drugs. *Chem Res Toxicol* 1994;7: 434–442.

20. Sandhu P, Baba T, Guengerich FP. Expression of modified cytochrome P450 2C10 (2C9) in *Escherichia coli,* purification, and reconstitution of catalytic activity. *Arch Biochem Biophys* 1993;306:443–450.

21. Richardson TH, Jung F, Griffin KJ, et al. A universal approach to the expression of human and rabbit cytochrome P450s of the 2C subfamily in *Escherichia coli. Arch Biochem Biophys* 1995;323:87–96.

22. Haining RL, Hunter AP, Veronese ME, Trager WF, Rettie AE. Allelic variants of human cytochrome P450 2C9: baculovirus-mediated expression, purification, structural characterization, substrate stereoselectivity, and prochiral selectivity of the wild-type and I359L mutant forms. *Arch Biochem Biophys* 1996;333:447–458.

23. Ong CE, Miners JO, Birkett DJ, Bhasker CR. Baculovirus-mediated expression of cytochrome P4502C8 and human NADPH-cytochrome P450 reductase: optimization of protein expression. *Xenobiotica* 1998;28:137–152.

24. Dehal SS, Kupfer D. CYP2D6 catalyzes tamoxifen 4-hydroxylation in human liver. *Cancer Res* 1997;57:3402–3406.

25. Goldstein JA, De M-SM. Biochemistry and molecular biology of the human CYP2C subfamily. *Pharmacogenetics* 1994;4:285–299.

26. Inoue K, Yamazaki H, Imiya K, Akasaka S, Guengerich FP, Shimada T. Relationship between CYP2C9 and 2C19 genotypes and tolbutamide methyl hydroxylation and S-mephenytoin 4′-hydroxylation activities in livers of Japanese and Caucasian populations. *Pharmacogenetics* 1997;7:103–113.

27. Lasker JM, Wester MR, Aramsombatdee E, Raucy JL. Characterization of CYP2C19 and CYP2C9 from human liver: respective roles in microsomal tolbutamide, S-mephenytoin, and omeprazole hydroxylations. *Arch Biochem Biophys* 1998;353:16–28.

28. Ibeanu GC, Goldstein JA. Transcriptional regulation of human CYP2C genes: functional comparison of CYP2C9 and CYP2C18 promoter regions. *Biochemistry* 1995;34:8028–8036.

29. Hellmold H, Rylander T, Magnusson M, Reihner E, Warner M, Gustafsson JA. Characterization of cytochrome P450 enzymes in human breast tissue from reduction mammaplasties. *J Clin Endocrinol Metab* 1998;83:886–895.

30. McFayden MC, Melvin WT, Murray GI. Regional distribution of individual forms of cytochrome P450 mRNA in normal adult human brain. *Biochem Pharmacol* 1998;55:825–830.

31. Hukkanen J, Hakkola J, Anttila S, et al. Detection of mRNA encoding xenobiotic-metabolizing cytochrome P450s in human bronchoalveolar macrophages and peripheral blood lymphocytes. *Mol Carcinog* 1997;20:224–230.

32. Hakkola J, Raunio H, Purkunen R, et al. Detection of cytochrome P450 gene expression in human placenta in first trimester of pregnancy. *Biochem Pharmacol* 1996;52:379–383.

33. Shimizu Y, Kusunose E, Kikuta Y, Arakawa T, Ichihara K, Kusunose M. Purification and characterization of two new cytochrome P-450 related to CYP2C subfamily from rabbit small intestine microsomes. *Biochim Biophys Acta* 1997;1339:268–276.

34. Klose TS, Blaisdell JA, Goldstein JA. Gene structure of CYP2C8 and extrahepatic distribution of the human CYP2Cs. *J Biochem Mol Toxicol* 1999;13(6):289–295.

35. Daikh BE, Lasker JM, Raucy JL, Koop DR. Regio- and stereoselective epoxidation of arachidonic acid by human cytochromes P450 2C8 and 2C9. *J Pharmacol Exp Ther* 1994;271:1427–1433.

36. Rifkind AB, Lee C, Chang TK, Waxman DJ. Arachidonic acid metabolism by human cytochrome P450s 2C8, 2C9, 2E1, and 1A2: regioselective oxygenation and evidence for a role for CYP2C enzymes in arachidonic acid epoxygenation in human liver microsomes. *Arch Biochem Biophys* 1995;320:380–389.

37. Bylund J, Kunz T, Valmsen K, Oliw EH. Cytochromes P450 with bisallylic hydroxylation activity on arachidonic and linoleic acids studied with human recombinant enzymes and with human and rat liver microsomes. *J Pharmacol Exp Ther* 1998;284:51–60.

38. Zeldin DC, DuBois RN, Falck JR, Capdevila JH. Molecular cloning, expression and characterization of an endogenous human cytochrome P450 arachidonic acid epoxygenase isoform. *Arch Biochem Biophys* 1995;322:76–86.

39. Karara A, Dishman E, Jacobson H, Falck JR, Capdevila JH. Arachidonic acid epoxygenase: stereochemical analysis of the endogenous epoxyeicosatrienoic acids of human kidney cortex. *FEBS Lett* 1990; 268:227–230.

40. Rahman A, Korzekwa KR, Grogan J, Gonzalez FJ, Harris JW. Selective biotransformation of taxol to 6 alpha-hydroxytaxol by human cytochrome P450 2C8. *Cancer Res* 1994;54:5543–5546.

41. Hamman MA, Thompson GA, Hall SD. Regioselective and stereoselective metabolism of ibuprofen by human cytochrome P450 2C. *Biochem Pharmacol* 1997;54:33–41.

42. Leo MA, Lasker JM, Raucy JL, Kim CI, Black M, Lieber CS. Metabolism of retinol and retinoic acid by human liver cytochrome P450IIC8. *Arch Biochem Biophys* 1989;269:305–312.

43. Relling MV, Aoyama T Gonzalez FJ, Meyer UA. Tolbutamide and mephenytoin hydroxylation by human cytochrome P450s in the CYP2C subfamily. *J Pharmacol Exp Ther* 1990;252:442–447.

44. Yun CH, Shimada T, Guengerich FP. Roles of human liver cytochrome

P4502C and 3A enzymes in the 3-hydroxylation of benzo(a)pyrene. *Cancer Res* 1992;52:1868–1874.

45. Kerr BM, Thummel KE, Wurden CJ, et al. Human liver carbamazepine metabolism: role of CYP3A4 and CYP2C8 in 10,11-epoxide formation. *Biochem Pharmacol* 1994;47:1969–1979.

46. Rettie AE, Korzekwa KR, Kunze KL, et al. Hydroxylation of warfarin by human cDNA-expressed cytochrome P-450: a role for P-4502C9 in the etiology of (*S*)-warfarin-drug interactions. *Chem Res Toxicol* 1992; 5:54–59.

47. Veronese ME, Mackenzie OI, Doecke CJ, McManus ME, Miners JO, Birkett DJ. Tolbutamide and phenytoin hydroxylations by cDNA-expressed human liver cytochrome P4502C9. *Biochem Biophys Res Commun* 1991;175:1112–1118.

48. Breckenridge A, Orme M, Wesseling H, Lewis RJ, Gibbons R. Pharmacokinetics and pharmacodynamics of the enantiomers of warfarin in man. *Clin Pharmacol Ther* 1974;15:424–430.

49. Toon S, Low LK, Gibaldi M, et al. The warfarin-sulfinpyrazone interaction: stereochemical considerations. *Clin Pharmacol Ther* 1986;39: 15–24.

50. Rettie AE, Eddy AC, Heimark LD, Gibaldi M, Trager WF. Characteristics of warfarin hydroxylation catalyzed by human liver microsomes. *Drug Metab Dispos* 1989;17:265–270.

51. Kunze KL, Eddy AC, Gibaldi M, Trager WF. Metabolic enantiomeric interactions: the inhibition of human (*S*)-warfarin-7-hydroxylase by (*R*)-warfarin. *Chirality* 1991;3:24–29.

52. Yamano S, Tatsuno J, Gonzalez FJ. The CYP2A3 gene product catalyzes coumarin 7-hydroxylation in human liver microsomes. *Biochemistry* 1990;29:1322–1329.

53. Sadeque AJM, Fisher MB, Korzekwa KR, Gonzalez FJ, Rettie AE. Human CYP2C9 and CYP2A6 mediate formation of the hepatotoxin 4-ene-valproic acid. *J Pharmacol Exp Ther* 1997;283:698–703.

54. Butler TC, Dudley KH, Johnson D, Roberts SB. Studies of the metabolism of 5,5-diphenylhydantoin relating principally to the stereoselectivity of the hydroxylation reactions in man and the dog. *J Pharmacol Exp Ther* 1976;199:82–92.

55. Fritz S, Lindner W, Roots I, Frey BM, Kupfer A. Stereochemistry of aromatic phenytoin hydroxylation in various drug hydroxylation phenotypes in humans. *J Pharmacol Exp Ther* 1987;241:615–622.

56. Bajpai M, Roskos LK, Shen DD, Levy RH. Roles of cytochrome P4502C9 and cytochrome P4502C19 in the stereoselective metabolism of phenytoin to its major metabolite. *Drug Metab Dispos* 1996; 24:1401–1403.

57. Ko JW, Desta Z, Flockhart DA. Human *N*-demethylation of (*S*)-mephenytoin by cytochrome P450s 2C9 and 2B6. *Drug Metab Dispos* 1998;26:775–778.

58. Schellens JH, van der Wart JH, Breimer DD. Relationship between mephenytoin oxidation polymorphism and phenytoin, methylphenytoin and phenobarbitone hydroxylation assessed in a phenotyped panel of healthy subjects. *Br J Clin Pharmacol* 1990;29:665–671.

59. Miners JO, Birkett DJ. Use of tolbutamide as a substrate probe for human hepatic cytochrome P450 2C9. *Methods Enzymol* 1996;272: 139–145.

60. Veronese ME, Doecke CJ, Mackenzie PI, et al. Site-directed mutation studies of human liver cytochrome P-450 isoenzymes in the CYP2C subfamily. *Biochem J* 1993;289:533–538.

61. Rettie AE, Wienkers LC, Gonzalez FJ, Trager WF, Korzekwa KR. Impaired (*S*)-warfarin metabolism catalysed by the R144C allelic variant of CYP2C9. *Pharmacogenetics* 1994;4:39–42.

62. Miners JO, Rees DL, Valente L, Veronese ME, Birkett DJ. Human hepatic cytochrome P450 2C9 catalyzes the rate-limiting pathway of torosemide metabolism. *J Pharmacol Exp Ther* 1995;272:1076–1081.

63. Miners JO, Birkett DJ. Cytochrome P4502C9: an enzyme of major importance in human drug metabolism. *Br J Clin Pharmacol* 1998;45: 525–538.

64. Mansuy D, Dansette PM. New biological reactive intermediates: metabolic activation of thiophene derivatives. *Adv Exp Med Biol* 1996;387:1–6.

65. Homberg JC, Andre C, Abuaf N. A new anti-liver-kidney microsome antibody (anti-LKM2) in tienilic acid-induced hepatitis. *Clin Exp Immunol* 1984;55:561–570.

66. Lecoeur S, Andre C, Beaune PH. Tienilic acid-induced autoimmune hepatitis: anti-liver and -kidney microsomal type 2 autoantibodies recognize a three-site conformational epitope on cytochrome P4502C9. *Mol Pharmacol* 1996;50:326–333.

67. Jean P, Lopez G-P, Dansette P, Mansuy D, Goldstein JL. Oxidation of tienilic acid by human yeast-expressed cytochromes P-450 2C8, 2C9, 2C18 and 2C19: evidence that this drug is a mechanism-based inhibitor specific for cytochrome P-450 2C9. *Eur J Biochem* 1996; 241:797–804.

68. Lopez-Garcia MP, Dansette PM, Mansuy D. Thiophene derivatives as new mechanism-based inhibitors of cytochromes P-450: inactivation of yeast-expressed human liver cytochrome P-450 2C9 by tienilic acid. *Biochemistry* 1994;33:166–175.

69. Leemann T, Kondo M, Zhao J, Transon C, Bonnabry P, Dayer P. (The biotransformation of NSAIDs: a common elimination site and drug interactions). *Schweiz Med Wochenschr* 1992;122:1897–1899.

70. Klose TS, Ibeanu GC, Ghanayem BI, et al. Identification of residues 286 and 289 as critical for conferring substrate specificity of human CYP2C9 for diclofenac and ibuprofen. *Arch Biochem Biophys* 1998; 357:240–248.

71. Tracy TS, Rosenbluth BW, Wrighton SA, Gonzalez SJ, Korzekwa KR. Role of cytochrome P450 2C9 and an allelic variant in the 4′-hydroxylation of (*R*)- and (*S*)-flurbiprofen. *Biochem Pharmacol* 1995;49: 1269–1275.

72. Korzekwa KR, Krishnamachary N, Shou M, et al. Evaluation of atypical cytochrome P450 kinetics with two-substrate models: evidence that multiple substrates can simultaneously bind to cytochrome P450 active sites. *Biochemistry* 1998;37:4137–4147.

73. Mancy A, Broto P, Dijols S, Dansette PM, Mansuy D. The substrate binding site of human liver cytochrome P450 2C9: an approach using designed tienilic acid derivatives and molecular modeling. *Biochemistry* 1995;34:10365–10375.

74. Jones BC, Hawksworth G, Horne VA, et al. Putative active site template model for cytochrome P4502C9 (tolbutamide hydroxylase). *Drug Metab Dispos* 1996;24:260–266.

75. Jones JP, He M, Trager WF, Rettie AE. Three-dimensional quantitative structure-activity relationship for inhibitors of cytochrome P4502C9. *Drug Metab Dispos* 1996;24:1–6.

76. Haining RL, Jones JP, Henne KR, et al. Enzymatic determinants of the substrate specificity of CYP2C9: role of B′-C loop residues in providing the pi-stacking anchor site for warfarin binding. *Biochemistry* 1999;38:3285–3292.

77. Jung F, Griffin KJ, Song W, Richardson TH, Yang M, Johnson EF. Identification of amino acid substitutions that confer a high affinity for sulfaphenazole binding and a high catalytic efficiency for warfarin metabolism to P450 2C19. *Biochemistry* 1998;37:16270–16279.

78. Jung F, Richardson TH, Raucy JL, Johnson EF. Diazepam metabolism by cDNA-expressed human 2C P450s: identification of P4502C18 and P4502C19 as low K(M) diazepam *N*-demethylases. *Drug Metab Dispos* 1997;25:133–139.

79. Pichard L, Curi P-R, Bonfils C. et al. Oxidative metabolism of lansoprazole by human liver cytochromes P450. *Mol Pharmacol* 1995;47: 410–418.

80. Karam WG, Goldstein JA, Lasker JM, Ghanayem BI. Human CYP2C19 is a major omeprazole 5-hydroxylase, as demonstrated with recombinant cytochrome P450 enzymes. *Drug Metab Dispos* 1996; 24:1081–1087.

81. Mancy A, Dijols S, Poli S, Guengerich P, Mansuy D. Interaction of sulfaphenazole derivatives with human liver cytochromes P450 2C: molecular origin of the specific inhibitory effects of sulfaphenazole on CYP 2C9 and consequences for the substrate binding site topology of CYP 2C9. *Biochemistry* 1996;35:16205–16212.

82. Bertilsson L. Geographical/interracial differences in polymorphic drug oxidation: current state of knowledge of cytochromes P450 (CYP) 2D6 and 2C19. *Clin Pharmacokinet* 1995;29:192–209.

83. Rost KL, Brockmoller J, Esdorn F, Roots I. Phenocopies of poor metabolizers of omeprazole caused by liver disease and drug treatment. *J Hepatol* 1995;23:268–277.

84. Chang M, Dahl ML, Tybring G, Gotharson E, Bertilsson L. Use of omeprazole as a probe for CYP2C19 phenotype in Swedish Caucasians: comparison with *S*-mephenytoin hydroxylation phenotype and CYP2C19 genotype. *Pharmacogenetics* 1995;5:358–363.

85. Pearce RE, Rodrigues AD, Goldstein JA, Parkinson A. Identification of the human P450 enzymes involved in lansoprazole metabolism. *J Pharmacol Exp Ther* 1996;277:805–816.

86. Ono S, Hatanaka T, Miyazawa S, et al. Human liver microsomal diazepam metabolism using cDNA-expressed cytochrome P450s: role of CYP2B6, 2C19 and the 3A subfamily. *Xenobiotica* 1996;26:1155–1166.

87. Somogyi AA, Reinhard HA, Bochner F. Pharmacokinetic evaluation of proguanil: a probe phenotyping drug for the mephenytoin hydroxylase polymorphism. *Br J Clin Pharmacol* 1996;41:175–179.
88. Basci NE, Bozkurt A, Kortunay S, Isimer A, Sayal A, Kayaalp SO. Proguanil metabolism in relation to *S*-mephenytoin oxidation in a Turkish population. *Br J Clin Pharmacol* 1996;42:771–773.
89. Ibeanu GC, Ghanayem BI, Linko P, Li L, Pederson LG, Goldstein JA. Identification of residues 99, 220, and 221 of human cytochrome P450 2C19 as key determinants of omeprazole activity. *J Biol Chem* 1996;271:12496–12501.
90. Kupfer A, Desmond PV, Schenker S, Branch RA. Stereoselective metabolism and disposition of the enantiomers of mephenytoin during chronic oral administration of the racemic drug in man. *J Pharmacol Exp Ther* 1982;221:590–597.
91. Kupfer A, Preisig R. Pharmacogenetics of mephenytoin: a new drug hydroxylation polymorphism in man. *Eur J Clin Pharmacol* 1984;26:753–759.
92. Kupfer A, Desmond P, Patwardhan R, Schenker S, Branch RA. Mephenytoin hydroxylation deficiency: kinetics after repeated doses. *Clin Pharmacol Ther* 1984;35:33–39.
93. Nakamura K, Goto F, Ray WA, et al. Interethnic differences in genetic polymorphism of debrisoquin and mephenytoin hydroxylation between Japanese and Caucasian populations. *Clin Pharmacol Ther* 1985;38:402–408.
94. Jurima M, Inaba T, Kadar D, Kalow W. Genetic polymorphism of mephenytoin p(4')-hydroxylation: difference between Orientals and Caucasians. *Br J Clin Pharmacol* 1985;19:483–487.
95. Wedlund PJ, Aslanian WS, McAllister CB, Wilkinson GR, Branch RA. Mephenytoin hydroxylation deficiency in Caucasians: frequency of a new oxidative drug metabolism polymorphism. *Clin Pharmacol Ther* 1984;36:773–780.
96. Inaba T, Jurima M, Nakano M, Kalow W. Mephenytoin and sparteine pharmacogenetics in Canadian Caucasians. *Clin Pharmacol Ther* 1984;36:670–676.
97. Wilkinson GR, Guengerich FP, Branch RA. Genetic polymorphism of *S*-mephenytoin hydroxylation. *Pharmacol Ther* 1989;43:53–76.
98. Srivastava PK, Yun CH, Beaune PH, Ged C, Guengerich FP. Separation of human liver microsomal tolbutamide hydroxylase and (*S*)-mephenytoin 4'-hydroxylase cytochrome P-450 enzymes. *Mol Pharmacol* 1991;40:69–79.
99. De M-SM, Wilkinson GR, Blaisdell J, Nakamura K, Meyer UA, Goldstein JA. The major genetic defect responsible for the polymorphism of *S*-mephenytoin metabolism in humans. *J Biol Chem* 1994;269:15419–15422.
100. De M-SM, Wilkinson GR, Blaisdell J, Meyer UA, Nakamura, Goldstein JA. Identification of a new genetic defect responsible for the polymorphism of (*S*)-mephenytoin metabolism in Japanese. *Mol Pharmacol* 1994;46:594–598.
101. Goldstein JA, Ishizaki T, Chiba K, et al. Frequencies of the defective CYP2C19 alleles responsible for the mephenytoin poor metabolizer phenotype in various Oriental, Caucasian, Saudi Arabian and American black populations. *Pharmacogenetics* 1997;7:59–64.
102. Ferguson RJ, De M-SM, Benhamou D, et al. A new genetic defect in human CYP2C19: mutation of the initiation codon is responsible for poor metabolism of *S*-mephenytoin. *J Pharmacol Exp Ther* 1998;284:356–361.
103. Ibeanu GC, Goldstein JA, Meyer U, et al. Identification of new human CYP2C19 alleles (CYP2C19*6 and CYP2C19*2B) in a Caucasian poor metabolizer of mephenytoin. *J Pharmacol Exp Ther* 1998;286:1490–1495.
104. Yasumori T, Kawano S, Nagata K, Shimada M, Yamazoe Y, Kato R. Nucleotide sequence of a human liver cytochrome P-450 related to the rat male specific form. *J Biochem (Tokyo)* 1987;102:1075–1082.
105. Sullivan-Klose TH, Ghanayem BI, Bell et al. The role of the CYP2C9-Leu359 allelic variant in the tolbutamide polymorphism. *Pharmacogenetics* 1996;6:341–349.
106. Crespi CL, Miller VP. The R144C change in the CYP2C9*2 allele alters interaction of the cytochrome P450 with NADPH:cytochrome P450 oxidoreductase. *Pharmacogenetics* 1997;7:203–210.
107. Steward DJ, Haining RL, Henne KR, et al. Genetic association between sensitivity to warfarin and expression of CYP2C9*3. *Pharmacogenetics* 1997;7:361–367.
108. Stearns RA, Chakravarty PK, Chen R, Chiu SH. Biotransformation of losartan to its active carboxylic acid metabolite in human liver micro-

somes: role of cytochrome P4502C and 3A subfamily members. *Drug Metab Dispos* 1995;23:207–215.
109. Spielberg S, McCrea J, Cribb A. et al. A mutation in CYP2C9 is responsible for decreased metabolism of losartan. *Clin Pharmacol Ther* 1996;59:215.
110. Takahashi H, Kashima T, Nomizo Y, et al. Metabolism of warfarin enantiomers in Japanese patients with heart disease having different CYP2C9 and CYP2C19 genotypes. *Clin Pharmacol Ther* 1998;63:519–528.
111. Leeder JS, Gaedigk A, Gupta G, et al. Determinants of warfarin S:R ratio in orthopedic surgery (OS) patients. *Clin Pharmacol Ther* 1999;65:194.
112. Furuya H, Fernandez S-P, Gregory W, et al. Genetic polymorphism of CYP2C9 and its effect on warfarin maintenance dose requirement in patients undergoing anticoagulation therapy. *Pharmacogenetics* 1995;5:389–392.
113. Komai K, Sumida K, Kaneko H, Nakatsuka I. Identification of a new non-functional CYP2C18 allele in Japanese: substitution of T204 to A in exon 2 generates a premature stop codon. *Pharmacogenetics* 1996;6:117–119.
114. Inoue K, Yamazaki H, Shimada T. Linkage between the distribution of mutations in the CYP2C18 and CYP2C19 genes in the Japanese and Caucasian. *Xenobiotica* 1998;28:403–411.
115. Cresteil T, Beaune P, Kremers P, Celier C, Guengerich FP, Leroux JP. Immunoquantification of epoxide hydrolase and cytochrome P-450 isozymes in fetal and adult human liver microsomes. *Eur J Biochem* 1985;151:345–350.
116. Ratanasavanh D, Beaune P, Morel F, Flinois JP, Guengerich FP, Guillouzo A. Intralobular distribution and quantitation of cytochrome P-450 enzymes in human liver as a function of age. *Hepatology* 1991;13:1142–1151.
117. Treluyer JM, Gueret G, Cheron G, Sonnier M, Cresteil T. Developmental expression of CYP2C and CYP2C-dependent activities in the human liver: in-vivo/in-vitro correlation and inducibility. *Pharmacogenetics* 1997;7:441–452.
118. Treluyer JM, Cheron G, Sonnier M, Cresteil T. Cytochrome P-450 expression in sudden infant death syndrome. *Biochem Pharmacol* 1996;52:497–504.
119. Heimark LD, Gibaldi M, Trager WF, O'Reilly RA, Goulart DA. The mechanism of the warfarin-rifampin drug interaction in humans. *Clin Pharmacol Ther* 1987;42:388–394.
120. Zhou HH, Anthony LB, Wood AJ, Wilkinson GR. Induction of polymorphic 4'-hydroxylation of *S*-mephenytoin by rifampicin. *Br J Clin Pharmacol* 1990;30:471–475.
121. Breckenridge A, Orme M. Clinical implications of enzyme induction. *Ann N Y Acad Sci* 1971;179:421–431.
122. Goldberg MR, Lo MW, Deutsch PJ, Wilson SE, McWilliams EJ, McCrea JB. Phenobarbital minimally alters plasma concentrations of losartan and its active metabolite E-3174. *Clin Pharmacol Ther* 1996;59:268–274.
123. Nation RL, Evans AM, Milne RW. Pharmacokinetic drug interactions with phenytoin (Part II). *Clin Pharmacokinet* 1990;18:131–350.
124. Nation RL, Evans AM, Milne RW. Pharmacokinetic drug interactions with phenytoin (Part I). *Clin Pharmacokinet* 1990;18:37–60.
125. Li AP, Maurel P, Gomez-Lechon MJ, Cheng LC, Jurima-Romet M. Preclinical evaluation of drug-drug interaction potential: present status of the application of primary human hepatocytes in the evaluation of cytochrome P450 induction. *Chem Biol Interact* 1997;107:5–16.
126. Ohmori S, Chiba K, Nakasa H, Horie T, Kitada M. Characterization of monkey cytochrome P450, P450 CMLd, responsible for *S*-mephenytoin 4-hydroxylation in hepatic microsomes of cynomolgus monkeys. *Arch Biochem Biophys* 1994;311:395–401.
127. Jones CR, Guengerich FP, Rice JM, Lubet RA. Induction of various cytochromes CYP2B, CYP2C and CYP3A by phenobarbitone in non-human primates. *Pharmacogenetics* 1992;2:160–172.
128. Mansuy D. Topology of the active sites of human cytochromes P450 of the 2C subfamily. *ISSX Proc* 1998;13:7.
129. Miners JO, Smith KJ, Robson RA, McManus ME, Veronese ME, Birkett DJ. Tolbutamide hydroxylation by human liver microsomes: kinetic characterisation and relationship to other cytochrome P-450 dependent xenobiotic oxidations. *Biochem Pharmacol* 1988;37:1137–1144.
130. Back DJ, Tjia JF, Karbwang J, Colbert J. In vitro inhibition studies of tolbutamide hydroxylase activity of human liver microsomes by azoles, sulphonamides and quinolines. *Br J Clin Pharmacol* 1988;26:23–29.

131. Lewis RJ, Trager WF, Chan KK, et al. Warfarin: stereochemical aspects of its metabolism and the interaction with phenylbutazone. *J Clin Invest* 1974;53:1607–1617.

132. Black DJ, Kunze KL, Wienkers LC, et al. Warfarin-fluconazole. II. A metabolically based drug interaction: in vivo studies. *Drug Metab Dispos* 1996;24:422–428.

133. Heimark LD, Wienkers L, Kunze K, et al. The mechanism of the interaction between amiodarone and warfarin in humans. *Clin Pharmacol Ther* 1992;51:398–407.

134. O'Reilly RA, Goulart DA, Kunze KL, et al. Mechanisms of the stereoselective interaction between miconazole and racemic warfarin in human subjects. *Clin Pharmacol Ther* 1992;51:656–667.

135. Anderson GD. A mechanistic approach to antiepileptic drug interactions. *Ann Pharmacother* 1998;32:554–563.

136. Wrighton SA, Vandenbranden M, Stevens JC, et al. In vitro methods for assessing human hepatic drug metabolism: their use in drug development. *Drug Metabol Rev* 1993;25:453–484.

137. Ono S, Hatanaka T, Hotta H, Satoh T, Gonzalez FJ, Tsutsui M. Specificity of substrate and inhibitor probes for cytochrome P450s: evaluation of in vitro metabolism using cDNA-expressed human P450s and human liver microsomes. *Xenobiotica* 1996;26:681–693.

138. Jeppesen U, Rasmussen BB, Brosen K. Fluvoxamine inhibits the CYP2C19-catalyzed bioactivation of chloroguanide. *Clin Pharmacol Ther* 1997;62:279–286.

139. Funck B-C, Becquemont L, Lenevu A, Roux Jaillon P, Beaune P. Inhibition by omeprazole of proguanil metabolism: mechanism of the interaction in vitro and prediction of in vivo results from the in vitro experiments. *J Pharmacol Exp Ther* 1997;280:730–738.

140. Levy RH. Cytochrome P450 isozymes and antiepileptic drug interactions. *Epilepsia* 1995;36(suppl 5):S8–S13.

141. Shimoji M, Yin H, Higgins L, Jones JP. Design of a novel P450: a functional bacterial-human cytochrome P450 chimera. *Biochemistry* 1998;37:8848–8852.

142. Von W-C, Richardson TH, Cosme J, Johnson EH. Microsomal P450 2C3 is expressed as a soluble dimer in *Escherichia coli* following modification of its N-terminus. *Arch Biochem Biophys* 1997;339:107–114.

CHAPTER 8

CYP2D6

Ulrich M. Zanger and Michel Eichelbaum

OVERVIEW

Cytochrome P450 2D6 belongs to the CYP2 family of P450s and is the only functionally active isozyme of the CYP2D subfamily in humans. The gene encoding its synthesis is located in the *CYP2D* locus (1) at q13.1 on the long arm of chromosome 22 (2–4). It is part of a gene cluster consisting of the two pseudogenes *CYP2D7P* and *CYP2D8P* (1). Like other members of the human *CYP2* gene family, the *CYP2D* genes consist of nine exons and eight introns.

The enzyme exhibits a common genetic polymorphism (5–7). It was the first cytochrome P450 enzyme for which a genetic polymorphism was demonstrated. Based on the two substrates that led to the discovery, it is also named debrisoquine/sparteine polymorphism (8,9). Depending on the metabolic handling of these two probe drugs, between 5% and 10% of subjects of European populations could be identified who had a severely impaired capacity to form the major metabolites 4-hydroxydebrisoquine and 2-dehydrosparteine. These subjects were designated as poor metabolizers (PMs), and the remainder of the population were so-called extensive metabolizers (EMs). The trait "poor metabolism" is inherited in an autosomal recessive fashion (i.e., PMs are carriers of two nonfunctional alleles). In addition to debrisoquine and sparteine, many other drugs are inefficiently metabolized in PM subjects, including antiarrhythmics, β-adrenergic receptor antagonists, antidepressants, neuroleptics, opioids, amphetamines, and others (5,10,11). In addition to nonfunctional alleles, several variant functional alleles occur at extremely variable frequencies in different populations.

U. M. Zanger and M. Eichelbaum: Dr. Margarete Fischer-Bosch Institute of Clinical Pharmacology, Auerbachstrasse 112, Stuttgart D70376, Germany

EXPRESSION IN LIVER AND IN EXTRAHEPATIC TISSUES

The fact that CYP2D6 is the only isozyme of the CYP2D subfamily that is expressed at the protein level permitted the development of specific monoclonal and polyclonal antibodies that can be used to quantitate the protein in liver microsomes rather accurately by Western blot analysis, as has been shown in protein–activity correlation studies (12–14). Compared with CYP2C and CYP3A isoenzymes, which constitute up to 20% and 30%, respectively, of the total hepatic cytochrome P450 content, CYP2D6 expression reaches on average only about 2% to 5% of the total P450 content (15, and own unpublished observations). However, its expression varies dramatically from person to person, ranging from undetectable in PM individuals, very low in so-called IMs (intermediate metabolizers) to more than 100-fold higher levels in the most active EMs (13,14,16).

Evidence for CYP2D6 protein expression also was presented for several extrahepatic tissues including the gastrointestinal (GI) tract (17), the brain (18), and lung (19); however, at much lower levels, and in some cases, contradicting results were obtained (20). The expression in the brain is of particular interest because this enzyme not only metabolizes many centrally active drugs but is also able to hydroxylate tryptamine to dopamine (21). Further indications for CYP2D6 expression in brain were obtained at the messenger RNA (mRNA) level (22,23), but enzymatic activity has not been demonstrated conclusively. CYP2D6 mRNA also was detected by reverse transcriptase–polymerase chain reaction (RT-PCR) in blood mononuclear cells (24), breast tissue and breast tumors (25,26), and bladder mucosa and tumor tissue (27). CYP2D6 protein and mRNA can also be demonstrated by immunohistochemical analysis and by in situ hybridization in various brain regions in neurons, in skin, in pancreas, and in reproductive tissues (own unpublished data).

SUBSTRATES, INHIBITORS, PROBE DRUGS

Although expressed at rather low levels compared with other human P450s, CYP2D6 belongs to the most important CYPs, together with CYP3A4, CYP2C, and CYP1A2, regarding the number of metabolic pathways of drugs and xenobiotics it catalyzes. Table 8-1 contains an updated list of substrates, most of which are in clinical use. For many of them, the CYP2D6-dependent pathway constitutes the major elimination route such that these drugs are inefficiently metabolized in PM subjects of debrisoquine or sparteine. They include antiarrhythmics, β-adrenergic receptor antagonists, tricyclic antidepressants, selective serotonin reuptake inhibitors (SSRIs), neuroleptics, opiates, anticancer agents, as well as amphetamines and many other drugs. Numerous case reports and clinical studies have demonstrated that for some of these drugs, the polymorphic oxidation has therapeutic consequences, either leading to a higher propensity to develop adverse reactions at conventional doses (28) or to decreased drug effects [e.g., absence of the analgesic effect of codeine in PMs (29)], or to therapeutic failure at normal antidepressant doses in ultrarapid metabolizers (30).

In Vivo Probe Drugs

Debrisoquine, dextromethorphan, metoprolol, and sparteine are the most widely used probe drugs to assess CYP2D6 function in vivo (e.g., to determine the phenotype of a subject). As an index of metabolic function, the metabolic ratio (MR) is used which is derived from the relative excretion of unchanged parent drug and metabolite in urine (amount of parent drug/amount of metabolite excreted) within a defined period. In the case of sparteine, this parameter is closely related to metabolic clearance (31). The structures and sites of oxygen attack by CYP2D6 for these various probe drugs are depicted in Fig. 8-1. The MRs of all these probe drugs show bimodal or trimodal distribution in European populations (Fig. 8-2). The antimodes used to discriminate between EMs and PMs are 20 or more for sparteine, 12.6 or more for debrisoquine, 0.3 for dextromethorphan, and 10.5 or more for metoprolol. In populations with low frequencies of nonfunctional alleles (i.e., Asian), this bimodal or trimodal distribution of MR is no longer apparent.

In Vitro Probe Drugs

The same substrates and metabolic reactions can be used to study CYP2D6-catalyzed biotransformation in vitro (32–36). In addition, propafenone 5'-hydroxylation is a metabolic pathway almost exclusively mediated by 2D6, and therefore this substrate is quite useful as an in vitro probe (37). The most commonly used in vitro probe

TABLE 8-1. *Drugs metabolized at least in part by CYP2D6*

Substrate	Pathway
Alprenolol	Aromatic hydroxylation
Amiflamine	N-Demethylation
Amitriptyline	Benzylic hydroxylation
Aprindine	Aromatic hydroxylation
Brofaromine	O-Demethylation
Bufuralol	Aliphatic I'- and aromatic hydroxylation
Bunitrolol	Hydroxylation
Bupranolol	Hydroxylation
Cinnarizine	Aromatic hydroxylation
Clomipramine	Aromatic hydroxylation
Codeine	O-Demethylation
Debrisoquine	4-Hydroxylation
Desipramine	Aromatic hydroxylation
Desmethylcitalopram	Demethylation
Dexfenfluramine	N-Dealkylation
Dextromethorphan	O-Demethylation
Dihydrocodeine	O-Demethylation
Dolasetron	Hydroxylation
Encainide	O-Demethylation
Ethylmorphine	O-Deethylation
Flecainide	O-Dealkylation
Flunarizine	Aromatic hydroxylation
Fluvoxamine	Unclear
Guanoxan	Aromatic hydroxylation
Haloperidol	N-Dealkylation
Hydrocodone	O-Demethylation
Indoramin	Aromatic hydroxylation
Imipramine	Aromatic hydroxylation
Maprotiline	Unclear
Methoxyamphetamine	O-Dealkylation
Methoxyphenamine	Aromatic hydroxylation and N-demethylation
Methylenedioxymeth-amphetamine ("ecstasy")	Demethylenation
Metoprolol	Aliphatic hydroxylation and O-dealkylation
Mexiletine	Hydroxylation
Mianserin	Hydroxylation
Minaprine	Hydroxylation
Norcodeine	O-Demethylation
Nortriptyline	Benzylic hydroxylation
N-Propylajmaline	Benzylic hydroxylation
Ondansetron	Hydroxylation
Oxycodone	O-Demethylation
Paroxetine	Demethylenation
Perhexiline	Aliphatic hydroxylation
Perphenazine	Unclear
Phenformin	Aromatic hydroxylation
Promethazine	Aromatic hydroxylation
Propafenone	Aromatic hydroxylation
Propranolol	Aromatic hydroxylation
Risperidone	Hydroxylation
Sparteine	Hydroxylation
Tamoxifen	Hydroxylation
Thioridazine	Side-chain sulfoxidation
Timolol	O-Dealkylation
Tomoxetine	
Tropisetron	Aromatic hydroxylation
Venlafaxine	O-Demethylation
Zuclopenthixol	

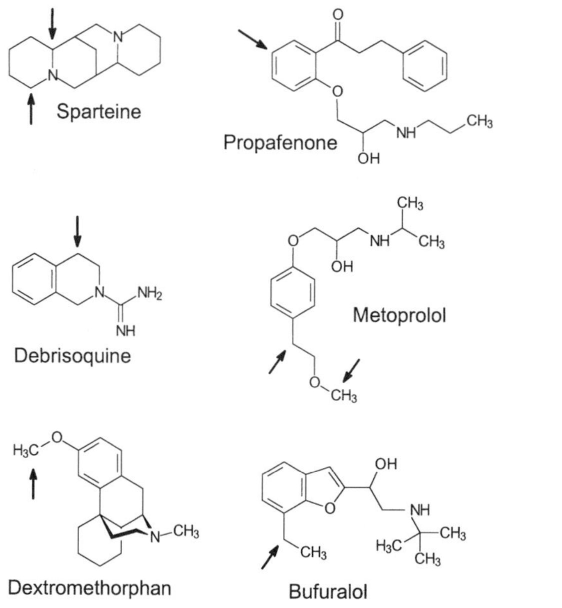

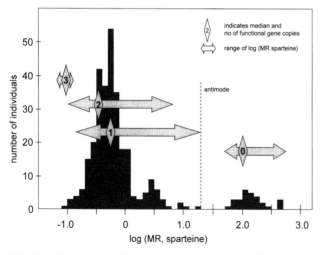

FIG. 8-1. Structures of drugs commonly used as *in vivo* and *in vitro* probe drugs for CYP2D6. The site of oxidative attack is indicated by an arrow.

drug is bufuralol, because of its fluorescent properties, which were used to develop a simple and highly sensitive high-performance liquid chromatography (HPLC) assay (32,36,38). The 1′-hydroxylation of bufuralol is catalyzed by CYP2D6 with a K_m in the low micromolar range, but other isozymes with higher K_m values contribute to the

FIG. 8-2. Frequency histogram of the metabolic ratio for sparteine in a European volunteer population (N = 316) that has been completely genotyped for 12 CYP2D6 alleles. The arrows indicate the metabolic ratio (MR) ranges within which homozygous poor metabolizers (PMs; 0), heterozygous (1), and homozygous (2) extensive metabolizers (EMs), and carriers of one normal and one duplicated allele of CYP2D6 (3) are found.

total activity of liver microsomes. If the reaction is supported by the artificial oxygen donor, cumene hydroperoxide, CYP2D6 becomes even more active, whereas other isozymes do not support this peroxygenase function, so that bufuralol is turned into a highly 2D6-selective *in vitro* probe drug (13). Although these assay conditions were shown to be useful for debrisoquine 4-hydroxylation as well, they have not been systematically investigated and should be used cautiously with other substrates (39).

Modulation of Activity and Expression by Substrates

The activity of a drug-metabolizing enzyme can be profoundly influenced by drugs and environmental substances either through direct inhibition at the active site or by modulation of gene expression. There are many examples in the case of CYP2D6 for competitive inhibition of substrate oxidation by another high-affinity substrate or a high-affinity inhibitor, which is not by itself an efficient substrate. Some of these drug interactions block the enzyme completely and result in the change of phenotype from EM to PM (phenocopying). Among others, this effect was demonstrated for the potent inhibitor quinidine (40), the SSRIs paroxetine (41), fluoxetine and fluvoxamine (42), the monoamine oxidase-A (MAO-A) inhibitor moclobemide (43), and the antiarrhythmic flecainide (44).

In contrast to all other CYPs involved in drug metabolism (1A1/2, 2B6, 2C8, 2C9, 2C18, 2C19, 2E1, and 3A4/5), which can be induced by a variety of xenobiotics, CYP2D6 cannot be induced significantly by antipyrine, phenobarbital, and rifampin (45). However, a limited increase in metabolism of metoprolol and dextromethorphan was found during pregnancy in women of the EM but not of the PM phenotype, indicating a possible regulation by induction (46,47).

Pharmacophore and Protein Models

Small-molecule models ("pharmacophores") predicting the CYP2D6 substrate features have been developed based on the observation that substrates of CYP2D6 have a basic nitrogen at a distance of 5 Å (e.g., debrisoquine) or 7 Å (e.g., dextromethorphan), respectively, from the site of oxidation (Fig. 8-3). The initial models, based on few substrates with these features, could, however, not explain the dichotomy of 5 Å and 7 Å substrates, and novel substrate predictions were not very accurate (48,49). An improved model that integrates both 5 Å and 7 Å substrates was derived from the assumption that an ion pair is formed between the substrate's basic nitrogen and the same acidic amino acid residue in the protein's active site, but that the interaction would take place either with the closer or with the more distant oxygen atom of

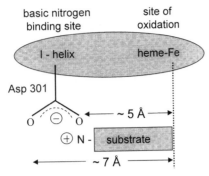

FIG. 8-3. Schematic representation of the structural requirements for CYP2D6 substrates and their steric position with respect to some identified protein determinants in the active site.

the carboxylate group, respectively. The improved predictive value of this model was experimentally tested and shown to be correct for 13 of 14 investigated metabolic pathways (50).

Three-dimensional models of the CYP2D6 protein were calculated by a process called "homology model building," which is based on the known crystal structure of another, sequence-related P450. This approach is severely limited by the fact that only some distantly related bacterial P450s have been crystallized to date. Furthermore, most bacterial P450s like the structurally first known CYP101 (P450$_{cam}$) from *Pseudomonas putida* use an iron–sulfur redoxin as a redox component, rather than a flavoprotein reductase as the membraneous mammalian P450s. The first such model for CYP2D6 contained only sequence fragments and residues that were conserved between CYP101 and CYP2D6 (51). By positioning the probe drugs debrisoquine and dextromethorphan into a planar pocket formed by residues Val^{370}, Pro^{371}, Leu^{372}, and Trp^{316} in the active site, Asp^{301} was identified as candidate for a carboxylate moiety interacting with the basic nitrogen of the substrate. Further improved models of the CYP2D6 three-dimensional structure were constructed by using the crystal structure of the heme moiety of the *Bacillus megaterium* form CYP102 (P450$_{bm3}$) as a template, which uses a flavoprotein reductase as redox partner and is therefore more closely related to the mammalian isoforms (52,53).

The contention that Asp^{301}, which is located within the strongly conserved I-helix is a critical substrate-contact residue, has been tested by site-directed mutagenesis (54). This study included substitutions with a negatively charged glutamic acid or neutral asparagine, alanine, or glycine in this position, and the deletion of Asp^{301}. The mutants containing neutral amino acids at position 301 showed marked reduction in catalytic activity. In the case of the deletion, the amount of holoprotein was significantly reduced or absent, relative to the amount of apoprotein pointing to restricted heme incorporation (54). It should be mentioned that several atypical reac-

tions were shown to be catalyzed by the wild-type enzyme, which does not fit the single model of substrates being fixed through Asp^{301} and oxidized at a certain distance. Examples are deprenyl *N*-demethylation (55), and even progesterone is hydroxylated by CYP2D6, although this steroid lacks a functional group with nitrogen (56).

MOLECULAR BIOLOGY AND GENETIC POLYMORPHISM

The unraveling of the molecular basis of the *CYP2D6* genetic polymorphism was started more than a decade ago by the two collaborating groups of Urs A. Meyer at the Biocenter of the University of Basle, Switzerland, and of Frank J. Gonzalez at the National Cancer Institute in Bethesda, Maryland, U.S.A. After the isolation of the full-length human cDNA (14), the *CYP2D* locus on chromosome 22 was characterized and shown to comprise the three highly homologous genes, *CYP2D8P, CYP2D7P,* and *CYP2D6,* which are located in this orientation (5' to 3') on a contiguous region of about 45 kb (1,57,58). *CYP2D8P* is a pseudogene that contains multiple deletions and insertions and therefore does not have an open reading frame encoding a full-length P450. The *CYP2D7P* gene is more similar to *CYP2D6* than to *CYP2D8P,* and its coding sequence indicates only a single inactivating mutation, an insertion of T226 in the first exon, causing a shift of the reading frame and premature translation stop. This mutation leads to the inactivation of *CYP2D6* in some alleles (see Fig. 8-4) which are hybrid forms between *CYP2D7P* and *CYP2D6* (59). No specific mRNA derived from *CYP2D7* was detected in human livers (1), but recently *CYP2D7P* transcripts were identified in human breast tissue (25), indicating that the gene is transcriptionally active at least in some tissues.

The systematic analysis of the *CYP2D6* gene in many individuals of the EM or PM phenotype led to the discovery of more than 50 mutations, which have been grouped into alleles and allele families according to the occurrence of key mutations with profound effect on expression or function (60). The allele frequencies in the European population and their association with phenotype have recently been determined in larger population studies (31,61,62).

Nonfunctional Alleles

Alleles that cause the PM phenotype in a homozygous situation or in combination with another nonfunctional allele are summarized in Fig. 8-4. Most of the inactivating key mutations of the various alleles cause a premature stop codon on the mRNA and lead to short and unstable protein products (63–72), or to the complete chromosomal deletion of the entire *CYP2D6* gene (73,74). The lack of CYP2D6 immunoreactivity observed in liver samples of PM subjects is a consequence of the fact that the most

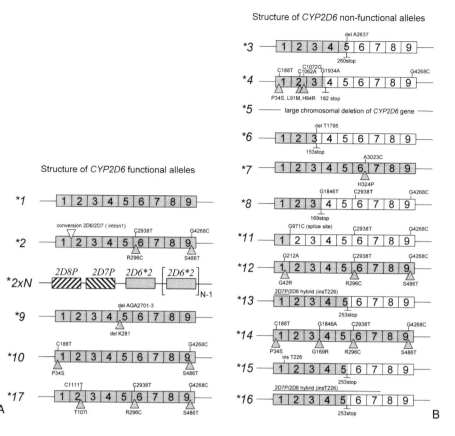

FIG. 8-4. Structure of CYP2D6 functional (A) and nonfunctional (B) alleles. The nine exons are indicated by numbered boxes. The positions of DNA mutations are indicated on top of each allele (del, deletion of base; ins, insertion of base) according to the accepted allele nomenclature (from Daly AK, Brockmöller J, Broly F, et al. Nomenclature for human CYP2D6 alleles. *Pharmacogenetics* 1996;6: 193–201, with permission). The consequences of the mutations are indicated at the bottom by the predicted amino acid change or the first occurrence of a stop codon. Open reading frames are indicated in grey. Silent mutations are not shown.

frequent nonfunctional alleles are of this type. The most frequent nonfunctional alleles in whites are the CYP2D6*4 and the CYP2D6*5 alleles, which are found with frequencies of about 20% and 3% to 5%, respectively. The key inactivating mutation of the CYP2D6*4 or "B-allele" affects the consensus acceptor splice site of the third intron, whereas the CYP2D6*5 or "D-allele" refers to the previously mentioned deletion allele. The structure of this allele was analyzed in genomic clones from a PM individual homozygous for the Xba I 11.5-kb haplotype, and shown to comprise the pseudogenes CYP2D8P and CYP2D7P, whereas the entire CYP2D6 coding sequence was deleted (73). Allele *7 is one of the two exceptions in which a full-length protein is predicted by the open reading frame. In this case, an amino acid substitution, H324P, is predicted in exon six (75). Expression of CYP2D6(324P) by recombinant baculovirus in insect cells resulted in comparable amounts of mutant and wild-type protein, but the 324P mutant lacked heme and was enzymatically inactive (76).

Simple PCR tests are now available to identify all of these mutations in a blood DNA sample, and it can be estimated that the sensitivity of predicting the PM phenotype by genotyping is now better than 99% (77–79). Population screening has shown that the frequencies of the various mutations are extremely different in different populations. Whereas the mutation due to a deletion of the complete functional gene occurs with similar fre-

quencies throughout the world, the *4 allele is rarely observed in Asians. The *3 mutation and most other nonfunctional alleles occur almost exclusively in Europeans.

Functional Alleles

Apart from alleles with total loss of function, several alleles are associated with impaired *in vivo* and *in vitro* metabolism. Among extensive metabolizers, the MR for sparteine varies almost 100-fold and to a similar extent for other substrates. The terms IM (for MR between 1 and 20) and "ultrarapid metabolizer" (for MR less than 0.1) have been used to describe these phenotypic subpopulations (80,81).

Some functional alleles can be correlated to decreased metabolic capacity and low CYP2D6 enzymatic activity. In CYP2D6*9, deletion of the three nucleotides representing codon 281 leads to loss of a lysine residue (82). The kinetic parameters determined with several substrates for the mutant enzyme expressed by recombinant vaccinia virus in HepG2 cells were comparable to those of the wild type. A family study including several members with the *5/*9 genotype allowed correlation between this allele and debrisoquine MRs, which are intermediate between the typical EM and the PM values (83).

The C188T mutation causes a Pro to Ser amino acid change at position 34 and occurs in a number of functional and nonfunctional alleles (see Fig. 8-4). It was shown by expression studies in COS cells to dramatically impair CYP2D6 enzyme function (64). Alleles harboring this mutation in the absence of further inactivating mutations are designated *10 alleles and lead to higher than normal (intermediate) MR values. In whites, these alleles are much less frequent than in Asian populations, where they exceed 50% allele frequency and therefore result in a shift in the median metabolic ratio of debrisoquine/sparteine and a lower metabolic clearance of CYP2D6 drugs in this population compared with that in whites (84–87). Pro34 is part of a proline-rich region that is highly conserved among microsomal P450s and may function as a hinge between the hydrophobic membrane anchor and the globular heme-binding portion of the enzyme. The *in vitro* enzymatic activity of COS cell-expressed P34S mutant in combination with a mutation in exon 9 (allele *10; see Fig. 8-4) was estimated to be about 5% of the wild-type activity (84). Nevertheless, individuals with a heterozygous genotype of one *10 and one nonfunctional allele are always EMs.

Similarly, the high frequency of the *17 allele in African populations, ranging from 9% to 34%, has been implicated as an explanation of why black Africans have a higher median MR of probe drugs (88–90). By using bufuralol 1'-hydroxylation as an index of CYP2D6 activity, the functional consequences of the *17 allele have been assessed (91). This allele has three mutations, of which only one (T107I) is specifically associated with the *17 allele, whereas the other mutations lead to amino acids exchanges R296C and S486T, which are also found in other alleles (see Fig. 8-4). No effect on activity was seen when only one substitution was tested. A combination of the T107I and R296C substitutions is required to alter catalytic properties. In comparison to the *1 allele, the *17 mutation has a very similar V_{max}; however, the affinity of substrate to the enzyme was substantially reduced with apparent K_m values at least five-fold higher than those observed with the *1 allele. As a consequence of this, intrinsic clearance of CYP2D6 *17 is only 20% of the *1 activity, which is in good agreement with the in vivo data. Because threonine 107 is located in the B' helix region of the molecule, which is known to be involved in substrate binding, substitution of the hydrophilic residue threonine by hydrophobic isoleucine is likely to affect substrate binding (91).

The ultrarapid metabolizer phenotype also was shown to have a genetic basis. It was first observed in a clinical environment in which two patients required antidepressants at unusually high doses ("megaprescribing") to attain therapeutic plasma levels (80). Both patients were subsequently shown to carry one normal allele and one novel allele harboring two head-to-tail oriented functional copies of CYP2D6*2. Multiple copies, as a result of germline gene amplifications by unequal crossover, have been found in a number of variants with up to 13 apparently functional gene copies (92,93). Alleles with ampli-

fied CYP2D6 (CYP2D6*2xN) were shown to occur with allele frequencies of about 1% to 2% in northern European populations (31,61,94), about 3.5% in Spanish populations (95), but appear to be much more common among northern African populations (96). Amplification of CYP2D6 involves the variant CYP2D6*2, which is distinct from the wild-type gene at several positions including a gene conversion with CYP2D7P in the first intron, which provides a convenient way of identifying *2 alleles by PCR (31) and two point mutations causing amino acid substitutions R296C and S486T. Correlation studies suggested that the *2 allele encodes a variant protein with more or less normal function, although position 296 maps to the vicinity of Asp_{301} in the I-helix.

REFERENCES

1. Kimura S, Umeno M, Skoda RC, Meyer UA, Gonzalez FJ. The human debrisoquine 4-hydroxylase (CYP2D) locus: sequence and identification of the polymorphic CYP2D6 gene, a related gene, and a pseudogene. *Am J Hum Genet* 1989;45:889–904.
2. Eichelbaum M, Baur MP, Dengler HJ, et al. Chromosomal assignment of human cytochrome P-450 (debrisoquine/sparteine type) to chromosome 22. *Br J Clin Pharmacol* 1987;23:455–458.
3. Gonzalez FJ, Vilbois F, Hardwick JP, McBride OW, et al. Human debrisoquine 4-hydroxylase (P450IID1): cDNA and deduced amino acid sequence and assignment of the CYP2D locus to chromosome 22. *Genomics* 1988;2:174–179.
4. Gough AC, Smith CA, Howell SM, Wolf CR, Bryant SP, Spurr NK. Localization of the CYP2D gene locus to human chromosome 22q13.1 by polymerase chain reaction, in situ hybridization, and linkage analysis. *Genomics* 1993;15:430–432.
5. Price-Evans DAP. *Genetic factors in drug therapy: clinical and molecular pharmacogenetics.* Cambridge: Cambridge University Press, 1993.
6. Daly AK. Molecular basis of polymorphic drug metabolism. *J Mol Med* 1995;173:539–553.
7. Meyer UA, Zanger UM. Molecular mechanisms of genetic polymorphisms of drug metabolism. *Annu Rev Pharmacol Toxicol* 1997;37:269–296.
8. Mahgoub A, Idle JR, Dring LG, Lancester R, Smith RL. Polymorphic hydroxylation of debrisoquine in man. *Lancet* 1977;2:584–586.
9. Eichelbaum M, Steincke B, Spannbrucker N, Dengler HJ. Defective N-oxidation of sparteine in man: a new pharmacogenetic defect. *Eur J Clin Pharmacol* 1979;16:183–187.
10. Eichelbaum M, Gross A S: The genetic polymorphism of debrisoquine/sparteine metabolism: clinical aspects. *Pharmacol Ther* 1990;46:377–394.
11. Brøsen K, Gram LF. Clinical significance of the sparteine/debrisoquine oxidation polymorphism. *Eur J Clin Pharmacol* 1989;36:537–547.
12. Zanger UM, Hauri HP, Loeper J, Homberg JC, Meyer UA. Antibodies against human cytochrome P-450db1 in autoimmune hepatitis type II. *Proc Natl Acad Sci USA* 1988;85:8256–8260.
13. Zanger UM, Vilbois F, Hardwick JP, Meyer UA. Absence of hepatic cytochrome P450bufI causes genetically deficient debrisoquine oxidation in man. *Biochemistry* 1988;27:5447–5454.
14. Gonzalez FJ, Skoda RC, Kimura S, et al. Characterization of the common genetic defect in humans deficient in debrisoquine metabolism. *Nature* 1988;331:442–446.
15. Shimada T, Yamazaki H, Mimura M, Inui Y, Guengerich FP. Interindividual variations in human liver cytochrome P-450 enzymes involved in the oxidation of drugs, carcinogens and toxic chemicals: studies with liver microsomes of 30 Japanese and 30 Caucasians. *J Pharmacol Exp Ther* 1994;270:414–423.
16. Zanger UM, Meyer UA. Absent, decreased or variant P450db1 in livers with poor capacity for debrisoquine metabolism. In: Schuster I, ed. *Cytochrome P450: biochemistry and biophysics.* London: Taylor & Francis, 1989:568.
17. Prueksaritanont T, Dwyer LM, Cribb AE. (+)-Bufuralol 1'-hydroxyla-

tion activity in human and rhesus monkey intestine and liver. *Biochem Pharmacol* 1995;50:1521–1525.

18. Fonne-Pfister R, Bargetzi MJ, Meyer UA. MPTP, the neurotoxin inducing Parkinson's disease, is a potent competitive inhibitor of human and rat cytochrome P450 isozymes (P450buff, P450db1) catalyzing debrisoquine 4-hydroxylation. *Biochem Biophys Res Commun* 1987;148:1144–1150.

19. Guidice JM, Marez D, Sabbagh N, et al. Evidence for CYP2D6 expression in human lung. *Biochem Biophys Res Commun* 1997;8:79–85.

20. Kivistö KT, Griese E-U, Stüven T, et al. Analysis of CYP2D6 expression in human lung: implications for the association between CYP2D6 activity and susceptibility to lung cancer. *Pharmacogenetics* 1997;7:295–302.

21. Hiroi T, Imaoka S, Funae Y. Dopamine formation from tyramine by CYP2D6. *Biochem Biophys Res Commun* 1998;249:838–843.

22. Tyndale RF, Sunahara R, Inaba T, Kalow W, Gonzalez FJ, Niznik HB. Neuronal cytochrome P450IID1 (debrisoquine/sparteine-type): potent inhibition of activity by (–)-cocaine and nucleotide sequence identity to human hepatic P450 gene CYP2D6. *Mol Pharmacol* 1991;40:63–68.

23. Gilham DE, Cairns W, Paine MJ, et al. Metabolism of MPTP by cytochrome P4502D6 and the demonstration of 2D6 mRNA in human foetal and adult brain by in situ hybridization. *Xenobiotica* 1997;27:111–125.

24. Carcillo JA, Parise RA, Adedoyin A, Frye R, Branch RA, Romkes M. CYP2D6 mRNA expression in circulating peripheral blood mononuclear cells correlates with in vivo debrisoquine hydroxylase activity in extensive metabolizers. *Res Commun Mol Pathol Pharmacol* 1996;91:149–159.

25. Huang Z, Fasco MJ, Kaminsky LS. Alternative splicing of CYP2D mRNA in human breast tissue. *Arch Biochem Biophys* 1997;343:101–108.

26. Huang Z, Fasco MJ, Figge HL, Keyomarsi K, Kaminsky LS. Expression of cytochromes P450 in human breast tissue and tumors. *Drug Metab Dispos* 1996;24:899–905.

27. Romkes-Sparks M, Mnuskin A, et al. Correlation of polymorphic expression of CYP2D6 mRNA in bladder mucosa and tumor tissue to in vivo debrisoquine hydroxylase activity. *Carcinogenesis* 1994;15:1955–1961.

28. Spina E, Gitto C, Avenoso A, Campo GM, Caputi AP, Perucca E. Relationship between plasma desipramine levels, CYP2D6 phenotype and clinical response to desipramine: a prospective study. *Eur J Clin Pharmacol* 1997;51:395–398.

29. Sindrup SH, Brosen K. The pharmacogenetics of codeine hypoalgesia. *Pharmacogenetics* 1995;5:335–346.

30. Bertilsson L, Dahl ML, Sjoqvist F, et al. Molecular basis for rational megaprescribing in ultrarapid hydroxylators of debrisoquine. *Lancet* 1993;341:63.

31. Griese U, Zanger UM, Brudermanns U, et al. Assessment of the predictive power of genotypes for the in-vivo catalytic function of CYP2D6 in a German population. *Pharmacogenetics* 1998;8:15–26.

32. Kronbach T, Mathys D, Gut J, Catin T, Meyer UA. High-performance liquid chromatographic assays for bufuralol 1′-hydroxylase, debrisoquine 4-hydroxylase, and dextromethorphan O-demethylase in microsomes and purified cytochrome P-450 isozymes of human liver. *Anal Biochem* 1987;162:24–32.

33. Osikowska-Evers B, Dayer P, Meyer UA, Robertz GM, Eichelbaum M. Evidence for altered catalytic properties of the cytochrome P-450 involved in sparteine oxidation in poor metabolizers. *Clin Pharmacol Ther* 1987;41:320–325.

34. Dayer P, Leemann T, Striberni R. Dextromethorphan O-demethylation in liver microsomes as a prototype reaction to monitor cytochrome P-450 db1 activity. *Clin Pharmacol Ther* 1989;45:34–40.

35. Ellis SW, Ching MS, Watson PF, et al. Catalytic activities of human debrisoquine 4-hydroxylase cytochrome P450 (CYP2D6) expressed in yeast. *Biochem Pharmacol* 1992;44:617–620.

36. Kronbach T. Bufuralol, dextromethorphan, and debrisoquine as prototype substrates for human P450IID6. *Methods Enzymol* 1991;206:509–517.

37. Kroemer HK, Mikus G, Kronbach T, Meyer UA, Eichelbaum M. In vitro characterization of the human cytochrome P-450 involved in polymorphic oxidation of propafenone. *Clin Pharmacol Ther* 1989;45:28–33.

38. Dayer P, Kronbach T, Eichelbaum M, Meyer UA. Enzymatic basis of the debrisoquine/sparteine-type genetic polymorphism of drug oxidation: characterization of bufuralol 1′- hydroxylation in liver microsomes of in vivo phenotyped carriers of the genetic deficiency. *Biochem Pharmacol* 1987;36:4145–4152.

39. Bichara N, Ching MS, Blake CL, Ghabrial H, Smallwood RA. Propranolol hydroxylation and N-desisopropylation by cytochrome P4502D6: studies using the yeast-expressed enzyme and NADPH/O2 and cumene hydroperoxide-supported reactions. *Drug Metab Dispos* 1996;24:112–118.

40. Brosen K, Gram LF, Haghfelt T, Bertilsson L. Extensive metabolizers of debrisoquine become poor metabolizers during quinidine treatment. *Pharmacol Toxicol* 1987;60:312–314.

41. Sindrup SH, Brosen K, Gram LF, et al. The relationship between paroxetine and the sparteine oxidation polymorphism. *Clin Pharmacol Ther* 1992;51:278–287.

42. Vandel S, Bertschy G, Baumann P, et al. Fluvoxamine and fluoxetine: interaction studies with amitriptyline, clomipramine and neuroleptics in phenotyped patients. *Pharmacol Res* 1995;31:347–353.

43. Gram LF, Brosen K. Moclobemide treatment causes a substantial rise in the sparteine metabolic ratio: Danish University Antidepressant Group. *Br J Clin Pharmacol* 1993;35:649–652.

44. Haefeli WE, Bargetzi MJ, Follath F, Meyer UA. Potent inhibition of cytochrome P450IID6 (debrisoquin 4-hydroxylase) by flecainide in vitro and in vivo. *J Cardiovasc Pharmacol* 1990;15:776–779.

45. Eichelbaum M, Mineshita S, Ohnhaus EE, Zekorn C. The influence of enzyme induction on polymorphic sparteine oxidation. *Br J Clin Pharmacol* 1986;22:49–53.

46. Hogstedt S, Lindberg B, Rane A. Increased oral clearance of metoprolol in pregnancy. *Eur J Clin Pharmacol* 1983;24:217–220.

47. Wadelius M, Darj E, Frenne G, Rane A. Induction of CYP2D6 in pregnancy. *Clin Pharmacol Ther* 1997;62:400–407.

48. Wolff T, Distlerath LM, Worthington MT, et al. Substrate specificity of human liver cytochrome P-450 debrisoquine 4-hydroxylase probed using immunochemical inhibition and chemical modeling. *Cancer Res* 1985;45:2116–2122.

49. Islam SA, Wolf CR, Lennard MS, Sternberg MJ. A three-dimensional molecular template for substrates of human cytochrome P450 involved in debrisoquine 4-hydroxylation. *Carcinogenesis* 1991;12:2211–2219.

50. Koymans L, Vermeulen NP, van Acker SA, et al. A predictive model for substrates of cytochrome P450-debrisoquine (2D6). *Chem Res Toxicol* 1992;5:211–219.

51. Koymans LMH, Vermeulen NPE, Baarslag A, Donné-Op den Kelder GM. A preliminary 3D model for cytochrome P450 2D6 constructed by homology model building. *J Comput Aided Mol Des* 1993;7:281–289.

52. Lewis DF, Eddershaw PJ, Goldfarb PS, Tarbit MH. Molecular modelling of cytochrome P4502D6 (CYP2D6) based on an alignment with CYP102: structural studies on specific CYP2D6 substrate metabolism. *Xenobiotica* 1997;27:319–339.

53. de Groot MJ, Vermeulen NP, Kramer JD, van Acker FA, Donne-Op den Kelder GM. A three-dimensional protein model for human cytochrome P450 2D6 based on the crystal structures of P450 101, P450 102, and P450 108. *Chem Res Toxicol* 1996;9:1079–1091.

54. Ellis SW, Hayhurst GP, Smith G, et al. Evidence that aspartic acid 301 is a critical substrate-contact residue in the active site of cytochrome P450 2D6. *J Biol Chem* 1995;270:29055–29058.

55. Grace JM, Kinter MT, Macdonald TL. Atypical metabolism of deprenyl and its enantiomer, (S)-(+)-N,alpha-dimethyl-N-propynylphenethylamine, by cytochrome P450 2D6. *Chem Res Toxicol* 1994;7:286–290.

56. Niwa T, Yabusaki Y, Honma K, et al. Contribution of human hepatic cytochrome P450 isoforms to regioselective hydroxylation of steroid hormones. *Xenobiotica* 1998;28:539–547.

57. Skoda RC, Gonzalez FJ, Demierre A, Meyer UA. Two mutant alleles of the human cytochrome P-450db1 gene (P450C2D1) associated with genetically deficient metabolism of debrisoquine and other drugs. *Proc Natl Acad Sci USA* 1988;85:5240–5243.

58. Heim MH, Meyer UA. Evolution of a highly polymorphic human cytochrome P450 gene cluster: CYP2D6. *Genomics* 1992;14:49–58.

59. Daly AK, Fairbrother KS, Andreassen OA, London SJ, Idle JR, Steen VM. Characterization and PCR-based detection of two different hybrid CYP2D7P/CYP2D6 alleles associated with the poor metabolizer phenotype. *Pharmacogenetics* 1996;6:319–328.

60. Daly AK, Brockmöller J, Broly F, et al. Nomenclature for human CYP2D6 alleles. *Pharmacogenetics* 1996;6:193–201.

61. Sachse C, Brockmöller J, Bauer S, Roots I. Cytochrome P450 2D6 variants in a Caucasian population: allele frequencies and phenotypic consequences. *Am J Hum Genet* 1997;60:284–295.

62. Marez D, Legrand M, Sabbagh N, et al. Polymorphism of the cytochrome P450 CYP2D6 gene in a European population: characterization of 48 mutations and 53 alleles, their frequencies and evolution. *Pharmacogenetics* 1997;7:193–202.

63. Hanioka N, Kimura S, Meyer UA, Gonzalez FJ. The human CYP2D locus associated with a common genetic defect in drug oxidation: a G1934-A base change in intron 3 of a mutant CYP2D6 allele results in an aberrant 3′ splice recognition site. *Am J Hum Genet* 1990;47:994–1001.

64. Kagimoto M, Heim M, Kagimoto K, Zeugin T, Meyer UA. Multiple mutations of the human cytochrome P450IID6 gene (CYP2D6) in poor metabolizers of debrisoquine: study of the functional significance of individual mutations by expression of chimeric genes. *J Biol Chem* 1990;265:17209–17214.

65. Evans WE, Relling MV. *Xba* I 16- plus 9-kilobase DNA restriction fragments identify a mutant allele for debrisoquine hydroxylase: report of a family study. *Mol Pharmacol* 1990;37:639–642.

66. Saxena R, Shaw GL, Reilling MV, et al. Identification of a new variant *CYP2D6* allele with a single base deletion in exon 3 and its association with the poor metabolizer phenotype. *Hum Mol Genet* 1994;3: 923–926.

67. Evert B, Griese EU, Eichelbaum M. Cloning and sequencing of a new non-functional *CYP2D6* allele: deletion of T1795 in exon 3 generates a premature stop codon. *Pharmacogenetics* 1994;4:271–274.

68. Broly F, Marez D, Sabbagh N, et al. An efficient strategy for detection of known and new mutations of the CYP2D6 gene using single strand conformation polymorphism analysis. *Pharmacogenetics* 1995;5:373–384.

69. Marez D, Sabbagh N, Legrand M, Lo-Guidice JM, Boone P, Broly F. A novel *CYP2D6* allele with an abolished splice site recognition site associated with the poor metabolizer phenotype. *Pharmacogenetics* 1995;5: 305–311.

70. Panserat S, Mura C, Gérard N, et al. An unequal cross-over event within the *CYP2D* gene cluster generates a chimeric *CYP2D7/CYP2D6* gene which is associated with the poor metabolizer phenotype. *Br J Clin Pharmacol* 1995;40:361–367.

71. Sachse C, Brockmöller J, Bauer S, Reum T, Roots I. A rare insertion of T226 in exon 1 of *CYP2D6* causes a frameshift and is associated with the poor metabolizer phenotype: *CYP2D6*15. Pharmacogenetics* 1996; 6:269–272.

72. Marez D, Legrand M, Sabbagh N, Lo-Guidice JM, Boone P, Broly F. An additional allelic variant of the *CYP2D6* gene causing impaired metabolism of sparteine. *Hum Genet* 1996;97:668–670.

73. Gaedigk A, Blum M, Gaedigk R, Eichelbaum M, Meyer UA. Deletion of the entire cytochrome P450 CYP2D6 gene as a cause of impaired drug metabolism in poor metabolizers of the debrisoquine/sparteine polymorphism. *Am J Hum Genet* 1991;48:943–950.

74. Steen VM, Andreassen OA, Daly AK, et al. Detection of the poor metabolizer-associated CYP2D6(D) gene deletion allele by long-PCR technology. *Pharmacogenetics* 1995;5:215–223.

75. Evert B, Griese EU, Eichelbaum M. A missense mutation in exon 6 of the CYP2D6 gene leading to a histidine 324 to proline exchange is associated with the poor metabolizer phenotype of sparteine. *Naunyn Schmiedebergs Arch Pharmacol* 1994;350:434–439.

76. Evert B, Eichelbaum M, Haubruck H, Zanger UM. Functional properties of CYP2D6 1 (wild-type) and CYP2D6 7 (His324Pro) expressed by recombinant baculovirus in insect cells. *Naunyn Schmiedebergs Arch Pharmacol* 1997;355:309–318.

77. Heim M, Meyer UA. Genotyping of poor metabolisers of debrisoquine by allele-specific PCR amplification. *Lancet* 1990;336:529–532.

78. Steen VM, Andreassen OA, Daly AK, et al. Detection of the poor metabolizer-associated CYP2D6(D) gene deletion allele by long-PCR technology. *Pharmacogenetics* 1995;5:215–223.

79. Stüven T, Griese EU, Kroemer HK, Eichelbaum M, Zanger UM. Rapid detection of *CYP2D6* null-alleles by long distance and multiplex polymerase chain reaction. *Pharmacogenetics* 1996;6:417–421.

80. Bertilsson L, Dahl ML, Sjoqvist F, et al. Molecular basis for rational megaprescribing in ultrarapid hydroxylators of debrisoquine. *Lancet* 1993;341:363.

81. Bock KW, Schrenk D, Froster A, et al. The influence of environmental and genetic factors on CYP2D6, CYP1A2 and UDP-glucuronosyl-transferases in man using sparteine, caffeine and paracetamol as probes. *Pharmacogenetics* 1994;4:209–218.

82. Tyndale RF, Aoyama T, Broly F, et al. Identification of a new variant CYP2D6 allele lacking the codon encoding Lys 281: possible association with the poor metabolizer phenotype. *Pharmacogenetics* 1991;1: 26–32.

83. Broly F, Meyer UA. Debrisoquine oxidation polymorphism: phenotypic consequences of a 3-base-pair deletion in exon 5 of the CYP2D6 gene. *Pharmacogenetics* 1993;3:123–130.

84. Johansson I, Oscarson M, Yue QY, Bertilsson L, Sjoqvist F, Ingelman Sundberg M. Genetic analysis of the Chinese cytochrome P4502D locus: characterization of variant CYP2D6 genes present in subjects with diminished capacity for debrisoquine hydroxylation. *Mol Pharmacol* 1994;6:452–459.

85. Wang SL, Huang JD, Lai MD, Liu BH, Lai ML. Molecular basis of genetic variation in debrisoquin hydroxylation in Chinese subjects: polymorphism in RFLP and DNA sequence of CYP2D6. *Clin Pharmacol Ther* 1993;53:410–418.

86. Armstrong M, Fairbrother K, Idle JR, Daly AK. The cytochrome P450 CYP2D6J allelic variant CYP2D6J and related polymorphisms in a European population. *Pharmacogenetics* 1994;4:73–81.

87. Yokota H, Tamura S, Furuya H, et al. Evidence for a new variant CYP2D6 allele CYP2D6J in a Japanese population associated with lower in vivo rates of sparteine metabolism. *Pharmacogenetics* 1993;3: 256–263.

88. Eichelbaum M, Woolhouse NM. Interethnic differences in sparteine oxidation among Ghanaians and Germans. *Eur J Clin Pharmacol*, 1985;28:79–83.

89. Masimirembwa C, Hasler J, Bertilsson L, Johansson I, Ekberg O, Ingelman-Sundberg M. Phenotype and genotype analysis of debrisoquine hydroxylase (CYP2D6) in a black Zimbabwean population: reduced enzyme activity and evaluation of metabolic correlation of CYP2D6 drugs. *Eur J Clin Pharmacol* 1996;51:117–122.

90. Masimirembwa C, Persson I, Bertilsson L, Hasler J, Ingelman-Sundberg M. A novel mutant variant of the CYP2D6 gene (CYP2D6*17) common in black African population: association with diminished debrisoquine hydroxylase activity. *Br J Clin Pharmacol* 1996;42: 713–719.

91. Oscarson M, Hidestrand M, Johansson I, Ingelman-Sundberg M. A combination of mutations in the CYP2D6*17 (CYP2D6Z) allele causes alterations in enzyme function. *Mol Pharmacol* 1997;52:1034–1040.

92. Johansson I, Lundqvist E, Bertilsson L, Dahl ML, Sjoqvist F, Ingelman Sundberg M. Inherited amplification of an active gene in the cytochrome P450 CYP2D locus as a cause of ultrarapid metabolism of debrisoquine. *Proc Natl Acad Sci USA* 1993;90:11825–11829.

93. Lundqvist E, Johansson I, Ingelman-Sundberg M. Genetic mechanisms for duplication and multiduplication of the human CYP2D6 gene and methods for detection of duplicated CYP2D6 genes. *Gene* 1999;226: 327–338.

94. Dahl ML, Johansson I, Bertilsson L, Ingelman Sundberg M, Sjoqvist F. Ultrarapid hydroxylation of debrisoquine in a Swedish population: analysis of the molecular genetic basis. *J Pharmacol Exp Ther* 1995; 274:516–520.

95. Agundez JA, Ledesma MC, Ladero JM, Benitez J. Prevalence of CYP2D6 gene duplication and its repercussion on the oxidative phenotype in a white population. *Clin Pharmacol Ther* 1995;57:265–269.

96. Aklillu E, Persson I, Bertilsson L, Johansson I, Rodrigues F, Ingelman-Sundberg M. Frequent distribution of ultrarapid metabolizers of debrisoquine in an Ethiopian population carrying duplicated and multiduplicated functional CYP2D6 alleles. *J Pharmacol Exp Ther* 1996; 278:441–446.

CHAPTER 9

CYP2E1

Judy Raucy and Susan P. Carpenter

The focus of this chapter is on the ethanol-inducible P450, *CYP2E1*. The importance of *CYP2E1* to human health and drug metabolism is described, including sections on regulation, polymorphisms, substrates, inhibitors, and drug interactions. Wherever possible, human studies are emphasized. However, in certain circumstances, investigations with human subjects were not ethical. In these instances, experimental animal studies are included to illustrate potential drug and/or chemical interactions that could occur in humans.

MOLECULAR BIOLOGY OF 2E1

Historical Perspective:
Discovery of the Ethanol-inducible P450 Enzyme

The first observation that ethanol promoted proliferation of smooth endoplasmic reticulum (SER) in rat liver was in 1966 (1). Because similar hepatic ultrastructural changes were seen with other compounds primarily metabolized by the CYP450 enzyme system, it was postulated that P450 was also involved in the metabolism of ethanol (2). This microsomal ethanol-oxidizing system, or MEOS as it was named, was found to be enhanced by prolonged ethanol feeding. The MEOS system required reduced nicotinamide adenine dinucleotide phosphate (NADPH) and molecular oxygen for activity, further suggesting the contribution of a P450 enzyme to this reaction. Evidence that ethanol induces a novel species of CYP450 was derived when the enzyme was purified and characterized (3,4). These studies included sodium dodecylsulfate–polyacrylamide gel electrophoresis (SDS-PAGE) analysis (3,5), spectral and catalytic characteristics, and production of monospecific antibodies and their subsequent use in immunoinhibition studies (6).

J. Raucy: La Jolla Institute for Experimental Medicine, 505 Coast Boulevard South, Suite 412, La Jolla, California 92037

S. P. Carpenter: Puracyp, 505 Coast Boulevard South, La Jolla, California 92037

Purification of the Ethanol-inducible CYP450

The ethanol-inducible form of CYP450 was first purified to homogeneity from hepatic microsomes of alcohol-treated rabbits (3). Based on its electrophoretic mobility, the purified protein was designated P450 LM-3a. The enzyme displayed an enhanced capacity to oxidize ethanol and other primary aliphatic alcohols to their corresponding aldehydes when compared with other purified rabbit P450 enzymes. In subsequent years, an homologous enzyme was purified from hepatic microsomes of isoniazid-treated rats and named P450j (4). Finally in 1987, the human protein was purified from a normal human liver (7) and from hepatic microsomes obtained from a recently drinking individual (8), by two separate laboratories. These enzymes were designated P450-ALC and P450HLj, respectively. P450-ALC was shown to oxidize ethanol and aniline and other primary alcohols at turnover rates 10 times greater than two other human P450 enzymes purified from the same liver (7). This purified enzyme was also shown to demethylate the nitrosamine, *N*-nitrosodimethylamine (NDMA) effectively at low substrate concentrations. Two years later, a systematic nomenclature was implemented, and the ethanol-inducible P450 was termed *CYP2E1* (2E1) (9).

CYP2E1 Gene

The human 2E1 cDNA and the full-length gene have been isolated, sequenced, and characterized. The encoded protein shares a common feature among the other 12 families of P450 enzymes, having a noncovalently bound heme associated with a conserved cysteine-containing peptide near the carboxy terminus of the enzyme (exon 9). Full-length *CYP2E1* spans 11,413 base pairs (bp) from the start site to the poly (A) addition site and is divided into nine exons by eight introns (10). The location of the introns within the gene is conserved, and the transcription start site is 23 bp downstream from a TATA box. A

CCATT box was detected at −144 bp from the start site. Moreover, the *CYP2E1* gene was mapped to chromosome 10 (10). Because of gene divergence, other members of the *CYP2* family, are localized to different chromosomes. For example 2A is located on chromosome 19 and 2D on chromosome 22 (10,11). Although only one *CYP2E1* gene is present in humans, gene duplication accounts for an additional gene, *CYP2E2*, in rabbits (12).

Subcellular, Cellular, and Tissue Localization

2E1 is expressed in many mammalian species and tissues (Table 9-1). Similar to other P450 enzymes engaged in xenobiotic metabolism, the highest concentrations of 2E1 are found in the liver. In humans, 2E1 composes approximately 6% of the total hepatic P450 and can vary up to 20-fold among individuals (13). 2E1 expression predominates among hepatocytes composing the perivenular zone of the liver acinus (2). This regiospecific pattern of 2E1 expression in liver has been invoked to explain the enhanced susceptibility of perivenular cells to damage from hepatotoxins. With regard to subcellular localization, 2E1 is present not only in the endoplasmic reticulum (ER; i.e., microsomes) but also in the plasma membrane of hepatocytes (14). In fact, purified preparations of plasma membranes demethylate NDMA at rates nearly one third of those obtained with microsomes, reflecting the difference in 2E1 content between the two organelles. 2E1 levels in the hepatocyte plasma membrane are inducible (14), an observation that may have toxicologic significance with regard to the production of acylated protein adducts on the cell surface. The formation of acylated 2E1 adducts in plasma membranes as a result of halocarbon bioactivation may, in turn, elicit the immunogenic (and toxic) response observed in certain types of drug-promoted hepatitis, such as that described for halothane.

It is now realized that 2E1 not only is expressed but also is induced in extrahepatic tissues including rat lung, kidney, and nasal epithelial microsomes (see Table 9-1). Most often, immunoblot analyses have been used to localize the enzyme in extrahepatic tissues. A more sensitive procedure, immunohistochemistry, reveals expression and ethanol-mediated induction of the enzyme in rat duodenal and jejunal villous cells, and in epithelial cells derived from the cheek mucosa, tongue, esophagus, fore stomach, and proximal colon (see Table 9-1). 2E1 is also present in rabbit kidney, nasal mucosa and, interestingly, bone marrow (15–17) (see Table 9-1). Treatment with ethanol or acetone induces the enzyme nearly five-fold in kidney and more than 12-fold in bone marrow, but these agents are without effect on 2E1 in nasal mucosa (15,16). The elevation of enzyme content in kidney and bone marrow was accompanied by a similar enhancement of 2E1-catalyzed activities (e.g., aniline and benzene hydroxylase) in these tissues (15,17). Within the kidney, 2E1 is present mainly in the proximal tubules. In contrast to the rat and rabbit homologs, however, mouse renal 2E1 is regulated in a sex-dependent manner. Kidney microsomes obtained from adult male mice possess substantial levels of immunoreactive 2E1 and also demethylate NDMA, whereas those obtained from female and immature male mice do not exhibit these characteristics (18,19). The role of testosterone in regulation of mouse renal 2E1 is evident by the appearance of a microsomal low K_m NDMA-demethylase as well as 2E1 messenger RNA (mRNA) in kidneys from female animals treated with the hormone.

Fetal and Placental 2E1 Expression

2E1 is present in rat (20) and human fetal liver (21) and human cephalic tissue (22) (see Table 9-1). Interestingly, ethanol-mediated induction of 2E1 from both fetal rat and human liver occurs *in vivo* and *in vitro*, respectively (20,21). In addition to embryonic tissues, 2E1 is localized

TABLE 9-1. *Species and tissue specificity of CYP2E1*

Tissue	Human Adult	Human Fetal	Rat Adult	Rat Fetal	Hamster Adult	Hamster Fetal	Mouse Adult	Rabbit Adult
Liver	7, 8*	21	112, 113	20	115, 117	115	114	3
Kidney	116		112, 113, 121		117		118	15
Lung	119		112		115, 117	115		120
Lymphocyte	60, 33		55					54
Nasal mucosa			113					15
Intestine			121, 122					
Placenta	23, 24							
Skin							123	
Brain		22	121, 124					
CNS		22	121					
Testes			113					
Ovary			113					
Bone marrow								17

CNS, central nervous system.
*Reference numbers.

in human placenta (23,24). Considering the significance of this enzyme to the bioactivation of ethanol and other agents, high levels of fetal and/or placental 2E1, caused by xenobiotic exposure, may exacerbate chemically mediated teratogenesis. This enhanced susceptibility to teratogens, due to increased formation of reactive metabolites, underlies the importance of identifying P450 enzymes in embryonic tissues.

Gene Methylation of 2E1

Expression of 2E1 in the human fetus is regulated by gestational age (21). The enzyme is not detectable in liver samples from fetuses younger than 16 weeks of gestation. This may be due to the methylation status of the *CYP2E1* gene. The methylation of DNA, causing inaccessibility to transcription factors and other proteins, plays an important role in the regulation of gene expression (25). Low-gestational-age human embryos (younger than 16 weeks) exhibit highly methylated *CYP2E1* DNA and undetectable levels of the enzyme in hepatic microsomes (26,27). DNA methylation also plays a role in tissue-specific expression of proteins. The human *CYP2E1* gene is differentially methylated in various tissues, which accounts for differences in expression (25). In contrast, hypoexpression of 2E1 in lung tumors corresponds to a hypomethylation of the *CYP2E1* gene (28).

Molecular Processing

CYP2E1 is encoded in the nucleus and synthesized on membrane-bound polyribosomes in the cytoplasm (Fig. 9-1). A segment of hydrophobic amino acids at the NH_2-terminus, called the signal-anchor sequence (29), directly interacts with a complex of proteins and RNA called the signal-recognition particle (SRP). This SRP functions to bind the nascent polypeptide and its associated ribosome to the ER membrane during translation (30). In this manner, the newly formed peptide is directly inserted into the membrane during the course of its synthesis with the NH_2-terminal sequence residing in the lipid bilayer and the majority of the 2E1 protein on the cytoplasmic surface of the ER. NADPH-P450 reductase also is anchored to the ER by a segment of hydrophobic residues at its amino terminus. Reductase is integral in microsomal metabolism by P450 enzymes, and thus the topology of this protein in the ER membrane is critical. Despite the importance of positioning, specific structural features required for a common mode of interaction between P450s and reductase molecules have yet to be elucidated (29).

Mechanisms of 2E1 Regulation

The modulation of cellular 2E1 levels by xenobiotics and physiological states occurs in several mammalian species including humans. However, mechanisms governing the regulation of this enzyme are complex, involving transcriptional, posttranscriptional, and posttranslational events (Fig. 9-2). These three mechanisms may act individually or in concert with each other to increase hepatic 2E1 content, leading to enhanced catalytic activities mediated by this P450. Species differences, and the

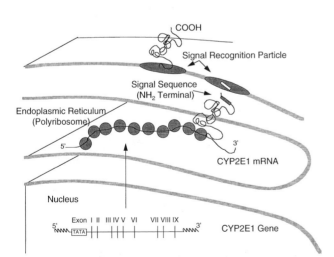

FIG. 9-1. Molecular processing of 2E1. 2E1 encoded in the nucleus is synthesized on polyribosomes located in the cytoplasm. The signal anchor sequence acts with the recognition particle to bind the nascent polypeptide to the endoplasmic reticular membrane during translation. The newly translated protein is then inserted into this membrane.

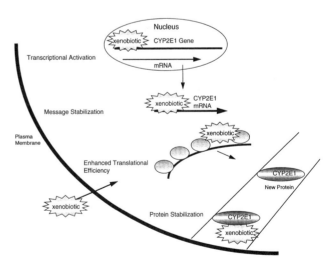

FIG. 9-2. Mechanisms of xenobiotic 2E1 regulation in hepatocytes. Four major mechanisms have been proposed for the regulation of this P450 by xenobiotics and include transcriptional activation occurring in the nucleus, stabilization of 2E1 transcripts in the cytosol, enhanced polyribosomal messenger RNA translational efficiency, and protein stabilization occurring in the endoplasmic reticulum. Any or all of these mechanisms may cause enhanced 2E1 expression when a cell is targeted by a drug or chemical.

particular regulator used, determine which mechanism predominates. In this section, we describe inducers and the various modes of regulation proposed for 2E1.

Xenobiotic Regulation

2E1 can be induced by a variety of compounds that are structurally diverse and include small-molecular-weight volatile molecules such as alcohols, aldehydes, ketones, halogenated and nonhalogenated alkanes and alkenes, and ethers (Table 9-2). Of these agents, the prevalence of alcohol abuse has rendered ethanol the most widely studied 2E1 inducer (31). That prolonged ethanol consumption induces 2E1 was initially observed when microsomes from rats exposed to alcohol exhibited increased ethanol oxidation (2). The P450 enzyme involved in this activity was initially characterized when it was purified from ethanol-treated rabbits (3).

2E1 in humans is similar to that of animals in that its content is increased in liver samples obtained from recently drinking alcoholics (32). Induction of this P450 was further supported in humans *in vivo* by the administration of a therapeutic probe specific for 2E1: the muscle-relaxant chlorzoxazone. When chlorzoxazone is given to alcoholics, altered pharmacokinetics are noted. Indeed, increases in clearance of the muscle-relaxant occur (33,34), and the area under the plasma concentration–time curve (AUC) for chlorzoxazone is reduced in alcoholics when compared with nonalcoholics (33–35). The mean plasma concentrations of the primary oxidative metabolite, 6-hydroxychlorzoxazone, reaches a peak approximately 30 minutes earlier in alcoholic when compared with nonalcoholic subjects (34), and the concentrations of the metabolite are higher in alcohol abusers (33).

TABLE 9-2. *Chemical inducers of CYP2E1*

Agent	Reference
Ethanol	2, 36
Isopropanol	125, 126
Isopentanol	127
Acetone	128
β-Hydroxybutyrate	128
Ether	129
Trichloroethylene	130
Pyridine	131
Myristicin	45
Isoniazid	2, 36
Pyrazole	132
4-Methylpyrazole	132
Acetylsalicylic acid	43
Clofibrate/Ciprofibrate	21, 44
Dexamethasone	123
Sulfur- and nitrogen-containing heterocycles	133
Xylene	38
Toluene	38
Benzene	38
Cigarette smoke	41, 42

Thus elevated 2E1 concentrations in hepatic microsomes caused by prolonged exposure to alcohol produces enhanced *in vivo* metabolism of chlorzoxazone.

In addition to ethanol, the nonhalogenated alkane, acetone, produces increases in rodent and rabbit 2E1 (36). The capacity for 2E1 to metabolize this compound led to the proposal that it plays a physiologic role in ketone disposition. Under conditions in which blood acetone levels are elevated (e.g., starvation and diabetic ketoacidosis), 2E1 may be induced in the liver, resulting in increased conversion of acetone to acetol and subsequent formation of methoxyglycol, two proposed gluconeogenic intermediates (36). This may represent a pathway that is an important source of glucose. It is noteworthy that acetone may be a significant gluconeogenic precursor, accounting for 10% of the glucose demands in humans fasted for 21 days (37). Other ketones, such as β-hydroxybutyrate, also induce 2E1 (2,36), further indicating a physiologic function in ketone disposition for this P450 enzyme.

Solvents including halogenated alkanes and alkenes and aromatic hydrocarbons such as benzene, toluene, and xylene induce 2E1 in animals (38) (see Table 9-2). Of the halogenated compounds, the common cleaning solvent, trichloroethylene enhances enzyme expression (31). Other than solvents, aromatic hydrocarbons including pyrazole, 4-methylpyrazole, and the antituberculin agent, isoniazid, also induce rodent and rabbit 2E1 (2,36) (see Table 9-2). Isoniazid also elevates 2E1 content in human liver (32,39), and the effects of this enhanced enzyme expression on subsequent drug therapy are similar to those observed for ethanol induction (33,34,40). Indeed, individuals exposed over the long term to isoniazid exhibit altered chlorzoxazone pharmacokinetic parameters, including greater clearance of chlorzoxazone when compared with that determined before isoniazid treatment (39).

Cigarette smoke induces 2E1 in rodents (see Table 9-2). Pulmonary microsomes from mice exposed to levels of cigarette smoke equivalent to three cigarettes per day for 4 or 8 days exhibit significant increases in 2E1 content, leading to corresponding increases in 2E1-mediated catalytic activity (41). In addition, cigarette smoke induces 2E1 activity, protein, and mRNA in mouse kidney (42). The induction of 2E1 in this latter tissue correlates with greater renal DNA single-strand breaks, suggesting a role for this P450 in carcinogenesis. Cigarette smoke contains several chemicals including pyridine, benzene, pyridizine, pyridazine, pyrimidine, thiophene, and triazole (2) (see Table 9-2), constituents that may be responsible for 2E1 induction observed in renal and pulmonary microsomes from tobacco smoke–exposed animals. Because this P450 has been found in human lung and kidney, 2E1 induction may also occur from cigarette smoke in these tissues.

Other agents modulating the expression of 2E1 in animals and potentially in humans include acetylsalicylic acid (43), the antihyperlipoproteinemic agents, clofibrate and ciprofibrate (21,44), and myristicin, a naturally occurring benzodioxole compound found in nutmeg, carrots, and flavoring agents, to name a few (45) (see Table 9-2). All of these structurally diverse agents increase hepatic 2E1 content significantly. The implications of such induction are altered pharmacokinetic parameters of subsequently administered therapeutic agents, such as those described earlier for ethanol-mediated induction of chlorzoxazone metabolism.

The mechanisms by which these xenobiotics induce 2E1 involve transcriptional and posttranscriptional events (see Fig. 9-2). Of the various treatments that increase hepatic 2E1 in rodents, ethanol and other agents (acetone, pyrazole, 4-methylpyrazole, and imidazole) have little effect on 2E1 transcript content (2,31,36). Indeed, numerous experimental studies have failed to document substantial increases in hepatic 2E1 mRNA after short- and/or long-term administration of ethanol or "ethanol-like" compounds (36). Moreover, the addition of ethanol for 2 days to HepG2 cells stably transfected with human 2E1 complementary DNA (cDNA) results in increased 2E1 content (46). In this situation, transcription would not occur because only the 2E1 cDNA was transfected. Such observations led to the consensus that induction of 2E1 caused by xenobiotics occurs through posttranscriptional mechanisms, primarily by protein stabilization against proteolytic degradation.

Decreased 2E1 protein degradation resulting from inducer-mediated enzyme stabilization was first noted in primary cultures of rat hepatocytes treated with isopropanol, dimethylsulfoxide, or imidazole (2,36). The inducers prevented the rapid decline in 2E1 generally detected when hepatocytes are cultured. A decrease in 2E1 protein degradation also was observed *in vivo* when rats were treated with acetone. In this situation, acetone prolonged the short half-life of 2E1 from 7 to 37 hours (47). The mechanism by which 2E1 degradation occurs is believed to involve ubiquitin-conjugation of the enzyme. Ubiquitination of proteins is an intracellular signal for proteolysis, and the inhibition of 2E1 degradation by inducers such as 4-methylpyrazole results from a decrease in formation of 2E1 ubiquitin conjugates (48) produced via the proteasome proteolytic pathway (49). Confirmation that 2E1 forms ubiquitin conjugates was established by using the suicide substrate, carbon tetrachloride (CCl_4). In these experiments, treatment of animals with this halogenated hydrocarbon resulted in the formation of high-molecular-weight ubiquitin–2E1 conjugates followed by rapid protein degradation (47,48). Ethanol treatment protected against the rapid CCl_4-mediated proteolysis (47).

In addition to the ubiquitin-dependent pathway for protein degradation, an independent pathway also exists and uses the 20S proteasome complex. The 20S proteasome is the catalytic core of the larger 26S complex (49).

This proteolytic pathway, requiring Mg^{2+} and adenosine triphosphate (ATP), proved to be the route of degradation for recombinant human 2E1 in transfected HepG2 cells (50). Addition of a proteasome inhibitor or 4-methylpyrazole to these transfected hepatoma cells prevents the rapid degradation of human 2E1. Other than ubiquitin targeting for rapid protein turnover, phosphorylation of 2E1 also increases the rate of its degradation. The cyclic adenosine monophosphate (cAMP)-dependent phosphorylation of 2E1-Ser[129] targets the enzyme for denaturation (2). This hormone-stimulated phosphorylation process is blocked by the addition of ethanol or imidazole to rat hepatocyte cultures, resulting in enhanced 2E1 content.

It is apparent from this discussion that several mechanisms are proposed for substrate-mediated stabilization of 2E1. To date, the exact mechanism by which chemical inducers are capable of preventing 2E1 degradation is unclear. However, considering the recent advances described earlier, it may be possible to resolve such issues in the near future. Collectively protein stabilization, which occurs by blocking proteolytic degradation of 2E1 with xenobiotics, causes accumulation of the enzyme. This accumulation ultimately results in greater rates of chemical oxidation mediated by 2E1.

Another mechanism of 2E1 induction by xenobiotics involves inducer-promoted increases in both 2E1 mRNA and protein synthesis (see Fig. 9-2). In contrast to previous investigations, recent studies demonstrated elevations in liver 2E1 mRNA content after the administration of xenobiotics in several species. In cultured rabbit hepatocytes, an increase in 2E1 transcripts was noted in cells treated with acetone for short periods (6 to 24 hours) (51). This paralleled the increase in newly synthesized 2E1 protein. Concomitant exposure of rabbit hepatocytes to acetone and α-amanitin, an inhibitor of gene transcription, blocked the increase of both 2E1 mRNA and protein produced by the former compound, suggesting that the enhanced rate of 2E1 protein synthesis found in acetone-treated rabbit hepatocytes may stem from increased transcription of the *CYP2E1* gene. Treatment with acetone appears to stimulate rates of 2E1 protein synthesis in rats as well (31). A single injection of acetone was found to increase aniline hydroxylation by liver microsomes both 30 minutes and 48 hours after administration. Regulation of 2E1 by transcriptional activation also occurs in hamsters and, importantly, in humans. Long-term ethanol and pyrazole given to hamsters resulted in an enhancement of hepatic 2E1 protein and translatable mRNA (2). More important, induction of human 2E1 protein occurring within the hepatic perivenular zone of ethanol-abusing subjects is accompanied by an increase in 2E1 transcripts within the same acinar zone (2). Furthermore, levels of 2E1 protein and mRNA in perivenular, pericentral, and periportal hepatocytes were significantly correlated among all patients studied.

Elevations of 2E1 mRNA and protein are reported in rats receiving continuous ethanol infusion (2,31). An interesting phenomenon was noted by using a continuous-infusion model of ethanol treatment. Despite the constant rate of intragastric infusion, blood ethanol levels were cyclical in nature, and ranged from 10 to 500 mg/dL over a 7-day period (52). Blood ethanol levels less than 250 mg/dL displayed a six-fold increase in hepatic 2E1 content, whereas at levels greater than 250 mg/dL, there was a 12-fold elevation of enzyme. A marked increase in 2E1 mRNA content also was observed. In addition, nuclear run-on experiments showed that the elevation of 2E1 mRNA when blood alcohol concentrations (BACs) were high occurred through transcription of the CYP2E1 gene (53). Interestingly, these types of pulsatile 2E1 and BACs also were noted in rabbits fed 10% or 15% ethanol in their drinking water (54). At the 10% dose, BAC and hepatic enzyme content increased above control at 3 days, decreased at 6 days, and then at 12 and 24 days, returned to levels originally observed at 3 days. When a 15% dose of ethanol was used, a time-dependent increase in BAC and hepatic 2E1 expression occurred up to and including 12 days. However, at 24 days, BAC and 2E1 content decreased, albeit remained elevated above control values. The mechanisms by which pulsatile blood alcohol levels and hence 2E1 content occur are unknown. However, it is clear that 2E1 content and BAC are highly correlated (53,54). One speculation is that 2E1 could be involved in altering BAC. Indeed, there is also a circadian variation of ethanol metabolism in the alcoholic (2), which may be related to a diurnal variation in the relative amounts of 2E1 within the hepatic lobule.

Translational control of protein synthesis also may play a role in the 2E1 induction process (see Fig. 9-2). For instance, pyridine and acetone increased hepatic 2E1 content not by enhancing levels of 2E1 transcripts, but by increasing the efficiency with which preexisting transcripts were translated (2,31). The two- to four-fold increase in 2E1 content noted 6 to 24 hours after a single pyridine injection could be completely blocked by prior administration of cycloheximide, whereas actinomycin D, an inhibitor of transcription, was without effect. The stimulation of mRNA translational efficiency by pyridine was attributed to a shift in 2E1 transcripts from light to heavy polyribosomes, which are more effective at protein synthesis.

Clearly, attempts to differentiate the mechanism by which xenobiotics induce 2E1 have produced several putative processes. The various mechanisms may stem in part from differences among species, the duration and/or manner of inducer treatment, and/or distinct mechanisms of induction by various compounds. Nevertheless, both protein stabilization and increased protein synthesis are thought to occur when animals or humans are exposed to agents that induce 2E1.

Regulation by Physiological States

Fasting/Diet/Obesity

Fasting markedly enhances microsomal 2E1-mediated drug metabolism in rats. These increases in enzyme activity are accompanied by parallel increases in hepatic 2E1 protein and its corresponding mRNA (31,36) (Table 9-3). More recently, lymphocytes isolated from rats fasted for 36 hours exhibited increased levels of both 2E1 protein and its transcript when compared with nonfasted animals (55). These findings paralleled those of rat hepatic 2E1 (56). Elevated 2E1 protein and mRNA in liver and kidney have also been observed in fasted rabbits, although renal 2E1 protein levels were enhanced more than hepatic levels of the enzyme (31,36). The molecular events underlying the elevation in 2E1 mRNA and protein that occurs during fasting are not clear. However, a number of studies have implicated pretranslational control that involves either CYP2E1 gene transcription or stabilization of 2E1 mRNA (55,56). Increased circulating ketone levels were the proposed cause for induction, because the administration of ketogenic compounds such as n-hexane, 2-hexanone, and acetonyl acetone increased 2E1 concentrations in the liver (2,31). Interestingly, prolonged fasting (38 hours) of human volunteers did not alter chlorzoxazone pharmacokinetic parameters (57). These findings demonstrate that 2E1 levels were similar among fasted and nonfasted subjects, suggesting a discordance between the effect of fasting on 2E1 concentrations in rodents and that observed in humans.

Dietary alterations may also result in the induction of 2E1 protein (see Table 9-3). Ketogenic diets fed to rats,

TABLE 9-3. *CYP2E1 regulators and mechanisms governing expression*

CYP2E1 regulators	Examples	Proposed mechanism of expression	Reference
Xenobiotics	Ethanol, imidazole, isoniazid, pyridine, pyrazole, halogenated hydrocarbons, acetone	Protein stabilization, increased translational efficiency, transcriptional activation	2, 31, 36
Physiological conditions	Diabetes, high-fat diet	mRNA stabilization	56, 58, 134
Starvation		Transcriptional activation	135
Hepatoprotectants	Malotilate, YH439, AS, AMS, AM	Decreased transcription	62–64
Hormones	Growth hormone	Decreased transcription	136

mRNA, messenger RNA; AM, allylmercaptan; AMS, allylmethylsulfide; AS, allyl sulfide.

including those deficient in carbohydrate or high in fat, are known to enhance metabolism of many halogenated hydrocarbons and nitrosodimethylamine (NDMA) (2,31,36). The higher rates of metabolism observed for these agents likely stem from the increase in 2E1-elicited by the high levels of circulating ketones attendant with the diets. Animals fed enriched-fat diets (20%) exhibited higher serum levels of acetone, β-hydroxybutyrate, and acetoacetate when compared with control animals. These levels correlated with increased content of 2E1 and its corresponding metabolic activity in liver microsomes (58). Both hepatic and renal 2E1 were induced by high-fat diets, and the increase in enzyme was accompanied by a three-fold increase in 2E1 mRNA (56). Such results indicate that high-fat diets can influence expression of 2E1, possibly in a manner similar to that observed with fasting (see Table 9-3). It also has been shown that high-fat diets potentiate 2E1 induction mediated by xenobiotics. Administration of ethanol to rats in liquid diets containing 35% fat resulted in a greater induction compared with that in animals fed ethanol in liquid diets containing 5% fat (2,31). In addition, the long-term (6 months) feeding of high-fat diets to render rats obese also results in induction of 2E1 protein and its corresponding catalytic activities (59). At present, it is unclear whether the ketogenic diet or obesity itself causes increases in 2E1 enzyme concentrations. The capacity of high-fat diets as well as obesity produced by these diets to elevate hepatic 2E1 content may have significant implications for humans; the obese individual could be at greater risk of drug-promoted toxicity. Indeed, enhanced biotransformation of halothane is observed in obese patients compared with nonobese patients (31). Furthermore, obesity resulted in altered pharmacokinetic parameters for chlorzoxazone. Oral clearance of the muscle relaxant was significantly higher in obese than in nonobese volunteers (57). Fractional clearance of 6-hydroxychlorzoxazone also is increased by obesity. Thus obesity in humans is associated with increased rates of dehalogenation of halothane and 6-hydroxylation of chlorzoxazone, consistent with induction of 2E1.

Diabetes

Chemically induced and spontaneous diabetes in rats are both conditions that may influence the outcome of exposure to substrates metabolized by 2E1. Uncontrolled diabetes results in a dramatic elevation of serum ketone levels (see Table 9-3). In fact, it has been shown in spontaneously diabetic rats (BB) that plasma β-hydroxybutyrate levels (but not those of glucose or insulin) correlated with microsomal 2E1 content and associated activities (31). Moreover, rats with chemically induced diabetes displayed elevations in 2E1 protein and mRNA similar to those in fasted rats. Interestingly, insulin treatment was found to reverse the induction of 2E1 caused by

diabetes. Furthermore, the elevations noted in 2E1 protein are reportedly due to 2E1 mRNA stabilization (36). Diabetes is also implicated as an inducer of 2E1 in humans. Indeed, insulin-dependent diabetes enhances the expression of lymphocyte 2E1 in juveniles when compared with that in nondiabetic children (60).

Suppression of 2E1

Several agents exhibit inhibitory properties toward 2E1-mediated activities and act by suppressing hepatic expression of the enzyme (see Table 9-3). Malotilate (MT), a hepatoprotectant, decreases rat microsomal metabolism of 2E1 substrates coincident with a decline in 2E1 protein levels (61). Nonetheless, 2E1 mRNA levels are unaffected by MT treatment, suggesting that MT suppresses 2E1 expression at the posttranscriptional level. Conversely, its structural analogue, YH439, which displays even more marked inhibition, acts by decreasing transcription of the CYP2E1 gene (62). Rats treated with YH439 exhibit a rapid decline in immunoreactive 2E1 and its corresponding activity in time- and dose-dependent manners as early as 2 hours. A single dose of YH439 also reduces the elevation of 2E1 activity, protein, and mRNA in starved rats, negating the inductive effect of starvation. Nuclear run-on transcription analysis confirms that inhibition of 2E1 by YH439 occurs at the transcriptional level.

Additional agents that suppress 2E1 enzyme levels include allylmercaptan (AM), allylmethylsulfide (AMS), and allyl sulfide (AS) (63). These agents decrease 2E1-mediated activity in a manner similar to that of MT. Immunoblot analyses of hepatic microsomes from rats treated with either AS, AM, or AMS reveal significant suppression of constitutive levels of 2E1 apoprotein in a time-dependent fashion. Furthermore, induction by pyridazine is completely blocked by treatment of rats with AS. Interestingly, no significant changes occur in 2E1 mRNA levels, suggesting that posttranscriptional regulation is associated with the suppression of 2E1 apoprotein (see Table 9-3).

2-Allylthiopyrazine (2-AP) substantially decreases both 2E1 activity and expression in rat liver. Moreover, 2-AP suppresses isoniazid-inducible hepatic 2E1 levels (64). Thus 2-AP was effective in suppressing both constitutive and inducible 2E1 expression. However, in contrast to MT or AS, 2-AP also suppresses 2E1 mRNA levels, suggesting that the decline in expression is due to a reduction in transcription of the CYP2E1 gene. Because of the ability of 2-AP to reduce hepatic 2E1 levels, marked reduction in hepatic injury occurs in rats treated with the toxins acetaminophen or CCl_4.

Phenethylisothiocyanate (PEITC), a dietary compound derived from cruciferous vegetables, also decreases 2E1 activity and in particular blocks DNA-adduct formation produced by metabolism of the carcinogen, NDMA (65).

In vitro PEITC acts by competitive inhibition of NDMA metabolism mediated by 2E1. However, *in vivo* pretreatment of rats with PEITC produces suppression of 2E1 apoprotein levels. The selective inhibition of 2E1 activity and suppression of its levels in microsomes indicates a role for PEITC as a chemoprotective agent against toxic or carcinogenic metabolites produced by this enzyme (see Table 9-3).

Polymorphism in Human 2E1

Various genetically linked polymorphisms in oxidative drug metabolism are described in humans. Such polymorphisms play an important role in the differences observed among individuals with regard to drug response as well as to drug toxicity. The open reading frame of the human *CYP2E1* gene is well conserved, and functional mutations are very rare, which may be due to its endogenous role in gluconeogenesis (66,67). Nevertheless, mutations in the human gene were discovered (2,31). One approach for identifying structural changes in P450 genes is restriction fragment length polymorphism (RFLP) analysis. Indeed, by using this technique, *Taq* I and *Dra* I RFLPs were found within intron 7 and intron 2, respectively, of the gene. Both are two-allele polymorphisms that occur with a frequency of 0.1 (*Taq* I) and 0.24 (*Dra* I). With regard to the *Dra* I polymorphism, it is caused by the presence or absence of a *Dra* I restriction digest site. The frequency of the *Dra* I RFLP is higher in the Japanese population (25%) than in the caucasian population (10%) (66). Whether *Taq* I or *Dra* I RFLPs have ramifications in terms of 2E1 protein expression or function is unknown.

More recently, two other RFLPs in the human 2E1 gene have been detected. *Pst* I and *Rsa* I polymorphisms are both found in the 5′-flanking (i.e., regulatory) region of the gene, are in complete linkage disequilibrium with each other, and occur with frequencies of 0.81 (c1, *Pst* I–, *Rsa* I+) and 0.19 (c2, *Pst* I+, *Rsa* I-) among unrelated Japanese subjects (68). The predominant homozygous allele, heterozygous allele, and the homozygous rare allele are designated type A (c1/c1), type B (c1/c2), and type C (c2/c2), respectively (68). Comparison of type A and type C gene structure reveals several point mutations within the 2E1 distal promoter region but no changes in the proximal promoter region of the gene. Nevertheless, these base substitutions have a marked effect on gene transcription. Indeed, the level of expression is 10-fold higher with the type C gene (68). The type C genotype gives rise to a phenotype that exhibits enhanced metabolism of 2E1 substrates. The rare allele incidence is much higher in the Japanese population than in whites or African-Americans. In Japanese, the occurrence of the *Pst* I allele (c2) is 24%, and the frequency of the *Rsa* I allele (c1) is 27%. In contrast, the frequency of the c2 allele is 2% and 5% in whites and in African-Americans,

respectively, whereas the c1 allele is 8% and 2%, respectively (69,70). Regardless of the lower frequency in whites or African-Americans, the identification of such genotypes may be important in predicting those subjects at greater risk of xenobiotic exposure.

Two additional 2E1 gene variants have been found with functional mutations; one (2E1*2) in which a point mutation $G^{1168}A$ in exon 2 caused an $R^{76}H$ amino acid substitution, and the other (2E1*3) in which a $G^{10059}A$ base substitution in exon 8 yielded a $V^{389}I$ amino acid exchange (71). When expressed in COS-1 cells, the 2E1*3 cDNA variant is indistinguishable from the wild-type cDNA, whereas the 2E1*2 cDNA, although yielding similar amounts of mRNA, produces only 37% of the protein and 36% of the catalytic activity when compared with wild-type cDNA. Results from population screening for these alleles suggest that they are very rare.

In summary, 2E1 content in various tissues is under the control of several factors, including xenobiotics such as ethanol, physiological states including diabetes and obesity, and genetic polymorphisms. Because of its important catalytic functions, altered expression of this P450 due to any of these factors can significantly affect the pharmacokinetics of an administered drug. Understanding molecular events associated with 2E1 expression and whether these differences are due to xenobiotic exposure or polymorphisms can lead to appropriate mechanisms for identifying individuals with reduced or enhanced capacity to metabolize drug substrates. In this manner, adverse drug reactions can be avoided by establishing appropriate dosing strategies for those therapeutic agents metabolized by 2E1. Table 9-3 summarizes the agents and conditions affecting 2E1 expression and the proposed mechanisms of regulation.

2E1 SUBSTRATES

The toxicologic significance of 2E1 results not only from the oxidation of substrates but also from the unique capacity of 2E1 to activate many xenobiotics to their toxic metabolites, often free radicals. Factors that affect the relative balance between activation and detoxification as catalyzed by 2E1 can affect the outcome of exposure to toxins. Among these factors is the alteration in enzyme expression, as previously discussed, occurring as a result of either genetic polymorphisms or exposure to compounds that induce the enzyme. Therefore from a quantitative standpoint, the formation of toxic metabolites depends on the concentrations of 2E1 present at the time of exposure.

With regard to substrates, 2E1 catalyzes the oxidation of a variety of compounds including drugs, solvents, small-molecular-weight volatile compounds, and environmental procarcinogens to cytotoxic and/or carcinogenic metabolites (2,31,72) (Table 9-4). Studies to date indicate that structural features of the substrate play a

TABLE 9-4. *CYP2E1 substrates*

Class	Substrate examples	Reference
Alcohols	Ethanol, isopropanolol	2
Aldehydes	Acetaldehyde	2
Fatty acids	Arachidonate, laurate	72
Alkanes and alkenes	Acetone, acetol, 1,3-butadiene	2, 72
Ethers	Diethyl ether	2
Halogenated hydrocarbons	Chloroform, enflurane, vinyl chloride, dichloromethane, halothane, carbon tetrachloride	31
Carcinogens	Azoxymethane, N-nitrosodimethylamine	137
Therapeutics	Acetaminophen, caffeine, chlorzoxazone, tamoxifen, disulfiram	2, 72
Aromatics	Styrene, toluene, benzene, capsaicin	2, 72
Metals	Chromium (VI)	2

critical role in determining whether catalysis by 2E1 will occur. The active-site cavity of human 2E1 is relatively open above pyrrole rings A and D, allowing substrate access, but is closed above pyrrole rings B and C (73,74), preventing large-molecular-weight chemicals from approaching the active site. In addition, for optimal interaction of a carboxylic acid moiety with the active site of 2E1, the hydrocarbon end of the molecule binds to the substrate binding site, leaving the carboxylic acid group outside of the proposed substrate access channel. The length of optimal substrates reflects the distance of the substrate access channel and the size of the active site, which has been estimated to be about 10 to 15 Å (73,74).

In addition to oxidative reactions, 2E1 also catalyzes the reduction of certain chemicals. The formation of trichloromethyl radicals from CCl_4 and reduction of hydroperoxide have been described (31,75). Included in the list of substrates for reductive reactions is molecular oxygen (2). When oxygen is reduced, peroxide formation is thought to occur by release and subsequent dismutation of superoxide. Direct release of peroxide from the two-electron reduced enzyme can also occur. Other substrates reduced by 2E1 include chromium (VI) (see Table 9-4), t-butylhydroperoxide, and cumyl hydroperoxide (2,72).

Of the various substrates oxidized by 2E1, ethanol is particularly important because of its prevalent abuse by humans. 2E1-mediated ethanol metabolism results in the formation of the primary metabolite, acetaldehyde (ACH). In tandem with aldehyde dehydrogenase, ACH is then further oxidized by 2E1 to acetic acid. The high K_m for ethanol metabolism (10 mM) indicates that 2E1 plays a major role when BACs are elevated (2).

In addition to ethanol, many other substrates for 2E1 have been identified and are provided in Table 9-4. Some of these are endogenous substrates such as acetone and fatty acids, but most are exogenous. Among the xenobiotics are halogenated hydrocarbons, such as CCl_4, vinyl chloride, vinyl bromide, trichlorethylene, and chloroform, and also the anesthetic agents halothane, enflurane, and isoflurane (31). Other halogenated hydrocarbons include the pesticide 1,2-dibromoethane and the lead scavenger, ethylene dibromide (31). Additional 2E1-mediated reactions include the demethylation of NDMA and the hydroxylation of p-nitrophenol. These latter reactions are most effective for monitoring the level of enzyme in vitro (i.e., in microsomes). In vivo, the 6-hydroxylation of chlorzoxazone has been suggested as a probe for 2E1 phenotyping, particularly in humans, because it is a relatively innocuous drug substrate. Other therapeutic agents also have been identified as 2E1 substrates and include aniline, acetaminophen, theophylline, tamoxifen, and isoniazid (2,72,76–78). Caffeine also has been proposed as a probe substrate for in vivo monitoring of 2E1 levels in humans (78,79). However, this methylxanthine is not metabolized exclusively by 2E1 (79).

Inhibitors

Several types of P450 inhibitors exist and can be classified as either competitive or mechanism based. Because of the many substrate interactions resulting from competitive inhibition, we limit our discussion to those agents classified as suicide- or mechanism-based inhibitors. Suicide enzyme inactivation occurs when a substrate is biotransformed by a P450 to a highly reactive metabolite that binds proteins, and in particular the P450 metabolizing the inhibitor. The levels of hepatic 2E1 decrease during microsomal catalysis of substrates such as CCl_4 (Table 9-5). The formation of reactive species at the active site directly inactivates the enzyme and also labilizes 2E1 for degradation by proteases. Studies in HepG2 cells transfected with human 2E1 cDNA confirmed that CCl_4 produced a 30% to 50% loss of both 2E1-mediated activity and protein (80).

Other mechanism-based inhibitors include disulfiram, which has been widely used in avoidance therapy for alcohol abuse and more recently investigated for its protective effect against chemically induced toxicity and carcinogenesis (81) (see Table 9-5). Disulfiram is reduced by 2E1 to diethyldithiocarbamate, which inhibits the hepatotoxicity of chloroform, CCl_4, acetaminophen, and NDMA. When disulfiram is given to rats, a very rapid decrease of NDMA demethylase activity is observed. This decrease is due to a loss of 2E1 protein.

TABLE 9-5. *CYP2E1 inhibitors*

Mechanism-based inhibitor (suicide substrates)	Chemical use	Mechanism of inhibition	Reference
3-Amino-1,2,4,-triazole	Agricultural chemical	N/D	47, 82
Carbon tetrachloride	Industrial solvent	Putative dichlorocarbene (:CCl₂) ligand responsible	80
Disulfiram and metabolites	Adjunct used in treatment of chronic ethanol abuse	N/D	138, 139
Carbon disulfide			
Diethyldithiocarbamate			
Diallylsulfide and metabolites	Component of garlic oil (hepatoprotectant)	N-alkylation of prosthetic heme groups	140, 141
Diallylsulfoxide			
Diallylsulfone			
Capsaicin	Topical analgesic	Binds to active site of CYP2E1	142
Halothane	Anesthetic	N/D	143, 144
Phenethyl isothiocyanate	Dietary compound derived from cruciferous vegetables	N/D	65
In vivo inhibitors			
2-(Allylthio)pyrazine	Chemoprotectant	Transcriptional inactivation	64
Chlormethiazole	Treatment of ethanol withdrawal states	Transcriptional inactivation	145
Malotilate and analog YH439	Hepatoprotectant	Posttranscriptional inactivation, transcriptional inactivation	61 62
4-Methylpyrazole and pyrazole	ADH inhibitor	Posttranscriptional inactivation	146

ADH, Alcohol dehydrogenase; N/D, not determined.

Diallyl sulfide (DAS), a component of garlic oil, exerts a potent inhibitory effect on the production of colon and liver cancer promoted by chemical carcinogens by inhibiting 2E1 activity (2) (see Table 9-5). Indeed, low doses of DAS inhibit hepatocarcinogenicity of 1,2-dimethylhydrazine in rats. As an *in vivo* inhibitor, microsomes prepared from rats 18 hours after treatment with DAS exhibited a marked decrease in NDMA activity and suppression of 2E1 protein. Another mechanism-based 2E1 inhibitor, 3-amino-1,2,4-triazole, decreases *p*-nitrophenol hydroxylase activity by hepatic microsomes in a time- and NADPH-dependent manner (82) (see Table 9-5). The loss of activity displays characteristics consistent with suicide inhibition of 2E1, including irreversibility, saturability, and protection by substrate. Other inhibitors are listed in Table 9-5, as well as their use and their mechanism of inhibition. Many can be used successfully *in vivo* as hepatoprotectants.

Diseases Associated with 2E1

Diseases identified to date that are associated with 2E1 are primarily those caused by metabolic activation of certain substrates. These diseases include alcoholic liver disease (ALD), carcinogenesis, and drug- or chemical-promoted hepatotoxicities. In addition, there is the potential for 2E1 to play a role in fetal alcohol syndrome (FAS). Because 2E1 also possesses several important physiologic roles (e.g., catalysis of arachidonate and acetone), it is anticipated that future research will identify disease processes involving these physiologic functions. For now,

this discussion focuses on the diseases mediated by 2E1 bioactivation reactions.

Alcoholic Liver Disease

Alcoholic liver injury is characterized by the predominance of lesions in the perivenular zone of the hepatic acinus (83). This is thought to be due to an increased oxygen consumption in this region caused by higher levels of 2E1. In addition, two of the earliest and most obvious features of hepatic damage produced by ethanol are the deposition of fat and the enlargement of the liver. Hepatomegaly has been ascribed primarily to accumulation of lipids, but another factor contributing to enlargement of hepatocytes involves the elevation of intracellular proteins and amino acids. Accumulation of proteins is due, in part, to impairment of protein secretion via microtubules. Indeed, hepatic microtubules are decreased in ALD. The deposition of proteins and lipids in hepatocytes produces two- to three-fold increases in diameter and a corresponding increase in volume of more than 10-fold. Other changes in the liver that are characteristic of ALD include alterations in mitochondria, such as swelling and abnormal cristae. These changes are associated with functional impairment including decreased oxidation of fatty acids and ACH. Liver injury triggers a fibrotic response in the perivenular region. This perivenular fibrosis occurs at the fatty-liver stage and progresses to cirrhosis. Cirrhosis is characterized by collagen deposition due to an increase in synthesis and a decrease in the degradation of this protein. Thus ALD progresses from various stages of fatty liver to perivenular fibrosis, to septal fibrosis, and finally to cirrhosis (2).

The capacity of 2E1 to generate reactive oxygen intermediates makes this P450 the primary culprit in the pathogenesis of ALD (2). During the oxidation of ethanol, lipid peroxidation occurs, which can be prevented by antioxidants (84) (Fig. 9-3). This suggests that lipid peroxidation results from the generation of oxygen radicals. Of the P450 enzymes, 2E1 is especially reactive in production of oxygen intermediates during substrate oxidation, and in particular, ethanol. This is because catalysis by this enzyme is a loosely coupled process resulting in "leaking" of hydrogen peroxide, superoxide, and hydroxyl radicals (2). These oxygen radicals produce oxidative stress within the hepatocyte. Furthermore, membranous lipids are targets of free radical attack, resulting in lipid peroxidation and cytotoxicity. Increased production of oxygen radicals and hence oxidative stress in the alcoholic is the result of induced levels of 2E1.

2E1 also metabolizes ethanol to the toxic metabolite ACH, which can be further metabolized by mitochondrial aldehyde dehydrogenase (ALDH) or 2E1 (see Fig. 9-3). However, in the alcoholic, there is a decreased capacity of ALDH to oxidize ACH, which is associated with enhanced rates of ethanol oxidation caused by induction of 2E1. This results in an imbalance between production and inactivation of ACH. Toxicity associated with ACH is partially due to its capacity to form protein adducts. Indeed, ACH binds covalently to liver microsomal proteins. This binding is significantly increased after long-term ethanol consumption and parallels 2E1 induction (83). Interestingly, ACH selectively forms stable adducts with 2E1 and also binds to hepatic macromolecules, circulating proteins, and cytoskeletal proteins, such as tubulin. ACH also produces impairment of the capacity of the liver to use oxygen. Moreover, ACH promotes glutathione depletion, collagen synthesis, and lipid peroxidation (2).

Nitrosamine-mediated Carcinogenesis

For many years, a correlation between alcohol abuse and an increased incidence of upper alimentary and respiratory tract cancers was known to exist (83,85). The relationship between alcohol and cancer occurs primarily in alcoholics who are also heavy cigarette smokers. Indeed, long-term ethanol consumption enhances the mutagenicity of tobacco-derived products (85). This synergism toward carcinogenesis is most likely due to the ability of ethanol to induce 2E1. As previously discussed in this chapter, 2E1 bioactivates many small-molecular-weight procarcinogens including those contained in tobacco smoke such as NDMA.

Metabolism of NDMA by 2E1 results in the formation of a methyl radical that can react with critical macromolecules including proteins and nucleic acids. Enhanced production of this radical results when 2E1 concentrations are elevated by attendant exposure to an inducing agent such as ethanol or tobacco-smoke constituents, such as pyridazine. The result of activation of tobacco-smoke–derived nitrosamines could eventually be manifested as lung and/or other respiratory tract cancers. In addition, nitrosamines are constituents of diet, and therefore induction of 2E1 in the alimentary tract can result in nitrosamine-promoted cancers (86). Indeed, the effect of nitrosamine activation is demonstrated primarily in those tissues that are at the principal portals of entry for tobacco smoke and dietary agents, and include not only lungs but also intestine and esophagus (85,86). Thus ethanol consumption increases the capacity for microsomal activation of nitrosamine carcinogens in various tissues. It is important to note here that the effect of ethanol

FIG. 9-3. Metabolic pathway for the oxidation of ethanol. Ethanol oxidation occurs in both the cytosol by the alcohol dehydrogenase (ADH) enzymes and in the endoplasmic reticulum by 2E1. The major intermediary metabolite produced is acetaldehyde, which is further oxidized to acetic acid by aldehyde dehydrogenases (ALDH) in the mitochondria or by 2E1. During 2E1-mediated oxidation of ethanol, oxygen radicals are formed, which may produce cellular damage when concentrations of the intermediates are high. Further injury can result when levels of acetaldehyde exceed those that can be efficiently detoxified. High levels of reactive oxygen species and/or acetaldehyde can occur when 2E1 is induced.

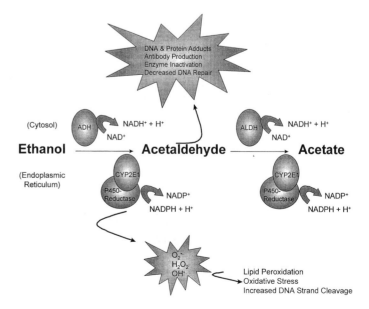

and other 2E1 inducers to increase the risk of cancer is influenced by other factors as well. These factors include the capacity of a tissue to detoxify the carcinogen and the length of time between exposure to an inducer and a carcinogen. Nevertheless, in the final analysis, induction of 2E1 can significantly increase the susceptibility to cancers promoted by nitrosamine bioactivation.

In addition to induction of 2E1 as a risk factor, another element that may play a role in enhanced susceptibility to carcinogens is polymorphic expression of this P450. Because a genetic polymorphism is associated with 2E1, susceptibility to carcinogenesis may be influenced by differences in 2E1 expression and/or function. In a Japanese population, there was a statistically significant association between the rare *Dra* I RFLP genotype and predisposition to lung cancer (87). However, the distribution of *Dra* I genotypes in lung cancer patients was not significantly different from that of healthy controls in a Finnish population (88). Another polymorphism in 2E1 that is detectable by the restriction enzymes *Rsa* I and *Pst* I may be functionally important because it is associated with higher levels of 2E1 transcription. It is conceivable that because 2E1 is involved in the metabolism of nitrosamines in tobacco smoke, the *Rsa* I/*Pst* I polymorphism might contribute to differences in susceptibility to lung cancer (69). Indeed, this polymorphism is linked with lung cancer as well as alcoholic liver disease in Japanese individuals. The *Pst* I mutation that causes overexpression of the 2E1 gene exhibits a higher frequency in individuals with adenocarcinomas of the lung (89). To date, the correlation between lung cancer and a 2E1 polymorphism is observed only in the Japanese population (70,90). No significant difference occurs in the distribution of polymorphic alleles between controls and lung cancer patients in the Swedish population (91), white Americans (69,70), or African Americans (69,70).

With regard to alcoholic liver disease, it was determined that Japanese volunteers exhibiting the c2/c2 or c1/c2 alleles of the *Rsa* I/*Pst* I polymorphism consumed more alcohol than those homozygous for the c1/c1 allele (92). Furthermore, alcoholic liver cirrhosis may be associated with the *Rsa* I/*Pst* I polymorphism in Japanese (93). Indeed, Japanese men with ALD exhibited a marked frequency of the c2 allele when compared with normal subjects (94).

Xenobiotic-promoted Hepatotoxicities and Hepatocarcinogenesis

In addition to ethanol and procarcinogens, 2E1 activates a number of xenobiotics to hepatotoxins. A well-known over-the-counter analgesic, acetaminophen (APAP), is bioactivated by 2E1 to the reactive intermediate *N*-acetyl-*p*-benzoquinone imine (NAPQI) (31). In general, metabolism of this analgesic by P450 is limited, and the major metabolites are the sulfate and glucuronide conjugates. However, in situations in which large doses of APAP (~20 to 25 g) are consumed or 2E1 is elevated, a greater portion of the drug is oxidatively metabolized by this P450. When elevation of 2E1 occurs, enhanced oxidation of APAP results in higher concentrations of NAPQI and ultimately occult liver injury. Indeed, therapeutic doses (2.5 to 4 g/day) of APAP can cause severe hepatotoxicity in alcoholics (95,96). These clinical observations are substantiated in experimental animals given ethanol for long periods (2). Hepatotoxicity occurs when APAP is administered to rats after ethanol is withdrawn and the analgesic is no longer competing for the same metabolic pathway as ethanol. Therefore alcoholics are most vulnerable to the toxic effects of APAP shortly after cessation of prolonged drinking, when 2E1 levels are still elevated. The significance of 2E1 as a major catalyst in APAP-mediated hepatotoxicity is further confirmed by studies with *Cyp2e1* knock-out mice (97). When these mice are challenged with toxic doses of APAP, less sensitivity to hepatotoxicity occurs when compared with that in wild-type mice.

Many halogenated hydrocarbons that are used clinically are also bioactivated by 2E1, and in situations in which 2E1 is induced, hepatotoxicity or hepatocarcinogenesis can occur. The trihalomethanes cause damage to both the liver and kidney and have been found to promote cancer in these organs (31). The most widely studied of this class of compounds is chloroform, which promotes hepatic centrilobular and renal proximal tubular necrosis in humans as well as in experimental animals. Monosubstituted haloethylenes, such as vinyl chloride and vinylidene chloride, are metabolized by 2E1 to compounds that are mutagenic and carcinogenic (31). The human carcinogenicity of vinyl chloride was established in 1974, when 50 cases of hepatic angiosarcoma were found within 1 year in workers exposed to this compound. Another halogenated hydrocarbon, trichloroethylene (TCE), which is a widely used organic solvent and general anesthetic, is weakly hepatocarcinogenic in B6C3F mice and hepatotoxic in rats and humans (31). TCE oxide has been detected as an oxidative metabolite, and 2E1 is the major TCE-metabolizing enzyme at physiologically relevant concentrations of this halogenated alkene.

The most widely used inhalation anesthetics are polyhaloalkanes or alkyl ethers containing fluorine. Most of these anesthetics are oxidized and/or reduced by 2E1 to reactive metabolites that can bind to proteins and lipids (31). This biotransformation of volatile anesthetics is of concern because it has been linked in a number of instances to toxic side effects, including hepatotoxicity and nephrotoxicity. The best-studied of the inhalation anesthetics is halothane, an agent that causes hepatotoxicity in humans and animals (98). Oxidative biotransformation of halothane is predominant in humans and results in lesions far more extensive than those produced by reductive metabolism (31). Metabolism of halothane produces either trifluoroacetyl chloride or bromide, which subsequently hydrolyze to trifluoroacetic acid and acylates proteins. A trifluoroacetyl-2E1 adduct has been detected on the outer cell surface of hepatocyte membranes after treatment with halothane (99,100). This acylated 2E1 ($M_r = 54,000$) may be immunogenic and promote the development of halothane hepatitis (99,101). Enflurane, methoxyflurane, and isoflurane are also oxidatively metabolized by 2E1 (31). Fluoride is released during metabolism of these compounds, and during prolonged anesthesia, enough fluoride ion is generated to produce subclinical nephrotoxicity.

Fetal Alcohol Syndrome

2E1 may also play an important role in FAS. The human fetus, through maternal exposure, is susceptible to teratogenesis from a variety of foreign chemicals. Many drugs are known to produce morphologic and/or neurologic abnormalities in the fetus. Among the most prevalent of teratogenic disorders are those associated with the maternal consumption of ethanol, which results in a broad spectrum of embryonic abnormalities called fetal alcohol effects (FAEs) and FAS (102). Resulting harmful effects range from gross morphologic defects to more subtle cognitive/behavioral dysfunctions. Central nervous system abnormalities also may occur, such as mental deficiency or developmental delay. Prenatal alcohol exposure is one of the leading known causes of mental retardation in developed countries (103). The capacity of 2E1 to metabolize ethanol could have serious consequences for the developing fetus. First, the primary metabolite produced during ethanol oxidation, ACH, can elicit tissue damage through protein adduct formation and may cause chromosomal damage (104,105). Second, oxygen radicals generated during ethanol metabolism may play an important role in the peroxidation of cell-membrane lipids (2). Thus the presence and inducibility of 2E1 in fetal tissues could have deleterious affects (106). Recently 2E1 was found in human liver samples from fetuses between 16 to 24 weeks of gestation (21). The enzyme also is functional, in that it metabolizes ethanol. In addition, ethanol induces the fetal form of 2E1 in isolated cultured hepatocytes. Because fetal 2E1 mediates ethanol metabolism, the enzyme may play a pivotal role in the local production of ACH and oxygen radicals, both of which could produce insidious effects on the developing fetus. The potential for ethanol to induce fetal 2E1 transplacentally is of concern, because this is the major route of fetal exposure. Interestingly, catalytic activities associated with 2E1 and the protein were elevated in rat liver microsomes from fetuses of dams exposed to a 5% ethanol diet throughout gestation (20). These latter findings demonstrate that maternal consumption of ethanol produces induction of 2E1 in the fetus.

Another factor that may contribute to FAS/FAE is the presence and inducibility of 2E1 in human placenta (23,24). Evidence for induction of placental 2E1 became clear when placental microsomes from women whose periconceptional average daily alcohol intake was greater than 1 ounce exhibited immunodetectable levels of 2E1 protein (24). Individual variation in the amount of placental 2E1 also was observed. 2E1 concentrations in placenta correlated significantly to morphologic changes in neonates born to drinking women, including a smaller headsize, birthweight, and birthlength when compared with neonates from nondrinking controls.

In summary, 2E1 and its induction by ethanol plays a crucial role in the pathogenesis of ALD through free radical and ACH generation. The formation of these toxic intermediates of metabolism leads to ACH-adduct formation, lipid peroxidation, and ultimately liver injury. Furthermore, characteristics associated with FAS/FAE may be caused by enhanced 2E1 expression in placenta and/or in the developing fetus. In addition, 2E1 plays a prominent role in the activation of carcinogens. Importantly, enhanced expression of the enzyme by alcohol or other agents leads to a synergistic effect toward promotion of carcinogenesis. Finally, many therapeutic agents are metabolized by 2E1 to reactive intermediates that can bind to cellular proteins and under optimal conditions produce toxicity. Elevation of 2E1 by inducers is a primary cause of drug-mediated toxicity because in most cases, there is a shift in the delicate balance from inactivation to activation. Accordingly, 2E1 inhibitors should be beneficial in preventing or improving ethanol-induced liver disorders, FAS/FAE, nitrosamine-promoted carcinogenesis, and drug-induced toxicities (2). With regard to 2E1 polymorphisms, links between various forms of cancer and/or alcoholic liver disease and RFLPs for the *CYP2E1* gene are inconclusive at present. The important toxicologic role of this enzyme still requires further investigations in the area of molecular epidemiology with respect to cancer and drug or alcohol toxicity. A major goal for future research might be to determine the role of polymorphically distributed alleles in relation to the inducibility of this P450.

Probes for 2E1 Phenotyping

Because 2E1 can activate many therapeutic agents and other xenobiotics to highly toxic metabolites, knowledge of the state of induction of 2E1 may have practical applications. For example, determining the extent of induction of 2E1 in heavy drinkers, individuals receiving isoniazid, or those exhibiting certain physiological characteristics (e.g., obesity) may curtail treatment with a potential hepatotoxin, preventing serious liver injury. In this manner, estimating the content of hepatic 2E1 would identify individuals at higher risk for these drug-promoted hepatotoxicities. Although direct hepatic 2E1 quantitation requires a liver biopsy, noninvasive approaches hold inherent appeal and would be of value.

One probe for ascertaining hepatic 2E1 levels is to measure the 6-hydroxychlorzoxazone metabolite in blood samples obtained from subjects administered chlorzoxazone. There are, however, limitations to this procedure. One limitation might be that other P450s contribute to the hydroxylation of chlorzoxazone. CYP1A1, CYP1A2, and CYP3A have each been shown to hydroxylate chlorzoxazone (107–109). Nonetheless, the contribution of these enzymes *in vivo* in human subjects has not been validated. Other limitations are associated with the use of chlorzoxazone as a probe. The application of this procedure may not be suitable in general clinical settings for screening large numbers of samples. It is also time consuming, costly, inconvenient, and requires subject compliance and catheterization for up to 12 hours.

An alternative approach is to measure 2E1 content in an easily accessible peripheral tissue that reflects the hepatic concentration of the enzyme. This may be feasible, given results recently obtained in animals (54,55). Expression of 2E1 in the lymphocyte fraction of white blood cells appears to be influenced by the same factors that affect the concentration of the hepatic enzyme, including xenobiotics and physiological states. Indeed, insulin-dependent diabetes enhances the expression of lymphocyte 2E1 in humans (60), and starvation increases the expression of 2E1 protein and mRNA in rodent lymphocytes (55). With regard to xenobiotics, ethanol produced a 10-fold enrichment of lymphocyte 2E1 in rabbits compared with their control counterparts (54). Interestingly, 2E1 induction by either ethanol (54) or fasting (55) occurred in both liver and lymphocytes in a parallel manner. In a recent report (33) involving human subjects, pharmacokinetic parameters for chlorzoxazone hydroxylation were compared with 2E1 expression in blood. Human peripheral blood lymphocyte (HPBL) microsomes were isolated from blood samples obtained from alcoholics and nonalcoholics, and 2E1 content assessed. In alcoholic subjects, an increase in lymphocyte 2E1 content coincided with a similar increase in chlorzoxazone clearance and decrease in the AUC for chlorzoxazone. An important correlation was observed between 2E1 content in lymphocytes and chlorzoxazone clearance rates. Thus monitoring for lymphocyte 2E1 expression may provide a noninvasive alternative for estimating hepatic activity of this P450.

DRUG INTERACTIONS

As with other human P450 enzymes, serious drug interactions can occur with 2E1. These interactions are largely due to the ability of the enzyme to bioactivate many substrates. The toxic consequences associated with multiple chemical exposures for this P450 reside at the level of induction. Probably the most well-known example is that interaction associated with ethanol and acetaminophen previously described here. Other clinical examples in which exposure of individuals to one chemical has resulted in toxicity from another include the interaction described here for ethanol and tobacco smoke. In this case, a higher incidence of alimentary- and/or respiratory-tract cancers were observed in alcoholic smokers than nonalcoholic tobacco users. Physiological conditions in which 2E1 is elevated, resulting in toxicity from exposure to a drug, represent another form of drug interaction. An example might be greater metabolism of halothane in obese subjects, resulting in a greater susceptibility to halothane-mediated hepato- and nephrotoxicity. From the discussion presented here, and considering the multitude of inducers and substrates for this P450, it is not difficult to envision many putative interactions that could result in serious consequences.

Other than drug interactions involving 2E1 induction, the simultaneous exposure of two xenobiotics metabolized by this P450 can result in an altered pharmacologic response for one of the agents. When 2E1 is involved, this competitive inhibition of metabolism may produce an hepatoprotective response or toxicity, depending on the pharmacologic agent being inhibited. For example, DAS inhibits colon and liver cancer mediated by chemical carcinogens such as *N*-nitrosodimethylamine (2). However, if the agent produces a pharmacologic response before metabolism, inhibition can exaggerate that response. An example of such a situation might be combination therapy of chlorzoxazone and enflurane. Such a drug interaction could enhance the anesthetic effect of enflurane, which could potentially be fatal. Collectively, drug interactions involving 2E1 can occur when the enzyme is induced by one agent with subsequent metabolism of another. Interactions also can occur when two agents that are 2E1 substrates are administered simultaneously. Either situation could have serious consequences or side affects depending on the drugs involved.

An area of considerable current interest for the development of new drugs is the assignment of human P450 enzymes to specific metabolic functions (110). This knowledge provides a basis for determining the potential for drug–drug interactions. Several approaches are used to assign substrate specificities to P450 enzymes. Heterologous expression of these enzymes allows catalytic properties to be examined and is one commonly used approach. *In vitro* studies using heterologously expressed 2E1 indicate substrate specificity and enhance our understanding of metabolism mediated by this enzyme. 2E1 was cloned and expressed in a number of systems for this purpose. The cDNA-directed expression of 2E1 is somewhat complicated because of intrinsic properties of the enzyme. In addition to the general requirements for P450 expression and catalysis, such as noncovalently bound heme (iron-protoporphyrin IX), lipid environment for stability, and NADPH P450 reductase, 2E1 also requires

TABLE 9-6. *Heterologous CYP2E1 expression systems*

Expression system	Promoter	Expression vector	Host cell	Comments	Expected yield	Ref.
Viral Vaccinia virus	Vaccinia early gene	pSC11	TK 143, HepG2	P450 reductase and b_5 present, special utility in mutagenicity studies, human virus is a biohazard, low enzyme expression, transient	36 pmol/mg microsomal protein	147
Baculovirus	Polyhedrin gene	pVL1393	SF9, *T. ni*	High yields purified protein, hemin, and reductase required	50–100 nM	148
Bacterial *Escherichia coli*	*tac, trc*	pCW, pSE420	*Escherichia coli*	Easy manipulation, low cost, many choices for cloning vectors, requires reductase	160 nM	149, 150
Mammalian COS 1 cells	N/A	p91023(B)	COS 1	Utility in multiple cDNA co-transfections, low enzyme expression, transient	N/A	10
Chinese hamster cells	SV40 early gene	pSV450	V79 Chinese hamster	Extremely useful for mutagenicity studies	50 pmol/10^7 cells	151
PC-12	RSV	RSVβ-globin	PC-12	P450 reductase and b_5 present, stable transfection, low enzyme expression	2.5 pmol/mg total protein	152
Human B lymphoblastoid	HSVtk	pEBVHistK	AHH-1TK+/–	Useful for *in situ* toxicity, drug metabolism studies, low enzyme expression	1 pmol/mg total protein	153
HepG2	Thymidine kinase (TK)	pMV7	HepG2	Liver-specific cell functions, P450 reductase & b_5 present, stable transfection	10 pmol/mg microsomal protein	84
Yeast *Saccharomyces cerevisiae*	Metallothionein gene	YEp13	*S. cerevisiae*	Large-scale preps, low cost, requires reductase	8 nM	154

N/A, not applicable.

cytochrome b_5 in the same lipid bilayer (111). These enzyme characteristics require expression systems that have available heme, sufficient amounts of ER, adequate quantities of components required for insertion of 2E1 into the lipid bilayer, such as SRP, and the appropriate membrane receptors. To date, expression systems that have been successfully used to support production of 2E1 are listed in Table 9-6 and include viral, bacterial, yeast, and mammalian systems. Also included in this table are the promoters, expression vectors, host cells used, any pertinent comments, and anticipated yields.

CONCLUDING REMARKS

In this chapter, we emphasized the importance of the ethanol-inducible P450, 2E1, in the metabolism of drugs and chemicals to which humans are routinely exposed. The presence of the enzyme in humans can predict various pathologic disorders that stem from 2E1-mediated metabolism of a variety of chemicals including ethanol. Of the many factors that affect bioactivation and resultant toxicity, the most prominent is variations in 2E1 content. If conversion of a particular substrate to its toxic metabolite is limited by the amount of enzyme present, then enzyme induction may markedly enhance toxicity of the compound. From experimental studies, it is apparent that the regulation of 2E1 expression by both endogenous and exogenous compounds is complex and involves at least three distinct mechanisms operating at the level of transcription, translation, or posttranslation. Age, diet, and hormonal and physiological status are among the endogenous factors affecting 2E1 enzyme levels. Also important are tissue distribution and the various responses of 2E1 within a particular organ to endogenous factors. Of the exogenous factors, alcohol abuse is the most important because of its prevalence. Prolonged ethanol consumption enhances hepatotoxicity and/or hepatocarcinogenesis from numerous agents. In addition, many 2E1 substrates can induce their own bioactivation (e.g., trichloroethylene and ethanol), increasing susceptibility to organ toxicity.

2E1 substrates, for the most part, exhibit similar structural characteristics, being small-molecular-weight compounds with some being volatile in nature. Therapeutic agents that constitute the list of 2E1 substrates are either aromatic, alkanes or alkenes, or halogenated hydrocarbons. Several substrates for 2E1 can act as suicide inhibitors such as the therapeutic agent, disulfiram. These suicide inactivators can result in either a reduction or potentiation of xenobiotic-promoted toxicities. In the case of several environmental agents (e.g., NDMA) that require bioactivation by 2E1, toxicity would be reduced (hepatoprotection), whereas those drugs (e.g., chlorzoxazone) normally converted by the enzyme to an inactive product would exhibit an exaggerated therapeutic response.

Genetic variability in 2E1 expression is also a factor that can influence the outcome of chemical exposure. If it is determined that inheritable polymorphisms within the *CYP2E1* gene affect the expression or function of the encoded protein, then individuals expressing high levels of 2E1 would exhibit enhanced metabolism of 2E1 substrates to reactive intermediates, and as a result, enhanced susceptibility to their cytotoxic effects. New methods are currently being developed to phenotype individuals for hepatic 2E1 expression and hence susceptibility to chemical-mediated toxicities. Among these procedures are the ability to use HPBLs to detect hepatic 2E1 expression. This method alleviates the need for invasive liver biopsies or metabolic studies with a probe drug, such as chlorzoxazone. Monitoring 2E1 expression in HPBLs provides a noninvasive, convenient, and less costly procedure for estimating hepatic activity of this P450. Defining 2E1-catalyzed activities and estimating hepatic concentrations can help to avoid serious drug interactions involving this P450.

REFERENCES

1. Iseri OA, Gottlieb LS, Lieber CS. The ultrastructure of fatty liver induced by prolonged ethanol ingestion. *Am J Pathol* 1966;48:535–555.
2. Lieber CS. Cytochrome P-4502E1: its physiological and pathological role. *Physiol Rev* 1997;77:517–544.
3. Koop DR, Morgan ET, Tarr GE, Coon MJ. Purification and characterization of a unique isozyme of cytochrome P-450 from liver microsomes of ethanol-treated rabbits. *J Biol Chem* 1982;257:8472–8480.
4. Ryan DE, Ramanathan L, Iida S, et al. Characterization of a major form of rat hepatic microsomal cytochrome P-450 induced by isoniazid. *J Biol Chem* 1985;260:6385–6393.
5. Ryan DE, Levin W. Purification and characterization of hepatic microsomal cytochrome P-450. *Pharmacol Ther* 1990;45:153–239.
6. Ryan DE, Koop DR, Thomas PE, Coon MJ, Levin W. Evidence that isoniazid and ethanol induce the same microsomal cytochrome P-450 in rat liver, an isozyme homologous to rabbit liver cytochrome P-450 isozyme 3a. *Arch Biochem Biophys* 1986;246:633–644.
7. Lasker JM, Raucy JL, Kubota S, Bloswick BP, Black M, Lieber CS. Purification and characterization of human liver cytochrome P450-ALC. *Biochem Biophys Res Commun* 1987;148:232–238.
8. Wrighton SA, Thomas PE, Ryan DE, et al. Purification and characterization of ethanol-inducible human hepatic cytochrome P-450HLj. *Arch Biochem Biophys* 1987;258:292–297.
9. Nebert DW, Nelson DR, Adesnik M, et al. The P450 superfamily: updated listing of all genes and recommended nomenclature for the chromosomal loci. *DNA* 1989;8:1–13.
10. Umeno M, McBride OW, Yang CS, Gelboin HV Gonzalez FJ. Human ethanol-inducible P450IIE1: complete gene sequence, promoter characterization, chromosome mapping, and cDNA-directed expression. *Biochemistry* 1988;27:9006–9013.
11. Gonzalez FJ. The molecular biology of cytochrome P450s. *Pharmacol Rev* 1989;40:243–288.
12. Khani SC, Porter TD, Fujita VS, Coon MJ. Organization and differential expression of two highly similar genes in the rabbit alcohol-inducible cytochrome P-450 subfamily. *J Biol Chem* 1988;263:7170–7175.
13. Shimada T, Yamazaki H, Mimura M, Inui Y, Guengerich FP. Interindividual variations in human liver cytochrome P-450 enzymes involved in the oxidation of drugs, carcinogens and toxic chemicals: studies with liver microsomes of 30 Japanese and 30 Caucasians. *J Pharmacol Exp Ther* 1994;270:414–423.
14. Wu D, Cederbaum AI. Presence of functionally active cytochrome P-450IIE1 in the plasma membrane of rat hepatocytes. *Hepatology* 1992;15:515–524.

15. Ding X, Koop DR, Crump BL, Coon MJ. Immunochemical identification of cytochrome P450-3a (P450ALC) in rabbit nasal and kidney microsomes and evidence for differential induction by alcohol. *Mol Pharmacol* 1986;30:370–378.

16. Ding X, Coon MJ. Induction of cytochrome P450 isozyme 3a (P450IIE1) in rabbit olfactory mucosa by ethanol and acetone. *Drug Metab Dispos* 1990;18:742–745.

17. Schnier GG, Laethem CL, Koop DR. Identification and induction of cytochrome P450, P450IIE1 and P450IA1, in rabbit bone marrow. *J Pharmacol Exp Ther* 1989;251:790–796.

18. Hong JY, Pan J, Ning SM, Yang CS. Molecular basis for the sex-related difference in renal *N*-nitrosodimethylamine demethylase in C3H/HeJ mice. *Cancer Res* 1989;49:2973–2977.

19. Mohla S, Ahir S, Ampy FR. Tissue specific regulation of renal *N*-nitrosodimethylamine-demethylase activity by testosterone in BALB/c mice. *Biochem Pharmacol* 1988;37:2697–2702.

20. Carpenter SP, Savage DD, Schultz ED, Raucy JL. Ethanol-mediated transplacental induction of CYP2E1 in fetal rat liver. *J Pharmacol Exp Ther* 1997;282:1028–1036.

21. Carpenter SP, Lasker JM, Raucy JL. Expression, induction, and catalytic activity of the ethanol-inducible cytochrome P450 (CYP2E1) in human fetal liver and hepatocytes. *Mol Pharmacol* 1996;49:260–268.

22. Boutelet-Bochan H, Huang Y, Juchau MR. Expression of *CYP2E1* during embryogenesis and fetogenesis in human cephalic tissues: implications for the fetal alcohol syndrome. *Biochem Biophys Res Commun* 1997;238:443–447.

23. Hakkola J, Pasanen M, Hukkanen J, et al. Expression of xenobiotic-metabolizing cytochrome P450 forms in human full-term placenta. *Biochem Pharmacol* 1996;51:403–411.

24. Rasheed A, Hines RN, McCarver-May DG. Variation in induction of human placental CYP2E1: possible role in susceptibility to fetal alcohol syndrome? *Toxicol Appl Pharmacol* 1997;144:396–400.

25. Botto F, Seree E, Khyari SE, et al. Tissue-specific expression and methylation of the human *CYP2E1* gene. *Biochem Pharmacol* 1994;48:1095–1103.

26. Vieira I, Sonnier M, Cresteil T. Developmental expression of CYP2E1 in the human liver: hypermethylation control of gene expression during the neonatal period. *Eur J Biochem* 1996;238:476–483.

27. Jones SM, Boobis AR, Moore GE, Stanier PM. Expression of CYP2E1 during human fetal development: methylation of the CYP2E1 gene in human fetal and adult liver samples. *Biochem Pharmacol* 1992;43:1876–1879.

28. Botto F, Seree E, El Khyari S, et al. Hypomethylation and hypoexpression of human *CYP2E1* gene in lung tumors. *Biochem Biophys Res Commun* 1994;205:1086–1092.

29. Tukey RH, Johnson EF. Molecular aspects of regulation and structure of the drug-metabolizing enzymes. In: Pratt WB, Taylor P, eds. *Principles of drug action: the basis of pharmacology.* New York: Churchill Livingstone, 1990:423–467.

30. Sakaguchi M, Mihara K, Sato R. Signal recognition particle is required for co-translational insertion of cytochrome P450 into microsomal membranes. *Proc Natl Acad Sci USA* 1984;81:3361–3364.

31. Raucy JL, Kraner JC, Lasker JM. Bioactivation of halogenated hydrocarbons by cytochrome P4502E1. *Crit Rev Toxicol* 1993;23:1–20.

32. Wrighton SA, Thomas PE, Molowa DT, et al. Characterization of ethanol-inducible human liver *N*-nitrosodimethylamine demethylase. *Biochemistry* 1986;25:6731–6735.

33. Raucy JL, Schultz ED, Wester MR, et al. Human lymphocyte cytochrome P450 2E1: a putative marker for alcohol-mediated changes in hepatic chlorzoxazone activity. *Drug Metab Dispos* 1997;25:1429–1435.

34. Girre C, Lucas D, Hispard E, Menez C, Dally S, Menez JF. Assessment of cytochrome P4502E1 induction in alcoholic patients by chlorzoxazone pharmacokinetics. *Biochem Pharmacol* 1994;47:1503–1508.

35. Lucas D, Menez C, Girre C, et al. Cytochrome P450 2E1 genotype and chlorzoxazone metabolism in healthy and alcoholic Caucasian subjects. *Pharmacogenetics* 1995;5:298–304.

36. Koop DR, Tierney DJ. Multiple mechanisms in the regulation of ethanol-inducible cytochrome P450IIE1. *Bioessays* 1990;12:429–435.

37. Reichard GA, Haff AC, Skutches CL, Paul P, Holroyde CP, Owen OE. Plasma acetone metabolism in the fasting human. *J Clin Invest* 1979;63:619–626.

38. Kim SK, Kim YC. Effect of a single administration of benzene, toluene or m-xylene on carboxyhaemoglobin elevation and metabolism of dichloromethane in rats. *J Appl Toxicol* 1996;16:437–444.

39. Zand R, Nelson SD, Slattery JT, et al. Inhibition and induction of cytochrome P4502E1-catalyzed oxidation by isoniazid in humans. *Clin Pharmacol Ther* 1993;54:142–149.

40. Lucas D, Menez C, Girre C, Bodenez P, Hispard E, Menez JF. Decrease in cytochrome P4502E1 as assessed by the rate of chlorzoxazone hydroxylation in alcoholics during the withdrawal phase. *Alcohol Clin Exp Res* 1995;19:362–366.

41. Villard PH, Seree E, Lacarelle B, et al. Effect of cigarette smoke on hepatic and pulmonary cytochromes P450 in mouse: evidence for CYP2E1 induction in lung. *Biochem Biophys Res Commun* 1994;202:1731–1737.

42. Seree EM, Villard PH, Re JL, et al. High inducibility of mouse renal CYP2E1 gene by tobacco smoke and its possible effect on DNA single strand breaks. *Biochem Biophys Res Commun* 1996;219:429–434.

43. Damme B, Darmer D, Pankow D. Induction of hepatic cytochrome P4502E1 in rats by acetylsalicylic acid or sodium salicylate. *Toxicology* 1996;106:99–103.

44. Zangar RC, Woodcroft KJ, Kocarek TA, Novak RF. Xenobiotic-enhanced expression of cytochrome P450 2E1 and 2B1/2B2 in primary cultured rat hepatocytes. *Drug Metab Dispos* 1995;23:681–687.

45. Jeong HG, Yun CH. Induction of rat hepatic cytochrome P450 enzymes by myristicin. *Biochem Biophys Res Commun* 1995;217:966–971.

46. Carroccio A, Wu D, Cederbaum AI. Ethanol increases content and activity of human cytochrome P4502E1 in a transduced HepG2 cell line. *Biochem Biophys Res Commun* 1994;203:727–733.

47. Tierney DJ, Haas AL, Koop DR. Degradation of cytochrome P450 2E1: selective loss after labilization of the enzyme. *Arch Biochem Biophys* 1992;293:9–16.

48. Roberts BJ, Song BJ, Soh Y, Park SS, Shoaf SE. Ethanol induces CYP2E1 by protein stabilization: role of ubiquitin conjugation in the rapid degradation of CYP2E1. *J Biol Chem* 1995;270:29632–29635.

49. Roberts BJ. Evidence of proteasome-mediated cytochrome P-450 degradation. *J Biol Chem* 1997;272:9771–9778.

50. Yang M-X, Cederbaum AI. Role of the proteasome complex in degradation of human CYP2E1 in transfected HepG2 cells. *Biochem Biophys Res Commun* 1996;226:711–716.

51. Kraner JC, Lasker JM, Corcoran GB, Ray SD, Raucy JL. Induction of P4502E1 by acetone in isolated rabbit hepatocytes: role of increased protein and mRNA synthesis. *Biochem Pharmacol* 1993;45:1483–1492.

52. Badger TM, Crouch J, Irby D, Hakkak R, Shahare M. Episodic excretion of ethanol during chronic intragastric ethanol infusion in the male rat: continuous vs. cyclic ethanol and nutrient infusions. *J Pharmacol Exp Ther* 1993;264:938–943.

53. Badger TM, Huan J, Ronis M, Lumpkin CK. Induction of cytochrome P4502E1 during chronic ethanol exposure occurs via transcription of the CYP2E1 gene when blood alcohol concentrations are high. *Biochem Biophys Res Commun* 1993;190:780–785.

54. Raucy JL, Curley G, Carpenter SP. The use of lymphocytes for assessing ethanol-mediated alterations in the expression of hepatic CYP2E1. *Alcohol Clin Exp Res* 1995;19:1369–1375.

55. Soh Y, Rhee HM, Sohn DH, Song BJ. Immunological detection of CYP2E1 in fresh rat lymphocytes and its pretranslational induction by fasting. *Biochem Biophys Res Commun* 1996;227:541–546.

56. Yun Y-P, Casazza JP, Sohn DH, Veech RL, Song BJ. Pretranslational activation of cytochrome P450IIE1 during ketosis induced by a high fat diet. *Mol Pharmacol* 1992;41:474–479.

57. O'Shea D, Davis SN, Kim RB, Wilkinson GR. Effect of fasting and obesity in humans on the 6-hydroxylation of chlorzoxazone: a putative probe of CYP2E1 activity. *Clin Pharmacol Ther* 1994;56:359–367.

58. Yoo JS, Ning SM, Pantuck CB, Pantuck EJ, Yang CS. Regulation of hepatic microsomal cytochrome P450IIE1 level by dietary lipids and carbohydrates in rats. *J Nutr* 1991;121:959–965.

59. Raucy JL, Lasker JM, Kraner JC, Salazar DE, Lieber CS, Corcoran GB. Induction of P450IIE1 in the obese overfed rat. *Mol Pharmacol* 1991;39:275–280.

60. Song BJ, Veech RL, Saenger P. Cytochrome P450IIE1 is elevated in lymphocytes from poorly controlled insulin-dependent diabetics. *J Clin Endocrinol Metab* 1990;71:1036–1040.

61. Kim SG, Kwak JY, Lee JW, Novak RF, Park SS, Kim ND. Malotilate, a hepatoprotectant, suppresses CYP2E1 expression in rats. *Biochem Biophys Res Commun* 1994;200:1414–1420.

62. Jeong K-S, Lee IJ, Roberts BJ, et al. Transcriptional inhibition of cytochrome P4502E1 by a synthetic compound, YH439. *Arch Biochem Biophys* 1996;326:137–144.

63. Kwak MK, Kim SG, Kwak JY, Novak RF, Kim ND. Inhibition of cytochrome P4502E1 expression by organosulfur compounds allylsulfide, allylmercaptan and allylmethylsulfide in rats. *Biochem Pharmacol* 1994;47:531–539.

64. Kim ND, Kwak MK, Kim SG. Inhibition of cytochrome P450 2E1 expression by 2-(allylthio)pyrazine, a potential chemoprotective agent: hepatoprotective effects. *Biochem Pharmacol* 1997;53:261–269.

65. Ishizaki H, Brady JF, Ning SM, Yang CS. Effect of phenethylisothiocyanate on microsomal *N*-nitrosodimethylamine metabolism and other monooxygenase activities. *Xenobiotica* 1990;20:255–264.

66. Nedelcheva V, Persson I, Ingelman-Sundberg M. Genetic polymorphism of human cytochrome P450 2E1. *Methods Enzymol* 1996;272: 218–225.

67. Ingelman-Sundberg M. Genetic polymorphism of drug metabolizing enzymes: implications for toxicity of drugs and other xenobiotics. *Arch Toxicol Suppl* 1997;19:3–13.

68. Hayashi S, Watanabe J, Kawajiri K. Genetic polymorphisms in the 5'-flanking region change transcriptional regulation of the human cytochrome P450IIE1 gene. *J Biochem (Tokyo)* 1991;110:559–565.

69. London SJ, Daly AK, Cooper J, et al. Lung cancer risk in relation to the *CYP2E1 Rsa* I genetic polymorphism among African-Americans and Caucasians in Los Angeles County. *Pharmacogenetics* 1996;6: 151–158.

70. Kato SS, Shields PG, Caporaso NE, et al. Cytochrome P450IIE1 genetic polymorphism, racial variation and lung cancer risk. *Cancer Res* 1992;52:6712–6715.

71. Hu Y, Oscarson M, Johansson I, et al. Genetic polymorphism of human *CYP2E1*: characterization of two variant alleles. *Mol Pharmacol* 1997;51:370–376.

72. Koop DR. Oxidative and reductive metabolism by cytochrome P450 2E1. *FASEB J* 1992;6:724–730.

73. Mackman R, Guo Z, Guengerich FP, Ortiz de Montellano P. Active site topology of human cytochrome P450 2E1. *Chem Res Toxicol* 1996;9:223–226.

74. Swanson BA, Dutton DR, Lunetta JM, Yang CS, Ortiz de Montellano PR. The active sites of cytochromes P450 1A1, IIB1, IIB2, and IIE1: topological analysis by *in situ* rearrangement or phenyl-iron complexes. *J Biol Chem* 1991;266:19258–19264.

75. Reinke LA, Lai EK, McCay PB. Ethanol feeding stimulates trichloromethyl radical formation from carbon tetrachloride in liver. *Xenobiotica* 1988;18:1311–1318.

76. Raucy JL, Lasker JM, Lieber CS, Black M. Acetaminophen activation by human liver cytochromes P450IIE1 and P450IA2. *Arch Biochem Biophys* 1989;271:270–283.

77. Raucy J, Fernandes P, Black M, Yang SL, Koop DR. Identification of a human liver cytochrome P450 exhibiting catalytic and immunochemical similarities to cytochrome P450 3a of rabbit liver. *Biochem Pharmacol* 1987;36:2921–2916.

78. Gu L, Gonzalez FJ, Kalow W, Tang BK. Biotransformation of caffeine, paraxanthine, theobromine and theophylline by cDNA-expressed human CYP1A2 and CYP2E1. *Pharmacogenetics* 1992;2: 73–77.

79. Tassaneeyakul W, Birkett DJ, McManus ME, et al. Caffeine metabolism by human hepatic cytochromes P450: contributions of 1A2, 2E1 and 3A isoforms. *Biochem Pharmacol* 1994;47:1767–1776.

80. Dai Y, Cederbaum AI. Inactivation and degradation of human cytochrome P4502E1 by CCl_4 in a transfected HepG2 cell line. *J Pharmacol Exp Ther* 1995;275:1614–1622.

81. Lauriault VV, Khan S, O'Brien PJ. Hepatocyte cytotoxicity induced by various hepatotoxins mediated by cytochrome P-450IIE1: protection with diethyldithiocarbamate administration. *Chem Biol Interact* 1992; 81:271–289.

82. Koop DR. Inhibition of ethanol-inducible cytochrome P450IIE1 by 3-amino-1,2,4-triazole. *Chem Res Toxicol* 1990;3:377–383.

83. Lieber CS. Biochemical and molecular basis of alcohol-induced injury to liver and other tissues. *N Engl J Med* 1988;319: 1639–1650.

84. Dai Y, Rashba-Step J, Cederbaum AI. Stable expression of human cytochrome P4502E1 in HepG2 cells: characterization of catalytic activities and production of reactive oxygen intermediates. *Biochemistry* 1993;32:6928–6937.

85. Lieber CS, Garro A, Leo MA, Mak LM, Worner T. Alcohol and cancer. *Hepatology* 1986;6:1005–1019.

86. Garro AJ, Lieber CS. Alcohol and cancer. *Annu Rev Pharmacol Toxicol* 1990;30:219–249.

87. Uematsu F, Kikuchi H, Motomiya M, et al. Association between restriction fragment length polymorphism of the human cytochrome P450IIE1 gene and susceptibility to lung cancer. *Jpn J Cancer Res* 1991;82:254–256.

88. Hirvonen A, Husgafvel-Pursiainen K, Anttila S, Karjalainen A, Vainio H. The human CYP2E1 gene and lung cancer: *Dra* I and *Rsa* I restriction fragment length polymorphisms in a Finnish study population. *Carcinogenesis* 1993;14:85–88.

89. El-Zein RA, Zwischenberger JB, Abdel-Rahman SZ, Sankar AB, Au WW. Polymorphism of metabolizing genes and lung cancer histology: prevalence of CYP2E1 in adenocarcinoma. *Cancer Lett* 1997;112: 71–78.

90. Oyama T, Kawamoto T, Mizoue T, et al. Cytochrome P450 2E1 polymorphism as a risk factor for lung cancer: in relation to p53 gene mutation. *Anticancer Res* 1997;17:583–587.

91. Persson I, Johansson I, Bergling H, et al. Genetic polymorphism of cytochrome P4502E1 in a Swedish population: relationship to incidence of lung cancer. *FEBS Lett* 1993;319:207–211.

92. Iwahashi K, Nakamura K, Suwaki H, Matsuo Y, Ichikawa Y. Relationship between genetic polymorphism of CYP2E1 and ALDH2, and possible susceptibility to alcoholism. *Alcohol Alcohol* 1994;29: 639–642.

93. Maezawa Y, Yamauchi M, Toda G. Association between restriction fragment length polymorphism of the human cytochrome P450IIE1 gene and susceptibility to alcoholic liver cirrhosis. *Am J Gastroenterol* 1994;89:561–565.

94. Tanaka F, Shiratori Y, Yokosuka O, Imazeki F, Tsukada Y, Omata M. Polymorphism of alcohol-metabolizing genes affects drinking behavior and alcoholic liver disease in Japanese men. *Alcohol Clin Exp Res* 1997;21:596–601.

95. Seeff LB, Cuccherini BA, Zimmerman HJ, Alder E, Benjamin SB. Acetaminophen hepatotoxicity in alcoholics. *Ann Intern Med* 1986; 104:399–404.

96. Black M, Raucy JL. Acetaminophen, alcohol, and cytochrome P450. *Ann Intern Med* 1986;104:427–429.

97. Lee SST, Buters JTM, Pineau T, Fernandez-Salguero P, Gonzalez FJ. Role of CYP2E1 in the hepatotoxicity of acetaminophen. *J Biol Chem* 1996;271:12063–12067.

98. Kharasch ED, Hankins D, Mautz D, Thummel KE. Identification of the enzyme responsible for oxidative halothane metabolism: implications for prevention of halothane hepatitis. *Lancet* 1996;347: 1367–1371.

99. Bourdi M, Chen W, Peter RM, et al. Human cytochrome P450 2E1 is a major autoantigen associated with halothane hepatitis. *Chem Res Toxicol* 1996;9:1159–1166.

100. Eliasson E, Kenna JG. Cytochrome P450 2E1 is a cell surface autoantigen in halothane hepatitis. *Mol Pharmacol* 1996;50:573–582.

101. Kitteringham NR, Kenna JG, Park BK. Detection of autoantibodies directed against human hepatic endoplasmic reticulum in sera from patients with halothane-associated hepatitis. *Br J Clin Pharmacol* 1995;40:379–386.

102. Jones KL, Smith DW. Recognition of the fetal alcohol syndrome in early infancy. *Lancet* 1973;2:999–1001.

103. Abel EL, Sokol RJ. Incidence of fetal alcohol syndrome and economic impact of FAS-related anomalies. *Drug Alcohol Depend* 1987; 19:51–70.

104. Lieber CS. Metabolic effects of acetaldehyde. *Biochem Soc Trans* 1988;16:241–247.

105. Ristow H, Seyfarth A, Lochmann E-R. Chromosomal damages by ethanol and acetaldehyde in *Saccharomyces cerevisiae* as studied by pulsed field gel electrophoresis. *Mutat Res* 1995;326:165–170.

106. Raucy JL, Carpenter SJ. The expression of xenobiotic-metabolizing cytochromes P450 in fetal tissues. *J Pharmacol Toxicol Methods* 1993;29:121–128.

107. Gorski JC, Jones DR, Wrighton SA, Hall SD. Contribution of human CYP3A subfamily members to the 6-hydroxylation of chlorzoxazone. *Xenobiotica* 1997;27:243–256.

108. Carriere V, Goasduff T, Ratanasavanh D, et al. Both cytochromes P450 2E1 and 1A1 are involved in the metabolism of chlorzoxazone. *Chem Res Toxicol* 1993;6:852–857.

109. Ono S, Hatanaka T, Hotta H, Tsutsui M, Satoh T, Gonzalez FJ. Chlorzoxazone is metabolized by human CYP1A2 as well as by human CYP2E1. *Pharmacogenetics* 1995;5:143–150.

110. Peck CC, Temple R, Collins SM. Understanding the consequences of concurrent therapies. *JAMA* 1993;269:1550–1552.

111. Gonzalez FJ, Aoyama T, Gelboin HV. Heterologous expression. *Methods Enzymol* 1991;206:85–145.

112. Zerilli A, Lucas D, Amet Y, et al. Cytochrome P-450 2E1 in rat liver, kidney and lung microsomes after chronic administration of ethanol either orally or by inhalation. *Alcohol Alcohol* 1995;30:357–365.

113. Yang CS, Patten CJ, Ishizaki H, Yoo JH. Induction, purification, and characterization of cytochrome P450IIE1. *Methods Enzymol* 1991; 206:595–603.

114. Yang CS, Koop DR, Wang T, Coon MJ. Immunochemical studies on the metabolism of nitrosamines by ethanol-inducible cytochrome P-450. *Biochem Biophys Res Commun* 1985;2:1007–1013.

115. Miller MS, Warner SP, Jorquera R, Castonguay A, Schuller HM. Expression of the cytochrome P4502E and 2B gene families in the lungs and livers of nonpregnant, pregnant, and fetal hamsters. *Biochem Pharmacol* 1992;44:797–803.

116. Amet Y, Berthou F, Fournier G, et al. Cytochrome P450 4A and 2E1 expression in human kidney microsomes. *Biochem Pharmacol* 1997; 53:765–771.

117. Ueng T-H, Tsai J-N, Ju J-M, et al. Effects of acetone administration on cytochrome P450-dependent monooxygenases in hamster liver, kidney, and lung. *Arch Toxicol* 1991;65:45–51.

118. Davis JF, Felder MR. Mouse ethanol-inducible cytochrome P450 (P450IIE1): characterization of cDNA clones and testosterone induction in kidney tissue. *J Biol Chem* 1993;268:16584–16589.

119. Wheeler CW, Wrighton SA, Guenthner TM. Detection of human lung cytochromes P450 that are immunochemically related to cytochrome P450IIE1 and cytochrome P450IIIA. *Biochem Pharmacol* 1992;44: 183–187.

120. Ueng TH, Friedman FK, Miller H, Park SS, Gelboin HV, Alvares AP. Studies on ethanol-inducible cytochrome P-450 in rabbit liver, lungs and kidneys. *Biochem Pharmacol* 1987;36:2689–2691.

121. Roberts BJ, Shoaf SE, Jeong K-S, Song BJ. Induction of CYP2E1 in liver, kidney, brain and intestine during chronic ethanol administration and withdrawal: evidence that CYP2E1 possesses a rapid phase half-life of 6 hours or less. *Biochem Biophys Res Commun* 1994;205: 1064–1071.

122. Shimizu M, Lasker JM, Tsutsumi M, Lieber CS. Immunohistochemical localization of ethanol-inducible P450IIE1 in the rat alimentary tract. *Biochem Biophys Res Commun* 1990;99:1044–1050.

123. Sampol E, Mirrione A, Villard PH, et al. Evidence for a tissue-specific induction of cutaneous CYP2E1 by dexamethasone. *Biochem Biophys Res Commun* 1997;235:557–561.

124. Warner M, Gustafsson JA. Effect of ethanol on cytochrome P450 in the rat brain. *Proc Natl Acad Sci U S A* 1994;91:1019–1023.

125. Sipes IG, Stripp B, Krishna G, Maling HM, Gillette JR. Enhanced hepatic microsomal activity by pretreatment of rats with acetone or isopropanol. *Proc Soc Exp Biol Med* 1973;142:237–240.

126. Tu YY, Peng R, Chang ZF, Yang CS. Induction of a high affinity nitrosamine demethylase in rat liver microsomes by acetone and isopropanol. *Chem Biol Interact* 1983;44:247–260.

127. Kostrubsky VE, Strom SC, Wood SG, Wrighton SA, Sinclair PR, Sinclair JF. Ethanol and isopentanol increase CYP3A and CYP2E in primary cultures of human hepatocytes. *Arch Biochem Biophys* 1995;322:516–520.

128. Brady JF, Li D, Ishizaki H, et al. Induction of cytochromes P450IIE1 and P450IIB1 by secondary ketones and the role of the P450IIE1 in chloroform metabolism. *Toxicol Appl Pharmacol* 1989;100:342–349.

129. Brady JF, Lee MJ, Li M, Ishizaki H, Yang CS. Diethyl ether as a substrate for acetone/ethanol-inducible cytochrome P-450 and as an inducer for cytochrome(s) P-450. *Mol Pharmacol* 1988;33:148–154.

130. Koop DR, Crump BL, Nordblom GD, Coon MJ. Immunochemical evidence for induction of the alcohol-oxidizing cytochrome P-450 of rabbit liver microsomes by diverse agents: ethanol, imidazole, trichloroethylene, acetone, pyrazole, and isoniazid. *Proc Natl Acad Sci USA* 1985;82:4065–4069.

131. Novak RF, Kaul KL, Kim SG. Induction of the alcohol-inducible form of cytochrome P-450 by nitrogen-containing heterocycles: effects on pyridine *N*-oxide production. *Drug Metab Rev* 1989;20:781–792.

132. Winters DK, Cederbaum AI. Time course characterization of the induction of cytochrome P450 2E1 by pyrazole and 4-methylpyrazole. *Biochim Biophys Acta* 1992;1117:15–24.

133. Kim SG, Novak RF. The induction of cytochrome P4502E1 by nitrogen- and sulfur-containing heterocycles: expression and molecular regulation. *Toxicol Appl Pharmacol* 1993;120:257–265.

134. Song BJ, Matsunaga T, Hardwick JP, et al. Stabilization of cytochrome P450j messenger ribonucleic acid in the diabetic rat. *Mol Endocrinol* 1987;1:542–547.

135. Johansson I, Lindros KO, Eriksson H, Ingelman-Sundberg M. Transcriptional control of CYP2E1 in the perivenous liver region and during starvation. *Biochem Biophys Res Commun* 1990;173:331–338.

136. Yamazoe Y, Murayama N, Shimada M, Imaoka S, Funae Y, Kato R. Suppression of hepatic levels of an ethanol-inducible P450DM/j by growth hormone: relationship between the increased level of P450DM/j and depletion of growth hormone in diabetes. *Mol Pharmacol* 1989;36:716–722.

137. Guengerich FP, Kim DH, Iwasaki M. Role of human cytochrome P-450 IIE1 in the oxidation of many low molecular weight cancer suspects. *Chem Res Toxicol* 1991;4:168–179.

138. Brady JF, Xiao F, Wang MH, et al. Effects of disulfiram on hepatic P450IIE1, other microsomal enzymes, and hepatotoxicity in rats. *Toxicol Appl Pharmacol* 1991;108:366–373.

139. Chang TKH, Gonzalez FJ, Waxman DJ. Evaluation of triacetyloleandomycin: α-naphthoflavone and diethyldithiocarbamate as selective chemical probes for inhibition of human cytochromes P450. *Arch Biochem Biophys* 1994;311:437–442.

140. Brady JF, Ishizaki H, Fukuto JM, et al. Inhibition of cytochrome P-450 2E1 by diallyl sulfide and its metabolites. *Chem Res Toxicol* 1991;4:642–647.

141. Chen L, Lee M, Hong J-Y, Huang W, Wang E, Yang CS. Relationship between cytochrome P450 2E1 and acetone catabolism in rats as studied with diallyl sulfide as an inhibitor. *Biochem Pharmacol* 1994;48: 2199–2205.

142. Surh YJ, Lee RC, Park KK, Mayne ST, Liem A, Miller JA. Chemoprotective effects of capsaicin and diallyl sulfide against mutagenesis or tumorigenesis by vinyl carbamate and *N*-nitrosodimethylamine. *Carcinogenesis* 1995;16:2467–2471.

143. Manno M, Cazzaro S, Rezzadore M. The mechanism of the suicidal reductive inactivation of microsomal cytochrome P-450 by halothane. *Arch Toxicol* 1991;65:191–198.

144. Manno M, Ferrara R, Cazzaro S, Rigotti P, Ancona E. Suicidal inactivation of human cytochrome P-450 by carbon tetrachloride and halothane *in vitro*. *Pharmacol Toxicol* 1992;70:13–18.

145. Hu Y, Mishin V, Johansson I, et al. Chlormethiazole as an efficient inhibitor of cytochrome P450 2E1 expression in rat liver. *J Pharmacol Exp Ther* 1994;269:1286–1291.

146. Wu D, Cederbaum AI. Induction of liver cytochrome P4502E1 by pyrazole and 4-methylpyrazole in neonatal rats. *J Pharmacol Exp Ther* 1993;264:1468–1473.

147. Patten CJ, Ishizaki H, Aoyama T, et al. Catalytic properties of the human cytochrome P450 2E1 produced by cDNA expression in mammalian cells. *Arch Biochem Biophys* 1992;299:163–171.

148. Grogan J, Shou M, Andrusiak EA, et al. Cytochrome P450 2A1, 2E1, and 2C9 cDNA-expression by insect cells and partial purification using hydrophobic chromatography. *Biochem Pharmacol* 1995;50: 1509–1515.

149. Gillam EM, Guo Z, Guengerich FP. Expression of modified human cytochrome P450 2E1 in *Escherichia coli*, purification, and spectral and catalytic properties. *Arch Biochem Biophys* 1994;312:59–66.

150. Winters DK, Cederbaum AI. Expression of a catalytically active human cytochrome P4502E1 in *Escherichia coli*. *Biochim Biophys Acta* 1992;1156:43–49.

151. Schmalix WA, Barrenscheen M, Landsiedel R, et al. Stable expression of human cytochrome P450 2E1 in V79 Chinese hamster cells. *Eur J Pharmacol* 1995;293:123–131.

152. Mapoles J, Berthou F, Alexander A, Simon F, Menez J-F. Mammalian PC-12 cell genetically engineered for human cytochrome P4502E1 expression. *Eur J Biochem* 1993;214:735–745.

153. Crespi CL, Langenbach R, Penman BW. Human cell lines, derived from AHH-1 TK+/– human lymphoblasts, genetically engineered for expression of cytochromes P450. *Toxicology* 1993;82:89–104.

154. Pernecky SJ, Porter TD, Coon MJ. Expression of rabbit cytochrome P-450IIE2 in yeast and stabilization of the enzyme by 4-methylpyrazole. *Biochem Biophys Res Commun* 1990;172:1331–1337.

CHAPTER 10

CYP3A

Steven A. Wrighton and Kenneth E. Thummel

The CYP3A subfamily of cytochromes P450 in humans is composed of several enzymes that catalyze the metabolism of an amazingly large number of structurally diverse xenobiotics and endobiotics (1–4). Studies to date indicate that the CYP3A P450s are the dominant oxidative enzymes in human drug metabolism. Estimates suggest that CYP3A forms participate in the metabolism of more than 50% of all drugs for which the P450s responsible for their metabolism are known (5). Thus, factors that alter the catalytic activity of the forms of P450 in the CYP3A subfamily contribute to the variability observed in the metabolic clearance of a large number of drugs in patients. In addition to interindividual differences that are related to constitutive expression of these enzymes, there can be wide swings in the metabolic clearance of CYP3A substrates as a result of enzyme induction and inhibition. Indeed, as is described later in this chapter, drugs that affect CYP3A function cause some of the most profound and clinically significant interactions reported with modern drug therapy.

HUMAN CYP3A ENZYMES

CYP3A3 and CYP3A4

The first CYP3A subfamily member isolated from human liver was at the time termed $P450_5$ (6). However, little characterization of this P450 was reported. Watkins and colleagues isolated and characterized a human liver P450 termed HLp, which was immunochemically and structurally related to rat CYP3A1 (7). Shortly after the isolation of HLp, the isolation and characterization of a P450 capable of oxidizing nifedipine, termed P450NF,

was reported (8). All three of these P450s were related in that antibodies raised against $P450_5$ were strongly cross reactive to each protein. Monoclonal antibodies recognizing $P450_5$ and HLp were used to screen a human liver cDNA expression library. This screening resulted in the isolation of three overlapping cDNA clones, which yielded a sequence then known as CYP3A3 (9,10). Beaune and colleagues screened the same human liver cDNA expression library with a polyclonal anti-P450$_{NF}$ antibody and obtained a full-length cDNA termed NF25 (11). The sequence obtained from NF25, currently termed CYP3A4 (10), was found to differ from that reported for CYP3A3 by 14 nucleotide positions, including a three-base frameshift. The deduced amino acid sequences from these two cDNAs are 97% similar.

Until recently, it was thought that CYP3A3 and CYP3A4 represented separate genes, despite their close similarity. However, a considerable number of studies have been performed in a number of different laboratories investigating the relative expression of CYP3A3 and CYP3A4 in human tissues. The expression of an mRNA encoding CYP3A3 has not been detected when the polymerase chain reaction was used with primers specific for CYP3A3 (12). As the result of such studies, the existence of CYP3A3 as a gene separate from CYP3A4 is in doubt (1,10,12). Therefore, when publications discuss the CYP3A subfamily, the reader should keep in mind that CYP3A3 and CYP3A4, and thus HLp and P450NF, are considered to be the same P450.

CYP3A4 Tissue Distribution

The most prominently expressed P450 in the human liver is CYP3A4. In a study examining the relative expression of the various P450s in 60 human livers, CYP3A4 was found to account for, on average, 29% of the total P450 present (13). As much as 60% of the P450 present in microsomes from an exceptional human liver was found to be CYP3A4 (14). Furthermore, the levels of CYP3A4

S. A. Wrighton: Department of Drug Disposition, Eli Lilly & Co., Lilly Research Laboratories, Mail Drop 0825, Indianapolis, Indiana 46285

K. E. Thummel: Department of Pharmaceutics, University of Washington, Box 357610, H272 Health Sciences Building, Seattle, Washington 98195-7610

determined immunochemically in a bank of human liver samples exhibited a 20-fold range (1). CYP3A4 is also the dominant microsomal P450 in the mucosal epithelial barrier of the small intestine (15,16). Its expression is higher in the proximal (duodenum-jejunum) small bowel, in comparison to the distal (ileum) bowel (15,17). The mean level of duodenal mucosal microsomal CYP3A in a bank of human small intestines was found to be approximately 44% of that in the human liver, but like the liver, individual levels varied more than 20-fold (18). Whereas some of the intestinal variability may be the result of *ex vivo* enzyme degradation, much of it is likely to result from the effects of endogenous and exogenous factors.

There are several mechanisms that may account for widely varying expression of hepatic CYP3A4. The levels of CYP3A4 are induced or increased by exposure of the patient to a number of drugs. The levels of CYP3A4 are also decreased by a number of mechanism-based or suicidal inhibitors. In addition, basal expression of the enzyme may be under the control of endogenous circulating hormones.

CYP3A4 Gene Regulation

As previously discussed, the levels of hepatic and intestinal CYP3A4 are induced by the exposure of patients to a number of structurally diverse agents. Inducing agents include glucocorticoids (e.g., dexamethasone), carbamazepine, phenobarbital, and rifampin (1,4). A more thorough discussion of inducers and the clinical significance of induction occurs later in this chapter. The mechanism by which inducers increase the expression of CYP3A4 in human liver is not completely understood. However, there has been extensive recent progress using animal models to examine the induction of CYP3A forms by glucocorticoids. Initial studies by Schuetz and colleagues (19,20) demonstrated that induction of rat CYP3A by glucocorticoids occurred by a mechanism separate from that for classic glucocorticoid-responsive genes such as tyrosine amino transferase (TAT). These investigators demonstrated that rat CYP3A induction differed from TAT induction by (a) time course of induction, (b) concentration of steroid necessary to achieve a response, (c) structure–activity relationship of the responses to glucocorticoid and related steroids, and (d) response to the antiglucocorticoid pregnenolone 16α-carbonitrile (PCN). Specifically, PCN did induce CYP3A expression and, as predicted for an antiglucocorticoid, inhibited the induction of TAT by dexamethasone. Therefore, the glucocorticoid inducers of rat CYP3A appeared to be acting through a nonclassic glucocorticoid receptor or the glucocorticoid receptor in a nonclassic fashion, resulting in increased transcription of the CYP3A gene.

Several recent studies have shed some light on the mechanism by which at least glucocorticoids activate the transcription of CYP3A genes. Using a number of molec-

ular biologic techniques, including reporter systems linked to the 5'-regulatory regions of the CYP3A genes, DNAase footprinting, mutation analyses, and gel mobility shifts, these studies demonstrated that several *cis*-acting elements in the rat CYP3A genes are involved in the response of CYP3A to glucocorticoids (21–23). These dexamethasone-responsive elements are different in DNA sequence than the classic glucocorticoid-responsive elements and do not appear to bind the glucocorticoid receptor. Recently, however, an orphan nuclear receptor termed the pregnane X receptor (PXR) in mice was found to be activated by both glucocorticoids and the antiglucocorticoid PCN (24). After activation by dexamethasone or PCN, mPXR was shown to bind as a heterodimer with 9-*cis* retinoic acid receptor to the dexamethasone-responsive elements, discussed earlier, of the CYP3A genes (24).

Although the dexamethasone-responsive elements and the mPXR were identified in investigations using experimental animal models, a similar mechanism for the induction of CYP3A4 in humans by glucocorticoids would be expected. This was demonstrated when a reporter system containing the 5'-regulatory region of the human CYP3A4 gene was transfected into rat hepatocytes and inducers of CYP3A4 were found to trigger the expression of the reporter gene (25). In addition, rifampin was shown to displace dexamethasone from the human glucocorticoid receptor (26), suggesting that rifampin is a nonsteroidal ligand of the human PXR. This was confirmed definitively with the identification and characterization of hPXR, the human ortholog to the mouse nuclear receptor (27). Like mPXR, hPXR forms a heterodimer with 9-*cis* retinoic acid receptor, which binds to the dexamethasone response element in the promoter region of the CYP3A4 gene. Furthermore, hPXR was shown to be activated by several of the compounds known to induce CYP3A4 transcription in hepatocytes (i.e., dexamethasone, rifampin, clotrimazole, and phenobarbital) and, more notably, was only weakly activated by PCN, a compound that is a potent inducer of rat CYP3A but not human hepatocellular CYP3A. Finally, Northern blot analysis indicated selective expression of hPXR in human liver and intestine, tissues with abundant CYP3A4 protein and catalytic activity. Thus, glucocorticoids and other nonsteroidal inducers of CYP3A4 may transcriptionally regulate the expression of CYP3A4 *in vivo* by the same mechanism.

The source of constitutive variability in CYP3A4 expression remains largely a mystery. In the rat, hepatic CYP3A2 is regulated by circulating levels of growth hormone (28). A similar mechanism for humans has not been demonstrated to date, although growth hormone has a stimulatory effect on CYP3A4 expression in primary hepatocyte culture (29). In addition, another circulating hormone, triiodothyronine, appears to have the opposite effect on CYP3A4 expression in human hepatocyte culture, reducing mRNA levels well below that of untreated controls (29). It is possible that homeostatic or pathophysiologic variability in the circulating concentrations of these and other hormones contributes to interindividual differences in hepatic CYP3A4 expression.

Recent findings from studies with Caco-2 cell monolayers raise the possibility that yet another hormone, $1\alpha,25$-dihydroxy vitamin D_3, may influence the expression of intestinal CYP3A4. Produced by the liver and kidney, $1\alpha,25$-dihydroxy vitamin D_3 is a known modulator of cell function throughout the body and it exerts profound effects on epithelial cells of the small intestine (30,31). When added to confluent Caco-2 cell monolayers, the hormone stimulates the expression of CYP3A4 and increases CYP3A4 catalytic activity by 50-fold (32). The relative magnitude of effect of $1\alpha,25$-dihydroxy vitamin D_3, 25-hydroxy vitamin D_3, and vitamin D_3 on CYP3A4 catalytic function in Caco-2 cells is consistent with their ability to interact with the vitamin D receptor (32). Thus, it is possible that $1\alpha,25$-dihydroxy vitamin D_3 exerts a similar regulatory effect on CYP3A4 expression in mucosal epithelial cells of the human small intestine *in vivo*.

CYP3A5 Tissue Distribution, Regulation, and Function

The second functional member of the human CYP3A subfamily is CYP3A5 (10). This P450 was first isolated from human liver and demonstrated to have a distinct molecular weight and amino terminal amino acid sequence as compared to CYP3A4 (33). The cDNA sequence of CYP3A5 was found to be 88% similar to that of CYP3A4 (34). Interestingly, unlike CYP3A4, which appears to be expressed in all livers, CYP3A5 was detected by immunochemical methods in only about 30% of livers (33,35). Furthermore, in those livers in which CYP3A5 was detected, it was usually expressed at levels significantly lower than those of CYP3A4 (33,35), although it is the major CYP3A form in approximately one of 20 livers (18). Recent work indicates that CYP3A5 may be expressed in the liver more often than originally suggested, but at levels that are near the limits of detection of immunochemical methods (36).

A polymorphic pattern of "readily detectable" CYP3A5 expression has also been observed with microsomes isolated from human intestinal mucosa (18). However, low levels of the protein can be found along the entire gastrointestinal tract, most notably in the epithelial barrier of the stomach and large intestine (12). As is discussed in greater detail later in this chapter, CYP3A5 is the dominant CYP3A form in the human kidney, where it may play a role in the hydroxylation of endogenous molecules such as cortisol (37,38). CYP3A5 has also been detected at trace levels in other extrahepatic sites, including lung (39,40) and pancreas (12).

The regulation of CYP3A5 expression is not as well understood as that of CYP3A4. The reason for the unusual expression of CYP3A5 in the liver has been investigated.

One potential explanation arises from the identification of an allelic variant of CYP3A5, which has a point mutation that may result in the expression of an unstable protein (36). The level of expression of CYP3A5 in the liver does not appear to be directly related to the expression of CYP3A4. Several studies have indicated that, in those livers with high levels of CYP3A4 as a result of induction by dexamethasone or barbiturates, CYP3A5 levels are not necessarily elevated (33,35,41). However, Schuetz and colleagues (42), in examining the 5'-regulatory region of the CYP3A5 gene, found that it contained a novel dexamethasone-responsive element and that transcriptional activation of the CYP3A5 gene was dependent on the glucocorticoid receptor. In addition, recent work in cultures of primary human hepatocytes has shown that CYP3A5 is induced by rifampin and phenobarbital treatment (V. Kostrubsky, University of Pittsburgh, *personal communication*, 1998). In order to determine whether these *in vitro* findings concerning the factors that influence CYP3A5 expression have any meaning *in vivo*, more sensitive methods for the detection of CYP3A5 are required.

The substrate specificity of CYP3A5 in general appears to be similar to that of CYP3A4. That is, CYP3A5 has been shown to be capable of metabolizing most substrates of CYP3A4 (33,35). For some substrates, the rates of metabolism by CYP3A5 are reported to be slower in comparison to that seen with CYP3A4 (35,43,44). However, more recent reports suggest that conditions for enzyme reconstitution can have a profound effect on CYP3A5 catalytic activity (45). For example, erythromycin, the classic substrate of CYP3A4, was found not to be metabolized by CYP3A5 when reconstituted in phosphate buffer with human liver lipid extract and CHAPS or with DLPC (35), yet CYP3A5 was more active toward erythromycin than CYP3A4 when reconstituted with a phospholipid mixture and cholate in HEPES [*N*-(2-hydroxyethyl)piperazine-*N'*-2-ethanesulphonic acid] buffer (45). Similarly, the rate of testosterone 6β-hydroxylation was found to be much slower for CYP3A5 than CYP3A4 by Wrighton and colleagues (35), yet comparable rates were reported by Gillam and colleagues (45). For some reactions, such as midazolam 1'-hydroxylation, CYP3A5 has been found consistently to catalyze a more rapid rate of metabolism than that of CYP3A4 (46,47). Nonetheless, because of a lower expression level and a narrower spectrum of substrates, the role of CYP3A5 in hepatic drug clearance is generally regarded to be significantly less than that of CYP3A4, although in certain extrahepatic organs, CYP3A5 may contribute significantly to the metabolism of some substrates, such as midazolam and endobiotics.

CYP3A7

The human fetal liver is capable of metabolizing a wide array of endobiotics and xenobiotics. This is unlike the fetal liver from experimental animal models (48). To investigate the great metabolic capacity of the human fetal liver, Kitada and co-workers purified the major P450 found in the fetal liver and termed it HFLa (49). The initial characterization of the substrate specificity and structure of HFLa suggested that it was related to the CYP3A subfamily. Wrighton and VandenBranden isolated and characterized another P450 from human fetal liver that was immunochemically related to CYP3A4 and termed this P450 HLp2 (50). The N-terminal amino acid sequence of HLp2 was found to be 78% homologous to CYP3A4 through the first 29 residues. Subsequent amino acid sequence information from HFLa (51) indicated that HLp2 and HFLa were the same P450 that is currently termed CYP3A7 (10). The cDNA encoding CYP3A7 has been isolated and its deduced amino acid sequence is 88% similar to that of CYP3A4 (52).

Although CYP3A7 represents about 50% of the total P450 expressed in the human fetal liver, it is not present in significant levels in the adult liver (53). Total fetal liver CYP3A7 levels (nmol/g liver) (54) appear to be somewhat comparable to total CYP3A levels found in adult liver (13). In addition to the fetal liver, CYP3A7 has also been identified in human endometrium and placenta (55). Total levels at these sites appear to be lower than that found in fetal liver, but they are still appreciable.

There have been only a limited number of investigations of the metabolic capabilities of CYP3A7 and these have been conducted *in vitro* (48). Results from these studies suggest that the metabolic capabilities of CYP3A7 are similar to the related forms CYP3A4 and CYP3A5. Importantly, CYP3A7 has been shown to be responsible for the 16α-hydroxylation of dehydroepiandrosterone 3-sulfate (DHEA-sulfate), a reaction that occurs at a much greater rate in human fetal liver samples compared with adult liver samples (56). This reaction has physiologic importance in that it is the major pathway leading to estriol production in the maternal-fetal pair (57).

The overall role of CYP3A7 in drug clearance in the adult appears to be limited. However, the role of CYP3A7 in drug–drug and drug–endobiotic interactions that may occur in the fetus is of potential importance and has not yet been examined.

IN VITRO PROBES OF CYP3A FUNCTION

As previously discussed, the number of molecules that have been shown to be metabolized by CYP3A are numerous. Not surprisingly, an equally impressive number of compounds have been used over the years as marker substrates of CYP3A function with various *in vitro* incubation systems. The choice of one compound over another is often made on the basis of convenience and local experience, although the sensitivity of the assay and minimum amounts of active enzyme required can enter into the decision.

Regardless of the choice of substrate, enzyme-selectivity is essential for incubations with a system that contains more than one catalytically functional enzyme (i.e., liver microsomes). It is not necessary that the substrate be converted to a single product, but the enzyme must be the only or overwhelmingly dominant source of the product of interest. In the case of CYP3A, there are several substrate–product pairs that appear to fit this criterion. The N-demethylation of erythromycin (7), the ring oxidation of nifedipine (8), the 6β-hydroxylation of testosterone (58), and the primary oxidations of cyclosporine (59,60) were each used for the characterization of CYP3A4 purified from human liver, and they continue to find extensive use in the characterization of drug–drug interactions that involve CYP3A (14,61–64). Another CYP3A-specific substrate–product pair that has garnered considerable attention is the 1'-hydroxylation of midazolam (65,66). Like erythromycin, midazolam can be used as both an *in vitro* (67–71) and *in vivo* probe for studies of drug–CYP3A interactions.

The use of a nonspecific CYP3A substrate is also acceptable when probing the function of a single purified or cDNA-expressed enzyme. For example, Crespi and coworkers have describe the use of the benzyl ether of resorufin for rapid, high-throughput screening for CYP3A4 inhibitors with their commercially available expressed enzymes (72). In adapting the incubation conditions for a 96-well plate format, the investigators chose as their CYP3A substrate a compound whose metabolism could be monitored by a highly sensitive automated fluorescence plate reader. In this application, the need for enzyme selectivity was rendered moot because only a single enzyme at a time was overexpressed in the microsomal preparation.

A truly selective CYP3A5 probe has yet to be identified, although it has been suggested that 1'-/4-hydroxymidazolam product ratios can be followed as a marker for significant CYP3A5 activity (46), because the product ratio is greater for CYP3A5 than for CYP3A4. As mentioned earlier, DHEA-sulfate is a selective substrate for CYP3A7. CYP3A4 and CYP3A5 can catalyze the reaction (35), but at a much lower rate than CYP3A7 (56). The use of DHEA-sulfate for evaluating fetal drug–drug interaction potential is largely unexplored. However, the need for a selective probe may not be great because CYP3A7 is the dominant P450 and CYP3A form in human fetal liver (48), and it can metabolize other more conventional CYP3A substrates such as (R)-warfarin (73) and midazolam (74).

IN VIVO PROBES OF CYP3A FUNCTION

Because of the recognized importance of CYP3A in drug metabolism, there has been a great deal of interest in the development of an *in vivo* probe to characterize interindividual variability in protein expression and function under actual therapeutic conditions. One of the earliest CYP3A substrates identified, nifedipine (8), was used to probe the absence or presence of a functionally significant genetic polymorphism. The nifedipine data from healthy volunteers (75,76) revealed either skewed or unimodal distribution in oral nifedipine area under the concentration-time curve (AUC), the AUC ratio of nifedipine and its ring oxidized metabolite, and the percent of dose excreted into urine as the CYP3A-catalyzed ring oxidized metabolite in 8 hours. There was no evidence of a significant functional polymorphism. Recent studies suggest that because of a significant first pass effect, the observed nifedipine AUC or the fraction metabolized to dehydronifedipine may be determined by intestinal as well as hepatic enzyme activity, particularly after coadministration of a CYP3A inducer (77).

Several other compounds have been examined for their suitability as an *in vivo* CYP3A probe, including cortisol, erythromycin, midazolam, dapsone, and dextromethorphan. The merits of each and the extent of validation have been reviewed by Watkins (78) and are discussed briefly here. An important consideration in the use of any *in vivo* CYP3A probe is the phenomenon of intestinal first pass metabolism. Probes that can be administered by the intravenous route, such as erythromycin and midazolam, appear to be metabolized primarily by hepatic enzyme. In contrast, an orally dosed CYP3A probe is subject to both hepatic and intestinal first pass metabolism. The contribution of intestinal enzyme to the bioavailability of an orally administered substrate has yet to be evaluated for more than a few compounds (77,79–82) and its relative importance, in comparison to liver, is still a matter of debate. In addition, recent studies suggest that, for some substrates, such as cyclosporine, intestinal first pass metabolism may be mediated through a complicated interplay between CYP3A and the apical membrane countertransporter, P-glycoprotein (83). Because the dependence of oral bioavailability on P-glycoprotein function may vary with the CYP3A substrate, it would be ideal that the CYP3A4 probe not be a substrate for P-glycoprotein or any other epithelial transporter. Such a probe might be valuable for characterization of CYP3A regulation and function, but perhaps not as useful as a predictor of the oral clearance of another CYP3A substrate with a more complicated picture of intestinal bioavailability (i.e., subject to countertransport processes).

6β-Hydroxycortisol

One of the first truly noninvasive *in vivo* measures of human cytochrome P450–dependent oxidative metabolism to appear in the literature was the quantitation of 6β-hydroxycortisol/free cortisol ratio in urine. It was recognized in the early 1960s that hepatic microsomal enzymes catalyze the 6β-hydroxylation of cortisol. Because cortisol is produced endogenously, it was suggested that

hepatic mixed function oxidase activity could be assessed indirectly by monitoring the product/substrate ratio in urine (84). Day-to-day variability in the production of cortisol could be accounted for by normalization of 6β-hydroxycortisol excretion with the excretion of unconjugated cortisol or mitochondrial cortisol products, 17-hydroxycorticosteroids. Potential applications, such as a characterization of the effect of important therapeutic agents like anticonvulsants and rifampin on drug metabolism, were obvious. The test would provide a window on hepatic enzyme regulation in an unobtrusive, noninvasive manner. Indeed, clinical studies revealed that the production of 6β-hydroxycortisol was markedly elevated by therapy with phenytoin, phenobarbital, the phenobarbital prodrug primidone, carbamazepine, and rifampin in adult and pediatric patients (84–86).

It was shown later that the hepatic microsomal 6β-hydroxylation of steroids (87), including cortisol (88), is catalyzed predominantly by CYP3A. Furthermore, the induction of cortisol metabolism by anticonvulsants and rifampin was shown to be mediated through an increase in hepatic expression of CYP3A4 (88). Thus, it was proposed that the 6β-hydroxycortisol test could also be applied as an *in vivo* probe of interindividual hepatic CYP3A variability in the absence of enzyme induction (89,90). However, it was noted previously (88) that there was no correlation between hepatic biopsy CYP3A level and 6β-hydroxycortisol test, when data from control or induced subjects were compared separately. This suggests that even though the 6β-hydroxycortisol test responds appropriately to hepatic CYP3A4 induction, basal production of the metabolite might also be determined by extrahepatic catalytic activity.

The most obvious site for extrahepatic 6β-hydroxycortisol production is the kidney. CYP3A5 is expressed within proximal tubular epithelial cells, loop of Henle, cortical collecting ducts, and epithelial cells lining the renal pelvis (91,92), and it can catalyze the 6β-hydroxylation of cortisol (35). Unlike the liver, CYP3A5 is the dominant CYP3A form in human kidney (37,38). It has been suggested that intrarenal production of 6β-hydroxycortisol by CYP3A5 has a significant impact on the total excretion of 6β-hydroxycortisol into urine, despite the relatively low (compared to hepatic) level of enzyme expression, and that this may have pathophysiologic implications (37,38). Because renal cortisol metabolism would involve reuptake of the hormone from the glomerular filtrate, metabolism and reexcretion of metabolite into urine, its efficiency might not be readily apparent from the total kidney CYP3A5 content. Of more relevance, but difficult to quantitate, would be the relative CYP3A5 content in renal epithelial cells, in comparison to that in hepatocytes.

An attractive feature of the aforementioned hypothesis, is the observation that renal CYP3A5 protein expression and catalytic activity is highly variable (37,38). Many individuals would be expected to have a clear deficiency in renal 6β-hydroxycortisol production based on immunoblot analysis. Because renal activity would be unlikely to correlate with CYP3A4-dominated hepatic activity, it might be unrealistic to expect a good correlation between any other measure of hepatic CYP3A (direct or indirect) and the 6β-hydroxycortisol test.

Because of the minimum effort involved and proven sensitivity to hepatic CYP3A induction, Kovacs and colleagues have recommended that the 6β-hydroxycortisol test be conducted routinely for drugs under development, with the earliest repeated dose administration studies in humans (93). Relative potency could be assessed by comparison of new data with literature values for one of the most potent CYP3A inducers, rifampin. Positive findings could be followed up with more specific or clinically relevant CYP3A substrates. Negative findings could serve as a useful check on potentially spurious, positive findings of induction potential in animals (93).

Erythromycin Breath Test

A major route of erythromycin elimination in humans is N-demethylation (94,95). The majority of published *in vitro* data (7,16,70,95,96) indicates that the reaction is catalyzed selectively by CYP3A, although this has been called into question recently (13). With respect to *in vivo* erythromycin metabolism, Watkins and co-workers (95) showed that, when a tracer dose of erythromycin, labeled with carbon-14 at the metabolically sensitive methyl groups, was administered intravenously, the percent of labeled dose exhaled in breath as $^{14}CO_2$ increased with the pretreatment of rifampin and dexamethasone and decreased with troleandomycin. These *in vivo* effects were consistent with CYP3A modulating properties of the affecting drugs, that is, enzyme induction and mechanism-based inhibition, respectively. These investigators also found that erythromycin N-demethylation was dramatically reduced in patients with severe liver disease (97,98) and decreased to a negligible rate when the drug was administered to an anhepatic subject (98), demonstrating the importance of the liver to the metabolic process. Furthermore, *in vivo* erythromycin breath test (ERMBT) results were reasonably well correlated with the amount of CYP3A protein detected in hepatic biopsy specimens from study subjects (97). All of these data have been taken as prima facie evidence in support of the sensitivity and specificity of the ERMBT as an *in vivo* hepatic CYP3A probe.

The ERMBT has been used to characterize intersubject differences in hepatic CYP3A content between male and female volunteers (95,99) and between the young and elderly (99). The data indicate approximately six-fold interindividual variability in CYP3A metabolic activity in a "healthy" population and a slightly higher average demethylation rate for female subjects compared to male

subjects. However, because determination of the ERMBT parameter can also be affected by drug distribution, the observed sex-specific difference in the initial $^{14}CO_2$ excretion rate may simply reflect the recognized female–male difference in erythromycin volume of distribution (100).

The ERMBT has also been used to study the source of interpatient variability in oral cyclosporine A (83,101, 102) and cyclosporine G (103) kinetics. In general, the test explains roughly 30% to 60% of intersubject variability in oral cyclosporine clearance. The ERMBT was also predictive of a similar percentage of the variability in unbound systemic midazolam clearance (104). In another study, ERMBT results did not correlate with duodenal mucosal CYP3A content, although mucosal CYP3A midazolam 1′-hydroxylation activity was well correlated with mucosal CYP3A content, suggesting that hepatic and intestinal CYP3A expression are not coordinately regulated (105). When Lown and colleagues (83) examined relationships among the ERMBT, intestinal CYP3A, intestinal P-glycoprotein content, and oral cyclosporine clearance, they found that the breath test explained 56% of the variability in cyclosporine clearance and that consideration of intestinal P-glycoprotein content explained an additional 17% of the interindividual differences in cyclosporine clearance.

Comparisons between the intravenous ERMBT and other putative CYP3A tests have yielded mixed results. Correlation coefficients between ERMBT results and 6β-hydroxycortisol/cortisol ratio were reported to be very poor (106,107) or weakly significant (98). However, this general lack of agreement between the two probe tests may reflect incomplete specificity of one or both probes for CYP3A or significant extrahepatic formation of 6β-hydroxycortisol, as mentioned previously. A similarly poor correlation resulted from a comparison of ERMBT results and the dapsone recovery ratio, another putative CYP3A probe (see later text), in healthy volunteers. However, this discordance may be due to the contribution of non-CYP3A enzymes to the dapsone hydroxylation reaction (108,109).

Perceived limitations to the ERMBT include its unproven use as a probe for intestinal CYP3A and potential concerns over the administration of a radioisotope. The latter may be addressed with the use of stable isotope–labeled substrate. The issue of intestinal metabolism may be more problematic. Even though labeled erythromycin can be administered orally in a formulation that avoids nonenzymatic degradation, the fate of carbon-14 formaldehyde produced by N-demethylation within the enterocyte is unknown. It is possible that the conversion of intestinal formaldehyde to CO_2 may not follow a path that is kinetically identical to hepatically generated formaldehyde (110). Thus, if hepatic and intestinal CYP3A are not coordinately expressed, as the current data indicates, first pass erythromycin demethylation may not correlate with the recovery of labeled CO_2 in the breath. Studies that directly compare CO_2 production following intravenous and oral administration with independent measures of intestinal CYP3A content should clarify the issue.

Regardless of its ultimate utility for investigations of constitutive hepatic and intestinal CYP3A expression, the ERMBT has clearly demonstrated its value for examining drug–drug interactions. Two recent publications highlight the type of information that can be gained using the ERMBT. The first involved a determination of an *in vivo* K_i parameter for the established inhibitor ketoconazole (111) and the second, a characterization of the time-course of hepatic CYP3A induction and de-induction following a course of repeated delavirdine administration (112). In both studies, the ERMBT generated a relatively instantaneous measure of hepatic CYP3A activity that could be correlated directly with a measured level of modulator in blood. The data with ketoconazole demonstrated good agreement between the observed *in vivo* K_i, with respect to unbound plasma inhibitor concentration (111), and that obtained *in vitro* with microsomal incubations (47,61). Furthermore, because the ERMBT can be repeated a number of times in the same individual, one can obtain the full scope of the time and concentration dependency of a particular interaction, such as that exerted by delavirdine (112). Assuming that results with erythromycin can be extrapolated to other CYP3A substrates, the information could greatly aid in the development of strategies to avoid or minimize clinical interactions.

Midazolam Hydroxylation

The selectivity of midazolam as a CYP3A probe has also been investigated. The primary metabolite, 1'-hydroxymidazolam, and minor metabolites, 4-hydroxymidazolam and 1,4-dihydroxymidazolam, are all generated predominantly if not exclusively from CYP3A4/5 in the adult human (41,46,65,66,113,114). Unlike erythromycin, a majority of the intravenous or oral dose can be readily recovered in urine (115,116). Based on the recovery of a radioactive dose of midazolam in urine, the absorption of an oral midazolam dose is essentially complete (117). Assuming a systemic clearance of 0.25 to 0.66 L/min (118) and limited partitioning into red blood cells (119), midazolam can be classified as a medium hepatic extraction drug. The half-life of midazolam in blood is relatively short (approximately 60–90 minutes) and elimination of primary (120) and secondary metabolites (121) is formation rate limited. Together, these kinetic features are ideal for the conduct of a complete pharmacokinetic study in a 24-hour interval for determination of hepatic and intestinal CYP3A activity. Midazolam also exhibits one other property that can be viewed as advantageous for a CYP3A probe, that is, it does not appear to be a substrate for P-glycoprotein (32).

In a study conducted in liver transplant patients, Thummel and colleagues (113) showed that the systemic clearance of midazolam was strongly correlated with hepatic CYP3A content. An excellent correlation between midazolam clearance and cyclosporine clearance was also reported. In addition to these findings, the investigators reported an excellent correlation between the 1'-hydroxymidazolam/midazolam ratio measured 30 minutes after an intravenous midazolam dose given to organ donors and hepatic CYP3A content (41). Although the positive relationships generated in these studies were most likely strengthened by large interindividual differences in enzyme and substrate clearances, the results clearly demonstrated the potential utility of intravenous midazolam as an *in vivo* hepatic CYP3A probe.

Numerous drug–midazolam interaction studies have been reported over the past 10 years since the identification of CYP3A-dependent midazolam metabolism. All can be readily explained on the basis of the modulator's known effect on CYP3A expression or catalytic function. For example, chronic treatment with rifampin more than doubles the systemic clearance of midazolam (121). The effect of rifampin, phenytoin, and carbamazepine on the oral midazolam clearance (CL/F) is even more dramatically affected, a 15-fold increase (122,123), demonstrating the multiplicative effect of the induction of CYP3A4 within the liver and small intestine, as well as the importance of intestinal metabolism to the significant midazolam first pass effect. Similar in magnitude but opposing effects on intravenous midazolam clearance are found after treatment with the potent CYP3A inhibitors erythromycin (124), troleandomycin (121), and clarithromycin (125), and on oral midazolam clearance after administration of ketoconazole or itraconazole (126) and clarithromycin (125). More modest are the inhibitory effects of the CYP3A inhibitors verapamil and diltiazem (127), fluconazole (128), and grapefruit juice (129) on oral midazolam clearance. The selectivity of CYP3A-dependent midazolam is also indicated by the absence of an interaction between compounds that are relatively weak CYP3A inhibitors, such as azithromycin (130).

Unlike the ERMBT, midazolam has also been used successfully to probe intestinal CYP3A4-dependent metabolism. Paine and co-workers reported a substantial (43%) intestinal first pass extraction after intraduodenal administration in anhepatic liver transplant patients (82). This value is comparable to the predicted hepatic (44%) and intestinal (43%) extraction values in healthy volunteers (118). The intestinal first pass extraction was approximately five-fold higher than the intestinal midazolam extraction after intravenous drug administration (82), reflecting a fundamental difference in drug delivery to the enzymatic site and possibly the nonenzymatic variables controlling extraction efficiency (i.e., intracellular residence time). Both *in vivo* (82,118,125) and *in vitro* (18) studies suggest that mucosal CYP3A-dependent drug extraction can be quite variable, with some individuals exhibiting minimal activity and others profound activity as a consequence of highly variable CYP3A expression.

Simple oral administration of midazolam, or any other well-extracted CYP3A probe, will not give data that can be resolved into hepatic and intestinal components. However, one can use basic pharmacokinetic relationships for intravenous and oral administration (131,132), with an assumption of negligible intestinal contribution to systemic clearance, to obtain independent estimates of the hepatic and intestinal first pass extraction ratios. Assuming weight-normalized values for hepatic and intestinal (small) mucosal blood flow, independent organ extraction ratios can be calculated from the two unknown parameters—hepatic and intestinal intrinsic clearances.

The ideal study design involves simultaneous intravenous and oral administration of unlabeled and stable isotope–labeled substrate to control for intraindividual variability in splanchnic blood flow and CYP3A expression. Such an approach was used successfully by Gorski and colleagues to characterize the inhibitory effects of clarithromycin on hepatic and intestinal CYP3A enzymes (125). These investigators reported a 142% increase in midazolam oral bioavailability that was the result of a reduction in both intestinal and hepatic metabolic extraction. Most of the interindividual differences in oral bioavailability, under either control or clarithromycin treatment, could be explained by variability in the intestinal first pass extraction.

The most significant limitation to the use of midazolam as an *in vivo* CYP3A probe is the need for delivery of a pharmacologic dose to achieve adequate blood levels for quantitative analysis and intravenous administration for assessment of hepatic activity. This necessitates supervision of the kinetic study by trained personnel in a clinical setting, particularly if reduced drug clearance is expected.

Other CYP3A Probes

From a strictly pharmacokinetic perspective, any CYP3A4 substrate that exhibits low first pass extraction, no interactions with P-glycoprotein and essentially complete oral bioavailability would be better suited as an *in vivo* liver enzyme probe than a substrate that undergoes extensive first pass extraction. The confounding effect of first pass intestinal metabolism disappears and the AUC resulting from an oral or intravenous dose is simply a function of hepatic enzymatic activity. This presumably was behind the use of dextromethorphan *N*-demethylation as an *in vivo* index of hepatic CYP3A function (133–135). However, dextromethorphan metabolism is more commonly associated with the polymorphic CYP2D6-catalyzed *O*-demethylation reaction. Because this is a major parallel pathway to *N*-demethylation, and

because the metabolites of *N*- and *O*-demethylation undergo further metabolism to a common secondary metabolite (3-hydroxymorphinan), interpretation of urinary product ratios may not provide more than a qualitative picture of hepatic CYP3A activity.

Another molecule that has been investigated for potential use as a CYP3A probe is dapsone. Although dapsone metabolism is catalyzed by both conjugative (*N*-acetyltransferase) and oxidative enzymes, the latter process, which leads to the formation of a hydroxylamine metabolite, appears to account for much of the interindividual variability in drug clearance (136). Early investigations indicated that hepatic microsomal dapsone *N*-hydroxylation was catalyzed predominantly by CYP3A isozymes (137). On the basis of this *in vitro* finding and *in vivo* dapsone elimination kinetics (136), a urinary dapsone recovery ratio (dapsone hydroxylamine/dapsone hydroxylamine + dapsone, in 0- to 8-hr urine following a 100-mg oral dose) was proposed to be an *in vivo* probe of hepatic CYP3A population variability (138). However, recent *in vivo* and *in vitro* studies call into question the specificity of dapsone as a hepatic CYP3A probe. In two different studies, dapsone test results did not correlate with the ERMBT (107,139), nor with a cyclosporine blood level/dose ratio (139). Furthermore, other investigators have reported multienzyme kinetics for the formation of dapsone hydroxylamine in human liver microsomes. A member of the CYP2C subfamily (108,140) and CYP2E1 (109) appear also to contribute to product formation, particularly at low, more therapeutically relevant substrate concentrations. Thus, dapsone may be another molecule that will be sensitive to the effect of CYP3A inducers and inhibitors, but that might not be a truly selective CYP3A probe.

Lidocaine—MEGX Test

Although lidocaine is not metabolized exclusively by CYP3A isozymes, it is presented in this chapter as an *in vivo* probe because of its use to determine liver function. Bargetzi and colleagues (141) first demonstrated that the conversion of lidocaine to monoethylglycinexylidine (MEGX) in human liver was catalyzed in part by CYP3A4 (35%–65%) and by an as yet unidentified isozyme. At about the same time came reports on the measurement of MEGX formation following intravenous lidocaine administration as an indicator of pretransplant donor liver function (142,143) and residual liver function in patients with cirrhosis (144). Serum MEGX concentration measured 15 minutes after the lidocaine dose was shown to be a good prognostic indicator of postoperative graft function and short-term patient survival. From studies of cirrhotic patients (145–148), it appears that this simple test may be superior to conventional measures of liver function, such as the Pugh score, in identifying patients in imminent need of transplantation. Similarly, administration of the MEGX test to organ donors may provide a reliable means to screen out livers that have a high chance of primary failure following transplantation, as well as selecting those that are questionable on gross appearance but still retain good oxidative metabolic activity and would perform well after transplantation (149,150). It has been suggested that the MEGX test performs so well because it indirectly reflects the status of oxidative phosphorylation within the hepatocyte. The fact that CYP3A (and at least one other P450 isozyme) catalyzes this reaction may not be material to its success, except that the reaction proceeds with a relatively rapid turnover.

An expected range of MEGX test values for normal male and female subjects of varying ages has been described (151,152), paving the way for widespread usage in clinical practice. However, continued development of the rapid immunoassay for MEGX quantitation has not been pursued at this time by the original test manufacturer, forcing the need for conventional hospital analytic support if clinical use of the test is to continue.

MODULATORS OF CYP3A FUNCTION

Inducers

Induction of hepatic and possibly intestinal CYP3A4 forms the basis for many clinically significant drug–drug interactions. In the absence of evidence to the contrary, inducers of CYP3A4 are assumed to increase the total pool of functionally active enzyme within the liver or intestinal mucosa, without altering the rate constants for catalysis (e.g., K_m and k_{cat}). The outward pharmacokinetic effect of a CYP3A inducer that increases the enzyme pool by increased synthesis is to elevate the maximal capacity of the eliminating organ to metabolize a substrate (V_{max}) and, hence, increase the first order intrinsic metabolite formation clearance (V_{max}/K_m). A list of compounds found to induce human CYP3A protein, mRNA, or catalytic activity in vitro (primary hepatocytes or immortalized human cell lines) is presented in Table 10-1. Some compounds, such as the recently approved drug troglitazone (Rezulin®) (166) and antipyrine (167,168), are thought to induce CYP3A, based on observed increases in urinary 6β-hydroxycortisol excretion, but corroborative in vitro findings with the use of human tissues has not yet been reported.

When evaluating the literature on CYP3A inducers, it is important to distinguish between compounds that elevate enzyme levels and activity in vitro and those for which there is corroborative data in vivo. For many putative CYP3A inducers, conditions that elicited transcriptional gene activation or stabilization of mRNA or the enzyme are clearly suprapharmacologic. Therefore, conclusions with regard to the clinical relevance of an in vitro finding should be made with caution until clinical inter-

TABLE 10-1. *Human CYP3A induction* in vitro

Inducer	CYP3A protein/mRNA[a]	CYP3A activity[a]
Carbamazepine	62	
Clotrimazole	42, 153	
Dexamethasone	62, 154	29, 62, 155, 156
Erythromycin	42, 157	
Ethanol	158	
Lansoprazole	159	159, 160
Lovastatin	154	
Omeprazole	159	159, 160
Phenobarbital	62, 154	62, 156, 161
Phenylbutazone	62	62
Phenytoin	62	62
Prednisone	62, 155	62, 155
Reserpine	42	
Rifabutin	162	162
Rifapentine	162	162
Rifampin	42, 62, 163	62, 162, 164
Sulfadimidine	62	62
Sulfinpyrazone	62	62
Taxol	165	

[a]Based on results from experiments with isolated human hepatocytes or a human-derived, immortalized cell line.

action studies are performed. For example, some of the azole antifungals and macrolide antibiotics increase CYP3A protein levels in human cell culture (153,157,169) or in animal liver (170). However, the overall effect of these agents on the clearance of a CYP3A substrate appears to be exclusively one of inhibition rather than induction. In these cases, it is believed that CYP3A induction occurs in parallel to occupancy of the enzyme active site by inhibitor, such that the metabolism of a substrate is precluded. As a result, induced clearance will only be manifested when administration of the "inducer/inhibitor" is discontinued and the half-life of that molecule in the body is short relative to the CYP3A half-life, as has been demonstrated for isoniazid and CYP2E1 (171).

When considering the clinical effect of a CYP3A inducer on drug clearance, it is also important to understand the route of administration and basal intrinsic clearance of the enzyme substrate. For drugs that are eliminated exclusively by the liver, a CYP3A inducer should cause an increase in the total body clearance and a reduction in blood AUC of an orally administered substrate that is proportional to the magnitude of increase in the hepatic enzyme content. In contrast, the effect of an inducer on the clearance of an intravenously administered substrate can be partially or completely masked by a blood flow limitation to hepatic clearance, if the basal intrinsic clearance is similar to or exceeds hepatic blood flow. For example, treatment of healthy volunteers with rifampin was found to profoundly reduce the plasma AUC of midazolam, a selective CYP3A probe substrate, by more than 95% when the probe was given orally (122), but by only

62% when the probe was administered intravenously (121). This corresponds to an approximately 20-fold and 2.6-fold change in the apparent total body clearance of midazolam after oral and intravenous dosing, respectively. Similar findings have been reported for other highly extracted CYP3A substrates, including nifedipine (77) and verapamil (80).

Although there is a theoretic basis for the differential effect of a hepatic CYP3A inducer on oral and intravenous AUCs (modulation of the first pass effect), it has been suggested that for some drugs the route of administration-specific differences described in the literature are a consequence of the modulation of CYP3A expression in the gastrointestinal mucosa (77,80,172). Rifampin (173) and presumably other CYP3A4 inducers increase the level of intestinal CYP3A4 expression. Because of the sequential nature of intestinal and hepatic first-pass extraction, one would expect even greater reductions in the AUC of a CYP3A substrate when it is given orally, compared to intravenously, than if there were no intestinal metabolism. Application of a model-dependent pharmacokinetic analysis to intravenous and oral AUC data, before and during treatment with CYP3A inducers, implicates the intestinal mucosa as a major site of enzyme induction (77,80,172). However, as Lin and colleagues have pointed out (174), such analyses are based on the assumption that the intestinal mucosa does not contribute significantly to the systemic clearance of the CYP3A substrate. This assumption may be true under basal conditions (82), but might be inappropriate after treatment with the inducer, particularly if the inducer exerts a more profound effect on the gut wall enzyme in comparison to hepatic enzyme. In such circumstances, successive approximation of extraction ratios may be more appropriate. Nonetheless, it is clear that management of a drug–drug interaction with CYP3A inducers such as rifampin, phenytoin, and carbamazepine, will be more imperative for the high-clearance orally administered substrate, compared to the low-clearance substrate, and that up to 20- to 30-fold changes in blood AUC can be expected.

Inhibitors

Given the broad diversity of molecules that CYP3A will metabolize, it is not surprising to find that there are also many different inhibitors of the enzyme. Although there is no single structural feature that imparts the property of enzyme inhibition, most CYP3A inhibitors are relatively large lipophilic molecules (175). They can reduce enzyme-catalyzed drug metabolism by (a) direct, rapidly reversible binding of the inhibitor molecule to the enzyme (competitive or noncompetitive), (b) after conversion to a metabolite that either reversibly binds with high affinity to the enzyme immediately after formation or after accumulation in blood, (c) forming a stable metabolite-intermediate complex (MI inhibitor), or (d) forming an irreversible adduct (suicide inhibitor) with the enzyme. Table 10-2 lists compounds that have been shown to block CYP3A-dependent drug metabolism in vitro (human liver or intestinal microsomes or cDNA-expressed enzymes). Only those compounds for which the in vitro K_i was reported to be less than 100 μM are suspected of generating a stable enzyme-inhibitor complex, or that cause suicide inactivation of the enzyme are presented. Some compounds, such as erythromycin, can inhibit by both rapidly reversible (i.e., competitive) and time-dependent (i.e., formation of a MI complex) mechanisms. The same scenario applies to the time-dependent suicide inhibitors gestodene, ethinyl estradiol, and delavirdine.

The most potent of the reversible CYP3A inhibitors appear to be the azole-substituted antifungals (i.e., clotrimazole, $K_i \sim 250$ pM; ketoconazole, $K_i = 15$ nM; itraconazole, $K_i = 270$ nM), the first generation of human immunodeficiency virus (HIV) protease inhibitors (ritonavir, $K_i \sim 15$–70 nM; indinavir, $K_i \sim 200$ nM; saquinavir, $K_i \sim 700$ nM), some of the furanocoumarin dimers found in grapefruit juice (GF-I-1, $K_i = 50$ nM; GF-I-4, $K_i = 29$ nM), and the secondary metabolite of diltiazem (didesmethyl diltiazem, $K_i = 100$ nM). The remaining compounds listed, many of which are substrates for CYP3A, inhibit the enzyme with a binding constant in the low micromolar range. In some circumstances, a compound will not inhibit CYP3A in vivo, despite exhibiting an in vitro K_i of less than 100 μM for the enzyme. This appears to be the case for fluoxetine and its major metabolite norfluoxetine (fluoxetine, $K_i = 7.1$–66 μM; norfluoxetine, $K_i = 1.4$–19 μM), which do not appear to inhibit the metabolic clearance of the selective CYP3A substrates terfenadine (201), triazolam (202), and midazolam (203).

Although any CYP3A substrate is a potential inhibitor of the enzyme by virtue of its ability to compete with another substrate for the active site, in practice many are not. The basis for this observation can be found in the mathematic relationships for the different types of enzyme inhibition (204). For most substrates, the binding constant of the substrate/inhibitor for the enzyme is much higher than the unbound concentration of inhibitor encountered at the enzyme active site in vivo. For a substrate to be an effective competitive or noncompetitive enzyme inhibitor, it must at least partially saturate the enzyme active site or a second noncompetitive binding site that, when occupied, impedes substrate turnover. It is apparent that this does not always occur, because most CYP3A4 substrates do not display saturable, Michaelis-Menten kinetics in vivo. As is discussed in more detail later, an alternative way in which a CYP3A substrate may inhibit the enzyme is through time-dependent enzyme inactivation (205). Once again, one would expect to see a time-dependent (single dose versus multiple dose) and dose-dependent change in the elimination kinetics of the

TABLE 10-2. *Human CYP3A inhibition* in vitro

Inhibitor	Apparent K_i (µM)	Mechanism[a]	Selected references
Anastrozole	10–55	Mixed	176
Betamethasone	31	Undefined	177
Bromocriptine	7–8	Competitive	62, 178
Cimetidine	36–268	Competitive	179, 180
Clarithromycin	10–28	Competitive*	181, 182
Clotrimazole	0.00025–0.15	Mixed	153, 183
Cyclosporine	2–37	Competitive	67, 177, 178, 181
Delaverdine	22	Suicide	184
Desmethylsertraline	3.5–48	Mixed/competitive	71, 179
Dexamethasone	23–61	Competitive	155, 178, 185
Dihydroergotamine	7–23	Competitive	62, 67
Diltiazem	50–75	Competitive*	62
Desmethyldiltiazem	2	Competitive*	186
Didesmethyldiltiazem	0.1	Competitive*	186
Ergotamine	0.5–14	Competitive	62, 67, 178
Erythromycin	13–194	Competitive*	62, 63, 180, 181, 187
Ethinyl estradiol	34	Suicide	178, 188
Gestodene	5.6	Suicide	14, 177
Fluconazole	1.3–63	Competitive/noncompetitive	47, 69, 153, 189
Fluvoxamine	5.6	Competitive	179
Fluoxetine	7.1–66	Mixed/competitive	69, 71, 179
Furanocoumarins	0.029–59	Mixed*	190, 191
Indinavir	0.2–0.7	Competitive	192, 193
Itraconazole	0.27–11	Competitive	69, 181
Josamycin	12–21	Competitive/mixed	62, 63, 178
Ketoconazole	0.015–8	Mixed/noncompetitive	47, 61, 178, 180
Miconazole	0.9–1.3	Competitive	62, 153
Midazolam	40–63	Competitive	62, 70, 133
Mifepristone	3.5	Undefined/suicide?	194
Naringenin	22–70	Competitive	181, 195
Navelbine	11	Mixed	196
Nefazodone	0.6	Competitive	179
Nelfinavir	4.8	Competitive*	193
Nicardipine	8	Competitive	62
Nifedipine	5–22	Competitive	62, 67, 180, 197
Norfluoxetine	1.4–19	Mixed/competitive	69, 71, 179
Omeprazole	79	Competitive	178
Paroxetine	3.8	Competitive	179
Pimozide	77	Noncompetitive	198
Progesterone	8–45	Competitive	62, 178
Quercetin	14	Uncompetitive	70
Quinidine	3.6–10	Competitive	196, 197
Rapamycin	83	Competitive	178
Ritonavir	0.017–0.11	Mixed	64, 193
Rokitamycin	41	Competitive*	63
Roxithromycin	113	Competitive*	63
Saquinavir	0.7–4	Competitive	192, 193
Sertraline	3.5–64	Mixed/competitive	71, 179
Tamoxifen	100	Competitive	199
Terfenadine	28	Competitive	68
Troleandomycin	10–51	Competitive*	7, 62, 63, 178, 181
Valspodar	1.2	Mixed	200
Verapamil	24–82	Competitive/mixed	62, 178
Vinblastine	3.8	Mixed	196
Vincristine	19	Mixed	196

[a]Only compounds for which the K_i value was found to be ≤100 µM, or which are known or thought to undergo time-dependent formation of an enzyme-inhibitor complex (*) or suicide inactivation are shown.

substrate *in vivo* if the reaction leading to enzyme inactivation was significant. However, if the pathway of interest was a relatively minor route of elimination for the substrate, enzyme inhibition might occur in the absence of any apparent time-dependent or dose-dependent *in vivo* elimination kinetics.

Recent studies suggest that reversible interactions among inhibitor, substrate, and CYP3A may be more complex than previously thought. Koley and co-workers (206,207) have presented evidence for the existence of at least two conformations of CYP3A4 in the presence of an active site ligand. An allosteric change induced with the binding of ligand may influence the binding of a second molecule. In the case of a quinidine–nifedipine–CYP3A4 interaction (208), quinidine appears to act as an allosteric inhibitor. It produces noncompetitive inhibition of nifedipine oxidation by inducing a shift in CYP3A4 conformation that does not allow nifedipine oxidation. Nifedipine binding to the quinidine–CYP3A4 complex is improved, yielding a ternary complex that is more stable than the nifedipine–CYP3A4 binary complex. Thus, for some CYP3A4 inhibitors, the dissociation of the ternary complex may be a relatively slow process in comparison to the initial binding of inhibitor to enzyme.

Classification of CYP3A inhibitors into either rapidly reversible or mechanism-based groups emphasizes a practical difference between the inhibitors. The effect of a competitive or noncompetitive inhibitor *in vivo* should be more predictable from a knowledge of *in vitro* K_i than the effect of mechanism-based inhibitors. Assuming nonsaturable elimination kinetics for the substrate, the degree of inhibition for a competitive or noncompetitive inhibitor should depend only on the dose and elimination kinetics of the inhibitor and its affinity for the enzyme. However, the *in vivo* inhibitory effect of a mechanism-based inhibitor depends not only on these parameters but also on the rate of enzyme inactivation or complexation and the synthesis and degradation kinetics of the active enzyme (209).

Formation of Metabolite-Intermediate Complexes

Drugs that are *N*-alkyl substituted molecules (a common structural feature of CYP3A substrates) often behave as rapidly reversible inhibitors of CYP3A when co-incubated with substrate and enzyme, yet they are capable of inhibiting more effectively when preincubated with microsomes and nicotinamide adenine dinucleotide phosphate-reduced (NADPH). Many such molecules have been shown to undergo successive oxidations to a nitrosoalkane species that forms a slowly reversible complex (MI complex) with the one electron–reduced heme of CYP3A (7,170,210), producing a unique red shift in the P450 absorption spectrum (211). Multiple oxidation steps may be required for the conversion of a disubstituted amine to the nitroso species, some of which may involve product release and rebinding of metabolite. Compounds that generate MI complexes with either human or animal liver CYP3A include several of the macrolide antibiotics (see Table 10-2), triacetyloleandomycin (211), oleandomycin (212), erythromycin (213), clarithromycin (214), roxithromycin (215), the antibiotic tiamulin (216), some antidepressants such as fluoxetine (217,218), nortriptyline (219), desipramine (217,219), imipramine (217), as well as amiodarone (220), diltiazem (217), lidocaine (217), tamoxifen (217), and SKF525 (217).

Because the half-life of the complex can be relatively long, the effect of an MI complex–forming inhibitor may be sustained beyond the detectable presence of inhibitor in blood. In addition, effective inhibition *in vivo* may not require saturation of the enzyme but instead repeated exposure of the catalytic enzyme to inhibitor, accumulation of primary and secondary inhibitor metabolites and, ultimately, the enzyme–inhibitor complex (209).

Unless the conversion of an inhibitor to the nitroso metabolite is rapid and relatively efficient, it may be difficult to reveal, *in vitro*, a slowly reversible and perhaps more clinically relevant aspect of enzyme inhibition. For example, erythromycin is reported to be a modestly potent competitive inhibitor of CYP3A-dependent oxidations at $K_i = 16$–194 μM (62,63,178,180,196). Although erythromycin can be oxidized by human liver microsomes to yield an MI complex, the efficiency of complexation or stability of the complex is low in comparison to the more potent macrolide troleandomycin (187,213). *In vivo*, effective inhibition of CYP3A-dependent theophylline, cyclosporine, alfentanil, and terfenadine metabolism by erythromycin appears to require multiple doses (221–224). In addition, inhibition following repeated 500-mg doses occurs with a peak systemic erythromycin concentration (5–6 μM), which is well below the reported K_i values. Thus, it is generally accepted that the *in vivo* inhibitory effect of erythromycin is the result of MI complex formation rather than rapidly reversible binding to the enzyme. Whether this is also true for other CYP3A alkylamine inhibitors is unclear, but such a phenomenon might account for some observed *in vitro–in vivo* discrepancies in the potency of enzyme inhibition. Sutton and co-workers (186) have shown that the desmethyl and didesmethyl metabolites of diltiazem are much more potent reversible inhibitors of CYP3A4 than the parent compound, and have suggested that reversible inhibition *in vivo* by such metabolites, as they accumulate in the body, may be a more important mechanism than MI complex formation. Again, whether this also applies to other alkylamine inhibitors remains to be determined but research interest in this aspect of drug–drug interactions has been heightened.

Suicide Inhibitors

Mechanism-based suicide inactivation of CYP3A has been described for several compounds, some of which are structurally related. A number of 17α-ethinyl–substituted steroids (e.g., gestodene, ethinyl estradiol, and levonorgestrol) (14,188) irreversibly inactivate human CYP3A in an NADPH- and time-dependent manner (see Table 10-2). The new antigestational agent mifepristone also falls into the category of a 17α-ethinyl–substituted steroid that causes time-dependent inhibition of CYP3A (194), but whether it is a suicide inactivator of CYP3A has not been investigated. More recently, L-754,394, an analogue to the HIV protease inhibitor indinavir containing a fused furanopyridine ring, was found to be a highly potent and selective suicide inhibitor of CYP3A4 (223). A major component of grapefruit juice, 6′,7′-dihydroxybergamottin, selectively inhibits CYP3A4-catalyzed biotransformations (226) by initiating the autocatalytic destruction of intestinal enzyme both *in vitro* (191) and *in vivo* (227). Furanocoumarin dimers (GF-I-1 and GF-I-4), also found in grapefruit juice, are potent reversible inhibitors of CYP3A and also appear to cause time-dependent enzyme inactivation (190). A structurally related compound, 8-methoxypsoralen, is a suicide inactivator of rat CYP3A (228), but in humans it appears to be selective for CYP2A6 (229). Finally, delavirdine, the newly released nonnucleoside HIV-1 reverse transcriptase inhibitor has also been shown to cause irreversible inactivation of CYP3A in human liver microsomes (184) and it is an effective *in vivo* inhibitor of the metabolism of other CYP3A substrates as well as its own (dose-dependent clearance) (112).

The *in vivo* effectiveness of suicide inhibitors of CYP3A will depend to a great extent on the total amount of inhibitor administered, the amount of target CYP3A enzyme (intestinal or hepatic), and the partitioning of reactive product to an irreversible ligand, all relative to the resynthesis rate of new enzyme (209). From a review of the literature, it is apparent that some of the CYP3A suicide inhibitors can elicit an *in vivo* inhibitory effect (112,129,230–233). In the case of 6′,7′-dihydroxybergamottin, enzyme inactivation appears to be selective for the gastrointestinal tract. For reasons that are not fully understood, grapefruit juice alters the oral clearance but not systemic clearance of midazolam (129) and cyclosporine (233). It is also possible that the relatively low-dose acetylenic steroids selectively inhibit intestinal CYP3A-dependent first pass extraction but not hepatic extraction simply because there is far less total enzyme in the gastrointestinal mucosa (18).

Activators of CYP3A

Another interesting property of the human CYP3A isozymes is the ability to undergo an acceleration of substrate turnover, rather than inhibition, with the addition of a second molecule to an *in vitro* reaction mixture. It was recognized years ago that 7,8-benzoflavone could stimulate the metabolic activity of rat microsomal P450 toward different substrates (234,235). Positive cooperativity or activation of CYP3A-dependent metabolism by 7,8-benzoflavone was also described for human CYP3A4 (236). Other additional activators of human CYP3A have been reported, including other flavonoids (236,237), testosterone (238), and progesterone (239). Many CYP3A substrates are susceptible to activation. Those drugs that are activated include nifedipine (240), carbamazepine (239), acetaminophen (237), losartan (241), and diazepam (242). Furthermore, some substrates, such as carbamazepine (239), aflatoxin B_1 (243), amitriptyline, testosterone, and 17β-estradiol (242) activate their own metabolism. Other substrates, such as midazolam (46,66) and erythromycin (244), apparently cause an allosteric change in the CYP3A enzyme that leads to substrate inhibition of product formation (and possibly alters a product formation ratio) with increasing substrate concentration. Korzekwa and colleagues have recently proposed a two-binding site model that encompasses the different manifestations of atypical Michaelis-Menten kinetics observed with CYP3A and other human CYPs (140). In their model, the relative kinetic constants for the formation of the enzyme–substrate and enzyme–substrate–substrate complex and conversion of each to product dictates the type of substrate-velocity profile that is observed.

A major implication of CYP3A allosterism from the perspective of substrate elimination is that the intrinsic metabolic clearance may increase with an increase in activator concentration (140). In the case of a substrate that activates itself *in vitro* (e.g., carbamazepine), the phenomenon is manifested at low rather than high substrate concentrations (140,239,243), increasing the likelihood that it could occur *in vivo*. The phenomenon of P450 activation has been shown to occur *in vivo* in the rat (245). If CYP3A4 activation can occur in humans, it will greatly complicate the predictability of substrate bioavailability and systemic clearance, as well as inhibitory drug–drug interactions.

REFERENCES

1. Guengerich FP. In: Ortiz de Montellano PR, ed. *Human cytochrome P450 enzymes, Cytochrome P450.* New York, Plenum Press, 1995: 473–535.
2. Li AP, Kaminski DL, Rasmussen A. Substrates for human cytochrome P450 3A4. Toxicology 1995;104:1–8.
3. Parkinson A. An overview of current cytochrome P450 technology for assessing the safety and efficacy of new materials. *Toxicol Pathol* 1996;24:45–57.
4. Wrighton SA, Stevens JC. The human hepatic cytochromes P450 involved in drug metabolism. *Crit Rev Toxicol* 1992;22:1–21.
5. Benet LZ. In: Hardman JG, Molinoff PB, Ruddon RW, Gilman AG, eds. *Pharmacokinetics, Goodman and Gilman's. The Pharmacological Basis of Therapeutics.* New York: McGraw-Hill, 1996:14.

6. Wang PP, Beaune P, Kaminsky LS, et al. Purification and characterization of six cytochrome P-450 isozymes from human liver microsomes. *Biochemistry* 1983;22:5375–5383.

7. Watkins PB, Wrighton SA, Maurel P, et al. Identification of an inducible form of cytochrome P-450 in human liver. *Proc Natl Acad Sci* 1985;82:6310–6314.

8. Guengerich FP, Martin MV, Beaune PH, Kremers P, Wolff T, Waxman DJ. Characterization of rat and human liver microsomal cytochrome P450 forms involved in nifedipine oxidation, a prototype for genetic polymorphism in oxidative drug metabolism. *J Biol Chem* 1986;261: 5051–5060.

9. Molowa DT, Schuetz EG, Wrighton SA, et al. Complete cDNA sequence of a cytochrome P-450 inducible by glucocorticoids in human liver. *Proc Natl Acad Sci* 1986;83:5311–5315.

10. Nelson DR, Koymans L, Kamataki T, et al. P450 superfamily: update on new sequences, gene mapping, accession numbers and nomenclature. *Pharmacogenetics* 1996;6:1–42.

11. Beaune PH, Umbenhauer DR, Bork RW, Lloyd RS, Guengerich FP. Isolation and sequence determination of a cDNA clone related to human cytochrome P-450 nifedipine oxidase. *Proc Natl Acad Sci 1986;83:8064–8068.*

12. Kolars JC, Lown KS, Schmiedlin-Ren P, et al. CYP3A gene expression in human gut epithelium. *Pharmacogenetics* 1994;4:247–259.

13. Shimada T, Yamazaki H, Mimura M, Inui Y, Guengerich FP. Interindividual variations in human liver cytochrome P450 enzymes involved in the oxidation of drugs, carcinogens and toxic chemicals: studies with liver microsomes of 30 Japanese and 30 caucasians. *J Pharmacol Exp Ther* 1994;270:414–423.

14. Guengerich FP. Mechanism-based inactivation of human liver cytochrome P450 IIIA4 by gestodene. *Chem Res Toxicol* 1990;3:363–371.

15. DeWaziers I, Cugnenc PH, Yang CS, Leroux J-P, Beaune PH. Cytochrome P450 isoenzymes, epoxide hydrolase and glutathione transferases in rat and human hepatic and extrahepatic tissues. *J Pharmacol Exp Ther* 1990;253:387–394.

16. Watkins PB, Wrighton SA, Schuetz EG, Guzelian PS. Identification of glucocorticoid-inducible cytochromes P-450 in the intestinal mucosa of rats and man. *J Clin Invest* 1987;80:1029–1036.

17. Paine MF. *Intestinal Versus Hepatic CYP3A-Dependent First-Pass Metabolism, Pharmaceutical Sciences.* Seattle: University of Washington, 1997:207.

18. Paine MF, Khalighi M, Fisher JM, et al. Characterization of inter- and intra-intestinal differences in human CYP3A-dependent metabolism. *J Pharmacol Exp Ther* 1997;283:1552–1562.

19. Schuetz EG, Guzelian PS. Induction of cytochrome P-450 by glucocorticoids in rat liver. II. Evidence that glucocorticoids regulate induction of cytochrome P-450 by a non-classical receptor mechanism. *J Biol Chem* 1984;259:2007–2012.

20. Schuetz EG, Wrighton SA, Barwick JL, Guzelian PS. Induction of cytochrome P-450 by glucocorticoids in rat liver. I. Evidence that glucocorticoids and pregnenolone 16α-carbonitrile regulate de novo synthesis of a common form of cytochrome P-450 in cultures of adult rat hepatocytes and in the liver in vivo. *J Biol Chem* 1984;259:1999–2006.

21. Huss JM, Wang SI, Anstrom A, McQuiddy P, Kasper CB. Dexamethasone responsiveness of a major glucocorticoid-inducible CYP3A gene is mediated by elements unrelated to a glucocorticoid receptor binding motif. *Proc Natl Acad Sci* 1996;93:4666–4670.

22. Miyata M, Nagata K, Yamazoe Y, Kato R. Transcriptional elements directing a liver-specific expression of P450/6βA (CYP3A2) gene-encoding testosterone 6β-hydroxlase. *Arch Biochem Biophys* 1995; 318:71–79.

23. Quattrochi LC, Mills AS, Barwick JL, Yockey CB, Guzelian PS. A novel *cis*-element in a liver cytochrome P450 3A gene confers synergistic induction by glucocorticoids plus antiglucocorticoids. *J Biol Chem* 1995;270:28917–28923.

24. Kliewer SA, Moore JT, Wade L, et al. An orphan nuclear receptor activated by pregnanes defines a novel steroid signaling pathway. *Cell* 1998;92:73–82.

25. Barwick JL, Quattrochi LC, Mills AS, Potenza C, Tikey RH, Guzelian PS. Trans-species gene transfer for analysis of glucocorticoid-inducible transcriptional activation of transiently expressed human CYP3A4 and rabbit CYP3A6 in primary cultures of adult rat and rabbit hepatocytes. *Mol Pharmacol* 1996;50:10–16.

26. Calleja C, Pascussi JM, Mani JC, Maurel P, Vilaren MJ. The antibiotic rifampicin is a nonsteroidal ligand and activator of the glucocorticoid receptor. *Nat Med* 1998;4:92–96.

27. Lehmann JM, McKee DD, Watson MA, Willson TM, Moore JT, Kliewer SA. The human orphan nuclear receptor PXR is activated by compounds that regulate CYP3A4 gene expression and cause drug interactions. *J Clin Invest* 1998;102:1016–1023.

28. Waxman DJ. Interactions of hepatic cytochromes P-450 with steroid hormones. Regioselectivity and stereoselectivity of steroid metabolism and hormonal regulation of rat P-450 enzyme expression. *Biochem Pharmacol* 1988;37:71–88.

29. Liddle C, Goodwin B, George J, Tapner M, Farrell G. Separate and interactive regulation of cytochrome P450 by triiodothyronine, dexamethasone, and growth hormone in cultured hepatocytes. *J Clin Endocrinol Metab* 1998;83:2411–2416.

30. Kumar R. Vitamin D metabolism and mechanisms of calcium transport. *J Am Soc Nephrol* 1990;1:30–42.

31. Waserman RH, Fullmer CS. Vitamin D and intestinal calcium transport: facts, speculations and hypotheses. *J Nutr* 1995;125: 1971S–1979S.

32. Schmiedlin-Ren P, Thummel KE, Fisher JM, Paine MF, Lown KS, Watkins PB. Expression of enzymatically active CYP3A4 by Caco-2 cells grown on extracellular matrix-coated permeable supports in the presence of 1α,25-dihydroxyvitamin D_3. *Mol Pharmacol* 1997;51: 741–754.

33. Wrighton SA, Ring BJ, Watkins PB, VandenBranden M. Identification of a polymorphically expressed member of the human cytochrome P-450III family. *Mol Pharmacol* 1989;36:97–105.

34. Schuetz JD, Molowa DT, Guzelian PS. Characterization of a cDNA encoding a new member of the glucocorticoid-responsive cytochromes P450 in human liver. *Arch Biochem Biophys* 1989;274:355–365.

35. Wrighton SA, Brian WR, Sari M-A, et al. Studies on the expression and metabolic capabilities of human liver cytochrome P450IIIA5 (HLp3). *Mol Pharmacol* 1990;38:207–213.

36. Jounäidi Y, Hyrailles V, Gervot L, Maurel P. Detection of a CYP3A5 allelic variant: a candidate for the polymorphic expression of the protein? *Biochem Biophys Res Commun* 1996;221:466–470.

37. Haehner BD, Gorski JC, VandenBranden M, et al. Bimodal distribution of renal cytochrome P450 3A activity in humans. *J Pharmacol Exp Ther* 1996;50:52–59.

38. Schuetz EG, Schuetz JD, Grogan WM, et al. Expression of cytohrome P450 3A in amphibian, rat, and human kidney. *Arch Biochem Biophys* 1992;294:206–214.

39. Anttila S, Hukkanen J, Stejernvall T, et al. Expression and localization of CYP3A4 and CYP3A5 in human lung. *Am J Respir Cell Mol Biol* 1997;16:242–49.

40. Kivistö KT, Griese E-U, Fritz P, et al. Expression of cytochrome P450 3A enzymes in human lung: a combined RT-PCR and immunohistochemical analysis of normal and lung tumours. *Naunyn-Schmiedeberg's Archives of Pharmacology* 1996;353:207–212.

41. Thummel KE, Shen DD, Podoll TD, et al. RLC: Use of midazolam as a human cytochrome P450 3A probe: II. Characterization of inter- and intra-individual hepatic P4503A variability after liver transplantation. *J Pharmacol Exp Ther* 1994;271:557–566.

42. Schuetz JD, Schuetz EG, Thottassery JV, Guzelian PS, Strom S, Sun D. Identification of a novel dexamethasone responsive enhancer in the human CYP3A5 gene and its activation in human and rat liver cells. *Mol Pharmacol* 1996;49:63–72.

43. Aoyama T, Yamano S, Waxman DJ, et al. Cytochrome P-450 hPCN3, a novel cytochrome P-450IIIA gene product that is differentially expressed in adult human liver. cDNA and deduced amino acid sequence and distinct specificities of cDNA-expressed hPCN1 and hPCN3 for the metabolism of steroid hormones and cyclosporine. *J Biol Chem* 1989;264:10388–10395.

44. Waxman DJ, Lapenson DP, Aoyama T, Gelboin HV, Gonzalez FJ, Korzekwa K. Steroid hormone hydroxylase specificities of eleven cDNA-expressed human cytochrome P450s. *Arch Biochem Biophys* 1991;290:160–166.

45. Gillam EMJ, Guo Z, Ueng Y-F, et al. Expression of cytochrome P450 3A5 in *Escherichia coli*: effects of 5′ modification, purification, spectral characterization, reconstitution conditions, and catalytic activities. *Arch Biochem Biophys* 1995;317:374–384.

46. Gorski JC, Hall SD, Jones DR, VandenBranden M, Wrighton SA. Regioselective biotransformation of midazolam by members of the human cytochrome P450 3A (CYP3A) subfamily. *Biochem Pharmacol* 1994;47:1643–1653.

47. Gibbs MA, Thummel KE, Shen DD, Kunze KL. Inhibition of CYP3A in human intestinal and liver microsomes: comparison of Ki values

and impact of CYP3A5 expression. *Drug Metab Dispos* 1999;27:180–187.

48. Kitada M, Kamataki T. Cytochrome P450 in human fetal liver: significance and fetal-specific expression. *Drug Metab Rev* 1994;26:305–323.

49. Kitada K, Kamataki T, Itahashi K, Rikihisa T, Kato R, Kanakubo Y. Purification and properties of cytochrome P450 from homogenates of human fetal livers. *Arch Biochem Biophys* 1985;241:275–280.

50. Wrighton SA, VandenBranden M. Isolation and characterization of human fetal liver cytochrome P450HLp2: a third member of the P450III gene family. *Arch Biochem Biophys* 1989;268:144–151.

51. Kitada K, Taneda M, Itahashi K, Kamataki T. Four forms of cytochrome P-450 in human fetal livers: purification and their capacity to activate promutagens. *Jpn J Cancer Res* 1991;82:426–432.

52. Komori M, Nishio K, Ohi H, Kitada M, Kamataki T. Molecular cloning and sequence analysis of cDNA containing the entire coding region for human fetal liver cytochrome P-450. *J Biochem* 1989;105:161–163.

53. Wrighton SA, Molowa DT, Guzelian PS. Identification of a cytochrome P-450 in human fetal liver related to glucocorticoid-inducible cytochrome P-450HLp in the adult. *Biochem Pharmacol* 1988;37:3053–3055.

54. Kitada M, Kato T, Ohmori S, Kamataki T, Itahashi K, Guengerich FP, Rikihishi T, Kanakubo Y. Immunochemical characterization and toxicological significance of P-450HFLb purified from human fetal livers. *Biochim Biophys Acta* 1992;1117:301–305.

55. Schuetz JD, Kauma S, Guzelian PS. Identification of the fetal liver cytochrome CYP3A7 in human endometrium and placenta. *J Clin Invest* 1993;92:1018–1024.

56. Kitada M, Kamataki T, Itahashi K, Rikihisa T, Kanakubo Y. P-450 HFLa, a form of cytochrome P-450 purified from human fetal livers, is the 16α-hydroxylase of dehydroepiandrosterone 3-sulfate. *J Biol Chem* 1987;262:13534–13537.

57. Speroff L. The endocrinology of pregnancy. In: Speroff L, Glass R, Kase N, eds. *Clinical gynecologic endocrinology and infertility.* Baltimore: Williams & Wilkins, 1994:317–350.

58. Kawano S, Kamataki T, Yasumori T, Yamazoe Y, Kato R. Purification of human liver cytochrome P-450 catalyzing testosterone 6β-hydroxylation. *J Biochem* 1987;102:493–501.

59. Combalbert J, Fabre I, Fabre G, et al. Metabolism of cyclosporin A. IV. Purification and identification of the rifampin-inducible human liver cytochrome P-450 (cyclosporin A oxidase) as a product of P450IIIA gene family. *Drug Metab Dispos* 1989;17:197–207.

60. Shaw PM, Barnes TS, Cameron D, et al. Purification and characterization of an anticonvulsant-induced human cytochrome P-450 catalysing cyclosporin metabolism. *Biochem J* 1989;263:653–663.

61. Bourrie M, Meunier V, Berger Y, Fabre G. Cytochrome P450 isoform inhibitors as a tool for the investigation of metabolic reactions catalyzed by human liver microsomes. *J Pharmacol Exp Ther* 1996;277:321–332.

62. Pichard L, Fabre I, Fabre G, et al. Cyclosporin A drug interactions. Screening for inducers and inhibitors of cytochrome P-450 (cyclosporin A oxidase) in primary cultures of human hepatocytes and in liver microsomes. *Drug Metab Dispos* 1990;18:595–605.

63. Marre F, Sousa Gd, Orloff AM, Rahmani R. In vitro interaction between cyclosporin A and macrolide antibiotics. *Br J Clin Pharmacol* 1993;35:447–448.

64. Kumar GN, Rodrigues AD, Buko AM, Denissen JF. Cytochrome P450-mediated metabolism of the HIV-1 protease inhibitor ritonavir (ABT-538) in human liver microsomes. *J Pharmacol Exp Ther* 1996;277:423–431.

65. Fabre G, Rahmani R, Placidi M, et al. Characterization of midazolam metabolism using human hepatic microsomal fractions and hepatocytes in suspension obtained by perfusing whole human livers. *Biochem Pharmacol* 1988;37:4389–4397.

66. Kronbach T, Mathys D, Umeno M, Gonzalez FJ, Meyer UA. Oxidation of midazolam and triazolam by human liver cytochrome P450IIIA4. *Mol Pharmacol* 1989;36:89–96.

67. Gascon MP, Dayer P. In vitro forecasting of drugs which may interfere with the biotransformation of midazolam. *Eur J Clin Pharmacol* 1991;41:573–578.

68. Goldberg MJ, Ring B, DeSante K, et al. Effect of dirithromycin on human CYP3A in vitro and on pharmacokinetics and pharmacodynamics of terfenadine in vivo. *J Clin Pharmacol* 1996;36:1154–1160.

69. Moltke LLv, Greenblatt DJ, Schmider J, et al. Midazolam hydroxylation by liver microsomes in vitro: inhibition by fluoxetine, norfluoxe-

tine, and by azole antifungal agents. *J Clin Pharmacol* 1996;36:783–791.

70. Ring BJ, Parli CJ, George MC, Wrighton SA. In vitro metabolism of zatosetron. Interspecies comparison and role of CYP3A. *Drug Metab Dispos* 1994;22:352–357.

71. Ring BJ, Binkley SN, Roskos L, Wrighton SA. Effect of fluoxetine, norfluoxetine, sertraline and desmethyl sertraline on human CYP3A catalyzed 1′-hydroxy midazolam formation in vitro. *J Pharmacol Exp Ther* 1995;275:1131–1135.

72. Crespi CL, Miller VP, Penman BW. Microtiter plate assays for inhibition of human, drug-metabolizing cytochrome P450. *Anal Biochem* 1997;248:188–190.

73. Yang H-Y, Lee QP, Rettie AE, Juchau MR. Functional cytochrome P4503A isoforms in human embryonic tissues: expression during organogenesis. *Mol Pharmacol* 1994;46:922–928.

74. Li Y, Yokoi T, Sasaki M, Hattori K, Katsuki M, Kamataki T. Perinatal expression and inducibility of human CYP3A7 in C57BL/6N transgenic mice. *Biochem Biophys Res Commun* 1996;228:312–317.

75. Schellens JHM, Soons PA, Breimer DD. Lack of bimodality in nifedipine kinetics in a large population of healthy subjects. *Biochem Pharmacol* 1988;37:2507–2510.

76. Breimer DD, Schellens JHM, Soons PA. Nifedipine: variability in its kinetics and metabolism in man. *Pharmacol Ther* 1989;44:445–454.

77. Holtbecker N, Fromm M, Kroemer HK, Ohnhaus EE, Heidemann H. The nifedipine-rifampin interaction. Evidence for induction of gut wall metabolism. *Drug Metab Dispos* 1996;24:1121–1123.

78. Watkins PB. Noninvasive tests of CYP3A enzymes. *Pharmacogenetics* 1994;4:171–184.

79. Fleishaker JC, Pearson PG, Wienkers LC, Pearson LK, Graves GR. Biotransformation of tirilazad in humans: 2. Effect of ketoconazole on tirilazad clearance and oral bioavailability. *J Pharmacol Exp Ther* 1996;277:991–998.

80. Fromm MF, Busse D, Kroemer HK, Eichelbaum M. Differential induction of prehepatic and hepatic metabolism of verapamil by rifampin. *Hepatology* 1996;24:796–801.

81. Kolars JC, Awni WM, Merion RM, Watkins PB. First-pass metabolism of cyclosporin by the gut. *Lancet* 1991;338:1488–1490.

82. Paine MF, Shen DD, Kunze KL, et al. First-pass metabolism of midazolam by the human intestine. *Clin Pharmacol Ther* 1996;60:14–24.

83. Lown KS, Mayo RR, Leichtman AB, et al. Role of intestinal P-glycoprotein (mdr1) in interpatient variation in the oral bioavailability of cyclosporine. *Clin Pharmacol Ther* 1997;62:248–260.

84. Roots I, Holbe R, Hövermann W, Nigam S, Heinemeyer G, Hildebrabt AG. Quantitative determination by HPLC of urinary 6β-hydroxycortisol, an indicator of enzyme induction by rifampicin and antiepileptics. *Eur J Clin Pharmacol* 1979;16:63–71.

85. Saenger P. 6β-Hydroxycortisol in random urine samples as an indicator of enzyme induction. *Clin Pharmacol Ther* 1983;34:818–821.

86. Saenger P, Forster E, Kream J. 6β-Hydroxycortisol: a noninvasive indicator of enzyme induction. *J Clin Endocrinol Metab* 1981;52:381–384.

87. Waxman DJ, Attisano C, Guengerich FP, Lapenson DP. Human liver microsomal steroid metabolism: identification of the major microsomal steroid hormone 6β-hydroxylase cytochrome P-450 enzyme. *Arch Biochem Biophys* 1988;263:424–436.

88. Ged C, Rouillon JM, Pichard L, et al. The increase in urinary excretion of 6β-hydroxycortisol as a marker of human hepatic cytochrome P450IIIA induction. *Br J Clin Pharmacol* 1989;28:373–387.

89. Bienvenu T, Rey E, Pons G, D'Athis P, Olive G. A simple non-invasive procedure for the investigation of cytochrome P-450 IIIA dependent enzymes in humans. *Int J Clin Pharmacol Ther Toxicol* 1991;29:441–445.

90. Horsmans Y, Desager JP, Harvengt C. Absence of CYP3A genetic polymorphism assessed by urinary excretion of 6β-hydroxycortisol in 102 healthy subjects on rifampin. *Pharmacol Toxicol* 1992;71:258–261.

91. Murray GI, Barnes TS, Sewell HF, Ewen SWB, Melvin WT, Burke MD. The immunocytochemical localisation and distribution of cytochrome P-450 in normal hepatic and extrahepatic tissues with a monoclonal antibody to human cytcohrome P-450. *Br J Clin Pharmacol* 1988;25:465–475.

92. Leggat JE, Johnson KJ, Kolars JC, Schmiedlin-Ren P, Watkins PB, Leightman AB. Immunohistochemical localization of cytochrome P450 3A in normal and neoplastic kidney and urinary bladder epithelium. *J Am Soc Nephrol* 1994;5:786.

93. Kovacs SJ, Martin DE, Everitt DE, Patterson SD, Jorkasky DK. Urinary excretion of 6β-hydroxycortisol as an in vivo marker for CYP3A induction: applications and recommendations. *Clin Pharmacol Ther* 1998;63:617–622.

94. Wilson JT, Boxtel CJV. Pharmacokinetics of erythromycin in man. *Antibiot Chemother* 1978;25:181–203.

95. Watkins PB, Murray SA, Winkelman LG, Heuman DM, Wrighton SA, Guzelian PS. Erythromycin breath test as an assay of glucocorticoid-inducible liver cytochromes P-450. Studies in rats and patients. *J Clin Invest* 1989;83:688–697.

96. Iribarne C, Berthou F, Baird S, et al. Involvement of cytochrome P450 3A4 enzyme in the N-demethylation of methadone in human liver microsomes. *Chem Res Toxicol* 1996;9:365–373.

97. Lown K, Kolars J, Turgeon K, Merion R, Wrighton SA, Watkins PB. The erythromycin breath test selectively measures P450IIIA in patients with severe liver disease. *Clin Pharmacol Ther* 1992;51:229–238.

98. Watkins PB, Turgeon DK, Saenger P, et al. Comparison of urinary 6-β-cortisol and the erythromycin breath test as measures of hepatic P450IIIA (CYP3A) activity. *Clin Pharmacol Ther* 1992;52:265–273.

99. Hunt CM, Westerkam WR, Stave GM. Effect of age and gender on the activity of human hepatic CYP3A. *Biochem Pharmacol* 1992;44: 275–283.

100. Austin KL, Mather LE, Philpot CR, McDonald PJ. Intersubject and dose-related variability after intravenous administration of erythromycin. *Br J Clin Pharmacol* 1980;10:273–279.

101. Watkins PB, Hamilton TA, Annesley TM, Ellis CN, Kolars JC, Voorhees JJ. The erythromycin breath test as a predictor of cyclosporine blood levels. *Clin Pharmacol Ther* 1990;48:120–129.

102. Turgeon DK, Normolle DP, Leightman AB, Annesley TM, Smith DE, Watkins PB. Erythromycin breath test predicts oral clearance of cyclosporine in kidney transplant recipients. *Clin Pharmacol Ther* 1992; 52:471–478.

103. Turgeon DK, Leightman AB, Blake DS, et al. Prediction of interpatient and intrapatient variation in OG 37-325 dosing requirements by the erythromycin breath test. *Transplantation* 1994;57:1736–1741.

104. Lown KS, Thummel KE, Benedict PE, et al. The erythromycin breath test predicts the clearance of midazolam. *Clin Pharmacol Ther* 1995; 57:16–24.

105. Lown KS, Kolars JC, Thummel KE, et al. Interpatient heterogeneity in expression of CYP3A4 and CYP3A5 in small bowel: lack of prediction by the erythromycin breath test. *Drug Metab Dispos* 1994;22: 947–955.

106. Hunt CM, Watkins PB, Saenger P, et al. Heterogeneity of CYP3A isoforms metabolizing erythromycin and cortisol. *Clin Pharmacol Ther* 1992;51:18–23.

107. Kinirons MT, O'Shea D, Downing TE, et al. Absence of correlations among three putative in vivo probes of human cytochrome P4503A activity in young healthy men. *Clin Pharmacol Ther* 1993;54:621–629.

108. Gill HJ, Tingle MD, Park BK. N-Hydroxylation of dapsone by multiple enzymes of cytochrome P450: implications for inhibition of haemotoxicity. *Br J Clin Pharmacol* 1995;40:531–538.

109. Mitra AK, Thummel KE, Kalhorn TF, Kharasch ED, Unadkat JD, Slattery JT. Metabolism of dapsone to its hydroxylamine by CYP2E1 in vitro and in vivo. *Clin Pharmacol Ther* 1995;58:556–566.

110. Lane EA, Parashos I. Drug pharmacokinetics and the carbon dioxide breath test. *J Pharmacokinet Biopharm* 1985;14:29–49.

111. Jamis-Dow CA, Pearl ML, Watkins PB, Blake DS, Klecker RW, Collins JM. Predicting drug interactions in vivo from experiments in vitro. Human studies with paclitaxel and ketoconazole. *Am J Clin Oncol* 1997;20:592–599.

112. Cheng C-L, Smith DE, Carver PL, et al. Steady-state pharmacokinetics of delavirdine in HIV-positive patients: effect on erythromycin breath test. *Clin Pharmacol Ther* 1997;61:531–543.

113. Thummel KE, Shen DD, Podoll TD, et al. RLC. Use of midazolam as a human cytochrome P450 3A probe: I. In vitro-in vivo correlations in liver transplant patients. *J Pharmacol Exp Ther* 1994;271:549–556.

114. Ghosal A, Satoh H, Thomas PE, Bush E, Moore D. Inhibition and kinetics of cytochrome P4503A activity in microsomes from rat, human and cDNA-expressed human cytochrome P450. *Drug Metab Dispos* 1996;24:940–947.

115. Heizmann P, Eckert M, Ziegler WH. Pharmacokinetics and bioavailability of midazolam in man. *Br J Clin Pharmacol* 1983;16:43S–49S.

116. Dundee JW, Halliday NJ, Harper KW, Brogden RN. Midazolam. A review of its pharmacological properties and therapeutic use. *Drugs* 1984;28:519–543.

117. Heizmann P, Ziegler WH. Excretion and metabolism of 14C-midazolam in humans following oral dosing. *Arzneim-Forsch/Drug Res* 1981;31:2220–2223.

118. Thummel KE, O'Shea D, Paine MF, et al. Oral first-pass elimination of midazolam involves both gastrointestinal and hepatic CYP3A-mediated metabolism. *Clin Pharmacol Ther* 1996;59:491–502.

119. Smith MT, Eadie MJ, Brophy TOR. The pharmacokinetics of midazolam in man. *Eur J Clin Pharmacol* 1981;19:271–278.

120. Mandema JW, Tuk B, Steveninck ALv, Breimer DD, Cohen AF, Danhof M. Pharmacokinetic-pharmacodynamic modeling of the central nervous system effects of midazolam and its main metabolite α-hydroxymidazolam in healthy volunteers. *Clin Pharmacol Ther* 1992; 51:715–728.

121. Kharasch ED, Russell M, Mautz D, et al. The role of cytochrome P450 3A4 in alfentanil clearance. Implications for interindividual variability in disposition and perioperative drug interactions. *Anesthesiology* 1997;87:36–50.

122. Backman JT, Olkkola KT, Neuovnen PJ. Rifampin drastically reduces plasma concentrations and effects of oral midazolam. *Clin Pharmacol Ther* 1996;59:7–13.

123. Backman JT, Olkkola KT, Ojala M, Laaksovirta H, Neuvonen PJ. Concentrations and effects of oral midazolam are greatly reduced in patients treated with carbamazepine or phenytoin. *Epilepsia* 1996; 37:253–257.

124. Olkkola KT, Aranko K, Luuila H, et al. A potentially hazardous interaction between erythromycin and midazolam. *Clin Pharmacol Ther* 1993;53:298–305.

125. Gorski JC, Jones DR, Haehner-Daniels BD, Hamman MA, O'Mara EM, Hall SD. The contribution of intestinal and hepatic CYP3A to the interaction between midazolam and clarithromycin. *Clin Pharmacol Ther* 1998;64:133–143.

126. Olkkola KT, Backman JT, Neuoven PJ. Midazolam should be avoided in patients receiving the systemic antimycotics ketoconazole or itraconazole. *Clin Pharmacol Ther* 1994;55:481–485.

127. Backman JT, Olkkola KT, Aranko K, Himberg J-J, Neuvonen PJ. Dose of midazolam should be reduced during diltiazem and verapamil treatments. *Br J Clin Pharmacol* 1994;37:221–225.

128. Ahonen J, Olkkola KT, Neuvonen PJ. Effect of route of administration of fluconazole on the interaction between fluconazole and midazolam. *Eur J Clin Pharmacol* 1997;51:415–419.

129. Kupferschmidt HHT, Ha HR, Ziegler WH, Meier PJ, Krähenbühl S. Interaction between grapefruit juice and midazolam in humans. *Clin Pharmacol Ther* 1995;58:20–28.

130. Mattila MJ, Vanakoski J, Idänpään-Heikkilä JJ. Azithromycin does not alter the effects of oral midazolam on human performance. *Eur J Clin Pharmacol* 1994;47:49–52.

131. Gillette JR, Pang KS. Theoretical aspects of pharmacokinetic drug interactions. *Clin Pharmacol Ther* 1977;22:623–639.

132. Wu C-Y, Benet LZ, Hebert MF, Gupta SK, Rowland M, Gomez DY, Wacher VJ. Differentiation of absorption and first-pass gut and hepatic metabolism in humans: studies with cyclosporine. *Clin Pharmacol Ther* 1995;58:492–497.

133. Gorski JC, Jones DR, Wrighton SA, Hall SD. Characterization of dextromethorphan N-demethylation by human liver microsomes. Contribution of the cytochrome P450 3A (CYP3A) subfamily. *Biochem Pharmacol* 1994;48:173–182.

134. Jacqz-Aigrain E, Funck-Brentano C, Cresteil T. CYP2D6- and CYP3A-dependent metabolism of dextromethorphan in humans. *Pharmacogenetics* 1993;3:197–204.

135. Jones DR, Gorski C, Haehner BD, O'Mara EM, Hall SD. Determination of cytochrome P450 3A4/5 activity in vivo with dextromethorphan N-demethylation. *Clin Pharmacol Ther* 1996;60:374–384.

136. May DG, Porter JA, Uetrecht JP, Wilkinson GR, Branch RA. The contribution of N-hydroxylation and acetylation to dapsone pharmacokinetics in normal subjects. *Clin Pharmacol Ther* 1990;48:619–627.

137. Fleming CM, Branch RA, Wilkinson GR, Guengerich FP. Human liver microsomal N-hydroxylation of dapsone by cytochrome P-4503A4. *Mol Pharmacol* 1992;41:975–980.

138. May DG, Porter J, Wilkinson GR, Branch RA. Frequency distribution of dapsone N-hydroxylase, a putative probe for P4503A4 activity, in a white population. *Clin Pharmacol Ther* 1994;55:492–500.

139. Stein CM, Kinirons MT, Pincus T, Wilkinson GR, Wood AJJ. Comparison of the dapsone recovery ratio and the erythromycin breath test as in vivo probes of CYP3A activity in patients with rheumatoid arthritis receiving cyclosporine. *Clin Pharmacol Ther* 1996;59:47–51.

140. Korzekwa KR, Krishnamachary N, Shou M, et al. Evaluation of atypical cytochrome P450 kinetics with two-substrate-models: evidence that multiple substrates can simultaneously bind to cytochrome P450 active sites. *Biochemistry* 1998;37:4137–4147.

141. Bargetzi MJ, Aoyama T, Gonzalez FJ, Meyer UA. Lidocaine metabolism in human liver microsomes by cytochrome P450IIIA4. *Clin Pharmacol Ther* 1989;46:521–527.

142. Oellerich M, Burdelski M, Ringe B, et al. Lignocaine metabolite formation as a measure of pre-transplant liver function. *Lancet* 1989;1:640–642.

143. Schroeder TJ, Gremse DA, Mansour ME, et al. Lidocaine metabolism as an index of liver function in hepatic transplant donors and recipients. *Transplant Proc* 1989;21:2299–2301.

144. Oellerich M, Burdelski M, Lautz H-U, Schulz M, Schmidt F-W, Herrmann H. Lidocaine metabolite formation as a measure of liver function in patients with cirrhosis. *Ther Drug Monit* 1990;12:219–226.

145. Gremse DA, A-Kadar HH, Schroeder TJ, Balistreri WF. Assessment of lidocaine metabolite formation as a quantitative liver function test in children. *Hepatology* 1990;12:565–569.

146. Oellerich M, Burdelski M, Lautz H-U, Binder L, Pichlmayr R. Predictors of one-year pretransplant survival in patients with cirrhosis. *Hepatology* 1991;14:1029–1034.

147. Shiffman ML, Fisher RA, Sanyal AJ, et al. Hepatic lidocaine metabolism and complications of cirrhosis. Implications for assessing patient priority for hepatic transplantation. *Transplantation* 1993;55:830–834.

148. Arrigoni A, Gindro T, Aimo G, et al. Monoethylglicinexylidide test: a prognostic indicator of survival in cirrhosis. *Hepatology* 1994;20:383–387.

149. Adam R, Azoulay D, Astarcioglu I, Bao YM, Bonhomme L, Fredj G, Bismuth H. Reliability of the MEGX test in the selection of liver grafts. *Transplant Proc* 1991;23:2470–2471.

150. Burdelski M, Oellerich M, Bornscheuer A, et al. Donor rating in human liver transplantation: correlation of oxygen consumption after revascularization with MEGX formation in donors. *Transplant Proc* 1989;21:2392–2393.

151. Rossi SJ, Schroeder TJ, Vine WH, et al. Monoethylglycinexylide formation in assessing pediatric donor liver function. *Ther Drug Monit* 1992;14:452–456.

152. Oellerich M, Schütz E, Polzien F, Ringe B, Armstrong VW, Hartmann H, Burdelski M. Influence of gender on the monoethylglycinexylidide test in normal subjects and liver donors. *Ther Drug Monit* 1994;16:225–231.

153. Maurice M, Pichard L, Daujat M, Fabre I, Joyeux H, Domergue J, Maurel P. Effects of imidazole derivatives on cytochromes P450 from human hepatocytes in primary culture. *FASEB J* 1992;6:752–758.

154. Schuetz E, Schuetz J, Strom S, et al. Regulation of human liver cytochromes P-450 in family 3A in primary and continuous culture of human hepatocytes. *Hepatology* 1993;18:1254–1262.

155. Pichard L, Fabre I, Daujat M, Domergue J, Joyeux H, Maurel P. Effect of corticosteroids on the expression of cytochromes P450 and on cyclosporin A oxidase activity in primary cultures of human hepatocytes. *Mol Pharmacol* 1992;41:1047–1055.

156. Donato M, Castell J, Gomez-Lechon M. Effect of model inducers on cytochrome P450 activities of human hepatocytes in primary culture. *Drug Metab Dispos* 1995;23:553–558.

157. Guillouzo A, Begue J-M, Campion J-P, Gascoin M-N, Guguen-Guillouzo C. Human hepatocyte cultures: a model of pharmacological studies. *Xenobiotica* 1985;15:635–641.

158. Kostrubsky V, Strom S, Wood S, Wrighton S, Sinclair P, Sinclair J. Ethanol and isopentanol increase CYP3A and CYP2E in primary cultures of human hepatocytes. *Arch Biochem Biophys* 1995;322:516–520.

159. Curi-Pedrosa R, Daujat M, Pichard L, et al. Omeprazole and lansoprazole are mixed inducers of CYP1A and CYP3A in human hepatocytes in primary culture. *J Pharmacol Exp Ther* 1994;269:384–392.

160. Masubuchi N, Li A, Okazaki O. An evaluation of the cytochrome P450 induction potential of pantoprazole in primary human hepatocytes. *Chem Biol Interact* 1998;114:1–13.

161. Hassett C, Laurenzana E, Sidhu JS, Omiecinski C. Effects of chemical inducers on human microsomal epoxide hydrolase in primary hepatocyte cultures. *Biochem Pharmacol* 1998;55:1059–1069.

162. Li A, Reith M, Rasmussen A, et al. Primary human hepatocytes as a tool for the evaluation of structure-activity relationship in cytochrome P450 induction potential of xenobiotics: evaluation of rifampin, rifapentine and rifabutin. *Chem Biol Interact* 1997;107:17–30.

163. Mattes W, Li A. Quantitative reverse transcriptase/PCR assay for the

measurement of induction in cultured hepatocytes. *Chem Biol Interact* 1997;107:47–61.

164. Li A, Rasmussen A, Xu L, Kaminski D. Rifampicin induction of lidocaine metabolism in cultured human hepatocytes. *J Pharmacol Exp Ther* 1995;274:673–677.

165. Kostrubsky V, Lewis L, Strom S, et al. Induction of cytochrome P450 3A by taxol in primary cultures of human hepatocytes. *Arch Biochem Biophys* 1998;355:131–136.

166. Koup J, Anderson G, Loi C-M. Effect of troglitazone on urinary excretion of 6β-hydroxycortisol. *J Clin Pharmacol* 1998;38:815–818.

167. Ohnhaus E, Park B. Measurement of urinary 6-β-hydroxycortisol excretion as an in vivo parameter in clinical assessment of the microsomal enzyme-inducing capacity of antipyrine, phenobarbitone and rifampicin. *Eur J Clin Pharmacol* 1979;15:139–145.

168. Ohnhaus E, Breckenridge A, Park B. Urinary excretion of 6β-hydroxycortisol and the time course measurement of enzyme induction in man. *Eur J Clin Pharmacol* 1989;36:39–46.

169. Schuetz EG, Beck WT, Schuetz JD. Modulators and substrates of P-glycoprotein and cytochrome P4503A coordinately up-regulate these proteins in human colon carcinoma cells. *Mol Pharmacol* 1996;49:311–318.

170. Wrighton SA, Maurel P, Schuetz EG, Watkins PB, Young B, Guzelian PS. Identification of the cytochrome P-450 induced by macrolide antibiotics in rat liver as the glucocorticoid responsive cytochrome P-450p. *Biochemistry* 1985;24:2171–2178.

171. Chien JY, Peter RM, Nolan CM, et al. Influence of NAT2 phenotype on the inhibition and induction of acetaminophen bioactivation with chronic isoniazid. *Clin Pharmacol Ther* 1996;61:24–34.

172. Hebert MF, Roberts JP, Prueksaritanont T, Benet LZ. Bioavailability of cyclosporine with concomitant rifampin administration is markedly less than predicted by hepatic enzyme induction. *Clin Pharmacol Ther* 1992;52:453–457.

173. Kolars JC, Schmiedlin-Ren P, Schuetz JD, Fang C, Watkins PB. Identification of rifampin-inducible P450IIIA4 (CYP3A4) in human small bowel enterocytes. *J Clin Invest* 1992;90:1871–1878.

174. Lin JH, Chiba M, Baillie TA. In vivo assessment of intestinal drug metabolism. *Drug Metab Dispos* 1997;25:1107–1109.

175. Lewis DFV, Eddershaw PJ, Goldfarb PS, Tarbit MH. Molecular modelling of CYP3A4 from an allignment with CYP1O2: identification of key interactions between putative active site residues and CYP3A-specific chemicals. *Xenobiotica* 1996;26:1067–1086.

176. Grimm A, Dyroff M. Inhibition of human drug metabolizing cytochromes P450 by anastrozole, a potent and selective inhibitor of aromatase. *Drug Metab Dispos* 1997;25:598–602.

177. Abel A, Back D. Cortisol metabolism in vitro—III. Inhibition of microsomal 6β-hydroxylase and cytosolic 4-ene-reductase. *J Steroid Biochem Mol Biol* 1993;46:827–832.

178. Lampen A, Christians U, Guengerich FP, et al. Metabolism of the immunosuppressant tacrolimus in the small intestine: cytochrome P450, drug interactions, and interindividual variability. *Drug Metab Dispos* 1995;23:1315–1324.

179. Moltke LV, Greenblatt D, Harmatz J, et al. Triazolam biotransformation by human liver microsomes in vitro: effects of metabolic inhibitors and clinical confirmation of a predicted interaction with ketoconazole. *J Pharmacol Exp Ther* 1996;276:370–379.

180. Wrighton SA, Ring BJ. Inhibition of human CYP3A catalyzed 1'-hydroxymidazolam formation by ketoconzole, nifedipine, erythromycin, cimetidine, and nizatidine. *Pharm Res* 1994;11:921–923.

181. Jurima-Romet M, Crawford K, Cyr T, Inaba T. Terfenadine metabolism in human liver. In vitro inhibition by macrolide antibiotics and azole antifungals. *Drug Metab Dispos* 1994;22:849–857.

182. Iatsimirskaia E, Tulebaev S, Storozhuk E, et al. Metabolism of rifabutin in human enterocyte and liver microsomes: kinetic paramters, identification of enzyme systems, and drug interactions with macrolides and antifungal agents. *Clin Pharmacol Ther* 1997;61:554–562.

183. Gibbs M, Kunze K, Howald W, Thummel K. Effect of inhibitor depletion on inhibitory potency: tight binding inhibition of CYP3A by clotrimazole. *Drug Metab Dispos* 1999;27:596–599.

184. Voorman R, Maio S, Payne N, Zhao Z, Koeplinger K, Wang X. Microsomal metabolism of delavirdine: evidence for mechanism-based inactivation of human cytochrome P450 3A. *J Pharmacol Exp Ther* 1998;287:381–388.

185. Relling M, Nemec J, Schuetz E, Schuetz J, Gonzalez F, Korzekwa K. O-Demethylation of epipodophyllotoxins is catalyzed by human cytochrome P450 3A4. *Mol Pharmacol* 1994;45:352–358.

186. Sutton D, Butler A, Nadin L, Murray M. Role of CYP3A4 in human hepatic diltiazem N-demethylation: inhibition of CYP3A4 activity by oxidized diltiazem metabolites. *J Pharmacol Exp Ther* 1997;282:294–300.

187. Lindstrom TD, Hanssen BR, Wrighton SA. Cytochrome P-450 complex formation by dirithromycin and other macrolides in rats and human livers. *Antimicrob Agents Chemother* 1993;37:265–269.

188. Guengerich FP. Oxidation of 17α-ethynylestradiol by human liver cytochrome P-450. *Mol Pharmacol* 1988;33:500–508.

189. Kunze K, Wienkers L, Thummel K, Trager W. Warfarin-fluconazole I. Inhibition of the human cytochrome P450-dependent metabolism of warfarin by fluconazole: in vitro studies. *Drug Metab Dispos* 1996;24:414–421.

190. Fukuda K, Ohta T, Oshima Y, Ohashi N, Yoshikawa M, Yamazoe Y. Specific CYP3A4 inhibitors in grapefruit juice: furocoumarin dimers as components of drug interaction. *Pharmacogenetics* 1997;7:391–396.

191. Schmiedlin-Ren P, Edwards DJ, Fitzsimmons ME, et al. Mechanisms of enhanced oral availability of CYP3A4 substrates by grapefruit constituents: decreased enterocyte CYP3A4 concentration and mechanism-based inactivation by furanocoumarins. *Drug Metab Dispos* 1997;25:1228–1233.

192. Fitzsimmons ME, Collins JM. Selective biotransformation of the human immunodeficiency virus protease inhibitor saquinavir by human small-intestinal cytochrome P4503A4. *Drug Metab Dispos* 1997;25:256–266.

193. Lillibridge JH, Liang BH, Kerr BM, et al. Characterization of the selectivity and mechanism of human cytochrome P450 inhibition by the human immunodeficiency virus-protease inhibitor nelfinavir mesylate. *Drug Metab Dispos* 1998;26:609–616.

194. Jang G, Benet L. Antiprogestin-mediated inactivation of cytochrome P450 3A4. *Pharmacology* 1998;56:150–157.

195. Guengerich FP, Kim DH. In vitro inhibition of dihydropyridine oxidation and aflatoxin B1 activation in human liver microsomes by naringenin and other flavanoids. *Carcinogenesis* (Oxford) 1990;11:2275–2279.

196. Zhou X, Zhou-Pan X, Gauthier T, Placidi M, Maurel P, Rahmani R. Human liver microsomal cytochrome P450 3A isozymes mediated vindesine biotransformation. Metabolic drug reactions. *Biochem Pharmacol* 1993;45:853–861.

197. Guengerich FP, Müller-Enoch D, Blair IA. Oxidation of quinidine by human liver cytochrome P-450. *Mol Pharmacol* 1986;30:287–295.

198. Desta Z, Kerbusch T, Soukhova N, Richard E, Ko J-W, Flockhart DA. Identification and characterization of human cytochrome P450 isoforms interacting with pimozide. *J Pharmacol Exp Ther* 1998;285:428–437.

199. Jacolot F, Simon I, Dreano Y, Beaune P, Riche C, Berthou F. Identification of the cytochrome P450 IIIA family as the enzymes involved in the N-demethylation of tamoxifen in human liver microsomes. *Biochem Pharmacol* 1991;41:1911–1919.

200. Fischer V, Rodriguez-Gascon A, Heitz F, et al. The multidrug resistance modulator valspodar (PSC 833) is metabolized by human cytochrome P450 3A. Implications for drug-drug interactions and pharmacological activity of the main metabolite. *Drug Metab Dispos* 1998;26:802–811.

201. Bergstrom RF, Goldberg MJ, Cerimele BJ, Hatcher BL. Assessment of the potential for a pharmacokinetic interaction between fluoxetine and terfenadine. *Clin Pharmacol Ther* 1997;62:643–651.

202. Wright CE, Lasher-Sisson TA, Steenwyk RC, Swanson CN. A pharmacokinetic evaluation of the combined administration of triazolam and fluoxetine. *Pharmacotherapy* 1992;12:103–106.

203. Lam YW, Alfaro CL, Ereshefsky L, Miller M. Effect of antidepressants (AD) and ketoconazole (K) on oral midazolam (M) pharmacokinetics (PK). *Clin Pharmacol Ther* 1998;63:229(abst).

204. Segel IH. *Enzyme kinetics: behavior and analysis of rapid equilibrium and steady-state enzyme systems.* New York: John Wiley and Sons, 1975.

205. Guengerich FP. Role of cytochrome P450 enzymes in drug–drug interactions. *Adv Pharmacol* 1997;43:7–35.

206. Koley AP, Buters JTM, Robinson RC, Markowitz A, Friedman FK. CO binding kinetics of human cytochrome P450 3A4. Specific interaction of substrates with kinetically distinguishable conformers. *J Biol Chem* 1995;270:5014–5018.

207. Koley AP, Robinson RC, Friedman FK. Cytochrome P450 conformation and substrate interactions as probed by CO binding kinetics. *Biochimie* 1996;78:706–713.

208. Koley AP, Robinson RC, Markowitz A, Friedman FK. Drug-drug interactions: effect of quinidine on nifedipine binding to human cytochrome P450 3A4. *Biochem Pharmacol* 1997;53:455–460.

209. Gray MR, Tam YK. Pharmacokinetics of drugs that inactivate metabolic enzymes. *J Pharm Sci* 1991;80:121–127.

210. Watkins PB, Wrighton SA, Schuetz EG, Maurel P, Guzelian PS. Macrolide antibiotics inhibit the degradation of the glucocorticoid-responsive cytochrome P-450p in rat hepatocytes in vivo and in primary monolayer culture. *J Biol Chem* 1986;261:6264–6271.

211. Pessayre D, Descatoire V, Konstantinova-Mitcheva M, et al. Self-induction by triacetyloleandomycin of its own transformation into a metabolite forming a stable 456 nm-absorbing complex with cytochrome P-450. *Biochem Pharmacol* 1981;30:553–558.

212. Miura T, Iwasaki M, Komori M, et al. Decrease in a constitutive form of cytochrome P-450 by macrolide antibiotics. *J Antimicrob Chemother* 1989;24:551–559.

213. Babany G, Larrey D, Pessayre D. *Macrolide antibiotics as inducers and inhibitors of cytochrome P-450 in experimental animals and man.* London: Taylor & Francis, 1988.

214. Ohmori S, Ishii I, Kuriya SI, et al. Effects of clarithromycin and its metabolites on the mixed function oxidase system in hepatic microsomes of rats. *Drug Metab Dispos* 1993;21:358–363.

215. Tinel M, Descatoire V, Larrey D, Loeper J, Labbe G. Effects of clarithromycin on cytochrome P-450. Comparison with other macrolides. *J Pharmacol Exp Ther* 1989;250:746–751.

216. Witkamp RF, Nijmeijer SM, Monshouwer M, Van Miert AS. The antibiotic tiamulin is a potent inducer and inhibitor of cytochrome P4503A via the formation of a stable metabolic intermediate complex. Studies in primary hepatocyte cultures and liver microsomes of the pig. *Drug Metab Dispos* 1995;23:542–547.

217. Bensoussan C, Delaforge M, Mansuy D. Particular ability of cytochrome P450 3A to form inhibitory P450-iron-metabolite complexes upon metabolic oxidation of aminodrugs. *Biochem Pharmacol* 1995;49:591–602.

218. Franklin MR. Enhanced rates of cytochrome P450 metabolic-intermediate complex formation from nonmacrolide amines in rifampicin-treated rabbit liver microsomes. *Drug Metab Dispos* 1995;23:1379–1382.

219. Murray M, Field SL. Inhibition and metabolite complexation of rat hepatic microsomal cytochrome P450 by tricyclic antidepressants. *Biochem Pharmacol* 1992;43:2065–2071.

220. Larrey D, Tinel M, Letteron P, Geneve J, Descatoire V, Pessayre D. Formation of an inactive cytochrome P-450Fe(II)-metabolite complex after administration of amiodarone in rats, mice and hamsters. *Biochem Pharmacol* 1986;35:2213–2220.

221. Ludden TM. Pharmacokinetic interactions of the macrolide antibiotics. *Clin Pharmacokinet* 1985;10:63–79.

222. Bartkowski RR, Goldberg ME, Larijani GE, Boerner T. Inhibition of alfentanil metabolism by erythromycin. *Clin Pharmacol Ther* 1989;46:99–102.

223. Yee GC, McGuire TR. Pharmacokinetic drug interactions with cyclosporin (Part I). *Clin Pharmacokinet* 1990;19:319–332.

224. Honig P, Woosley R, Zamani K, Conner D Jr. Changes in the pharmacokinetics and electrocardiographic pharmacodynamics of terfenadine with concomitant administration of erythromycin. *Clin Pharmacol Ther* 1992;52:231–238.

225. Sahali-Sahly Y, Balani SK, Lin JH, Baillie TA. In vitro studies on the metabolic activation of the furanopyridine L-754,394, a highly potent and selective mechanism-based inhibitor of cytochrome P450 3A4. *Chem Res Toxicol* 1996;9:1007–1012.

226. Edwards DJ III, Woster PM. Identification of 6′,7′-dihydroxybergamottin, a cytochrome P450 inhibitor, in grapefruit juice. *Drug Metab Dispos* 1996;24:1287–1290.

227. Lown KS, Bailey DG, Fontana RJ, et al. Grapefruit juice increases felodipine oral availability in humans by increasing intestinal CYP3A protein expression. *J Clin Invest* 1997;99:2545–2553.

228. Labbe G, Descatoire V, Beaune P, Letteron P, Larrey D, Pessayre D. Suicide inactivation of cytochrome P-450 by methoxsalen. Evidence for the covalent binding of a reactive intermediate to the protein moiety. *J Pharmacol Exp Ther* 1989;250:1034–1042.

229. Koenigs LL, Peter RM, Thompson SJ, Rettie AE, Trager WF. Mechanism-based inactivation of human liver cytochrome P450 2A6 by 8-methoxypsoralen. *Drug Metab Dispos* 1997;25:1407–1415.

230. Back DJ, Orme MLE. Pharmacokinetic drug interactions with oral contraceptives. *Clin Pharmacokinet* 1990;18:472–484.

231. Pazzucconi F, Malavasi B, Galli G, Franceschini G, Calabresi L, Sirtori CR. Inhibition of antipyrine metabolism by low-dose contraceptives with gestodene and desogestrel. *Clin Pharmacol Ther* 1991; 49:278–284.

232. Bailey DG, Bend JR, Arnold JMO, Tran LT, Spence JD. Erythromycin-felodipine interaction: magnitude, mechanism, and comparison with grapefruit juice. *Clin Pharmacol Ther* 1996;60:25–33.

233. Ducharme MP, Warbasse LH, Edwards DJ. Disposition of intravenous and oral cyclosporine after administration with grapefruit juice. *Clin Pharmacol Ther* 1995;57:485–491.

234. Kapitulnik J, Poppers PJ, Buening MK, Fortner JG, Conney AH. Activation of monooxygenases in human liver by 7,8-benzoflavone. *Clin Pharmacol Ther* 1977;22:475–484.

235. Wiebel FJ, Leutz JC, Diamond L, Gelboin HV. Aryl hydrocarbon (benzo[a]pyrene) hydroxylase in microsomes from rat tissues: differential inhibition and stimulation by benzoflavones and organic solvents. *Arch Biochem Biophys* 1971;144:78–86.

236. Shou M, Grogan J, Mancewicz JA, et al. Activation of CYP3A4: evidence for the simultaneous binding of two substrates in a cytochrome P450 active site. *Biochemistry* 1994;33:6450–6455.

237. Li Y, Wang E, Patten CJ, Chen L, Yang CS. Effects of flavonoids on cytochrome P450-dependent acetaminophen metabolism in rats and human liver microsomes. *Drug Metab Dispos* 1994;22:566–571.

238. Kerlan V, Dreano Y, Bercovici JP, Beaune PH, Floch HH, Berthou F. Nature of cytochromes P450 involved in the 2-/4-hydroxylations of estradiol in human liver microsomes. *Biochem Pharmacol* 1992;44: 1745–1756.

239. Kerr BM, Thummel KE, Wurden CJ, et al. Human liver carbamazepine metabolism. Role of CYP3A4 and CYP2C8 in 10, 11-epoxide formation. *Biochem Pharmacol* 1994;47:1969–1976.

240. Shimada T, Guengerich FP. Evidence for cytochrome P-450NF, the nifedipine oxidase, being the principal enzyme involved in the bioactivation of aflatoxins in human liver. *Proc Natl Acad Sci USA* 1989;86: 462–465.

241. Yun C-H, Lee HS, Lee H, Rho JK, Jeong HG, Guengerich FP. Oxidation of the angiotensin II receptor antagonist losartan (DuP 753) in human liver microsomes. Role of cytochrome P4503A(4) in formation of the active metabolite EXP3174. *Drug Metab Dispos* 1995;23:285–289.

242. Ueng Y-F, Kuwabara T, Chun Y-J, Guengerich FP. Cooperativity in oxidations catalyzed by cytochrome P450 3A4. *Biochemistry* 1997;36: 370–381.

243. Gallagher EP, Kunze KL, Stapleton PL, Eaton DL. The kinetics of aflatoxin B1 oxidation by human cDNA-expressed and human liver microsomal cytochromes P450 1A2 and 3A4. *Toxicol Appl Pharmacol* 1996;141:595–606.

244. Riley RJ, Howbrook D. In vitro analysis of the activity of the major human hepatic CYP enzyme (CYP3A4) using [N-methyl-14C]-erythromycin. *J Pharmacol Toxicol Meth* 1998;38:189–193.

245. Lasker JM, Huang M-T, Conney AH. In vivo activation of zoxazolamine metabolism by flavone. *Science* 1982;216:1419–1421.

CHAPTER 11

P-Glycoprotein

Jeffrey A. Silverman

Active transport of drugs and their metabolites has been recently recognized as an important issue in pharmaceutics. Numerous transporters have been characterized in the liver, kidney, intestine, and lung, which serve diverse functions including ion, sugar, amino acid, and peptide transport as well as drug and metabolite disposition. This chapter focuses on one of these transporters, P-glycoprotein (P-gp), an adenosine triphosphate (ATP)-dependent drug transporter that has been extensively characterized for its role in multidrug resistance in cancer chemotherapy. Expression of this protein in tumors is associated with decreased intracellular accumulation of cytotoxic drugs, thereby enhancing cell survival in the presence of otherwise cytotoxic drug levels. P-gp is promiscuous in its ability to interact with a large number of structurally and mechanistically distinct drugs, resulting in tumors that are cross resistant to a diverse number of drugs, hence the term multidrug resistance.

One physiologic role of P-gp is to serve as a barrier to entry and as an efflux mechanism for xenobiotics and cellular metabolites. It has also been suggested that P-gp may limit intestinal drug absorption to constrain oral drug bioavailability. Since the discovery of the drug efflux activity of P-gp, numerous investigations have attempted to inhibit P-gp–mediated drug efflux with the ultimate goal of increasing the efficacy of cancer chemotherapy. Initial attempts used existing compounds; however, because of undesirable pharmacologic activities or limited success, ongoing investigations are using novel agents that are more specific and potent.

Recognition that P-gp is a critical determinant of oral drug bioavailability has generated an additional application for P-gp reversal. This chapter focuses on the role of P-gp in drug absorption and disposition and the potential consequences of drug interactions between substrates and/or inhibitors of this protein. This chapter briefly discusses the salient features of this transporter; for detailed information on the biology and molecular characterization of P-gp, refer to one of the numerous excellent reviews on this protein and its gene family (1–7).

MDR GENE FAMILY

P-gps are encoded by members of a small gene family referred to as the multidrug resistance (MDR) genes. Because of alternative naming schemes that evolved from the independent laboratories that isolated each of the cDNAs, the nomenclature of the MDR genes can be confusing. Table 11-1 summarizes the common nomenclature currently used. Humans and other primates have two members of this gene family, MDR1 and MDR2 (alternatively referred to as MDR3), whereas mice, hamsters, and rats have three (mdr1a, mdr1b and mdr2) (3,4,8–10). The MDR1 gene encodes a drug transporter that is capable of conveying resistance to a large number of compounds. In rodents, two genes—the mdr1a (pgp1, mdr3) and mdr1b (pgp2, mdr1)—correspond to the human MDR1 and encode drug transporters (11–14). In contrast, the MDR2 gene encodes a phospholipid transporter, which is not involved in drug absorption or disposition and is not discussed herein (15–17).

J. A. Silverman: Department of Molecular and Cellular Biology, AvMax Inc., 385 Oysterpoint Boulevard, Building #9A, South San Francisco, California 94080

TABLE 11-1. *Multidrug resistance gene nomenclature*

Species	Drug transporters		Phospholipid translocators
Human	MDR1		MDR2, MDR3
Mouse	mdr3/mdr1a	mdr1/mdr1b	mdr2
Hamster	pgp1	pgp2	pgp3
Rat	mdr1a	mdr1b	mdr2

STRUCTURE OF P-GLYCOPROTEIN

MDR1 is a large gene spanning more than 100 kb on chromosome 7, with 28 exons that are spliced into a 4.5-kb mRNA (18–20). The encoded P-gp is an integral membrane protein with a molecular weight of approximately 170 kDa. P-gp functions as an energy-dependent membrane pump, which extrudes generally cationic or neutral, hydrophobic drugs from cells (3,4,8,9).

P-gp is a member of the large, ATP-binding cassette (ABC) transporter family. Hundreds of these traffic ATPases have been identified in bacteria, plants, fungi, and animal cells and are important in the movement of a large number of nutrients and waste products (21). ABC transporters transport virtually any class of substrate, including ions, sugars, amino acids, peptides, and polysaccharides. These membrane transporters typically have four domains: two have up to six membrane-spanning regions and two, located at the cytoplasmic surface, bind ATP and couple its hydrolysis to substrate transport. Most notably in prokaryotes, these individual domains are encoded by separate genes; however, in mammals, they are often encoded by a large single gene such as MDR1. Examples of ABC transporters include the *Escherichia coli* MalEFGK gene, which imports maltose, the *Saccharomyces cervisiae* STE6, which exports the peptide a-mating factor, and the *Plasmodium falciparum* transporter *pfmdr*, which transports chloroquine and mediates drug resistance.

Sequence analysis revealed that P-gp is made up of 1,280 amino acids with roughly bilateral symmetry; the amino and carboxy halves of the protein each have six transmembrane domains and an ATP-binding region. This structural model for P-gp has been investigated using antibody mapping, site-directed mutagenesis, and biochemical analysis. Mapping epitope domains with MRK-16, an antihuman monoclonal antibody, demonstrated that the first and fourth predicted loops are extracellular (22). Similarly, antipeptide antibodies to Glu^{393}-Lys^{408} and Leu^{1206}-Thr^{1226} recognize their epitopes in permeabilized, but not intact, cells, confirming their predicted intracellular location (23). Mapping of the topology of cysteine residues into putative intracellular or extracellular loops provided further support for the 12-transmembrane domain model (24). Rosenberg and co-workers used high-resolution electron microscopy to present a model for P-gp that is consistent with the available immunologic and biochemical analysis (25). At 2.5-nM resolution, P-gp appears to function as a monomer and have a 5-nM central pore, which is closed on the cytoplasmic surface of the plasma membrane forming an aqueous compartment. Two 3-nM intracellular lobes were observed and are consistent with the predicted 200-amino acid nucleotide binding domains. These data agree with the hypothesis that substrate binding and cross-linking agents interact at the cytoplasmic face of the membrane (26). Biochemical analysis using nickel-chelate chromatography has also suggested that P-gp functions as a monomer (27). Sonveaux and colleagues examined the secondary and tertiary structure of P-gp using attenuated total reflection Fourier transform infrared spectroscopy (28). The secondary structure of P-gp was found to contain 32% α-helix, 26% β-sheet, 29% turns, and 13% random coil; no significant alterations in these parameters occurred upon binding of verapamil, ATP, or a nonhydrolyzable ATP analogue.

FUNCTION OF P-GLYCOPROTEIN

Unlike typical ABC transporters, which have a narrow, usually single, substrate range, a defining characteristic of P-gp is its ability to transport literally hundreds of compounds. A partial list of compounds that interact with P-gp is presented in Table 11-2. Increased expression of P-gp is associated with the multidrug-resistant phenotype in which cells become cross resistant to structurally and mechanistically distinct cytotoxic drugs. Demonstration that this protein is responsible for this phenotype comes most clearly from gene transfer experiments. Transfection of high–molecular-weight DNA isolated from drug-resistant cells confers a multidrug-resistant phenotype to previously drug-sensitive cells (29,30). Similarly, transfection of either the murine *mdr1* or human MDR1 cDNAs into drug-sensitive cells also results in a 200-fold increase in resistance to daunomycin and cross resistance

TABLE 11-2. *Representative list of P-gp substrates*

Anticancer agents		Other	
Actinomycin D	Teniposide	Celiprolol	Loperimide
Colchicine	Topotecan	Cortisol	Morphine
Daunorubicin	Vinblastine	Digoxin	Nifedipine
Docetaxel	Vincristine	Diltiazem	Nelfinavir
Doxorubicin	VP-16	Erythromycin	Progesterone
Etoposide		Estrogen glucuronide	Rifampicin
Mitomycin C		Gramicidin D	Saquinavir
Mitoxantrone		Indinavir	Terfenidine
Paclitaxel		Ivermectin	

to adriamycin, colchicine, vincristine, and vinblastine (31–33). The level of drug resistance in MDR1-transfected cells correlates with the expression of P-gp (34). Thus, transfer of the cDNA-encoding P-gp is in itself sufficient to confer a drug-resistant phenotype upon drug-resistant cells.

P-GLYCOPROTEIN EXPRESSION IN NORMAL TISSUES

P-gp is found in the epithelial cells lining the luminal surface of many organs often associated with an excretory or barrier function, that is, the hepatic bile canalicular membrane, renal proximal tubule, villus-tip enterocyte in the small intestine, and the endothelial cells making up the blood–brain and blood–testes barriers. Several approaches have been used to detect MDR mRNA or P-gp in many normal tissues in humans and other species. Immunohistochemical analysis using a monoclonal antibody against the MDR1-encoded P-gp MRK-16 demonstrated expression of P-gp in the biliary canaliculus of the liver, the proximal tubules of the kidney, the apical surface of enterocytes in the intestine, the ductules of the pancreas, and the adrenals (35,36). P-gp expression was also observed in endothelial cells making up the blood–brain and blood–testes barriers (37). Examination of mRNA levels using slot blot and reverse transcriptase polymerase chain reaction (RT-PCR) analysis have confirmed this pattern of expression. A high level of mRNA expression was observed in the kidney and adrenal gland; intermediate mRNA levels in the liver, lung, jejunum, colon, and rectum; and lower mRNA levels in the brain, prostate, muscle, skin, spleen, bone marrow, stomach, ovary, and esophagus (18,38–40). P-gp expression was also found at intermediate levels in the lymphoid bone marrow cells and T cells (41–44).

ROLE OF P-GLYCOPROTEIN IN DRUG ABSORPTION AND DISPOSITION

The role of P-gp in cancer chemotherapy is well established; however, recognition of its role in drug absorption, disposition, and potential drug interactions is more recent. P-gp can affect drug levels in several ways. For example, P-gp is expressed on the biliary canalicular membrane of hepatocytes facilitating the excretion of drugs, metabolites, and xenobiotics into the bile. Similarly, because of its expression on the apical surface of intestinal villus enterocytes, P-gp is well situated to affect the absorption of substrate drugs. A role for P-gp in detoxification pathways and limiting uptake of drugs and xenobiotics has long been postulated and has recently been substantiated by experimental observations using both in vitro and in vivo model systems.

A major contribution among the many models used to investigate the role of P-gp in drug absorption and dispo-

sition was the development of knockout mice in which the mdr1a alone or both the mdr1a and mdr1b genes have been functionally disrupted by homologous recombination (45,46). Using these mice, several studies have demonstrated a clear role for P-gp in the pharmacokinetics of drugs such as vinblastine, taxol, digoxin, and several cationic compounds. Mice lacking mdr1a exhibit reduced fecal elimination of vinblastine, digoxin, taxol, tri-n-butylmethylammonium (TbuMA), and azidoprocainamide methoiodide (APM) (45,47–51). These mice also exhibit increased accumulation of drugs in the liver, brain, and gall bladder, tissues which normally express P-gp. The serum terminal half-life of intravenously administered vinblastine was longer in the knockout mice than in wild-type animals, 3.6 versus 2.1 hours, respectively, and the fecal elimination was reduced from 20% to 25% to 9%. Vinblastine also accumulated in the brain, heart, and liver of the mdr1a-deficient animals. Similarly, reduced fecal and intestinal elimination and increased tissue accumulation of digoxin was observed in these animals (48,49). Thus, P-gp contributes substantially to the elimination of substrate drugs through both hepatic and intestinal secretion.

The mdr1a knockout mice have also been used to demonstrate a clear role of P-gp in drug absorption. Increased bioavailability and altered tissue distribution was observed for paclitaxel, loperamide, vinblastine, ivermectin, cyclosporin A (CsA), human immunodeficiency virus (HIV) protease inhibitors, TBuMA, and APM (45,49–54). Marked increases in accumulation of these drugs were observed in the brain, liver, intestine, and other tissues of the knockout versus wild-type animals. Oral administration of loperamide resulted in plasma levels that were two to three times higher in mdr1a knockout mice compared to wild-type mice (53). The lethal dose to wild-type mice was approximately 80 mg/kg, whereas, in the mdr1a-deficient mice, the lethal dose was 10 mg/kg. The knockout mice had clear central opiate effects, which were absent in the wild-type mice because of the low amount of this drug that normally crosses the blood–brain barrier. Similarly, a six-fold increase in the area under the plasma concentration versus time curve (AUC) and an 11-fold increase in C_{max} for orally administered paclitaxel was observed in the mdr1a deficient mice compared to the control animals (50). Consequently, the oral bioavailability of paclitaxel increased from 11% in wild-type mice to 35% in the knockout animals. Coadministration of the P-gp inhibitors PSC 833 or CsA with paclitaxel in wild-type animals resulted in a 10-fold increase in AUC, further supporting a role for P-gp in oral drug absorption (50,52,55,56). These data also clearly demonstrate the consequences of inhibition of P-gp on the pharmacokinetics of a coadministered drug. This increase is greater than that observed in the knockout mice and is likely due to inhibition of CYP3A in the intestine and liver, suggesting a combined role of P-gp and CYP3A in limiting oral bioavailability of substrate drugs.

Kim and co-workers recently observed that P-gp also limits the oral bioavailability of the HIV protease inhibitors indinavir, nelfinavir, and saquinavir, which suggests more effective treatment of this disease may be achieved by coadministration of a P-gp inhibitor with these agents (54). Administration of these protease inhibitors to *mdr1a*-deficient mice resulted in two- to five-fold higher plasma concentrations and a seven- to 36-fold increased brain accumulation of the drugs. These authors suggest that targeted inhibition of P-gp would result in higher protease inhibitor concentrations and more effective therapy.

The Caco-2 human intestinal cell line is a well-studied model for assessing drug absorption and investigation of mechanisms that affect oral bioavailability (57–59). Hunter and co-workers used immunofluorescence with the MRK16 antibody to demonstrate apical expression of P-gp in these cells (60). Using specialized dual-chamber tissue culture dishes, these authors observed transporter-mediated, directional, and saturable secretion of vinblastine from the basolateral toward the apical side of Caco-2 monolayers (60,61). This transport was inhibited by several P-gp modulators such as verapamil, MRK16, taxotere, 1,9-dideoxyforskolin, and nifedipine. Furthermore, this inhibition led to a dose-dependent increase in vinblastine absorptive flux. Similarly, P-gp mediated time and concentration dependent polarized efflux of CsA was observed in Caco-2 cells and was suggested to be a key physiologic determinant of CsA oral bioavailability (62). These data provided early support for the hypothesis that P-gp, located at the tip of the intestinal villus, is a barrier for drug absorption.

Intestinal absorption of β-adrenoreceptor antagonists (β-blockers) is variable and has been shown to be somewhat dependent on lipophilicity. Absorption of one such β-blocker, celiprolol, increases at high doses and is nonlinear in humans. Studies with Caco-2 cells show that celiprolol is actively and saturably effluxed but passively and nonsaturably absorbed, suggesting the involvement of an active transport mechanism (63). Celiprolol basolateral to apical (secretory) transport was inhibited by the P-gp substrate vinblastine as well as the P-gp reversal agents verapamil and quinidine. These data suggest that this transporter is involved in celiprolol absorption. Similarly, basolateral to apical transport of acebutolol is twofold greater than in the reverse direction (64). Intestinal absorption of acebutolol is increased 2.6-fold in the presence of CsA. Combined, these data as well as numerous additional investigations clearly demonstrate that P-gp is one factor important in determining drug absorption and elimination.

Recent studies have demonstrated that interaction between intestinal drug metabolism by cytochrome P450 3A and P-gp–mediated transport may contribute to the poor oral bioavailability and high interpatient and intrapatient variability in absorption of drugs (65,66). The liver has been classically viewed as the primary site of drug metabolism; recently, however, it has been recognized that a significant amount of drug metabolism occurs in the intestine and is mediated by CYP3A (67). Although the intestine does not quantitatively have as much CYP3A as the liver, the enzyme is located in the differentiated villus cells, which are the site of drug absorption. Greater than 50% of clinically important drugs are metabolized by CYP3A; thus, its location in the intestine suggests a critical role for it in oral drug bioavailability (66). Recently, a striking overlap between the substrates for P-gp and cytochrome P450 3A family members has been observed (65,68). Simultaneous expression of these proteins in the intestine suggests complementary roles that may limit drug absorption and increase disposition. Another potential function for P-gp in the intestine may be to transport compounds back into the lumen. This would establish a cyclic pathway for drugs as they transit the intestine, thereby increasing the exposure time of drugs to drug-metabolizing enzymes (e.g., CYP3A) to act. The cooperative nature of CYP3A and P-gp presents a unique opportunity to affect substrate absorption and a significant potential for drug interactions.

DRUG INTERACTIONS WITH P-GLYCOPROTEIN

A significant effort has been made to identify compounds that regulate the ability of P-gp to transport substrates (69,70). In effect, these investigations seek a directed drug interaction by using one agent to modify the response to a second drug through an effect on P-gp–mediated efflux. In cancer chemotherapy, these agents are used to increase the therapeutic effectiveness of cytotoxic anticancer drugs. More recently, P-gp reversal agents have been demonstrated to alter the pharmacokinetic properties of coadministered agents in therapeutic areas other than oncology (66,71).

Many of the initial compounds used to modify or reverse multidrug resistance including calcium channel blockers (verapamil, nifedipine), immunosuppresives (CsA, FK506) and antiarhythmic drugs (quinidine and amiodarone) (Table 11-3) were originally developed for alternative therapeutic reasons. The calcium channel blocker verapamil was one of the first compounds observed to be a P-gp reversal agent by its ability to increase the sensitivity of murine leukemia cells to vinblastine (72). Subsequently, many of these "first generation" reversal agents have been identified and some have progressed into human clinical trials (69,70,73,74). The mechanisms by which these compounds inhibit P-gp are diverse; in some cases, the inhibitor, such as CsA, is itself a substrate and, therefore, its activity may, in part, be due to competitive inhibition. The mechanisms of other rever-

TABLE 11-3. *Representative list of MDR reversal agents*

First generation	Second generation
Amiodarone	BIBW22
Cremophor EL	GG918 (GF120918)
Cyclosporin A	LY335979
FK506	PAK200
Trans-flupenthixol	PSC 833
Genistein	SDZ-280-446
Ketoconozole	VX-710
Progesterone	
Quercetin	
Quinidine	
Rapamycin	
Reserpine	
Staurosporine	
Tamoxifen	
TPGS	
Trifluoroperizine	
Verapamil	

sal agents remain unknown. Competition with photoaffinity-labeling agents suggests that some reversal agents share the same binding site as substrates (75,76). The affinity of these first generation reversal agents is low; thus, their clinical effectiveness is often limited by their pharmacologic activity. Dose-limiting toxicity of verapamil and CsA have each been observed (73,74). For example, the use of CsA as a reversal agent is limited by myelosuppression, hyperbilirubinemia, headache, hypomagnesemia, and mild hypertension (73).

Newer, "second generation" P-gp modulators have been and continue to be developed which specifically inhibit P-gp with high affinity and without undesired pharmacologic activities. One of these second generation P-gp reversal agents, GF120918, (also known as GG918) was discovered from a program aimed at identifying novel inhibitors of P-gp (77). In drug-resistant cell lines, 0.01 to 0.1 μM GF120918 blocks drug efflux and results in greater than 40-fold sensitization to drugs such as daunorubicin and mitoxantrone (77,78). At concentrations of 0.05 to 0.01 μM, GF120918 increased the sensitivity of drug-resistant MCF7/ADR cells to vincristine and competed with photoaffinity-labeling of P-gp (77). Thus, GF120918 is clearly effective at increasing the sensitivity of P-gp–expressing cell lines to cytotoxic drugs. Furthermore, coadministration of GF120918 with doxorubicin in isolated perfused rat liver also significantly decreases biliary excretion (79). Doxorubicin is primarily excreted by the liver; thus, altered hepatic function could significantly affect the pharmacokinetics of this drug. Inhibition of doxorubicin clearance by GF120918 in isolated livers clearly demonstrated that inhibition of P-gp significantly affects clearance of substrate such as doxorubicin and more generally suggests that this may be a source of drug interactions with other P-gp inhibitors and substrates (79).

PSC 833, a novel nonimmunosupressive cyclosporin D, is a potent and promising novel P-gp inhibitor (80,81). PSC 833 is an effective reversal agent *in vitro* at concentrations as low as 0.1 μM, more than ten-fold lower than CsA, making it a potent P-gp modulator (80–83). PSC 833 reduces intracellular accumulation of doxorubicin and vincristine in myelogenous leukemia cells three- to ten-fold more potently than CsA or verapamil, and it significantly enhances the lifespan of mice bearing adriamycin-resistant P388 tumors when coadministered with vinca alkaloids or doxorubicin. van Asperen and coworkers coadministered PSC 833 with paclitaxel in wildtype mice to clearly demonstrate inhibition of intestinal P-gp, which resulted in a 16-fold increase in serum paclitaxel AUC (56). Similarly, Mayer and colleagues observed that orally administered PSC 833 increased blood–brain penetration of digoxin (84). Early clinical data with this compound showed that it has a substantial effect on the pharmacokinetics of etoposide and paclitaxel; however, there is also a temporary ataxia associated with this treatment (85). Additional human trials are currently being undertaken to further determine the clinical value of this agent and P-gp modulation in cancer therapy.

The quest for novel, potent and specific P-gp reversal agents is ongoing and an important avenue of cancer research. For example, a recently described class of compounds suggested to be effective P-gp reversal agents are the ardeemins (86). Two hexacyclic indole alkaloids, 5-*N*-acetylardeemin and 5-*N*-acetyl-8-demethylardeemin enhance the cytotoxicity of doxorubicin and vinblastine *in vitro* and sensitize doxorubicin-resistant P388 tumors transplanted in mice. Low toxicity of these compounds suggest that they may be useful as P-gp–modulating agents in cancer chemotherapy. Similarly, 1,3-bis(9-oxo-acridin-10yl)propane (PBA) was recently observed to be a novel and potent modulator of P-gp. At 1 μM, PBA increased the accumulation of vinblastine approximately nine-fold in P-gp–expressing cells (87).

The cardiac glycoside digoxin is used to treat congestive heart failure. Its use, however, is problematic because of its narrow therapeutic index and interactions with many other drugs such as quinidine, amiodarone, and verapamil (88). Su and Huang recently observed that P-gp is involved in the absorption and elimination of digoxin in the intestine (89). Concomitant intravenous administration of digoxin with quinidine resulted in a doubling of plasma concentrations and a 40% decrease of digoxin in the intestine, which likely reflects decreased hepatic and renal clearance as well as an effect on intestinal secretion. The contribution of the intestine was further examined using everted intestinal sacs, which established that inhibitors of P-gp such as quinidine and the C219 antibody blocked the directional flux of digoxin. Cavet and co-workers also observed P-gp–mediated transport of digoxin in the Caco-2 intestinal epithelial cell line, further suggesting that the intestine is important in digoxin elimination (90). Mayer and colleagues observed that the intestine contributes significantly to elimination and to reuptake of biliary excreted digoxin (48). In *mdr1a*-deficient mice, a dramatic shift from fecal to urinary digoxin excretion occurred with both intravenous and orally administered drug. Intestinal excretion by P-gp accounted for approximately 16% of an intravenous dose within 90 minutes in the wild-type mouse, whereas, in the *mdr1a* knockout mouse, intestinal excretion was only 2%. Biliary excretion of digoxin was unchanged in the *mdr1a*-deficient mice, suggesting alternate transporters are also important for digoxin excretion in the liver. Combined, these data strongly suggest that P-gp is critical to the pharmacokinetics of digoxin and provide some insight into drug interactions that occur clinically.

A novel renal tubular cell model has recently been developed to investigate digoxin-drug interactions. Woodland and co-workers used this model to demonstrate interactions with drugs that have been established to have clinical interactions with digoxin, such as verapamil, CsA, quinidine, and vinca alkaloids (91). These drugs are all P-gp substrates or inhibitors. This model also detected a digoxin–itraconazole interaction. Itraconazole has only recently been identified as a P-gp substrate. In a small human trial, coadministration of itraconazole with digoxin resulted in a 50% increase in digoxin AUC and a 20% decrease in renal clearance (92). Similarly, Wakasugi and colleagues observed that clarithromycin inhibits P-gp–mediated digoxin transport *in vitro* (93). These authors also demonstrated decreased renal clearance of digoxin in two patients when coadministered with clarithromycin.

Numerous clinical drug interactions have been observed with digoxin, including quinidine, verapamil, CsA, amiodarone, diltiazem, and nifedipine (88). Each of these compounds has been observed to decrease digoxin clearance and cause increased blood levels. Interestingly these drugs are also substrates or inhibitors of P-gp. In light of the data discussed earlier, it is likely that inhibition of P-gp is, in part, responsible for the changes in digoxin pharmacokinetics, which occur with many drugs.

The recent development of HIV protease inhibitors has introduced a new and effective treatment for HIV-infected patients. Their use has produced dramatic reduction in viral load in plasma and tissues of HIV-infected patients; however, their long-term efficacy is unknown. Many of the currently available protease inhibitors have low oral absorption and poor tissue penetration, which may limit their efficacy. Recently, it has been observed that interaction with P-gp and drug-metabolizing enzymes are mechanisms that potentially determine their oral bioavailability (54,94–96). Cell-based assays have shown that ritonavir, saquinavir, and indinavir inhibit the transport of established P-gp substrates such as rhodamine 123 and bodipy-vinblastine as well as inhibit photoaffinity-labeling of P-gp with iodoarylazidoprazosin

(94,95). Specific directional transport of these drugs in P-gp–expressing epithelial cells in monolayer culture further established that protease inhibitors are substrates for this transporter. In mice, oral administration of indinavir, nelfinavir, and saquinavir to *mdr1a*-deficient animals resulted in plasma concentrations that were two to five times higher than in wild-type mice. The knockout animals also accumulated significantly higher amounts of these drugs in their brain tissue four hours following an intravenous dose. These data suggest that P-gp is important in limiting the oral bioavailability and tissue distribution of these compounds (54,94,95). Furthermore, higher doses of protease inhibitors are required to diminish reverse transcriptase activity in P-gp–expressing cells than in parental cells (95). In fact, the same extent of inhibition of reverse transcriptase activity was never achieved in the P-gp expressing cells. Furthermore, P-gp reversal agents such as quinidine, rapamycin, and PSC 833 increased the ability of the protease inhibitors to inhibit reverse transcriptase activity. Combined, these data suggest that the HIV protease inhibitors are substrates for P-gp and that this protein may limit their absorption and tissue distribution. The presence of P-gp in the intestine, the target T cells, and the blood–brain barrier may therefore reduce the effectiveness of these compounds. Coadministration of a P-gp inhibitor with these drugs may increase their oral bioavailability as well as increase their distribution into other tissues.

In studies on the pharmacokinetics of K02, a novel cysteine protease inhibitor, Zhang and associates observed the effect of ketoconazole on oral bioavailability (97). Ketoconazole has previously been described to be a P-gp reversal agent in drug-resistant cells (98). Coadministration of ketoconazole orally with KO2 increased the K02 AUC more than ten-fold and decreased plasma clearance to a similar extent. These data confirm that oral bioavailability of a P-gp substrate may be dramatically altered by coadministration of a P-gp reversal agent. Ketoconazole is also a potent inhibitor of cytochrome P450 3A; thus, the increased absorption of K02 in these experiments may additionally be due to inhibition of its metabolism in the intestine (97).

Ivermectin is the preferred drug for the control and treatment of a broad spectrum of parasitic nematode, arthropod infections of both animals and humans. It has proven to be extremely effective in the treatment of onchocerciasis, the filarial infection responsible for river blindness. Because of its low toxicity and interactions with P-gp, Pouliot and co-workers recently proposed that ivermectin is a suitable reversal agent (99). In drug-resistant cells, ivermectin modulates cytotoxicity to vinblastine and doxorubicin four- to nine-fold more potently than verapamil or CsA, respectively. Additionally, [³H] ivermectin is transported by P-gp *in vitro*. Schinkel and associates previously established increased absorption and tissue accumulation of ivermectin in *mdr1a* knockout mice versus control animals (45). Exposure of *mdr1a*-deficient mice to ivermectin results in significantly higher tissue and plasma levels compared to wild-type animals. Moreover, this compound is toxic in the knockout mice at doses that are innocuous to heterozygous and wild-type mice. These experiments also suggested a role for P-gp in the blood–brain barrier in that ivermectin accumulates in the brain of the *mdr1a*-deficient animals but not animals with an intact *mdr1a* gene. The knockout mice displayed systemic ivermectin toxicity at doses 50- to 100-fold less than wild-type mice. Death was due to central nervous system toxicity, which also occurred in wild-type animals, albeit at much higher doses. Clearly, P-gp plays a central role in the pharmacokinetics of this drug and changes in the activity of the transporter can dramatically alter its pharmacologic activity. Although not as effective as PSC 833 in reversing drug resistance, because of its low relatively toxicity, ivermectin may be an effective P-gp reversal agent (99).

P-gp may also have a role in steroid transport. Ueda and colleagues demonstrated specificity of P-gp–mediated transport for steroid hormones (100). P-gp transported cortisol, aldosterone, and dexamethasone but not progesterone. Progesterone does, however, interact with P-gp to reduce vinblastine binding (12,101). Recently, in a study on the absorption of steroid hormones, Saitoh and co-workers observed that P-gp likely limits the uptake of methylprednisolone but not prednisolone or hydrocortisone (102). An isolated intestinal loop technique was used to demonstrate that, in the presence of verapamil, quinidine, quinine, and methylpredisolone absorption increased 30% to 80% over that of control animals, suggesting a role for P-gp in limiting its absorption. In a study using multidrug-resistant MCF-7/ADR cells, Desai and associates observed that tamoxifen significantly enhanced the cytotoxicity of mitoxantrone (103). The effect was additive in the parental cells but synergistic in the P-gp–expressing subclone. Tamoxifen also increased mitoxantrone accumulation in the MCF-7 ADR cells relative to the parental cells. These data suggest that the combination of tamoxifen and mitoxantrone may be effective in treatment of P-gp–expressing tumors.

Despite the preponderance of evidence from *in vitro* and preclinical models, the true clinical importance of modulation of P-gp in cancer chemotherapy is still unclear. The ability of P-gp modulators to affect the pharmacokinetics of clinically used anticancer drugs is clearly demonstrated in a phase I trial in which CsA was coadministered with etoposide. Sixteen patients were administered 20 paired courses of etoposide or etoposide plus CsA (73,104). High CsA resulted in increased etoposide AUC, decreased total and renal clearance, and a two-fold increase in half-life. These data are consistent with inhibition of P-gp in tissues such as the kidney and liver, which are associated with etoposide disposition. An increased volume of distribution of etoposide in the

patients also given CsA further suggests inhibition of P-gp in additional organs. Because of the increased exposure to etoposide in the presence of CsA, Lum and colleagues advocated a 50% dose reduction of etoposide in patients receiving a P-gp modulator. Data from additional clinical trials with P-gp modulators have similarly demonstrated altered pharmacokinetic behavior of anticancer drugs such as doxorubicin, mitoxantrone, paclitaxel, and vinblastine (reviewed in (73,105). It is less clear, however, whether modulation of P-gp provides any advantage in improving the therapeutic index or efficacy beyond simple dose escalation (105). There are no data suggesting that P-gp function in tumors would be targeted by a reversal agent; thus, any pharmacokinetic alterations caused by P-gp reversal would likely affect normal as well as neoplastic tissues. Thus, the pharmacologic consequences of inhibition of P-gp in normal tissues (e.g., liver, blood–brain barrier, and intestine) must be considered. It is possible that increased toxicity of anticancer agents in sites other than the target tumor would occur.

Inhibition of P-gp in the endothelial cells at the blood–brain barrier may provide central nervous system access to many previously excluded drugs. Inhibition in the liver, kidney, and intestine may prolong drug clearance by lowering excretion. Another consequence of inhibition in those organs is altered bioavailability through increased drug absorption. Coadministration of a suboptimal dose of doxorubicin with CsA enhanced the effectiveness of doxorubicin chemotherapy to levels equivalent to a 25% higher dose (106). These authors, however, later suggested that addition of a reversal agent (e.g., CsA) significantly enhanced the toxic side effects equivalent to increasing the dose of the anticancer drug (107). New trials with controlled, crossover design using better P-gp modulators will provide further data to confirm or refute the role of P-gp reversal agents as a mechanism of enhancing cancer chemotherapy.

SUMMARY

P-gp is an important drug transporter located in the liver, intestine, kidney, blood–brain barrier, and other barrier epithelial tissues. P-gp was initially isolated and investigated for its role in multidrug resistance in tumors; however, it is increasingly evident that this protein also has a pivotal role in the pharmacokinetics of numerous drugs with many therapeutic indications. Investigations using *in vitro* and *in vivo* model systems have established that P-gp invluences the absorption and excretion of drugs such as vinblastine, taxol, etoposide, ivermectin, CsA, steroids, and digoxin. The very large and diverse number of compounds that interact with P-gp suggests that the potential for drug interactions to occur is significant. Clearly, inhibition of P-gp alters the pharmacokinetics of substrates in preclinical models. A review of known clinical drug-interactions involving established P-gp substrates and inhibitors is informative and, in some cases, suggests a mechanism for these interactions. With this knowledge, the molecular basis of these interactions can be specifically investigated. The therapeutic impact and clinical significance of these interactions, however, remain to be determined and is the focus of many ongoing human trials. It is likely that P-gp as well as additional drug transporters will have a significant role in interactions between substrate drugs.

REFERENCES

1. Sharom FJ. The P-glycoprotein efflux pump: how does it transport drugs. *J Membrane Biol* 1997;160:161–175.
2. Germann UA. P-glycoprotein—a mediator of multidrug resistance in tumour cells. *Eur J Cancer* 1996;32A:927–944.
3. Gottesman MM, Pastan I. Biochemistry of multidrug resistance mediated by the multidrug transporter. *Annu Rev Biochem* 1993;62:385–427.
4. Chin K-V, Pastan I, Gottesman MM. Function and regulation of the human multidrug resistance gene. *Adv Cancer Res* 1993;60:157–180.
5. Arceci RJ. Clinical significance of P-glycoprotein in multidrug resistance malignancies. *Blood* 1993;81:2215–2222.
6. Juranka PF, Zastawny RL, Ling V. P-glycoprotein: multidrug-resistance and a superfamily of membrane-associated transport proteins. *FASEB J* 1989;3:2583–2592.
7. van der Bliek AM, Borst P. Multidrug resistance. *Adv Cancer Res* 1989;52:165–203.
8. Endicott JA, Ling V. The biochemistry of P-glycoprotein mediated multidrug resistance. *Annu Rev Biochem* 1989;58:137–171.
9. Borst P, Schinkel AH, Smit JJM, et al. Classical and novel forms of multidrug resistance and the physiological functions of P-glycoproteins in mammals. *Pharmacol Ther* 1993;60:289–299.
10. Thorgeirsson SS, Silverman JA, Gant TW, Marino PA. Multidrug resistance gene family and chemical carcinogens. *Pharmacol Ther* 1991;49:283–292.
11. Hsu SI, Lothenstein L, Horwitz SB. Differential overexpression of three *mdr* gene family members in multidrug resistant J774.2 mouse cells. *J Biol Chem* 1989;264:12053–12062.
12. Yang C-PH, Cohen D, Greenberger LM, Hsu SI-H, Horwitz SB. Differential transport properties of two *mdr* gene products are distiguished by progesterone. *J Biol Chem* 1990;265:10282–10288.
13. Devault A, Gros P. Two members of the mouse *mdr* gene family confer multidrug resistance with overlapping but distinct drug specificities. *Mol Cell Biol* 1990;10:1652–1663.
14. Santoni-Rugiu E, Silverman JA. Functional characterization of the rat *mdr1b* encoded P-glycoprotein: not all inducing agents are substrates. *Carcinogenesis* 1997;18:2255–2263.
15. Smit JJM, Schinkel AH, Oude Elferink RPJ, et al. Homozygous disruption of the murine *mdr2* P-glycoprotein gene leads to a complete absence of phospholipid from bile and to liver disease. *Cell* 1993;75:451–462
16. Smith AJ, Timmermans-Hereijgers JLPM, Roelofsen B, et al. The human MDR3 P-glycoprotein promotes translocation of phosphotidylcholine through the plasma membrane of fibroblasts from transgenic mice. *FEBS Lett* 1994;354:263–266.
17. Ruetz S, Gros P. Phosphotidylcholine translocase: a physiological role for the *mdr2* gene. *Cell* 1994;77:1071–1081.
18. Chin JE, Soffir R, Noonan KE, Choi K, Roninson IB. Structure and expression of the human *MDR* (P-glycoprotein) gene family. *Mol Cell Biol* 1989;9:3808–3820.
19. Chen C-jie, Clark D, Ueda K, Pastan I, Gottesman MM, Roninson IB. Genomic organization of the human multidrug resistance (*MDR1*) gene and origin of P-glycoproteins. *J Biol Chem* 1990;265:506–514.
20. Fojo A, Lebo R, Shimizu N, et al. Localization of multidrug resistance-associated DNA sequences to human chromosome 7. *Somat Cell Mol Gen* 1986;12:415–420.
21. Higgins CF. ABC transporters: from microorganisms to man. *Annu Rev Cell Biol* 1992;8:67–113.
22. Georges E, Tsuruo T, Ling V. Topology of P-glycoprotein as determined by epitope mapping of MRK-16 monoclonal antibody. J Biol Chem 1993;268:1792–1798.
23. Yoshimura A, Kuwazuru Y, Sumizawa T, et al. Cytoplasmic orientation and two-domain structure of the multidrug transporter, P-glycoprotein, demonstrated with sequence-specific antibodies. *J Biol Chem* 1989;264:16282–16291.
24. Loo TW, Clarke DM. Membrane topology of a cysteine-less mutant of human P-glycoprotein. *J Biol Chem* 1995;270:843–848.
25. Rosenberg MF, Callaghan R, Ford RC, Higgins CF. Structure of the multidrug resistance P-glycoprotein to 2.5 nm resolution determined by electron microscopy and image analysis. *J Biol Chem* 1997;272:10685–10694.
26. Greenberger LM. Major photoaffinity drug labeling sites for iodaryl azidoprazosin in P-glycoprotein are within or immediately C-terminal to transmembrane domains 6 and 12. *J Biol Chem* 1993;268:11417–11425.
27. Loo TW, Clarke DM. The minimum functional unit of human P-glycoprotein appears to be a monomer. *J Biol Chem* 1996;271:27488–27492.
28. Sonveaux N, Shapiro AB, Goormaghtight E, Ling V, Ruysschaert J-M. Secondary and tertiary changes of reconstituted P-glycoprotein. *J Biol Chem* 1996;271:24617–24624.
29. Gros P, Fallows DA, Croop JM, Housman DE. Chromosome-mediated gene transfer of multidrug resistance. *Mol Cell Biol* 1986;6:3785–3790.
30. Roninson IB, Chin JE, Choi K, et al. Isolation of human mdr DNA sequences amplified in multidrug resistant KB carcinoma cells. *Proc Natl Acad Sci USA* 1986;83:4538–4542.
31. Gros P, Ben-Neriah Y, Croop JM, Housman DE. Isolation and expression of a complementary DNA that confers multidrug resistance. *Nature* 1986;323:728–731.
32. Hammond JR, Johnstone RM, Gros P. Enhanced efflux of 3-H-vinblastine from Chinese hamster ovary cells transfected with full length complementary DNA clone for the MDR1 gene. *Cancer Res* 1989;49:3867–3871.
33. Ueda K, Cardarelli C, Gottesman MM, Pastan I. Expression of a full length cDNA for the human "MDR1" gene confers resistance to colchicine, doxorubicin and vinblastine. *Proc Natl Acad Sci USA* 1987;84:3004–3008.
34. Choi K, Frommel THO, Stern RK, et al. Multidrug resistance after retroviral transfer of the human MDR1 gene correlates with P-glycoprotein density in the plasma membrane and is not affected by cytotoxic selection. *Proc Natl Acad Sci USA* 1991;88:7386–7390.
35. Thiebaut F, Tsuruo T, Hamada H, Gottesman MM, Pastan I, Willingham MC. Cellular localization of the multidrug resistance gene product P-glycoprotein in normal human tissues. *Proc Natl Acad Sci USA* 1987;84:7735–7738.
36. Thiebaut F, Tsuruo T, Hamada H, Gottesman MM, Pastan I, Willingham MC. Immunohistochemical localization in normal tissues of different epitopes in the multidrug transport protein P170: evidence for localization in brain capillaries and crossreactivity on one antibody with a muscle protein. *J Histochem Cytochem* 1989;37:159–164.
37. Cordon-Cardo C, O'Brien JP, Casals D, et al. Multidrug-resistance gene (P-glycoprotein) is expressed by endothelial cells at blood-brain barrier sites. *Proc Natl Acad Sci USA* 1989;86:695–698.
38. Fojo AT, Ueda K, Slamon DJ, Poplack DG, Gottesman MM, Pastan I. Expression of a multidrug-resistance gene in human tumors and tissues. *Proc Natl Acad Sci USA* 1987;84:265–269.
39. Bremer S, Hoof T, Wilke M, et al. Quantitative expression patterns of multidrug-resistance P-glycoprotein (MDR1) and differentially spliced cystic-fibrosis transmembrane-conductance regulator mRNA transcripts in human epithelia. *Eur J Biochem* 1992;206:137–149.
40. Croop JM, Raymond M, Haber D, et al. The three mouse multidrug resistance (*mdr*) genes are expressed in a tissue-specific manner in normal mouse tissues. *Mol Cell Biol* 1989;9:1345–1350.
41. Gupta S, Kim CH, Tsuruo T, Gollapudi S. Preferential expression and activity of multidrug resistance gene 1 product (P-glycoprotein), a functionally active efflux pump, in human CD8+ T cells: a role in cytotoxic effector function. *J Clin Immunol* 1992;12:451–458.
42. Gupta S, Gollapudi S. P-glycoprotein (MDR1 gene product) in cells of the immune system: Its possible physiologic role and alteration in aging and human immunodeficiency virus-1 (HIV-1) infection. *J Clin Immunol* 1993;13:289–301.
43. Chaudhary PM, Roninson IB. Expression and activity of P-glycopro-

tein, a multidrug efflux pump, in human and hematopoietic stem cells. *Cell* 1991;66:85–94.

44. Chaudhary PM, Metchener EB, Roninson IB. Expression and activity of the multidrug resistance P-glycoprotein in human peripheral blood lymphocytes. *Blood* 1992;80:2735–2739.

45. Schinkel AH, Smit JJM, van Tellingen O, et al. Disruption of the mouse *mdr1a* P-glycoprotein gene leads to a deficiency in the blood-brain barrier and to increased sensitivity to drugs. *Cell* 1994;77: 491–502.

46. Schinkel AH, Mayer U, Wagenaar E, et al. Normal viability and altered pharmacokinetics in mice lacking mdr1-type (drug transporting) P-glycoproteins. *Proc Natl Acad Sci USA* 1997;94:4028–4033.

47. van Asperen J, Schinkel AH, Beijnen JH, Nooijen WJ, Borst P, van Tellingen O. Altered pharmacokinetics of vinblastine in mdr1a P-glycoprotein-deficient mice. *J Natl Cancer Inst* 1996;88:994–999.

48. Mayer U, Wagenaar E, Beijnen JH, et al. Substantial excretion of digoxin via the intestinal mucosa and prevention of long-term digoxin accumulation in the brain by the mdr1a P-glycoprotein. *Br J Pharmacol* 1996;119:1038–1044.

49. Schinkel AH, Wagenaar E, van Deemter L, Mol CAAM, Borst P. Absence of the mdr1a P-glycoprotein in mice affects tissue distribution and pharmacokinetics of dexamethasone, digoxin and cyclosporine A. *J Clin Invest* 1995;96:1698–1705.

50. Sparreboom A, van Asperen J, Mayer U, et al. Limited oral bioavailability and active epithelial excretion of paclitaxel (Taxol) caused by P-glycoprotein in the intestine. *Proc Natl Acad Sci USA* 1997;94: 2031–2035.

51. Smit JW, Schinkel AH, Müller M, Weert B, Meijer DKF. Contribution of the murine mdr1a P-glycoprotein to hepatobiliary and intestinal elimination of cationic drugs as measured in mice with an *mdr1a* gene disruption. *Hepatology* 1998;27:1056–1063.

52. van Asperen J, van Tellingen O, Beijnen JH. The pharmacological role of P-glycoprotein in the intestinal epithelium. *Pharm Res* 1998;37: 429–435.

53. Schinkel AH, Wagenaar E, Mol CAAM, van Deemter L. P-glycoprotein in the blood-brain barrier of mice influences the brain penetration and pharmacological activity of many drugs. *J Clin Invest* 1996;97: 2517–2524.

54. Kim RB, Fromm MF, Wandel C, et al. The drug transporter P-glycoprotein limits oral absorption and brain entry of HIV-1 protease inhibitors. *J Clin Invest* 1998;101:289–294.

55. van Asperen J, van Tellingen O, Sparreboom A, et al. Enhanced oral bioavailability of paclitaxel in mice treated with the P-glycoprotein blocker SDZ PSC 833. *Br J Cancer* 1997;76:1181–1183.

56. van Asperen J, van Tellingen O, Sparreboom A, et al. Enhanced oral bioavailability of paclitaxel in mice treated with the P-glycoprotein blockers SDZ PSC 833 or cyclosporin A. *Proc Am Assoc Cancer Res* 1997;38:5.

57. Artursson P. Epithelial transport of drugs in cell culture. I: A model for studying the passive diffusion of drugs over intestinal absorbtive (Caco-2) cells. *J Pharm Sci* 1990;79:476–482.

58. Artursson P, Karlsson J. Correlation between oral drug absorption in humans and apparent drug permeability coefficients in human intestinal epithelial (Caco-2) cells. *Biochem Biophys Res Commun* 1991; 175:880–885.

59. Nerurkar MM, Burton PS, Borchardt RT. The use of surfactants to enhance the permeability of peptides through Caco-2 cells by inhibition of an apically polarized efflux system. *Pharm Res* 1996;13:528–534.

60. Hunter J, Jepson MA, Tsuruo T, Simmons NL, Hirst BH. Functional expression of P-glycoprotein in apical membranes of human intestinal Caco-2 cells. *J Biol Chem* 1993;268:14991–14997.

61. Hunter J, Hirst BH, Simmons NL. Drug absorption limited by P-glycoprotein-mediated secretory drug transport in human intestinal epithelial Caco-2 cell layers. *Pharm Res* 1993;10:743–749.

62. Augustijns PF, Bradshaw TP, Gan L-SL, Hendren RW, Thakker DR. Evidence for a polarized efflux system in Caco-2 cells capable of modulating cyclosporin A transport. *Biochem Biophys Res Commun* 1993;197:360–365.

63. Karlsson J, Kuo S-M, Ziemniak J, Artursson P. Transport of celiprolol across human intestinal epithelial (Caco-2) cells: mediation of secretion by multiple transporters including P-glycoprotein. *Br J Pharmacol* 1993;110:1009–1016.

64. Terao T, Hisanaga E, Sai Y, Tamai I, Tsuhi A. Active secretion of drugs from the small intestinal epithelium in rats by P-glycoprotein functioning as an absorption barrier. *J Pharm Pharmacol* 1996;48:1083–1089.

65. Wacher VJ, Wu C-Y, Benet LZ. Overlapping substrate specificities and tissue distribution of cytochrome P450 3A and P-glycoprotein: implications for drug delivery and activity in cancer chemotherapy. *Mol Carcinog* 1995;13:129–134.

66. Wacher VJ, Salphati L, Benet LZ. Active secretion and enterocytic drug metabolism barriers to drug absorption. *Adv Drug Del Rev* 1996; 20:99–112.

67. Watkins PB. Drug metabolism by cytochromes P450 in the liver and small bowel. *Gastrointest Pharmacol* 1992;21:511–526.

68. Schuetz EG, Beck WT, Schuetz JD. Modulators and substrates of P-glycoprotein and cytochrome p4503A coordinately up-regulate these proteins in human colon carcinoma cells. *Mol Pharmacol* 1996;49: 311–318.

69. Ford JM. Experimental reversal of P-glycoprotein-mediated multidrug resistance by pharmacological chemosensitizers. *Eur J Cancer* 1996; 32A:991–1001.

70. Ford JM, Hait WN. Pharmacology of drugs that alter multidrug resistance in cancer. *Pharmacol Rev* 1990;42:155–199.

71. Wacher VJ, Silverman JA, Zhang Y, Benet LZ. Role of P-glycoprotein and cytochrome P450 3A in limiting oral absorption of peptides and peptidomimetics. *J Pharm Sci* 1998;87:1322–1330.

72. Tsuruo T, Iida H, Tsukagoshi S, Sakurai Y. Overcoming of vincristine resistance in P388 leukemia *in vivo* and *in vitro* through enhanced cytotoxicity of vincristine and vinblastine by verapamil. *Cancer Res* 1981;41:1967–1972.

73. Lum BL, Gisher GA, Brophy NA, et al. Clincal trials of modulation of multidrug resistance. *Cancer Supplement* 1993;72:3502–3514.

74. Ferry DR, Traunecker H, Kerr DJ. Clinical trials of P-glycoprotein reversal in solid tumours. *Eur J Cancer* 1996;32A:1070–1081.

75. Akiyama S-I, Cornwell MM, Kuwano M, Pastan I, Gottesman MM. Most drugs that reverse multidrug resistance also inhibit photoaffinity labeling of P-glycoprotein by a vinblastine analog. *Mol Pharmacol* 1988;33:144–147.

76. Beck WT, Qian X-dong. Photoaffinity substrates for P-glycoprotein. *Biochem Pharmacol* 1992;43:89–93.

77. Hyafil F, Vergely C, Du Vignaud P, Grand-Perret T. In vitro and in vivo reversal of multidrug resistance by GF120918, an acridonecarboxamide derivative. *Cancer Res* 1993;53:4595–4602.

78. Zhou DC, Simonin G, Faussat AM, Zittoun R, Marie JP. Effect of the multidrug inhibitor GG918 on drug sensitivity of human leukemic cells. *Leukemia* 1997;11:1516–1522.

79. Booth CL, Brouwer KR, Brouwer KLR. Effect of multidrug resistance modulators on the hepatobiliary disposition of doxorubicin in the isolated perfused rat liver. *Cancer Res* 1998;58:3641–3648.

80. Jachez B, Nordmann R, Loor F. Restoration of taxol sensitivity of multidrug-resistant cells by the cyclosporine SDZ PSC 833 and the cyclopeptide SDZ 280–446. *J Natl Cancer Inst* 1993;85:478–483.

81. Keller RP, Altermatt HJ, Nooter K, et al. SDZ PSC833, a non-immunosuppressive cyclosporine: its potency in overcoming P-glycoprotein-mediated multidrug resistance of murine leukemia. *Int J Cancer* 1992;50:593–597.

82. Boesch D, Gaveriaux C, Jachez B, Pourtier-Manzanedo A, Bollinger P, Loor F. *In vivo* circumvention of P-glycoprotein-mediated multidrug resistance of tumor cells with SDZ PSC 833. *Cancer Res* 1991; 51:4226–4233.

83. Twentyman PR. Cyclosporins as drug resistance modifiers. *Biochem Pharmacol* 1992;43:109–117.

84. Mayer U, Wagenaar E, Dorobek B, Beijnen JH, Borst P, Schinkel AH. Full blockade of intestinal P-glycoprotein and extensive inhibition of blood-brain barrier P-glycoprotein by oral treatment of mice with PSC833. *J Clin Invest* 1997;100:2430–2436.

85. Fisher GA, Lum BL, Hausdorff J, Sikic BI. Pharmacological considerations in the modulation of multidrug resistance. *Eur J Cancer* 1996; 32A:1082–1088.

86. Chou T-C, Depew KM, Zheng Y-H, et al. Reversal of anticancer multidrug resistance by the ardeemins *Proc Natl Acad Sci USA* 1998;95: 8369–8374.

87. Horton J, Thimmaiah KN, Altenberg GA, et al. Characterization of a novel bisacridone and comparison with PSC833 as a potent and poorly reversible modulator of P-glycoprotein. *Mol Pharmacol* 1997;52: 948–957.

88. Kelly R, Smith TW. Pharmacological treatment of heart failure. In: Hardman JG, Limbird LE, Molinoff PB, Ruddon RW, Gilman AG, eds. *Goodman and Gilman's the pharmacological basis of therapeutics.* New York: McGraw-Hill, 1996:809–838.

89. Su S-F, Huang J-D. Inhibition of the intestinal digoxin absorption and exsorption by quinidine. *Drug Metab Dispos* 1996;24:142–147.

90. Cavet ME, West M, Simmons NL. Transport and epithelial secretion of the cardiac glycoside, digoxin, by human intestinal epithelial (Caco-2) cells. *Br J Pharmacol* 1996;118:1389–1396.

91. Woodland C, Ito C, Koren G. A model for the prediction of digoxin-drug interactions at the renal tubular cell level. *Ther Drug Monit* 1998; 20:134–138.

92. Jalava KM, Partanen J, Neuvonen PJ. Itraconazole decreases renal clearance of digoxin. *Ther Drug Monit* 1998;19:609–613.

93. Wakasugi H, Yano I, Ito T, et al. Effect of clarithromycin on renal excretion of digoxin: interaction with P-glycoprotein. *Clin Pharmacol Ther* 1998;64:123–128.

94. Kim AE, Dintaman JM, Waddell DS, Silverman JA. Saquinavir, an HIV protease inhibitor, is transported by P-glycoprotein. *J Pharm Exp Ther* 1998;286:1439–1445.

95. Lee CGL, Gottesman MM, Cardarelli CO, et al. HIV-1 protease inhibitors are substrates for the *MDR*1 multidrug transporter. *Biochemistry* 1998;37:3594–3601.

96. Fitzsimmons ME, Collins JM. Selective biotransformation of the human immunodeficiency virus protease inhibitor saquinavir by human small-intestinal cytochrome P4503A4. *Drug Metab Dispos* 1997;24:256–266.

97. Zhang Y, Hsieh Y, Izumi T, Lin ET, Benet LZ. Effects of ketoconazole on the intestinal metabolism, transport and oral bioavailability of K02, a novel vinylsulfone peptidomimetic cysteine protease inhibitor and a P450 3A, P-glycoprotein dual substrate, in male Sprague-Dawley rats. *J Pharm Exp Ther* 1998;287:246–252.

98. Siegsmund MJ, Cardarelli C, Aksentijevich I, Sugimoto Y, Pastan I, Gottesman MM. Ketoconazole effectively reverses multidrug resistance in highly resistant KB cells. *J Urol* 1994;151:485–491.

99. Pouliot J-F, L'Heureux F, Liu Z, Prichard RK, Georges E. Reversal of P-glycoprotein-associated multidrug resistance by ivermectin. *Biochem Pharmacol* 1997;53:17–25.

100. Ueda K, Okamura N, Hirai M, et al. Human P-glycoprotein transports cortisol, aldosterone and dexamethasone, but not progesterone. *J Biol Chem* 1992;267:24248–24252.

101. Yang C-PH, DePinho SG, Greenberger LM, Arceci RJ, Horwitz SB. Progesterone interacts with P-glycoprotein in multidrug resistant cells and in the endometrium of gravid uterus. *J Biol Chem* 1989;264: 782–788.

102. Saitoh H, Hatakeyama M, Eguchi O, Oda M, Takada M. Involvement of intestinal P-glycoprotein in the restricted absorption methylprednisolone from rat small intestine. *J Pharm Sci* 1998;87:73–75.

103. Desai PB, Bhardwaj R, Damle B. Effect of tamoxifen on mitoxantrone cytotoxicity in drug sensitive and multidrug-resistant MCF-7 cells. *Cancer Chemother Pharmacol* 1995;36:368–372.

104. Lum BL, Kaubisch S, Yahanda AM, et al. Alteration of etoposide pharmacokinetics and pharmacodynamics by cyclosporine in a phaseI trial to modulate multidrug resistance. *J Clin Oncol* 1992;10:1635–1642.

105. Relling MV. Are the major effects of P-glycoprotein modulators due to altered pharmacokinetics of anticancer drugs? *Ther Drug Monit* 1996;18:350–356.

106. van de Vrie W, Gheuens EE, Durante NM, et al. In vitro and in vivo chemosensitizing effect of cyclosporin A on an intrinsic multidrug-resistant rat colon tumour. *J Cancer Res Clin Oncol* 1993;119: 60–614.

107. van de Vrie W, Jonker AM, Marquet RL, Eggermont AMM. The chemosensitizer cyclosporin A enhances the toxic side-effects of doxorubicin in the rat. *J Cancer Res Clin Oncol* 1994;120:533–538.

CHAPTER 12

Other CYP: 2A6, 2B6, 4A

Michael P. Pritchard and C. Roland Wolf

CYP2A6

Molecular Biology

One of the first human P450 cDNAs to be isolated was a partial CYP2A cDNA clone described in 1985 (1). However, it was not until several years later that the first full-length human CYP2A cDNA sequence, originally termed CYP2A3 (2) but later renamed CYP2A6, was published independently by two research groups (3,4), and shortly after by a third group (5). Of these three clones, only one (4) was "full-length," because the other two sequences appeared to lack the first 15 nucleotides of coding sequence, starting instead with the methionine at amino-acid position 6. This was subsequently confirmed by N-terminal sequencing of the CYP2A6 protein purified from human liver (6,7).

The CYP2A6 cDNA has been expressed in active form in a number of different systems, including HepG2 cells (8), COS-7 cells (9,10), B-lymphoblastoid cells (5), C3H/10T1/2 cells (11), NIH 3T3 and HeLa cells (12), and, more recently, in insect cells (13–15), V79 cells (16), *Saccharomyces cerevisiae* (17), and *Escherichia coli* (18). Recombinant CYP2A6 exhibits the same molecular weight (49 kDa) on SDS-PAGE (sodium dodecylsulfate polyacrylamide electrophoresis) (9,10,12) as human liver CYP2A6 (6,8).

Early studies demonstrated that the CYP2A6 gene was located on the long arm of chromosome 19 (19), in close proximity to the CYP2B (3,20,21) and CYP2F (22) gene loci. Indeed, it has become clear that these three P450 subfamilies form a cluster spanning 350 kb at 19q13.2 (23–25), proximal to the apolipoprotein C1, C2, and E genes, and the myotonic dystrophy gene (26). Analysis of

this region has revealed the existence of three CYP2A genes (CYP2A6, CYP2A7, and CYP2A13) containing nine exons, plus two identical pseudogenes lacking exons 6 to 9, related to CYP2A7 (25). Little is known at present about the newly discovered CYP2A13, which shares 93% amino acid identity with CYP2A6 (25). CYP2A7 (originally named CYP2A4) shares 94% identity with CYP2A6 at the amino acid level (8), and exhibits the same molecular weight (49 kDa) as CYP2A6 on SDS-PAGE (10). However, the two proteins do not share the same catalytic properties, CYP2A7 being inactive toward the archetypal CYP2A6 substrate coumarin (8,10). The CYP2A7 mRNA is also found as an alternately spliced form, in which 163 bp of exon 2 are replaced with 10 bp of intron 1 (10), resulting in an in-frame deletion of 51 amino acids. Expression of this variant sequence in COS-7 cells led to the production of a 44-kDa protein with no discernible activity toward coumarin (10).

The expression of CYP2A6 in man is subject to genetic polymorphism, with four allelic variants having been described to date in addition to the wild type (25,27,28). The CYP2A6*2 allele differs from wild-type CYP2A6*1 by just two single nucleotide changes in the coding region (G60A and T488A), only one of which leads to an amino-acid change (Leu160 → His) (8,25). Expression of CYP2A6*2 in HepG2 cells results in the synthesis of a protein which is inactive toward coumarin (8). More recently, this finding has been confirmed by a phenotyping study, in which subjects homozygous for the CYP2A6*2 allele were shown to be poor metabolisers of coumarin (27). The CYP2A6*2 allele frequency, initially estimated to be 15–20% (25), was found to be only 1–3% in caucasians and 0% in Chinese, using an improved genotyping method which avoids co-amplification of homologous genes (27). Applying this method, allele CYP2A6*3, described as resulting from multiple gene conversion events between CYP2A6 and CYP2A7 in exons 3, 6 and 8 (25), was not

M. P. Pritchard and C. R. Wolf: Biomedical Research Centre, University of Dundee, Level 5, Ninewells Hospital and Medical School, Dundee DD1 9SY Scotland, United Kingdom.

found in either caucasians or Chinese (28). Allele CYP2A6*4, a deletion of the entire gene leading to a failure to express functional CYP2A6 protein, was found with allele frequencies of 0.5% in caucasians and 15% in Chinese (28). In CYP2A6*5, a single nucleotide change (G1436T) causes an enzyme-inactivating amino-acid change (Gly479 → Leu). To date, this allele has only been found in Chinese, at a frequency of 1% (28).

Ontogeny, Tissue Distribution, and Sexual Differentiation

CYP2A6 is essentially absent from fetal liver (31–33), but can be detected 16 to 20 weeks after birth (5). Two *in vitro* studies have found no effect of age on CYP2A6 levels in liver microsomal samples from donors aged 8 to 73 years (29,34). Although one study found the elimination of coumarin *in vivo* to be significantly impaired in healthy elderly (older than 65 years) subjects, compared with their younger (younger than 25 years) counterparts (35), another found no effect of age in the range 19 to 56 years (36). Taken together, these data suggest that CYP2A6 appears in the liver around the time of birth and is maintained throughout adult life.

Both CYP2A6 and CYP2A7 mRNA species can be detected in adult liver (3,8,10,32), with the ratio of the two messages showing considerable variation (10). CYP2A6 protein represents about 1% to 14% of the total hepatic P450 (6,7,29). In normal liver, CYP2A6 is distributed uniformly throughout the acinus (37,38). However, expression increases markedly in hepatocytes adjacent to areas of fibrosis and inflammation, for example, in cirrhosis (37), viral hepatitis (38), or liver fluke infection (39). In contrast, CYP2A6 protein could not be detected in a series of liver tumor samples (40).

In contrast to the liver, placenta is devoid of CYP2A6-associated enzyme activity (41), immunoreactive protein (7), and mRNA (42, 43). CYP2A6 protein is also undetectable (<0.2 pmol/mg) in breast, colon, and kidney (7), although a recent report has shown that the oxidative defluorination of the anesthetic methoxyflurane, catalyzed by recombinant CYP2A6, can be inhibited by coumarin in kidney microsomes (44). CYP2A6 protein and activity are also virtually undetectable in lung (7,33), and low levels of CYP2A6 protein have been found in larynx (45). Of greater interest is the discovery of a CYP2A-related protein in human olfactory mucosa and, to a lesser extent, respiratory mucosa by immunohistochemistry (46). More recently, primer-specific polymerase chain reaction (PCR) was used to demonstrate the presence of the CYP2A6 mRNA in nasal mucosa (47). This may have toxicologic significance, given that CYP2A6 can catalyze the metabolic activation of olfactory-specific toxicants such as 2,6-dichlorobenzonitrile (48). Finally, CYP2A6 mRNA is not detectable in pri-

mary cultures of human oral or cervical epithelial cells (49), in the uterine tumor-derived HeLa cell line (12), or in HepG2 hepatoma cells (49).

Evidence suggests that CYP2A6 expression is not sexually differentiated in humans. For example, levels of immunoreactive CYP2A protein are similar in liver microsomes from male and female subjects (29,34), as is coumarin 7-hydroxylase activity (34). This is supported by studies showing no effect of gender on coumarin elimination *in vivo* (35,50).

Interindividual Variability

Even before the molecular basis of the genetic polymorphism of CYP2A6 expression was discovered (see earlier discussion), it was clear that this enzyme exhibited enormous interindividual variability in expression. Levels of immunodetectable CYP2A protein in liver microsomes varied up to 100-fold between individuals (6,7,9,34,40, 51). Indeed, in some samples, particularly those from Japanese subjects (29,30), CYP2A protein was undetectable. The CYP2A6 content of human liver microsomes has been estimated to range from less than 0.1 to 60 pmol/mg protein (30). The origin of this large interindividual variability appears to be pretranslational, in that CYP2A6 mRNA levels also vary widely between liver samples (3,8,10,52). Perhaps not surprisingly, coumarin 7-hydroxylase activity in human liver microsomes also shows significant variability (Table 12-1), ranging from 0

TABLE 12-1. *Coumarin 7-hydroxylase activity in human liver microsomes*

Activity range[a]	n	Ref.
160–650	28	55
0–496	32	201
430–2070	8	202
150–491	4	63
25–1675	12	9
31–1350	12	8
187–730	9	203
0–2600	60	6
14–2330	20	7
110–940	14	51
13–69	12	52
370–890	7	75
280–4750	22	34
<1–117	12	84
100–1350	10	88
190–710	4	31
<1–50	18	154
119–2366	10	129
307–3950	10	142
100–2260	33	118
2–524[b]	10	30
179–2470[b]	11	76
120–1360	11	82

[a]Activity in pmol/min/mg microsomal protein
[b]Denotes V_{max} values.

to 4,750 pmol/min/mg protein. Similar results have been observed in phenotyping studies looking at the elimination of coumarin *in vivo* (Table 12-2). Whereas most humans excrete approximately 50% to 70% of an oral dose of coumarin within 4 hours by CYP2A6-mediated conversion to 7-hydroxycoumarin and excretion into the urine as glucuronide conjugates, individual subjects can vary from 0% to 100% of the dose excreted (see Table 12-2). Indeed, in one study looking at a Thai population (39), five individuals were found who were unable to eliminate coumarin by this route. Although DNA analysis revealed mutations in the CYP2A6 gene in these individuals, no details were given as to the precise genetic defects found.

Coumarin phenotyping studies have also permitted investigations into the influence of disease and lifestyle status on CYP2A6 metabolic capacity (see Table 12-2). For example, the elimination of coumarin is significantly impaired in severe and, to a lesser extent, in moderate alcoholic liver disease, but not in mild alcoholic liver disease (53), or in fatty liver or chronic active hepatitis (54). Interestingly, in a previous *in vitro* study, the rate of coumarin 7-hydroxylation was found to be severely reduced in chronic active hepatitis (55). Subjects testing positive for hepatitis A infection also have a reduced capacity to metabolize coumarin (56). Urinary 7-hydroxycoumarin excretion is also reduced in kidney disease (53), although this presumably is a reflection of compromised renal function rather than any effect on CYP2A6.

With regard to lifestyle influences, coumarin 7-hydroxylase activity *in vitro* is similar in liver microsomal samples from smokers and nonsmokers (57), but *in vivo*, elimination of coumarin in smokers is significantly reduced (36). As to potential dietary effectors of CYP2A6, grapefruit juice has been shown to delay the excretion of 7-hydroxycoumarin (58,59), whereas no difference was found between vegans and their matched omnivorous controls (60).

Substrates

CYP2A6 is the major, if not the only, coumarin 7-hydroxylase in human liver (61). Evidence for this conclusion is provided by correlation analysis, immunoinhibition experiments, and cDNA-directed expression. First, a high degree of correlation exists between the level of CYP2A-immunoreactive protein and coumarin 7-hydroxylase activity in human liver microsomes (6–9,29,30,34,62). Anti-CYP2A antibody is able to inhibit coumarin

TABLE 12-2. In vivo *studies of coumarin metabolism in man*

Study group	Oral dose (mg)	n	Sampling time (h)	Urinary 7-OHC excretion (% dose)		Ref.
				Mean±SD	Range	
Healthy	200	8	0–24	79±9	68–92	70
?	200	7	0–24	63.4		72
Healthy	1000	10	0–48	36	20–39	204
Control	5	17	0–4	57.2±10.2		54
Liver cirrhosis	5	13	0–4	46.6±13.4		54
Healthy	2	64	0–8	86±24	10–116	73
Healthy + "patients"	5	110	0–4	65±15	20–100	50
Healthy + "patients"	5				0–100	205
Healthy	10	13	0–24	63.7±12.0		58
Healthy (control)	5	5	0–4	73.4±9.6	61–87	115
Healthy (methoxsalen treated)	5	5	0–4	40.6±16.5	19–63	115
Healthy	5	100	0–8	58.6±22.2	17–100	36
Control	5	20	0–2	56.2±11.6		53
Severe alcoholic liver disease	5	12	0–2	18.0±10.3		53
Moderate alcoholic liver disease	5	12	0–2	34.2±15.6		53
Mild alcoholic liver disease	5	12	0–2	49.7±19.0		53
Kidney disease	5	12	0–2	27.8±15.7		53
Epilepsy	5	12	0–2	69.5±13.2		53
Healthy	10	12	0–12		67–76	206
Omnivores	5	20	0–6	64.0±16.0	39–92	60
Vegans	5	20	0–6	58.2±17.2	23–85	60
Young men(<25 y)	5	10	0–2	68.1±13.1		35
Young women (<25 y)	5	10	0–2	65.0±18.3		35
Elderly men (>65 y)	5	10	0–2	46.5±16.3		35
Elderly women (>65 y)	5	10	0–2	44.8±18.3		35
Control/liver fluke infection	15	91	0–4	41	0–71	39
Hepatitis A–positive children	5	11	0–2	12.9±12.5		56
Healthy children	5	10	0–2	62.0±27.9		56
Hepatitis A–positive adults	5	9	0–2	45.6±30.2		56
Healthy adults	5	20	0–2	61.5±14.4		56

7-hydroxylation *in vitro* by 91% to 100% (5,6,8,9, 12,34,62–64), as is specific anti-CYP2A6 IgG (7,30). Second, recombinant CYP2A6 expressed in a variety of cell types displays activity toward coumarin (5,8–18,65). As mentioned previously, neither CYP2A6*2 (8) nor CYP2A7 (8,10) have coumarin 7-hydroxylase activity. Experiments using other cDNA-expressed P450s suggest that this activity is specific for CYP2A6 (66), although in another study, CYP2B6 was also shown to catalyze this reaction, albeit at a rate some 20-fold lower than CYP2A6 (65).

Apparent kinetic parameters for the 7-hydroxylation of coumarin in human liver microsomes have been determined. Two sets of V_{max} values are given in Table 12-1 and reflect the wide interindividual variability in CYP2A6 expression (see earlier text). K_m values are remarkably consistent between different microsome preparations and different research groups (Table 12-3), and are typically of the order of 1 to 2 μM, similar to the 1.2 ± 0.1 μM determined for CYP2A6 purified from human liver (30). K_m values for recombinant CYP2A6 also generally fall within this range (see Table 12-3). Purified human liver CYP2A6 catalyzes coumarin 7-hydroxylation with a turnover ranging from 1.40 (30) to 2.09 min^{-1} (7). Turnovers for recombinant CYP2A6 range from 2.14 min^{-1} for baculovirus-mediated expression in insect cells (14) to 13 to 15 min^{-1} for vaccinia virus–mediated expression in HepG2 cells (8,66).

As well as being a suitable *in vitro* probe, coumarin is useful in phenotyping studies *in vivo* (see Table 12-2 and earlier text). Although coumarin was banned as a food flavoring agent in 1954 because of resulting hepatotoxicity in experimental animals (67,68), cases of liver toxicity in humans are exceedingly rare and idiosyncratic (69). Coumarin is metabolized in humans almost exclusively by CYP2A6-mediated 7-hydroxylation (68%–92% of the dose), with only a small proportion (1%–6%) being converted to *o*-hydroxyphenylacetic acid (70). A similar pattern of metabolite formation is also seen *in vitro* (71). The 7-hydroxycoumarin formed is excreted in the urine, predominantly as glucuronide conjugate, where it can be quantitated (72,73).

With coumarin being such a good substrate for CYP2A6, the most important potential drug–drug interaction is with coumarin anticoagulants such as dicumarol and warfarin. However, dicumarol metabolism by human liver microsomes correlates neither with coumarin 7-hydroxylase activity nor with immunodetectable CYP2A6 (34). In addition, dicumarol is only a weak inhibitor of coumarin 7-hydroxylation (34,74). Warfarin, too, does not appear to be a substrate of CYP2A6, because warfarin biotransformation *in vitro* is not consistently inhibited by anti-CYP2A antibody and does not correlate with coumarin metabolism (75). Furthermore, warfarin does not inhibit coumarin 7-hydroxylation (34,74–76).

CYP2A6 does, however, catalyze the C-oxidation of nicotine to form nicotine-$\Delta^{1'(5')}$-iminium ion (51,77–79), which is further oxidized by aldehyde oxidase to cotinine (51). These data are in contrast to an earlier report using recombinant P450s expressed in HepG2 cells, which suggested that CYP2B6 was the major catalyst of nicotine C-oxidation in human liver and that CYP2A6 was barely active (80). In the presence of exogenously added aldehyde oxidase, cotinine formation correlates both with immunodetectable CYP2A6 (51,78,79) and with coumarin 7-hydroxylase activity in human liver microsomes (51,78), and is inhibited by both coumarin (78,79) and anti-CYP2A antibody (78,79). Finally, recombinant CYP2A6 expressed in B-lymphoblastoid cells catalyzes cotinine formation from nicotine (78,79) with a K_m (47 μM) similar to that observed in human liver microsomes (64.9 ± 32.7 μM) (79). Among other cDNA-expressed P450s, only CYP2B6 and CYP2D6 catalyzed nicotine C-oxidation at rates ten- and 20-fold less than CYP2A6, respectively (78).

In addition to the C-oxidation of nicotine, CYP2A6 also catalyzes the stereospecific 3'-hydroxylation of cotinine to form *trans*-3'-hydroxycotinine, a major metabolite of nicotine in humans (81). Cotinine 3'-hydroxylation *in vitro* correlates both with immunoreactive CYP2A6 and with coumarin 7-hydroxylase activity, and is inhibited by both coumarin and anti-CYP2A antibody (81). Of a series of recombinant P450s expressed in B-lymphoblastoid cells, only CYP2A6 catalyzed this reaction, with a K_m (265 μM) similar to that determined in human liver microsomes (235 ± 27 μM) (81). CYP2A6, therefore, plays a pivotal role in the disposition of nicotine in humans, given that the two major urinary metabolites excreted following a dose of nicotine are cotinine (10%–15%) and *trans*-3'-hydroxycotinine (20%–30%) (51). The other major route of nicotine metabolism is to nicotine *N'*-oxide, catalyzed by flavin-containing monooxygenase (51).

Another related compound metabolized by CYP2A6 is the carcinogen *N'*-nitrosonornicotine, which is converted to an unstable 5'-hydroxylated metabolite, which, in turn,

TABLE 12-3. *Apparent K_m values for the 7-hydroxylation of coumarin by human liver and recombinant CYP2A6*

Source	n	K_m (μM) Mean ± SD	Range	Ref.
Human liver	5	1.63	0.37–3.57	114
Human liver	2	2.3		8
Human liver	22		0.1–0.9	34
Human liver	1	13.0		112
Human liver	10	2.1 ± 0.7	1.1–3.3	30
Human liver	2	0.34		118
Human liver	9	0.57 ± 0.07	0.50–0.70	76
Recombinant	2		3.6–7.1	8
Recombinant	—	1.4		5
Recombinant		6		14
Recombinant		0.62		76

decomposes to form 4-hydroxy-4-(3-pyridyl)butanal (82). Formation of this metabolite correlates with coumarin 7-hydroxylase activity, is inhibited by coumarin and anti-CYP2A6 monoclonal antibody, and is catalyzed specifically by recombinant CYP2A6, with a K_m (2.1 ± 0.6 µM) similar to that determined in a sample of human liver microsomes high in CYP2A6 activity (5 µM) (82). It should be noted that the 2'-hydroxylation of N'-nitrosonornicotine is catalyzed by CYP3A4 (82).

Other substrates for CYP2A6 have been elucidated using the methods described. For example, CYP2A6 probably plays a major role in the metabolism of the tobacco carcinogen 4-(methylnitrosamino)-1-(3-pyridyl)-1-butanone (NNK) (11,83–87), the mutagens N-nitrosodiethylamine (NDEA) (5,84,85,88) and quinoline (89), the anticonvulsant losigamone (90), and the PAF receptor antagonist (+)-cis-3,5-dimethyl-2-(3-pyridyl) thiazolidin-4-one hydrochloride (91). A recent paper has also implicated CYP2A6, along with CYP2C9, in the terminal desaturation of the anticonvulsant valproic acid, to form the hepatotoxin 4-ene-valproic acid (92). CYP2A6 may make a minor contribution to the sulfoxidation of S-methyl-N,N-diethylthiolcarbamate (93), the reductive metabolism of halothane, along with CYP3A4 (94), to antipyrine 4-hydroxylation (95,96), and to the N-oxidation of 4,4'-methylene-bis(2-chloroaniline) (7,97). Although CYP2A6 can catalyze the metabolic activation of aflatoxin B₁ (7,12,98,99), this reaction is carried out at much higher rates by CYP1A2 and CYP3A4 (100). CYP2A6 is therefore unlikely to make a significant contribution, except in a small number of cases (101).

One striking feature of many substrates of CYP2A6 is that they are also substrates for CYP2E1, often to the virtual exclusion of any other P450. Examples of these common CYP2A6/CYP2E1 substrates include N-nitrosodimethylamine and N-nitrosodiethylamine (5,84), 1,3-butadiene (102,103) and butadiene monoxide (104), N-nitrosopyrrolidine (105), methoxyflurane and sevoflurane (with CYP3A4) (44), 1,2-dibromoethane (with CYP2B6) (106), 2,6-dichlorobenzonitrile (48), 4-nitrophenol (14), 4-nitroanisole (107), and methyl tert-butyl ether (108).

Among other probe substrates commonly used in the determination of P450 activities, 7-ethoxycoumarin is metabolized by CYP2A6 (6–8,12,65,109,110), with the exception of one study using the enzyme purified from human liver (111). However, this reaction is by no means specific, being catalyzed by many other P450s (65,109, 111). CYP2A6 has no detectable activity toward testosterone (7,12,14,17,65,112), unlike certain CYP2A proteins from other animal species (61). A molecular model attempting to rationalize the difference in substrate specificity between different CYP2A isoforms has been described (113). Other compounds that do not appear to be substrates for CYP2A6 include 7-ethoxyresorufin (12,66), debrisoquine (17), caffeine, theophylline, tolbu-

tamide, phenytoin, S-mephenytoin, bufuralol, dextromethorphan, chlorzoxazone, aniline, and diazepam (66).

Inducers and Inhibitors

One of the first investigations into the possible effect of "inducing drugs" on CYP2A6 looked at coumarin 7-hydroxylation in liver homogenates prepared from biopsy samples (114). No difference was observed between "control" and "treated" patients, suggesting that CYP2A6 was not induced. However, subsequent experiments have indicated that CYP2A6 is inducible to some extent. The level of CYP2A6 protein in primary cultures of human hepatocytes is increased by treatment with phenobarbital, dexamethasone, and rifampicin (6,62). Coumarin 7-hydroxylation and cotinine formation from nicotine in vitro were found to be increased in samples from barbiturate-treated subjects (51,77). Finally, one in vivo study found a significantly increased urinary excretion of 7-hydroxycoumarin in patients with epilepsy (53), presumably as a result of treatment with anticonvulsive drugs.

One problem with the study of CYP2A6 has been the lack of a suitable specific inhibitor. For this reason, coumarin has often been used to act as a competitive inhibitor of CYP2A6-mediated reactions (78,79,81,82). However, this approach is not without limitations, because, although coumarin clearly is a substrate for CYP2A6 in human liver, it is also metabolized to other products (70) by P450s, which may not be CYP2A6. Competitive inhibition by coumarin may not, therefore, be specific to CYP2A6-catalyzed reactions. Not surprisingly, other substrates of CYP2A6, such as nicotine and 4-nitrophenol, can also be used as competitive inhibitors (76).

The furanocoumarin derivative 8-methoxypsoralen, or methoxsalen, is one of the most potent inhibitors of coumarin 7-hydroxylase activity in human liver microsomes (74,76). This inactivation of CYP2A6 by methoxsalen occurs extremely rapidly and noncompetitively, with a K_i in the range 0.3 to 1.5 µM (76,115). Methoxsalen also strongly inhibits recombinant CYP2A6 expressed in NIH 3T3 cells (12), but, strangely, is apparently only a weak inhibitor of CYP2A6 expressed in insect cells (14). In a more clinically relevant study, the urinary excretion of 7-hydroxycoumarin by five volunteers was reduced almost 50% when 45 mg methoxsalen was taken 1 hour before the dose of coumarin (see Table 12-2) (115), demonstrating that this inhibition can also occur in vivo. However, methoxsalen is not a specific inhibitor of CYP2A6, in that, at 10 µM, it also reduces the activity of recombinant CYP1A2, CYP3A4, and CYP3A5 expressed in HepG2 cells (66). Among other closely related compounds, psoralen itself is only a weak inhibitor of CYP2A6, and 5-methoxypsoralen and 5,8-dimethoxypsoralen are noninhibitory (74).

Among competitive inhibitors of CYP2A6, the most potent found to date is probably the monoamine oxidase inhibitor tranylcypromine, which has a K_i of 0.04 μM (76). However, at higher concentrations, this compound inhibits reactions mediated by other P450s, such as the 4'-hydroxylation of mephenytoin ($K_i = 8$ μM) (116), and at very high concentrations, tranylcypromine becomes extremely nonspecific (66). Another strong competitive inhibitor of CYP2A6 is pilocarpine, with a K_i of 1 to 4 μM in human liver microsomes (117,118). Although little is known about the specificity of pilocarpine, it is a weak inhibitor of testosterone 6β-hydroxylation (suggesting CYP3A4) (119) and tolbutamide 4-methylhydroxylation (suggesting CYP2C9) (118). The remaining competitive inhibitors of CYP2A6 ($K_i < 100$ μM) characterized to date, such as menadione (74), miconazole and clotrimazole (74,76), and ketoconazole (66,76,120), are often strong inhibitors of other P450s. The CYP1A2 inhibitor α-naphthoflavone is also an inhibitor of CYP2A6 at a concentration of 10 μM (76,84,114,121), but this effect is almost completely abolished when the concentration is reduced to 1 μM (66,84,121). Data concerning the effects of another CYP1A2 inhibitor, ellipticine, on CYP2A6 are contradictory, with one study (76) finding strong competitive inhibition ($K_i \approx 10$ μM) and another (66) finding almost no effect at the same concentration.

The other major inhibitor of CYP2A6 is diethyldithiocarbamate (66,76,84,121), but this also inactivates CYP2E1 (122) and has effects on several other P450s (66,121). Chlorophyllin is another nonspecific inhibitor of CYP2A6 (123), as is diallyldisulfide (118). Other common P450 inhibitors, such as metyrapone and SKF-525A, have relatively weak effects on CYP2A6 (14,66,74,76,114). Among the compounds that have little or no inhibitory effect on CYP2A6 in vitro ($K_i > 200$ μM), are caffeine, chlorzoxazone, cimetidine, dextromethorphan, diazepam, diclofenac, erythromycin, ethinylestradiol, fluconazole, furafylline, hexobarbital, itraconazole, mephenytoin, methimazole, metronidazole, naringenin, nifedipine, norfloxacin, orphenadrine, papaverine, pyrimethamine, quinidine, phenacetin, ranitidine, spironolactone, sulfaphenazole, sulfinpyrazone, testosterone, tolbutamide, troleandomycin, and warfarin (66,76,118,121,124,125). Dextromethorphan and mephenytoin have also been shown not to interact with coumarin disposition in vivo (126). Finally, CYP2A6 is also inhibited by a number of organic solvents at a final concentration of 1% (v/v), including tetrahydrofuran and dioxane, and to a lesser extent, acetonitrile, acetone, and ethanol (76).

CYP2B6

Molecular Biology

Full-length CYP2B6 cDNA was first described in 1989 (127), following an earlier account of the isolation of two partial CYP2B6 cDNA clones (20). The deduced amino acid sequence of the CYP2B6 protein showed 76% similarity with rat CYP2B1 (127). A second full-length CYP2B cDNA, which is currently known as CYP2B7, was also isolated, sharing similarities to CYP2B6 of 95% and 93% at the nucleotide and amino acid levels, respectively (127). This transcript contained an internal TGA stop codon at position 1148, as a result of a C→T transition, and was therefore expected to encode a truncated protein, which, lacking the critical heme-coordinating cysteine residue, would be nonfunctional (127). In contrast, the CYP2B6 cDNA was expressed and shown to be both spectrally and catalytically active (127).

Owing to problems of low expression levels, it was several years before CYP2B6 was partially purified from human liver (128), and the N-terminal amino acid sequence shown to be identical to that deduced from the cDNA sequence (127). Purified human liver CYP2B6 has an apparent molecular weight of approximately 48 kDa on SDS-PAGE (128). A similar size has also been found for CYP2B6 detected by immunoblotting in human liver microsomes (29) and for recombinant CYP2B6 purified from S. cerevisiae (17). However, other studies have put the molecular weight of CYP2B6 at 51.5 (52), 52 (127), and even 54 kDa (129). This discrepancy probably reflects slightly differing experimental conditions for the gel electrophoresis, rather than any gross effect on the CYP2B6 protein.

It was realized early on that the CYP2B gene subfamily was located very close to the CYP2A genes, on the long arm of chromosome 19 (3,20,21). Indeed, it has come to be known that the CYP2A, CYP2B, and CYP2F genes are organized into a single gene cluster at 19q13.2 (23), as is discussed earlier. At the center of this cluster are located the two complete CYP2B genes—CYP2B6 and CYP2B7—plus a CYP2B7-like pseudogene, termed CYP2B7P, which lacks the 3'-untranslated region and possibly also exon 9 (23).

Unlike CYP2A6, no evidence has yet come to light for the possible existence of allelic variants of CYP2B6. However, one potential source of interindividual variability in CYP2B6 expression comes from alternative splicing of the CYP2B6 mRNA (20), leading to the generation of variant transcripts. To date, three such splice variants have been isolated from human liver. In one case, the use of a cryptic exon within intron 3 and an alternative splice acceptor site within exon 4 leads to the generation of an aberrant mRNA species in which the first 29 nucleotides of exon 4 are replaced by 44 nucleotides of intron 3 (127,130). The other two splice variants, one containing intron 5 but lacking exon 8, and another in which exon 8 was replaced by a cryptic exon 8A found within intron 8, were identified in all 15 liver samples tested (20,131), suggesting that alternative splicing of CYP2B6 mRNA is a common event.

The discovery of significant correlations between the expression of CYP2B6 and CYP2A6 at both the mRNA

(3) and protein level (52), coupled with the close association of the two genes on chromosome 19 (see earlier text), has led to the suggestion that the expression of these two enzymes may share some degree of coordinate regulation (3,52). In support of this theory, a more recent study found a strong correlation ($r = 0.91$) between S-mephenytoin N-demethylase activity (thought to be catalyzed by CYP2B6) and CYP2A6-dependent coumarin 7-hydroxylase activity in human liver microsomes (132). Similarly, two studies have found a good correlation ($r = 0.88$) between CYP2B6-dependent 7-ethoxy-4-trifluoromethylcoumarin (7-EFC) O-deethylase and coumarin 7-hydroxylase activities (99,133).

Ontogeny, Tissue Distribution, and Sexual Differentiation

Little is known at present about the ontogeny of CYP2B6 expression in humans. However, CYP2B6 mRNA is detectable in adult, but not in fetal liver (32). In addition, immunoblotting using anti–monkey CYP2B antibody found a relatively high level of CYP2B protein in a sample of liver microsomes from a subject aged 4 months (29). The same study also found no effect of age on CYP2B6 levels in adult liver microsomes. It is likely, therefore, that, in the liver at least, CYP2B6 appears around the time of birth and is then maintained throughout adult life.

Both CYP2B6 (3,32,52,127,134) and CYP2B7 (134) mRNA can be identified in liver, CYP2B7 being present at less than 10% of the level of CYP2B6 (134). Immunodetection of CYP2B6 protein in liver has been somewhat hampered in certain cases by the lack of a suitable specific antibody. For example, a widely used commercially available rabbit anti–rat CYP2B antibody has been shown to cross-react with other members of the CYP2 family (135). Nonetheless, CYP2B6 protein can be detected immunologically in liver microsomes (17,29,40, 52,99,127,128,136), where it is said to represent no more than 1% of the total P450 (29,128). In healthy liver, CYP2B6 has a uniform distribution throughout the acinus (37,38). However, expression of CYP2B6 appears to be increased in hepatocytes adjacent to areas of fibrosis (37,38).

In contrast to liver, CYP2B6 mRNA is not detectable in either placenta (42,43) or lung (134,137). CYP2B7 mRNA, however, is detectable in lung (134,137), where it is found in bronchial epithelial cells, but not in alveolar macrophages (138). CYP2B7 mRNA is also found in the majority of lung tumors (134). CYP2B6 mRNA is not detectable in primary cultures of umbilical vein endothelial cells (139) and is barely detectable in cultured oral or cervical epithelial cells (49). Finally, CYP2B6 protein has been identified in esophagus (140), but is undetectable in gingiva (141).

There is little information available on the effect of gender on CYP2B6 expression. One *in vitro* study has reported no significant difference in levels of immunodetectable CYP2B6 in liver microsomes from male and female subjects (29).

Interindividual Variability

As with CYP2A6, the expression of CYP2B6 in humans is subject to wide interindividual variability. Estimates of CYP2B6 content in panels of human liver microsomes are <0.5 to 7 (128), < 0.5 to 17 (17), and 0.3 to 74 (99) pmol/mg protein. Indeed, in a number of livers, CYP2B6 is almost undetectable by immunochemical means (29,40,52,99). Again as with CYP2A6, CYP2B6 expression appears to be lower in Japanese than in caucasians (29). The source of this variability appears to be pretranslational, in that CYP2B6 mRNA levels also vary widely between individuals (3,52,127). In one study, seven of 13 samples of total liver RNA contained very low or undetectable levels of CYP2B6 mRNA (127).

Substrates

One of the problems associated with the study of CYP2B6 , apart from the generally low level of expression, has been the lack of a suitable specific substrate. One of the activities used in the assessment of CYP2B6 activity is the O-deethylation of 7-EFC, which is catalyzed by recombinant CYP2B6 expressed in B-lymphoblastoid cells with a K_m of 1.7 to 2.9 µM (99,135) and a turnover of 1.6 to 2.5 min^{-1} (99,135,142). However, CYP1A1 and CYP1A2, and to a lesser extent CYP2C19 and CYP2E1, also catalyze this reaction (99,135,142). Although CYP1A1 is unlikely to make a substantial contribution to the overall rate of 7-EFC metabolism in human liver microsomes, the contribution of the other P450s, particularly CYP1A2, may be significant. Indeed, the best correlation between immunodetectable CYP2B6 and 7-EFC O-deethylase activity ($r^2 = 0.80$) was obtained when the incubations were carried out in the presence of a mixture of anti-CYP1A, anti-CYP2C, and anti-CYP2E1 antibodies (99).

CYP2B6 also catalyzes the O-deethylation of 7-ethoxycoumarin (65,109–111,127), leading to the use of this activity as a marker for CYP2B6 *in vitro* (129). However, 7-ethoxycoumarin is a substrate for a number of other P450s, particularly CYP2E1 (65,109–111), and so is not specific. Data concerning CYP2B6 and 7-benzyloxyresorufin O-dealkylation are contradictory, with one group demonstrating participation of most P450s in this reaction (65) and another indicating strong specificity for CYP2B6 (66). A recent study has also found correlation between levels of CYP2B and pentoxyresorufin O-dealkylation in liver microsomes (136).

To date, CYP2B6 has been implicated in the metabolism of very few therapeutic agents. Reactions that appear to involve a contribution from CYP2B6 include the *N*-demethylation of *S*-mephenytoin (132), the diphenylmethyl *p*-hydroxylation of cinnarizine (143), the cyclopentyl *trans*-hydroxylation of the phosphodiesterase IV inhibitor RP 73401 (133), and to a lesser extent, the *N*-deethylation of lidocaine (with CYP1A2 and CYP3A4) (17), the *N*-demethylation of diazepam and temazepam (with CYP2C19, CYP2C9, and CYP3A4) (144), and possibly the *N*-demethylation of mianserin (with CYP2C19, CYP1A2, and CYP3A4) (145). In addition, correlation analysis has implicated CYP2B6 in the metabolic activation of tamoxifen (146).

The role of CYP2B6 in the metabolic activation of the anticancer alkylating prodrug cyclophosphamide, via the formation of 4-hydroxycyclophosphamide, is a matter of contention. Recombinant CYP2B6 catalyzes this reaction *in vitro*, although the process is characterized by a high K_m (109). In addition, B-lymphoblastoid cells expressing CYP2B6 are more sensitive to the cytotoxicity and mutagenicity of cyclophosphamide than the parental cell line (99,109). Furthermore, anti-CYP2B IgG inhibits cyclophosphamide 4-hydroxylation in human liver microsomes by 40% (109). However, other P450s, notably CYP2C8 and CYP2C9 (low K_m) and CYP3A4 (high K_m), can catalyze this reaction (109), and given the relative levels of expression of these enzymes in human liver compared with CYP2B6 (29), it might be expected that they make a major contribution to cyclophosphamide activation *in vivo*. Indeed, a recent study suggests that CYP2C9 and CYP3A are the major P450 forms catalyzing cyclophosphamide 4-hydroxylation at low and high therapeutic concentrations, respectively (147). Nonetheless, CYP2B6 probably plays a significant minor role in this process, particularly at higher cyclophosphamide concentrations, and in those patients in whom CYP2B6 levels are elevated, perhaps as a result of concomitant treatment with inducing drugs (see later text).

Recently, CYP2B6 has been implicated in the 16α- and 16β-hydroxylation of testosterone (17), analogous to rat CYP2B1. However, this is in complete contrast to an earlier study, which found CYP2B6 to be "essentially inactive" toward testosterone, androstenedione, and progesterone (65). CYP2B6 does appear to catalyze the 4-hydroxylation of antipyrine (96), but is unlikely to contribute substantially to the overall rate of this reaction, given the significant input of CYP1A2, CYP2C, and CYP3A4 (96). Other reactions in which CYP2B6 is thought to be involved include the ring hydroxylation and *O*-demethylation of methoxychlor (148), the defluorination of 2-chloro-1,1-difluoroethene (129), the 3-hydroxylation of 2,4,5,2′,4′,5′-hexachlorobiphenyl (149), and, together with CYP1A2 and CYP2E1, the conversion of styrene to styrene glycol (150) and of toluene to benzyl alcohol and *p*-cresol (151). CYP2B6 may also play a role

in the conversion of isoprene to 3,4-epoxy-3-methyl-1-butene, although the major catalyst for this reaction is CYP2E1 (142). As with CYP2A6, the activation of aflatoxin B_1 to genotoxic metabolites catalyzed by CYP2B6 (98,99) is unlikely to be significant, given the much greater activities of CYP1A2 and CYP3A4 (100). Finally, CYP2B6 demonstrates activity toward a range of polycyclic aromatic hydrocarbons, in some cases carrying out metabolic activation to species that are precursors of known ultimate carcinogens. Thus, CYP2B6 (along with CYP2C9 and CYP1A2) can activate benzo(a)pyrene to the 7,8-epoxide (152), and dibenzo(a,h)anthracene to the 3,4-epoxide (153), and may play a role in the activation of 6-aminochrysene (128,154,155), a reaction which is also catalyzed by CYP3A4 and CYP1A2. Other reactions of this type catalyzed by CYP2B6 include the 9,10-epoxidation of phenanthrene (156), the 5,6-epoxidation of 7,12-dimethylbenz(a)anthracene (157), the direct 3-hydroxylation as well as the 4,5-epoxidation of benzo(a)pyrene (152), and to a lesser extent, the 11,12-epoxidation of dibenzo(a,l)pyrene (158) and the 9,10-epoxidation of benzo(a)pyrene (152).

Inducers and Inhibitors

Unlike the rat, very little is known about the induction of CYP2B in humans. Although one study found a high level of CYP2B6 mRNA in liver from a subject who had received phenytoin and phenobarbital, no significant effect of drug treatment was observed overall in the 13 livers tested (127). In another approach, immune-deficient mice were used as carriers of xenograft human colon tumors. Treatment of such animals with either 3-methylcholanthrene or 1,4-*bis*-2-(3,5-dichloropyridyloxy)benzene (TCPOBOP) resulted in a large induction of CYP2B mRNA in the tumor (159). A more recent study has shown that exposure of primary cultures of human hepatocytes to phenobarbital, dexamethasone, or rifampicin leads to an increase in immunoreactive CYP2B6 (160). Finally, two studies compared the levels of CYP2B7 mRNA in lung (134) and in bronchial epithelial cells (161) from smokers and nonsmokers and found no statistically significant difference.

To date, very few inhibition studies relating to CYP2B6 have been carried out. Part of the reason for this has been the lack of a specific substrate, making interpretation of human liver microsome data difficult. With the ready availability of cDNA-expressed CYP2B6, this area is beginning to be investigated. Probably one of the first inhibitors of CYP2B6 to become established, following a description of its effect on cyclophosphamide 4-hydroxylation in human liver microsomes, was orphenadrine (109). This has been shown to inhibit both *S*-mephenytoin *N*-demethylation (132), and 7-EFC *O*-deethylation (125,135) by human liver and recombinant CYP2B6. However, similar concentrations of orphenadrine inhibit other P450s, particularly CYP2D6 (125), and so it cannot be described as specific. Substrates of CYP2B6, such as S-mephenytoin and methoxychlor, can also be used as inhibitors (135), but this approach has limitations, particularly because S-mephenytoin is a substrate of CYP2C19 (162).

Nonspecific inhibitors of CYP2B6 include diethyldithiocarbamate, tranylcypromine, quercetin, ketoconazole, methimazole, SKF-525A, piperonyl butoxide, and high concentrations of α-naphthoflavone (66,121,125, 135). Compounds that have little or no inhibitory effect on CYP2B6 include triacetyloleandomycin, sulfaphenazole, and quinidine (66,121,135).

CYP4A

Two P450 genes, namely CYP4A9 and CYP4A11, have been assigned to the human CYP4A subfamily (163). However, the nature of CYP4A9 is unknown, given that no sequence data are available (163) and no publications relating to CYP4A9 can be found. This section, therefore, deals with the current state of knowledge relating to CYP4A11.

Molecular Biology

The full-length CYP4A11 cDNA was initially isolated from kidney by two independent research groups (164, 165). This sequence shared approximately 80% amino acid similarity with four members of the rabbit CYP4A subfamily. Subsequently, a third group isolated the same clone from liver (166). Despite an assertion from the authors that the liver sequence differs from that in the kidney by one amino acid residue (Ala → Leu at position 144) (166), the two cDNA sequences, as written in the respective publications and as deposited in the GenBank Database, are in fact identical in the coding region apart from a single silent nucleotide change (T → C) at position 1374 (Ile^{458}). A partial CYP4A11 clone has also been isolated from liver by a fourth group (167). The CYP4A11 gene has been assigned to chromosome 1 (167), where it exists in a cluster with the CYP4B1 gene (168).

A variant full-length sequence, termed CYP4A11v, has been found in kidney (165). This cDNA is identical to CYP4A11 apart from a single base deletion at position 1540 in the coding region and eight base changes in the 3'-noncoding region. The frameshift resulting from the single base deletion creates an extended reading frame, generating a protein with an additional 72 C-terminal amino acids, but retaining the key heme-coordinating cysteine residue (165). However, a PCR-based assay failed to detect this variant sequence in DNA from 15 subjects, leading the authors to conclude that CYP4A11v constituted a rare allele (165). Expression of CYP4A11v

in recombinant systems led to the synthesis of an unstable and poorly functional protein (165).

A protein has been purified from human liver (166,169), which, apart from missing the first four amino acid residues, shares the same N-terminal amino acid sequence as CYP4A11. This protein exhibits a molecular weight of 52 kDa on SDS-PAGE—identical to recombinant CYP4A11 expressed in yeast (166) and to a CYP4A protein in human liver (166,169,170) and kidney (171) microsomes, which appears to correspond to CYP4A11. A CYP4A protein of 52 kDa has also been purified by two groups from kidney (172,173). However, the sequence of one of these proteins differs at one position (Ala → Val) from that deduced from the CYP4A11 cDNA.

Ontogeny, Tissue Distribution, and Sexual Differentiation

Little is known about the ontogeny of CYP4A expression in humans, although lauric acid 12-hydroxylase activity, indicative of CYP4A, can be detected in fetal liver microsomes (174). Analysis of infant and adult liver microsomes using an anti–rat CYP4A1 antibody indicated that CYP4A was present less than 24 hours after birth (175). Indeed, levels of CYP4A were found to be generally higher in infants than in adults in this study. Interestingly, sudden infant death syndrome was associated with a significant reduction in CYP4A expression (175).

CYP4A11 mRNA (164,166,167) and protein (166, 170,176) can both be detected in liver. Given that the CYP4A11 cDNA was first isolated from kidney, it is perhaps not surprising that mRNA (164,166,177) and protein (171) can also be detected in kidney, at levels at least as high as those seen in liver. CYP4A in kidney is found in the cortex (178), but the precise localization is still unknown. CYP4A11 mRNA is markedly decreased in renal adenocarcinoma (177), although it appears to increase in the cells immediately surrounding the tumor (177) compared with normal kidney. CYP4A11 mRNA is not expressed in lung, skin, colon, ileum, small intestine, stomach, mammary artery, cervix, ovary, uterus, testes, or adrenal (164).

To date, there is no evidence for any effect of gender on CYP4A expression in humans. No significant differences between male and female subjects have been found in lauric acid ω-hydroxylase activity in liver (170,176) and kidney (171) microsomes.

Interindividual Variability

The degree of interindividual variability in CYP4A11 expression appears to be less than that seen with certain other P450s. Microsomal lauric acid ω-hydroxylase activity varies only up to 11-fold between individuals

(Table 12-4), and a similar variability has been observed for immunoquantified microsomal CYP4A protein (169–171,176).

Substrates

The activity most commonly associated with CYP4A is the ω- or 12-hydroxylation of lauric acid. However, until recently, it had proved difficult to demonstrate a clear association between this activity and CYP4A11 in human liver microsomes. For example, two studies found virtually no correlation between laurate ω-hydroxylase activity and CYP4A protein detected immunochemically using anti–rat CYP4A antibodies (170,176). Despite this lack of correlation, the same antibody was able to immunoinhibit lauric acid ω-hydroxylation in liver microsomes by 60% to 65% (170), suggesting either that the reaction was catalyzed by another human CYP4A protein that was not detected by the anti–rat CYP4A antibody, or that the antibody was not specific.

Analysis of the ω-hydroxylation of lauric acid by human liver microsomes revealed biphasic kinetics for seven of the eight livers tested (179). The high-affinity component ($K_m = 22 \pm 12$ µM) did not correlate with levels of CYP 1A2, 2A6, 2C, 2D6, 2E1, or 3A, and was presumed to be catalyzed by CYP4A. The low-affinity component ($K_m = 550 \pm 310$ µM) was highly correlated ($r = 0.97$) with cyclosporine oxidation, indicative of CYP3A. It was therefore suggested that the lack of correlation seen between immunodetectable CYP4A and laurate ω-hydroxylation was due to the contribution of CYP3A to this activity (179). More recently, however, links have been found between immunodetectable CYP4A and laurate ω-hydroxylation. In one study, using specific anti-CYP4A11 IgG, immunodetectable CYP4A was found to correlate highly ($r = 0.89$) with this activity in liver microsomes, and immunoinhibition of 80% to 85% could be achieved (169). In a second study, CYP4A protein measured in kidney microsomes using anti–rat CYP4A antibody was also shown to correlate ($r = 0.86$) with laurate ω-hydroxylase activity (171), and immunoinhibition of 60% was observed.

Most convincing are the data obtained using purified and recombinant systems (Table 12-5). The two CYP4A proteins purified from liver, with identical N-terminal amino acid sequences to CYP4A11, both catalyze the ω-hydroxylation of lauric acid (166,169), as does recombinant CYP4A11 expressed in *E. coli* (164), insect cells and COS-7 cells (165), and *S. cerevisiae* (166). Finally, the specificity of this reaction for CYP4A has been demonstrated using a panel of purified yeast-expressed P450s, with no activity being detected with CYP 2A6, 2B6, 2C8, 2C9, 2C18, 2D6, or 2E1 (17).

Although hydroxylation at the ω-position is strongly preferred, CYP4A11 also catalyzes the (ω-1)- or 11-hydroxylation of lauric acid (see Table 12-5). However, data obtained using both purified human liver P450s (169) and purified recombinant P450s (17) show that this reaction is also catalyzed by CYP2C9 and CYP2E1. Indeed, lauric acid (ω-1)-hydroxylation has been proposed as a specific marker for CYP2E1 (170,179,180).

Another activity expected to be catalyzed by human CYP4A is the ω-hydroxylation of arachidonic acid, given that CYP4A proteins from other animal species, such as rat CYP4A2 (181) and rabbit CYP4A4, CYP4A6, and CYP4A7 (182) perform this reaction. The metabolite formed by this process, 20-hydroxyeicosatetraenoic acid, is particularly interesting, because it has been implicated in a number of physiologic processes, such as renal function (183,184) and the control of vascular tone (185), and it is produced *in vivo*, in that it can be detected as a glucuronide conjugate in human urine (186).

However, data concerning the role of CYP4A11 in the ω-hydroxylation of arachidonic acid are somewhat contradictory. For example, recombinant CYP4A11 catalyzes this reaction when expressed in *E. coli* (164), but not when expressed in insect cells (165) or yeast (166). This may reflect the different lipid environments encountered by the P450 in each of the expression hosts. Interestingly, a similar effect has been observed with the human liver leukotriene B_4 ω-hydroxylase CYP4F2 (187), which apparently catalyzes arachidonate ω-hydroxylation when expressed in insect cells (188), but not when expressed in yeast (187). Another paper discusses a meet-

TABLE 12-4. *Lauric acid ω-hydroxylase activity in human liver and kidney microsomes*

Tissue source	n	Activity (nmol/min/mg protein)	Fold variation	Ref.
Liver	7	0.86–3.52	4.1	178
Liver	13	0.60–1.95	3.3	176
Liver	8	0.63–3.67[a,b]	5.8	179
Liver	5	0.8–4.1[a]	5.1	180
Liver	14	0.83–1.40	1.7	170
Liver	11	1.2 ± 0.4		169
Kidney	7	0.10–0.28	2.8	178
Kidney	18	0.51–5.78	11.3	171

[a]Denotes V_{max} values
[b]Low K_m component only

TABLE 12-5. *Lauric acid ω and (ω-1) hydroxylation by purified and recombinant CYP4A11*

Protein	Source	[laurate] (µM)	−b_5			+b_5			Ref.
			ω	(ω − 1)	ω/(ω − 1)	ω	(ω − 1)	ω/(ω − 1)	
Purified	Kidney	400	13.1	0.5	26	25.1	1.0	25	172
Purified[a]	Kidney	167				4.06	0.24	17	173
Purified	Liver	100				1.8	0.4	4.5	166
Purified	Liver	100	16.1	1.8	8.9	45.7	5.4	8.5	169
Recombinant	Kidney	400	10.11[b]	0.99[b]	10				165
Recombinant	Kidney	25	4.0	0.27	15	9.8	0.51	19	164
Recombinant	Liver	100	14.8[b]	1.0[b]	15				166

[a]Different N-terminal amino-acid sequence from CYP4A11.
[b]Addition of cytochrome b_5 had no effect on activity.
Activities are expressed as nmol product formed/min/nmol P450.

ing abstract that discloses that purified liver CYP4A11 catalyzes arachidonate ω-hydroxylation (169). Furthermore, correlations have been found between arachidonate ω-hydroxylase and both immunodetectable CYP4A ($r = 0.75$) and laurate ω-hydroxylase ($r = 0.68$) in human kidney (171). Finally, the decreased levels of CYP4A11 mRNA seen in renal adenocarcinoma are mirrored by a decrease in arachidonate ω-hydroxylase activity (177). Taken together, these data indicate that the ω-hydroxylation of arachidonic acid probably is catalyzed by CYP4A in humans, but exactly which proteins are involved remains a matter of contention.

Human CYP4A enzymes presumably also play a role in the ω-hydroxylation of other simple fatty acids, as well as prostaglandins, but as with arachidonate, the data are contradictory. For example, palmitic acid is ω-hydroxylated by recombinant CYP4A11 when expressed in *E. coli* (164), but not when expressed in yeast (166). However, a purified kidney CYP4A protein, with one amino acid change from CYP4A11 in the N-terminal sequence, does catalyze this activity (173). Given the current confusion regarding the involvement of particular human CYP4A proteins in these various reactions, it is wise to leave the discussion of substrate specificity to a future date.

Inducers and Inhibitors

The mechanism of induction most commonly associated with proteins of the CYP4A subfamily is that caused by peroxisome proliferators (189–192), acting through the peroxisome proliferator–activated receptor, or PPAR (193–196). Recombinant human PPARα has been shown to be an efficient *trans*-activator of genes containing the PPAR response element, such as rabbit CYP4A6 (197), and yet humans seem to be refractory to the effects of peroxisome proliferators (198). One possible explanation for this discrepancy may be that there is a much lower level of PPARα in human liver compared with mouse liver (199).

The mechanism-based suicide inhibitors 11-dodecynoic acid and 10-undecynoic acid inhibit lauric acid hydroxylation in rat liver microsomes (200). Their mode of action suggests that they are also likely to inhibit CYP4A in man, although this has not yet been tested. Both compounds, however, inhibit (ω-1)-hydroxylation as well as ω-hydroxylation, suggesting that CYP2E1 may be affected, although this requires confirmation. Among the more commonly used inhibitors of P450, ketoconazole, furafylline, quinidine, sulfaphenazole, diethyldithiocarbamate (179), and metyrapone (178) have no significant effect on hepatic CYP4A activity, but SKF-525A is reported to be a specific inhibitor of hepatic CYP4A, having no effect on laurate ω-hydroxylation in the kidney (178).

ACKNOWLEDGMENT

The authors would like to acknowledge financial support from the Imperial Cancer Research Fund (CRW), the Biotechnology and Biological Sciences Research Council, the UK Department of Trade and Industry, and the LINK consortium of pharmaceutical companies: Astra, Glaxo-Wellcome, Janssen Pharmaceutica, Lilly, Novo Nordisk, Parke-Davis, Pfizer, Roche Products, Sanofi-Winthrop, Servier, Smith-Kline Beecham, Wyeth-Ayerst, and Zeneca.

REFERENCES

1. Phillips IR, Shephard EA, Ashworth A, Rabin BR. Isolation and sequence of a human cytochrome P-450 cDNA clone. *Proc Natl Acad Sci USA* 1985;82:983–987.
2. Nebert DW, Nelson DR, Coon MJ, et al. The P450 superfamily: update on new sequences, gene mapping, and recommended nomenclature. *DNA Cell Biol* 1991;10:1–14.
3. Miles JS, Bickmore W, Brook JD, McLaren AW, Meehan R, Wolf CR. Close linkage of the human cytochrome P450IIA and P450IIB gene subfamilies: implications for the assignment of substrate specificity. *Nucl Acids Res* 1989;17:2907–2917.
4. Yamano S, Nagata K, Yamazoe Y, Kato R, Gelboin HV, Gonzalez FJ. cDNA and deduced amino acid sequences of human P450 IIA3 (CYP2A3). *Nucl Acids Res* 1989;17:4888.

5. Crespi CL, Penman BW, Leakey JA, et al. Human cytochrome P450IIA3: cDNA sequence, role of the enzyme in the metabolic activation of promutagens, comparison to nitrosamine activation by human cytochrome P450IIE1. *Carcinogenesis* 1990;11:1293–1300.

6. Maurice M, Emiliani S, Dalet Beluche I, Derancourt J, Lange R. Isolation and characterization of a cytochrome P450 of the IIA subfamily from human liver microsomes. *Eur J Biochem* 1991;200:511–517.

7. Yun CH, Shimada T, Guengerich FP. Purification and characterization of human liver microsomal cytochrome P-450 2A6. *Mol Pharmacol* 1991;40:679–685.

8. Yamano S, Tatsuno J, Gonzalez FJ. The CYP2A3 gene product catalyzes coumarin 7-hydroxylation in human liver microsomes. *Biochemistry* 1990;29:1322–1329.

9. Miles JS, McLaren AW, Forrester LM, Glancey MJ, Lang MA, Wolf CR. Identification of the human liver cytochrome P-450 responsible for coumarin 7-hydroxylase activity. *Biochem J* 1990;267:365–371.

10. Ding S, Lake BG, Friedberg T, Wolf CR. Expression and alternative splicing of the cytochrome P-450 CYP2A7. *Biochem J* 1995;306: 161–166.

11. Tiano HF, Hosokawa M, Chulada PC, et al. Retroviral mediated expression of human cytochrome P450 2A6 in C3H/10T1/2 cells confers transformability by 4-(methylnitrosamino)-1-(3-pyridyl)-1-butanone (NNK). *Carcinogenesis* 1993;14:1421–1427.

12. Salonpää P, Hakkola J, Pasanen M, et al. Retrovirus-mediated stable expression of human CYP2A6 in mammalian cells. *Eur J Pharmacol* 1993;248:95–102.

13. Nanji M, Clair P, Shephard EA, Phillips IR. Expression in a baculovirus system of a cDNA encoding human CYP2A6. *Biochem Soc Trans* 1994;22:122s.

14. Liu C, Zhuo X, Gonzalez FJ, Ding X. Baculovirus-mediated expression and characterization of rat CYP2A3 and human CYP2A6: role in metabolic activation of nasal toxicants. *Mol Pharmacol* 1996;50: 781–788.

15. Chen L, Buters JTM, Hardwick JP, et al. Coexpression of cytochrome P4502A6 and human NADPH-P450 oxidoreductase in the baculovirus system. *Drug Metab Dispos* 1997;25:399–405.

16. Street JC, Lee JS, Jarema MAC. Study of coumarin metabolism by Chinese hamster lung fibroblasts expressing a human cytochrome P450 using ^{1}H-nmr. *Xenobiotica* 1996;26:447–457.

17. Imaoka S, Yamada T, Hiroi T, et al. Multiple forms of human P450 expressed in *Saccharomyces cerevisiae*. Systematic characterization and comparison with those of the rat. *Biochem Pharmacol* 1996;51: 1041–1050.

18. Pritchard MP, Ossetian R, Li DN, et al. A general strategy for the expression of recombinant human cytochrome P450s in *Escherichia coli* using bacterial signal peptides: expression of CYP3A4, CYP2A6 and CYP2E1. *Arch Biochem Biophys* 1997;345:342–354.

19. Davis MB, West LF, Shephard EA, Phillips IR. Regional localization of a human cytochrome P450 (CYP1) to chromosome 19q13.1-13.3. *Ann Hum Genet* 1986;50:237–240.

20. Miles JS, Spurr NK, Gough AC, et al. A novel human cytochrome P450 gene (P450IIB): chromosomal localization and evidence for alternative splicing. *Nucl Acids Res* 1988;16:5783–5795.

21. Santisteban I, Povey S, Shephard EA, Phillips IR. The major phenobarbital-inducible cytochrome P-450 gene subfamily (P450IIB) mapped to the long arm of human chromosome 19. *Ann Hum Genet* 1988;52:129–135.

22. Bale AE, Mitchell AL, Gonzalez FJ, McBride OW. Localization of CYP2F1 multipoint linkage analysis and pulse-field gel electrophoresis. *Genomics* 1991;10:284–286.

23. Hoffman SM, Fernandez Salguero P, Gonzalez FJ, Mohrenweiser HW. Organization and evolution of the cytochrome P450 CYP2A-2B-2F subfamily gene cluster on human chromosome 19. *J Mol Evol* 1995; 41:894–900.

24. Fernandez-Salguero P, Gonzalez FJ. The CYP2A gene subfamily: species differences, regulation, catalytic activities and role in chemical carcinogenesis. *Pharmacogenetics* 1995;5:S123–128.

25. Fernandez-Salguero P, Hoffman SMG, Cholerton S, et al. A genetic polymorphism in coumarin 7-hydroxylation: sequence of the human CYP2A genes and identification of variant CYP2A6 alleles. *Am J Hum Genet* 1995;57:651–660.

26. Walsh KV, Harley HG, Brook JD, et al. Linkage relationships of the apolipoprotein C1 gene and a cytochrome P450 gene (CYP2A) to myotonic dystrophy. *Hum Genet* 1990;85:305–310.

27. Oscarson M, Gullstén H, Rautio A, et al. Genotyping of human cytochrome P450 2A6 (CYP2A6), a nicotine C-oxidase. *FEBS Lett* 1998;438:201–205.

28. Oscarson M, McLellan RA, Gullstén H, et al. Identification and characterisation of novel polymorphisms in the CYP2A locus: implications for nicotine metabolism. *FEBS Lett* 1999;460:321–327.

29. Shimada T, Yamazaki H, Mimura M, Inui Y, Guengerich FP. Interindividual variations in human liver cytochrome P-450 enzymes involved in the oxidation of drugs, carcinogens and toxic chemicals: studies with liver microsomes of 30 Japanese and 30 caucasians. *J Pharmacol Exp Ther* 1994;270:414–423.

30. Shimada T, Yamazaki H, Guengerich FP. Ethnic-related differences in coumarin 7-hydroxylation activities catalyzed by cytochrome P4502A6 in liver microsomes of Japanese and caucasian populations. *Xenobiotica* 1996;26:395–403.

31. Mäenpää J, Rane A, Raunio H, Honkakoski P, Pelkonen O. Cytochrome P450 isoforms in human fetal tissues related to phenobarbital-inducible forms in the mouse. *Biochem Pharmacol* 1993;45:899–907.

32. Hakkola J, Pasanen M, Purkunen R, et al. Expression of xenobiotic-metabolizing cytochrome P450 forms in human adult and fetal liver. *Biochem Pharmacol* 1994;48:59–64.

33. Shimada T, Yamazaki H, Mimura M, et al. Characterization of microsomal cytochrome P450 enzymes involved in the oxidation of xenobiotic chemicals in human fetal liver and adult lungs. *Drug Metab Dispos* 1996;24:515–522.

34. Pearce R, Greenway D, Parkinson A. Species differences and interindividual variation in liver microsomal cytochrome P450 2A enzymes: effects on coumarin, dicumarol, and testosterone oxidation. *Arch Biochem Biophys* 1992;298:211–225.

35. Sotaniemi EA, Lumme P, Arvela P, Rautio A. Age and CYP3A4 and CYP2A6 activities marked by the metabolism of lignocaine and coumarin in man. *Therapie* 1996;51:363–366.

36. Iscan M, Rostami H, Iscan M, Guray T, Pelkonen O, Rautio A. Interindividual variability of coumarin 7-hydroxylation in a Turkish population. *Eur J Clin Pharmacol* 1994;47:315–318.

37. Palmer CN, Coates PJ, Davies SE, Shephard EA, Phillips IR. Localization of cytochrome P-450 gene expression in normal and diseased human liver by in situ hybridization of wax-embedded archival material. *Hepatology* 1992;16:682–687.

38. Kirby GM, Batist G, Alpert L, Lamoureux E, Cameron RG, Alaoui Jamali MA. Overexpression of cytochrome P-450 isoforms involved in aflatoxin B1 bioactivation in human liver with cirrhosis and hepatitis. *Toxicol Pathol* 1996;24:458–467.

39. Satarug S, Lang MA, Yongvanit P, et al. Induction of cytochrome P450 2A6 expression in humans by the carcinogenic parasite infection, opisthorchiasis viverrini. *Cancer Epidemiol Biomarkers Prev* 1996;5: 795–800.

40. Kirby GM, Wolf CR, Neal GE, et al. In vitro metabolism of aflatoxin B1 by normal and tumorous liver tissue from Thailand. *Carcinogenesis* 1993;14:2613–2620.

41. Pelkonen O, Moilanen ML. The specificity and multiplicity of human placental xenobiotic-metabolizing monooxygenase system studied by potential substrates, inhibitors and gel electrophoresis. *Med Biol* 1979;57:306–312.

42. Hakkola J, Pasanen M, Hukkanen J, et al. Expression of xenobiotic-metabolizing cytochrome P450 forms in human full-term placenta. *Biochem Pharmacol* 1996;51:403–411.

43. Hakkola J, Raunio H, Purkunen R, et al. Detection of cytochrome P450 gene expression in human placenta in first trimester of pregnancy. *Biochem Pharmacol* 1996;52:379–383.

44. Kharasch ED, Hankins DC, Thummel KE. Human kidney methoxyflurane and sevoflurane metabolism. Intrarenal fluoride production as a possible mechanism of methoxyflurane nephrotoxicity. *Anesthesiology* 1995;82:689–699.

45. Degawa M, Stern SJ, Martin MV, et al. Metabolic activation and carcinogen-DNA adduct detection in human larynx. *Cancer Res* 1994; 54:4915–4919.

46. Getchell ML, Chen Y, Ding X, Sparks DL, Getchell TV. Immunohistochemical localization of a cytochrome P-450 isozyme in human nasal mucosa: age-related trends. *Ann Otol Rhinol Laryngol* 1993; 102:368–374.

47. Su T, Sheng JJ, Lipinskas TW, Ding X. Expression of CYP2A genes in rodent and human nasal mucosa. *Drug Metab Dispos* 1996;24: 884–890.

48. Ding X, Spink DC, Bhama JK, Sheng JJ, Vaz AD, Coon MJ. Metabolic activation of 2,6-dichlorobenzonitrile, an olfactory-specific toxicant, by rat, rabbit, and human cytochromes P450. *Mol Pharmacol* 1996; 49:1113–1121.

49. Farin FM, Bigler LG, Oda D, McDougall JK, Omiecinski CJ. Expression of cytochrome P450 and microsomal epoxide hydrolase in cervical and oral epithelial cells immortalized by human papillomavirus type 16 E6/E7 genes. *Carcinogenesis* 1995;16:1391–1401.

50. Rautio A, Kraul H, Kojo A, Salmela E, Pelkonen O. Interindividual variability of coumarin 7-hydroxylation in healthy volunteers. *Pharmacogenetics* 1992;2:227–233.

51. Cashman JR, Park SB, Yang ZC, Wrighton SA, Jacob PD, Benowitz NL. Metabolism of nicotine by human liver microsomes: stereoselective formation of trans-nicotine N'-oxide. *Chem Res Toxicol* 1992;5: 639–646.

52. Forrester LM, Henderson CJ, Glancey MJ, et al. Relative expression of cytochrome P450 isoenzymes in human liver and association with the metabolism of drugs and xenobiotics. *Biochem J* 1992;281:359–368.

53. Sotaniemi EA, Rautio A, Bäckstrom M, Arvela P, Pelkonen O. CYP3A4 and CYP2A6 activities marked by the metabolism of lignocaine and coumarin in patients with liver and kidney diseases and epileptic patients. *Br J Clin Pharmac* 1995;39:71–76.

54. Kraul H, Truckenbrodt J, Otto A, Brix R, Hoffman A. Elimination of coumarin (Venalot) in patients with different degrees of liver disease. *Naunyn-Schmiedeberg's Arch Pharmacol* 1991;344:R95.

55. Kratz F. Coumarin-7-hydroxylase activity in microsomes from needle biopsies of normal and diseased human liver. *Eur J Clin Pharmacol* 1976;10:133–137.

56. Pasanen M, Rannala Z, Tooming A, Sotaniemi EA, Pelkonen O, Rautio A. Hepatitis A impairs the function of human hepatic CYP2A6 *in vivo*. *Toxicology* 1997;123:177–184.

57. Pelkonen O, Pasanen M, Kuha H, et al. The effect of cigarette smoking on 7-ethoxyresorufin O-deethylase and other monooxygenase activities in human liver: analyses with monoclonal antibodies. *Br J Clin Pharmacol* 1986;22:125–134.

58. Merkel U, Sigusch H, Hoffmann A. Grapefruit juice inhibits 7-hydroxylation of coumarin in healthy volunteers. *Eur J Clin Pharmacol* 1994;46:175–177.

59. Runkel M, Tegtmeier M, Legrum W. Metabolic and analytical interactions of grapefruit juice and 1,2-benzopyrone (coumarin) in man. *Eur J Clin Pharmacol* 1996;50:225–230.

60. Rauma AL, Rautio A, Pasanen M, Pelkonen O, Törrönen R, Mykkänen H. Coumarin 7-hydroxylation in long-term adherents of a strict uncooked vegan diet. *Eur J Clin Pharmacol* 1996;50:133–137.

61. Chang TKH, Waxman DJ. The CYP2A subfamily. In: Ioannides C, ed. *The CYP2A subfamily*. Boca Raton: CRC Press, 1996:99–134.

62. Dalet-Beluche I, Boulenc X, Fabre G, Maurel P, Bonfils C. Purification of two cytochrome P450 isozymes related to CYP2A and CYP3A gene families from monkey (baboon, *Papio papio*) liver microsomes. Cross reactivity with human forms. *Eur J Biochem* 1992;204: 641–648.

63. Raunio H, Syngelma T, Pasanen M, et al. Immunochemical and catalytical studies on hepatic coumarin 7-hydroxylase in man, rat, and mouse. *Biochem Pharmacol* 1988;37:3889–3895.

64. Raunio H, Valtonen J, Honkakoski P, et al. Immunochemical detection of human liver cytochrome P450 forms related to phenobarbital-inducible forms in the mouse. *Biochem Pharmacol* 1990;40: 2503–2509.

65. Waxman DJ, Lapenson DP, Aoyama T, Gelboin HV, Gonzalez FJ, Korzekwa K. Steroid hormone hydroxylase specificities of eleven cDNA-expressed human cytochrome P450s. *Arch Biochem Biophys* 1991;290:160–166.

66. Ono S, Hatanaka T, Hotta H, Satoh T, Gonzalez FJ, Tsutsui M. Specificity of substrate and inhibitor probes for cytochrome P450s: evaluation of in vitro metabolism using cDNA-expressed human P450s and human liver microsomes. *Xenobiotica* 1996;26:681–693.

67. Egan D, O'Kennedy R, Moran E, Cox D, Prosser E, Thornes RD. The pharmacology, metabolism, analysis, and applications of coumarin and coumarin-related compounds. *Drug Metab Rev* 1990;22:503–529.

68. Fentem JH, Fry JR. Species differences in the metabolism and hepatotoxicity of coumarin. *Comp Biochem Physiol C* 1993;104:1–8.

69. Cox D, O'Kennedy R, Thornes RD. The rarity of liver toxicity in patients treated with coumarin (1,2-benzopyrone). *Hum Toxicol* 1989; 8:501–506.

70. Shilling WH, Crampton RF, Longland RC. Metabolism of coumarin in man. *Nature* 1969;221:664–665.

71. van Iersel ML, Henderson CJ, Walters DG, Price RJ, Wolf CR, Lake BG. Metabolism of [3-14C] coumarin by human liver microsomes. *Xenobiotica* 1994;24:795–803.

72. Moran E, O'Kennedy R, Thornes RD. Analysis of coumarin and its urinary metabolites by high-performance liquid chromatography. *J Chromatogr* 1987;416:165–169.

73. Cholerton S, Idle ME, Vas A, Gonzalez FJ, Idle JR. Comparison of a novel thin-layer chromatographic-fluorescence detection method with a spectrofluorometric method for the determination of 7-hydroxy-coumarin in human urine. *J Chromatogr* 1992;575:325–330.

74. Mäenpää J, Sigusch H, Raunio H, et al. Differential inhibition of coumarin 7-hydroxylase activity in mouse and human liver microsomes. *Biochem Pharmacol* 1993;45:1035–1042.

75. Honkakoski P, Arvela P, Juvonen R, Lang MA, Kairaluoma M, Pelkonen O. Human and mouse liver coumarin 7-hydroxylases do not metabolize warfarin in vitro. *Br J Clin Pharmac* 1992;33:313–317.

76. Draper AJ, Madan A, Parkinson A. Inhibition of coumarin 7-hydroxylase activity in human liver microsomes. *Arch Biochem Biophys* 1997; 341:47–61.

77. Berkman CE, Park SB, Wrighton SA, Cashman JR. In vitro-in vivo correlations of human (S)-nicotine metabolism. *Biochem Pharmacol* 1995;50:565–570.

78. Nakajima M, Yamamoto T, Nunoya K-I, et al. Role of human cytochrome P4502A6 in C-oxidation of nicotine. *Drug Metab Dispos* 1996;24:1212–1217.

79. Messina ES, Tyndale RF, Sellers EM. A major role for CYP2A6 in nicotine C-oxidation by human liver microsomes. *J Pharmacol Exp Ther* 1997;282:1608–1614.

80. Flammang AM, Gelboin HV, Aoyama T, Gonzalez FJ, McCoy GD. Nicotine metabolism by cDNA-expressed human cytochrome P-450s. *Biochem Arch* 1992;8:1–8.

81. Nakajima M, Yamamoto T, Nunoya K, et al. Characterization of CYP2A6 involved in 3'-hydroxylation of cotinine in human liver microsomes. *J Pharmacol Exp Ther* 1996;277:1010–1015.

82. Patten CJ, Smith TJ, Friesen MJ, Tynes RE, Yang CS, Murphy SE. Evidence for cytochrome P450 2A6 and 3A4 as major catalysts for N'-nitroso-nornicotine α-hydroxylation by human liver microsomes. *Carcinogenesis* 1997;18:1623–1630.

83. Smith TJ, Guo Z, Gonzalez FJ, Guengerich FP, Stoner GD, Yang CS. Metabolism of 4-(methylnitrosamino)-1-(3-pyridyl)-1-butanone in human lung and liver microsomes and cytochromes P-450 expressed in hepatoma cells. *Cancer Res* 1992;52:1757–1763.

84. Yamazaki H, Inui Y, Yun CH, Guengerich FP, Shimada T. Cytochrome P450 2E1 and 2A6 enzymes as major catalysts for metabolic activation of N-nitrosodialkylamines and tobacco-related nitrosamines in human liver microsomes. *Carcinogenesis* 1992;13:1789–1794.

85. Nesnow S, Beck S, Rosenblum S, et al. N-nitrosodiethylamine and 4-(methylnitrosamino)-1-(3-pyridyl)-1-butanone induced morphological transformation of C3H/10T1/2CL8 cells expressing human cytochrome P450 2A6. *Mutat Res* 1994;324:93–102.

86. Smith TJ, Stoner GD, Yang CS. Activation of 4-(methylnitrosamino)-1-(3-pyridyl)-1-butanone (NNK) in human lung microsomes by cytochromes P450, lipoxygenase, and hydroperoxides. *Cancer Res* 1995;55:5566-5573.

87. Patten CJ, Smith TJ, Murphy SE, et al. Kinetic analysis of the activation of 4-(methylnitrosamino)-1-(3-pyridyl)-1-butanone by heterologously expressed human P450 enzymes and the effect of P450-specific chemical inhibitors on this activation in human liver microsomes. *Arch Biochem Biophys* 1996;333:127–138.

88. Camus AM, Geneste O, Honkakoski P, et al. High variability of nitrosamine metabolism among individuals: role of cytochromes P450 2A6 and 2E1 in the dealkylation of N-nitrosodimethylamine and N-nitrosodiethylamine in mice and humans. *Mol Carcinog* 1993;7:268–275.

89. Reigh G, McMahon H, Ishizaki M, et al. Cytochrome P450 species involved in the metabolism of quinoline. *Carcinogenesis* 1996;17: 1989–1996.

90. Torchin CD, McNeilly PJ, Kapetanovic IM, Strong JM, Kupferberg HJ. Stereoselective metabolism of a new anticonvulsant drug candidate, losigamone, by human liver microsomes. *Drug Metab Dispos* 1996;24:1002–1008.

91. Nunoya K, Yokoi Y, Kimura K, et al. (+)-cis-3,5-dimethyl-2-(3-pyridyl) thiazolidin-4-one hydrochloride (SM-12502) as a novel sub-

strate for cytochrome P450 2A6 in human liver microsomes. *J Pharmacol Exp Ther* 1996;277:768–774.

92. Sadeque AJM, Fisher MB, Korzekwa KR, Gonzalez FJ, Rettie AE. Human CYP2C9 and CYP2A6 mediate formation of the hepatotoxin 4-ene-valproic acid. *J Pharmacol Exp Ther* 1997;283:698–703.

93. Madan A, Parkinson A, Faiman MD. Identification of the human and rat P450 enzymes responsible for the sulfoxidation of S-methyl N,N-diethylthiolcarbamate (DETC-ME). The terminal step in the bioactivation of disulfiram. *Drug Metab Dispos* 1995;23:1153–1162.

94. Spracklin DK, Thummel KE, Kharasch ED. Human reductive halothane metabolism in vitro is catalyzed by cytochrome P450 2A6 and 3A4. *Drug Metab Dispos* 1996;24:976–983.

95. Sharer JE, Wrighton SA. Identification of the human hepatic cytochromes P450 involved in the in vitro oxidation of antipyrine. *Drug Metab Dispos* 1996;24:487–494.

96. Engel G, Hofmann U, Heidemann H, Cosme J, Eichelbaum M. Antipyrine as a probe for human oxidative drug metabolism: identification of the cytochrome P450 enzymes catalyzing 4-hydroxyantipyrine, 3-hydroxymethylantipyrine, and norantipyrine formation. *Clin Pharmac Ther* 1996;59:613–623.

97. Yun CH, Shimada T, Guengerich FP. Contributions of human liver cytochrome P450 enzymes to the N-oxidation of 4,4′-methylene-bis(2-chloroaniline). *Carcinogenesis* 1992;13:217–222.

98. Aoyama T, Yamano S, Guzelian PS, Gelboin HV, Gonzalez FJ. Five of 12 forms of vaccinia virus-expressed human hepatic cytochrome P450 metabolically activate aflatoxin B1. *Proc Natl Acad Sci U S A* 1990; 87:4790–4793.

99. Code EL, Crespi CL, Penman BW, Gonzalez FJ, Chang TKH, Waxman DJ. Human cytochrome P4502B6. Interindividual hepatic expression, substrate specificity, and role in procarcinogen activation. *Drug Metab Dispos* 1997;25:985–993.

100. Mace K, Aguilar F, Wang J-S, et al. Aflatoxin B1-induced DNA adduct formation and p53 mutations in CYP450-expressing human liver cell lines. *Carcinogenesis* 1997;18:1291–1297.

101. Forrester LM, Neal GE, Judah DJ, Glancey MJ, Wolf CR. Evidence for involvement of multiple forms of cytochrome P-450 in aflatoxin B₁ metabolism in human liver. *Proc Natl Acad Sci USA* 1990;87: 8306–8310.

102. Duescher RJ, Elfarra AA. Human liver microsomes are efficient catalysts of 1,3-butadiene oxidation: evidence for major roles by cytochromes P450 2A6 and 2E1. *Arch Biochem Biophys* 1994;311: 342–349.

103. Elfarra AA, Krause RJ, Selzer RR. Biochemistry of 1,3-butadiene metabolism and its relevance to 1,3-butadiene-induced carcinogenicity. *Toxicology* 1996;113:23–30.

104. Krause RJ, Elfarra AA. Oxidation of butadiene monoxide to *meso*- and (+)-diepoxybutane by cDNA-expressed human cytochrome P450s and by mouse, rat, and human liver microsomes: evidence for preferential hydration of *meso* diepoxybutane in rat and human liver microsomes. *Arch Biochem Biophys* 1997;337:176–184.

105. Flammang AM, Gelboin HV, Aoyama T, Gonzalez FJ, McCoy GD. N-nitrosopyrrolidine metabolism by cDNA-expressed human cytochrome P-450s. *Biochem Arch* 1993;9:197–204.

106. Wormhoudt LW, Ploemen JH, de Waziers I, et al. Inter-individual variability in the oxidation of 1,2-dibromoethane: use of heterologously expressed human cytochrome P450 and human liver microsomes. *Chem Biol Interact* 1996;101:175–192.

107. Jones BC, Tyman CA, Smith DA. Identification of the cytochrome P450 isoforms involved in the O-demethylation of 4-nitroanisole in human liver microsomes. *Xenobiotica* 1997;27:1025–1037.

108. Hong JY, Yang CS, Lee M, et al. Role of cytochromes P450 in the metabolism of methyl tert-butyl ether in human livers. *Arch Toxicol* 1997;71:266–269.

109. Chang TK, Weber GF, Crespi CL, Waxman DJ. Differential activation of cyclophosphamide and ifosphamide by cytochromes P-450 2B and 3A in human liver microsomes. *Cancer Res* 1993;53:5629–5637.

110. Butler AM, Murray M. Biotransformation of parathion in human liver: participation of CYP3A4 and its inactivation during microsomal parathion oxidation. *J Pharmacol Exp Ther* 1997;280:966–973.

111. Yamazaki H, Inoue K, Mimura M, Oda Y, Guengerich FP, Shimada T. 7-Ethoxycoumarin O-deethylation catalyzed by cytochromes P450 1A2 and 2E1 in human liver microsomes. *Biochem Pharmacol* 1996; 51:313–319.

112. Yamazaki H, Mimura M, Sugahara C, Shimada T. Catalytic roles of rat and human cytochrome P450 2A enzymes in testosterone 7 alpha- and coumarin 7-hydroxylations. *Biochem Pharmacol* 1994;48:1524–1527.

113. Lewis DF, Lake BG. Molecular modelling of members of the P4502A subfamily: application to studies of enzyme specificity. *Xenobiotica* 1995;25:585–598.

114. Pelkonen O, Sotaniemi EA, Ahokas JT. Coumarin 7-hydroxylase activity in human liver microsomes. Properties of the enzyme and interspecies comparisons. *Br J Clin Pharmacol* 1985;19:59–66.

115. Mäenpää J, Juvonen R, Raunio H, Rautio A, Pelkonen O. Metabolic interactions of methoxsalen and coumarin in humans and mice. *Biochem Pharmacol* 1994;48:1363–1369.

116. Inaba T, Jurima M, Mahon WA, Kalow W. *In vitro* inhibition studies of two isozymes of human liver cytochrome P-450. *Drug Metab Dispos* 1985;13:443–448.

117. Kinonen T, Pasanen M, Gynther J, et al. Competitive inhibition of coumarin 7-hydroxylation by pilocarpine and its interaction with mouse CYP 2A5 and human CYP 2A6. *Br J Pharmacol* 1995;116: 2625–2630.

118. Bourrié M, Meunier V, Berger Y, Fabre G. Cytochrome P450 isoform inhibitors as a tool for the investigation of metabolic reactions catalyzed by human liver microsomes. *J Pharmacol Exp Ther* 1996;277: 321–332.

119. Kimonen T, Juvonen RO, Alhava E, Pasanen M. The inhibition of CYP enzymes in mouse and human liver by pilocarpine. *Br J Pharmacol* 1995;114:832–836.

120. Maurice M, Pichard L, Daujat M, et al. Effects of imidazole derivatives on cytochromes P450 from human hepatocytes in primary culture. *FASEB J* 1992;6:752–758.

121. Chang TK, Gonzalez FJ, Waxman DJ. Evaluation of triacetyloleandomycin, alpha-naphthoflavone and diethyldithiocarbamate as selective chemical probes for inhibition of human cytochromes P450. *Arch Biochem Biophys* 1994;311:437–442.

122. Koop DR. Oxidative and reductive metabolism by cytochrome P450 2E1. *FASEB J* 1992;6:724–730.

123. Yun CH, Jeong HG, Jhoun JW, Guengerich FP. Non-specific inhibition of cytochrome P450 activities by chlorophyllin in human and rat liver microsomes. *Carcinogenesis* 1995;16:1437–1440.

124. Puurunen J, Sotaniemi E, Pelkonen O. Effect of cimetidine on microsomal drug metabolism in man. *Eur J Clin Pharmac* 1980;18: 185–187.

125. Guo Z, Raeissi S, White RB, Stevens JC. Orphenadrine and methimazole inhibit multiple cytochrome P450 enzymes in human liver microsomes. *Drug Metab Dispos* 1997;25:390–393.

126. Endres HG, Henschel L, Merkel U, Hippius M, Hoffmann A. Lack of pharmacokinetic interaction between dextromethorphan, coumarin and mephenytoin in man after simultaneous administration. *Pharmazie* 1996;51:46–51.

127. Yamano S, Nhamburo PT, Aoyama T, et al. cDNA cloning and sequence and cDNA-directed expression of human P450 IIB1: identification of a normal and two variant cDNAs derived from the CYP2B locus on chromosome 19 and differential expression of the IIB mRNAs in human liver. *Biochemistry* 1989;28:7340–7348.

128. Mimura M, Baba T, Yamazaki H, et al. Characterization of cytochrome P-450 2B6 in human liver microsomes. *Drug Metab Dispos* 1993;21:1048–1056.

129. Baker MT, Olson MJ, Wang Y, Ronnenberg WC Jr, Johnson JT, Brady AN. Isoflurane-chlorodifluoroethene interaction in human liver microsomes. Role of cytochrome P4502B6 in potentiation of haloethene metabolism. *Drug Metab Dispos* 1995;23:60–64.

130. Miles JS, McLaren AW, Gonzalez FJ, Wolf CR. Alternative splicing in the human cytochrome P450IIB6 gene: use of a cryptic exon within intron 3 and splice acceptor site within exon 4. *Nucl Acids Res* 1990; 18:189.

131. Miles JS, McLaren AW, Wolf CR. Alternative splicing in the human cytochrome P450IIB6 gene generates a high level of aberrant messages. *Nucl Acids Res* 1989;17:8241–8255.

132. Heyn H, White RB, Stevens JC. Catalytic role of cytochrome P4502B6 in the N-demethylation of S-mephenytoin. *Drug Metab Dispos* 1996;24:948–954.

133. Stevens JC, White RB, Hsu SH, Martinet M. Human liver CYP2B6-catalyzed hydroxylation of RP 73401. *J Pharmacol Exp Ther* 1997; 282:1389–1395.

134. Czerwinski M, McLemore TL, Gelboin HV, Gonzalez FJ. Quantification of CYP2B7, CYP4B1, and CYPOR messenger RNAs in normal human lung and lung tumors. *Cancer Res* 1994;54:1085–1091.

135. Ekins S, VandenBranden M, Ring BJ, Wrighton SA. Examination of purported probes of human CYP2B6. *Pharmacogenetics* 1997;7:165–179.

136. Shimada T, Mimura M, Inoue K, et al. Cytochrome P450-dependent drug oxidation activities in liver microsomes of various animal species including rats, guinea pigs, dogs, monkeys, and humans. *Arch Toxicol* 1997;71:401–408.

137. Gonzalez FJ, Crespi CL, Czerwinski M, Gelboin HV. Analysis of human cytochrome P450 catalytic activities and expression. *Tohoku J Exp Med* 1992;168:67–72.

138. Willey JC, Coy E, Brolly C, et al. Xenobiotic metabolism enzyme gene expression in human bronchial epithelial and alveolar macrophage cells. *Am J Respir Cell Mol Biol* 1996;14:262–271.

139. Farin FM, Pohlman TH, Omiecinski CJ. Expression of cytochrome P450s and microsomal epoxide hydrolase in primary cultures of human umbilical vein endothelial cells. *Toxicol Appl Pharmacol* 1994;124:1–9.

140. Nakajima T, Wang RS, Nimura Y, et al. Expression of cytochrome P450s and glutathione S-transferases in human esophagus with squamous-cell carcinomas. *Carcinogenesis* 1996;17:1477–1481.

141. Zhou LX, Pihlstrom B, Hardwick JP, Park SS, Wrighton SA, Holtzman JL. Metabolism of phenytoin by the gingiva of normal humans: the possible role of reactive metabolites of phenytoin in the initiation of gingival hyperplasia. *Clin Pharmacol Ther* 1996;60:191–198.

142. Bogaards JJP, Venekamp JC, van Bladeren PJ. The biotransformation of isoprene and the two isoprene monoepoxides by human cytochrome P450 enzymes, compared to mouse and rat liver microsomes. *Chem Biol Interact* 1996;102:169–182.

143. Kariya S, Isozaki S, Uchino K, Suzuki T, Narimatsu S. Oxidative metabolism of flunarizine and cinnarizine by microsomes from B-lymphoblastoid cell lines expressing human cytochrome P450 enzymes. *Biol Pharm Bull* 1996;19:1511–1514.

144. Ono S, Hatanaka T, Miyazawa S, et al. Human liver microsomal diazepam metabolism using cDNA-expressed cytochrome P450s—role of CYP2B6, 2C19 and the 3A subfamily. *Xenobiotica* 1996;26:1155–1166.

145. Koyama E, Chiba K, Tani M, Ishizaki T. Identification of human cytochrome P450 isoforms involved in the stereoselective metabolism of mianserin enantiomers. *J Pharmacol Exp Ther* 1996;278:21–30.

146. White IN, De Matteis F, Gibbs AH, et al. Species differences in the covalent binding of [14C]tamoxifen to liver microsomes and the forms of cytochrome P450 involved. *Biochem Pharmacol* 1995;49:1035–1042.

147. Ren S, Yang J-S, Kalhorn TF, Slattery JT. Oxidation of cyclophosphamide to 4-hydroxycyclophosphamide and deschloroethylcyclophosphamide in human liver microsomes. *Cancer Res* 1997;57:4229–4235.

148. Dehal SS, Kupfer D. Metabolism of the proestrogenic pesticide methoxychlor by hepatic P450 monooxygenases in rats and humans. Dual pathways involving novel ortho ring-hydroxylation by CYP2B. *Drug Metab Dispos* 1994;22:937–946.

149. Ariyoshi N, Oguri K, Koga N, Yoshimura H, Funae Y. Metabolism of highly persistent PCB congener, 2,4,5,2′,4′,5′-hexachlorobiphenyl, by human CYP2B6. *Biochem Biophys Res Commun* 1995;212:455–460.

150. Nakajima T, Elovaara E, Gonzalez FJ, et al. Styrene metabolism by cDNA-expressed human hepatic and pulmonary cytochromes P450. *Chem Res Toxicol* 1994;7:891–896.

151. Nakajima T, Wang R-S, Elovaara E, et al. Toluene metabolism by cDNA-expressed human hepatic cytochrome P450. *Biochem Pharmacol* 1997;53:271-277.

152. Shou M, Korzekwa KR, Crespi CL, Gonzalez FJ, Gelboin HV. The role of 12 cDNA-expressed human, rodent, and rabbit cytochromes P450 in the metabolism of benzo[a]pyrene and benzo[a]pyrene trans-7,8-dihydrodiol. *Mol Carcinog* 1994;10:159–168.

153. Shou M, Krausz KW, Gonzalez FJ, Gelboin HV. Metabolic activation of the potent carcinogen dibenzo[a,h]anthracene by cDNA-expressed human cytochromes P450. *Arch Biochem Biophys* 1996;328:201–207.

154. Yamazaki H, Mimura M, Oda Y, et al. Roles of different forms of cytochrome P450 in the activation of the promutagen 6-aminochrysene to genotoxic metabolites in human liver microsomes. *Carcinogenesis* 1993;14:1271–1278.

155. Yamazaki H, Mimura M, Oda Y, et al. Activation of trans-1,2-dihydro-1,2-dihydroxy-6-aminochrysene to genotoxic metabolites by rat and human cytochromes P450. *Carcinogenesis* 1994;15:465–470.

156. Shou M, Korzekwa KR, Krausz KW, Crespi CL, Gonzalez FJ, Gelboin HV. Regio- and stereo-selective metabolism of phenanthrene by twelve cDNA-expressed human, rodent, and rabbit cytochromes P-450. *Cancer Lett* 1994;83:305–313.

157. Shou M, Korzekwa KR, Krausz KW, et al. Specificity of cDNA-expressed human and rodent cytochrome P450s in the oxidative metabolism of the potent carcinogen 7,12-dimethylbenz[a]anthracene. *Mol Carcinog* 1996;17:241–249.

158. Shou M, Krausz KW, Gonzalez FJ, Gelboin HV. Metabolic activation of the potent carcinogen dibenzo[a,l]pyrene by human recombinant cytochrome P450, lung and liver microsomes. *Carcinogenesis* 1996;17:2429–2433.

159. Smith G, Harrison DJ, East N, Rae F, Wolf H, Wolf CR. Regulation of cytochrome P450 gene expression in human colon and breast tumour xenografts. *Br J Cancer* 1993;68:57–63.

160. Chang TKH, Yu L, Maurel P, Waxman DJ. Enhanced cyclophosphamide and ifosfamide activation in primary human hepatocyte cultures: response to cytochrome P-450 inducers and autoinduction by oxazaphosphorines. *Cancer Res* 1997;57:1946–1954.

161. Willey JC, Coy EL, Frampton MW, et al. Quantitative RT-PCR measurement of cytochromes P450 1A1, 1B1, and 2B7, microsomal epoxide hydrolase, and NADPH oxidoreductase expression in lung cells of smokers and nonsmokers. *Am J Respir Cell Mol Biol* 1997;17:114–124.

162. Goldstein JA, Faletto MB, Romkes-Sparks M, et al. Evidence that CYP2C19 is the major (S)-mephenytoin 4′-hydroxylase in humans. *Biochemistry* 1994;33:1743–1752.

163. Nelson DR, Koymans L, Kamataki T, et al. P450 superfamily: update on new sequences, gene mapping, accession numbers and nomenclature. *Pharmacogenetics* 1996;6:1–42.

164. Palmer CN, Richardson TH, Griffin KJ, et al. Characterization of a cDNA encoding a human kidney, cytochrome P-450 4A fatty acid omega-hydroxylase and the cognate enzyme expressed in Escherichia coli. *Biochim Biophys Acta* 1993;1172:161–166.

165. Imaoka S, Ogawa H, Kimura S, Gonzalez FJ. Complete cDNA sequence and cDNA-directed expression of CYP4A11, a fatty acid omega-hydroxylase expressed in human kidney. *DNA Cell Biol* 1993;12:893–899.

166. Kawashima H, Kusunose E, Kikuta Y, et al. Purification and cDNA cloning of human liver CYP4A fatty acid omega-hydroxylase. *J Biochem Tokyo* 1994;116:74–80.

167. Bell DR, Plant NJ, Rider CG, et al. Species-specific induction of cytochrome P-450 4A RNAs: PCR cloning of partial guinea-pig, human and mouse CYP4A cDNAs. *Biochem J* 1993;294:173–180.

168. Heng YM, Kuo C-WS, Jones PS, et al. A novel murine P-450 gene, Cyp4a14, is part of a cluster of Cyp4a and Cyp4b, but not of CYP4F, genes in mouse and humans. *Biochem J* 1997;325:741–749.

169. Powell PK, Wolf I, Lasker JM. Identification of CYP4A11 as the major lauric acid omega-hydroxylase in human liver microsomes. *Arch Biochem Biophys* 1996;335:219–226.

170. Castle PJ, Merdink JL, Okita JR, Wrighton SA, Okita RT. Human liver lauric acid hydroxylase activities. *Drug Metab Dispos* 1995;23:1037–1043.

171. Amet Y, Berthou F, Fournier G, et al. Cytochrome P450 4A and 2E1 expression in human kidney microsomes. *Biochem Pharmacol* 1997;53:765–771.

172. Imaoka S, Nagashima K, Funae Y. Characterization of three cytochrome P450s purified from renal microsomes of untreated male rats and comparison with human renal cytochrome P450. *Arch Biochem Biophys* 1990;276:473–480.

173. Kawashima H, Kusunose E, Kubota I, Maekawa M, Kusunose M. Purification and NH2-terminal amino acid sequences of human and rat kidney fatty acid ω-hydroxylases. *Biochim Biophys Acta* 1992;1123:156–162.

174. Cresteil T, Beaune P, Kremers P, Celier C, Guengerich FP, Leroux JP. Immunoquantification of epoxide hydrolase and cytochrome P-450 isozymes in fetal and adult human liver microsomes. *Eur J Biochem* 1985;151:345–350.

175. Treluyer JM, Cheron G, Sonnier M, Cresteil T. Cytochrome P-450 expression in sudden infant death syndrome. *Biochem Pharmacol* 1996;52:497–504.

176. Dirven HA, Peters JG, Gibson GG, Peters WH, Jongeneelen FJ. Lauric acid hydroxylase activity and cytochrome P450 IV family proteins in human liver microsomes. *Biochem Pharmacol* 1991;42:1841–1844.

177. Goodman AI, Choudhury M, da Silva JL, Schwartzman ML, Abraham NG. Overexpression of the heme oxygenase gene in renal cell carcinoma. *Proc Soc Exp Biol Med* 1997;214:54–61.

178. Okita RT, Jakobsson SW, Prough RA, Masters BSS. Lauric acid hydroxylation in human liver and kidney cortex microsomes. *Biochem Pharmacol* 1979;28:3385–3390.

179. Clarke SE, Baldwin SJ, Bloomer JC, Ayrton AD, Sozio RS, Chenery RJ. Lauric acid as a model substrate for the simultaneous determination of cytochrome P450 2E1 and 4A in hepatic microsomes. *Chem Res Toxicol* 1994;7:836–842.

180. Amet Y, Berthou F, Baird S, Dreano Y, Bail JP, Menez JF. Validation of the (ω-1) hydroxylation of lauric acid as an *in vitro* substrate probe for human liver CYP2E1. *Biochem Pharmacol* 1995;50:1775–1782.

181. Wang M-H, Stec DE, Balazy M, et al. Cloning, sequencing, and cDNA-directed expression of the rat renal CYP4A2: arachidonic acid ω-hydroxylation and 11,12-epoxidation by CYP4A2 protein. *Arch Biochem Biophys* 1996;336:240–250.

182. Roman LJ, Palmer CNA, Clark JE, et al. Expression of rabbit cytochromes P4504A which catalyze the ω-hydroxylation of arachidonic acid, fatty acids, and prostaglandins. *Arch Biochem Biophys* 1993;307:57–65.

183. Schwartzman ML, Martasek P, Rios AR, et al. Cytochrome P450-dependent arachidonic acid metabolism in human kidney. *Kidney Int* 1990;37:94–99.

184. Laniado-Schwartzman M, Abraham NG. The renal cytochrome P-450 arachidonic acid system. *Pediatr Nephrol* 1992;6:490–498.

185. Harder DR, Campbell WB, Roman RJ. Role of cytochrome P-450 enzymes and metabolites of arachidonic acid in the control of vascular tone. *J Vasc Res* 1995;32:79–92.

186. Prakash C, Zhang JY, Falck JR, Chauhan K, Blair IA. 20-hydroxy-eicosatetraenoic acid is excreted as a glucuronide conjugate in human urine. *Biochem Biophys Res Comm* 1992;185:728–733.

187. Kikuta Y, Kusunose E, Kondo T, Yamamoto S, Kinoshita H, Kusunose M. Cloning and expression of a novel form of leukotriene B$_4$ ω-hydroxylase from human liver. *FEBS Lett* 1994;348:70–74.

188. Chen L, Hardwick JP. The human CYP4F2 gene cDNA sequence and catalytic activity of baculovirus-infected insect cells. *FASEB J* 1994; 8:A1257.

189. Reddy JK, Lalwani ND. Carcinogenesis by hepatic peroxisome proliferators: evaluation of the risk of hypolipidemic drugs and industrial plasticizers to humans. *CRC Crit Rev Toxicol* 1983;12:1–58.

190. Hardwick JP, Song B, Huberman E, Gonzalez FJ. Isolation, complementary cDNA sequence, and regulation of rat hepatic lauric acid ω-hydroxylase. *J Biol Chem* 1987;262:801–810.

191. Sharma R, Lake BG, Gibson GG. Co-induction of microsomal cytochrome P-452 and the peroxisomal fatty acid β-oxidation pathway in the rat by clofibrate and di-(2-ethylhexyl)phthalate. *Biochem Pharmacol* 1988;37:1203–1206.

192. Lock EA, Mitchell AM, Elcombe CR. Biochemical mechanisms of induction of hepatic peroxisome proliferation. *Annu Rev Pharmacol Toxicol* 1989;29:145–163.

193. Issemann I, Green S. Activation of a member of the steroid hormone receptor superfamily by peroxisome proliferators. *Nature* 1990;347:645–650.

194. Tugwood JD, Issemann I, Anderson RG, Bundell KR, McPheat WL, Green S. The mouse peroxisome proliferator activated receptor recognizes a response element in the 5′ flanking sequence of the rat acyl CoA oxidase gene. *EMBO J* 1992;11:433–439.

195. Muerhoff AS, Griffin KJ, Johnson EF. The peroxisome proliferator-activated receptor mediates the induction of CYP4A6, a cytochrome P450 fatty acid ω-hydroxylase, by clofibric acid. *J Biol Chem* 1992; 267:19051–19053.

196. Johnson EF, Palmer CNA, Griffin KJ, Hsu M-H. Role of the peroxisome proliferator-activated receptor in cytochrome P450 4A gene regulation. *FASEB J* 1996;10:1241–1248.

197. Sher T, Yi H-F, McBride OW, Gonzalez FJ. cDNA cloning, chromosomal mapping, and functional characterization of the human peroxisome proliferator activated receptor. *Biochemistry* 1993;32:5598–5604.

198. Green S. Receptor-mediated mechanisms of peroxisome proliferators. *Biochem Pharmacol* 1992;43:393–401.

199. Palmer CNA, Hsu M-H, Griffin KJ, Raucy JL, Johnson EF. Peroxisome proliferator activated receptor α (PPARα) expression in human liver. *Mol Pharmacol* 1998;53:14–22.

200. Ortiz de Montellano PR, Reich NO. Specific inactivation of hepatic fatty acid hydroxylases by acetylenic fatty acids. *J Biol Chem* 1984; 259:4136–4141.

201. Kapitulnik J, Poppers PJ, Conney AH. Comparative metabolism of benzo[a]pyrene and drugs in human liver. *Clin Pharmac Ther* 1977; 21:166–176.

202. Kapitulnik J, Poppers PJ, Buening MK, Fortner JG, Conney AH. Activation of monooxygenases in human liver by 7,8-benzoflavone. *Clin Pharmac Ther* 1977;22:475–484.

203. Mäenpää J, Syngelmä T, Honkakoski P, Lang MA, Pelkonen O. Comparative studies on coumarin and testosterone metabolism in mouse and human livers. Differential inhibitions by the anti-P450Coh antibody and metyrapone. *Biochem Pharmacol* 1991;42:1229–1235.

204. Sharifi S, Lotterer E, Michaelis HC, Bircher J. Pharmacokinetics of coumarin and its metabolites after intravenous and peroral administration of high dose coumarin in normal human volunteers. *Naunyn-Schmiedeberg's Arch Pharmacol* 1991;344(suppl):R95.

205. Pelkonen O, Rautio A, Raunio H, Mäenpää J, Hakkola J. Regulation of coumarin 7-hydroxylation in man. *J Cancer Res Clin Oncol* 1994; 120:S30–S31.

CHAPTER 13

UDP-Glucuronosyltransferases

Thomas R. Tephly and Mitchell D. Green

The UDP-glycosyltranferases (UGTs) are a superfamily of enzymes that catalyze the addition of the glycosyl group from a nucleotide sugar to an acceptor molecule (aglycone). A second review on a nomenclature system for the UGT gene superfamily based on divergent evolution has been published (1). Thirty-three UGT gene families have been identified as related in animals, yeast, plants, and bacteria. Within this superfamily of proteins are a subset of enzymes called the UDP-glucuronosyltransferases (UDPGTs; EC 2.4.1.17), which catalyze the glucuronidation of a wide array of endobiotics and xenobiotics. The UDPGTs have been assigned to the UGT1 and UGT2 gene families (1). The gene products of the two families are less than 50% identical in primary amino acid sequence, yet the UGT1 and UGT2 gene products exhibit significant overlap in their substrate specificities.

Glucuronidation occurs at nucleophilic functional groups of oxygen (e.g., hydroxyl groups or carboxylic acids), nitrogen (e.g., amines), sulfur (e.g., thiols), and carbon (2). Glucuronidation represents an important metabolic elimination pathway for endogenous compounds and xenobiotics whereby many lipid-soluble substances are rendered more water soluble and become more readily excreted by renal or biliary routes. UDPGTs catalyze the SN_2 reaction of the acceptor group of a substrate (represented by a generic alcohol in Fig. 13-1) on the C1 of the pyranose acid ring of UDP-glucuronic acid. The reaction products are the glucuronide (a β-D glucopyranosiduronic acid conjugate), UDP, and water. Important endogenous compounds such as androgens, estrogens, progestins, bilirubin, and retinoids are substrates for UDPGTs. Many compounds of environmental [e.g., benzo(a)pyrenes (BaP)] and dietary (flavonoids and sapogenins) origins, as well as important pharmacologic

agents [e.g., nonsteroidal antiinflammatory drugs (NSAIDs), opioids, antihistaminics, antipsychotics, and antidepressants] are substrates for these enzymes.

There are two important points concerning glucuronidation reactions. First, glucuronidation is not strictly a phase II conjugation reaction in that most substrates do not require phase I metabolism before they can undergo glucuronidation. Many endobiotics (e.g., testosterone, androsterone, estrone, retinoic acid, and bilirubin) and xenobiotics (e.g., acetaminophen, amitriptyline, chloramphenicol, morphine, and oxazepam) are conjugated without prior conversion to products of oxidative, reductive, or hydrolytic enzymes. Second, although, in general, glucuronidation results in the formation of water-soluble inactive metabolites, active and reactive glucuronide metabolites have been described. For example, morphine is metabolized in humans to morphine-3-glucuronide and morphine-6-glucuronide (3). Morphine-6-glucuronide has been shown to be at least 50 times more potent than morphine as an antinociceptive agent (4–6). Even though morphine-3-glucuronide does not possess analgesic activity, it has been reported to be an antagonist of morphine at opioid receptors (7,8). It has also been shown that D-ring glucuronides of steroids such as testosterone and estriol cause cholestasis (9,10), in contrast to A-ring glucuronides, which are inactive (11). Acyl glucuronidation of zomepirac, clofibrate, and valproate has been implicated in adverse drug reactions whereby acyl migration leads to the production of reactive metabolites that bind to cellular and serum proteins and may lead to the development of immunotoxicity (12–15). Glucuronides are also seriously being considered as prodrugs in certain disease states. The use of budesonide β-D-glucuronide in ulcerative colitis (16) and retinoyl-β-glucuronide in acne (17,18) have been suggested and may have substantial pharmacologic effectiveness.

A generally accepted model of UDPGT structure has been proposed (19) whereby the UDPGT proteins are

T. R. Tephly and M. D. Green: Department of Pharmacology, University of Iowa, 2-512 Bowen Science Building, Iowa City, Iowa 52242

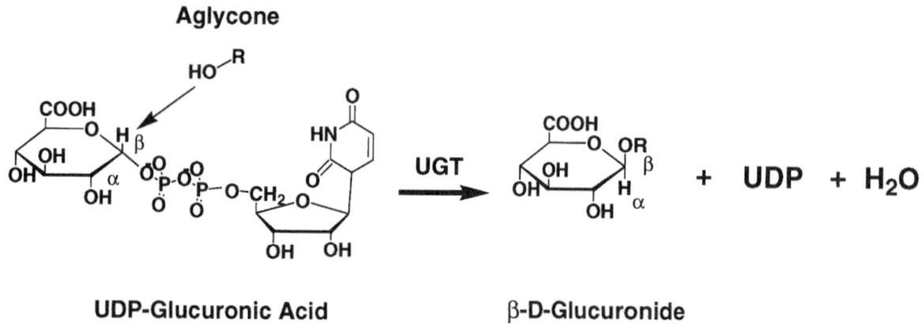

FIG. 13-1. Glucuronidation reaction showing the reaction of UDP-glucuronic acid with an aglycone (ROH) resulting in the formation of a glucuronide, UDP, and water.

considered to be localized on the luminal side of the endoplasmic reticulum membrane. The phenomenon of latency (1), which is observed with these proteins, is partially based on this property. Most UDPGTs possess hydrophobic signal sequences (which are cleaved during processing) and a highly hydrophobic sequence in the C-terminal region of the protein. This is characteristic of the stop-transfer signals of transmembrane proteins and anchors the protein to the membrane of the endoplasmic reticulum. Despite the differences in primary amino acid sequences between the UGT1 and UGT2 proteins, the C-terminal domains of the proteins have quite high sequence identity, suggesting a conserved function—probably UDP-glucuronic acid binding (20). The N-terminal binding domain of the UDPGTs are least conserved and are thought to provide the specificity of aglycone substrate binding.

The following discussion considers the UDPGTs (those which use UDP-glucuronic acid as substrate) in animals and primarily those characterized in humans, which catalyze the glucuronidation of xenobiotic and endobiotic substances. The molecular biology involved in characterizing the protein products are noted and the substrate specificity is reviewed. In certain cases, laboratories that have studied expressed UGT cDNAs have found different substrate reactivities. Certain differences in the analytic methods may account for some of the variable results and an interlaboratory comparison of much of the earlier expression work reflects the fact that reaction conditions were not always kinetically favorable. In this review, specific substrates for various UDPGTs are noted, and there is discussion of the overlap in substrate reactivities for these enzymes. The two UGT gene families are discussed based on the nomenclature system suggested by Mackenzie and colleagues (1).

THE UGT1 FAMILY

The structure of the human UGT1 gene was first reported by Ritter and colleagues (21). This gene is highly unusual in that it contains at least 12 first exons, which appear to be capable of splicing with common exons 2 through 5, leading to proteins with different N-terminal sequences but identical C-terminal domains. An identical UGT1 gene structure has been shown to exist in

the rat (22), and experimental evidence from mouse (23,24) and rabbit (23,25) suggest that a similar UGT1 gene structure also exists in those species. It has been suggested that each UGT1 first exon has its own promoter elements upstream of their individual TATAA boxes (21) and that the expression of each UGT1A protein is individually controlled. Strassburg and colleagues (26,27) have recently shown using reverse transcriptase polymerase chain reaction (RT-PCR) that only UGT1A1, 1A3, 1A4, 1A6, and 1A9 are expressed in human liver. Other evidence for the regulation of UGT1A proteins is discussed in subsequent paragraphs.

UGT1A1

Ritter and colleagues (28) reported on the isolation and characterization of two human cDNA clones—HUG-Br1 (UGT1A1) and HUG-Br2 (UGT1A4)—which, when expressed in COS-1 cells, catalyzed the glucuronidation of bilirubin. This was the first demonstration of cDNAs that encode for proteins that react with bilirubin. It is currently accepted that UGT1A1 is the only physiologically significant enzyme involved in bilirubin glucuronidation in humans (29). Ritter and colleagues (28) also showed that, in the monkey, expression of UGT1A1 is not inducible by phenobarbital administration. Therefore, it is probable that the beneficial effects of phenobarbital administration to patients with Crigler-Najjar type II is independent of its effect on expression of UGT1A1.

Using human UGT1A1 stably expressed in Chinese hamster V79 cells, Senafi and colleagues (30) studied more than 100 compounds, including bilirubin, and found that a number of other endobiotics and xenobiotics from various chemical classes were substrates for the enzyme (Table 13-1). Kinetic studies showed that the apparent K_m for bilirubin was 20 μM. In addition to UDP-glucuronic acid, expressed UGT1A1 was also shown to react with UDP-xylose and UDP-glucose as cosubstrates. Using bilirubin as the aglycone, the apparent K_m values of the UDP sugars were found to be 0.41 mM, 0.32 mM and 3.80 mM for the glucuronic acid, xylose, and glucose derivatives, respectively (30). The authors point out that, because the level of bilirubin glucuronides is 20-fold higher in bile than that of bilirubin xylosides, and because efficiency values are very similar

TABLE 13-1. *Substrates for human UGT1A proteins*

Substrate class	UGT1A1	UGT1A3	UGT1A4	UGT1A6	UGT1A9
Morphinan opioids	+	+	0	0	0
Oripavine opioids	+++	++	0	?	?
Primary amines	0	+	+++	+	+
Tertiary amines	0	+	++	0	0
Monoterpenoid alcohols	0	0	+	0	0
Anthraquinones	+++	+++	0	0	+++
3-Hydroxy androgens	0	0	+	0	0
17-Hydroxy androgens	0	0	+	0	+
Estrone	0	++	0	0	+
Catechol estrogens	++	++	0	?	++
Estriol	0	+	+	0	0
Progestins	0	0	++	?	?
Bilirubin	++	0	0	0	0
Sapogenins	0	0	+	0	0
Profen nonsteroidal antiinflammatory drugs	0	++	0	0	+
7-Hydroxy coumarins	++	+++	0	++	+
Simple phenols	+	++	+	+++	++
Propofol	0	0	0	0	+++
Flavonoids	++	+++	0	0	+++
Hydroxy benzo[a]pyrene	?	+	?	+	?

0 = no detectable activity, + <50 pmol/min/mg protein, ++ 50–500 pmol/min/mg protein, +++ >500 pmol/min/mg protein

in kinetic studies, the concentration of UDP-xylose in human liver must be low in comparison to that of UDP-glucuronic acid. Expressed human UGT1A1 was also found to have glucuronidation activity toward endogenous estrogenic substrates; estriol, 17β-estradiol, and 2-hydroxyestriol. Xenobiotic substrates such as phenols, anthraquinones, and flavonoids were also found to be quite reactive with UGT1A1; especially octylgallate, 4-nitrophenol, 1-naphthol, eugenol, anthraflavic acid, quercetin, fisetin, and naringenin (30). Another study using stably expressed UGT1A1 showed that thyroid hormones, T_4 and reverse T_3, were glucuronidated but T_3 was not glucuronidated (31).

Coffman and colleagues (32) first isolated a cDNA for rat UGT1A1 and showed that the encoded protein, stably expressed in human embryonic kidney 293 (HK293) cells, catalyzed the glucuronidation of bilirubin and opioids. This was the first demonstration that a UGT1 could catalyze the glucuronidation of opioids. King and colleagues (33) compared the substrate specificity of rat and human UGT1A1 and concluded that the proteins are functionally similar. In addition to the substrates studied by Senafi and colleagues (30), both proteins were extremely reactive with opioids of the oripavine class (e.g., buprenorphine). Interestingly, the efficiency of the reactivity of UGT1A1 with buprenorphine was found to be of the same order of magnitude as that of bilirubin, which is considered to be the major substrate for this UGT. In addition to buprenorphine, UGT1A1 also reacted with nalorphine, naltrexone, and morphine, although at rates much less than those obtained with buprenorphine. King and colleagues (33) also compared buprenorphine and naltrexone glucuronidation activities

in normal human liver microsomes and in liver microsomes from two patients with Crigler-Najjar type I. Buprenorphine glucuronidation activity in Crigler-Najjar type I liver was only 25% of that in normal human liver, whereas naltrexone glucuronidation activities were about the same in both preparations. These results demonstrate that UGT1A1 has a major role in the glucuronidation of buprenorphine in human liver.

Stably expressed rat UGT1A1 has been shown to react with quite high efficiency with retinoic acid derivatives such as all-*trans*-retinoic acid (atRA) and 5,6-epoxy-atRA (34). [11,12-³H]atRA also served as a photolabel of UGT1A1. Liver microsomes from Gunn rats, which lack all UGT1 isoforms (34), still displayed significant activity toward atRA, suggesting that enzymes outside the UGT1 family also catalyze the glucuronidation of retinoids.

Polymorphisms have been described for human UGT1A1 (1), many of which lead to protein products that are inactive (leading to Crigler-Najjar type I hyperbilirubinemia), or only partially active (Crigler-Najjar type II and Gilbert's disease). If defects in the human UGT1 gene occur in the first exon or its promoter region, only UGT1A1 expression is affected and these patients would be expected to have normal expression of other members of the UGT1 gene family. On the other hand, genetic defects in any of the common second through fifth exons should lead to inactive or reduced activity in all UGT1 gene products.

The genetic defect that produces the hyperbilirubinemic Gunn rat strain has been shown to be the result of a −1 frameshift mutation in the third exon of the UGT1 gene, resulting in the expression of a truncated protein

(35). Thus, Gunn rats are unable to express any of the UGT1 gene family isoforms. King and colleagues (36) used hepatic microsomes from Gunn rats to show that 75% of the buprenorphine glucuronidation activity in these preparations is catalyzed by UGT1 gene products, presumably UGT1A1. Interestingly, hepatic microsomal rates of morphine glucuronidation in Gunn rat liver microsomes were the same as morphine glucuronidation rates in Wistar rat liver microsomes, demonstrating that UGT1A1 does not contribute significantly to hepatic morphine glucuronidation in rats.

A recent review on UGT nomenclature (1) lists 30 defects in the human UGT1 gene locus that have been shown to be associated with defective bilirubin glucuronidation. Whereas point mutations in the UGT1A1 gene are most commonly associated with the hyperbilirubinemic diseases, frameshift mutations, amino acid deletions, and promotor region alterations of the gene have been described. One mutation that has been described for two patients with Crigler-Najjar II relates to a leucine to arginine transition (UGT1A1*30), which disrupts the hydrophobic core of the signal peptide of UGT1A1 and leads to a markedly decreased efficiency of expression of the protein (37).

Gilbert's disease represents a benign hyperbilirubinemia, which is common in the human population (2%–12%) and is characterized by a slight, but significant, elevation in serum bilirubin levels. Two explanations for reduced UGT1A1 activity in these patients have been reported. Bosma and colleagues (38) have shown that many patients with Gilbert's disease have an abnormal TATAA element at the 5′ promoter region of the UGT1A1 gene; A(TA)$_7$TAA rather than the normal A(TA)$_6$TAA. The frequency of the abnormal allele in normal subjects was 40%. By linking the abnormal A(TA)$_7$TAA promoter element to a reporter gene it was possible to show greatly reduced expression of the reporter gene product (38). The authors concluded that reduced expression of UGT1A1 activity resulting from perturbation of the promoter region of the gene appears to be necessary but may not be sufficient for the complete manifestation of the syndrome. Monaghan and colleagues (39) studied serum bilirubin levels and genotypes in a Scottish population. The 7/7 genotype was associated with individuals with higher bilirubin levels than those who had the 6/7 or 6/6 promoter region genotype, provided that the subjects were fasted and not exposed to known inducers of the UGT1A1 isoform such as alcohol and drugs. These data suggest that differences in the promoter region of the UGT1A1 gene contributes, at least in part, to the manifestation of Gilbert's syndrome.

Koiwai and colleagues (40) studied patients with hyperbilirubinemia in the range of 31 to 86 µmol/L and found a variety of missense mutations in the coding region of the UGT1A1 gene and that the mutations were heterozygous. This would lead to expression of a mixture of normal UGT1A1 and mutated UGT1A1 (that is inactive or has greatly reduced activity) and would result in an overall reduction in bilirubin glucuronidation. Koiwai and colleagues (40) studied patients with a more severe hyperbilirubinemia than those investigated by Bosma and colleagues (38) and Monaghan and colleagues (39). Thus, it would appear that the presence of one mutated allele in the coding region leads to more severe hyperbilirubinemia and that homozygosity for these mutations leads to either Crigler-Najjar syndrome type I or type II.

One major point about UGT1A1 that has generally escaped the attention of clinicians interested primarily in bilirubin glucuronidation is that UGT1A1 catalyzes the glucuronidation of many xenobiotics (see Table 13-1). Monaghan and colleagues (39) emphasize the fact that patients with diseases related to the hyperbilirubinemias may also be at risk for xenobiotic-related toxicities caused by the interaction of xenobiotics with UGT1A1-catalyzed glucuronidation of bilirubin. They cite the reaction of UGT1A1 with ethynylestradiol as a major example of an agent that is glucuronidated by UGT1A1 and is widely taken as a drug. However, this is only one of a large number of substrates that have been shown to react with high affinity with UGT1A1. Another example is the use of opioid antagonists such as naltrexone or buprenorphine in the treatment of alcohol and narcotic addictions (41), where it is possible that, in certain individuals, a drug-endobiotic interaction may occur and a development of hyperbilirubinemia may be anticipated. UGT1A1 was recently shown to react with the active metabolite (SN-38) of the antitumor agent irinotecan (42). SN-38 is excreted in the bile as the glucuronide that limits the toxicity (diarrhea) of irinotecan. Thus, in patients with low levels of UGT1A1 activity, one might expect the possibility of increased risk of irinotecan toxicity. Indeed, a recent case report has appeared that described severe irinotecan toxicity in two patients with Gilbert's syndrome (43).

UGT1A2

Catalytically active UGT1A2 protein is not expressed in humans because there is a premature stop codon in the first exon of this gene product, giving rise to a pseudogene product (21). In the rat, UGT1A2 has been found to catalyze the glucuronidation of bilirubin (44); however, its reactivity with other substrates is not known. Thus, it appears that the rat expresses two proteins that can catalyze bilirubin glucuronidation: UGT1A1 and UGT1A2.

UGT1A3, UGT1A4, and UGT1A5

Of the human UGT1A proteins, UGT1A3, 1A4, and 1A5 are the most similar to each other based on primary amino acid sequence (>90% identical). To date, cloning or tissue expression of human UGT1A5 has not been described, but UGT1A3 and UGT1A4 have been studied extensively for their substrate specificities and expression (28,45–48). A comparison of the substrate specificities of UGT1A3 and 1A4 (see Table 13-1) shows that the expressed proteins exhibit some similarities but also some very different reactivities toward compounds from many chemical classes.

The first isolation and cloning of UGT1A4 (HUG Br 2) was reported by Ritter and colleagues (28) who also showed that, in monkey, UGT1A4 mRNA levels are elevated after phenobarbital treatment. UGT1A4 expressed in COS-1 cells was found to have low activity toward bilirubin glucuronidation and, for this reason, UGT1A4 was considered a "minor" and insignificant UGT protein. However, Green and colleagues (45) showed that it was a major catalyst in the conversion of many tertiary amines to quaternary ammonium glucuronides. There are a number of important tertiary amine-containing pharmacologic agents that are converted to quaternary ammonium-linked glucuronides in humans. This is a relatively unique and important metabolic pathway for these compounds, which include such pharmacologic agents as antihistamines, antiepileptics, anxiolytics, tricyclic antidepressants, and antipsychotics. In addition to important pharmacologically active tertiary amines such as imipramine, doxepin, amitryptyline, and chlorpromazine, potentially carcinogenic primary amines such as α- and β-naphthylamines, benzidine, aniline, and 4-aminobiphenyl are also substrates for expressed UGT1A4 (45,46). In general, reactivity of amines with UGT1A4 is characterized by low apparent K_m values for the aglycones and high glucuronidation efficiencies (46). Rabbit UGT1A4 has been cloned and the expressed protein was also found to catalyze the glucuronidation of tertiary amines to form quaternary ammonium-linked glucuronides (25). The reactivity of the expressed rabbit enzyme is also characterized by low apparent K_m values for amine substrates. UGT1A4 is a pseudogene in the rat (22), which probably accounts for the lack of quaternary ammonium glucuronidation in this species.

Recently, human UGT1A3 has also been shown to catalyze the glucuronidation of primary and tertiary amines (47). In contrast to UGT1A4, reactivity of amines with UGT1A3 is characterized by high apparent K_m values for the aglycones and low glucuronidation efficiencies.

Aside from their ability to catalyze quaternary ammonium glucuronide formation and despite their high degree of primary amino acid sequence identity, expressed human UGT1A3 and UGT1A4 exhibit very different substrate specificities for other classes of compounds. In general, expressed UGT1A4 does not catalyze glucuronidation of aromatic phenols, but displays significant activity toward compounds with aliphatic hydroxyl groups such as monoterpenoid alcohols, androgens, progestins, and plant sterols (sapogenins). Indeed, the best substrates for UGT1A4 found thus far are progestins and

sapogenins. It has been suggested that sapogenins may be specific substrates for human UGT1A4 (46). In contrast, UGT1A3 does not react with either progestins or sapogenins, but reacts very well with many compounds that UGT1A4 does not react with, such as estrone, flavonoids, 7-hydroxycoumarins, 2-hydroxyestrogens, and anthraquinones (47). UGT1A3 also catalyzes the glucuronidation of hydroxylated BaP metabolites and hydroxylated 2-acetylaminofluorene metabolites (48).

Another remarkable difference between expressed UGT1A3 and UGT1A4 is the glucuronidation activity toward NSAIDs and opioids exhibited by UGT1A3. In this respect, the activity of UGT1A3 with opioids and NSAIDs is similar to that observed for UGT2B7, which also catalyzes the glucuronidation of these substrates. This is an excellent example of the unpredicted overlapping substrate specificity of two proteins from different UGT families that have less than 45% identity in primary amino acid sequence.

UGT1A6

Whereas UGT1A1 is arguably the most studied UDPGT in humans, UGT1A6 is the most studied UDPGT enzyme in laboratory animals. A 3-methylcholanthrene (3-MC)–inducible rat phenol UDPGT was originally purified to apparent homogeneity by Falany and Tephly (49). This purified protein (later shown to be UGT1A6) catalyzed the glucuronidation of planar phenols, but not androgens (e.g., testosterone and androsterone) or estrone. Expressed UGT1A6 has also been shown to react primarily with planar phenols (50) and has no activity with bulky phenolic compounds, except for 2-hydroxybiphenyl, which has been shown to react with the expressed rabbit and mouse isoforms (23). Gschaidmeier and colleagues (51) have shown that human UGT1A6 catalyzes monoglucuronide formation of planar polyaromatic hydrocarbon quinols but not diglucuronide formation. Acetaminophen has been shown to react with UGT1A6 and this substrate has been suggested as a possible probe of UGT1A6 activity *in vivo* (52,53). UGT1A6 is likely to be functionally orthologous across species because its reactivity with simple phenols has been shown to be similar for rat, rabbit, mouse, and humans (23,50,52).

4-Nitrophenol has long been used as a substrate that investigators have used to serve as a substrate for UDPGTs. Its limitations in this regard have been discussed previously by Tephly and Burchell (19). 4-Nitrophenol glucuronidation activity is markedly enhanced in hepatic microsomes obtained from rats treated with 3-MC because of the induction of UGT1A6 in rat liver. However, in the liver from untreated rats, UGT2B3 is the main catalyst for 4-nitrophenol glucuronidation (49). Similarly, many human UGTs have been shown to react with this phenolic substrate, and it is unlikely that 4-nitrophenol is a good indicator of UGT1A6 abundance in human liver.

Emi and colleagues (22,54) have identified a xenobiotic responsive element–mediated transcriptional activation related to UGT1A6 in rat liver. These workers identified a *cis*-acting element in the promoter region of the UGT1A6 locus by using a DNA fragment carrying 1,100 nucleotides derived from the 5'-flanking region of the UGT1A6 gene and coupling it to a chloramphenicol acetyltransferase gene. Transfection of rat liver hepatocytes with the construct and treatment with 3-MC led to induction of UGT1A6. Deletion analysis of the region revealed one xenobiotic response element, TGCGTG, between −134 and −129, and 3-MC–inducible binding of the nuclear Ah receptor–ligand complex to this element was observed. The induction of UGT1A6 by TCDD has also been shown in mice but not in rabbits (23). The Ah receptor was involved in the TCDD-mediated induction of mouse UGT1A6, but the UGT1A6 gene in rabbits does not respond to Ah receptor interactions, even though CYP1A1 mRNA levels are dramatically enhanced by TCDD (23). Münzel and colleagues (55) have shown that UGT1A6 mRNA is inducible by TCDD in human-derived Caco-2 cells, but not in lung carcinoma A549 cells. They also showed that UGT1A6 is inducible by TCDD in primary cell cultures of human hepatocytes. These results suggest that species differences occur in the regulation of UGT1A6 expression and that the expression of the gene product may not always be mediated simply by Ah receptor–ligand interactions.

Masmoudi and colleagues (56) have reported on the transcriptional regulation of UGT1A6 by triiodothyronine (T_3) and have shown that T_3 induction is prevented by cycloheximide in primary hepatic cell cultures whereas 3-MC stimulation is only partially affected after treatment. They suggest that 3-MC induction is the result of a direct action of the Ah receptor complex whereas T_3 requires de novo protein synthesis. They indicate that T_3 may be promoting the synthesis of a factor, which, in turn, regulates the transcription of UGT1A6. This interesting possibility merits further study.

Bock and colleagues have explored the regulation of UGT1A6 in rat liver cancer prestages such as hepatocyte foci (57) and hepatocyte nodules (58). They have observed that mRNA for UGT1A6 was preferentially increased in preneoplastic nodules and carcinomas produced by feeding 2-acetylaminofluorene or *N*-nitrosomorpholine. A persistent expression of UGT1A6 was described in these conditions. Recently, Strassburg and colleagues (26) showed that UGT1A1, UGT1A3, UGT1A4, and UGT1A9 are significantly downregulated in malignant hepatocellular carcinoma and its premalignant precursor, hepatic adenoma, but that UGT1A6 is not significantly regulated in liver tumors. These results are strikingly similar to those reported from Bock's laboratory with respect to the "persistence" of UGT1A6 in the face of modulatory events perturbing other loci at the UGT1A locus.

UGT1A7

UGT1A7 has been identified in rat, human, and, tentatively, in rabbit liver. Strassburg and colleagues (27) have identified the presence of mRNA for UGT1A7 in human biliary and gastric tissue. To date, no activity has been identified for the human isoform.

Grove and colleagues (59) have isolated and stably expressed rat UGT1A7 and have shown that it catalyzes the glucuronidation of a number of BaP metabolites. Apparent K_m values for *trans* benzo(a)pyrene-7,8-diol (BPD) and 3-OH-BaP were low. This isoform in rat liver is highly induced by oltipraz, a chemopreventive agent that has been shown to induce BPD activity and may be an important agent in enhancing the metabolism of other carcinogenic BaP metabolites.

Bruck and colleagues (25) have cloned and expressed a cDNA from rabbit liver, which has been tentatively identified as UGT1A7. It is 77% and 81% similar to the rat and human sequences, respectively, which encode the seventh first exon of the UGT1A locus. Activity toward a number of simple phenols was observed in transfected COS-1 cells. Of some interest is the reactivity of this protein with the tertiary amine, imipramine, to form the quaternary ammonium-linked glucuronide. A comparison of rabbit UGT1A7 with rabbit UGT1A4 showed that UGT1A7 was less efficient than UGT1A4 in catalyzing quaternary ammonium glucuronidation.

UGT1A9

Human UGT1A9, previously known as UGT1*02, bulky phenol UGT, HP4, and UGT1*7, was cloned and stably expressed by Burchell's laboratory (50). This UDPGT seems to be a relatively abundant hepatic UGT, which accepts a diverse group of substrates, including bulky phenols, anthraquinones, flavones, aliphatic alcohols, aromatic carboxylic acids, steroids, and a variety of drugs (e.g., propofol) (see Table 13-1). Activity toward *N*-hydroxy arylamines and *N*-hydroxy-naphthylamine was also shown by Bock's laboratory (60).

UGT1A10

Recently, Mojarrabi and Mackenzie (61) cloned UGT1A10 from human colon and showed it to be about 90% similar in amino acid sequence to UGT1A9. The enzyme, as expressed in COS-7 cells, was active toward mycophenolic acid, an antineoplastic and immunosuppressive agent. Strassburg and colleagues (27) have identified the presence of mRNA for UGT1A10 in biliary and gastric tissue but not in liver.

THE UGT2 FAMILY

The gene structure for the UGT2 gene family is different than that described for the UGT1 gene family. UGT2 mRNAs are transcribed from individual genes. The gene structures for rat UGT2B2 (62), human UGT2B4 (63), and UGT2B17 (64) have been described, and each UGT2 gene product appears to be encoded by six exons. Even though human UGT2 proteins are encoded by separate genes, many human UGT2 genes appear to be closely clustered on chromosome 4 (63,64).

UGT2A1

UGT2A1 was isolated from rat and bovine olfactory epithelium and may be specifically expressed in that tissue because expression was not detected in liver, kidney, lung, brain, or intestine (65). Expressed UGT2A1 catalyzes the glucuronidation of monoterpenoid alcohols, simple phenols, and coumarins, many of which have odorant properties. It has been suggested that olfactory-specific expression of UGT2A1 may be involved in odorant signal termination (65). To date, expression of a similar protein has not been identified in human olfactory epithelium.

Rat UGT2B1, UGT2B2, UGT2B3, and UGT2B12

These proteins were originally purified and characterized from rat liver (49,66,67). Two of these proteins were shown to be specific for androsterone and testosterone glucuronidation and were termed the 3α-hydroxysteroid (UGT2B2) and 17β-hydroxysteroid (UGT2B3) UDP-glucuronosyltransferases, respectively. cDNAs for these UGTs were cloned and sequenced by several laboratories and the substrate specificities were determined in COS cells (68–73). The substrate specificities for expressed UGT2B2 and UGT2B3 agree well with those described for the purified proteins. Both proteins are constituitively expressed in rat liver and do not appear to be inducible (69,70,74). Expression of UGT2B2 has been shown to be age dependent, that is, low at birth and increasing post-natally to adult levels by puberty (74).

UGT2B1 was cloned by Mackenzie (70) and its expression in rat liver was shown to be induced by phenobarbital treatment. UGT2B1 was expressed in COS cells and the expressed protein catalyzed the glucuronidation of testosterone and chloramphenicol. Coffman and colleagues (66) purified this protein to apparent homogeneity from rat liver microsomes and showed its reaction with morphine. Pritchard and colleagues (71) stably expressed UGT2B1 in V79 cells and showed that it catalyzed the glucuronidation of a variety of xenobiotics and endobiotics. The most interesting of the xenobiotic substrates that reacted with the expressed protein were morphine (which was converted to morphine-3-glucuronide) and acidic substrates such as NSAIDs and

clofibric acid. An extensive study has been done by King and colleagues (36) using rat UGT2B1 and UGT1A1 stably expressed in HK293 cells to investigate their capacity to catalyze the glucuronidation of a number of opioid agonists, antagonists, and partial agonists. It was shown that rat UGT2B1 and UGT1A1 are quite similar to human counterparts UGT2B7 and UGT1A1 with an important exception: Rat UGT2B1 catalyzes only morphine 3-glucuronide formation, whereas human UGT2B7 catalyzes morphine glucuronidation to form both the 3- and 6-glucuronide.

A cDNA encoding for rat UGT2B12 was isolated, cloned, and stably expressed in HK293 cells (73). UGT2B12 catalyzed the glucuronidation of a large number of xenobiotic substrates, especially monoterpenoid alcohols, and essentially no endobiotic compounds. Natural products such as borneol, menthol, citronellol, coumarins, and flavonoids were efficient substrates as was hexafluoro-2-propanol, the major metabolite of the general anesthetic agent sevoflurane. Hepatic UGT2B12 expression is induced in rat liver with phenobarbital treatment (73).

Human UGT2B4

UGT2B4 has been cloned and expressed in three different laboratories. Fournel-Gigleux and colleagues (75,76) have cloned and studied the expressed enzyme in both COS-7 and V79 cells and have shown activity toward the 6α-hydroxy group of the bile acid, hyodeoxycholic acid (Table 13-2). In stably expressed V79 cell homogenates, UGT2B4 was expressed at levels approaching that found in a human liver microsomal preparation. An apparent K_m of 0.27 mM was found for hyodeoxycholic acid but, even in this system, a relatively low efficiency was observed. Furthermore, no activity was found when other bile acids, androgens, estrogens, serotonin, and chloramphenicol were employed as substrates.

Ritter and colleagues (77,78) cloned and expressed UGT2B4 in COS-1 cells. These authors showed that UGT2B4 is a relatively inefficient UGT in catalyzing glucuronidation of hyodeoxycholic acid, estriol, and 4-hydroxyestrone (see Table 13-2). They also showed that UGT2B4 is expressed in human liver but not in human kidney, a finding that correlates with tissue studies on the microsomal UGT activity toward hyodeoxycholic acid glucuronidation.

Jin and colleagues (79) studied UGT2B4 expressed in COS-7 cells. They showed glucuronidation activity toward estrogens and catechol estrogens, phenolic xenobiotics, and the monoterpenoid alcohol menthol, but, interestingly, no activity was found with hyodeoxycholic acid. A more recent study from this group has shown that expressed UGT2B4 has low glucuronidation activity toward 3α-hydroxysteroids (see Table 13-2).

TABLE 13-2. *Substrates for Human UGT2B proteins*

Substrate class	UGT2B4	UGT2B7	UGT2B15	UGT2B17
Morphinan opioids	?	+++	0	?
Oripavine opioids	?	+++	0	?
Primary amines	0	?	0	?
Tertiary amines	0	?	0	0
Monoterpenoid alcohols	+	++	0	?
Anthraquinones	?	?	+	?
3-Hydroxy androgens	+	+++	0	+
17-Hydroxy androgens	0	+	+	+
Estrone	0	0	0	0
Catechol estrogens	+	++	+	0
Estriol	+	++	0	0
Progestins	0	++	?	0
Bilirubin	0	0	0	0
Sapongenins	?	?	0	?
Profen nonsteroidal antiinflammatory drugs	?	++	0	?
7-Hydroxy coumarins	0	+	++	?
Simple phenols	+	++	++	+
Propofol	?	?	0	?
Flavonoids	?	?	++	?
Hydroxy benzo[a]pyrene	?	?	?	?
Bile acids	+	++	0	0

0 = no detectable activity, + <50 pmol/min/mg protein, ++ 50–500 pmol/min/mg/protein, +++ >500 pmol/min/mg protein

In summary, the aforementioned results suggest that UGT2B4 has a specific catalytic glucuronidating activity toward the 6α-hydroxy group of hyodeoxycholic acid. This has been verified by Pillot and colleagues (80) who have used immunoinhibition of 6α-hydroxy glucuronidation of hyodeoxycholic acid with a specific polyclonal antibody. This antibody was raised against a protein A fusion protein containing a variable region of UGT2B4. Studies using human liver microsomes showed marked inhibition of hyodeoxycholic acid 6-O-glucuronidation with no effect on the glucuronidation of phenols, bilirubin, other bile acids, or estrogenic steroids. Thus, UGT2B4 seems to have a specific substrate activity that can distinguish it from other UGTs in human liver. However, its activity with regard to other substrates tested thus far appears to be unremarkable.

Human UGT2B7

UGT2B7 is one of the most important human UGT isoforms. It is highly active toward a variety of endobiotics and xenobiotics and is a polymorphic UGT isoform. Although it has been studied by several laboratories, its full importance has yet to be completely understood. UGT2B7 has a wide substrate specificity and efficiently mediates the glucuronidation of a large variety of xenobiotics and endobiotics of different chemical classes. These include phenolic and aliphatic alcoholic agents and carboxylic acid substances. Tetrazoles, which are chemically similar to carboxylic acids, are also likely to be substrates for UGT2B7 because losartan, an angiotensin II receptor antagonist, serves as a relatively good substrate (81).

Much more work is needed to determine its extent of importance using stably expressed isoforms with high levels of expression.

Ritter and colleagues (77) were the first to clone and express UGT2B7. They characterized the expressed protein in COS-1 cells as a 52-kDa protein that is glycosylated and reactive with catechol estrogens, estrogens and several androgenic substrates. They observed no activity toward 4-nitrophenol, 1-naphthol, 4-methylumbelliferone, morphine, testosterone, or androsterone. Substrates that were most reactive with UGT2B7 were estrogen catechols, especially 4-hydroxy estrone. They observed an apparent K_m for 4-hydroxyestrone of 0.13 mM. In a later publication, results compared the reactivity of UGT2B7 with UGT2B4, which share 86% sequence identity (78). Although both UGTs catalyze hyodeoxycholate glucuronidation, UGT2B7 has about 100 times higher activity compared to UGT2B4. In addition, UGT2B7 catalyzes glucuronidation of bile acids at the 3-hydroxyl and carboxylic acid moieties, whereas UGT2B4 catalyzed bile acid glucuronidation at the 6α-hydroxyl group (80).

Jin and colleagues (82) cloned a form of UGT2B7 that differed from the deduced sequence isolated by Ritter and colleagues (77) in a single amino acid at position 268 (tyrosine for histidine). These investigators expressed UGT2B7(Y), the tyrosine variant, transiently in COS-7 cells and found that it had activity toward a number of carboxyl-containing xenobiotics such as NSAIDs, clofibric acid, and valproic acid. R- and S-enantiomers of ibuprofen were studied and a glucuronidation ratio of 1.62 (S/R) was obtained. Glucuronidation of enantiomers of ketoprofen and naproxen showed no selective rates.

Although 4-hydroxyestrone and hyodeoxycholic acid glucuronidation rates were high, they also observed activity toward androsterone, 4-nitrophenol, and menthol. Interestingly, no activity was found for morphine, lorazepam, or zidovudine.

In another study, Jin and colleagues (83) compared the activity of UGT2B7(Y) in COS-7 cells with UGT1A6, an isoform that is generally associated with the catalysis of carcinogenic polycyclic hydrocarbons such as hydroxylated BaP metabolites. UGT2B7(Y) catalyzed the glucuronidation of a wide range of hydroxylated BaP derivatives as well as the 4,5- and 7,8-dihydrodiols. Its activity toward the 4,5-diol was two to seven times that of its activity toward other substrates. UGT1A6 had no activity toward the dihydrodiols and glucuronidated only a limited range of monophenols. Hydroxylated metabolites of 2-acetylaminofluorene (AAF) were also studied. Both UGT2B7(Y) and UGT1A6 glucuronidated *N*-, 1-, 3-, and 8-hydroxy AAF, but 5-hydroxy AAF was glucuronidated only by UGT1A6. This suggests that cell content and organ distribution of either UGT2B7 or UGT1A6 may play an important role in the metabolism of these metabolites of carcinogens.

Coffman and colleagues (84) cloned a cDNA from a human liver cDNA library that proved to be identical to UGT2B7(Y). It was stably expressed in HK293 cells and tested for its activity toward opioids such as morphine and codeine. Expressed UGT2B7(Y) was found to have high glucuronidation activity for these compounds and was shown to catalyze both 3-glucuronide and 6-glucuronide formation. Its glucuronidation efficiency (V_m/K_m) was also very high when nalorphine and buprenorphine were studied as substrates. This finding was surprising in that other laboratories that had expressed UGT2B7(H) or UGT2B7(Y) had specifically reported no morphine glucuronidation in transient COS cell expression systems. Recently, our laboratory has shown that losartan, the tetrazole-containing angiotensin II antagonist and antihypertensive agent, is glucuronidated by UGT2B7(H) and (Y) (81). Apparent K_m values obtained were 43 μM and 83 μM, for UGT2B(Y) and (H), respectively. RT-PCR analysis with subsequent restriction enzyme digestion was performed on tissue samples from 27 individuals. Three of 27 were homozygous for H, 10 were homozygous for Y, and 14 were heterozygous (81).

Table 13-3 shows a comparison of morphinan and oripavine opioids in their reactivity with UGT2B7(Y) and UGT2B7(H). In general, there is little difference between the activity of the (H) and (Y) isoforms, either with respect to K_m values or efficiency for these compounds. It is clear that substitutions at the N-position influence the apparent K_m values obtained for opioids. Lower apparent K_m values are favored by the aliphatic chain substitutions over the cyclic, and apparent K_m values are higher when methyl group substitution is present. The presence of a

TABLE 13-3. *Comparison of the glucuronidation efficiencies of expressed UGT2B7(Y) and UGT2B7(H) for opioids and androsterone*

Substrate	UGT2B7(Y)	UGT2B7(H)
Morphine		
3-O glucuronide	1,150[a]	850
6-O glucuronide	110	170
Codeine	40	16
Nalorphine	3,500	2,800
Naloxone	6,900	8,100
Naltrexone	600	1,000
Hydromorphone	350	410
Oxymorphone	500	1,250
Buprenorphine	19,400	1,840
Androsterone	10,000	7,800

[a]Average glucuronidation efficiencies (V_{max}/K_m) from two experiments using approximately equivalent amounts of the expressed UGT2B7 isoforms.

14-hydroxy group yields values of higher apparent K_m, and increases the V_{max} (oxymorphone versus hydromorphone). The methoxy substitution at the 3-O position influences the V_{max} rates obtained because morphine-6-glucuronide V_{max} rates are higher than codeine-6-glucuronidation rates.

Glucuronidation of (+) and (−) menthol and androsterone was studied by Coffman and colleagues (85) and found to be catalyzed in a similar fashion by both forms. However, efficiency for androsterone glucuronidation was so high as to suggest that UGT2B7 is the major isoform catalyzing 3α-hydroxysteroids, a finding also reported by Jin and colleagues (86). No activity was observed toward testosterone although epitestosterone (17 α-ol) displayed high activity.

Patel and colleagues (87) have proposed that the two forms of UGT2B7 accounted for differences in two human populations with respect to differences in the ratio of R- and S-oxazepam glucuronides excreted in the urine when a racemic mixture of oxazepam was administered orally. The involvement of UGT2B7(Y) and UGT2B7(H) in this observation seems not to be valid. First, oxazepam is glucuronidated by expressed UGT2B7(H) and UGT2B7(Y) at very low rates (82,85). In fact, the rates were so low that it was impossible to determine glucuronidation kinetics with accuracy. Second, no differences in glucuronidation rates for oxazepam were observed between the two expressed isoforms (85). Thus, there must be another UGT isoform involved in oxazepam glucuronidation because oxazepam glucuronidation rates obtained from human liver microsomes are much higher than can be accounted for using expressed UGT2B7(Y) or (H).

It is well known that rats do not convert morphine to morphine-6-glucuronide and that they only glucuronidate morphine to the 3-O glucuronide (36). This can be explained because UGT2B1 and UGT1A1, the isoforms that catalyze morphine glucuronidation in rats, only mediate formation of the 3-O glucuronide. Humans form morphine 3-O and 6-O glucuronides after administration of morphine and, because UGT1A1 does not catalyze formation of the 6-O glucuronide (33), the role of UGT2B7 in morphine glucuronidation is most important in the metabolism of this opioid. As would be expected, UGT2B7 also catalyzes formation of the major codeine metabolite, codeine 6-O glucuronide. UGT2B7 is the only human UDPGT that has been shown to catalyze morphinan 6-O glucuronidation.

Monkey UGT2B9

Recently a cDNA for UGT2B9 has been isolated from cynomolgus monkey (88). The expressed protein was shown to catalyze the glucuronidation of a number of endobiotics, and, like human UGT2B7, monkey UGT2B9 catalyzes the 3-O and 6-O glucuronidation of morphine (89). The substrate specificities of the expressed human and monkey proteins have been shown to be very similar for endobiotics and xenobiotics. The major difference in substrate specificity between the UGT2B7 and UGT2B9 is the ability of the monkey UGT to catalyze the glucuronidation of 17-hydroxylated androgens such as testosterone and dihydrotestosterone (88).

Human UGT2B10

A cDNA encoding for a UGT termed UGT2B10 has been cloned and expressed in COS cells (79). To date, no glucuronidation activity has been found for this UGT.

Human UGT2B15

Chen and colleagues (90) cloned UGT2B15 and expressed the protein in COS-1 cells. Glucuronidation activity toward phenolphthalein, dihydrotestosterone, 5α-androstane-3α,17β-diol and 4-hydroxybiphenyl was observed. Northern blot analysis showed that mRNA encoding UGT2B15 was present in liver, prostate, and testis. These authors found that UGT2B15 mRNA was absent in the liver of a patient with benign prostatic hyperplasia and suggested that depressed glucuronidation of dihydrotestosterone denotes a critical role for this UGT in benign prostatic hyperplasia. Recently, Chang and colleagues (91) have shown that UGT2B15 is expressed in androgen-independent LNCaP cells and that its expression is downregulated by androgens and 1,25-dihydroxy vitamin D_3.

Green and colleagues (92) cloned and expressed a cDNA for UGT2B15, which was identical to that isolated by Chen and colleagues (90), and stably expressed this cDNA in HK293 cells. More than 100 compounds were tested for activity with expressed UGT2B15. Activity was observed toward several classes of substrates, including phenols, 7-hydroxylated coumarins, flavonoids, anthraquinones, and drugs and their hydroxylated metabolites. The expressed enzyme also catalyzed glucuronidation of endogenous catechol estrogens, dihydrotestosterone, and testosterone. To date, this is the only human UGT that has been found to catalyze the glucuronidation of testosterone, although several glucuronidate dihydrotestosterone. This protein has the highest efficiency toward eugenol, naringenin, and 5α-androstane-3α,17β-diol. Of interest is the fact this expressed UGT as did not catalyze the glucuronidation of estriol which one might have expected based on the results obtained with the pI 7.4 protein preparation purified by Irshaid and Tephly (93) and Coffman and colleagues (94). Because the glucuronidation activity obtained toward estriol in those preparations was low, it is likely that another UGT with high activity but low abundance must have been present in the purified enzyme preparations. The high activity of UGT2B15 toward natural products such as flavonoids (citrus fruits), eugenol (cloves), apigenin (parsley), genistein (pea pods) and quercetin point out the important nature of the UGTs that have evolved in mammals in response to dietary impact pressures.

Polymorphism of the UGT2B15 gene has been described by Lévesque and colleagues (95). UGT2B15 exists as either UGT2B15(D85), which was shown previously (90,92), or as UGT2B15(Y85). The genomic DNA of 27 individuals were analyzed by direct sequencing of PCR products and it was shown that UGT2B15(D) and UGT2B15(Y) are encoded by variant alleles prevalent in the caucasian population. Interestingly, both stably expressed proteins possessed similar substrate specificity and efficiency toward phenols, coumarins, flavonoids, and steroid. However, UGT2B15(Y) had a higher V_{max} toward the androgenic steroid substrates than UGT2B15(D). RT-PCR analyses revealed that the UGT2B15 gene was expressed in a wide range of tissues including human liver, kidney, testis, mammary gland, placenta, adipose, skin, uterus, prostate, and lung. This observation further suggests the important role of UGT2B15 in the detoxification of xenobiotic and certain endobiotic substances.

Human UGT2B17

Beaulieu and colleagues (96) isolated a cDNA clone from human prostate and LNCaP cell cDNA libraries that was 95% identical with UGT2B15 and that had a substrate specificity similar to that of UGT2B15. Major substrates were found to be eugenol, 4-methylumbelliferone, dihydrotestosterone, testosterone, and androsterone. RT-PCR analysis showed a tissue distribution similar to that of UGT2B15. Although UGT2B17 protein reacts with androsterone, recent studies show that UGT2B7 reacts with this steroid with very high efficiency (96). Guillemette and colleagues (97) showed that, in androgen-dependent LNCaP cells, UGT2B17 was downregulated by dihydrotestosterone and epidermal growth factor, whereas the level of UGT2B15 mRNA was not affected.

Rabbit UGT2B13, UGT2B14, and UGT2B16

Three UGTs of the UGT2 family have been cloned and expressed by Tukey and co-workers (98,99). UGT2B13 and UGT2B16 are 78% identical in primary amino acid sequence the expressed proteins with 4-hydroxybiphenyl. UGT2B16 also reacts with 4-hydroxyestrone and 4-tert-butylphenol, substrates that are not glucuronidated well by UGT2B13. UGT2B14 has not been found to react with any substrate at this time. UGT2B13 expression was found to be primarily in adult rabbits; however, UGT2B13 mRNA expression in neonatal rabbits was increased as was 4-hydroxybiphenyl glucuronidation by treatment with dexamethasone or rifampin.

SUMMARY

Glucuronide formation is an important conjugation reaction that is catalyzed by proteins in the endoplasmic reticulum. Two gene families have been identified that encode for the different UDPGT isoforms. The UGT1 gene complex has been shown to be structurally similar in rodents and humans, in that multiple unique first exons exist and the gene products arise from alternate splicing of single first exons with shared exons two to 5. As a result, the human UGT1 gene complex codes for 12 proteins with variable amino acid sequences in their N-terminal region and identical C-termini. Whereas much overlap in substrate specificities has been observed for human UGT1A proteins (see Table 13-1), it has also been possible to identify specific substrates for some of these gene products (Table 13-4). UGT1A1 catalyzes the glucuronidation of many xenobiotics (especially buprenorphine) but is specific for bilirubin (see Table 13-4). UGT1A4 has been identified as a major, but not exclusive, catalyst for the formation of quaternary ammonium-linked glucuronides from a number of therapeutically important drugs and for the formation of amine glucuronides from carcinogenic primary amines. Experimental evidence suggests that sapogenins, such as hecogenin or tigogenin, may be specific substrates for this

UDPGT isoform. UGTs 1A6 and 1A9 display broad substrate reactivities toward many simple phenolic compounds, but only UGT1A9 appears to catalyze the glucuronidation of propofol.

UDPGT proteins encoded by the UGT2 family are derived from unique genes, although many of these genes have been shown to be closely clustered on the same chromosome (chromosome 4 in humans). Similar to the UGT1 proteins, isoforms of UGT2 have broadly overlapping substrate reactivities (see Table 13-2), but specific substrates have also been identified. Although both UGT2B4 and UGT2B7 have been shown to catalyze the glucuronidation of hyodeoxycholate, only UGT2B4 specifically catalyzes hyodeoxycholic acid glucuronidation at the 6α-hydroxyl position on the steroid B-ring. Three UDPGTs have been shown to catalyze the glucuronidation of morphinan-type opioids; however, only UGT2B7 has been shown to catalyze opioid glucuronidation at the 6-hydroxyl position. Therefore, codeine (which has only a 6-hydroxyl group) is an ideal compound to assess UGT2B7 activity.

Polymorphic forms of UGT2B7 and 2B15 have been identified, but it does not appear that the single amino acid differences between the isoforms results in significant differences in the glucuronidation rates of the xenobiotics and endobiotics studied to date. In contrast, mutations in the UGT1A1 gene lead to either moderate or complete loss of the ability to conjugate bilirubin with glucuronic acid. In humans, this results in hyperbilirubinemias associated with Gilbert's syndrome or Crigler-Najjar type I or type II disease.

With the availability of cloned and expressed UDPGT isoforms, it will be possible to predict potential drug–drug, drug–endobiotic, and other xenobiotic–drug interactions. Further studies are needed to determine the relative hepatic abundance and tissue distributions of these proteins.

REFERENCES

1. Mackenzie PI, Owens IS, Burchell B, et al. The UDP glycosyltransferase gene superfamily: recommended nomenclature update based on evolutionary divergence. *Pharmacogenetics* 1997;7:255–269.
2. Dutton GJ. *Glucuronidation of drugs and other compounds.* Boca Raton, FL: CRC Press, 1980.
3. Oguri K, Ida S, Yoshimura H, Tsukamoto H. Metabolism of drugs LXIX. Studies on the urinary metabolites of morphine in several mammalian species. *Chem Pharm Bull* 1970;18:2414–2419.
4. Abbott FV, Palmour RM. Morphine-6-glucuronide: analgesic effects and receptor binding profile in rats. *Life Sci* 1988;43:1685–1695.
5. Paul D, Standifer KM, Inturrisi CE, Pasternak GW. Pharmacological characterization of morphine-6β-glucuronide, a very potent morphine metabolite. *J Pharmacol Exp Ther* 1989;240:890–894.
6. Frances B, Gout R, Monsarrat B, Cros J, Zajac J-M. Further evidence that morphine-6β-glucuronide is a more potent opioid agonist than morphine. *J Pharmacol Exp Ther* 1992;262:25–31.
7. Smith MT, Watt JA, Cramond T. Morphine-3-glucuronide—a potent antagonist of morphine analgesia. *Life Sci* 1990;47:579–585.
8. Gong Q-L, Hedner J, Björkman R, Hedner T. Morphine-3-glucuronide may functionally antagonize morphine-6-glucuronide induced antinociception and ventilatory depression in the rat. *Pain* 1992;48: 249–255.

TABLE 13-4. *Specific substrates for human UGTs*

UGT isoform	Substrate
UGT1A1	Bilirubin
UGT1A4	Tigogenin
UGT1A9	Propofol
UGT1A10	Mycophenolic acid
UGT2B4	Hyodeoxycholic acid (6α-hydroxyl position)
UGT2B7	Codeine

9. Meyers M, Slikker W, Vore M. Steroid D-ring glucuronides: characterization of a new class of cholestatic agents in the rat. *J Pharmacol Exp Ther* 1981;218:63–73.

10. Vore M, Liu Y, Huang L. Cholestatic properties and hepatic transport of steroid glucuronides. *Drug Metab Rev* 1997;29:183–203.

11. Slikker W, Vore M, Bailey JR, Meyers M, Montgomery C. Hepatotoxic effects of estradiol-17-β-D-glucuronide in the rat and monkey. *J Pharmacol Exp Ther* 1983;225:138–143.

12. Sinclair KA, Caldwell J. The formation of β-glucuronidase resistant glucuronides by the intramolecular rearrangement of glucuronic acid conjugates at mild alkaline pH. *Biochem Pharmacol* 1982;31:953–957.

13. Smith PC, Hasegawa J, Langendijk PNJ, Benet LZ. Stability of acyl glucuronides in blood, plasma and urine: studies with zomepirac. *Drug Metab Dispos* 1985;13:110–112.

14. Rowe BJ, Meffin PJ. Diisopropylfluorophosphate increases clofibric acid clearance: supporting evidence for a futile cycle. *J Pharmacol Exp Ther* 1984;230:237–241.

15. Williams AM, Worral S, de Jersey J, Dickinson RG. Studies on the reactivity of acyl glucuronides-III glucuronide-derived adducts of valproic acid and plasma protein and anti-adduct antibodies in humans. *Biochem Pharmacol* 1992;43:745–755.

16. Nolen H, Fedorak RN, Friend DR. Budesonide-β-D-glucuronide: a potential prodrug for treatment of ulcerative colitis. *J Pharm Sci* 1995;84:677–681.

17. Gunning DB, Barua AB, Lloyd R, Olson JA. Retinoyl-β-glucuronide: a nontoxic retinoid for the topical treatment of acne. *J Dermatol Treat* 1994;5:181–185.

18. Barua AB. Retinoyl β-glucuronide: a biologically active form of vitamin A. *Nutr Rev* 1997;55:259–267.

19. Tephly TR, Burchell B. UDP-glucuronosyltransferases: a family of detoxifying enzymes. *TIPS* 1990;11:276–279.

20. Mackenzie PI. Expression of chimeric cDNAs in cell culture defines a region of UDP-glucuronosyltransferase involved in substrate selection. *J Biol Chem* 1990;265:3432–3435.

21. Ritter JK, Chen F, Sheen YY, et al. A novel complex locus *UGT1* encodes human bilirubin, phenol and other UDP-glucuronosyltransferase isozymes with identical carboxyl termini. *J Biol Chem* 1992; 267:3257–3261.

22. Emi Y, Ikushiro S, Iyanagi T. Drug-responsive and tissue-specific alternative expression of multiple first exons in rat UDP-glucuronosyltransferase family 1 (*UGT1*) gene complex. *J Biochem* 1995;117:392–399.

23. Lamb JG, Straub P, Tukey RH. Cloning and characterization of cDNAs encoding mouse Ugt1.6 and rabbit UGT1.6: differential induction by 2,3,7,8-tetrachlorodibenzo-*p*-dioxin. *Biochemistry* 1994;33: 10513–10520.

24. Kong A-NT, Ma M, Tao D, Yang L. Molecular cloning of two cDNAs encoding the mouse bilirubin/phenol family of UDP-glucuronosyltransferases (*mUGT*$_{br/p}$). *Pharm Res* 1993;10:461–465.

25. Bruck M, Li Q, Lamb JG, Tukey RH. Characterization of rabbit UDP-glucuronosyltransferase UGT1A7: tertiary amine glucuronidation is catalyzed by UGT1A7 and UGT1A4. *Arch Biochem Biophys* 1997;344: 357–364.

26. Strassburg CP, Manns MP, Tukey RH. Differential down-regulation of the *UDP-glucuronosyltransferase 1A* locus is an early event in human liver and biliary cancer. *Cancer Res* 1997;57:2979–2985.

27. Strassburg CP, Oldhafer K, Manns MP, Tukey RH. Differential expression of the *UGT1A* locus in human liver, biliary and gastric tissue: identification of *UGT1A7* and *UGT1A10* transcripts in extrahepatic tissue. *Mol Pharmacol* 1997;52:212–220.

28. Ritter JK, Crawford JM, Owens IS. Cloning of two human liver bilirubin UDP-glucuronosyltransferase cDNAs with expression in COS-1 cells. *J Biol Chem* 1991;266:1043–1047.

29. Bosma PJ, Seppen J, Goldhoorn B, et al. Bilirubin UDP-glucuronosyltransferase 1 is the only relevant bilirubin glucuronidating isoform in man. *J Biol Chem* 1994;269:17960–19764.

30. Senafi SB, Clarke DJ, Burchell B. Investigation of the substrate specificity of a cloned expressed human bilirubin UDP-glucuronosyltransferase: UDP-sugar specificity and involvement in steroid and xenobiotic glucuronidation. *Biochem J* 1994;303:233–240.

31. Visser TJ, Kaptein E, Gijzel AL, et al. Glucuronidation of thyroid hormone by human bilirubin and phenol UDP-glucuronosyltransferase isoenzymes. *FEBS Let* 1993;324:358–360.

32. Coffman BL, Green MD, King CD, Tephly TR. Cloning and stable expression of a cDNA encoding a rat liver UDP-glucuronosyltransferase (UDP-glucuronosyltransferase 1.1) that catalyzes the glu-curonidation of opioids and bilirubin. *Mol Pharmacol* 1995;47: 1101–1105.

33. King CD, Green MD, Rios GR, et al. The glucuronidation of exogenous and endogenous compounds by stably expressed rat and human UDP-glucuronosyltransferase 1A1. *Arch Biochem Biophys* 1996;332: 92–100.

34. Radominska A, Little JM, Lehman PA, et al. Glucuronidation of retinoids by rat recombinant UDP-glucuronosyltransferase 1.1 (bilirubin UGT). *Drug Metab Dispos* 1997;25:889–892.

35. Iyanagi T. Molecular basis of multiple UDP-glucuronosyltransferase isoenzyme deficiencies in the hyperbilirubinemic rat (Gunn rat). *J Biol Chem* 1991;266:24048–24052.

36. King CD, Rios GR, Green MD, Mackenzie PI, Tephly TR. Comparison of stably expressed rat UGT1.1 and UGT2B1 in the glucuronidation of opioid compounds. *Drug Metab Dispos* 1997;25:251–255.

37. Seppen J, Steenken E, Lindhout D, Bosma PJ, Oude Elferink RPL. A mutation which disrupts the hydrophobic core of the signal peptide of bilirubin UDP-glucuronosyltransferase, an endoplasmic reticulum membrane protein, causes Crigler-Najjar type II. *FEBS Lett* 1996;390: 294–298.

38. Bosma PJ, Roy Chowdhury J, Bakker C, et al. The genetic basis of the reduced expression of bilirubin UDP-glucuronosyltransferase 1 in Gilbert's syndrome. *N Engl J Med* 1995;333:1171–1175.

39. Monaghan G, Ryan M, Seddon R, Hume R, Burchell B. Genetic variation in bilirubin UDP-glucuronosyltransferase gene promoter and Gilbert's syndrome. *Lancet* 1996;347:578–581.

40. Koiwai O, Nishizawa M, Hasada K, et al. Gilbert's syndrome is caused by a heterozygous missense mutation in the gene for bilirubin UDP-glucuronosyltransferase. *Hum Mol Genet* 1995;4:1183–1186.

41. Cowan A, Lewis JW, eds. *Buprenorphine: combating drug abuse with a unique opioid.* New York: Wiley-Liss, 1995.

42. Iyer L, King CD, Whitington PF, et al. Genetic predisposition to the metabolism of irinotecan (CPT-11): role of UGT isoform 1A1 (UGT1A1) in the glucuronidation of its active metabolite (SN-38) in human liver microsomes. *J Clin Invest* 1998;101:847–854.

43. Wasserman E, Myara A, Lokiec F, et al. Severe CPT-11 toxicity in patients with Gilbert's syndrome: two case reports. *Ann Oncol* 1997;8: 1049–1051.

44. Sato H, Koiwai O, Tanabe K, Kashiwamata S. Isolation and sequencing of rat liver bilirubin UDP-glucuronosyltransferase cDNA: possible alternate splicing of a common primary transcript. *Biochem Biophys Res Commun* 1990;169:260–264.

45. Green MD, Bishop WP, Tephly TR. Expressed human UGT1.4 protein catalyzes the formation of quaternary ammonium-linked glucuronides. *Drug Metab Dispos* 1995;23:299–302.

46. Green MD, Tephly TR. Glucuronidation of amines and hydroxylated xenobiotics and endobiotics catalyzed by expressed human UGT1.4 protein. *Drug Metab Dispos* 1996;24:356–363.

47. Green MD, King CD, Mojarrabi B, Mackenzie PI, Tephly TR. Glucuronidation of amines and other xenobiotics catalyzed by expressed human UDP-glucuronosyltransferase 1A3. *Drug Metab Dispos* 1998; 26:507–512.

48. Mojarrabi B, Butler R, Mackenzie PI. cDNA cloning and characterization of the human UDP-glucuronosyltransferase, UGT1A3. *Biochem Biophys Res Commun* 1996;225:785–790.

49. Falany CN, Tephly TR. Separation, purification and characterization of three isoforms of UDP-glucuronosyltransferase from rat liver microsomes. *Arch Biochem Biophys* 1983;227:248–258.

50. Ebner T, Burchell B. Substrate specificities of two stably expressed human liver UDP-glucuronosyltransferases of the *UGT1* gene family. *Drug Metab Dispos* 1993;21:50–55.

51. Gschaidmeier H, Seidel A, Burchell B, Bock KW. Formation of mono- and diglucuronides and other glycosides of benzo(a)pyrene-3,6-quinol by V79 cell-expressed human phenol UDP-glucuronosyltransferases of the UGT1 gene complex. *Biochem Pharmacol* 1995;49:1601–1606.

52. Bock KW, Forster A, Gschaidmeier H, et al. Paracetamol glucuronidation by recombinant rat and human phenol UDP-glucuronosyltransferases. *Biochem Pharmacol* 1993;45:1809–1814.

53. Bock KW, Schrenk D, Forster A, et al. The influence of environmental and genetic factors on CYP2D6, CYP1A2, and UDP-glucuronosyltransferases in man using sparteine, caffeine and paracetamol as probes. *Pharmacogenetics* 1994;4:209–218.

54. Emi Y, Ikushiro S-I, Iyanagi T. Xenobiotic responsive element-mediated transcriptional activation in the UDP-glucuronosyltransferase family 1 gene complex. *J Biol Chem* 1996;271:3952–3958.

55. Münzel PA, Bookjans G, Mehner G, Lehmköster T, Bock KW. Tissue-specific 2,3,7,8-tetrachlorodibenzo-*p*-dioxin-inducible expression of human UDP-glucuronosyltransferase UGT1A6. *Arch Biochem Biophys* 1996;335:205–210.

56. Masmoudi T, Hihi AK, Vázquez M, et al. Transcriptional regulation by triiodothyronine of the UDP-glucuronosyltransferase family 1 gene complex in rat liver. *J Biol Chem* 1997;272:17171–17175.

57. Bock KW, Kobusch A-B, Fischer G. Heterogeneous alterations of UDP-glucuronosyltransferases in mouse hepatic foci. *J Cancer Res Clin Oncol* 1989;115:285–289.

58. Bock KW, Münzel PA, Röhrdanz E, Schrenk D, Eriksson LC. Persistently increased expression of a 3-methycholanthrene-inducible phenol uridine diphosphate-glucuronosyltransferase in rat hepatocyte nodules and hepatocellular carcinomas. *Cancer Res* 1990;50:3569–3573.

59. Grove AD, Kessler FK, Metz BP, Ritter JK. Identification of a rat oltipraz-inducible UDP-glucuronosyltransferase (UGT1A7) with activity towards benzo(a)pyrene-7,8-dihydrodiol. *J Biol Chem* 1997;272:1621–1627.

60. Orzechowski A, Schrenk D, Bock-Henning BS, Bock KW. Glucuronidation of carcinogenic arylamines and their N-hydroxy derivatives by rat and human phenol UDP-glucuronosyltransferases of the UGT1 gene complex. *Carcinogenesis* 1994;15:1549–1553.

61. Mojarrabi B, Mackenzie PI. The human UDP glucuronosyltransferase, UGT1A10, glucuronidates mycophenolic acid. *Biochem Biophys Res Commun* 1997;238:775–778.

62. Mackenzie PI, Rodbourn L. Organization of the rat UDP-glucuronosyltransferase, UDPGTr-2 gene and characterization of its promoter. *J Biol Chem* 1990;265:11328–11332.

63. Monaghan G, Burchell B, Boxer M. Structure of the human UGT2B4 gene encoding a bile acid UDP-glucuronosyltransferase. *Mamm Genome* 1997;8:692–694.

64. Beaulieu M, Lévesque E, Tchernof A, Beatty BG, Bélanger A, Hum DW. Chromosomal localization, structure and regulation of the *UGT2B17* gene, encoding a C19 steroid metabolizing enzyme. *DNA Cell Biol* 1997;16:1143–1153.

65. Lazard D, Zupko K, Poria Y, et al. Odorant signal termination by olfactory UDP-glucuronosyltransferase. *Nature* 1991;349:790–793.

66. Coffman BL, Rios GR, Tephly TR. Purification and properties of two rat liver phenobarbital-inducible UDP-glucuronosyltransferases that catalyze the glucuronidation of opioids. *Drug Metab Dispos* 1996;24:329–333.

67. Styczynski P, Green M, Puig J, Coffman B, Tephly T. Purification and properties of a rat liver phenobarbital-inducible 4-hydroxybiphenyl UDP-glucuronosyltransferase. *Mol Pharmacol* 1991;40:80–84.

68. Mackenzie PI. Rat liver UDP-glucuronosyltransferase: sequence and expression of a cDNA encoding a phenobarbital-inducible form. *J Biol Chem* 1986;261:6119–6125.

69. Mackenzie PI. Rat liver UDP-glucuronosyltransferase: cDNA sequence and expression of a form glucuronidating 3-hydroxyandrogens. *J Biol Chem* 1986;261:14112–14117.

70. Mackenzie PI. Rat liver UDP-glucuronosyltransferase: identification of cDNAs encoding two enzymes which glucuronidate testosterone, dihydrotestosterone, and β-estradiol. *J Biol Chem* 1987;262:9744–9749.

71. Pritchard M, Fournel-Gigleux S, Siest G, Mackenzie P, Magdalou J. A recombinant phenobarbital-inducible rat liver UDP-glucuronosyltransferase 2B1 stably expressed in V79 cells catalyzes the glucuronidation of morphine, phenols and carboxylic acids. *Mol Pharmacol* 1994;45:42–50.

72. Harding D, Wilson SM, Jackson MR, et al. Nucleotide and deduced amino acid sequence of rat liver 17β-hydroxysteroid UDP-glucuronosyltransferase. *Nucl Acids Res* 1987;15:3936.

73. Green MD, Clarke DJ, Oturu EM, et al. Cloning and expression of a rat liver phenobarbital-inducible UDP-glucuronosyltransferase (2B12) with specificity for monoterpenoid alcohols. *Arch Biochem Biophys* 1995;322:460–468.

74. Haque SJ, Petersen DD, Nebert DW, Mackenzie PI. Isolation, sequence and developmental expression of rat UGT2B2: the gene encoding a constitutive UDP-glucuronosyltransferase that metabolizes etiocholanolone and androsterone. *DNA Cell Biol* 1991;10:515–524.

75. Fournel-Gigleux S, Jackson MR, Wooster R, Burchell B. Expression of a human liver cDNA encoding a UDP-glucuronosyltransferase catalysing the glucuronidation of hyodeoxycholic acid in cell culture. *FEBS Lett* 1989;243:119–122.

76. Fournel-Gigleux S, Sutherland L, Sabolovic N, Burchell B, Siest G. Stable expression of two human UDP-glucuronosyltransferase cDNAs in V79 cell cultures. *Mol Pharmacol* 1991;39:177–183.

77. Ritter JK, Sheen YY, Owens IS. Cloning and expression of human liver UDP-glucuronosyltransferase in COS-1 cells. *J Biol Chem* 1990;265:7900–7906.

78. Ritter JK, Chen F, Sheen YY, Lubet RA, Owens IS. Two human liver cDNAs encode UDP-glucuronosyltransferases with 2 log differences in activity toward parallel substrates including hyodeoxycholic acid and certain estrogen derivatives. *Biochemistry* 1992;31:3409–3414.

79. Jin C-J, Miners JO, Lillywhite KJ, Mackenzie PI. cDNA cloning and expression of two new members of the human liver UDP-glucuronosyltransferase 2B subfamily. *Biochem Biophys Res Commun* 1993;194:496–503.

80. Pillot T, Ouzzine M, Fournel-Gigleux S, et al. Glucuronidation of hyodeoxycholic acid in human liver. Evidence for a selective role of UDP-glucuronosyltransferase 2B4. *J Biol Chem* 1993;268:25636–25642.

81. Rios GR, Green MD, Schuetz E, Tephly TR. Metabolism of losartan by polymorphic human UDP-glucuronosyltransferase (UGT) 2B7. *FASEB J* 1998;12:A962.

82. Jin C-J, Miners JO, Lillywhite KJ, Mackenzie PI. Complementary deoxyribonucleic acid cloning and expression of a human liver uridine diphosphate-glucuronosyltransferase glucuronidating carboxylic acid-containing drugs. *J Pharmacol Exp Ther* 1993;264:475–479.

83. Jin C-J, Miners JO, Burchell B, Mackenzie PI. The glucuronidation of hydroxylated metabolites of benzo[a]pyrene and 2-acetylaminofluorene by cDNA-expressed human UDP-glucuronosyltransferases. *Carcinogenesis* 1993;14:2637–2639.

84. Coffman BL, Rios GR, King CD, Tephly TR. Human UGT2B7 catalyzes morphine glucuronidation. *Drug Metab Dispos* 1997;25:1–4.

85. Coffman BL, King CD, Rios GR, Tephly TR. The glucuronidation of opioids, other xenobiotics and androgens by human UGT2B7Y(268) and UGT2B7H(268). *Drug Metab Dispos* 1998;26:73–77.

86. Jin C-J, Mackenzie PI, Miners JO. The regio- and stereo-selectivity of C19 and C21 hydroxysteroid glucuronidation by UGT2B7 and UGT2B11. *Arch Biochem Biophys* 1997;341:207–211.

87. Patel M, Tang BK, Grant DM, Kalow W. Interindividual variability in the glucuronidation of (S) oxazepam contrasted with that of (R) oxazepam. *Pharmacogenetics* 1995;5:287–297.

88. Bélanger G, Beaulieu M, Lévesque E, Hum DW, Bélanger A. Expression and characterization of a novel UDP-glucuronosyltransferase, UGT2B9, from cynomolgus monkey. *DNA Cell Biol* 1997;16:1195–1205.

89. Green MD, Bélanger G, Hum DW, Bélanger A, Tephly TR. Glucuronidation of opioids, carboxylic acid-containing drugs, and hydroxylated xenobiotics catalyzed by expressed monkey UDP-glucuronosyltransferase 2B9 protein. *Drug Metab Dispos* 1997;25:1389–1394.

90. Chen F, Ritter JK, Wang MG, et al. Characterization of a cloned human dihydrotestosterone/androstanediol UDP-glucuronosyltransferase and its comparison to other steroid isoforms. *Biochemistry* 1993;32:10648–10657.

91. Chang GTG, Blok LJ, Steenbeek M, et al. Differentially expressed genes in androgen-dependent and -independent prostate carcinomas. *Cancer Res* 1997;57:4075–4081.

92. Green MD, Oturu EM, Tephly TR. Stable expression of human liver UDP-glucuronosyltransferase (UGT2B15) with activity toward steroid and xenobiotic substrates. *Drug Metab Dispos* 1994;22:799–805.

93. Irshaid YM, Tephly TR. Isolation and purification of two human liver UDP-glucuronosyltransferases. *Mol Pharmacol* 1987;32:27–34.

94. Coffman BL, Tephly TR, Irshaid YM, et al. Characterization and primary sequence of a human hepatic microsomal estriol UDP-glucuronosyltransferase. *Arch Biochem Biophys* 1990;281:170–175.

95. Lévesque E, Beaulieu M, Green MD, Tephly TR, Bélanger A, Hum DW. Isolation and characterization of UGT2B15(Y[85]): a UDP-glucuronosyltransferase encoded by a polymorphic gene. *Pharmacogenetics* 1997;7:317–325.

96. Beaulieu M, Lévesque E, Hum DW, Bélanger A. Isolation and characterization of a novel cDNA encoding a human UDP-glucuronosyltransferase active on C19 steroids. *J Biol Chem* 1996;271:22855–22862.

97. Guillemette C, Lévesque E, Beaulieu M, Turgeon D, Hum DW, Bélanger A. Differential regulation of two uridine diphospho-glucuronosyltransferases, UGT2B15 and UGT2B17, in human prostate LNCaP cells. *Endocrinology* 1997;138:2998–3005.

98. Tukey RH, Pendurthi UR, Nguyen NT, Green MD, Tephly TR. Cloning and characterization of rabbit liver UDP-glucuronosyltransferase cDNAs. Developmental and inducible expression of 4-hydroxybiphenyl UGT2B13. *J Biol Chem* 1993;268:15260–15266.

99. Li QL, Lou X, Peyronneau M-A, Obermayer Straub P, Tukey RH. Expression and functional domains of rabbit liver UDP-glucuronosyltransferase 2B16 and 2B13. *J Biol Chem* 1997;272:3272–3279.

CHAPTER 14

Glutathione S-Transferases

David L. Eaton and Theo K. Bammler

HISTORICAL PERSPECTIVE

Originally in 1961, Booth and co-workers (1) described an enzymatic activity present in rat liver cytosol that catalyzed the conjugation of glutathione (GSH) with 1,2-dichloro-4-nitrobenzene (DCNB). In the following years of that decade, many different glutathione S-transferase (GST) substrates were identified (2), and evidence for the existence of several distinct isoenzymes began to emerge (3,4). Early attempts to classify enzymes displaying GST activity were based on the chemical structure of the electrophilic substrates and resulted in names such as aryl-, alkyl-, alkene-, and epoxide-transferases (2,5,6). Investigators from Jakoby's laboratory were the first to report the successful purification of GSTs from rat liver (3,4). Subsequently, characterization of homogeneous enzyme preparations confirmed the existence of several catalytically distinct GSTs (4). In addition to catalyzing the conjugation of reduced glutathione with numerous electrophilic compounds, GSTs were shown to possess ligandin (7,8), selenium-independent peroxidase (9), and ketosteroid isomerase activity (10).

Sodium dodecylsulfate–polyacrylamide gel electrophoresis (SDS-PAGE) analysis (11) and reversible denaturation experiments (12) of individual rat GSTs revealed the existence of homo- and heterodimeric isoenzymes and provided the basis for dividing GSTs into structurally distinct groups. More recently the isolation of different cDNA clones provided the ultimate proof that GST subunits with distinct electrophoretic behavior were indeed the products of distinct genes (13–16).

Catalytic, immunochemical, and N-terminal sequence analyses indicated that certain GST isoenzymes isolated from different species (e.g., mouse, rat, human) were more similar than were distinct GSTs from the same species. This observation led Mannervik et al. (17) to propose a species-independent classification system, according to which mammalian cytosolic GSTs were grouped into three classes termed alpha, mu, and pi. In more recent years, two additional classes of mammalian cytosolic GSTs have been identified and designated theta (18) and zeta (19).

Since the initial pioneering work by Jakoby et al. (3,7), a large number of GSTs have been isolated and purified from bacteria, yeast, nematodes, insects, fish, birds, mammals, and plants (20). The ubiquitous occurrence suggests that GSTs play an important role in protecting organisms from the potentially devastating effects caused by chemical insult.

In 1991, Reinemer et al. (21) were the first to report the three-dimensional structure of a pi-class GST isolated from pig lung. Since then, the structures of alpha (22), mu (23), and further pi class GSTs (24,25) have been resolved [for recent review, see (26)].

CLASSIFICATION AND NOMENCLATURE

Based on nucleotide and amino acid sequence similarities, mammalian cytosolic GSTs (EC 2.5.1.18) are grouped into five subfamilies named alpha, mu, pi, theta, and zeta (17–19,27). Members of the same subfamily share more than 40% sequence identity, whereas members of distinct subfamilies possess less than 30% identity. In addition to the cytosolic GSTs, three membrane-associated forms have been isolated and are referred to as microsomal GSTs (28–33). Amino acid sequence comparison revealed that the microsomal GSTs share no homology with the cytosolic isoenzymes, suggesting that both groups evolved through independent pathways. The scope of this review does not allow including a discussion of the microsomal GSTs.

D. L. Eaton and T. K. Bammler: Department of Environmental Health, University of Washington, 4225 Roosevelt Way NE, Suite 100, Seattle, Washington 98195-7610

Historically, the nomenclature of GSTs has been problematic, as different investigators have developed their own independent designations. The lack of a commonly used nomenclature system often resulted in multiple names for the same GST enzyme, confusing the matter. To resolve this problem, Mannervik et al. (27) proposed a unifying nomenclature for human cytosolic GSTs. These investigators suggested using upper-case Roman letters to indicate the class (A, alpha; M, mu; P, pi; T, theta; Z, zeta) and Arabic numerals separated by a hyphen to specify the subunit composition. Arabic numerals are assigned to the subunits, on the basis of the chronologic order of discovery. Allelic variants are represented by lower-case Roman letters (e.g., GSTM1a-1a). The corresponding gene loci also are named according to this system, with the modification that only one letter is used. As the microsomal forms are not members of the cytosolic GSTs, no change in the nomenclature of these enzymes has been proposed. In addition, Mannervik et al. (27) suggested extension of this system for naming GSTs from other mammalian species by using an appropriate lower-case letter prefix to indicate the origin (e.g., h, human; r, rat; m, mouse). A detailed review and assignment of nomenclature for human and other mammalian GSTs can be found in (34).

REGULATION OF GSTS

The regulation of cytosolic GSTs is subject to a complex set of endogenous and exogenous parameters. These include developmental, sex- (35,36), and tissue-specific factors (37), as well as a large number of xenobiotic inducing agents such as polycyclic aromatic hydrocarbons (PAH), phenolic antioxidants, Michael acceptors, reactive oxygen species, organic isothiocyanates, trivalent arsenicals, barbiturates, and synthetic glucocorticoids [for recent reviews, see (34,38)]. Northern blot analyses and nuclear run-on experiments demonstrated that induction occurs at the transcriptional level (39). The structural diversity of the compounds that induce or enhance the expression of GSTs suggests that multiple mechanisms are involved in their regulation, some of which have been identified and are described later.

Most of the mechanistic studies on transcriptional regulation of GSTs have used rodents. Therefore to provide an overview of GST regulation, both the rodent and the human data are discussed.

Transcriptional Regulation of Rodent Alpha Class GST Genes

Pickett et al. (37) identified five distinct cis-acting elements in the 5′-flanking region of the rat *GSTA2* gene (previously named Ya). Two of these contain core DNA sequences that are recognized by the liver-specific transcription factors HNF1 and HNF4 (hepatocyte nuclear factors 1 and 4), and are required for maximal basal-level expression. In addition, a glucocorticoid-response element (GRE), a xenobiotic-response element (XRE; also named the dioxin response element, DRE), and an antioxidant-response element (ARE) were identified (37,40). The GRE is likely to mediate induction of the rat *GSTA2* gene through the synthetic glucocorticoid dexamethasone (41).

The XRE core sequence (5′-GCGTG-3′) (42) has also been identified in the 5′-regulatory regions of both the rat and mouse cytochrome P450 *1A1* genes, and interacts with the aryl hydrocarbon (Ah)-receptor complex. The Ah receptor is required for transcriptional activation of the rat *GSTA2* gene by planar aromatic compounds such as β-naphthoflavone (β-NF), 3-methylcholanthrene (3-MC), and 2,3,7,8-tetrachlorodibenzo-p-dioxin (TCDD) (37).

In addition to the XRE-mediated transcriptional activation of the rat *GSTA2* gene, which requires a functional Ah receptor, a novel Ah receptor–independent mechanism has been identified (37,43). Pickett et al. (43) showed that phenolic antioxidants such as *tert*-butylhydroquinone or 3,5-di-*tert*-butylcatechol activated transcription in cells lacking a functional Ah receptor. A cis-acting element was identified that was required for transcriptional activation of the rat *GSTA2* gene by phenolic antioxidants and, hence, was named the ARE. Subsequent point-mutation analysis established that the minimal ARE consensus sequence required for inducible activity was 5′-TGACNNNGC-3′ (N, any nucleotide). It was later noted that a common characteristic of the phenolic antioxidants that induced *GSTA2* expression through the ARE was their ability to undergo or otherwise stimulate redox cycling, potentially generating superoxide anions and hydrogen peroxide. Consistent with this observation, it was shown that hydrogen peroxide was a potent inducer of transcription through the ARE (43).

Friling et al. (44,45) analyzed the 5′-flanking region of the mouse *GstA1* gene (previously named Ya gene) and identified a 41-bp sequence that mediates transcriptional activation by electrophilic compounds (e.g., *trans*-4-phenyl-3-butene-2-one). Therefore the enhancer core sequence, 5′-TGACATTGCNNNNNNNTGACAAAGC-3′, contained in this region, was named the electrophile-response element (EpRE). Subsequently it was found that the EpRE conferred inducibility to a wide range of chemicals including β-NF and 3-MC. Sequence analysis revealed that the murine gene contains the ARE sequence, 5′-TGACAAAGC-3′, identical to that found in the rat *GSTA2* gene, as well as an additional ARE consensus sequence, 5′-TGACATTGC-3′, located 6 bp upstream. Although the mouse EpRE and the rat ARE function in a similar manner, it has been proposed that the presence of an additional ARE consensus sequence found in the EpRE makes this enhancer more responsive to certain inducers (46). Indeed, a recent literature review by Hayes and Pulford (34) suggested that the EpRE is 500-fold more responsive to β-NF than is the ARE.

Recently Wasserman and Fahl (46) found that additional nucleotides outside of the core ARE sequence defined initially by Pickett et al. (43) were important for the degree of inducibility. The extended ARE consensus sequence is 5′-TMANNRTGAYNNNGCRWWWW-3′ (M, A or C; R, A or G; Y, C or T; W, A or T; N, any nucleotide).

Wasserman and Fahl also identified seven ARE-binding proteins (termed ARE-BP-1 through -7) (47). Although these researchers provided evidence for the involvement of several *trans*-acting factors in the ARE-mediated induction process, they concluded that ARE-BP-1 played a predominant role in the unique ARE responsiveness to chemoprotective agents.

Transcriptional Regulation of Human Alpha Class GST Genes

The research groups led by Peters and van Bladeren explored induction of human GSTs *in vivo* (48,49). These investigators measured a 1.4-fold increase of alpha class GSTs in the plasma of healthy volunteers after consumption of 300 g brussels sprouts for 3 weeks (49). It was concluded that the increase in plasma GST was due to *de novo* synthesis rather than to liver toxicity. In addition, rectal biopsies from volunteers consuming 300 g brussels sprouts daily for 1 week showed a 1.3-fold increase in alpha class GST compared with the control group (48). Brussels sprouts contain high amounts of allyl isothiocyanates and goitrin, both of which are known to induce GSTs in rodents.

Morel et al. (50) exposed human primary hepatocytes to various chemical compounds and found that the dithiolthiones 1,2-dithiol-3-thione and oltipraz increased alpha class GST (A1 and/or A2) mRNA levels significantly. Phenobarbital and 3-MC also induced alpha class GST levels in some but not all individuals and were less potent inducers than the dithiolthiones. GSTM1 mRNA levels were modestly increased in certain samples after treatment with these inducers (50,51). In contrast, none of these compounds induced GSTP1, which remained undetectable in all samples.

Suzuki et al. (52) cloned and sequenced both the human *GSTA1* and *GSTA2* genes and found that they share 95% sequence identity between nucleotides −1301 and +500. Deletion analysis of the human *GSTA1* gene revealed a negative regulatory element(s) between −694 and −336 and an enhancer element between −336 and −232. However, in contrast to the rat *GSTA2* and the mouse *GstA1* genes, no XRE or ARE sequence elements were found between −1301 and +755. Consistent with the lack of these elements, this region did not mediate transcriptional activation by PAHs such as β-NF and 3-MC,

or phenolic antioxidants such as *tert*-butylhydroquinone. These results suggest that the regulation of the human *GSTA1* and *GSTA2* genes may be significantly different from that of the rat *GSTA2* and the mouse *GstA1* genes. Further studies are needed to investigate whether regions upstream of −1301 contain XRE and/or ARE elements that mediate transcriptional activation of the human genes by xenobiotics (48–50).

Transcriptional Regulation of the Rat *GSTP1* Gene

The regulation of pi class GSTs is of interest because their expression is significantly increased (a) in many tumors (53), (b) in cell lines made resistant to chemotherapeutic agents (53), and (c) during hepatocarcinogenesis in the rat (54).

In the rat *GSTP1* gene, Muramatsu et al. (55,56) identified two enhancing elements, termed GPEI and GPEII (*GSTP1* enhancer I and II), located approximately 2.5 kb and 2.2 kb upstream from the transcriptional start site, respectively. GPEI was found to be the dominant *cis*-acting element controlling *GSTP1* expression. They found that the transcription factors *Jun* and *Fos* and other as yet unidentified *trans*-acting elements interact with GPEI (57).

Transcriptional Regulation of the Human *GSTP1* Gene

Moffat et al. (58) used promoter-deletion analysis to demonstrate that transcriptional activity was the major mechanism responsible for increased GSTP1-1 levels in the multidrug-resistant cell line, VCREMS (derived from the MCF7 breast cancer cell line). A putative AP-1 response element (5′-TGACTCA-3′) was identified between nucleotides −69 and −63, and point-mutation analysis and preincubation of the nuclear extracts with antisera raised against either human c-*Jun* or c-*Fos* demonstrated that a *Jun–Fos* heterodimer complex was binding to the promoter region (−73 to −54) in VCREMS cells but not MCF7 cells (58–60). Promoter-deletion analysis also indicated that a negative regulatory element mediated suppression of *GSTP1* transcription in MCF7 cells (61).

Two potential Sp1 binding sites (5′-GGGGCGGA-3′) in the 5′ regulatory region of *hGSTP1* gene also were identified, and it was found that SP1 bound to this promoter region in three different cell lines (MCF7, VCREMS, and EJ, a bladder carcinoma cell line) (62). Sp1 binding was required for optimal levels of *GSTP1* expression, suggesting that this *trans*-activating factor plays an important role in regulating basal levels of *GSTP1* transcription (62).

In addition to AP-1 and SP1 regulatory elements, other studies have demonstrated that insulin activates (63) and that retinoic acid (64) suppresses transcription of the *hGSTP1* gene. A putative insulin response element (63) has been identified in the *hGSTP1* regulatory region.

Xia et al. (63) reported that H_2O_2 induces transcription of the human *GSTP1* gene, suggesting regulation of this gene by the redox status of the cell. In addition, these researchers provided evidence that the induction by H_2O_2 is mediated by the *trans*-acting factor NF-κB (nuclear factor kappa B), via a putative NF-κB site in the *GSTP1* promoter.

Posttranscriptional Regulation of the Human *GSTP1* Gene

Posttranscriptional mechanisms also are involved in regulating human GSTP1-1 protein levels (65–67). For example, Moffat et al. (66) demonstrated that mRNA stability was the predominant mechanism explaining differences in expression of the *GSTP1* gene in different cell lines. Other investigators have shown that *GSTP1* is highly expressed in estrogen receptor–negative (ER–) but not in ER+ human breast cancer cell lines, and that this difference is largely due to the extraordinary stability of GSTP1 mRNA in ER– cells, rather than differences in transcriptional activation (65,67).

The Role of Methylation in the Regulation of the Human *GSTP1* Gene

Intriguingly, Lee et al. (68) found that the regulatory sequences of the *GSTP1* gene were hypermethylated in all 20 human prostatic carcinoma specimens studied, but not in normal tissue or tissue exhibiting benign prostatic

hyperplasia. In addition, hypermethylation was associated with a drastic decrease in *GSTP1* expression in prostatic carcinoma samples. Furthermore, a human prostatic cancer cell line containing exclusively hypermethylated *GSTP1* promoter sequences did not express any GSTP1-1 as judged by both the mRNA and the protein level.

Regulation of mu, theta, and zeta Class GSTs

The regulation of mu, theta, and zeta class GSTs is poorly understood, and studies designed to elucidate the molecular mechanisms governing the expression of these GST classes are eagerly awaited.

TISSUE-SPECIFIC EXPRESSION OF HUMAN GSTS

Regulation of GST expression differs among tissues, such that not all GST isoforms are expressed in every tissue. Furthermore, as discussed in detail in the subsequent section, Polymorphisms in the Human Glutathione S-Transferases, some GSTs are polymorphic, and in the case of both *GSTM1* and *GSTT1*, gene deletions are quite prevalent in the human population. Thus individuals homozygous for the *GSTM1* deletion polymorphism (approximately 50% of the population) will lack expression of this enzyme in any tissue in the body. Because of such interindividual genetic differences, and because of the complex tissue-specific expression of GSTs and their inducibility by diet and xenobiotics, it is difficult to predict accurately the extent of expression of any GST gene in a given tissue. Shown in Table 14-1 are estimates of

TABLE 14-1. *Tissue distribution of human GSTs determined with antisera raised against different GSTs*

	hGSTA1-2	rGSTA4-4	hGSTM1a-1a	hGSTM3-3	rGSTP1-1	hGSTT1-1	hGSTZ1-1
Liver	+++++	+	++++	—	—	++++	+++
Kidney	+++++	++	—	+	+	+++++	++
Small intestine	+	++++	++	+++	++	+++	NA
Pancreas	+	+	+	+	+	+	NA
Lung	—	+	—	—	++	+	NA
Spleen	—	+++	++	—	++	++	NA
Cerebrum	—	+	+++	++++	+++	+++	NA
Prostate	+	++	+++	++	++	++	NA
Testis	+++++	++	++++	+++++	+	++	NA
Heart	—	+	+	++	++	++	NA
Skeletal muscle	—	+	++++	++	?	++	+

Immunoblot analysis of alpha, mu, pi, theta, and zeta class GSTs of human tissues based on the organs of a single 73-year-old man, who was positive for both GSTM1 and GSTT1, as reported by Sherratt PJ, Pulford DJ, Harrison DJ, Green T, Hayes JD. Evidence that human class theta glutathione *S*-transferase T1-1 can catalyse the activation of dichloromethane, a liver and lung carcinogen in the mouse: comparison of the tissue distribution of GST T1-1 with that of classes alpha, mu and pi GST in human. *Biochem J* 1997;326:837–846, with permission. Data for hGSTZ1-1 are from Board P, Baker R, Chelvanayagam G, Jermiin L. Zeta, a novel class of glutathione transferases in a range of species from plants to humans. *Biochem Pharmacol* 1997;328:929–935, with permission. Number of + indicate the intensity of the signal seen on immunoblots of cytosol from a variety of human tissues probed with antisera raised against native hGSTA1-2, rat GSTA4-4 (previously named YkYk), native hGSTM1a-1a, native human GSTM3-3, native rat GSTP1-1, and recombinant hGSTT1-1 and hGSTZ1-1.

—, not detected; ?, a band was visible with a significantly higher molecular weight than the standard.

tissue distribution of various GSTs in one human who possessed both *GSTM1* and *GSTT1* genes, based on immunoblot analysis by using various GST antibodies (69). In this individual, alpha class GSTs are, in general, relatively highly expressed in liver, kidney, and testis, but not lung, whereas GSTP1-1 is expressed in lung but not in liver (see Table 14-1). Limited studies from other sources of human tissues agree in general with the pattern of tissue expression of GSTs shown for this individual in Table 14-1.

SUBSTRATES AND INHIBITORS OF GSTS

GST Substrates and Their Specificity

Clinically Useful Drugs as GST Substrates

In contrast to a substantial number of industrial chemicals, pesticides, and natural products, surprisingly few drugs of therapeutic importance have been identified as GST substrates (the upper half of Table 14-2). The reac-

TABLE 14-2. *Drugs and chemicals of clinical or environmental importance that are GST substrates (either directly, or as metabolites of other biotransformation reactions)*

Therapeutic agents that are GST substrates
  Ethacrynic acid
  Melphalan
  Busulfan
  Chlorambucil
  BCNU (bis-chloronitrosourea)
  Cyclophosphamide
  Mechlorethamine
  Paracetamol (acetaminophen)
  Nitroglycerin
  Menadione (vitamin K$_3$)
  α-bromoisovalerylurea
  Bromosulfophthalein
  Thiotepa
  Mitozantrone
  Bromisoval
  Adriamycin (doxorubicin)
Putative environmental/occupational carcinogens
    that are GST substrates
  PAH-epoxides (e.g., benzo(a)pyrene-4,5-oxide;
    benzo(a)pyrene-7,8-dihydrodiol-9,10-epoxide)
  PAH-hydroxysulfate esters
    (e.g., 5-hydroxymethylchrysene-sulfate)
  Nitropyrene-epoxides
  Aflatoxin-8,9-epoxide
  PhIP [2-amino-1-methyl-6-phenylimidazo (4,5b) pyridine]
  Styrene oxide
  N,N'-dimethylaminoazobenzene
  2-Acetylaminofluorene
  Ethylene dibromide
  Ethylene oxide
  Dichloromethane
  Butadiene mono- and diepoxides

tive intermediate of acetaminophen, *N*-acetyl-*p*-benzoquinonimine (NAPQI), is effectively detoxified by conjugation with glutathione, which may occur both enzymatically and nonenzymatically. Several bifunctional alkylating agents that are widely used as chemotherapeutic drugs, including melphalan, busulfan, and chlorambucil, also are detoxified by GSTs. Recent studies demonstrated that human GSTA1-1 is the most catalytically efficient form of GST for GSH conjugation of busulfan (70). The nitrosourea alkylating agent bischloroethylnitrosourea (BCNU) undergoes GSH-dependent deactivation by two distinct mechanisms, both of which are catalyzed by GSTs (71). Another chemotherapeutic agent, cyclophosphamide, is metabolized to the cytotoxic acrolein, which can be detoxified by GSTs. Other drugs and potentially important chemicals found in the workplace and general environment that serve as GST substrates are listed in the lower half of Table 14-2 (34,71,72). No studies have evaluated whether genetic polymorphisms of the various GST isoforms (see Polymorphisms in the Human Glutathione S-Transferases) might be clinically important determinants of either efficacy or toxicity from these drugs. However, numerous studies have been conducted to evaluate whether genetic differences in GSTs might contribute to increased risk for chronic diseases in populations exposed to environmental or occupational chemicals that serve as substrates for GSTs.

Nondrug Substrates

Individual GSTs belonging to different classes display overlapping substrate specificities (Table 14-3). For example, 1-chloro-2,4-dinitrobenzene (CDNB) is a popular GST substrate, because it is metabolized by members of all classes with the exception of the theta and zeta classes. However, despite a certain degree of overlap in substrate specificities, each GST has a characteristic profile of substrates. In addition, certain substrates are, within reason, considered diagnostic for each GST class. High activity toward cumene hydroperoxide is indicative of alpha-class GSTs, whereas *trans*-stilbene oxide and *trans*-4-phenyl-3-butene-2-one are characteristic substrates for the mu class (73). Ethacrynic acid has been shown to be a typical substrate for the pi class (73), whereas 1-menaphthyl sulfate and 1,2-epoxy-3-(*p*-nitrophenoxy)propane are metabolized by members of the theta class (18,74). However, it must be emphasized that very few substrates are truly specific for a certain class of GSTs or an individual GST. For example, whereas human alpha class GSTs exhibit high catalytic activities toward cumene hydroperoxide, GSTs belonging to the theta and zeta classes (especially hGSTT2-2) also metabolize this substrate (see Table 14-3).

TABLE 14-3. *Specific activities (μmol/min/mg) of human glutathione S-transferase isoenzymes*

	Substrates								
	CDNB	DCNB	EA	CH	MS	Δ^5AD	ENPP	tPBO	TSO
hGSTA1-1	82.0	0.25	0.1	3.1	ND	4.0	BD	BD	BD
hGSTA1-2	ND	0.8	ND	9.2	ND	ND	ND	BD	BD
hGSTA2-2	80.0	0.9	0.1	10.4	ND	ND	BD	BD	BD
hGSTA4-4	12.5	0.91	0.1	0.6	ND	BD	2.4	ND	ND
hGSTM1b-1b	107.4	0.7	0.9	BD	ND	ND	BD	0.06	10.5
hGSTM2-2	186.4	3.4	3.2	BD	ND	ND	7.0	0.07	BD
hGSTM3-3	6.0	0.1	0.06	BD	ND	ND	BD	BD	BD
hGSTM4-4	1.3	BD	0.04	BD	ND	ND	BD	BD	BD
hGSTM5-5	52.6	ND	ND	ND	ND	ND	ND	ND	ND
hGSTP1-1	103.0	0.1	1.2	0.03	ND	ND	0.5	0.02	ND
hGSTT1-1[a]	BD	ND	BD	2.8	BD	ND	18.0	BD	ND
hGSTT2-2	BD	ND	ND	6.9	0.5	ND	BD	ND	ND
hGSTZ1-1	BD	BD	0.05	0.16	BD	ND	ND	BD	ND

ND, not determined; BD, below detection limit. The data are compiled from Sherratt PJ, Pulford DJ, Harrison DJ, Green T, Hayes JD. Evidence that human class theta glutathione *S*-transferase T1-1 can catalyse the activation of dichloromethane, a liver and lung carcinogen in the mouse: comparison of the tissue distribution of GST T1-1 with that of classes alpha, mu and pi GST in human. *Biochem J* 1997;326:837–846, Ross VL, Board PG. Molecular cloning and heterologous expression of an alternatively spliced human mu class glutathione *S*-transferase transcript. *Biochem J* 1993;294:373–380, Guthenberg C, Mannervik B. Glutathione *S*-transferase (transferase pi) from human placenta is identical or closely related to glutathione *S*-transferase (transferase rho) from erythrocytes. *Biochem Biophys Acta* 1981;661:255–260, Hussey AJ, Hayes JD. Characterization of a human class-theta glutathione *S*-transferase with activity towards 1-menaphthyl sulphate. *Biochem J* 1992;286:929–935, Stockman PK, McLellan LI, Hayes JD. Characterization of the basic glutathione *S*-transferase B1 and B2 subunits from human liver. *Biochem J* 1987;244:55–61, and Board P, Baker R, Chelvanayagam G, Jermiin L. Zeta, a novel class of glutathione transferases in a range of species from plants to humans. *Biochem Pharmacol* 1997;328:929–935, with permission.

[a]Catalytic activities are given for recombinant His-tagged GSTT1-1 as described by Sherratt et al.

CDNB activity data for hGSTM5-5 are unpublished data generated by the authors in collaboration with Dr. Irving Listowsky. CDNB, 1-chloro-2,4-dinitrobenzene; DCNB, 1,2-dichloro-4-nitrobenzene; EA, ethacrynic acid; CH, cumene hydroperoxide; MS, 1-menaphthyl sulfate; Δ^5AD, Δ^5 androstene-3,17-dione; ENPP, 1,2-epoxy-3-(*p*-nitrophenoxy)propane; tBPO, *trans*-4-phenyl-3-buten-2-one.

Inhibitors of GSTs

GST activity has been implicated in the resistance of tumor cells against chemotherapeutic agents (75,76). One strategy to sensitize tumor cells to the toxic effects of cytostatic compounds is the development of GST-specific inhibitors. Despite a considerable effort, so far the only *in vivo* active inhibitors of GSTs are ethacrynic acid and a number of glutathione-derived structures [(77), for recent review see (78)]. However, GST inhibitors that are clinically safe, active *in vivo*, and isoenzyme specific have not yet been developed.

A number of inhibitors have been reported to be suitable for *in vitro* experiments. These include ethacrynic acid (79), the antibiotic calvatic acid (80), curcumin (81,82), haloenol lactone (83), and disulfiram (84). It must be pointed out that the isoenzyme selectivity of most of these inhibitors is limited.

POLYMORPHISMS IN THE HUMAN GLUTATHIONE S-TRANSFERASES

Four human GSTs, *hGSTM1, hGSTM3, hGSTT1,* and *hGSTP1,* are polymorphic in the human population.

Because these enzymes are involved in the detoxification of a wide variety of potentially toxic and carcinogenic substances, numerous molecular epidemiology studies have examined the association between GST polymorphisms and increased risk for disease, especially cancer. The potential functional significance of these polymorphisms in terms of increased cancer risk may provide the foundation to explore functional consequences of these polymorphisms in enhancing susceptibility to drug–drug and/or drug–environment interactions.

GSTM1 Polymorphism

In 1985 Seidegard et al. (85,86) first described a human genetic polymorphism in lymphocytic GST activity when measured toward the substrate, *trans*-stilbene oxide (TSO). Individuals with little or no activity toward TSO were later shown to be homozygous for a deletion of a major portion of the *GSTM1* gene (87,88). It is now recognized that this homozygous deletion is quite common in the population, and that significant ethnic differences in gene frequency are evident (Table 14-4).

TABLE 14-4. *Frequency of the GSTM1 gene deletion in various ethnic groups*

Ethnic group	GSTM1*0/GSTM1*0 genotype
Micronesian/Polynesian	64%–100%
Chinese	35%–63%
Caucasian	38%–67%
Japanese	48%–51%
French national	43%
African American	28%–35%
Hispanic	49%–53%
Indian	33%
Nigerians	22%

From Hayes JD, Pulford DJ. The glutathione *S*-transferase supergene family: regulation of GST and the contribution of the isoenzymes to cancer chemoprotection and drug resistance. *Crit Rev Biochem Mol Biol* 1995;30:445–600, Chen H, Sandler D, Taylor J, Shore D, Liu E, Bloomfield C, Bell D. Increased risk for myelodysplastic syndromes in individuals with glutathione transferase theta 1 (*GSTT1*) gene defect. *Lancet* 1996;347:295–297, Rebbeck TR. Molecular epidemiology of the human glutathione *S*-transferase genotypes GSTM1 and GSTT1 in cancer susceptibility. *Cancer Epidemiol Biomarkers Prev* 1997;6:733–743, and Zhao B, Lee EJ, Wong JY, Yeoh PN, Gong NH. Frequency of mutant CYP1A1, NAT2 and GSTM1 alleles in normal Indians and Malays. *Pharmacogenetics* 1995;5:275–280, with permission.

There are actually three allelic variants of the *GSTM1* gene, referred to as *GSTM1*A, *GSTM1*B, and *GSTM1*0, with the latter representing the deleted, or null, allele. *GSTM1*A and *GSTM1*B differ only in the amino acid present at position 173 and have essentially identical catalytic activities toward substrates examined thus far. Most epidemiologic studies have used phenotyping (activity toward TSO) or genotyping polymerase chain reaction (PCR)-based assays that do not distinguish between the M1*A and M1*B allelic variants, or distinguish heterozygotes (*GSTM1/GSTM1*0) from homozygotes for the active allele (*GSTM1/GSTM1*).

Functional Significance of the GSTM1 *Polymorphism*

GSTM1-1 is active in the detoxification of a variety of epoxides, including oxidative products of some known carcinogens such as benzo(a)pyrene (89), a polyaromatic hydrocarbon present as a combustion by-product in cigarette smoke and in some occupational environments, and aflatoxin B₁ (90), a fungal toxin contaminant of peanuts and corn (see Table 14-2).

Some, but not all, *in vitro* studies with human cells and/or body fluids have suggested that *GSTM1*-deficient individuals may be more susceptible to the genotoxic actions of epoxide carcinogens. For example, it was found that urine from smokers with the *GSTM1*0/GSTM1*0 genotype was about 3 times more mutagenic in the Ames test than urine from smokers with one or two active *GSTM1* alleles (91). Other studies have found that lymphocyte sister chromatid exchange rate, but not

micronuclei formation, is increased in *GSTM1*-deficient smokers compared with *GSTM1*-positive smokers (92,93). However, DNA adduct levels in nontarget tissue such as lymphocytes may not be reflective of adduct levels in target tissue such as lung. For example, when PAH-DNA adducts were examined directly in lymphocytes from smokers, no association between adduct levels and *GSTM1* alleles was found (94), whereas a significant increase (OR, 8.6) in PAH-DNA adducts was found in lung tissue in *GSTM1*-deficient samples compared with *GSTM1*-positive controls (95). Such differences could result from differences in the type and/or level of expression of individual GST isoforms, and/or tissue-specific differences in activity of oxidative enzymes necessary to form the epoxide that serves as the GST substrate. Obviously, the lack of a functional GST allele will have no consequence in tissues that are incapable of forming an epoxide substrate because of lack of expression of the particular cytochrome P450 necessary to form the epoxide.

Cancer Susceptibility for the GSTM1 *Polymorphism*

Numerous molecular epidemiology studies have examined the potential significance of the *GSTM1* polymorphism as a susceptibility factor for environmentally and/or occupationally related cancers. Positive associations (absence of both alleles conferring increased risk) have been convincingly found for lung and bladder cancers, with limited evidence for an association with several other types of cancer.

Lung Cancer

More than a dozen molecular epidemiology studies have examined whether the absence of the *GSTM1* gene places individuals, especially smokers, at increased risk for lung cancer (96–112). Although not all studies have found a statistically significant association between the *GSTM1* null genotype and increased risk for lung cancer (99,101,109,111,113), most have at least suggested a trend for such an association. A meta-analysis of 11 studies completed prior to 1995 found a composite odds ratio (OR) for an association between the *GSTM1* null genotype and lung cancer risk of 1.6 (114). When these studies were controlled for smoking by using only incident cases and healthy controls, the composite OR increased slightly to 1.76 (114). Several studies have suggested that Japanese populations with the *GSTM1* null genotype might be at especially high risk for lung cancer when combined with other susceptibility genotypes such as the *CYP1A1MspI* variant allele (100,105,115), although a recent study in the United States found only a two-fold increased risk for lung cancers in the combined *CYP1A1-GSTM1* genotype group (113). Absence of the *GSTM1* gene also has been associated with a slightly elevated risk for developing emphysema among smokers (116), suggesting that the protective effects of this enzyme in the lung may extend beyond lung cancer.

Thus there is substantial support for the hypothesis that the *GSTM1* null genotype is a significant determinant of lung cancer risk in smokers, especially when combined with other susceptibility genotypes. As both the gene frequency for this deletion and the prevalence of lung cancer are quite common, Caporaso et al. (117) estimated that an increased risk of 60% to 70% associated with the GST null genotype in smokers would result in an attributable risk because of this one gene that would exceed the total population cancer risks of the breast cancer (BRCA1) gene and the human nonadenoma polyposis carcinoma (HNPCC) gene combined.

Bladder Cancer

More than a dozen studies have examined the relationship between the *GSTM1* null genotype and bladder cancer, and most have demonstrated a significant association (118–131). A meta-analysis of six studies in caucasians completed prior to 1995 found an aggregate OR of 1.54 (114). Based on only two studies with a small sample size, a similar association was found for African Americans (OR, 1.41) (119,128) and Asians (OR, 2.40) (123,128). The attributable risk for total bladder cancers for the *GSTM1* polymorphism has been estimated to range from 17% to 25% (119,121).

Because smoking is associated with bladder cancer, it is not surprising that the strongest association has been identified in smokers, although several studies also found increased risk among nonsmokers. Individuals (both smokers and nonsmokers) with the null *GSTM1* genotype have a higher level of 3- and 4-aminobiphenyl hemoglobin adducts (132), lending biologic plausibility to such an association. In one relatively large case–control study, no statistically significant overall association between the *GSTM1* null genotype and bladder cancer was found (OR, 1.33), but a significant relationship was found when surviving cases were examined (129).

Stomach and Colorectal Cancers

Several studies have suggested that the *GSTM1* null genotype is associated with increased risk for stomach cancer (133–135), although other studies have failed to find an association (136,137). All of the studies to date have been relatively small, and further research is necessary to determine whether the GSTM1 null polymorphism is a significant risk factor for stomach cancer.

Several case control studies on *GSTM1* genotype and colon cancer have been completed, again with mixed findings. Two initial studies both suggested an approximate increase in risk of 60% to 70% for the null genotype (131,135), but more recent studies (136–138) have not found a significant overall association. No association was found between anal cancer and the GST null genotype in a population-based case–control study (139).

Other Cancers

Case–control studies on the association between *GSTM1* null genotype and breast (131,133,140,141), brain (142,143), skin (144–147), ovarian (148), cervical (149), and oral (136,150) cancers, and myelodysplastic syndromes (151), have been negative, although in a few instances, a trend was noticed, or subclassification resulted in marginally significant associations. A strong association (OR, 12.7) was found for esophageal cancer risk in smokers when the *GSTM1* null genotype was combined with the cytochrome P450 *1A1 MspI* polymorphism (152). One small study on head and neck cancers (153) found an OR of 3.1 when compared with matched controls for the *GSTM1* null genotype. No association between the *GSTM1* null genotype and liver cancer was found in two studies (132,154), but *GSTM1* null individuals exposed to aflatoxin B_1 in the diet may be at slightly increased risk relative to *GSTM1*-positive individuals (155,156).

GSTM3 Polymorphism

A more recently described *GSTM3* polymorphism has been shown to have a frequency of 16% in the caucasian population and is in linkage disequilibrium with the *GSTM1*A* deletion polymorphism (157). This polymorphism has been associated with an increased risk of cutaneous basal cell carcinomas (147) and laryngeal carcinomas (158), but no association was found for astrocytomas (143) and pharyngeal carcinomas (158).

GSTT1 Polymorphism

A polymorphism for the theta class GSTT1 enzyme in humans was first described in 1994 (159). Like the *GSTM1* polymorphism, the *GSTT1* polymorphism also occurs because of a deletion of a substantial part of the gene, and thus individuals who are homozygous for the deleted form lack GSTT1 activity in all tissues. The frequency of the homozygous *GSTT1*0* genotype is quite variable among different ethnic groups, ranging from 12% to 62% (Table 14-5).

This enzyme is of particular functional significance because it is involved in both the activation and detoxification of a variety of oxidative metabolites of important industrial chemicals, including methylene chloride, ethylene dichloride (EDC), methyl bromide, ethylene oxide, and 1,3-butadiene (see Table 14-2) (34,160). Because of the dichotomous role in activation and detoxification, the gene deletion could conceivably decrease risk from some exposures (e.g., EDC; the GSTT1 enzyme activates EDC

TABLE 14-5. *Ethnic variability in the frequency of the GSTT1*0 genotype (homozygous null)*

Ethnic group	Frequency of GSTT1*0 genotype
Caucasian	
English	16%
Germans	12%
U.S.–"nationwide"	24%
U.S.–New England	16%
U.S.–general	15%
Asian	
Japanese	45%
Chinese	58%–62%
Blacks	
African American	24%

Data from Nelson HH, Wiencke JK, Christiani DC, et al. Ethnic differences in the prevalence of the homozygous deleted genotype of glutathione, *S*-transferase theta. *Carcinogenesis* 1995;16:1243–1245, and Lee EJ, Wong JY, Yeoh PN, Gong NH. Glutathione *S* transferase-theta (GSTT1) genetic polymorphism among Chinese, Malays and Indians in Singapore. *Pharmacogenetics* 1995;5:332–334, with permission.

to a genotoxic metabolite) while increasing risk from other chemicals (e.g., butadiene; GSTT1 detoxifies butadiene epoxides). The significance of the deletion toward a particular substrate will also depend on the level of expression of other GSTs that may act on the same substrate. Thus interpretation of epidemiologic studies on the relationship between disease end points and the *GSTT1* null genotype is greatly complicated under circumstances in which mixed exposures to potential GSTT1 substrates occur.

The potential significance of GSTT1 as a detoxification enzyme is suggested by several studies on butadiene exposed workers. *GSTT1*-null individuals occupationally exposed to butadiene demonstrated a 16-fold increase in sister chromatid exchange compared with *GSTT1*-positive individuals with similar exposures (161). Chromosomal aberrations in butadiene workers also were significantly higher in *GSTT1*-null individuals compared with *GSTT1*-positives (162).

Relatively few molecular epidemiology studies have been completed on the relationship between the *GSTT1* deletion and chronic diseases such as cancer. No association was found between the *GSTT1* deletion polymorphism and increased risk for lung cancer in smokers (136,163). However, in Hispanic and African-American populations, the GST theta deletion, when combined with the *GSTM1* deletion, produced a significant, three-fold increase in risk in both ethnic groups (163). The *GSTT1* deletion polymorphism has been associated with increased risk for brain astrocytoma [OR, 2.7 (142)] and meningioma [OR, 4.5 (142)], although the sample size was small. A recent study (164) found a significant, 4.3-fold increase in risk for myelodysplastic diseases among individuals homozygous for the theta deletion. An asso-

ciation between colon cancer and the *GSTT1* null allele was found in one study [OR 1.88 (136)], but not another (137). A third study of colon cancer patients found that, although the frequency was not significantly different between cases and controls, *GSTT1* null homozygotes were more common in patients who were diagnosed before age 70 years (138). The authors suggested from this that the *GSTT1* genotype might influence the age of onset of colorectal cancer (138).

No association between *GSTT1* null genotype and skin cancer was found in one study (145), but a longitudinal study suggested that accrual of basal cell carcinomas occurred at a significantly greater rate in *GSTT1* null individuals [rate ratio, 2.15 (146)]. *GSTT1* deletion was associated with a 2.6-fold increased risk for bladder cancer in nonsmokers, but not in intermediate or heavy smokers (120). Other studies on oral (136) and gastric (136,137) cancers have failed to find any statistically significant association with the *GSTT1* null genotype. However, very few epidemiology studies of adequate power have been completed for the *GSTT1* polymorphism, and the significance of this polymorphism will require further study.

GSTP1 Polymorphism

The gene encoding GSTP1 is located on chromosome 11 (34,165), and the enzyme appears to be the most widely abundant form found in many tissues (165). Although members of all GST classes are normally expressed in the human lung (166), GSTP1 is the predominant form, accounting for most of the immunohistochemical GST staining (166) and 90% to 97% of GST activity (167–169). GSTP1-1 also has the highest specific activity toward the active benzo(a)pyrene metabolite of tobacco smoke, benzo(a)pyrene-7,8-dihydrodiol-9,10-epoxide (BPDE), and is almost exclusively active toward the (+)-enantiomer of anti-BPDE (89,170), which is believed to be the ultimate mutagenic form of benzo(a)pyrene (see Table 14-2). Thus GSTP1-1 conceptually could be even more important than GSTM1-1 in preventing tobacco-induced lung cancer.

Recently two genetic polymorphisms in the human *GSTP1* gene have been identified (171,172). Two variant alleles have been described. *GSTP1*B* results from a transition mutation in codon 104 (nucleotide +313) that changes Ile to Val, and *GSTP1*C* has the same codon 104 as *GSTP1*B*, but also has a second transition mutation in codon 113 that changes Ala to Val (171). The codon 113 change has not been identified as an allele by itself, although only a relatively small number of samples (75) have been examined (171). Molecular modeling studies have shown that the amino acids at both codons 104 and 113 lie in the hydrophobic binding site for electrophilic substrates and would be expected to affect substrate binding (171). In fact, cDNA-expressed GSTP1b-1b and

GSTP1c-1c proteins have altered enzymatic activity when compared with the wild-type GSTP1a-1a protein (171). The catalytic efficiency (K_{cat}/K_m) of both variant enzymes for CDNB is about three-fold to four-fold lower than that of the wild-type protein (171). Catalytic differences between these variants have been shown for the carcinogenic (+)-anti-BPDE, such that the variant enzyme (104 Val) exhibits a V_{max} 3.4-fold higher than the V_{max} for the common (104 Ile) form (173). The allele frequency for the combined GSTP1*B + GSTP1*C variant alleles is about 30% (171,172), and homozygotes for the variant B + C alleles occurred in 6.5% (172) and 12% of samples examined (171). Ali-Osman et al. (171) found that the GSTP1*C allele was four-fold higher in cells obtained from malignant gliomas than in those from normal tissue, although it was not possible to tell whether this was due to differences in the subjects' genotypes or to loss of heterozygosity or other genetic changes that may have occurred in the tumor tissue.

Harries et al. (172) examined the association between the GSTP1*B gene and a variety of cancers. The authors did not distinguish between GSTP1*B and GST1*C alleles, but the method they used would have measured both variant alleles (*B + *C) if Ali-Osman et al. (171) were correct in noting that all GSTP1*C alleles also carry the GSTP1*B allele change. Harries et al. (172) found statistically significant associations between homozygotes for the variant allele(s) and testicular (OR, 3.3) and bladder (OR, 3.6) cancers, and teratomas (OR, 3.4), but not for breast or colon cancer. A nonsignificant increase in lung cancer (OR, 1.9) was suggested. Although the sample size was small and the results were not statistically significant, a protective effect for prostate cancer was suggested (OR, 0.4).

Clearly, additional studies are needed to clarify the significance of the polymorphism identified in human GSTP1.

CONCLUSIONS

In contrast to other multigene families of drug-metabolizing enzymes such as the cytochromes P450, the clinical importance of the glutathione S-transferases as a site of drug–drug interactions are poorly studied, and there are currently few documented examples in which one drug enhances the toxicity (or increases the efficacy) of another drug solely through drug-induced inhibition or induction of GST enzymes. However, because of the high prevalence in the human population of genetic polymorphisms for various GSTs, and because of the putative role of these enzymes in the detoxification of a variety of environmental and occupational carcinogens, there has been a very high level of interest in these enzymes as determinants of chronic disease susceptibility in exposed populations. Although many of these epidemiologic studies have failed to identify significant increased cancer

risks associated with GST gene variants in populations with known carcinogen exposure (e.g., cigarette smokers), risk of lung and bladder cancer among smokers does appear to be influenced by GST genotype.

As more is learned about the role of GSTs in the biotransformation (both activation and detoxification) of clinically useful therapeutic agents, it is likely that important metabolic drug interactions with this broad class of biotransformation enzymes will be discovered. For example, it is known that relatively high doses of acetaminophen deplete hepatic stores of reduced glutathione, enhancing the hepatotoxicity of subsequent doses of the same drug. It is reasonable to assume that acetaminophen-induced depletion of GSH could also enhance the toxicity of other drugs that are detoxified by GSTs. Indeed, studies in animal models have demonstrated that sympathomimetic drugs such as phenylpropanolamine can potentiate the hepatotoxicity of acetaminophen and other hepatotoxicants that are detoxified through GSH-dependent pathways, apparently by adrenergic-stimulated depression of hepatic GSH (174,175). Similar drug–drug interactions that involve the glutathione metabolic pathway in general, and glutathione S-transferases specifically, may plausibly occur in humans.

REFERENCES

1. Booth J, Boyland E, Sims P. An enzyme from rat liver catalysing conjugations with glutathione. *Biochem J* 1961;79:516–524.
2. Boyland E, Chasseaud LF. The role of glutathione and glutathione S-transferases in mercapturic acid biosynthesis. *Adv Enzymol Relat Areas Mol Biol* 1969;32:173–219.
3. Fjellstedt TA, Allen RH, Duncan BK, Jakoby WB. Enzymatic conjugation of epoxides with glutathione. *J Biol Chem* 1973;248: 3702–3707.
4. Habig WH, Pabst MJ, Jakoby WB. Glutathione S-transferases: the first enzymatic step in mercapturic acid formation. *J Biol Chem* 1974; 249:7130–7139.
5. Johnson MK. Studies on glutathione S-alkyltransferase of the rat. *Biochem J* 1966;98:44–56.
6. Chasseaud LF. The nature and distribution of enzymes catalyzing the conjugation of glutathione with foreign compounds. *Drug Metab Rev* 1973;2:185–220.
7. Habig WH, Pabst MJ, Fleischner G, Gatmaitan Z, Arias IM, Jakoby WB. The identity of glutathione S-transferase B with ligandin, a major binding protein of liver. *Proc Natl Acad Sci USA* 1974;71: 3879–3882.
8. Kaplowitz N, Percy Robb IW, Javitt NB. Role of hepatic anion-binding protein in bromsulphthalein conjugation. *J Exp Med* 1973;138: 483–487.
9. Prohaska JR, Ganther HE. Glutathione peroxidase activity of glutathione-s-transferases purified from rat liver. *Biochem Biophys Res Commun* 1976;76:437–445.
10. Benson AM, Talalay P, Keen JH, Jakoby WB. Relationship between the soluble glutathione-dependent delta 5-3-ketosteroid isomerase and the glutathione S-transferases of the liver. *Proc Natl Acad Sci USA* 1977;74:158–162.
11. Bass NM, Kirsch RE, Tuff SA, Marks I, Saunders SJ. Ligandin heterogeneity: evidence that the two non-identical subunits are the monomers of two distinct proteins. *Biochim Biophys Acta* 1977;492: 163–175.
12. Hayes JD, Strange RC, Percy Robb IW. A study of the structures of the YaYa and YaYc glutathione S-transferases from rat liver cytosol: evidence that the Ya monomer is responsible for lithocholate-binding activity. *Biochem J* 1981;197:491–502.

13. Lai HC, Li N, Weiss MJ, Reddy CC, Tu CP. The nucleotide sequence of a rat liver glutathione S-transferase subunit cDNA clone. *J Biol Chem* 1984;259:5536–5542.

14. Lai HC, Grove G, Tu CP. Cloning and sequence analysis of a cDNA for a rat liver glutathione S-transferase Yb subunit. *Nucleic Acids Res* 1986;14:6101–6114.

15. Pickett CB, Telakowski Hopkins CA, Ding GJ, Argenbright L, Lu AY. Rat liver glutathione S-transferases: complete nucleotide sequence of a glutathione S-transferase mRNA and the regulation of the Ya, Yb, and Yc mRNAs by 3-methylcholanthrene and phenobarbital. *J Biol Chem* 1984;259:5182–5188.

16. Telakowski Hopkins CA, Rodkey JA, Bennett CD, Lu AY, Pickett CB. Rat liver glutathione S-transferases: construction of a cDNA clone complementary to a Yc mRNA and prediction of the complete amino acid sequence of a Yc subunit. *J Biol Chem* 1985;260:5820–5825.

17. Mannervik B, Alin P, Guthenberg C, et al. Identification of three classes of cytosolic glutathione transferase common to several mammalian species: correlation between structural data and enzymatic properties. *Proc Natl Acad Sci USA* 1985;82:7202–7206.

18. Meyer DJ, Coles B, Pemble SE, Gilmore KS, Fraser GM, Ketterer B. Theta, a new class of glutathione transferases purified from rat and man. *Biochem J* 1991;274:409–414.

19. Board P, Baker R, Chelvanayagam G, Jermiin L. Zeta: a novel class of glutathione transferases in a range of species from plants to humans. *Biochem Pharmacol* 1997;328:929–935.

20. Buetler TM, Eaton DL. Glutathione S-transferases: amino acid sequence comparison, classification and phylogenetic relationship. *Environ Carcinog Ecotox Rev* 1992;C10:181–203.

21. Reinemer P, Dirr HW, Ladenstein R, Schaffer J, Gallay O, Huber R. The three-dimensional structure of class pi glutathione S-transferase in complex with glutathione sulfonate at 2.3 Å resolution. *EMBO J* 1991;10:1997–2005.

22. Sinning I, Kleywegt GJ, Cowan SW, et al. Structure determination and refinement of human alpha class glutathione transferase A1-1, and a comparison with the mu and pi class enzymes. *J Mol Biol* 1993;232: 192–212.

23. Ji X, Zhang P, Armstrong RN, Gilliland GL. The three-dimensional structure of a glutathione S-transferase from the mu gene class: structural analysis of the binary complex of isoenzyme 3-3 and glutathione at 2.2-Å resolution. *Biochemistry* 1992;31:10169–10184.

24. Reinemer P, Dirr HW, Ladenstein R, et al. Three-dimensional structure of class pi glutathione S-transferase from human placenta in complex with S-hexylglutathione at 2.8 Å resolution. *J Mol Biol* 1992; 227:214–226.

25. Garcia SaI, P'Arraga A, Phillips MF, Mantle TJ, Coll M. Molecular structure at 1.8 Å of mouse liver class pi glutathione S-transferase complexed with S-(*p*-nitrobenzyl)glutathione and other inhibitors. *J Mol Biol* 1994;237:298–314.

26. Armstrong RN. Structure, catalytic mechanism, and evolution of the glutathione transferases. *Chem Res Toxicol* 1997;10:2–18.

27. Mannervik B, Awasthi YC, Board PG, et al. Nomenclature for human glutathione transferases [Letter]. *Biochem J* 1992;282:305–306.

28. Morgenstern R, DePierre JW. Microsomal glutathione transferase: purification in unactivated form and further characterization of the activation process, substrate specificity and amino acid composition. *Eur J Biochem* 1983;134:591–597.

29. Morgenstern R, DePierre JW, Jornvall H. Microsomal glutathione transferase: primary structure. *J Biol Chem* 1985;260:13976–13983.

30. Jakobsson PJ, Mancini JA, Riendeau D, Ford Hutchinson AW. Identification and characterization of a novel microsomal enzyme with glutathione-dependent transferase and peroxidase activities. *J Biol Chem* 1997;272:22934–22939.

31. Jakobsson PJ, Mancini JA, Ford Hutchinson AW. Identification and characterization of a novel human microsomal glutathione S-transferase with leukotriene C_4 synthase activity and significant sequence identity to 5-lipoxygenase-activating protein and leukotriene C4 synthase. *J Biol Chem* 1996;271:22203–22210.

32. Lam BK, Penrose JF, Freeman GJ, Austen KF. Expression cloning of a cDNA for human leukotriene C_4 synthase, an integral membrane protein conjugating reduced glutathione to leukotriene A_4. *Proc Natl Acad Sci USA* 1994;91:7663–7667.

33. Welsch DJ, Creely DP, Hauser SD, Mathis KJ, Krivi GG, Isakson PC. Molecular cloning and expression of human leukotriene-C_4 synthase. *Proc Natl Acad Sci USA* 1994;91:9745–9749.

34. Hayes JD, Pulford DJ. The glutathione S-transferase supergene family: regulation of GST and the contribution of the isoenzymes to cancer chemoprotection and drug resistance. *Crit Rev Biochem Mol Biol* 1995;30:445–600.

35. Hatayama I, Satoh K, Sato K. Developmental and hormonal regulation of the major form of hepatic glutathione S-transferase in male mice. *Biochem Biophys Res Commun* 1986;140:581–588.

36. Mera N, Ohmori S, Itahashi K, Kiuchi M, Igarashi T, Kitada M. Immunochemical evidence for the occurrence of mu class glutathione S-transferase in human fetal livers. *J Biochem (Tokyo)* 1994;116: 315–320.

37. Rushmore TH, Pickett CB. Transcriptional regulation of the rat glutathione S-transferase Ya subunit gene: characterization of a xenobiotic-responsive element controlling inducible expression by phenolic antioxidants. *J Biol Chem* 1990;265:14648–14653.

38. Daniel V. Glutathione S-transferases: gene structure and regulation of expression. *Crit Rev Biochem Mol Biol* 1993;28:173–207.

39. Ding VD, Pickett CB. Transcriptional regulation of rat liver glutathione S-transferase genes by phenobarbital and 3-methylcholanthrene. *Arch Biochem Biophys* 1985;240:553–559.

40. Paulson KE, Darnell JE Jr, Rushmore T, Pickett CB. Analysis of the upstream elements of the xenobiotic compound-inducible and positionally regulated glutathione S-transferase Ya gene. *Mol Cell Biol* 1990;10:1841–1852.

41. Rushmore TM, Nguyen T, Pickett CB. ARE and XRE mediated induction of the glutathione S-transferase Ya subunit gene: induction by planar aromatic compounds and phenolic antioxidants. In: Tew KD, Pickett CB, Mantle TJ, Mannervik B, Hayes JD, eds. *Structure and function of glutathione transferases*. Boca Raton, FL: CRC Press, 119–128.

42. Fujisawa Sehara A, Sogawa K, Yamane M, Fujii Kuriyama Y. Characterization of xenobiotic responsive elements upstream from the drug-metabolizing cytochrome P-450c gene: a similarity to glucocorticoid regulatory elements. *Nucleic Acids Res* 1987;15:4179–4191.

43. Rushmore TH, Morton MR, Pickett CB. The antioxidant responsive element: activation by oxidative stress and identification of the DNA consensus sequence required for functional activity. *J Biol Chem* 1991;266:11632–11639.

44. Friling RS, Bensimon A, Tichauer Y, Daniel V. Xenobiotic-inducible expression of murine glutathione S-transferase Ya subunit gene is controlled by an electrophile-responsive element. *Proc Natl Acad Sci USA* 1990;87:6258–6262.

45. Friling RS, Bergelson S, Daniel V. Two adjacent AP-1-like binding sites form the electrophile-responsive element of the murine glutathione S-transferase Ya subunit gene. *Proc Natl Acad Sci USA* 1992;89:668–672.

46. Wasserman WW, Fahl WE. Functional antioxidant responsive elements. *Proc Natl Acad Sci USA* 1997;94:5361–5366.

47. Wasserman WW, Fahl WE. Comprehensive analysis of proteins which interact with the antioxidant responsive element: correlation of ARE-BP-1 with the chemoprotective induction response. *Arch Biochem Biophys* 1997;344:387–396.

48. Nijhoff WA, Grubben MJ, Nagengast FM, et al. Effects of consumption of brussels sprouts on intestinal and lymphocytic glutathione S-transferases in humans. *Carcinogenesis* 1995;16:2125–2128.

49. Bogaards JJ, Verhagen H, Willems MI, van Poppel G, van Bladeren PJ. Consumption of brussels sprouts results in elevated alpha-class glutathione S-transferase levels in human blood plasma. *Carcinogenesis* 1994;15:1073–1075.

50. Morel F, Fardel O, Meyer DJ, et al. Preferential increase of glutathione S-transferase class alpha transcripts in cultured human hepatocytes by phenobarbital, 3-methylcholanthrene, and dithiolethiones. *Cancer Res* 1993;53:231–234.

51. Langouet S, Coles B, Morel F, et al. Inhibition of CYP1A2 and CYP3A4 by oltipraz results in reduction of aflatoxin B_1 metabolism in human hepatocytes in primary culture. *Cancer Res* 1995;55: 5574–5579.

52. Suzuki T, Smith S, Board PG. Structure and function of the 5′ flanking sequences of the human alpha class glutathione S-transferase genes. *Biochem Biophys Res Commun* 1994;200:1665–1671.

53. Black SM, Wolf CR. The role of glutathione-dependent enzymes in drug resistance. *Pharmacol Ther* 1991;51:139–154.

54. Sato K, Kitahara A, Satoh K, Ishikawa T, Tatematsu M, Ito N. The placental form of glutathione S-transferase as a new marker protein for

preneoplasia in rat chemical hepatocarcinogenesis. *Gann* 1984;75: 199–202.

55. Sakai M, Okuda A, Muramatsu M. Multiple regulatory elements and phorbol 12-*O*-tetradecanoate 13-acetate responsiveness of the rat placental glutathione transferase gene. *Proc Natl Acad Sci USA* 1988;85: 9456–9460.

56. Okuda A, Imagawa M, Maeda Y, Sakai M, Muramatsu M. Structural and functional analysis of an enhancer GPEI having a phorbol 12-*O*-tetradecanoate 13-acetate responsive element-like sequence found in the rat glutathione transferase P gene. *J Biol Chem* 1989;264: 16919–16926.

57. Diccianni MB, Imagawa M, Muramatsu M. The dyad palindromic glutathione transferase P enhancer binds multiple factors including AP1. *Nucleic Acids Res* 1992;20:5153–5158.

58. Moffat GJ, McLaren AW, Wolf CR. Involvement of Jun and Fos proteins in regulating transcriptional activation of the human pi class glutathione S-transferase gene in multidrug-resistant MCF7 breast cancer cells. *J Biol Chem* 1994;269:P16397–16402.

59. Morrow CS, Goldsmith ME, Cowan KH. Regulation of human glutathione S-transferase pi gene transcription: influence of 5′-flanking sequences and *trans*-activating factors which recognize AP-1-binding sites. *Gene* 1990;88:215–225.

60. Xia CL, Cowell IG, Dixon KH, Pemble SE, Ketterer B, Taylor JB. Glutathione transferase pi: its minimal promoter and downstream *cis*-acting element. *Biochem Biophys Res Commun* 1991;176:233–240.

61. Moffat GJ, McLaren AW, Wolf CR. Functional characterization of the transcription silencer element located within the human pi class glutathione S-transferase promoter. *J Biol Chem* 1996;271:20740–20747.

62. Moffat GJ, McLaren AW, Wolf CR. Sp1-mediated transcriptional activation of the human pi class glutathione S-transferase promoter. *J Biol Chem* 1996;271:P1054–1060.

63. Xia C, Hu J, Ketterer B, Taylor JB. The organization of the human GSTP1-1 gene promoter and its response to retinoic acid and cellular redox status. *Biochem J* 1996;313:155–161.

64. Xia C, Taylor JB, Spencer SR, Ketterer B. The human glutathione S-transferase P1-1 gene: modulation of expression by retinoic acid and insulin. *Biochem J* 1993;292:845–850.

65. Morrow CS, Chiu J, Cowan KH. Posttranscriptional control of glutathione S-transferase pi gene expression in human breast cancer cells. *J Biol Chem* 1992;267:10544–10550.

66. Moffat GJ, McLaren AW, Wolf CR. Transcriptional and post-transcriptional mechanisms can regulate cell-specific expression of the human pi-class glutathione S-transferase gene. *Biochem J* 1997; 324:91–95.

67. Jhaveri MS, Stephens TE, Morrow CS. Role of posttranscriptional processes in the regulation of glutathione S-transferase P1 gene expression in human breast cancer cells. *Biochem Biophys Res Commun* 1997;237:729–734.

68. Lee WH, Morton RA, Epstein JI, et al. Cytidine methylation of regulatory sequences near the pi-class glutathione S-transferase gene accompanies human prostatic carcinogenesis. *Proc Natl Acad Sci USA* 1994;91:11733–11737.

69. Sherratt PJ, Pulford DJ, Harrison DJ, Green T, Hayes JD. Evidence that human class theta glutathione S-transferase T1-1 can catalyse the activation of dichloromethane, a liver and lung carcinogen in the mouse: comparison of the tissue distribution of GST T1-1 with that of classes alpha, mu and pi GST in human. *Biochem J* 1997;326: 837–846.

70. Czwerwinski M, Gibbs JP, Slattery JT. Busulfan conjugation by glutathione S-transferases alpha, mu, and pi. *Drug Metab Dispos* 1996; 24:1015–1019.

71. Beckett GJ, Hayes JD. Glutathione S-transferases: biomedical applications. *Adv Clin Chem* 1993;30:281–380.

72. Mulders TM, Bergman DJ, Poll TBT, et al. Abnormal glutathione conjugation in patients with tyrosinaemia type I. *J Inherit Metab Dis* 1997;20:473–485.

73. Mannervik B, Danielson UH. Glutathione transferases—structure and catalytic activity. *CRC Crit Rev Biochem* 1988;23:283–337.

74. Hiratsuka A, Sebata N, Kawashima K, et al. A new class of rat glutathione S-transferase Yrs-Yrs inactivating reactive sulfate esters as metabolites of carcinogenic arylmethanols. *J Biol Chem* 1990;265: 11973–11981.

75. Tew KD. Glutathione-associated enzymes in anticancer drug resistance. *Cancer Res* 1994;54:4313–4320.

76. O'Brien ML, Tew KD. Glutathione and related enzymes in multidrug resistance. *Eur J Cancer* 1996;32A:967–978.

77. Morgan AS, Ciaccio PJ, Tew KD, Kauvar LM. Isozyme-specific glutathione S-transferase inhibitors potentiate drug sensitivity in cultured human tumor cell lines. *Cancer Chemother Pharmacol* 1996;37: 363–370.

78. Mulder GJ, Ouwerkerk Mahadevan S. Modulation of glutathione conjugation in vivo: how to decrease glutathione conjugation in vivo or in intact cellular systems in vitro. *Chem Biol Interact* 1997;105:17–34.

79. Ploemen JH, van Ommen B, van Bladeren PJ. Inhibition of rat and human glutathione S-transferase isoenzymes by ethacrynic acid and its glutathione conjugate. *Biochem Pharmacol* 1990;40:1631–1635.

80. Antonini G, Pitari G, Caccuri AM, et al. Inhibition of human placenta glutathione transferase P1-1 by the antibiotic calvatic acid and its diazocyanide analogue—evidence for multiple catalytic intermediates. *Eur J Biochem* 1997;245:663–667.

81. Iersel ML, Ploemen JP, Struik I, et al. Inhibition of glutathione S-transferase activity in human melanoma cells by alpha, beta-unsaturated carbonyl derivatives: effects of acrolein, cinnamaldehyde, citral, crotonaldehyde, curcumin, ethacrynic acid, and trans-2-hexenal. *Chem Biol Interact* 1996;102:117–132.

82. Oetari S, Sudibyo M, Commandeur JN, Samhoedi R, Vermeulen NP. Effects of curcumin on cytochrome P450 and glutathione S-transferase activities in rat liver. *Biochem Pharmacol* 1996;51:39–45.

83. Zheng J, Hammock BD. Development of polyclonal antibodies for detection of protein modification by 1,2-naphthoquinone. *Chem Res Toxicol* 1996;9:904–909.

84. Ploemen JP, van Iersel ML, Wormhoudt LW, Commandeur JN, Vermeulen NP, van Bladeren PJ. In vitro inhibition of rat and human glutathione S-transferase isoenzymes by disulfiram and diethyldithiocarbamate. *Biochem Pharmacol* 1996;52:197–204.

85. Seidegard J, Pero RW. The hereditary transmission of high glutathione transferase activity towards *trans*-stilbene oxide in human mononuclear leukocytes. *Hum Genet* 1985;69:66–68.

86. Seidegard J, DePierre JW, Pero RW. Hereditary interindividual differences in the glutathione transferase activity towards *trans*-stilbene oxide in resting human mononuclear leukocytes are due to a particular isozyme(s). *Carcinogenesis* 1985;6:1211–1216.

87. Seidegard J, Vorachek WR, Pero RW, Pearson WR. Hereditary differences in the expression of the human glutathione transferase active on *trans*-stilbene oxide are due to a gene deletion. *Proc Natl Acad Sci USA* 1988;85:7293–7297.

88. Seidegard J, Pero RW, Stille B. Identification of the *trans*-stilbene oxide-active glutathione transferase in human mononuclear leukocytes and in liver as GST1. *Biochem Genet* 1989;27:253–261.

89. Robertson IGC, Guthenberg C, Mannervik B, Jernstrom B. Differences in stereoselectivity and catalytic efficiency of three human glutathione transferases in the conjugation of glutathione with 7b, 8a-dihydroxy-9a, 10a-oxy-7,8,9,10-tetrahydrobenzo(a)pyrene. *Cancer Res* 1986;46:2220–2224.

90. Raney KD, Meyer DJ, Ketterer B, Harris TM, Guengerich FP. Glutathione conjugation of aflatoxin B_1 exo- and endo-epoxides by rat and human glutathione S-transferases. *Chem Res Toxicol* 1992;5: 470–478.

91. Hirvonen A, Nylund L, Kociba P, Husgafvel P-K, Vainio H. Modulation of urinary mutagenicity by genetically determined carcinogen metabolism in smokers. *Carcinogenesis* 1994;15:813–815.

92. Cheng TJ, Christiani DC, Wiencke JK, Wain JC, Xu X, Kelsey KT. Comparison of sister chromatid exchange frequency in peripheral lymphocytes in lung cancer cases and controls. *Mutat Res* 1995; 348:75–82.

93. van Poppel G, Verhagen H, van't Veer P, van Bladeren PJ. Markers for cytogenetic damage in smokers: associations with plasma antioxidants and glutathione S-transferase mu. *Cancer Epidemiol Biomarkers Prev* 1993;2:441–447.

94. Rothman N, Shields PG, Poirier MC, Harrington AM, Ford DP, Strickland PT. The impact of glutathione s-transferase M1 and cytochrome P450 1A1 genotypes on white-blood-cell polycyclic aromatic hydrocarbon-DNA adduct levels in humans. *Mol Carcinog* 1995;14:63–68.

95. Kato S, Bowman ED, Harrington AM, Blomeke B, Shields PG. Human lung carcinogen-DNA adduct levels mediated by genetic polymorphisms in vivo [see comments]. *J Natl Cancer Inst* 1995; 87:902–907.

96. Alexandrie AK, Sundberg MI, Seidegard J, Tornling G, Rannug A.

Genetic susceptibility to lung cancer with special emphasis on CYP1A1 and GSTM1: a study on host factors in relation to age at onset, gender and histological cancer types. *Carcinogenesis* 1994;15: 1785–1790.

97. Anttila S, Luostarinen L, Hirvonen A, et al. Pulmonary expression of glutathione S-transferase M3 in lung cancer patients: association with GSTM1 polymorphism, smoking, and asbestos exposure. *Cancer Res* 1995;55:3305–3309.

98. Bell DA, Thompson CL, Taylor J, et al. Genetic monitoring of human polymorphic cancer susceptibility genes by polymerase chain reaction: application to glutathione transferase mu. *Environ Health Perspect* 1992;98:113–117.

99. Brockmoller J, Kerb R, Drakoulis N, Nitz M, Roots I. Genotype and phenotype of glutathione S-transferase class isoenzymes mu and psi in lung cancer patients and controls. *Cancer Res* 1993;53:1004–1011.

100. Hayashi S, Watanabe J, Kawajiri K. High susceptibility to lung cancer analyzed in terms of combined genotypes of P450IA1 and Mu-class glutathione S-transferase genes. *Jpn J Cancer Res* 1992;83:866–870.

101. Heckbert SR, Weiss NS, Hornung SK, Eaton DL, Motulsky AG. Glutathione S-transferase and epoxide hydrolase activity in human leukocytes in relation to risk of lung cancer and other smoking-related cancers. *J Natl Cancer Inst* 1992;84:414–422.

102. Hirvonen A, Husgafvel-Pursiainen K, Anttila S, Karjalainen A, Vainio H. The human CYP2E1 gene and lung cancer: *Dra* I and *Rsa* I restriction fragment length polymorphisms in a Finnish study population. *Carcinogenesis* 1993;14:85–88.

103. Kawajiri K, Eguchi H, Nakachi K, Sekiya T, Yamamoto M. Association of CYP1A1 germ line polymorphisms with mutations of the p53 gene in lung cancer. *Cancer Res* 1996;56:72–76.

104. Kawajiri K, Watanabe J, Eguchi H, Hayashi S. Genetic polymorphisms of drug-metabolizing enzymes and lung cancer susceptibility. *Pharmacogenetics* 1995;S70–S73.

105. Kihara M, Kihara M, Noda K. Risk of smoking for squamous and small cell carcinomas of the lung modulated by combinations of CYP1A1 and GSTM1 gene polymorphisms in a Japanese population. *Carcinogenesis* 1995;16:2331–2336.

106. Kihara M, Noda K, Kihara M. Distribution of GSTM1 null genotype in relation to gender, age and smoking status in Japanese lung cancer patients. *Pharmacogenetics* 1995;S74–S79.

107. Kihara M, Kihara M, Noda K. Lung cancer risk of GSTM1 null genotype is dependent on the extent of tobacco smoke exposure. *Carcinogenesis* 1994;15:415–418.

108. Liu L, Wang LH. Correlation between lung cancer prevalence and activities of aryl hydrocarbon hydroxylase and glutathione S-transferase in human lung tissues. *Biomed Environ Sci* 1988;1:277–282.

109. London SJ, Daly AK, Fairbrother KS, et al. Lung cancer risk in African-Americans in relation to a race-specific CYP1A1 polymorphism. *Cancer Res* 1995;55:6035–6037.

110. London SJ, Daly AK, Cooper J, et al. Lung cancer risk in relation to the CYP2E1 *Rsa* I genetic polymorphism among African-Americans and Caucasians in Los Angeles County. *Pharmacogenetics* 1996;6: 151–158.

111. Zhong S, Howie AF, Ketterer B, et al. Glutathione S-transferase mu locus: use of genotyping and phenotyping assays to assess association with lung cancer susceptibility. *Carcinogenesis* 1991;12:1533–1537.

112. Sun GF, Shimojo N, Pi JB, Lee S, Kumagai Y. Gene deficiency of glutathione S-transferase mu isoform associated with susceptibility to lung cancer in a Chinese population. *Cancer Lett* 1997;113:169–172.

113. Garcia-Closas M, Kelsey KT, Wiencke JK, Xu X, Wain JC, Christiani DC. A case-control study of cytochrome P450 1A1, glutathione S-transferase M1, cigarette smoking and lung cancer susceptibility (Massachusetts, United States). *Cancer Causes Control* 1997;8: 544–553.

114. d'Errico A, Taioli E, Chen X, Vineis P. Genetic metabolic polymorphisms and the risk of cancer: a review of the literature. *Biomarkers* 1996;1:149–173.

115. Nakachi K, Imai K, Hayashi S, Kawajiri K. Polymorphisms of the CYP1A1 and glutathione S-transferase genes associated with susceptibility to lung cancer in relation to cigarette dose in a Japanese population. *Cancer Res* 1993;53:2994–2999.

116. Harrison DJ, Cantlay AM, Rae F, Lamb D, Smith CA. Frequency of glutathione S-transferase M1 deletion in smokers with emphysema and lung cancer. *Hum Exp Toxicol* 1997;16:356–360.

117. Caporaso N, DeBaun MR, Rothman N. Lung cancer and CYP2D6

118. Anwar WA, Abdel Rahman SZ, El Zein RA, Mostafa HM, Au WW. Genetic polymorphism of GSTM1, CYP2E1 and CYP2D6 in Egyptian bladder cancer patients. *Carcinogenesis* 1996;17:1923–1929.

119. Bell DA, Taylor JA, Paulson DF, Robertson CN, Mohler JL, Lucier GW. Genetic risk and carcinogen exposure: a common inherited defect of the carcinogen-metabolism gene glutathione S-transferase M1 (GSTM1) that increases susceptibility to bladder cancer. *J Natl Cancer Inst* 1993;85:1159–1164.

120. Brockmoller J, Cascorbi I, Kerb R, Roots I. Combined analysis of inherited polymorphisms in arylamine *N*-acetyltransferase 2, glutathione S-transferases M1 and T1, microsomal epoxide hydrolase, and cytochrome P450 enzymes as modulators of bladder cancer risk. *Cancer Res* 1996;56:3915–3925.

121. Brockmoller J, Kerb R, Drakoulis N, Staffeldt B, Roots I. Glutathione S-transferase M1 and its variants A and B as host factors of bladder cancer susceptibility: a case control study. *Cancer Res* 1994;53: 1004–1011.

122. Daly AK, Thomas DJ, Cooper J, Pearson WR, Neal WR, Idle JR. Homozygous deletion of gene for glutathione S-transferase M1 in bladder cancer. *Br Med J* 1993;307:481–482.

123. Katoh T, Inatomi H, Nagaoka A, Sugita A. Cytochrome P4501A1 gene polymorphism and homozygous deletion of the glutathione S-transferase M1 gene in urothelial cancer patients. *Carcinogenesis* 1995;16:655–657.

124. Lafuente A, Giralt M, Cervello I, Pujol F, Mallol J. Glutathione-S-transferase activity in human superficial transitional cell carcinoma of the bladder: comparison with healthy controls. *Cancer* 1990;65: 2064–2068.

125. Lafuente A, Pujol F, Carretero P, Villa JP, Cuchi A. Human glutathione S-transferase mu (GST mu) deficiency as a marker for the susceptibility to bladder and larynx cancer among smokers. *Cancer Lett* 1993; 68:49–54.

126. Lafuente A, Zakahary MM, ElAziz MAA, et al. Influence of smoking in the glutathione-S-transferase M1 deficiency-associated risk for squamous cell carcinoma of the bladder in schistosomiasis patients in Egypt. *Br J Cancer* 1996;74:836–838.

127. Lin HJ, Han CY, Bernstein DA, Hsiao W, Lin BK, Hardy S. Ethnic distribution of the glutathione S-transferase M1-1 (GSTM1) null genotype in 1473 individuals and application to bladder cancer. *Carcinogenesis* 1993;15:1077–1081.

128. Lin HJ, Han CY, Lin BK, Hardy S. Ethnic distribution of slow acetylator mutations in the polymorphic *N*-acetyltransferase (NAT2) gene. *Pharmacogenetics* 1994;4:125–134.

129. Okkels H, Sigsgaard T, Wolf H, Autrup H. Glutathione S-transferase mu as a risk factor in bladder tumours. *Pharmacogenetics* 1996;6: 251–256.

130. Rothman N, Hayes RB, Zenser TV, et al. The glutathione S-transferase M1 (GSTM1) null genotype and benzidine-associated bladder cancer, urine mutagenicity, and exfoliated urothelial cell DNA adducts. *Cancer Epidemiol Biomarkers Prev* 1996;5:979–983.

131. Zhong S, Wyllie AH, Barnes D, Wolf CR, Spurr NK. Relationship between the GSTM1 genetic polymorphism and susceptibility to bladder, breast and colon cancer. *Carcinogenesis* 1993;14:1821–1824.

132. Yu MC, Ross RK, Chan KK, et al. Glutathione S-transferase M1 genotype affects aminobiphenyl-hemoglobin adduct levels in white, black and Asian smokers and non-smokers. *Cancer Epidemiol Biomarkers Prev* 1995;4:861–864.

133. Harada S, Misawa S, Nakamura T, Tanaka N, Ueno E, Mutzumi N. Detection of GST1 gene deletion by polymerase chain reaction and its possible correlation with stomach cancer in Japanese. *Hum Genet* 1992;90:62–64.

134. Kato S, Onda M, Matsukura N, et al. Genetic polymorphisms of the cancer related gene and Helicobacter pylori infection in Japanese gastric cancer patients: an age and gender matched case-control study. *Cancer* 1996;77:1654–1661.

135. Strange RC, Matharoo B, Faulder GC, et al. The human glutathione S-transferase: a case control study of the incidence of the GST 10 phenotype in patients with adenocarcinoma. *Carcinogenesis* 1991;12:25–28.

136. Deakin M, Elder J, Hendrickse C, et al. Glutathione S-transferase GSTT1 genotypes and susceptibility to cancer: studies of interactions with GSTM1 in lung, oral, gastric and colorectal cancers. *Carcinogenesis* 1996;17:881–884.

(the debrisoquine polymorphism): sources of heterogeneity in the proposed association. *Pharmacogenetics* 1995;5:S129–S134.

137. Katoh T, Nagata N, Kuroda Y, et al. Glutathione S-transferase M1 (GSTM1) and T1 (GSTT1) genetic polymorphism and susceptibility to gastric and colorectal adenocarcinoma. *Carcinogenesis* 1996;17: 1855–1859.

138. Chenevix T-G, Young J, Coggan M, Board P. Glutathione S-transferase M1 and T1 polymorphisms: susceptibility to colon cancer and age of onset. *Carcinogenesis* 1995;16:1655–1657.

139. Chen C, Madeleine MM, Lubinski C, Weiss NS, Tickman EW, Daling JR. Glutathione S-transferase M1 genotypes and the risk of anal cancer: a population-based case-control study. *Cancer Epidemiol Biomarkers Prev* 1996;5:985–991.

140. Ambrosone CB, Freudenheim JL, Graham S, et al. Cytochrome P4501A1 and glutathione S-transferase (M1) genetic polymorphisms and postmenopausal breast cancer risk. *Cancer Res* 1995;55: 3483–3485.

141. Fontana X, Peyrotte I, Valente E, et al. (Glutathione S-transferase mu 1 (GSTM1): susceptibility gene of breast cancer). *Bull Cancer* 1997; 84:35–40.

142. Elexpuru C-J, Buxton N, Kandula V, et al. Susceptibility to astrocytoma and meningioma: influence of allelism at glutathione S-transferase (GSTT1 and GSTM1) and cytochrome P-450 (CYP2D6) loci. *Cancer Res* 1995;55:4237–4239.

143. Hand PA, Inskip A, Gilford J, et al. Allelism at the glutathione S-transferase GSTM3 locus: Interactions with GSTM1 and GSTT1 as risk factors for astrocytoma. *Carcinogenesis* 1996;17:1919–1922.

144. Heagerty A, Fitzgerald D, Smith A, et al. Glutathione S-transferase GSTM1 phenotypes and protection against cutaneous tumours. *Lancet* 1994;343:266–268.

145. Heagerty A, Smith A, English J, et al. Susceptibility to multiple cutaneous basal cell carcinomas: significant interactions between glutathione S-transferase GSTM1 genotypes, skin type and male gender. *Br J Cancer* 1996;73:44–48.

146. Lear JT, Heagerty AHM, Smith A, et al. Multiple cutaneous basal cell carcinomas: glutathione S-transferase (GSTM1, GSTT1) and cytochrome P450 (CYP2D6, CYP1A1) polymorphisms influence tumour numbers and accrual. *Carcinogenesis* 1996;17:1891–1896.

147. Yengi L, Inskip A, Gilford J, et al. Polymorphism at the glutathione S-transferase locus GSTM3: Interactions with cytochrome P450 and glutathione S-transferase genotypes as risk factors for multiple cutaneous basal cell carcinoma. *Cancer Res* 1996;56:1974–1977.

148. Sarhanis P, Redman C, Perrett C, et al. Epithelial ovarian cancer: influence of polymorphism at the glutathione S-transferase GSTM1 and GSTT1 loci on p53 expression. *Br J Cancer* 1996;74:1757–1761.

149. Warwick AP, Redman CW, Jones PW, et al. Progression of cervical intraepithelial neoplasia to cervical cancer: interactions of cytochrome P450 CYP2D6 EM and glutathione s-transferase GSTM1 null genotypes and cigarette smoking. *Br J Cancer* 1994;70:704–708.

150. Katoh T. Application of molecular biology to occupational health field—the frequency of gene polymorphism of cytochrome P450 1A1 and glutathione S-transferase M1 in patients with lung, oral and urothelial cancer. *Sangyo Ika Daigaku Zasshi* 1995;17:271–278.

151. Cheng TJ, Christiani DC, Xu X, Wain JC, Wiencke JK, Kelsey KT. Increased micronucleus frequency in lymphocytes from smokers with lung cancer. *Mutat Res* 1996;349:43–50.

152. Nimura Y, Yokoyama K, Fujimori M, et al. Genotyping of the CYP1A1 and GSTM1 genes in esophageal carcinoma patients with special reference to smoking. *Cancer* 1997;80:852–857.

153. Trizna Z, Clayman GL, Spitz MR, Briggs KL, Goepfert H. Glutathione s-transferase genotypes as risk factors for head and neck cancer. *Am J Surg* 1995;170:499–501.

154. Hsieh LL, Huang RC, Yu MW, Chen CJ, Liaw YF. L-*myc*, GST M1 genetic polymorphism and hepatocellular carcinoma risk among chronic hepatitis B carriers. *Cancer Lett* 1996;103:171–176.

155. Chen CJ, Yu MW, Liaw YF, et al. Chronic hepatitis B carriers with null genotypes of glutathione S-transferase M1 and T1 polymorphisms who are exposed to aflatoxin are at increased risk of hepatocellular carcinoma. *Am J Hum Genet* 1996;59:128–134.

156. McGlynn KA, Rosvold EA, Lustbader ED, et al. Susceptibility to hepatocellular carcinoma is associated with genetic variation in enzymatic detoxification of aflatoxin B$_1$. *Proc Natl Acad Sci USA* 1995; 92:2384–2387.

157. Inskip A, Elexpuru C-J, Buxton N, et al. Identification of polymorphism at the glutathione S-transferase, GSTM3 locus: evidence for linkage with GSTM1*A. *Biochem J* 1995;312:713–716.

158. Jahnke V, Matthias C, Fryer A, Strange R. Glutathione S-transferase and cytochrome P-450 polymorphism as risk factors for squamous cell carcinoma of the larynx. *Am J Surg* 1996;172:671–673.

159. Pemble S, Schroeder KR, Spencer SR, et al. Human glutathione S-transferase theta (GSTT1): cDNA cloning and the characterization of a genetic polymorphism. *Biochem J* 1994;300:271–276.

160. Guengerich FP, Thier R, Persmark M, Taylor JB, Pemble SE, Ketterer B. Conjugation of carcinogens by theta class glutathione s-transferases: mechanisms and relevance to variations in human risk. *Pharmacogenetics* 1995;S103–S107.

161. Wiencke JK, Pemble S, Ketterer B, Kelsey KT. Gene deletion of glutathione S-transferase theta: correlation with induced genetic damage and potential role in endogenous mutagenesis. *Cancer Epidemiol Biomarkers Prev* 1995;4:253–259.

162. Sorsa M, Osterman Golkar S, Peltonen K, Saarikoski ST, Sram R. Assessment of exposure to butadiene in the process industry. *Toxicology* 1996;113:77–83.

163. Kelsey KT, Spitz MR, Zuo ZF, Wiencke JK. Polymorphisms in the glutathione S-transferase class mu and theta genes interact and increase susceptibility to lung cancer in minority populations (Texas, United States). *Cancer Causes Control* 1997;8:554–559.

164. Chen H, Sandler D, Taylor J, et al. Increased risk for myelodysplastic syndromes in individuals with glutathione transferase theta 1 (*GSTT1*) gene defect. *Lancet* 1996;347:295–297.

165. Suzuki T, Coggan M, Shaw DC, Board PG. Electrophoretic and immunological analysis of human glutathione S-transferase isoenzymes. *Ann Hum Genet* 1987;51:95–106.

166. Awasthi Y, Singh S, Ahmad H, Moller PC. Immunohistochemical evidence for the expression of GST1, GST2, and GST3 gene loci for glutathione S-transferase in human lung. *Lung* 1987;195:323–332.

167. Di Ilio C, DelBoccio G, Aceto A, Casaccia R, Mucilli F. Elevation of glutathione S-transferase activity in human lung tumor. *Carcinogenesis* 1988;9:355–340.

168. Koskelo K, Valmet E, Tenhunen R. Purification and characterization of an acid glutathione S-transferase from human lung. *Scan J Clin Lab Invest* 1981;41:683–689.

169. Partridge CA, Dao DD, Awasthi YC. Glutathione S-transferase of lung: purification and characterization of human lung glutathione S-transferases. *Lung* 1984;162:27–36.

170. Jernstrom B, Dock L, Hall M, Mannervik B, Tahir MK, Grover PL. Glutathione transferase catalyzed conjugation of benzo(a)pyrene 7,8-diol 9,10-epoxide with glutathione in human skin. *Chem Biol Interact* 1989;70:173–180.

171. Ali-Osman F, Akande O, Antoun G, Mao JX, Boulamwini J. Molecular cloning, characterization, and expression in *Escherichia coli* of full-length cDNAs of three human glutathione S-transferase pi gene variants. *J Biol Chem* 1997;272:10004–10012.

172. Harries LW, Stubbins MJ, Forman D, Howard GC, Wolf CR. Identification of genetic polymorphisms at the glutathione S-transferase pi locus and association with susceptibility to bladder, testicular and prostate cancer. *Carcinogenesis* 1997;18:641–644.

173. Hu X, O'Donnell R, Srivastava SK, et al. Active site architecture of polymorphic forms of human glutathione S-transferase P1-1 accounts for their enantioselectivity and disparate activity in the glutathione conjugation of 7-beta,8-alpha-dihydroxy-9-alpha,10-alpha-oxy-7,8,9,10-tetrahydrobenzo(a)pyrene. *Biochem Biophys Res Commun* 1997; 235:424–428.

174. Roberts S, DeMott RP, James RC. Adrenergic modulation of hepatoxicity. *Drug Metab Rev* 1997;29:329–353.

175. James RC, Harbison RD, Roberts SM. Phenylpropanolamine potentiation of acetaminophen-induced hepatotoxicity: evidence for a glutathione-dependent mechanism. *Toxicol Appl Pharmacol* 1993;118: 159–168.

176. Ross VL, Board PG. Molecular cloning and heterologous expression of an alternatively spliced human mu class glutathione S-transferase transcript. *Biochem J* 1993;294:373–380.

177. Guthenberg C, Mannervik B. Glutathione S-transferase (transferase pi) from human placenta is identical or closely related to glutathione S-transferase (transferase rho) from erythrocytes. *Biochim Biophys Acta* 1981;661:255–260.

178. Hussey AJ, Hayes JD. Characterization of a human class-theta glutathione S-transferase with activity towards 1-menaphthyl sulphate. *Biochem J* 1992;286:929–935.

179. Stockman PK, McLellan LI, Hayes JD. Characterization of the basic glutathione S-transferase B1 and B2 subunits from human liver. *Biochem J* 1987;244:55–61.

180. Rebbeck TR. Molecular epidemiology of the human glutathione S-transferase genotypes GSTM1 and GSTT1 in cancer susceptibility. *Cancer Epidemiol Biomarkers Prev* 1997;6:733–743.
181. Zhao B, Lee EJ, Wong JY, Yeoh PN, Gong NH. Frequency of mutant CYP1A1, NAT2 and GSTM1 alleles in normal Indians and Malays. *Pharmacogenetics* 1995;5:275–280.
182. Nelson HH, Wiencke JK, Christiani DC, et al. Ethnic differences in the prevalence of the homozygous deleted genotype of glutathione S-transferase theta. *Carcinogenesis* 1995;16:1243–1245.
183. Lee EJ, Wong JY, Yeoh PN, Gong NH. Glutathione S transferase-theta (GSTT1) genetic polymorphism among Chinese, Malays and Indians in Singapore. *Pharmacogenetics* 1995;5:332–334.

CHAPTER 15

Sulfotransferases and Methyltransferases

Richard M. Weinshilboum and Rebecca B. Raftogianis

INTRODUCTION

Sulfation and methylation are important pathways in the biotransformation of many drugs and other xenobiotics (1,2). Our understanding of the sulfotransferase and methyltransferase enzymes that catalyze these reactions has increased dramatically in recent years as a result of application of the techniques of molecular biology to study these two enzyme families. That molecular information has complemented a knowledge base developed by decades of biochemical experiments. Because of the importance of these recent advances, the subsequent discussion focuses on newer information with regard to these two large and growing families of drug- and xenobiotic-metabolizing enzymes. Although the abbreviation "ST" was often used previously to refer to sulfotransferase enzymes, a recent International Workshop on Sulfotransferase Enzyme Nomenclature proposed that the abbreviation "SULT" be applied to these enzymes to conform with international guidelines for gene nomenclature. Therefore throughout this chapter, SULT is used as an abbreviation for sulfotransferase, and MT is used as an abbreviation for methyltransferase.

Although the SULTs and MTs are similar in many ways, they also display significant differences. Most members of both of these families of phase II enzymes are cytosolic, but although the majority of MTs are monomeric, most of the cytosolic SULTs are dimers. Both families of enzymes use high-energy donor cosubstrates derived from adenosine triphosphate (ATP). 3'-Phosphoadenosine 5'-phosphosulfate (PAPS) is the "sulfate donor" for SULTs, and S-adenosyl-L-methionine (AdoMet) is the "methyl donor" for virtually all MTs that participate in drug

metabolism (1,2). Both families of enzymes have signature amino acid sequence motifs that have been shown to be involved in the binding of their cosubstrates, PAPS or AdoMet, respectively (3–5). For both SULTs and MTs, concentrations of either the sulfate- or methyl-donor cosubstrate can be limiting under certain circumstances. Reaction products derived from these donor cosubstrates, PAP and S-adenosyl-L-homocysteine (AdoHcy), are competitive inhibitors of their respective reactions (2,6). Both the SULTs and MTs participate in the biotransformation, not only of exogenous compounds such as drugs and other xenobiotics, but also of endogenous compounds such as neurotransmitters and hormones. Finally, the physical consequences of the conjugation reactions catalyzed by these two classes of enzymes are quite different. Sulfation results in a striking enhancement of the water solubility of the substrate, whereas methylation is one of the few pathways of xenobiotic biotransformation that usually decreases water solubility of the reaction product.

Although our understanding of both the SULTs and MTs has been advanced significantly by application of the techniques of molecular biology, the conceptual impact of that information has differed for these two families of drug-metabolizing enzymes. The application of molecular approaches to study the SULTs has resulted in what can only be described as an explosive increase in the number of these enzymes identified and characterized. The total number of SULT cDNAs presently cloned is more than 30, with seven cloned from humans alone. That information, in turn, has made it possible to begin to define a SULT gene superfamily that is assumed to have arisen by divergent evolution (5)—a superfamily similar to that which has been defined for the cytochromes P450 (7). Although our understanding of the MTs has also been advanced significantly by these techniques, no all-encompassing gene superfamily analogous to that which has helped to bring order to the classification of other drug-metabolizing enzymes has yet emerged. Therefore

R. M. Weinshilboum: Department of Pharmacology, Mayo Medical School, 200 First Street SW, Rochester, Minnesota 55905
R.B. Raftogianis: Department of Pharmacology, Fox Chase Cancer Center, 7701 Burholme Avenue, Philadelphia, Pennsylvania 19111

in the subsequent description of the SULTs, the discussion begins with a sketch of the emerging SULT gene superfamily. The classification scheme for this superfamily is based on the degree of amino acid sequence identity among these proteins. That classification provides an "ordering principle" for the subsequent discussion. However, because no such overarching classification of the MTs has yet been developed, the portion of this chapter that deals with MTs is organized along the more traditional lines of enzyme substrate specificities, with molecular information integrated into the discussion of each individual enzyme. This contrasting organization demonstrates that molecular information can alter the way in which we think about drug-metabolizing enzymes. In addition, because the purpose of this volume is to focus on drug interactions, emphasis is placed on SULTs and MTs that are expressed in human tissues, and data from other species is described only when it serves to clarify the function of these enzymes in humans. Finally, because this brief chapter includes a description of two very large families of drug-metabolizing enzymes, it must be selective rather than encyclopedic in scope. As a result, although general classes of substrate are described for each enzyme, no attempt is made to discuss every known substrate or inhibitor for each enzyme. However, references are provided to reviews in which more detailed information can be obtained.

SULFOTRANSFERASES

Sulfate conjugation is an important metabolic pathway for many drugs, other xenobiotics, neurotransmitters, and hormones—especially steroid hormones (2,8). As mentioned previously, the cosubstrate for all of these reactions is PAPS (Fig. 15-1). In prokaryotes, the synthesis of PAPS is catalyzed by two separate enzymes, ATP sulfurylase and adenosine 5'-phosphosulfate (APS) kinase, with the formation of one mole of PAPS from one mole of inorganic sulfate and two moles of ATP (9). However, a single, bifunctional enzyme catalyzes PAPS synthesis in higher organisms (Fig. 15-1) (10,11). Strictly speaking, the reaction catalyzed by the SULTs is not "sulfation" because it involves the transfer of an SO_3^-, rather than a "sulfate" group (2). However, for historical reasons, we will continue to use the term sulfation throughout this chapter.

SULTs can be either membrane bound or cytosolic, but it is the cytosolic enzymes that are thought to catalyze the sulfation of drugs, xenobiotics, neurotransmitters, and hormones. Membrane-bound SULTs catalyze the sulfation of carbohydrate groups on compounds such as heparan, as well as the sulfate conjugation of proteins (12,13). However, these enzymes have very different amino acid sequences from those of the cytosolic SULTs. Because this chapter involves drug metabolism, the subsequent discussion focuses entirely on the cytosolic

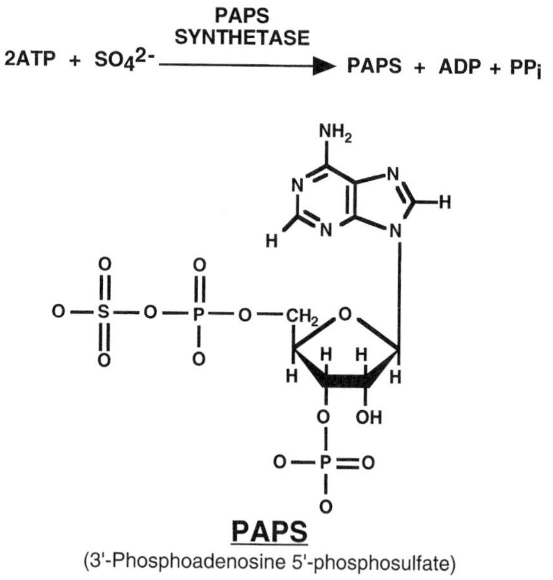

FIG. 15-1. 3'-Phosphoadenosine 5'-phosphosulfate (PAPS) synthesis in higher organisms. **(Top)** Reaction catalyzed by PAPS synthetase and the **(Bottom)** structure of PAPS.

SULTs. Although sulfate conjugation usually serves to "inactivate" the acceptor molecule by increasing its polarity, thus facilitating its excretion, sulfation can also "activate" drugs such as the antihypertensive agent minoxidil or procarcinogens such as *N*-hydroxy-2-acetylaminofluorene (14–16). The subsequent discussion begins with a brief description of SULT molecular biology because the molecular data provide an organizational structure for our approach to these enzymes.

Molecular Biology

cDNAs for more than 30 cytosolic SULTs from eight species have been cloned and characterized (5,17–20). Many of the genes encoding those cDNAs also have been cloned and structurally characterized (5). The dendrogram in Fig. 15-2 shows the relationships among the amino acid sequences of the proteins encoded by these cDNAs. Those relationships are presumed to have arisen as a result of divergent evolution. The dendrogram also makes it possible to subdivide this gene superfamily into phenol SULT and hydroxysteroid SULT families in mammals and a flavonol SULT family in plants. Proteins that share 45% or greater amino acid sequence identity have been classified as members of the same family, and those that share 60% or greater identity constitute subfamilies, specifically the phenol and estrogen SULT subfamilies (see Fig. 15-2). These criteria are similar to those that have been used successfully to classify the cytochromes P450 (7). Seven cytosolic SULTs are presently known to be expressed in human tissues ("circled" enzymes in Fig. 15-2), including three phenol SULTs (previously abbrevi-

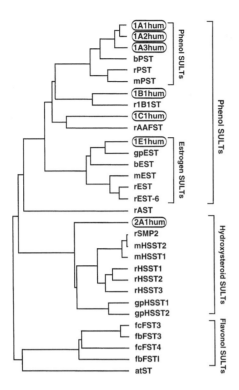

FIG. 15-2. Dendrogram depicting the relative identities among sulfotransferase (SULT) amino acid sequences. This dendrogram was generated with the Pileup Program of GCG, version 9.0, with the "oldpep.cmp" matrix. The human SULT isoforms are circled. Abbreviations for human SULT isoforms are those listed in Table 15-1. The abbreviations for isoforms in other species have been described elsewhere (From Weinshilboum RM, Otterness DM, Aksoy IA, Wood TC, Her C, Raftogianis RB. Sulfotransferase molecular biology: cDNAs and genes. *FASEB J* 1997;11:3–14; and Yoshinari K, Nagata K, Ogino M, et al. Molecular cloning and expression of an amine sulfotransferase cDNA: a new gene family of cytosolic sulfotransferases in mammals. *J Biochem* 1998; 123:479–486, with permission).

ated PSTs), SULT1A1, SULT1A2, and SULT1A3; a thyroid hormone SULT (1B1); a possible human orthologue for a rat *N*-hydroxy-2-acetylaminofluorene SULT (1C1); an estrogen SULT (1E1); and a hydroxysteroid SULT (2A1). Because the nomenclature for human cytosolic

SULTs is presently in a state of "evolution," both previous and proposed nomenclatures for human SULT isoforms, as well as "prototypic" substrates for these enzymes, are listed in Table 15-1. SULT isoforms display significant overlap in their substrate specificities, so several different isoforms may participate in the biotransformation of any given substrate (2). The phenol SULTs are the isoforms that are most likely to participate in the sulfate conjugation of small molecules such as drugs. The reaction catalyzed by a phenol SULT is depicted schematically in Fig. 15-3.

Alignment of the amino acid sequences encoded by all known cytosolic SULTs revealed four regions of conserved sequence, two of which (regions I and IV) were particularly striking (2,5,21). Those two regions have been shown by site-directed mutagenesis to be involved in PAPS binding (21,22). Region I, located near the amino terminus, has the consensus sequence YPKS-GTxW, in which "x" can represent any amino acid. The sequence of region IV, located near the carboxyl terminus of these proteins, is RKGxxGDWKNxFT (2,5). The crystal structure for a mouse estrogen SULT was recently solved (23). Analysis of that structure confirmed that both regions I and IV might be involved in the binding of PAPS. It also suggested that His108, Lys106, and Lys48 in this particular mouse enzyme might participate in the transfer of the SO_3^- group from PAPS to the sulfate-acceptor substrate.

Genes have been cloned for five of the seven known human SULTs (*1A1*, *1A2*, *1A3*, *1E1*, and *2A1*; see Table 15-1 and Fig. 15-4) (5). The structures of those genes are very similar. The phenol and estrogen SULT genes (Family 1) have seven exons that encode amino acid sequence, and the locations of exon–intron splice junctions are highly conserved among these genes (see Fig. 15-4) (5). The human hydroxysteroid *SULT2A1* gene has six exons that encode amino acid sequence (24), and the locations of splice junctions for exons III through VI are also highly conserved when compared with those of exons V through VIII of the phenol SULT family (Family 1). The only human SULT gene presently known to contain a TATA box is *SULT1E1* (25). The human phenol SULT

TABLE 15-1. *Human SULT isoforms*

| | Human SULT enzymes | | |
SULT family or subfamily	Proposed SULT nomenclature	Previous nomenclature	Prototypic substrate
	SULT1A1	TS OR P PST1	4-Nitrophenol 4 μM
Phenol SULTs	SULT1A2	TS or P PST2	4-Nitrophenol 100 μM
	SULT1A3	TL or M PST	Dopamine 60 μM
Other SULTs	SULT1B1	—	Triiodothyronine
	SULT1C1	—	?
Estrogen SULT	SULT1E1	EST	Estrone, 17 βOH-estradiol
Hydroxysteroid SULT	SULT2A1	DHEA ST	DHEA

Previous and proposed nomenclatures for these enzymes as well as examples of prototypic substrates for each isoform are listed.

DHEA, dehydroepiandrosterone.

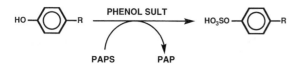

FIG. 15-3. Phenol sulfation catalyzed by a phenol sulfotransferase (SULT).

TABLE 15-2. *Common human SULT1A1 allozymes and allele frequencies in caucasians*

| Allozyme | Amino acid | | Allele frequency[a] |
	213	223	
1	Arg	Met	0.67
2	His	Met	0.31
3	Arg	Val	0.01

[a]Values for allele frequencies do not add up to 1.0 because of the existence of less frequent variant allozymes not included in the table.

genes (*1A1*, *1A2*, and *1A3*) all display alternative transcription initiation, with different exons encoding alternative 5′-untranslated region sequences (26–28). The biologic importance of alternative transcription initiation for these genes is not known.

Chromosomal localizations also have been determined for all of the human SULT genes that have been characterized. The three human *SULT1A*s map to a gene complex located on the short arm of chromosome 16, from 16p12.1 to 16p11.2 (27,28). That information, plus the very high degree of structural homology among these genes (see Fig. 15-4) and the fact that the proteins that they encode are more than 90% identical in amino acid sequence, all suggest that these three genes arose as a result of gene duplication events. *SULT1C1* maps to a region between chromosome bands 2q11.1 and 2q11.2 (18); *SULT1E1* maps to chromosome 4q13.1 (25); and *SULT2A1* has been localized to human chromosome 19q13.3 (29).

Interindividual variation in the "activities" of the PSTs in humans was shown by biochemical genetic studies to be controlled in part by inheritance as a result of genetic polymorphisms (30,31). Those biochemical "pharmacogenetic" data, data obtained during experiments performed with blood platelets, were recently extended to the molecular level by the identification of common genetic polymorphisms within *SULT1A1* that alter the

amino acid sequences of the encoded proteins (32). The different amino acid sequences and the frequencies of allozymes encoded by the most common alleles for *SULT1A1* in caucasians are listed in Table 15-2. Furthermore, the human *SULT1A1* genotype is functionally correlated with both level of enzyme activity and enzyme thermal stability in the blood platelet when 4 μM 4-nitrophenol is used as a substrate (Fig. 15-5). Figure 15-5 shows that subjects homozygous for the SULT1A1 allozyme encoding His213 uniformly had low levels of enzyme activity as well as low thermal stability in their platelets (32). The figure shows also that this genetic polymorphism was only responsible for a portion of the individual variation in this activity. Of most importance for the subject of this chapter, the level of human platelet SULT1A1 activity measured with 4 μM 4-nitrophenol as a substrate is correlated with the relative level of that activity in tissues with relevance for drug metabolism such as the liver, small intestine, and brain (33–36).

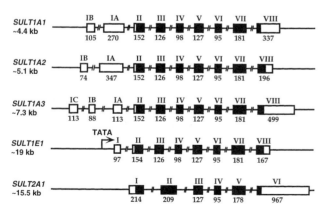

FIG. 15-4. Human sulfotransferase (SULT) gene structures. Black rectangles represent coding regions of exons; open rectangles represent untranslated regions of exons. Numbers beneath exons represent their lengths in bp, and numbers beneath gene designations represent approximate gene lengths, in kb, from the initial through the final exon.

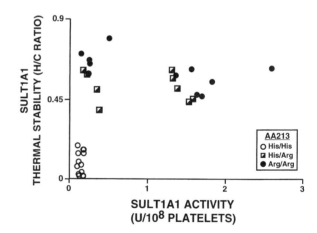

FIG. 15-5. Human platelet *SULT1A1* activity plotted versus enzyme thermal stability measured as a heated/control (H/C) ratio. The amino acid at position 213 is indicated for each sample (see Table 15-2). Reproduced from Raftogianis RB, Wood TC, Otterness DM, Van Loon JA, Weinshilboum RM. Phenol sulfotransferase pharmacogenetics in humans: association of common *SULT1A1* alleles with TS PST phenotype. *Biochem Biophys Res Commun* 1997;239:298–304, with permission.

There also are common genetic polymorphisms for the hydroxysteroid *SULT2A1* gene (36). However, unlike the genotype–phenotype correlation for SULT1A1 depicted in Fig. 15-5, *SULT2A1* genotype does not correlate with individual variation in the sulfation of the prototypic hydroxysteroid SULT substrate dehydroepiandrosterone (DHEA) in human liver biopsy samples (36). The remaining human SULT isoforms also can be studied for possible functionally significant genetic polymorphisms because their cDNA and gene sequences are now known. Finally, a cDNA for human PAPS synthetase has recently been cloned (11), opening the way for molecular genetic studies of the regulation of PAPS synthesis in humans.

Biochemistry

Cytosolic SULTs catalyze the sulfation of a wide variety of both exogenous and endogenous substrates (see Tables 15-1 and 15-3). Prototypic substrates that have been used most often to study SULT isoforms are 4-nitrophenol and dopamine for the phenol SULTs, 17β-estradiol for estrogen SULTs, and DHEA for hydroxysteroid SULTs (2). Most SULTs are active only as dimers (2,8), presumably homodimers, although it has been reported that phenol SULT heterodimers may exist in the rat (37). SULT monomer M_r values range from approximately 30 to 35 kDa. Endogenous substrates for these enzymes include steroid hormones, catecholamines, and thyroid hormones (2). Many of these endogenous substrates also are administered as drugs. Included among the hundreds of drugs that undergo sulfate conjugation in humans are acetaminophen, β-adrenergic agonists, and minoxidil (8). As mentioned previously, minoxidil is a prodrug, and it is the sulfate conjugate of this compound that is responsible for its antihypertensive activity as well as its ability to stimulate hair growth (38). Many other drugs are sulfated after initially undergoing oxidation catalyzed by phase I enzymes such as the cytochromes P450 (2,8). Sulfation

also can result in the metabolic activation of procarcinogens such as N-hydroxy-2-acetylaminofluorene and other hydroxylamines to produce carcinogens (16). The biochemical properties of each of the known human SULT isoforms are described briefly in the subsequent paragraphs.

The three human SULT1A isoforms catalyze the sulfation of phenolic and catechol compounds and represent the isoforms most likely to be involved in the metabolism of drugs other than steroids (2,8). Biochemical experiments performed during the past two decades led to the definition of two "PST" isoforms in human tissues (39–42). Both of those activities were expressed in a variety of tissues including liver, jejunum, kidney, lung, brain, and—of importance for pharmacogenetic studies—the blood platelet (39–44). The biochemically defined "thermostable," or TS, form of PST preferentially catalyzed the sulfation of small planar phenols such as 4-nitrophenol at micromolar concentrations and was sensitive to inhibition by the SULT inhibitor 2,6-dichloro-4-nitrophenol (DCNP). TS PST also has been referred to as the phenol-preferring (P) form of the enzyme, and the prototypic substrate used to measure TS PST activity in human tissue has been 4 μM 4-nitrophenol (2). A separate "thermolabile" (TL) isoform of PST preferentially catalyzed the sulfation of micromolar concentrations of catechol monoamines such as dopamine and was relatively resistant to DCNP inhibition. The prototypic substrate for "TL PST activity," also referred to as the monoamine-preferring, or M isoform, was 60 μM dopamine. Those biochemical experiments demonstrated that TS PST could catalyze the sulfation of dopamine, but with a K_m value in the millimolar range, approximately three orders of magnitude higher than the apparent K_m of the TL isoform (2). Conversely, the TL isoform could catalyze the sulfate conjugation of 4-nitrophenol, but with an apparent K_m value approximately three orders of magnitude higher than that of the TS isoform.

TABLE 15-3. *Selected substrates for human SULT isoforms*

Substrate	Recombinant SULT isoform						
	1A1	1A2	1A3	1B1	1C1	1E1	2A1
4-Nitrophenol	++++ (100)	+++ (46)	+ (100,101)	+++ (17)	N.S.	++ (Aksoy and Weinshilboum, unpublished data)	— (8)
Dopamine	++ (100)	N.S.	+++ (100,101)	++ (17)	N.S.	— (102)	— (8)
3,3′,5-Triidothyrine	++ (17)	N.S.	++ (17)	+++ (17)	N.S.	N.S.	N.S.
Estradiol	+++ (103)	N.S.	— (101)	— (17)	N.S.	++++ (102)	+++ (103)
DHEA	— (104)	N.S.	— (101)	— (17)	N.S.	++++ (49)	+++ (36)
Acetaminophen	++ (99)	N.S.	++ (106)	N.S.	N.S.	N.S.	N.S.
Minoxidil	+ (107)	N.S.	+ (107)	N.S.	N.S.	++ (108)	+ (107)

(+), the relative ability of the SULT isoform to catalyze the sulfation of that substrate based on apparent K_m values; (—), the isoform was tested and did not catalyze sulfate conjugation of that substrate; N.S., the SULT isoform has not been studied with that substrate. References for the data used to construct the table are shown in parentheses beneath each symbol.

Therefore, even though these biochemically defined isoforms displayed overlapping substrate specificities, their apparent K_m values for prototypic substrates differed dramatically. As described in the preceding paragraphs, gene-cloning experiments have demonstrated that there are at least three phenol SULTs in humans (26–28). *SULT1A1* and *SULT1A2* exhibit "TS PST-like" activity, and biochemical characterization of recombinant proteins encoded by these genes has shown that *SULT1A1* is most likely to be responsible for the sulfation of 4 μM 4-nitrophenol (32,45,46). The *SULT1A3* gene encodes the enzyme that catalyzes TL PST activity. *SULT1A1* can also catalyze the sulfation of estrogens such as estrone and 17β-estradiol (2,8,47).

A SULT1B1 cDNA has only recently been cloned (17,20). The protein encoded by this cDNA was able to catalyze the sulfation of thyroid hormones such as 3,3′,5-triiodothyronine (T_3). Sulfate conjugation is thought to contribute to the regulation of the physiologic activities of thyroid hormones. Recombinant human SULT1B1 also could catalyze the sulfation of 4-nitrophenol and dopamine, but not that of 17β-estradiol or DHEA (17,20).

SULT1C1 in the rat has been shown to catalyze the sulfation of the procarcinogen *N*-hydroxy-2-acetylaminofluorene (48). Recently a cDNA that may represent a human orthologue of SULT1C1 was cloned from a human fetal liver/spleen cDNA library (18). However, the substrate specificity of the protein encoded by that cDNA has not been reported. Dot blot and Northern blot analyses demonstrated that human SULT1C1 was expressed in the kidney, stomach, and thyroid gland, but not in the adult liver (18).

SULT1E1 preferentially catalyzes the sulfation of estrogens, although several other human SULT isoforms also can catalyze the sulfate conjugation of those compounds (see Table 15-3) (2,8,49). Recombinant SULT1E1 catalyzes the sulfation of both estrone and 17β-estradiol with K_m values in the nanomolar range, whereas SULT1A1 and SULT2A1 have K_m values for these substrates in the low micromolar range. SULT1E1 also can catalyze the sulfation of DHEA, pregnenolone, equilenin, 17α-ethinylestradiol, and 4-hydroxytamoxifen, as well as that of many small phenols and phytoestrogens (2,8,49). This enzyme has been reported to be expressed in human liver, small intestine, testis, endometrium, and in primary cultures of mammary epithelial cells, but not in breast cancer cell lines (2,8,49).

SULT2A1 was the first human SULT for which a cDNA was cloned (50). DHEA is the prototypic substrate for this and other hydroxysteroid SULTs, but SULT2A1 also can catalyze the sulfation of bile acids and estrogens (2,8). Although sulfate conjugation is usually regarded as a reaction that facilitates excretion, DHEA sulfate is excreted approximately 100-fold more slowly than is DHEA, and DHEA can be regenerated from DHEA sulfate by enzymatic hydrolysis of the sulfate conjugate catalyzed by sulfatase(s) (51). SULT2A1 is expressed in human liver, adrenal cortex, and small intestine (50,52).

The synthetic SULT inhibitors that have been studied most frequently are DCNP and pentachlorophenol (39,53). However, all SULTS also display profound substrate inhibition, perhaps because of their high affinity for PAP and the formation of an enzyme–PAP substrate complex (2,54). Sulfation can be regulated *in vivo* by the availability of either inorganic sulfate or the cosubstrate, PAPS (9). PAPS can be synthesized rapidly in the liver, but it can also be rapidly depleted. The availability of inorganic sulfate required for PAPS synthesis (see Fig. 15-1) is critical for the maintenance of adequate levels of PAPS (9,55). Therefore the *in vivo* rate of drug sulfation can potentially be affected by a low-sulfate diet or by the ingestion of multiple SULT substrates.

In summary, the SULTs represent an expanding gene superfamily of enzymes that participate in the phase II biotransformation of a very large number of both exogenous and endogenous phenolic and catechol compounds. The coadministration of two competing substrates for any one isoform could, theoretically, result in clinically significant drug interactions. Furthermore, the activities of these enzymes can be affected by the concentration of the sulfate donor cosubstrate, PAPS. Therefore the SULTs represent a potentially fertile area for future studies of clinically relevant drug interactions.

METHYLTRANSFERASES

MT enzymes catalyze the methyl conjugation of "small molecules" such as drugs, hormones, and neurotransmitters, as well as macromolecules such as proteins, RNA, and DNA. The most recent edition of the International Union of Biochemistry and Molecular Biology reference volume, *Enzyme Nomenclature*, lists 113 MT enzymes, approximately evenly divided between activities that catalyze small-molecule and macromolecule methylation (56). However, it has been estimated that hundreds of additional MT genes remain to be identified in the human genome. The majority of these enzymes use AdoMet as a methyl donor. AdoMet is synthesized from ATP and methionine by methionine adenosyltransferase (MAT, EC 2.5.1.6; Fig. 15-6) (57). There are two separate MAT genes in mammals. One of these genes is expressed predominantly in the liver, whereas the other is expressed primarily in extrahepatic tissue. In humans, the amino acid sequences of the proteins encoded by these two genes are approximately 84% identical. MAT is active as either a homotetramer or a homodimer, but the apparent K_m value of the tetramer for methionine is lower than is that of the dimer (57).

Most AdoMet-dependent MTs have two common amino acid signature sequences, one of which has been shown by site-directed mutagenesis to be involved in

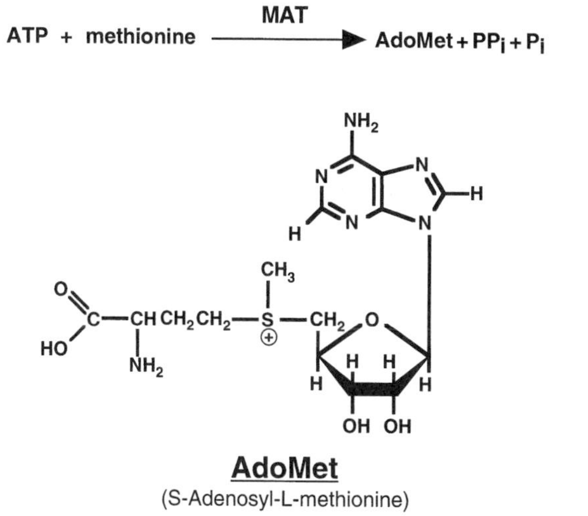

ATP + methionine $\xrightarrow{\text{MAT}}$ AdoMet + PP$_i$ + P$_i$

AdoMet
(S-Adenosyl-L-methionine)

FIG. 15-6. *S*-Adenosyl-L-methionine (AdoMet) synthesis. **(Top)** A Reaction catalyzed by methionine adenosyltransferase (MAT) and the **(Bottom)** structure of AdoMet is shown.

AdoMet binding (3,4). Although our understanding of small-molecule MTs has benefited greatly from application of the techniques of molecular biology, that information has not yet provided an overall organizational structure for the classification of these enzymes as it has for the SULTs. Therefore the subsequent discussion uses a "conventional" approach to the classification of these enzymes based on the general class of their substrates and the type of reaction that they catalyze—*O*-methylation, *S*-methylation, or *N*-methylation. In each case, a "prototypic" enzyme of importance for drug metabolism is described to illustrate general principles and other examples of MTs that catalyze methylation of the same heteroatom, *O*-, *S*-, or *N*-, may be mentioned briefly. The MTs also represent a group of enzymes that has been studied intensively for possible pharmacogenetic variation, and a series of clinically significant genetic polymorphisms for these enzymes has been described (1). Because abbreviations for the names of these enzymes can quickly become an "alphabet soup" of MTs for those who do not work with them regularly, Table 15-4 lists the major enzymes discussed in this chapter as well as abbreviations and prototypic substrates for each enzyme.

O-Methyltransferases

It seems appropriate to begin a discussion of MT enzymes with catechol *O*-methyltransferase (COMT, EC 2.1.1.6). The discovery of COMT (58), like that of many of the other MTs described subsequently, was made possible by the identification, isolation, and subsequent availability of AdoMet. This methyl donor was then radioactively labeled for use as a cosubstrate to identify MT activities that could then be purified and studied. COMT was one of the first of these enzymes to be characterized biochemically; it plays an important role in the biotransformation of both endogenous and exogenous compounds; and it recently became the first of the small-molecule MTs for which a crystal structure was solved (59). This enzyme was discovered initially because of its role in the biotransformation of catecholamine neurotransmitters such as dopamine, norepinephrine, and epinephrine (58) (Fig. 15-7).

COMT was originally described as a cytosolic monomeric enzyme with an M_r value of approximately 25 kDa (58). However, for many years, there was debate with regard to whether a separate, membrane-bound form of COMT might exist, and, if so, whether it was the product of the same or a separate gene. Cloning of the COMT gene has now answered that question, and it is clear that a single gene with two different sites of transcription initiation encodes both cytosolic and membrane-bound forms of this enzyme, forms that differ only at their amino termini (60). The membrane-bound form of COMT includes an additional 50-amino-acid hydrophobic segment at the N-terminus that is not present in the cytosolic enzyme. Human tissues such as liver and kidney appear to express mainly the cytosolic form of the enzyme, whereas the membrane-bound form is highly expressed in the brain (60). Biochemically, COMT has an absolute requirement for the catechol structure and will not catalyze the methylation of monophenols. It also is dependent on Mg^{2+} for enzymatic activity (58). Substrates include not only the catecholamine neurotransmitters, but also drugs that contain the catechol structure such as the anti–Parkinson's disease agent L-dopa, the antihypertensive methyldopa, and the antiasthmatic drug isoproterenol (1). COMT also participates in the biotransformation of endogenous compounds that are not biogenic amines, compounds like the catechol estrogens

TABLE 15-4. *Selected MT enzymes*

Enzyme	Abbreviation	Substrate
Catechol *O*-methyltransferase	COMT	Catecholamines
Thiopurine methyltransferase	TPMT	6-Mercaptopurine
Thiol methyltransferase	TMT	2-Mercaptoethanol
Nicotinamide *N*-methyltransferase	NNMT	Nicotinamide
Histamine *N*-methyltransferase	HNMT	Histamine

Abbreviations and prototypic substrates for the enzymes highlighted in this chapter are listed.

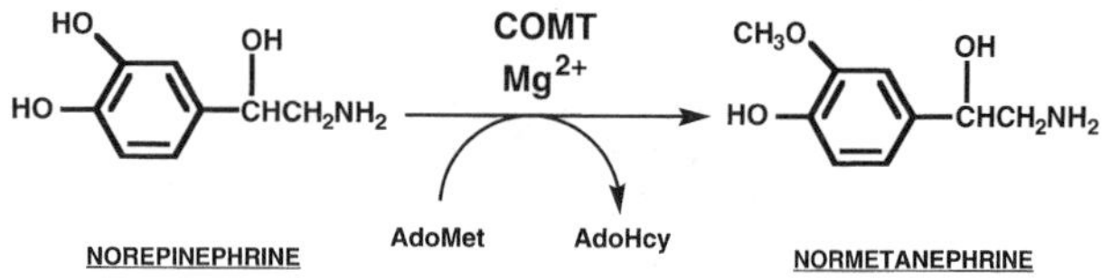

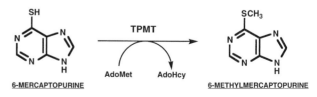

FIG. 15-7. Catechol *O*-methyltransferase (COMT)-catalyzed *O*-methylation of norepinephrine.

that can be formed *in vivo* from estrone and 17β-estradiol (61). Although COMT inhibitors such as tropolone have been available for decades, those early compounds were much too toxic for clinical use. Several nontoxic COMT inhibitors such as nitecapone have recently been developed for use as adjuncts during the L-dopa therapy of patients with Parkinson's disease (62).

COMT also was the first of the MT enzymes to be subjected to pharmacogenetic analysis. There is a well-defined common genetic polymorphism for this enzyme in humans (63). This polymorphism was defined initially by measuring human red blood cell (RBC) COMT activity. RBC COMT activity varied among individuals over a five-fold range and had a well-defined bimodal frequency distribution, with approximately 25% of white subjects homozygous for the inherited trait of low level of enzyme activity (63). Subsequent studies demonstrated that RBC COMT activity was correlated with the level of COMT activity in other human tissues and organs such as liver, kidney, and lung (1). The COMT genetic polymorphism also was found to be correlated with individual differences in the biotransformation of catechol drugs such as L-dopa and methyldopa (1). This genetic polymorphism was recently reported to represent a risk factor for the occurrence of breast cancer (61), perhaps because of its role in the biotransformation of catechol estrogens. Cloning of the human COMT cDNA and gene (60) also made it possible to demonstrate that the COMT genetic polymorphism results from a Val → Met change in amino acid at codon 108/158 (depending on whether the soluble or membrane-bound form of the enzyme is encoded) (64). The "low-activity" form of the enzyme contains methionine at codon 108/158. This sequence of events, identification of a genetic polymorphism at the biochemical level—often in an easily accessible tissue such as the RBCs—followed by functional characterization (i.e., determination of the influence of the polymorphism on individual variation in drug or endogenous compound metabolism), and finally, determination of the molecular mechanism responsible for the polymorphism, is a paradigm that also has been applied to several other human MT enzymes.

S-Methyltransferases

S-Methylation is an important reaction for the biotransformation of sulfur-containing compounds, particularly sulfhydryls (65). Included among drugs that contain

sulfhydryl groups are the antineoplastic and immune-suppressant thiopurine drugs, 6-mercaptopurine (6-MP), 6-thioguanine, and azathioprine; the aliphatic antihypertensive sulfhydryl captopril, and the sulfhydryl-containing antiinflammatory agent D-penicillamine. All of these drugs have been shown to undergo *S*-methylation in humans (65). Three separate MTs are known to catalyze *S*-methylation in mammals. Thiopurine methyltransferase (TPMT, EC 2.1.1.67) catalyzes the *S*-methylation of aromatic and heterocyclic sulfhydryl compounds including 6-MP and other thiopurines (Fig. 15-8); thiol methyltransferase (TMT, EC 2.1.1.9) catalyzes the *S*-methylation of captopril, D-penicillamine, and other aliphatic sulfhydryl compounds; and thioether methyltransferase (TEMT, EC 2.1.1.96), an enzyme studied thus far only in the mouse, catalyzes the *S*-methylation of thioethers (65,66). Two of these enzymes, TPMT and TMT, have been shown to be genetically polymorphic in humans (67,68). Because TEMT has not yet been characterized in human tissues, the subsequent discussion focuses on TPMT and TMT.

TPMT is a cytosolic monomeric AdoMet-dependent MT that uses aromatic and heterocyclic sulfhydryl compounds as substrates (see Fig. 15-8) (69,70). It is inhibited noncompetitively by benzoic acid derivatives (70), an observation of importance with regard to a clinically significant drug interaction described subsequently. TPMT is widely expressed in human tissues, with high levels of expression in human kidney, liver, and gut (71). It catalyzes a major pathway for the biotransformation of thiopurine drugs, a pathway that is in competition with a bioactivation pathway that converts 6-MP, itself a prodrug, into 6-thioguanine nucleotides (6-TGN), which can then be incorporated into DNA. RBC 6-TGN concentrations are highly correlated with both the therapeutic efficacy and toxicity of thiopurine drugs (72). Therefore subjects with inherited low levels of TPMT might theoretically be at risk for the occurrence of high 6-TGN concentrations and thus for thiopurine drug-induced toxicity. That is exactly what clinical studies have demonstrated (73). Those studies showed that genetically determined variation in TPMT activity is an important risk factor for differences among individual patients in both the therapeutic efficacy and toxicity of thiopurine drugs (74).

The TPMT genetic polymorphism was first described by measuring the enzyme activity in an easily accessible

FIG. 15-8. Thiopurine methyltransferase (TPMT)-catalyzed *S*-methylation of 6-mercaptopurine.

tissue, the RBC, by using an approach analogous to that used to discover the COMT genetic polymorphism. Approximately 89% of randomly selected white subjects were homozygous for the trait of high RBC TPMT activity, approximately 11% were heterozygous and had intermediate activity, and one of every 300 subjects was homozygous for the inherited trait of extremely low or undetectable activity (Fig. 15-9) (67). Furthermore, levels of TPMT activity in the RBC were highly correlated with levels of this enzyme activity in other human tissues such as liver and kidney (74). As previously described, clinical studies then demonstrated that subjects homozygous for the trait of low or absent TPMT activity were at greatly increased risk for life-threatening thiopurine toxicity such as myelosuppression when exposed to "standard" doses of these drugs (73–75). Those patients could be treated with thiopurines, but the dose had to be reduced to 1/10 to 1/15 of usual doses, and the patient had to be monitored carefully for signs of toxicity. There is also preliminary evidence that patients with very high levels of TPMT activity might be undertreated with standard doses of thiopurine drugs (75). As a result of these reports, the TPMT genetic polymorphism, as measured phenotypically in the RBC, has become one of the first pharmacogenetic diagnostic tests to enter standard clinical practice.

The observation that TPMT can be inhibited by benzoic acid derivatives (70) has recently been extended to include inhibition by the aminosalicylic acid compounds that are used to treat inflammatory bowel disease (76). Those in vitro experiments raised the possibility of a clinically significant drug interaction in patients with inflammatory bowel disease treated simultaneously with thiopurines and aminosalicylic acid derivatives. Clinical case reports of serious adverse responses to that drug combination have recently begun to appear (77). It is unclear whether the 10% of white patients with "intermediate" TPMT activity, those who are heterozygous for the genetic polymorphism (see Fig. 15-9), might be particularly susceptible to this drug interaction.

A cDNA for TPMT, a processed pseudogene located on human chromosome 18, and, finally, the active gene located on the short arm of chromosome 6, have all been cloned in an attempt to determine the molecular basis for the TPMT genetic polymorphism (71,78,79). The human TPMT gene is approximately 34 kb in length and consists of 10 exons, eight of which encode protein. The most common variant allele for very low TPMT activity in whites, TPMT*3A, has two separate polymorphisms, one located within exon VII that changes the amino acid encoded by codon 154 from Ala to Thr, and a second polymorphism in exon X, which alters the amino acid encoded by codon 240 from Tyr to Cys (Fig. 15-10) (79). Each of these two polymorphisms can also exist separately. The most common variant allele in whites, TPMT*3A, has not been reported among Asians, but the exon X variant alone, TPMT*3C, has been observed in Asian subjects (see Fig. 15-10) (80). At least eight separate polymorphisms associated with very low TPMT activity have been reported, seven of which alter encoded amino acid sequence, and one that involves a mutation at the 3′-acceptor splice site between TPMT intron IX and exon X (79–81). These observations are similar to those made for other genetically polymorphic human drug-metabolizing enzymes. In most cases, these polymorphisms display allelic heterogeneity, but only a few of the variant alleles are observed frequently. In the case of TPMT, the *3A allele accounts for 55% to 70% of all variant alleles in whites (80). Ethnic variation in the frequencies or presence of variant alleles also is common among genetically polymorphic drug-metabolizing enzymes (82). Clarification of the molecular basis for the

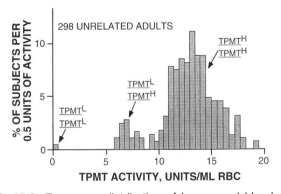

FIG. 15-9. Frequency distribution of human red blood cell (RBC) thiopurine methyltransferase (TPMT) activity. Apparent genotypes for the "trait" of level of RBC TPMT activity in 298 randomly selected white adults also are indicated. TPMT^L is the allele or alleles for the trait of "low," and TPMT^H is the allele or alleles for the trait of "high" activity. Reproduced from Weinshilboum RM, Sladek SL. Mercaptopurine pharmacogenetics: monogenic inheritance of erythrocyte thiopurine methyltransferase activity. Am J Hum Genet 1980;32:651–662, with permission.

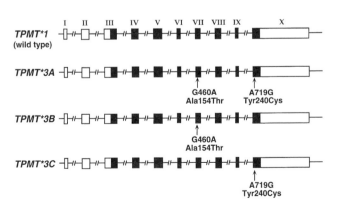

FIG. 15-10. Selected human thiopurine methyltransferase (TPMT) alleles. Black rectangles represent coding regions of exons; open rectangles represent untranslated regions of exons.

TPMT genetic polymorphism now raises the possibility that DNA-based diagnostic tests might be developed either to supplement or to replace the present phenotypic test, in which TPMT activity is measured in the RBCs.

The other biochemically well-characterized sulfhydryl MT expressed in human tissues is TMT. TMT, unlike most other AdoMet-dependent small-molecule MTs, is membrane bound (65). This enzyme has a relative specificity for aliphatic sulfhydryl compounds, rather than the aromatic and heterocyclic sulfhydryls that are the preferred substrates for TPMT. 2-Mercaptoethanol (2-ME) is the prototypic substrate that has been used most often to measure TMT activity. However, TMT also can catalyze the S-methylation of a variety of drugs, including captopril, D-penicillamine, and N-acetylcysteine (65). TMT, unlike TPMT, has not yet been purified, so TMT activity has been characterized only with membrane preparations, including human hepatic microsomes and, for pharmacogenetic studies, human RBC membranes. Kinetic studies performed with 2-ME and a variety of other substrates have demonstrated biphasic substrate kinetics for this enzyme. For example, the enzyme displays two apparent K_m values for 2-ME that differ by approximately three orders of magnitude, 9.0 μM and 20 mM (83). Those observations have been interpreted to indicate either the existence of two separate membrane-bound MTs that catalyze the S-methylation of aliphatic sulfhydryls, or substrate-dependent alteration in the kinetic behavior of a single enzyme. Most data seem to favor the latter interpretation (67). Individual variations in levels of human RBC TMT have been shown to be primarily regulated by inheritance, with a heritability of 0.98 [i.e., 98% of the approximately five-fold individual variation in level of activity is due to the effects of inheritance (68,84)]. Future pharmacogenetic studies will require the purification of TMT as well as the cloning of its cDNA and gene, followed by studies of the molecular basis for the genetic regulation of this drug-metabolizing MT enzyme.

N-Methyltransferases

N-Methylation is a common metabolic pathway for endogenous neurotransmitters and hormones. For example, phenylethanolamine N-methyltransferase (PNMT, EC 2.1.1.28) catalyzes the N-methylation of the neurotransmitter norepinephrine to form epinephrine (85). However, PNMT is found only in the adrenal medulla and in a few nuclei in the central nervous system (CNS). Therefore it can play little, if any, role in the biotransformation of exogenously administered drugs or other xenobiotics. However, some N-MTs are expressed in organs such as the liver and gut, which could participate in the biotransformation of exogenously administered compounds. Two of these enzymes are nicotinamide N-methyltransferase (NNMT, EC 2.1.1.1) and histamine N-methyltransferase (HNMT, EC 2.1.1.8).

NNMT catalyzes the N-methylation of nicotinamide and structurally related pyridine compounds to form positively charged pyridinium ions. NNMT is a monomeric cytosolic AdoMet-dependent enzyme that is highly expressed in the human liver (86). NNMT participates in the biotransformation of at least one commonly used drug, nicotinic acid. Nicotinic acid is converted to nicotinamide in vivo. Because NNMT catalyzes the biotransformation of nicotinamide, a substrate required for the formation of nicotinamide adenine dinucleotide (NAD), it is potentially in a position to contribute to the regulation of NAD-dependent reactions. Therefore understanding the regulation of NNMT activity in humans could have functional significance that extends well beyond its role in the metabolism of xenobiotics such as nicotinic acid. Human liver-biopsy samples display wide individual variation in NNMT activity, with an apparent subgroup of approximately 25% of subjects who have high levels of activity (86). Because those observations raised the possibility that this enzyme might also be genetically polymorphic, cDNAs and genes for NNMT have been cloned and characterized for both humans and mice (87–89). Mice were studied because of the presence of large, strain-dependent—therefore presumably genetic—variations in levels of NNMT activity in the mouse liver (90). However, unlike the situation for COMT and TPMT, no functionally important genetic polymorphisms at the nucleotide level have yet been observed for NNMT in humans (L. Yan and R.M. Weinshilboum, unpublished observation).

Histamine, discovered and characterized early in this century by Sir Henry Dale and his colleagues (91), may play a role in the pathophysiology of a variety of human diseases including allergy, asthma, and peptic ulcer disease. HNMT catalyzes one of two major pathways for histamine biotransformation and is the only process available for termination of the neurotransmitter actions of histamine in the mammalian CNS (92). HNMT is a cytosolic monomeric AdoMet-dependent enzyme that catalyzes the N^t-methylation of histamine on the heterocyclic ring (93). Levels of HNMT activity in human tissues, like those of COMT and TPMT, have been shown to be regulated by a common genetic polymorphism (94,95). Initial pharmacogenetic studies of HNMT, like those of COMT and TPMT, involved measurements of the enzyme activity in the human RBC (94). Large individual variations in levels of this enzyme activity in the RBC were found to be regulated predominantly by inheritance as a result of a common genetic polymorphism. The cDNA and gene for HNMT in humans have now been cloned (96,97), and common polymorphisms at the DNA level that are associated with variations in levels of HNMT activity have recently been described (98). The functional implications of those observations in the pathophysiology of human disease or in response to drug therapy remain to be determined.

CONCLUSIONS

Sulfation and methylation, like other pathways for the biotransformation of drugs and other xenobiotics, also participate in the metabolism of endogenous compounds such as hormones and neurotransmitters. Our understanding of both of these phase II enzyme families has recently increased as a result of the application of molecular biology techniques. Those techniques have helped to identify and characterize enzymes that were previously unknown and to make it possible to study the molecular basis for the regulation of the expression of these enzymes. The continuation of this process will be essential if we are ultimately to understand, predict, and prevent drug interactions. The thiopurine–aminosalicylate interaction that occurs in patients with inflammatory bowel disease who are treated with these two agents offers a glimpse of that future. That interaction was predicted (76) before it was recognized in the clinic (77). Furthermore, understanding the critical role of genetic variation in TPMT activity in determining individual differences in response to thiopurine drugs has been an important advance in our ability to use these beneficial, but potentially toxic, pharmacologic agents. In summary, our evolving understanding of the SULT and MT enzymes demonstrates that it may eventually become possible to anticipate and avoid many adverse drug reactions and to move toward the goal of individualization of pharmacologic therapy for every patient.

ACKNOWLEDGMENT

We thank Luanne Wussow and Diane Otterness for their assistance with the preparation of this manuscript. This study was supported in part by National Institutes of Health grants RO1 GM28157 (R.M.W.) and RO1 GM35720 (R.M.W.) as well as NRSA (NIH) Individual Postdoctoral Fellowship GM18800 (R.B.R.).

REFERENCES

1. Weinshilboum R. Methyltransferase pharmacogenetics. *Pharmacol Ther* 1989;43:77–90.
2. Weinshilboum RM, Otterness DM. Sulfotransferase enzymes. In: Kaufmann FC, ed. *Conjugation-deconjugation reactions in drug metabolism and toxicity: handbook of experimental pharmacology.* Vol 112. Berlin: Springer-Verlag, 1994:45–78.
3. Ingrosso D, Fowler AV, Bleibaum J, Clarke S. Sequence of the D-aspartyl/L-isoaspartyl protein methyltransferase from human erythrocytes: common sequence motifs for protein, DNA, RNA and small molecule S-adenosylmethionine-dependent methyltransferases. *J Biol Chem* 1989;264:20131–20139.
4. Fujioka M. Mammalian small molecule methyltransferases: their structural and functional features. *Int J Biochem* 1992;24:1917–1924.
5. Weinshilboum RM, Otterness DM, Aksoy IA, Wood TC, Her C, Raftogianis RB. Sulfotransferase molecular biology: cDNAs and genes. *FASEB J* 1997;11:3–14.
6. Borchardt RT. Synthesis and biological activity of analogs of adenosylhomocysteine as inhibitors of methyltransferases. In: Salvatore F, Borek E, Zappia V, Williams-Ashman HG, Schlenk F, eds. *Biochemistry of adenosylmethionine.* New York: Columbia University Press, 1977:151–171.
7. Nelson DR, Koymans L, Kamataki T, et al. P450 superfamily: update on new sequences, gene mapping, accession numbers and nomenclature. *Pharmacogenetics* 1996;6:1–42.
8. Falany CN. Enzymology of human cytosolic sulfotransferase. *FASEB J* 1997;11:206–216.
9. Klassen CD, Boles JW. The importance of 3′-phosphoadenosine-5′-phosphosulfate (PAPS) in the regulation of sulfation. *FASEB J* 1997;11:404–418.
10. Konstantinidus AK, Schwartz NB. The isolation and characterization of cDNA encoding the mouse bifunctional ATP sulfurylase-adenosine 5′-phosphosulfate kinase. *J Biol Chem* 1995;270:29453–29459.
11. Girard J-P, Baekkevold ES, Amalric F. Sulfation in high endothelial venules: cloning and expression of the human PAPS synthetase. *FASEB J* 1998;12:603–612.
12. Hashimoto Y, Orellana A, Gil G, Hirschberg CB. Molecular cloning and expression of rat liver *N*-heparan sulfate sulfotransferase. *J Biol Chem* 1992;267:15744–15750.
13. Ouyang YB, Lane WS, Moore KL. Tyrosylprotein sulfotransferase: purification and molecular cloning of an enzyme that catalyzes tyrosine *O*-sulfation, a common posttranslational modification of eukaryotic proteins. *Proc Natl Acad Sci USA* 1998;95:2896–2901.
14. Falany CN, Kerl EA. Sulfation of minoxidil by human liver phenol sulfotransferase. *Biochem Pharmacol* 1990;40:1027–1032.
15. Kudlecek PE, Clemens DL, Anderson RJ. Characterization of recombinant human liver thermolabile phenol sulfotransferase with minoxidil as the substrate. *Biochem Biophys Res Commun* 1995;210:363–369.
16. Glatt H. Bioactivation of mutagens via sulfation. *FASEB J* 1997;11:314–321.
17. Fujita K, Nagata K, Ozawa S, Sasano H, Yamazoe Y. Molecular cloning and characterization of rat ST1B1 and human ST1B2 cDNAs, encoding thyroid hormone sulfotransferases. *J Biochem* 1997;122:1052–1061.
18. Her C, Kaur GP, Athwal RS, Weinshilboum RM. Human sulfotransferase SULT1C1: cDNA cloning, tissue-specific expression and chromosomal localization. *Genomics* 1997;41:467–470.
19. Yoshinari K, Nagata K, Ogino M, et al. Molecular cloning and expression of an amine sulfotransferase cDNA: a new gene family of cytosolic sulfotransferases in mammals. *J Biochem* 1998;123:479–486.
20. Wang J, Falany JL, Falany CN. Expression and characterization of a novel thyroid hormone-sulfating form of cytosolic sulfotransferase from human liver. *Mol Pharmacol* 1998;53:274–282.
21. Marsolais F, Varin L. Identification of amino acid residues critical to catalysis and cosubstrate binding in the flavonol 3-sulfotransferase. *J Biol Chem* 1995;270:30458–30463.
22. Komatsu K, Driscoll WJ, Koh Y, Strott CA. A P-loop related motif (GxxGxxK) highly conserved in sulfotransferases is required for binding the activated sulfate donor. *Biochem Biophys Res Commun* 1994;204:1178–1185.
23. Kakuta Y, Pedersen LG, Carter CW, Negishi M, Pedersen LC. Crystal structure of estrogen sulphotransferase. *Nat Struct Biol* 1997;4:904–908.
24. Otterness DM, Her C, Aksoy S, Kimura S, Wieben ED, Weinshilboum RM. Human dehydroepiandrosterone sulfotransferase gene: molecular cloning and structural characterization. *DNA Cell Biol* 1995;14:331–341.
25. Her C, Aksoy IA, Kimura S, Brandriff BF, Wasmuth JJ, Weinshilboum RM. Human estrogen sulfotransferase gene (STE): cloning, structure and chromosomal localization. *Genomics* 1995;29:16–23.
26. Aksoy IA, Weinshilboum RM. Human thermolabile phenol sulfotransferase gene (STM): molecular cloning and structural characterization. *Biochem Biophys Res Commun* 1995;208:786–795.
27. Her C, Raftogianis R, Weinshilboum RM. Human phenol sulfotransferase *STP2* gene: molecular cloning, structural characterization and chromosomal localization. *Genomics* 1996;33:409–420.
28. Raftogianis R, Her C, Weinshilboum RM. Human phenol sulfotransferase pharmacogenetics: *STP1* gene cloning and structural characterization. *Pharmacogenetics* 1996;6:473–487.
29. Otterness DM, Mohrenweiser HW, Brandriff BF, Weinshilboum RM. Dehydroepiandrosterone sulfotransferase gene (STD): localization to human chromosome 19q13.3. *Cytogenet Cell Genet* 1995;70:45–47.
30. Price RA, Cox NJ, Spielman RS, Van Loon J, Maidak BL, Weinshilboum RM. Inheritance of human platelet thermolabile phenol sulfotransferase (TL PST) activity. *Genet Epidemiol* 1988;5:1–15.
31. Price RA, Spielman RS, Lucena AL, Van Loon JA, Maidak BL,

Weinshilboum RM. Genetic polymorphism for human platelet thermostable phenol sulfotransferase (TS PST) activity. *Genetics* 1989; 122:905–914.

32. Raftogianis RB, Wood TC, Otterness DM, Van Loon JA, Weinshilboum RM. Phenol sulfotransferase pharmacogenetics in humans: association of common *SULT1A1* alleles with TS PST phenotype. *Biochem Biophys Res Commun* 1997;239:298–304.

33. Campbell NRC, Weinshilboum R. Human phenol sulfotransferase (PST): correlation of liver and platelet activities. *Can Soc Clin Invest* 1986;9(suppl):A14.

34. Young WF Jr, Laws ER Jr, Sharbrough FW, Weinshilboum RM. Human phenol sulfotransferase: correlation of brain and platelet activities. *J Neurochem* 1985;44:1131–1137.

35. Sundaram RS, Van Loon JA, Tucker R, Weinshilboum RM. Sulfation pharmacogenetics: correlation of human platelet and small intestinal phenol sulfotransferase. *Clin Pharmacol Ther* 1989;46:501–509.

36. Wood TC, Her C, Aksoy IA, Otterness DM, Weinshilboum RM. Human dehydroepiandrosterone sulfotransferase pharmacogenetics: quantitative Western analysis and gene sequence polymorphisms. *J Steroid Biochem Mol Biol* 1996;59:467–478.

37. Kiehlbauch CC, Lam YF, Ringer DP. Homodimeric and heterodimeric aryl sulfotransferases catalyze the sulfuric acid esterification of *N*-hydroxyl-2-acetylaminofluorene. *J Biol Chem* 1995;270: 18941–18947.

38. McCall JM, Aiken JW, Chidester CG, DuCharme DW, Wendling MG. Pyrimidine and triazine 3-oxide sulfates: a new family of vasodilators. *J Med Chem* 1983;26:1791–1793.

39. Rein G, Glover V, Sandler M. Multiple forms of phenolsulfotransferase in human tissues: selective inhibition by dichloronitrophenol. *Biochem Pharmacol* 1982;31:1893–1897.

40. Reiter C, Mwaluko G, Dunnette J, Van Loon J, Weinshilboum R. Thermolabile and thermostable human platelet phenol sulfotransferase: substrate specificity and physical separation. *Naunyn Schmiedebergs Arch Pharmacol* 1983;324:140–147.

41. Campbell NRC, Van Loon JA, Weinshilboum RM. Human liver phenol sulfotransferase: assay conditions, biochemical properties and partial purification of isozymes of the thermostable form. *Biochem Pharmacol* 1987;36:1435–1446.

42. Sundaram RS, Szumlanski C, Otterness D, Van Loon JA, Weinshilboum RM. Human intestinal phenol sulfotransferase: assay conditions, activity levels and partial purification of the thermolabile (TL) form. *Drug Metab Dispos* 1989;17:255–264.

43. Hart RF, Renskers KJ, Nelson EB, Roth JA. Localization and characterization of phenol sulfotransferase in human platelets. *Life Sci* 1979; 24:125–130.

44. Young WF Jr, Okazaki H, Laws ER Jr, Weinshilboum RM. Human brain phenol sulfotransferase: biochemical properties and regional localization. *J Neurochem* 1984;43:706–715.

45. Ozawa SH, Nagata K, Shimada M, Ueda M, Tsuzuki T, Yamazoe Y, Kato R. Primary structures and properties of two related forms of aryl sulfotransferase in human liver. *Pharmacogenetics* 1995;5: S135–S140.

46. Zhu X, Veronese ME, Iocco P, McManus ME. cDNA cloning and expression of a new form of human aryl sulfotransferase. *Int J Biochem Cell Biol* 1996;28:565–571.

47. Hernández JS, Watson RWG, Wood TC, Weinshilboum RM. Sulfation of estrone and 17β-estradiol in human liver: catalysis by thermostable phenol sulfotransferase and by dehydroepiandrosterone sulfotransferase. *Drug Metab Dispos* 1992;20:413–422.

48. Nagata K, Ozawa S, Miyata M, et al. Isolation and expression of a cDNA encoding a male-specific rat sulfotransferase that catalyzes activation of *N*-hydroxy-2-acetylaminofluorene. *J Biol Chem* 1993; 268:24720–24725.

49. Aksoy IA, Wood TC, Weinshilboum RM. Human liver estrogen sulfotransferase: cDNA cloning, expression and biochemical characterization. *Biochem Biophys Res Commun* 1995;200:1621–1629.

50. Otterness DM, Wieben ED, Wood TC, et al. Human liver dehydroepiandrosterone sulfotransferase: molecular cloning and expression of cDNA. *Mol Pharmacol* 1992;41:865–872.

51. Hobkirk R. Steroid sulfation. *Trends Endocrinol Metab* 1993;4:69–74.

52. Otterness DM, Weinshilboum R. Human dehydroepiandrosterone sulfotransferase: molecular cloning of cDNA and genomic DNA. *Chem Biol Interact* 1994;92:145–159.

53. Mulder GJ, Scholtens E. Phenol sulphotransferase and uridine diphosphate glucuronyltransferase from rat liver in vivo and vitro: 2,6-dichloro-4-nitrophenol as selective inhibitor of sulphation. *Biochem J* 1977;165:553–559.

54. Rens-Domiano SS, Roth JA. Inhibition of M and P phenol sulfotransferase by analogues of 3'-phosphoadenosine-5'-phosphosulfate. *J Neurochem* 1987;48:1411–1415.

55. Levy G. Sulfate conjugation in drug metabolism: role of inorganic sulfate. *Fed Proc* 1986;45:2235–2240.

56. Nomenclature Committee of the International Union of Biochemistry and Molecular Biology. *Enzyme nomenclature: recommendations of the Nomenclature Committee of the International Union of Biochemistry and Molecular Biology on the nomenclature and classification of enzymes.* Prepared for NC-IUBMB by Edwin C. Webb. New York: Academic Press, 1992.

57. Kotb M, Geller AM. Methionine adenosyltransferase: structure and function. *Pharmacol Ther* 1993;59:125–143.

58. Axelrod J, Tomchick R. Enzymatic *O*-methylation of epinephrine and other catechols. *J Biol Chem* 1958;233:702–705.

59. Vidgren J, Svensson LA, Liljas A. Crystal structure of catechol *O*-methyltransferase. *Nature* 1994;368:354–358.

60. Tenhunen J, Salminen M, Lundstrom K, Kiviluoto T, Savolainen R, Ulmanen I. Genomic organization of the human catechol-*O*-methyltransferase gene and its expression from two distinct promoters. *Eur J Biochem* 1994;223:1049–1059.

61. Lavigne JA, Helzlsouer KJ, Huang H-Y, et al. An association between the allele coding for a low activity variant of catechol *O*-methyltransferase and the risk for breast cancer. *Cancer Res* 1997;57:5493–5497.

62. LeWitt PA. New options for treatment of Parkinson's disease. *Baillieres Clin Neurol* 1997;6:109–123.

63. Weinshilboum RM, Raymond FA. Inheritance of low erythrocyte catechol-*O*-methyltransferase activity in man. *Am J Hum Genet* 1977;29: 125–135.

64. Lachman HM, Papolos DF, Saito T, Yu Y-M, Szumlanski CL, Weinshilboum RM. Human catechol *O*-methyltransferase pharmacogenetics: description of a functional polymorphism and its potential application to neuropsychiatric disorders. *Pharmacogenetics* 1996;6: 243–250.

65. Weinshilboum R. Thiol S-methyltransferases I. Biochemistry. In: Damani LA, ed. *Sulphur-containing drugs and related organic chemicals: chemistry, biochemistry and toxicology.* Vol 2, Pt A. Chichester, UK: Ellis Horwood, 1989:121–142.

66. Mozier NM, McConnell KP, Hoffman JL. *S*-Adenosyl-L-methionine: thioether *S*-methyltransferase, a new enzyme in sulfur and selenium metabolism. *J Biol Chem* 1988;263:4527–4531.

67. Weinshilboum RM, Sladek SL. Mercaptopurine pharmacogenetics: monogenic inheritance of erythrocyte thiopurine methyltransferase activity. *Am J Hum Genet* 1980;32:651–662.

68. Price RA, Keith RA, Spielman RS, Weinshilboum RM. Major gene polymorphism for human erythrocyte (RBC) thiol methyltransferase (TMT). *Genet Epidemiol* 1989;6:651–662.

69. Woodson LC, Weinshilboum RM. Human kidney thiopurine methyltransferase: purification and biochemical properties. *Biochem Pharmacol* 1983;32:819–826.

70. Woodson LC, Ames MM, Selassie CD, Hansch C, Weinshilboum RM. Thiopurine methyltransferase: aromatic thiol substrates and inhibition by benzoic acid derivatives. *Mol Pharmacol* 1983;24:471–478.

71. Lee D, Szumlanski C, Houtman J, et al. Thiopurine methyltransferase pharmacogenetics: cloning of human liver cDNA and presence of a processed pseudogene on human chromosome 18q21.1. *Drug Metab Dispos* 1995;23:398–405.

72. Lennard L, Lilleyman JS. Variable 6-mercaptopurine metabolism and treatment outcome in childhood lymphoblastic leukemia. *J Clin Oncol* 1989;7:1816–1823.

73. Lennard L, Van Loon JA, Weinshilboum RM. Pharmacogenetics of acute azathioprine toxicity: relationship to thiopurine methyltransferase genetic polymorphism. *Clin Pharmacol Ther* 1989;46:149–154.

74. Weinshilboum RM. Methylation pharmacogenetics: thiopurine methyltransferase as a model system. *Xenobiotica* 1992;22:1055–1071.

75. Lennard L, Lilleyman JS, Van Loon J, Weinshilboum RM. Genetic variation in response to 6-mercaptopurine for childhood acute lymphoblastic leukaemia. *Lancet* 1990;336:225–229.

76. Szumlanski C, Weinshilboum RM. Sulphasalazine inhibition of thiopurine methyltransferase: possible mechanism for interaction with 6-mercaptopurine and azathioprine. *Br J Clin Pharmacol* 1995;39: 456–459.

77. Lewis LD, Benin A, Szumlanski C, et al. Olsalazine and 6-mercaptopurine-related hematologic suppression: a possible drug-drug interaction. *Clin Pharmacol Ther* 1997;62:464–475.

78. Honchel R, Aksoy I, Szumlanski C, et al. Human thiopurine methyltransferase: molecular cloning and expression of T84 colon carcinoma cell cDNA. *Mol Pharmacol* 1993;43:878–887.

79. Szumlanski C, Otterness D, Her C, et al. Thiopurine methyltransferase pharmacogenetics: human gene cloning and characterization of a common polymorphism. *DNA Cell Biol* 1996;15:17–30.

80. Otterness D, Szumlanski C, Lennard L, et al. Human thiopurine methyltransferase pharmacogenetics: gene sequence polymorphisms. *Clin Pharmacol Ther* 1997;62:60–73.

81. Otterness DM, Szumlanski CL, Wood TC, Weinshilboum RM. Human thiopurine methyltransferase pharmacogenetics: kindred with a terminal exon splice junction mutation that results in loss of activity. *J Clin Invest* 1998;101:1036–1044.

82. Kalow W. Pharmacoanthropology and the genetics of drug metabolism. In: Kalow W, ed. *Pharmacogenetics of drug metabolism*. New York: Pergamon Press, 1992:865–877.

83. Glauser TA, Kerremans AL, Weinshilboum RM. Human hepatic microsomal thiol methyltransferase: assay conditions, biochemical properties and correlation studies. *Drug Metab Dispos* 1992;20:247–255.

84. Keith RA, Van Loon J, Wussow LF, Weinshilboum RM. Thiol methylation pharmacogenetics: heritability of human erythrocyte thiol methyltransferase activity. *Clin Pharmacol Ther* 1983;34:521–528.

85. Axelrod J. Purification and properties of phenylethanolamine *N*-methyltransferase. *J Biol Chem* 1962;237:1657–1660.

86. Rini J, Szumlanski C, Guerciolini R, Weinshilboum RM. Human liver nicotinamide *N*-methyltransferase: ion-pairing radiochemical assay, biochemical properties and individual variation. *Clin Chim Acta* 1989;186:359–374.

87. Aksoy S, Szumlanski CL, Weinshilboum RM. Human liver nicotinamide *N*-methyltransferase: cDNA cloning, expression and biochemical characterization. *J Biol Chem* 1994;265:14835–14840.

88. Yan L, Otterness DM, Craddock TL, Weinshilboum RM. Mouse liver nicotinamide *N*-methyltransferase: cDNA cloning, expression and nucleotide sequence polymorphisms. *Biochem Pharmacol* 1997;54:1139–1149.

89. Yan L, Otterness DM, Kozak CA, Weinshilboum RM. Mouse nicotinamide *N*-methyltransferase gene: molecular cloning, structural characterization and chromosomal localization. *DNA Cell Biol* 1998;17:659–667.

90. Scheller T, Orgacka H Szumlanski CL, Weinshilboum RM. Mouse liver nicotinamide *N*-methyltransferase pharmacogenetics: biochemical properties and variation in activity among inbred strains. *Pharmacogenetics* 1996;6:43–53.

91. Dale HH, Laidlaw PP. The physiological action of β-iminazolyethylamine. *J Physiol* 1910;41:318–344.

92. Schwartz JC. Histaminergic mechanisms in brain. *Annu Rev Pharmacol Toxicol* 1977;17:325–339.

93. Brown DD, Axelrod J, Tomchick R. Enzymatic *N*-methylation of histamine. *Nature* 1959;183:680.

94. Scott MC, Van Loon JA, Weinshilboum RM. Pharmacogenetics of *N*-methylation: heritability of human erythrocyte histamine *N*-methyltransferase activity. *Clin Pharmacol Ther* 1988;43:256–262.

95. Price RA, Scott MC, Weinshilboum RM. Genetic segregation analysis of red blood cell (RBC) histamine *N*-methyltransferase (HNMT) activity. *Genet Epidemiol* 1993;10:123–131.

96. Girard B, Otterness DM, Wood TC, Honchel R, Wieben ED, Weinshilboum RM. Human histamine *N*-methyltransferase pharmacogenetics: cloning and expression of kidney cDNA. *Mol Pharmacol* 1994;45:461–468.

97. Aksoy S, Raftogianis R, Weinshilboum R. Human histamine *N*-methyltransferase gene: structural characterization and chromosomal localization. *Biochem Biophys Res Commun* 1996;219:548–554.

98. Preuss CV, Wood TC, Szumlanski CL, et al. Human histamine *N*-methyltransferase pharmacogenetics: common genetic polymorphisms that alter activity. *Mol Pharmacol* 1998;53:708–717.

99. Lewis AJ, Kelly MM, Walle UK, Eaton EA, Falany CN, Walle T. Improved bacterial expression of the human P form phenolsulfotransferase. *Drug Metab Dispos* 1996;24:1180–1185.

100. Veronese ME, Burgess W, Zhu X, McManus ME. Functional characterization of two human sulphotransferase cDNAs that encode monoamine- and phenol-sulphating forms of phenol sulphotransferase: substrate kinetics, thermal-stability and inhibitor-sensitivity studies. *Biochem J* 1994;302:497–502.

101. Wood TC, Aksoy IA, Aksoy S, Weinshilboum RM. Human liver thermolabile phenol sulfotransferase: cDNA cloning, expression and characterization. *Biochem Biophys Res Commun* 1994;198:1119–1127.

102. Falany CN, Krasnykh V, Falany JL. Bacterial expression and characterization of a cDNA for human liver estrogen sulfotransferase. *J Steroid Biochem Mol Biol* 1995;52:529–539.

103. Falany CN, Wheeler J, Falany JL. Steroid sulfation by expressed human cytosolic sulfotransferases. *J Steroid Biochem Mol Biol* 1994;48:369–375.

104. Jones AL, Hagen M, Coughtrie MWH, Roberts RC, Glatt H. Human platelet phenolsulfotransferase: cDNA cloning, stable expression in V79 cells and identification of a novel allelic variant of the phenolsulfating form. *Biochem Biophys Res Commun* 1995;208:855–862.

105. Aksoy S, Brandriff BF, Ward V, Little PFR, Weinshilboum RM. Human nicotinamide *N*-methyltransferase gene: molecular cloning, structural characterization, and chromosomal localization. *Genomics* 1995;29:555–561.

106. Reiter C, Weinshilboum RM. Acetaminophen and phenol: substrates for both a thermostable and a thermolabile form of human platelet phenol sulfotransferase. *J Pharmacol Exp Ther* 1982;221:43–51.

107. Kudlacek P, Clemens DL, Halgard CM, Anderson RJ. Characterization of recombinant human liver dehydroepiandrosterone sulfotransferase with minoxidil as the substrate. *Biochem Pharmacol* 1997;53:215–221.

108. Kudlacek P, Clemens DL, Anderson RJ. Characterization of recombinant human liver estrogen sulfotransferase (EST) with minoxidil as the substrate. *ISSX Proc* 1997;12:191.

CHAPTER 16

Epoxide Hydrolases

Curtis J. Omiecinski

OVERVIEW

Epoxide derivates are often chemically reactive species and unstable in aqueous environments. Epoxide intermediates are frequently generated *in situ* through oxidative metabolic processes. These intermediates may function as critical initiators of cellular damage, damage that includes protein and RNA adduction with the epoxide as well as genetic mutation (1-2) In this context, epoxide metabolites have been identified as ultimate carcinogenic reaction products (1-4). The epoxide hydrolases (EHs; EC3.3.2.3) are a family of enzymes that function to hydrate simple epoxides to vicinal diols and arene oxides to *trans*-dihydrodiols. These enzymes represent one category of the broader group of hydrolytic enzymes, which include esterases, proteases, dehalogenases, and lipases (5). The epoxide hydrolases, in particular, the microsomal form of the hydrolase, have been associated historically with the metabolism of xenobiotic chemicals, including pharmaceuticals. Xenobiotic metabolism results principally in detoxication. However, in certain instances, bioactivated and highly toxic intermediates are generated in the metabolic process. In this context, microsomal EH has been implicated in both detoxication and bioactivation reactions. The bioactivation role of the microsomal enzyme is perhaps most clearly illustrated in the metabolism of the procarcinogenic polyaromatic hydrocarbons to highly reactive and mutagenic bay region diol-epoxides (1,6). Although exposure to xenobiotic epoxides can occur directly, for example, to styrene oxide (7), many epoxide substrates are generated *in situ* by the cytochrome P450 monooxygenases (8,9) and other oxidative enzymes in mammalian cells (10). The soluble form of EH also participates in xenobiotic metabolism, with a preference for *trans*-substituted epoxides such as *trans*-stilbene oxide (8,9).

Several forms of EH are now recognized for their roles in the metabolism of endogenous substances, for example, epoxides of steroids and arachidonic acid derivatives (11,12) and leukotrienes (13). Structural and regulatory information on the various EH family members is accumulating at a rapid rate. These data include primary sequences of the respective EH genes and proteins, and identification of genetic polymorphism for certain family members (5,14). Although not so expansive in number or nomenclature as the P450s, glutathione S-transferases, uridine diphosphate (UDP)-glucuronosyl transferases, or sulfotransferases, the EHs are nevertheless very important enzymes that direct biotransformation processes for a wide variety of substances.

CLASSES OF EPOXIDE HYDROLASE

Five classes of mammalian EH have been characterized. These include (a) a microsomal enzyme exhibiting a specific substrate preference for cholesterol 5,6-oxide (15); (b) a membrane-associated hepoxilin A_3 hydrolase (16); (c) a leukotriene A_4 hydrolase (17); and two xenobiotic-metabolizing enzymes; (d) a soluble form (18); and (e) the microsomal EH (19). The foregoing classes of EH are immunologically and structurally distinct (5). An overview for each of the first four classes of EH is provided below, followed with a more detailed review on the xenobiotic metabolizing microsomal EH.

Cholesterol Oxide Hydrolase

Molecular Biology/Regulation

This microsomal enzyme exhibits a specific substrate preference for cholesterol epoxides. The gene or cDNA encoding this enzyme has not been cloned. Therefore primary sequence data or detailed attributes of the corresponding protein are not available. Cholesterol oxide

C. J. Omiecinski: Department of Environmental Health, University of Washington, 4225 Roosevelt Way NE, Seattle, Washington 98105-6099

hydrolase is distinct from oxidosqualene cyclase (20). The oxidation of cholesterol occurs during the lipid peroxidation process in membranes. Several oxidized products characteristic of a free-radical mechanism are formed and may serve as indicators of the nature and extent of cholesterol oxidation and lipid peroxidation in general. Common products of lipid peroxide–dependent propagation reactions are the enantiomeric 5,6-epoxides and 7-ketocholestanol (15). Conversion of cholesterol epoxides to cholestane triol may occur in cells possessing cholesterol epoxide hydrolase (15). In general, the cholesterol oxidation products possess significant cytotoxicity, in part because of effects on the plasma membrane, resulting in increases in intracellular calcium. The cholesterol epoxides also are weakly mutagenic, although the mechanism accounting for the mutagenicity is unclear. This property is in contrast to other lipid epoxides normally encountered in tissues, chiefly fatty acid epoxides, which do not appear to be mutagenic and are less toxic than the oxysterols (21). The cholesterol EH is inducible in rodent tissues by phenoxyacetate hypolipidic drugs such as clofibrate and ciprofibrate (22). Among tissues studied for cholesterol EH activity (i.e., liver, kidney, lung, testis, spleen, brain, and intestinal epithelium), the highest levels were detected in liver microsomes, in which the activities were at least five-fold greater than in other microsomal preparations (23).

Substrates and Products

Cholestane 3β, 5α, 6β-triol has been identified as the exclusive product formed on hydration of cholesterol 5,6α- and 5,6β-oxide catalyzed by cholesterol oxide hydrolase in liver microsomes obtained from five mammalian species (20). Both acid- and base-catalyzed hydrolysis of these two epoxides produce this product, apparently due to preference for pseudo-axial opening of the oxirane ring to form product with a *trans*-AB ring junction. Although the β-oxide is more reactive than the α-oxide on acid-catalyzed hydration, the α-oxide is a 4.5-fold better substrate than the β-oxide, as indicated by values of V_{max}/K_m (24). Several imino compounds are competitive inhibitors for the enzyme from rat liver, the most effective being 5,6α-iminocholestanol (K_i, 0.085 μM) (24). Inhibition by the aziridines is consistent with the participation of acid catalysis mechanism of enzymatic action (20). The cholesterol EH does not share a similar mechanism of reaction with the microsomal and soluble EHs and is not likely to be structurally related to these latter forms (25).

Hepoxilin A₃ Hydrolase

Molecular Biology/Regulation

Hepoxilin A₃ hydrolase (HA3H) is a cytosolic enzyme participating in arachidonic acid metabolism in the cen-

tral nervous system and in vascular cells, although the enzyme is expressed in many different cell types (16). The gene encoding HA3H has not been characterized, but the protein has been purified and possesses a molecular mass value of 53 kDa (16). The M_r, pI, and substrate specificity of HA3H indicate that this enzyme is distinct from leukotriene A₄ hydrolase (16). The biologic effects of the hepoxilins appear to include changes in intracellular concentrations of ions such as calcium and potassium ions as well as changes in second-messenger systems. Available experimental evidence suggests that the biologic actions of the hepoxilins are receptor mediated because the existence of hepoxilin-specific binding proteins in human neutrophils has been detected (26). These data further implicate the association of G proteins in hepoxilin-binding together with hepoxilin action (26). Other investigators have reported that plasma volume expansion triggers the formation and release of hepoxilin A₃ from intact human platelets, indicating that hepoxilin plays a role in blood-volume regulation (27). Details of hepoxilin biosynthesis have been reviewed recently (28).

Substrates and Products

The purified protein uses hepoxilin A₃ (8-hydroxy-11,12-epoxyeicosa-(5Z,9E,14Z)-trienoic acid) as preferred substrate, converting it to trioxilin A₃. The enzyme is only marginally active toward other epoxides such as leukotriene A₄ and styrene oxide (16). Incubation of (8R)- and (8S)-[1-¹⁴C]hepoxilin A₃ and glutathione with homogenates of rat brain hippocampus results in products that were identified as the (8R) and (8S) diastereomers of 11-glutathionyl hepoxilin A₃ (29). Evidence exists for the function of these products as neuromodulators (29). Results of activity assays have demonstrated that the pineal gland possesses HA3H, which hydrolyzed hepoxilin A₃ to trioxilin A₃ (30). The hydrolysis was inhibited by 1 μM 3,3,3-trichloropropene-1,2-oxide and resulted in decreased production of cyclic adenosine monophosphate (AMP) in cultured organ rat pineals after stimulation with 5'-N-ethylcarboxamidoadenosine, an α_1/α_2 adenosine receptor agonist (30). This latter effect was stereospecific because the (8S)-enantiomer was much more active in decreasing cyclic AMP production than was the (8R)-enantiomer (30).

Leukotriene A₄ Hydrolase

Molecular Biology/Regulation

Leukotrienes are products of arachidonic acid metabolism derived through the action of the 5-lipoxygenase enzyme pathway. The leukotriene A₄ (LTA4) hydrolase is a bifunctional Zn^{2+}-containing enzyme exhibiting aminopeptidase activity with the ability to convert LTA4 to LTB4, a proinflammatory mediator (13). LTA4 is a cytosolic enzyme expressed in many human tissues, including endothelial cells, neutrophils, erythrocytes, lung, liver, and keratinocytes (17,31–33). The human enzyme has been purified and exhibits an apparent molecular mass of approximately 54 kDa, an isoelectric point of 4.9, an apparent K_m of from 7 to 36 μM for enzymatic hydration of leukotriene A$_4$, and a pH optimum ranging from 7 to 8 (31). The human gene structure for LTA4 hydrolase has been characterized. The gene is more than 35 kbp and contains 19 exons (34). The essential zinc-binding histidine residues and glutamate residue, delineating the zinc-binding domain required for both enzyme activities of LTA4 hydrolase, are located in exons 10 and 11 (34). The human LTA4 hydrolase gene was localized to chromosome 12q22 and is a single-copy gene (34). No genetic polymorphisms have yet been reported at this locus, although evidence for alternative mRNA splicing for the LTA4 hydrolase has been presented (35). The available gene-sequence data are not supportive of an evolutionary relationship between the LTA4 hydrolase and the microsomal or soluble hydrolases (5).

LTA4 hydrolase is regulated by phosphorylation status. LTA4 hydrolase is phosphorylated at serine 415 under basal conditions in human endothelial cells and, in the phosphorylated state, does not exhibit LTA4 to LTB4 epoxide hydrolase activity (32). LTA4 hydrolase purified from endothelial cells is efficiently dephosphorylated by incubation with protein phosphatase-1 in the presence of an LTA4 hydrolase peptide substrate but not in the absence of substrate. Under conditions that lead to dephosphorylation, protein phosphatase-1 activates the EH activity of the LTA4 enzyme (32).

Substrates and Products

From sequence comparisons with aminopeptidases, a tyrosine at position 383 in LTA4 hydrolase was suggested as a possible catalytic amino acid, where it may act as a proton donor in a general base mechanism (36). However, the available data do not support a similar involvement for this position in the hydrolysis of LTA4 into LTB4 (36). Other results, from using the model substrate, alanine-4-nitroanilide, indicate that under physiologic conditions, chloride ions may selectively stimulate the peptidase activity of LTA4 hydrolase (37). In contrast to these effects on the peptidase activity, no chloride stimulation is detected for LTA4 hydrolase activity of the enzyme (37). Recent studies have indicated that LTB4 is of significance in the pathogenesis of psoriasis, and efforts are under way to develop potent LTA4 hydrolase inhibitors for treatment of this syndrome (38). A systematic study on the enzyme specificity and the inhibition of its amidase activity with more than 30 synthetic inhibitors has led to the development of an α-keto-β-amino ester and a thioamine as tight-binding, competitive-type transition-state analog inhibitors of the aminopeptidase activity, with K_i values of 46 and 18 nM, respectively (39). Both

compounds also inhibit the epoxide hydrolase activity, with the median inhibitory concentration (IC$_{50}$) values of 1 μM and 0.1 μM for these reagents, respectively (39). The design and synthesis of a number of potent β-amino hydroxylamine and amino hydroxamic acid inhibitors of the aminopeptidase and hydrolase activities of the enzyme also have been described (40).

Soluble Epoxide Hydrolase

Molecular Biology/Regulation

The xenobiotic-metabolizing soluble, or cytosolic, form of EH metabolizes various *trans*-epoxides, such as *trans*-stilbene oxide, as well as several endogenous arachidonate and prostaglandin-derived epoxide intermediates (41). The purified mammalian proteins exhibit an apparent molecular mass of approximately 62 kDa and contain an apparently imperfect peroxisomal targeting signal of Ser-Lys-Met at the carboxy terminus (18,42,43). The enzyme appears to be expressed in all tissues and is distributed preferentially in the cytosolic compartment of the cell, but also is localized to the peroxisomes (44,45). Sequences for the human, rat, mouse, and potato soluble EH cDNAs or genes have been published (18,46–49). The human gene consists of 19 exons and encompasses approximately 45 kb (49). By sequence analysis, soluble EH and microsomal EH are marginally related (19% to 25% sequence identities) to each other and to a bacterial haloacid dehalogenase (5). The soluble EH gene has been localized to the human chromosomal region 8p21-p12 (50).

Preliminary data for genetic polymorphism for the human form of the enzyme has been presented recently (51), although characterization details have not yet been published. In past investigations, researchers have attempted to determine whether genetic mechanisms account for the rather large (11-fold) variation in soluble EH activity observed in unstimulated lymphocytes from normal human subjects (52). Soluble EH activity was measured in monozygotic (MZ) twins, dizygotic (DZ) twins, families, and 100 unrelated male subjects. The twin and family studies indicated predominantly genetic control of soluble EH expression, consistent with either monogenic or polygenic control mechanisms (52).

The soluble form of EH is inducible in several tissues of rodent species by pretreatment with peroxisomal proliferator agents, such as 2,4-dichlorophenoxyacetic acid and Wyeth 14.643, and hypolipidemic drugs, such as clofibrate (53–57). These changes appear to parallel the induction of peroxisomal β-oxidation activity in affected tissues (58,59). The molecular mechanisms responsible for the genetic induction of soluble EH have not been elucidated but are likely to involve upregulation through the peroxisome proliferator-activated receptor α pathway.

Substrates and Products

The substrate specificity of the soluble EH is distinct from that of the other EH forms. Classically, microsomal and cytosolic epoxide hydrolase are distinguished through differences in substrate specificity; for example, styrene-7,8-oxide, benzo(a)pyrene 4,5-oxide, and *cis*-stilbene oxide are preferentially hydrolyzed by the microsomal EH, whereas *trans*-stilbene oxide is the preferred substrate for soluble EH (53). More recently, a series of specific soluble EH substrates have been developed. These include epoxy esters or carbonate-derivatives that cyclize spontaneously during hydrolysis of the epoxide moiety, releasing an alcohol that can be assayed directly or by coupling to a second reaction (60). The resulting alcohol, or its secondary reaction products, can be selected to give an absorption in the visible or near-UV range of the spectrum. This allows the synthesis of a variety of useful spectrophotometric substrates specific for soluble EH, for example, 4-nitrophenyl (2*S*,3*S*)-2,3-epoxy-3-phenylpropyl carbonate (60). Additionally, sensitive radiometric substrates specific for the soluble enzyme have been developed, including [^{14}C]*cis*-9,10-epoxystearic acid and [2-^{3}H]*trans*-1,3-diphenyl-propene oxide, which are hydrolyzed at rates substantially higher than those of *trans*-stilbene oxide (61). Catalytically, experimental results implicate the involvement of aspartic acid-333 and histidine-523 of the soluble EH in a catalytic mechanism similar to that of other α/β hydrolase fold enzymes, including the bacterial haloalkane dehalogenases (62,63). Chalcone oxides have been tested and characterized as potent inhibitors of the soluble EH enzyme (64).

A large number of studies have demonstrated that various diepoxy fatty methylesters and endogenous arachidonate epoxides (epoxyeicosatrienoic acids) are substrates of the soluble EH (11,12,65). These observations argue for an important role of this enzyme in endogenous metabolism of fatty acid and membrane lipid-derived epoxides. A provocative study by Hammock et al. (66) demonstrated that leukotoxin, a linoleic acic oxide produced by leukocytes that has been associated with the multiple organ failure and adult respiratory distress syndrome seen in some severe burn patients, can be bioactivated by soluble EH to diol products. These products are apparently the ultimate cytotoxic derivatives of the parent compound because the diol metabolite of leukotoxin is toxic to pulmonary alveolar epithelial cells (66).

Microsomal Epoxide Hydrolase

Molecular Biology/Regulation

The microsomal form of the enzyme (mEH) was the initial member of the EH family characterized. Microsomal EH catalyzes the *trans*-addition of water to a broad range of epoxides and arene oxides, including oxides of the carcinogenic polycyclic aromatic hydrocarbons (3,67). In concert with the cytochrome P450s, mEH has been implicated in generating highly reactive diol-epoxides (67). Thus in certain instances, mEH is involved in bioactivation processes. However, mEH also plays a pivotal role in the deactivation of epoxide intermediates, such that in most scenarios, mEH catalysis is considered a detoxifying event (3,67,68). Consequently, mEH is widely recognized for its important role in drug and foreign-compound biotransformation. Although epoxide derivatives of certain steroids (e.g., estroxide) have been identified as endogenous substrates of microsomal EH (69–71), another potential biologic function of microsomal EH is that of a sodium-dependent bile acid transporter (72). However, the precise nature of mEH to endogenous metabolism, transport, or cellular homeostasis is not well elucidated.

Primary coding sequence data for mEH are available for several mammalian species (5,19,73). The mEH protein comprises 455 amino acids, exhibits an apparent molecular mass of approximately 49 kDa, and is highly conserved (5,73). The enzyme appears to be expressed in all tissues and cell types (3,74). The enzyme's mechanism of action likely proceeds through a generalized base pathway favoring nucleophilic attack of water (75,76), involving a histidine-431 as part of a catalytic triad together with aspartic acid-226 and glutamic acid-404 residue at or near the active site (77).

Gene Structure

Results obtained from Southern hybridization, cloning, and sequencing experiments have demonstrated that human mEH exists as a single gene in the haploid genome (19,78). Thus in contrast to the complexities of the cytochrome P450 and glutathione S-transferase gene families, mEH presents itself as a very tractable system for assessment of individual gene variation. The coding region of the human mEH gene [also termed HYL1 (5)] is contained within approximately 20 kb and comprises nine exons, with exon 1 being noncoding (14,78). A high concentration of repetitive *Alu* elements exists within four introns of the human mEH gene, together with an approximately 200-bp inverted repetitive unit in the 5′-flanking region (78). The biologic implications, if any, of these repetitive regions are presently unknown. The gene for human mEH has been mapped with *in situ* hybridization to chromosome 1q42.1 (79).

Genetic Polymorphism

With the characterization of the human gene and cDNA structures for mEH, the existence of genetic polymorphism for the enzyme has been established (14,78,80). Two genetic polymorphisms have been characterized in the gene's coding region. One polymorphism exists within exon 3 and results in either a His or a Tyr substitution in amino acid position 113; another polymorphism occurs in exon 4, resulting in either a His or an Arg substitution at amino acid position 139 (14,80). Tyr is the predominant amino acid at the 113 position in white populations, with His more common at the 139 position (14). The allelic distributions exist in Hardy–Weinberg equilibrium. The individual haplotypes have been expressed *in vitro* from cDNA constructs and assayed for mEH activity, by using benzo(a)pyrene-4,5-oxide as substrate. The resulting activities ranged approximately two-fold when values were normalized to either total cellular S9 protein, or cellular EH RNA content. In this comparison the Tyr[113]/Arg[139] construct exhibited the highest overall activity, whereas the His[113]/His[139] allele exhibited the lowest (14). However, specific activities, expressed as enzymatic activities per unit mEH protein, also were measured in this study, and these activities differed only marginally (14). These observations, together with results obtained by examining the half-lives of the respective variant proteins, indicate that altered protein stability may contribute to the altered levels of allelic expression (81). Evidence indicating the contribution of posttranscriptional regulatory control of mEH expression has been provided in several other studies (14,82,83). In addition to the coding region polymorphisms, seven additional 5'-region noncoding polymorphisms also have been identified, with certain of these moderately affecting transcriptional activity of the mEH gene (84).

Genetics of Disease Susceptibility

Although the function of mEH is primarily one of detoxication of xenobiotic epoxides, its participation in the bioactivation of carcinogenic polyaromatic hydrocarbons has been well characterized (67). Results from several investigations have indicated a potential association of mEH genotype and altered disease susceptibility. Several studies have examined the relationship between cancer susceptibility and EH genotype. McGlynn et al. (85) examined a Chinese population and reported that individuals with at least one His[113] allele exhibited a 3.3-fold increased risk of developing hepatocellular carcinoma, when considered independent of glutathione transferase M1 genotype or hepatitis B virus exposure. Individuals with both viral infection and the high-risk EH genotype exhibited greater than 77 times the risk of disease compared with individuals with neither factor (85). A 3.8-fold odds ratio [95% confidence interval (CI), 1.8–8.0] was reported for increased risk of colon cancer in individuals with a His[113] genotype (86). In contrast to these findings, a study by Lancaster et al. (87) concluded that an increased risk for ovarian cancer was associated with the Tyr[113] EH allele, with an associated odds ratio of 2.6 (95% CI, 1.3–5.0). Another investigation examined bladder cancer relative risk and concluded that mEH allelic

status was not associated with disease incidence (88). Most recently, a report in *Lancet* concluded that individuals homozygous for mEH His[113] exhibited increased likelihood of pulmonary disorders with odds ratios of 4.1 (95% CI, 1.8–9.7) for chronic obstructive pulmonary disease and 5.0 (95% CI, 2.3–10.9) for emphysema (89). Additional studies examining potential relationships between EH allelic status and risk of disease development will be required to evaluate these associations definitively, with an emphasis toward large, well-controlled epidemiologic investigations and combined analyses with other potential risk determinants. The contribution of altered microsomal EH, cytochrome P450, glutathione S-transferase, and *N*-acetyltransferase genetic polymorphism to alteration in disease incidence has been reviewed recently (90).

Developmental Regulation

Microsomal EH gene expression in humans and rodents appears developmentally regulated (82,91,92). Of the human fetal tissues surveyed, the liver and adrenal glands exhibited the highest levels of detectable mEH RNA, followed by the lung and kidney (82,91,92). In fetal hepatic tissues, both enzymatic levels and immunodetectable protein levels of mEH were strongly correlated with increasing gestational age (82). However, mEH enzymatic activity in the fetal lung did not exhibit similar concordance nor did measured RNA levels appear to correlate with enzymatic activity levels in fetal or adult tissue samples (82). Low levels of mEH functional activity in early-stage fetal liver tissues may represent a risk factor contributing to developmental abnormalities consequent to toxicant exposures; however, additional studies will be required more thoroughly to investigate specific relationships.

Enzyme Induction

A review of the effects of chemical inducers on mEH expression presents a mixed picture. *In vivo* studies in animals exposed to prototypic inducers such as phenobarbital, 2(3)-tert-butyl-4-hydroxyanisole (BHA), β-naphthoflavone, or polyaromatic hydrocarbons demonstrated modest increases in mEH expression relative to control values, and did not exceed 6.5-fold induction (93,94). However, *in vivo* exposures to imidazole compounds such as ketoconazole and miconazole in rats have been reported to induce mEH approximately 10-fold (95). In recent studies using cultured primary human hepatocytes from seven different donors, only relatively small alterations in mEH mRNA or protein levels were detected, with the maximal increase detected at 3.5-fold after Arochlor 1254 exposure (96). No induction of human mEH was noted with exposures to imidazole compounds in these experiments, despite marked induction responses achieved with prototypic agents for various cytochrome P450 genes (96). In human population studies in which blood lymphocyte mEH activities were examined within the same subjects several months apart, a relatively stable profile of intraindividual activity was noted (74). Although the data available are limited regarding human mEH induction parameters, it appears that the human gene is not modulated to any major extent by chemical exposures. An interesting mode of regulation for human microsomal EH has been suggested by a recent report from Gaedigk et al. (97), demonstrating the use of tissue-specific alternative promoters and RNA splicing events for this gene. Details of these molecular controls must be further explored.

Substrates and Products

Microsomal EH exhibits broad substrate specificity. An endogenous role for the enzyme has been postulated for metabolism of androstene oxide and estroxide (98). However, its major function has been related to the hydrolysis of epoxides derived from xenobiotics, resulting in the formation of dihydrodiol products. The bay-region diol epoxide derivatives of the ubiquitous polyaromatic hydrocarbons have been implicated as ultimate mutagenic and carcinogenic products of microsomal enzyme metabolism (67). It is noteworthy that the bay-region diol epoxides are resistant to hydrolytic inactivation by mEH, yet this enzyme is required for their bioactivation (1). Historically, diagnostic substrates of the enzyme have included epoxide derivatives of the polyaromatic hydrocarbons [e.g., benzo(a)pyrene 4,5-oxide (74,99)]. In addition, many other substrate probes for mEH have been detailed and are used routinely in experimental assays. Perhaps most notable in this regard are styrene oxide (7,75,100,101) and cis-stilbene oxide (53,70,102). Other xenobiotic epoxide substrates that have been characterized include epoxide derivatives of 1,3-butadiene (103,104), benzene (105,106), aflatoxin B_1 (107), carbamazepine (108,109), chrysene (110), 1-nitropyrene (111), naphthalene and anthracene (112), and several additional polyaromatic hydrocarbon epoxides (113). The epoxide substrates of mEH are normally quite specific, exhibiting only minimal or no cross-reactivity with purified enzymes from the other classes of EH (62,102). 1,1,1-Trichloropropene oxide and cyclohexene oxide have been used as an effective in vitro inhibitors of the enzyme (70,114).

Individual Variation

Population variation in mEH activity may be an important determinant of drug or xenobiotic toxicity. Estimates of activity variation in the human population vary, and range up to 63-fold (74,109,115). Recent studies performed on transplant-quality liver tissues from 40 indi-

viduals, by using benzo(a)pyrene 4,5-oxide as substrate, indicated a range of approximately eight-fold both for activity and for immunodetectable level of protein in this population (83). Other investigators have investigated mEH enzyme kinetics comparatively in six different species, including humans (108). In this study, activity was measured by using the substrates, cis-stilbene oxide, carbamazepine 10,11-epoxide, and naphthalene 1,2-epoxide. Marked substrate-dependent species variation in enzyme activity was reported, with cis-stilbene oxide being rapidly hydrolyzed by microsomes from all species, in the rank order, human > rabbit > dog > rat > hamster > mouse (108). In contrast, hydrolysis of carbamazepine 10,11-epoxide was observed only in the human samples. Activity variation in humans ranged from two- to seven-fold, depending on the substrate probes used (108). In the latter study, and the report by Hassett et al. (83), correlation of activity and genotype for the amino acid 113 or 139 coding positions was not clearly identified. However, these analyses are complicated because of heterozygosity of many of the individuals in the study, and by evidence suggesting that 5' gene regulatory region polymorphisms may affect expression of mEH (84).

Anticonvulsant Agents and Developmental Abnormalities

Microsomal EH likely plays an important role in the disposition of several anticonvulsant medications. Antiepileptic agents such as phenobarbital, phenytoin, and carbamazepine are oxidatively metabolized through the cytochrome P450 monooxygenase system to epoxide intermediates that have been implicated in teratogenic events and other developmental abnormalities in offspring whose mothers were treated with these agents while pregnant (116–120). Because the epoxide metabolites of these drugs are substrates for mEH, it appears logical to implicate EH enzymatic status as a potential risk factor for the drug-induced developmental syndromes. Attempts to identify at-risk fetuses prenatally on the basis of low or deficient EH activity have met with only limited success (117,118). Genetic studies assessing mEH allelic status as a prognosticator of developmental outcome in women treated with anticonvulsant medications have not been conducted. The potential relationships are likely to be confounded by polymorphism at cytochrome P450 gene loci as well as the interactive potential of combination anticonvulsant drug strategies on mEH activity (90,121,122).

Hypersensitivity Reactions

The aromatic anticonvulsant agents (e.g., phenytoin, phenobarbital, and carbamazepine) also are associated with a hypersensitivity syndrome that manifests with fever, rash, lymphadenopathy, and hepatitis as potential outcomes (123). The mechanism of these reactions is poorly understood, but evidence from *in vitro* lymphocyte toxicity tests and enzyme-inhibitor studies suggested that an inherited defect in mEH function may be responsible for the enhanced drug toxicity observed in affected individuals (124). However, Green et al. (125) studied 10 carbamazepine-hypersensitive patients and 10 healthy volunteers but found no association of mEH coding regions genotype and disease incidence. Twenty-six subjects with a history of hypersensitivity reactions to carbamazepine were studied for mEH genetic determinants by Gaedigk et al. (80), and no associations with disease incidence could be determined. Circulating cytochrome P450 autoantibodies have been detected in patients exhibiting the idiosyncratic hypersensitivity response, thus implicating an immunologic disease mechanism (126).

Drug–Drug Interactions

Valpromide and valproic acid represent a class of branched-chain fatty acid–like antiepileptic compounds that are effective against both generalized and partial epilepsies, and therefore are considered broad-spectrum anticonvulsants (127). On the basis of drug interactions with carbamazepine 10,11-epoxide, it has been hypothesized that these agents are inhibitors of mEH (128). Therapeutic concentrations of valproic acid (less than 1 mM) and valpromide (less than 10 μM) were found to inhibit hydrolysis of carbamazepine 10,11-epoxide and styrene oxide in human liver microsomes and in preparations of purified human liver microsomal epoxide hydrolase, with valpromide being approximately 100 times more potent than valproic acid (122). After administration of carbamazepine epoxide to volunteers, the transdihydrodiol formation clearance was decreased 20% by valproic acid (blood concentration, approximately 113 μM) and 67% by valpromide (blood concentration, less than 10 μM), correlating well with *in vitro* measures (122). These drugs were the first shown to inhibit mEH at therapeutic concentrations (122,127).

Another antiepileptic compound, progabide, was investigated as a potential inhibitor of mEH after reports of elevated levels of carbamazepine 10,11-epoxide subsequent to coadministration of progabide and carbamazepine to patients with epilepsy. The formation and clearance of carbamazepine transdihydrodiol after administration of carbamazepine 10,11-epoxide to healthy volunteers was decreased 26% by progabide (121). Therapeutic concentrations of progabide also inhibited styrene oxide hydrolysis in human liver microsomes and with purified human liver mEH preparations (121). The excellent agreement between the *in vivo* and *in vitro* inhibitory potencies of progabide suggested that potential inhibitors of this important detoxification enzyme can be predicted *in vitro* (121).

Interactions between carbamazepine and loxapine, an antipsychotic agent, have been investigated. Plasma car-

bamazepine and carbamazepine 10,11-epoxide concentrations were prospectively monitored in a single patient during and after discontinuation of loxapine comedication (129). Additionally, four patients who had received concomitant therapy with these agents were assessed retrospectively (129). Individuals receiving concomitant loxapine–carbamazepine therapy all had unusually elevated carbamazepine epoxide/carbamazepine plasma concentration ratios, suggesting an interaction between these two compounds *in vivo*, likely due to the inhibition of mEH by loxapine (129).

In another study, six patients stabilized with carbamazepine therapy received an 8-day "add-on" supplement of valnoctamide, a tranquilizer that exhibits anticonvulsant activity in animal models and is available over the counter (OTC) in several European countries (130). During valnoctamide intake, serum levels of the carbamazepine 10,11-epoxide metabolite increased approximately five-fold in these individuals (130). In four of the patients, the increase in serum carbamazepine 10,11-epoxide levels was associated with clinical signs of carbamazepine intoxication, and carbamazepine 10,11-epoxide levels returned to baseline after valnoctamide therapy was discontinued (130). This interaction appears similar to that described for patients treated with carbamazepine and valpromide combinations, thus implicating valnoctamide-based inhibition of mEH.

SUMMARY AND CONCLUSIONS

The EH proteins represent an interesting and important group of biotransformation enzymes. Five classes of EH enzyme have been described, and the diversity of substrates metabolized by these proteins is quite large, encompassing many xenobiotic and endogenous epoxide derivatives. Regulatory schemes, genetic features, and clinical ramifications of these systems are only beginning to be investigated. The distinctive functional properties and regulatory schemes controlling expression of these genes will continue to attract the attention of researchers and clinicians for many years to come.

REFERENCES

1. Sayer JM, Yagi H, van Bladeren PJ, Levin W, Jerina DM. Stereoselectivity of microsomal epoxide hydrolase toward diol epoxides and tetrahydroepoxides derived from benz[a]anthracene. *J Biol Chem* 1985;260:1630–1640.
2. Adams JD Jr, Yagi H, Levin W, Jerina DM. Stereo-selectivity and regio-selectivity in the metabolism of 7,8-dihydrobenzo[a]pyrene by cytochrome P450, epoxide hydrolase and hepatic microsomes from 3-methylcholanthrene-treated rats. *Chem Biol Interact* 1995;95:57–77.
3. Guengerich FP. Epoxide hydrolase: properties and metabolic roles. *Rev Biochem Toxicol* 1982;4:5–30.
4. Thakker DR, Levin W, Yagi H, et al. Stereoselective metabolism of the (+)-(S,S)- and (−)-(R,R)- enantiomers of trans-3,4-dihydroxy-3,4-dihydrobenzo[c]-phenanthrene by rat and mouse liver microsomes and by a purified and reconstituted cytochrome P-450 system. *J Biol Chem* 1986;261:5404–5413.
5. Beetham JK, Grant D, Arand M, et al. Gene evolution of epoxide

hydrolases and recommended nomenclature. *DNA Cell Biol* 1995;14:61–71.

6. Wood AW, Chang RL, Levin W, et al. Bacterial and mammalian cell mutagenicity of four optically active bay-region 3,4-diol-1,2-epoxides and other derivatives of the nitrogen heterocycle dibenz[c,h]acridine. *Cancer Res* 1986;46:2760–2766.

7. Rappaport SM, Yeowell-O'Connell K, Bodell W, Yager JW, Symanski E. An investigation of multiple biomarkers among workers exposed to styrene and styrene-7,8-oxide. *Cancer Res* 1996;56:5410–5416.

8. Bauer E, Guo Z, Ueng YF, Bell LC, Zeldin D, Guengerich FP. Oxidation of benzo[a]pyrene by recombinant human cytochrome P450 enzymes. *Chem Res Toxicol* 1995;8:136–142.

9. Bjelogrlic NM, Makinen M, Stenback F, Vahakangas K. Benzo[a]pyrene-7,8-diol-9,10-epoxide-DNA adducts and increased p53 protein in mouse skin. *Carcinogenesis* 1994;15:771–774.

10. Gasser R. The flavin-containing monooxygenase system. *Exp Toxicol Pathol* 1996;48:467–470.

11. Zeldin DC, Kobayashi J, Falck JR, et al. Regio- and enantiofacial selectivity of epoxyeicosatrienoic acid hydration by cytosolic epoxide hydrolase. *J Biol Chem* 1993;268:6402–6407.

12. Zeldin DC, Wei S, Falck JR, Hammock BD, Snapper JR, Capdevila JH. Metabolism of epoxyeicosatrienoic acids by cytosolic epoxide hydrolase: substrate structural determinants of asymmetric catalysis. *Arch Biochem Biophys* 1995;316:443–451.

13. Haeggstrom JZ, Wetterholm A, Medina JF, Samuelsson B. Novel structural and functional properties of leukotriene A4 hydrolase: implications for the development of enzyme inhibitors. *Adv Prostaglandin Thromboxane Leukot Res* 1994;22:3–12.

14. Hassett C, Aicher L, Sidhu JS, Omiecinski CJ. Human microsomal epoxide hydrolase: genetic polymorphism and functional expression in vitro of amino acid variants. *Hum Mol Genet* 1994;3:421–428.

15. Sevanian A, McLeod LL. Catalytic properties and inhibition of hepatic cholesterol: epoxide hydrolase. *J Biol Chem* 1986;261:54–59.

16. Pace Asciak CR, Lee WS. Purification of hepoxilin epoxide hydrolase from rat liver. *J Biol Chem* 1989;264:9310–9313.

17. Fu JY, Haeggstrom J, Collins P, Meijer J, Radmark O. Leukotriene A4 hydrolase: analysis of some human tissues by radioimmunoassay. *Biochim Biophys Acta* 1989;1006:121–126.

18. Beetham JK, Tian T, Hammock BD. cDNA cloning and expression of a soluble epoxide hydrolase from human liver. *Arch Biochem Biophys* 1993;305:197–201.

19. Skoda RC, Demierre A, McBride OW, Gonzalez FJ, Meyer UA. Human microsomal xenobiotic epoxide hydrolase: complementary DNA sequence, complementary DNA-directed expression in COS-1 cells, and chromosomal localization. *J Biol Chem* 1988;263:1549–1554.

20. Nashed NT, Michaud DP, Levin W, Jerina DM. Properties of liver microsomal cholesterol 5,6-oxide hydrolase. *Arch Biochem Biophys* 1985;241:149–162.

21. Sevanian A, Peterson AR. The cytotoxic and mutagenic properties of cholesterol oxidation products. *Food Chem Toxicol* 1986;24:1103–1110.

22. Finley BL, Hammock BD. Increased cholesterol epoxide hydrolase activity in clofibrate-fed animals. *Biochem Pharmacol* 1988;37:3169–3175.

23. Astrom A, Eriksson M, Eriksson LC, Birberg W, Pilotti A, DePierre JW. Subcellular and organ distribution of cholesterol epoxide hydrolase in the rat. *Biochim Biophys Acta* 1986;882:359–366.

24. Nashed NT, Michaud DP, Levin W, Jerina DM. 7-Dehydrocholesterol 5,6 beta-oxide as a mechanism-based inhibitor of microsomal cholesterol oxide hydrolase. *J Biol Chem* 1986;261:2510–2513.

25. Muller F, Arand M, Frank H, et al. Visualization of a covalent intermediate between microsomal epoxide hydrolase, but not cholesterol epoxide hydrolase, and their substrates. *Eur J Biochem* 1997;245:490–496.

26. Pace-Asciak CR. Hepoxilins: a review on their cellular actions. *Biochim Biophys Acta* 1994;1215:1–8.

27. Margalit A, Sofer Y, Grossman S, Reynaud D, Pace-Asciak CR, Livne AA. Hepoxilin A3 is the endogenous lipid mediator opposing hypotonic swelling of intact human platelets. *Proc Natl Acad Sci USA* 1993;90:2589–2592.

28. Pace-Asciak CR, Reynaud D, Demin P. Mechanistic aspects of hepoxilin biosynthesis. *J Lipid Mediat Cell Signal* 1995;12:307–311.

29. Pace-Asciak CR, Laneuville O, Su WG, et al. A glutathione conjugate of hepoxilin A3: formation and action in the rat central nervous system. *Proc Natl Acad Sci USA* 1990;87:3037–3041.

30. Reynaud D, Delton I, Gharib A, et al. Formation, metabolism, and action of hepoxilin A3 in the rat pineal gland. *J Neurochem* 1994;62:126–133.

31. McGee J, Fitzpatrick F. Enzymatic hydration of leukotriene A4: purification and characterization of a novel epoxide hydrolase from human erythrocytes. *J Biol Chem* 1985;260:12832–12837.

32. Rybina IV, Liu H, Gor Y, Feinmark SJ. Regulation of leukotriene A4 hydrolase activity in endothelial cells by phosphorylation. *J Biol Chem* 1997;272:31865–31871.

33. Iversen L, Kristensen P, Nissen JB, Merrick WC, Kragballe K. Purification and characterization of leukotriene A4 hydrolase from human epidermis. *FEBS Lett* 1995;358:316–322.

34. Mancini JA, Evans JF. Cloning and characterization of the human leukotriene A4 hydrolase gene. *Eur J Biochem* 1995;231:65–71.

35. Jendraschak E, Kaminski WE, Kiefl R, von Schacky C. The human leukotriene A4 hydrolase gene is expressed in two alternatively spliced mRNA forms. *Biochem J* 1996;314:733–737.

36. Blomster M, Wetterholm A, Mueller MJ, Haeggstrom JZ. Evidence for a catalytic role of tyrosine 383 in the peptidase reaction of leukotriene A4 hydrolase. *Eur J Biochem* 1995;231:528–534.

37. Wetterholm A, Haeggstrom JZ. Leukotriene A4 hydrolase: an anion activated peptidase. *Biochem Biophys Acta* 1992;1123:275–281.

38. Iversen L, Kragballe K, Ziboh VA. Significance of leukotriene-A4 hydrolase in the pathogenesis of psoriasis. *Skin Pharmacol* 1997;10:169–177.

39. Yuan W, Munoz B, Wong CH, Haeggstrom JZ, Wetterholm A, Samuelsson B. Development of selective tight-binding inhibitors of leukotriene A4 hydrolase. *J Med Chem* 1993;36:211–220.

40. Hogg JH, Ollmann IR, Haeggstrom JZ, Wetterholm A, Samuelsson B, Wong CH. Amino hydroxamic acids as potent inhibitors of leukotriene A4 hydrolase. *Bioorg Med Chem* 1995;3:1405–1415.

41. Meijer J, DePierre JW. Cytosolic epoxide hydrolase. *Chem Biol Interact* 1988;64:207–249.

42. Arand M, Knehr M, Thomas H, Zeller HD, Oesch F. An impaired peroxisomal targeting sequence leading to an unusual bicompartmental distribution of cytosolic epoxide hydrolase. *FEBS Lett* 1991;294:19–22.

43. Thomas H, Schladt L, Doehmer J, Knehr M, Oesch F. Rat and human liver cytosolic epoxide hydrolases: evidence for multiple forms at level of protein and mRNA. *Environ Health Perspect* 1990;88:49–55.

44. Schladt L, Worner W, Setiabudi F, Oesch F. Distribution and inducibility of cytosolic epoxide hydrolase in male Sprague-Dawley rats. *Biochem Pharmacol* 1986;35:3309–3316.

45. Eriksson AM, Zetterqvist MA, Lundgren B, Andersson K, Beije B, DePierre JW. Studies on the intracellular distributions of soluble epoxide hydrolase and of catalase by digitonin-permeabilization of hepatocytes isolated from control and clofibrate-treated mice. *Eur J Biochem* 1991;198:471–476.

46. Grant DF, Storms DH, Hammock BD. Molecular cloning and expression of murine liver soluble epoxide hydrolase. *J Biol Chem* 1993;268:17628–17633.

47. Knehr M, Thomas H, Arand M, Gebel T, Zeller HD, Oesch F. Isolation and characterization of a cDNA encoding rat liver cytosolic epoxide hydrolase and its functional expression in *Escherichia coli*. *J Biol Chem* 1993;268:17623–17627.

48. Stapleton A, Beetham JK, Pinot F, et al. Cloning and expression of soluble epoxide hydrolase from potato. *Plant J* 1994;6:251–258.

49. Sandberg M, Meijer J. Structural characterization of the human soluble epoxide hydrolase gene (EPHX2). *Biochem Biophys Res Commun* 1996;221:333–339.

50. Larsson C, White I, Johansson C, Stark A, Meijer J. Localization of the human soluble epoxide hydrolase gene (EPHX2) to chromosomal region 8p21-p12. *Hum Genet* 1995;95:356–358.

51. Sandberg M, Hassett C, Meijer J, Omiecinski CJ. Human soluble epoxide hydrolase genetic polymorphisms. *Toxicol Lett* 2000 (*in press*).

52. Vesell ES. Genetic factors that regulate cytosolic epoxide hydrolase activity in normal human lymphocytes. *Ann Genet* 1991;34:167–172.

53. Oesch F, Schladt L, Hartmann R, Timms C, Worner W. Rat cytosolic epoxide hydrolase. *Adv Exp Med Biol* 1986;197:195–201.

54. Lundgren B, Meijer J, DePierre JW. Induction of cytosolic and microsomal epoxide hydrolases and proliferation of peroxisomes and mitochondria in mouse liver after dietary exposure to p-chlorophenoxyacetic

acid, 2,4-dichlorophenoxyacetic acid and 2,4,5-trichlorophenoxyacetic acid. *Biochem Pharmacol* 1987;36:815–821.

55. Lundgren B, Meijer J, Birberg W, Pilotti A, DePierre JW. Induction of cytosolic and microsomal epoxide hydrolases in mouse liver by peroxisome proliferators, with special emphasis on structural analogues of 2-ethylhexanoic acid. *Chem Biol Interact* 1988;68:219–240.

56. Lundgren B, DePierre JW. Proliferation of peroxisomes and induction of cytosolic and microsomal epoxide hydrolases in different strains of mice and rats after dietary treatment with clofibrate. *Xenobiotica* 1989;19:867–881.

57. Johansson C, Stark A, Sandberg M, Ek B, Rask L, Meijer J. Tissue specific basal expression of soluble murine epoxide hydrolase and effects of clofibrate on the mRNA levels in extrahepatic tissues and liver. *Arch Toxicol* 1995;70:61–63.

58. Oesch F, Schladt L. Coordinate induction of peroxisomal beta-oxidation activity and cytosolic epoxide hydrolase activity. *Pharmacol Ther* 1987;33:29–35.

59. Oesch F, Hartmann R, Timms C, et al. Time-dependence and differential induction of rat and guinea pig peroxisomal beta-oxidation, palmitoyl-CoA hydrolase, cytosolic and microsomal epoxide hydrolase after treatment with hypolipidemic drugs. *J Cancer Res Clin Oncol* 1988;114:341–346.

60. Dietze EC, Kuwano E, Hammock BD. Spectrophotometric substrates for cytosolic epoxide hydrolase. *Anal Biochem* 1994;216:176–187.

61. Borhan B, Mebrahtu T, Nazarian S, Kurth MJ, Hammock BD. Improved radiolabeled substrates for soluble epoxide hydrolase. *Anal Biochem* 1995;231:188–200.

62. Arand M, Grant DF, Beetham JK, Friedberg T, Oesch F, Hammock BD. Sequence similarity of mammalian epoxide hydrolases to the bacterial haloalkane dehalogenase and other related proteins: implication for the potential catalytic mechanism of enzymatic epoxide hydrolysis. *FEBS Lett* 1994;338:251–256.

63. Pinot F, Grant DF, Beetham JK, et al. Molecular and biochemical evidence for the involvement of the Asp-333-His-523 pair in the catalytic mechanism of soluble epoxide hydrolase. *J Biol Chem* 1995;270:7968–7974.

64. Miyamoto T, Silva M, Hammock BD. Inhibition of epoxide hydrolases and glutathione S-transferases by 2-, 3-, and 4-substituted derivatives of 4'-phenylchalcone and its oxide. *Arch Biochem Biophys* 1987;254:203–213.

65. Nourooz Zadeh J, Uematsu T, Borhan B, Kurth MJ, Hammock BD. Characterization of the cytosolic epoxide hydrolase-catalyzed hydration products from 9,10:12,13-diepoxy stearic esters. *Arch Biochem Biophys* 1992;294:675–685.

66. Moghaddam MF, Grant DF, Cheek JM, Greene JF, Williamson KC, Hammock BD. Bioactivation of leukotoxins to their toxic diols by epoxide hydrolase [Comments]. *Nat Med* 1997;3:562–566.

67. Shou M, Gonzalez FJ, Gelboin HV. Stereoselective epoxidation and hydration at the K-region of polycyclic aromatic hydrocarbons by cDNA-expressed cytochromes P450 1A1, 1A2, and epoxide hydrolase. *Biochemistry* 1996;35:15807–15813.

68. Armstrong RN. Enzyme-catalyzed detoxication reactions: mechanisms and stereochemistry. *Crit Rev Biochem* 1987;22:39–88.

69. Fandrich F, Degiuli B, Vogel Bindel U, Arand M, Oesch F. Induction of rat liver microsomal epoxide hydrolase by its endogenous substrate 16 alpha, 17 alpha-epoxyestra-1,3,5-trien-3-ol. *Xenobiotica* 1995;25:239–244.

70. Papadopoulos D, Seidegard J, Georgellis A, Rydstrom J. Subcellular distribution, catalytic properties and partial purification of epoxide hydrolase in the human adrenal gland. *Chem Biol Interact* 1985;55:249–260.

71. Seidegard J, DePierre JW, Guenthner TM, Oesch F. The effects of metyrapone, chalcone epoxide, benzil, clotrimazole and related compounds on the activity of microsomal epoxide hydrolase in situ, in purified form and in reconstituted systems towards different substrates. *Eur J Biochem* 1986;159:415–423.

72. von Dippe P, Amoui M, Stellwagen RH, Levy D. The functional expression of sodium-dependent bile acid transport in Madin-Darby canine kidney cells transfected with the cDNA for microsomal epoxide hydrolase. *J Biol Chem* 1996;271:18176–18180.

73. Hassett C, Turnblom SM, DeAngeles A, Omiecinski CJ. Rabbit microsomal epoxide hydrolase: isolation and characterization of the xenobiotic metabolizing enzyme cDNA. *Arch Biochem Biophys* 1989;271:380–389.

74. Omiecinski CJ, Aicher L, Holubkov R, Checkoway H. Human peripheral lymphocytes as indicators of microsomal epoxide hydrolase activity in liver and lung. *Pharmacogenetics* 1993;3:150–158.

75. Dansette PM, Makedonska VB, Jerina DM. Mechanism of catalysis for the hydration of substituted styrene oxides by hepatic epoxide hydrase. *Arch Biochem Biophys* 1978;187:290–298.

76. Armstrong RN. Kinetic and chemical mechanism of epoxide hydrolase. *Drug Metab Rev* 1999;31:71–86.

77. Arand M, Muller F, Mecky A, et al. Catalytic triad of microsomal epoxide hydrolase: replacement of Glu404 with Asp leads to a strongly increased turnover rate. *Biochem J* 1999;337(Pt 1):37–43.

78. Hassett C, Robinson KB, Beck NB, Omiecinski CJ. The human microsomal epoxide hydrolase gene (EPHX1): complete nucleotide sequence and structural characterization. *Genomics* 1994;23:433–442.

79. Hartsfield JK Jr, Sutcliffe MJ, Everett ET, Hassett C, Omiecinski CJ, Saari JA. Assignment of microsomal epoxide hydrolase (EPHX1) to human chromosome 1q42.1 by in situ hybridization. *Cytogenet Cell Genet* 1998;83:44–45.

80. Gaedigk A, Spielberg SP, Grant DM. Characterization of the microsomal epoxide hydrolase gene in patients with anticonvulsant adverse drug reactions. *Pharmacogenetics* 1994;4:142–153.

81. Laurenzana EM, Hassett C, Omiecinski CJ. Post-transcriptional regulation of human microsomal epoxide hydrolase. *Pharmacogenetics* 1998;8:157–167.

82. Omiecinski CJ, Aicher L, Swenson L. Developmental expression of human microsomal epoxide hydrolase. *J Pharmacol Exp Ther* 1994;269:417–423.

83. Hassett C, Lin J, Carty CL, Laurenzana EM, Omiecinski CJ. Human hepatic microsomal epoxide hydrolase: comparative analysis of polymorphic expression. *Arch Biochem Biophys* 1997;337:275–283.

84. Raaka S, Hassett C, Omiencinski CJ. Human microsomal epoxide hydrolase: 5'-flanking region genetic polymorphisms. *Carcinogenesis* 1998;19:387–393.

85. McGlynn KA, Rosvold EA, Lustbader ED, et al. Susceptibility to hepatocellular carcinoma is associated with genetic variation in the enzymatic detoxification of aflatoxin B_1. *Proc Natl Acad Sci USA* 1995;92:2384–2387.

86. Harrison DJ, Hubbard AL, MacMillan J, Wyllie AH, Smith CA. Microsomal epoxide hydrolase gene polymorphism and susceptibility to colon cancer. *Br J Cancer* 1999;79:168–171.

87. Lancaster JM, Brownlee HA, Bell DA, et al. Microsomal epoxide hydrolase polymorphism as a risk factor for ovarian cancer. *Mol Carcinog* 1996;17:160–162.

88. Brockmoller J, Cascorbi I, Kerb R, Roots I. Combined analysis of inherited polymorphisms in arylamine N-acetyltransferase 2, glutathione S-transferases M1 and T1, microsomal epoxide hydrolase, and cytochrome P450 enzymes as modulators of bladder cancer risk. *Cancer Res* 1996;56:3915–3925.

89. Smith CA, Harrison DJ. Association between polymorphism in gene for microsomal epoxide hydrolase and susceptibility to emphysema. *Lancet* 1997;350:630–633.

90. Wormhoudt LW, Commandeur JN, Vermeulen NP. Genetic polymorphisms of human N-acetyltransferase, cytochrome P450, glutathione-S-transferase, and epoxide hydrolase enzymes: relevance to xenobiotic metabolism and toxicity. *Crit Rev Toxicol* 1999;29:59–124.

91. Cresteil T, Beaune P, Kremers P, Celier C, Guengerich FP, Leroux JP. Immunoquantification of epoxide hydrolase and cytochrome P-450 isozymes in fetal and adult human liver microsomes. *Eur J Biochem* 1985;151:345–350.

92. Simmons DL, Kasper CB. Quantitation of mRNAs specific for the mixed-function oxidase system in rat liver and extrahepatic tissues during development. *Arch Biochem Biophys* 1989;271:10–20.

93. Meijer J, DePierre JW. Hepatic levels of cytosolic, microsomal and "mitochondrial" epoxide hydrolases and other drug-metabolizing enzymes after treatment of mice with various xenobiotics and endogenous compounds. *Chem Biol Interact* 1987;62:249–269.

94. Hammock BD, Ota K. Differential induction of cytosolic epoxide hydrolase, microsomal epoxide hydrolase, and glutathione S-transferase activities. *Toxicol Appl Pharmacol* 1983;71:254–265.

95. Kim SG. Transcriptional regulation of rat microsomal epoxide hydrolase gene by imidazole antimycotic agents. *Mol Pharmacol* 1992;42:273–279.

96. Hassett C, Laurenzana EM, Sidhu JS, Omiecinski CJ. Effects of

chemical inducers on human microsomal epoxide hydrolase in primary hepatocyte cultures. *Biochem Pharmacol* 1998;55:1059–1069.

97. Gaedigk A, Leeder JS, Grant DM. Tissue-specific expression and alternative splicing of human microsomal epoxide hydrolase. *DNA Cell Biol* 1997;16:1257–1266.

98. Vogel BU, Bentley P, Oesch F. Endogenous role of microsomal epoxide hydrolase: ontogenesis, induction inhibition, tissue distribution, immunological behaviour and purification of microsomal epoxide hydrolase with 16 alpha, 17 alpha-epoxyandrostene-3-one as substrate. *Eur J Biochem* 1982;126:425–431.

99. Jerina DM, Dansette PM, Lu AYH, Levin W. Hepatic microsomal epoxide hydrase: a sensitive radiometric assay for hydration of arene oxides of carcinogenic aromatic hydrocarbons. *Mol Pharmacol* 1977;13:342–351.

100. Lu AYH, Jerina DM, Levin W. Liver microsomal epoxide hydrase: hydration of alkene and arene oxides by membrane-bound and purified enzymes. *J Biol Chem* 1977;252:3715–3723.

101. Mendrala AL, Langvardt PW, Nitschke KD, Quast JF, Nolan RJ. In vitro kinetics of styrene and styrene oxide metabolism in rat, mouse, and human. *Arch Toxicol* 1993;67:18–27.

102. Gill SS, Ota K, Hammock BD. Radiometric assays for mammalian epoxide hydrolases and glutathione S-transferases. *Anal Biochem* 1983;131:273–282.

103. Himmelstein MW, Turner MJ, Asgharian B, Bond JA. Comparison of blood concentrations of 1,3-butadiene and butadiene epoxides in mice and rats exposed to 1,3-butadiene by inhalation. *Carcinogenesis* 1994;15:1479–1486.

104. Krause RJ, Elfarra AA. Oxidation of butadiene monoxide to meso- and (±)-diepoxybutane by cDNA-expressed human cytochrome P450s and by mouse, rat, and human liver microsomes: evidence for preferential hydration of meso-diepoxybutane in rat and human liver microsomes. *Arch Biochem Biophys* 1997;337:176–184.

105. Lindstrom AB, Yeowell-O'Connell K, Waidyanatha S, Golding BT, Tornero VR, Rappaport SM. Measurement of benzene oxide in the blood of rats following administration of benzene. *Carcinogenesis* 1997;18:1637–1641.

106. Snyder R, Chepiga T, Yang CS, Thomas H, Platt K, Oesch F. Benzene metabolism by reconstituted cytochromes P450 2B1 and 2E1 and its modulation by cytochrome b5, microsomal epoxide hydrolase, and glutathione transferases: evidence for an important role of microsomal epoxide hydrolase in the formation of hydroquinone. *Toxicol Appl Pharmacol* 1993;122:172–181.

107. Walters JM, Combes RD. Activation of benzo[a]pyrene and aflatoxin B₁ to mutagenic chemical species by microsomal preparations from rat liver and small intestine in relation to microsomal epoxide hydrolase. *Mutagenesis* 1986;1:45–48.

108. Kitteringham NR, Davis C, Howard N, Pirmohamed M, Park BK. Interindividual and interspecies variation in hepatic microsomal epoxide hydrolase activity: studies with *cis*-stilbene oxide, carbamazepine 10,11-epoxide and naphthalene. *J Pharmacol Exp Ther* 1996;278:1018–1027.

109. Kroetz DL, Kerr BM, McFarland LV, Loiseau P, Wilensky AJ, Levy RH. Measurement of in vivo microsomal epoxide hydrolase activity in white subjects. *Clin Pharmacol Ther* 1993;53:306–315.

110. Yang SK, Bao ZP. Stereoselective formations of K-region and non-K-region epoxides in the metabolism of chrysene by rat liver microsomal cytochrome P-450 isozymes. *Mol Pharmacol* 1987;32:73–80.

111. Heflich RH, Thornton Manning JR, Kinouchi T, Beland FA. Muta-genicity of oxidized microsomal metabolites of 1-nitropyrene in Chinese hamster ovary cells. *Mutagenesis* 1990;5:151–157.

112. van Bladeren PJ, Sayer JM, Ryan DE, Thomas PE, Levin W, Jerina DM. Differential stereoselectivity of cytochromes P-450b and P-450c in the formation of naphthalene and anthracene 1,2-oxides: the role of epoxide hydrolase in determining the enantiomer composition of the 1,2-dihydrodiols formed. *J Biol Chem* 1985;260:10226–10235.

113. Yang SK. Stereoselectivity of cytochrome P-450 isozymes and epoxide hydrolase in the metabolism of polycyclic aromatic hydrocarbons. *Biochem Pharmacol* 1988;37:61–70.

114. Prestwich GD, Lucarelli I, Park SK, Loury DN, Moody DE, Hammock BD. Cyclopropyl oxiranes: reversible inhibitors of cytosolic and microsomal epoxide hydrolases. *Arch Biochem Biophys* 1985;237:361–372.

115. Mertes I, Fleischmann R, Glatt HR, Oesch F. Interindividual variations in the activities of cytosolic and microsomal epoxide hydrolase in human liver. *Carcinogenesis* 1985;6:219–223.

116. Strickler SM, Dansky LV, Miller MA, Seni MH, Andermann E, Spielberg SP. Genetic predisposition to phenytoin-induced birth defects. *Lancet* 1985;2:746–749.

117. Finnell RH, Buehler BA, Kerr BM, Ager PL, Levy RH. Clinical and experimental studies linking oxidative metabolism to phenytoin-induced teratogenesis. *Neurology* 1992;42:25–31.

118. Buehler BA, Delimont D, van Waes M, Finnell RH. Prenatal prediction of risk of the fetal hydantoin syndrome [Comments]. *N Engl J Med* 1990;322:1567–1572.

119. Buehler BA, Rao V, Finnell RH. Biochemical and molecular teratology of fetal hydantoin syndrome. *Neurol Clin* 1994;12:741–748.

120. Lindhout D. Pharmacogenetics and drug interactions: role in antiepileptic-drug-induced teratogenesis. *Neurology* 1992;42:43–47.

121. Kroetz DL, Loiseau P, Guyot M, Levy RH. In vivo and in vitro correlation of microsomal epoxide hydrolase inhibition by progabide. *Clin Pharmacol Ther* 1993;54:485–497.

122. Kerr BM, Rettie AE, Eddy AC, et al. Inhibition of human liver microsomal epoxide hydrolase by valproate and valpromide: in vitro/in vivo correlation. *Clin Pharmacol Ther* 1989;46:82–93.

123. Leeder JS, Riley RJ, Cook VA, Spielberg SP. Human anti-cytochrome P450 antibodies in aromatic anticonvulsant-induced hypersensitivity reactions. *J Pharmacol Exp Ther* 1992;263:360–367.

124. Shear NH, Spielberg SP. Anticonvulsant hypersensitivity syndrome: in vitro assessment of risk. *J Clin Invest* 1988;82:1826–1832.

125. Green VJ, Pirmohamed M, Kitteringham NR, et al. Genetic analysis of microsomal epoxide hydrolase in patients with carbamazepine hypersensitivity. *Biochem Pharmacol* 1995;50:1353–1359.

126. Leeder JS, Gaedigk A, Lu X, Cook VA. Epitope mapping studies with human anti-cytochrome P450 3A antibodies. *Mol Pharmacol* 1996;49:234–243.

127. Bialer M. Clinical pharmacology of valpromide. *Clin Pharmacokinet* 1991;20:114–122.

128. Pisani F, Fazio A, Oteri G, Ruello C, Gitto C, Russo F, Perucca E. Sodium valproate and valpromide: differential interactions with carbamazepine in epileptic patients. *Epilepsia* 1986;27:548–552.

129. Collins DM, Gidal BE, Pitterle ME. Potential interaction between carbamazepine and loxapine: case report and retrospective review. *Ann Pharmacother* 1993;27:1180–1187.

130. Pisani F, Haj Yehia A, Fazio A, et al. Carbamazepine-valnoctamide interaction in epileptic patients: in vitro/in vivo correlation. *Epilepsia* 1993;34:954–959.

Drugs as Substrates of Metabolic Enzymes

CHAPTER 17

Anticonvulsants

Gary G. Mather and René H. Levy

The therapeutic armamentarium for the long-term treatment of epilepsy has until recently included only a small number of effective agents with narrow therapeutic ranges. Even after the introduction of several new agents within the last 5 years, these same few drugs still account for the majority of prescriptions for antiepileptic drugs (AEDs) on a world-wide basis. Treatment of epilepsy often includes polypharmacy and drug interactions among AEDs are common. Induction of metabolic enzymes associated with drugs such as phenytoin (PHT), carbamazepine (CBZ), phenobarbital (PB), or primidone may lead to decreased plasma concentrations of other AEDs and loss of seizure control. Conversely, inhibition-based interactions may increase plasma concentrations and result in toxicities and adverse effects such as dizziness, somnolence, blurred vision, and so on.

The majority of commonly used AEDs are metabolized by the cytochrome P450 mixed-function oxidases. The clearances of several drugs of this class (PHT, CBZ, PB) are dependent on the formation of a major oxidative metabolite and are subject to variability arising from various factors including age, genotype, and induction status. Thus dosages necessary to achieve seizure control may vary substantially and need to be individualized. Numerous studies have shown that identification of metabolic enzymes aids in the rational understanding and prediction of drug–drug interactions (1–4). In the case of AEDs, identity of the isoforms responsible for their metabolism has until recently been limited to PHT and CBZ.

In this review, anticonvulsants are discussed as substrates of metabolic enzymes and are divided into three

groups: (a) drugs that have been recently introduced; (b) established drugs commonly used in clinical practice; and (c) drugs used less frequently or for which little information is available. The clinical pharmacokinetics of each drug in the first two groups is reviewed, and the primary route(s) of elimination are summarized along with the evidence supporting the identification of the enzymes responsible for the drug's clearance. Thereafter, known interactions with each drug are discussed and placed within the context of the isozymes of clearance. Drugs in the third group are discussed only when information is available and pertinent to the understanding of a specific interaction.

DRUGS RECENTLY INTRODUCED IN CLINICAL PRACTICE: FELBAMATE, GABAPENTIN, LAMOTRIGINE, OXCARBAZEPINE, TIAGABINE, TOPIRAMATE, VIGABATRIN, AND ZONISAMIDE

Felbamate

Approximately 90% to 95% of an administered oral dose of felbamate (FBM) is absorbed from the gastrointestinal (GI) tract (5), and absorption is not affected by food (6). After single doses of FBM (100–1,200 mg) in healthy volunteers, maximal plasma concentrations are achieved in 2 to 5 hours. The half-life is approximately 20 hours in healthy volunteers, and the kinetics are linear through most of the therapeutic range (7). Some evidence of nonlinearity exists with doses greater than 1,600 mg/day (8). The drug is excreted in the urine of healthy volunteers appreciably as unchanged drug (40% to 65%). In induced patients, the amount of unchanged drug excreted is reduced to 14% to 29% (9). Early studies identified urinary metabolites as 2-hydroxy-felbamate, p-hydroxy-felbamate, and the monocarbamate derivative or their conjugates. However, recent identification of a secondary metabolite of the monocarbamate derivative

G. G. Mather: CEDRA Corporation, 8609 Cross Park Drive, Austin, Texas 78754

R. H. Levy: Departments of Pharmaceutics and Neurological Surgery, Box 357610, H272 Health Sciences Building, University of Washington, Seattle, Washington 98195-7610

(3-carbamoyloxy-2-phenylproprionic acid; CPPA) suggests that enzymatic hydrolysis to the monocarbamate is a primary metabolic pathway (10). Although the enzymes involved in the oxidative formation of the 2-hydroxy- and p-hydroxy-metabolites have been identified as CYP3A4 and CYP2E1 (11,12), enzymes forming the monocarbamate and its subsequent oxidation to CPPA have not been identified.

Interactions Resulting in Increased Plasma Concentrations

In a study of 12 volunteers with epilepsy, FBM kinetics were not changed significantly by coadministration of erythromycin [333 mg q8h (13)]. This is consistent with the fact that in healthy subjects, oxidative metabolites of FBM account for less than half of the total clearance of FBM, and CYP3A4 mediates only a portion of this oxidative clearance; therefore, inhibition of CYP3A4 appears to have only minimal effects on the overall clearance of the drug. Coadministration of gabapentin appears to decrease the clearance of FBM. In 40 patients treated with monotherapy, the measured clearance was 0.67 L/kg/day, and the calculated half-life was 24 hours, whereas in seven patients treated with FBM and gabapentin, clearance and half-life were 0.42 L/kg/day and 35 hours, respectively (14). It has been speculated that this interaction represents a competition at the level of a transporter for renal excretion rather than an enzymatic interaction. Coadministration of valproic acid (VPA) did not result in changes in pharmacokinetic parameters or plasma concentrations of FBM (15).

Interactions Associated with Enzyme Inducers

The clearance of FBM is increased and the half-life decreased to approximately 14 hours by coadministration of the enzyme-inducing drugs PHT, CBZ, and PB (9,16). In a controlled discontinuation trial, FBM clearance decreased 22% as PHT was removed from cotherapy and by 16.5% when CBZ doses were decreased (17). These findings are consistent with induction of CYP3A4 and/or CYP2E1 by PHT and CBZ and demonstrate the increased importance of oxidative pathways in patients treated with inducing drugs.

Gabapentin

Absorption of gabapentin is mediated by the saturable L system amino acid transporter (18), and its bioavailability is dependent on the dose administered. In healthy volunteers, bioavailability has been estimated at approximately 60% and 40% after single doses of 300 and 600 mg, respectively (19). Bioavailability was further reduced to approximately 35% in subjects taking 1,600 mg t.i.d. (20). As anticipated, the plasma concentration is nonlinear with respect to dose, increasing less than proportionately at higher doses. Absorption is not affected by food.

Gabapentin is not metabolized and is excreted mostly unchanged in urine (21) with a half-life of between 5 and 9 hours in healthy volunteers. Clearance of gabapentin is dependent on renal function and is strongly correlated with clearance of creatinine. As creatinine clearance decreases, the corresponding half-life of gabapentin increases (22).

Effects of Inducers/Inhibitors

Because gabapentin is not metabolized, interactions through these mechanisms seem unlikely. The standard AEDs PB (23), CBZ and VPA (24), and PHT (25,26) do not affect the pharmacokinetics of gabapentin.

Other Interactions

Administration of aluminum hydroxide or magnesium hydroxide antacid to healthy volunteers either concomitantly or 2 hours after a dose of 400 mg gabapentin reduced bioavailability by 20%.

Lamotrigine

Lamotrigine (LTG) is well absorbed from the GI tract, with absolute bioavailability estimated at 98% in a combined oral and intravenous administration study (27). Peak plasma concentrations are generally attained in 2.5 to 3 hours (28,29), and linear kinetics are observed within the therapeutic range (30). The half-life in healthy volunteers is approximately 24 hours. Lamotrigine is extensively metabolized, and 70% to 90% of the administered dose can be recovered in urine (28,31). Glucuronide conjugates formed by uridine diphosphate (UDP)-glucuronyl transferases account for nearly 90% of urinary products. The 2-N-glucuronide is the major metabolite, whereas the 5-N-glucuronide and parent drug account for smaller fractions of urinary products (32–34).

Interactions Associated with Increased Plasma Concentrations

Because the primary route of elimination is through glucuronidation, inhibition of this pathway can be expected to decrease LTG clearance and increase plasma concentrations. Furthermore, LTG clearance should not be affected by inhibitors of P450 oxidative enzymes. Valproic acid also is eliminated by the glucuronyl transferase system, and VPA coadministration results in significant increases in the half-life of LTG (35). Short-term administration of VPA reduced the total clearance by 21% in a study of six healthy volunteers (36). In a larger study, the steady-state half-life of LTG was increased to nearly 70 hours when coadministered with VPA (500 mg b.i.d.)

(37). There have also been two reports of interaction in patients with epilepsy treated with LTG involving sertraline (38). In the first case, toxicity was observed and LTG levels were doubled 6 weeks after the addition of sertraline, 25 mg/day, to the treatment regimen. Conversely, a 25-mg reduction in the total daily dose of sertraline, in a second case, resulted in reduction of LTG levels to nearly half, even though the LTG dose was increased by 33%. FBM increased the C_{max} and AUC_{0-12} of LTG by 13% and 14%, respectively, in a crossover study in 21 healthy volunteers. These effects were not expected to be clinically significant (39).

Interactions Associated with Decreased Plasma Concentrations

The rate of elimination of LTG is increased substantially in patients receiving treatment with inducing agents such as PHT, CBZ, PB, and primidone, with corresponding half-lives reduced to 14 to 15 hours compared with 24 hours for healthy volunteers (40–42). Discontinuation of concomitant enzyme-inducing AEDs resulted in a decrease of more than 50% in the mean systemic clearance of LTG with an associated two-fold increase in LTG plasma concentrations (43). These interactions are consistent with induction of UDP-glucuronyl transferase activities by PHT, CBZ, and PB; thus higher doses of LTG are required to maintain therapeutic levels when it is coadministered with these drugs. Coadministration of escalating doses of topiramate (TPM) in a group of 25 patients resulted in only slight decreases in average LTG levels compared with baseline without TPM. However, LTG levels were decreased 20% to 30% in three of the patients, indicating that this interaction may reach clinical significance in some patients (44). Because acetaminophen also is glucuronidated to a substantial degree, Depot et al. (45) examined the effects of acetaminophen (900 mg, t.i.d., for 11 days) on the pharmacokinetics of a single oral dose of LTG (300 mg) in healthy volunteers. Both AUC_{0-8} and half-life were decreased by 20% and 15%, respectively, by coadministration of acetaminophen, apparently through activation of transferase activity (46). This change is not likely to be significant clinically with occasional acetaminophen doses.

Oxcarbazepine

Oxcarbazepine (OXC) is essentially a prodrug that, when given orally, is almost completely absorbed and rapidly reduced by the action of cytosolic arylketone reductase to the active metabolite, 10,11-dihydro-10-hydroxy-5H-dibenzo[b,f]azepine-5-carboxamide (MHD). Maximal plasma concentrations of MHD are generally reached within 4 hours (47). Plasma concentration of MHD is linearly related to OXC dose within the therapeutic range (48). MHD has an elimination half-life of 8 to 10 hours (49) and is excreted primarily in the urine as free MHD or as its glucuronide conjugate (50,51). Although MHD may also be oxidized to 10,11-dihydro-10,11-dihydroxycarbamazepine (DHD), the contribution of this pathway to total MHD elimination appears to be minimal [approximately 5% in healthy volunteers (52)].

Interactions Associated with Increased Plasma Concentrations

Because OXC and MHD are excreted primarily through nonoxidative pathways, significant interactions resulting from metabolic inhibition seem unlikely. However, inhibition of the formation of DHD may cause relatively small increases in the plasma concentration of MHD in some patients. Viloxazine (100 mg, b.i.d., for 10 days) increased the plasma concentration of MHD by 11% and decreased the DHD levels by 31% in a group of six patients with epilepsy treated with OXC (53,54). Verapamil (120 mg), either as a single dose or as a b.i.d. treatment for 6 days, decreased the AUC of DHD by 20% and 50%, respectively (55). Similarly, the steady-state C_{max}, C_{min}, and AUC_{0-24} for DHD were all lower when dextropropoxyphene (65 mg, t.i.d., for 8 days) was added to the treatment regimen of eight patients stabilized with OXC (56). Due to the small contribution of this pathway, no significant effects were seen in pharmacokinetic parameters of OXC or MHD. Neither cimetidine nor erythromycin (500 mg, b.i.d., for 7 days) in groups of eight healthy volunteers coadministered OXC altered the kinetics of MHD (52,57). No differences were noted in the metabolic clearance of MHD between groups of patients treated with OXC monotherapy ($n = 63$) compared with OXC and VPA combined therapy ($n = 10$) (58). Similarly, addition of FBM (2,400 mg/day for 10 days) to OXC treatment (1,200 mg/day) did not result in significant changes in plasma concentrations or urinary pharmacokinetics of MHD in healthy volunteers (59).

Interactions Associated with Reduced Plasma Concentrations

Although the formation of MHD is refractory to the effects of classic enzyme-inducing drugs, McKee and Brodie (60) reported that MHD concentrations were significantly lower in 12 CBZ-treated patients compared with seven untreated controls. Likewise, Kumps and Wurth (61) demonstrated increased levels of DHD, the oxidative metabolite of MHD, in six patients treated with PHT and PB when standardized to a constant OXC dose. Although these studies indicate that elimination of MHD through the DHD pathway can be induced, this effect does not appear to be clinically significant.

Tiagabine

Tiagabine is quickly absorbed after oral administration to healthy volunteers and reaches maximal plasma concentrations within 1 hour, with secondary peaks suggestive of enterohepatic circulation (62). The rate, but not the extent, of absorption is affected by concomitant food ingestion (63). The absolute oral bioavailability was 90% in a study of eight healthy volunteers (64). Its half-life is 5 to 13 hours without dose dependency over the therapeutic range (40–80 mg/day) (65).

Tiagabine is extensively metabolized with only 1% to 2% excreted unchanged (62). Consistent with significant biliary recirculation, 25% of the total dose was recovered in urine and 63% in the feces after administration of ^{14}C-labeled tiagabine (66). The primary metabolic pathway involves oxidation of the thiophene ring, resulting in two 5-oxo-tiagabine isomers (66,67), which account for approximately 22% of the total dose. Correlation and inhibition studies suggested that this reaction is mediated by the CYP3A subfamily, and subsequently, the formation of the 5-oxo metabolites has been demonstrated in incubations with expressed CYP3A4 (68). Tiagabine clearance appears to be independent of renal function and exhibits similar pharmacokinetics in healthy volunteers and subjects with varying degrees of renal impairment (69).

Interactions Associated with Increased Plasma Concentrations

Because tiagabine clearance is mediated partially by CYP3A4, interactions resulting in decreased clearance and increased plasma concentrations may be anticipated when it is coadministered with CYP3A4 inhibitors. However, coadministration of cimetidine (400 mg, b.i.d.) caused only marginal (5%) increases in tiagabine plasma concentration in 12 healthy volunteers (70), and coadministration of erythromycin (500 mg, b.i.d., for 4 days) did not alter the C_{max}, AUC, or half-life of tiagabine in a study in 13 healthy volunteers (71). These data must be interpreted with caution, particularly when treating patients coadministered enzyme-inducing drugs in whom the oxidative pathways may play a substantially more important role.

Interactions Associated with Decreased Plasma Concentrations

The mean AUC of tiagabine was significantly lower in groups of four patients taking CBZ and PHT, CBZ and primidone, or CBZ and vigabatrin, compared with that in patients treated with VPA monotherapy or compared with a group of 30 healthy volunteers (72). The half-life of tiagabine is reduced to 2 to 5 hours and plasma concentrations reduced to one half to one third of those observed in patients not comedicated with enzyme-inducing drugs (73).

Topiramate

Oral doses of TPM are well absorbed, and maximal plasma concentrations are reached in 2 to 4 hours (74). Absorption is delayed by concomitant ingestion of food,

but the extent of absorption is unchanged (75). Topiramate is primarily (80%) excreted unchanged in the urine of healthy volunteers, with an elimination half-life of approximately 20 to 30 hours. Increases in plasma concentration are linear but less than proportional up to single doses of 1,200 mg (74) and up to 200 mg/day in multiple-dose studies (75,76). Neither the identification of oxidative metabolites nor the enzymes responsible for their formation have been reported.

Interactions Associated with Increased Plasma Concentrations

Because metabolism is of minor importance in the overall clearance of TPM, significant interactions resulting from inhibition are unlikely.

Interactions Associated with Decreased Plasma Concentrations

Topiramate metabolic clearance is increased by CBZ (77), PHT (78), and PB, and the corresponding plasma concentrations and half-lifes are decreased. Topiramate clearance is twofold to threefold greater when administered in combination with PHT. The importance of inductive interactions is apparent in three patients whose plasma levels increased by 70% when CBZ was discontinued from their treatment regimen. When TPM was studied in a crossover design with VPA, topiramate C_{max} and AUC_{0-12} were slightly higher (17%, $n = 8$) during TPM monotherapy than during concomitant VPA therapy (79).

Vigabatrin

Vigabatrin is administered as a racemic mixture with pharmacologic activity residing in the S(+) enantiomer. In a study of six healthy volunteers, the clearance of S(+)-vigabatrin was not affected by the R(−) enantiomer, and no chiral inversion was detected (80). After administration, peak plasma concentration is reached within 0.5 to 2.0 hours, and the mean terminal half-life is about 6 hours (75). No metabolites have been identified, and renal clearance of the unchanged compound accounts for 70% of the total clearance.

Because the clearance of vigabatrin is primarily mediated through renal excretion of unchanged drug, metabolic interactions altering the clearance of vigabatrin are unlikely. In a study of 18 healthy subjects, coadministration of FBM (1,200 mg, b.i.d., for 8 days) resulted in a small (13%) increase in the AUC_{0-12} of active S(+)-vigabatrin, whereas R(−)-vigabatrin was unchanged (81). The mechanism for this interaction is not fully understood.

Zonisamide

Zonisamide (ZNS) is almost completely absorbed after oral dosing, generally reaches maximal plasma concentrations in 2 to 5 hours (82–84), and may be administered without regard to the timing of meals (85). Plasma levels of ZNS are linearly related to dose within the range of normal therapeutic use [10–15 mg/kg/day (86)]; however, some evidence of nonlinearity was reported in a study of 10 adult patients with corresponding in vivo K_m values averaging 25.1 µg/mL (87). The elimination half-life reported in studies of healthy volunteers ranged from 57 to 68 hours (83,88). Like other sulfonamide derivatives, ZNS is markedly bound by erythrocytes, with resultant total blood concentrations significantly higher than plasma concentrations (82).

The largest part of an oral dose of ZNS is excreted in the urine as unchanged ZNS, 2-sulfamoylacetylphenol (SMAP), and SMAP conjugates (83). The open-ring metabolite SMAP has been shown to be the product of reductive P450 metabolism, catalyzed largely by CYP3A4 (89). The in vitro K_m describing this reaction has been estimated at approximately 325 µM (90). It has recently been reported that the expressed enzymes CYP2C19 and CYP3A5 are also capable of catalyzing ZNS reduction (91). However, the intrinsic clearance of CYP3A4 is much higher than those of CYP2C19 and CYP3A5. Therefore, from the point of view of enzyme quantity and relative intrinsic clearances, it is suggested that CYP3A4 is mainly responsible for ZNS metabolism in vivo.

Interactions Resulting in Increased Plasma Concentrations

Because a primary route of metabolic clearance of ZNS is catalyzed by CYP3A4, it can be anticipated that inhibitors of this enzyme may decrease ZNS clearance and increase its plasma concentrations; however, no studies demonstrating these effects have been reported. Administration of cimetidine, 300 mg, q.i.d., did not result in changes in the pharmacokinetic profile of single doses of 300 mg ZNS in a study of eight healthy volunteers (92). Although unlikely to involve inhibition of CYP3A4, plasma concentrations of ZNS were increased from 27 µg/mL and 33 µg/mL to 62 µg/mL and 66 µg/mL, respectively, in two patients previously stabilized on ZNS therapy when LTG was added. Signs and symptoms of toxicity appeared as LTG doses reached 400 mg/day and resolved as the dose was decreased (93). The mechanism for this interaction remains unexplained.

Interactions Resulting in Decreased Plasma Concentrations

It also can be anticipated that drugs capable of inducing metabolic enzymes will increase the clearance of ZNS and reduce its plasma concentration. The AEDs PHT, CBZ, and PB have all been shown to alter ZNS pharmacokinetics. Zonisamide half-life was 36.4 hours in

six patients with epilepsy coadministered CBZ and 27.1 hours in six patients treated with PHT (84) compared with about 60 hours in healthy volunteers (83). Furthermore, the ZNS plasma concentration-to-dose ratios were reduced in eight patients coadministered PB, 10 patients coadministered PHT, and 15 patients coadministered CBZ compared with 26 patients treated with ZNS monotherapy (94). Coadministration of clonazepam to seven patients had no effect on the plasma concentration-to-dose ratio of ZNS. Although the ZNS concentration-to-dose ratio demonstrated significant negative correlations with VPA dose and VPA plasma concentration, the overall difference in ratio between ZNS monotherapy and ZNS with VPA was not significant (91,94).

ESTABLISHED DRUGS COMMONLY USED IN CLINICAL PRACTICE: PHENOBARBITAL, CARBAMAZEPINE, PHENYTOIN, AND VALPROIC ACID

Phenobarbital

Most studies of PB demonstrate high bioavailability (less than 80%) and rapid absorption, with the average time to peak plasma concentrations occurring approximately 2 hours after dosing, although considerable variation exists between patients. Concentrations are linearly related to dose within a wide range of doses (95). Phenobarbital half-life is the longest among commonly used AEDs, ranging from 75 to 126 hours after single doses and even longer in newborn infants. Several studies have demonstrated that approximately 22% to 25% of a dose is excreted unchanged in the urine. It has also been shown that metabolic formation of p-hydroxyphenobarbital (PBOH) represents a major elimination pathway, accounting for 10% to 35% of the administered dose. An average of 56% of the PBOH formed is excreted as the O-glucuronide. The N-glucoside of PB also has been identified as a major metabolite, representing 26% of the PB dose in a study of five healthy volunteers. PB dihydrodiol and its corresponding catechol and m-hydroxyphenobarbital also have been identified as minor metabolites. The enzymes responsible for the metabolic clearance of PB have not been completely elucidated; however, in vitro studies in human liver microsomes or expressed enzymes suggest that CYP2C9 and CYP2C19 contribute substantially to the formation of PBOH (96).

Interactions Resulting in Increased Plasma Concentrations

Accumulation of PB caused by VPA is among the most likely and most clinically relevant interactions with PB. The mechanistic etiology of this interaction is most probably polymorphic. VPA inhibition of CYP2C9 (97), resulting in decreased PB clearance through p-hydroxylation, is likely to be one of the factors and is consistent with a role for CYP2C9 in PB metabolism. Consistent with this theory, the amount of PBOH was reduced by 30% after VPA administration in a study by Kapetanovic and Kupferberg (98). Although highly variable, plasma concentrations of PB may increase as much as twofold with addition of VPA. PHT also may increase PB levels in some patients (99). Because therapeutic levels of PHT are above its K_m for CYP2C9 (i.e., the enzyme is saturated), the mechanism for the PHT interaction with PB is likely also to be inhibition of CYP2C9. The degree of change and the clinical significance appear to be related to PB dose and concentration when PHT is added. In patients taking primidone, both VPA and PHT were associated with increased ratios of derived PB to dose when compared with patients taking primidone alone (100). Similarly, when methsuximide was administered to patients with petit mal seizures treated with PB or primidone, serum concentrations of PB increased by 38% and 40%, respectively (101). The precise mechanisms of these interactions have not been investigated. Dextropropoxyphene (65 mg, t.i.d., for 6 days) resulted in modest (10% to 15%) elevations of PB plasma concentrations (102), as did administration of acetazolamide (103) and phenylethylacetylurea (104).

Interactions Resulting in Decreased Plasma Concentrations

CBZ and PHT, among the most potent inducers known, have little effect on PB metabolism and usually do not alter plasma PB levels (104,105). Furthermore, there is little clinical or laboratory evidence that PB induces its own metabolism, even though PB is also a potent inducer. Inclusion of the psychotropic drug thioridazine in the therapy of patients also treated with PB was associated with a lower PB level-to-dose ratio compared with patients treated with PB alone (106).

Carbamazepine

The rate of CBZ absorption from the GI tract varies considerably between patients, but maximal plasma concentrations are generally reached 4 to 8 hours after ingestion. However, peaks as late as 24 hours have been reported (107). Estimates of bioavailability derived from administration of [^{14}C]CBZ range from 75% to 85% (108). The rate of disappearance from plasma also is variable. The half-life of CBZ after a single dose in healthy volunteers is 18 to 55 hours, but with repeated administration is reduced to 5 to 26 hours (107).

CBZ undergoes nearly complete biotransformation with only 2% to 5% of a given dose excreted unchanged (109,110). A large number of metabolites are formed by parallel or consecutive reactions. The enzymatic formation of carbamazepine 10,11-epoxide (CBZE) is quantitatively the most important metabolic pathway, accounting for 40% to 60% of the dose. Investigations with human liver microsomes, purified or expressed enzymes have identified two of the isoforms catalyzing the formation of CBZE as CYP3A4 and CYP2C8 (111). CBZE is subsequently hydrolyzed to CBZ DHD through the activity of microsomal epoxide hydrolase (mEH) and excreted largely in conjugated forms. Formation of 9-hydroxymethyl-10-carbamoylacridine and oxidation of the aromatic rings represent additional pathways of CBZ metabolism, which collectively represent an additional 10% to 25% of the total dose. Several CYP enzymes are probably involved in the formation of the phenolic metabolites that are subsequently excreted primarily as glucuronide conjugates. Because of the multiplicity of enzymes involved, these pathways will most likely contribute substantially to drug interactions only in the presence of broad-spectrum inhibitors.

Interactions Resulting in Increased Plasma Concentrations

A sizeable list of drugs from several therapeutic classes have been reported to interact with CBZ and increase its plasma concentration. Because the principal metabolic pathway (i.e., epoxidation to CBZE) is catalyzed primarily by CYP3A4, coadministration of any drug that inhibits CYP3A4 can be expected to decrease clearance of CBZ and increase plasma concentration. Inhibition of minor isoforms of CBZ clearance also may alter CBZ clearance but would be expected to be less significant clinically. Those drugs capable of inhibiting several enzymes at therapeutic concentrations, and therefore, multiple metabolic pathways, are most likely to cause interactions with CBZ. The clearance of CBZE, mediated by mEH, is also subject to inhibition, and adverse effects have been reported after addition of mEH inhibitors to treatment regimens using CBZ.

Increased CBZ plasma concentrations resulting in toxicity have been reported after coadministration of the calcium channel blockers diltiazem and verapamil (112–114). In a case described by Maoz et al. (115), a patient with epilepsy controlled with CBZ developed neurotoxicity after being given an increased dosage of diltiazem as adjunctive therapy. Abrupt discontinuation of diltiazem reduced CBZ plasma concentrations and resulted in loss of seizure control. In other cases (116), CBZ plasma levels have been increased approximately 200% after addition of diltiazem (120 mg/day) to stable CBZ monotherapy. Although diltiazem and verapamil are known to be substrates of CYP3A4 (4,117), the inhibition constants (K_i) determined in vitro for their inhibition of CYP3A4 are considerably higher than therapeutic concentrations. This suggests that diltiazem or verapamil do not inhibit by a simple competitive mechanism involving only the parent drug. The respective metabolites of diltiazem and verapamil may also inhibit CYP3A4, as demonstrated in vitro by Tsao et al. (118).

Inhibition of CBZ metabolism associated with macrolide antibiotics has been reported repeatedly and is among the most important drug interactions. Listed in decreasing order of tendency to inhibit CYP3A4 *in vitro*, troleandomycin (TAO), erythromycin, clarithromycin, roxithromycin, azithromycin, ponsinomycin, flurithromycin, josamycin, and spiramycin also inhibit the formation of CBZE and result in increased plasma concentrations of CBZ (119). Both TAO and erythromycin form a tight complex with CYP3A4, resulting in loss of enzyme activity (120). Addition of TAO (8–33 mg/kg/day) to the therapy of 17 patients on CBZ resulted in toxicity within 24 to 48 hours. Symptoms of toxicity disappeared 2 to 3 days after TAO was discontinued (121). Similarly, the clearance of CBZ was reduced 17% in healthy volunteers by erythromycin (250 mg every 6 hours for 8 days) (122). Numerous case reports have been published documenting the clinical significance of the erythromycin–CBZ interaction. Many of the newer macrolide antibiotics form weaker heme complexes with cytochrome P450, but nevertheless cause clinically relevant increases in CBZ plasma concentration (123). Even though CBZ dose was reduced approximately 22%, CBZ plasma levels increased by 50% when clarithromycin (500 mg/day) was added to the therapy of one patient with epilepsy (124). Similarly, josamycin (2 g daily for 1 week) decreased CBZ clearance by 17% (125). Flurithromycin and ponsinomycin are both newer macrolide antibiotics not known to inactivate heme complexes *in vitro* (126); however, both resulted in significant increases in the AUC of single doses of CBZ in healthy volunteers (127,128).

The effects of ketoconazole (200 mg/day orally for 10 days) on the plasma concentrations of CBZ and CBZE were assessed in eight patients with epilepsy receiving stable CBZ therapy. Consistent with inhibition of CYP3A4 by ketoconazole, CBZ plasma levels increased from 5.6 µg/mL to 7.2 µg/mL when ketoconazole was added (129), but a more pronounced effect was expected. Data with other antifungals are lacking.

The synthetic androgen danazol, used to treat endometriosis, increases steady-state plasma levels of CBZ 50% to 100% through inhibition of the epoxide-transdiol pathway (130). CBZ plasma concentrations reached 76 µ*M* in one patient 4 days after addition of danazol to previously stable CBZ therapy (1,400 mg/day) (131). Signs of toxicity resolved after discontinuation of danazol.

In a group of eight patients stabilized with CBZ therapy, toxicity was manifest, and trough plasma concentrations were increased from 6 to 11.7 µg/mL to 13.8 to 45 µg/mL after administration of propoxyphene. Symptoms resolved, and CBZ levels returned to baseline in all cases when propoxyphene administration was discontinued (132). The clinical importance of this interaction was evaluated by using population kinetics in a group of elderly patients ($n = 7,263$) who were part of a drug-dis-

pensing program in Sweden. In patients taking both CBZ and dextropropoxyphene, dosages for both drugs were lower and plasma levels higher than those in patients taking either drug alone. Plasma levels of the metabolite CBZE were lower in the combination group, indicating inhibition of the epoxide metabolic pathway (133).

Cimetidine has been noted to result in increased plasma concentrations of CBZ when coadministered to healthy volunteers (134). Although cimetidine has been shown to decrease the activity of CYP3A4 *in vitro,* thus suggesting an influence on this metabolic pathway *in vivo,* cimetidine also is known to inhibit CYP2C19 (135). This interaction appears to have only modest clinical significance, and increases in CBZ plasma concentrations in patients receiving long-term therapy may be compensated for by the inductive effects of additional CBZ (136).

Coadministration of the antidepressants fluoxetine and fluvoxamine has been reported to result in increased plasma concentrations and toxicity. In six healthy subjects taking CBZ (400 mg/day), addition of fluoxetine (20 mg for 7 days) decreased CBZ oral clearance from 3.87 ± 0.68 L/h to 2.98 ± 0.26 L/h and increased plasma concentrations of CBZ and CBZE approximately 30% (137). Additional studies also have demonstrated that both CBZ and CBZE are increased in the presence of fluoxetine, suggesting that this interaction is more complex than simple inhibition of CYP3A4-mediated epoxide formation (138). Consistent with this suggestion, the enantiomers of fluoxetine and their metabolites are known inhibitors of CYP2C19 and CYP2D6 (139) but affect CYP3A4 *in vitro* only at concentrations 20 times therapeutic concentrations (140). Fluvoxamine also has been implicated in decreasing the clearance of CBZ (141–143). Plasma concentrations of CBZ were increased from 7.3 µg/mL to 12.4 µg/mL after addition of 600 mg/day fluvoxamine to the regimen of a patient previously maintained with CBZ (143). Viloxazine (300 mg/day for 3 weeks), added to the regimen of six patients, increased CBZ concentrations from 7.5 ± 3.2 µg/mL to 11.6 ± 4.8 µg/mL (144). The concentration of CBZE also increased 16% in these subjects. Although the mechanisms responsible for these interactions are not completely understood, it should be noted that fluoxetine and its metabolites, fluvoxamine and viloxazine, are all potent inhibitors of CYP2C19. However, a substantial role for CYP2C19 in the clearance of CBZ has not been elucidated.

Isoniazid and nicotinamide also have been shown to decrease CBZ clearance and increase plasma concentrations; however, the enzymatic mechanisms for these interactions are less clear (145–147).

Interactions Resulting in Increased Plasma Concentrations of Carbamazepine 10,11-Epoxide

Plasma concentrations of the metabolite CBZE are approximately 10% to 30% of the parent drug in patients with epilepsy, and the unbound fraction of CBZE is larger than that of CBZ; thus CBZE contributes to both to pharmacologic and toxicologic activities. Because CBZE is cleared from plasma through the activity of mEH, inhibition of this enzyme can be expected to increase plasma concentrations of CBZE. The most notable interactions mediated through this pathway are the interactions with valpromide, VPA, and progabide. Meijer et al. (148) reported increased CBZE concentrations in patients treated with CBZ when VPA was replaced with valpromide. This suggested that valpromide was a potent mEH inhibitor. In a study of healthy volunteers, the half-life of a single oral dose of CBZE (100 mg) was compared in a control state and after administration of VPA (500 mg, b.i.d., for 6 days). The CBZE half-life was increased from 6.3 hours to 9.0 hours in the presence of VPA, and clearance was reduced by one third (149). Kerr et al. (149a) provided experimental evidence by evaluating the K_i values of VPA and valpromide toward mEH in human liver microsomes and in purified enzymes. Similar interactions have been reported when CBZ is administered with progabide (150,151).

Interactions Resulting in Decreased Plasma Concentrations

The metabolism of CBZ is highly inducible, most probably through induction of CYP3A4. Clearance is increased by the anticonvulsants PHT, PB, primidone, and FBM (129,152,153) and by rifampin (154). Moreover, CBZ induces its own metabolism. This factor complicates many inhibition studies in that, as CBZ levels increase as a result of inhibition, metabolism is increased, and plasma levels decrease as a new steady state is approached.

Phenytoin

Phenytoin is a prochiral compound that is slowly but almost completely absorbed. The drug undergoes extensive metabolism, with less than 5% of a given dose being excreted unchanged in urine. The principal urinary products are the glucuronide conjugates of p-hydroxyphenytoin (pHPPH), which exists as the (R) and (S) enantiomers. CYP2C9 has been identified as a primary isozyme in pHPPH formation (155,156). Stereoselectivity of metabolism and contribution of a second enzyme was suggested by the fact that urinary ratios of (S)-pHPPH to (R)-pHPPH decrease with increasing PHT plasma concentration (157). Based on this observation and the fact that pHPPH formation can be reduced by drugs known not to interact with CYP2C9, CYP2C19 was identified as a second contributor to pHPPH formation (158). Additional evidence of the contribution by CYP2C19 was generated in poor and extensive metabolizers of (S)-mephenytoin (159) in which the primary

change observed in poor metabolizers was a decrease in the formation of (R)-pHPPH, whereas excretion of (S)-pHPPH was unchanged. These observations are clarified by the fact that CYP2C9 forms predominantly the S-enantiomer (S/R ratio of 43), whereas CYP2C19 forms nearly equal amounts of both enantiomers (S/R ratio, 1.2) (158). The K_m estimates for PHT hydroxylation in expressed CYP2C9 and CYP2C19 were 5.5 μM and 70 μM, respectively. Thus therapeutic concentrations of PHT (up to 80 μM) should readily saturate CYP2C9, resulting in increasing fractional contribution by CYP2C19 as PHT plasma concentrations increase. Because of the saturability of biotransformation, the overall clearance of PHT is concentration dependent.

Interactions Resulting in Increased Plasma Levels

Because CYP2C9 and CYP2C19 both participate in the metabolism of PHT, it can be predicted that drugs inhibiting CYP2C9 or CYP2C19 at therapeutic concentrations will decrease PHT clearance and increase plasma concentrations. The extent of change in PHT clearance in any one individual depends, not only on the potency of the inhibitor and its plasma concentration, but also on the initial PHT concentration and the degree to which CYP2C9 and CYP2C19 contribute to the overall clearance. This information will be used to try to classify PHT drug interactions in two mechanistic groups: (a) those interactions involving inhibition of the primary CYP2C9, and (b) those interactions compatible with inhibition of CYP2C19. Inhibitors of CYP2C9 such as amiodarone, phenylbutazone, and fluconazole are also known to decrease the clearances of other CYP2C9 substrates such as S-warfarin and/or tolbutamide, whereas inhibitors of CYP2C19, such as cimetidine, FBM, and fluoxetine have no effect on warfarin and/or tolbutamide.

Interactions Consistent with Inhibition of CYP2C9

Amiodarone

After case reports of an interaction between amiodarone and PHT (92,160,161), healthy volunteers were given intravenous PHT before and after 3 weeks of oral amiodarone (200 mg/day). PHT half-life was increased from 16.1 to 22.6 hours in the presence of amiodarone (162). Subsequently, steady-state pharmacokinetic parameters were determined after 14 days of oral PHT (2–4 mg/kg/day) before and after amiodarone (200 mg daily for 6 weeks). In this case, amiodarone decreased the oral clearance of PHT from 1.29 ± 0.30 L/h to 0.93 ± 0.25 L/h and reduced the excretion of pHPPH by 33% (163).

Azapropazone and Phenylbutazone

Inhibition of PHT metabolism by the pyrazole nonsteroidal antiinflammatory drugs (NSAIDS) azapropazone and phenylbutazone is well documented (164,165). When azapropazone (600 mg, b.i.d.) was added to the therapy of five healthy volunteers stabilized with long-term oral PHT, plasma concentrations of PHT doubled, and urinary *p*HPPH/PHT ratios decreased, indicating inhibition of the *p*-hydroxylation pathway (166). Resolution of toxicity and decreased PHT concentrations were observed when azapropazone therapy was discontinued in patients with epilepsy (165). Similar interactions have been observed with coadministration of PHT and phenylbutazone, a drug no longer in clinical use (167).

Disulfiram

Increased concentrations of PHT were noted by Olesen (168) in patients treated concurrently with disulfiram (400 mg/day). In subsequent studies, PHT half-life was increased from 11 to 19 hours, and PHT clearance was reduced from 51.2 mL/min to 34 mL/min in the presence of disulfiram (169).

Antifungal Agents

Several reports in the literature described PHT toxicities in the presence of the antifungal agents fluconazole and miconazole (170,171). In healthy volunteers treated with 200 mg/day fluconazole, the AUC_{0-24} of intravenous PHT (250 mg) was increased 75%, and trough concentrations increased 125% over comparable parameters in a control (untreated) phase (172). In a similar study, PHT plasma concentrations were increased 132% by fluconazole (400 mg/day), whereas no effect was observed with treatment with ketoconazole (200 mg. b.i.d.), a compound with no CYP2C9-inhibiting activity. It should be noted that fluconazole has subsequently been shown to inhibit both CYP2C9 (K_i, 7–8 μM) and CYP2C19 (K_i, 2–6 μM) (2); consequently the mechanism of the interaction between fluconazole and PHT probably involves both enzymes. Intravenous miconazole, 500 mg q8h, for treatment of a fungal infection in a patient with epilepsy controlled with PHT (300 mg/day), resulted in nystagmus and ataxia with a concurrent twofold increase in PHT concentration (171). Coadministration of another imidazole antibiotic, metronidazole, has been shown to result in modest alterations in PHT metabolism. Clearance of intravenous PHT (300 mg) was reduced by 15%, and PHT half-life increased from 16 to 23 hours in the presence of metronidazole treatment (250 mg, t.i.d.) in healthy volunteers (173). Because miconazole and metronidazole also inhibit the clearance of warfarin, these interactions can be attributed to inhibition of CYP2C9 (174).

Isoniazid noncompetitively inhibits PHT metabolism and has resulted in significant PHT accumulation in 10% to 15% of patients using these drugs. The inhibitory effects of isoniazid are more serious in subjects identified as slow acetylators of isoniazid, in whom isoniazid levels are higher. This interaction is observed frequently in countries such as South Africa, where roughly 50% of the population are slow acetylators, and the incidence of tuberculosis is high (175).

Hansen et al. (176) demonstrated that sulfaphenazole, sulfadiazine, sulfamethizole, sulfamethoxazole, and cotrimoxazole all increased the half-life of an intravenous dose of PHT. Sulfaphenazole decreased PHT clearance by 67% and increased plasma concentrations by a factor of 2. There are additional case reports of PHT intoxication in patients coadministered cotrimoxazole (177). Because these agents also inhibit the metabolism of either (S)-warfarin or tolbutamide or both, these interactions can be attributed to inhibition of CYP2C9. Additionally, sulfaphenazole and cotrimoxazole are demonstrated inhibitors of CYP2C9 *in vitro*.

Coadministration of dicoumarol or phenprocoumon with PHT has been reported to cause elevation of plasma PHT levels in some patients, whereas warfarin and phenindione appear to have no effect on PHT (178).

Interactions Consistent with Inhibition of CYP2C19
Cimetidine

The inhibitory effects of cimetidine on PHT metabolism are well established (179–182). Addition of cimetidine, 900 to 1,200 mg/day, to the therapy of patients taking PHT reduces PHT clearance approximately 15% to 20% and concomitantly increases PHT plasma levels 13% to 60% (179,180,183,184).

Felbamate

Felbamate has been shown to inhibit CYP2C19 *in vitro* with an inhibition constant within the therapeutic range (K_i, 225 μM) (12). When FBM was added in a stepwise fashion from 0 to 400 to 600 mg, t.i.d., to the therapeutic regimen of patients with epilepsy previously treated with PHT monotherapy, PHT plasma concentrations increased, and PHT clearance decreased from 18 to 14 to 12 mL/h/kg in a dose-dependent manner (185).

Fluoxetine

After anecdotal observations from 23 cases, the interaction between fluoxetine and PHT was investigated. Fluoxetine was known to inhibit CYP2D6 and CYP3A4, but interactions with CYP2C9 or CYP2C19 had not been elucidated at that time. Two cases of toxicity were reported in patients with stable PHT (300 and 400 mg/day) monotherapy after addition of fluoxetine (40 and 20 mg/day) to their treatment. PHT levels in both cases increased to more than two-fold the levels with the same PHT dose without fluoxetine. Fluoxetine and its metabolite norfluoxetine have subsequently been shown to inhibit CYP2C19 *in vitro* (139,140).

Omeprazole

Although the AUC_{0-72h} of a single 300-mg dose of PHT was increased by 25% when healthy volunteers were comedicated with 40 mg/day omeprazole (186), a similar study using a lower dose (20 mg/day) failed to demonstrate any effect (187). Thus it appears that inhibition of PHT metabolism by omeprazole may be dependent on both omeprazole and PHT dose. Omeprazole is a substrate of CYP2C19 and inhibits this enzyme *in vitro*.

Ticlopidine

Increases in PHT plasma concentration and PHT-associated toxicity after the addition of the platelet antiaggregant ticlopidine to stable PHT therapy have been documented in several recent case reports (188–192). In one patient, acute symptomatic PHT toxicity was manifest, along with a serum concentration of 46.5 μg/mL, 25 days after addition of ticlopidine (193). These same researchers determined *in vitro* constants (K_i) of 3.7 μ*M* and 39 μ*M* for ticlopidine inhibition of CYP2C19 and CYP2C9, respectively, thus suggesting that this interaction results primarily from inhibition of CYP2C19.

Viloxazine

The effect of viloxazine (150–300 mg daily for 21 days) on plasma PHT levels at steady state was examined in 10 patients with epilepsy stabilized on a fixed PHT dose. After starting viloxazine treatment, plasma PHT concentrations increased 37% on average (range, 7% to 94%) during the last week of combined therapy (194). Although the mechanism for this interaction cannot be verified because specific urinary metabolites were not measured, inhibition of CYP2C19 is probably involved because viloxazine is known to inhibit this enzyme.

Topiramate and Zonisamide

In an add-on study, TPM was added to PHT therapies in doses up to 800 mg/day. Although the average change in PHT clearance among all patients was not significant, modest increases (up to 25%) in PHT plasma concentrations were observed in six of 12 patients treated with combined therapy, and PHT dose reductions were necessary (78). Addition of ZNS decreased the K_m observed for patients treated also with PHT (195). This is suggestive of modest inhibition of CYP2C19. Although TPM and ZNS have both been examined for their potential to inhibit the cytochromes P450 *in vitro*, inhibition of CYP2C19 was observed only at concentrations significantly higher than those achieved therapeutically. Significant inhibition of other P450 enzymes was not observed (3,90).

Other Interactions

Methylphenidate

It appears that methylphenidate may also inhibit PHT metabolism, although this interaction was not observed in healthy volunteers in a study by Mirkin and Wright (196). One case report documents an increase in PHT plasma concentration from 11.9 μg/mL to 56 μg/mL in a young patient treated with PHT when methylphenidate (10 mg, b.i.d.) was added. Signs of toxicity disappeared, and PHT levels returned to normal levels when methylphenidate was discontinued (197).

To study the pharmacokinetic interaction between PHT and methsuximide, PHT levels were measured in a group of patients with petit mal epilepsy. When methsuximide was given to patients taking PHT, the mean concentration of PHT increased by 78% (101). Although this interaction appears to result from metabolic inhibition, the isoform(s) involved have not been investigated.

Vigabatrin is associated with approximately 20% reductions of PHT steady-state serum concentrations, although the mechanism underlying this effect is unknown (198,199).

Valproic Acid

Valproic acid is rapidly and almost completely absorbed from the GI tract (200). The time to peak plasma concentration is generally 2 to 5 hours, dependent on gastric emptying time and the dissolution rate of the formulation. Clearance of VPA is mediated almost exclusively by hepatic metabolism, with less than 5% of an administered dose excreted unchanged. The half-life in healthy volunteers and in adult patients treated with monotherapy is 12 to 16 hours. Although the half-life is longer (up to 40 hours) in neonates (0–2 months), it is reduced to 8 to 10 hours in children (2 months to 10 years). Urinary metabolites account for greater than 85% of a given dose (201). VPA undergoes metabolism by a variety of processes including conjugation, acyl CoA formation, β-oxidation and other oxidative pathways, and desaturation. VPA glucuronide and 3-oxo-VPA are quantitatively the most abundant metabolites found in urine, followed by the conjugates of several hydroxylation products and the 4-oxo-derivative. Although unimportant quantitatively, the metabolite Δ^4-VPA is of interest because of its properties as a hepatotoxin. CYP2A6 and CYP2C9 have recently been identified as oxidative isozymes capable of forming Δ^4-VPA in humans (202).

Interactions Resulting in Increased Plasma Concentrations

Because of the multiplicity of pathways of VPA metabolism, drug interactions resulting in increased plasma concentrations are complex and often multifactorial. The enzymes mediating glucuronidation are most important quantitatively, followed by enzymes of β-oxidation and the CYP enzymes, so inhibition of any of these specific pathways may decrease VPA clearance and increase VPA plasma concentrations. Administration of FBM to patients treated with VPA has been shown to result in a 28% to 54% decrease in VPA clearance and concurrent increase in VPA plasma concentration (203). The effects of felbamate on the disposition of VPA were assessed in healthy volunteers who received VPA (400 mg/day) for 21 days (204). Felbamate was added in doses up to 3,600 mg/day. Plasma concentrations of VPA were increased by approximately 50% in the presence of FBM. Recovery of 3-oxo-VPA was reduced by FBM in a dose-dependent fashion, thus indicating inhibition of the β-oxidation pathway. A recent population-based pharmacokinetic study has also identified a significant reduction of the apparent clearance of VPA when coadministered with clobazam (205).

Addition of fluoxetine to stable VPA therapy has been reported to increase VPA plasma concentrations up to 150% compared with VPA alone. Although fluoxetine and its metabolite norfluoxetine are known to inhibit CYP2D6 and CYP2C19 at therapeutic concentrations of fluoxetine (139), the mechanism of the fluoxetine/VPA interaction is unclear. Preliminary clinical observations suggest a similar but unexplained decrease in VPA clearance in the presence of isoniazid (206,207) and guanfacine (208). VPA plasma level decreased 41% as guanfacine was discontinued in one patient and rapidly increased with addition of guanfacine in another. The inhibitory spectra of isoniazid and guanfacine have not been established.

Interactions Resulting in Decreased Plasma Concentrations

Reduction of VPA half-life and decreased VPA plasma concentrations are well-known phenomena when VPA is coadministered with the AEDs PHT, CBZ, and PB. Population-based investigations indicated that coadministration of these drugs with VPA increases relative VPA clearance compared with monotherapy (209). The magnitude of the change appears to be maximal (54%) in children coadministered CBZ (210). Typically, the half-life of VPA is reduced to 5 to 9 hours in patients treated concomitantly with these drugs, and VPA plasma concentrations are reduced 30% to 50% (200,211). Similarly, coadministration of ethosuximide and VPA in a group of children resulted in a 28% reduction in VPA serum concentration. Conversely, when ethosuximide was discontinued, VPA levels increased by 36.7% (212). Although not mediated through induction of oxidative enzymes, a small but significant decrease in steady-state VPA plasma concentration was noted after addition of LTG to VPA (500 mg, b.i.d.) in a group of healthy volunteers (213).

The AUC_{0-12} of VPA decreased 11.3% with the addition of TPM (400 mg, b.i.d.) (79).

Decreases in VPA levels due to concomitant administration of drugs other than anticonvulsants are less common. However, acyclovir has been reported to reduce plasma levels of PHT and VPA, resulting in loss of seizure control (214).

DRUGS USED LESS FREQUENTLY: ETHOSUXIMIDE, METHSUXIMIDE, BENZODIAZEPINES, AND RELATED AEDS

Ethosuximide

Ethosuximide is eliminated by hepatic enzymes (more than 90%) to one or two primary oxidative metabolites, which are subsequently excreted in the urine as their respective glucuronide conjugates. Although the isoforms involved in the metabolism of ethosuximide in humans have not been definitively characterized, the drug appears to exhibit a pattern of interactions including both induction and inhibition. Increased clearance of ethosuximide and reduction of its half-life have been reported with concomitant administration of CBZ, PB, and rifampin (215,216). Conversely, coadministration of VPA has been reported to prolong ethosuximide half-life and increase plasma concentrations. Mattson and Cramer (217) described a mean increase of 53% in the plasma level of ethosuximide in five patients when VPA was added. Similar results have been observed in healthy volunteers (218). It has also been suggested that isoniazid may inhibit the metabolism of ethosuximide, but evidence for this interaction is inconclusive (219).

Methsuximide has a short half-life and is quickly converted to its N-desmethyl metabolite from which the pharmacologic activity is derived. This active metabolite has a half-life of 28 to 36 hours (after a single dose) and is prolonged to 34 to 80 hours in adults with prolonged treatment (220). In a study of 94 hospitalized patients, higher N-desmethyl-methsuximide serum concentrations were observed in patients comedicated with PB or PHT (101). The mechanism of this interaction has not been elucidated.

Evidence exists suggesting that metabolism of the benzodiazepines diazepam, clonazepam, nitrazepam, clorazepate, and clobazam can be induced and the corresponding clearances increased by comedication with potent inducing drugs such as CBZ, PB, PHT, and rifampin. The metabolism of diazepam is mediated primarily by CYP2C19, and clearance may be reduced by inhibitors of this enzyme such as omeprazole, cimetidine, and FBM (221). CYP3A4 also participates in the hydroxylation of diazepam and its metabolite nordiazepam, but significant interactions mediated through inhibition of these pathways have not been reported. Lorazepam is eliminated primarily by glucuronidation

(222), and its clearance is relatively refractory to the effects of metabolic induction; however, coadministration of VPA reduced lorazepam clearance by approximately 40% through inhibition of glucuronyltransferases (223).

REFERENCES

1. Black DJ, Kunze KL, Wienkers LC, et al. Warfarin-fluconazole. II. A metabolically based drug interaction: in vivo studies. *Drug Metab Dispos* 1996;24:422–428.
2. Kunze KL, Wienkers LC, Thummel KE, Trager WF. Warfarin-fluconazole. I: inhibition of the human cytochrome P450-dependent metabolism of warfarin by fluconazole: in vitro studies. *Drug Metab Dispos* 1996;24:414–421.
3. Mather GG, Levy RH. Pharmacokinetics of polypharmacy: prediction of drug interactions. *Epilepsy Res Suppl* 1996;11:113–121.
4. Pichard L, Fabre I, Fabre G, et al. Cyclosporin A drug interactions: screening for inducers and inhibitors of cytochrome P-450 (cyclosporin A oxidase) in primary cultures of human hepatocytes and in liver microsomes. *Drug Metab Dispos* 1990;18:595–606.
5. Shumaker RC, Fantel C, Kelton E, Wong K, Weliky I. Evaluation of the elimination of (^{14}C) felbamate in healthy men. *Epilepsia* 1990;31:642.
6. Gudipati RM, Raymond RH, Ward DL, Shumaker RC, Perhach JL. Effect of food on the absorption of felbamate in healthy male volunteers. *Neurology* 1992;42(suppl 3):332.
7. Perhach JL, Weliky I, Newton JJ, Sofia RD, Romanyshyn WM, Arndt WFJ. Felbamate. In: Meldrum BS, Porter RJ, eds. *New anticonvulsant drugs.* London: John Libbey, 1986:117–123.
8. Sofia RD, Kramer L, Perhach JL, Rosenberg A. Felbamate. *Epilepsy Res Suppl* 1991;3:103–108.
9. Wilensky AJ, Friel PN, Ojemann LM, Kupferberg HJ, Levy RH. Pharmacokinetics of W-554 (ADD 03055) in epileptic patients. *Epilepsia* 1985;26:602–606.
10. Adusumalli VE, Choi YM, Romanyshyn LA, et al. Isolation and identification of 3-carbamoyloxy-2-phenylpropionic acid as a major human urinary metabolite of felbamate. *Drug Metab Dispos* 1993; 21:710–716.
11. Racha JK, Mather GG, Bishop FE, Kunze KL, Levy RH. Involvement of CYP3A4 and CYP2E1 in the metabolism of felbamate in human liver microsomes. In: *ISSX Proceedings; 7th North American ISSX Meeting; San Diego.* Bethesda, MD: International Society for the Study of Xenobiotics, 1996:370.
12. Glue P, Banfield CR, Perhach JL, Mather GG, Racha JK, Levy RH. Pharmacokinetic interactions with felbamate: in vitro-in vivo correlation. *Clin Pharmacokinet* 1997;33:214–224.
13. Montgomery PA, Sachdeo RJ, Narang-Sachdea SK, Rosenberg A, Perhach JL. Felbamate pharmacokinetics after coadministration of erythromycin. *Epilepsia* 1994;35(suppl 8):113.
14. Hussein G, Troupin AS, Montouris G. Gabapentin interaction with felbamate. *Neurology* 1996;47:1106.
15. Ward DL, Wagner ML, Perhach JL, et al. Felbamate steady-state pharmacokinetics during coadministration of valproate. *Epilepsia* 1991;32 (suppl 3):8.
16. Wagner ML, Leppik IE, Graves NM, Remme RP, Campbell JI. Felbamate serum concentrations: effect of valproate, carbamazepine, phenytoin and phenobarbital. *Epilepsia* 1990;31:642.
17. Wagner ML, Graves NM, Marienau K, Holmes GB, Remmel RP, Leppik IE. Discontinuation of phenytoin and carbamazepine in patients receiving felbamate. *Epilepsia* 1991;32:398–406.
18. Stewart BH, Kugler AR, Thompson PR, Bockbrader HN. A saturable transport mechanism in the intestinal absorption of gabapentin is the underlying cause of the lack of proportionality between increasing dose and drug levels in plasma. *Pharmacol Res* 1993;10:276–281.
19. Vollmer KO, Turck D, Wagner F, Jahnchen E, Anhut H, Thomman P. Multiple dose pharmacokinetics of the new anticonvulsant gabapentin. *Eur J Clin Pharmacol* 1989;36:A-310.
20. McLean MJ. Gabapentin. *Epilepsia* 1995;36(suppl 2):S73–S86.
21. Vollmer KO, von Hodenberg A, Kolle EU. Pharmacokinetics and metabolism of gabapentin in rat, dog and man. *Arzneimittelforschung* 1986;36:830–839.
22. Comstock TJ, Sica DA, Bockbrader HN, Underwood BA, Sedman AJ. Gabapentin pharmacokinetics in subjects with various degrees of renal function. *J Clin Pharmacol* 1990;30:862.
23. Hooper WD, Kavanagh MC, Herkes GK, Eadie MJ. Lack of a pharmacokinetic interaction between phenobarbitone and gabapentin. *Br J Clin Pharmacol* 1991;31:171–174.
24. Radulovic LL, Wilder BJ, Leppik IE, et al. Lack of interaction of gabapentin with carbamazepine or valproate [published erratum appears in *Epilepsia* 1994;35:707]. *Epilepsia* 1994;35:155–161.
25. Graves NM, Leppik IE, Wagner ML, Spencer MM, Erdmann GR. Effect of gabapentin on carbamazepine. *Epilepsia* 1990;31:644.
26. Crawford P, Ghadiali E, Lane R, Blumhardt L, Chadwick D. Gabapentin as an antiepileptic drug in man. *J Neurol Neurosurg Psychiatry* 1987;50:682–686.
27. Yuen AWC, Peck AW. Lamotrigine pharmacokinetics: oral and i.v. infusion in man. *Br J Clin Pharmacol* 1988;26:242P.
28. Peck AW. Clinical pharmacology of lamotrigine. *Epilepsia* 1991;32 (suppl 2):S9–S12.
29. Yuen AWC. Lamotrigine: interactions with other drugs. In: Levy RH, Mattson RH, Meldrum BS, ed. *Antiepileptic drugs.* 4th ed. New York: Raven Press, 1995:883–887.
30. Yau MK, Garnett WR, Wargin WA, Pellock JM. A single dose, dose proportionality, and bioequivalence study of lamotrigine in normal volunteers. *Epilepsia* 1991;32(suppl 3):8.
31. Cohen AF, Land GS, Breimer DD, Yuen WC, Winton C, Peck AW. Lamotrigine: a new anticonvulsant: pharmacokinetics in normal humans. *Clin Pharmacol Ther* 1987;42:535–541.
32. Sinz MW, Remmel RP. Analysis of lamotrigine and lamotrigine 2-*N*-glucuronide in guinea pig blood and urine by reserved-phase ion-pairing liquid chromatography. *J Chromatogr* 1991;571:217–230.
33. Doig MV, Clare RA. Use of thermospray liquid chromatography-mass spectrometry to aid in the identification of urinary metabolites of a novel antiepileptic drug, lamotrigine. *J Chromatogr* 1991;554:181–189.
34. Dickins M, Sawyer DA, Morley TJ, Parsons DN. Lamotrigine: chemistry and biotransformation. In: Levy RH, Mattson RH, Meldrum BS, eds. *Antiepileptic drugs.* 4th ed. New York: Raven Press, 1995:871–875.
35. Binnie CD, van Emde Boas W, Kasteleijn-Nolste-Trenite DG, et al. Acute effects of lamotrigine (BW430C) in persons with epilepsy. *Epilepsia* 1986;27:248–254.
36. Yuen AW, Land G, Weatherley BC, Peck AW. Sodium valproate acutely inhibits lamotrigine metabolism. *Br J Clin Pharmacol* 1992; 33:511–513.
37. Yau MK, Wargin WA, Wolf KB, et al. Effect of valproate on the pharmacokinetics of lamotrigine (Lamictal) at steady state. *Epilepsia* 1992;33:82.
38. Kaufman KR, Gerner R. Lamotrigine toxicity secondary to sertraline. *Seizure* 1998;7:163–165.
39. Colucci R, Glue P, Holt B, et al. Effect of felbamate on the pharmacokinetics of lamotrigine. *J Clin Pharmacol* 1996;36:634–638.
40. Binnie CD, Debets RM, Engelsman M, et al. Double-blind crossover trial of lamotrigine (Lamictal) as add-on therapy in intractable epilepsy. *Epilepsy Res* 1989;4:222–229.
41. Jawad S, Yuen WC, Peck AW, Hamilton MJ, Oxley JR, Richens A. Lamotrigine: single-dose pharmacokinetics and initial 1 week experience in refractory epilepsy. *Epilepsy Res* 1987;1:194–201.
42. Ramsay RE, Pellock JM, Garnett WR, et al. Pharmacokinetics and safety of lamotrigine (Lamictal) in patients with epilepsy. *Epilepsy Res* 1991;10:191–200.
43. Bass J, Matsuo F, Leroy RF, et al. Lamotrigine monotherapy in patients with partial epilepsies. *Epilepsia* 1990;31:643–644.
44. Berry DJ, Besag FMC, Pool F, Natarajan J, Doose D, Johnson RW. Does topiramate change lamotrigine serum concentrations when added to treatment? An audit of a dose-escalation study. *Epilepsia* 1998;39(suppl 6):56.
45. Depot M, Powell JR, Messenheimer JA Jr, Cloutier G, Dalton MJ. Kinetic effects of multiple oral doses of acetaminophen on a single oral dose of lamotrigine. *Clin Pharmacol Ther* 1990;48:346–355.
46. Thorgeirsson SS, Mitchell JR, Sasame HA, Potter WZ. Biochemical changes after hepatic injury by allyl alcohol and *N*-hydroxy-2-acetylaminofluorene. *Chem Biol Interact* 1976;15:139–147.
47. Dam M, Ostergaard LH. Other antiepileptic drugs: oxcarbazepine. In: Levy RH, Mattson RH, Meldrum BS, eds. *Antiepileptic drugs.* 4th ed. New York: Raven Press, 1995:987–995.

48. Augusteijn R, van Parys JAP. Oxcarbazepine (Trileptal, OXC): dose-concentration relationship in patients with epilepsy. *Acta Neurol Scand* 1990;82(suppl 133):37.

49. Dickinson RG, Hooper WD, Dunstan PR, Eadie MJ. First dose and steady-state pharmacokinetics of oxcarbazepine and its 10-hydroxy metabolite. *Eur J Clin Pharmacol* 1989;37:69–74.

50. Feldmann KF, Dorhofer G, Faigle JW, Imhof P. Pharmacokinetics and metabolism of GP 47 779, the main human metabolite of oxcarbazepine (GP 47 680) in animals and healthy volunteers. In: Dam M, Gram L, Penry JK, eds. *Advances in epileptology: XIIth epilepsy international symposium.* New York: Raven Press, 1981:89–96.

51. Schutz H, Feldmann KF, Faigle JW, Kriemler HP, Winkler T. The metabolism of ¹⁴C-oxcarbazepine in man. *Xenobiotica* 1986;16:769–778.

52. Keranen T, Jolkkonen J, Jensen PK, Menge GP, Andersson P. Absence of interaction between oxcarbazepine and erythromycin. *Acta Neurol Scand* 1992;86:120–123.

53. Pisani F, Fazio A, Oteri G, et al. Effects of the antidepressant drug viloxazine on oxcarbazepine and its hydroxylated metabolites in patients with epilepsy. *Acta Neurol Scand* 1994;90:130–132.

54. Pisani F, Oteri G, Russo M, et al. Double-blind, within-patient study to evaluate the influence of viloxazine on the steady-state plasma levels of oxcarbazepine and its metabolites. *Epilepsia* 1991;32(suppl 1):70.

55. Kramer G, Tettenborn B, Flesch G. Oxcarbazepine-verapamil drug interaction in healthy volunteers. *Epilepsia* 1991;32(suppl 1):70.

56. Mogensen PH, Jorgensen L, Boas J, et al. Effects of dextropropoxyphene on the steady-state kinetics of oxcarbazepine and its metabolites. *Acta Neurol Scand* 1992;85:14–17.

57. Keranen T, Jolkkonen J, Klosterskov-Jensen P, Menge GP. Oxcarbazepine does not interact with cimetidine in healthy volunteers. *Acta Neurol Scand* 1992;85:239–242.

58. Arnoldussen W, Hulsman J, Rentmeester T. Oxcarbazepine interactive with valproate? A clinical and pharmacokinetic study in several patient groups. *Epilepsia* 1992;33(suppl 3):111.

59. Rentmeester TW, Hulsman JARJ, Glue P, Banfield C. Effects of felbamate on the pharmacokinetics of oxcarbazepine. *Epilepsia* 1995;36(suppl 3):S160.

60. McKee PJW, Brodie MJ. Pharmacokinetic interactions with antiepileptic drugs. In: Trimble MR, ed. *New anticonvulsants: advances in the treatment of epilepsy.* Chichester: John Wiley and Sons, 1994:1–33.

61. Kumps A, Wurth C. Oxcarbazepine disposition: preliminary observations in patients. *Biopharmacol Drug Dispos* 1990;11:365–370.

62. Gustavson LE, Mengel HB. Pharmacokinetics of tiagabine, a gamma-aminobutyric acid-uptake inhibitor, in healthy subjects after single and multiple doses. *Epilepsia* 1995;36:605–611.

63. Inami M, Watanabe H, Takahashi A, Fujiwara H, Jansen NA, Murasaki M. Tiagabine in healthy Japanese subjects: single- and multiple-dose study. *Epilepsia* 1995;36(suppl 3):S158.

64. Jansen JA, Oliver S, Dirach J, B. MH. Absolute bioavailability of tiagabine. *Epilepsia* 1995;36(suppl 3):S159.

65. Mengel HB, Pierce MW, Mant T, Christensen MS, Gustavson L. Tiagabine: safety and tolerance during 2-week multiple dosing to healthy volunteers. *Epilepsia* 1991;32(suppl 1):99.

66. Bopp BA, Gustavson LE, Johnson MK, et al. Disposition and metabolism of orally administered ¹⁴C-tiagabine in humans. *Epilepsia* 1992;33(suppl 3):83.

67. Bopp B, Gustavson L, Johnson M, et al. Pharmacokinetics and metabolism of [¹⁴C]tiagabine HCl after oral administration to human subjects. *Epilepsia* 1995;36(suppl 3):S158.

68. Bopp BA, Nequist GE, Rodrigues AD, et al. Role of the cytochrome P450 3A subfamily in the metabolism of (¹⁴C)-tiagabine by human hepatic microsomes. *Epilepsia* 1995;36(suppl 3):S159.

69. Cato A, Qian JX, Gustavson LE, et al. Pharmacokinetics and safety of tiagabine in subjects with various degrees of renal function. *Epilepsia* 1995;36(suppl 3):S159.

70. Snel S, Jonkman JHG, van Heiningen PNM, Jansen JA, Mengel HG. Tiagabine: evaluation of interaction with cimetidine in healthy male volunteers. *Epilepsia* 1994;35(suppl 7):74.

71. Thomsen MS, Groes L, Agerso H, Kruse T. Lack of pharmacokinetic interaction between tiagabine and erythromycin. *J Clin Pharmacol* 1998;38:1051–1056.

72. Richens A, Gustavson LE, McKelvy JF, Mengel H, Deaton R, Pierce MW. Pharmacokinetics and safety of single-dose tiagabine HCl in epileptic patients chronically treated with four other antiepileptic drug regimens. *Epilepsia* 1991;32(suppl 3):12.

73. So EL, Wolff D, Graves NM, et al. Pharmacokinetics of tiagabine as add-on therapy in patients taking enzyme-inducing antiepilepsy drugs. *Epilepsy Res* 1995;22:221–226.

74. Easterling DE, Zaksewski T, Moyer MD, Margul BL, Marriott TB, Nayak RK. Plasma pharmacokinetics of topiramate, a new anticonvulsant in humans. *Epilepsia* 1988;29:662.

75. Ben-Menachem E. Vigabatrin. *Epilepsia* 1995;36(suppl 2):S95–S104.

76. Doose DR, Scott VV, Margul BL, Marriott TB, Nayak RK. Multiple dose pharmacokinetics of topiramate in healthy male subjects. *Epilepsia* 1988;29:662.

77. Doose DR, Walker SA, Sachdeo R, Kramer LD, Nayak RK. Steady-state pharmacokinetics of Tegretol (carbamazepine) and Topamax (topiramate) in patients with epilepsy on monotherapy, and during combination therapy. *Epilepsia* 1994;35(suppl 8):54.

78. Gisclon LG, Curtin CR, Kramer LD. The steady-state (SS) pharmacokinetics (PK) of phenytoin (Dilantin) and topiramate (Topamax) in epileptic patients on monotherapy, and during combination therapy. *Epilepsia* 1994;35(suppl 8):54.

79. Rosenfeld WE, Liao S, Kramer LD, et al. Comparison of the steady-state pharmacokinetics of topiramate and valproate in patients with epilepsy during monotherapy and concomitant therapy. *Epilepsia* 1997;38:324–333.

80. Haegele KD, Schechter PJ. Kinetics of the enantiomers of vigabatrin after an oral dose of the racemate or the active S-enantiomer. *Clin Pharmacol Ther* 1986;40:581–586.

81. Reidenberg P, Glue P, Banfield C, et al. Pharmacokinetic interaction studies between felbamate and vigabatrin. *Br J Clin Pharmacol* 1995;40:157–160.

82. Sackellares JC, Donofrio PD, Wagner JG, Abou-Khalil B, Berent S, Aasved-Hoyt K. Pilot study of zonisamide (1,2-benzisoxazole-3-methanesulfonamide) in patients with refractory partial seizures. *Epilepsia* 1985;26:206–211.

83. Ito T, Yamaguchi T, Miyazaki H, et al. Pharmacokinetic studies of AD-810, a new antiepileptic compound: Phase I trials. *Arzneimittelforschung* 1982;32:1581–1586.

84. Ojemann LM, Shastri RA, Wilensky AJ, et al. Comparative pharmacokinetics of zonisamide (CI-912) in epileptic patients on carbamazepine or phenytoin monotherapy. *Ther Drug Monit* 1986;8:293–296.

85. Shellenberger K, Wallace J, Groves L. Effect of food on pharmacokinetics of zonisamide in healthy volunteers. *Epilepsia* 1998;39(suppl 6):191.

86. Mimaki T. Clinical pharmacology and therapeutic drug monitoring of zonisamide [In Process Citation]. *Ther Drug Monit* 1998;20:593–597.

87. Wagner JG, Sackellares JC, Donofrio PD, Berent S, Sakmar E. Nonlinear pharmacokinetics of CI-912 in adult epileptic patients. *Ther Drug Monit* 1984;6:277–283.

88. Matsumoto K, Miyazaki H, Fujii T, Kagemoto A, Maeda T, Hashimoto M. Absorption, distribution and excretion of 3-(sulfamoyl[¹⁴C]methyl)-1,2-benzisoxazole (AD-810) in rats, dogs and monkeys and of AD-810 in men. *Arzneimittelforschung* 1983;33:961–968.

89. Nakasa H, Komiya M, Ohmori S, Rikihisa T, Kiuchi M, Kitada M. Characterization of human liver microsomal cytochrome P450 involved in the reductive metabolism of zonisamide. *Mol Pharmacol* 1993;44:216–221.

90. Mather GG, Carlson S, Trager WF, Buchanan RA, Levy RH. Prediction of zonisamide interactions based on metabolic isozymes. *Epilepsia* 1997;38(suppl 8):108.

91. Nakasa H, Nakamura H, Ono S, et al. Prediction of drug-drug interactions of zonisamide metabolism in humans from in vitro data. *Eur J Clin Pharmacol* 1998;54:177–183.

92. Groves L, Wallace J, Shellenberger K. Effect of cimetidine on zonisamide pharmacokinetics in healthy volunteers. *Epilepsia* 1998;39(suppl 6):191.

93. McJilton J, DeToledo J, DeCerce J, Huda S, Abubakr A, Ramsay RE. Cotherapy of lamotrigine/zonisamide results in significant elevation of zonisamide levels. *Epilepsia* 1996;37(suppl 5):173.

94. Shinoda M, Akita M, Hasegawa M, Hasegawa T, Nabeshima T. The necessity of adjusting the dosage of zonisamide when coadministered with other anti-epileptic drugs. *Biol Pharm Bull* 1996;19:1090–1092.

95. Dodson WE, Rust RS. Phenobarbital: absorption, distribution, and excretion. In: Levy RH, Mattson RH, Meldrum BS, eds. *Antiepileptic drugs.* 4th ed. New York: Raven Press, 1995:379–387.

96. Hargreaves JA, Howald WN, Racha JK, Levy RH. Identification of enzymes responsible for the metabolism of phenobarbital. In: *ISSX Proceedings; 7th North American ISSX Meeting; San Diego.* Bethesda, MD: International Society for the Study of Xenobiotics, 1996:259.

97. Hurst S, Labroo R, Carlson S, Mather G, Levy R. In vitro inhibition profile of valproic acid for cytochrome P450. In: *ISSX Proceedings; 8th North American ISSX Meeting; Hilton Head, SC.* Bethesda, MD: International Society for the Study of Xenobiotics, 1997:64.

98. Kapetanovic IM, Kupferberg HJ. Stable isotope methodology and gas chromatography mass spectrometry in a pharmacokinetic study of phenobarbital. *Biomed Mass Spectrom* 1980;7:47–52.

99. Morselli PL, Rizzo M, Garattini S. Interaction between phenobarbital and diphenylhydantoin in animals and in epileptic patients. *Ann NY Acad Sci* 1971;179:88–107.

100. Yukawa E, Higuchi S, Aoyama T. The effect of concurrent administration of sodium valproate on serum levels of primidone and its metabolite phenobarbital. *J Clin Pharm Ther* 1989;14:387–392.

101. Rambeck B. Pharmacological interactions of methsuximide with phenobarbital and phenytoin in hospitalized epileptic patients. *Epilepsia* 1979;20:147–156.

102. Dam M, Christiansen JM, Brandt J, et al. Antiepileptic drugs: interaction with dextropropoxyphene. In: Johannessen SI, Morselli PL, Pippenger CE, Richens A, Schmidt D, Meinardi HH, eds. *Antiepileptic therapy: advances in drug monitoring.* New York: Raven Press, 1980: 299–304.

103. Kelly WN, Richardson AP, Mason MF, Rector FC. Acetazolamide in phenobarbital intoxication. *Arch Intern Med* 1966;117:64–69.

104. Perucca E. Pharmacokinetic interactions with antiepileptic drugs. *Clin Pharmacokinet* 1982;7:57–84.

105. Kutt H. Interactions between anticonvulsants and other commonly prescribed drugs. *Epilepsia* 1984;25(suppl 2):S118–S131.

106. Gay PE, Madsen JA. Interaction between phenobarbital and thioridazine. *Neurology* 1983;33:1631–1632.

107. Morselli PL. Carbamazepine: absorption, distribution, and excretion. In: Levy RH, Mattson RH, Meldrum BS, ed. *Antiepileptic drugs.* 4th ed. New York: Raven Press, 1995:515–528.

108. Faigle JW, Feldmann KF. Pharmacokinetic data of carbamazepine and its major metabolites in man. In: Schneider H, et al., eds. *Clinical pharmacology of anti-epileptic drugs.* Berlin: Springer, 1975:159–165.

109. Eichelbaum M, Tomson T, Tybring G, Bertilsson L. Carbamazepine metabolism in man: induction and pharmacogenetic aspects. *Clin Pharmacokinet* 1985;10:80–90.

110. Faigle JW, Feldmann KF. Antiepileptic drugs. In: Levy RH, Mattson RH, Melrum BS, eds. *Antiepileptic drugs.* 4th ed. New York: Raven Press, 1995:499–513.

111. Kerr BM, Thummel KE, Wurden CJ, et al. Human liver carbamazepine metabolism: role of CYP3A4 and CYP2C8 in 10,11-epoxide formation. *Biochem Pharmacol* 1994;47:1969–1979.

112. Brodie MJ, MacPhee GJ. Carbamazepine neurotoxicity precipitated by diltiazem. *Br Med J* 1986;292:1170–1171.

113. Gadde K, Calabrese JR. Diltiazem effect on carbamazepine levels in manic depression. *J Clin Psychopharmacol* 1990;10:378–379.

114. Bahls FH, Ozuna J, Ritchie DE. Interactions between calcium channel blockers and the anticonvulsants carbamazepine and phenytoin. *Neurology* 1991;41:740–742.

115. Maoz E, Grossman E, Thaler M, Rosenthal T. Carbamazepine neurotoxic reaction after administration of diltiazem. *Arch Intern Med* 1992;152:2503–2504.

116. Ahmad S. Diltiazem-carbamazepine interaction [Letter]. *Am Heart J* 1990;120:1485–1486.

117. Kroemer HK, Gautier JC, Beaune P, Henderson C, Wolf CR, Eichelbaum M. Identification of P450 enzymes involved in metabolism of verapamil in humans. *Naunyn Schmiedebergs Arch Pharmacol* 1993; 348:332–337.

118. Tsao SC, Dickinson TH, Abernethy DR. Metabolite inhibition of parent drug biotransformation: studies of diltiazem. *Drug Metab Dispos* 1990;18:180–182.

119. Ketter TA, Post RM, Worthington K. Principles of clinically important drug interactions with carbamazepine: part I. *J Clin Psychopharmacol* 1991;11:198–203.

120. Lindstrom TD, Hanssen BR, Wrighton SA. Cytochrome P-450 com-

121. Mesdjian E, Dravet C, Cenraud B, Roger J. Carbamazepine intoxication due to triacetyloleandomycin administration in epileptic patients. *Epilepsia* 1980;21:489–496.

122. Pessayre D, Larrey D, Funck-Brentano C, Benhamou JP. Drug interactions and hepatitis produced by some macrolide antibiotics. *J Antimicrob Chemother* 1985;16(suppl A):181–194.

123. Tinel M, Descatoire V, Larrey D, et al. Effects of clarithromycin on cytochrome P-450: comparison with other macrolides. *J Pharmacol Exp Ther* 1989;250:746–751.

124. Albani F, Riva R, Baruzzi A. Clarithromycin-carbamazepine interaction: a case report. *Epilepsia* 1993;34:161–162.

125. Vincon G, Albin H, Demotes-Mainard F, Guyot M, Bistue C, Loiseau P. Effects of josamycin on carbamazepine kinetics. *Eur J Clin Pharmacol* 1987;32:321–323.

126. Larrey D, Tinel M, Pessayre D. Formation of inactive cytochrome P-450 Fe(II)-metabolite complexes with several erythromycin derivatives but not with josamycin and midecamycin in rats. *Biochem Pharmacol* 1983;32:1487–1493.

127. Couet W, Istin B, Ingrand I, Girault J, Fourtillan JB. Effect of ponsinomycin on single-dose kinetics and metabolism of carbamazepine. *Ther Drug Monit* 1990;12:144–149.

128. Barzaghi N, Gatti G, Crema F, et al. Effect of flurithromycin, a new macrolide antibiotic, on carbamazepine disposition in normal subjects. *Int J Clin Pharmacol Res* 1988;8:101–105.

129. Spina E, Arena D, Scordo MG, Fazio A, Pisani F, Perucca E. Elevation of plasma carbamazepine concentrations by ketoconazole in patients with epilepsy. *Ther Drug Monit* 1997;19:535–538.

130. Kramer G, Theisohn M, von Unruh GE, Eichelbaum M. Carbamazepine-danazol drug interaction: its mechanism examined by a stable isotope technique. *Ther Drug Monit* 1986;8:387–392.

131. Hayden M, Buchanan N. Danazol-carbamazepine interaction [Letter]. *Med J Aust* 1991;155:851.

132. Oles KS, Mirza W, Penry JK. Catastrophic neurologic signs due to drug interaction: tegretol and darvon. *Surg Neurol* 1989;32: 144–151.

133. Bergendal L, Friberg A, Schaffrath AM, Holmdahl M, Landahl S. The clinical relevance of the interaction between carbamazepine and dextropropoxyphene in elderly patients in Gothenburg, Sweden. *Eur J Clin Pharmacol* 1997;53:203–206.

134. Christiansen J, Dam M. Drug interaction in epileptic patients. In: Schneider H, Janz D, Gardner-Thorpe C, Meinardi H, Sherwin AL, eds. *Clinical pharmacology of anti-epileptic drugs.* Berlin: Springer-Verlag, 1975:197–200.

135. Knodell RG, Browne DG, Gwozdz GP, Brian WR, Guengerich FP. Differential inhibition of individual human liver cytochromes P-450 by cimetidine. *Gastroenterology* 1991;101:1680–1691.

136. Levine M, Jones MW, Sheppard I. Differential effect of cimetidine on serum concentrations of carbamazepine and phenytoin. *Neurology* 1985;35:562–565.

137. Grimsley SR, Jann MW, Carter JG, D'Mello AP, D'Souza MJ. Increased carbamazepine plasma concentrations after fluoxetine coadministration. *Clin Pharmacol Ther* 1991;50:10–15.

138. Gidal BE, Anderson GD, Seaton TL, Miyoshi HR, Wilenksy AJ. Evaluation of the effect of fluoxetine on the formation of carbamazepine epoxide. *Ther Drug Monit* 1993;15:405–409.

139. Preskorn SH. *Clinical pharmacology of selective serotonin reuptake inhibitors.* Caddo, OK: Professional Communications, 1996.

140. Ring BJ, Binkley SN, Roskos L, Wrighton SA. Effect of fluoxetine, norfluoxetine, sertraline and desmethyl sertraline on human CYP3A catalyzed 1'-hydroxy midazolam formation in vitro. *J Pharmacol Exp Ther* 1995;275:1131–1135.

141. Martinelli V, Bochetta A, Palmas AM, Del Zompo M. An interaction between carbamazepine and fluvoxamine. *Br J Clin Pharmacol* 1993; 36:615–616.

142. Fritze J, Unsorg B, Lanczik M. Interaction between carbamazepine and fluvoxamine. *Acta Psychiatr Scand* 1991;84:583–584.

143. Bonnet P, Vandel S, Nezelof S, Sechter D, Bizouard P. Carbamazepine, fluvoxamine: is there a pharmacokinetic interaction? [Letter]. *Therapie* 1992;47:165.

144. Pisani F, Fazio A, Oteri G, et al. Carbamazepine-viloxazine interaction in patients with epilepsy. *J Neurol Neurosurg Psychiatry* 1986;49: 1142–1145.

145. Block SH. Carbamazepine-isoniazid interaction. *Pediatrics* 1982;69: 494–495.
146. Fleenor ME, Harden JW, Curtis G. Interaction between carbamazepine and antituberculosis agents [Letter]. *Chest* 1991;99:1554.
147. Bourgeois BF, Dodson WE, Ferrendelli JA. Interactions between primidone, carbamazepine, and nicotinamide. *Neurology* 1982;32: 1122–1126.
148. Meijer JW, Binnie CD, Debets RM, van Parys JA, de Beer-Pawlikowski NK. Possible hazard of valpromide-carbamazepine combination therapy in epilepsy [Letter]. *Lancet* 1984;1:802.
149. Pisani F, Caputo M, Fazio A, et al. Interaction of carbamazepine-10,11-epoxide, an active metabolite of carbamazepine, with valproate: a pharmacokinetic study. *Epilepsia* 1990;31:339–342.
149a. Kerr BM, Rettie AE, Eddy AC, et al. Inhibition of human liver microsomal epoxide hydrolase by valproate and valpromide: *in vitro/in vivo* correlation. *Clin Pharmacol Ther* 1989;46:82–93.
150. Bianchetti G, Padovani P, Thenot JP, Thiercelin JF, Morselli PL. Pharmacokinetic interactions of progabide with other antiepileptic drugs. *Epilepsia* 1987;28:68–73.
151. Graves NM, Fuerst RH, Cloyd JC, Brundage RC, Welty TE, Leppik IE. Progabide-induced changes in carbamazepine metabolism. *Epilepsia* 1988;29:775–780.
152. Albani F, Theodore WH, Washington P, et al. Effect of felbamate on plasma levels of carbamazepine and its metabolites. *Epilepsia* 1991; 32:130–132.
153. Graves NM, Holmes GB, Fuerst RH, Leppik IE. Effect of felbamate on phenytoin and carbamazepine serum concentrations. *Epilepsia* 1989; 30:225–229.
154. Bachmann KA, Jauregui L. Use of single sample clearance estimates of cytochrome P450 substrates to characterize human hepatic CYP status in vivo. *Xenobiotica* 1993;23:307–315.
155. Doecke CJ, Veronese ME, Pond SM, et al. Relationship between phenytoin and tolbutamide hydroxylations in human liver microsomes. *Br J Clin Pharmacol* 1991;31:125–130.
156. Veronese ME, Mackenzie PI, Doecke CJ, McManus ME, Miners JO, Birkett DJ. Tolbutamide and phenytoin hydroxylations by cDNA-expressed human liver cytochrome P4502C9 [published erratum appears in *Biochem Biophys Res Commun* 1991;180:1527]. *Biochem Biophys Res Commun* 1991;175:1112–1118.
157. Fritz S, Lindner W, Roots I, Frey BM, Kupfer A. Stereochemistry of aromatic phenytoin hydroxylation in various drug hydroxylation phenotypes in humans. *J Pharmacol Exp Ther* 1987;241:615–622.
158. Bajpai M, Roskos LK, Shen DD, Levy RH. Roles of cytochrome P4502C9 and cytochrome P4502C19 in the stereoselective metabolism of phenytoin to its major metabolite. *Drug Metab Dispos* 1996;24: 1401–1403.
159. Ieiri I, Mamiya K, Urae A, et al. Stereoselective 4′-hydroxylation of phenytoin: relationship to (S)-mephenytoin polymorphism in Japanese. *Br J Clin Pharmacol* 1997;43:441–445.
160. McGovern B, Geer VR, LaRaia PJ, Garan H, Ruskin JN. Possible interaction between amiodarone and phenytoin. *Ann Intern Med* 1984; 101:650–651.
161. Shackleford EJ, Watson FT. Amiodarone–phenytoin interaction [Letter]. *Drug Intell Clin Pharmacol* 1987;21:921.
162. Nolan PE Jr, Marcus FI, Hoyer GL, Bliss M, Gear K. Pharmacokinetic interaction between intravenous phenytoin and amiodarone in healthy volunteers. *Clin Pharmacol Ther* 1989;46:43–50.
163. Nolan PE Jr, Erstad BL, Hoyer GL, Bliss M, Gear K, Marcus FI. Steady-state interaction between amiodarone and phenytoin in normal subjects [Comments]. *Am J Cardiol* 1990;65:1252–1257.
164. Roberts CJ, Daneshmend TK, Macfarlane D, Dieppe PA. Anticonvulsant intoxication precipitated by azapropazone. *Postgrad Med J* 1981; 57:191–192.
165. Geaney DP, Carver JG, Aronson JK, Warlow CP. Interaction of azapropazone with phenytoin. *Br Med J* 1982;284:1373.
166. Geaney DP, Carver JG, Davies CL, Aronson JK. Pharmacokinetic investigation of the interaction of azapropazone with phenytoin. *Br J Clin Pharmacol* 1983;15:727–734.
167. Andreasen PB, Froland A, Skovsted L, Andersen SA, Hauge M. Diphenylhydantoin half-life in man and its inhibition by phenylbutazone: the role of genetic factors. *Acta Med Scand* 1973;193:561–564.
168. Olesen OV. Disulfiram (Antabuse) as inhibitor of phenytoin metabolism. *Acta Pharmacol Toxicol* 1966;24:317–322.
169. Svendsen TL, Kristensen MB, Hansen JM, Skovsted L. The influence of disulfiram on the half life and metabolic clearance rate of diphenylhydantoin and tolbutamide in man. *Eur J Clin Pharmacol* 1976;9: 439–441.
170. Cadle RM, Zenon GJ III, Rodriguez-Barradas MC, Hamill RJ. Fluconazole-induced symptomatic phenytoin toxicity. *Ann Pharmacother* 1994;28:191–195.
171. Rolan PE, Somogyi AA, Drew MJ, Cobain WG, South D, Bochner F. Phenytoin intoxication during treatment with parenteral miconazole. *Br Med J* 1983;287:1760.
172. Blum RA, Wilton JH, Hilligoss DM, et al. Effect of fluconazole on the disposition of phenytoin. *Clin Pharmacol Ther* 1991;49:420–425.
173. Blyden GT, Scavone JM, Greenblatt DJ. Metronidazole impairs clearance of phenytoin but not of alprazolam or lorazepam. *J Clin Pharmacol* 1988;28:240–245.
174. O'Reilly RA. The stereoselective interaction of warfarin and metronidazole in man. *N Engl J Med* 1976;295:354–357.
175. Walubo A, Aboo A. Phenytoin toxicity due to concomitant antituberculosis therapy. *S Afr Med J* 1995;85:1175–1176.
176. Hansen JM, Kampmann JP, Siersbaek-Nielsen K, et al. The effect of different sulfonamides on phenytoin metabolism in man. *Acta Med Scand Suppl* 1979;624:106–110.
177. Gillman MA, Sandyk R. Phenytoin toxicity and co-trimoxazole [Letter]. *Ann Intern Med* 1985;102:559.
178. Skovsted L, Kristensen M, Hansen M, Siersbaek-Nielsen K. The effect of different oral anticoagulants on diphenylhydantoin (DPH) and tolbutamide metabolism. *Acta Med Scand* 1976;199:513–515.
179. Algozzine GJ, Stewart RB, Springer PK. Decreased clearance of phenytoin with cimetidine [Letter]. *Ann Intern Med* 1981;95:244–245.
180. Hetzel DJ, Bochner F, Hallpike JF, Shearman DJ, Hann CS. Cimetidine interaction with phenytoin. *Br Med J* 1981;282:1512.
181. Phillips P, Hansky J. Phenytoin toxicity secondary to cimetidine administration [Letter]. *Med J Aust* 1984;141:602.
182. Salem RB, Breland BD, Mishra SK, Jordan JE. Effect of cimetidine on phenytoin serum levels. *Epilepsia* 1983;24:284–288.
183. Neuvonen PJ, Tokola RA, Kaste M. Cimetidine-phenytoin interaction: effect on serum phenytoin concentration and antipyrine test. *Eur J Clin Pharmacol* 1981;21:215–220.
184. Sambol NC, Upton RA, Chremos AN, Lin ET, Williams RL. A comparison of the influence of famotidine and cimetidine on phenytoin elimination and hepatic blood flow. *Br J Clin Pharmacol* 1989;27:83–87.
185. Sachdeo RC, Padela MF. The effect of felbamate on phenobarbital serum concentrations. *Epilepsia* 1994;35(suppl 8):94.
186. Prichard PJ, Walt RP, Kitchingman GK, et al. Oral phenytoin pharmacokinetics during omeprazole therapy. *Br J Clin Pharmacol* 1987;24: 543–545.
187. Andersson T, Lagerstrom PO, Unge P. A study of the interaction between omeprazole and phenytoin in epileptic patients. *Ther Drug Monit* 1990;12:329–333.
188. Lopez-Ariztegui N, Ochoa M, Sanchez-Migallon MJ, Nevado C, Martin M. [Acute phenytoin poisoning secondary to an interaction with ticlopidine]. *Rev Neurol* 1998;26:1017–1018.
189. Rindone JP, Bryan G II. Phenytoin toxicity associated with ticlopidine administration [Letter]. *Arch Intern Med* 1996;156:1113.
190. Riva R, Cerullo A, Albani F, Baruzzi A. Ticlopidine impairs phenytoin clearance: a case report. *Neurology* 1996;46:1172–1173.
191. Klaassen SL. Ticlopidine-induced phenytoin toxicity. *Ann Pharmacother* 1998;32:1295–1298.
192. Privitera M, Welty TE. Acute phenytoin toxicity followed by seizure breakthrough from a ticlopidine-phenytoin interaction. *Arch Neurol* 1996;53:1191–1192.
193. Donahue SR, Flockhart DA, Abernethy DR, Ko JW. Ticlopidine inhibition of phenytoin metabolism mediated by potent inhibition of CYP2C19. *Clin Pharmacol Ther* 1997;62:572–577.
194. Pisani F, Fazio A, Artesi C, et al. Elevation of plasma phenytoin by viloxazine in epileptic patients: a clinically significant drug interaction. *J Neurol Neurosurg Psychiatry* 1992;55:126–127.
195. Odani A, Hashimoto Y, Takayanagi K, et al. Population pharmacokinetics of phenytoin in Japanese patients with epilepsy: analysis with a dose-dependent clearance model. *Biol Pharm Bull* 1996;19:444–448.
196. Mirkin BL, Wright F. Drug interactions: effect of methylphenidate on the disposition of diphenylhydantoin in man. *Neurology* 1971;21: 1123–1128.
197. Ghofrani M. Possible phenytoin-methylphenidate interaction [Letter]. *Dev Med Child Neurol* 1988;30:267–268.

198. Rimmer EM, Richens A. Interaction between vigabatrin and phenytoin. *Br J Clin Pharmacol* 1989;27(suppl 1):27S–33S.

199. Rimmer EM, Richens A. Double-blind study of gamma-vinyl GABA in patients with refractory epilepsy. *Lancet* 1984;1:189–190.

200. Levy RH, Shen DD. Valproic acid: absorption, distribution, and excretion. In: Levy RH, Mattson RH, Meldrum BS, eds. *Antiepileptic drugs*. 4th ed. New York: Raven Press, 1995:605–619.

201. Baillie TA, Sheffels PR. Valproic acid: chemistry and biotransformation. In: Levy RH, Mattson RH, Meldrum BS, eds. *Antiepileptic drugs*. 4th ed. New York: Raven Press, 1995:589–604.

202. Sadeque AJM, Fisher MB, Korzekwa KR, Gonzalez FJ, Rettie AE. Human CYP2C9 and CYP2A6 mediate formation of the hepatotoxin 4-ene-valproic acid. *J Pharmacol Exp Ther* 1997;283:698–703.

203. Wagner ML, Graves NM, Leppik IE, et al. The effect of felbamate on valproic acid disposition. *Clin Pharmacol Ther* 1994;56:494–502.

204. Hooper WD, Franklin ME, Glue P, et al. Effect of felbamate on valproic acid disposition in healthy volunteers: inhibition of beta-oxidation. *Epilepsia* 1996;37:91–97.

205. Theis JG, Koren G, Daneman R, et al. Interactions of clobazam with conventional antiepileptics in children. *J Child Neurol* 1997;12:208–213.

206. Jonville AP, Gauchez AS, Autret E, et al. Interaction between isoniazid and valproate: a case of valproate overdosage [Letter]. *Eur J Clin Pharmacol* 1991;40:197–198.

207. Dockweiler U. Isoniazid-induced valproic-acid toxicity, or vice versa [Letter]. *Lancet* 1987;2:152.

208. Ambrosini PJ, Sheikh RM. Increased plasma valproate concentrations when coadministered with guanfacine. *J Child Adolesc Psychopharmacol* 1998;8:143–147.

209. Yukawa E, To H, Ohdo S, Higuchi S, Aoyama T. Population-based investigation of valproic acid relative clearance using nonlinear mixed effects modeling: influence of drug-drug interaction and patient characteristics. *J Clin Pharmacol* 1997;37:1160–1167.

210. Yukawa E, To H, Ohdo S, Higuchi S, Aoyama T. Detection of a drug-drug interaction on population-based phenobarbitone clearance using nonlinear mixed-effects modeling. *Eur J Clin Pharmacol* 1998;54:69–74.

211. Scheyer RD, Mattson RH. Valproic acid: interactions with other drugs. In: Levy RH, Mattson RH, Meldrum BS, eds. *Antiepileptic drugs*. 4th ed. New York: Raven Press, 1995:621–631.

212. Salke-Kellermann RA, May T, Boenigk HE. Influence of ethosuximide on valproic acid serum concentrations. *Epilepsy Res* 1997;26:345–349.

213. Anderson GD, Yau MK, Gidal BE, et al. Bidirectional interaction of valproate and lamotrigine in healthy subjects. *Clin Pharmacol Ther* 1996;60:145–156.

214. Parmeggiani A, Riva R, Posar A, Rossi PG. Possible interaction between acyclovir and antiepileptic treatment. *Ther Drug Monit* 1995;17:312–315.

215. Pisani F, Bialer M. Ethosuximide: chemistry and biotransformation. In: Levy RH, Mattson RH, Meldrum BS, eds. *Antiepileptic drugs*. 4th ed. New York: Raven Press, 1995:655–658.

216. Bialer M, Xiaodong S, Perucca E. Ethosuximide: absorption, distribution, and excretion. In: Levy RH, Mattson RH, Meldrum BS, eds. *Antiepileptic drugs*. 4th ed. New York: Raven Press, 1995:659–666.

217. Mattson RH, Cramer JA. Valproic acid and ethosuximide interaction. *Ann Neurol* 1980;7:583–584.

218. Pisani F, Narbone MC, Trunfio C, et al. Valproic acid-ethosuximide interaction: a pharmacokinetic study. *Epilepsia* 1984;25:229–233.

219. van Wieringen A, Vrijlandt CM. Ethosuximide intoxication caused by interaction with isoniazid. *Neurology* 1983;33:1227–1228.

220. Browne TR. Methsuximide. In: Levy RH, Mattson RH, Meldrum BS, eds. *Antiepileptic drugs*. 4th ed. New York: Raven Press, 1995:681–688.

221. Yasumori T, Nagata K, Yang SK, et al. Cytochrome P450 mediated metabolism of diazepam in human and rat: involvement of human CYP2C in *N*-demethylation in the substrate concentration-dependent manner. *Pharmacogenetics* 1993;3:291–301.

222. Homan RW, Treiman DM. Lorazepam. In: Levy RH, Mattson RH, Meldrum BS, eds. *Antiepileptic drugs*. 4th ed. New York: Raven Press, 1995:779–790.

223. Anderson GD, Gidal BE, Kantor ED, Wilensky AJ. Lorazepam-valproate interaction: studies in normal subjects and isolated perfused rat liver. *Epilepsia* 1994;35:221–225.

CHAPTER 18

Antidepressants

Kan Chiba and Kaoru Kobayashi

Tricyclic antidepressants have been widely used for the treatment of major depression since the early 1960s (1). The mechanism of their action has been accounted for by the inhibition of neuronal reuptake of biogenic amines. Tricyclic antidepressants with a tertiary amine side chain, such as imipramine, have an effect on the reuptake of norepinephrine and serotonin. On the other hand, those with a secondary amine side chain, such as desipramine, are highly selective for the reuptake of norepinephrine. Recently, a series of new antidepressants with diverse chemical structures designated as selective serotonin reuptake inhibitors (SSRIs) have emerged (1). They have a great affinity for the reuptake carrier of serotonin and much less affinity for that of norepinephrine. In addition to tricyclic antidepressants and SSRIs, atypical antidepressants with less defined pharmacologic characters as well as monoamine oxidase inhibitors have been used.

During the course of antidepressant therapy, metabolic drug interactions are often a problem that may modify the outcome of treatment (2–5). For example, certain SSRIs increase plasma concentration of tricyclic antidepressants and may potentiate their effects. On the other hand, anticonvulsants and cigarette smoking decrease plasma concentration of tricyclic antidepressants and may reduce their effects. These drug interactions are caused by the inhibition or induction of hepatic cytochrome P450 (CYP) involved in the metabolism of antidepressants.

In the past decade, considerable advances have been made in the area of drug metabolism, particularly human CYPs and related areas (6–8). Much information has been accumulated regarding which isoform of CYP is responsible for the metabolism of therapeutic agents, and which drugs inhibit or induce specific isoforms of CYP (8). This kind of knowledge may allow one to understand and predict drug–drug interactions of antidepressants that may occur through the modification of CYP-related drug metabolism.

This chapter describes the interactions of antidepressants, focusing on the modification of CYP-dependent metabolism of antidepressants by other drugs and that of other drugs by antidepressants. Also described is the CYP-catalyzed metabolism of the antidepressants, which is essential to understanding the metabolic interactions of the antidepressants.

METABOLISM OF ANTIDEPRESSANTS

Tertiary amine tricyclics are metabolized by way of demethylation to secondary amine tricyclics (Fig. 18-1). Tertiary amine and secondary amine tricyclics are also metabolized by way of hydroxylation (see Fig. 18-1). Hydroxylation of tertiary and secondary amine tricyclics is mediated exclusively by CYP2D6, whereas demethylation of tertiary amine tricyclics is catalyzed by multiple forms of CYP including CYP2C19, CYP1A2, and CYP3A4 (see Fig. 18-1). SSRIs undergo extensive oxidative metabolism catalyzed by CYP. The metabolism of fluoxetine and paroxetine is predominantly catalyzed by CYP2D6 whereas both CYP2D6 and CYP1A2 appear to be involved in the metabolism of fluvoxamine. N-Demethylation of citalopram is mediated by CYP2C19 and CYP3A4.

Tricyclics

Imipramine and Desipramine

Imipramine is exclusively metabolized in the liver. Major metabolic pathways of imipramine are 2-hydroxylation and demethylation to form an active metabolite, desipramine (see Fig. 18-1). Desipramine is further oxidized to 2-hydroxydesipramine (see Fig. 18-1). 2-Hydroxymetabolites of imipramine and desipramine

K. Chiba and K. Kobayashi: Laboratory of Biochemical Pharmacology and Toxicology, Department of Pharmaceutical Sciences, Chiba University, 1-33 Yayoi-cho, Inage-ku, Chiba-shi, Chiba 263-8522, Japan

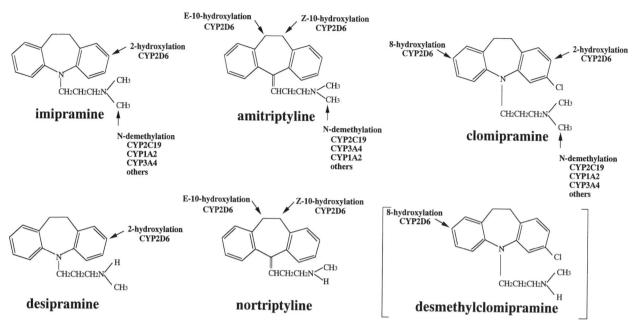

FIG. 18-1. The structures of tricyclic antidepressants (imipramine, desipramine, amitriptyline, nortriptyline, clomipramine, and its metabolite, desmethylclomipramine), the sites of metabolism, and the CYP isoforms involved.

retain some ability to block the uptake of amines and may have cardiac depressant actions (9). They are excreted in urine predominantly as glucuronide conjugates. *In vitro* and *in vivo* studies have clearly demonstrated that 2-hydroxylation of imipramine and desipramine is mainly catalyzed by CYP2D6 (10–12), whereas *N*-demethylation of imipramine is mediated by CYP2C19 (13,14). *In vitro* studies have also shown that CYP1A2 and CYP3A4 are involved in the *N*-demethylation of imipramine as the second and third enzymes, respectively (15,16).

Amitriptyline and Nortriptyline

The predominant metabolic process of amitriptyline is aliphatic hydroxylation in position 10 of the central ring and *N*-demethylation to form an active metabolite, nortriptyline (see Fig. 18-1). Nortriptyline is further oxidized to 10-hydroxynortriptyline (see Fig. 18-1). Because of asymmetry on the side chains of amitriptyline and nortriptyline, the genometric isomers of 10-hydroxy metabolites—E- and Z-10-hydroxyamitriptyline and E- and Z-10-hydroxynortriptyline—are formed. The formation is stereoselective with E-10-hydroxy metabolites exceeding the Z-configured metabolites in quantity (17). These 10-hydroxymetabolites may have some biologic activity but are less cardiotoxic than 2-hydroxy metabolites of imipramine or desipramine (18). *In vitro* and *in vivo* studies have shown that the formation of E-10-hydroxymetabolites of amitriptyline and nortriptyline are mediated by CYP2D6, whereas CYP2C19 is involved in the

N-demethylation of amitriptyline (19–21). *In vitro* studies also have shown that CYP3A4, CYP1A2, CYP2D6, and CYP2C9 catalyze the *N*-demethylation of amitriptyline (20,21).

Clomipramine

Clomipramine undergoes extensive metabolism in humans. Side chain *N*-demethylation leads to the formation of an active metabolite, desmethylclomipramine (see Fig. 18-1). Both clomipramine and desmethylclomipramine are hydroxylated in the aromatic position of 8, leading to the formation of 8-hydroxyclomipramine and 8-hydroxydesmethylclomipramine, respectively (see Fig. 18-1). Clomipramine is also hydroxylated to form 2-hydroxyclomipramine (see Fig. 18-1). *In vitro* and *in vivo* studies showed that the major isoform of CYP involved in the 2- and 8-hydroxylation of clomipramine and 8-hydroxylation of desmethylclomipramine is CYP2D6 (22, 23), while *N*-demethylation of clomipramine is catalyzed by CYP2C19 (22, 23). An *in vitro* study also suggests that multiple isoforms of CYP including CYP3A4 and CYP1A2 are involved in the *N*-demethylation of clomipramine in addition to CYP2C19 (23).

Amoxapine

Amoxapine is oxidized predominantly to 8-hydroxyamoxapine with some production of a 7-hydroxy metabolite. 7-Hydroxyamoxapine is pharmacologically active, probably with an antagonistic action for the dopamine D_2 receptor (24). There are no published data on which isoform of CYP is involved in 7- and 2-hydroxylation of amoxapine.

Maprotyline

Little information is available on the metabolism of maprotiline in humans. However, a human panel study showed that the mean area under the plasma concentration–time curve (AUC) is 3.5 times greater in poor metabolizers of debrisoquine than in extensive metabolizers, suggesting that approximately 70% of maprotiline clearance is explainable by metabolism through CYP2D6 (25).

Mianserin

Mianserin is administered as the racemic mixture of R-(−)- and S-(+)-mianserin. The S-(+)-enantiomer is much more pharmacologically active than the R-(−)-enantiomer (26). R-(−)- and S-(+)-mianserin are metabolized extensively in the liver and their major metabolic pathways are 8-hydroxylation, N-demethylation and N-oxidation. Previous in vivo studies suggested that 8-hydroxylation of S-(+)-mianserin is mediated by CYP2D6 and other processes are not (27). More recently, an in vitro study showed that 8-hydroxylation of both enatiomers of mianserin is mainly catalyzed by CYP2D6, whereas N-demethylation of both enantiomers and N-oxidation of S-(+)-mianserin is mainly mediated by CYP1A2 (28). The study also showed that CYP3A4 is responsible for each of the metabolic processes of mianserin enantiomers to a certain extent (28).

Selective Serotonin Reuptake Inhibitors

Fluoxetine

Fluoxetine is extensively metabolized and a very small fraction of an ingested dose appears as unchanged drug in urine (29). The major route of metabolism is N-demethylation to the active metabolite, norfluoxetine. Because the steady-state concentration of norfluoxetine approximates that of the parent compound, it is likely that this metabolite contributes significantly to the observed therapeutic or toxic effects of the medication (30). The formation of norfluoxetine from fluoxetine is considered to be predominantly catalyzed by CYP2D6, in that the partial metabolic clearance of fluoxetine to norfluoxetine is ten-fold less in poor metabolizers than in extensive metabolizers of debrisoquine (31). The finding indicates that 90% of the metabolic clearance of fluoxetine N-demethylation is mediated by CYP2D6. No published data are available regarding which isoform of CYP is involved in the further metabolism of norfluoxetine in humans.

Paroxetine

Paroxetine is almost completely metabolized in the liver. At least 85% of an oral dose of paroxetine is metabolized to a catechol intermediate, which undergoes subsequent methylation and conjugation to highly polar glucuronide or sulfate metabolites (32). Pharmacokinetic studies of paroxetine showed that there is considerable interindividual variation in plasma levels of paroxetine (33). For example, there is a 25-fold difference in steady-state plasma levels of paroxetine after repeated oral doses of 30 mg/day (34). This extreme variation is at least partially due to the polymorphism of CYP2D6 (35) and nonlinear elimination processes of paroxetine metabolism which consist of high-affinity but saturable and low-affinity but linear processes (34). The enzyme responsible for the high-affinity but saturable process is CYP2D6 because poor metabolizers of debrisoquine lack this process (34). However, no data are currently available regarding which enzyme is involved in the low-affinity process of paroxetine metabolism.

Sertraline

Sertraline is extensively metabolized in the liver and less than 0.2% of unchanged drug appears in the urine within 48 hours of administration (36). The primary metabolite of sertraline is N-desmethysertraline, which is one-tenth as potent as sertraline itself (37). Because no significant differences were found in the pharmacokinetics of sertraline and N-desmethysertraline between extensive and poor metabolizers of debrisoquine, CYP2D6 does not appear to play a major role in the metabolism of sertraline (31). An in vitro study using human liver microsomes and recombinant CYP indicated that multiple isoforms of CYP are involved in the demethylation of sertraline, including CYP2B6, CYP2C9, CYP2C19, CYP2D6, and CYP3A4 (38).

Fluvoxamine

Fluvoxamine is eliminated predominantly by oxidation in the liver (39). Numerous metabolites have been found in plasma and urine, although they appear to be devoid of significant pharmacologic activity (40). The main route of metabolism begins with the elimination of a methoxy group. Although the isoforms of CYP involved in the metabolism have not yet been identified, it has been reported that smokers have lower serum concentrations of fluvoxamine than nonsmokers (41,42). In addition, serum concentrations of fluvoxamine are higher in poor metabolizers of debrisoquine than in extensive metabolizers (43,44). The findings suggest that CYP1A2 and CYP2D6 play an important role in the metabolism of fluvoxamine in vivo.

Citalopram

Citalopram is metabolized by *N*-demethylation to desmethylcitalopram, which is further metabolized to didesmethylcitalopram and a propionic acid derivative (45). Twelve percent of administered dose is recovered as unchanged form, 12% as *N*-desmethylcitalopram, 1.5% as propionic acid metabolite, and 4.3% as conjugated propionic acid metabolite in human urine (45). *In vitro* and *in vivo* studies have suggested that CYP2C19 and CYP3A4 are involved in the *N*-demethylation of citalopram (46–48), whereas CYP2D6 mainly catalyzes further desmethylation of *N*-desmethylcitalopram (46).

Others

Trazodone

Trazodone is *N*-dealkylated to form *m*-chlorophenylpiperadine, an active metabolite with serotonergic activity (49). Previous *in vivo* studies suggested that CYP2D6 and CYP1A2 are involved in the metabolism of trazodone, because concurrent administration of thioridazine or fluoxetine increased the plasma concentration of trazodone, and smokers had lower plasma concentration of trazodone (50,51). However, a recent *in vitro* study using human liver microsomes and recombinant human CYPs indicated that the formation of *m*-chlorophenylpiperadine from trazodone is mainly catalyzed by CYP3A4 (52). Metabolic processes other than *N*-dealkylation might be mediated by CYP2D6 or CYP1A2.

Nefazodone

Nefazodone undergoes extensive presystemic metabolism mediated by CYP3A4 (53). Three active metabolites are formed—hydroxynefazodone, *m*-chlorophenylpiperadine, and triazoledione—which are thought to contribute to adverse events (54).

DRUG INTERACTIONS RESULTING FROM MODIFICATION OF ANTIDEPRESSANT METABOLISM BY OTHER DRUGS

Drug interactions of antidepressants that are caused by the modification of their metabolism are predominantly caused by the inhibition or induction of CYP. The major isoforms of human CYPs involved in the metabolism of antidepressants are CYP2D6, CYP2C19, CYP1A2, and CYP3A4. Inhibition of the enzymes results in increased plasma concentrations and may potentiate pharmacologic effects of antidepressants. Common side effects of antidepressants are anticholinergic effects, cardiovascular symptoms, increased risk of tonic-clonic seizures, and confusion or delirium secondary to central anticholinergic activity (1). These side effects may be more common for tricyclic antidepressants than for SSRIs, because of their wider therapeutic range (55). Therefore, clinically important interactions of antidepressants resulting from the inhibition of CYP-dependent metabolism are apparently limited to those of tricyclic antidepressants.

Enzyme induction leads to decreased plasma concentrations of parent drugs and may attenuate the effects of tricyclic antidepressants. However, when administration of the inducer is discontinued, plasma concentration of tricyclics can elevate and may lead to intoxication of tricyclic antidepressants. Among the isoforms of CYP involved in the metabolism of antidepressants in humans, CYP3A4, CYP2C19, and CYP1A2 are inducible forms (6–8).

Inhibition of CYP

CYP2D6

Because CYP2D6 is a key enzyme in the metabolism of antidepressants, coadministration of a drug with an inhibitory potency against CYP2D6 is expected to increase the plasma concentration of tricyclic antidepressants and may potentiate their effects. Many case studies and clinical trials have shown that inhibitors or substrates of CYP2D6 increase the plasma concentration of tricyclic antidepressants when they are administered concurrently (2–5). For example, Linnolia and colleagues (56) reported that patients receiving amitriptyline or nortriptyline in combination with perfenazine have up to 70% higher antidepressant plasma levels than patients receiving antidepressants alone. Brøsen and Gram (57) also reported that the total oral clearances of imipramine and desipramine were reduced by 35% and 85%, respectively, by the concurrent administration of quinidine in healthy volunteers. Certain SSRIs such as fluoxetine, paroxetine, and sertraline were also shown to increase plasma concentration of tricyclic antidepressants (2–5). These drugs (described earlier) are substrates or inhibitors of CYP2D6 (6–8). Other drugs that may inhibit CYP2D6 *in vivo* are neuroleptics, such as chlorpromazine (58), levomepromazine (59), thioridazine (60), and haloperidol (61); beta blockers, such as labetalol (62) and propranolol (63); and antiarrhythmic drugs, such as propafenone (64).

The extent of increase in the plasma concentration of tricyclic antidepressants caused by the inhibition of CYP2D6 depends on several factors, including the importance of CYP2D6 in the overall elimination of a tricyclic antidepressant from the body and the inhibitory potency of the concurrently administered drug against CYP2D6 (65). As described earlier, tertiary amine tricyclics are metabolized by way of hydroxylation catalyzed by CYP2D6 and demethylation processes mediated by multiple isoforms of CYP, whereas secondary amine tricyclics are metabolized only by way of hydroxylation catalyzed by CYP2D6. Therefore, when CYP2D6 is inhibited, the extent of increase in the plasma concentrations of antidepressants is expected to be more pronounced with secondary amine tricyclics than with tertiary amine tricyclics. This appears to be reflected on the interaction of imipramine and desipramine with quinidine, which causes three- and six-fold increases in the plasma levels of imipramine and desipramine, respectively (57).

With respect to the inhibitory potency of the concurrently administered drugs against CYP2D6, the most potent inhibitor of CYP2D6 reported previously is quinidine, which has a K_i value of 30 nM in human liver microsomes (66,67). Fluoxetine and paroxetine are other potent inhibitors of CYP2D6, with K_i values of less than 1 µM (67). When these drugs are coadministered with desipramine, plasma concentration of desipramine increases by six-fold, three- to four-fold, and three-fold by quinidine (57), fluoxetine (68,69), and paroxetine (70,71), respectively. On the contrary, fluvoxamine produces a minimal change in the plasma concentration of desipramine when it is administered concurrently (72,73). The K_i value of fluvoxamine against CYP2D6 is 8.2 µM in human liver microsomes (67). The findings suggest that the extent of increase in the plasma concentration of secondary amine tricyclics by the inhibitor of CYP2D6 corresponds well with their *in vitro* inhibitory potency against CYP2D6. However, *in vivo* inhibition of CYP2D6 is dependent not only on *in vitro* K_i value but also on other factors such as free drug concentration in the liver, the saturable kinetics of CYP2D6, and the presence of some metabolites that may inhibit CYP2D6 (65). Therefore, it is important to balance *in vitro* inhibitory potency and *in vivo* factors that may influence the disposition of the drug and its metabolites that may inhibit CYP2D6.

CYP2D6 is a classical isoform of CYP that shows the genetic polymorphism (74); approximately 7% of caucasians are defective in enzymatic activity (74). Genetic factors may also affect the magnitude of CYP2D6-dependent interaction of tricyclic antidepressants. For example, paroxetine decreases the clearance of desipramine in extensive metabolizers but not in poor metabolizers of debrisoquine (70), suggesting that coadministration of an inhibitor or substrate of CYP2D6 does not affect the clearance of secondary amine tricyclics in the subjects with the CYP2D6 deficiency. Similarly, CYP2D6-dependent interaction of tricyclic antidepressants may be attenuated in the intermediate metabolizers of CYP2D6 (who are heterozygous for the defective allele or homozygous for the Ch mutant allele) compared with extensive metabolizers who are homozygous for the wild-type allele. However, there is little information available regarding this topic.

CYP2C19

The demethylation process of tertiary amine tricyclics is mediated by multiple forms of CYP. However, CYP2C19 is the predominant enzyme responsible for this metabolic process of tricyclics; CYP2C19 accounts for approximately 50% of the demethylation of imipramine (75). Thus, coadministration of an inhibitor of CYP2C19 is expected to elevate plasma concentrations of imipramine and other tertiary amine tricyclics. In fact, fluvoxamine increases the plasma concentration of imipramine by three- to four-fold without affecting the concentration of desipramine, probably through the inhibition of CYP2C19 (72). Similarly, coadministration of fluoxetine with imipramine or desipramine results in three- to four-fold increase in AUC for both imipramine and desipramine (68,69). The increase in the imipramine concentration in plasma appears to be accounted for by the inhibition of imipramine *N*-demethylation by fluoxetine and norfluoxetine, because these compounds exhibit a significant inhibitory effect on the activity of CYP2C19 *in vitro* (76).

Among the substrates of CYP2C19, omeprazole may interact with tertiary amine tricyclics because omeprazole has been reported to increase the plasma concentration of diazepam in extensive metabolizers but not in poor metabolizers of mephenytoin, suggesting that omeprazole inhibits CYP2C19 *in vivo* (77).

CYP1A2 and CYP3A4

CYP1A2 and CYP3A4 may be partially involved in the demethylation of tertiary amine tricyclics *in vivo*. However, to what extent these enzymes are involved in other metabolic processes of tertiary amine tricyclics remains unclear. Recent studies using ketoconazole, a relatively specific inhibitor of CYP3A enzymes, showed that oral clearance of imipramine decreases by 20% with the administration of ketoconazole and that ketoconazole inhibits *N*-demethylation of imipramine without affecting 2-hydroxylation (78). Similarly, coadministration of troleandomycin, a specific inhibitor of CYP3A enzymes, decreases the oral clearance of imipramine by 30% in healthy volunteers (79). The findings suggest that inhibition of CYP3A4 does not produce a remarkable change in the plasma concentration of tricyclic antidepressants. Little information is available on the effects of the substrates or inhibitors of CYP1A2 on the disposition of antidepressants *in vivo*.

Others

Valproamide, or valproic acid, is used for treatment of affective disorders; therefore, it may be coadministered with tricyclic antidepressants. When they are administered concurrently, 50% to 60% increases in the plasma level of amitriptyline and nortriptyline have been reported (80,81). However, the particular CYP isoforms involved in this interaction remain unclear.

Cimetidine has been reported to increase the plasma concentration of tricyclic antidepressants 1.8- to 2.7-fold

(82,83). The effect of cimetidine is thought to be a general inhibition of CYP by the binding of an imidazole ring to the heme moiety of CYP.

Induction of CYP

CYP3A4 and CYP2C19

Important inducers of CYP3A4 are rifampicin and anticonvulsants (84,85). These drugs also induce CYP2C19 (86). Because CYP2C19 and CYP3A4 are involved in the demethylation process of tertiary amine tricyclics, plasma concentrations of tertiary amine tricyclics are expected to decrease in patients taking rifampicin or anticonvulsants. Brown and colleagues (87) reported that the dose of imipramine in patients given carbamazepine is significantly higher than when imipramine is given alone. Moreover, the plasma concentration of imipramine was significantly lower in patients given carbamazepine despite their receiving larger doses of imipramine (87). Similar findings were also reported for amitriptyline and other tertiary amine tricyclics (88). Therefore, coadministration of rifampicin or anticonvulsants such as carbamazepine, phenobarbital, and phenytoin may decrease the plasma concentration of tertiary amine tricyclic antidepressants and may attenuate their effects.

CYP1A2

Cigarette smoking induces CYP1A2 (84,85). CYP1A2 is partially involved in the demethylation pathway of imipramine and other tertiary amine tricyclics; therefore, the metabolism of these antidepressants can be accelerated by the smoking habit. Several reports have indicated that plasma concentrations of imipramine and other tertiary amine antidepressants are significantly lower in smokers than in nonsmokers (89–91). Recently, some proton-pump inhibitors, including omeprazole, were reported to induce CYP1A2 (92). Therefore, long-term administration of omeprazole may decrease the plasma concentration of tertiary amine tricyclic antidepressants.

Others

Anticonvulsants and rifampicin have been reported to increase the clearance of secondary amine tricyclics of which metabolism is predominantly catalyzed by CYP2D6. For example, Spina and colleagues (93,94) reported that the oral clearance of desipramine is increased by 70% in patients with epilepsy who are routinely given phenobarbital and by 40% in healthy volunteers given carbamazepine. These findings may be contradicted by the observation that a 7-day treatment of subjects with phenobarbital or rifampicin caused only 30% increase in the clearance of sparteine, a specific substrate of CYP2D6, suggesting that CYP2D6 is relatively resistant to the inducing effects of rifampicin and phenobarbital (95). Although the precise mechanism of the induction of the metabolism of secondary amine tricyclics remains controversial, larger doses of secondary amine tricyclics may be necessary for patients taking anticonvulsants or rifampicin.

MODIFICATION OF OTHER DRUGS' METABOLISM BY ANTIDEPRESSANTS

Newer antidepressants including SSRIs are potent inhibitors of several different isoforms of CYP (96–100). Fluoxetine substantially inhibits CYP2D6 and probably CYP2C9, moderately inhibits CYP2C19, and mildly inhibits CYP3A4. Paroxetine substantially inhibits CYP2D6 but does not appear to inhibit other isoforms of CYP. Sertraline produces moderate inhibition of CYP2D6 but has little effect on CYP1A2, CYP2C9, CYP2C19, or CYP3A4. Fluvoxamine inhibits CYP1A2 and CYP2C19 and may inhibit CYP3A4. Citalopram produces mild inhibition of CYP2D6. Nefazodone is a potent inhibitor of CYP3A4 and a weak inhibitor of CYP1A2 and CYP2D6. Venlafaxine does not seem to inhibit these isoforms of CYP. Inhibitory potencies of SSRIs on the individual isoforms of CYP are summarized in Table 18-1.

Antidepressants do not appear to induce CYP except that sertraline may be a weak inducer of CYP3A4 *in vivo*

TABLE 18-1. *Inhibitory potency of selective serotonin reuptake inhibitors and nefazodone on the individual isoforms of CYP*

	CYP1A2	CYP2C9	CYP2C19	CYP2D6	CYP3A4
Fluoxetine	−	++	++	+++	+/−
Fluvoxamine	+++	(+)	+++	−	+/−
Sertraline	−	(−)	(+)	+	(+)
Paroxetine	−	(−)	−	+++	(+)
Citalopram	−	NA	−	+	NA
Nefazodone	(−)	NA	NA	(−)	+++

+++, potent inhibition; ++, moderate inhibition; +, mild inhibition; −, no effect; +/−, contradicted; NA, not available *in vitro* and *in vivo*; (+), (−), based on *in vitro* studies.

(101). However, the inducing effect of sertraline on CYP3A4 is unlikely to be of clinical importance.

CYP2D6

Clinical and pharmacokinetic studies have shown substantial increases in plasma concentrations of tricyclic antidepressants associated with signs of toxicity when tricyclic antidepressants are coadministered with fluoxetine (68,69). This interaction seems to arise from the inhibition of CYP2D6 by fluoxetine or its active metabolite norfluoxetine, because *in vitro* studies using human liver microsomes demonstrated that fluoxetine and its metabolite norfluoxetine are potent inhibitors of CYP2D6 (67). Elimination half-life of norfluoxetine is much longer than fluoxetine, and significant levels of norfluoxetine continue to be detected in plasma 2 weeks after cessation of fluoxetine administration (30).

Similarly, paroxetine was reported to produce a remarkable increase in the plasma concentration of perfenazine associated with central nervous system side effects such as extrapyramidal symptoms and impairment of psychomotor performance (102). Because perfenazine is mainly metabolized by CYP2D6 (103), paroxetine is considered to be an inhibitor of CYP2D6 *in vivo* at a standard therapeutic dose. CYP2D6 metabolizes many useful therapeutic agents, including some tricyclic antidepressants, neuroleptics, beta-blockers, type Ic antiarrhythmics, and morphine derivatives (6–8). Therefore, dosage of these drugs should be reduced when fluoxetine or paroxetine is administered concurrently, particularly when patients are taking CYP2D6 substrates with a narrow therapeutic window.

Treatment of subjects with 50 mg/day of sertraline for 10 days increases plateau concentrations of desipramine in plasma by 44% and AUC by 37% (71). Because this increase in plasma levels of desipramine is much lower than those reported for fluoxetine or paroxetine (three- to four-fold increase), sertraline appears to be a modest inhibitor of CYP2D6 *in vivo*.

Fluvoxamine and citalopram do not show a remarkable effect on the disposition of drugs metabolized by CYP2D6 (72,73). The administration of citalopram causes a modest increase in sparteine metabolic ratio, an index of CYP2D6 activity *in vivo*. However, the extent of increase is small and phenotype does not change from extensive to poor metabolizers of debrisoquine (104).

CYP1A2

Fluvoxamine is a potent inhibitor of CYP1A2, whereas other SSRIs are weak inhibitors of the enzyme *in vitro* (105). In accordance with the *in vitro* findings, concomitant administration of fluvoxamine increases plasma concentrations of theophylline (106,107) and caffeine (108), both of which are representative substrates of CYP1A2 (6–8). Fluvoxamine was also reported to elevate the plasma concentration of imipramine (72) and clozapine (109), which are partially metabolized by CYP1A2 (6–8).

Other SSRIs including fluoxetine, paroxetine, citalopram, and sertraline did not change the metabolic ratio of caffeine (104,110).

CYP2C9

There are a few case reports indicating that clearance of phenytoin is reduced when it is coadministered with fluoxetine (111–114). Because the clearance of phenytoin predominantly depends on CYP2C9-mediated metabolism (115), it was thought that fluoxetine has the potential to inhibit CYP2C9. This idea was confirmed in *in vitro* studies showing that fluoxetine, particularly its *R*-enantiomer, and norfluoxetine inhibit *p*-hydroxylation of phenytoin in human liver microsomes (116). Similarly, fluvoxamine was reported to produce 65% increase in a plasma concentration of warfarin and increase anticoagulant effects (117). Because warfarin is mainly metabolized by CYP2C9 (118), this interaction is considered to be produced by the inhibitory effects of fluvoxamine on CYP2C9. CYP2C9 metabolizes various drugs with narrow therapeutic ranges, such as phenytoin, warfarin, tolbutamide, and some nonsteroidal antiinflammatory drugs (6–8). Careful monitoring of plasma levels or caution should be exercised when these drugs are administered with fluoxetine or fluvoxamine.

In vitro and *in vivo* studies have suggested that sertraline is a weak inhibitor of CYP2C9 in humans. A pharmacokinetic study showed a small but statistically significant decrease (16%) in the clearance of tolbutamide in patients receiving the maximum recommended dosage of sertraline (119). Sertraline also produced a small increase in the free fraction of warfarin and a modest increase in the prothrombin time, although it is considered to be clinically insignificant (120). These *in vivo* findings are consistent with the *in vitro* observation that sertraline and desmethylsertraline are relatively weak inhibitors of CYP2C9 in human liver microsomes (116). There are no *in vivo* data showing the inhibitory effects of paroxetine and citalopram on CYP2C9-mediated drug metabolism, although *in vitro* data suggest that paroxetine may inhibit CYP2C9 (116).

CYP2C19

S to *R* ratio of mephenytoin, an indicator of CYP2C19 activity *in vivo*, increases significantly after the administration of fluoxetine (104). However, because phenotype of subjects does not change from extensive to poor metabolizer of mephenytoin, fluoxetine appears to be a moderate inhibitor of CYP2C19 *in vivo* (104). This is consistent with the *in vitro* finding that fluoxetine shows a modest inhibition of CYP2C19 activity in human liver microsomes (76). It may be noteworthy that norfluoxetine is a more potent inhibitor of CYP2C19 than its parent compound, fluoxetine, in human liver microsomes (14). Norfluoxetine appears to contribute to some extent to the inhibitory effects of fluoxetine on CYP2C19 *in vivo*. Because phenytoin is also partly metabolized by CYP2C19 (121), inhibition of this enzyme may also explain the fluoxetine-phenytoin interaction.

Therapeutic doses of fluvoxamine administered for 2 weeks caused a significant increase in the *S/R* ratio of mephenytoin (73). In addition, partial clearance of chloroguanide to form cycloguanil, its active metabolite, decreases significantly during fluvoxamine intake in extensive metabolizers but not in poor metabolizers of mephenytoin (122). Moreover, fluvoxamine markedly inhibits the *N*-demethylation of imipramine without affecting 2-hydroxylation of imipramine (72). The findings suggest that fluvoxamine is an effective inhibitor of CYP2C19 *in vivo*.

Sertraline appears to exhibit a weak inhibitory effect on CYP2C19 *in vivo*. For example, a pharmacokinetic study indicated that the systemic clearance of diazepam decreased by 13% as compared to placebo when sertraline was administered repeatedly, although this decrease in diazepam clearance is not clinically meaningful (123).

Citalopram is a weak inhibitor of (*S*)-mephenytoin 4′-hydroxylation *in vitro* (76), but no significant increase in *S/R* ratio of mephenytoin is seen after a usual dose of citalopram to healthy volunteers (104). Paroxetine does not appear to inhibit CYP2C19 because the *S/R* ratio of mephenytoin does not change during the concurrent administration of paroxetine (104).

CYP3A4

CYP3A4 metabolizes a number of drugs including alprazolam, triazolam, midazolam, terfenadine, astemizole, carbamazepine, calcium channel blockers, cyclosporine, erythromycin, and others (6–8). In this regard, CYP3A4 is the most important isoform of CYP in relation to the occurrence of drug–drug interactions. Among the clinically used antidepressants, nefazodone is the most potent inhibitor of CYP3A4; it is contraindicated with concurrent administration of terfenazine, astemizole, and cisapride (100,124).

Fluvoxamine appears to inhibit CYP3A4 moderately. *In vitro* studies showed that fluvoxamine inhibits the metabolism of alprazolam (125), terfenazine (126), and triazolam (127), which are predominantly metabolized by CYP3A4. In accordance with the *in vitro* findings, an *in vivo* study showed a decrease in the clearance of alprazolam by 55% during the treatment with fluvoxamine (128). A case report also showed that the trough levels of carbamazepine in plasma increased two-fold with the addition of fluvoxamine (129), although another report showed that metabolism of carbamazepine was not affected by fluvoxamine administration (130).

In vitro studies using human liver microsomes showed that fluoxetine and norfluoxetine are inhibitors of CYP3A4. However, their potencies are approximately 100-fold less than that of ketoconazole (126,127,131). In accordance with the *in vitro* findings, there is no change in the plasma concentration of carbamazepine in patients given fluoxetine (130). However, another study showed a 33% decrease in the intrinsic clearance of carbamazepine by the concurrent administration of fluoxetine in healthy volunteers (132). Similarly, fluoxetine does not produce a remarkable change in the pharmacokinetics of terfenadine in healthy volunteers (133), whereas a case report indicated that cardiac abnormalities developed after the addition of fluoxetine to terfenadine (134). Therefore, whether fluoxetine impairs the drug metabolism catalyzed by CYP3A4 *in vivo* remains controversial.

In vitro studies showed that sertraline and desmethylsertraline inhibit the metabolism of CYP3A4 substrates, triazolam, and midazolam (127,131). However, little information is available on the *in vivo* inhibition of CYP3A4 by sertraline. Similarly, there are no published data on the inhibitory effects of paroxetine and citalopram on the activity of CYP3A4.

REFERENCES

1. Baldessarini RJ. Drugs and the treatment of psychiatric disorders. In: Hardman JG, Molinoff PB, Ruddon RW, Goodman Gilman A, eds. *Goodman & Gilman's The pharmacological basis of therapeutics,* 9th ed. New York: McGraw-Hill, 1996.
2. Ketter TA, Flockhart DA, Post RM, et al. The emerging role of cytochrome P450 3A in psychopharmacology. *J Clin Psychopharmacol* 1995;15:387–398.
3. Meyer UA, Amrein R, Balant LP, et al. Antidepressants and drug metabolizing enzymes—expert group report. *Acta Psychiatr Scand* 1996;93:71–79.
4. Cohen LJ, DeVane CL. Clinical implications of antidepressant pharmacokinetics and pharmacogenetics. *Ann Pharmacother* 1996;3: 1471–1480.
5. Nemeroff CB, DeVane CL, Pollock BG. Newer antidepressants and cytochrome P450 system. *Am J Psychiatry* 1996;153:311–320.
6. Slaughter RL, Edwards DJ. Recent advances: the cytochrome P450 enzymes. *Pharmacotherapy* 1995;29:619–624.
7. Wrighton SA, Vander Branden M, Ring BJ. The human drug metabolizing cytochrome P450. *J Pharmacokinet Biopharm* 1996;24:461–473.
8. Rendic S, Di Carlo FJ. Human cytochrome P450 enzymes: a status report summarizing their reactions, substrates, inducers, and inhibitors. *Drug Metab Rev* 1997;29:413–580.
9. Kutcher SP, Reid K, Dubbin JD, Shulman KI. Electrocardiogram changes and therapeutic desipramine and 2-hydroxy-desipramine concentrations in elderly depressives. *Br J Psychiatry* 1986;148:676–679.
10. Brøsen K, Otton SV, Gram LF. Imipramine demethylation and hydroxylation phenotype. *Clin Pharmacol Ther* 1986;40:544–549.
11. Brøsen K, Gram LF. First-pass metabolism of imipramine and desipramine: impact of the sparteine oxidation phenotype. *Clin Pharmacol Ther* 1988;43:400–406.
12. Brøsen K, Zeugin T, Meyer UA. Role of P450 IID6, the target of the sparteine-debrisoquin oxidation polymorphism, in the metabolism of imipramine. *Clin Pharmacol Ther* 1991;49:609–617.
13. Skjelbe E, Gram LF, Brosen K. The *N*-demethylation of imipramine correlates with the oxidation of *S*-mephenytoin (S/R-ratio). A population study. *Br J Clin Pharmacol* 1993;35:331–334.
14. Chiba K, Saitoh A, Koyama E, Tani M, Hayashi M, Ishizaki T. The role of *S*-mephenytoin 4′-hydroxylase in imipramine metabolism by human liver microsomes: a two-enzyme kinetic analysis of *N*-demethylation and 2-hydroxylation. *Br J Clin Pharmacol* 1994;37:237–242.

15. Lemoine A, Gautier JC, Azoulay D, et al. Major pathway of imipramine metabolism is catalyzed by cytochrome P-450 1A2 and P-450 3A4 in human liver. *Mol Pharmacol* 1993;43:827–832.

16. Koyama E, Chiba K, Tani M, Ishizaki T. Reappraisal of human CYP isoforms involved in imipramine *N*-demethylation and 2-hydroxylation: a study using microsomes obtained from putative extensive and poor metabolizers of *S*-mephenytoin and eleven recombinant human CYPs. *J Pharmacol Exp Ther* 1997;281:1199–1210.

17. Nusser E, Nill K, Breyer-Pfaff U. Enantioselective formation and disposition of (E)- and (Z)-10-hydroxynortriptyline. *Drug Metab Dispos* 1988;16:509–511.

18. Polloch BG, Perel JM. Hydroxy metabolites of tricyclic antidepressants: evaluation of relative cardiotoxicity. In: Dahl SG, Gram LF, eds. *Clinical pharmacology in psychiatry: from molecular studies to clinical reality*. Berlin: Springer-Verlag, 1989.

19. Breyer-Pfaff U, Pfandl B, Nill K, et al. Enantioselective amitriptyline metabolism in patients phenotyped for two cytochrome P450 isozymes. *Clin Pharmacol Ther* 1992;52:350–358.

20. Venkatakrishnan K, Greenblatt DJ, von Moltke LL, Schmider J, Harmatz JS, Shader RI. Five distinct human cytochromes mediate amitriptyline *N*-demethylation in vitro: dominance of CYP 2C19 and 3A4. *J Clin Pharmacol* 1998;38:112–121.

21. Olesen OV, Linnet K. Metabolism of the tricyclic antidepressant amitriptyline by cDNA-expressed human cytochrome P450 enzymes. *Pharmacology* 1997;55:235–243.

22. Kramer Nielsen K, Brosen K, Hansen MGJ, Gram LF. Single-dose kinetics of clomipramine: relationship to the sparteine and *S*-mephenytoin oxidation polymorphisms. *Clin Pharmacol Ther* 1994;55:518–527.

23. Kramer Nielsen K, Flinois JP, Beaune P, Brosen K. The biotransformation of clomipramine in vitro, identification of the cytochrome P450s responsible for the separate metabolic pathways. *J Pharmacol Exp Ther* 1996;277:1659–1664.

24. Jue SG, Dawson GW, Brogden RN. Amoxapine: a review of its pharmacology and efficacy in depressed states. *Drugs* 1982;24:1–23.

25. Firkusny L, Gleiter CH. Maprotiline metabolism appears to co-segregate with the genetically-determined CYP2D6 polymorphic hydroxylation of debrisoquine. *Br J Clin Pharmacol* 1994;37:383–388.

26. Pinder RM, van Delft AML. The potential therapeutic role of the enantiomers and metabolites of mianserin. *Br J Clin Pharmacol* 1983;15:269s–276s.

27. Dahl M-L, Tybring G, Elwin C-E, et al. Stereoselective disposition of mianserin is related to debrisoquin hydroxylation polymorphism. *Clin Pharmacol Ther* 1994;56:176–183.

28. Koyama E, Chiba K, Tani M, Ishizaki T. Identification of human cytochrome P450 isoforms involved in the stereoselective metabolism of mianserin enantiomers. *J Pharmacol Exp Ther* 1996;278:21–30.

29. Benfield P, Heel RC, Lewis SP. Fluoxetine. A review of its pharmacodynamic and pharmacokinetic properties, and therapeutic efficacy in depressive illness. *Drugs* 1986;32:481–508.

30. Greenblatt DJ, Preskorn SH, Cotreau MM, Horst WD, Harmatz JS. Fluoxetine impairs clearance of alprazolam but not of clonazepam. *Clin Pharmacol Ther* 1992;52:479–486.

31. Hamelin BA, Turgeon J, Vallée F, Bélanger P-M, Paquet F, LeBel M. The disposition of fluoxetine but not sertraline is altered in poor metabolizers of debrisoquin. *Clin Pharmacol Ther* 1996;60:512–521.

32. Kaye CM, Haddock RE, Langley PF, et al. A review of the metabolism and pharmacokinetics of paroxetine in man. *Acta Psychiatr Scand* 1989;80:60–75.

33. Brøsen K. The pharmacogenetics of the selective serotonin reuptake inhibitors. *Clin Invest* 1993;71:1002–1009.

34. Sindrup SH, Brøsen K, Gram LF, et al. The relationship between paroxetine and the sparteine oxidation polymorphism. *Clin Pharmacol Ther* 1992;51:278–287.

35. Sindrup SH, Brøsen K, Gram LF. Pharmacokinetics of the selective serotonin reuptake inhibitor paroxetine: nonlinearity and relation to the sparteine oxidation polymorphism. *Clin Pharmacol Ther* 1992;51:288–295.

36. Murdoch D, McTavish D. Sertraline. A review of its pharmacodynamic and pharmacokinetic properties, and therapeutic potential in depression and obsessive-compulsive disorder. *Drugs* 1992;44:604–624.

37. Sprouse J, Clarke T, Reynolds L, Heym J, Rollema H. Comparison of the effects of sertraline and its metabolite desmethylsertraline on blockade of central 5-HT reuptake in vivo. *Neuropsychopharmacology* 1996;14:225–231.

38. Kobayashi K, Ishizuka T, Shimada N, Yosimura Y, Kamijima K, Chiba K. Sertraline *N*-demethylation is catalyzed by multiple isoforms of human cytochrome P450 in vitro. Drug Metab Dispos 1999;27: 763–766.

39. Overmars H, Scherpenisse PM, Post LC. Fluvoxamine maleate: metabolism in man. *Eur J Drug Metab Pharmacokinet* 1983;8: 269–280.

40. Benfield P, Ward A. Fluvoxamine. A review of its pharmacodynamic and pharmacokinetic properties, and therapeutic efficacy in depressive illness. *Drugs* 1986;32:313–334.

41. Spigset O, Carleborg L, Hedenmalm K, Dahlqvist R. Effect of cigarette smoking on fluvoxamine pharmacokinetics in humans. *Clin Pharmacol Ther* 1995;58:399–403.

42. Sesardic D, Boobis AR, Edwards RJ, Davies DS. A form of cytochrome P450 in man, orthologous to form d in the rat, catalyses the *O*-deethylation of phenacetin and is inducible by cigarette smoking. *Br J Clin Pharmacol* 1988;26:363–372.

43. Carrillo JA, Dahl M-L, Svensson J-O, Alm C, Rodríguez I, Bertilsson L. Disposition of fluvoxamine in humans is determined by the polymorphic CYP2D6 and also by the CYP1A2 activity. *Clin Pharmacol Ther* 1996;60:183–190.

44. Spigset O, Granberg K, Hägg S, Norström Å, Dahlqvist R. Relationship between fluvoxamine pharmacokinetics and CYP2D6/CYP2C19 phenotype polymorphisms. *Eur J Clin Pharmacol* 1997;52:129–133.

45. Øyehaug E, Østensen ET. High-performance liquid chromatographic determination of citalopram and four of its metabolites in plasma and urine samples from psychiatric patients. *J Chromatogr* 1984;308: 199–208.

46. Sindrup SH. Brøsen K, Hansen MGJ, Aaes-Jørgensen T, Overø KF, Gram LF. Pharmacokinetics of citalopram in relation to the sparteine and the mephenytoin oxidation polymorphisms. *Ther Drug Monit* 1993;15:11–17.

47. Kobayashi K, Chiba K, Yagi T, et al. Identification of cytochrome P450 isoforms involved in citalopram *N*-demethylation by human liver microsomes. *J Pharmacol Exp Ther* 1997;280:927–933.

48. Rochat B, Amey M, Gillet M, Meyer UA, Baumann P. Identification of three cytochrome P450 isozymes involved in *N*-demethylation of citalopram enantiomers in human liver microsomes. *Pharmacogenetics* 1997;7:1–10.

49. Smith TM, Suckow RF. Trazodone and m-chlorophenylpiperazine. Concentration in brain and receptor activity in regions in the brain associated with anxiety. *Neuropharmacology* 1985;24:1067–1071.

50. Mihara K, Otani K, Suzuki A, et al. Relationship between the CYP2D6 genotype and the steady-state plasma concentrations of trazodone and its active metabolite m-chlorophenylpiperazine. *Psychopharmacology (Berl)* 1997;133:95–98.

51. Ishida M, Otani K, Kaneko S, et al. Effects of various factors on steady state plasma concentrations of trazodone and its active metabolite m-chlorophenylpiperazine. *Int Clin Psychopharmacol* 1995;10: 143–146.

52. Rotzinger S, Fang J, Baker GB. Trazodone is metabolized to m-chlorophenylpiperazine by CYP3A4 from human sources. *Drug Metab Dispos* 1998;26:572–575.

53. Greene DS, Barbhaiya RH. Clinical pharmacokinetics of nefazodone. *Clin Pharmacokinet* 1997;33:260–275.

54. Davis R, Whittington R, Bryson HM. Nefazodone. A review of its pharmacology and clinical efficacy in the management of major depression. *Drugs* 1997;53:608–636.

55. Preskorn SH. Recent pharmacological advances in antidepressant therapy for the elderly. *Am J Med* 1993;94[Suppl 5A]:13–23.

56. Linnolia M, George L, Guthrie S. Interaction between antidepressants and perfenazine in psychiatric inpatients. *Am J Psychiatry* 1982;139: 1329–1331.

57. Brøsen K, Gram LF. Qunidine inhibits the 2-hydroxylation of imipramine and desipramine but not the demethylation of imipramine. *Eur J Clin Pharmacol* 1989;37:155–160.

58. Dayer P, Desmeules J, Striberni R. In vitro forecasting of drugs that may interfere with codeine bioactivation. *Eur J Drug Metab Pharmacokinet* 1992;17:115–120.

59. Balant-Gorgia AE, Balant LP, Genet CH, Dayer P, Aeschlimann JM, Garrone G. Importance of oxidative polymorphism and levomepromazine treatment on the steady-state blood concentration of clomipramine and its major metabolites. *Eur J Clin Pharmacol* 1986; 31:449–455.

60. Yasui N, Tybring G, Otani K, et al. Effects of thioridazine, an inhibitor of CYP2D6, on the steady-state plasma concentrations of the enantiomers of mianserin and its active metabolite, desmethylmianserin, in depressed Japanese patients. *Pharmacogenetics* 1997;7:369–374.

61. Gram LF, Overo KF. Drug interaction: inhibitory effect of neuroleptics on metabolism of tricyclic antidepressants in man. *BMJ* 1972; 1:463–465.

62. Hermann DJ, Krol TF, Dukes GE, et al. Comparison of verapamil, diltiazem, and labetalol on the bioavailability and metabolism of imipramine. *J Clin Pharmacol* 1992;32:176–183.

63. Gillette DW, Tannery LP. Beta blocker inhibits tricyclic metabolism. *J Am Acad Child Adolesc Psychiatry* 1994;33:223–224.

64. Wagner F, Kalusche D, Trenk D, Jahnchen E, Roskamm H. Drug interaction between propafenone and metoprolol. *Br J Clin Pharmacol* 1987;24:213–220.

65. Sproule BA, Naranjo CA, Bremmer KE, Hassan PC. Selective serotonin reuptake inhibitors and CNS drug interactions. A critical review of the evidence. *Clin Pharmacokinet* 1997;33:454–471.

66. Ching MS, Blake CL, Ghabrial H, et al. Potent inhibition of yeast-expressed CYP2D6 by dihydroquinidine, quinidine, and its metabolites. *Biochem Pharmacol* 1995;50:833–837.

67. Crewe HK, Lennard MS, Tucker GT, Wood FR, Haddock RE. The effect of selective serotonin re-uptake inhibitors on cytochrome P4502D6 (CYP2D6) activity in human liver microsomes. *Br J Clin Pharmacol* 1992;34:262–265.

68. Bergstrom RF, Peyton AL, Lemberger L. Quantification and mechanism of the fluoxetine and tricyclic antidepressant interaction. *Clin Pharmacol Ther* 1992;51:239–248.

69. Preskorn SH, Alderman J, Chung M, Harrison W, Messig M, Harris S. Pharmacokinetics of desipramine coadministered with sertraline and fluoxetine. *J Clin Psychopharmacol* 1994;14:90–98.

70. Brøsen K, Hansen JG, Nielsen KK, Sindrup SH, Gram LF. Inhibition by paroxetine of desipramine metabolism in extensive but not in poor metabolizers of sparteine. *Eur J Clin Pharmacol* 1993;44:349–355.

71. Alderman J, Preskorn SH, Greenblatt DJ, et al. Desipramine pharmacokinetics when coadministered with paroxetine or sertraline in extensive metabolizers. *J Clin Psychopharmacol* 1997;17:284–291.

72. Spina E, Pollicino AM, Avenoso A, Campo GM, Perucca E, Caputi AP. Effect of fluvoxamine on the pharmacokinetics of imipramine and desipramine in healthy subjects. *Ther Drug Monit* 1993;15:243–246.

73. Xu Z-H, Xie H-G, Zhou H-H. In vivo inhibition of CYP2C19 but not CYP2D6 by fluvoxamine. *Br J Clin Pharmacol* 1996;42:518–521.

74. Eichelbaum M, Gross AS. The genetic polymorphism of debrisoquine/sparteine metabolism-clinical aspects. *Pharmacol Ther* 1990; 46:377–394.

75. Skjelbo E, Brøsen K, Hallas J, Gram LF. The mephenytoin oxidation polymorphism is partially responsible for the *N*-demethylation of imipramine. *Clin Pharmacol Ther* 1991;49:18–23.

76. Kobayashi K, Yamamoto T, Chiba K, Tani M, Ishizaki T, Kuroiwa Y. The effects of selective serotonin reuptake inhibitors and their metabolites on *S*-mephenytoin 4′-hydroxylase activity in human liver microsomes. *Br J Clin Pharmacol* 1995;40:481–485.

77. Ishizaki T, Chiba K, Manabe K, et al. Comparison of the interaction potential of a new proton pump inhibitor, E3810, versus omeprazole with diazepam in extensive and poor metabolizers of *S*-mephenytoin 4′-hydroxylation. *Clin Pharmacol Ther* 1995;58:155–164.

78. Spaina E, Avenoso A, Campo GM, Caputi AP, Perucca E. Effect of ketoconazole on the pharmacokinetics of imipramine and desipramine in healthy subjects. *Br J Clin Pharmacol* 1997;43:315–318.

79. Wang JS, Wang W, Xie HG, Huang SL, Zhou HH. Effect of troleandomycin on the pharmacokinetics of imipramine in Chinese: the role of CYP3A. *Br J Clin Pharmacol* 1997;44:195–198.

80. Bertschy G, Vandel S, Jounet JM, Allers G. Valproamide-amitriptyline interaction. Increase in the bioavailability of amitriptyline and nortriptyline caused by valproamide. *Encephale* 1990;16:43–45.

81. DeToledo JC, Haddad H, Ramsay RE. Status epilepticus associated with the combination of valproic acid and clomipramine. *Ther Drug Monit* 1997;19:71–73.

82. Well BG, Pieper JA, Self TH, et al. The effect of ranitidine and cimetidine on imipramine disposition. *Eur J Clin Pharmacol* 1986;31: 285–290.

83. Abernethy DR, Greenblatt DJ, Shader RI. Imipramine-cimetidine interaction: impairment of clearance and enhanced absolute bioavailability. *J Pharmacol Exp Ther* 1984;229:702–705.

84. Barry M, Feely J. Enzyme induction and inhibition. *Pharmacol Ther* 1990;48:71–94.

85. Park BK, Kitteringham NR, Pirmohamed M, Tucker GT. Relevance of induction of human drug-metabolizing enzymes: pharmacological and toxicological implications. *Br J Clin Pharmacol* 1996;41:477–491.

86. Wilkinson GR, Guengerich FP, Branch R. Genetic polymorphism of *S*-mephenytoin hydroxylation. *Pharmacol Ther* 1989;43:53–76.

87. Brown CS, Wells BG, Cold JA, Froemming JH, Self TH, Jabbour JT. Possible influence of carbamazepine on plasma imipramine concentrations in children with attention deficit hyperactivity disorder. *J Clin Psychopharmacol* 1990;10:359–362.

88. Leinonen E, Lillsunde P, Laukkanen V, Ylitalo P. Effects of carbamazepine on serum antidepressant concentration in psychiatric patients. *J Clin Psychopharmacol* 1991;11:313–318.

89. Madsen H, Nielsen KK, Brøsen K. Imipramine metabolism in relation to the sparteine and mephenytoin oxidation polymorphisms—a population study. *Br J Clin Pharmacol* 1995;39:433–439.

90. Balant-Gorgia AE, Gex-Fabry M, Balant LP. Clinical pharmacokinetics of clomipramine. *Clin Pharmacokinet* 1991;20:447–462.

91. Edelbroek PM, Zitman FG, Knoppert-van der Klein EA, van Putten PM, de Wolff FA. Therapeutic drug monitoring of amitriptyline: impact of age, smoking and contraceptives on drug and metabolite levels in bulimic women. *Clin Chim Acta* 1987:165:177–187.

92. Rost KL, Brosicke H, Brockmoller J, Scheffler M, Helge H, Roots I. Increase of cytochrome P450IA2 activity by omeprazole: evidence by the 13C-[*N*-3-methyl]-caffeine breath test in poor and extensive metabolizers of *S*-mephenytoin. *Clin Pharmacol Ther* 1992;52:170–180.

93. Spina E, Avenoso A, Campo GM, Caputi AP, Perucca E. Phenobarbital induces the 2-hydroxylation of desipramine. *Ther Drug Monit* 1996;18:60–64.

94. Spina E, Avenoso A, Campo GM, Caputi AP, Perucca E. The effect of carbamazepine on the 2-hydroxylation of desipramine. *Psychopharmacology* 1995;117:413–416.

95. Eichelbaum M, Mineshita S, Ohnhaus EE, Zekorn C. The influence of enzyme induction on polymorphic sparteine oxidation. *Br J Clin Pharmacol* 1986;22:49–53.

96. Ereshefsky L, Riesenman C, Lam YW. Serotonin selective reuptake inhibitor drug interactions and the cytochrome P450 system. *J Clin Psychiatry* 1996;57[Suppl 8]:17–24.

97. Ereshefsky L. Drug-drug interactions involving antidepressants: focus on venlafaxine. *J Clin Psychopharmacol* 1996;16[Suppl 2]:37–50.

98. Richelson E. Pharmacokinetic drug interactions of new antidepressants: a review of the effects on the metabolism of other drugs. *Mayo Clin Proc* 1997;72:835–847.

99. Preskorn SH. Clinically relevant pharmacology of selective serotonin reuptake inhibitors. An overview with emphasis on pharmacokinetics and effects on oxidative drug metabolism. *Clin Pharmacokinet* 1997; 32[Suppl 1]1–21.

100. Owen JR, Nemeroff CB. New antidepressants and the cytochrome P450 system: focus on venlafaxine, nefazodone, and mirtazapine. *Depress Anxiety* 1998;7[Suppl 1]:24–32.

101. Warrington SJ. Clinical implications of the pharmacology of sertraline. *Int Clin Psychopharmacol* 1991;6:11–21.

102. Özdemir V, Naranjo CA, Herrmann N, et al. Paroxetine potentiates the central nervous system side effects of perphenazine: contribution of cytochrome P4502D6 inhibition in vivo. *Clin Pharmacol Ther* 1997; 62:334–347.

103. Dahl-Puustinen M-L, Lidén A, Alm C, Nordin C, Bertilsson L. Disposition of perfenazine is related to polymorphic debrisoquin hydroxylation in human beings. *Clin Pharmacol Ther* 1989;46:78–81.

104. Jeppesen U. Gram LF, Vistisen K, Loft S, Poulsen HE, Brøsen K. Dose-dependent inhibition of CYP1A2, CYP2C19 and CYP2D6 by citalopram, fluoxetine, fluvoxamine and paroxetine. *Eur J Clin Pharmacol* 1996;51:73–78.

105. Brøsen K, Skjelbo E, Rasmussen BB, Poulsen HE, Loft S. Fluvoxamine is a potent inhibitor of cytochrome P4501A2. *Biochem Pharmacol* 1993;45:1211–1214.

106. Sperber AD. Toxic interaction between fluvoxamine and sustained release theophylline in an 11-year-old boy. *Drug Safety* 1991;6: 460–462.

107. Thomson AH, McGovern EM, Bennie P, Caldwell G, Smith M. Interaction between fluvoxamine and theophylline. *Pharm J* 1992;249:137.

108. Jeppesen U, Loft S, Poulsen HE, Brøsen K. A fluvoxamine-caffeine interaction study. *Pharmacogenetics* 1996;6:213–222.

109. Jerling M, Lindström L, Bondesson U, Bertilsson L. Fluvoxamine inhibition and carbamazepine induction of the metabolism of clozapine: evidence from a therapeutic drug monitoring service. *Ther Drug Monit* 1994;16:368–374.

110. Ozdemir V, Naranjo CA, Hermann N, et al. The extent and determinants of changes in CYP2D6 and CYP1A2 activities with therapeutic doses of sertraline. *J Clin Psychopharmacol* 1998;18:55–61.

111. Jalil P. Toxic reaction following the combined administration of fluoxetine and phenytoin: two case reports. *J Neurol Neurosurg Psychiatry* 1992;55:412–413.

112. Shader RI, Greenblatt DJ, von Moltke LL. Fluoxetine inhibition of phenytoin metabolism. *J Clin Psychopharmacol* 1994;14:375–376.

113. Woods DJ, Coulter DM, Pillans P. Interaction of phenytoin and fluoxetine. *N Z Med J* 1994;107:19.

114. Darley J. Interaction between phenytoin and fluoxetine. *Seizure* 1994;3:151–152.

115. Veronese ME, Mackenzie PI, Doecke CJ, McManus ME, Miner JO, Birkett DJ. Tolbutamide and phenytoin hydroxylations by cDNA-expressed human liver cytochrome P4502C9. *Biochem Biophys Res Commun* 1991;175:1112–1118.

116. Schmider J, Greenblatt DJ, von Moltke LL, Karsov D, Shader RI. Inhibition of CYP2C9 by selective serotonin reuptake inhibitors *in vitro*: studies of phenytoin *p*-hydroxylation. *Br J Clin Pharmacol* 1997;44:495–498.

117. Duncan D, Sayal K, McConnell H, Taylor D. Antidepressant interactions with warfarin. *Int Clin Psychopharmacol* 1998;13:87–94.

118. Kaminsky LS, Zhang Z-Y. Human P450 metabolism of warfarin. *Pharmacol Ther* 1997;73:67–74.

119. Tremaine LM, Wilner KD, Preskorn SH. A study of the potential effect of sertraline on the pharmacokinetics and protein binding of tolbutamide. *Clin Pharmacokinet* 1997;32[Suppl 1]:31–36.

120. Apseloff G, Wilner KD, Gerber N, Tremaine LM. Effect of sertraline on protein binding of warfarin. *Clin Pharmacokinet* 1997;32[Suppl 1]:37–42.

121. Bajpai M, Roskos LK, Shen DD, Levy RH. Roles of cytochrome P4502C9 and P4502C19 in the stereoselective metabolism of phenytoin to its major metabolite. *Drug Metab Dispos* 1996;24:1401–1403.

122. Jeppesen U, Rasmussen BB, Brøsen K. Fluvoxamine inhibits the CYP2C19-catalyzed bioactivation of chloroguanide. *Clin Pharmacol Ther* 1997;62:279–286.

123. Gardner MJ, Baris BA, Wilner KD, Preskorn SH. Effect of sertraline on the pharmacokinetics and protein binding of diazepam in healthy volunteers. *Clin Pharmacokinet* 1997;32[Suppl 1]:43–49.

124. Greene DS, Barbhaiya RH. Clinical pharmacokinetics of nefazodone. *Clin Pharmacokinet* 1997;33:260–275.

125. von Moltke LL, Greenblatt DJ, Court MH, Duan SX, Harmatz JS, Shader RI. Inhibition of alprazolam and desipramine hydroxylation *in vitro* by paroxetine and fluvoxamine: comparison with other selective serotonin reuptake inhibitor antidepressants. *J Clin Psychopharmacol* 1995;15:125–131.

126. von Moltke LL, Greenblatt DJ, Duan SX, Harmatz JS, Wright CE, Shader BI. Inhibition of terfenadine metabolism *in vitro* by azole antifungal agents and by selective serotonin reuptake inhibitor antidepressants: relation to pharmacokinetic interactions *in vivo*. *J Clin Psychopharmacol* 1996;16:104–112.

127. von Moltke LL, Greenblatt DJ, Harmatz JS, et al. Triazolam biotransformation by human liver microsomes *in vitro*: effects of metabolic inhibitors and clinical confirmation of a predicted interaction with ketoconazole. *J Pharmacol Exp Ther* 1996;276:370–379.

128. Fleishaker JC, Hulst LK. A pharmacokinetic and pharmacodynamic evaluation of the combined administration of alprazolam and fluvoxamine. *Eur J Clin Pharmacol* 1994;46:35–39.

129. Martinelli V, Bocchetta A, Palmas AM, Delzompo M. An interaction between carbamazepine and fluvoxamine. *Br J Clin Pharmacol* 1993;36:615–616.

130. Spina E, Avenoso A, Pollicino AM, Caputi AP, Fazio A, Pisani F. Carbamazepine coadministration with fluoxetine or fluvoxamine. *Ther Drug Monit* 1993;15:247–250.

131. Ring BJ, Binkley SN, Roskos L, Wrighton SA. Effect of fluoxetine, norfluoxetine, sertraline and desmethyl sertraline on human CYP3A catalyzed 1′-hydroxy midazolam formation *in vitro*. *J Pharmacol Exp Ther* 1995;275:1131–1135.

132. Grimsley SR, Jann MW, Carter JG, D'Mello AP, D'Souza MJ. Increased carbamazepine plasma concentrations after fluoxetine coadministration. *Clin Pharmacol Ther* 1991;50:10–15.

133. Bergstrom RF, Goldberg MJ, Cerimele BJ, Hatcher BL. Assessment of the potential for a pharmacokinetic interaction between fluoxetine and terfenadine. *Clin Pharmacol Ther* 1997;62:643–651.

134. Swims MP. Potential terfenadine-fluoxetine interaction. *Ann Pharmacother* 1993;27:1404–1405.

CHAPTER 19

Antipsychotics

C. Lindsay DeVane and John S. Markowitz

Drugs from a variety of chemical classes comprise the therapeutic class known as antipsychotics. They are indicated for the management of the manifestations of psychotic illness and are the most effective medications for the treatment of schizophrenia (1). Table 19-1 lists the antipsychotic drugs currently available in the United States or that are in advanced stages of clinical development.

In 1988, the designation "atypical" was applied to the antipsychotic clozapine. This drug was shown to be superior to other antipsychotics in patients who had inadequately responded to previous treatments. Until that time, the phenothiazines and other conventional antipsychotics were regarded as interchangeable therapeutically. Subsequently, several atypical antipsychotics were developed for clinical use. The term has come to be widely used to denote drugs that have specific behavioral and neurochemical differences from the conventional drugs. These characteristics include a lower propensity to cause extrapyramidal side effects such as pseudoparkinsonism, an improved efficacy for symptom control, and a neuroreceptor binding profile, which includes affinity for the serotonin type 2A (5-HT$_{2A}$) postsynaptic receptors in the frontal cortex. These atypical drugs are rapidly supplanting the clinical use of the older antipsychotics (see Table 19-1).

The atypical antipsychotics were the focus of research during the 1990s, and interest in these drugs as substrates of metabolic enzymes has been high. It is likely that they will continue to be prototypes for development of subsequent antipsychotic compounds. This chapter focuses on the atypical antipsychotics and haloperidol. Haloperidol continues to be used extensively clinically and is widely used as a comparative compound in phase II and III clinical trials for drug development of new antipsychotics.

Because of the recent development of atypical antipsychotics, a substantial amount of information is available regarding the metabolic pathways in contrast to the relatively sparse knowledge related to the enzymes that metabolize the conventional phenothiazines (see Table 19-1). This chapter focuses on the atypical antipsychotics.

C. L. DeVane: Department of Psychiatry and Behavioral Sciences, Medical University of South Carolina, 67 President Street, Charleston, South Carolina 29425

J. S. Markowitz: Department of Pharmaceutical Sciences, College of Pharmacy, Medical University of South Carolina, 171 Ashley Avenue, Charleston, South Carolina 29425

TABLE 19-1. *Antipsychotic drugs currently available in the United States*

Traditional antipsychotics	Atypical antipsychotics
Phenothiazines	Dibenzodiazepines
Chlorpromazine	Clozapine
Thioridazine	Benzisoxazoles
Mesoridazine	Risperidone
Acetophenazine	Thienobenzodiazepines
Prochlorperazine	Olanzapine
Perphenazine	Dibenzothiazepines
Trifluoperazine	Quetiapine
Triflupromazine	Benzisothiazoyl piperazine
Fluphenazine	Ziprasidone
Thioxanthenes	
Thiothixene	
Chlorprothixene	
Dibenzoxazepines	
Loxapine	
Dihydroindolones	
Molindone	
Butyrophenones	
Haloperidol	

HALOPERIDOL

Haloperidol (HAL), chemically known as 4-[-(p-chlorophenyl])-4-hydroxy-piperidinol]-4'-fluorobutyrophenone, has the structural formula and metabolic profile shown in Fig. 19-1. It has been considered to have the least complicated metabolism of the traditional antipsychotics with fewer pharmacologically active metabolites.

The metabolism of haloperidol has been studied for more than 30 years (2). Early studies using tritium-labeled compounds suggested the existence of several metabolites. Since Forsman and Larsson (3) reported that reduced haloperidol (RHAL) was a major metabolite in human plasma, RHAL has been the focus of research for more than 20 years. Furthermore, the concentration of RHAL could occasionally exceed that of HAL. This finding was potentially significant for the therapeutic drug monitoring of haloperidol because one animal study indicated this metabolite possessed 10% to 20% of the pharmacologic activity of the parent drug (4) and human studies reported correlations between plasma concentrations of RHAL and clinical outcome (5,6).

An additional complexity emerged as the results from several studies revealed RHAL was interconverted with HAL (7,8). Variability in this reaction has been used by various authors to explain the apparent curvilinear response between haloperidol plasma concentration and therapeutic effects observed in some patients. Several pharmacokinetic studies of reduced haloperidol have been performed, but its pharmacologic significance is still unclear.

A more complete profile of the metabolism of haloperidol has been defined in recent years. Gorrod and Fang (10) used hepatic microsomes harvested from four animal species (rat, hamster, rabbit, guinea pig) to identify additional metabolites of haloperidol. The proposed pathways are shown in Figure 19-1. Haloperidol is N-dealkylated to form 3-(p-fluorobenzoyl)propionic acid (FBPA) and 4-(p-chlorophenyl)-4-hydroxypiperidene (CPHP). An additional pathway involves enzymatic dehydration to form the 1,2,3,6-tetrahydropyridine analogue (HTP). HTP is further converted to haloperidol pyridinium (HP+), a reversible N-oxide (HTPNO), or its N-dealkylation product (CPTP). It has been hypothesized that the formation of HP+ may be involved in the neurotoxicity of haloperidol (11,12). Apart from the activity of reduced haloperidol, none of the remaining metabolites have been proposed to have therapeutic activity.

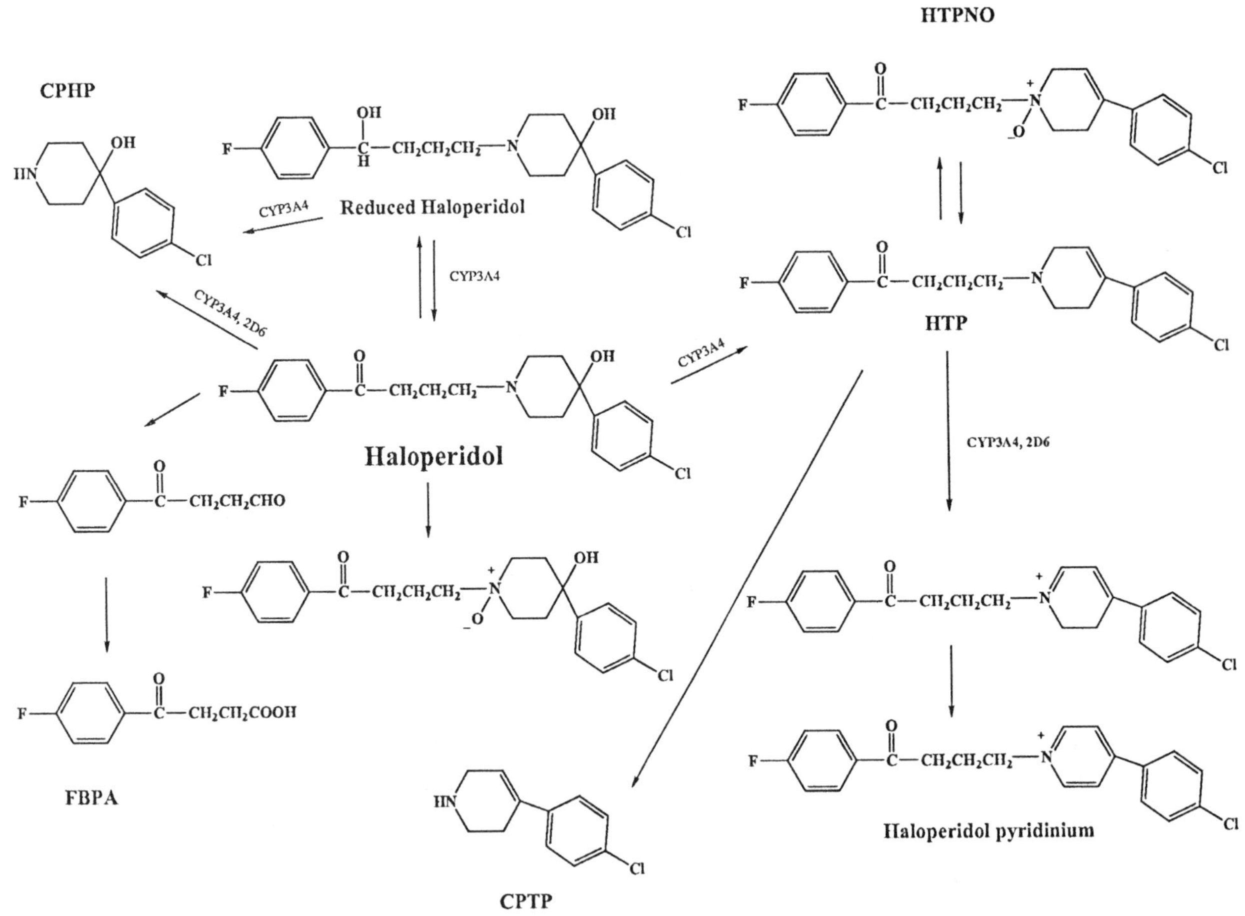

FIG. 19-1. Metabolic profile of haloperidol. Abbreviations are given in the text.

The interconversion of HAL and RHAL was initially hypothesized to involve CYP2D6 based on evidence that HAL is apparently a CYP2D6 inhibitor *in vitro* and *in vivo* (13,14). Additional support was provided by *in vitro* data that the oxidation of RHAL to HAL was inhibited by quinidine (15). A study by Young and colleagues (16) appears to refute the contention that CYP2D6 is involved in the HAL to RHAL interconversion. These investigators administered both haloperidol and reduced haloperidol to 13 volunteers phenotyped for CYP2D6 with and without quinidine. The interconversion was unaffected, indicating that CYP2D6 is probably not linked in this metabolic process. This continues to be a discrepancy in the literature. Llerena and colleagues (17) reported that the plasma concentrations of reduced haloperidol were significantly higher in poor metabolizers compared to extensive metabolizers of debrisoquine. Lane and colleagues (18) found similar results in schizophrenic patients phenotyped as poor or extensive metabolizers of dextromethorphan. It is likely that CYP2D6 is at least involved in the reoxidation of reduced haloperidol to haloperidol.

There is evidence that CYP3A4 is involved in the metabolism of haloperidol. Kim and colleagues (19) found substantial decreases, up to 63%, in the plasma concentration of haloperidol in patients administered rifampin compared to pretreatment concentration values. Haloperidol concentration increased after discontinuation of rifampin. This finding suggests the involvement of CYP3A4, which is induced by rifampin, but this anticonvulsant may also induce isozymes in the CYP2C subfamily. Reduced haloperidol was not measured in this study.

Other drug interaction studies have been insightful. Vandel and colleagues (20) found that fluvoxamine induced a moderate increase in the plasma concentration of haloperidol in patients; however, fluvoxamine is a known inhibitor of CYP1A2, CYP2C19, and CYP3A4, with negligible effects on CYP2D6. Avenoso and colleagues (21) studied the interaction between fluoxetine and haloperidol and found a 35% increase in haloperidol concentrations in 13 schizophrenic patients given concomitant antidepressants. Whereas the major effect of fluoxetine is to inhibit CYP2D6, its metabolite, norfluoxetine, has the potential, when dosed to steady-state, to competitively inhibit CYP3A4 (22). A relatively pure CYP3A4 inhibitor, nefazodone, was combined with haloperidol and found to induce a 36% increase in the area under the plasma concentration versus time curve (AUC) of haloperidol in 12 healthy men (23). These data would seem to confirm the involvement of CYP3A4 to form one or more metabolites.

The *in vitro* data of Fang and colleagues (24) using cytochrome isoenzymes expressed in a human cell line found that CYP3A4 catalyzed the conversion of haloperidol to HTP (see Fig. 19-1). CYP3A4 and CYP2D6 were both involved in the formation of the pyridium metabolite and *N*-dealkylation of haloperidol.

In addition, CYP3A4 catalyzed the oxidation of reduced haloperidol back to haloperidol. In summary, a variety of *in vivo* and *in vitro* evidence indicates the involvement of cytochrome P450 enzymes in the oxidation of haloperidol. CYP2D6 and CYP3A4 are the principal enzymes, but their relative importance for some pathways is unclear.

CLOZAPINE

Clozapine, chemically known as 8-chloro-11-(4-0-methyl-1-piperazinyl)-5H-dibenzo[b,e] [1,4] diazepine, has the structural formula and metabolic profile shown in Fig. 19-2. The drug was first synthesized more than 30 years ago as a dibenzodiazepine derivative (25). It is currently recognized as the prototypic atypical antipsychotic, representing the first major advance in antipsychotic drug therapy in nearly 25 years. Clozapine became widely available for use in the United States in 1990. The unique pharmacology of clozapine conveys advantages over conventional antipsychotics because of its effectiveness in treatment-resistant patients and its relative lack of neurologic side effects, including tardive dyskinesia. These properties are thought to be a result of its high affinity for and blockade of D_1 and D_4 dopaminergic receptors with relatively low D_2 receptor binding. Additionally, there is high affinity for serotonergic receptor subtypes ($5-HT_{2A}$, $5-HT_{2C}$, $5-HT_{3C}$) (26), which is increasingly viewed as an important property for antipsychotic effectiveness (27). Significant antagonism of histaminergic, α-adrenergic, and muscarinic receptors occurs, but these properties appear to be related more to adverse events than to therapeutic effects. Despite these advantages over conventional antipsychotics, the use of clozapine is associated with a high incidence (0.8%–1.3%) of agranulocytosis. This hazard curtails its wider use and necessitates frequent hematologic monitoring (28).

Clozapine undergoes extensive hepatic metabolism in humans (25) (see Fig. 19-2). Although greater than 10 metabolites have been identified in humans, the major biotransformation products are *N*-desmethylclozapine, which may exceed plasma concentrations of clozapine, and clozapine-*N*-oxide, which can be reduced back to the parent compound *in vivo* (29). Clozapine-*N*-oxide is devoid of activity at serotonin or dopaminergic receptors, whereas *N*-desmethylclozapine appears to have similar D_2 and $5-HT_2$ receptor affinity to the parent compound (30). This metabolite has been associated with toxicity to hemopoietic precursors (31). Other metabolites identified in human urine include 8-hydroxy-deschloro-desmethylclozapine, 7-hydroxy-8-chloro-desmethylclozapine sulfate (32), as well as other methiolated (33) and glucuronidated metabolites (25,32,34). Recently, the formation of cytotoxic nitrenium intermediate products and glutathionyl conjugates have been observed *in vitro* (35).

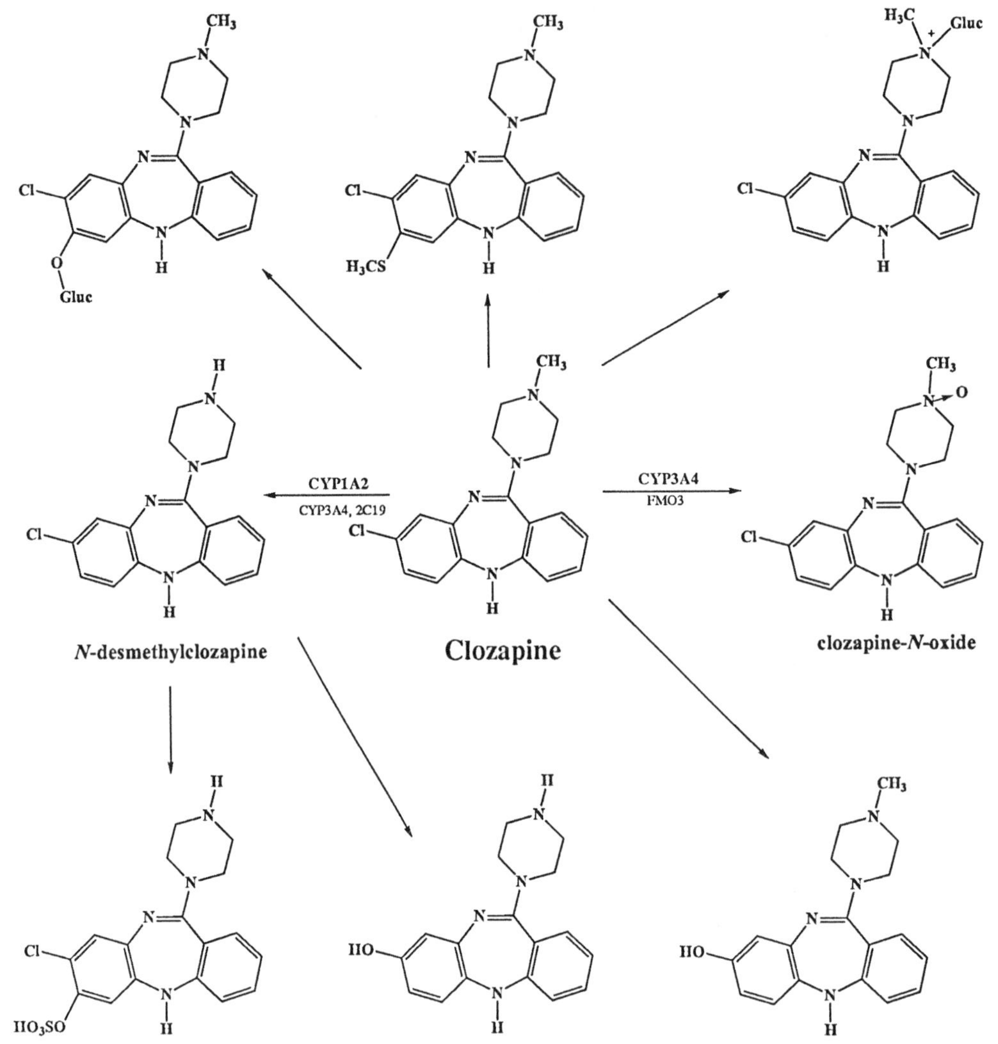

FIG. 19-2. Metabolic profile of clozapine.

Thus, clozapine appears to produce one pharmacologically active metabolite whose plasma concentration may be useful in therapeutic drug monitoring. Measurements of plasma clozapine have been suggested to be of value in evaluating nonresponse to usual doses. Although a "therapeutic window" has not been established, the majority of studies support a threshold concentration of 350 to 420 ng/mL (36).

Results from both *in vivo* and *in vitro* studies suggest multiple CYP isoforms are involved in the oxidative metabolism of clozapine. However, the two prominent hepatic cytochrome P450 isoforms mediating the metabolism of clozapine appear to be CYP1A2 and CYP3A4. Pirmohamed and co-workers (37) investigated clozapine metabolism using human liver microsomes and found that clozapine demethylation is mediated through CYP1A2 and suggested that *N*-oxidation proceeded through CYP2E1 and CYP2C9/CYP2C10. Subsequent *in vitro* studies using human liver microsome incubations

corroborated a major role for CYP1A2 in clozapine *N*-demethylation whereas *N*-oxidation was found to be exclusively catalyzed by CYP3A4 with little role for CYP2E1 found in the formation of either metabolite.(38,39). It has been proposed that as much as 45% of the hepatic metabolism of clozapine may be mediated by CYP3A4 (38).

In vivo human studies and drug interaction reports (40) also suggest an important role for CYP1A2 and CYP3A4. Clozapine disposition was found to co-vary with CYP1A2 activity as determined by *N*-3-demethylation of caffeine (41). Additionally, numerous case reports (40) and at least two studies (42,43) have found that robust increases in clozapine and desmethylclozapine plasma concentrations occur following the coadministration of fluvoxamine, a known potent inhibitor of CYP1A2 (44). However, it must not be overlooked that fluvoxamine strongly inhibits CYP2C19, moderately inhibits CYP3A4, and to a very minor extent CYP2D6

(45,46). These isoforms also appear to be implicated in clozapine metabolism (38).

Additional evidence for CYP1A2 involvement is provided by induction of clozapine metabolism by aryl hydrocarbon exposure from smoking and rifampicin (induction) coadministration, which induces CYP1A2 and CYP3A4 (40,47). Also, modulation of clozapine plasma concentrations based on caffeine consumption have been noted (40). Lastly, limited data suggest that clozapine plasma concentrations are increased following coadministration of the fluoroquinolone antibiotic ciprofloxacin, a known potent inhibitor of CYP1A2 (47,48).

Several clinical reports of drug interactions with clozapine give conflicting accounts with respect to the role of CYP3A4 in the *in vivo* metabolism of clozapine. For example, at least two cases have been reported in which coadministration of the antimicrobial erythromycin, which is a relatively specific inhibitor of CYP3A4, resulted in significant increases in clozapine plasma concentrations, a finding that supports *in vitro* findings (40). Additionally, coadministration of clozapine with the known inducers of CYP3A4—carbamazepine (43) and rifampicin (47)—has been shown to result in diminution of clozapine plasma concentrations.

Interestingly, a recent double-blind, randomized study found no significant effects on clozapine or desmethyl-clozapine plasma concentrations following the addition of the antimycotic itraconazole, a potent inhibitor of CYP3A4, which has been shown to have greater inhibitory capacity than erythromycin with respect to a number of other CYP3A4 substrates (49). Based on current *in vitro* data, a modest inhibitory effect on clozapine plasma concentration would have been predicted. Clozapine-*N*-oxide concentrations were not measured in the itraconazole study.

Studies of CYP2D6 involvement in clozapine metabolism have been conflicting. An initial *in vitro* investigation suggested that CYP2D6 was one of the major isoforms involved in clozapine metabolism (50). Subsequent studies reported either an absent or only minor role for CYP2D6 in the *N*-demethylation or *N*-oxidation of clozapine (37–39). Additionally, *in vivo* studies have not supported a significant role for CYP2D6. A lack of association with debrisoquine polymorphism indicated that CYP2D6 was not the major metabolizing enzyme (51). Furthermore, in a study of 123 schizophrenic patients receiving clozapine, no correlation between poor or extensive metabolizers of CYP2D6 and drug response were found (52).

In general, data from clinical experience does not support the participation of CYP2D6 inhibitors with significant drug interactions. Limited published data involving the coadministration of the serotonin selective reuptake inhibitor (SSRI) antidepressant fluoxetine and clozapine has been conflicting, with reports showing either an inhibitory effect (53) or no effect (54) on clozapine

plasma concentrations. The interpretation of fluoxetine data is complicated because evidence exists that this antidepressant may have inhibitory effects on multiple isoforms, specifically CYP2C19 and CYP3A4 in addition to the well-characterized inhibition of CYP2D6 (55). Additionally, coadministration of the SSRI paroxetine, a potent and relatively selective inhibitor of CYP2D6, has been demonstrated to minimally affect clozapine plasma concentrations (42).

In vitro investigations have indicated that the isoform CYP2C9 occupies only a minor role in clozapine *N*-demethylation (37–39), whereas at least one study (38) demonstrated that CYP2C19 was involved in *N*-demethylation of clozapine. Furthermore, the investigators suggest that, when taking into account the abundance of each isoform in the liver, CYP2C19 may account for as much as 30% of the oxidative metabolism of clozapine. This observation is significant in that CYP2C19 has a genetic polymorphism. However, no association has been detected between clozapine metabolic rate and the (S)-mephenytoin phenotype (51).

Recently, the flavin-containing monooxygenase FMO3 has been shown to catalyze the *in vitro* formation of clozapine-*N*-oxide (56). This finding is not consistent with those reported from an earlier study (37). Further evaluation of the role of FMO3 in the metabolism of clozapine seems warranted.

In summary, current *in vitro* data suggest primary roles for CYP1A2 and CYP3A4 in the formation of *N*-desmethylclozapine and clozapine-*N*-oxide, respectively. The isoforms CYP3A4, and CYP2C19 may also have significant effects on clozapine *N*-demethylation, whereas CYP2C9 and CYP2D6 appear to have minor effects. Additionally, FMO3 may effect the formation of clozapine-*N*-oxide.

RISPERIDONE

Risperidone, known chemically as 3-[2-[4-(6-fluoro-1,2-benzisoxazol-3-yl)-1-piperidinyl]ethyl]-6,7,8,9-tetrahydro-2-methyl-4H-pyrido[1,2a]pyrimidin-4-one, has a chemical structure and metabolic profile as shown in Fig. 19-3. Since its introduction into clinical practice, it has become an extensively used drug for the treatment of psychotic symptoms in adults and in elderly patients (57). Despite its extensive use, there is little published information related to its metabolism and enzyme-mediated pathways.

Risperidone is principally metabolized by aliphatic hydroxylation and oxidative *N*-dealkylation (58,59). Its metabolism and excretion have been studied in various species. The principal metabolites in humans are 9-hydroxy-risperidone and 7-hydroxy-risperidone (see Fig. 19-1). The 9-hydroxy metabolite is the predominant species in urine and accounts for more than 32% of an

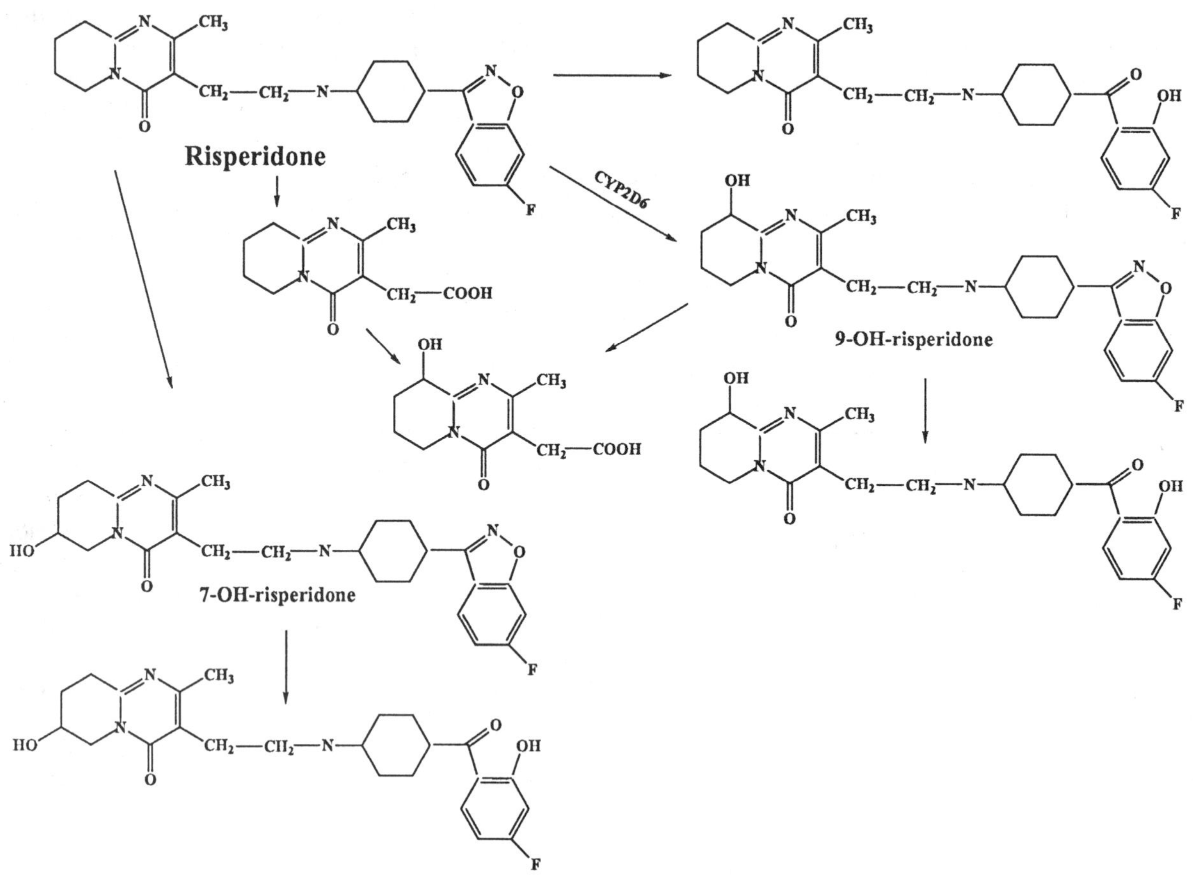

FIG. 19-3. Metabolic profile of risperidone.

administered dose (59). The 7-hydroxy metabolite accounted for 1% to 5% of an administered dose. The 9-hydroxy metabolite also predominates in plasma in patients taking risperidone (60). It appears to be equipotent with the parent drug as an antipsychotic compound in terms of dopamine receptor affinity (61,62).

The metabolism of risperidone to 9-hydroxy-risperidone is mediated by CYP2D6 (58). Its formation was highly correlated with the dextromethorphan phenotype status of healthy volunteers. The pharmacokinetics of combined risperidone plus 9-hydroxy-risperidone varied little between subjects who were extensive or poor metabolizers. Drug interaction studies have contributed little to the further understanding of specific enzymes involved in the metabolism of risperidone (63).

OLANZAPINE

Olanzapine is a thienobenzodiaepine derivative and structural analogue of clozapine (64). Of the available atypical antipsychotic agents, olanzapine has the most similar *in vitro* receptor binding profile to clozapine without its apparent propensity to induce agranulocytosis. Olanzapine has a broad binding profile with significant affinity for D_1, D_2, D_4, $5-HT_{2C}$, $5-HT_{2A}$, $5-HT_3$,

α_1-adrenergic, histaminergic, and muscarinic receptors (62).

Olanzapine undergoes extensive hepatic metabolism with at least ten metabolites identified in humans (Fig. 19-4). The four dominant metabolic pathways are N-glucuronidation, allylic hydroxylation, N-oxidation, and N-demethylation (65). Major metabolites in the plasma include the 10-N-glucuronide, which may be present at 44% of circulating olanzapine concentrations, and 4-N-desmethylolanzapine, which has been detected at 31% of the plasma concentration of the parent compound. Other metabolites detected in plasma include N-desmethyl, 2-hydroxymethyl, and olanzapine-N-oxide (65). None of these metabolites appear to have central nervous system activity (64). Metabolites detected in urine in order of abundance include 10-N-glucuronide, 2-carboxy olanzapine, olanzapine-N-oxide, N-desmethylolanzapine, and a number of glucuronides including a quaternary N-linked 4'-N-glucuronide (65).

In vitro data indicate that, analogous to the metabolism of clozapine, the major oxidative metabolite N-desmethylolanzapine is predominantly formed by CYP1A2 and to a lesser degree by CYP3A4 (66). FMO3 is the dominant pathway responsible for olanzapine-N-oxide formation with small contributions from CYP3A4, CYP1A2,

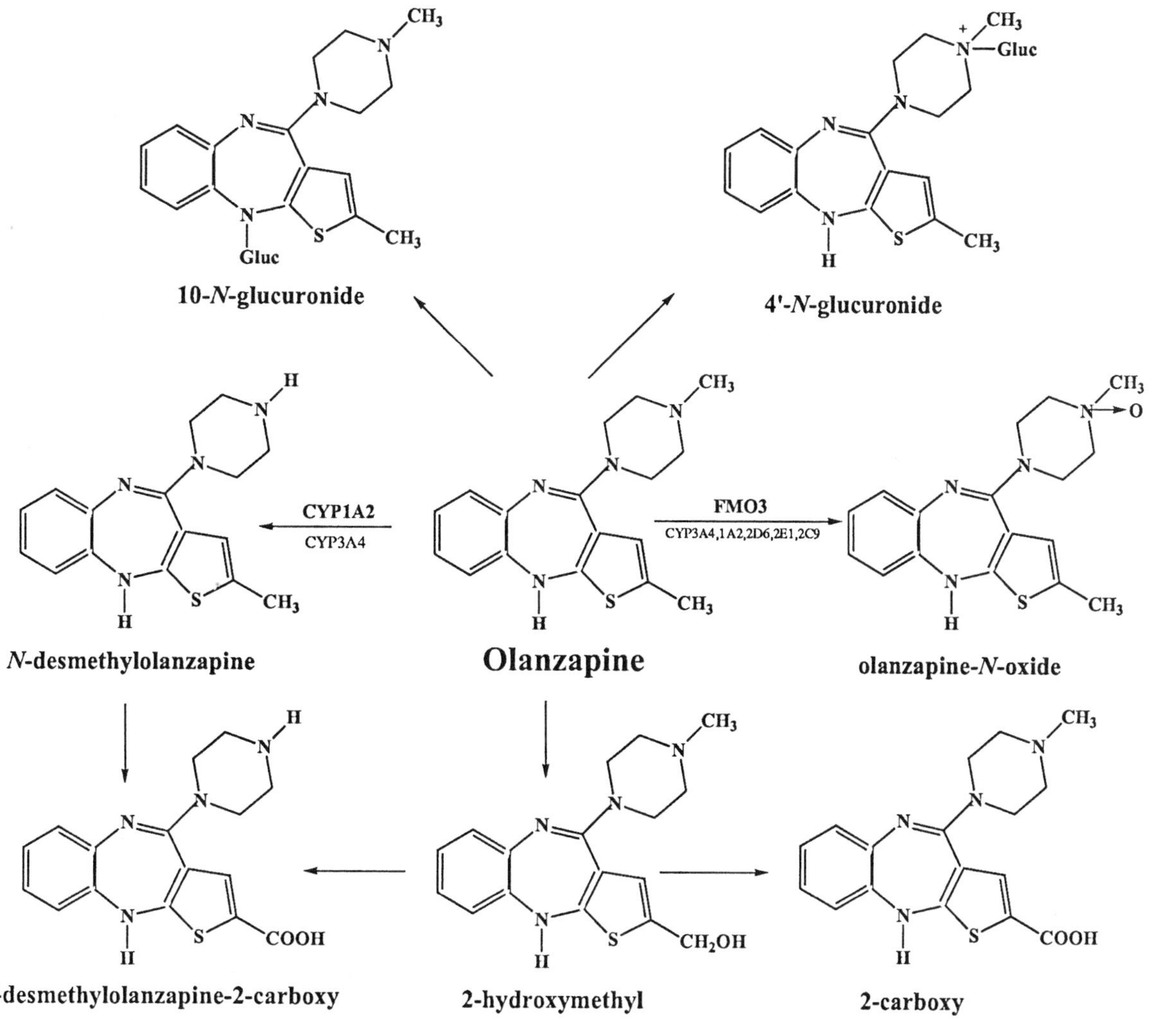

FIG. 19-4. Metabolic profile of olanzapine.

CYP2D6, CYP2E1, and CYP2C9 (66). Additionally, CYP1A2 appears to be involved in the formation of 7-hydroxy olanzapine, a metabolite yet to be identified *in vivo*. The formation of a less abundant metabolite, 2-hydroxy olanzapine, appears to be mediated by CYP2D6 (66). Although therapeutic drug monitoring of olanzapine is not a routine clinical procedure, preliminary data suggest that a plasma concentration of at least 9 ng/mL is predictive of a favorable response (67).

Olanzapine has been systematically assessed *in vitro* to determine its potential to inhibit the cytochrome P450s CYP2C9, CYP2C19, CYP2D6, and CYP3A (68). After determining the percent inhibition by olanzapine of substrates metabolized by these cytochromes, it appears that therapeutic doses of olanzapine would be unlikely to significantly inhibit coadministered substrates of these isozymes (68). CYP1A2 was not evaluated in this study. However, a drug interaction study has been performed in which olanzapine and the tricyclic antidepressant imipramine were administered alone and in combination to healthy subjects (69). The pharmacokinetics of imipramine were unaltered, suggesting that olanzapine is not a potent inhibitor of CYP1A2, CYP2D6, or CYP3A *in vivo*.

It is unclear how the disposition of olanzapine is affected by coadministered inhibitors of isozymes such as CYP1A2. It is known that smoking, through induction of CYP1A2, increases the clearance of olanzapine and may reduce olanzapine half-life by as much as 50% (70). Although no reports are currently available, it is likely that concurrent use of drugs that inhibit CYP1A2 activity, such as fluvoxamine or ciprofloxacin, could result in decreased clearance of olanzapine. Conversely, inducers of CYP1A2 such as carbamazepine or rifampicin may lead to increased clearance of olanzapine. For example, relatively low doses of carbamazepine (400 mg/day) have resulted in a 50% increase in olanzapine clearance (71). Given the abundance of phase II elimination products, such as the 10-*N*-glucuronide, it is possible that inducers or inhibitors of glucuronosyltransferase (UDGPT) enzymes may affect the clearance of olanzapine.

QUETIAPINE

Quetiapine is a dibenzothiazepine derivative with a broad spectrum of receptor affinity. Quetiapine has moderate affinity for 5-HT$_{2A}$, α_1, muscarinic, and histaminergic receptors. It has only minor affinity for D$_2$ and 5-HT$_{1A}$ receptors, and very low affinity for 5-HT$_{2C}$, α_2, and D$_1$ receptors (72). The ratio of 5-HT$_2$ to D$_2$ antagonism appears similar to that of clozapine.

Quetiapine undergoes extensive hepatic biotransformation with less than 1% excreted as unchanged drug in the urine (72). Principal elimination pathways include sulfoxidation, oxidation of the terminal alcohol to the corresponding carboxylic acid, hydroxylation of the dibenzothiazepine ring, O-dealkylation, N-dealkylation,

and phase II conjugation (Fig. 19-5) (73). A number of metabolites have been tested both *in vitro* and *in vivo* for affinity for 5-HT$_2$ and D$_1$ and D$_2$ receptors. These studies indicate that the primary sulfoxide metabolite is pharmacologically inactive, whereas both the 7-hydroxy and 7-hydroxy-N-dealkylated metabolites display activity similar to the parent compound. These latter two metabolites account for only 5% and 2%, respectively, of the plasma quetiapine concentration at steady-state.

In vitro studies indicate that CYP3A4 is the primary isozyme involved in the metabolism of quetiapine to its major sulfoxide metabolite. A lesser role is found for CYP2D6, which is thought to contribute to the hydroxylation pathway (74). Coadministration of the CYP3A4 inducer phenytoin resulted in a five-fold increase in the

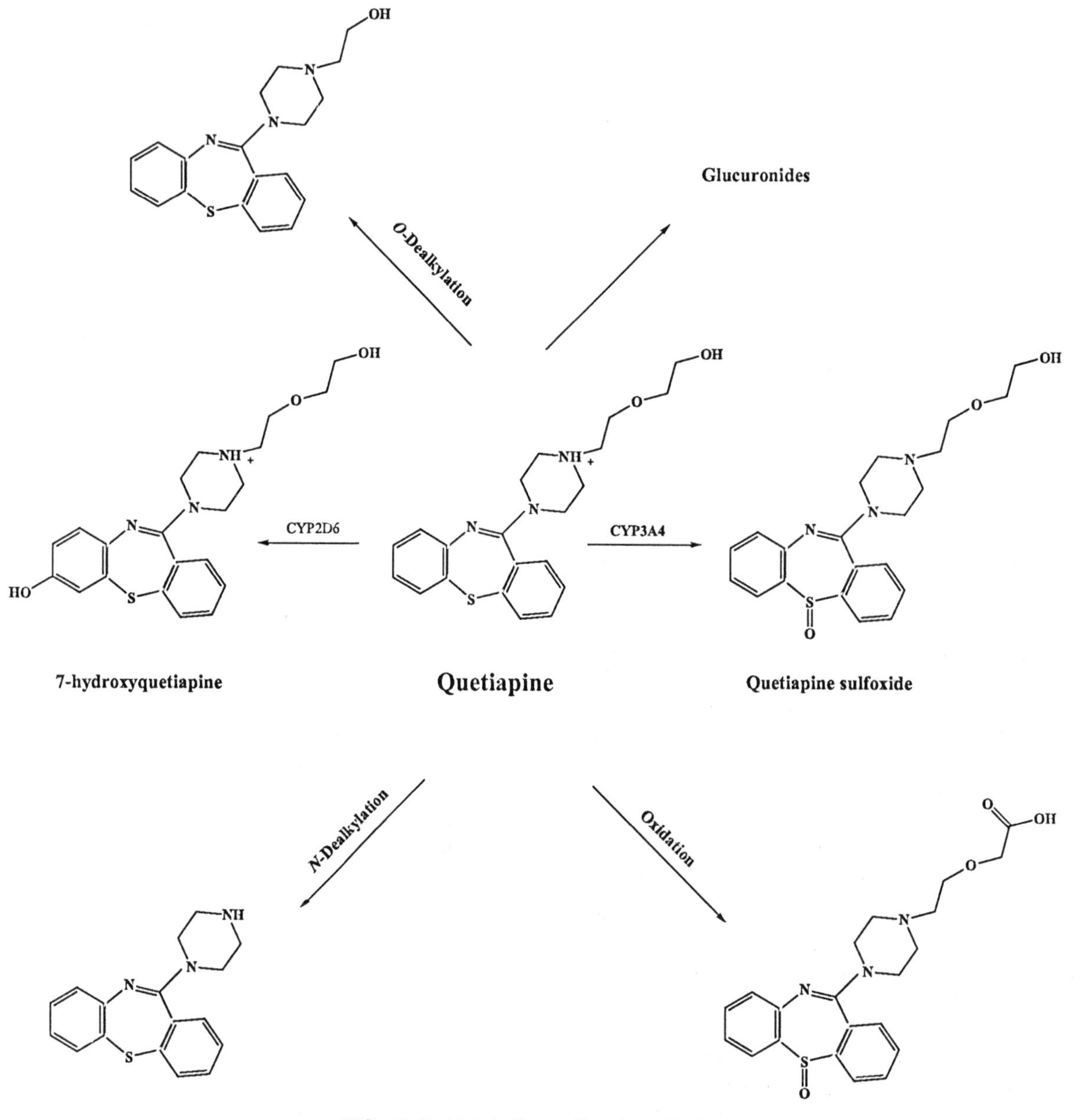

FIG. 19-5. Metabolic profile of quetiapine.

clearance of quetiapine. However, coadministration of cimetidine did not significantly affect the steady-state pharmacokinetics of quetiapine. Additionally, coadministration of quetiapine with the phenothiazine thioridazine resulted in a 65% increase in the oral clearance of quetiapine and significant decreases in AUC, C_{max}, and C_{min}, suggesting thioridazine induction of quetiapine metabolism (74).

ZIPRASIDONE

Ziprasidone is a benzisothiazoyl piperazine antipsychotic currently undergoing late phase III clinical trials. Ziprasidone has high affinity for D_2, 5-HT_{2A}, 5-HT_{2C}, 5-HT_{1D}, and α_1-adrenergic receptors. It has moderate affinity for D_1 and D_4 receptors and little activity at β-adrenergic, muscarinic, or histaminergic receptors (75).

Ziprasidone is highly metabolized with at least 12 metabolites identified in humans and only minor amounts excreted unchanged in urine (Fig. 19-6). Ziprasidone sulfoxide and sulfone are the most abundant metabolites detected in the serum (76). These metabolites have low affinity for 5-HT_2 and D_2 receptors relative to the parent drug and are thought to be unlikely to contribute therapeutic effects. Major urinary metabolites identified include oxindole-acetic acid—its glucuronide—benzisothiazole-3-yl-piperazine (BITP), BITP-sulfoxide, BITP-sulfone, and its lactam (76).

At present there is little information available regarding the isoforms responsible for the formation of the

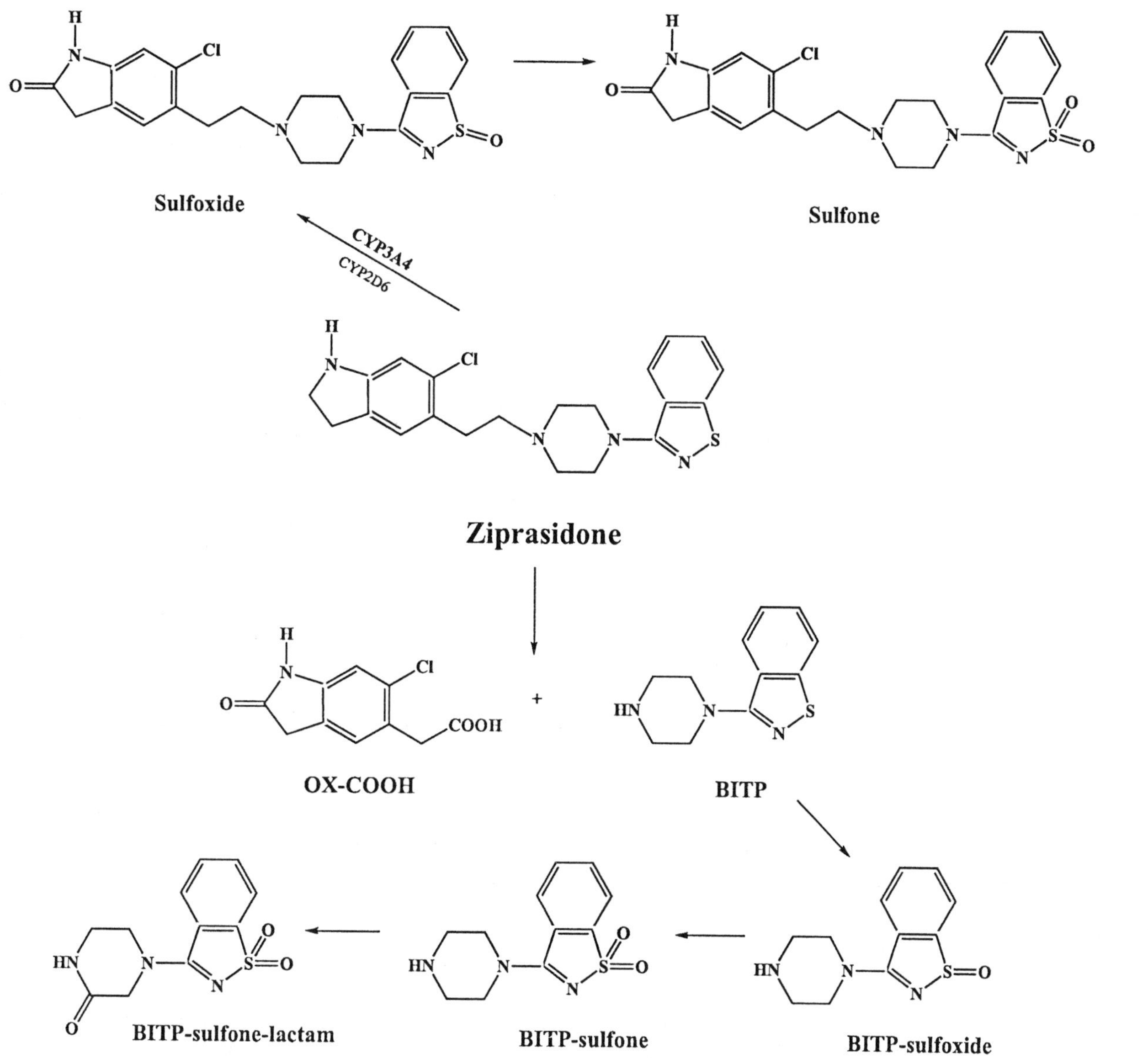

FIG. 19-6. Metabolic profile of ziprasidone.

major metabolites of ziprasidone. It appears that the formation of the sulfoxide and sulfone metabolites is mediated by CYP3A4 with little contribution by CYP2D6 (76).

PHENOTHIAZINES AND CONVENTIONAL ANTIPSYCHOTICS

Following the introduction of chlorpromazine in 1952 and ensuing structural analogues, the phenothiazines rapidly became the mainstay treatments for schizophrenia and other psychotic disorders (1). Although these medications continue to be in wide use, they are being supplanted by the atypical antipsychotics for clinical use. The phenothiazines and other conventional antipsychotics possess significant side effect liabilities and limited efficacy in the treatment of the negative or deficit symptoms of schizophrenia (1).

As a class, the phenothiazines are extensively metabolized in humans by numerous pathways including aromatic hydroxylation, N-dealkylation, N-oxidation, and S-oxidation. Additionally, they are subject to a number of conjugation reactions with glucuronic acid, sulphuric acid, and glutathione (77,78). A large interindividual variability in phenothiazine plasma concentrations is well recognized.

Chlorpromazine is regarded as the prototypic phenothiazine antipsychotic agent. Its biotransformation is probably the most extensively studied of the antipsychotics, and thin layer chromatography has revealed the presence of as many as 75 urinary metabolites of chlorpromazine (79,80), 45 of which have been identified in humans. Major metabolites include N-desmethylchlorpromazine, chlorpromazine-N-oxide, chlorpromazine sulfoxide, N,N-didesmethylchlorpromazine, and 7-hydroxychlorpromazine. This latter metabolite is equipotent to the parent compound (81). Plasma concentrations of 7-hydroxy metabolite may exceed those of the parent compound and potentially contribute to chlorpromazine-induced toxicity (79).

An in vitro investigation using human liver microsomal preparations suggested that N-oxidation is catalyzed by FMO form II whereas ring S-oxidation is catalyzed by CYP3A4 with possible contributions from CYP2A6, CYP2C8, and CYP2D6 (82). Although both in vitro and in vivo studies have suggested that chlorpromazine may be a substrate of CYP2D6, it has been demonstrated that coadministration of quinidine with chlorpromazine in subjects phenotyped with methoxyphenamine as poor metabolizers does not increase plasma concentrations of the parent compound. However, quinidine was found to inhibit the 7-hydroxylation pathway, which appears to lead to compensatory increases in amounts of chlorpromazine sulfoxide, N-desmethylchlorpromazine, and N,N-didesmethylchlorpromazine excreted in the urine (83).

Thioridazine is another well-known phenothiazine antipsychotic undergoing extensive biotransformation

(see Table 19-1). Primary metabolites include thioridazine-2-sulfoxide, sulforidazine, mesoridazine (separately marketed as the preformed antipsychotic), thioridazine 2-sulfone, and thioridazine 5-sulfoxide. Mesoridazine and sulforidazine are therapeutically active (79,84), whereas thioridazine 5-sulfoxide has little therapeutic activity and may contribute to the toxicity of the parent drug (85). Thioridazine contains an asymmetric carbon. Oxidation of the ring sulfur atom and the side chain forming the 5-sulfoxide and mesoridazine, respectively, results in the formation of two additional chiral centers. As a consequence, the drug has been the object of studies addressing the stereoselective pharmacology of the various enantiomers. For instance, Svendsen and coworkers (86) have demonstrated that the thioridazine enantiomers exhibit significant differences in D_1 and D_2 receptor affinity.

In studies using both human volunteers and patients who had been phenotyped as either poor or extensive metabolizers of CYP2D6 and CYP2C19 substrates, it has been shown that the formation of mesoridazine, thioridazine 2-sulfoxide, and possibly thioridazine 5-sulfoxide, but not thioridazine 2-sulfone, is catalyzed by CYP2D6 (87,88). Additionally, significant differences in thioridazine AUC has been found between poor and extensive metabolizers administered the drug (87). It has also been suggested that CYP2C19 could possibly play a role in the formation of some identified metabolites (88).

Perphenazine is another phenothiazine antipsychotic that has been used extensively in the treatment of psychotic disorders and is also marketed in fixed combinations with the tricyclic antidepressant amitriptyline. Like other members of this drug class, perphenazine undergoes extensive metabolism with perphenazine sulfoxide and a dealkylated metabolite among the most abundantly formed metabolites reported (89). Neither is believed to be therapeutically significant. Currently, most investigations have pointed toward a prominent role for CYP2D6 in the disposition of perphenazine. Dahl-Puustinen and co-workers (90) found the AUC of perphenazine in poor metabolizers to be 4.1 times that of extensive metabolizers of debrisoquine. Furthermore, a three-fold difference in perphenazine clearance was found between genotyped extensive metabolizers and poor metabolizers (91). In one study (92), it was found that genotyped patients who were poor metabolizers had median perphenazine plasma concentration per dose approximately twice that of extensive metabolizers. However, significant interindividual differences in perphenazine concentrations were found in both groups, leading the investigators to conclude that other factors such as a prominent first pass effect may contribute greater variability to perphenazine disposition than metabolic status.

In a study in which elderly patients receiving perphenazine were prospectively phenotyped (93), it was found that poor metabolizers of CYP2D6 had significantly greater drug side effects such as sedation and extrapyramidal effects. The investigators concluded that prospective monitoring of CYP2D6 status may have clinical utility in the elderly population receiving antipsychotics metabolized by CYP2D6.

Because perphenazine is commonly coadministered with other therapeutic agents, it is not unlikely that significant drug–drug interaction could occur if an inhibitor of CYP2D6 is given concurrently with perphenazine. A recent double-blind study demonstrated that extensive metabolizers of CYP2D6 substrates experienced robust increases in perphenazine plasma concentrations as well as dose-related side effects following the addition of the SSRI paroxetine, a known inhibitor of CYP2D6, to clinically relevant doses of perphenazine (94).

SUMMARY

As a therapeutic drug class, the antipsychotics represent a chemically and pharmacologically diverse group of compounds. All of the agents are noted to undergo extensive biotransformation by both phase I and II processes. Oxidative metabolism is represented most prominently by CYP3A4, CYP1A2, CYP2D6, FMO, and to a lesser extent, by other isozymes. Regarding phase II metabolism, extensive glucuronidation is in evidence. Although specific isoforms of UDGPT that mediate the metabolism of antipsychotics have not been identified, recent evidence suggests UGT1.4 participates in the glucuronidation of a number of tertiary amine psychotropic agents, including clozapine (95).

REFERENCES

1. Kane JM. Schizophrenia. *New Engl J Med* 1996;334:34–41.
2. Soudijn W, Van Wijngaarden L, Allewijn F. Distribution, excretion and metabolism of neuroleptics of the butyrophenone type I. Excretion and metabolism of haloperidol and nine related butyrophenone derivatives in the Wistar rat. *Eur J Pharmacol* 1967;1:47–57.
3. Forsman A, Larsson M. Metabolism of haloperidol. *Curr Ther Res* 1978;24:567–568.
4. Korpi JR, Wyatt RJ. Reduced haloperidol: effects on striatal dopamine metabolism and conversion to haloperidol in the rat. *Psychopharmacologia* 1984;83:34–37.
5. Ereshefsky L, Davis CM, Harrington CA, et al. Haloperidol and reduced haloperidol plasma levels in selected schizophrenic patients. *J Clin Psychopharmacol* 1984;4:138–142.
6. Altamura AC, Mauri MC, Cavallaro R, Gorni A. Haloperidol metabolism and antipsychotic effect in schizophrenia. *Lancet* 1987;1:814–815.
7. Korpi ER, Costakos DT, Wyatt JR. Interconversions of haloperidol and reduced haloperidol in guinea pig and rat liver microsomes. *Biochem Pharmacol* 1985;34:2923–2927.
8. Midha KK, Hawes EM, Hubbard JW, Korchinski ED, McKay G. Interconversion between haloperidol and reduced haloperidol in humans. *J Clin Psychopharmacol* 1987;7:362–364.
9. Lane HY, Lin HN, Hu OY, Chen CC, Jann MW, Chang WH. Blood levels of reduced haloperidol versus clinical efficacy and extrapyramidal side effects of haloperidol. *Prog Neuropsychopharmacol Biol Psychiatry* 1997;21:299–311.
10. Gorrod JW, Fang J. On the metabolism of haloperidol. *Xenobiotica* 1993;23:495–508.
11. Fang J, Zuo DM, Yu PH. A comparison of a quaternary pyridinium metabolite of haloperidol (HP+) with the neurotoxin N-methyl-4-phenylpyridinium (MPP+) towards cultured dopaminergic neuroblastoma cells. *Psychopharmacology* 1995;121:373–378.
12. Rollema H, Skonik M, d'Engelbronner J, Igarashi K, Usuki E, Castagnoli N Jr. MPP+-like neurotoxicity of a pyridinium metabolite derived from haloperidol: in vivo microdialysis and in vitro mitochondrial studies. *J Pharmacol Exp Ther* 1994;268:380–387.
13. Inaba T, Jurima M, Mahon WA, Kalow W. In vitro inhibition studies of two isozymes of human liver cytochrome P-450: mephenytoin p-hydroxylase and sparteine monooxygenase. *Drug Metab Dispos* 1985;13:443–448.
14. Spina E, Martines C, Caputi AP, et al. Debrisoquin oxidation phenotype during neuroleptic monotherapy. *Eur J Clin Pharmacol* 1991;41:467–470.
15. Tyndale RF, Kalow W, Inaba T. Oxidation of reduced haloperidol to haloperidol: involvement of P450IID6 (sparteine/debrisoquine monooxygenase). *Br J Clin Pharmacol* 1991;31:655–660.
16. Young D, Midha KK, Fossler MJ, et al. Effect of quinidine on the interconversion kinetics between haloperidol and reduced haloperidol in humans: implications for the involvement of cytochrome P450II2D6. *Eur J Clin Pharmacol* 1993;44:433–438.
17. Llerena A, Dahl M-L, Ekqvist B, Bertilsson L. Haloperidol disposition is dependent on the debrisoquine hydroxylation phenotype: increased plasma levels of the reduced metabolite in poor metabolizers. *Ther Drug Monitor* 1992;14:261–264.
18. Lane H-Y, Hu O Y-P, Jann MW, Deng H-C, L H-N, Chang W-H. Dextromethorphan phenotyping and haloperidol disposition in schizophrenic patients. *Psych Res* 1997;69:105–111.
19. Kim Y-H, Cha I-J, Shim J-C, et al. Effect of rifampin on the plasma concentration and the clinical effect of haloperidol concomitantly administered to schizophrenic patients. *J Clin Psychopharmacol* 1996;16:247–252.
20. Vandel S, Bertschy G, Baumann P, et al. Fluvoxamine and fluoxetine: interaction studies with amitriptyline, clomipramine and neuroleptics in phenotyped patients. *Pharmacol Res* 1995;31:347–353.
21. Avenoso A, Spine E, Campo G, et al. Interaction between fluoxetine and haloperidol: pharmacokinetic and clinical implications. *Pharm Res* 1997;35:335–339.
22. Von Moltke LL, Greenblatt DJ, Cotreau-Bibbo MM, et al. Inhibition of desipramine hydroxylation in vitro by serotonin-reuptake inhibitor antidepressants, and by quinidine and ketoconazole: a model system to predict drug interactions in vivo. *J Pharmacol Exp Ther* 1994;268:1278–1283.
23. Barbhajya RH, Shukla UA, Greene D, Breuel H-P, Midha KK. Investigation of pharmacokinetic and pharmacodynamic interactions after coadministration of nefazodone and haloperidol. *J Clin Psychopharmacol* 1996;16:26–34.
24. Fang J, Baker GB, Silverstone PH, Coutts RT. Involvement of CYP3A4 and CYP21D6 in the metabolism of haloperidol. *Cell Mol Neurobiol* 1997;17:227–233.
25. Gauch R, Michaelis W. The metabolism of 8-chloro-11-(4-methyl-1-piperazinyl)-5H-dibenzo[b,e,] [1,4] diazepine (clozapine) in mice, dogs and human subjects. *Farm Ed Pract* 1971;26:667–681.
26. Tandon R, Kane JM. Neuropharmacological basis of clozapine's unique profile. *Arch Gen Psychiatry* 1993;50:157–159.
27. Kapur S, Remington G. Serotonin-dopamine interaction and its relevance to schizophrenia. *Am J Psychiatry* 1996;153:466–476.
28. Alvir JMJ, Lieberman JA. A reevaluation of the clinical characteristics of clozapine-induced agranulocytosis in light of the United States experience. *J Clin Psychopharmacol* 1994;14:87–89.
29. Jann MW, Lam LY, Chang WH. Rapid formation of clozapine in guinea-pigs and man following clozapine-N-oxide administration. *Arch Int Pharmacodyn Ther* 1994;328:243–250.
30. Kuoppamäki M, Syvalahti E, Hietala J. Clozapine and N-desmethylclozapine are potent 5-HT1c antagonists. *Eur J Pharmacol* 1993;245:179–182.
31. Gerson SL, Arce C, Meltzer HY. N-desmethylclozapine: a clozapine metabolite that suppresses haemopoiesis. *Br J Haematol* 1994;86:555–561.
32. Dain JG, Nicoletti J, Ballard F. Biotransformation of clozapine in humans. *Drug Metab Dispos* 1997;25:603-609.
33. Stock VB, Spiteller G, Heipertz R. Austausch aromatisch gehinderter halogens gegen OH-and SCH3-bei der metabolisierung des clozapine in minschlichen korper. *Arzneim Forsch* 1977;27:982–990.
34. Luo H, McKay G, Midha KK. Identification of clozapine N-glu-

curonide in the urine of patients treated with clozapine using electrospray mass spectrometry. *Biol Mass Spectrom* 1994;23:147–148.

35. Williams DP, Pirmohamed M, Naisbitt DJ, Maggs JL, Park BK. Neutrophil cytotoxicity of the chemically reactive metabolite(s) of clozapine: possible role in agranulocytosis. *J Pharmacol Exp Ther* 1997; 283:1375–1382.

36. Cooper TB. Clozapine plasma level monitoring: current status. *Psychiatr Q* 1996;67:297–311.

37. Pirmohamed M, Williams D, Madden S, Templeton E, Park BK. Metabolism and bioactivation of clozapine by human liver in vitro. *J Pharmacol Exp Ther* 1995;272:984–990.

38. Linnet K, Olesen OV. Metabolism of clozapine by cDNA-expressed human cytochrome P450 enzymes. *Drug Metab Dispos* 1997;25: 1379–1382.

39. Eierman B, Engel G, Johansson I, Zanger UM, Bertilsson L. The involvement of CYP1A2 and CYP3A4 in the metabolism of clozapine. *Br J Clin Pharmacol* 1997;44:439–446.

40. Edge SC, Markowitz JS, DeVane CL. Clozapine drug-drug interactions: a review of the literature. *Hum Psychopharmacol* 1997;12:5–20.

41. Bertilsson L, Carrillo JA, Dahl M-L, et al. Clozapine disposition covaries with CYP1A2 activity determined by the caffeine test. *Br J Clin Pharmacol* 1994;38:471–473.

42. Wetzel H, Anghelescu I, Szegedi A, et al. Pharmacokinetic interactions of clozapine with selective serotonin reuptake inhibitors: differential effects of fluvoxamine and paroxetine in a prospective study. *J Clin Psychopharmacol* 1998;18:2–9.

43. Jerling M, Lindström L, Bertilsson L. Fluvoxamine inhibition and carbamazepine induction of the metabolism of clozapine: evidence from a therapeutic drug monitoring service. *Ther Drug Monit* 1994;16:368–374.

44. Brøsen K, Skjelbo E, Rasmussen BB, Poulsen He, Loft S. Fluvoxamine is a potent inhibitor of cytochrome P450 1A2. *Biochem Pharmacol* 1994;45:1211–1214.

45. Xu Z-H, Xie H-G, Zhou H-H. *In vivo* inhibition of CYP2C19 but not CYP2D6 by fluvoxamine. *Br J Clin Pharmacol* 1996;42:518–521.

46. von Moltke LL, Greenblatt DJ, Court MH, Duan SX, Harmatz JS, Shader RJ. Inhibition of alprazolam and desipramine hydroxylation in vitro by paroxetine and fluvoxamine: comparison with other selective serotonin reuptake inhibitor antidepressants. *J Clin Psychopharmacol* 1995;15:125–131.

47. Joos AAB, Frank UG. Pharmacokinetic interaction of clozapine and rifampicin in a forensic patient with an atypical mycobacterial infection. *J Clin Psychopharmacol* 1998;18:83–85.

48. Markowitz JS, Gill HS, DeVane CL, Mintzer J. Fluoroquinolone-mediated inhibition of clozapine metabolism. *Am J Psychiatry* 1997;153:881.

49. Raaska K, Neuvonen PJ. Serum concentrations of clozapine and N-desmethylclozapine are unaffected by the potent CYP3A4 inhibitor itraconazole. *Eur J Clin Pharmacol* 1998;54:167–170.

50. Fisher V, Vogels B, Maurer G, Tynes, R. The antipsychotic clozapine is metabolized by the polymorphic human microsomal and recombinant cytochrome P450 2D6. *J Pharmacol Exp Ther* 1992;260:1355–1360.

51. Dahl M-L, Llerena A, Bondesson U, Lindström L, Bertilsson L. Disposition of clozapine in man: lack of an association with debrisoquine and S-mephenytoin hydroxylation polymorphisms. *Br J Clin Pharmacol* 1994;37:71–74.

52. Arranz MJ, Dawson E, Shaikh S, et al. Cytochrome P4502D6 does not determine response to clozapine. *Br J Clin Pharmacol* 1995;39: 417–420.

53. Centorrino F, Baldessarini RJ, Kando J, et al. Serum concentration of clozapine and its major metabolite effects of cotherapy with fluoxetine or valproate. *Am J Psychiatry* 1994;151:123–125.

54. Eggert AC, Crismon ML, Dovjon PG. Lack of effect with fluoxetine on plasma clozapine concentration. *J Clin Psychiatry* 1994;55:454–455.

55. Nemeroff CB, DeVane CL, Pollack BG. Newer antidepressants and the cytochrome P450 system. *Am J Psychiatry* 1996;153:311–320.

56. Tugnait M, Hawes EM, McKay G, Rettie AE, Haining RL, Midha KK. N-oxidation of clozapine by flavin-containing monooxygenases. *Drug Metab Dispos* 1997;25:524–527.

57. Kane J. Risperidone. *Am J Psychiatry* 1994;151:802.

58. Huang ML, Van Peer A, Woestenborghs R, et al. Pharmacokinetics of the novel antipsychotic agent risperidone and the prolactin response in healthy subjects. *Clin Pharmacol Ther* 1993;54:257–268.

59. Mannens GM, Huang M-L, Meuldermans W, Hendrickx J, Woestenborghs R, Heykants J. Absorption, metabolism, and excretion of risperidone in humans. *Drug Metab Dispos* 1993;21:1134–1141.

60. Ereshefsky L, Anderson CB, True J, et al. Plasma concentration of oral risperidone and active metabolite in schizophrenics. *Pharmacotherapy* 1993;13:292(abst).

61. Janssen PAJ, Niemegeers CJE, Awouters F, Schellekens KHL, Megens AAHP, Meert TF. Risperidone a new antipsychotic with serotonin-S1 and dopamine-D2 antagonistic properties. *J Pharm Exp Ther* 1988; 244:685–693.

62. Schotte A, Janssen PFM, Gommeren W, et al. Risperidone compared with new and reference antipsychotic drugs: in vitro and in vivo receptor binding. *Psychopharmacology* 1996;124:57–73.

63. Byerly MJ, DeVane CL. Pharmacokinetics of clozapine and risperidone: a review of recent literature. *J Clin Psychopharmacol* 1996;16: 177–187.

64. Fulton B, Goa KL. Olanzapine: a review of its pharmacological properties and therapeutic efficacy in the management of schizophrenia and related psychosis. *Drugs* 1997;53:281–298.

65. Kassahun K, Mattiuz E, Nyhart E, et al. Disposition and biotransformation of the antipsychotic agent olanzapine in humans. *Drug Metab Dispos* 1997;25:81–93.

66. Ring BJ, Catlow J, Linday TJ, et al. Identification of the human cytochromes P450 responsible for the *in vitro* formation of the major oxidative metabolites of the antipsychotic agent olanzapine. *J Pharmacol Exp Ther* 1996;276:658–666.

67. Perry PJ, Sanger T, Beasley C. Olanzapine plasma concentrations and clinical response in acutely ill schizophrenic patients. *J Clin Psychopharmacol* 1997;17:472–477.

68. Ring BJ, Binkley SN, Vandenbranden M, Wrighton SA. *In vitro* interaction of the antipsychotic agent olanzapine with human cytochromes P450 CYP2C9, CYP2C19, CYP2D6 and CYP3A. *Br J Clin Pharmacol* 1996;41:181–186.

69. Callaghan JT, Cerimele BJ, Kassahun KJ, Nyhart EH, Hoyes-Beehler PJ, Kondraske GV. Olanzapine: interaction study with imipramine. *J Clin Pharmacol* 1997;37:971–978.

70. Ereshefsky L. Pharmacokinetics and drug interactions: update for new antipsychotics. *J Clin Psychiatry* 1996;57:12–25.

71. Zyprexa (olanzapine) prescribing information. Eli Lilly, 1998.

72. Seroquel (quetiapine) prescribing information. Zeneca Pharmaceuticals, 1998.

73. Wong YWF, Ewing BJ, Thyrum PT, et al. The effect of phenytoin and cimetidine on the pharmacokinetics of Seroquel (quetiapine). Presented at the American Psychiatric Association Annual Meeting, San Diego, CA, May 17–22, 1997.

74. Grimm SW, Stams KR, Bui K. In vitro prediction of potential metabolic drug interactions for Seroquel (quetiapine). Presented at the American Psychiatric Association Annual Meeting, San Diego, CA, May 17–22, 1997.

75. Seeger TF, Seymour PA, Schmidt AW, et al. Ziprasidone (CP-88,059): a new antipsychotic with combined dopamine and serotonin receptor antagonist activity. *J Pharmacol Exp Ther* 1995;275:1995;101–113.

76. Prakash C, Kamel A, Gummerus J, Wilner K. Metabolism of a new antipsychotic drug, ziprasidone, in humans. *Drug Metab Dispos* 1997; 25:863–872.

77. Curry SH. Phenothiazines: metabolism and pharmacokinetics. In: Burrows GD, Norman TR, Davies B, eds. *Antipsychotics*. Amsterdam: Elsevier, 1985:79–97.

78. Hubbard JW, Midha KK, Hawes EM, McKay G, Marder SR, Aravagiri M, Korchinski ED. Metabolism of phenothiazine and butyrophenone antipsychotic drugs: a review of some recent findings and clinical implications. *Br J Psychiatry* 1993;163:19–24.

79. Patrick KS. Effect of metabolism on the response to dopamine agonists and antagonists. *Am J Pharm Ed* 1993;53:163–168.

80. Yeung PK-F, Hubbard JW, Korchinski ED, Midha KK. Pharmacokinetics of chlorpromazine and key metabolites. *Eur J Clin Pharmacol* 1993;45:563–569.

81. Creese I, Manian AA, Prosser TD, Snyder SH. ^{3}H-Haloperidol binding to dopamine receptors in rat corpus striatum: influence of chlorpromazine metabolites and derivatives. *Eur J Pharmacol* 1978;47:291–296.

82. Cashman JR, Yung Z, Yang L, Wrighton SA. Stereo and regioselective N- and S-oxidation of tertiary amines and sulfides in the presence of adult human liver microsomes. *Drug Metab Dispos* 1993;21:492–501.

83. Muralidharan G, Cooper JK, Hawes EM, Korchinski ED, Midha KK. Quinidine inhibits the 7-hydroxylation of chlorpromazine in extensive metabolizers of debrisoquine. *Eur J Clin Pharmacol* 1996;50:121–128.

84. Niedzwiecki DM, Cubeddu LX, Mailman RB. Comparative anti-

dopaminergic properties of thioridazine, mesoridazine, and sulforidazine on the corpus striatum. *J Pharmacol Exp Ther* 1989;250:117–125.

85. Dahl SG. Active metabolites of neuroleptic drugs: possible contribution to therapeutic and toxic effects. *Ther Drug Monit* 1982;4:33–40.

86. Svendsen CN, Froimowitz W, Hrbek C, et al. Receptor affinity, neurochemistry and behavioral characteristics of the enantiomers of thioridazine: evidence of different stereoselectivities at D1 and D2 receptors in rat brain. *Neuropharmacology* 1988;27:1117–1124.

87. Von Bahr C, Movin G, Nordin C, et al. Plasma levels of thioridazine and metabolites are influenced by the debrisoquin hydroxylation phenotype. *Clin Pharmacol Ther* 1991;49:234–240.

88. Eap CB, Guentert TW, Schaublin-Loidl M, et al. Plasma levels of the enantiomers of thioridazine, thioridazine 2-sulfoxide, thioridazine 2-sulfone, and thioridazine 5-sulfoxide in poor and extensive metabolizers of dextromethorphan and mephenytoin. *Clin Pharmacol Ther* 1996; 59:322–331.

89. Larsen NE, Hansen LB, Knudsen P. Quantitative determination of perphenazine and its dealkylated metabolite using high-performance liquid chromatography. *J Chromatogr* 1985;341:244–250.

90. Dahl-Puustinen ML, Lidén A, Alm C, Nordin C, Bertilsson L. Disposition of perphenazine is related to polymorphic debrisoquine hydroxylation in human beings. *Clin Pharmacol Ther* 1989;46:78–81.

91. Jerling M, Dahl ML, Åbergwistedt A, et al. The CYP2D6 genotype predicts the oral clearance of the neuroleptic agents perphenazine and zuclopenthixol. *Clin Pharmacol Ther* 1996;59:423–428.

92. Linnet K, Wilborg O. Steady-state concentrations of the neuroleptic perphenazine in relation to CYP2D6 genetic polymorphism. *Clin Pharmacol Ther* 1996;60:41–47.

93. Pollock BG, Mulsant BH, Sweet RA, Rosen J, Altieri LP, Perel JM. Prospective cytochrome P450 phenotyping for neuroleptic treatment in dementia. *Psychopharmacol Bull* 1995;31:327–331.

94. Özdemir V, Naranjo CA, Herrman N, Reed K, Sellers EM, Kalow W. Paroxetine potentiates the central nervous system side effects of perphenazine: contribution of cytochrome P4502D6 inhibition in vivo. *Clin Pharmacol Ther* 1997;62:334–347.

95. Green MD, Tephly TR. Glucuronidation of amines and hydroxylated xenobiotics and endobiotics catalyzed by expressed human UGT1.4 protein. *Drug Metab Dispos* 1996;24:356–363.

CHAPTER 20

Sedative-Hypnotic and Anxiolytic Agents

David J. Greenblatt and Lisa L. von Moltke

The sedative-hypnotic class of medications includes those drugs used to treat anxiety, panic disorder, and sleep disorders (Table 20-1). For practical purposes, the benzodiazepine derivatives account for the majority of sedative-hypnotics used throughout the world (1–4). Since 1995, the imidazopyridine hypnotic agent zolpidem also has gained widespread acceptance in the treatment of sleep disorders (5–8). Because anxiety and insomnia commonly coexist with other medical and psychiatric diseases, pharmacokinetic and pharmacodynamic interactions with sedative-hypnotics is of ongoing medical and scientific concern. Of particular concern in the context of drug interactions are the medications used to treat human immunodeficiency virus (HIV) infection and its complications. The availability of these drugs (including the viral protease inhibitors, nonnucleoside reverse transcriptase inhibitors, and azole antifungal agents) has greatly improved survival in HIV-infected individuals (9–13). However, the medications also have the capacity to inhibit and/or induce the activity of human cytochrome P450 (CYP) enzymes, with the consequent possibility of pharmacokinetic drug interactions (14,15). In a number of cases, these interactions are very large in magnitude and of major clinical importance.

BIOTRANSFORMATION OF SEDATIVE-HYPNOTICS: ROLE OF CYP3A

The CYP3A subfamily of drug-metabolizing enzymes assumes (16) central importance for the under-standing of drug interactions with sedative-hypnotics, since most of these medications are partial or complete substrates for CYP3A (see Table 20-1). As such, the drug interaction profiles are largely consistent with the established patterns of susceptibility of CYP3A to inhibition or induction by various foreign chemicals (17–20). The pertinent properties of CYP3A, extensively reviewed in Chapter 10 and elsewhere in the lit-

TABLE 20-1. *Sedative-hypnotic and anxiolytic medications in common clinical use in North America*

Substrate	Enzymes mediating biotransformation
Primary clinical use for anxiety or panic disorder	
Diazepam	CYP3A (also CYP2C19)
Desmethyldiazepam[a]	CYP3A (also CYP2C19)
Oxazepam	Glucuronyl transferase
Lorazepam	Glucuronyl transferase
Alprazolam	CYP3A
Clonazepam	?CYP3A
Chlordiazepoxide	Not established
Buspirone	CYP3A
Primary clinical use for sleep disorder	
Flurazepam[b]	Not established
Triazolam	CYP3A
Temazepam	Glucuronyl transferase
Quazepam[b]	Not established
Estazolam	Not established
Zolpidem	CYP3A, CYP2C9 (also CYP1A2)
Midazolam[c]	CYP3A
Zaleplon	?CYP3A

[a]Administered as precursor or prodrugs: clorazepate or prazepam.
[b]Prodrugs for desalkylflurazepam.
[c]Oral midazolam not approved in the United States; parenteral midazolam used in anesthetic practice.

D. J. Greenblatt: Department of Pharmacology and Experimental Therapeutics, Tufts University School of Medicine, 136 Harrison Avenue, and General Clinical Research Center, New England Medical Center, Boston, Massachusetts 02111

L. L. von Moltke: Department of Pharmacology and Experimental Therapeutics, Tufts University School of Medicine, 136 Harrison Avenue, and Department of Medicine, New England Medical Center, Boston, Massachusetts 02111

TABLE 20-2. *Inhibitors and inducers of CYP3A activity in humans*

CYP3A inhibitors	CYP3A inducers
Ketoconazole	Carbamazepine
Itraconazole	Rifampin
Fluconazole	Ritonavir
Erythromycin	Dexamethasone
Troleandomycin	Nevirapine
Clarithromycin	
Ritonavir	
Indinavir	
Delavirdine	
Norfluoxetine	
Fluvoxamine	
Nefazodone	
Grapefruit juice[a]	

[a]May inhibit gastrointestinal CYP3A.

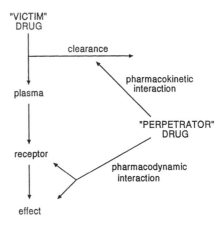

FIG. 20-1. Schematic representation of pharmacokinetic and pharmacodynamic drug interactions. A pharmacokinetic interaction occurs when the perpetrator either decreases or increases the clearance of the victim, correspondingly changing the plasma concentration, receptor availability, and clinical effect of the victim drug. A pharmacodynamic interaction occurs when the perpetrator either potentiates or antagonizes the clinical effect of the victim by acting on the same receptor system, or on another receptor system that yields similar or identical clinical actions.

erature (16–20), include high relative abundance in human liver, quantitatively important presence in gastrointestinal tract, lack of a genetic polymorphic pattern of expression and activity, and an established list of probable inhibitors and inducers (Table 20-2). As discussed later, the pharmacokinetic and pharmacodynamic consequences of inhibition or induction of a CYP3A substrate drug are likely to be greatest for those substrates that ordinarily undergo moderate or extensive presystemic extraction after oral dosage. Three commonly used benzodiazepine derivatives—oxazepam, lorazepam, and temazepam—are biotransformed mainly by glucuronide conjugation (21–23) (see Chapter 12), mediated by one or more glucuronyl transferases. Patterns of drug interactions with these three compounds differ greatly from the CYP3A substrates. In general, glucuronide conjugation is uninfluenced or minimally influenced by factors that alter CYP3A-mediated metabolism.

NOMENCLATURE FOR DRUG INTERACTIONS

The agent causing the drug interaction is called the "perpetrator," whereas the drug being affected by the interaction is called the "victim" (Fig. 20-1). A pharmacokinetic drug interaction implies that the perpetrator causes a change in the metabolic clearance of the victim, in turn either increasing or decreasing concentrations of the victim drug in plasma and presumably also at the site of action. This change may alter the clinical activity of the victim drug, but this is not always the case. An interesting pharmacokinetic interaction "variant" is one in which the perpetrator does not change the systemic clearance of the victim, but rather modifies the access of the victim to its pharmacologic receptor site. A familiar example is the antagonism of benzodiazepine activity by flumazenil; not so familiar is benzodiazepine receptor antagonism by ketoconazole (24).

A pharmacodynamic interaction involves either antagonism or enhancement of the clinical effects of the victim drug as a consequence of similar or identical end-organ actions. Examples are the enhancement or antagonism of the sedative-hypnotic actions of benzodiazepines due to coadministration of ethanol or caffeine, respectively.

INHIBITION VERSUS INDUCTION OF METABOLISM

Fundamentally different processes are involved in drug interactions involving inhibition as opposed to induction of metabolism mediated by CYP enzymes (Table 20-3). Chemical inhibition (25,26) is an immediate phenomenon. The effect is evident as soon as the inhibitor comes in contact with the enzyme, and is in principle reversible when the inhibitor is no longer present (an exception is "mechanism-based" inhibition). In general, the magnitude of inhibition—that is, the size of the interaction—depends on the concentration of the inhibitor at the site of the enzyme relative to the intrinsic potency of the inhibitor. The latter can be measured using *in vitro* systems yielding quantitative inhibitory potency estimates such as the inhibition constant (K_i) or the 50% inhibitory concentration (IC_{50}). Methods of calculating K_i and IC_{50}, including the limitations and drawbacks inherent in the calculations, are reviewed elsewhere (25–27). Current technologic capacity to determine K_i or IC_{50} using *in vitro* systems is more advanced than current understanding of how to apply the numbers to quantitative predictions of drug interaction *in*

TABLE 20-3. *Comparison of pharmacokinetic inhibition and induction*

	Inhibition	Induction
Mechanism	Direct inhibition of metabolizing enzyme	Increased quantities of metabolizing enzyme
Onset	Rapid	Slow
Reversibility	Rapid	Slow
Current exposure needed	Yes	No
Prior exposure needed	No	Yes
In vitro models	Yes	Yes (intact cells)
Quantitative indexes of potency	Yes	No

vivo. Such predictions require knowledge of the effective concentration of inhibitor that is available to the enzyme (17,19,28–30). No generally applicable scheme is currently available to relate total or unbound plasma concentrations of inhibitor to effective enzyme-available concentration. However, it has become clear, based on numerous counterexamples, that the theoretic assumption of equality of unbound plasma concentrations and enzyme-available intrahepatic concentrations is incorrect in reality, and will frequently tend to underestimate observed *in vivo* drug interactions by as much as an order of magnitude or more (29–31).

Induction of CYP-mediated metabolism requires prior exposure of the CYP-synthesis mechanism of the hepatocyte to a chemical inducer, which signals the synthetic mechanisms to upregulate the production of one or more CYP isoforms (32–35). This takes time. Consequently, evidence of increased CYP activity is of slow onset following initiation of exposure to the inducer; conversely, activity slowly reverts to baseline after the inducer is removed. Enhanced CYP expression or activity due to chemical induction, therefore, reflects prior but not necessarily current exposure to the inducer. In general, the quantitative extent of CYP induction depends on the dosage (concentration) of the inducer and on the duration of exposure. In contrast to inhibition, induction is not straightforwardly studied *in vitro*, since induction requires intact cellular protein synthesis mechanisms as available in cell culture models (36).

Inducers and inhibitors of CYP3A can be expected to influence both hepatic and gastrointestinal CYP3A, although not necessarily to the same extent. However, profound changes in both hepatic and gastrointestinal CYP3A will be caused by potent inhibitors (such as ketoconazole) or strong inducers (such as rifampin).

INHIBITION OF SEDATIVE-HYPNOTIC CLEARANCE

The medical literature contains extensive documentation on inhibitory interactions with various sedative-hypnotics, causing reduced clearance, increased plasma concentrations, and in some cases enhanced pharmacodynamic effects of the victim drug. This discussion focuses mainly on interactions that have been described during the past

decade, with abbreviated discussion on well-recognized inhibitory interactions such as those involving cimetidine. Most of the interactions influence the clearance of drugs with partial or complete CYP3A-mediated clearance, whereas the clearance of lorazepam, oxazepam, and temazepam—mediated through glucuronyl transferase—is generally unaffected.

H₂ Antagonists: Cimetidine

Impairment of CYP3A-mediated metabolism by cimetidine has been recognized for nearly two decades (37–39). Inhibition is presumed to be "mechanism based" (40), involving production of a metabolite of cimetidine that inactivates the CYP enzyme (41,42). For this reason, *in vitro* determinations of inhibitory K_i or IC_{50} values for cimetidine probably are of little help in predicting the magnitude of actual clinical interactions.

In general, cimetidine is a quantitatively modest *in vivo* inhibitor of CYP3A-mediated clearance, producing decrements in clearance in the range of 50% (Table 20-4). Clearance of benzodiazepines transformed by glucuronide conjugation is unaffected by cimetidine. Other H₂ antagonists—ranitidine and famotidine—have minimal influence on CYP3A-mediated metabolism (45,63–65).

TABLE 20-4. *Effect of cimetidine on clearance of sedative-hypnotics and anxiolytics*

Victim drug	References for inhibition by cimetidine	References for lack of inhibition by cimetidine
Diazepam	43–46	
Desmethyldiazepam	47, 48	
Chlordiazepoxide	49	
Alprazolam	50, 51	
Triazolam	50–52	
Midazolam	53–55	56
Desalkylflurazepam	57	
Nitrazepam	58	
Oxazepam		47, 57, 59
Lorazepam		45, 57, 59
Temazepam		60
Zolpidem	61	
Buspirone		62

Macrolide and Related Antimicrobials

Troleandomycin (TAO), erythromycin, and clarithromycin are moderately potent mechanism-based inhibitors (40,66) of CYP3A-mediated clearance of a number of psychotropic drugs (Table 20-5). The structurally related azalide derivative, azithromycin, has minimal CYP3A-inhibitory activity. As in the case of cimetidine, *in vitro* K_i or IC_{50} values do not directly predict the magnitude of all *in vivo* interactions. However, relative inhibitory potencies *in vitro* do in fact correspond to relative inhibitory activity in clinical studies (70) (Fig. 20-2). It appears that macrolides impair both the hepatic and gastrointestinal component of CYP3A-mediated metabolism (78).

TABLE 20-5. *Effect of macrolide and related antimicrobials on clearance of sedative-hypnotics and anxiolytics*

Perpetrator drug	Victim drug	References for inhibition	References for lack of inhibition
Erythromycin or troleandomycin	Alprazolam	67	
	Triazolam	68–70	
	Midazolam	71	
	Buspirone	74	
	Diazepam	75	
	Flunitrazepam	75	
	Nitrazepam	76	
	Temazepam		77
Clarithromycin	Triazolam	70	
	Midazolam	71, 72, 78	
Azithromycin	Triazolam		70
	Midazolam		71, 73

α-OH-TRIAZOLAM FORMATION

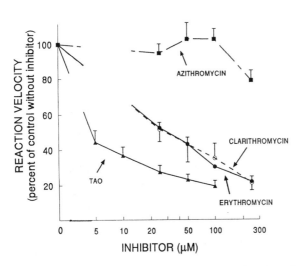

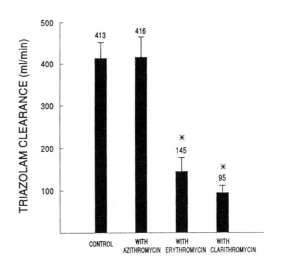

FIG. 20-2. Left: Effect of coaddition of troleandomycin (TAO), erythromycin, clarithromycin, or azithromycin on the formation of α-hydroxytriazolam from triazolam by human liver microsomes *in vitro*. Inhibitors were preincubated before addition of the substrate, triazolam (250 µM). Reaction velocities with inhibitor present are expressed as a percentage ratio versus the control velocity without inhibitor. Each point is the mean (±SE) of four separate microsomal preparations. Note that TAO (mean IC_{50} = 3.9 µM), erythromycin (IC_{50} = 33 µM), and clarithromycin (IC_{50} = 31.4 µM) are significant inhibitors of triazolam hydroxylation *in vitro*, whereas azithromycin produces minimal inhibition even at concentrations of 250 µM. **Right:** Mean (±SE) values of triazolam oral clearance in a clinical study in which triazolam, 0.125 mg, was given to volunteer subjects in the control condition, and with coadministration of therapeutic doses of erythromycin, clarithromycin, or azithromycin. Asterisk (*) indicates a significant decrement in clearance compared to the control value.
See reference 70 for details of this study.

Azole Antifungal Agents

Inhibition of CYP3A-mediated sedative-hypnotic clearance by azole antifungal agents can be quantitatively large and of major clinical importance. The relative order of inhibitory potency *in vitro* is ketoconazole > itraconazole > fluconazole (79–81) (Fig. 20-3). The same order appears to hold *in vivo*. Fluconazole also has significant inhibitory activity against CYP2C9.

CYP3A inhibition by azoles is consistent with a competitive inhibitory mechanism, or at least has a significant competitive component (19,80). Hydroxyitraconazole, a hydroxylated metabolite of itraconazole, appears in plasma in concentrations exceeding those of the parent drug (82). Both itraconazole and hydroxyitraconazole have essentially identical inhibitory capacity against CYP3A activity *in vitro* (81), but the contributions of the hydroxy metabolite to inhibition *in vivo* cannot be estimated without data on its relative intrahepatic availability.

In vitro-in vivo scaling procedures for some azole derivatives as CYP3A inhibitors demonstrate the nonvalidity of the assumption that the unbound plasma concentration equals the enzyme-available unbound intrahepatic concentration. For example, both ketoconazole and itraconazole are more than 99% bound to plasma components in humans (83). Total hepatic concentrations of ketoconazole are similar to or higher than total concentrations in plasma (29,30,84), while hepatic levels of itraconazole are 10 to 20 times higher than those in plasma

(85,86). Based on *in vitro* K_i values for itraconazole versus midazolam hydroxylation as an example (80), predicted inhibition greatly underestimates actual *in vivo* inhibition (87–90) using the unbound concentration partition assumption (Fig. 20-4). This indicates that enzyme-available intrahepatic levels of inhibitor considerably exceed unbound plasma levels.

Azole antifungal agents inhibit both the hepatic and gastrointestinal components of CYP3A activity. The interactions are most dramatic after oral dosage of sedative-hypnotics that are relatively pure CYP3A substrates and that ordinarily undergo extensive presystemic extraction. Examples include triazolam, midazolam, and buspirone; coadministration of usual therapeutic doses of azoles may cause a decrease in clearance (increase in AUC) of tenfold or more after oral administration of these substrate drugs (Table 20-6). For zolpidem, only a

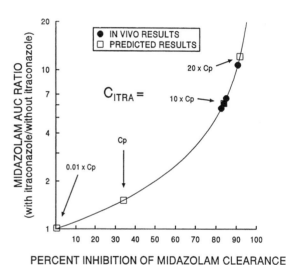

FIG. 20-4. The solid line represents the general functional relationship between the fractional decrement in clearance of a substrate caused by coadministration of an inhibitor (x axis) and the consequent increment in area under the plasma concentration curve (AUC) at steady-state (y-axis), calculated as AUC with inhibitor present divided by AUC in the control condition without inhibitor. (See reference 19 for derivation.)

Solid circles represent mean results of four different clinical studies in which the clearance of oral midazolam was determined with and without coadministration of itraconazole (87–90). Also shown are values predicted (open squares) based on *in vitro* data, assuming a K_i value of 0.275 µM for itraconazole versus midazolam α-hydroxylation (80). Given typical minimum steady-state plasma itraconazole concentrations (Cp) of 0.1 µg/mL (0.14 µM) and an expected plasma protein binding of 99% (free fraction = 0.01), the predicted degree of *in vivo* inhibition is estimated at only 0.5% if the enzyme-available inhibitor concentration (C_{ITRA}) is assumed to equal the free concentration in plasma (0.01 × Cp). *In vivo* inhibition is also underestimated if C_{ITRA} is assumed to equal Cp. Reasonable predictions are achieved only if C_{ITRA} is assumed to be 10 to 20 times Cp; this is consistent with studies of liver to plasma partitioning of itraconazole in experimental animals (85,86).

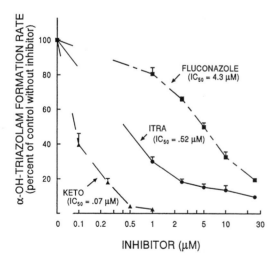

FIG. 20-3. Effect of coaddition of ketoconazole, itraconazole, or fluconazole on formation of α-hydroxytriazolam from triazolam by human liver microsomes *in vitro*. Relative reaction velocities are determined as described in Figure 20-2. Mean (±SE, n = 4) IC_{50} values are also shown. The order of inhibitory potency is ketoconazole > itraconazole > fluconazole. Not shown are data for inhibition by hydroxyitraconazole, an *in vivo* metabolite of itraconazole that has inhibitory potency nearly identical to itraconazole. See reference 81 for details.

TABLE 20-6. *Effect of azole antifungal agents on clearance of sedative-hypnotics and anxiolytics*

Victim drug	References for inhibition by		
	Ketoconazole	Itraconazole	Fluconazole
Midazolam	87	87–90	89, 91
Triazolam	84, 92, 93	92, 94	95, 96
Alprazolam	93	97	
Diazepam		98	
Chlordiazepoxide	99		
Zolpidem	82	82[a]	82[a]
Buspirone		74	

[a]A small degree of inhibition demonstrated.

partial CYP3A substrate with presystemic extraction of about 30% (100), azole coadministration produced a relatively small decrement in clearance (82).

Antidepressants

Nefazodone, a mixed mechanism antidepressant, is a strong CYP3A inhibitor (101), causing large and clinically important interactions with triazolam and alprazolam (102–104), but not with lorazepam (105). *In vitro* studies demonstrate that nefazodone and a major hydroxylated metabolite share similar CYP3A inhibiting activity; two other clinically relevant metabolites—a triazoledione derivative and metachlorophenylpiperazine (mCPP)—produce minimal CYP3A inhibition *in vitro* (106). Trazodone, although structurally related to nefazodone, does not inhibit CYP3A *in vitro*.

Among selective serotonin reuptake inhibitor antidepressants (27), norfluoxetine (the principal metabolite of fluoxetine) and fluvoxamine are modest CYP3A inhibitors *in vitro* (107–109). Coadministration of fluoxetine or fluvoxamine (as perpetrators) with CYP3A substrate drugs alprazolam or diazepam (as victims) has caused significantly impaired clearance of the victim drugs (110–114). However, inhibitory effect of fluoxetine *in vivo* is not consistent, since fluoxetine only slightly impaired triazolam clearance *in vivo* (115). A concurrent induction effect of fluoxetine is possible and cannot be ruled out. Sertraline and desmethylsertraline are weak CYP3A inhibitors *in vitro* (108,109); sertraline coadministration did not alter alprazolam clearance in clinical studies (116). *In vitro* studies of other antidepressants (paroxetine, venlafaxine and metabolites, mirtazapine, citalopram and metabolites) suggest that they are weak or negligible CYP3A inhibitors (27).

Antiretroviral Agents

The viral protease inhibitors (VPIs) ritonavir and indinavir are highly potent CYP3A inhibitors *in vitro* (117–122). It has been assumed that coadministration of ritonavir with sedative-hypnotics whose clearance is mediated by CYP3A will cause large and clinically

important impairment of clearance of such drugs. Ritonavir strongly inhibits CYP3A-mediated triazolam hydroxylation *in vitro* (117); in a clinical study, coadministration of low-dose ritonavir on a short-term basis (200 mg twice daily for 2 days) caused approximately a 20-fold impairment of clearance (increase in AUC) of orally administered triazolam (122a). However, the net influence of ritonavir administration for longer periods of time at higher daily dosages is more difficult to predict, since ritonavir also has significant CYP3A-inducing properties (Fig. 20-5). A study of 10 days of pretreatment with ritonavir, 500 mg twice daily, demonstrated a small net increase in clearance of alprazolam, probably explained by a balance of the induction effects of pretreatment together with the acute inhibitory effect (123). This outcome led to the unwise removal of warnings against ritonavir plus alprazolam cotreatment in the product labeling for ritonavir. Ritonavir is a potent inhibitor of alprazolam hydroxylation *in vitro* (122a). Until clinical data prove otherwise, a significant and potentially hazardous impairment of alprazolam clearance by short-term low-dose ritonavir must be assumed. It is of interest that impairment of clearance of the VPI saquinavir (also a CYP3A substrate) by ritonavir (124) persists despite continued exposure to ritonavir (125). This is probably explained by the persistent and concurrent inhibition by

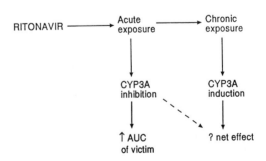

FIG. 20-5. Schematic diagram of the effect of ritonavir on CYP3A-mediated sedative-hypnotic clearance. Initial administration of ritonavir is likely to impair clearance. However, the net outcome of chronic administration is difficult to predict, due to the opposing effects of inhibition and induction.

ritonavir of the action of gastrointestinal CYP3A4 P-glycoprotein (P-gp), which contributes to poor bioavailability of oral saquinavir.

The nonnucleoside reverse transcriptase inhibitor (NNRTI) delavirdine also is a strong CYP3A inhibitor (126,127). Significant impairment by delavirdine of clearance of sedative-hypnotics metabolized by CYP3A should be anticipated, although no clinical studies are available. Nevirapine, also an NNRTI, has minimal CYP3A-inhibiting activity.

Probenecid

The uricosuric agent probenecid impairs clearance of lorazepam and acetaminophen, apparently by impairing formation of the ether glucuronide conjugates of these compounds (128). There is no evidence that probenecid significantly impairs CYP activity in humans.

Ethanol

It is usually assumed that acute ethanol ingestion has the capacity to inhibit CYP3A activity, while chronic exposure to ethanol may produce induction. Studies of acute coadministration of ethanol and benzodiazepines have yielded inconsistent results regarding the net effect on the kinetics of the "victim" benzodiazepine, although pharmacodynamic additivity is a common outcome (129–141). Inducing effects of ethanol during chronic exposure have been difficult to assess in controlled studies.

Other inhibitors

A number of studies have evaluated possible alterations in clearance of some sedative-hypnotics and anxiolytics by agents such as oral contraceptive preparations (141–146), propranolol (146–148), propoxyphene (149), isoniazid (150), or calcium channel blockers (151,152). However, the outcomes of these studies are inconsistent, and when metabolic inhibition is demonstrated, the magnitude is generally small.

INDUCTION OF SEDATIVE-HYPNOTIC CLEARANCE

Coadministration of inducing agents as perpetrators will increase clearance of the victim drug and reduce AUC. This interaction, in general, is likely to reduce clinical activity of the victim, if activity is attributable to the parent compound. However, the net clinical effect of induction is less predictable if a metabolite of the victim drug contributes to clinical efficacy or toxicity.

Rifampin

The antituberculous agent rifampin is a powerful inducer of CYP3A and possibly other cytochromes. Both hepatic and gastrointestinal CYP3A are induced by rifampin. For sedative-hypnotic medications that ordinarily undergo substantial presystemic extraction after oral dosage, and for which CYP3A in the gastrointestinal tract contributes to oral clearance (e.g., triazolam, midazolam, and buspirone), rifampin pretreatment may reduce AUC by more than ten-fold (90,153–155). Rifampin also increases clearance of sedative-hypnotics with lower hepatic clearance, such as zolpidem (156), diazepam (157,158), and alprazolam (158a). When clinical circumstances indicate a need for treatment with rifampin, major changes in plasma concentration and clinical activity of other coadministered CYP3A substrate drugs can be anticipated.

Carbamazepine

Carbamazepine is an established CYP3A inducer, although not as powerful as rifampin. Enhanced clearance of alprazolam (159) and clonazepam (160) by carbamazepine has been demonstrated in clinical studies. Carbamazepine itself is a CYP3A substrate (161) and may be a victim in drug interactions. Coadministration of fluoxetine (as perpetrator) significantly increases plasma AUC of carbamazepine (27%) (as victim) (162). The interaction probably is attributable to the modest CYP3A inhibitory effects of norfluoxetine, the principal metabolite of fluoxetine (107) or inhibition of nonepoxide pathways such as phenol formation (161). Carbamazepine also produces induction of its own metabolism (163).

Ritonavir

As discussed earlier, ritonavir is a CYP3A inducer, in addition to being a CYP3A inhibitor after acute exposure. The net clinical effect on the clearance of a CYP3A substrate drug as victim may be difficult to predict, particularly if that substrate is also a P-gp substrate. A further complication is that ritonavir itself is a CYP3A substrate and induces its own metabolism (15).

CLINICAL IMPORTANCE OF PHARMACOKINETIC INTERACTIONS

Given the prevalence of polypharmacy in contemporary therapeutics, the number of possible drug interactions is huge. This is especially true for individuals with serous illness, such as HIV infection or severe cardiovascular disease, who are on multiple drug regimens for the underlying illness as well as treatments for complicating or coincident disorders.

Most drugs do not interact when given together. Of these interactions that can be detected under well-controlled conditions, the majority are small enough in magnitude, or are so highly variable in occurrence, that they are not ordinarily detectable in clinical practice when superimposed on the intrinsic variability in response. A few interactions are clinically important and require close monitoring or adjustment in dosage of perpetrator or victim drugs. Least common are drug interactions that are so large or so hazardous as to make cotreatment with the two medications unsafe or unfeasible.

Drug interactions are most likely to be important when they are large in magnitude. For inhibitory interactions due to coadministration of reversible inhibitors such as ketoconazole, the relative increase in AUC of the victim drug (i.e., AUC during inhibition divided by AUC without inhibitor) is approximately given by $K_i/(K_i + I)$, where I is the concentration of inhibitor available to the enzyme (19). In the case of ketoconazole, typical K_i values versus CYP3A substrates are less than 0.1 μM, while total plasma concentrations of ketoconazole usually exceed 1.0 μM. Thus the relation of I to K_i for ketoconazole is consistent with observed AUC increments of ten-fold or more when ketoconazole is coadministered with CYP3A substrates such as triazolam or midazolam.

The clinical consequences of an interaction also depend on the pharmacokinetic properties of the victim drug. When the victim drug ordinarily undergoes extensive presystemic extraction after oral dosage, impairment of clearance will cause reduction in presystemic extraction, increased peak plasma concentration, and increased AUC. This pattern may well enhance the single-dose pharmacodynamic effects of the victim, as well as increase steady-state plasma concentrations during multiple dosage. When the victim drug ordinarily undergoes minimal presystemic extraction after oral dosage, impairment of clearance will prolong elimination half-life, increase AUC, and increase steady-state plasma concentrations during chronic therapy. However, a change in peak plasma concentrations after single doses is less likely and therefore it is also less likely that the interaction will enhance pharmacodynamic effects of the victim drug after single doses. This distinction is illustrated in kinetic-dynamic studies (93) in which ketoconazole is coadministered with triazolam (which undergoes moderate presystemic extraction) or alprazolam (which undergoes minimal presystemic extraction) (Fig. 20-6).

Finally, the clinical importance of a pharmacokinetic interaction depends on the inherent concentration-response relationship of the victim drug. Potential interactions are of more concern when the therapeutic range of the victim is narrow, and a change in clearance is likely to move plasma concentrations into the range of potential toxicity or ineffectiveness. As examples, drug interactions with coumarin anticoagulants or with anticonvulsant drugs are of concern, since the therapeutic range is narrow, and the consequences of toxicity or ineffectiveness are important. In contrast, interactions with penicillin antimicrobials are of less concern, since the range of effective doses and plasma concentrations is very large.

COMMENT

Rational clinical therapeutics depends on identification and understanding of clinically important drug interactions. Because time and resources available for clinical studies of drug interactions are always limited, it is

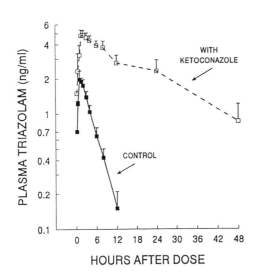 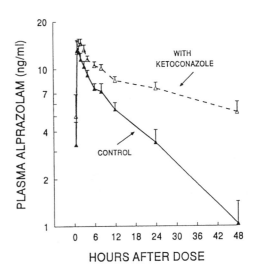

FIG. 20-6. Effect of ketoconazole (200 mg twice daily) on the kinetics of a single 0.25-mg oral dose of triazolam **(left)**, or a single 1.0-mg oral dose of alprazolam **(right)**. Each point is the mean (±SE) value for a series of healthy volunteers. In the case of triazolam, having moderate presystemic extraction, ketoconazole prolongs elimination half-life, reduces presystemic extraction, and increases peak plasma concentrations. For alprazolam, having minimal presystemic extraction, ketoconazole prolongs elimination half-life, but has little effect on peak plasma concentration. Adapted in part from reference 93.

inevitable that some drug interactions will not be identified during clinical development of a new therapeutic entity. The use of *in vitro* models to identify likely drug interactions *in vivo*, or rule out interactions that are unlikely, has increased substantially during the past decade (28–30). Such models may allow more judicious targeting of resources allocated to clinical studies. Delineation of the value and limitations of *in vitro* models will be a topic of ongoing research during the next decade.

ACKNOWLEDGMENTS

This work was supported in part by Grants MH-34233 and DA-05258 from the Department of Health and Human Services, and by Grant RR-00054 supporting the General Clinical Research Center, Tufts University School of Medicine and New England Medical Center Hospital. Dr. von Moltke is the recipient of a Scientist Development Award (K21-MH-01237) from the Department of Health and Human Services. The authors are grateful for the collaboration of Richard I. Shader and Jerold S. Harmatz.

REFERENCES

1. Shader RI, Greenblatt DJ. Use of benzodiazepines in anxiety disorders. *N Engl J Med* 1993;328:1398–1405.
2. Hollister LE, Müller-Oerlinghausen B, Rickels K, Shader RI. Clinical uses of benzodiazepines. *J Clin Psychopharmacol* 1993;13 [Suppl 1]:1S–169S.
3. Greenblatt DJ. Benzodiazepine hypnotics: sorting the pharmacokinetic facts. *J Clin Psychiatry* 1991;52[9, Suppl]:4–10.
4. Greenblatt DJ. Pharmacology of benzodiazepine hypnotics. *J Clin Psychiatry* 1992:53[6, Suppl]:7–13.
5. Nowell PD, Mazumdar S, Buysse DJ, Dew MA, Reynolds CF, Kupfer DJ. Benzodiazepines and zolpidem for chronic insomnia: a meta-analysis of treatment efficacy. *JAMA* 1997;278:2170–2176.
6. Langtry HD, Benfield P. Zolpidem: a review of its pharmacodynamic and pharmacokinetic properties and therapeutic potential. *Drugs* 1990;40:291–313.
7. Hoehns JD, Perry PJ. Zolpidem: a nonbenzodiazepine hypnotic for treatment of insomnia. *Clin Pharmacy* 1993;12:814–828.
8. Roth T, Puech AJ, Paiva T. Zolpidem—place in therapy. In: Freeman H, Puech AJ, Roth T, eds. *Zolpidem: an update of its pharmacological properties and thereapeutic place in the management of insomnia.* Paris: Elsevier, 1996:215–230.
9. Kakuda TN, Struble KA, Piscitelli SC. Protease inhibitors for the treatment of human immunodeficiency virus infection. *Am J Health-System Pharmacy* 1998;55:233–254.
10. Barry M, Mulcahy F, Back DJ. Antiretroviral therapy for patients with HIV disease. *Br J Clin Pharmacol* 1998;45:221–228.
11. Flexner C. HIV-protease inhibitors. *N Engl J Med* 1998;338:1281–1292.
12. Carpenter CCJ, Fischl MA, Hammer SM, et al. Antiretroviral therapy for HIV infection in 1998: updated recommendations of the International AIDS Society—USA Panel. *JAMA* 1998;280:78–86.
13. Moyle GJ, Gazzard BG, Cooper DA, Gatell J. Antiretroviral therapy for HIV infection. *Drugs* 1998;55:383–404.
14. Barry M, Gibbons S, Back D, Mulcahy F. Protease inhibitors in patients with HIV disease. Clinically important pharmacokinetic considerations. *Clin Pharmacokinet* 1997;32:194–209.
15. Hsu A, Granneman GR, Bertz RJ. Ritonavir. Clinical pharmacokinetics and interactions with other anti-HIV agents. *Clin Pharmacokinet* 1998;35:275–291.
16. Maurel P. The CYP3A family. In: Ionnides C, ed. *Cytochromes P450.* Boca Raton, FL: CRC Press, 1996:241–270.

17. Thummel KE, Wilkinson GR. In vitro and in vivo drug interactions involving human CYP3A. *Ann Rev Pharmacol Toxicol* 1998;38:389–430.
18. Wilkinson GR. Cytochrome P4503A (CYP3A) metabolism: prediction of in vivo activity in humans. *J Pharmacokinet Biopharm* 1996;24:475–490.
19. von Moltke LL, Greenblatt DJ, Schmider J, Harmatz JS and Shader RI. Metabolism of drugs by Cytochrome P450 3A isoforms: implications for drug interactions in psychopharmacology. *Clin Pharmacokinet* 1995;29[Suppl 1]:33–43.
20. Thummel KE, Kunze KL, Shen DD. Enzyme-catalyzed processes of first-pass hepatic and intestinal drug extraction. *Adv Drug Del Rev* 1997;27:99–127.
21. Greenblatt DJ, Schillings RT, Kyriakopoulos AA, et al. Clinical pharmacokinetics of lorazepam. I. Absorption and disposition of oral 14C-lorazepam. *Clin Pharmacol Ther* 1976;20:329–341.
22. Greenblatt DJ. Clinical pharmacokinetics of oxazepam and lorazepam. *Clin Pharmacokinet* 1981;6:88–105.
23. Locniskar A, Greenblatt DJ. Oxidative versus conjugative biotransformation of temazepam. *Biopharm Drug Dispos* 1990;11:499–506.
24. Fahey JM, Pritchard GA, von Moltke LL, et al. The effects of ketoconazole on triazolam pharmacokinetics, pharmacodynamics and benzodiazepine receptor binding in mice. *J Pharmacol Exp Ther* 1998;285:271–276.
25. Halpert JR. Structural basis of selective cytochrome P450 inhibition. *Ann Rev Pharmacol Toxicol* 1995;35:29–53.
26. Segel IH. *Enzyme kinetics.* New York: John Wiley and Sons, 1975.
27. Greenblatt DJ, von Moltke LL, Harmatz JS, Shader RI. Drug interactions with newer antidepressants: role of human cytochromes P450. *J Clin Psychiatry* 1998;59[Suppl 15]:19–27.
28. Bertz RJ, Granneman GR. Use of in vitro and in vivo data to estimate the likelihood of metabolic pharmacokinetic interactions. *Clin Pharmacokinet* 1997;32:210–258.
29. Greenblatt DJ, von Moltke LL. Can in vitro models predict drug interactions in vivo? A review of methods, problems, and successes. In: Hori W, ed. *Drug-drug interactions: analyzing in vitro-in vivo correlations.* Southboro, MA: International Business Communications, 1997:2.2.1–2.2.28.
30. von Moltke LL, Greenblatt DJ, Schmider J, Wright CE, Harmatz JS, Shader RI. In vitro approaches to predicting drug interactions in vivo. *Biochem Pharmacol* 1998;55:113–122.
31. von Moltke LL, Greenblatt DJ, Duan SX, Daily JP, Harmatz JS, Shader RI. Inhibition of desipramine hydroxylation (cytochrome P450-2D6) in vitro by quinidine and by viral protease inhibitors: relation to drug interactions in vivo. *J Pharm Sci* 1998;87:1184–1189.
32. Park BK, Kitteringham NR, Piromohamed M, Tucker GT. Relevance of induction of human drug-metabolizing enzymes: pharmacological and toxicological implications. *Br J Clin Pharmacol* 1996;41:477–491.
33. Waxman DJ, Azaroff L. Phenobarbital induction of cytochrome P-450 gene expression. *Biochem J* 1992;281:577–592.
34. Bock KW, Lipp H-P, Bock-Hennig BS. Induction of drug-metabolizing enzymes by xenobiotics. *Xenobiotica* 1990;20:1101–1111.
35. Denison MS, Whitlock JP. Xenobiotic-inducible transcription of cytochromes P450 genes. *J Biol Chem* 1995;270:18175–18178.
36. Li AP, Jurima-Romet M. Applications of primary human hepatocytes in the evaluation of pharmacokinetic drug-drug interactions: evaluation of model drugs terfenadine and rifampin. *Cell Biol Toxicol* 1997;13:365–374.
37. Sedman AJ. Cimetidine-drug interactions. *Am J Med* 1984;76:109–114.
38. Somogyi A, Gugler R. Drug interactions with cimetidine. *Clin Pharmacokinet* 1982;7:23–41.
39. Powell JR, Donn KH. Histamine H2-antagonist drug interactions in perspective: mechanistic concepts and clinical implications. *Am J Med* 1984;77[Suppl 5B]:57–84.
40. Silverman R. Mechanism-based enzyme inactivators. *Methods Enzymol* 1992;249:241–282.
41. Knodell RG, Holtzman JL, Crankshaw DL, Steele NM, Stanley LN. Drug metabolism by rat and human hepatic microsomes in response to interaction with H2-receptor antagonists. *Gastroenterology* 1982;82:84–88.
42. Rendić S, Kažfe F, Ruf H-H. Characterization of cimetidine, ranitidine, and related structures' interaction with cytochrome P450. *Drug Metab Dispos* 1983;11:137–142.

43. Klotz U, Reimann I. Delayed clearance of diazepam due to cimetidine. *N Engl J Med* 1980;302:1012–1014.

44. Klotz U, Reimann I. Elevation of steady-state diazepam levels by cimetidine. *Clin Pharmacol Ther* 1981;30:513–517.

45. Abernethy DR, Greenblatt DJ, Divoll M, Ameer B, Shader RI. Differential effect of cimetidine on drug oxidation (antipyrine and diazepam) versus conjugation (acetaminophen and lorazepam): prevention of acetaminophen toxicity by cimetidine. *J Pharmacol Exp Ther* 1983; 224:508–513.

46. Greenblatt DJ, Abernethy DR, Morse DS, Shader RI, Harmatz JS. Clinical importance of the interaction of diazepam and cimetidine. *N Engl J Med* 1984;310:1639–1643.

47. Klotz U, Reimann I. Influence of cimetidine on the pharmacokinetics of desmethyldiazepam and oxazepam. *Eur J Clin Pharmacol* 1980;18: 517–520.

48. Divoll M, Greenblatt DJ, Abernethy DR, Shader RI. Cimetidine impairs clearance of antipyrine and desmethyldiazepam in the elderly. *J Am Geriatr Soc* 1982;30:684–689.

49. Desmond PV, Patwardhan RV, Schenker S, Speeg KV. Cimetidine impairs elimination of chlordiazepoxide (Librium) in man. *Ann Intern Med* 1980;93:266–268.

50. Abernethy DR, Greenblatt DJ, Divoll M, Moschitto LJ, Harmatz JS, Shader RI. Interaction of cimetidine with the triazolobenzodiazepines alprazolam and triazolam. *Psychopharmacology* 1983;80:275–278.

51. Pourbaix S, Desager JP, Hulhoven R, Smith RB, Harvengt C. Pharmacokinetic consequences of long term coadministration of cimetidine and triazolobenzodiazepines, alprazolam and triazolam, in healthy subjects. *Int J Clin Pharmacol Ther Toxicol* 1985;23:447–451.

52. Cox SR, Kroboth PD, Anderson PH, Smith RB. Mechanism for the interaction between triazolam and cimetidine. *Biopharm Drug Dispos* 1986;7:567–575.

53. Fee JP, Collier PS, Howard PJ, Dundee JW. Cimetidine and ranitidine increase midazolam bioavailability. *Clin Pharmacol Ther* 1987;41: 80–84.

54. Elliott P, Dundee JW, Elwood RJ, Collier PS. The influence of H2 receptor antagonists on the plasma concentrations of midazolam and temazepam. *Eur J Anaesthesiol* 1984;1:245–251.

55. Klotz U, Arvela P, Rosenkranz B. Effect of single doses of cimetidine and ranitidine on the steady-state plasma levels of midazolam. *Clin Pharmacol Ther* 1985;38:652–655.

56. Greenblatt DJ, Locniskar A, Scavone JM, et al. Absence of interaction of cimetidine and ranitidine with intravenous and oral midazolam. *Anesth Analg* 1986;65:176–180.

57. Greenblatt DJ, Abernethy DR, Koepke HH, Shader RI. Interaction of cimetidine with oxazepam, lorazepam, and flurazepam. *J Clin Pharmacol* 1984;24:187–193.

58. Ochs HR, Greenblatt DJ, Gugler R, Müntefering G, Locniskar A, Abernethy DR. Cimetidine impairs nitrazepam clearance. *Clin Pharmacol Ther* 1983;34:227–230.

59. Patwardhan RV, Yarborough GW, Desmond PV, Johnson RF, Schenker S, Speeg KV. Cimetidine spares the glucuronidation of lorazepam and oxazepam. *Gastroenterology* 1980;79:912–916.

60. Greenblatt DJ, Abernethy DR, Divoll M, Locniskar A, Harmatz JS, Shader RI. Noninteraction of temazepam and cimetidine. *J Pharm Sci* 1984;73:399–401.

61. Hulhoven R, Desager JP, Harvengt C, Hermann P, Guillet P, Thiercelin JF. Lack of interaction between zolpidem and H2 antagonists, cimetidine and ranitidine. *Int J Clin Pharm Res* 1988;8:471–476.

62. Gammans RE, Pfeffer M, Westrick ML, Faulkner HC, Rehm KD, Goodson PJ. Lack of interaction between cimetidine and buspirone. *Pharmacotherapy* 1987;7:72–79.

63. Abernethy DR, Greenblatt DJ, Eshelman FN, Shader RI. Ranitidine does not impair oxidative or conjugative metabolism: noninteraction with antipyrine, diazepam, and lorazepam. *Clin Pharmacol Ther* 1984;35:188–192.

64. Locniskar A, Greenblatt DJ, Harmatz JS, Zinny MA, Shader RI. Interaction of diazepam with famotidine and cimetidine, two H-2 receptor antagonists. *J Clin Pharmacol* 1986;26:299–303.

65. Kirch W, Hoensch H, Janisch HD. Interactions and non-interactions with ranitidine. *Clin Pharmacokinet* 1984;9:493–510.

66. Gillum JG, Israel DS, Polk RE. Pharmacokinetic drug interactions with antimicrobial agents. *Clin Pharmacokinet* 1993;25:450–482.

67. Yasui N, Otani K, Kaneko S, et al. A kinetic and dynamic study of oral alprazolam with and without erythromycin in humans: in vivo evidence for the involvement of CYP3A4 in alprazolam metabolism. *Clin Pharmacol Ther* 1996;59:514–519.

68. Phillips JP, Antal EJ, Smith RB. A pharmacokinetic drug interaction between erythromycin and triazolam. *J Clin Psychopharmacol* 1986; 6:297–299.

69. Warot D, Bergougnan L, Lamiable D, et al. Troleandomycin-triazolam interaction in healthy volunteers: pharmacokinetic and psychometric evaluation. *Eur J Clin Pharmacol* 1987;32:389–393.

70. Greenblatt DJ, von Moltke LL, Harmatz JS, et al. Inhibition of triazolam clearance by macrolide antimicrobial agents: in vitro correlates and dynamic consequences. *Clin Pharmacol Ther* 1998;64: 278–285.

71. Yeates RA, Laufen H, Zimmermann T, Schumacher T. Pharmacokinetic and pharmacodynamic interaction study between midazolam and the macrolide antibiotics, erythromycin, clarithromycin, and the azalide azithromycin. *Int J Clin Pharmacol Ther* 1997;35:577–579.

72. Olkkola KT, Aranko K, Luurila H, et al. A potentially hazardous interaction between erythromycin and midazolam. *Clin Pharmacol Ther* 1993;53:298–305.

73. Backman JT, Olkkola KT, Neuvonen PJ. Azithromycin does not increase plasma concentrations of oral midazolam. *Int J Clin Pharmacol Ther* 1995;33:356–359.

74. Kivistö KT, Lamberg TS, Kantola T, Neuvonen PJ. Plasma buspirone concentrations are greatly increased by erythromycin and itraconazole. *Clin Pharmacol Ther* 1997;62:348–354.

75. Luurila H, Olkkola KT, Neuvonen PJ. Interaction between erythromycin and the benzodiazepines diazepam and flunitrazepam. *Pharmacol Toxicol* 1996;78:117–122.

76. Luurila H, Olkkola KT, Neuvonen PJ. Interaction between erythromycin and nitrazepam in healthy volunteers. *Pharmacol Toxicol* 1995;76:255–258.

77. Luurila H, Olkkola KT, Neuvonen PJ. Lack of interaction of erythromycin with temazepam. *Ther Drug Monit* 1994;16:548–551.

78. Gorski JC, Jones DR, Haehner-Daniels BD, Hamman MA, O'Mara EM, Hall SD. The contribution of intestinal and hepatic CYP3A to the interaction between midazolam and clarithromycin. *Clin Pharmacol Ther* 1998;64:133–143.

79. Back DJ, Tjia JF. Comparative effects of the antimycotic drugs ketoconazole, fluconazole, itraconazole and terbinafine on the metabolism of cyclosporin by human liver microsomes. *Br J Clin Pharmacol* 1991;32:624–626.

80. von Moltke LL, Greenblatt DJ, Schmider J, et al. Midazolam hydroxylation by human liver microsomes in vitro: inhibition by fluoxetine, norfluoxetine, and by azole antifungal agents. *J Clin Pharmacol* 1996; 36:783–791.

81. von Moltke LL, Greenblatt DJ, Duan SX, Harmatz JS, Shader RI. Inhibition of triazolam hydroxylation by ketoconazole, itraconazole, hydroxyitraconazole and fluconazole in vitro. *Pharm Pharmacol Commun* 1998;4:443–445.

82. Greenblatt DJ, von Moltke LL, Harmatz JS, et al. Kinetic and dynamic interaction study of zolpidem with ketoconazole, itraconazole, and fluconazole. *Clin Pharmacol Ther* 1998;64:661–671.

83. Como JA, Dismukes WE. Oral azole drugs as systemic antifungal therapy. *N Engl J Med* 1994;330:263–272.

84. von Moltke LL, Greenblatt DJ, Harmatz JS, et al. Triazolam biotransformation by human liver microsomes in vitro: effects of metabolic inhibitors, and clinical confirmation of a predicted interaction with ketoconazole. *J Pharmacol Exp Ther* 1996;276:370–379.

85. Heykants J, van Peer A, van de Velde V, et al. The clinical pharmacokinetics of itraconazole: an overview. *Mycoses* 1989;32[Suppl 1]: 67–87.

86. Heykants J, Michiels M, Meuldermans W, et al. The pharmacokinetics of itraconazole in animals and man: an overview. In: Fromtling R, ed. *Recent Trends in the discovery, development and evaluation of antifungal agents.* Barcelona: JR Prous Science Publishers, 1987: 223–249.

87. Olkkola KT, Backman JT, Neuvinen PJ. Midazolam should be avoided in patients receiving the systemic antimycotics ketoconazole or itraconazole. *Clin Pharmacol Ther* 1994;55:481–485.

88. Ahonen J, Olkkola K, Neuvonen P. Effect of itraconazole and terbinafine on the pharmacokinetics and pharmacodynamics of midazolam in healthy volunteers. *Br J Clin Pharmacol* 1995;40:270–272.

89. Olkkola K, Ahonen J, Neuvonen P. The effect of the systemic antimycotics, itraconazole and fluconazole, on the pharmacokinetics and

pharmacodynamics of intravenous and oral midazolam. *Anesth Analg* 1996;82:511–516.

90. Backman JT, Kivistö KT, Olkkola KT, Neuvonen PJ. The area under the plasma concentration-time curve for oral midazolam is 400-fold larger during treatment with itraconazole than with rifampicin. *Eur J Clin Pharmacol* 1998;54:53–58.

91. Ahonen J, Olkkola KT, Neuvonen PJ. Effect of route of administration of fluconazole on the interaction between fluconazole and midazolam. *Eur J Clin Pharmacol* 1997;51:415–419.

92. Varhe A, Olkkola KT, Neuvonen PJ. Oral triazolam is potentially hazardous to patients receiving systemic antimycotics ketoconazole or itraconazole. *Clin Pharmacol Ther* 1994;56:601–607.

93. Greenblatt DJ, Wright CE, von Moltke LL, et al. Ketoconazole inhibition of triazolam and alprazolam clearance: differential kinetic and dynamic consequences. *Clin Pharmacol Ther* 1998;64:237–247.

94. Neuvonen PJ, Varhe A, Olkkola KT. The effect of ingestion time interval on the interaction between itraconazole and triazolam. *Clin Pharmacol Ther* 1996;60:326–331.

95. Varhe A, Olkkola KT, Neuvonen PJ. Fluconazole, but not terbinafine, enhances the effects of triazolam by inhibiting its metabolism. *Br J Clin Pharmacol* 1996;41:319–323.

96. Varhe A, Olkkola KT, Neuvonen PJ. Effect of fluconazole dose on the extent of fluconazole-triazolam interaction. *Br J Clin Pharmacol* 1996;42:465–470.

97. Yasui N, Kondo T, Otani K, et al. Effect of itraconazole on the single oral dose pharmacokinetics and pharmacodynamics of alprazolam. *Psychopharmacology* 1998;139:269–273.

98. Ahonen J, Olkkola KT, Neuvonen PJ. The effect of the antimycotic itraconazole on the pharmacokinetics and pharmacodynamics of diazepam. *Fundam Clin Pharmacol* 1996;10:314–318.

99. Brown MW, Maldonado AL, Meredith CG, Speeg KV. Effect of ketoconazole on hepatic oxidative drug metabolism. *Clin Pharmacol Ther* 1985;37:290–297.

100. Patat A, Trocherie S, Thebault JJ, et al. EEG profile of intravenous zolpidem in healthy volunteers. *Psychopharmacology* 1994;114:138–146.

101. Greene DS, Barbhaiya RH. Clinical pharmacokinetics of nefazodone. *Clin Pharmacokinet* 1997;4:260–275.

102. Barbhaiya RH, Shukla UA, Kroboth PD, Greene DS. Coadministration of nefazodone and benzodiazepines: II. A pharmacokinetic interaction study with triazolam. *J Clin Psychopharmacol* 1995;15:320–326.

103. Greene DS, Salazar DE, Dockens RC, Kroboth P, Barbhaiya RH. Coadministration of nefazodone and benzodiazepines: III. A pharmacokinetic interaction study with alprazolam. *J Clin Psychopharmacol* 1995;15:399–408.

104. Rickels K, Schweizer D, Case WG, et al. Nefazodone in major depression: adjunctive benzodiazepine therapy and tolerability. *J Clin Psychopharmacol* 1998;18:145–153.

105. Greene DS, Salazar DE, Dockens RC, Kroboth P, Barbhaiya RH. Coadministration of nefazodone and benzodiazepines: IV. A pharmacokinetic interaction study with lorazepam. *J Clin Psychopharmacol* 1995;15:409–416.

106. von Moltke LL, Greenblatt DJ, Schmider J, Harmatz JS, Shader RI. Nefazodone in vitro: metabolic conversions, and inhibition of P450-3A isoforms. *Clin Pharmacol Ther* 1996;59:176.

107. Greenblatt DJ, von Moltke LL, Schmider J, Harmatz JS, Shader RI. Inhibition of human cytochrome P450-3A isoforms by fluoxetine and norfluoxetine: in vitro and in vivo studies. *J Clin Pharmacol* 1996;36:792–798.

108. von Moltke LL, Greenblatt DJ, Cotreau-Bibbo MM, Harmatz JS, Shader RI. Inhibitors of alprazolam metabolism in vitro: effect of serotonin-reuptake-inhibitor antidepressants, ketoconazole and quinidine. *Br J Clin Pharmacol* 1994;38:23–31.

109. von Moltke LL, Greenblatt DJ, Court MH, Duan SX, Harmatz JS, Shader RI. Inhibition of alprazolam and desipramine hydroxylation in vitro by paroxetine and fluvoxamine: comparison with other selective serotonin reuptake inhibitor antidepressants. *J Clin Psychopharmacol* 1995;15:125–131.

110. Greenblatt DJ, Preskorn SH, Cotreau MM, Horst WD, Harmatz JS. Fluoxetine impairs clearance of alprazolam but not of clonazepam. *Clin Pharmacol Ther* 1992;52:479–486.

111. Lasher TA, Fleishaker JC, Steenwyk RC, Antal EJ. Pharmacokinetic pharmacodynamic evaluation of the combined administration of alprazolam and fluoxetine. *Psychopharmacology* 1991;104:323–327.

112. Lemberger L, Rowe H, Bosomworth JC, Tenbarge JB, Bergstrom RF. The effect of fluoxetine on the pharmacokinetics and psychomotor responses of diazepam. *Clin Pharmacol Ther* 1988;43:412–419.

113. Fleishaker JC, Hulst LK. A pharmacokinetic and pharmacodynamic evaluation of the combined administration of alprazolam and fluvoxamine. *Eur J Clin Pharmacol* 1994;46:35–39.

114. Perucca E, Gatti G, Cipolla G, et al. Inhibition of diazepam metabolism by fluvoxamine: a pharmacokinetic study in normal volunteers. *Clin Pharmacol Ther* 1994;56:471–476.

115. Wright CE, Lasher-Sisson TA, Steenwyk RC, Swanson CN. A pharmacokinetic evaluation of the combined administration of triazolam and fluoxetine. *Pharmacotherapy* 1992;12:103–106.

116. Preskorn SH, Alderman J, Greenblatt DJ, Horst WD. Sertraline does not inhibit cytochrome P450 3A-mediated drug metabolism *in vivo*. *Psychopharmacol Bull* 1997;33:659–665.

117. von Moltke LL, Greenblatt DJ, Grassi JM, et al. Protease inhibitors as inhibitors of human cytochromes P450: high risk associated with ritonavir. *J Clin Pharmacol* 1998;38:106–111.

118. Eagling VA, Back DJ, Barry MG. Differential inhibition of cytochrome P450 isoforms by the protease inhibitors, ritonavir, saquinavir and indinavir. *Br J Clin Pharmacol* 1997;44:190–194.

119. Iribarne C, Berthou F, Carlhant D, et al. Inhibition of methadone and buprenorphine N-dealkylations by three HIV-1 protease inhibitors. *Drug Metab Dispos* 1998;26:257–260.

120. Inaba T, Fischer NE, Riddick DS, Stewart DJ, Hidaka T. HIV protease inhibitors, saquinavir, indinavir and ritonavir: inhibition of CYP3A4-mediated metabolism of testosterone and benzoxazinorifamycin, KRM-1648, in human liver microsomes. *Toxicol Lett* 1997;93:215–219.

121. Lillibridge JH, Liang BH, Kerr BM, Webber S, Quart B, Shetty BV, Lee CA. Characterization of the selectivity and mechanism of human cytochrome P450 inhibition by the human immunodeficiency virus-protease inhibitor nelfinavir mesylate. *Drug Metab Dispos* 1998;26:609–616.

122. Koudriakova T, Iatsimirskaia E, Utkin I, et al. Metabolism of the human immunodeficiency virus protease inhibitors indinavir and ritonavir by human intestinal microsomes and expressed cytochrome P4503A4/3A5: mechanism-based inactivation of cytochrome P4503A by ritonavir. *Drug Metab Dispos* 1998;26:552–561.

122a.Greenblatt DJ, von Moltke LL, Daily JP, Harmatz JS, Shader RI. Extensive impairment of triazolam and alprazolam clearance by short-term low-dose ritonavir: the clinical dilemma of concurrent inhibition and induction. *J Clin Psychopharmacol* 1999;19:293–296.

123. Frye R, Bertz R, Granneman GR, Qian J, Lamm J, Dennis S, Valdes J. Effect of ritonavir on the pharmacokinetics and pharmacodynamics of alprazolam (abstr A-59). 37th Interscience Conference on Antimicrobial Agents and Chemotherapy, Toronto, Canada 1997;37:12.

124. Merry C, Barry MG, Mulcahy F, et al. Saquinavir pharmacokinetics alone and in combination with ritonavir in HIV-infected patients. *AIDS* 1997;11:F29–F33.

125. Lorenzi P, Yerly S, Abderrakim K, et al. Toxicity, efficacy, plasma drug concentrations and protease mutations in patients with advanced HIV infection treated with ritonavir plus saquinavir. *AIDS* 1997;11:F95–F99.

126. Cheng C-L, Smith DE, Carver PL, et al. Steady-state pharmacokinetics of delavirdine in HIV-positive patients: effect on erythromycin breath test. *Clin Pharmacol Ther* 1997;61:531–543.

127. Voorman RL, Maio SM, Payne NA, Zhao Z, Koeplinger KA, Wang X. Microsomal metabolism of delavirdine: evidence for mechanism-based inactivation of human cytochrome P450 3A. *J Pharmacol Exp Ther* 1998;287:381–388.

128. Abernethy DR, Greenblatt DJ, Ameer B, Shader RI. Probenecid impairment of acetaminophen and lorazepam clearance: direct inhibition of ether glucuronide formation. *J Pharmacol Exp Ther* 1985;234:345–349.

129. Divoll M, Greenblatt DJ. Alcohol does not enhance diazepam absorption. *Pharmacology* 1981;22:263–268.

130. Greenblatt DJ, Shader RI, Weinberger DR, Allen MD, MacLaughlin DS. Effect of a cocktail on diazepam absorption. *Psychopharmacology* 1978;57:199–203.

131. Ochs HR, Greenblatt DJ, Arendt RM, Hübbel W, Shader RI. Pharmacokinetic noninteraction of triazolam and ethanol. *J Clin Psychopharmacol* 1984;4:106–107.

132. Linnoila M, Stapleton JM, Lister R, et al. Effects of adinazolam and diazepam, alone and in combination with ethanol, on psychomotor and cognitive performance and on autonomic nervous system reactivity in healthy volunteers. *Eur J Clin Pharmacol* 1990;39:21–28.

133. Desmond PV, Patwardhan RV, Schenker S, Hoyumpa AM. Short-term ethanol administration impairs the elimination of chlordiazepoxide (Librium) in man. *Eur J Clin Pharmacol* 1980;18:272–278.

134. Sellers EM, Greenblatt DJ, Zilm DH, Degani N. Decline in chlordiazepoxide plasma levels during fixed-dose therapy of alcohol withdrawal. *Br J Clin Pharmacol* 1978;6:370–372.

135. Whiting B, Lawrence JR, Skellern GG, Meier J. Effect of acute alcohol intoxication on the metabolism and plasma kinetics of chlordiazepoxide. *Br J Clin Pharmacol* 1979;7:95–100.

136. Wills RJ, Crouthamel WG, Iber FL, Perkal MB. Influence of alcohol on the pharmacokinetics of diazepm controlled-release formulation in healthy volunteers. *J Clin Pharmacol* 1982;22:557–561.

137. Hoyumpa AM, Patwardhan R, Maples M, Desmond PV, Johnson RF, Sinclair AP, Schenker S. Effect of short-term ethanol administration on lorazepam clearance. *Hepatology* 1981;1:47–53.

138. Laisi U, Linnoila M, Seppälä T, Himberg J-J, Mattila MJ. Pharmacokinetic and pharmacodynamic interactions of diazepam with different alcoholic beverages. *Eur J Clin Pharmacol* 1979;16:263–270.

139. Dorian P, Sellers EM, Kaplan HL, Hamilton C, Greenblatt DJ, Abernethy D. Triazolam and ethanol interaction: kinetic and dynamic consequences. *Clin Pharmacol Ther* 1985;37:558–562.

140. Bond A, Silveira JC, Lader M. Effects of single doses of alprazolam and alcohol alone and in combination on psychological performance. *Hum Psychopharmacol* 1991;6:219–228.

141. Scavone JM, Greenblatt DJ, Harmatz JS, Shader RI. Kinetic and dynamic interaction of brotizolam and ethanol. *Br J Clin Pharmacol* 1986;21:197–204.

142. Stoehr GP, Kroboth PD, Juhl RP, Wender DB, Phillips JP, Smith RB. Effect of oral contraceptives on triazolam, temazepam, alprazolam, and lorazepam kinetics. *Clin Pharmacol Ther* 1984;36:683–690.

143. Abernethy DR, Greenblatt DJ, Divoll M, Arendt R, Ochs HR, Shader RI. Impairment of diazepam metabolism by low-dose estrogen oral contraceptive steroids. *N Engl J Med* 1982;306:791–792.

144. Abernethy DR, Greenblatt DJ, Ochs HR, et al. Lorazepam and oxazepam kinetics in women on low-dose oral contraceptives. *Clin Pharmacol Ther* 1983;33:628–632.

145. Scavone JM, Greenblatt DJ, Locniskar A, Shader RI. Alprazolam pharmacokinetics in women on low-dose oral contraceptives. *J Clin Pharmacol* 1988;28:454–457.

146. Ochs HR, Greenblatt DJ, Friedman H, et al. Bromazepam pharmacokinetics: influence of age, gender, oral contraceptives, cimetidine, and propranolol. *Clin Pharmacol Ther* 1987;41:562–570.

147. Ochs HR, Greenblatt DJ, Verburg-Ochs B. Propranolol interactions with diazepam, lorazepam, and alprazolam. *Clin Pharmacol Ther* 1984;36:451–455.

148. Friedman H, Greenblatt DJ, Burstein ES, Scavone JM, Harmatz JS, Shader RI. Triazolam kinetics: interaction with cimetidine, propranolol, and the combination. *J Clin Pharmacol* 1988;28:228–233.

149. Abernethy DR, Greenblatt DJ, Morse DS, Shader RI. Interaction of propoxyphene with diazepam, alprazolam, and lorazepam. *Br J Clin Pharmacol* 1985;19:51–57.

150. Ochs HR, Greenblatt DJ, Knüchel M. Differential effect of isoniazid on triazolam oxidation and oxazepam conjugation. *Br J Clin Pharmacol* 1983;16:743–746.

151. Backman JT, Olkkola KT, Aranko K, Himberg J-J, Neuvonen PJ. Dose of midazolam should be reduced during diltiazem and verapmil treatments. *Br J Clin Pharmacol* 1994;37:221–225.

152. Varhe A, Olkkola KT, Neuvonen PJ. Diltiazem enhances the effects of triazolam by inhibiting its metabolism. *Clin Pharmacol Ther* 1996;59:369–375.

153. Villikka K, Kivistö KT, Backman JT, Olkkola KT, Neuvonen PJ. Triazolam is ineffective in patients taking rifampin. *Clin Pharmacol Ther* 1997;61:8–14.

154. Backman JT, Olkkola KT, Neuvonen PJ. Rifampin drastically reduces plasma concentrations and effects of oral midazolam. *Clin Pharmacol Ther* 1996;59:7–13.

155. Lamberg TS, Kivistö KT, Neuvonen PJ. Concentrations and effects of busipirone are considerably reduced by rifampicin. *Br J Clin Pharmacol* 1998;45:381–385.

156. Villikka K, Kivistö KT, Luurila H, Neuvonen PJ. Rifampin reduces plasma concentrations and effects of zolpidem. *Clin Pharmacol Ther* 1997;62:629–634.

157. Ohnhaus EE, Brockmeyer N, Dylewicz P, Habicht H. The effect of antipyrine and rifampin on the metabolism of diazepam. *Clin Pharmacol Ther* 1987;42:148–156.

158. Ochs HR, Greenblatt DJ, Roberts GM, Dengler JH. Diazepam interaction with antituberculosis drugs. *Clin Pharmacol Ther* 1981;29:671–678.

158a. Schmider J, Brockmöller J, Arold G, Bauer S, Roots I. Simultaneous assessment of CYP3A4 and CYP1A2 activity *in vivo* with alprazolam and caffeine. *Pharmacogenetics* 1999;9:725–734.

159. Furukori H, Otani K, Yasui N, et al. Effect of carbamazepine on the single oral dose pharmacokinetics of alprazolam. *Neuropsychopharmacology* 1998;18:364–369.

160. Lai AA, Levy RH, Cutler RE. Time-course of interaction between carbamazepine and clonazepam in normal man. *Clin Pharmacol Ther* 1978;24:316–323.

161. Kerr BM, Thummel KE, Wurden CJ, et al. Human liver carbamazepine metabolism: role of CYP3A4 and CYP2C8 in 10,11-epoxide formation. *Biochem Pharmacol* 1994;47:1969–1979.

162. Grimsley SR, Jann MW, Carter JG, D'Mello AP, D'Souza MJ. Increased carbamazepine plasma concentrations after fluoxetine coadministration. *Clin Pharmacol Ther* 1991;50:10–15.

163. Bernus I, Dickinson RG, Hooper WD, Eadie MJ. Early stage autoinduction of carbamazepine metabolism in humans. *Eur J Clin Pharmacol* 1994;47:355–360.

CHAPTER 21

Volatile, Intravenous, and Local Anesthetics

Evan D. Kharasch and Andra E. Ibrahim

Anesthetics constitute a broad class of drugs, including halogenated volatile ether and alkane anesthetics, local anesthetics, and a diverse group of intravenous anesthetics. Members of this broad drug class are extensively biotransformed to active, inactive, or toxic metabolites. This chapter reviews metabolic-based drug interactions involving anesthetics, with a specific focus on those occurring in humans. Pharmacokinetic interactions resulting from altered absorption, distribution, and protein binding are not discussed; they are described elsewhere (1–6).

VOLATILE ANESTHETICS

Currently used volatile anesthetics include halothane, enflurane, isoflurane, desflurane, and sevoflurane. Methoxyflurane, although no longer used clinically, is nonetheless historically important because of its metabolism-based toxicity. These drugs are administered by inhalation and are eliminated both by exhalation and by P450-catalyzed biotransformation, with varying extents of metabolism: methoxyflurane (75%), halothane (46%), enflurane (8%), sevoflurane (3%–5%), isoflurane (0.2%–2%), and desflurane (0.02%) (7). The liver is the primary site of metabolism, although methoxyflurane (but not sevoflurane, and presumably not the other ether anesthetics) is also metabolized in the kidney (8).

Halothane

Halothane undergoes both oxidative and reductive metabolism (Fig. 21-1) (9). Oxidation forms trifluo-

E. D. Kharasch: Department of Anesthesiology, University of Washington, 1959 NE Pacific Street, Box 356540, Seattle, Washington 98195-6540 and Anesthesiology Service, Puget Sound Veterans Affairs Medical Center, Seattle, Washington 98108

A. E. Ibrahim: Department of Anesthesiology, University of Washington, 1959 NE Pacific, Box 356540, Seattle, Washington 98195

roacetyl chloride, which leads to trifluoroacetic acid, but more importantly to trifluoroacetylation of hepatic proteins. These proteins can stimulate the formation of antibodies, which, upon subsequent exposure to halothane or other structural congeners (enflurane, isoflurane, or desflurane), mediate an immune response, causing fulminant hepatic necrosis (10,11). Halothane is reduced anaerobically to a radical that may form 2-chloro-1,1,1-trifluoroethane (CTE), undergo further reduction to 2-chloro-1,1-difluoroethylene (CDE), initiate lipid peroxidation, or bind covalently to microsomal phospholipids, proteins, or P450, causing suicide inactivation (9,12,13). Sequelae of halothane reduction are clinically insignificant, except for altered postoperative mixed function oxidase activity (14).

Halothane is unique, in that oxidation and reduction are mediated by different P450 isoforms. Human halothane oxidation by hepatic microsomes *in vitro,* and in patients *in vivo,* is catalyzed predominantly by CYP2E1 (K_m 30 μM, clinical halothane concentration typically > 400 μM) (15–17). At high halothane concentrations present only during anesthesia, oxidation is also catalyzed by CYP2A6 (K_m 600–800 μM) *in vitro* and *in vivo* (17,18). In contrast, human hepatic microsomal halothane reduction is catalyzed principally by CYP2A6 and CYP3A4 as the low K_m (approximately 15 μM) and high K_m (100–300 μM) enzymes, respectively; both are thought to metabolize halothane during clinical anesthesia (19,20).

Alterations in P450 activity produce corresponding changes in halothane metabolism. Human liver microsomal halothane oxidation was diminished by the CYP2E1 inhibitors 4-methylpyrazole and diethyldithiocarbamate, and to a lesser extent by the CYP2A6 inhibitor 8-methoxypsoralen (17). Human halothane oxidation *in vivo* to trifluoroacetyl chloride was diminished 85% to 90% by treatment before surgery with the CYP2E1 inhibitor disulfiram (21) evidenced by significantly diminished plasma and urine concentrations of trifluoroacetic acid (Fig. 21-2) (15). Disulfiram was therefore

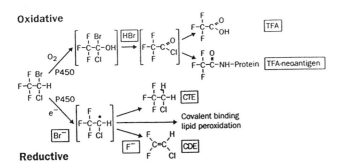

Oxidative

Reductive

FIG. 21-1. Pathways of oxidative and reductive halothane metabolism. Trifluoroacetic acid (TFA) results exclusively from oxidative metabolism. Fluoride, and the volatile metabolites chlorotrifluoroethane (CTE) and chlorodifluoroethylene (CDE), result exclusively from reductive metabolism. Bromide results from both oxidative and reductive metabolism. From Kharasch ED, Hankins D, Mautz D, Thummel KE. Identification of the enzyme responsible for oxidative halothane metabolism: implications for prevention of halothane hepatitis. *Lancet* 1996;347:1367–1371, with permission.

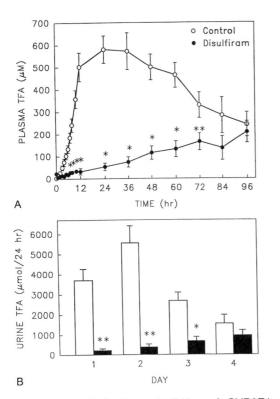

FIG. 21-2. Effect of disulfiram inhibition of CYP2E1 on halothane metabolism in humans. **(A)** Plasma metabolite concentration. **(B)** Urinary metabolite excretion. Significant differences between controls and disulfiram-treated patients are shown (*$p < 0.05$, **$p < 0.01$). Redrawn from Kharasch ED, Hankins D, Mautz D, Thummel KE. Identification of the enzyme responsible for oxidative halothane metabolism: implications for prevention of halothane hepatitis. *Lancet* 1996;347:1367–1371, with permission.

recommended as a possible prophylactic agent against CYP2E1-mediated halothane toxification, or as treatment or prophylaxis against other CYP2E1 substrates (environmental toxins or therapeutic drugs) whose bioactivation results in toxicity (15). At high halothane concentrations only, oxidation in humans *in vivo* was also decreased by 8-methoxypsoralen. Obesity increased human halothane oxidation *in vivo* (22,23) and is a risk factor for fulminant hepatic necrosis (24), consistent with its known induction of CYP2E1 activity (25). Cimetidine did not diminish human clinical halothane metabolism (26), although it did inhibit rat halothane oxidation in microsomes (27) and *in vivo* (28). Human liver microsomal halothane reduction was diminished by the CYP2A6 inhibitors coumarin and 8-methoxypsoralen, and the CYP3A4 inhibitors ketoconazole and troleandomycin (19,20). Human halothane reduction during surgery was enhanced in patients taking the CYP3A4 inducer phenytoin (29), and the incidence of mild liver injury was significantly higher in patients taking phenobarbital (30). However neither 8-methoxypsoralen nor troleandomycin diminished halothane reduction in humans *in vivo*.

Halothane is known to alter the metabolism of numerous drugs by reduction of hepatic blood flow or inhibition of P450-mediated biotransformation (2). Halothane consistently decreases portal blood flow, whereas hepatic arterial flow is variably diminished and to a lesser extent (31,32). Halothane is a suicide substrate for hepatic microsomal P450, forming a catalytically inactive metabolite complex (12,33–35). In humans, antipyrine clearance measured 48 hours after halothane anesthesia was decreased 30% compared with preanesthesia clearance (14). Halothane also substantially diminished the plasma clearance of fentanyl, a high-extraction drug, but effects were not attributed to changes in intrinsic clearance or hepatic blood flow (36). Halothane had no effect on the systemic clearance of propofol, another high-extraction drug (37). Most investigations, however, have studied halothane effects on drug disposition in animals (2). For example, halothane inhibited the metabolism of enflurane in rats and reduced by 30% the clearance of chlorzoxazone in rabbits (both CYP2E1 substrates), but did not alter lidocaine clearance (CYP3A4 activity) in rabbits (38,39). In rats *in vivo*, halothane significantly decreased the plasma clearance and systemic metabolism, and increased brain concentrations of the intravenous anesthetic ketamine, and noncompetitively inhibited ketamine *N*-demethylation by liver microsomes *in vitro* (40,41). In dogs, halothane decreased the systemic clearance of racemic propranolol by 40%, attributed somewhat to changes in hepatic blood flow but primarily to inhibition of hepatic intrinsic clearance, which was decreased by 62% (42). Halothane effects were subsequently shown to be somewhat stereoselective, with the intrinsic clearance of (−)-propranolol decreased significantly more than that of (+)-propranolol (73% ± 5% versus 62% ± 3%) (43). The clearance of fentanyl (2), theophylline (44), and lidocaine (45) was decreased to half that in awake dogs during halothane anesthesia. Similarly, halothane diminished verapamil clearance to half that in awake dogs, attributed to changes in both hepatic blood flow and oxidative biotransformation (46), and reduced meperidine systemic clearance, hepatic extraction ratio, hepatic clearance, and hepatic intrinsic clearance to 44%, 94%, 60%, and 16% of awake values (47). Morphine systemic clearance was decreased 40% by halothane, attributed to diminished hepatic blood flow, because hepatic intrinsic clearance was not significantly decreased (48). Halothane may have less effect on phase II compared with phase I metabolism. In rats, halothane decreased hepatic UDP-glucuronic acid content and diminished biliary excretion of acetaminophen glucuronide and sulfate conjugates, while increasing biliary acetaminophen-glutathione excretion (49). Halothane had no effect on morphine 3-glucuronidation in dogs or humans and increased 6-glucuronidation in humans (48,50). More detailed reviews of halothane effects on drug disposition are available (2,5).

Fluorinated Ethers

The halogenated ether anesthetics methoxyflurane, enflurane, isoflurane, sevoflurane, and desflurane (Fig. 21-3) are exclusively oxidized, forming inorganic and organic fluoride metabolites (7). Like halothane, the metabolism of enflurane, isoflurane, and desflurane to trifluoroacetyl chloride can form trifluoroacetylated liver proteins and cause fulminant hepatic necrosis mediated by antitrifluoroacetylated protein antibodies (51–53). Metabolism of methoxyflurane has been of considerable

interest, because this drug caused postoperative renal failure, the incidence and severity of which were directly related to the extent of metabolic defluorination (54). Enflurane, isoflurane, sevoflurane, and desflurane also undergo P450-mediated metabolism, releasing inorganic fluoride; however, they do not cause clinical renal toxicity (7,8). This may relate to the observation that only methoxyflurane undergoes human intrarenal defluorination (7,8).

P450 isoforms responsible for halogenated ether oxidation and attendant drug interactions have been identified. Human liver microsomal metabolism of enflurane, isoflurane, sevoflurane, and probably desflurane is catalyzed predominantly if not exclusively by CYP2E1 (55,56). Human methoxyflurane defluorination *in vitro* is also catalyzed predominantly by CYP2E1; however, P450s 2A6, 3A4, 3A5, and possibly 2C9/10 and 2D6 also participate (7,56). Human enflurane, isoflurane, and sevoflurane metabolism *in vivo* is also catalyzed predominantly by CYP2E1. In surgical patients, CYP2E1 induction by isoniazid (57,58) increased the metabolism of enflurane and isoflurane, resulting in increased plasma fluoride concentrations (Fig. 21-4) (59,60). In contrast, inhibition by disulfiram markedly diminished enflurane, sevoflurane, and isoflurane metabolism, causing decreased plasma and urine metabolite concentrations (61–63). Sevoflurane metabolism was also found to be proportional to CYP2E1 activity (64).

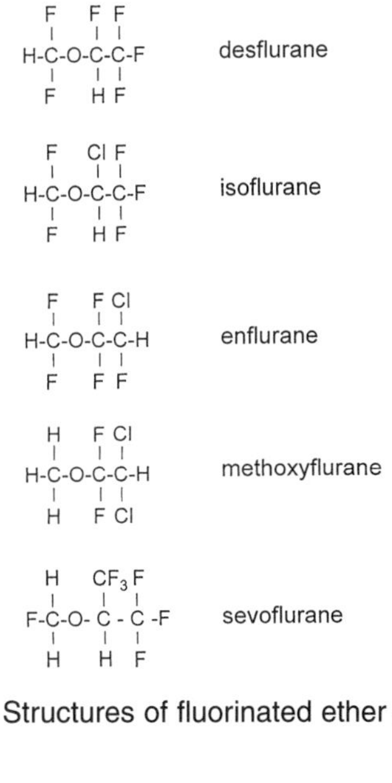

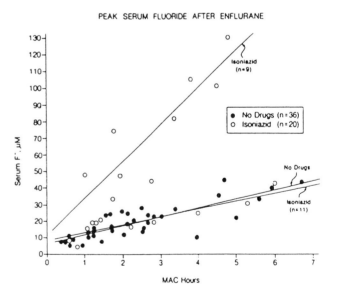

FIG. 21-3. Structures of fluorinated ether anesthetics.

FIG. 21-4. Isoniazid effect on isoflurane metabolism in humans. Shown are peak serum F⁻ levels for individual patients and the linear regression lines for the two isoniazid-treated subgroups and the control group. Isoniazid treatment enhanced defluorination in 9 of 20 subjects. The isoniazid (n = 9) group is different than the other two groups (*p* < 0.001). From Mazze RI, Woodruff RE, Heerdt ME. Isoniazid-induced enflurane defluorination in humans. *Anesthesiology* 1982;57: 5–8, with permission.

Obesity enhanced the microsomal metabolism of enflurane (65) and increased the metabolism of methoxyflurane, enflurane, isoflurane, and sevoflurane in surgical patients (22,66–68), most likely resulting from increases in CYP2E1 activity (69). Cimetidine had no effect on enflurane metabolism (70,71). In contrast to isoniazid, barbiturates and phenytoin do not increase anesthetic defluorination (72,73), because these drugs do not induce CYP2E1. This differs from effects in rats and rabbits, in which phenobarbital and phenytoin induction does increase enflurane, sevoflurane, and isoflurane metabolism (74–76) because CYP2B-mediated metabolism plays a prominent role in these species (7,56). However, barbiturates do induce human methoxyflurane defluorination (77), consistent with its metabolism by P450s 2C and 3A.

Compared with halothane, considerably less has been published regarding the effects of enflurane, isoflurane, sevoflurane, and desflurane on drug metabolism. This is most likely because of lesser effects on hepatic blood flow and P450-mediated biotransformation. Enflurane, isoflurane, and sevoflurane preserve hepatic blood flow, in comparison with halothane (31,78). Unlike halothane, there is no evidence that enflurane, isoflurane, sevoflurane, or desflurane are suicide substrates for P450. In humans, enflurane, unlike halothane, had no effect on postoperative mixed function oxidase activity (antipyrine clearance) (14). In rats, enflurane and isoflurane did not inhibit aminopyrine clearance (79). In dogs, however, enflurane and isoflurane did diminish the clearance of verapamil and propranolol, as a result of decreases in intrinsic clearance (46,80).

INTRAVENOUS ANESTHETICS

Barbiturates

Barbiturates were first used as anesthetics in the 1920s and 1930s, after oral barbiturates used as sedatives were reformulated as sodium salts for intravenous use (81,82). The oxybarbiturate pentobarbital was the first widely used barbiturate in anesthesia; however, this drug and its congeners had a slow onset of action. Hexobarbital, introduced in 1932, was the first rapidly acting intravenous anesthetic, a property conferred by 1-methylation of the barbiturate ring. Methylation, however, also caused involuntary muscle movement, which was undesirable, and, upon introduction of subsequent barbiturates, hexobarbital use in anesthesia was vanquished. Nevertheless, hexobarbital is addressed herein because of its historical significance and long use as an *in vivo* probe of drug oxidation. The first thiobarbiturate, thiopental, was introduced into clinical practice in 1934 (81) and was the predominant anesthetic barbiturate for half a century. Methohexital, first used in 1956, gained popularity and is still used because it has a shorter duration of action than thiopental; however, pain on injection and involuntary muscle movement have limited its use (81,83). Barbiturate structures are shown in Fig. 21-5.

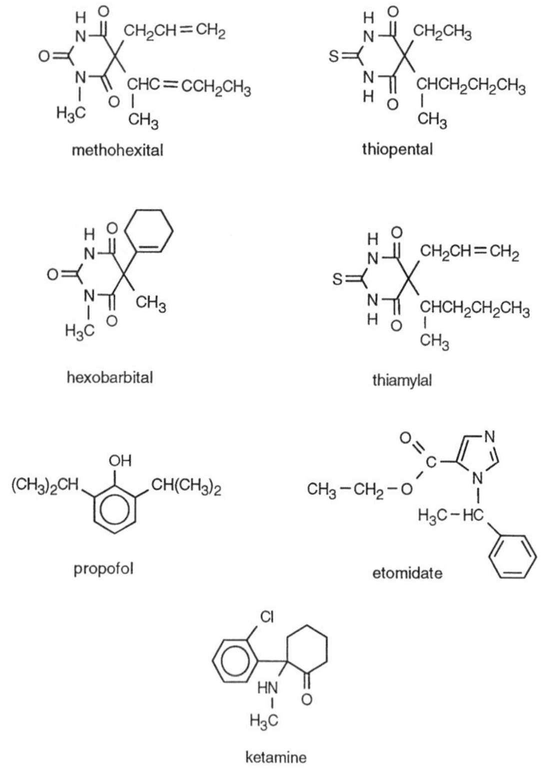

FIG. 21-5. Structures of intravenous anesthetics.

Thiopental

Thiopental, until recently, was the preeminent drug for intravenous induction of anesthesia. Thiopental is extensively metabolized, with less than 1% being excreted unchanged in urine (84,85). The major metabolite in human urine is the (carboxypropyl) carboxylic acid, whereas desulphuration to pentobarbital, which is pharmacologically active, accounts for 2% to 4% of the dose (84). Thiopental is slowly eliminated from the body—clearance averages 2 to 3 mL/kg/min (86–88), and the hepatic extraction ratio is 0.1 to 0.2, suggesting that systemic clearance is dependent on intrinsic clearance (86,89,90). Thiopental is used clinically as the racemate. Although the systemic clearance of R-thiopental averaged 6% to 25% greater than that of S-thiopental after racemate administration, this was attributed to stereoselective protein binding, with no stereoselectivity in intrinsic clearance and, hence, hepatic metabolism (85,91). The human enzymes responsible for thiopental metabolism have not been identified.

Despite undergoing extensive biotransformation, thiopental drug interactions have been rarely reported. This is probably because redistribution from the central compartment terminates (after 5–10 min) the pharmacologic effects, by which time metabolism is still negligible (87, 89,92). During the long elimination phase (12-hour half-life), plasma thiopental concentrations are subtherapeutic and detection of drug interactions based on clinical signs is therefore unlikely. In addition, after thiopental bolus, concentrations of the active metabolite pentobarbital were only one-tenth those of the parent drug—too low to exert significant pharmacologic effects (91). During prolonged, high-dose thiopental infusions, however, pentobarbital formation may be relevant (93,94). Formal pharmacokinetic studies have detected a few thiopental metabolic interactions. Phenobarbital may increase the clearance of thiopental in humans (88). Systemic clearance was increased by 45% in patients with chronic alcoholism, attributed to hepatic enzyme induction (95); however, a subsequent investigation found no difference in clearance, perhaps because subjects were evaluated 1 to 2 weeks after cessation of drinking, by which time enzyme deinduction had occurred (96). In animals, neither inhibition nor phenobarbital induction of hepatic microsomal enzymes altered sleep duration after thiopental (97,98). Volatile (halothane and isoflurane) and certain other anesthetics (the α_2 agonist dexmedetomidine) do alter thiopental kinetics, but this appears to involve distribution rather than altered metabolism (99–101). Barbiturates are known microsomal enzyme inducers. Thiopental increased rat liver microsomal P450 content and ethylmorphine N-demethylase and aniline hydroxylase activities, although the degree of induction was much less than that by phenobarbital (102).

Methohexital

Methohexital is eliminated from the body more quickly than thiopental. Clearance is three-fold greater (9–11 mL/kg/min) and the terminal half-life is one-third that of thiopental (2–4 hours) (92,103,104). Methohexital is extensively metabolized in humans, with less than 1% excreted unchanged in urine (105). The major route of metabolism is allylic oxidation to 4′-hydroxymethohexital (106). Plasma 4′-hydroxymethohexital concentrations quickly exceed those of the parent drug (107). The metabolite is only one-tenth as potent as the parent drug and therefore does not contribute to methohexital clinical effects (108). In rats, 4′-hydroxymethohexital is also the major metabolite, whereas N-demethylation accounts for less than 1% of metabolism (105). Methohexital is used clinically as the racemate; however, metabolism of the individual enantiomers has not been reported.

Clinical drug interactions with methohexital have not been reported. Even though the drug undergoes greater metabolic clearance than thiopental, redistribution still terminates the pharmacologic effects, at which time metabolism is minor (92). Because methohexital is a high-extraction drug, with a hepatic extraction ratio of 0.7 to 0.9 (109), metabolic drug interactions would theoretically be unlikely (110).

Hexobarbital

Hexobarbital is no longer used clinically in anesthesia, but it has been used extensively as a model substrate to study animal and human drug metabolism *in vitro* and *in vivo* (111). Systemic clearance in humans averages 3 to 5 mL/kg/min (111). In rats, hexobarbital is a high-extraction drug; comparable data in humans are not available (111). Hexobarbital undergoes essentially complete metabolism by way of several P450-mediated pathways (Fig. 21-6): allylic oxidation forms 3′-hydroxyhexobarbital, which may be subsequently dehydrogenated to 3′-ketohexobarbital; 1′,2′-epoxidation followed by hydrolysis and decomposition forms 1,5-dimethylbarbituric acid; N-dealkylation forms small amounts of norhexobarbital; and 6′-ketoxyhexobarbital is an additional minor pathway (111,112). In humans, after administration of racemic hexobarbital, urinary recovery of 3′-hydroxyhexobarbital, 3′-ketohexobarbital, and 1,5-dimethylbarbituric acid constituted 5% to 10%, 30% to 45%, and 10% to 20% of the dose, respectively (111). Subsequently, collection of urine for longer intervals (72 hours) showed that 1,5-dimethylbarbituric acid was the major metabolite (average 37% of the dose) and that 3′-oxidation (3′-hydroxyhexobarbital and 3′-ketohexobarbital) and 1,5-dimethylbarbituric acid together accounted for more than 90% of recovered drug (50%–70% of the dose) (112). Knodell and co-workers first showed that human liver microsomal hexobarbital 3′-hydroxylation *in vitro* was catalyzed by the S-mephenytoin 4′-hydroxylase (CYP2C19) and that hexobarbital 3′-oxidation *in vivo* cosegregated with polymorphic S-mephenytoin 4′-hydroxylase activity (113).

Hexobarbital is used in humans as the racemic mixture, and exhibits stereoselectivity in clearance (112,114, 115) and hepatic metabolism (116–118). In subjects phenotyped as extensive metabolizers of S-mephenytoin, oral clearance of R(−)-hexobarbital averaged six to nine times greater than that of S(+)-hexobarbital, due primarily to 5- to 15-fold greater R(−)- versus S(+)- hexobarbi-

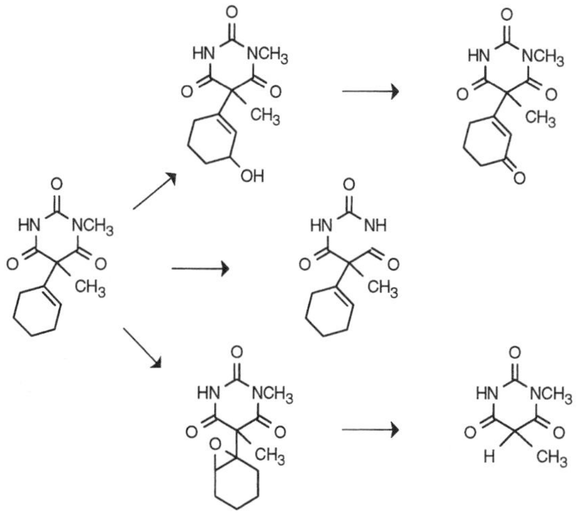

FIG. 21-6. Pathways of hexobarbital metabolism. Based on data in Ref. 111.

tal 3'-oxidation and 1,5-dimethylbarbituric acid formation (112,115). Minor, 6'-oxidation was also stereoselective whereas N-demethylation was not (112). Based on differences between extensive and poor S-mephenytoin metabolizers, in hexobarbital enantiomers metabolism, it appears that 3'-oxidation, 6'-oxidation, and 1,5-dimethylbarbituric acid formation from both enantiomers cosegregates with the mephenytoin polymorphism (112). In vitro, R(−)-hexobarbital, 3'α-hydroxylation, and S(+)-hexobarbital 3'β-hydroxylation were clearly catalyzed predominantly by CYP2C19, whereas CYP2C19 and other enzymes participated in 3'α-hydroxy-S(+)-hexobarbital and 3'β-hydroxy-R(−)-hexobarbital formation (116–118). Thus human hexobarbital metabolism is catalyzed by CYP2C19, but with stereoselective differences in the extent of involvement. In contrast, hexobarbital is metabolized by CYP2B1/2 in rats and exhibits opposite (R versus S) stereoselectivity compared with humans (113,119).

Drug interactions with hexobarbital have been widely reported, owing to its wide use as a probe for drug metabolism (120). Initial studies evaluated hexobarbital metabolism without stereoselective assays. In humans, induction of hepatic enzymes by rifampin caused a three-fold increase in the plasma clearance of intravenous hexobarbital, and increased urinary 3'-ketohexobarbital excretion in most subjects (121). Similarly, phenobarbital, phenytoin, and pentobarbital induction caused a two- to threefold increase in intravenous hexobarbital plasma clearance, although urinary metabolite excretion was not evaluated (122,123). These results are consistent with known barbiturate induction of CYP2C activity. In contrast, 10-day pretreatment with prednisone had no effect on hexobarbital clearance (124). In rats, phenobarbital but not 3-methylcholanthrene increased hexobarbital metabolism in vitro and in vivo (111). Co-induction with phenobarbital and calcium channel antagonists (nifedipine, verapamil, or diltiazem) further shortened hexobarbital sleeping times compared with phenobarbital induction alone, whereas acute treatment with calcium channel antagonists increased hexobarbital sleeping times, suggesting inhibition of hexobarbital metabolism (125). The H_2-receptor antagonist cimetidine, but not ranitidine or famotidine, prolonged hexobarbital sleeping times in rats (126), and cimetidine, mifentidine, and structural analogues but not famotidine caused dose-dependent increases in hexobarbital sleeping times in mice (127). In mice, fluoxetine and norfluoxetine enantiomers were said to stereospecifically inhibit hexobarbital metabolism, based on brain racemic hexobarbital concentrations (128), which is consistent with their effects on CYP2C.

Later investigations studied hexobarbital drug interactions using stereoselective assays. The effect of rifampin induction on the disposition of hexobarbital enantiomers after oral racemate administration was studied in young (mean 29 years) and old (mean 71 years) men (129). In young subjects, rifampin caused six- and 89-fold increases in the oral clearance of S(+)- and R(−)- hexobarbital, respectively. Although there were no age-dependent differences in the clearance of either hexobarbital enantiomer, induction effects were stereoselectively attenuated in the elderly, who showed only six- and 19-fold increases in the oral clearance of S(+)- and R(−)-hexobarbital, respectively. These effects were attributed to rifampin induction of CYP2C19 (129). Although not specifically studied, it can be predicted that other known modulators of CYP2C19 activity (inhibitors, alternate substrates) will correspondingly affect hexobarbital disposition (130). In rats, phenobarbital induction induced the metabolism of both hexobarbital enantiomers, but appeared to have differential effects on S(+)- and R(−)-hexobarbital plasma clearance and metabolite excretion (131).

Propofol

Propofol (2,6-diisopropylphenol) (see Fig. 21-5) is administered as a bolus for induction of anesthesia and as an infusion for maintenance of anesthesia or for sedation (perioperative or intensive care unit) (132–135). It has largely supplanted thiopental for inducing anesthesia. Propofol exhibits rapid redistribution and a high systemic clearance (which exceeds hepatic blood flow and persists during the anhepatic phase of liver transplantation, indicating extrahepatic clearance), which rapidly terminate the therapeutic effect. Propofol is rapidly and extensively metabolized, with less than 1% excreted unchanged (132,134). Approximately 50% to 70% of the dose is excreted as propofol glucuronide, whereas the remainder is 4-hydroxylated to 2,6-diisopropyl-1,4-quinol and excreted as the 1-glucuronide, 4-glucuronide, and 4-sulfate conjugates (136,137). Human liver microsomal propofol oxidation exhibits little (i.e., two-fold) interindividual variability and has been suggested to be catalyzed by numerous P450 isoforms including CYP2C9 as well as CYPs 1A2, 2A6, 2C8, 2C18, and 2C19 (but not 2E1 or 3A4), even though oxidation shows single-enzyme kinetics with a K_m (18 µM) approximating therapeutic concentrations (10–40 µM) (137). Propofol glucuronidation was catalyzed predominantly by uridine diphosphate glucuronosyltransferase I family enzymes (UGT HP4; UGT1.8/9) (138), although participation of another isoform was also suggested (139). Identities of the P450 and UGT enzymes responsible for human propofol metabolism in vivo are not available.

Some in vitro propofol drug interactions have been identified; however, the data are conflicting. Therapeutically relevant propofol concentrations (up to 50 µM) caused modest inhibition of CYP2B but not CYP2E1 activity in rat liver microsomes (140), and only 5% to 20% inhibition of CYP1A, 2B, and 2E1 activities in hamster liver microsomes (141), but they did cause greater

(30% to 70%) inhibition of human liver microsomal metabolism of benzo(a)pyrene, benzphetamine, and aniline (142). Human liver microsomal metabolism of the CYP3A substrates alfentanil and sufentanil (143–146) was inhibited 50% by 50 to 60 μM propofol (147), whereas that of midazolam (148) was unaffected by concentrations less than 100 μM (149). Reasons for these discrepancies are not apparent, but in general, propofol is not a potent P450 inhibitor. In contrast, human liver microsomal propofol glucuronidation *in vitro* was inhibited by riluzole (IC$_{50}$ = 19 μM), which is used to treat patients with amyotrophic lateral sclerosis (150), and by enalapril, acetylsalicylic acid, chloramphenicol, ketoprofen, oxazepam, and fentanyl, albeit at substantially higher concentrations (K$_i$ 1–5 mM) (139).

The only clinical propofol drug interactions noted in humans have been with opioids, and these are mild (5,151,152). Propofol infusions achieving concentrations of 0.4 and 0.8 μg/mL in plasma and 1 to 3 μg/mL in blood caused 10%, 15%, and 20% increases, respectively, in plasma concentrations of alfentanil, although the mechanism of the interaction was not evaluated (153, 154). Alfentanil infusions achieving 40 to 80 ng/mL caused 20% increases in plasma propofol concentrations in two investigations (152,154); however, a third study found no effect of higher alfentanil concentrations (300–500 ng/mL) on propofol concentrations or pharmacokinetic parameters. The interaction between propofol and fentanyl is even less than that between propofol and alfentanil, if existent at all. An initial investigation suggested that a single, small fentanyl bolus (1.5 μg/kg) caused a sustained (8 hour) doubling of propofol blood concentrations and a 30% decrease in propofol systemic clearance (37). Subsequent studies, however, showed no effect of fentanyl (1.5 or 5 μg/kg) on the blood concentration of propofol administered either by bolus or computer-controlled infusion (155,156). Propofol clearance was unaffected by concurrent halothane anesthesia (37). In animals, propofol decreased meperidine hepatic clearance in sheep by 20% without changing the extraction ratio (157), and produced 40% and 65% decreases, respectively, in the intrinsic and free drug clearances of propranolol in dogs, suggesting some inhibition of hepatic metabolism (158). In summary, the clinical significance of propofol pharmacokinetic drug interactions appears modest, particularly in comparison with the more prominent and clinically important pharmacodynamic interactions (151,152).

Etomidate

Etomidate is an imidazole ester (see Fig. 21-5) administered by intravenous bolus for induction of anesthesia; it was formerly used for continuous sedation by intravenous infusion. Etomidate is a high-extraction drug, with systemic clearance 18 to 22 mL/kg/min (approach-

ing hepatic blood flow) and a hepatic extraction ratio of 0.7 to 1.0 (159–161). Etomidate undergoes extensive metabolism, with 90% recovered as metabolites in 24-hour urine and only trace amounts (2%) excreted unchanged (162,163). The drug is principally metabolized by ester hydrolysis to a carboxylic acid metabolite, mainly by nonspecific hepatic esterases (164). *N*-dealkylation is a minor route of metabolism, and all metabolites are inactive (164).

The most important etomidate metabolic interaction is not a drug–drug interaction, but rather an interaction with endogenous steroidogenesis. Etomidate infusions for sedation of intensive care patients were associated with increased mortality rate and low plasma cortisol concentrations (165,166). Subsequently, both an etomidate bolus and a chronic infusion were shown to cause adrenocortical suppression, with decreased plasma cortisol and aldosterone and increased 11-deoxycortisol and 11-deoxycorticosterone (the cortisol precursor) concentrations, resulting from high-affinity etomidate binding to P450 isoforms responsible for steroidogenesis (167–170). After these studies, the use of etomidate infusions ceased. Somewhat similar inhibitory effects on P450-dependent steroidogenesis has been reported for other imidazoles, such as ketoconazole, cloconazole, and clotrimazole, resulting from interaction of the imidazole ring with the heme iron of P450 (171). Investigation of human adrenal steroid biosynthesis *in vitro* revealed etomidate inhibition of 11β-hydroxylase activity, suppressing formation of corticosterone from 11-deoxycorticosterone (IC$_{50}$ 30 nM) (172). By comparison, the IC$_{50}$ for ketoconazole inhibition of 11β-hydroxylase activity was 15 μM, although it was a potent inhibitor of C17, 20-desmolase-catalyzed synthesis of androstenedione (whereas etomidate had negligible effects) (172). Both drugs weakly and similarly inhibited 17α-hydroxylase (IC$_{50}$ 6–18 μM) and 16α-hydroxylase (IC$_{50}$ 4–8 μM) activities, and had no effect on 21-hydroxylase (172). In isolated rat adrenal cells and adrenal mitochondria, etomidate caused a concentration-dependent inhibition of mitochondrial P450s 11-β-hydroxylase (P450$_{11β}$) and cholesterol side chain cleavage (P450scc), without significant effect on microsomal enzymes in the glucocorticoid pathway (21-hydroxylase, 3β-hydroxysteroid dehydrogenase, ^{Δ5}-3 oxosteroid isomerase) (167). Using pig testis P450sccII and its reductase *in vitro*, etomidate was shown to inhibit the C21-steroid 17α-hydroxylase-17,20 activity without interfering with 17α-hydroxylase activity (173). Further *in vitro* studies revealed etomidate inhibition of bovine adrenal gland NADPH–cytochrome P450–phenylisocyanide complex reductase and cholesterol side chain cleavage (P450scc) (171). Etomidate adrenocortical suppression may be stereoselective, because *dl*- and *d*- but not *l*-etomidate decreased plasma steroid concentrations (174).

Etomidate has also been shown to perturb some P450-mediated drug metabolism. Etomidate infusion mildly decreased the clearance (11%) and prolonged the half-life (18%) of antipyrine in humans, but had no effect on the metabolism or clearance of high extraction drugs such as ketamine, fentanyl, and meperidine (175). An interaction between etomidate and alfentanil was postulated in a human study, which reported possible shortening of the half-life of etomidate in the presence of alfentanil (176); however, this contention was not well-founded. Etomidate did cause dose-dependent inhibition of human liver microsomal ketamine N-demethylation *in vitro,* and elicited a type II spectrum upon binding to microsomal P450 (175). In rabbit liver microsomes, etomidate reversibly inhibited P450 activity, with competitive inhibition of aniline p-hydroxylation and mixed-type inhibition of ketamine N-demethylation, meperidine N-demethylation, and p-nitroanisole O-demethylation (177). Although initial speculation was that the inhibitory effects of commercial etomidate (Amidate) on drug biotransformation were related to the solvent (propylene glycol) rather than etomidate itself (178), subsequent studies reported decreased clearance of antipyrine by etomidate (175) but not by propylene glycol (179).

Ketamine

The dissociative anesthetic ketamine (see Fig. 21-5) is administered by intravenous (or rarely intramuscular) bolus for anesthetic induction, and, more recently, has been used as an infusion for prolonged surgical anesthesia or sedation, either alone or in combination with other intravenous agents (180–183). Oral administration results in diminished and erratic plasma concentrations because of significant first-pass clearance and low (16%) oral bioavailability (184). Ketamine is used clinically as the racemic mixture of S(+) and R(−) enantiomers, which differ in their pharmacokinetic and pharmacodynamic

properties, although the single S(+)-enantiomer was recently introduced in Europe (185). The analgesic and hypnotic potency of S(+)-ketamine is approximately four times greater than that of the antipode (186,187). Cessation of ketamine effects is influenced both by redistribution and metabolism (188–191). Termination of hypnosis occurs at high plasma concentrations, primarily because of redistribution from the brain, although there is a contribution of metabolic clearance. Termination of analgesia occurs at lower plasma concentrations, resulting predominantly from biotransformation.

Ketamine is cleared almost exclusively by hepatic metabolism (extraction ratio 0.8) and subsequent renal excretion of primary and secondary metabolites, with less than 3% of the dose eliminated unchanged (189). The major biotransformation products in humans *in vivo* are norketamine ("metabolite I" in early publications) and several hydroxylated norketamine metabolites (Fig. 21-7). Early investigations reported the formation of 5,6-dehydronorketamine ("metabolite II") (189,192–194), which are currently known to be not a metabolite but rather an artifact of the original plasma extraction and gas chromatography assay. Metabolite II is thus a "pseudometabolite," derived from nonenzymatic dehydration of hydroxynorketamine metabolites, specifically 5-hydroxynorketamine (195,196). Quantification of 5,6-dehydronorketamine is still used, however, as an indirect measure of 5-hydroxynorketamine formation (197–202). In humans, 80% of the dose is excreted as glucuronic acid conjugates of hydroxynorketamine metabolites, with norketamine and 5,6-dehydronorketamine constituting 2% and 16%, respectively (189,194). The liver is the primary site of metabolism, although there is evidence for pulmonary but not brain metabolism (203,204).

Hepatic microsomal ketamine metabolism *in vitro* has been studied extensively in animals and humans (195,

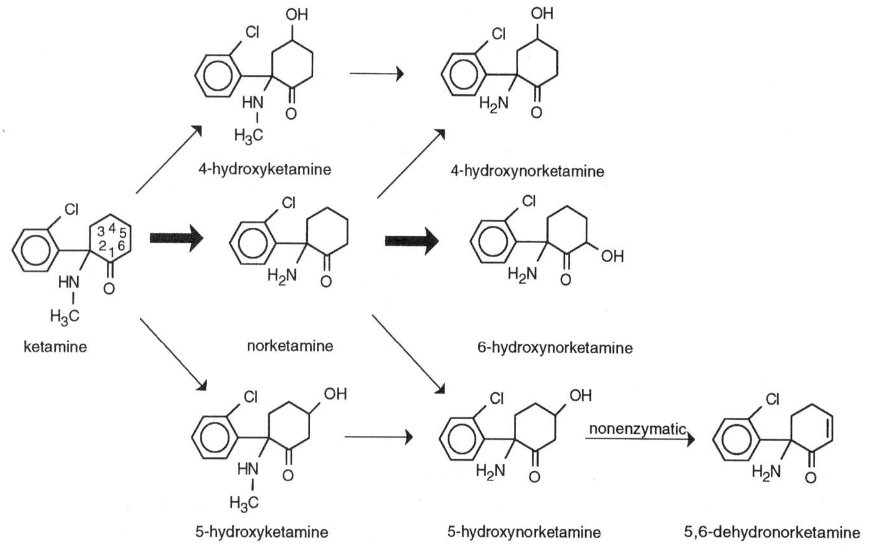

FIG. 21-7. Pathways of ketamine metabolism.

205–208). *N*-demethylation to norketamine is the major pathway. Norketamine undergoes further hydroxylation on the cyclohexanone ring forming 4-, 5-, and 6-hydroxynorketamine. Human and rodent liver microsomes preferentially hydroxylate norketamine at the 6 position, forming 6-hydroxynorketamine as the major hydroxylated ketamine metabolite (195,196). Ketamine itself can be hydroxylated on the cyclohexanone ring, forming 4-, 5-, and 6-hydroxyketamine. Human and rat liver microsomes preferentially form 4- and 5-hydroxyketamine, respectively; however ketamine hydroxylation is clinically a quantitatively insignificant pathway (195,196). Hydroxylation on the cyclohexanone ring introduces a second chiral center, and both 5-hydroxynorketamine isomers are formed by rodent and human liver microsomes (195,196). In contrast, norketamine 6-hydroxylation is stereoselective, forming exclusively (Z)-6-hydroxynorketamine (the *cis*-diastereomer) but not the (E)- or *trans*-diastereomer). Ketamine is not metabolized on the aromatic ring, and phenolic metabolites are not formed. In human liver microsomes, there are at least two isoforms of P450 that catalyze ketamine *N*-demethylation, with the activity of one isoform predominating at therapeutic drug concentrations, although the identity of these P450 isoforms is not yet known (207).

Alterations in hepatic microsomal enzyme activity influence ketamine disposition and duration of effect, even though ketamine is a high extraction drug and clearance, therefore, is theoretically dependent on hepatic blood flow (110). Benzodiazepine pretreatment is used to ameliorate the psychomimetic side effects and emergence delirium of ketamine (180,209), but also results in altered ketamine metabolism, which is the best characterized ketamine metabolic drug interaction. Patients pretreated with intravenous diazepam before induction with intravenous ketamine bolus showed higher plasma ketamine concentrations for the 30 minutes following induction and slightly diminished clearance compared to untreated controls (198). Rectal diazepam given 1 hour before intravenous ketamine (bolus and infusion) in adults diminished ketamine metabolism and prolonged the plasma half-life compared with untreated controls (197). Pediatric patients receiving intramuscular diazepam (or secobarbital) before induction with intramuscular ketamine had a longer duration of hypnosis and longer ketamine half-life compared with untreated controls (210). Midazolam effects on ketamine disposition have been examined more recently. Ketamine half-life was significantly shorter in patients receiving a midazolam-ketamine infusion compared with a diazepam-ketamine infusion (211), suggesting that midazolam may have less of an effect on the metabolism and disposition of ketamine. Indeed, the kinetics of a ketamine infusion with midazolam did not differ significantly from that of a bolus (182,212). In humans, enzyme induction by chronic phenobarbital or diazepam treatment reduced the elimination half-life of ketamine and increased metabolism, evidenced by higher plasma hydroxynorketamine concentrations (197) or shorter ketamine half-life (210). Ketamine infusions administered to phenobarbital-induced patients resulted in steady-state plasma ketamine concentrations one-third of those in uninduced control subjects (201).

Animal data also demonstrate ketamine metabolic interactions. Halothane noncompetitively inhibited ketamine *N*-demethylation *in vitro*, increased ketamine brain and plasma half-lives *in vivo*, and prolonged the pharmacologic effect (40). Etomidate also inhibited ketamine metabolism *in vitro*, but had no effect on ketamine disposition *in vivo* (175,177). Enzyme induction by chronic phenobarbital treatment in rats increased ketamine *N*-demethylation *in vitro*, diminished brain and plasma ketamine concentrations *in vivo*, and shortened the duration of pharmacologic effect (188,213). Ketamine may also induce its own metabolism (188) and that of other drugs (214,215).

Another type of interaction is the metabolic enantiomeric interaction between S(+)- and R(−)-ketamine observed in humans. After administration of the racemate, S(+)-ketamine clearance was significantly (15%) greater than that of R(−)-ketamine (216), and when injected individually, S(+)-ketamine clearance was 22% greater than that of the R(−)-enantiomer (186). Recovery from racemic ketamine was significantly slower than that from either of the individual enantiomers, leading to the suggestion that R(−)-ketamine could inhibit S(+)-ketamine metabolism and delay recovery from the more potent S(+)-enantiomer, accounting for the longer recovery from the racemate compared with S(+)-ketamine alone (186). Subsequently, human hepatic microsomes were found to catalyze ketamine enantiomer demethylation at different rates, with S(+)-ketamine demethylation being 15% to 30% faster than that of R(−)-ketamine, accounting for the clinical observations (207). Furthermore, the rate of racemic ketamine demethylation was significantly less than that expected by summing the rates for the individual enantiomers, strongly suggesting a metabolic enantiomeric interaction in which each ketamine enantiomer inhibited the metabolism of its antipode. The ketamine metabolic enantiomeric interaction may provide an explanation for the prolongation of recovery from racemic compared with S(+)-ketamine (186).

LOCAL ANESTHETICS

Local anesthetics block the generation and propagation of impulses in excitable neural and cardiac tissues. All local anesthetics contain a hydrophilic amine residue and a lipophilic domain separated by an intermediate alkyl chain (Fig. 21-8). The intermediate chain contains either an ester or an amide linkage, which subdivides the clinically useful local anesthetics into two main groups: the aminoesters, which are metabolized by plasma

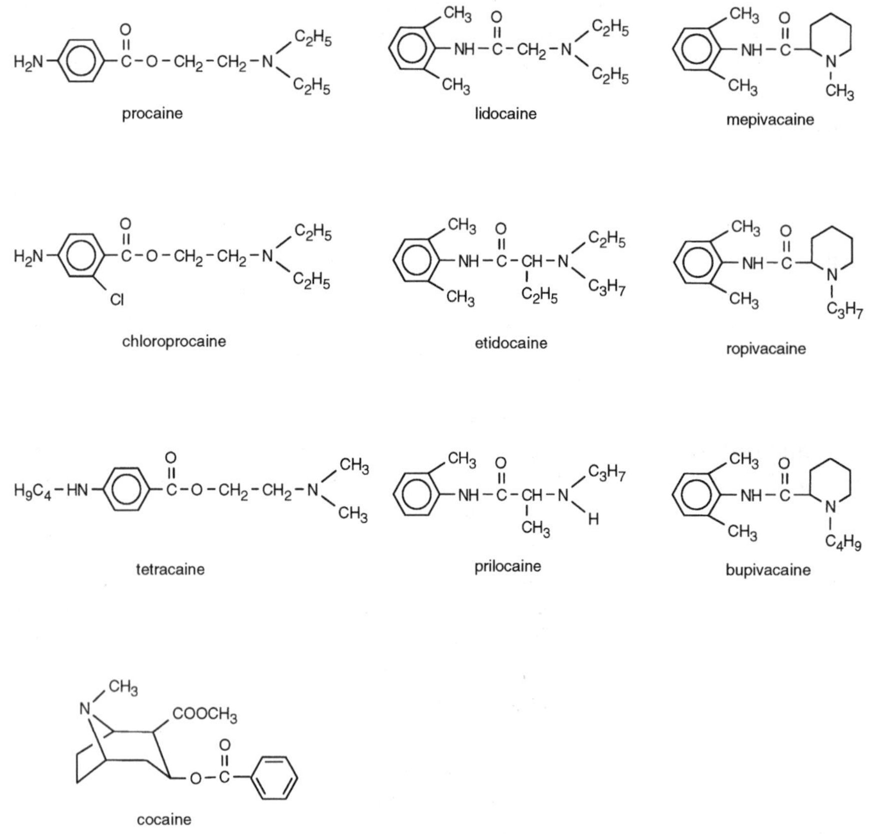

FIG. 21-8. Structures of local anesthetics.

cholinesterase (cocaine, procaine, chloroprocaine, amethocaine, tetracaine), and the aminoamides (lidocaine, prilocaine, mepivacaine, bupivacaine, ropivacaine, etidocaine), which are metabolized in the liver.

Amide Local Anesthetics

Lidocaine

Lidocaine is the most commonly used local anesthetic, administered intravenously as an antiarrhythmic, applied topically, or injected for neural blockade. It is rapidly eliminated, with systemic clearance averaging 1 L/min and half-life of 1.6 hours, predominantly by hepatic metabolism, with a hepatic extraction ratio of 0.6 to 0.7 (217,218). Lidocaine is extensively metabolized in humans, with less than 3% excreted unchanged in 24-hour urine (219). Metabolites (and their percentage elimination in urine) include monoethylglycinexylidide (MEGX) (3.7%), glycinexylidide (GX) (2.3), 2,6-xylidide (2,6-dimethylaniline) (1.0), 4-hydroxy-2,6-dimethylaniline (73), 3-hydroxy-lidocaine (1.1), and 3-hydroxy-MEGX (0.3) (219). The predominant route of metabolism is N-deethylation to MEGX, which, in turn, may undergo further N-deethylation to either GX, 3'-hydroxylation, or mostly amide hydrolysis to 2,6-xylidide, which is then 4'-hydroxylated to 4-hydroxy-2,6-dimethylaniline (217). MEGX metabolism is extensive,

with only 12% of an injected dose recovered unchanged (220). Tucker and Mather suggested that direct amide hydrolysis of lidocaine is a minor pathway (217), although a more recent investigation showed that both lidocaine and MEGX were equally hydrolyzed by human liver slices (but only lidocaine was hydrolyzed by human liver microsomes or homogenates) (221). Lidocaine metabolites are pharmacologically active. MEGX has the same degree of central nervous and cardiovascular system toxicity as lidocaine, and a slightly longer half-life with steady-state unbound plasma concentrations about 70% those of lidocaine. GX has weak local anesthetic, antiarrhythmic, and central nervous system depressant effects, although no convulsant effect in animals, and has a half-life of approximately 10 hours (222–224). MEGX formation has been observed in an anhepatic female following surgical hepatectomy, demonstrating extrahepatic lidocaine metabolism, possibly in intestine or kidney, but not in heart, lungs, or skeletal muscle (225).

The human liver microsomal P450 isoforms catalyzing lidocaine metabolism have been identified (226,227). N-deethylation was biphasic, indicating involvement of two isoforms (high-affinity K_m 8-130 μM, V_{max} 0.08–2.5 nmol/min/mg; low-affinity K_m 1.4–1.9 mM, V_{max} 7–11 nmol/min/mg), with activity of the high-affinity isoform predominating (84%–99%) (226). A subsequent investigation reported only one lidocaine deethylase (K_m 1.9 mM, V_{max} 7.1 nmol/min/mg) (221). The predominant low-affinity isoform catalyzing lidocaine *N*-deethylation was identified as CYP3A4, based on chemical and antibody inhibition, correlation with immunoreactive CYP3A4, and the activity of purified and cDNA-expressed CYP3A4 (226,227). Expressed CYP3A5 also catalyzed lidocaine *N*-deethylation, with specific activity approximately half that of CYP3A4 (226). Formation of the other lidocaine metabolite found in human liver microsomes, 3-hydroxylidocaine, was catalyzed by purified CYP1A2 (227). Somewhat similar isoform specificities were found with rat liver microsomes and purified P450s, demonstrating lidocaine *N*-deethylation by CYP3A, CYP2B1, and CYP2C11, and 3-hydroxylation by CYP1A2 (228,229), although evidence for lidocaine 3-hydroxylation by rat CYP2D has also been provided (230,231). In rats *in vivo*, phenobarbital induction experiments showed that MEGX formation was catalyzed by hepatic CYP3A2 or CYP2B1 (232). Extrahepatic lidocaine metabolism has been examined in rat tissues, which formed MEGX (lung, kidney) and 3-hydroxylidocaine (lung), with highest activity in pulmonary microsomes, and catalyzed predominantly by CYP2B1 (229,233). Intestinal lidocaine metabolism was not examined, however.

Lidocaine clearance and, in particular, MEGX production have been evaluated and used as putative quantitative indicators of hepatic function in liver disease and in pretransplant and posttransplant patients (234–237). It was originally anticipated that the MEGX test would reflect both hepatic blood flow (because lidocaine is an intermediate- to high-extraction drug) and hepatic oxidative capacity (specifically CYP3A4-mediated activity) (234). Clinically, MEGX formation was found to be inversely proportional to the severity of histologic liver disease in patients with chronic hepatitis or cirrhosis, to reflect improvement or progression of liver disease, and to predict morbidity and mortality related to complications of chronic liver disease (Fig. 21-9) (235,238–240). In liver transplant recipients, MEGX formation was lowest in patients with the poorest clinical outcome (i.e., sensitive), although not specific (236). The donor MEGX test, in which lidocaine is administered to organ donors to (hopefully) predict graft function in recipients, although initially appearing promising (241), has not been found to predict early graft function, graft survival, or patient survival (237,242). Consistent with its liver blood flow–dependent clearance (243,244), lidocaine is a remarkably sensitive indicator of disturbed liver blood flow, for instance, hepatic artery thrombosis and hepatic ischemia, potential complications of liver transplantation (236). In contrast, the MEGX test does not appear to be an accurate indicator of CYP3A4-mediated liver function (see later text) (245–247).

Lidocaine drug interactions *in vivo* and *in vitro* have been extensively studied, both in humans and rats. Although lidocaine has been used extensively for decades, effects of classic enzyme inducers and inhibitors on lidocaine disposition have only recently been clarified.

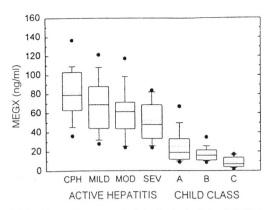

FIG. 21-9. Hepatic monoethylglycinexylodide (MEGX) production in patients with chronic hepatitis and cirrhosis. The boxes represent the 25th and 75th percentiles, capped bars the 10th and 90th percentiles, and filled circles the 5th and 95th percentiles. The solid line within each box is the 50th percentile. The dotted line represents the mean. Patients with cirrhosis had significantly ($p < 0.05$) lower mean MEGX than patients without cirrhosis. CPH, chronic persistent hepatitis. From Shiffman ML, Luketic VA, Sanyal AJ, Thompson EB. Use of hepatic lidocaine metabolism to monitor patients with chronic liver disease. *Ther Drug Monit* 1996;18:372–377, with permission.

In rats *in vivo*, phenobarbital pretreatment, which caused a five-fold induction in hepatic CYP2B1 and 3A2 contents, had no effect on systemic lidocaine clearance but significantly increased plasma MEGX concentrations (four-fold increase in AUC) while decreasing those of 3-hydroxylidocaine (232). In liver microsomes from phenobarbital-induced rats, lidocaine *N*-deethylation was increased five-fold whereas 3-hydroxylation was unaffected (232). In humans, an early investigation showed that phenytoin and phenobarbital pretreatment decreased plasma lidocaine concentrations by 30% to 40% after intravenous injection (248). Similarly, in patients taking epileptic drugs, including phenytoin, phenobarbitone, primidone, and carbamazepine, apparent oral clearance of lidocaine was significantly higher than in normal subjects (7.0 ± 4.8 versus 2.5 ± 1.2 L/kg/hr), with 50% to 60% reduction in oral lidocaine bioavailability (249). These effects were attributed to enzyme induction and enhanced lidocaine metabolism (248,249). In contrast, more recently, plasma MEGX concentrations were surprisingly lower in patients taking antiepileptic drugs known to induce CYP3A4 (carbamazepine, or phenobarbital plus phenytoin) (245). In human liver microsomes, lidocaine and the CYP3A4 substrate cyclosporine were mutual inhibitors of each other's metabolism, with cyclosporine inhibiting MEGX formation (IC_{50} 0.2 μM) and lidocaine inhibiting cyclosporine metabolism (IC_{50} 950 μM) (250). In cultured human hepatocytes, the CYP3A4 inducer rifampin caused a dose-dependent (up to six-fold) increase in lidocaine *N*-deethylation to MEGX, consistent with induction of CYP3A4 activity (Fig. 21-10) (251,252). In marked contrast, however,

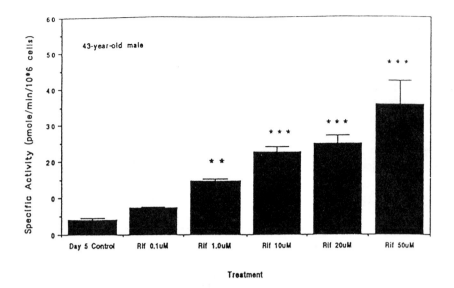

FIG. 21-10. Rifampin induction of lidocaine metabolism in primary human hepatocytes. Hepatocytes were cultured for 3 days before a 2-day treatment with rifampin at the concentrations indicated (mean ± SEM, n = 3). ** $p < 0.01$; *** $p < 0.001$. From Li AP, Rasmussen A, Xu L, Kaminski DL. Rifampicin induction of lidocaine metabolism in cultured human hepatocytes. *J Pharmacol Exp Ther* 1995;274:673–677, with permission.

rifampin induction of CYP3A4 activity in humans (four-fold) resulted in only 15% increases in plasma MEGX concentrations (statistically insignificant) and lidocaine clearance (Fig. 21-11) (246). This small change was attributed to rifampin-related increases in hepatic perfusion rather than to lidocaine metabolism. Similarly, in humans *in vivo*, pretreatment with erythromycin or itraconazole for 4 days, both known to substantially inhibit CYP3A4 activity, had no effect (itraconazole) or actually increased (erythromycin) plasma MEGX concentrations and had no effect on lidocaine clearance (247). These investigations suggest that although the predominant route of lidocaine metabolism in humans is catalyzed by hepatic CYP3A4, *in vivo* alterations in enzyme activity have minimal effects on lidocaine metabolism and clearance, possibly reflecting principal dependence of clearance on hepatic blood flow (243,244). Phenobarbital

effects on lidocaine clearance may reflect known increases in hepatic blood flow (253,254).

Lidocaine metabolic interactions with other cardioactive drugs have also been of particular interest. Several investigations have shown that lidocaine clearance in animals (255) and humans (256) is significantly reduced by β-adrenergic antagonists. Ochs and co-workers first observed in humans that propranolol (80 mg every 8 hours for 3 days) reduced the clearance of lidocaine administered by bolus (10.7 ± 3.1 versus 18.0 ± 7.6 mL/min/kg) or infusion (6.4 ± 1.3 versus 8.5 ± 2.1 mL/min/kg) (257). Subsequent investigations confirmed the 16% to 47% decrease by propranolol in oral, bolus, and steady-state lidocaine clearance (Fig. 21-12) (258–261). More variable results have been obtained with less lipophilic β-adrenergic antagonists. For example, one investigation found that lidocaine plasma clearance was

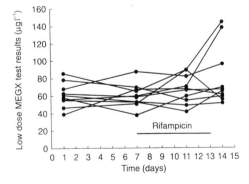

FIG. 21-11. Rifampin effects on lidocaine metabolism in humans. Low dose MEGX test results before, during and after P450 induction with rifampicin are shown as data points (*filled circles*). The results of each healthy volunteer are connected with lines. From Reichel C, Skodra T, Nacke A, Spengler U, Sauerbruch T. The lignocaine metabolite (MEGX) liver function test and P-450 induction in humans. *Br J Clin Pharmacol* 1998;46:535–539, with permission.

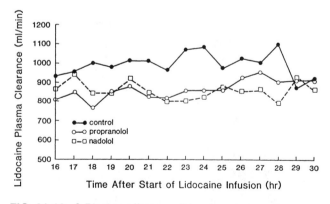

FIG. 21-12. β-Blocker effects on lidocaine plasma clearance during lidocaine infusion in humans. From 259. Schneck DW, Luderer JR, Davis D, Vary J. Effects of nadolol and propranolol on plasma lidocaine clearance. *Clin Pharmacol Ther* 1984;36:584–587, with permission.

moderately reduced (31%) by 1-day pretreatment with metoprolol (258), whereas others found no effect of metoprolol, even after multiple doses (262,263). Nadolol slightly (17%) diminished lidocaine clearance (259), whereas atenolol, the most hydrophilic β-blocker, had no effect (263).

The mechanism of propranolol alteration of lidocaine clearance is somewhat unresolved. Theoretically, decreased clearance could result from diminished hepatic blood flow, plasma protein binding, or oxidative metabolism (260,261). Early investigations attributed the effect, at least in part, to diminished hepatic blood flow (257–259), because propranolol and nadolol decreased hepatic blood flow by 25% without altering lidocaine intrinsic clearance (259). The second mechanism was discounted because propranolol did not alter lidocaine plasma protein binding (260). More evidence exists for the third mechanism, a direct effect on lidocaine metabolism. This was supported, in part, because observed decreases in lidocaine clearance exceeded the reduction in hepatic blood flow (257,258,260,261). In addition, propranolol, and to a lesser extent, metoprolol, but not atenolol, inhibited human liver microsomal lidocaine metabolism (Fig. 21-13) (260). The correlation between inhibition of lidocaine metabolism and β-blocker lipophilicity was even greater in rat liver microsomes (264,265). Rat studies must be evaluated cautiously, however, because the primary route of metabolism, and the

one most inhibited by propranolol, was CYP2D6 and/or CYP1A2-mediated 3-hydroxylation (competitive, K_i = 0.096 ± 0.013 μM), whereas N-deethylation (the predominant pathway in humans) was not affected by propranolol (264–266). Perfused rat liver studies support the theory of propranolol inhibition of intrinsic clearance, because propranolol reduced lidocaine clearance, metabolism, and the hepatic extraction ratio even when perfusion was held constant (244). Thus, particularly in conjunction with recent results with CYP3A4 inhibitors, it appears that lipophilic β-blockers diminish lidocaine elimination *in vivo* by reducing hepatic blood flow (and possibly lidocaine oxidation), whereas hydrophilic β-blockers clearly have no effect on metabolism and only minor effects on hepatic blood flow and lidocaine elimination.

The interaction between lidocaine and the antiarrhythmic agent amiodarone, a known CYP3A4 substrate (267,268), has been recently characterized. The first description was a case report of a patient receiving a lidocaine infusion in whom seizures, toxic lidocaine plasma concentrations, and reduced lidocaine systemic clearance developed 65 hours after amiodarone therapy was initiated (269). Prospective evaluation in humans *in vivo* showed that amiodarone increased the serum lidocaine AUC (112 ± 23 to 135 ± 33 mg/mL/min), decreased the MEGX AUC (19 ± 6 to 16 ± 8 mg/mL/min), and decreased lidocaine systemic clearance by 20% (7.7 ± 1.8 to 6.3 ± 2.2 mL/kg/min) (270). These effects were attributed to inhibition of lidocaine N-deethylation by amiodarone or its N-deethylated metabolite, because amiodarone was a competitive inhibitor of human liver microsomal lidocaine N-deethylation (K_i 47 μM), and N-deethylamiodarone also inhibited lidocaine N-deethylation in a concentration-dependent manner (270). In contrast, another investigation found no significant effect of amiodarone on lidocaine disposition in humans *in vivo* (271).

A possible interaction between lidocaine and the antiarrhythmic agent mexiletine has also been suggested. Administration of oral viscous lidocaine to a patient undergoing long-term treatment with mexiletine, who also had impaired liver function and congestive heart failure, resulted in a toxic serum lidocaine concentration and signs of lidocaine toxicity (272). Whether this effect represents a metabolic interaction between mexiletine, a known CYP2D6 substrate (273,274), and lidocaine has not been evaluated.

Addition of the α_2 adrenoceptor agonist clonidine to lidocaine is known to prolong the duration of local anesthetic action, but clonidine effects on lidocaine systemic disposition are unresolved. Plasma lidocaine concentrations were increased by clonidine plus lidocaine for epidural anesthesia, suggesting altered lidocaine metabolism (275). In mice and rats, subcutaneous clonidine administered before intravenous lidocaine increased

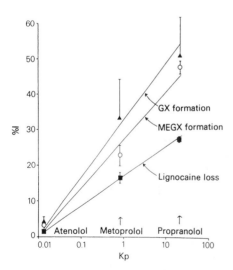

FIG. 21-13. β-Blocker effects on human liver microsomal lidocaine metabolism. Shown is the relationship between inhibition of lidocaine (42.7 μM) metabolism (%*I*) and octanol/pH 7.4 buffer partition coefficient (*K*p) for three β-blockers (50 μM). Controls showed 43% to 47% metabolism of lidocaine. Points represents the mean from two livers, and bars represent ranges. From Tucker GT, Max NDS, Lennard MS, Al-Asadt S, Bharaj HS, Woods HF. Effects of β-adrenoceptor antagonists on the pharmacokinetics of lignocaine. *Br J Clin Pharmacol* 1984;17:21S–28S, with permission.

plasma lidocaine concentrations and transiently lowered MEGX and GX concentrations (276). Apparent inhibition of lidocaine metabolism was reversed by the α_2-adrenoceptor antagonist, yohimbine, suggesting mediation by α_2-adrenoceptors, although further mechanisms were not explored (276). Opposite results were observed, however, in another investigation in patients in which clonidine did not alter systemic lidocaine elimination after epidural anesthesia (277).

A metabolic drug interaction was found when lidocaine was co-infused with the calcium channel antagonist diltiazem in isolated perfused rat liver (278). Lidocaine addition at steady-state diltiazem initially increased the perfusate diltiazem concentration, attributed to diltiazem displacement from tissue-binding sites. This was followed by a new and higher steady-state diltiazem concentration, attributed to the inhibition by lidocaine of diltiazem hepatic clearance, intrinsic clearance, N-oxidation, and O-demethylation (and some unknown primary metabolic pathways). Similarly, co-infusion of lidocaine and diltiazem resulted in lower concentrations of MEGX and 3-hydroxylidocaine, suggesting diltiazem inhibition of both N-dealkylation and aromatic hydroxylation of lidocaine (278). These results are consistent with mutual interaction of lidocaine and diltiazem, a known CYP3A4 substrate (279), with CYP3A4.

Lidocaine interactions with histamine H_2-receptor antagonists have been repeatedly evaluated, with generally consistent results but conflicting interpretations. Cimetidine decreased the average systemic clearance of intravenous lidocaine by 20% to 30%, and increased the incidence of lidocaine toxicity, although some individuals showed no effect (Fig. 21-14) (280–283). A single cimetidine dose had no effect on epidural lidocaine clearance

(284). Oral lidocaine clearance was inhibited to a greater extent than intravenous lidocaine clearance (42% ± 7% versus 21% ± 6%) (282). Initial investigations attributed cimetidine effects to diminished hepatic blood flow (280,281), whereas others suggested that diminished clearance was due exclusively to reduced lidocaine extraction and impaired metabolism (282,283). Ranitidine consistently had no significant effect on lidocaine disposition, generally attributed to a lack of ranitidine effect on lidocaine metabolism (283–285). Pretreatment with the proton pump inhibitor omeprazole for 1 week had no effect on lidocaine disposition, clearance, or the formation of MEGX (286).

Other lidocaine interactions have also been studied. In humans, general anesthesia with halothane and nitrous oxide reduced intravenous lidocaine clearance by 34% compared with a balanced technique of thiopental, fentanyl, and nitrous oxide (287). In contrast, no significant difference was found in the effect of residual diethyl ether, methoxyflurane, or sodium pentobarbital anesthesia on lidocaine metabolism by isolated perfused rat livers, suggesting no residual P450 inhibition (288). In humans, propafenone, a known CYP2D6 substrate and inhibitor, had a negligible effect on the clearance of continuously infused lidocaine (289). In mice in vivo, intravenous and subcutaneous morphine, fentanyl, and meperidine increased plasma lidocaine concentrations and reduced MEGX and GX concentrations, possibly by reducing hepatic blood flow (276,290).

Etidocaine

Etidocaine is a lidocaine analogue with systemic clearance approaching hepatic blood flow (1.2 L/min) and hepatic extraction ratio (0.7–0.8) exceeding those of lidocaine (217,220,291). The drug is extensively biotransformed, with less than 1% excreted unchanged in urine (217). More than 20 metabolites have been identified, yet still only 40% of the dose is accounted for (217,292–294). Unlike for lidocaine, N-dealkylation is a minor route of metabolism, with secondary and primary amines accounting for 1% and 10% of the dose, respectively. Amide hydrolysis (via either etidocaine or its N-dealkylated metabolites) to 2,6-xylidide accounts for 9% of the dose. Cyclic imidazolinone and hydantoin metabolites, arising by way of intramolecular cyclization of N-dealkylated carbiinolamine intermediates, account for an additional 12% and 10% of the dose (293). P450 isoforms catalyzing etidocaine metabolism are unknown. Metabolic interactions have not been reported, but would not be expected unless hepatic blood flow were significantly reduced.

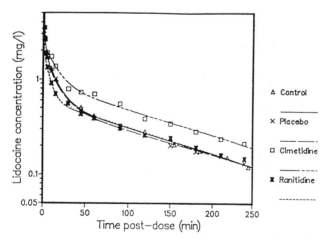

FIG. 21-14. Effect of histamine H_2-receptor antagonists on lidocaine disposition. Shown are plasma concentration-time curves from a typical subject. From Jackson JE, Bentley JB, Glass SJ, Fukui T, Gandolfi AJ, Plachetka JR. Effects of histamine-2 receptor blockade on lidocaine kinetics. *Clin Pharmacol Ther* 1985;37:544–548, with permission.

Prilocaine

Prilocaine has a high systemic clearance in excess of liver blood flow (2.4 L/min), suggesting extrahepatic metabolism (218). It undergoes amide hydrolysis to *N*-propylalamine and to *o*-toluidine, which are in turn 4- and 6-hydroxylated, probably by rearrangement of an *N*-hydroxy intermediate, which has been implicated in methemoglobinemia and cyanosis after large prilocaine doses (217). Prilocaine is used clinically as the racemate, and there is considerable stereoselectivity in the rates of enantiomer hydrolysis (295,296), but this appears to have little implications for prilocaine toxicity. Significant drug interactions with prilocaine are not apparent.

Bupivacaine

Bupivacaine (see Fig. 21-8) is used exclusively for neural blockade. It is more slowly eliminated than lidocaine, with systemic clearance averaging 0.5 L/min and half-life of 2 to 3 hours, predominantly by hepatic metabolism, with an hepatic extraction ratio of 0.3 to 0.4 (217,218,291,297). Bupivacaine is extensively metabolized in humans, with less than 6% excreted unchanged in 24-hour urine (298,299). Metabolites in humans include 2,6-pipecoloxylidide (desbutylbupivacaine, 5% of the dose), 4'-hydroxybupivacaine, and pipecolic acid, but these constitute only a small fraction of the dose excreted in urine, and the majority of parent drug remains unaccounted for. Both 2,6-pipecoloxylidide and 4'-hydroxybupivacaine can be detected in plasma, but concentrations are less than one-tenth those of bupivacaine (299–302). The predominant route of metabolism in humans is *N*-dealkylation to desbutylbupivacaine, which, in turn, may undergo amide hydrolysis to pipecolic acid and 2,6-xylidide, although the extent of hydrolysis (50%) is less than that for the corresponding lidocaine metabolite, MEGX (298). Bupivacaine, used clinically as a racemate, undergoes stereoselective elimination in humans, with clearance of R(+)-bupivacaine averaging 37% higher than that of S(+)-bupivacaine, although stereoselectivity of hepatic microsomal metabolism has not been reported (303). In rats, a large proportion of a dose is excreted as 3'-hydroxybupivacaine, whereas the monkey excretes predominantly pipecolic acid (304). P450 isoforms catalyzing human bupivacaine metabolism have not been reported.

A few bupivacaine metabolic drug interactions have been reported. Propranolol reduced the systemic clearance of intravenous bupivacaine by 35% (0.33 ± 0.12 versus 0.21 ± 0.12 L/min) and prolonged the elimination half-life (2.6 versus 4.9 hours) (305). In another investigation, patients receiving a variety of β-blockers had higher mean plasma bupivacaine concentrations, compared with a group in whom β-blockers had been withdrawn, but the differences were not statistically significant (306). Propranolol has been shown to decrease first pass pulmonary extraction of bupivacaine by about 10% in rabbits, presumably by competing for tissue binding sites. Cimetidine, in most investigations, had no effect on the clearance of epidural bupivacaine (307–309) and

there was no effect of cimetidine on the clearance of intramuscular bupivacaine, or on the excretion of bupivacaine metabolites (300). One limited investigation did suggest that oral cimetidine decreased the total body clearance of intravenous bupivacaine (310). In rat liver microsomes and hepatocytes, cimetidine noncompetitively inhibited bupivacaine metabolism (K_i 220 μM) demonstrating a reduction in intrinsic clearance (311). In monkeys *in vivo*, cimetidine had no significant effect on bupivacaine clearance, because decreases in intrinsic clearance were offset by changes in protein binding (311). Ranitidine consistently had no effect on epidural or intravenous bupivacaine pharmacokinetics in humans (308–310,312). In children, diazepam increased the peak plasma concentration and the area under the plasma concentration-time curve of bupivacaine, but not lidocaine, following caudal injection of a mixture of these drugs (313). In mice, clonidine doubled the plasma bupivacaine AUC and halved the clearance, apparently by inhibiting hepatic bupivacaine metabolism, because the plasma desbutylbupivacaine to bupivacaine AUC ratio was substantially diminished (0.22 ± 0.02 versus 0.42 ± 0.03) (314). In contrast, nicorandil, a potassium-channel agonist, decreased the bupivacaine plasma AUC and increased the clearance, with increased hepatic metabolism suggested by an increase in the plasma desbutylbupivacaine to bupivacaine AUC ratio (315).

Mepivacaine

Mepivacaine is the monomethyl analogue of bupivacaine (see Fig. 21-8). It is eliminated more rapidly than bupivacaine, with systemic clearance averaging 0.8 L/min and half-life of 2 hours, predominantly by hepatic metabolism, with a hepatic extraction ratio of 0.5 (217,218,220). Mepivacaine is extensively metabolized in humans, with less than 1% excreted unchanged, but more than 50% of the dose still remains unaccounted for (220,298). Metabolites in humans, and their percentage of the dose recovered in urine, include 3-hydroxymepivacaine (15%–20%), 4-hydroxymepivacaine (10%–14%), and the *N*-demethylated metabolite 2,6-pipecoloxylidide (1%). Other metabolites include 6-oxopipecolo-2,6-xylidide, 1-methyl-6-oxopipecolo-2,6-xylidide, and a piperidine ring-hydroxylated derivative of the latter. Mepivacaine, used clinically as a racemate, undergoes stereoselective elimination in humans, with clearance of R(+)-mepivacaine approximately 50% greater than that of S(+)-mepivacaine, although stereoselectivity of hepatic metabolism has not been reported (316). The P450 isoforms catalyzing mepivacaine metabolism, and mepivacaine metabolic interactions, have not been reported.

Ropivacaine

Ropivacaine is the propyl analogue of bupivacaine (see Fig. 21-8), used exclusively as the single S(−)-enantiomer, and is the most recently introduced local anesthetic (218,317). Plasma clearance (0.4–0.5 L/min) and half-life (2 hours) are similar to those of mepivacaine (318–320). Ropivacaine is a low- to intermediate-extraction drug, with a hepatic extraction ratio of 0.2 to 0.6 (321,322); it is extensively metabolized in humans, with 1% excreted unchanged in 96-hour urine (320). Metabolites in humans (and their percentage elimination in urine) include 3-hydroxyropivacaine (37%), 2-hydroxymethylropivacaine (18%), 4-hydroxyropivacaine (0.4%), and the N-dealkylated metabolites 2,6-pipecoloxylidide (3%) and 3-hydroxy-2,6-pipecoloxylidide (2%) (320). Ropivacaine undergoes biotransformation by human liver microsomes to ten metabolites, of which four (3-hydroxyropivacaine, 4-hydroxyropivacaine, 2,6-pipecoloxyli-

dide, 2-hydroxymethylropivacaine) have been identified (321,323). Unlike metabolism in vivo, in which aromatic hydroxylation predominates, 2,6-pipecoloxylidide is the predominant metabolite in vitro, particularly at higher substrate concentrations (321,323). Kinetic parameters for human liver microsomes are (K_m and V_{max}) 3-hydroxyropivacaine (16 µM, 46 pmol/min/mg), 4-hydroxyropivacaine (393 µM, 105 pmol/min/mg), 2,6-pipecoloxylidide (406 µM, 1,847 pmol/min/mg), and 2-hydroxymethylropivacaine (485 µM, 9 pmol/min/mg), with therapeutic concentrations of 2 to 8 µM. Based on correlations with microsomal protein content and catalytic activity, chemical and immunoinhibition, and activity of cDNA-expressed enzymes, CYP1A2 was identified as the predominant catalyst of 3-hydroxyropivacaine formation, whereas CYP3A4 was the major isoform forming 2,6-pipecoloxylidide, 4-hydroxyropivacaine, and 2-hydroxymethylropivacaine (321,323).

One ropivacaine metabolic interaction has been reported, which confirmed the in vivo role of CYP1A2 and CYP3A4 in ropivacaine metabolism in humans (Fig. 21-15) (322). Coadministration with the CYP1A2 inhibitor fluvoxamine increased plasma ropivacaine concentrations, decreased plasma clearance by 68% (from 0.35 ± 0.11 to 0.11 ± 0.03 L/min), doubled the half-life, decreased urine 3-hydroxyropivacaine excretion from 39% to 13% of the dose, and was accompanied by metabolic switching, with increased 2,6-pipecoloxylidide plasma concentrations and urinary excretion (from 1% to 17% of the dose). Coadministration with the CYP3A4 inhibitor ketoconazole had comparatively minor effects, but still demonstrated the in vivo role for this isoform. Plasma ropivacaine clearance was decreased by 15%, while plasma and urine 2,6-pipecoloxylidide concentrations were substantially reduced.

Ester Local Anesthetics

Ester local anesthetics (see Fig. 21-8) undergo hydrolysis by plasma pseudocholinesterase, red cell esterases, and nonspecific esterases in the liver (217,218). Only small amounts of unchanged drug are eliminated in urine. In vitro hydrolysis rates of ester-type agents are rapid for chloroprocaine and procaine (in vitro half-life less than 1 minute) and somewhat longer for tetracaine. The clinical implication of these rapid clearances is that, if a toxic concentration is attained, the ensuing reaction should be relatively short-lived. If, however, the esterase becomes saturated or substrate inhibited, because of a very high concentration of drug, or if the enzyme is genetically atypical, then toxicity may be prolonged.

Procaine is metabolized by ester hydrolysis to para-aminobenzoate and diethylaminoethanol (324,325). Significant procaine esterase activity is found in washed erythrocytes and this activity is completely inhibited by acetazolamide, but not by sodium fluoride, suggesting

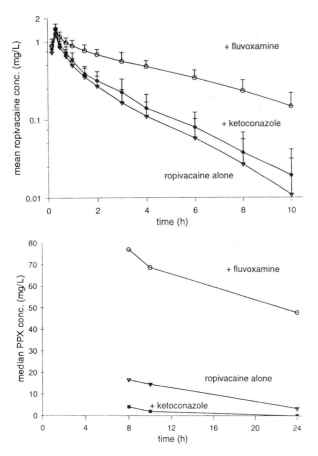

FIG. 21-15. Effect of CYP1A2 or CYP3A4 inhibition on ropivacaine disposition in humans. Subjects were administered either fluvoxamine (25 mg twice daily for 2 days) or ketoconazole (100 mg twice daily for 2 days) before 40 mg ropivacaine (20-minute intravenous infusion) in a crossover study. (Top) Plasma ropivacaine concentrations (mean ± SD). (Bottom) Median plasma (S)-2',6'-pipecoloxylidide (PPX) metabolite concentrations. From Arlander E, Ekström G, Alm C, et al. Metabolism of ropivacaine in humans is mediated by CYP1A2 and to a minor extent by CYP3A4: an interaction study with fluvoxamine and ketoconazole as in vivo inhibitors. Clin Pharmacol Ther 1998;64:484–491, with permission.

that erythrocyte carbonic anhydrase may be the enzyme involved (325). Diethylaminoethanol is further metabolized by alcohol dehydrogenase to diethylglycine. Hydrolysis products of procaine and 2-chloroprocaine have been measured in human plasma and are thought to be pharmacologically inactive, although the aminobenzoic acids may contribute to the rare allergic reaction (217,218). Most of the chlorobenzoic acid formed from 2-chloroprocaine is further metabolized and excreted as the N-acetyl derivative (326).

Drug interactions with ester local anesthetics are relatively unusual, owing to the ubiquitous nature of esterases. Inhibition of plasma esterases by eserine, ecothiophate, and sodium fluoride impaired procaine hydrolysis in vitro, as did acetazolamide inhibition of red blood cell esterases (325). Ecothiophate inhibition of plasma cholinesterase activity could theoretically impair hydrolysis of other ester-type local anesthetics; however, chloroprocaine was used without incident in a patient using ecothiophate eye drops for several years (327). Chloroprocaine hydrolysis in human serum was inhibited 38% and 21%, respectively, by bupivacaine and etidocaine, whereas mepivacaine, lidocaine, MEGX, and glycinexylidide were inhibitory only at concentrations higher than those occurring clinically (328).

Cocaine

Although cocaine is still used clinically as a local anesthetic, most current interest in cocaine metabolism emanates from its recreational use. The main routes of cocaine biotransformation are (329,330): (a) methyl ester hydrolysis to benzoylecgonine, which occurs both nonenzymatically at neutral pH and catalyzed by hepatic esterases; (b) benzoyl ester hydrolysis catalyzed by serum and hepatic esterases yielding ecgonine methylester, with further hydrolysis of both ecgonine methylester and benzoylecgonine to ecgonine; (c) arylhydroxylation with subsequent methylation, glucuronidation, or sulfation; and (d) N-demethylation to norcocaine, which may undergo an analogous series of hydrolysis steps or further sequential metabolism to N-hydroxynorcocaine, norcocaine nitroxide, and possibly norcocaine nitrosonium ion (329–331). The N-oxidation pathway is thought to mediate the hepatotoxicity of cocaine.

Cocaine hydrolysis to inactive benzoylecgonine (30%–45%), ecgonine methylester (15%–35%), and ecgonine accounts for 90% to 95% of the dose in human urine. Methyl ester hydrolysis to benzoylecgonine is catalyzed regioselectively by carboxylesterase hCE-1 (332–334). Benzoyl ester hydrolysis to ecgonine methylester is catalyzed regioselectively by hepatic carboxylesterase hCE-2 and by plasma cholinesterase (pseudocholinesterase), currently referred to as butyrylcholinesterase (332,335). Drug interactions with cocaine hydrolysis are limited, but have recently been revisited

with the aim of therapeutic intervention. The organophosphate esterase inhibitor diazinon markedly potentiated the hepatotoxicity of cocaine, norcocaine, and norcocaine nitroxide in mice in vivo, presumably by inhibiting hydrolysis to nontoxic metabolites with concomitant metabolic switching toward the N-oxidation pathway (331,336). Hepatic cocaine esterase activity in mice in vivo was substantially (>11-fold) increased by dexamethasone, which may have protected against cocaine and norcocaine hepatotoxicity by increasing hydrolysis, despite more modest increases in P450 activity (see later text) (337). A more unconventional metabolic interaction concerns the use of butyrylcholinesterase itself as a drug (338,339). In rats and cats, administration of human butyrylcholinesterase markedly (>80%) reduced plasma and brain cocaine concentrations and decreased plasma norcocaine concentrations to undetectable levels, with concomitant increase in plasma ecgonine methylester concentrations (338). Butyrylcholinesterase administration also decreased the hypertensive, arrhythmogenic and locomotor hyperactive effects of cocaine and reduced the incidence of seizures and death.

Cocaine is often coabused with ethanol, and numerous interactions, some metabolic, have been observed (330). Ethanol potentiates cocaine hepatotoxicity. In the presence of ethanol, hepatic carboxylesterase hCE-1 also catalyzes the ethyl transesterification of cocaine to cocaethylene, in preference to benzoylecgonine formation by hydrolysis, as well as the transesterification of norcocaine to cocaethylene (332–334). Cocaethylene is pharmacologically active, appears more lethal than cocaine, and also causes hepatotoxicity (332,340). In vitro, ethanol decreased cocaine metabolism to benzoylecgonine by human liver 60,000 g supernatant, and by rat hepatocytes, with concomitant formation of cocaethylene (340,341). In vivo in rats, ethanol diminished cocaine hydrolysis, with two- to three-fold decreases in benzoylecgonine hepatic concentration and plasma AUC, with concomitant increases in cocaine, ecgonine methylester, and norcocaine (341).

Cocaine N-oxidation accounts for approximately 5% to 10% of metabolism, is catalyzed by both flavin monooxygenases and P450, and is the most toxicologically meaningful metabolic pathway (329,330). Norcocaine has significant adrenergic activity (342). In addition, norcocaine and its daughter metabolites are considered to mediate cocaine hepatotoxicity. Human liver microsomes catalyze cocaine N-demethylation (K_m 2.3–2.9 mM), with a predominant role for CYP3A4 identified based on chemical inhibition and the activity of cDNA-expressed CYP3A4, with similar results obtained for mouse liver (337,343,344). In contrast, rat liver CYP2B1, 2B2, and CYP3A all N-demethylated cocaine, whereas expressed human CYP2B6 had no activity (345,346). Subsequent metabolism of norcocaine is less well characterized, in part owing to apparent species differences. Expressed human CYP3A4 did not catalyze norcocaine hydroxylation to N-hydroxynorcocaine (343), and CYP3A enzymes did not appear involved in norcocaine toxification in rat hepatocytes (346), whereas CYP3A did appear to catalyze norcocaine hydroxylation in mouse liver microsomes (337). CYP2Bs did appear to mediate norcocaine toxification in rats (346). Norcocaine nitroxide undergoes further oxidation, catalyzed by P450, with preliminary evidence suggesting a role for CYP2B and 3A isoforms in mouse liver (336). Norcocaine nitroxide can also be reduced, by flavoproteins, back to N-hydroxynorcocaine, with futile redox cycling between these two metabolites (330,336).

Metabolic drug interactions with cocaine N-oxidation have been used to identify relevant enzymes, with concomitant effects on hepatotoxicity. Phenobarbital increased cocaine toxicity in rat hepatocytes, induced mouse liver microsomal cocaine N-demethylation and norcocaine hydroxylation (337), and increased the hepatotoxicity of cocaine, norcocaine, and N-hydroxynorcocaine, but not norcocaine nitroxide in mice in vivo (331,336,337). Chloramphenicol inhibition of CYP2B1/2 activity diminished cocaine N-demethylation and hepatotoxicity in rat liver slices and hepatocytes (346,347). In human liver microsomes, troleandomycin and gestodene inhibited cocaine N-demethylation (343,344). Although ethanol increased cocaine hepatotoxicity, this effect was not mediated by CYP2E1 (348).

REFERENCES

1. Halsey MJ. Drug interactions in anaesthesia. Br J Anaesth 1987;59:112–123.
2. Wood M. Pharmacokinetic drug interactions in anaesthetic practice. Clin Pharmacokinet 1991;21:285–307.
3. Christensen LQ, Bonde J, Kampmann JP. Drug interactions with inhalational anaesthetics. Acta Anaesthesiol Scand 1993;37:231–244.
4. Christensen LQ, Bonde J, Kampmann JP. Drug interactions with intravenous and local anaesthetics. Acta Anaesthesiol Scand 1994;38:15–29.
5. Naguib M, Magboul MMA, Jaroudi R. Clinically significant drug interactions with general anaesthetics—incidence, mechanisms and management. CNS Drugs 1997;8:51–78.
6. Naguib M, Magboul MMA, Samarkandi AH, Attia M. Adverse effects and drug interactions associated with local and regional anaesthesia. Drug Safety 1998;18:221–250.
7. Kharasch ED. Biotransformation of sevoflurane. Anesth Analg 1995;81:S27–S38.
8. Kharasch ED, Hankins DC, Thummel KE. Human kidney methoxyflurane and sevoflurane metabolism: intrarenal fluoride production as a possible mechanism of methoxyflurane nephrotoxicity. Anesthesiology 1995;82:689–699.
9. Ray DC, Drummond GB. Halothane hepatitis. Br J Anaesth 1991;67:84–99.
10. Pohl LR, Kenna JG, Satoh H, Christ DD, Martin JL. Neoantigens associated with halothane-hepatitis. Drug Metab Rev 1989;20:203–217.
11. Gut J, Christen U, Huwyler J. Mechanisms of halothane toxicity: novel insights. Pharmac Ther 1993;58:133–155.
12. Baker MT, Vasquez MT, Chiang C-K. Evidence for the stability and cytochrome P450 specificity of the phenobarbital-induced reductive halothane-cytochrome P450 complex formed in rat hepatic microsomes. Biochem Pharmacol 1991;41:1691–1699.
13. Awad JA, Horn J-L, Roberts J II, Franks JJ. Demonstration of halothane-induced hepatic lipid peroxidation in rats by quantification of F2-isoprostanes. Anesthesiology 1996;84:910–916.

14. Cousins MJ, Gourlay GK, Knights KM, Hall PM, Lunam CA, O'Brien P. A randomized prospective controlled study of the metabolism and hepatotoxicity of halothane in humans. Anesth Analg 1987;66:299–308.
15. Kharasch ED, Hankins D, Mautz D, Thummel KE. Identification of the enzyme responsible for oxidative halothane metabolism: implications for prevention of halothane hepatitis. Lancet 1996;347:1367–1371.
16. Madan A, Parkinson A. Characterization of the NADPH-dependent covalent binding of [^{14}C]halothane to human liver microsomes. A role for cytochrome P4502E1 at low substrate concentrations. Drug Metab Dispos 1996;24:1307–1313.
17. Spracklin D, Hankins DC, Fisher JM, Thummel KE, Kharasch ED. Cytochrome P450 2E1 is the principal catalyst of human oxidative halothane metabolism. J Pharmacol Exp Ther 1997;281:400–411.
18. Kharasch ED, Hankins DC, Fenstamaker K, Cox K. Human halothane metabolism and cytochromes P4502A6 and P4503A4. J Pharmacol Exp Ther 1999 (in press).
19. Spracklin D, Thummel KE, Kharasch ED. Human reductive halothane metabolism in vitro is catalyzed by cytochrome P450 2A6 and 3A4. Drug Metab Dispos 1996;24:976–983.
20. Spracklin D, Kharasch ED. Human halothane reduction in vitro by cytochrome P450 2A6 and 3A4: identification of low and high K_m isoforms. Drug Metab Dispos 1998;26:605–608.
21. Kharasch ED, Thummel K, Mhyre J, Lillibridge J. Single-dose disulfiram inhibition of chlorzoxazone metabolism: a clinical probe for P450 2E1. Clin Pharmacol Ther 1993;53:643–650.
22. Young SR, Stoelting RK, Peterson C, Madura JA. Anesthetic biotransformation and renal function in obese patients during and after methoxyflurane or halothane anesthesia. Anesthesiology 1975;42:451–457.
23. Bentley JB, Vaughan RW, Gandolfi AJ, Cork RC. Halothane biotransformation in obese and nonobese patients. Anesthesiology 1982;57:94–97.
24. Cousins MJ, Plummer JL, Hall PM. Risk factors for halothane hepatitis. Aust N Z J Surg 1989;59:5–14.
25. O'Shea D, Davis SN, Kim RB, Wilkinson GR. Effect of fasting and obesity in humans on the 6-hydroxylation of chlorzoxazone: a putative probe of CYP2E1 activity. Clin Pharmacol Ther 1994;56:359–367.
26. Ray DC, Howie AF, Beckett GJ, Drummond GB. Preoperative cimetidine does not prevent subclinical halothane hepatotoxicity in man. Br J Anaesth 1989;63:531–535.
27. Loesch J, Siegers C-P, Younes M. Influence of cimetidine and diethyldithiocarbamate on the metabolism of halothane and methoxyflurane in vitro. Pharmacol Res Commun 1987;19:395–403.
28. Wood M, Uetrecht J, Phythyon JM, et al. The effect of cimetidine on anesthetic metabolism and toxicity. Anesth Analg 1986;65:481–488.
29. Jenner MA, Plummer JL, Cousins MJ. Halothane reductive metabolism in an adult surgical population. Anaesth Intens Care 1990;18:395–399.
30. Nomura F, Hatano H, Ohnishi K, Akikusa B, Okuda K. Effect of anticonvulsant agents on halothane-induced liver injury in human subjects and experimental animals. Hepatology 1986;6:952–956.
31. Gelman S. General anesthesia and hepatic circulation. Can J Physiol Pharmacol 1987;65:1762–1779.
32. Kanaya N, Nakayama M, Fujita S, Namiki A. Comparison of the effects of sevoflurane, isoflurane and halothane on indocyanine green clearance. Br J Anaesth 1995;74:164–167.
33. Brown BR. The diphasic action of halothane on the oxidative metabolism of drugs by the liver: an in-vitro study in the rat. Anesthesiology 1971;35:241–246.
34. Manno M, Cazzaro S, Rezzadore M. The mechanism of the suicidal reductive inactivation of microsomal cytochrome-P-450 by halothane. Arch Toxicol 1991;65:191–198.
35. Manno M, Ferrara R, Cazzaro S, Rigotti P, Ancona E. Suicidal inactivation of human cytochrome P-450 by carbon tetrachloride and halothane in vitro. Pharmacol Toxicol 1992;70:13–18.
36. Lehmann KA, Weski C, Hunger L, Heinrich C, Daub D. Biotransformation von fentanyl II. Akute arzneimittelinteraktionen—untersuchungen bei ratten und mensch. Anaesthesist 1982;31:221–227.
37. Cockshott ID, Briggs LP, Douglas EJ, White M. The pharmacokinetics of propofol in female patients. Studies using single bolus injections. Br J Anaesth 1987;59:1103–1110.
38. Fish KJ, Rice SA. Halothane inhibits metabolism of enflurane in Fischer 344 rats. Anesthesiology 1983;59:417–420.

39. Tateishi T, Watanabe M, Nakura H, et al. Halothane inhalation inhibits the metabolism of chlorzoxazone, a substrate for CYP2E1, in rabbits. *Anesth Analg* 1997;85:199–203.

40. White PF, Marietta MP, Pudwill CR, Way WL, Trevor AJ. Effects of halothane anesthesia on the biodisposition of ketamine in rats. *J Pharmacol Exp Ther* 1976;196:545–555.

41. White PF, Johnston RR, Pudwill CR. Interaction of ketamine and halothane in rats. *Anesthesiology* 1975;42:179–186.

42. Reilly CS, Wood AJJ, Koshakji RP, Wood M. The effect of halothane on drug disposition: contribution of changes in intrinsic drug metabolizing capacity and hepatic blood flow. *Anesthesiology* 1985;63:70–76.

43. Whelan E, Wood AJJ, Koshakji RP, Shay S, Wood M. Halothane inhibition of propranolol metabolism is stereoselective. *Anesthesiology* 1989;71:561–564.

44. Nakatsu K. Anesthetics and theophylline metabolism. *Anesth Analg* 1985;64:460–462.

45. Boyce JR, Cervenko FW, Wright FJ. Effects of halothane on the pharmacokinetics of lidocaine in digitalis-toxic dogs. *Can Anaesth Soc J* 1978;25:323–328.

46. Chelly JE, Hysing ES, Abernethy DR, Doursout M-F, Merin RG. Effects of inhalational anesthetics on verapamil pharmacokinetics in dogs. *Anesthesiology* 1986;65:266–271.

47. Mather LE, Runciman WB, Ilsley AH, Carapetis RJ, Upton RN. A sheep preparation for studying interactions between blood flow and drug disposition. V: The effects of general and subarachnoid anaesthesia on blood flow and pethidine disposition. *Br J Anaesth* 1986;58:888–896.

48. Merrell WJ, Gordon L, Wood AJ, Shay S, Jackson EK, Wood M. The effect of halothane on morphine disposition: relative contributions of the liver and kidney to morphine glucuronidation in the dog. *Anesthesiology* 1990;72:308–314.

49. Watkins JB III. Exposure of rats to inhalational anesthetics alters the hepatobiliary clearance of cholephilic xenobiotics. *J Pharmacol Exp Ther* 1989;250:421–427.

50. Sear JW, Hand CW, Moore RA, McQuay HJ. Studies on morphine disposition: influence of general anaesthesia on plasma concentrations of morphine and its metabolites. *Br J Anaesth* 1989;62:22–27.

51. Christ DD, Satoh H, Kenna JG, Pohl LR. Potential metabolic basis for enflurane hepatitis and the apparent cross-sensitization between enflurane and halothane. *Drug Metab Dispos* 1988;16:135–140.

52. Martin JL, Plevak DJ, Flannery KD, et al. Hepatotoxicity after desflurane anesthesia. *Anesthesiology* 1995;83:1125–1129.

53. Njoku D, Laster MJ, Gong DH, Eger EI II, Reed GF, Martin JL. Biotransformation of halothane, enflurane, isoflurane, and desflurane to trifluoroacetylated liver proteins: association between protein acylation and hepatic injury. *Anesth Analg* 1997;84:173–178.

54. Mazze RI. Fluorinated anaesthetic nephrotoxicity: an update. *Can Anaesth Soc J* 1984;31:S16–S22.

55. Thummel KE, Kharasch ED, Podoll T, Kunze K. Human liver microsomal enflurane defluorination catalyzed by cytochrome P-450 2E1. *Drug Metab Dispos* 1993;21:350–357.

56. Kharasch ED, Thummel KE. Identification of cytochrome P450 2E1 as the predominant enzyme catalyzing human liver microsomal defluorination of sevoflurane, isoflurane and methoxyflurane. *Anesthesiology* 1993;79:795–807.

57. Zand R, Nelson SD, Slattery JT, et al. Inhibition and induction of cytochrome P4502E1-catalyzed oxidation by isoniazid in humans. *Clin Pharmacol Ther* 1993;54:142–149.

58. O'Shea D, Kim RB, Wilkinson GR. Modulation of CYP2E1 activity by isoniazid in rapid and slow N-acetylators. *Br J Clin Pharmacol* 1997;43:99–103.

59. Mazze RI, Woodruff RE, Heerdt ME. Isoniazid-induced enflurane defluorination in humans. *Anesthesiology* 1982;57:5–8.

60. Gauntlett IS, Koblin DD, Fahey MR, et al. Metabolism of isoflurane in patients receiving isoniazid. *Anesth Analg* 1989;69:245–249.

61. Kharasch ED, Thummel KE, Mautz D, Bosse S. Clinical enflurane metabolism by cytochrome P450 2E1. *Clin Pharmacol Ther* 1994;55:434–440.

62. Kharasch ED, Armstrong AS, Gunn K, Artru A, Cox K. Clinical sevoflurane metabolism and disposition: II. The role of cytochrome P450 2E1 in fluoride and hexafluoroisopropanol formation. *Anesthesiology* 1995;82:1379–1388.

63. Kharasch ED, Hankins DC, Cox K. Clinical isoflurane metabolism by cytochrome P450 2E1. *Anesthesiology* 1999;90:766–771.

64. Wandel C, Neff S, Keppler G, et al. The relationship between cytochrome P4502E1 activity and plasma fluoride levels after sevoflurane anesthesia in humans. *Anesth Analg* 1997;85:924–930.

65. Yoo JSH, Ning SM, Pantuck CB, Pantuck EJ, Yang CS. Regulation of hepatic microsomal cytochrome–P450IIE1 level by dietary lipids and carbohydrates. *J Nutr* 1991;121:959–965.

66. Miller MS, Gandolfi AJ, Vaughan RW, Bentley JB. Disposition of enflurane in obese patients. *J Pharmacol Exp Ther* 1980;215:292–296.

67. Strube PJ, Hulands GH, Halsey MJ. Serum fluoride levels in morbidly obese patients: enflurane compared with isoflurane anesthesia. *Anaesthesia* 1987;42:685–689.

68. Higuchi H, Satoh T, Arimura S, Kanno M, Endoh R. Serum inorganic fluoride levels in mildly obese patients during and after sevoflurane anesthesia. *Anesth Analg* 1993;77:1018–1021.

69. Raucy JL, Lasker JM, Kraner JC, Salazar DE, Lieber CS, Corcoran GB. Induction of cytochrome-P450IIE1 in the obese overfed rat. *Mol Pharmacol* 1991;39:275–280.

70. Yeager MP, Coombs DW, Dodge CP, Maloney LL. Effect of cimetidine on biotransformation of enflurane in man. *Can Anaesth Soc J* 1986;33:466–470.

71. Oikkonen M, Rosenberg PH, Saarnivaara L. Cimetidine and ranitidine do not affect enflurane metabolism in surgical patients. *Acta Anaesthesiol Scand* 1989;33:129–131.

72. Dooley JR, Mazze RI, Rice SA, Borel JD. Is enflurane defluorination inducible in man? *Anesthesiology* 1979;50:213–217.

73. Apfelbaum JL, Zacny JP, Lichtor JL, et al. Phenobarbital and the defluorination of sevoflurane in healthy male volunteers. *Anesthesiology* 1994;81:A364.

74. Mazze RI. Metabolism of the inhaled anaesthetics: implications of enzyme induction. *Br J Anaesth* 1984;56:27S–41S.

75. Rice SA, Talcott RE. Effects of isoniazid treatment on selected hepatic mixed-function oxidases. *Drug Metab Dispos* 1979;7:260–262.

76. Waskell L, Canova-Davis E, Philpot R, Parandoush Z, Chiang JYL. Identification of the enzymes catalyzing metabolism of methoxyflurane. *Drug Metab Dispos* 1986;14:643–648.

77. Cousins MJ, Mazze RI. Methoxyflurane nephrotoxicity: a study of dose response in man. *JAMA* 1973;225:1611–1616.

78. Frink EJ Jr, Morgan SE, Coetzee A, Conzen PF, Brown BR Jr. The effects of sevoflurane, halothane, enflurane, and isoflurane on hepatic blood flow and oxygenation in chronically instrumented greyhound dogs. *Anesthesiology* 1992;76:85–90.

79. Wood M, Wood AJJ. Contrasting effects of halothane, isoflurane, and enflurane on in vivo drug metabolism in the rat. *Anesth Analg* 1984;63:709–714.

80. Reilly CS, Merrell J, Wood AJJ, Koshakji RP, Wood M. Comparison of the effects of isoflurane or fentanyl-nitrous oxide anaesthesia on propranolol disposition in dogs. *Br J Anaesth* 1988;60:791–796.

81. Dundee JW, McIlroy PDA. The history of the barbiturates. *Anaesthesia* 1982;37:726–734.

82. Ghoneim MM, Korttila K. Pharmacokinetics of intravenous anaesthetics: implications for clinical use. *Clin Pharmacokinet* 1977;2:344–372.

83. Whitwam JG. Methohexitone. *Br J Anaesth* 1976;48:617–619.

84. Carroll FI, Smith D, Mark LC, Brand L, Perel JM. Determination of optically active thiopental, thiamylal, and their metabolites in human urine. *Drg Metab Dispos* 1977;5:177.

85. Cordato DJ, Gross AS, Herkes GK, Mather LE. Pharmacokinetics of thiopentone enantiomers following intravenous injection or prolonged infusion of *rac*-thiopentone. *Br J Clin Pharmacol* 1997;43:355–562.

86. Morgan DJ, Blackman GL, Paull JD, Wolf LJ. Pharmacokinetics and plasma binding of thiopental. I: Studies in surgical patients. *Anesthesiology* 1981;54:468–473.

87. Burch PG, Stanski DR. The role of metabolism and protein binding in thiopental anesthesia. *Anesthesiology* 1983;58:146–152.

88. Russo H, Brès J, Duboin M-P, Roquefeuil B. Variability of thiopental clearance in routine critical care patients. *Eur J Clin Pharmacol* 1995;48:479–487.

89. Mark L, Brand L, Kamvyssi S, et al. Thiopental metabolism by human liver *in vivo* and *in vitro*. *Nature* 1965;206:1117–1119.

90. Pandele G, Chaux F, Salvadori C, Farinotti M, Duvaldestin P. Thiopental pharmacokinetics in patients with cirrhosis. *Anesthesiology* 1983;59:123–126.

91. Nguyen KT, Stephens DP, McLeish MJ, Crankshaw DP, Morgan DJ.

Pharmacokinetics of thiopental and pentobarbital enantiomers after intravenous administration of racemic thiopental. *Anesth Analg* 1996; 83:552–558.

92. Hudson RJ, Stanski DR, Burch PG. Pharmacokinetics of methohexital and thiopental in surgical patients. *Anesthesiology* 1983;59: 215–219.

93. Stanski DR, Mihm FG, Rosenthal MH, Kalman SM. Pharmacokinetics of high-dose thiopental used in cerebral resuscitation. *Anesthesiology* 1980;53:169–171.

94. Chan HNJ, Morgan DJ, Crankshaw DP, Boyd MD. Pentobarbitone formation during thiopentone infusion. *Anaesthesia* 1985;40:1155–1159.

95. Couderc E, Ferrier C, Haberer JP, Henzel D, Duvaldestin P. Thiopentone pharmacokinetics in patients with chronic alcoholism. *Br J Anaesth* 1984;56:1393–1397.

96. Swerdlow BN, Holley FO, Maitre PO, Stanski DR. Chronic alcohol intake does not change thiopental anesthetic requirement, pharmacokinetics, or pharmacodynamics. *Anesthesiology* 1990;72:455–461.

97. Novelli GP, Marsili M, Lorenzi P. Influence of liver metabolism on the actions of althesin and thiopentone. *Br J Anaesth* 1975;47:913–916.

98. Reiche R, Frey H-H. Interactions between chloramphenicol and intravenous anesthetics. *Anaesthesist* 1981;30:504–507.

99. Büch U, Altmayer P, Isenberg JC, Büch HP. Increase of thiopental concentration in rat tissues due to anesthesia with isoflurane. *Meth Find Exp Clin Pharmacol* 1991;13:687–691.

100. Büch U, Altmayer P, Isenberg JC, Büch HP. Increase of thiopental concentration in tissues of the rat due to an anesthesia with halothane. *Arzneimittel Forschung* 1991;41:363–366.

101. Bührer M, Mappes A, Lauber R, Stanski DR, Maitre PO. Dexmedetomidine decreases thiopental dose requirement and alters distribution pharmacokinetics. *Anesthesiology* 1994;80:1216–1227.

102. Valerino DM, Vesell ES, Aurori KC, Johnson AO. Effects of various barbiturates on hepatic microsomal enzymes: a comparative study. *Drug Metab Dispos* 1974;2:448–457.

103. Duvaldestin P, Chauvin M, Lebrault C, Bertrand F, Karolak FT, Farinotti R. Effect of upper abdominal surgery and cirrhosis upon the pharmacokinetics of methohexital. *Acta Anaesthesiol Scand* 1991;35: 159–163.

104. Ghoneim MM, Chiang CK, Schoenwald RD, Lilburn JK, Dhanaraj J. The pharmacokinetics of methohexital in young and elderly subjects. *Acta Anaesthesiol Scand* 1985;29:480–482.

105. Murphy PJ. Biotransformation of methohexital. *Int Aneshesiol Clin* 1974;12:139–143.

106. Heusler H, Epping J, Heusler S, Richter E, Vermeulen NPE, Breimer DD. Simultaneous determination of blood concentrations of methohexital and its hydroxy metabolite by gas chromatography and identification of 4'-hydroxymethohexital by combined gas-liquid chromatography-mass spectrometry. *J Chromatogr* 1981;226:403–412.

107. Engelhardt W, Ebert W, Rietbrock I, Richter E. Dosis-wirkungsbeziehung und serumkonzentrationen von methohexital und hydroxymethohexital nach rektaler anaesthesieeinleitung mit 1%iger und 5%iger methohexitösung bei kindern. *Anaesthesist* 1986;35:491–495.

108. Korttila K, Ghoneim MM, Chiang C-K, Nuotto E, Fischer LJ. Metabolites of methohexitone do not contribute to its prolonged action on the central nervous system. *Acta Anaesthesiol Scand* 1990; 34:55–58.

109. Lange H, Stephan H, Brand C, Zielmann S, Sonntag H. Hepatic disposition of methohexitone in patients undergoing coronary bypass surgery. *Br J Anaesth* 1992;69:478–481.

110. Wilkinson GR, Shand DG. A physiologic approach to hepatic drug clearance. *Clin Pharmacol Ther* 1975;18:377–390.

111. van der Graaff M, Vermeulen NP, Breimer DD. Disposition of hexobarbital: 15 years of an intriguing model substrate. *Drug Metab Rev* 1988;19:109–164.

112. Adedoyin A, Prakash C, O'Shea D, Blair A, Wilkinson GR. Stereoselective disposition of hexobarbital and its metabolites: relationship to the S-mephenytoin polymorphism in caucasian and Chinese subjects. *Pharmacogenetics* 1994;4:27–38.

113. Knodell RG, Dubey RK, Wilkinson GR, Guengerich FP. Oxidative metabolism of hexobarbital in human liver: relationship to polymorphic S-mephenytoin 4-hydroxylation. *J Pharmacol Exp Ther* 1988; 245:845–849.

114. Breimer DD, van Rossum JM. Pharmacokinetics of (+)-, (−)- and (±)- hexobarbitone in man after oral administration. *J Pharm Pharmacol* 1973;25:762–764.

115. Chandler MHH, Scott SR, Blouin RA. Age-associated stereoselective alterations in hexobarbital metabolism. *Clin Pharmacol Ther* 1988; 43:436–441.

116. Yasumori T, Murayama N, Yamazoe Y, Kato R. Polymorphism in hydroxylation of mephenytoin and hexobarbital stereoisomers in relation to hepatic P-450 human-2. *Clin Pharmacol Ther* 1990;47: 313–322.

117. Yasumori T, Yamazoe Y, Kato R. Cytochrome P-450 human-2 (P-450IIC9) in mephenytoin hydroxylation polymorphism in human livers: differences in substrate and stereoselectivities among microheterogeneous P-450IIC species expressed in yeasts. *J Biochem* 1991; 109:711–717.

118. Kato R, Yamazoe Y, Yasumori T. Polymorphism in stereoselective hydroxylations of mephenytoin and hexobarbital by Japanese liver samples in relation to cytochrome P-450 human-2 (IIC9). *Xenobiotica* 1992;22:1083–1092.

119. Ryan DE, Thomas PE, Reik LM, Levin W. Purification, characterization and regulation of five rat hepatic microsomal cytochrome P-450 isozymes. *Xenobiotica* 1982;12:727–744.

120. Groen K, Breimer DD. Antipyrine theophylline, and hexobarbital as *in vivo* P450 probe drugs. *Methods Enzymol* 1996;272:169–177.

121. Zilly W, Breimer DD, Richter E. Induction of drug metabolism in man after rifampicin treatment measured by increased hexobarbital and tolbutamide clearance. *Eur J Clin Pharmacol* 1975;9:219–227.

122. Richter E, Breimer DD, Zilly W. Disposition of hexobarbital in intra- and extrahepatic cholestasis in man and the influence of drug metabolism-inducing agents. *Eur J Clin Pharmacol* 1980;17:197–202.

123. Heinemeyer G, Gramm H-J, Simgen W, Dennhardt R, Roots I. Kinetics of hexobarbital and dipyrone in critical care patients receiving high-dose pentobarbital. *Eur J Clin Pharmacol* 1987;32:273–277.

124. Breimer DD, Zilly W, Richter E. Influence of corticosteroid on hexobarbital and tolbutamide disposition. *Clin Pharmacol Ther* 1978;24: 208–212.

125. Koleva MR, Stoychev TS. Effect of nifedipine, verapamil and diltiazem on the enzyme-inducing activity of phenobarbital and beta-naphthoflavone. *Gen Pharmac* 1995;26:225–228.

126. Lin JH, Cocchetto DM, Yeh KC, Duggan DE. Comparative effects of H₂-receptor antagonists on drug interaction in rats. *Drug Metab Dispos* 1986;14:649–653.

127. Kim DH, Kim EJ, Han SS, Roh JK, Jeong TC, Park JH. Inhibitory effects of H₂-receptor antagonists on cytochrome P450 in male ICR mice. *Hum Exp Toxicol* 1995;14:623–629.

128. Fuller RW, Perry KW. Comparison of fluoxetine and norfluoxetine enantiomers as inhibitors of hexobarbitone metabolism in mice. *J Pharm Pharmacol* 1992;44:1041–1042.

129. Smith DA, Chandler MHH, Shedlofsky SI, Wedlund PJ, Blouin RA. Age-dependent stereoselective increase in the oral clearance of hexobarbitone isomers caused by rifampicin. *Br J Clin Pharmacol* 1991; 32:735–739.

130. Flockhart DA. Drug interactions and the cytochrome P450 system: The role of cytochrome P450 2C19. *Clin Pharmacokinet* 1995;29:45–52.

131. Groen K, Breimer DD, Jansen EJ, Van Bezooijen CFA. The influence of aging on the metabolism of simultaneously administered hexobarbital enantiomers and antipyrine before and after phenobarbital induction in male rats: a longitudinal study. *J Pharmacol Exp Ther* 1994; 268:531–536.

132. Sebel PS, Lowdon JD. Propofol: a new intravenous anesthetic. *Anesthesiology* 1989;71:260–277.

133. Shafer SL. Advances in propofol pharmacokinetics and pharmacodynamics. *J Clin Anesth* 1993;5[Suppl 1]:14S–21S.

134. White PF. Propofol: pharmacokinetics and pharmacodynamics. *Semin Anesth* 1988;7[Suppl 1]:4–20.

135. Bryson HM, Fulton BR, Faulds D. Propofol. An update of its use in anaesthesia and conscious sedation. *Drugs* 1995;50:513–559.

136. Simons PJ, Cockshott ID, Douglas EJ, Gordon EA, Hopkins K, Rowland M. Disposition in male volunteers of a subanesthetic intravenous dose of an oil in water emulsion of ¹⁴C-propofol. *Xenobiotica* 1988; 18:429–440.

137. Guitton J, Buronfosse T, Desage M, et al. Possible involvement of multiple human cytochrome P450 isoforms in the liver metabolism of propofol. *Br J Anaesth* 1998;80:788–795.

138. Ebner T, Burchell B. Substrate specificities of two stably expressed human liver UDP-glucuronosyltransferases of the UGT1 gene family. *Drug Metab Dispos* 1993;21:50–55.

139. Le Guellec C, Lacarelle B, Villard PH, Point H, Catalin J, Durand A. Glucuronidation of propofol in microsomal fractions from various tissues and species including humans: effect of different drugs. *Anesth Analg* 1995;81:855–861.

140. Baker MT, Chadam MV, Ronnenberg WC. Inhibitory effects of propofol on cytochrome P450 activities in rat hepatic microsomes. *Anesth Analg* 1993;76:817–821.

141. Chen TL, Wang MJ, Huang CH, Liu CC, Ueng TH. Difference between *in vivo* and *in vitro* effects of propofol on defluorination and metabolic activities of hamster hepatic cytochrome P450-dependent mono-oxygenases. *Br J Anaesth* 1995;75:462–466.

142. Chen TL, Ueng TH, Chen SH, Lee PH, Fan SZ, Liu CC. Human cytochrome P450 mono-oxygenase system is suppressed by propofol. *Br J Anaesth* 1995;74:558–562.

143. Yun C-H, Wood M, Wood AJJ, Guengerich FP. Identification of the pharmacogenetic determinants of alfentanil metabolism: cytochrome P450 3A4. *Anesthesiology* 1992;77:467–474.

144. Kharasch ED, Thummel K. Human alfentanil metabolism by cytochrome P450 3A3/4. An explanation for the interindividual variability in alfentanil clearance? *Anesth Analg* 1993;76:1033–1039.

145. Labroo RB, Thummel KE, Kunze KL, Podoll T, Trager WF, Kharasch ED. Catalytic role of cytochrome P4503A4 in multiple pathways of alfentanil metabolism. *Drug Metab Dispos* 1995;23:490–496.

146. Tateishi T, Krivoruk Y, Ueng Y-F, Wood AJJ, Guengerich FP, Wood M. Identification of human liver cytochrome P-450 3A4 as the enzyme responsible for fentanyl and sufentanil N-dealkylation. *Anesth Analg* 1996;82:167–172.

147. Janicki PK, James MFM, Erskine WAR. Propofol inhibits enzymatic degradation of alfentanil and sufentanil by isolated liver microsomes in vitro. *Br J Anaesth* 1992;68:311–312.

148. Kronbach T, Mathys D, Umeno M, Gonzalez FJ, Meyer UA. Oxidation of midazolam and triazolam by human liver cytochrome P450IIIA4. *Mol Pharmacol* 1989;36:89–96.

149. Leung BP, Miller E, Park GR. The effect of propofol on midazolam metabolism in human liver microsome suspension. *Anaesthesia* 1997;52:945–948.

150. Sanderink G-J, Bournique B, Stevens J, Petry M, Martinet M. Involvement of human CYP1A isoenzymes in the metabolism and drug interactions of riluzole *in vitro*. *J Pharmacol Exp Ther* 1997;282: 1465–1472.

151. Vuyk J. Pharmacokinetic and pharmacodynamic interactions between opioids and propofol. *J Clin Anesth* 1997;9:23S–26S.

152. Vuyk J. TCI: supplementation and drug interactions. *Anaethesia* 1998; 53:35–41.

153. Gepts E, Jonckheer K, Maes V, Sonck W, Camu F. Disposition kinetics of propofol during alfentanil anaesthesia. *Anaesthesia* 1988;43 [Suppl]:8–13.

154. Pavlin DJ, Coda B, Shen D, et al. Effects of combining propofol and alfentanil on ventilation, analgesia, sedation, and emesis in human volunteers. *Anesthesiology* 1996;84:23–37.

155. Dixon J, Roberts FL, Tackley RM, Lewis GTR, Connell H, Prys-Roberts C. Study of the possible interaction between fentanyl and propofol using a computer-controlled infusion of propofol. *Br J Anaesth* 1990;64:142–147.

156. Gill SS, Wright EM, Reilly CS. Pharmacokinetic interaction of propofol and fentanyl: single bolus injection study. *Br J Anaesth* 1990;65: 760–765.

157. Mather LE, Selby DG, Runciman WB. Effects of propofol and of thiopentone anaesthesia on the regional kinetics of pethidine in the sheep. *Br J Anaesth* 1990;65:365–372.

158. Perry SM, Whelan E, Shay S, Wood AJJ, Wood M. Effect of i.v. anaesthesia with propofol on drug distribution and metabolism in the dog. *Br J Anaesth* 1991;66:66–72.

159. Schüttler J, Wilms M, Lauven PM, Stoeckel H, Koenig A. Pharmakokinetische untersuchungen über etomidat beim menschen. *Anaethesist* 1980;29:658–661.

160. Arden JR, Holley FO, Stanski DR. Increased sensitivity to etomidate in the elderly: initial distribution versus altered brain response. *Anesthesiology* 1986;65:19–27.

161. Henthorn TK. Pharmacokinetics of intravenous induction agents. In: Bowdle TA, Horita A, Kharasch ED, eds. *The pharmacologic basis of anesthesiology*. New York: Churchill Livingstone, 1994:307–318.

162. Heykants JJP, Meuldermans WEG, Michiels LJM, Lewi PJ, Janssen PAJ. Distribution, metabolism and excretion of etomidate, a short-act-ing hypnotic drug, in the rat. Comparative study of (R)-(+) and (S)-(−) etomidate. *Arch Int Pharmacodyn* 1975;216:113–129.

163. Van Hamme MJ, Ghoneim MM, Ambre JJ. Pharmacokinetics of etomidate, a new intravenous anesthetic. *Anesthesiology* 1978;49: 274–277.

164. Ghoneim MM, Van Hamme MJ. Hydrolysis of etomidate. *Anesthesiology* 1979;30:227–229.

165. Ledingham IM, Watt I. Influence of sedation on mortality in critically ill multiple trauma patients. *Lancet* 1983;1:1270.

166. Ledingham IM, Finlay WEI, Watt I, McKee JI. Etomidate and adrenocortical function. *Lancet* 1983;1:1434.

167. Wagner RL, White PF, Kan PB, Rosenthal MH, Feldman D. Inhibition of adrenal steroidogenesis by the anesthetic etomidate. *N Engl J Med* 1984;310:1415–1421.

168. Fragen RJ, Shanks CA, Molteni A, Avram MJ. Effects of etomidate on hormonal responses to surgical stress. *Anesthesiology* 1984;61: 652–656.

169. de Jong FH, Mallios C, Jansen C, Scheck PAE, Lamberts SWJ. Etomidate suppresses adrenocortical function by inhibition of 11β-hydroxylation. *J Clin Endocrinol Metab* 1984;59:1143–1147.

170. Allolio B, Dörr H, Stuttmann R, Knorr D, Engelhardt D, Winkelmann W. Effect of a single bolus of etomidate upon eight major corticosteroid hormones and plasma ACTH. *Clin Endocrinol* 1985;22: 281–286.

171. Kurokohchi K, Nishioka M, Ichikawa Y. Inhibition mechanism of reconstituted cytochrome P-450scc-linked monooxygenase system by antimycotic reagents and other inhibitors. *J Steroid Biochem Molec Biol* 1992;42:287–292.

172. Weber MM, Lang J, Abedinpour F, Zeilberger K, Adelmann B, Engelhardt D. Different inhibitory effect of etomidate and ketoconazole on the human adrenal steroid biosynthesis. *Clin Invest* 1993;71:933–938.

173. Nagai K, Miyamori I, Takeda R, Suhara K. Effect of ketoconazole, etomidate and other inhibitors of steroidogenesis on cytochrome P-450sccII-catalyzed reactions. *J Steroid Biochem* 1987;28:333–336.

174. Vacca M, Cerrito F, Preziosi P. Effect of etomidate enantiomers on CRH-ACTH and prolactin release. *Arch Int Pharmacodyn Ther* 1983; 263:328–330.

175. Atiba JO, Horai Y, White PF, Trevor AJ, Blaschke TF, Sung M-L. Effect of etomidate on hepatic drug metabolism in humans. *Anesthesiology* 1988;68:920–924.

176. Richter O, Klatte A, Abel J, Freye E, Haag W, Hartung E. Pharmacokinetic data analysis of alfentanil after multiple injections and etomidate-infusion in patients undergoing orthopedic surgery. *Int J Clin Pharm Ther Toxicol* 1985;23:11–15.

177. Horai Y, White PF, Trevor AJ. Effect of etomidate on rabbit liver microsomal drug metabolism *in vitro*. *Drug Metab Dispos* 1985;13: 364–367.

178. Margary J, Rice SA, Fish KJ. Propylene glycol and amidate inhibit enflurane metabolism in Fischer 344 rats. *Anesthesiology* 1986;65: A249.

179. Nelson EB, Egan JM, Abernethy DR. The effect of propylene glycol on antipyrine clearance in humans. *Clin Pharmacol Ther* 1987;41: 571–573.

180. Reich DL, Silvay G. Ketamine: an update on the first twenty-five years of clinical experience. *Can J Anaesth* 1989;36:186–197.

181. White PF. Use of continuous infusion versus intermittent bolus administration of fentanyl or ketamine during outpatient anesthesia. *Anesthesiology* 1983;59:294–300.

182. Kudo T, Kudo M, Ishihara H, Kotani N, Matsuki A. Clinical study on total intravenous anesthesia with droperidol, fentanyl and ketamine— 3. Pharmacokinetics during prolonged continuous ketamine infusion. *Masui* 1991;40:179–183.

183. Mayer M, Ochmann O, Doenicke A, Angster R, Suttmann H. The effect of propofol-ketamine anesthesia on hemodynamics and analgesia in comparison with propofol-fentanyl. *Anaesthesist* 1990;39:609–616.

184. Grant IS, Nimmo WS, Clements JA. Pharmacokinetics and analgesic effects of i.m. and oral ketamine. *Br J Anaesth* 1981;53:805–810.

185. Adams HA, Bauer R, Gebhardt B, Menke W, Baltes-Gotz B. TIVA mit S-(+)-ketamin in der orthopadischen alterschirurgie. Endokrine streβreaktion, kreislauf—und aufwachverhalten. *Anaesthetist* 1994;43: 92–100.

186. White PF, Schüttler J, Shafer A, Stanski DR, Horai Y, Trevor AJ. Comparative pharmacology of the ketamine isomers. *Br J Anaesth* 1985; 57:197–203.

187. Schüttler J, Stanski DR, White PF, et al. Pharmacodynamic modeling of the EEG effects of ketamine and its enantiomers in man. *J Pharmacokinet Biopharm* 1987;15:241–253.

188. Marietta MP, White PF, Pudwill CR, Way WL, Trevor AJ. Biodisposition of ketamine in the rat: self-induction of metabolism. *J Pharmacol Exp Ther* 1976;196:536–544.

189. Wieber J, Gugler R, Hengstmann JH, Dengler HJ. Pharmacokinetics of ketamine in man. *Anaesthesist* 1975;24:260–263.

190. Domino EF, Zsigmond EK, Domino LE, Domino KE, Kothary SP, Domino SE. Plasma levels of ketamine and two of its metabolites in surgical patients using a gas chromatographic mass fragmentographic assay. *Anesth Analg* 1982;61:87–92.

191. White PF, Dworsky WA, Horai Y, Trevor AJ. Comparison of continuous infusion fentanyl or ketamine versus thiopental—determining the mean effective serum concentrations for outpatient surgery. *Anesthesiology* 1983;59:564–569.

192. Little B, Chang T, Chucot L, et al. Study of ketamine as an obstetric anesthetic agent. *Am J Obstet Gynecol* 1972;113:247–260.

193. Chang T, Glazko AJ. A gas chromatographic assay for ketamine in human plasma. *Anesthesiology* 1972;36:401–404.

194. Chang T, Glazko AJ. Biotransformation and disposition of ketamine. *Int Anesthesiol Clin* 1974;12:157–177.

195. Adams JD Jr, Baillie TA, Trevor AJ, Castagnoli N Jr. Studies on the biotransformation of ketamine. 1—Identification of metabolites produced in vitro from rat liver microsomal preparations. *Biomed Mass Spectrom* 1981;8:527–538.

196. Woolf TF, Adams JD. Biotransformation of ketamine, (Z)-6-hydroxyketamine, and (E)-6-hydroxyketamine by rat, rabbit, and human liver microsomal preparations. *Xenobiotica* 1987;17:839–847.

197. Idvall J, Aronsen KF, Stenberg P, Paalzow L. Pharmacodynamic and pharmacokinetic interactions between ketamine and diazepam. *Eur J Clin Pharmacol* 1983;24:337–343.

198. Domino EF, Domino SE, Smith RE, et al. Ketamine kinetics in unmedicated and diazepam-premedicated subjects. *Clin Pharmacol Ther* 1984;36:645–653.

199. Pedraz JL, Lanao JM, Dominguez-Gil A. Kinetics of ketamine and its metabolites in rabbits with normal and impaired renal function. *Eur J Drug Metab Pharmacokinet* 1985;10:33–39.

200. Pedraz JL, Lanao JM, Calvo MB, Muriel C, Hernandez-Arbeiza J, Dominguez-Gil A. Pharmacokinetic and clinical evaluation of ketamine administered by i.v. and epidural routes. *Int J Clin Pharmacol Ther Toxicol* 1987;25:77–80.

201. Koppel C, Arndt I, Ibe K. Effects of enzyme induction, renal and cardiac function on ketamine plasma kinetics in patients with ketamine long-term analgosedation. *Eur J Drug Metab Pharmacokinet* 1990;15:259–263.

202. Pedraz JL, Calvo MB, Gascon AR, et al. Pharmacokinetics and distribution of ketamine after extradural administration to dogs. *Br J Anaesth* 1991;67:310–316.

203. Pedraz JL, Lanao JM, Hdez JM, Dominguez-Gil A. The biotransformation kinetics of ketamine "in vitro" in rabbit liver and lung microsome fractions. *Eur J Drug Metab Pharmacokinet* 1986;11:9–16.

204. Cohen ML, Chan S-L, Way WL, Trevor AJ. Distribution in the brain and metabolism of ketamine in the rat after intravenous administration. *Anesthesiology* 1973;39:370–376.

205. Trevor AJ, Woolf TF, Baillie TA, Adams JD, Castagnoli N. Stereoselective metabolism of ketamine enantiomers. In: Kamenka JM, Domino EF, Geneste P, eds. *Phencyclidine and related arylcyclohexylamines: Present and future applications.* Ann Arbor: NPP Books, 1983:279–289.

206. Trevor AJ. Biotransformation of ketamine. In: Domino EF, ed. *Status of ketamine in anesthesiology.* Ann Arbor: NPP Books, 1990:93–100.

207. Kharasch ED, Labroo R. Metabolism of ketamine stereoisomers by human liver microsomes. *Anesthesiology* 1992;77:1201–1207.

208. Kharasch ED, Herrmann S, Labroo R. Ketamine as a probe for medetomidine stereoisomer inhibition of human liver drug metabolism. *Anesthesiology* 1992;77:1208–1214.

209. White PF, Way WL, Trevor AJ. Ketamine—its pharmacology and therapeutic uses. *Anesthesiology* 1982;56:119–136.

210. Lo JN, Cumming JF. Interaction between sedative premedicants and ketamine in man and in isolated perfused rat livers. *Anesthesiology* 1975;43:307–312.

211. Toft P, Romer U. Comparison of midazolam and diazepam to supplement total intravenous anaesthesia with ketamine for endoscopy. *Can J Anaesth* 1987;34:466–469.

212. Matsuki A, Ishihara H, Kotani N, Takahashi S, Ogasawara E, Kudo T. A clinical study on total intravenous anesthesia with droperidol, fentanyl and ketamine—2. Pharmacokinetics following the end of continuous ketamine infusion. *Masui* 1991;40:61–65.

213. Cohen ML, Trevor AJ. On the cerebral accumulation of ketamine and the relationship between metabolism of the drug and its pharmacological effects. *J Pharmacol Exp Ther* 1974;189:351–358.

214. Marietta MP, Vore ME, Way WL, Trevor AJ. Characterization of ketamine induction of hepatic microsomal drug metabolism. *Biochem Pharmacol* 1977;26:2451–2453.

215. Kammerer RC, Schmitz DA, Hwa JJ, Cho AK. Induction of phencyclidine metabolism by phencyclidine, ketamine, ethanol, phenobarbital and isosafrole. *Biochem Pharmacol* 1984;33:599–604.

216. Geisslinger G, Menzel-Soglowek S, Kamp H-D, Brune K. Stereoselective high-performance liquid chromatographic determination of the enantiomers of ketamine and norketamine in plasma. *J Chromatogr* 1991;568:165–176.

217. Tucker GT, Mather LE. Absorption and disposition of local anesthetics: pharmacokinetics. In: Cousins MJ, Bridenbaugh PO, eds. *Neural blockade in clinical anesthesia and the management of pain.* Philadelphia: Lippincott-Raven, 1980:45–85.

218. Tucker GT, Mather LE. Properties, absorption, and disposition of local anesthetic agents. In: Cousins MJ, Bridenbaugh PO, eds. *Neural blockade in clinical anesthesia and the management of pain.* Philadelphia: Lippincott-Raven, 1998:55–96.

219. Keenaghan JB, Boyes RN. The tissue distribution, metabolism and excretion of lidocaine in rats, guinea pigs, dogs and man. *J Pharmacol Exp Ther* 1972;180:454–463.

220. Boyes RN. A review of the metabolism of amide local anaesthetic agents. *Br J Anaesth* 1975;47:225–230.

221. Parker RJ, Collins JM, Strong JM. Identification of 2,6-xylidine as a major lidocaine metabolite in human liver slices. *Drug Metab Dispos* 1996;24:1167–1173.

222. Collinsworth KA, Strong JM, Atkinson AJ Jr, Winkle RA, Perlroth F, Harrison DC. Pharmacokinetics and metabolism of lidocaine in patients with renal failure. *Clin Pharmacol Ther* 1975;18:59–64.

223. Blumer J, Strong JM, Atkinson AJ Jr. The convulsant potency of lidocaine and its N-dealkylated metabolites. *J Pharmacol Exp Ther* 1973;186:31–36.

224. Burney RG, DiFazio CA, Peach MJ, Petrie KA, Silvester MJ. Antiarrhythmic effects of lidocaine metabolites. *Am Heart J* 1974;88:765–769.

225. Sallie RW, Tredger JM, Williams R. Extrahepatic production of the lignocaine metabolite monoethylglycinexylidide (MEGX). *Biopharm Drug Dispos* 1992;13:555–558.

226. Bargetzi MJ, Aoyama T, Gonzalez FJ, Meyer UA. Lidocaine metabolism in human liver microsomes by cytochrome P450IIIA4. *Clin Pharmacol Ther* 1989;46:521–527.

227. Imaoka S, Enomoto K, Oda Y, et al. Lidocaine metabolism by human cytochrome P-450s purified from hepatic microsomes: comparison of those with rat hepatic cytochrome P-450s. *J Pharmacol Exp Ther* 1990;255:1385–1391.

228. Oda Y, Imaoka S, Nakahira Y, et al. Metabolism of lidocaine by purified rat liver microsomal cytochrome P-450 isozymes. *Biochem Pharmacol* 1989;38:4439–4444.

229. Hanna IH, Roberts ES, Hollenberg PF. Molecular basis for the differences in lidocaine binding and regioselectivity of oxidation by cytochromes P450 2B1 and 2B2. *Biochemistry* 1998;37:311–318.

230. Masubuchi Y, Umeda S, Igarashi S, Fujita S, Narimatsu S, Suzuki T. Participation of the CYP2D subfamily in lidocaine 3-hydroxylation and formation of a reactive metabolite covalently bound to liver microsomal protein in rats. *Biochem Pharmacol* 1993;46:1867–1869.

231. Ohishi N, Imaoka S, Suzuki T, Funae Y. Characterization of two P-450 isozymes placed in the rat CYP2D subfamily. *Biochim Biophys Acta* 1993;1158:227–236.

232. Nakamoto T, Oda Y, Imaoka S, Funae Y, Fujimori M. Effect of phenobarbital on the pharmacokinetics of lidocaine, monoethylglycinexylidide and 3-hydroxylidocaine in the rat: correlation with P450 isoform levels. *Drug Metab Dispos* 1997;25:296–300.

233. Tanaka K, Oda Y, Asada A, Fujimori M, Funae Y. Metabolism of lidocaine by rat pulmonary cytochrome P450. *Biochem Pharmacol* 1994;47:1061–1066.

234. Oellerich M, Raude E, Burdelski M, et al. Monoethylglycinexylidide formation kinetics: a novel approach to assessment of liver function. *J Clin Chem Clin Biochem* 1987;25:845–853.

235. Shiffman ML, Luketic VA, Sanyal AJ, Thompson EB. Use of hepatic lidocaine metabolism to monitor patients with chronic liver disease. *Ther Drug Monit* 1996;18:372–377.

236. Potter JM, Hickman PE, Henderson A, Balderson GA, Lynch SV, Strong RW. The use of the lidocaine-monoethylglycinexylidide test in the liver transplant recipient. *Ther Drug Monit* 1996;18:383–387.

237. Zotz RB, von Schönfeld J, Erhard J, et al. Value of an extended monoethylglycinexylidide formation test and other dynamic liver function tests in liver transplant donors. *Transplantation* 1997;63:538–541.

238. Oellerich M, Burdelski M, Lautz H-U, Schulz M, Schmidt F-W, Herrmann H. Lidocaine metabolite formation as a measure of liver function in patients with cirrhosis. *Ther Drug Monit* 1990;12:219–226.

239. Shiffman ML, Luketic VA, Sanyal AJ, et al. Hepatic lidocaine metabolism and liver histology in patients with chronic hepatitis and cirrhosis. *Hepatology* 1994;19:933–940.

240. Testa R, Campo N, Caglieris S, et al. Lidocaine elimination and monoethylglycinexylidide formation in patients with chronic hepatitis or cirrhosis. *Hepatogastroenterology* 1998;45:154–159.

241. Oellerich M, Burdelski M, Ringe B, et al. Lignocaine metabolite formation as a measure of pre-transplant liver function. *Lancet* 1989;1: 640–642.

242. Dette K, Knoop M, Langrehr JM, et al. Donor MEGX test fails to predict graft functioN after orthotopic liver transplant. *Transplant Proc* 1997;29:376–377.

243. Stenson RE, Constantino RT, Harrison DC. Interrelationships of hepatic blood flow, cardiac output, and blood levels of lidocaine in man. *Circulation* 1971;43:205–211.

244. Vu VT, Chen CP. Effects of *dl*-propranolol on lidocaine disposition in the perfused rat liver. *Drug Metab Dispos* 1982;10:350–355.

245. Sotaniemi EA, Rautio A, Backstrom M, Arvela P, Pelkonen O. CYP3A4 and CYP2A6 activities marked by the metabolism of lignocaine and coumarin in patients with liver and kidney diseases and epileptic patients. *Br J Clin Pharmacol* 1995;39:71–76.

246. Reichel C, Skodra T, Nacke A, Spengler U, Sauerbruch T. The lignocaine metabolite (MEGX) liver function test and P-450 induction in humans. *Br J Clin Pharmacol* 1998;46:535–539.

247. Isohanni MH, Neuvonen PJ, Palkama VJ, Olkkola KT. Effect of erythromycin and itraconazole on the pharmacokinetics of intravenous lignocaine. *Eur J Clin Pharmacol* 1998;54:561–565.

248. Heinonen J, Takki S, Jarho L. Plasma lidocaine levels in patients treated with potential inducers of microsomal enzymes. *Acta Anaesth Scand* 1970;14:89–95.

249. Perucca E, Hedges A, Makki KA, Richens A. A comparative study of antipyrine and lignocaine disposition in normal subjects and in patients treated with enzyme-inducing drugs. *Br J Clin Pharmacol* 1980;10:491–497.

250. Christians U, Kohlhaw K, Esselmann H, et al. The yin and yang of lidocaine and cyclosporine metabolism in liver graft recipients. *Transplant Proc* 1994;26:2827–2828.

251. Li AP, Rasmussen A, Xu L, Kaminski DL. Rifampicin induction of lidocaine metabolism in cultured human hepatocytes. *J Pharmacol Exp Ther* 1995;274:673–677.

252. Li AP, Jurima-Romet M. Applications of primary human hepatocytes in the evaluation of pharmacokinetic drug–drug interactions: evaluation of model drugs terfenadine and rifampin. *Cell Biol Toxicol* 1997;13:365–374.

253. Ohnhaus EE, Locher JT. Liver blood flow and blood volume following chronic phenobarbitone administration. *Eur J Pharmacol* 1975; 31:161–165.

254. McDevitt DG, Nies AS, Wilkinson GR. Influence of phenobarbital on factors responsible for hepatic clearance of indocyanine green in the rat: relative contributions of induction and altered liver blood flow. *Biochem Pharmacol* 1977;26:1247–1250.

255. Branch RA, Shand DG, Wilkinson GR, Nies AS. The reduction of lidocaine clearance by *dl*–propranolol: an example of hemodynamic drug interaction. *J Pharmacol Exp Ther* 1973;184:515–519.

256. Nattel S, Gagne G, Pineau M. The pharmacokinetics of lignocaine and β-adrenoceptor antagonists in patients with acute myocardial infarction. *Clin Pharmacokinet* 1987;13:293–316.

257. Ochs HRl, Carstens G, Greenblatt DJ. Reduction in lidocaine clearance during continuous infusion and by coadministration of propranolol. *N Engl J Med* 1980;303:373–377.

258. Conrad KA, Byers JM, Finley PR, Burnham L. Lidocaine elimination: effects of metoprolol and of propranolol. *Clin Pharmacol Ther* 1983; 33:133–138.

259. Schneck DW, Luderer JR, Davis D, Vary J. Effects of nadolol and propranolol on plasma lidocaine clearance. *Clin Pharmacol Ther* 1984; 36:584–587.

260. Tucker GT, Max NDS, Lennard MS, Al-Asadt S, Bharaj HS, Woods HF. Effects of β-adrenoceptor antagonists on the pharmacokinetics of lignocaine. *Br J Clin Pharmacol* 1984;17:21S–28S.

261. Bax NDS, Tucker GT, Lennard MS, Woods HF. The impairment of lignocaine clearance by propranolol—major contribution from enzyme inhibition. *Br J Clin Pharmac* 1985;19:597–603.

262. Jordö L, Johnsson G, Lundborg P, Regardh CG. Pharmacokinetics of lidocaine in healthy individuals pretreated with multiple doses of metoprolol. *Int J Clin Pharmacol Ther Toxicol* 1984;22:312–315.

263. Miners JO, Wing LM, Lillywhite KJ, Smith KJ. Failure of "therapeutic" doses of beta-adrenoceptor antagonists to alter the disposition of tolbutamide and lignocaine. *Br J Clin Pharmacol* 1984;18:853–860.

264. Bax NDS, Lennard MS, Al-Asady S, Deacon CS, Tucker GT, Woods HF. Inhibition of drug metabolism by β-adrenoceptor antagonists. *Drugs* 1983;25[Suppl 2]:121–126.

265. Ahokas JT, Davies C, Ravenscroft PJ. Comparison of β-adrenoceptor antagonists as modulators of drug metabolism: effect of lipophilicity on microsomal phase I and II reactions. *Br J Clin Pharmac* 1984; 17:103S–105S.

266. Suzuki T, Ishida R, Matsui S, Masubuchi Y, Narimatzu S. Kinetic analysis of mutual metabolic inhibition of lidocaine and propranolol in rat liver microsomes. *Biochem Pharmacol* 1993;45:1528–1530.

267. Fabre G, Julian B, Saint-Aubert B, Joyeux H, Berger Y. Evidence for CYP3A-mediated N-deethylation of amiodarone in human liver microsomal fractions. *Drug Metab Dispos* 1993;21:978–985.

268. Trivier J-M, Libersa C, Belloc C, Lhermitte M. Amiodarone N-deethylation in human liver microsomes: involvement of cytochrome P450 3A enzymes. *Life Sci* 1993;52:91–96.

269. Siegmund JB, Wilson JH, Imhoff TE. Amiodarone interaction with lidocaine. *J Cardiovasc Pharmacol* 1993;21:513–515.

270. Ha HR, Candinas R, Stieger B, Meyer UA, Follath F. Interaction between amiodarone and lidocaine. *J Cardiovasc Pharmacol* 1996;28: 533–539.

271. Nattel S, Talajic M, Beaudoin D, Matthews C, Roy D. Absence of pharmacokinetic interaction between amiodarone and lidocaine. *Am J Cardiol* 1994;73:92–94.

272. Geraets DR, Scott SD, Ballew KA. Toxicity potential of oral lidocaine in a patient receiving mexiletine. *Ann Pharmacother* 1992;26:1380.

273. Broly F, Libersa C, Lhermitte M, Dupuis B. Inhibitory studies of mexiletine and dextromethorphan oxidation in human liver microsomes. *Biochem Pharmacol* 1990;39:1045–1053.

274. Turgeon J, Fiset C, Giguere R, et al. Influence of debrisoquine phenotype and of quinidine on mexiletine disposition in man. *J Pharmacol Exp Ther* 1991;259:789–798.

275. Nishikawa T, Dohi S. Clinical evaluation of clonidine added to lidocaine solution for epidural anesthesia. *Anesthesiology* 1990;73: 853–859.

276. Garty M, Ben-Zvi Z, Hurwitz A. Interaction of clonidine and morphine with lidocaine in mice and rats. *Toxicol Appl Pharmacol* 1989;101:255–260.

277. Mazoit JX, Benhamou D, Veillette Y, Samii K. Clonidine and or adrenaline decrease lignocaine plasma peak concentration after epidural injection. *Br J Clin Pharmacol* 1996;42:242–245.

278. Delwar Hussain M, Tam YK, Gray MR, Coutts RT. Kinetic interactions of lidocaine, diphenhydramine, and verapamil with diltiazem: a study using isolated perfused rat liver. *Drug Metab Dispos* 1994;22: 530–536.

279. Pichard L, Gillet G, Fabre I, et al. Identification of the rabbit and human cytochromes P-450IIIA as the major enzymes involved in the N-demethylation of diltiazem. *Drug Metab Dispos* 1990;18:711–719.

280. Feely J, Wilkinson R, McAllister CB, Wood AJJ. Increased toxicity and reduced clearance of lidocaine by cimetidine. *Ann Intern Med* 1982;96:592–594.

281. Bauer LA, Edwards WAD, Randolph FP, Blouin RA. Cimetidine-induced decrease in lidocaine metabolism. *Am Heart J* 1984;108: 413–415.

282. Wing LM, Miners JO, Birkett DJ, Foenander T, Lillywhite K, Wanwimolruk S. Lidocaine disposition—sex differences and effects of cimetidine. *Clin Pharmacol Ther* 1984;35:695–701.

283. Jackson JE, Bentley JB, Glass SJ, Fukui T, Gandolfi AJ, Plachetka JR. Effects of histamine-2 receptor blockade on lidocaine kinetics. *Clin Pharmacol Ther* 1985;37:544–548.

284. Flynn RJ, Moore J, Collier PS, Howard PJ. Single dose oral H_2-antagonists do not affect plasma lidocaine levels in the parturient. *Acta Anaesthesiol Scand* 1989;33:593–596.

285. Feely J, Guy E. Lack of effect of ranitidine on the disposition of lignocaine. *Br J Clin Pharmac* 1983;15:378–379.

286. Noble DW, Bannister J, Lamont M, Andersson T, Scott DB. The effect of oral omeprazole on the disposition of lignocaine. *Anaesthesia* 1994;49:497–500.

287. Bentley JB, Glass S, Gandolfi AJ. The influence of halothane of lidocaine pharmacokinetics in man. *Anesthesiology* 1983;59:A246.

288. Ngo LY, Tam YK, Coutts RT. Lack of residual effects of diethyl ether, methoxyflurane, and sodium pentobarbital on lidocaine metabolism in a single-pass isolated rat liver perfusion system. *Drug Metab Dispos* 1995;23:525–528.

289. Ujhelyi MR, O'Rangers EA, Fan C, Kluger J, Pharand C, Chow MSS. The pharmacokinetic and pharmacodynamic interaction between propafenone and lidocaine. *Clin Pharmacol Ther* 1993;53:38–48.

290. Garty M, Ben-Zvi Z, Hurwitz A. Opioid effects on lidocaine disposition and toxicity in mice. *J Pharmacol Exp Ther* 1985;234:391–394.

291. Tucker GT, Wiklund L, Berlin-Wahlen A, Mather LE. Hepatic clearance of local anesthetics in man. *J Pharmacokinet Biopharm* 1977;5:111–122.

292. Thomas J, Morgan D, Vine J. Metabolism of etidocaine in man. *Xenobiotica* 1976;6:39–48.

293. Morgan DJ, Smyth MP, Thomas J, Vine J. Cyclic metabolites of etidocaine in humans. *Xenobiotica* 1977;7:365–375.

294. Vine J, Morgan D, Thomas J. The identification of eight hydroxylated metabolites of etidocaine by chemical ionization mass spectrometry. *Xenobiotica* 1978;8:509–513.

295. Åkerman B, Ross S. Stereospecificity of the enzymatic biotransformation of the enantiomers of prilocaine (Citanest). *Acta Pharmacol Toxicol* 1970;28:445–453.

296. Tucker GT, Mather LE, Lennard MS, Gregory A. Plasma concentrations of the stereoisomers of prilocaine after administration of the racemate: impications for toxicity? *Br J Anaesth* 1990;65:333–336.

297. Burm AGL, de Boer AG, van Kleef JW, et al. Pharmacokinetics of lidocaine and bupivacaine and stable isotope labelled analogues: a study in healthy volunteers. *Biopharm Drug Dispos* 1988;9:85–95.

298. Reynolds F. Metabolism and excretion of bupivacaine in man: a comparison with mepivacaine. *Br J Anaesth* 1971;43:33–37.

299. Lindberg RLP, Kanto JH, Pihlajamaki KK. Simultaneous determination of bupivacaine and its two metabolites, desbutyl- and 4'-hydroxy-bupivacaine, in human serum and urine. *J Chromatogr* 1986;383:357–364.

300. Pihlajamaki KK, Lindberg RLP, Jantunen ME. Lack of effect of cimetidine on the pharmacokinetics of bupivacaine in healthy subjects. *Br J Clin Pharmacol* 1988;26:403–406.

301. Rosenberg PH, Pere P, Hekali R, Tuominen M. Plasma concentrations of bupivacaine and two of its metabolites during continuous interscalene brachial plexus block. *Br J Anaesth* 1991;66:25–30.

302. Pere P, Tuominen M, Rosenberg PH. Cumulation of bupivacaine, desbutylbupivacaine and 4-hydroxybupivacaine during and after continuous interscalene brachial plexus block. *Acta Anaesthesiol Scand* 1991;35:647–650.

303. Mather LE, McCall P, McNicol PL. Bupivacaine enantiomer pharmacokinetics after intercostal neural blockade in liver transplantation patients. *Anesth Analg* 1995;80:328–335.

304. Goehl TJ, Davenport JB, Stanley MJ. Distribution, biotransformation and excretion of bupivacaine in the rat and the monkey. *Xenobiotica* 1973;3:761–772.

305. Bowdle TA, Freund PR, Slattery JT. Propranolol reduces bupivacaine clearance. *Anesthesiology* 1987;66:36–38.

306. Pontén J, Biber B, Henriksson B-Å, Jonsteg C. Bupivacaine for intercostal nerve blockade in patients on long-term β-receptor blocking therapy. *Acta Anaesth Scand* 1982;76:70–77.

307. Kuhnert BR, Zuspan KJ, Kuhnert PM, Syracuse CD, Brashear WT, Brown DE. Lack of influence of cimetidine on bupivacaine levels during parturition. *Anesth Analg* 1987;66:986–990.

308. O'Sullivan GM, Smith M, Morgan B, Brighouse D, Reynolds F. H_2 antagonists and bupivacaine clearance. *Anaesthesia* 1988;43:93–95.

309. Flynn RJ, Moore J, Collier PS, McClean E. Does pretreatment with cimetidine and ranitidine affect the disposition of bupivacaine? *Br J Anaesth* 1989;62:87–91.

310. Noble DW, Smith KJ, Dundas CR. Effects of H-2 antagonists on the elimination of bupivacaine. *Br J Anaesth* 1987;59:735–737.

311. Thompson GA, Myers JA, Turner PA, Denson DD, Coyle DE, Ritschel WA. Influence of cimetidine on bupivacaine disposition in rat and monkey. *Drug Metab Dispos* 1984;12:625–630.

312. Brashear WT, Zuspan KJ, Lazebnik N, Kuhnert BR, Mann LI. Effect of ranitidine on bupivacaine disposition. *Anesth Analg* 1991;72:369–376.

313. Giaufre E, Bruguerolle B, Morisson-Lacombe G, Rousset-Rouviere B. The influence of diazepam on the plasma concentrations of bupivacaine and lignocaine after caudal injection of a mixture of the local anaesthetics in children. *Br J Clin Pharmacol* 1988;26:116–118.

314. Bruguerolle B, Attolini L, Lorec AM, Gantenbein M. Kinetics of bupivacaine after clonidine pretreatment in mice. *Can J Anaesth* 1995;42:434–437.

315. Gantenbein M, Attolini L, Bruguerolle B. Kinetics of bupivacaine after nicorandil treatment in mice. *J Pharm Pharmacol* 1996;48:749–752.

316. Vree TB, Beumer EMC, Lagerwerf AJ, Simon MAM, Gielen MJM. Clinical pharmacokinetics of R(+)- and S(-)-mepivacaine after high doses of racemic mepivacaine with epinephrine in the combined psoas compartment/sciatic nerve block. *Anesth Analg* 1992;75:75–80.

317. McClure JH. Ropivacaine. *Br J Anaesth* 1996;76:300–307.

318. Lee A, Fagan D, Lamont M, Tucker GT, Halldin M, Scott DB. Disposition kinetics of ropivacaine in humans. *Anesth Analg* 1989;69:736–738.

319. Erichsen CJ, Sjövall J, Kehlet H, Hedlund C, Arvidsson T. Pharmacokinetics and analgesic effect of ropivacaine during continuous epidural infusion for postoperative pain relief. *Anesthesiology* 1996;84:834–842.

320. Halldin MM, Bredberg E, Angelin B, et al. Metabolism and excretion of ropivacaine in humans. *Drug Metab Dispos* 1996;24:962–968.

321. Ekström G, Gunnarsson U-B. Ropivacaine, a new amide-type local anesthetic agent, is metabolized by cytochromes P450 1A and 3A in human liver microsomes. *Drug Metab Dispos* 1996;24:955–961.

322. Arlander E, Ekström G, Alm C, et al. Metabolism of ropivacaine in humans is mediated by CYP1A2 and to a minor extent by CYP3A4: an interaction study with fluvoxamine and ketoconazole as in vivo inhibitors. *Clin Pharmacol Ther* 1998;64:484–491.

323. Oda Y, Furuichi K, Tanaka K, et al. Metabolism of a new local anesthetic, ropivacaine, by human hepatic cytochrome P450. *Anesthesiology* 1995;82:214–220.

324. Kalow W. Hydrolysis of local anesthetics by human serum cholinesterase. *J Pharmacol Exp Ther* 1952;104:122–134.

325. Calvo R, Carlos R, Erill S. Effects of disease and acetazolamide on procaine hydrolysis by red blood cell enzymes. *Clin Pharmacol Ther* 1980;27:179–183.

326. Krohg K, Jellum E. Urinary metabolites of chloroprocaine studied by combined gas chromatography–mass spectrometry. *Anesthesiology* 1981;54:329–332.

327. Brodsky JB, Campos FA. Chloroprocaine analgesia in a patient receiving echothiophate iodide eye drops. *Anesthesiology* 1978;48:288–289.

328. Lalka D, Vicuna N, Burrow SR, et al. Bupivacaine and other amide local anesthetics inhibit the hydrolysis of chloroprocaine by human serum. *Anesth Analg* 1978;57:534–539.

329. Pasanen M, Pellinen P, Stenbäck F, Juvonen RO, Raunio H, Pelkonen O. The role of CYP enzymes in cocaine-induced liver damage. *Arch Toxicol* 1995;69:287–290.

330. Boelsterli UA, Göldlin C. Biomechanisms of cocaine-induced hepatocyte injury mediated by the formation of reactive metabolites. *Arch Toxicol* 1991;65:351–360.

331. Thompson ML, Shuster L, Shaw K. Cocaine-induced hepatic necrosis in mice—the role of cocaine metabolism. *Biochem Pharmacol* 1979;28:2389–2395.

332. Dean RA, Christian CD, Sample RHB, Bosron WF. Human liver cocaine esterases: ethanol-mediated formation of ethylcocaine. *FASEB J* 1991;5:2735–2739.

333. Brzezinski MR, Abraham TL, Stone CL, Dean RA, Bosron WF. Purification and characterization of a human liver cocaine carboxylesterase that catalyzes the production of benzoylecgonine and the formation of cocaethylene from alcohol and cocaine. *Biochem Pharmacol* 1994;48:1747–1755.

334. Brzezinski MR, Spink BJ, Dean RA, Berkman CE, Cashman JR, Bosron WF. Human liver carboxylesterase hCE-1: binding specificity for cocaine, heroin, and their metabolites and analogs. *Drug Metab Dispos* 1997;25:1089–1096.

335. Pindel EV, Kedishvili NY, Abraham TL, et al. Purification and cloning of a broad substrate specificity human liver carboxylesterase that catalyzes the hydrolysis of cocaine and heroin. *J Biol Chem* 1997; 272:14769–14775.

336. Ndikum-Moffor FM, Schoeb TR, Roberts SM. Liver toxicity from norcocaine nitroxide, an N-oxidative metabolite of cocaine. *J Pharmacol Exp Ther* 1998;284:413–419.

337. Bornheim LM. Effect of cytochrome P450 inducers on cocaine-mediated hepatotoxicity. *Toxicol Appl Pharmacol* 1998;150:158–165.

338. Mattes CE, Lynch TJ, Singh A, et al. Therapeutic use of butyrylcholinesterase for cocaine intoxication. *Toxicol Appl Pharmacol* 1997; 145:372–380.

339. Gorelick DA. Enhancing cocaine metabolism with butyrylcholinesterase as a treatment strategy. *Drug Alcohol Depend* 1997;48:159–165.

340. Figliomeni ML, Abdel-Rahman MS. Role of ethanol exposure on cocaine metabolism in rat hepatocytes. *J Appl Toxicol* 1997;17:105–112.

341. Roberts SM, Harbison RD, James RC. Inhibition by ethanol of the metabolism of cocaine to benzoylecgonine and ecgonine methyl ester in mouse and human liver. *Drug Metab Dispos* 1993;21:537–541.

342. Hawks RL, Kopin IJ, Colburn RW, Thoa NB. Norcocaine: a pharmacologically active metabolite of cocaine found in brain. *Life Sci* 1974;15:2189–2195.

343. LeDuc BW, Sinclair PR, Shuster L, Sinclair JF, Evans JE, Greenblatt DJ. Norcocaine and N-hydroxynorcocaine formation in human liver microsomes: role of cytochrome P-450 3A4. *Pharmacology* 1993;46: 294–300.

344. Pellinen P, Honkakoski P, Stenbäck F, et al. Cocaine N-demethylation and the metabolism-related hepatotoxicity can be prevented by cytochrome P450 3A inhibitors. *Eur J Pharmacol Environ Toxic* 1994; 270:35–43.

345. Boelsterli UA, Lanzotti A, Göldlin C, Oertle M. Identification of cytochrome P-450IIB1 as a cocaine-bioactivating isoform in rat hepatic microsomes and in cultured rat hepatocytes. *Drug Metab Dispos* 1992;20:96–101.

346. Poet TS, McQueen CA, Halpert JR. Participation of cytochromes P4502 and P4503A in cocaine toxicity in rat hepatocytes. *Drug Metab Dispos* 1996;24:74–80.

347. Poet TS, Brendel K, Halpert JR. Inactivation of cytochromes P450 2B protects against cocaine-mediated toxicity in rat liver slices. *Toxicol Appl Pharmacol* 1994;126:26–32.

348. Boelsterli UA, Atanasoski S, Göldlin C. Ethanol-induced enhancement of cocaine bioactivation and irreversible protein binding: evidence against a role of cytochrome P-450IIE1. *Alcohol Clin Exp Res* 1991;15:779–784.

CHAPTER 22

Opioid Analgesics

Evan D. Kharasch

Analgesic opioids include the naturally occurring opiate alkaloids, semisynthetic and synthetic potent opioids, and agonist/antagonist opioids. Opioids and opiates are biotransformed to both active and inactive metabolites, and there are important therapeutic consequences of altered metabolism due either to genetic variability and/or to drug interactions. The synthetic opioids are used parenterally, and numerous other opioids are ingested orally, the latter portending the possibility of intestinal as well as hepatic drug interactions. This chapter reviews metabolic-based drug interactions with opioid analgesics, with a specific focus on those occurring in humans. Pharmacokinetic interactions resulting from altered absorption, distribution, and protein binding are not covered and have been described elsewhere (1).

ALKALOID OPIATES AND SEMISYNTHETIC OPIOIDS

The natural alkaloid and semisynthetic opioids include the plant alkaloids codeine and morphine, the morphinan dextromethorphan, the semisynthetic opioids dihydrocodeine, hydrocodone, oxycodone, and the structurally unrelated synthetic drug tramadol (Fig. 22-1). These drugs are extensively biotransformed by oxidation and conjugation, subject to polymorphic metabolism, susceptible to metabolic drug interactions, and some in particular demonstrate the clinical consequence of such drug interactions.

Dextromethorphan

Dextromethorphan is the nonopioid, nonanalgesic *d*-isomer of *N*-methyl-methoxymorphinan and is used

E.D. Kharasch: Department of Anesthesiology, University of Washington, 1959 NE Pacific Street, Box 356540, Seattle, Washington 98195-6540 and Anesthesiology Service, Puget Sound Veterans Affairs Medical Center, Seattle, Washington 98108

widely as a nonprescription antitussive, where it is approximately half as effective as codeine. There has been considerable basic and clinical research interest in the metabolism of dextromethorphan, because it is an excellent *in vitro* and *in vivo* probe for CYP2D6 activity, as well as that of CYP3A4/5, and is subject to, and an excellent probe for, CYP2D6 polymorphic metabolism.

Dextromethorphan undergoes extensive biotransformation, with less than 2% eliminated unchanged in urine and oral bioavailability only 1% to 2% in extensive metabolizers (2,3). Metabolite concentrations in plasma markedly exceed those of the parent drug, which has a plasma half-life of 1 to 4 hours (3–6). The predominant dextromethorphan metabolites are *O*-demethylated dextrorphan, *N*-demethylated 3-methoxymorphinan, and *N,O*-didemethylated 3-hydroxymorphinan (Fig. 22-2). The latter is thought to arise primarily by *N*-demethylation of dextrorphan (2). Dextrorphan and 3-hydroxymorphinan circulate in plasma and are excreted in urine predominantly as glucuronide and sulfate conjugates (4,5). With conventional (0 to 8 hour) urine collections, in extensive metabolizers, dextrorphan, 3-methoxymorphinan, and 3-hydroxymorphinan accounted for 64% to 74%, 0.2% or less, and 25% to 35% of metabolites excreted, with total recovery averaging 29% to 42% of the dose (7,8). When extended urine collections were performed (72 or 168 hours), these metabolites accounted for 66% to 78%, 0.2% or less, and 21% to 39% of the total recovered, which was 41% to 73% of the dose (2,3,6). Biotransformation *in vivo* is most commonly expressed as the 0- to 8-hour urinary dextromethorphan/dextrorphan metabolic ratio, which is less than 0.3 in extensive metabolizers (9), but also has been expressed as (dextrorphan + 3-hydroxymorphinan)/(3-methoxymorphinan + dextromethorphan) (8). Jones et al. (2) also found a significant correlation between the two metabolic ratios that reflect *O*-demethylation (dextromethorphan/dextrorphan and 3-methoxymorphinan/3-hydroxymor-

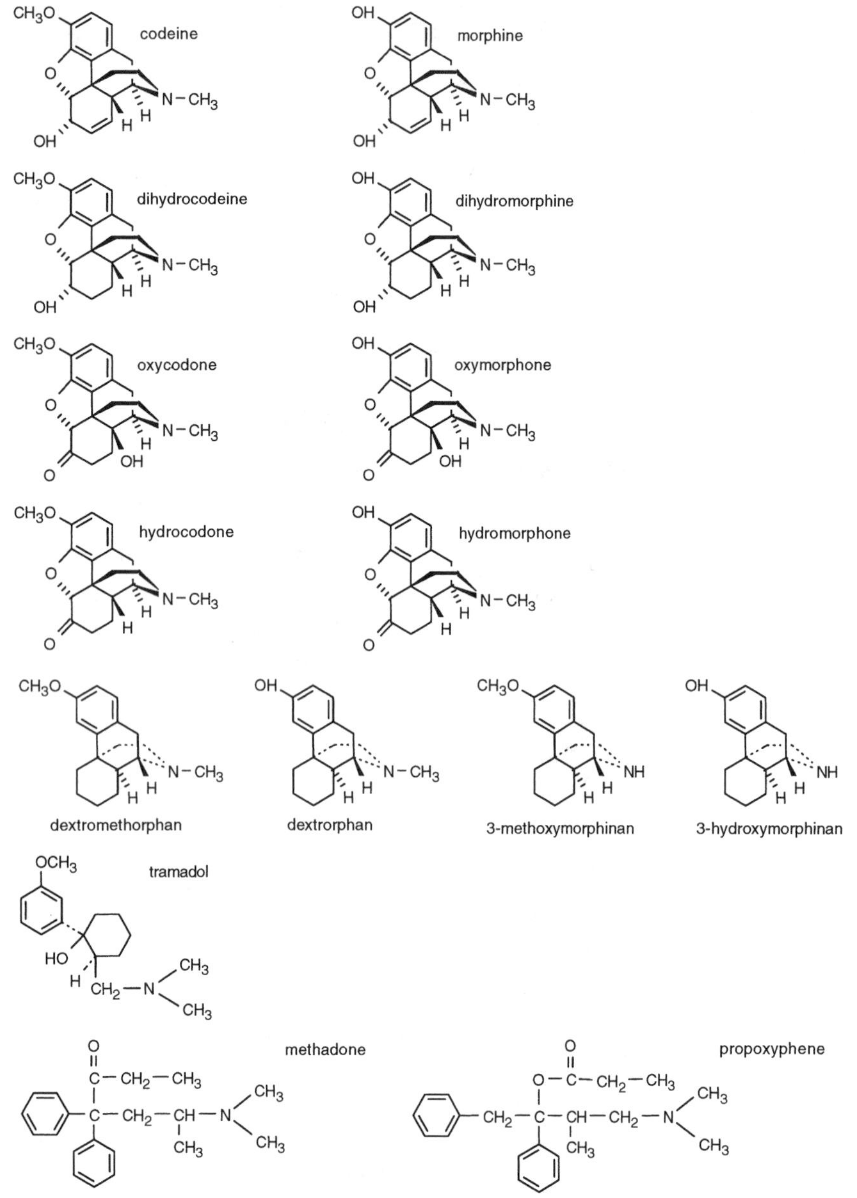

FIG. 22-1. Structures of alkaloid opiates, diphenylpropylamine synthetic opioids, and tramadol.

phinan), and between the dextromethorphan/dextrorphan and dextromethorphan/3-hydroxymorphinan metabolic ratios.

Approximately 5% to 10% of whites are poor metabolizers of dextromethorphan (4,9). In these individuals, approximately 23% of the parent drug was eliminated unchanged in urine, and the oral bioavailability reached 80% (2,3). Mean plasma 0- to 24-hour area under the curve (AUC) values for dextromethorphan, dextrorphan, and 3-hydroxymorphinan were seven-fold higher, 17-fold lower, and 11-fold lower, respectively, in poor metabolizers than in extensive metabolizers, and the urinary dextromethorphan/dextrorphan and dextromethorphan/3-hydroxymorphinan metabolic ratios were 352 and 338 times greater than in extensive metabolizers (4). Similar results also were obtained in subsequent investigations

(2,3,6,7,10). The 0- to 8-hour urinary dextromethorphan/dextrorphan metabolic ratio is greater than 0.3 in poor metabolizers (9). N-Demethylation of dextromethorphan and dextrorphan do not appear significantly different in poor metabolizers, although 3-methoxymorphinan excretion may be increased because further O-demethylation to 3-hydroxymorphinan is impaired (2–7,10,11).

Several investigations have characterized human hepatic microsomal dextromethorphan metabolism *in vitro* (Table 22-1). O-Demethylation of dextromethorphan was biphasic, catalyzed by at least two isoforms in extensive metabolizers, with the high-affinity form (K_m, ~5 μM) accounting for greater than 90% of total activity, based on *in vitro* clearance estimates (7,11–14). In poor metabolizers, dextromethorphan O-demethylation was

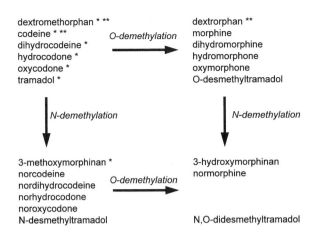

FIG. 22-2. *O*-Demethylation and *N*-demethylation of alkaloid opiates and semisynthetic opioids. Pathways known to be catalyzed by CYP2D6 and CYP3A4 are indicated by * and **, respectively.

monophasic (11,15), with only the low-affinity enzyme (K_m, ~100 μM) active. Based on cosegregation with debrisoquine hydroxylation *in vitro* and *in vivo*, chemical and antibody inhibition experiments, combination genotype/phenotype analysis, and the activity of purified or expressed enzyme, CYP2D6 was identified as the high-affinity dextromethorphan *O*-demethylase (9,11,15–20). The low-affinity dextromethorphan *O*-demethylase has not been identified; however, ketoconazole partially inhibited the reaction in liver microsomes from a poor metabolizer, suggesting that CYP3A4 may participate (21). In contrast to dextromethorphan *O*-demethylation, 3-methoxymorphinan *O*-demethylation to 3-hydroxymorphinan was monophasic in liver microsomes from

both extensive (K_m, 7–10 μM; V_{max}, 120–470 pmol/min/mg) and poor (K_m, 0.2–0.3 mM; V_{max}, 20–72 pmol/min/mg) metabolizers (11). Based on the higher K_m values in poor metabolizers, a strong correlation between dextromethorphan and 3-methoxymorphinan *O*-demethylase activities, chemical and antibody inhibition experiments, CYP2D6 was identified as the 3-methoxymorphinan *O*-demethylase (11). Thus CYP2D6 catalyzes both dextromethorphan *O*-demethylation reactions.

Dextromethorphan *N*-demethylation is a comparatively minor pathway, with *in vitro* clearance estimates 1/100 to 1/5 those for *O*-demethylation (11,14), and *in vivo* *N*-demethylation accounting for 21% to 39% of dextromethorphan metabolites recovered in urine (2,3,6–8). *N*-Demethylation is monophasic *in vitro* (see Table 22-1) (7,11,14,22) and does not cosegregate with *O*-demethylation *in vitro* or *in vivo* (2–7,10). Based on chemical and immunoinhibition experiments and correlation analysis with CYP3A4 protein content and catalytic activity in a bank of human microsomes, as well as the activity of purified or expressed enzyme, CYP3A4 and, to a lesser extent, CYP3A5 were identified as the primary catalysts of dextromethorphan *N*-demethylation (7,14,22). One investigation suggested the participation of a second isoform with similar K_m (14), although this is not supported by other studies (22).

Consistent with CYP2D6-catalyzed *O*-demethylation and CYP3A4/5-catalyzed *N*-demethylation, numerous drug interactions with dextromethorphan have been reported. *In vitro*, the prototypic CYP2D6 inhibitor quinidine was a potent competitive inhibitor of the high-affinity component of *O*-demethylation by microsomal and *expressed CYP2D6 (Table 22-2)* (11,12,14,15,19,21,23). *O*-Demethylation also was inhibited by dihydroquinidine,

TABLE 22-1. *Kinetic constants for human dextromethorphan metabolism*

Enzyme	Dextromethorphan *O*-demethylation				Dextromethorphan *N*-demethylation		Reference
	K_m (μM)	V_{max} (pmol/min/mg)	K_m (μM)	V_{max} (pmol/min/mg)	K_m (mM)	V_{max} (nmol/min/mg)	
EM	5 ± 2 (2–8)	70 ± 58 (18–155)	107 ± 31; (82–150)	85 ± 80 (22–202)			12,13
EM	3 ± 1 (2–5)	170 ± 88 (68–292)					15
EM	7 ± 3	70 ± 50	~74	Not determined	0.4–0.8	0.08–0.15	7
EM	5 ± 4 (2–9)	140 ± 95 (70–230)	133 ± 151 (56–307)	256 ± 58 (200–317)	0.85 ± 0.19 (0.6–1.0)	0.44 ± 0.01 (0.43–0.45)	11
EM	6	98					19
EM	3 ± 2 (1–4)	210 ± 100 (90–280)	196 ± 81 (140–290)	630 ± 120 (510–750)	(0.2–0.3)	6 ± 2 (3–7)	14
EM					(0.5–0.7)	(0.4–0.8)	22
PM			(157–560)	(132–167)	(0.68–0.74)	0.2	11
PM			48	37			15
Yeast CYP2D6	5	8					19

EM, human liver microsomes from extensive metabolizer; PM, human liver microsomes from poor metabolizer; ranges are shown in parentheses.

TABLE 22-2. *Inhibition constants for human hepatic dextromethorphan metabolism*

Enzyme	Inhibitor	Mode	K_i	Reference
O-demethylation to dextrorphan				
HLM	Quinidine	Competitive	25 ± 8 nM (15–39)	12
			15 nM	15
			28 nM	19
			0.1 μM	11
			0.1 ± 0.13 μM	14,23
HLM	Dihydroquinidine	Competitive	13 nM	19
HLM	Paroxetine	Competitive	65 nM	217
HLM	Fluoxetine	Competitive	0.1 ± 0.09 μM	23
			0.17 μM	25
			0.15 μM	217
HLM	SKF-525	Competitive	100 nM	15
HLM	Norfluoxetine	Competitive	0.19 μM	25
HLM	± Perhexiline	Competitive	0.4 μM	11
HLM	Sertraline	Competitive	1.5 μM	25
			1.2 μM	217
HLM	S(+)-Fenfluramine	Competitive	1.8 μM	25
HLM	Ritanserin	Competitive	1.8 μM	25
HLM	Fluvoxamine	Competitive	1.8 μM	25
HLM	± Methadone	Competitive	3–4 μM	8
			86 μM	11
HLM	(–)-Nicardipine	Competitive	3 μM	15
HLM	Dextropropoxyphene	Competitive	6 μM	11
HLM	(+)-Bufuralol	Competitive	8 μM	15
HLM	Trazodone	Competitive	9 μM	25
HLM	3-Methoxymorphinan	Competitive	15 μM	11
HLM	Mexiletine	Competitive	18 μM	13
HLM	Venlafaxine	Competitive	20 μM	217
HLM	Debrisoquine	Competitive	25 μM	15
HLM	Nefazodone	Competitive	26 ± 24 μM	23
HLM	Cimetidine	Competitive	40 μM	15
HLM	Sparteine	Competitive	45 μM	15
HLM	Ketanserin	Competitive	220 μM	25
HLM	Codeine	Competitive	230 μM	15
HLM	4-Hydroxydebrisoquine	Competitive	600 μM	24
CYP2D6	Quinidine	Competitive	27 nM	19
CYP2D6	Quinidine	Competitive	70 nM	21
CYP2D6	Dihydroquinidine	Competitive	14 nM	19
CYP2D6	3-Hydroxyquinidine	Competitive	2.3 μM	19
CYP2D6	Quinidine N-oxide	Competitive	0.44 μM	19
CYP2D6	O-Desmethylquinidine	Competitive	1.3 μM	19
CYP2D6	Quinine	Competitive	2.3 μM	19
CYP2D6	Dexmedetomidine	Mixed	0.4 μM	21
N-Demethylation to 3-methoxymorphinan				
HLM	Ketoconazole	Competitive	0.37 ± 0.07 μM	14,23
HLM	Midazolam	Competitive	54 μM	22
HLM	Nefazodone	Competitive	21 ± 1 μM	23
HLM	± Perhexiline	Competitive	65 μM	11
HLM	Dextropropoxyphene	Competitive	193 μM	11

HLM, human liver microsomes; CYP2D6, cDNA-expressed enzyme; ranges are shown in parentheses.

fluoxetine, SKF-525, norfluoxetine, ±perhexiline, sertraline, Σ(+)-fenfluramine, ritanserin, fluvoxamine, ±methadone, (-)-nicardipine, dextropropoxyphene, (+)-bufuralol, trazodone, 3-methoxymorphinan, mexiletine, debrisoquine, nefazodone, cimetidine, sparteine, ketanserin, codeine, 4-hydroxydebrisoquine, 3-hydroxyquinidine, quinidine N-oxide, O-desmethylquinidine, dexmedetomidine, flecainide, thebaine, and quinine (8,11,13,15,19,23–25), whereas other P450 isoform–selective inhibitors such as

phenacetin, tolbutamide, π-nitrophenol, erythromycin, a-naphthoflavone, sulfaphenazole, ketoconazole, and troleandomycin had no significant effect (14,19). N-Demethylation in vitro was competitively inhibited by ketoconazole and midazolam, prototypic CYP3A4/5 inhibitor and alternative substrate, respectively (see Table 22-2) (14,22,23). N-Demethylation also was inhibited by troleandomycin, nefazodone, ±perhexiline, and dextropropoxyphene (14,22,23), whereas other P450 isoform–selective inhibitors such as α-naphthoflavone, furafylline, coumarin, sulfaphenazole, mephenytoin, and quinidine had no significant effect (14,22). Diethyldithiocarbamate was inhibitory in one (14) but not another (22) investigation.

Inhibition of CYP2D6 and CYP3A4 in humans *in vivo* has been used to verify unequivocally the role of these isoforms in dextromethorphan *O*-demethylation and *N*-demethylation and systemic clearance. Quinidine daily for 1 week caused a dose-dependent increase in plasma dextromethorphan concentrations and the urine dextromethorphan metabolic ratio (18). For example, 60 mg dextromethorphan resulted in plasma dextromethorphan concentrations of 12 ± 13 ng/ml and 241 ± 94 before and after 75 mg quinidine, respectively, and 150 mg quinidine daily increased the urine metabolic ratio from 0.015 ± 0.061 to 1.9 ± 1.6, with all but one subject converted to a phenotypically poor metabolizer (metabolic ratio >0.3; Fig. 22-3) (18). Similarly, a single 100-mg oral quinidine dose administered 12 hours before dextromethorphan, or 50 mg, 1 hour before dextromethorphan, increased plasma parent drug concentrations, prolonged the dextromethorphan half-life, diminished plasma dextrorphan and 3-hydroxymorphinan concentrations, diminished urinary dextrorphan excretion, and increased urinary dextromethorphan excretion, with quinidine-treated subjects resembling known poor metabolizers (Fig. 22-4) (3,6). Methadone-treated subjects tended to excrete less dextrorphan and 3-hydroxymorphinan and more dextrorphan and 3-hydroxymorphinan and more dex-

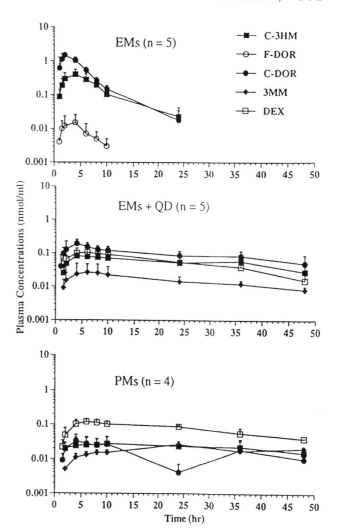

FIG. 22-4. Influence of CYP2D6 activity on dextromethorphan metabolism. Shown are plasma concentrations (mean ± SD) of dextromethorphan (DEX) and metabolites (conjugated 3-hydroxymorphinan (C-3HM), free dextrorphan (F-DOR), conjugated dextrorphan (C-DOR), and 3-methoxymorphinan (3MM)) in five extensive metabolizers (EMs) with and without quinidine (QD; 100 mg) pretreatment, and four poor metabolizers (PMs), after oral dextromethorphan. Reproduced from Schadel M, Wu D, Otton SV, Kalow W, Sellers EM. Pharmacokinetics of dextromethorphan and metabolites in humans: influence of the CYP2D6 phenotype and quinidine inhibition. *J Clin Psychopharmacol* 1995;15: 263–269, with permission.

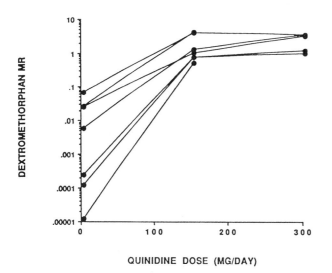

FIG. 22-3. Effect of quinidine on dextromethorphan *O*-demethylation. Shown are the dextromethorphan urinary metabolic ratios (MRs) in seven subjects before and after 1-week quinidine pretreatment. Reproduced from Zhang Y, Britto MR, Valderhaug KL, Wedlund PJ, Smith RA. Dextromethorphan: enhancing its systemic availability by way of low-dose quinidine-mediated inhibition of cytochrome P4502D6. *Clin Pharmacol Ther* 1992;51:647–655, with permission.

tromethorphan, suggesting methadone inhibition of dextromethorphan metabolism and CYP2D6 activity (8). Similar results were obtained after manipulation of CYP3A4 activity. In both extensive and poor (CYP2D6) metabolizers, CYP3A induction with rifampin and CYP3A inhibition with erythromycin (7 days each, in separate experiments) caused an eight-fold decrease, and a threefold increase, respectively, in the 0- to 72-hour (and 0- to 24-hour and 0- to 48-hour) urinary dextromethorphan/3-methoxymorphinan metabolic ratios (Fig. 22-5)

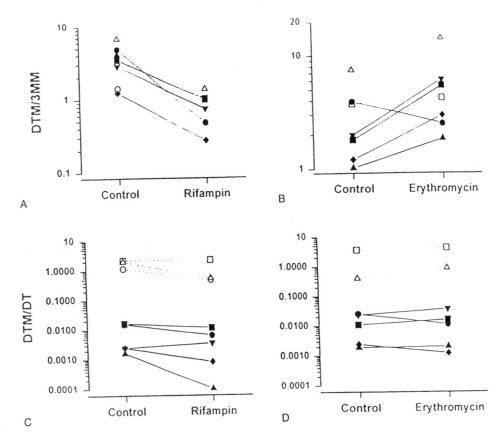

FIG. 22-5. Effects of CYP3A4 induction and inhibition on dextromethorphan metabolism. Shown are the dextromethorphan/3-methoxymorphinan (DTM/3MM) and dextromethorphan/dextrorphan (DTM/DT) 0-to 72-hour metabolic ratios (MRs) in extensive metabolizers (solid symbols) and poor metabolizers (open symbols) of CYP2D6. **A:** Effect of rifampin on the DTM/3MM MR. **B:** Effect of erythromycin on the DTM/3MM MR. **C:** Effect of rifampin on the DTM/DT MR. **D:** Effect of erythromycin on the DTM/DT MR. Reproduced from Jones DR, Gorski JC, Haehner BD, O'Mara EM, Hall SD. Determination of cytochrome P450 3A4/5 activity in vivo with dextromethorphan *N*-demethylation. *Clin Pharmacol Ther* 1996;60:374–384, with permission.

(2). Erythromycin (3 days) also caused a two-fold increase in the dextromethorphan/3-methoxymorphinan metabolic ratio in a 4-hour spot urine, whereas coingestion of grapefruit juice, a known inhibitor of intestinal CYP3A, produced a 15-fold increase in the urine dextromethorphan/3-methoxymorphinan metabolic ratio (10). Rifampin, erythromycin, and grapefruit juice had no effect on the dextromethorphan/dextrorphan metabolic ratios in either investigation, consistent with lack of effect on CYP2D6 activity (2,10). Dextromethorphan *N*-demethylation in humans *in vivo* was positively correlated with *N*-demethylation of both verapamil and tamoxifen, known CYP3A4 substrates, further supporting the role of CYP3A4 in dextromethorphan *N*-demethylation (10). Thus drug interactions both *in vitro* and *in vivo* have been used to identify the human P450 isoforms responsible for dextromethorphan metabolism, and to develop dextromethorphan as an *in vivo* probe for both CYP2D6 and CYP3A4 activities.

Codeine

Codeine (see Fig. 22-1) is a naturally occurring alkaloid opiate, widely used as an antitussive and a mild analgesic. The metabolism and pharmacology of codeine have recently been reviewed (26). Codeine is considered to be a prodrug whose pharmacologic effects are mediated by the minor metabolite morphine (and its glucuronide); thus metabolism is requisite for clinical analgesia. Because codeine, like dextromethorphan, is metabolized by CYP2D6 and CYP3A4/5, codeine disposition is subject to pharmacogenetic variability and drug interactions. Polymorphic metabolism and drug interactions have substantial implications for codeine analgesia and other opioid receptor–mediated effects; thus codeine metabolism and pharmacodynamic consequences have been extensively studied, and offer excellent examples of pharmacokinetic–pharmacodynamic analysis of metabolic interactions.

Codeine undergoes extensive biotransformation, with less than 10% eliminated unchanged in urine in poor, extensive, and ultrarapid CYP2D6 metabolizers, with no difference between groups (26–29). Plasma clearance and half-life after parenteral administration were 12 ± 2 mL/kg/min and 3.3 ± 0.4 hour, respectively, and oral bioavailability averaged 53% (42% to 71%) (30). Intestinal and hepatic first-pass metabolism are the cause of the 40% to 80% bioavailability, because absorption is complete (26). Codeine 6-glucuronidation is the predominant route of metabolism, with metabolite concentrations markedly exceeding those of codeine in plasma (Fig. 22-6), and accounting for 50% to 60% of administered drug recovered in urine (31–38). Other codeine metabolites include O-demethylated morphine and its 3- and 6-glucuronides, N-demethylated norcodeine and norcodeine 6-glucuronide, and N,O-didemethylated normorphine. Typical urinary recoveries in extensive metabolizers are (percentage of the dose) codeine (5–10), codeine 6-glucuronide (55–63), norcodeine (2–3), norcodeine 6-glucuronide (2–4), morphine (0.1–0.8), morphine 3-glucuronide (2–6), morphine 6-glucuronide (0.4–1.4), and normorphine (0.8–2), regardless of whether 8- or 48-hour urine collections were used (31–36). Thus approximately 2% to 8% of the prodrug is converted to the active metabolite, morphine, which is also reflected in morphine plasma and cerebrospinal fluid concentrations, which are approximately 1/50 to 1/20 those of codeine (33,34,37,39–42). Analogous to dextromethorphan, codeine biotransformation in vivo has also been expressed as the various urinary metabolite/codeine metabolic ratios (31,32,37,43). There was a significant correlation between the two metabolic ratios that reflect O-demethylation (codeine/morphine and norcodeine/normorphine), however the correlation between the two N-demethylation metabolic ratios (codeine/norcodeine and morphine/normorphine), was less strong and nonsignificant (37).

Genetic variability in codeine metabolism confers consequent variability in therapeutic efficacy and also serves as an excellent model for drug interactions that diminish codeine O-demethylation. Approximately 5% to 10% of

whites are poor metabolizers (O-demethylation) of codeine and have markedly diminished or absent morphine formation and analgesia (26). Poor metabolizers excrete substantially less morphine (and metabolites) than do extensive metabolizers [0.1% to 0.3% vs. 4% to 8% (28,32,33,36,38,43,44)], and have usually undetectable or markedly diminished plasma concentrations of morphine and its metabolites (see Fig. 22-6) (33,36,38,41,44–46), whereas plasma concentrations and excretion of codeine and codeine glucuronide are unchanged, as are codeine plasma clearance and N-demethylated metabolite formation clearances (28,33, 36,38,44). The urine metabolic ratio for codeine O-demethylation (codeine/morphine + metabolites) was 0.4 to 5.5 and 8.3 to 55.1 in extensive and poor metabolizers, respectively (32). Genetic deficiency in codeine O-demethylation resulting in diminished morphine formation, which may also be considered a model for CYP2D6 interactions resulting in diminished codeine demethylation, resulted in markedly reduced opioid analgesia (sharp pain, cold pressor pain; Fig. 22-7) (45). Other opioid effects, such as respiratory depression, pupillary constriction, psychomotor performance, and possibly gastrointestinal motility, also were significantly diminished in deficient codeine O-demethylators (28,36,38,41,44,46). More recently, individuals have been identified with CYP2D6 gene amplification and/or duplication, conferring ultrarapid debrisoquine metabolism and codeine O-demethylation (29). Ultrarapid codeine metabolizers excreted 15% $\pm$ 9% of the dose as morphine (and glucuronides), compared with 2% to 9% in extensive metabolizers and less than 0.4% in poor metabolizers, whereas N-demethylation was unchanged.

Several investigations have described human hepatic microsomal codeine metabolism in vitro. Dayer et al. (47) reported O-demethylation in extensive (K_m, 149 μM; V_{max}, 293 pmol/min/mg) and poor (K_m, more than 1,000 μM; V_{max}, 27 pmol/min/mg) debrisoquine metabolizers. Codeine N-demethylation exceeds that of O-demethylation, with in vitro clearance estimates approximately seven-fold greater (29). N-Demethylation was monopha-

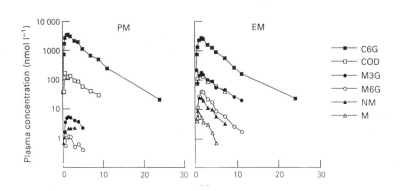

FIG. 22-6. Influence of CYP2D6 activity on codeine disposition. Shown are plasma concentration–time curves of codeine and metabolites (codeine-6-glucuronide, morphine-3-glucuronide, morphine-6-glucuronide, normorphine, and morphine) in a poor metabolizer (PM) and extensive metabolizer (EM) of debrisoquine after oral 50-mg codeine phosphate. (Data for norcodeine and norcodeine glucuronide were excluded for clarity). Reproduced from Yue QY, Hasselström J, Svensson JO, Säwe J. Pharmacokinetics of codeine and its metabolites in Caucasian healthy volunteers: comparisons between extensive and poor hydroxylators of debrisoquine. *Br J Clin Pharmacol* 1991;31:635–642, with permission.

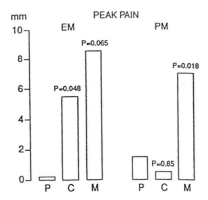

FIG. 22-7. Influence of CYP2D6 activity on codeine analgesia. Shown are the median of the peak changes in peak pain during the cold-pressor test in extensive (EM) and poor (PM) metabolizers of sparteine who received placebo (P), codeine (C), or morphine (M). Plasma codeine concentrations were not different in PMs and EMs; however, morphine and morphine-6-glucuronide were undetectable in plasma of PMs. Reproduced from Poulsen L, Brøsen K, Arendt-Nielsen L, Gram LF, Elbæk K, Sindrup SH. Codeine and morphine in extensive and poor metabolizers of sparteine: pharmacokinetics, analgesic effect and side effects. *Eur J Clin Pharmacol* 1996;51:289–295, with permission.

sic, with K_m and V_{max} averaging 1.3 mM and 1.7 nmol/min/mg in an initial report (48), and 2.0 mM and 3.3 nmol/min/mg in a more recent investigation, which also suggested the possibility of biphasic kinetics (29). CYP2D6 was identified as the codeine O-demethylase in humans, *in vitro* and *in vivo*, based on correlation of metabolism with debrisoquine hydroxylation, dextromethorphan O-demethylation, or immunoreactive CYP2D6 in microsomes *in vitro*, cosegregation with debrisoquine hydroxylation or dextromethorphan O-demethylation *in vivo*, and antibody and chemical inhibition experiments *in vitro* and *in vivo* (32–34,36,41–43, 45,47,49–52). CYP3A was identified as the codeine N-demethylase in humans, based on correlation of metabolism with dextromethorphan N-demethylation, nifedipine oxidation, or immunoreactive CYP3A, and antibody and chemical inhibition in microsomes *in vitro*, and by induction studies *in vivo* (35,44,48,52). Similar experiments support the role of CYP2D1, the rat orthologue of the human enzyme, in rat liver microsomal codeine O-demethylation (53,54). Rat brain can also catalyze codeine O-demethylation, suggesting that morphine formation may occur locally within the central nervous system (55).

Drug interactions can alter codeine O- or N-demethylation, consistent with CYP2D6- and CYP3A-mediated metabolism. *In vitro*, quinidine was a potent competitive inhibitor of human liver microsomal codeine O-demethylation (K_i, 15 nM), as were chlorpromazine (K_i, 0.5 μM), and clomipramine (K_i, 7 μM). Other tricyclic antidepressants were also potent inhibitors, as were methadone, dex-

tropropoxyphene, and metoprolol, whereas diazepam, midazolam, carbamazepine, phenytoin, erythromycin, theophylline, and nonsteroidal antiinflammatory drugs were not (47,52,56). In rat liver microsomes, dextromethorphan (K_i, 3 μM), propafenone (K_i, 0.6 μM), ± methadone (K_i, 0.3 μM), and quinine (K_i, 0.07 μM), were competitive inhibitors of O-demethylation (53,54). Human liver microsomal N-demethylation was inhibited by midazolam, cyclosporine, troleandomycin, erythromycin, gestodene, and ketoconazole, but not by α-naphthoflavone, theophylline, sulfaphenazole, quinidine, metoprolol, or diethyldithiocarbamate (48,52,57). O-Demethylation was more susceptible to inhibition by methadone and dextropropoxyphene than was N-demethylation (52).

In vivo drug interactions in humans, resulting from altered CYP2D6 and CYP3A4 activity, have confirmed the role of these isoforms in codeine biotransformation. Furthermore, altered demethylation caused attendant changes in codeine pharmacologic effects, thereby confirming codeine bioactivation to morphine as a critical determinant of codeine analgesia and other opioid receptor–mediated effects. Quinidine (50–200 mg orally) administered 0.5 to 10 hours before oral codeine markedly inhibited codeine O-demethylation in extensive metabolizers (36,42,50,51). Plasma morphine concentrations were undetectable, or nearly so, after quinidine pretreatment, and urinary recovery of morphine and morphine metabolites was reduced 15-fold. Quinidine decreased partial metabolic clearance by O-demethylation 10-fold, but had no effect on partial metabolic clearance by N-demethylation or glucuronidation (Fig. 22-8A) (36). In contrast, quinidine had no such effect in poor metabolizers, consistent with a deficiency of CYP2D6 to inhibit (36). Quinidine inhibition of morphine formation *in vivo* was associated with diminished codeine analgesia, measured by reduced tolerance to electrical or laser stimulation of the skin (50,51). In addition, in extensive but not poor metabolizers, quinidine significantly diminished codeine-dependent changes in spontaneous respiration, ventilatory response to carbon dioxide, psychomotor performance, and pupillary diameter (see Fig. 22-8B) (36). Perhaps more important, morphine concentrations in cerebrospinal fluid were also profoundly diminished by quinidine (1/15 those of untreated controls), which was interpreted to suggest that quinidine blocked codeine conversion to morphine in the brain (Fig. 22-9) (42). Thus inhibition of CYP2D6 activity diminishes codeine bioactivation and pharmacologic effects.

Drug-interaction studies with codeine and CYP3A4 in humans *in vivo* are limited to CYP3A4 induction. Three weeks of daily carbamazepine treatment before oral codeine in extensive CYP2D6 metabolizers significantly induced N-demethylation, evidenced by a doubling of norcodeine and normorphine urinary excretion, whereas O-demethylation was unchanged (35). Three weeks of daily rifampin treatment before oral codeine also induced

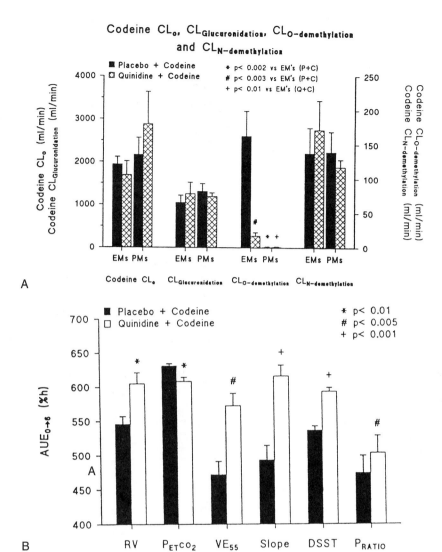

FIG. 22-8. Influence of CYP2D6 activity on codeine metabolism and pharmacologic effects. **A:** Mean (±SEM) codeine (C) clearance (Clo) and the partial metabolic clearances by glucuronidation, *O*-demethylation, and *N*-demethylation after the administration of placebo plus codeine (solid bars) or quinidine plus codeine (hatched bars) to CYP2D6 extensive (EMs) and poor (PMs) metabolizers. **B:** Mean (±SEM) respiratory, psychomotor, and pupillary area under the percentage of baseline effect curve at 0 to 6 hours (AUE$_{0\rightarrow6}$) in the EM subjects after administration of placebo plus codeine (solid bars) or quinidine plus codeine (open bars). RV, resting minute ventilation; P$_{ET}$CO$_2$, resting end-tidal carbon dioxide concentration; VE$_{55}$, minute ventilation at end-tidal CO$_2$, 55 mm Hg; Slope, slope of the CO$_2$–response curve; DSST, digit symbol substitution test; P$_{RATIO}$, pupil-to-iris diameter ratio. Reproduced from Caraco Y, Sheller J, Wood AJ. Pharmacogenetic determination of the effects of codeine and prediction of drug interactions. *J Pharmacol Exp Ther* 1996;278: 1165–1174, with permission.

N-demethylation, increasing norcodeine and norcodeine glucuronide plasma concentrations and causing profound increases in partial metabolic clearance by *N*-demethylation, consistent with known rifampin induction of CYP3A4 (Fig. 22-10A) (44). As expected, CYP2D6 metabolizer status did not influence rifampin induction of CYP3A4-mediated codeine *N*-demethylation, which was 20-fold and 17-fold, respectively, in extensive and poor CYP2D6 metabolizers. Rifampin mildly induces CYP2D6 activity (58), and rifampin also increased codeine partial metabolic clearance by *O*-demethylation by two- to 12-fold in extensive metabolizers (but had no effect in poor metabolizers) (44). However, CYP3A4 induction exceeded that of CYP2D6, metabolic clearance by *N*-demethylation was increased more than that by *O*-demethylation, and plasma concentrations of *O*-demethylated morphine and morphine glucuronides were actually diminished to half their control values by rifampin pretreatment (44). These reductions in active metabolite concentrations were reflected by commensurate decreases in codeine-dependent changes in spontaneous respiration, ventilatory response to carbon dioxide, psychomotor performance, and pupillary diameter (see Fig. 22-10B) (44). Thus despite enhanced rates of codeine *O*-demethylation, rifampin induction actually preferentially shunted codeine metabolism by *N*-demethylation and diminished morphine and morphine glucuronides plasma concentrations and codeine pharmacologic effects. Interestingly therefore, both quinidine and rifampin, albeit through opposite mechanisms (inhibition vs. induction of metabolism), inhibited codeine bioactivation to morphine and reduced its pharmacologic effects (44). Other CYP3A4 modulators might be expected to exert similar effects.

An apparent hormonally based drug interaction with codeine also was described (59). Somatostatin analogues, administered to extensive CYP2D6 metabolizers for 3 days, caused average 44% and 35% decreases in partial metabolic clearance by *N*- and *O*-demethylation, respec-

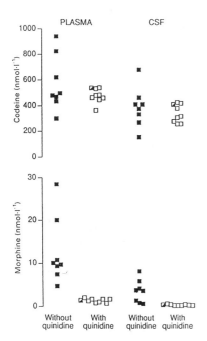

FIG. 22-9. Individual plasma and cerebrospinal fluid (CSF) concentrations of codeine and morphine in 17 patients 2 hours after 125 mg oral codeine without (solid bars) or with (open bars) oral pretreatment with 200 mg quinidine. One patient was a poor metabolizer of sparteine (diagonal half-filled square), and 16 were extensive metabolisers (solid, open). Reproduced from Sindrup SH, Hofmann U, Asmussen J, et al. Impact of quinidine on plasma and cerebrospinal fluid concentrations of codeine and morphine after codeine intake. *Eur J Clin Pharmacol* 1996;49:503–509, with permission.

tively, after intravenous codeine injection, with no effect on codeine glucuronidation. These effects were attributed to somatostatin inhibition of pituitary growth hormone secretion (59).

Codeine interactions with the metabolism of other substrates are rarely reported. Codeine has been shown to inhibit the CYP2D6-mediated metabolism, *in vitro*, of dextromethorphan and sparteine, with K_i values of 230 and 90 μM, respectively (8).

Compared with codeine oxidation, codeine conjugation is less well characterized. As described earlier, 6-glucuronidation is the predominant route of codeine biotransformation. Human liver and kidney microsomal codeine glucuronidation exhibited Michaelis–Menten kinetics, with K_m values for codeine and uridine diphosphoglucuronic acid of 2.2 and 1.4 mM, respectively, in liver, and codeine appeared to be glucuronidated by the same enzyme as was morphine (60). Human UGT2B7 was recently shown to catalyze codeine glucuronidation (K_m, 0.2–1.8 mM), with an efficiency approximately one tenth that of morphine (61,62). In human liver microsomes, morphine, probenecid, and amitriptyline were competitive inhibitors of codeine glucuronidation, with K_i values of 3.6, 1.7, and 0.13 mM, respectively, whereas chloramphenicol and diazepam were noncompetitive inhibitors, with K_i values of 0.27 and 0.18 mM, respectively (60). The clinical effects of these drugs on codeine disposition have not been reported.

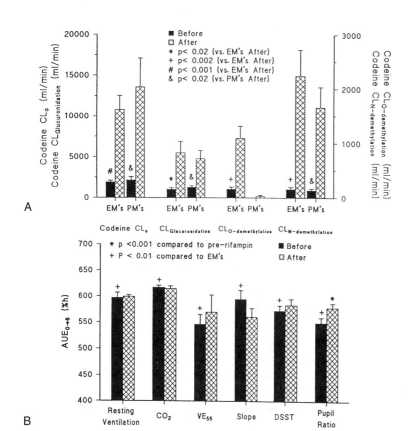

FIG. 22-10. Influence of CYP3A4 activity on codeine metabolism and pharmacologic effects. **A:** Mean (±SEM) codeine clearance and the partial metabolic clearances by glucuronidation, *O*-demethylation, and *N*-demethylation before (solid bars) and after (hatched bars) rifampin in CYP2D6 extensive (EMs) and poor (PMs) metabolizers. **B:** Mean (±SEM) respiratory, psychomotor, and pupillary area under the percentage baseline effect curve (0–6h; $AUE_{0\rightarrow6}$) in the EM subjects before (solid bars) and after (hatched bars) rifampin. $AUE_{0\rightarrow6}$, area under the percentage of baseline effect curve at 0 to 6 hours; CO_2, resting end-tidal carbon dioxide concentration; CO_2 Slope, the slope of the CO_2–response curve; DSST, digit symbol substitution test; Pupil Ratio, the ratio of pupil to iris diameter). Reproduced from Caraco Y, Sheller J, Wood AJJ. Pharmacogenetic determinants of codeine induction by rifampin: the impact on codeine's respiratory, psychomotor and miotic effects. *J Pharmacol Exp Ther* 1997;281:330–336, with permission.

Morphine

Morphine, a naturally occurring alkaloid opiate, is the prototypic μ-receptor opioid and the most widely used analgesic in the world. Morphine undergoes extensive biotransformation, with less than 10% eliminated unchanged in urine (63–67). Plasma clearance and half-life after parenteral administration are typically 9 to 28 ml/kg/min and 1.5 to 3.5 hours, respectively, with variable oral bioavailability (19% to 47%) owing to intestinal and hepatic first-pass metabolism (66,67). Morphine 3-glucuronidation is the predominant route of metabolism, with plasma metabolite concentrations at least an order of magnitude greater those of morphine after oral, intravenous, or other parenteral routes of administration. Morphine 6-glucuronidation is the next most important route of metabolism, with plasma concentrations approximately one-fifth those of morphine 3-glucuronide (66). Approximately 55% and 15% of morphine is metabolized to 3- and 6-glucuronides. In cerebrospinal fluid, however, glucuronide concentrations are substantially less (68). Other minor morphine metabolites include the 3,6-diglucuronide, morphine-3-ethereal sulfate, N-demethylated normorphine, normorphine-3-glucuronide, normorphine-6-glucuronide, and N,O-didemethylated normorphine (63–65).

Morphine glucuronidation is clinically significant, because the metabolites have vastly different pharmacologic effects (67,69,70). Morphine-6-glucuronide binds avidly to the μ-opioid receptor, produces analgesia, respiratory depression, and other classic opioid effects, and is considered to mediate, in part, the pharmacologic effects of morphine. Impaired morphine-6-glucuronide elimination in renal failure can cause signs of overdose (71,72). In contrast, morphine-3-glucuronide has minimal μ-opioid receptor binding, produces no analgesia or other opioid effects, and may antagonize the opioid effects of morphine or morphine-6-glucuronide (67).

Human liver, kidney, and brain microsomes catalyze both morphine 3- and 6-glucuronidation, with the former approximately tenfold greater at saturating substrate concentrations (73–76). Recently human UGT2B7 was shown to catalyze both morphine 3- and 6-glucuronidation, with similar K_m values (0.4–1 mM), although the V_{max} was tenfold greater for morphine 3-glucuronide (61,62).

Some drug interactions with morphine glucuronidation have been identified. Human liver microsomal morphine 3- and 6-glucuronidation was inhibited by the benzodiazepines diazepam, nitrazepam, lorazepam, and oxazepam (73), and by the tricyclic antidepressants clomipramine (competitive or mixed), amitriptyline (competitive or mixed), and nortriptyline (noncompetitive; K_i, 0.090, 0.160, and 0.033 mM, respectively, for 3-glucuronidation, and 0.056, 0.080, and 0.027 mM, respectively, for 6-glucuronidation) (77). Naloxone, which also undergoes 3-glucuronidation, was a competitive inhibitor (K_i, 0.6 mM) of morphine 3-glucuronidation (76). Neither cimetidine nor ranitidine affected morphine glucuronidation by rat liver microsomes in vitro (78). In humans, in vivo, chlorimipramine and, to a lesser extent, amitriptyline, but not nortriptyline, increased plasma concentrations of unconjugated morphine (79), and ranitidine had no apparent effect on morphine glucuronidation (80).

Dihydrocodeine

Dihydrocodeine (see Fig. 22-1) is a semisynthetic codeine analogue, used as a mild analgesic and antitussive. It is extensively metabolized, with low (21%) oral bioavailability, although pharmacokinetic data are limited (81–83). Dihydrocodeine is metabolized by N- and O-demethylation, to nordihydrocodeine, dihydromorphine, and nordihydromorphine, which are excreted as glucuronide and/or sulfate conjugates (see Fig. 22-2). All metabolites are pharmacologically active (84). Urinary recovery (percentage of dose) in normal subjects was dihydrocodeine (31%), dihydrocodeine-6-glucuronide (28%), nordihydrocodeine (including conjugates, 26%), dihydromorphine (less than 1% to 2%), and dihydromorphine conjugates (8%) (82,83). By extrapolation from codeine, dihydrocodeine O-demethylation to dihydromorphine was initially considered to be requisite for pharmacologic effect (83,85). Therefore recent investigations have focused on the O-demethylation pathway.

In human liver microsomes, N-demethylation to nordihydrocodeine was monophasic (K_m, 9,500 μM; V_{max}, 3.9 μmol/min/mg; Cl$_{int}$, 0.48 ml/min/g) and predominated over O-demethylation to dihydromorphine, which was also monophasic (K_m, 980 μM; V_{max}, 0.18 μmol/min/mg; Cl$_{int}$, 0.19 ml/min/g), although two enzymes with similar K_m values were suggested (84). N- and O-demethylation were catalyzed by CYP3A4 and CYP2D6, respectively, identified by using isoform-selective inhibitors and a CYP2D6 poor-metabolizer liver (84). O-Demethylation by CYP2D6 in humans in vivo was established from diminished dihydromorphine plasma concentrations and urinary excretion (1% vs. 9% of the dose) in poor versus extensive metabolizers of sparteine, and a strong correlation between the dihydromorphine and sparteine urinary metabolic ratios (82,83). Not surprisingly, there was no evidence for CYP2D6 participation in in vivo N-demethylation (83).

A few dihydrocodeine drug interactions consistent with metabolism by CYPs 2D6 and 3A4 have been reported. In human liver microsomes from extensive metabolizers, O-demethylation was competitively inhibited by quinidine (K_i, 16 nM) and quinine (K_i, 3.6 μM), and N-demethylation was inhibited by troleandomycin and erythromycin and activated by α-naphthoflavone (84). In humans in vivo, quinidine significantly reduced (three- to five-fold) dihydromorphine formation, based on urine metabolite excretion (82,86,87). Although dihydromorphine was initially speculated to be the active metabolite of dihydrocodeine and necessary for analgesia (83,85), this has not been substantiated. Quinidine premedication did not change dihydrocodeine analgesia in volunteers, measured by increased pain-tolerance thresholds, despite diminishing dihydromorphine formation, suggesting that dihydrocodeine analgesia is independent of dihydromorphine formation (87). This was corroborated in animals, in which intrathecal dihydrocodeine and dihydromorphine were equieffective, and inhibition of O-demethylation by metyrapone or cimetidine failed to diminish dihydrocodeine analgesia. Thus dihydrocodeine O- and N-demethylation will likely be susceptible to typical CYP2D6 and CYP3A drug interactions, although a significant clinical effect on drug efficacy does not seem likely.

Glucuronidation to dihydrocodeine-6-glucuronide is the major route of dihydrocodeine metabolism (82,83). Human liver microsomal dihydrocodeine glucuronidation was recently described and was attributed to uridine diphosphate (UDP)-glucuronosyltransferase isoform UGT2B7 (88). Dihydrocodeine-6-glucuronide formation was potently inhibited by diclofenac (70% inhibition at 50 μM), whereas amitriptyline, oxazepam, naproxen, chloramphenicol, and probenecid were inhibitory at higher (500 μM) concentrations (88). The clinical significance of these effects is unknown, because *in vivo* interactions have not been reported.

Hydrocodone

Hydrocodone is a semisynthetic analgesic and antitussive analogue of codeine, with similar effects. It is metabolized by O-demethylation to hydromorphone, N-demethylation to norhydrocodone, C6-keto reduction to form 6-α-hydrocol and 6-β-hydrocol equally, and hydromorphol formation from O-demethylation of hydrocodol or C6-keto reduction of hydromorphone (89). Urinary recovery in normal subjects was 6% to 14% hydromorphone, 20% norhydrocodone, 14% hydrocol, and approximately 45% hydrocodone (89,90). Hydromorphone (Dilaudid) is a potent analgesic, widely prescribed, and, like hydrocodeine, was initially speculated to be the active hydrocodone metabolite that conferred clinical analgesia (90). Therefore recent investigations have focused on the O-demethylation pathway.

In normal human liver microsomes, O-demethylation to hydromorphone was monophasic (K_m, 300 μM; V_{max}, 50 pmol/min/mg) and catalyzed by CYP2D6, with this identification based on negligible metabolism by a CYP2D6 poor-metabolizer liver and effect of isoform-selective inhibitors (90). CYP2D6 participation in humans *in vivo* was shown by decreased hydromorphone plasma concentrations and urinary excretion (1% vs. 6% of the dose) in poor versus extensive metabolizers of dextromethorphan (90). The only currently reported hydrocodone drug interaction is with quinidine, which was a competitive inhibitor of human liver microsomal O-demethylation *in vitro* (K_i, 15 nM) and reduced hydromorphone plasma concentrations and urinary excretion (1% vs. 6% of the dose) in humans *in vivo* (90,91).

There appears to be no pharmacologic consequence to hydrocodone–CYP2D6 drug interactions, even though O-demethylation to hydromorphone was initially thought to be important. Extensive and poor CYP2D6 metabolizers did not differ in their response to hydrocodone, measured by pupil diameter and subjective effects, nor did quinidine inhibition of hydromorphone formation alter hydrocodone effects (91). Similar absence of effect of CYP2D inhibition was observed in rats (92). Thus although hydrocodone is metabolized to the more active metabolite hydromorphone, the extent of this conversion is small, contributes little to hydrocodone clinical effects, and clinically significant CYP2D6 drug interactions seem unlikely.

Oxycodone

Oxycodone is a semisynthetic codeine analogue, which is a strong analgesic. It is metabolized by O-demethylation to oxymorphone, N-demethylation to noroxycodone, and C6-keto reduction to 6-oxycodol (93). Noroxycodone is the major metabolite, with plasma AUCs similar to those of oxycodone, whereas the AUC for oxymorphone is only 1% to 12% that of oxycodone (93). Oxymorphone is a potent analgesic and was speculated to be the active oxycodone metabolite that conferred analgesia (94). Recent investigations have focused on the O-demethylation pathway.

Human liver microsomal oxycodone O-demethylation to oxymorphone was described by Otton et al. (25), and the role of CYP2D6 established by diminished activity in microsomes from a CYP2D6 poor metabolizer. Oxymorphone formation *in vitro* was inhibited by quinidine [median inhibitory concentration (IC$_{50}$), 50 nM], fluoxetine (IC$_{50}$, 0.7 μM), and norfluoxetine (IC$_{50}$, 0.7 μM) (25). Human *in vivo* oxycodone drug interactions have not been reported. Hydromorphone does not appear to mediate, or significantly contribute to, the analgesic effects of oxycodone, which appears to be the active compound (93,94). Therefore like hydrocodone and unlike the prodrug codeine, there may be no pharmacologic consequence to CYP2D6 drug interactions with oxycodone.

Tramadol

Tramadol (see Fig. 22-1) is a mild analgesic originally marketed in Germany in 1977 and approved for use in the United States nearly two decades later, producing analgesia equivalent to that of codeine with either acetaminophen or aspirin (95,96). Tramadol has two chiral centers, and the clinical preparation is a 1:1 mixture of (+) (1R,2R) and (–) (1S,2S) enantiomers. Tramadol is metabolized (see Fig. 22-2) predominantly to *O*-desmethyltramadol (M1), *N*-desmethyltramadol, and di-*N,O*-desmethyltramadol, which are excreted in urine as the glucuronide and sulfate conjugates (97). Oral bioavailability is about 75%, and the half-lives of parent drug and metabolite M1 (the only active metabolite) are 5 to 6 and 7 to 9 hours, respectively (95,96). Tramadol analgesia is considered to result from both a μ-opioid receptor effect exerted by the metabolite (+)-*O*-desmethyltramadol (which has μ-opioid receptor affinity 200-fold greater than the parent) and inhibition of norepinephrine and serotonin reuptake by both (+) and (−) tramadol (96,98).

Human liver microsomal tramadol metabolism to *O*-desmethyltramadol exhibited monophasic kinetics and was stereoselective, with a two-fold difference [(−) greater than (+)] in V_{max} and similar a K_m (210 μ*M*) for both enantiomers (99). *N*-Demethylation showed opposite stereoselectivity [(+) greater than (−)] and exhibited biphasic kinetics, with higher apparent K_m values for both enzymes (99,100). In human liver microsomes, tramadol *O*-demethylation to M1 is catalyzed by CYP2D6 (99). In humans *in vivo*, *O*-demethylation of both (+) and (−) tramadol is catalyzed by CYP2D6, evidenced by altered disposition in poor metabolizers of sparteine (98,100). *N*-Demethylation is not catalyzed by CYP2D6, although the active isoform has not yet been identified (99).

Relatively few tramadol drug interactions have been reported, in part because analgesia is only partially mediated by biotransformation. Human liver microsomal *O*-demethylation of both tramadol enantiomers was competitively inhibited by quinidine (K_i, 15 n*M*) and propafenone (K_i, 34 n*M*), indicating metabolism by CYP2D6 (99). Quinidine also inhibited tramadol-induced miosis in humans *in vivo*, further indicating CYP2D6-mediated metabolism (101). Although quinidine suppressed tramadol miosis in extensive metabolizers, there was no effect on analgesia (101). Similarly, tramadol analgesia was only somewhat diminished in poor metabolizers (98). These results are consistent with a major nonopioid effect exerted by parent tramadol in the absence of *O*-desmethyltramadol formation. Thus metabolic interactions with CYP2D6 appear unlikely to alter tramadol analgesia significantly. Tramadol metabolism has been reported to be markedly increased by daily carbamazepine (possibly CYP3A-mediated *N*-demethylation), but not affected by cimetidine (95). Tramadol potentiation of warfarin has been reported; however, the mechanism of this interaction is presently unknown (102).

PHENYLPIPERIDINE SYNTHETIC OPIOIDS

The phenylpiperidine synthetic opioids include meperidine (pethidine), fentanyl and its analogues sufentanil and alfentanil, and the newest analogue, remifentanil (Fig. 22-11). All are exclusively administered parenter-

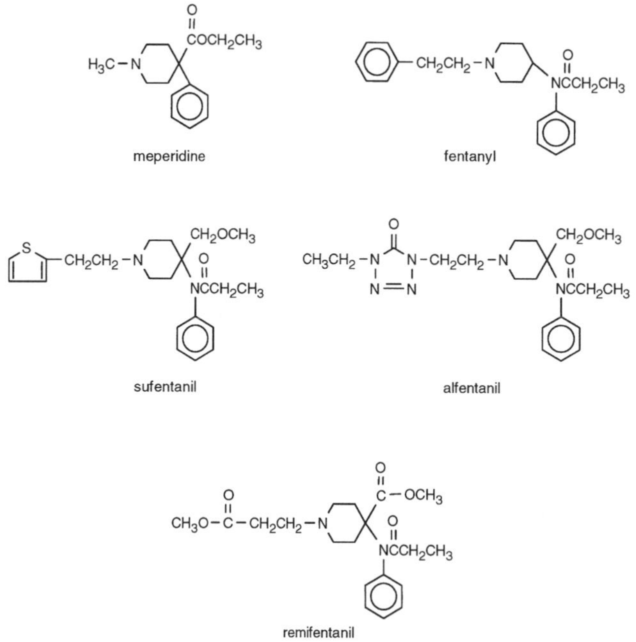

FIG. 22-11. Structures of phenylpiperidine synthetic opioids.

ally, except meperidine, which is also available for oral use. The phenylpiperidines all undergo extensive metabolism to multiple metabolites, with *N*-dealkylation predominant for all.

Meperidine

Meperidine was the first synthetic opioid and is widely used for treating acute and postoperative pain. Plasma clearance averages 12 mL/kg/min; half-life is 3 to 5 hours; oral bioavailability is 56%; and approximately 5% is eliminated unchanged in urine (unless the urine is alkaline, in which case, as much as 25% is excreted unchanged) (103,104).

The primary route of meperidine metabolism is *N*-demethylation to normeperidine (5% to 30% of the dose excreted in urine), and both parent and metabolite also undergo hydrolysis to meperidinic and normeperidinic acid, which are excreted as conjugates (103,105). Other metabolites include *p*-hydroxymeperidine, meperidine-*N*-oxide, hydroxymethoxymeperidine, *N*-hydroxynormeperidine, and *p*-hydroxynormeperidine, although only normeperidine is detected in blood (103,105). Normeperidine is not analgesic, but is a potent excitatory central nervous system toxin, causing nervousness, tremors, multifocal myoclonus, and grand mal seizures (106,107). It is eliminated more slowly (24-hour half-life) than meperidine and accumulates in patients with renal failure, who are more susceptible to (nor)meperidine toxicity (103,106).

Identification of the P450 isoforms responsible for human meperidine metabolism has not been reported.

Drug interactions have, however, been reported. Phenobarbital induction in humans increased meperidine plasma clearance from 1.5 to 1.8 L/min, increased urinary excretion of normeperidine and normeperidinic acid by approximately 50%, and reduced unchanged meperidine excretion, suggesting increased N-demethylation (108). A potential for increased risk of normeperidine toxicity after phenobarbital induction was suggested (108,109). Similarly, phenytoin induction increased systemic clearance from 1.0 to 1.3 L/min and the normeperidine 0- to 24-hour plasma AUC from 380 to 590 ng/h/mL after intravenous meperidine, and decreased bioavailability from 61% to 43% and increased the normeperidine AUC from 590 to 740 ng/h/mL after oral dosing (110). These studies indicate possible involvement of CYP2C and/or 3A isoforms in meperidine N-demethylation. Simultaneous injection of chlorpromazine, although not altering systemic meperidine disposition, did increase urine normeperidine and normeperidinic acid excretion, by an unknown mechanism (111). Cimetidine decreased intravenous meperidine plasma clearance by 22% and normeperidine 0- to 24-hour plasma AUC by 23% in humans, suggesting inhibition of N-demethylation (112), and was a competitive inhibitor of meperidine N-demethylation by human and rat liver microsomes (K_i, 0.45 mM) (78). In contrast, ranitidine had no effect on human meperidine metabolism *in vivo* (meperidine systemic clearance and normeperidine AUC were unchanged) or in human or rat liver microsomes *in vitro* (78,113). A recent investigation in rats suggested that meperidine can alter drug disposition (114). Daily meperidine injection increased hepatic liver microsomal activity of P450s 1A2, 2B1, 2C6, 2C7, 3A, and 4A1 but not 2C11 and 2E1, and increased N-demethylation but not O-demethylation of codeine and ethylmorphine. These effects were attributed to a nonopioid suprapituitary mechanism of action (114), and no human correlates are known. Meperidine does exhibit a very significant interaction with monoamine oxidase inhibitors, which can impair meperidine elimination (115). Nonetheless, the severe central nervous system excitation, which makes concomitant use absolutely contraindicated, has a pharmacodynamic rather than a pharmacokinetic etiology.

Alfentanil

Alfentanil is a relatively short-acting synthetic opioid used for surgical analgesia, introduced after and eliminated more rapidly than fentanyl and sufentanil (see later). It is administered exclusively by intravenous bolus and/or infusion. Alfentanil plasma clearance averages 2 to 5 mL/kg/min; however, there is considerable (10-fold) interindividual variability in clearance (104,116–118). It is a low-extraction drug, but elimination half-life is only 1.5 to 2 hours because of a small volume of distribution (104). Alfentanil is extensively metabolized in humans, with less than 1% of the dose recovered intact in urine (119).

The predominant route of metabolism in humans *in vitro* and *in vivo* is piperidine N-dealkylation to noralfentanil, in which it accounts for one third of the dose recovered in humans (119–122). The second most abundant microsomal metabolite *in vitro* is N-phenylpropionamide, resulting from N-dealkylation at the amide nitrogen (120–122). This metabolite is not found *in vivo,* possibly because of rapid further metabolism, yet isolation of abundant secondary phenolic metabolites (one fourth of the dose) demonstrates the existence and importance of the amide N-dealkylation pathway *in vivo* (119). Minor metabolites include desmethylalfentanil and desmethylnoralfentanil. N-Phenylpropionamide is derived directly from alfentanil, rather than from N-dealkylation of noralfentanil, so there are two primary routes of alfentanil metabolic inactivation (122).

Human liver microsomal alfentanil metabolism, as well as piperidine N-dealkylation to noralfentanil and amide N-dealkylation to N-phenylpropionamide, are catalyzed predominantly by CYP3A4 (122–125). Other hepatic isoforms, including expressed CYP3A5, do not show significant catalytic activity toward alfentanil (122,123,125). Expressed CYP1A1 was reported to catalyze alfentanil metabolism, but this is of unknown clinical significance (125). Kinetic parameters for human liver microsomal alfentanil metabolism were K_m, 23 μM and V_{max}, 3.9 nmol/min/mg (120), and K_m, 31 μM, and V_{max}, 7.6 nmol/min/mg (125). Alfentanil systemic clearance in humans *in vivo* is also highly dependent on CYP3A4 activity, shown by highly significant correlations between alfentanil clearance and CYP3A4 activity, assessed by midazolam clearance (126,127). There was no correlation, however, between alfentanil clearance and the erythromycin breath test (128), perhaps because of the narrow range of clearances measured.

Alfentanil metabolic drug interactions *in vitro* have been assessed by using human liver microsomes (122–125). CYP3A4 inhibitors troleandomycin, ketoconazole, erythromycin, midazolam, erythromycin, gestodene, and benzoflavone significantly inhibited alfentanil disappearance and/or formation of noralfentanil and N-phenylpropionamide.

Pharmacokinetic theory predicts that systemic clearance of alfentanil, a low-extraction drug, is independent of hepatic blood flow but dependent on intrinsic clearance (129). This has been confirmed. Alfentanil clearance was not affected by changes in hepatic blood flow (130,131) but was exquisitely sensitive to changes in CYP3A4 activity and drug interactions (127). Indeed, alfentanil clearance was suggested as an excellent probe for CYP3A4 activity (127). Effects of CYP3A4 induction by rifampin, and inhibition by troleandomycin, on human alfentanil disposition are shown in Fig. 22-12. Interpersonal differ-

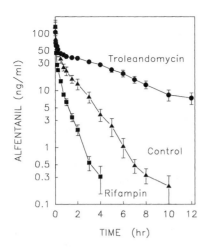

FIG. 22-12. Effect of CYP3A4 activity on alfentanil disposition. Shown are plasma concentrations in subjects receiving nothing (diamonds), rifampin for 5 days (squares), or troleandomycin 3 hours (circles) before a single i.v. alfentanil bolus. Clearance (mean ±SD) in the three groups was 5.3 ± 2.3 mL/kg/min, 14.6 ± 3.8 mL/kg/min, and 1.1 ± 0.5 mL/kg/min. Reproduced from Kharasch ED, Russell M, Mautz D, et al. The role of cytochrome P450 3A4 in alfentanil clearance: implications for interindividual variability in disposition and perioperative drug interactions. *Anesthesiology* 1997;87:36–50, with permission.

ences in CYP3A4 activity, caused by genetic variability and CYP3A4 drug interactions, are thought to underlie the extreme clinical variability in alfentanil disposition (123,124,127). Other clinical drug interactions with CYP3A4 substrates are known. Erythromycin treatment for 7 days, but not a single dose, decreased alfentanil clearance from 3.9 ± 0.8 mL/kg/min to 2.9 ± 1.2 mL/kg/min (132). Pretreatment for 2 days with intravenous cimetidine, but not ranitidine, significantly diminished alfentanil clearance (1.3 ± 0.5 mL/kg/min vs. 3.6 ± 1.2 mL/kg/min) (133). Both oral and intravenous fluconazole, after a single dose, diminished alfentanil plasma clearance (to 1.4 ± 0.4 mL/kg/min and 1.3 ± 0.3 mL/kg/min, respectively, from 3.1 ± 1.1 mL/kg/min), consistent with known fluconazole inhibition of CYP3A4 (134). Infusion of diltiazem, a CYP3A4 substrate, also diminished alfentanil clearance (135). Increased alfentanil plasma concentrations in subjects receiving erythromycin or fluconazole were associated with greater opioid-related respiratory depression (134,136), demonstrating the clinical significance of alfentanil drug interactions. As described earlier, propofol moderately increased plasma alfentanil concentrations, although the mechanism is unknown (137,138). Although midazolam inhibits alfentanil metabolism in human liver microsomes, midazolam premedication did not alter alfentanil systemic clearance *in vivo*, perhaps because concentrations were low (126). In summary, alfentanil clearance, and hence pharmacologic effects, are highly dependent on CYP3A4 activity and

exquisitely susceptible to CYP3A4 drug interactions. Drugs known to alter human CYP3A4 activity will likely influence alfentanil disposition.

Fentanyl

Fentanyl is the most commonly used opioid for surgery. The predominant route of administration is intravenous, although a transdermal patch and a lozenge designed for oral transmucosal absorption (and gastrointestinal absorption of swallowed drug) are available. Fentanyl is a high-extraction drug (ER, 0.9 or more), with plasma clearance averaging 12 mL/kg/min, and elimination half-life, 4 to 8 hours (104,139,140). It is extensively metabolized in humans, with only 2% to 6% excreted unchanged and more than 80% recovered in urine as metabolites. The primary route of human metabolism, *in vivo* and in liver microsomes *in vitro*, is N-dealkylation to norfentanyl (125,140–146). Minor metabolites include hydroxy(propyl)fentanyl, despropionylfentanyl, hydroxy-(propyl)norfentanyl, piperidine ring-hydroxylated fentanyl, and phenoxyethyl fentanyl, but not all studies have found all metabolites (125,141,142,145). Fentanyl metabolites possess no significant pharmacologic activity (147).

Human fentanyl N-dealkylation to norfentanyl is catalyzed predominantly by CYP3A4 in liver microsomes (125,144,145,148). One investigation showed that cDNA-expressed CYP3A5 also catalyzed fentanyl metabolism, with activity equal to that of CYP3A4, as did CYP1A1, although the clinical significance of the latter observation is unknown (125). Evidence for multiple, non-CYP3A P450 isoform involvement in hepatic microsomal fentanyl metabolism was reported in one (125), but not other investigations (145,148). Fentanyl N-dealkylation in human intestinal microsomes also is catalyzed predominantly by CYP3A isoform(s) (145). Kinetic parameters reported for human liver microsomal fentanyl metabolism were K_m, 36 μM, and V_{max}, 3.6 nmol/min/mg (125).

Metabolic drug interactions with fentanyl metabolism by human liver microsomes have been demonstrated *in vitro* (125,144,145,148). CYP3A4 inhibitors troleandomycin, erythromycin, midazolam, gestodene, and ketoconazole markedly decreased norfentanyl formation or fentanyl disappearance. Despite the predominant role of CYP3A in fentanyl metabolism and intrinsic clearance and the extensive clinical use of fentanyl, clinical metabolic drug interactions in humans have not been reported (140). Pharmacokinetic theory predicts that the systemic clearance of fentanyl, a high-extraction drug, is more dependent on hepatic blood flow than on intrinsic clearance (149). This may explain the absence of reported drug interactions. Nevertheless, and in contrast to alfentanil and sufentanil, relationships between P450 3A activity and metabolism and clearance of fentanyl have not been evaluated. One report suggests that changes in CYP3A activity and intrinsic clearance can affect fentanyl disposition (150). Patients receiving the anticonvulsants carbamazepine, carbamazepine and either valproic acid or phenytoin, and carbamazepine, valproic acid, and either phenytoin or primidone had increasing fentanyl requirements during surgery (150). However, a pharmacokinetic analysis was not performed. Because about 75% of fentanyl administered by oral transmucosal lozenge is swallowed (151), significant first pass intestinal metabolism likely occurs, and coadministration of drugs known to affect intestinal P450 3A activity will probably also affect fentanyl lozenge bioavailability. This has not, however, been evaluated.

Sufentanil

Sufentanil is also used for intraoperative anesthesia, with administration predominantly by intravenous injection, although epidural use in labor is not uncommon. Sufentanil is a high extraction drug (ER, 0.7–0.9), with plasma clearance averaging 12 to 18 mL/kg/min, and elimination half-life, 3 to 4 hours (104,152–156). Extrahepatic clearance has been suggested in some investigations (155,157). Because of the high potency of sufentanil (typical doses are 0.2–1 µg/kg) and consequent analytic constraints, scant information is available regarding sufentanil metabolism in humans (152,158,159). In animals, there is extensive metabolism, with little sufentanil excreted unchanged (160). Compared with alfentanil, there is greater biliary and less urinary metabolite excretion (160). The primary route of metabolism, in human liver microsomes, is piperidine N-dealkylation to norsufentanil (structurally identical to noralfentanil), accounting for 40% of metabolites (161). Amide N-dealkylation to N-phenylpropionamide formed 20% of metabolites detected, with O-demethylation to desmethylsufentanil and desmethylnorsufentanil constituting minor pathways (161). In humans, norsufentanil and desmethylsufentanil have been detected in plasma and/or urine *in vivo* (152,158,159).

Human sufentanil metabolism, in liver microsomes, is catalyzed predominantly by CYP3A4 (125,148). Both piperidine and amide N-dealkylation to norsufentanil and N-phenylpropionamide, respectively, were catalyzed predominantly by microsomal and recombinant CYP3A4 (148). Unlike fentanyl, sufentanil was not significantly metabolized by cDNA-expressed CYP3A5 (125). Both investigations suggested involvement of multiple, non-CYP3A P450 isoforms, in hepatic microsomal sufentanil metabolism (125,148). Kinetic parameters reported for human liver microsomal sufentanil metabolism were K_m, 15 and 34 µM, and V_{max}, 6 and 10 nmol/min/mg, in initial (161) and later (125) studies, respectively.

Sufentanil metabolic drug interactions in human liver microsomes have been reported *in vitro* (125,148).

CYP3A4 inhibitors troleandomycin, erythromycin, midazolam, and gestodene diminished norsufentanil formation or sufentanil disappearance. Although CYP3A4 is responsible for sufentanil metabolism and intrinsic clearance, human *in vivo* sufentanil metabolic drug interactions are not apparent. Volatile anesthetics (halothane, enflurane, isoflurane) had no effect on sufentanil disposition (154). Under conditions known to inhibit hepatic CYP3A4 activity and alfentanil clearance, erythromycin had no effect on sufentanil clearance (162). This result, the absence of reported interactions with known CYP3A4 substrates and inhibitors, and unchanged sufentanil clearance, even in patients with cirrhosis (163), have been attributed to the high extraction ratio (ER) of sufentanil and hence its dependence theoretically on hepatic blood flow rather than on intrinsic clearance, as well as to possible extrahepatic clearance (157).

Remifentanil

Remifentanil is the synthetic opioid most recently introduced for intraoperative use (164). Although structurally similar to fentanyl, sufentanil, and alfentanil, incorporation of a propanoic methyl ester in the alkyl side-chain substituent on the piperidine nitrogen rendered remifentanil susceptible to rapid hydrolysis by nonspecific esterases (165). Remifentanil plasma clearance in humans is 25 to 40 mL/kg/min, and the terminal half-life averages 10 to 15 min (166–171). Thus remifentanil has a very short clinical duration of effect and is used exclusively by infusion (164,169). Remifentanil in humans is extensively metabolized to one predominant metabolite, the carboxylic acid (165,166). N-Dealkylation is a minor route of metabolism in humans (166). Hydrolysis is catalyzed by nonspecific blood and tissue esterases, and not by pseudocholinesterase (164). The N-demethylase has not been identified. Owing to hydrolysis by multiple tissue and blood esterases (but not by cholinesterase, which is susceptible to drug interactions), remifentanil metabolic drug interactions would not be expected and have not been reported (164). Plasma clearance is unchanged in patients with severe liver disease (170).

DIPHENYLPROPYLAMINE SYNTHETIC OPIOIDS

The diphenylpropylamines are another group of synthetic opioids. These include methadone and propoxyphene (see Fig. 22-1). Both are administered orally, and methadone also is used intravenously. The diphenylpropylamines undergo extensive biotransformation to multiple metabolites.

Methadone

Methadone is an extremely long-acting opioid used for anesthesia, acute and chronic pain treatment, cancer pain, and substitution therapy for heroin dependence (172–175). Plasma clearance averages 2 to 3 mL/kg/min, and the elimination half-life is 20 to 40 hours (increasing with age), although there is extreme interindividual variability in clearance (23–2,100 mL/min) and half-life (4–130 hours), which is exaggerated with oral dosing (172,176–179). The hepatic extraction ratio is less than 0.1, and oral bioavailability averages 80% (176,177). Methadone is used clinically as the racemate, although pharmacologic efficacy resides almost exclusively with the (R)-enantiomer (180). Stereoselective differences in methadone enantiomer clearance and plasma disposition have been suggested by some but not all investigations (180–182).

Methadone is extensively metabolized, with approximately 5% to 10% eliminated unchanged in urine (177). The primary route of metabolism and inactivation is N-demethylation and spontaneous cyclization to form 2-ethylidene-1,5-dimethyl-3,3-diphenylpyrrolidine (EDPP), which is further N-demethylated to form the monomethyl analogue EMDP (176,183,184). These metabolites have been recovered in plasma and urine (184,185). Nevertheless, they constitute a small fraction of the dose recovered in urine, so other routes of metabolism must exist, including methadol and normethadol (176,185). Formation of EDPP, but not EMDP, by human liver microsomes in vitro has also been demonstrated (184,186,187).

Human hepatic microsomal N-demethylation of racemic methadone was found to be catalyzed predominantly by CYP3A (187,188). Single-enzyme kinetics were suggested, with K_m and V_{max} reported to be 545 μM and 2.8 nmol/min/mg (187) or 755 μM and 1.2 nmol/min/mg (188). Rates were correlated with CYP3A4 activity, and metabolism was diminished by CYP3A4 antibody and inhibitors, although minor participation of other CYP isoforms was suggested. Expressed CYP3A5 was devoid of methadone N-demethylase activity; however, expressed CYP2C18 and CYP2D6 exhibited turnover numbers exceeding that for CYP3A4. Furthermore, the CYP2C and 2D6 inhibitors sulfaphenazole and quinidine partially inhibited microsomal methadone N-demethylation in some livers.

Some methadone metabolic interactions in vitro have recently been reported. In liver microsomes from rats induced with phenobarbital or pregnenolone, methadone metabolism was increased two-fold (187). In vitro, human liver microsomal methadone N-demethylation was diminished by the CYP3A4 inhibitors troleandomycin, gestodene, ketoconazole, quercetin, dihydroergotamine, and by diazepam (competitive; K_i, 50 μM) (187,188). The selective serotonin reuptake inhibitors fluoxetine, norfluoxetine, and fluvoxamine (mixed inhibition; K_i, 55, 13, and 7 μM, respectively) also inhibited racemic methadone N-demethylation (188,189). The human immunodeficiency virus (HIV) protease inhibitors indinavir (noncompetitive; K_i, 3 μM), saquinavir (mixed inhibition; K_i 15 μM), and most

potently rotinavir (competitive; K_i, 50 nM) all inhibited human liver microsomal methadone metabolism (190).

Metabolic drug interactions are a major contributor to variable methadone elimination, and to clinical treatment failures (183,191,192). Increased methadone clearance occurs in opioid addicts and cancer pain patients treated with rifampin, barbiturates, phenytoin, and verapamil, and can precipitate withdrawal (178,184,192). For example, initiation of rifampin therapy in patients maintained with methadone caused acute withdrawal and substantially decreased plasma methadone concentrations while increasing urinary EDPP and EMDP excretion, consistent with induction of CYP3A4 and N-demethylase (183). Similar clinical and metabolic effects were seen with phenytoin (193). Although rifampin and rifabutin are structurally similar, prolonged therapy with the latter had no effect on methadone plasma concentrations or clearance, consistent with lesser or no induction of P450 (194). Fluconazole, another well-known P450 inhibitor, caused a 35% increase in methadone AUC and a 24% decrease in methadone oral clearance; however, inhibition of specific P450 isoform(s) could not be implicated because of the broad inhibitory character of fluconazole (195). Fluconazole effects did not elicit clinical signs of methadone overdose (195). Animal studies showed that prolonged ethanol treatment increased methadone metabolism and reduced plasma concentrations in vivo, whereas high ethanol concentrations inhibit methadone metabolism (192). The mechanism and clinical relevance of this interaction are not apparent, however, because CYP2E1 did not catalyze human methadone N-demethylation in vitro (187), and the CYP2E1 inhibitor disulfiram (196) did not inhibit human methadone metabolism in vivo (197). Diazepam was a competitive inhibitor of human liver microsomal methadone N-demethylation in vitro (187), and animal studies showed diazepam inhibition of methadone N-demethylation in vitro and in vivo (198). Nevertheless, long-term diazepam administration (0.3 mg/kg/day) had no effect on methadone disposition in humans in vivo, as assessed by blood and urine parent and EDDP concentrations (198,199).

Effects of selective serotonin reuptake inhibitors on clinical methadone disposition can be compared with in vitro effects. Based on in vitro K_i values and in vivo inhibitor and methadone concentrations, Iribarne et al. (189) predicted that fluvoxamine would inhibit in vivo methadone demethylation by 12%. In vivo, fluvoxamine, a strong CYP1A2 and 2C19 inhibitor, moderate CYP3A4 inhibitor, and weak CYP2D6 inhibitor (200), increased plasma concentrations of both methadone enantiomers 30% to 50% (191,201). Similarly, Iribarne et al. (189) predicted that fluoxetine would have no effect on racemic methadone metabolism in vitro. This prediction was confirmed. Fluoxetine, a strong CYP2D6 and moderate CYP3A4 inhibitor (200), had no effect on plasma racemic methadone concentrations (201–203). However, fluoxetine did increase (approximately 25%) plasma concentrations of R- but not S-methadone (201). These effects were attributed to methadone metabolism by both CYP1A2 and CYP2D6, with preferential metabolism of R- versus S-methadone by CYP2D6, and fluoxetine and fluvoxamine inhibition of CYP2D6 and CYP1A2 (201). Nevertheless, fluoxetine, norfluoxetine, and fluvoxamine inhibition of microsomal methadone N-demethylation (189) suggests a role for CYP3A4 inhibition (in addition to, or in place of CYPs 2D6 and 1A2) in the in vivo effects of these drugs on methadone clearance. A better understanding of these interactions may await identification of the P450s catalyzing metabolism of individual methadone enantiomers. Based on in vitro studies, Iribarne et al. (190) predicted that rotinavir would completely inhibit methadone metabolism in vivo, whereas neither indinavir nor saquinavir would inhibit in vivo. This prediction awaits clinical confirmation. These investigations, in general, suggest that known inhibitors of CYP3A4 activity in vivo will likely inhibit methadone metabolism and elimination, with the potential risk for relative overdose. A possibility for CYP2D6 interactions cannot be excluded. Methadone dosing must be carefully adjusted when initiating or discontinuing drugs affecting CYP3A4 activity.

Methadone effects on the phase I and II disposition of other drugs also have been described. Methadone was a competitive inhibitor of human liver microsomal dextromethorphan O-demethylation (CYP2D6; K_i, 4–8 μM) (8,11), and clinical reports of increased desipramine concentrations by methadone coadministration were attributed to inhibition of CYP2D6-catalyzed desipramine 2-hydroxylation (8). Methadone was a mixed inhibitor (K_i, 100 μM) of CYP3A4-catalyzed nifedipine oxidation (188). Consistent with these observations, methadone inhibition of human liver microsomal codeine O-demethylation (CYP2D6) was greater than that of N-demethylation (CYP3A4) (52). An explanation for greater methadone effects on CYP2D6, despite methadone being a CYP3A4 substrate, is not apparent. Mechanism-based inactivation of CYP3A4 by methadone has been reported (187); however, the clinical significance of this latter observation is unknown. In contrast, methadone had no effect on human liver microsomal CYP 1A2, 2B, 2C9, and 2E1 activities (188). Although zidovudine (AZT) had no effect on methadone disposition, methadone did significantly increase serum zidovudine concentrations and AUC in humans (204). This was not attributed to diminished zidovudine glucuronidation, which was unchanged in vivo and either unchanged (204) or inhibited only at very high methadone concentrations (IC_{50}, 8 μg/mL) in vitro (205), and the mechanism remains unknown.

Propoxyphene

Propoxyphene is a mild analgesic widely used for pain treatment. It contains two chiral centers and is used clinically as the (2S,3R) isomer (dextropropoxyphene). Propoxyphene is extensively metabolized by N-demethylation (mono and di), aromatic hydroxylation, and ester hydrolysis, as well as N-acetylation of N-demethylated metabolites (206). Norpropoxyphene, which is pharmacologically active, is the predominant metabolite, reaching plasma concentrations that markedly exceed those of the parent drug (207). Norpropoxyphene and dinorpropoxyphene are eliminated more slowly than the parent drug (206,207).

Human P450 isoforms responsible for dextropropoxyphene metabolism have not been identified, and there are few studies of human microsomal dextropropoxyphene metabolism. Nevertheless, there are numerous reports of dextropropoxyphene metabolic interactions. Dextropropoxyphene was a competitive inhibitor of human liver microsomal desipramine 2-hydroxylation (K_i, 2.5 μM) (208), and O-demethylation of both dextromethorphan (K_i, 6 μM) and 3-methoxymorphinan (11), demonstrating an interaction with CYP2D6. Dextropropoxyphene was an effective inhibitor of CYP2D6 in vivo, evidenced by increased debrisoquine metabolic ratios (209,210). It had no effect on CYP2C19 (209). Dextropropoxyphene was a weak competitive inhibitor (K_i, 1 mM) of human liver microsomal theophylline N-demethylation and 8-hydroxylation (CYP1A2) and tolbutamide hydroxylation (CYP2C9; K_i, 225 μM) in vitro (211,212). More recently, propoxyphene was shown to inhibit human liver microsomal metabolism of phenytoin, warfarin, and tolbutamide (CYP2C9) (213). In humans in vivo, dextropropoxyphene caused only a minor 17% reduction in theophylline 8-hydroxylation, and had no effect on theophylline 1- or 3-demethylation or on tolbutamide hydroxylation in vivo (214). Dextropropoxyphene interacts clinically with carbamazepine, markedly increasing plasma carbamazepine concentrations, decreasing those of the active metabolite (catalyzed by CYP3A4) carbamazepine 10,11-epoxide, and causing carbamazepine toxicity (215,216). Thus it appears that dextropropoxyphene interacts predominantly with CYP2D6 and CYP3A4. The in vivo inhibition of carbamazepine metabolism has led to the suggestion that the dextropropoxyphene–carbamazepine combination be avoided (216).

REFERENCES

1. Wood M. Pharmacokinetic drug interactions in anaesthetic practice. Clin Pharmacokinet 1991;21:285–307.
2. Jones DR, Gorski JC, Haehner BD, O'Mara EM, Hall SD. Determination of cytochrome P450 3A4/5 activity in vivo with dextromethorphan N-demethylation. Clin Pharmacol Ther 1996;60:374–384.
3. Capon DA, Bochner F, Kerry N, Mikus G, Danz C, Somogyi AA. The influence of CYP2D6 polymorphism and quinidine on the disposition and antitussive effect of dextromethorphan in humans. Clin Pharmacol Ther 1996;60:295–307.
4. Vetticaden SJ, Cabana BE, Prasad VK, et al. Phenotypic differences in dextromethorphan metabolism. Pharmacol Res 1989;6:13–19.
5. Chen ZR, Somogyi AA, Bochner F. Simultaneous determination of

dextromethorphan and three metabolites in plasma and urine using high-performance liquid chromatography with application to their disposition in man. *Ther Drug Monit* 1990;12:97–104.

6. Schadel M, Wu D, Otton SV, Kalow W, Sellers EM. Pharmacokinetics of dextromethorphan and metabolites in humans: influence of the CYP2D6 phenotype and quinidine inhibition. *J Clin Psychopharmacol* 1995;15:263–269.

7. Jacqz-Aigrain E, Funck-Brentano C, Cresteil T. CYP2D6-dependent and CYP3A-dependent metabolism of dextromethorphan in humans. *Pharmacogenetics* 1993;3:197–204.

8. Wu D, Otton SV, Sproule BA, et al. Inhibition of human cytochrome P450 2D6 (CYP2D6) by methadone. *Br J Clin Pharmacol* 1993;35: 30–34.

9. Schmid B, Bircher J, Preisig R, Kupfer A. Polymorphic dextromethorphan metabolism: co-segregation of oxidative O-demethylation with debrisoquin hydroxylation. *Clin Pharmacol Ther* 1985;38: 618–624.

10. Ducharme J, Abdullah S, Wainer IW. Dextromethorphan as an in vivo probe for the simultaneous determination of CYP2D6 and CYP3A activity. *J Chromatogr B* 1996;678:113–128.

11. Kerry NL, Somogyi AA, Bochner F, Mikus G. The role of CYP2D6 in primary and secondary oxidative metabolism of dextromethorphan: *in vitro* studies using human liver microsomes. *Br J Clin Pharmacol* 1994;38:243–248.

12. Broly F, Libersa C, Lhermitte M, Bechtel P, Dupuis B. Effect of quinidine on dextromethorphan O-demethylase activity of microsomal fractions from human liver. *Br J Clin Pharmacol* 1989;28:29–36.

13. Broly F, Libersa C, Lhermitte M, Dupuis B. Inhibitory studies of mexiletine and dextromethorphan oxidation in human liver microsomes. *Biochem Pharmacol* 1990;39:1045–1053.

14. Schmider J, Greenblatt DJ, Fogelman SM, von Moltke LL, Shader RI. Metabolism of dextromethorphan in vitro: involvement of cytochromes P450 2D6 and 3A3/4, with a possible role of 2E1. *Biopharmacol Drug Dispos* 1997;18:227–240.

15. Dayer P, Leemann T, Striberni R. Dextromethorphan O-demethylation in liver microsomes as a prototype reaction to monitor cytochrome P-450 db1 activity. *Clin Pharmacol Ther* 1989;45:34–40.

16. Gut J, Catin T, Dayer P, Kronbach T, Zanger U, Meyer U-A. Debrisoquine/sparteine-type polymorphism of drug oxidation: purification and characterization of two functionally different human liver cytochrome P-450 isozymes involved in impaired hydroxylation of the prototype substrate bufuralol. *J Biol Chem* 1986;261: 11734–11743.

17. Evans WE, Relling MV. Concordance of P450 2D6 (debrisoquine hydroxylase) phenotype and genotype: inability of dextromethorphan metabolic ratio to discriminate reliably heterozygous and homozygous extensive metabolizers. *Pharmacogenetics* 1991;1:143–148.

18. Zhang Y, Britto MR, Valderhaug KL, Wedlund PJ, Smith RA. Dextromethorphan: enhancing its systemic availability by way of low-dose quinidine-mediated inhibition of cytochrome P4502D6. *Clin Pharmacol Ther* 1992;51:647–655.

19. Ching MS, Blake CL, Chabrial H, et al. Potent inhibition of yeast-expressed CYP2D6 by dihydroquinidine, quinidine and its metabolites. *Biochem Pharmacol* 1995;50:833–837.

20. Ono S, Hatanaka T, Hotta H, Satoh T, Gonzalez FJ, Tsutsui M. Specificity of substrate and inhibitor probes for cytochrome P450s: evaluation of in vitro metabolism using cDNA-expressed human P450s and human liver microsomes. *Xenobiotica* 1996;26:681–693.

21. Rodrigues AD, Roberts EM. The in vitro interaction of dexmedetomidine with human liver microsomal cytochrome P4502D6 (CYP2D6). *Drug Metab Dispos* 1997;25:651–655.

22. Gorski JC, Jones DR, Wrighton SA, Hall SD. Characterization of dextromethorphan N-demethylation by human liver microsomes: contribution of the cytochrome P450 3A (CYP3A) subfamily. *Biochem Pharmacol* 1994;48:173–182.

23. Schmider J, Greenblatt DJ, von Moltke LL, Harmatz J, Shader RI. Inhibition of cytochrome P450 by nefazodone in vitro: studies of dextromethorphan O- and N-demethylation. *Br J Clin Pharmacol* 1996; 41:339–343.

24. Jaruratanasirikul S, Cooper AD, Blaschke TF. Inhibition of debrisoquin clearance in perfused rat livers and inhibition of dextromethorphan metabolism in human liver microsomes by 4-hydroxydebrisoquin or other metabolites of debrisoquin. *Drug Metab Dispos* 1992; 20:379–382.

25. Otton SV, Wu DF, Joffe RT, Cheung SW, Sellers EM. Inhibition by fluoxetine of cytochrome P450 2D6 activity. *Clin Pharmacol Ther* 1993; 53:401–409.

26. Sindrup SH, Brøsen K. The pharmacogenetics of codeine hypoalgesia. *Pharmacogenetics* 1995;5:335–346.

27. Adler TK, Fujimoto JM, Way EL, Baker EM. The metabolic fate of codeine in man. *J Pharmacol Exp Ther* 1955;114:251–262.

28. Hasselström J, Yue QY, Säwe J. The effect of codeine on gastrointestinal transit in extensive and poor metabolisers of debrisoquine. *Eur J Clin Pharmacol* 1997;53:145–148.

29. Yue QY, Alm C, Svensson JO, Säwe J. Quantification of the O- and N-demethylated and the glucuronidated metabolites of codeine relative to the debrisoquine metabolic ratio in urine in ultrarapid, rapid, and poor debrisoquine hydroxylators. *Ther Drug Monit* 1997;19:539–542.

30. Findlay JWA, Butz RF, Welch RM. Codeine kinetics as determined by radioimmunoassay. *Clin Pharmacol Ther* 1977;22:439–446.

31. Yue QY, Svensson J-O, Alm C, Sjoqvist F, Sawe J. Interindividual and interethnic differences in the demethylation and glucuronidation of codeine. *Br J Clin Pharmacol* 1989;28:629–637.

32. Yue QY, Svensson J-O, Alm C, Sjoqvist F, Sawe J. Codeine O-demethylation co-segregates with polymorphic debrisoquine hydroxylation. *Br J Clin Pharmacol* 1989;28:639–645.

33. Yue QY, Hasselström J, Svensson JO, Säwe J. Pharmacokinetics of codeine and its metabolites in Caucasian healthy volunteers: comparisons between extensive and poor hydroxylators of debrisoquine. *Br J Clin Pharmacol* 1991;31:635–642.

34. Chen ZR, Somogyi AA, Reynolds G, Bochner F. Disposition and metabolism of codeine after single and chronic doses in one poor and seven extensive metabolisers. *Br J Clin Pharmacol* 1991;31:381–390.

35. Yue QY, Tomson T, Säwe J. Carbamazepine and cigarette smoking induce differentially the metabolism of codeine in man. *Pharmacogenetics* 1994;4:193–198.

36. Caraco Y, Sheller J, Wood AJ. Pharmacogenetic determination of the effects of codeine and prediction of drug interactions. *J Pharmacol Exp Ther* 1996;278:1165–1174.

37. Hedenmalm K, Sundgren J, Granberg K, Spigset O, Dahlqvist R. Urinary excretion of codeine, ethylmorphine, and their metabolites: relation to the CYP2D6 activity. *Ther Drug Monit* 1997;19:643–649.

38. Mikus G, Trausch B, Rodewald C, et al. Effect of codeine on gastrointestinal motility in relation to CYP2D6 phenotype. *Clin Pharmacol Ther* 1997;61:459–466.

39. Findlay JWA, Jones EC, Butz RF, Welch RM. Plasma codeine and morphine concentrations after therapeutic oral doses of codeine-containing analgesics. *Clin Pharmacol Ther* 1978;24:60–68.

40. Hull JH, Findlay JWA, Rogers JF, Welch RM, Butz RF, Bustrack JA. An evaluation of the effects of smoking on codeine pharmacokinetics and bioavailability in normal human volunteers. *Drug Intell Clin Pharmacol* 1982;16:849–854.

41. Sindrup SH, Brosen K, Bjerring P, et al. Codeine increases pain thresholds to copper vapor laser stimuli in extensive but not poor metabolizers of sparteine. *Clin Pharmacol Ther* 1990;48:686–693.

42. Sindrup SH, Hofmann U, Asmussen J, et al. Impact of quinidine on plasma and cerebrospinal fluid concentrations of codeine and morphine after codeine intake. *Eur J Clin Pharmacol* 1996;49:503–509.

43. Chen ZR, Somogyi AA, Bochner F. Polymorphic O-demethylation of codeine. *Lancet* 1988;2:914–915.

44. Caraco Y, Sheller J, Wood AJJ. Pharmacogenetic determinants of codeine induction by rifampin: the impact on codeine's respiratory, psychomotor and miotic effects. *J Pharmacol Exp Ther* 1997;281: 330–336.

45. Poulsen L, Brøsen K, Arendt-Nielsen L, Gram LF, Elbæk K, Sindrup SH. Codeine and morphine in extensive and poor metabolizers of sparteine: pharmacokinetics, analgesic effect and side effects. *Eur J Clin Pharmacol* 1996;51:289–295.

46. Eckhardt K, Li S, Ammon S, Schänzle G, Mikus G, Eichelbaum M. Same incidence of adverse drug events after codeine administration irrespective of the genetically determined differences in morphine formation. *Pain* 1998;76:27–33.

47. Dayer P, Desmeules J, Leemann T, Striberni R. Bioactivation of the narcotic drug codeine in human liver is mediated by the polymorphic monooxygenase catalyzing debrisoquine 4-hydroxylation (cytochrome P-450 dbl/bufI). *Biochem Biophys Res Commun* 1988;152: 411–416.

48. Ladona MG, Lindström B, Thyr C, Dun-Ren P, Rane A. Differential

foetal development of the O-demethylation and N-demethylation of codeine and dextromethorphan in man. *Br J Clin Pharmacol* 1991; 32:295–302.

49. Mortimer O, Persson K, Ladona MG, et al. Polymorphic formation of morphine from codeine in poor and extensive metabolizers of dextromethorphan: relationship to the presence of immunoidentified cytochrome P-450IID1. *Clin Pharmacol Ther* 1990;47:27–35.

50. Desmeules J, Gascon MP, Dayer P, Magistris M. Impact of environmental and genetic factors on codeine analgesia. *Eur J Clin Pharmacol* 1991;41:23–26.

51. Sindrup SH, Arendt-Nielsen L, Brosen K, et al. The effect of quinidine on the analgesic effect of codeine. *Eur J Clin Pharmacol* 1992; 42:587–592.

52. Yue QY, Säwe J. Different effects of inhibitors on the O- and N-demethylation of codeine in human liver microsomes. *Eur J Clin Pharmacol* 1997;52:41–47.

53. Mikus G, Somogyi AA, Bochner F, Eichelbaum M. Codeine O-demethylation: rat strain differences and the effects of inhibitors. *Biochem Pharmacol* 1991;41:757–762.

54. Xu BQ, Aasmundstad TA, Christorphersen AS, Mørland J, Bjørneboe A. Evidence for CYP2D1-mediated primary and secondary O-dealkylation of ethylmorphine and codeine in rat liver microsomes. *Biochem Pharmacol* 1997;53:603–609.

55. Chen ZR, Irvine RJ, Bochner F, Somogyi AA. Morphine formation from codeine in rat brain: a possible mechanism of codeine analgesia. *Life Sci* 1990;46:1067–1074.

56. Dayer P, Desmeules J, Striberni R. In vitro forecasting of drugs that may interfere with codeine bioactivation. *Eur J Drug Metab Pharmacokinet* 1992;17:115–120.

57. Caraco Y, Tateishi T, Guengerich FP, Wood AJ. Microsomal codeine N-demethylation: cosegregation with cytochrome P4503A4 activity. *Drug Metab Dispos* 1996;24:761–764.

58. Eichelbaum M, Mineshita S, Ohnhaus EE, Zekorn C. The influence of enzyme induction on polymorphic sparteine oxidation. *Br J Clin Pharmacol* 1986;22:49–53.

59. Rasmussen E, Eriksson B, Öberg K, Bondesson U, Rane A. Selective effects of somatostatin analogs on human drug-metabolizing enzymes. *Clin Pharmacol Ther* 1998;64:150–159.

60. Yue Q, von Bahr C, Odar-Cederlof I, Sawe J. Glucuronidation of codeine and morphine in human liver and kidney microsomes: effect of inhibitors. *Pharmacol Toxicol* 1990;66:221–226.

61. Coffman BL, Rios GR, King CD, Tephly TR. Human UGT2B7 catalyzes morphine glucuronidation. *Drug Metab Dispos* 1997;25:1–4.

62. Coffman BL, King CD, Rios GR, Tephly TR. The glucuronidation of opioids, other xenobiotics, and androgens by human UGT2B7Y(268) and UGT2B7H(268). *Drug Metab Dispos* 1998;26:73–77.

63. Way EL, Adler TK. The biological disposition of morphine and its surrogates: 2. *Bull WHO* 1962;26:51–66.

64. Oguri K, Ida S, Yoshimura H, Tsukamoto H. Metabolism of drugs. LXIX. Studies on the urinary metabolites of morphine in several mammalian species. *Chem Pharmacol Bull Tokyo* 1970;18: 2414–2419.

65. Yeh SY, Gorodetzky CW, Krebs HA. Isolation and identification of morphine 3- and 6-glucuronides, morphine 3,6-diglucuronide, morphine 3-ethereal sulfate, normorphine, and normorphine 6-glucuronide as morphine metabolites in humans. *J Pharmacol Sci* 1977;66:1288–1293.

66. Osborne R, Joel S, Trew D, Slevin M. Morphine and metabolite behavior after different routes of morphine administration: demonstration of the importance of the active metabolite morphine-6-glucuronide. *Clin Pharmacol Ther* 1990;47:12–19.

67. Christup LL. Morphine metabolites. *Acta Anaesthesiol Scand* 1997; 41:116–122.

68. Samuelsson H, Hedner T, Venn R, Michalkiewicz A. CSF and plasma concentrations of morphine and morphine glucuronides in cancer patients receiving epidural morphine. *Pain* 1993;52:179–185.

69. Paul D, Standifer KM, Inturrisi CE, Pasternak GW. Pharmacological characterization of morphine-6β-glucuronide: a very potent morphine metabolite. *J Pharmacol Exp Ther* 1989;251:477–483.

70. Grace D, Fee JP. A comparison of intrathecal morphine-6-glucuronide and intrathecal morphine sulfate as analgesics for total hip replacement. *Anesth Analg* 1996;83:1055–1059.

71. Osborne R, Joel S, Grebenik K, Trew D, Slevin M. The pharmacokinetics of morphine and morphine glucuronides in kidney failure. *Clin Pharmacol Ther* 1993;54:158–167.

72. Portenoy RK, Foley KM, Stulman J, et al. Plasma morphine and morphine-6-glucuronide during chronic morphine therapy for cancer pain: plasma profiles, steady-state concentrations and the consequences of renal failure. *Pain* 1991;47:13–19.

73. Rane A, Säwe J, Pacifici GM, Svensson J-O, Kager L. Regioselective glucuronidation of morphine and interactions with benzodiazepines in human liver. *Adv Pain Res Ther* 1986;8:57–64.

74. Wahlström A, Winblad B, Bixo M, Rane A. Human brain metabolism of morphine and naloxone. *Pain* 1988;35:121–127.

75. Coughtrie MWH, Ask B, Rane A, Burchell B, Hume R. The enantioselective glucuronidation of morphine in rats and humans: evidence for the involvement of more than one UDP-glucuronosyltransferase isoenzyme. *Biochem Pharmacol* 1989;38:3273–3280.

76. Wahlström A, Persson K, Rane A. Metabolic interaction between morphine and naloxone in human liver: a common pathway to glucuronidation? *Drug Metab Dispos* 1989;17:218–220.

77. Wahlström A, Lenhammar L, Ask B, Rane A. Tricyclic antidepressants inhibit opioid receptor binding in human brain and hepatic morphine glucuronidation. *Pharmacol Toxicol* 1994;75:23–27.

78. Knodell RG, Holtzman JL, Crankshaw DL, Steele NM, Stanley LN. Drug metabolism by rat and human hepatic microsomes in response to interaction with H₂-receptor antagonists. *Gastroenterology* 1982; 82:82–88.

79. Ventafridda V, Bianchi M, Ripamonti C, et al. Studies on the effects of antidepressant drugs on the antinociceptive action of morphine and on plasma morphine in rat and man. *Pain* 1990;43:155–162.

80. Aasmundstad TA, Størset P. Influence of ranitidine on the morphine-3-glucuronide to morphine-6-glucuronide ratio after oral administration of morphine in humans. *Hum Exp Toxicol* 1998;17:347–352.

81. Rowell FJ, Seymour RA, Rawlins MD. Pharmacokinetics of intravenous and oral dihydrocodeine and its acid metabolites. *Eur J Clin Pharmacol* 1983;25:419–424.

82. Hufschmid E, Theurillat R, Martin U, Thormann W. Exploration of the metabolism of dihydrocodeine via determination of its metabolites in human urine using micellar electrokinetic capillary chromatography. *J Chromatogr B Biomed Appl* 1995;668:159–170.

83. Fromm MF, Hofmann U, Griese E-U, Mikus G. Dihydrocodeine: a new opioid substrate for the polymorphic CYP2D6 in humans. *Clin Pharmacol Ther* 1995;58:374–382.

84. Kirkwood LC, Nation RL, Somogyi AA. Characterization of the human cytochrome P450 enzymes involved in the metabolism of dihydrocodeine. *Br J Clin Pharmacol* 1997;44:549–555.

85. Jurna I, Kömen W, Balduf J, Fleischer W. Analgesia by dihydrocodeine is not due to formation of dihydromorphine: evidence from nociceptive activity in rat thalamus. *J Pharmacol Exp Ther* 1997; 281:1164–1170.

86. Hufschmid E, Theurillat R, Wilder-Smith CH, Thormann W. Characterization of the genetic polymorphism of dihydrocodeine O-demethylation in man via analysis of urinary dihydrocodeine and dihydromorphine by micellar electrokinetic capillary chromatography. *J Chromatogr B Biomed Appl* 1996;678:43–51.

87. Wilder-Smith CH, Hufschmid E, Thormann W. The visceral and somatic antinociceptive effects of dihydrocodeine and its metabolite, dihydromorphine: a cross-over study with extensive and quinidine-induced poor metabolizers. *Br J Clin Pharmacol* 1998;45:575–581.

88. Kirkwood LC, Nation RL, Somogyi AA. Glucuronidation of dihydrocodeine by human liver microsomes and the effect of inhibitors. *Clin Exp Pharmacol Physiol* 1998;25:266–270.

89. Cone EJ, Darwin WD, Gorodetzky CW, Tan T. Comparative metabolism of hydrocodone in man, rat, guinea pig, rabbit, and dog. *Drug Metab Dispos* 1978;6:488–493.

90. Otton SV, Schadel M, Cheung SW, Kaplan HL, Busto UE, Sellers EM. CYP2D6 phenotype determines the metabolic conversion of hydrocodone to hydromorphone. *Clin Pharmacol Ther* 1993;54: 463–472.

91. Kaplan HL, Busto UE, Baylon GJ, et al. Inhibition of cytochrome P450 2D6 metabolism of hydrocodone to hydromorphone does not importantly affect abuse liability. *J Pharmacol Exp Ther* 1997;281:103–108.

92. Tomkins DM, Otton SV, Joharchi N, et al. Effect of cytochrome P450 2D1 inhibition on hydrocodone metabolism and its behavioral consequences in rats. *J Pharmacol Exp Ther* 1997;280:1374–1382.

93. Kaiko RF, Benziger DP, Fitzmartin RD, Burke BE, Reder RF, Goldenheim PD. Pharmacokinetic-pharmacodynamic relationships of controlled-release oxycodone. *Clin Pharmacol Ther* 1996;59:52–61.

94. Cleary J, Mikus G, Somogyi A, Bochner F. The influence of pharmacogenetics on opioid analgesia: studies with codeine and oxycodone in the Sprague-Dawley/Dark Agouti rat model. *J Pharmacol Exp Ther* 1994;271:1528–1534.

95. Gibson TP. Pharmacokinetics, efficacy, and safety of analgesia with a focus on tramadol HCl. *Am J Med* 1996;101:47S–53S.

96. Dayer P, Desmeules J, Collart L. Pharmacologie du tramadol. *Drugs* 1997;53:18–24.

97. Paar WD, Frankus P, Dengler HJ. High-performance liquid chromatographic assay for the simultaneous determination of tramadol and its metabolites in microsomal fractions of human liver. *J Chromatogr B Biomed Appl* 1996;686:221–227.

98. Poulsen L, Arendt-Nielsen L, Brøsen K, Sindrup SH. The hypoalgesic effect of tramadol in relation to CYP2D6. *Clin Pharmacol Ther* 1996; 60:636–644.

99. Paar WD, Frankus P, Dengler HJ. The metabolism of tramadol by human liver microsomes. *Clin Invest* 1992;70:708–710.

100. Paar WD, Poche S, Gerloff J, Dengler HJ. Polymorphic CYP2D6 mediates *O*-demethylation of the opioid analgesic tramadol. *Eur J Clin Pharmacol* 1997;53:235–239.

101. Collart L, Luthy C, Favario-Constantin C, Dayer P. Dualité de l'effet analgésique du tramadol chez l'homme (Duality of the analgesic effect of tramadol in humans). *Schweiz Med Wochenschr* 1993;123: 2241–2243.

102. Sabbe JR, Sims PJ, Sims MH. Tramadol-warfarin iteration. *Pharmacotherapy* 1998;18:871–873.

103. Edwards DJ, Svensson CK, Visco JP, Lalka D. Clinical pharmacokinetics of pethidine: 1982. *Clin Pharmacokinet* 1982;7:421–433.

104. Bovill JG. Pharmacokinetics of opioids. In: Bowdle TA, Horita A, Kharasch ED, eds. *The pharmacologic basis of anesthesiology*. New York: Churchill Livingstone, 1994:37–85.

105. Yeh SY. Metabolism of meperidine in several animal species. *J Pharmacol Sci* 1984;73:1783–1787.

106. Kaiko RF, Foley KM, Grabinski PY, et al. Central nervous system excitatory effects of meperidine in cancer patients. *Ann Neurol* 1983; 13:180–185.

107. Plummer JL, Gourlay GK, Cmielewski PL, Odontiadis J, Harvey I. Behavioural effects of norpethidine, a metabolite of pethidine, in rats. *Toxicology* 1995;95:37–44.

108. Stambaugh JE Jr, Wainer IW, Schwartz I. The effect of phenobarbital on the metabolism of meperidine in normal volunteers. *J Clin Pharmacol* 1978;18:482–490.

109. Stambaugh JE, Hemphill DM, Wainer IW, Schwartz I. A potentially toxic drug interaction between pethidine (meperidine) and phenobarbitone. *Lancet* 1977;1:398–399.

110. Pond SM, Kretschzmar KM. Effect of phenytoin on meperidine clearance and normeperidine formation. *Clin Pharmacol Ther* 1981;30: 680–686.

111. Stambaugh JE Jr, Wainer IW. Drug interaction: meperidine and chlorpromazine, a toxic combination. *J Clin Pharmacol* 1981;21:140–146.

112. Guay DRP, Meatherall RC, Chalmers JL, Grahame GR. Cimetidine alters pethidine disposition in man. *Br J Clin Pharmacol* 1984;18: 907–914.

113. Guay DRP, Meatherall RC, Chalmers JL, Grahame GR, Hudson RJ. Ranitidine does not alter pethidine disposition in man. *Br J Clin Pharmacol* 1985;20:55–59.

114. Rane A, Liu Z, Henderson CJ, Wolf CR. Divergent regulation of cytochrome P450 enzymes by morphine and pethidine: a neuroendocrine mechanism? *Mol Pharmacol* 1995;47:57–64.

115. Browne B, Linter S. Monoamine oxidase inhibitors and narcotic analgesics: a critical review of the implications for treatment. *Br J Psychiatry* 1987;151:210–212.

116. Bovill JG, Sebel PS, Blackburn CL, Heykants J. The pharmacokinetics of alfentanil (R39209): a new opioid analgesic. *Anesthesiology* 1982;57:439–443.

117. Maitre PO, Vozeh S, Heykants J, Thomson DA, Stanski DR. Population pharmacokinetics of alfentanil: the average dose-plasma concentration relationship and interindividual variability in patients. *Anesthesiology* 1987;66:13–16.

118. Scholz J, Steinfath M, Schulz M. Clinical pharmacokinetics of alfentanil, fentanyl and sufentanil: an update. *Clin Pharmacokinet* 1996; 4:275–292.

119. Meuldermans W, Van Peer A, Hendrickx J, et al. Alfentanil pharmacokinetics and metabolism in humans. *Anesthesiology* 1988;69:527–534.

120. Lavrijsen KLM, Van Houdt JMG, Van Dyck DMJ, et al. Is the metabolism of alfentanil subject to debrisoquine polymorphism? *Anesthesiology* 1988;69:535–540.

121. Labroo RB, Kharasch ED. Gas chromatographic-mass spectrometric analysis of alfentanil metabolites: application to human liver microsomal alfentanil biotransformation. *J Chromatogr B* 1994;660:85–94.

122. Labroo RB, Thummel KE, Kunze KL, Podoll T, Trager WF, Kharasch ED. Catalytic role of cytochrome P4503A4 in multiple pathways of alfentanil metabolism. *Drug Metab Dispos* 1995;23:490–496.

123. Yun C-H, Wood M, Wood AJJ, Guengerich FP. Identification of the pharmacogenetic determinants of alfentanil metabolism: cytochrome P450 3A4. *Anesthesiology* 1992;77:467–474.

124. Kharasch ED, Thummel K. Human alfentanil metabolism by cytochrome P450 3A3/4. An explanation for the interindividual variability in alfentanil clearance? *Anesth Analg* 1993;76:1033–1039.

125. Guitton J, Buronfosse T, Désage M, Lepape A, Brazier JL, Beaune P. Possible involvement of multiple cytochrome P450s in fentanyl and sufentanil metabolism as opposed to alfentanil. *Biochem Pharmacol* 1997;53:1613–1619.

126. Raeder JC, Nilsen OG, Hole A. Pharmacokinetics of midazolam and alfentanil in outpatient general anesthesia: a study with concomitant thiopentone, flumazenil or placebo administration. *Acta Anaesthesiol Scand* 1988;32:467–472.

127. Kharasch ED, Russell M, Mautz D, et al. The role of cytochrome P450 3A4 in alfentanil clearance: implications for interindividual variability in disposition and perioperative drug interactions. *Anesthesiology* 1997;87:36–50.

128. Krivoruk Y, Kinirons MT, Wood AJ, Wood M. Metabolism of cytochrome P4503A substrates *in vivo* administered by the same route: lack of correlation between alfentanil clearance and erythromycin breath test. *Clin Pharmacol Ther* 1994;56:608–614.

129. Wilkinson GR. Clearance approaches in pharmacology. *Pharmacol Rev* 1987;39:1–47.

130. Bower S, Sear JW, Roy RC, Carter RF. Effects of different hepatic pathologies on disposition of alfentanil in anaesthetized patients. *Br J Anaesth* 1992;68:462–465.

131. Henthorn TK, Avram MJ, Krejcie TC. Alfentanil clearance is independent of the polymorphic debrisoquin hydroxylase. *Anesthesiology* 1989;71:635–639.

132. Bartkowski RR, Goldberg ME, Larijani GE, Boerner T. Inhibition of alfentanil metabolism by erythromycin. *Clin Pharmacol Ther* 1989; 46:99–102.

133. Kienlen J, Levron J-C, Aubas S, Roustan J-P, du Cailar J. Pharmacokinetics of alfentanil in patients treated with either cimetidine or ranitidine. *Drug Invest* 1993;6:257–262.

134. Palkama VJ, Isohanni MH, Neuvonen PJ, Olkkola KT. The effect of intravenous and oral fluconazole on the pharmacokinetics and pharmacodynamics of intravenous alfentanil. *Anesth Analg* 1998;87: 190–194.

135. Ahonen J, Olkkola KT, Salmenpera M, Hynynen M, Neuvonen PJ. Effect of diltiazem on midazolam and alfentanil disposition in patients undergoing coronary artery bypass grafting. *Anesthesiology* 1996;85: 1246–1252.

136. Bartkowski RR, McDonnell TE. Prolonged alfentanil effect following erythromycin. *Anesthesiology* 1990;73:566–568.

137. Gepts E, Jonckheer K, Maes V, Sonck W, Camu F. Disposition kinetics of propofol during alfentanil anaesthesia. *Anaesthesia* 1988;43 (suppl):8–13.

138. Pavlin DJ, Coda B, Shen D, et al. Effects of combining propofol and alfentanil on ventilation, analgesia, sedation, and emesis in human volunteers. *Anesthesiology* 1996;84:23–37.

139. Bower S, Hull CJ. Comparative pharmacokinetics of fentanyl and alfentanil. *Br J Anaesth* 1982;54:871–877.

140. Mather LE. Clinical pharmacokinetics of fentanyl and its newer derivatives. *Clin Pharmacokinet* 1983;8:422–446.

141. Van Rooy HH, Vermeulen NPE, Bovill JG. The assay of fentanyl and its metabolites in plasma of patients using gas chromatography with alkali flame ionisation detection and gas chromatography-mass spectrometry. *J Chromatogr* 1981;223:85–93.

142. Goromaru T, Matsuura H, Yoshimura N, et al. Identification and quantitative determination of fentanyl metabolites in patients by gas chromatography-mass spectrometry. *Anesthesiology* 1984;61:73–77.

143. Tateishi T, Wood AJJ, Guengerich FP, Wood M. Biotransformation of tritiated fentanyl in human liver microsomes: monitoring metabolism

using phenylacetic acid and 2-phenylethanol. *Biochem Pharmacol* 1995;50:1921–1924.

144. Feierman E, Lasker JM. Metabolism of fentanyl: a synthetic opioid analgesic, by human liver microsomes: role of CYP3A4. *Drug Metab Dispos* 1996;24:932–939.

145. Labroo RB, Paine ME, Thummel KE, Kharasch ED. Fentanyl metabolism by human hepatic and intestinal cytochrome P450 3A4: implications for interindividual variability in disposition, efficacy and drug interactions. *Drug Metab Dispos* 1997;25:1072–1080.

146. Guitton J, Désage M, Alamercery S, et al. Gas chromatographic-mass spectrometry and gas chromatographic-Fourier transform infrared spectroscopy assay for the simultaneous identification of fentanyl metabolites. *J Chromatogr B* 1997;59:59–70.

147. Schneider E, Brune K. Opioid activity and distribution of fentanyl metabolites. *Naunyn Schmiedebergs Arch Pharmacol* 1986;334:267–274.

148. Tateishi T, Krivoruk Y, Ueng Y-F, Wood AJJ, Guengerich FP, Wood M. Identification of human liver cytochrome P-450 3A4 as the enzyme responsible for fentanyl and sufentanil N-dealkylation. *Anesth Analg* 1996;82:167–172.

149. Haberer JP, Schoeffler P, Couderc E, Duvaldestin P. Fentanyl pharmacokinetics in anaesthetized patients with cirrhosis. *Br J Anaesth* 1982;54:1267–1270.

150. Tempelhoff R, Modica PA, Spitznagel EL. Anticonvulsant therapy increases fentanyl requirements during anaesthesia for craniotomy. *Can J Anaesth* 1990;37:327–332.

151. Streisand JB, Varvel JR, Stanski DR, et al. Absorption and bioavailability of oral transmucosal fentanyl citrate. *Anesthesiology* 1991;75:223–229.

152. Monk JP, Beresford R, Ward A. Sufentanil: a review of its pharmacological properties and therapeutic use. *Drugs* 1988;36:286–313.

153. Hudson RJ, Bergstrom RG, Thompson IR, Sabourin MA, Rosenbloom M, Strunin L. Pharmacokinetics of sufentanil in patients undergoing abdominal aortic surgery. *Anesthesiology* 1989;70:426–431.

154. Lehmann KA, Sipakis K, Gasparini R, Vanpeer A. Pharmacokinetics of sufentanil in general surgical patients under different conditions of anaesthesia. *Acta Anaesthesiol Scand* 1993;37:176–180.

155. Lange H, Stephan H, Zielmann S, Sonntag H. Hepatic disposition of sufentanil in patients undergoing coronary bypass surgery. *Acta Anaesthesiol Scand* 1993;37:154–158.

156. Gepts E, Shafer SL, Camu F, et al. Linearity of pharmacokinetics and model estimation of sufentanil. *Anesthesiology* 1995;83:1194–1204.

157. Raucoules-Aimé M, Kaidomar M, Levron J-C, et al. Hepatic disposition of alfentanil and sufentanil in patients undergoing orthotopic liver transplantation. *Anesth Analg* 1997;84:1019–1024.

158. Weldon ST, Perry DF, Cork RC, Gandolfi AJ. Detection of picogram levels of sufentanil by capillary gas chromatography. *Anesthesiology* 1985;63:684–687.

159. Heykants J, Woestenborghs R, Timmerman P. Reliability of sufentanil plasma level assays in patients. *Anesthesiology* 1986;65:112–113.

160. Meuldermans W, Hendrickx J, Lauwers W, et al. Excretion and biotransformation of alfentanil and sufentanil in rats and dogs. *Drug Metab Dispos* 1987;15:905–913.

161. Lavrijsen K, Van Houdt J, Van Dyck D, et al. Biotransformation of sufentanil in liver microsomes of rats, dogs, and humans. *Drug Metab Dispos* 1990;18:704–710.

162. Bartkowski RR, Goldberg ME, Huffnagle S, Epstein RH. Sufentanil disposition: is it affected by erythromycin administration? *Anesthesiology* 1993;78:260–265.

163. Chauvin M, Ferrier C, Haberer JP, et al. Sufentanil pharmacokinetics in patients with cirrhosis. *Anesth Analg* 1989;68:1–4.

164. Bürkle H, Dunbar S, Van Aken H. Remifentanil: a novel, short-acting, μ-opioid. *Anesth Analg* 1996;83:646–651.

165. Feldman PL, James MK, Brackeen MF, et al. Design, synthesis, and pharmacological evaluation of ultrashort-acting to long-acting opioid analgetics. *J Med Chem* 1991;34:2202–2208.

166. Westmoreland CL, Hoke JF, Sebel PS, Hug CC, Muir KT. Pharmacokinetics of remifentanil (GI87084B) and its major metabolite (GI90291) in patients undergoing elective inpatient surgery. *Anesthesiology* 1993;79:893–903.

167. Glass PSA, Hardman D, Kamiyama Y, et al. Preliminary pharmacokinetics and pharmacodynamics of an ultra-short-acting opioid: remifentanil (GI87084B). *Anesth Analg* 1993;77:1031–1040.

168. Kapila A, Glass PSA, Jacobs JR, et al. Measured context-sensitive half-times of remifentanil and alfentanil. *Anesthesiology* 1995;83:968–975.

169. Egan TD, Minto CF, Hermann DJ, Barr J, Muir KT, Shafer SL. Remifentanil versus alfentanil: comparative pharmacokinetics and pharmacodynamics in healthy adult male volunteers. *Anesthesiology* 1996;84:821–833.

170. Dershwitz M, Hoke JF, Rosow CE, et al. Pharmacokinetics and pharmacodynamics of remifentanil in volunteer subjects with severe liver disease. *Anesthesiology* 1996;84:812–820.

171. Minto CF, Schnider TW, Egan TD, et al. Influence of age and gender on the pharmacokinetics and pharmacodynamics of remifentanil. I. Model development. *Anesthesiology* 1997;86:10–23.

172. Gourlay GK, Wilson PR, Glynn CJ. Pharmacodynamics and pharmacokinetics of methadone during the perioperative period. *Anesthesiology* 1982;57:458–467.

173. Gourlay GK, Willis RJ, Wilson PR. Postoperative pain control with methadone: influence of supplementary methadone doses and blood concentration-response relationships. *Anesthesiology* 1984;61:19–26.

174. Kreek MJ. Long-term pharmacotherapy for opiate (primarily heroin) addiction: opioid agonists. *Handbook Exp Pharmacol* 1996;118:487–562.

175. Ripamonti C, Zecca E, Bruera E. An update on the clinical use of methadone for cancer pain. *Pain* 1997;70:109–115.

176. Säwe J. High-dose morphine and methadone in cancer patients: clinical pharmacokinetic considerations of oral treatment. *Clin Pharmacokinet* 1986;11:87–106.

177. Inturrisi CE, Colburn WA, Kaiko RF, Houde RW, Foley KM. Pharmacokinetics and pharmacodynamics of methadone in patients with chronic pain. *Clin Pharmacol Ther* 1987;41:392–401.

178. Plummer JL, Gourlay GK, Cherry DA, Cousins MJ. Estimation of methadone clearance: application in the management of cancer pain. *Pain* 1988;33:313–322.

179. Inturrisi CE, Portenoy RK, Max MB, Colburn WA, Foley KM. Pharmacokinetic-pharmacodynamic relationships of methadone infusions in patients with cancer pain. *Clin Pharmacol Ther* 1990;47:565–577.

180. Olsen GD, Wendel HA, Livermore JD, Leger RM, Lynn RK, Gerber N. Clinical effects and pharmacokinetics of racemic methadone and its optical isomers. *Clin Pharmacol Ther* 1976;21:147–157.

181. Kristensen K, Blemmer T, Angelo HR, et al. Stereoselective pharmacokinetics of methadone in chronic pain patients. *Ther Drug Monit* 1996;18:221–227.

182. Eap CB, Finkbeiner T, Gastpar M, Scherbaum N, Powell K, Baumann P. Replacement of (R)-methadone by a double dose of (R,S)-methadone in addicts: interindividual variability of the (R)/(S) ratios and evidence of adaptive changes in methadone pharmacokinetics. *Eur J Clin Pharmacol* 1996;50:385–389.

183. Kreek MJ, Gutjahr CL, Garfield JW, Bowen DV, Field FH. Drug interactions with methadone. *Ann NY Acad Sci* 1976;281:350–371.

184. de Vos JW, Geerlings PJ, van den Brink W, Ufkes JGR, van Wilgenburg H. Pharmacokinetics of methadone and its primary metabolite in 20 opiate addicts. *Eur J Clin Pharmacol* 1995;48:361–366.

185. Inturrisi CE, Verebely K. A gas-liquid chromatographic method for the quantitative determination of methadone in human plasma and urine. *J Chromatogr* 1972;65:361–369.

186. Alburges ME, Huang W, Foltz RL, Moody DE. Determination of methadone and its N-demethylation in biological specimens by GC-PICI-MS. *J Anal Toxicol* 1996;20:362–368.

187. Iribarne C, Berthou F, Baird S, et al. Involvement of cytochrome P450 3A4 enzyme in the N-demethylation of methadone in human liver microsomes. *Chem Res Toxicol* 1996;9:365–373.

188. Iribarne C, Dréano Y, Bardou LG, Ménez JF, Berthou F. Interaction of methadone with substrates of human hepatic cytochrome P450 3A4. *Toxicology* 1997;117:13–23.

189. Iribarne C, Picart D, Dréano Y, Berthou F. In vitro interactions between fluoxetine or fluvoxamine and methadone or buprenorphine. *Fund Clin Pharmacol* 1998;12:194–199.

190. Iribarne C, Berthou F, Carlhant D, et al. Inhibition of methadone and buprenorphine N-dealkylations by three HIV-1 protease inhibitors. *Drug Metab Dispos* 1998;26:257–260.

191. Bertschy G, Baumann P, Eap CB, Baettig D. Probable metabolic interaction between methadone and fluvoxamine in addict patients. *Ther Drug Monit* 1994;16:42–45.

192. Kreek MJ. Drug interactions in humans related to drug abuse and its treatment. *Mod Methods Pharmacol* 1990;6:265–282.

193. Tong TG, Pond SM, Kreek MJ, Jaffery NF, Benowitz NL. Phenytoin-induced methadone withdrawal. *Ann Intern Med* 1981;94:349–351.

194. Brown LS, Sawyer RC, Li R, Cobb MN, Colborn DC, Narang PK. Lack of a pharmacologic interaction between rifabutin and methadone in HIV-infected former injecting drug users. *Drug Alcohol Depend* 1996;43:71–77.

195. Cobb MN, Desai J, Brown JLS, Zannikos PN, Rainey PM. The effect of fluconazole on the clinical pharmacokinetics of methadone. *Clin Pharmacol Ther* 1998;63:655–662.

196. Kharasch ED, Thummel K, Mhyre J, Lillibridge J. Single-dose disulfiram inhibition of chlorzoxazone metabolism: a clinical probe for P450 2E1. *Clin Pharmacol Ther* 1993;53:643–650.

197. Tong TG, Benowitz NL, Kreek MJ. Methadone-disulfiram interaction during methadone maintenance. *J Clin Pharmacol* 1980;20:506–513.

198. Pond SM, Tong TG, Benowitz NL, Jacob P III, Rigod J. Lack of effect of diazepam on methadone metabolism in methadone-maintained addicts. *Clin Pharmacol Ther* 1982;31:139–143.

199. Preston KL, Griffiths RR, Cone EJ, Darwin WD, Gorodetzky CW. Diazepam and methadone blood levels following concurrent administration of diazepam and methadone. *Drug Alcohol Depend* 1986;18:195–202.

200. Lane RM. Pharmacokinetic drug interaction potential of selective serotonin reuptake inhibitors. *Int Clin Psychopharmacol* 1996;11:31–61.

201. Eap CB, Bertschy G, Powell K, Baumann P. Fluvoxamine and fluoxetine do not interact in the same way with the metabolism of the enantiomers of methadone. *J Clin Psychopharmacol* 1997;17:113–117.

202. Batki SL, Manfredi LB, Jacob P III, Jones RT. Fluoxetine for cocaine dependence in methadone maintenance: quantitative plasma and urine cocaine/benzoylecgonine concentrations. *J Clin Psychopharmacol* 1993;13:243–250.

203. Bertschy G, Eap CB, Powell K, Baumann P. Fluoxetine addition to methadone in addicts: pharmacokinetic aspects. *Ther Drug Monit* 1996;18:570–572.

204. Schwartz EL, Brechbühl A-B, Kahl P, Miller MA, Selwyn PA, Friedland GH. Pharmacokinetic interactions of zidovudine and methadone in intravenous drug-using patients with HIV infection. *J Acquired Immune Def* 1992;5:619–626.

205. Trapnell CB, Klecker RW, Jamis-Dow C, Collins JM. Glucuronidation of 3'-azido-3'-deoxythymidine (zidovudine) by human liver microsomes: relevance to clinical pharmacokinetic interactions with ato-vaquone, fluconazole, methadone, and valproic acid. *Antimicrob Agents Chemother* 1998;42:1592–1596.

206. Due SL, Sullivan HR, McMahon RE. Propoxyphene: pathways of metabolism in man and laboratory animals. *Biomed Mass Spectrom* 1976;3:217–225.

207. Inturrisi CE, Colburn WA, Verebey K, Dayton HE, Woody GE, O'Brien CP. Propoxyphene and norpropoxyphene kinetics after single and repeated doses of propoxyphene. *Clin Pharmacol Ther* 1982;31:157–167.

208. Henthorn TK, Spina E, Dumont E, von Bahr C. In vitro inhibition of a polymorphic human liver P-450 isozyme by narcotic analgesics. *Anesthesiology* 1989;70:339–342.

209. Sanz EJ, Bertilsson L. *d*-Propoxyphene is a potent inhibitor of debrisoquine metabolism, but not S-mephenytoin 4-hydroxylation *in vivo*. *Ther Drug Monit* 1990;12:297–299.

210. Beyeler C, Daly AK, Armstrong M, Astbury C, Bird HA, Idle JR. Phenotype/genotype relationships for the cytochrome P450 enzyme CYP2D6 in rheumatoid arthritis: influence of drug therapy and disease activity. *J Rheumatol* 1994;21:1034–1039.

211. Robson RA, Miners JO, Matthews AP, et al. Characterisation of theophylline metabolism by human liver microsomes. *Biochem Pharmacol* 1988;37:1651–1659.

212. Miners JO, Smith KJ, Robson RA, McManus ME, Veronene ME, Birkett DJ. Tolbutamide hydroxylation by human liver microsomes: kinetic characterisation and relationship to other cytochrome P-450 dependent xenobiotic oxidations. *Biochem Pharmacol* 1988;37:1137–1144.

213. Levy RH. Cytochrome P450 isozymes and antiepileptic drug interactions. *Epilepsia* 1995;36:S8–S13.

214. Robson RA, Miners JO, Whitehead AG, Birkett DJ. Specificity of the inhibitory effect of dextropropoxyphene on oxidative drug metabolism in man: effects on theophylline and tolbutamide disposition. *Br J Clin Pharmacol* 1987;23:772–775.

215. Spina E, Pisani F, Perucca E. Clinically significant pharmacokinetic drug interactions with carbamazepine: an update. *Clin Pharmacokinet* 1996;31:198–214.

216. Bergendal L, Friberg A, Schaffrath AM, Holmdahl M, Landahl S. The clinical relevance of the interaction between carbamazepine and dextropropoxyphene in elderly patients in Gothenburg, Sweden. *Eur J Clin Pharmacol* 1997;53:203–206.

217. Otton SV, Ball SE, Cheung SW, Inaba T, Sellers EM. Comparative inhibition of the polymorphic enzyme CYP2D6 by venlafaxine and other 5HT uptake inhibitors. *Clin Pharmacol Ther* 1994;55:141.

CHAPTER 23

Agents for the Treatment of Migraine, Parkinson's, and Alzheimer's Diseases

Tina M. deVries and S. Thomas Forgue

ALZHEIMER'S DISEASE

Tacrine

The clinical pharmacokinetics of tacrine (Cognex; 1,2,3,4-tetrahydro-9-aminoacridine monohydrochloride monohydrate) have been extensively reviewed (1,2). After oral administration, tacrine is rapidly and extensively absorbed with peak plasma concentrations (C_{max}) achieved within 0.5 to 3 hours after a single oral dose. Tacrine has a large volume of distribution (V_d, 350 L), suggesting extensive distribution within the body. Tacrine is rapidly and extensively metabolized in humans both systemically and presystemically. Even at early (0.5 hour) sampling times after oral dosing, monohydroxylated metabolite concentrations in plasma exceed those of tacrine. Low absolute bioavailability after oral dosing is attributable to extensive first pass metabolism that undoubtedly contributes to high between-patient variability (70-fold range) in plasma concentrations (2,3). Estimates of absolute bioavailability for individual subjects range from 3% to 65% (4–6). Bioavailability of a 10-mg dose is disproportionately low relative to higher doses, suggesting that a larger proportion of the 10-mg dose undergoes presystemic metabolism. For example, mean C_{max} values of 5.1, 20.7, and 33.9 ng/mL were reported after repeated, q6h dosing of 10-mg, 20-mg, and 30-mg doses, respectively (3). Presystemic metabolism can be partially circumvented by alternative routes of administration. When tacrine was given to patients with Alzheimer's disease (AD) as a rectal suppository, extent

of absorption was nearly twice that for an oral dose (7,8). Total plasma clearance after intravenous dosing is high, averaging about 150 L/h (2,500 mL/min). Clearance is almost entirely due to oxidative metabolism; a negligible amount of unchanged drug is recovered in urine. The elimination half-life ($t_{1/2}$) is short (less than 4 hours), and a q.i.d. dosing schedule is recommended. Steady-state plasma concentrations in AD patients were stable for up to 31 months of treatment (9). This indication that tacrine does not induce its own metabolism is consistent with the finding of insignificant induction potential in rats (10).

Metabolite Identification

Tacrine is extensively oxidized to a wide variety of monohydroxylated and dihydroxylated metabolites, a dihydrodiol, and possibly a quinone methide. These primary metabolites can be conjugated with glucuronic acid or glutathione, be further oxidized, or be cleared by the kidney. The 1-hydroxytacrine is the major metabolite, although no single compound accounts for more than 10% of radioactivity after administration of [^{14}C]tacrine to healthy subjects. In 1993, Woolf et al. (11) reported that on incubation with human microsomes, tacrine was extensively metabolized to 1-hydroxytacrine with small amounts of the 2-, 4-, and 7-hydroxy tacrine isomer present. Subsequently, Pool et al. (12) demonstrated that every position of the alicyclic ring can be hydroxylated by identifying 3-hydroxytacrine in human urine. After this metabolite was identified in rat urine by mass spectral and COSY nuclear magnetic resonance (NMR) analysis, it was synthesized to aid identification in human urine. They extended this work to a comprehensive ^{14}C-metabolism study that provided evidence for additional hydroxylated and conjugated metabolites (13). After administration of a single oral dose of [^{14}C]tacrine to

T.M. deVries: Research and Development, Warner Chilcott Laboratories, 100 Enterprise Drive, Suite 280, Rockaway, New Jersey 07866

S.T. Forgue: Lilly Laboratory for Clinical Research, 550 North University Boulevard, Indianapolis, Indiana 46202

321

healthy male subjects, most of the radiolabel was absorbed, and most of the absorbed material was eliminated renally, with no single compound constituting more than 10% of total recovered radioactivity. In addition to the various monohydroxy isomers, the 1,3-dihydroxy derivative, a dihydrodiol, and a phenol glucuronide of 7-hydroxytacrine were isolated and identified.

Hydroxylation of the aliphatic ring introduces a chiral center. Approximately 94% of the 1-hydroxytacrine recovered in urine of healthy elderly subjects administered 40 mg tacrine was the dextrorotatory isomer, a finding that corroborates stereoselectivity shown with human liver microsomes (14). Thus, the major metabolite arising from administration of tacrine to humans is distinct from velnacrine, the racemic mixture of 1-hydroxytacrine enantiomers (previously investigated for antidementia activity). Metabolites of velnacrine itself reflect hydroxylation of either the alicyclic or aromatic rings in a pattern analogous to that for tacrine (15).

There is substantial, unequivocal evidence from experiments with human liver microsomes, rat hepatocyte suspensions, and perfused rat liver that oxidation of tacrine produces one or more reactive electrophilic intermediates that bind irreversibly to cellular proteins (11,16–19). Associations between this bioactivation and elevations of serum alanine aminotransferase has been an important question because of a high incidence of reversible hepatic injury in patients initially treated with tacrine. Mechanisms by which sequential oxidation of the aliphatic and aromatic rings can lead to a reactive quinone methide intermediate have been elucidated (11,17,19).

Predominant Role of CYP1A2

A preponderance of metabolic and pharmacokinetic data indicate that cytochrome P450 1A2 (CYP1A2) is responsible for virtually all oxidative metabolism of tacrine. Spaldin et al. (20) used tacrine as a specific substrate to measure CYP1A2 activity *in vitro*. Rates of formation of 1-, 2-, 4-, and 7-hydroxytacrine were significantly correlated with CYP1A2 apoprotein content in 16 human liver samples quantified with a monospecific antibody. The total rate of formation of tacrine metabolites was significantly correlated with rate of 3-methylxanthine formation from theophylline, a reaction distinguishing the CYP1A2 isoform. Experiments with perfused livers from rats pretreated with 3-methylcholanthrene (3-MC) helped to corroborate the predominant role of CYP1A2 in tacrine metabolism (21). Pretreatment with this potent CYP1A2 (ortholog) inducer led to a seven-fold increase in tacrine clearance from the perfusate. Furafylline, a specific inhibitor of CYP1A2, markedly inhibited tacrine-derived protein binding in hepatocytes obtained from induced rats.

A clinically useful measure of CYP1A2 activity, the caffeine breath test, was investigated as a means of identifying patients most susceptible to tacrine-induced liver toxicity (22). Before the beginning of tacrine therapy, the test was administered to 37 AD patients. Caffeine demethylation rate was not correlated with peak serum transaminase levels; thus the breath test was not useful for predicting tacrine-induced injury. Caffeine-demethylation rate was correlated ($r^2 = 0.69$; $p = 0.003$) with the logarithm of steady-state plasma tacrine concentration in 10 patients, a result consistent with the premise that tacrine metabolic clearance is due to CYP1A2.

The researchers at Parke-Davis Pharmaceutical Research and at the University of Liverpool have accrued convincing evidence indicating that it is the CYP1A2 isoform that produces the tacrine metabolites that bind irreversibly to cellular proteins (14,16,17,20,21). In the presence of human liver microsomes, tacrine underwent reduced nicotinamide adenine dinucleotide phosphate (NADPH)-dependent bioactivation to compounds toxic to human lymphocytes. Enoxacin and furafylline, highly specific inhibitors of the CYP1A2 isoform, significantly inhibited bioactivation and production of all monitored tacrine metabolites (16,17,21). A strong and significant correlation between aromatic and alicyclic hydroxylation rates was consistent with the premise that both reactions proceeded through CYP1A2 (20).

Clinical Drug Interactions

Drug interactions affecting tacrine pharmacokinetics reported to date can be understood in terms of inhibition of hepatic CYP1A2, leading to reduced presystemic and systemic clearance. Anecdotal clinical reports of interactions between tacrine and ibuprofen (23) or haloperidol (24) may have a pharmacodynamic basis. Fluvoxamine, a selective serotonin reuptake inhibitor for antidepressant therapy, is a potent CYP1A2 inhibitor that has been coadministered with tacrine to patients with Alzheimer's dementia. In 1996, Becquemont et al. (25) demonstrated that fluvoxamine inhibited the metabolism of tacrine in vitro, and in 1997, they reported (26) the clinical significance of this interaction. In a double-blind, crossover study, 13 healthy volunteers received either fluvoxamine (100 mg/day) or placebo for 6 days, and pharmacokinetics of a single 40-mg dose of tacrine were determined. Fluvoxamine coadministration caused an eight-fold decrease in tacrine oral clearance (CL/F) with a corresponding eight-fold increase in systemic exposure, as assessed by area-under-the-curve (AUC) values. A statistically significant increase in AUC values for 1-, 2-, and 4-hydroxytacrine and a three-fold increase in urinary recovery of tacrine and these metabolites was observed. It is noteworthy that clearance of these primary metabolites, as well as metabolic clearance of tacrine itself, was diminished by fluvoxamine, presumably because all these reactions are CYP1A2 dependent.

In a study by Forgue et al. (27), 12 healthy elderly subjects received 40 mg tacrine either alone or during multiple-dose cimetidine (300 mg, q.i.d.) administration. Cimetidine is a nonspecific inhibitor of cytochrome P450 isoforms including CYP1A2. After cimetidine coadministration, systemic exposure to tacrine was about 33% higher than that after administration of tacrine alone. Although the CL/F value was reduced by 30%, elimination $t_{1/2}$ values for the two treatments were equivalent, suggesting no change in tacrine systemic clearance. This pattern has been reported repeatedly for coadministration of cimetidine with other drugs subject to high hepatic extraction (e.g., ref. 28). Rapid and extensive absorption can lead to high drug concentrations in the portal vein, partial saturation of first pass hepatic extraction in the presence of cimetidine, and hence an increase in oral bioavailability.

Polycyclic aromatic hydrocarbons in cigarette smoke are well-known inducers of CYP1A2; thus it is hardly surprising that plasma tacrine concentrations in smokers are markedly lower than those in nonsmokers (29). During early clinical development of tacrine, the possibility that CYP2D6 was involved in metabolism and that polymorphic expression of this isoform might be partially responsible for high between-patient variability was investigated by deVries et al. (30). Quinidine is a potent and selective inhibitor of CYP2D6. Coadministration of a single, 40-mg tacrine dose during repeated (100 mg every 8 hours) quinidine dosing had no consistent effect on noncompartmental parameters, indicating little if any role of this isoform in tacrine metabolism.

Tacrine can alter the pharmacokinetics of other drugs. Because of extensive metabolism and/or a narrow therapeutic index, deVries et al. (31) investigated whether tacrine affected the disposition of theophylline, diazepam, and digoxin. Lack of an effect on plasma concentrations of either diazepam or digoxin is consistent with an absence of any known role of CYP1A2 in their clearance. In contrast, theophylline is well characterized as a CYP1A2 substrate. Coadministration of tacrine (20 mg every 6 hours) with a 200-mg aminophylline tablet single dose increased the mean AUC value by 86% and nearly doubled the half-life. Excretion of unchanged theophylline was accompanied by significant decreases of 72% and 91% in excretion of 1-methyl uric acid and 3-methylxanthine, whereas excretion of 1,3-dimethyl uric acid was only slightly affected. This pattern is consistent with the contribution of CYP1A2 in the metabolic pathways of theophylline.

Donepezil

After oral administration, donepezil hydrochloride (Aricept, (R,S)-1-benzyl-4-[(5,6-dimethoxy-1-indanon)-2-yl] methylpiperidine hydrochloride, E2020) is rapidly and completely absorbed, with the C_{max} occurring approximately 3 hours after a single oral dose (32,33). Neither food nor administration time of day influenced the rate or extent of absorption (32,33). Time to C_{max} was shorter after multiple-dose administration as compared with single doses; this was postulated to be due to the pharmacologic action (increased motility) of donepezil on the gastrointestinal tract. Pharmacokinetics after oral doses of from 2 to 10 mg were adequately described by using a two-compartment open, linear pharmacokinetic model (32). Donepezil does not undergo presystemic metabolism (bioavailability is 100%). The α-phase and elimination $t_{1/2}$ values for donepezil are about 1.5 hours and approximately 70 hours, respectively, and mean (±SD) CL/F value is 9.1 (±3.2) L/h (32,34). After multiple-dose administration, donepezil accumulated 450%, and steady state was achieved after about 2 weeks. Clearance estimates after single and multiple doses were in good agreement with each other, consistent with linear kinetics. That is, neither autoinduction nor end-product inhibition of donepezil metabolism was apparent. Donepezil is about 95% bound to plasma albumin (about 75%) and α_1-acid glycoprotein (about 21%) over the therapeutic concentration range of 2 to 1,000 ng/mL (32,33). Donepezil, a highly lipid soluble drug, has a large volume of distribution (800 to 1,000 L; 12 L/kg), reflecting extensive distribution throughout the body (32,34). V_d value in elderly subjects (age 65–82 years) was about 40% higher than that in younger individuals. Although body-fat measurements were not reported, Ohnishi et al. (34) attributed this increase to a higher percentage of body fat in older subjects. Values for CL/F were similar, and $t_{1/2}$ values were prolonged in the elderly as compared with younger individuals. As such, similar steady-state concentrations will be achieved in younger and elderly patients, but it may take as long as 3 weeks to reach steady state in older patients. Renal elimination of unchanged drug accounts for only about 10% of total clearance (32,34). A study of four patients with moderate to severe renal impairment (CL_{cr}, less than 22 mL/min/1.73 m^2) revealed that clearance did not differ from results in four age- and sex-matched healthy subjects (33).

Metabolism

Donepezil is extensively metabolized to four major and a number of minor metabolites, not all of which have been identified (32,33,35,36). Identified metabolites include the 6-demethyl- (M1), the 5-demethyl- (M2), the 4′-hydroxy- (M3), and debenzyl-donepezil (M4), as well as a cis-N-oxide (M6), and the glucuronide conjugates of M1 and M2 (35,36). M1 inhibits acetylcholinesterase to the same extent as does donepezil in vitro (33). M2 should also bind to the acetylcholinesterase inhibition site and is presumably pharmacologically active (37,38). After single oral doses of up to 10 mg and multiple-dose administration of 2 mg per day, metabolite plasma concentrations were less than 0.5 ng/mL, the assay limit

(32,35,36). Mihara et al. (32) characterized the urinary and fecal recovery of donepezil and its metabolites. As expected with this long-half-life drug, excretion was not complete in 264 hours. Mean fecal excretion was 8.6%, and total recovery in urine and feces 264 hours after the dose was 45% of the dose. After administration of [^{14}C]donepezil, plasma radioactivity was present primarily as intact donepezil (33). Plasma M1 concentrations were about 20% of those for donepezil (33). Of the total radioactivity administered 57% was recovered in urine and 15% in feces over a 10-day period. Approximately 17% of the dose was recovered in the urine as unchanged donepezil. Donepezil is metabolized by CYP2D6 and CYP3A4 (33). In vitro studies show low-affinity binding to these enzymes (K_i is 50–130 μM). Therapeutic concentrations almost 1,000-fold lower (164 nM) than these K_i values suggest a low likelihood of a clinically important interference.

A study in patients with stable alcoholic cirrhosis revealed that donepezil clearance was 20% lower than that for healthy age-matched and sex-matched subjects (33). Whereas decreases on the order of 20% are usually considered not be clinically significant, it should be noted that for this long-$t_{1/2}$ compound, a 20% decrease in clearance would prolong the elimination $t_{1/2}$ by 20 hours, assuming a constant V_d.

Clinical Drug Interactions

Clinically important drug–drug interactions could arise from interference with protein binding or metabolic clearance of donepezil. In vitro drug-displacement studies were conducted between donepezil and other highly bound drugs (33). Donepezil concentrations of 0.3 to 10 μg/mL did not affect the binding of furosemide, digoxin, and warfarin to human albumin. Similarly, donepezil binding to human albumin was not affected by furosemide, digoxin, and warfarin. Furthermore, in pharmacokinetic studies of potential interactions between donepezil and warfarin or digoxin, no significant effects were observed (33). In studies evaluating the potential of donepezil for interaction with theophylline (a CYP1A2 substrate), cimetidine (a nonspecific inhibitor of various CYP450 isoforms), no significant effects were observed (33). Clinical trials investigating the effect of donepezil on the clearance of drugs metabolized by CYP3A4 (cisapride, terfenadine) or by CYP2D6 (e.g., imipramine) have not been reported. Although ketoconazole (CYP3A4 inhibitor) and quinidine (CYP2D6 inhibitor) inhibit donepezil metabolism in vitro, no clinically important interactions with these inhibitors have been reported. Inducers of CYP3A4 (e.g., phenytoin, carbamazepine, and phenobarbital) could increase donepezil clearance. There are no known inducers of CYP2D6.

MIGRAINE

Sumatriptan

After subcutaneous injection, sumatriptan (Imitrex; 3-[2-dimethoamino) ethyl]-N-methyl-1H-indole-5-methanesulfonamide succinate is rapidly and completely absorbed (39,40). After oral administration, sumatriptan also is rapidly absorbed, but bioavailability is low (about 14%). C_{max} values are achieved within 20 minutes after subcutaneous dosing and about 1 hour after a 100-mg single oral dose. The apparent absorption rate decreased with increasing dose; average t_{max} values increased from 1 to 3 hours as oral doses increased from 100 mg to 400 mg. However, multiple plasma peaks were evident, especially at doses greater than 100 mg. Increased t_{max} values reflect the subsequent peaks, as initial peak concentration was achieved in less than 1 hour. As such, the apparent decreased absorption rate probably reflects a prolonged absorption phase for the larger doses. Absolute oral bioavailability (F_{abs}) was low (14%) and variable; the coefficient of variation for C_{max} was 60% for oral doses, whereas that for subcutaneous doses was only 20% (39–41). Lower F_{abs} values also may be due to incomplete absorption, as almost 10% of an oral dose is excreted unchanged in the feces. Sumatriptan pharmacokinetics are not affected by food (39). Extent of absorption was linear up to 16-mg subcutaneous doses and up to 400-mg oral doses. Low and variable F_{abs} values suggest presystemic metabolism in the gastrointestinal tract and/or the liver. Plasma protein binding is low (16%), and V_d is large, 170 L, indicating extensive tissue distribution of the compound (39–41). The elimination $t_{1/2}$ is about 2 hours, and total plasma clearance is about 1.2 L/min. Although renal clearance (CL_r) is only 20% of total clearance, sumatriptan is actively secreted by the renal tubules. The primary process of elimination is metabolism, and the hepatic extraction ratio is 0.59.

Metabolism

Sumatriptan undergoes oxidative N-deamination of the N-dimethyl side chain to form the primary metabolite, the (inactive) indole acetic acid analogue (39–43). The majority of the dose is recovered as the indole acetic acid analogue. After oral and subcutaneous doses, 2% and 22% of the dose is recovered in urine as the parent compound, and 35% and 41% of the dose is recovered urine as the major metabolite, respectively (39). Relatively high (6 to 7 times parent) plasma concentrations of the major metabolite are consistent with extensive presystemic metabolism. Metabolite and parent $t_{1/2}$ values are also similar, indicating that metabolite clearance is formation rate limited (39). A minor metabolite, the ester glucuronide conjugate of the primary metabolite, also has been recovered from human urine (40).

Predominant Role of Monoamine Oxidase-A

Investigations by Dixon et al. (43) revealed that sumatriptan is primarily metabolized by monoamine oxidase-A (MAO-A). By using human liver *in vitro* ($n = 4$), Dixon et al. investigated the potential involvement of the cytochrome P450 and MAO enzyme systems to determine their role in the metabolism of sumatriptan. Sumatriptan metabolism was independent of NADPH. By using [^{14}C]testosterone as a probe, these investigators found no evidence to indicate that cytochrome P450 is involved. Both MAO inhibitors clorgyline (MAO-A) and deprenyl (MAO-B) inhibited sumatriptan metabolism, with clorgyline being a more effective inhibitor (more than 92% inhibition at concentrations of 2 to 200 μ*M*).

Clinical Drug Interactions

Coadministration of MAO inhibitors such as tranylcypromine sulfate (antidepressant), furazolidone (broad-spectrum antibiotic), isocarboxazid, pargyline, phenelzine (antidepressant), and procarbazine will significantly affect the pharmacokinetics of sumatriptan. By decreasing clearance and significantly increasing oral bioavailability, MAO-inhibitor coadministration will increase the systemic exposure of sumatriptan. After pretreatment with an MAO-A inhibitor and subcutaneous sumatriptan administration, both AUC and $t_{1/2}$ values increased markedly; clearance value decreased markedly (44). More significant changes are expected with oral sumatriptan administration. No significant effect was observed with the MAO-B inhibitor (44).

Because of the likelihood of coadministration of drugs commonly used for prophylaxis of migraine, interactions with propranolol, butorphanol, flunarizine, and pizotifen were investigated (45–48). No significant interactions were found. The lack of interaction with propranolol, a CYP2D6 substrate and known inhibitor of oxidative metabolism, is consistent with the previous conclusion that cytochrome P450 is not involved in sumatriptan metabolism (49).

Zolmitriptan

After oral administration, zolmitriptan (Zomig; (S)-4[[3-2-(dimethylamino)ethyl]-1H-indol-5-yl]methyl2-oxazolidinone) is rapidly absorbed; bioavailability is about 40% (50–52). C_{max} is achieved within 2 hours after an oral dose. Zolmitriptan pharmacokinetics are linear (51). Zolmitriptan plasma concentrations and its metabolites were decreased during a migraine attack; this was attributed to decreased absorption resulting from temporary gastric stasis during the migraine attack (50). Plasma protein binding is relatively low (25%), and V_d value is large, 140 L (52). Total plasma clearance is approximately 2 L/min; CL_r is greater than glomerular filtration rate. Thus as with sumatriptan, naratriptan, and rizatriptan, zolmitriptan undergoes renal tubular secretion. The apparent elimination $t_{1/2}$ of zolmitriptan is about 3 hours.

Metabolite Identification

Zolmitriptan is metabolized to one active, *N*-desmethyl-, and two inactive metabolites, *N*-oxide- and indole acetic acid-zolmitriptan (50,51). Active metabolite concentration relative to parent is 50% to 80%. Relative concentrations of the inactive *N*-oxide are 40% to 80% of parent and those for the indole acetic acid metabolite are up to double that for parent (51). Relatively high metabolite concentrations suggest that zolmitriptan undergoes presystemic metabolism. Elimination $t_{1/2}$ values for the metabolites are similar to those of the parent (3 hours), indicating that metabolite clearance is formation rate limited. The majority of a ^{14}C-labeled dose is recovered as the indole acetic acid analogue (31%); 3%, 4%, and 8% is recovered as *N*-oxide-, *N*-desmethyl, and zolmitriptan, respectively (52). Investigations identifying the enzyme system(s) responsible for zolmitriptan metabolism have not been reported. However, some insight can be drawn from drug-interaction study results.

Clinical Drug Interactions

Acetaminophen, a substrate for multiple CYP isoforms, did not affect zolmitriptan or *N*-desmethyl zolmitriptan pharmacokinetics (52). After administration of cimetidine, a nonspecific inhibitor of CYP isoforms, $t_{1/2}$ and AUC values of zolmitriptan and *N*-desmethyl-zolmitriptan doubled. Zolmitriptan pharmacokinetics were not affected by coadministration of the CYP2D6 inhibitor, fluoxetine. However, they were affected (50% increase in plasma concentrations) after 1 week of dosing with propranolol. Retrospective analysis across studies revealed that zolmitriptan plasma concentrations are 30% to 50% higher in women taking oral contraceptives. Although it appears that CYP2D6 is not responsible for zolmitriptan metabolism, these results suggest that other CYP isoforms play a role. Coadministration of the specific MAO-A inhibitor, meclobemide, resulted in a 25% increase in plasma concentrations of zolmitriptan, whereas plasma concentrations of *N*-desmethyl zolmitriptan increased 300%. Coadministration of the selective MAO-B inhibitor, selegiline, did not affect zolmitriptan or its active metabolite pharmacokinetics. These clinical drug-interaction studies reveal that MAO-A and CYP isoforms metabolize zolmitriptan. There is no evidence that MAO-B and CYP2D6 contribute.

Rizatriptan

After oral administration, rizatriptan (Maxalt; *N,N*-dimethyl-2-[5-(1,2,4-triazol-1-ylmethyl)-1H-indol-3-yl]ethylamine benzoate) is rapidly absorbed (53–55). C_{max} values are achieved within 1 to 1.5 hours after oral administration. Oral bioavailability after a 10-mg oral dose was estimated at 40%. Rizatriptan pharmacokinetics are linear for intravenous (i.v.) doses less than 5 mg and oral doses up to 20 mg; at i.v. doses greater than 5 mg and at oral doses of 40 and 60 mg, rizatriptan behaves nonlinearly (53,54). Mean AUC value for a 40-mg oral dose was 5.3 times that for a 10-mg dose. As with sumatriptan, rizatriptan protein binding is low (14%), and V_d value is large, 140 L (male subjects), indicating extensive tissue distribution of the compound (55). The elimination $t_{1/2}$ is about 2 hours, and total plasma clearance is about 2 L/min (53,54). The primary process of elimination is metabolism, and rizatriptan undergoes substantial first pass metabolism (55). Plasma concentrations were not changed for patients with mild hepatic impairment but were increased 30% for patients with moderate hepatic impairment. CL_R is only about 20% of total clearance, and rizatriptan (a weak base) is actively renally secreted by the renal tubules. The AUC value was not changed in patients with renal impairment (creatinine clearance, 10–60 mL/min/1.73 m^2) as compared with that of healthy subjects, but it was increased 44% for hemodialysis patients.

Metabolite Identification

Rizatriptan undergoes oxidative deamination to form the primary metabolite, the (inactive) indole acetic acid analogue (55). After oral administration of [^{14}C]rizatriptan, 51% of the dose was excreted in urine as the primary metabolite, whereas only 14% was recovered as unchanged drug. A minor metabolite, *N*-monodesmethyl-rizatriptan, has similar activity to that of the parent. Plasma concentrations are about 14% of those for parent, and elimination rates are similar. Other identified minor (inactive) metabolites include the *N*-oxide, the 6-hydroxy-rizatriptan, and its sulfate conjugate.

Predominant Role of MAO-A

As with sumatriptan, investigators found no significant role of cytochrome P450 in rizatriptan metabolism. Rizatriptan does not inhibit the activity of human liver cytochrome P450 isoforms CYP3A4/5, CYP1A2, CYP2C9, CYP2C19, or CYP2E1 (55). Although rizatriptan does competitively inhibit CYP2D6 (K_i, 1,400 nM), this was only at clinically irrelevant concentrations. MAO-A is responsible for rizatriptan metabolism (55).

Clinical Drug Interactions

Drug interactions are expected with MAO-A and non-selective MAO inhibitors such as isocarboxazid, pargy-line, phenelzine, and tranylcypromine. Coadministration of the selectively reversible MAO-A inhibitor, meclobemide, resulted in an 119% and 400% increase in AUC values for rizatriptan and *N*-monodesmethyl-rizatriptan, respectively (55). A greater change in pharmacokinetics is expected with an irreversible inhibitor. A study in 18 women revealed that rizatriptan did not affect plasma concentrations of ethinyl estradiol or norethindrone (55). Because of the likelihood of coadministration of drugs commonly used for prophylaxis of migraine, interactions with propranolol, nadolol, metoprolol, and paroxetine were investigated (55). No significant interactions were found with nadolol, metoprolol, and paroxetine. A significant interaction was observed with concurrent administration of 240 mg/day propranolol and 10 mg rizatriptan. Mean rizatriptan plasma AUC increased 70% (400% in one subject); the AUC of the active *N*-desmethyl metabolite was not changed. Data were not provided for the major metabolite. Although in the *in vitro* studies, rizatriptan inhibited CYP2D6 only at clinically irrelevant concentrations, these clinical results suggest that CYP2D6 may play a role in rizatriptan metabolism. It is interesting to note that propranolol did not affect sumatriptan (45). Further investigation is needed to elucidate the role CYP2D6 in rizatriptan metabolism.

Naratriptan

Very little has been published on the metabolism of naratriptan (Amerge; *N*-methyl-3-1-(1-methyl-4-piperidinyl)-1H-indole-5 ethanesulfonamide monohydrochloride). After oral administration, naratriptan is well absorbed; bioavailability is about 70% (56). C_{max} values are achieved 2 to 3 hours after an oral dose, and pharmacokinetics are linear over the therapeutic dose range. Plasma concentrations in women are higher than those for men. Plasma protein binding is relatively low (30%), and V_d value is large, 170 L (56). Total plasma clearance is 0.5 L/min; CL_R (220 mL/min) greater than glomerular filtration rate indicates that naratriptan undergoes renal tubular secretion. The apparent elimination $t_{1/2}$ of naratriptan is 6 hours. Smoking increased the naratriptan clearance by 30%. As smoking is known to induce CYP1A2, the role of CYP1A2 in naratriptan metabolism should be evaluated (29). Naratriptan is eliminated primarily in the urine; urinary recovery of parent drug and metabolites is 50% and 30%, respectively. Naratriptan is metabolized into a number of inactive metabolites by a wide range of cytochrome P450 isoenzymes.

Population pharmacokinetic analysis indicated that naratriptan clearance was not affected by fluoxetine (a CYP2D6 inhibitor), β-blockers, or tricyclic antidepressants. Coadministration of naratriptan with oral contraceptives resulted in decreased (32%) naratriptan clearance; this may be due to competitive inhibition of CYP1A2 or CYP3A4.

Methysergide

Ergot alkaloids such as methysergide, ergotamine, and dihydroergotamine are used in the treatment of migraine headaches. Oral bioavailability of methysergide maleate (Sansert; 9,10-didehydro-N-[1-(hydroxymethyl)propyl]-1,6-dimethylergoline-8-carboxamide maleate) is about 13%. Methysergide undergoes extensive first pass metabolism to form methylergometrine, the primary metabolite (57,58). Two other potential metabolites have been observed in human plasma (57). Methylergometrine plasma concentrations exceed those of methysergide within 1 hour of dosing. Methylergometrine C_{max} values were 3 times higher, and AUC values were 10 times higher than those for methysergide. After oral administration, the plasma $t_{1/2}$ value for the metabolite is much longer than that for parent drug (4 hours vs. 1 hour) (58). Experiments in conscious dogs confirmed that methysergide is rapidly and extensively metabolized (by N-demethylation at the 1 position of the indole) to methylergometrine (59). Both compounds were equally active venoconstrictor agents after oral administration; methylergometrine is the primary active component in the therapeutic effectiveness of methysergide (59).

Dihydroergotamine

Oral bioavailability of dihydroergotamine mesylate (DHE) is very low (less than 1%) (60,61). After intramuscular (i.m.) injection, C_{max} values are achieved within 30 minutes (62). After intravenous injection, Little et al. (61) estimated plasma clearance as 1 L/min; α- and β-$t_{1/2}$ values were 0.2 hour and 2.4 hours, respectively; $V_{d\beta}$ was 14.5 L/kg. Kanto et al. (63) reported a similar clearance value, but β-$t_{1/2}$ and $V_{d\beta}$ values were smaller, 0.5 hours and 0.63 L/kg. Kanto characterized the plasma concentration–time profile for only 4 hours after the dose. As Little et al. characterized the DHE profile for 8 hours after the dose, theirs may be a better estimation. About 7% of an i.m. dose is excreted in the urine; the majority of the dose is excreted in the feces after biliary excretion of unchanged drug and metabolites (64). The pharmacologic effect is sustained longer than plasma concentrations of parent or metabolites and is thought to be due to drug/metabolite(s) deposition in a peripheral-effect compartment (vascular smooth-muscle cells) (65,66).

Metabolite Identification

The metabolism profile of DHE was characterized after oral administration of [³H]dihydroergotamine to six healthy male volunteers (67). In vitro hepatic biotransformation also was investigated; microsomes were obtained from the livers of adult postmortem donors, male Han–Wistar rat livers, and male cynomolgus monkeys. The chromatographic properties of the primary metabolite (metabolite 4, M4) were similar to those of DHE (67).

The ultraviolet (UV) spectrum in methanol for DHE and for M4 also were identical. Results indicated that the indole structure was intact in M4. Amino-acid analysis indicated that the only amino acid present was phenylalanine. Mass spectral data revealed that the dihydrolysergic acid amide moiety was intact. Major evidence for the proposed structure was obtained from the 1H-NMR spectrum. The triplet of only one H-C8' was found; it corresponded to the signal of H-C8' of 8'β-hydroxy-DHE. M4 is a mixture (30:70) of 8'α-and 8'β-hydroxy-DHE. Seven metabolites formed through the following four pathways were proposed for biotransformation in humans: (a) hydroxylation or dihydroxylation of the proline ring: metabolites 4 and 5 (8'-hydroxy-DHE and 8',10'-dihydroxy-DHE); (b) oxidation of 8'-hydroxy-DHE to the carboxylic acid derivative (metabolite 3); (c) oxidative hydrolysis of the amide bond, leading to the dihydrolysergic acid and its amide: metabolites 1 and 2 [9,10-dihydrolysergic acid (DH-LS) and 9,10-dihydro-lysergic acid amide (DH-LSA)]; and (d) oxidation of the indole ring: metabolites 6 and 7 [2,3 seco,N(1)formyl,3-keto,8'-hydroxy-DHE and 2,3 seco,N(1)formyl,3-keto,8',10'-dihydroxy-DHE] (67). In humans, DHE, 8'-dihydroxy-DHE, DH-LS, and DH-LSA were detected and quantified in plasma and urine (67). In plasma and urine samples, 29% to 76% of radioactivity were identified compounds. DHE was present in very low concentrations (3% to 14% of plasma radioactivity). Almost half (44%) of the plasma radioactivity at 0 to 2 hours after the dose was identified as 8'-dihydroxy-DHE. Concentrations in urine for all identified compounds were less than 0.2%; the most prominent compound was the 8'-dihydroxy-DHE (0.18% of dose). Several more polar components were present but could not be identified. In vitro, the only metabolite that could be detected was 8'-dihydroxy-DHE (67). Its formation rate was similar to the disappearance rate of DHE.

Receptor binding studies performed with mammalian brain preparations revealed that the activity of the major metabolite, 8'-dihydroxy-DHE, was similar to that of DHE (67). More extensive studies of DHE, 8'-OH-DHE, 8',10'-dihydroxy-DHE, 8'-OH,N(1)formyl-DHE, DH-LSA, and DH-LS were conducted on human and canine veins in vitro, on canine veins in situ, and on rats in vivo (68). In the experimental rat model, results indicated that an intact ergoline moiety was essential, as DH-LS, DH-LSA, and 8'-OH,N(1)formyl-DHE lacked venoconstriction activity. DHE, 8'-hydroxy-, and 8',10'-dihydroxy-DHE had venoconstrictor activity. The major metabolite, 8'-hydroxy-DHE, is at least as potent as DHE, and is present in concentrations several times that of DHE.

Predominant Role of CYP3A4

Reported clinical drug interactions between macrolide antibiotics and ergot alkaloids led to the further investigation of DHE metabolism. In 1983, Martinet and Kiechel (69) found that coadministration of triacetyloleandomycin and DHE (oral and hepatoportal administration) in mini-pigs resulted in significantly increased AUC values; thus the interaction was at the hepatic site and was not due to altered absorption.

In 1989 Delaforge et al. (70) conducted more extensive studies with microsomes from male Sprague–Dawley rats pretreated with phenobarbitone (PB), 3-MC, troleandomycin (TAO), or pregnenolone 16α-carbonitrile (PCN). DHE elicited a type I spectral interaction with hepatic microsomes from control and pretreated rats. Results confirmed that DHE binds to the same cytochrome P450 as that complexed with TAO metabolite. DHE also interacted strongly with microsomes from PCN-treated rats. Mean (n = 3) dissociation constant (K_s) values for TAO- and PCN-treated rats were 2.3 to 2.9×10^{-6} M. Results with PB-treated rats were less marked, consistent with their CYP3A isozyme content. Regression analysis between DHE binding and TAO-metabolite complex formation revealed that the same amounts of the same isozymes were involved in DHE binding and macrolide binding and metabolism. Four metabolites were observed in the rat hepatic microsomal incubations; the major metabolite was 8′-hydroxy-DHE. Microsomes from the PB- and PCN-treated rats had much higher metabolizing activity than those for control and 3-MC–treated rats (70). Pretreatment with TAO led to inhibition (70%) of DHE metabolism; however, activity was restored after treatment with ferricyanide. Whereas more than one cytochrome P450 isozyme may be induced in rats after PCN treatment, these experiments revealed that the same isozymes were involved in macrolide–cytochrome P450 complex formation and DHE metabolism.

Peyronneau et al. (71) reported that P450s 3A exhibited a high affinity for DHE. Rats were pretreated with a variety of enzyme inducers including TAO and dexamethasone (strong inducers of CYP3A4). As expected, a strong spectral interaction was seen between DHE and dexamethasone and DHE- and TAO-derived (treated with K ferricyanide) microsomes. Addition of DHE to microsomes of yeast producing either allelic form of human CYP3A4 (P450 NF25 or P450 hPCN1) also led to a type-1 difference visible spectrum with a K_s value around 0.7 μM. In both pretreated rat microsomes and yeast-derived human P450s, the lysergic acid derivatives (DH-LS and DH-LSA) failed to produce a spectral interaction (71). Thus the tripeptide moiety was essential for the interaction with the CYP3A active site.

Clinical Drug Interactions

Drug interactions with ergotamine derivatives and macrolide antibiotics have been reported (72,73). Coadministration of erythromycin and ergotamine was associated with the induction of ischemia and peripheral vasospasm (73). Given the central role of CYP3A4 in

DHE metabolism, drug interactions resulting in increased DHE concentrations (decreased DHE metabolism) may be anticipated with CYP3A4 inhibitors such as ketoconazole, macrolide antibiotics, fluconazole, and cimetidine. CYP3A4 inducers such as dexamethasone, barbiturates, carbamazepine, and phenytoin may cause decreased DHE concentrations (increased DHE metabolism). One also must consider the contribution of the major (active) metabolite when speculating about drug interactions of DHE. Whereas the metabolism of 8′-hydroxy-DHE has not been defined, it is likely that the CYP3A4 plays an important role. Any drug inhibiting DHE metabolism would probably also inhibit 8′-hydroxy-DHE metabolism.

Ergotamine

Assay-sensitivity limitations have hampered the characterization of ergotamine pharmacokinetics. Several investigators have studied oral, intravenous, intramuscular, rectal, and buccal absorption (63,74–85). Ergotamine oral absorption is highly variable and low. The most complete characterization was by Sanders et al. (83), who characterized ergotamine plasma concentrations after oral and rectal (with caffeine) administration with a triple-sector mass spectrometric technique. Oral bioavailability was estimated as 5%, and CL/F, V_d, and $t_{1/2}$ values were 2.8 L/h, 550 L, and 3.3 hours after rectal administration, respectively. Ergotamine appears to be well absorbed but undergoes first pass metabolism. Analytic methods used previously may not have the specificity of the mass spectrometric assay and probably included metabolite(s) in the ergotamine quantitation. As with DHE, the pharmacologic effect is sustained longer than ergotamine plasma concentrations (81). The sustained effect may be due to active metabolites and/or tissue binding (peripheral compartment). Caffeine has been reported to increase the rate and extent of ergotamine absorption (85). Caffeine was coadministered with ergotamine in other studies, but assay sensitivity prevented delineation of caffeine's role in ergotamine absorption.

Metabolism: Predominant Role of CYP3A4

After oral administration of [³H]ergotamine, cumulative urinary excretion of radioactivity in 24 hours was about 2% of the dose (85). Here again, limited assay sensitivity hampered characterization and quantitation of ergotamine. As with DHE, CYP3A4 appears to be responsible for ergotamine metabolism. In experiments with rat liver microsomes, ergotamine had a high affinity for macrolide- or PCN-induced cytochromes P450; ergotamine was poorly recognized by other isoforms (86).

Clinical Drug Interactions

Drug interactions with ergotamine derivatives and macrolide antibiotics have been reported (72,73). Coadministration of erythromycin and ergotamine was associated with the induction of ischemia and peripheral vasospasm (73). Cyclosporine, metabolized by CYP3A4, interacted with ergotamine in vitro and would be expected to interact in vivo (88). Although ergotamine metabolism has not been characterized as well as that for DHE, similar drug interactions would be expected. Increased ergotamine and metabolite concentrations may be anticipated with CYP3A4 inhibitors such as ketoconazole, macrolide antibiotics, fluconazole, and cimetidine. CYP3A4 inducers such as dexamethasone, barbiturates, carbamazepine, and phenytoin may cause increased ergotamine metabolism.

PARKINSON'S DISEASE

Levodopa

In the brain, levodopa, $(-)$-L-α-amino-β-(3,4-dihydroxybenzene) propanoic acid, is decarboxylated to form dopamine, which is responsible for the therapeutic effect in Parkinson's disease (89,90). Dopamine does not cross the blood–brain barrier and extra–central nervous system (CNS) conversion of levodopa to dopamine contributes only to side effects, particularly nausea. After oral administration, levodopa is absorbed in the proximal small intestine through the large neutral amino acid active transport system. About 30% of a dose reaches the circulation intact because of first pass metabolism in the gut (primarily) and liver by aromatic L-amino acid decarboxylase (AAAD), and only about 1% reaches the brain because of metabolism by circulating enzymes. The plasma elimination $t_{1/2}$ is only 1 to 3 hours.

Metabolism

The four pathways for levodopa metabolism are decarboxylation, O-methylation, transamination, and oxidation (89,90). Decarboxylation through AAAD is the major pathway, as about 70% of the dose recovered in the urine are dopamine and its metabolites. Dopamine is metabolized by MAO and catechol-O-methyltransferase (COMT) to form homovanillic acid (HVA). (In the brain, MAO-B is the prominent isoform.) Methoxylation by COMT to form 3-O-methyldopa accounts for about 10% of levodopa metabolism. The major end products of transamination are vanillpyruvate, vanillacetate, and 2,4,5-trihydroxyphenylacetic acid. The finding of cysteinyldopa in urine is suggestive of oxidation through a dopa quinone intermediate (89).

Carbidopa Coadministration

Because of the extensive peripheral metabolism, levodopa is most often administered with the potent inhibitor of extracerebral AAAD, carbidopa [$(-)$-L-α-hydrazino-3,4-dihydroxy-α-methylbenzenepropanoic acid monohydrate] (89–91), so the levodopa–carbidopa combination is a planned metabolic drug interaction. Carbidopa does not cross the blood–brain barrier; it inhibits only peripheral AAAD. With carbidopa coadministration, peripheral conversion of levodopa to dopamine is significantly reduced, leading to decreased nausea and increased availability of levodopa to be transported into the brain (92). Formation of HVA also was reduced. Carbidopa coadministration (more than 75 mg) permits the use of lower levodopa doses. Oral bioavailability of carbidopa is about 50% (93–95). After administration of radiolabeled carbidopa, one third of that recovered in urine was parent compound (94,95). Carbidopa undergoes aromatic dehydroxylation to form α-methyl-3-(3-hydroxyphenyl)propionic acid (10%) and side-chain degradation to form α-methyl-3-(3-methoxy-4-hydroxyphenyl) propionic acid (10%–14%), α-methyl-3-4(3,4-dihydroxyphenyl)propionic acid (10%), and 3,4-dihydroxyphenylacetone (5%), which are excreted as glucuronide conjugates.

Pyridoxine

Pyridoxine coadministration significantly affects levodopa metabolism; dopamine plasma concentrations decreased 70%, and HVA concentrations increased (92). However, with carbidopa coadministration, pyridoxine had no significant effect (92,93).

Drug Interactions

Drug interactions with levodopa can be due to interference with absorption or transport, to pharmacologic interaction, and to metabolic interaction (96–98). Prolongation of gastric residence time increases levodopa exposure to gastric AAAD and may increase its conversion to dopamine. Coadministration with food and anticholinergics cause decreased gastric transit and could decrease levodopa bioavailability. Coadministration of the tricyclic antidepressant, imipramine, also has been reported to decrease levodopa bioavailability by delaying gastric emptying. Interactions due to pharmacologic interaction can result from many agents, including conventional antipsychotics, reserpine, methyldopa, and metoclopramide. Numerous agents have been reported to induce parkinsonism, including calcium antagonists, amiodarone, anticonvulsants, cytosine arabinoside, methotrexate, dacarbazine, fluorouracil, and amoxapine. Nonspecific MAO inhibitors, such as phenelzine, isocarboxazide, and pargyline, inhibit MAO-mediated metabolism of levodopa and catecholamines and can lead to hypertensive crisis. MAO inhibitors are contraindicated with levodopa and should be discontinued 2 weeks before levodopa therapy; this does not apply to the MAO-B inhibitor, selegiline.

Selegiline

Selegiline (*l*-deprenyl, Eldepryl; (R)-(−)-*N*-2-dimethyl-*N*-2-propenylphen-ethylamine hydrochloride) is a selective irreversible inhibitor of MAO-B and is used as an adjunct to levodopa for the treatment of Parkinson's disease (99). After oral administration, selegiline is rapidly absorbed but undergoes extensive presystemic metabolism in the gut and liver. Plasma concentrations vary highly between individuals. Absolute oral bioavailability is not known; relative bioavailability is increased three- to four-fold when administered with food. Pharmacokinetics during multiple doses are not predictable from single-dose pharmacokinetics; elimination $t_{1/2}$ is only 2 hours for single- and 10 hours for multiple-dose administration. Multiple-dose plasma concentrations are 4 times that for single dose.

Metabolism

Selegiline is rapidly metabolized to form the active major metabolite *N*-desmethylselegiline (DMS) and the inactive major metabolites L-methamphetamine (MET) and amphetamine (AMP) (100,101). [MET and AMP concentrations are considered too low to produce clinically important effects (99).] Six additional metabolites have been identified in urine: (1S,2R)-norephedrine, (1R,2R)-norpseudoephedrine, (1S,2R)-ephedrine, (1R,2R)-pseudoephedrine, (R)-*p*-hydroxyamphetamine, and (R)-*p*-hydroxymethamphetamine (100). Studies by Grace et al. (102) revealed that selegiline *N*-demethylation to form DMS and *N*-depropargylation to form MET were mediated by CYP2D6. DMS formation was favored 13:1 over MET formation. The k_{cat} value for formation of DMS was about 8.2 nmol of DMS/min/nmol of P450; the K_m and k_{cat} values for MET were 56 μM and 0.63 nmol of MET/min/nmol P450 (102). CYP3A4 also is involved in selegiline metabolism (103).

Drug Interactions

As with the previously discussed example of carbidopa and levodopa, coadministration of selegiline with levodopa is a planned metabolic drug interaction. By inhibiting MAO-B in the brain, metabolism of dopamine (the active metabolite of levodopa) is reduced, and the therapeutic action of levodopa is enhanced. At therapeutic doses (less than 10 mg/day), selegiline is selective for MAO-B, and dietary restrictions common to nonselective MAO inhibitors are not required. Interaction between meperidine and MAO inhibitors characterized as "central excitatory syndrome" is known; life-threatening adverse reactions between selegiline and meperidine have been reported (96). A similar syndrome may result from coadministration of conventional antidepressants (both tricyclics and selective serotonin reuptake inhibitors). This syndrome has been reported with selegiline coadministration with sertraline, paroxetine, and amitriptyline (96). It has been suggested that the potential for interaction with fluoxetine is reduced. However, fluoxetine is a CYP2D6 inhibitor, and there have been two clinical reports of fluoxetine–selegiline interactions (104,105).

REFERENCES

1. Wagstaff AJ, McTavish D. Tacrine: a review of its pharmacodynamic and pharmacokinetic properties and therapeutic potential in Alzheimer's disease. *Drugs Aging* 1994;4:1–31.
2. Madden S, Spaldin V, Park BK . Clinical pharmacokinetics of tacrine. *Clin Pharmacokinet* 1995;28:449–457.
3. Cutler NR, Sedman AJ, Prior P, et al. Steady-state pharmacokinetics of tacrine in patients with Alzheimer's disease. *Psychopharmacol Bull* 1990;26:231–234.
4. Forsyth DR, Wilcock GK, Morgan RA, Truman CA, Ford JM, Roberts CJ. Pharmacokinetics of tacrine hydrochloride in Alzheimer's disease. *Clin Pharmacol Ther* 1989;46:634–641.
5. Hartvig P, Askmark H, Aquilonius SM, Wiklund L, Lindstrom B. Clinical pharmacokinetics of intravenous and oral 9-amino-1,2,3,4-tetrahydroacridine, tacrine. *Eur J Clin Pharmacol* 1990;38:259–263.
6. Ahlin A, Adem A, Junthe T, Ohman G, Nyback H. Pharmacokinetics of tetrahydroaminoacridine: relations to clinical and biochemical effects in Alzheimer's patients. *Int Clin Psychopharmacol* 1992;7:29–36.
7. Ahlin A, Hassan M, Junthe T, Nyback H. Tacrine in Alzheimer's disease: pharmacokinetic and clinical comparison of oral and rectal administration. *Int Clin Psychopharmacol* 1994;9:263–270.
8. Nyback H, Hassan M, Junthe T, Ahlin A. Clinical experiences and biochemical findings with tacrine (THA). *Acta Neurol Scand Suppl* 1993;149:36–38.
9. Johansson M, Hellstrom-Lindahl E, Nordberg A. Steady-state pharmacokinetics of tacrine in long-term treatment of Alzheimer patients. *Dementia* 1996;7:111–117.
10. Sinz MW, Woolf TF. Characterization of the induction of rat microsomal cytochrome P450 by tacrine. *Biochem Pharmacol* 1997;54:425–427.
11. Woolf TF, Pool WF, Bjorge SM, et al. Bioactivation and irreversible binding of the cognition activator tacrine using human and rat liver microsomal preparations: species differences. *Drug Metab Dispos* 1993;21:874–882.
12. Pool WF, Woolf TF, Reily MD, Caprathe BW, Emmerling MR, Jaen JC. Identification of a 3-hydroxylated tacrine metabolite in rat and man: metabolic profiling implications and pharmacology. *J Med Chem* 1996;39:3014–3018.
13. Pool WF, Reily MD, Bjorge SM, Woolf TF. Metabolic disposition of the cognition activator tacrine in rats, dogs, and humans: species comparisons. *Drug Metab Dispos* 1997;25:590–597.
14. Hooper WD, Pool WF, Woolf TF, Gal J. Stereoselective hydroxylation of tacrine in rats and humans. *Drug Metab Dispos* 1994;22:719–724.
15. Turcan RG, Hillbeck D, Hartley TE, et al. Disposition of [^{14}C]velnacrine maleate in rats, dogs, and humans. *Drug Metab Dispos* 1993;21:1037–1047.
16. Madden S, Woolf TF, Pool WF, Park BK. An investigation into the formation of stable, protein-reactive and cytotoxic metabolites from tacrine in vitro: studies with human and rat liver microsomes. *Biochem Pharmacol* 1993;46:13–20.
17. Spaldin V, Madden S, Pool WF, Woolf TF, Park BK. The effect of enzyme inhibition on the metabolism and activation of tacrine by human liver microsomes. *Br J Clin Pharmacol* 1994;38:15–22.
18. Kukan M, Bezek S, Pool WF, Woolf TF. Metabolic disposition of tacrine in primary suspensions of rat hepatocyte and in single-pass perfused liver: in vitro/in vivo comparisons. *Xenobiotica* 1994;24:1107–1117.
19. Madden S, Spaldin V, Hayes RN, Woolf TF, Pool WF, Park BK. Species variation in the bioactivation of tacrine by hepatic microsomes. *Xenobiotica* 1995;25:103–116.
20. Spaldin V, Madden S, Adams DA, Edwards RJ, Davies DS, Park BK. Determination of human hepatic cytochrome P4501A2 activity in

vitro use of tacrine as an isoenzyme-specific probe. *Drug Metab Dispos* 1995;23:929–934.
21. Bezek S, Kukan M, Pool WF, Woolf TF. The effect of cytochromes P4501A induction and inhibition on the disposition of the cognition activator tacrine in rat hepatic preparations. *Xenobiotica* 1996;26:935–946.
22. Fontana RJ, Turgeon DK, Woolf TF, Knapp MJ, Foster NL, Watkins PB. The caffeine breath test does not identify patients susceptible to tacrine hepatotoxicity. *Hepatology* 1996;1429–1435.
23. Hooten WM, Pearlson G. Delirium caused by tacrine and ibuprofen interaction. *Am J Psychiatry* 1996;153:842.
24. Maany I. Adverse interaction of tacrine and haloperidol. *Am J Psychiatry* 1996;153:1504.
25. Becquemont L, Le Bot MA, Riche C, Beaune P. Influence of fluvoxamine on tacrine metabolism in vitro: potential implication for the hepatotoxicity in vivo. *Fund Clin Pharmacol* 1996;10:156–157.
26. Becquemont L, Ragueneau I, Le Bot MA, Riche C, Funck-Brentano C, Jaillon P. Influence of the CYP1A2 inhibitor fluvoxamine on tacrine pharmacokinetics in humans. *Clin Pharmacol Ther* 1997;61:619–627.
27. Forgue ST, Reece PA, Sedman AJ, deVries TM. Inhibition of tacrine oral clearance by cimetidine. *Clin Pharmacol Ther* 1996;59:444–449.
28. Toon S, Davidson EM, Garstang FM, Batra J, Bowes RJ, Rowland M. The racemic metoprolol H₂-antagonist interaction. *Clin Pharmacol Ther* 1988;43:283–289.
29. Schein JR. Cigarette smoking and clinically significant drug interactions. *Ann Pharmacother* 1995;29:1139–1148.
30. deVries TM, O'Connor-Semmes RL, Guttendorf RJ, et al. Effect of cimetidine and low-dose quinidine on tacrine pharmacokinetics in humans. *Pharm Res* 1993;10:S–337.
31. deVries TM, Siedlik PH, Smithers JA, et al. Effect of multiple-dose tacrine administration of single-dose pharmacokinetics of digoxin, diazepam, and theophylline. *Pharm Res* 1993;10:S–333.
32. Mihara M, Ohnishi A, Tomono Y, et al. Pharmacokinetics of E2020, a new compound for Alzheimer's disease, in healthy male volunteers. *Int J Clin Pharmacol Ther Toxicol* 1993;31:223–229.
33. Pfizer Inc. Aricept® (donepezil hydrochloride) tablets, *Physicians' Desk Reference*. Medical Economics Co., Montvale NJ, 1998.
34. Ohnishi A, Mihara M, Kamakura H, et al. Comparison of the pharmacokinetics of E2020: a new compound for Alzheimer's disease, in healthy young and elderly subjects. *J Clin Pharmacol* 1993;33:1086–1091.
35. Oda Y, Ohs H, Eustace N, Acedia Y, Sat T, Nakagawa T. Resolution of 1-benzyl-4-[5,6-dimethoxy-1-indanon)-2-yl] methylpiperidine hydrochloride enantiomers in plasma by high-performance liquid chromatography with direct injection into avidin-conjugated column. *J Liquid Chromatogr* 1992;15:2997–3012.
36. Matsui K, Oda Y, Ohe H, Tanaka S, Asakawa N. Direct determination of E2020 enantiomers in plasma by liquid chromatography-mass spectrometry and column-switching techniques. *J Chromatogr* 1995;694:209–218.
37. Sugimoto H, Iimura Y, Yamanishi Y, Yamatsu K. Synthesis and structure-activity relationships of acetylcholinesterase inhibitors: 1-benzyl-4-[(5,6-dimethoxy-1-oxoindan-2-yl)methyl]piperidine hydrochloride and related compounds. *J Med Chem* 1995;38:4821–4829.
38. Inoue A, Kawai T, Wakita M, Iimura Y, Sugimoto H, Kawakami Y. The simulated binding of (±)-2,3-dihydro-5,6-dimethoxy-2-[[1-(phenylmethyl)-4-piperidinyl]methyl]-1H-inden-1-one hydrochloride (E2020) and related inhibitors to free and acylated acetylcholinesterases and corresponding structure-activity analyses. *J Med Chem* 1996;39:4460–4470.
39. Fowler PA, Lacey LF, Thomas M, Keene ON, Tanner RJN, Baber NS. The clinical pharmacology, pharmacokinetics, and metabolism of sumatriptan. *Eur Neurol* 1991;31:291–294.
40. Lacey LF, Hussey EK, Fowler PA. Single dose pharmacokinetics of sumatriptan in healthy volunteers. *Eur J Clin Pharmacol* 1995;47:543–548.
41. Dixon CM, Saynor DA, Andrew PD, Oxford J, Bradbury A, Tarbit MH. Disposition of sumatriptan in laboratory animals and humans. *Drug Metab Disp* 1993;21:761–769.
42. Andrew PD, Birch HL, Phillpot DA. Determination of sumatriptan succinate in plasma and urine by high-performance liquid chromatography with electrochemical detection. *J Pharma Sci* 1993;82:73–76.
43. Dixon CM, Park GR, Tarbit MH. Characterization of the enzyme responsible for the metabolism of sumatriptan in human liver. *Biochem Pharmacol* 1994;47:1253–1257.
44. Glaxo Wellcome Inc., Imitrex® (sumatriptan succinate), *Physicians' Desk Reference*, Medical Economics Co., Montvale NJ 1998.
45. Scott AK, Walley T, Breckenridge AM, Lacey LF, Fowler PA. Lack of an interaction between propranolol and sumatriptan. *Br J Clin Pharmacol* 1991;32:581–584.
46. Srinivas NR, Shyu WC, Upmalis D, Lee JS, Barbhaiya RH. Lack of pharmacokinetic interaction between butorphanol tartrate nasal spray and sumatriptan succinate. *J Clin Pharmacol* 1995;35:432–437.
47. Van Hecken AM, Depre M, DeSchepper PJ, Fowler PA, Lacey LF, Durham JM. Lack of effect of flunarizine on the pharmacokinetics and pharmacodynamics of sumatriptan in healthy volunteers. *Br J Clin Pharmacol* 1992;34:82–84.
48. Dechant KL, Clissold SP. Sumatriptan: a review of its pharmacodynamic and pharmacokinetic properties, and therapeutic efficacy in the acute treatment of migraine and cluster headache. *Drugs* 1992;43:776–798.
49. Guengerich P. Human cytochrome P450 enzymes. In: Ortiz de Montellano PR, ed. *Cytochrome P450, structure, mechanism and biochemistry*. New York: Plenum Press, 1995:473–535.
50. Thomsen LL, Dixon R, Lassen LH, et al. 311C90 (Zolmitriptan), a novel centrally and peripheral acting oral 5-hydroxytryptamine-1D agonist: a comparison of its absorption during a migraine attack and in a migraine-free period. *Cephalalgia* 1996;16:270–275.
51. Dixon R, Gillotin C, Gibbens M, Posner J, Peck RW. The pharmacokinetics and effects on blood pressure of multiple doses of the novel anti-migraine drug zolmitriptan (311C90) in healthy volunteers. *Br J Clin Pharmacol* 1997;43:273–281.
52. Zeneca Pharmaceuticals, Zomig® (zolmitriptan) tablets, *Physicians' Desk Reference*, Medical Economics Co., Montvale NJ 1999.
53. Cheng H, Polvino WJ, Sciberras D, et al. Pharmacokinetics and food interaction of MK-462 in healthy males. *Biopharmacol Drug Dispos* 1996;17:17–24.
54. Sciberras DG, Polvino WJ, Gertz BJ, et al. Initial human experience with MK-462 (rizatriptan): a novel 5-HT1D agonist. *Br J Clin Pharmacol* 1997;43:49–54.
55. Merck & Co., Maxalt® (rizatriptan benzoate) tablets, *Physicians' Desk Reference*, Medical Economics Co., Montvale NJ 1999.
56. Glaxo Wellcome Inc., Amerge® (naratriptan hydrochloride) tablets, *Physicians' Desk Reference*, Medical Economics Co., Montvale NJ 1999.
57. Smith HT, Molinaro NC. High-performance liquid chromatographic method for the determination of methysergide and methylergonovine in human plasma. *J Chromatogr* 1988;424:416–423.
58. Bredberg U, Eyjolfsdottir GS, Paalzow L, Tfelt-Hansen P, Trfelt-Hansen V. Pharmacokinetics of methysergide and its metabolite methylergometrine in man. *Eur J Clin Pharmacol* 1986;30:75–77.
59. Müller-Schweinitzer E, Tapparelli C. Methylergometrine, an active metabolite of methysergide. *Cephalalgia* 1986;6:35–41.
60. Bobik A, Jennings G, Skews H, Esler M, McLean A. Low oral bioavailability of dihydroergotamine and first-pass extraction in patients with orthostatic hypotension. *Clin Pharmacol Ther* 1981;30:673–679.
61. Little PJ, Jennings GL, Skews H, Bobik A. Bioavailability of dihydroergotamine in man. *Br J Clin Pharmacol* 1982;13:785–790.
62. Hilke H, Kanto J, Kleimola T, Mäntylä R. Intramuscular absorption of dihydroergotamine in man. *Int J Clin Pharmacol* 1978;16:277–278.
63. Kanto J, Allonen H, Koski K, et al. Pharmacokinetics of dihydroergotamine in healthy volunteers and in neurological patients after a single intravenous injection. *Int J Clin Pharmacol Ther Toxicol* 1981;19:127–130.
64. Silberstein S. The pharmacology of ergotamine and dihydroergotamine. *Headache* 1997;S15–S25.
65. Müller-Schweinitzer E. What is known about the action of dihydroergotamine on the vasculature in man? *Int J Clin Pharmacol Ther Toxicol* 1984;22:677–682.
66. de Marées H, Welzel D, de Marées A, Klotz U, Tiedjen KU, Knaup G. Relationship between the venoconstrictor activity of dihydroergotamine and its pharmacokinetics during acute and chronic oral dosing. *Eur J Clin Pharmacol* 1986;30:685–689.
67. Maurer G, Frick W. Elucidation of the structure and receptor binding studies of the major, primary, metabolite of dihydroergotamine in man. *Eur J Clin Pharmacol* 1984;26:463–470.

68. Müller-Schweinitzer E. Pharmacological actions of the main metabolites of dihydroergotamine. *Eur J Clin Pharmacol* 1984;26:699–705.

69. Martinet M, Kiechel JR. Interaction of dihydroergotamine and triacetyloleandomycin in the minipig. *Eur J Drug Metab Pharmacokinet* 1983;8:261–267.

70. Delaforge M, Rivière R, Sartori E, Doignon JL, Grognet JM. Metabolism of dihydroergotamine by a cytochrome P-450 similar to that involved in the metabolism of macrolide antibiotics. *Xenobiotica* 1989;19:1285–1295.

71. Peyronneau M-A, Delaforge M, Rivière R, Renaud J-P, Mansuy D. High affinity of ergopeptides for cytochromes P450 3A. *Eur J Biochem* 1994;223:947–956.

72. Stahlmann R, Lode H. Macrolides: tolerability and interactions with other drugs. *Antiinfect Drugs Chemother* 1996;14:155–162.

73. Novartis Pharmaceuticals Corp. DHE 45®, (dihydroergotamine mesylate), *Physicians' Desk Reference,* Medical Economics Co., Montvale NJ 1998.

74. Sutherland JM, Hooper WD, Eadie MJ, Tyrer JH. Buccal absorption of ergotamine. *J Neurol Neurosurg Psychiatry* 1974;37:1116–1120.

75. Ala-Hurula, Myllylä VV, Arvela P, Kärki NT, Hokkanen E. Systemic availability of ergotamine tartrate after three successive doses and during continuous medication. *Eur J Clin Pharmacol* 1979;16:355–360.

76. Ala-Hurula, Myllylä VV, Arvela P, Heikkilä J, Kärki NT, Hokkanen E. Systemic availability of ergotamine tartrate after oral, rectal and intramuscular administration. *Eur J Clin Pharmacol* 1979;15:51–55.

77. Ala-Hurula, Myllylä VV, Arvela P, Kärki NT, Hokkanen E. Systemic availability of ergotamine tartrate in healthy subjects after single and repeated oral doses. *Uppsala J Med Sci Suppl* 1980;31:7–9.

78. Ekbom K, Paalzow L, Waldenlind E. Low biological availability of ergotamine tartrate after oral dosing in cluster headache. *Cephalalgia* 1981;1:203–207.

79. Ibraheem JJ, Paalzow L, Tfelt-Hansen P. Kinetics of ergotamine after intravenous and intramuscular administration to migraine sufferers. *Eur J Clin Pharmacol* 1982;23:235–240.

80. Ibraheem JJ, Paalzow L, Tfelt-Hansen P. Low bioavailability of ergotamine tartrate after oral and rectal administration in migraine sufferers. *Eur J Clin Pharmacol* 1983;16:695–699.

81. Tfelt-Hansen P, Paalzow L. Intramuscular ergotamine: plasma levels and dynamic activity. *Clin Pharmacol Ther* 1985;37:29–35.

82. Ibraheem JJ, Paalzow L, Tfelt-Hansen P. Linear pharmacokinetics of intravenous ergotamine tartrate. *Eur J Clin Pharmacol* 1985;29:61–66.

83. Sanders SW, Haering N, Mosberg H, Jaeger H. Pharmacokinetics of ergotamine in healthy volunteers following oral and rectal dosing. *Eur J Clin Pharmacol* 1986;30:331–334.

84. Perrin VL. Clinical pharmacokinetics of ergotamine in migraine and cluster headache. *Clin Pharmacokinet* 1985;10:334–352.

85. Schmidt R, Fanchamps A. Effect of caffeine on intestinal absorption of ergotamine in man. *Eur J Clin Pharmacol* 1974;7:213–216.

86. Sartori E, Delaforge M. Specific drug binding to rat liver cytochrome P-450 isozymes induced by pregnenolone-16α-carbonitrile and macrolide antibiotics: implications for drug interactions. *Chem Biol Interact* 1990;73:297–307.

87. Stahlmann R, Lode H. Macrolides: tolerability and interactions with other drugs. *Antiinfect Drugs Chemother* 1996;14:155–162.

88. Lampen A, Christians U, Bader A, Hackbarth I, Sewing K-F. Drug interactions and interindividual variability of cyclosporin metabolism in the small intestine. *Pharmacology* 1996;52:159–168.

89. Nutt JG, Fellman JH. Review: pharmacokinetics of levodopa. *Clin Neuropharmacol* 1984;7:35–49.

90. Juncos J. Parkinson's disease, levodopa: pharmacology, pharmacokinetics and pharmacodynamics. *Neurol Clin* 1992;10:487–509.

91. Pinder RM, Brogden RN, Sawyer PR, Speight TM, Avery GS. Levodopa and decarboxylase inhibitors: a review of their clinical pharmacology and use in the treatment of parkinsonism. *Drugs* 1976;11:329–377.

92. Mars H. Metabolic interactions of pyridoxine, levodopa, and carbidopa in Parkinson's disease. *Trans Am Neurol Assoc* 1973;98:241–245.

93. Mars H. Levodopa, carbidopa, and pyridoxine in Parkinson disease: metabolic interactions. *Arch Neurol* 1974;30:444–447.

94. Vickers S, Stuart EK, Bianchine JR, Hucker HB, Jaffe ME, Rhodes RE. Metabolism of carbidopa [L-(−)-α-hydrazino-3,4-dihydroxy-α-methylhydrocinnamic acid monohydrate], an aromatic amino acid decarboxylase inhibitor in the rat, dog, rhesus monkey, and man. *Drug Metab Dispos* 1974;2:9–22.

95. Vickers S, Stuart EK, Hucker HB. Further studies on the metabolism of carbidopa (−)-L-α-hydrazino-3,4-dihydroxy-α-methylbenzenepropanoic acid monohydrate, in the human, rhesus monkey, dog and rat. *J Med Chem* 1975;18:134–138.

96. Pfeiffer RF. Antiparkinsonian agents: drug interactions of clinical significance. *Drug Safety* 1996;14:343–354.

97. Bianchine JR. Drugs for Parkinson's disease; centrally acting muscle relaxants. In: Gilman AG, Goodman LS, Gilman A, eds. *Goodman & Gilman's the pharmacological basis of therapeutics.* 6th ed. New York: Macmillan, 1980:475–493.

98. Standaert DG, Young AB. Treatment of central nervous system degenerative disorders. In: Hardman JG, Limbird LE, eds. *Goodman & Gilman's the pharmacological basis of therapeutics.* 9th ed. New York: McGraw-Hill, 1996:503–519.

99. Somerset Pharmaceuticals Inc., Eldepryl® (selegiline hydrochloride) capsules, *Physicians' Desk Reference,* Medical Economics Co., Montvale NJ 1998.

100. Mascher HJ, Kikuta C, Millendorfer A, Schiel H, Ludwig G. Pharmacokinetics and bioequivalence of the main metabolites of selegiline: desmethylselegiline, methamphetamine and amphetamine after oral administration of selegiline. *Int J Clin Pharmacol Ther* 1997;35:9–13.

101. Shin H-S. Metabolism of selegiline in humans, identification, excretion and stereochemistry of urine metabolites. *Drug Metab Dispos* 1997;25:657–662.

102. Grace JM, Kinter MT, Macdonald TL. Atypical metabolism of deprenyl and its enantiomer, (S)-(+)N, alpha-dimethyl-N-propynylphenthylamine, by cytochrome P450 2D6. *Chem Res Toxicol* 1994;72:286–290.

103. Barrett JS, Szego P, Rohatagi S, et al. Absorption and presystemic metabolism of selegiline hydrochloride at different regions in the gastrointestinal tract in healthy males. *Pharmacol Res* 1996;13:1535–1540.

104. Jermain DM, Hughes PL, Follender AB. Potential fluoxetine-selegiline interaction. *Ann Pharmacother* 1992;26:1300.

105. Montastruc JL, Chamontin B, Senard JM, et al. Pseudopheochromocytoma in parkinsonian patient treated with fluoxetine plus selegiline. *Lancet* 1993;341:555.

CHAPTER 24

Calcium Channel Blockers

David R. Jones and Stephen D. Hall

INTRODUCTION

The calcium channel blockers share the ability to inhibit the influx of calcium into smooth muscle and myocardial cells through "slow" calcium channels. As a consequence of this reduced calcium influx, there is a reduced tone of coronary and peripheral arterioles and negative chronotropic and inotropic effects. Calcium channel blockers are therefore primarily used therapeutically as antihypertensive agents and in the treatment of angina pectoris. The clinically useful calcium channel blockers are diverse in chemical structure but may be conveniently classified as dihydropyridines (e.g., nifedipine) or nondihydropyridines (e.g., verapamil, diltiazem) on a pharmacologic basis. Dihydropyridines selectively exert their pharmacologic activity on vascular smooth muscle, whereas the nondihydropyridines are selective for the sinus and atrioventricular nodes and therefore find some use as antiarrhythmic agents for the treatment of supraventricular arrhythmias.

In general, the calcium channel blockers undergo extensive biotransformation when administered to humans and often exhibit short half-lives and low to moderate bioavailability. Inappropriately high or low plasma concentrations of these drugs therefore stem from drug–drug interactions at the enzyme level or from altered regulation of the biotransforming enzymes by genetic and/or environmental factors. For a number of calcium channel blockers, there is a direct relation between plasma drug concentration and therapeutic effect, and therefore low concentrations necessarily result in therapeutic failure (1,2). Similarly, elevated plasma drug concentrations lead to significant morbidities such as hypotension and impairment of cardiac conduction. Inappropriately high

D. R. Jones and S. D. Hall: Department of Medicine, Division of Clinical Pharmacology, Indiana University School of Medicine, Wishard Memorial Hospital, OPW 320, 1001 West 10th Street, Indianapolis, Indiana 46202

plasma concentrations of calcium channel blockers may be particularly prevalent in elderly patients who require numerous other drug therapies and who may be intrinsically more susceptible to drug–drug interactions.

In this chapter we present both *in vivo* and *in vitro* evidence to support the involvement of specific drug-metabolizing enzymes in the biotransformation of the clinically useful calcium channel blockers. In turn, this database provides a rational basis for understanding known interactions with these drugs and predicting interactions with new therapeutic agents.

DIHYDROPYRIDINES

The dihydropyridines are a group of calcium channel blockers that share the same structural nucleus but have different substituents at the 2-, 3-, 4-, and 5- positions of the dihydropyridine ring (Fig. 24-1). This structural similarity results in a similar biotransformation pattern for most of the dihydropyridines. In general, this class of calcium channel blocker undergoes oxidative aromatization of the dihydropyridine nucleus, hydroxylation of the 2- or 5-methyl substituent, and deesterification at the 3- or 5- positions to give carboxylic acids (see Fig. 24-1). Loss of the dihydropyridine configuration is generally considered to be the primary metabolic route, and this leads to the loss of calcium channel blocking activity. It should be noted that, with the exception of nifedipine, all other dihydropyridines (calcium channel blockers) are chiral and thus may undergo a stereoselective metabolism.

Nifedipine

The prototype of the clinically useful dihydropyridines was nifedipine, and it remains one of the most widely prescribed drugs in this class. Nifedipine [1,4-dihydro-2,6-dimethyl-4-(2-nitrophenyl)-3,5-pyridinedicarboxylic acid dimethyl ester] has a short elimination half-life of 1.3 to

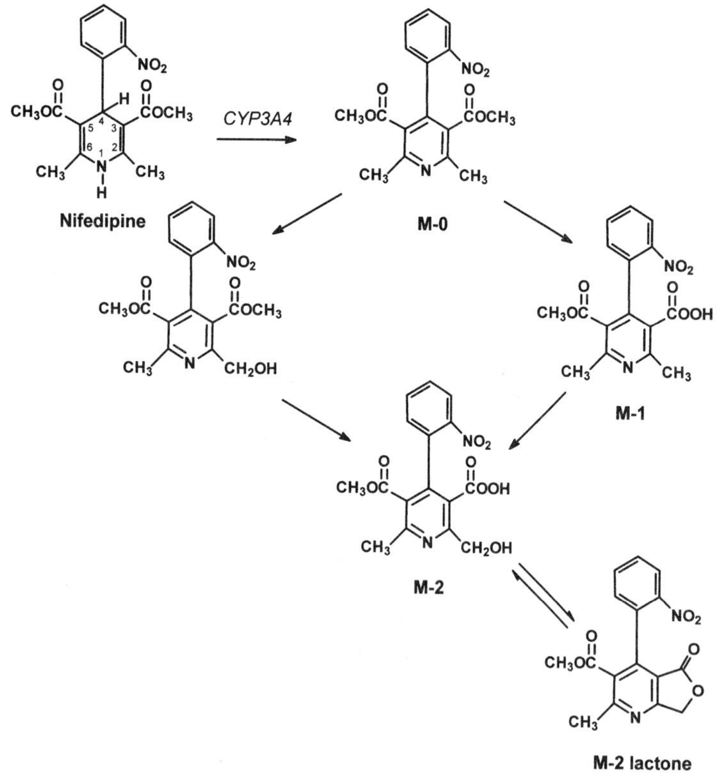

FIG. 24-1. Major pathways of nifedipine biotransformation in humans. Analogous pathways feature in the biotransformation of numerous other dihydropyridines. M-0 (primary pyridine metabolite) formation catalyzed primarily by CYP3A enzymes, but catalysts of the other pathways are undefined.

1.9 hours in humans and is therefore administered most commonly as a slow-release formulation (3,4). The clearance of nifedipine after intravenous administration was approximately 0.4 L/h/kg (3,4), and there is some evidence to suggest that sites other than the liver may make a significant contribution to this clearance (5). Absorption of nifedipine from an oral dose is essentially complete, but based on a comparison of area under the curve (AUC) after oral and intravenous administration, the bioavailability of nifedipine is approximately 45% to 55%, suggesting that extensive first-pass elimination occurs (3,6,7). After intraaortic nifedipine administration and sampling from the hepatic vein, the hepatic extraction was estimated at 64%, suggesting that hepatic elimination is the dominant component of the first-pass effect (5).

When nifedipine was administered orally or intravenously to human volunteers, 70% to 80% of the dose was excreted into the urine and 20% to 30% in the feces in the form of the metabolites, with only traces of the parent compound (3). The major metabolites of nifedipine identified in human urine (see Fig. 24-1) were the carboxylic acid (M-1) and the 2-methoxy (M-2) derivatives of the primary pyridine metabolite (3); M-1 constituted more than 90% of the urinary metabolites. Thus oxidative metabolism of nifedipine is the principal mechanism of elimination in humans.

After oral administration of nifedipine, plasma concentrations of M-0 reached a peak earlier than either M-1 or M-2 (3,4). Thus in the formation of the major terminal metabolite M-1 *in vivo,* the initial step appears to be oxidation to the pyridine, M-0 (see Fig. 24-1). The maximal plasma concentration of nifedipine was approximately 3 times greater than that of M-0 after oral dosage, but M-0 was present at very low concentrations in plasma after intravenous nifedipine administration, suggesting that sites other than the liver contribute to the first-pass metabolism of nifedipine (4). No significant calcium channel–blocking activity is associated with any of the major metabolites of nifedipine (3).

The oxidation of nifedipine to the pyridine metabolite (M-0; see Fig. 24-1) is primarily catalyzed by cytochrome P450 (CYP) 3A4/5 in human liver microsomes *in vitro.* This was conclusively demonstrated by Guengerich et al. (8–10), who demonstrated that (a) inhibitory CYP3A antibodies blocked M-0 formation; (b) gestodene, a mechanistic inhibitor of CYP3A, inhibited M-0 formation; and (c) M-0 formation was catalyzed by cDNA-expressed CYP3A4 in yeast. Hydroxylation of nifedipine at the 2-methyl group of M-0 and deesterification of the pyridine to M-1 appear to be mediated by one or more unidentified CYPs, but these metabolite reactions have not been reported to occur for the dihydropyridines *per se* (11,12).

Drug Interactions In Vivo

As expected from the *in vitro* data, several well-defined inhibitors of CYP3A4 impaired the metabolism of nifedipine *in vivo*. Diltiazem pretreatment for 3 days resulted in an increase in the nifedipine half-life from 2.5 to 3.4 hours and a two- to three-fold increase in oral area under the plasma concentration–time curve (AUC; 13). A reduction in the formation of M-0 but no change in apparent hepatic blood flow accompanied these changes. Similarly quinidine coadministration caused a 40% increase in nifedipine half-life ($t_{1/2}$) with a 40% decrease in the clearance to M-0 (14,15). Cimetidine increased the oral AUC of nifedipine by 100% and, in a single patient, itraconazole therapy resulted in a five-fold increase in nifedipine plasma concentrations and significant ankle edema (16,17). Coadministration of regular or slow-release nifedipine tablets with grapefruit juice resulted in a 50% to 100% increase in AUC but no change in $t_{1/2}$ (18,19). The pharmacokinetics of intravenously administered nifedipine were unaffected by grapefruit juice (19). Thus in contrast to the drug interactions, the interaction with grapefruit juice appears to be limited to the first-pass effect at the intestinal wall that is relatively modest for nifedipine. Rifampin, a potent inducer of human CYP3A4, increased the apparent oral clearance from 1.5 to 20.9 L/min and reduced the systemic availability of nifedipine from 41% to 5% (20). Significant drug interactions should be expected for other CYP3A inhibitors and inducers.

Amlodipine

Amlodipine [(R,S)-2-[(2-aminoethoxy) methyl]-4-(2-chlorophenyl) - 1, 4 - dihydro - 6 - methyl - 3 , 5-pyridine-dicarboxylic acid 3-ethyl 5-methyl ester] is atypical of the dihydropyridine calcium channel blockers because it exhibits a relatively long $t_{1/2}$ of approximately 35 hours and slow absorption with peak plasma concentrations at 6 to 9 hours (21,22). After intravenous dosing, amlodipine is efficiently cleared at 7 mL/min/kg, indicating that the long half-life reflects a large volume of distribution (21 L/kg) (21). After oral administration, amlodipine displayed a systemic availability of approximately 64% (21–23). Absorption from the gastrointestinal tract was essentially complete based on recovery of radiolabeled metabolites in urine and feces, and less than 10% of an oral dose of radiolabeled amlodipine was excreted unchanged (24). Metabolism is therefore the primary elimination pathway, and in contrast to most dihydropyridines, first-pass extraction accounts for only a third of the dose.

After oral dosing to humans, all the urinary metabolites of amlodipine contained the pyridine nucleus (24). Major secondary metabolites resulting from oxidative deamination of the 2-aminoethoxymethyl moiety or esterolysis at the 5-methoxycarbonyl group accounted for approximately 60% of the urinary metabolites (24). Plasma metabolites consisted entirely of pyridine derivatives that were devoid of pharmacologic activity (24).

Oxidative aromatization therefore appears to be the dominant pathway in the elimination of amlodipine in humans.

Amlodipine is used clinically as a racemic mixture in which the S-enantiomer is responsible for the calcium channel–blocking activity, and the R-isomer is essentially inactive. Plasma concentrations of amlodipine were slightly enriched in the S-enantiomer because of the lower clearance of this isomer (25).

The identity of the enzyme(s) responsible for the biotransformation of amlodipine has not been determined, but it is tacitly assumed that CYP3A4 is the major catalyst for the primary aromatization step, as noted for other dihydropyridines. Support for this assumption is provided by the observation that simultaneous administration of 250 mL of grapefruit juice and 5 mg of amlodipine orally resulted in a 20% increase in AUC and maximal plasma concentrations (C_{max}) relative to control (26). The modest effect of grapefruit juice is consistent with a relatively small intestinal first-pass effect for amlodipine (*vide supra*).

Drug Interactions In Vivo

No significant changes in amlodipine pharmacokinetics due to concomitant therapy have been reported, but altered plasma concentrations should be expected when potent inhibitors or inducers of CYP3A are coadministered.

Felodipine

Felodipine, [(R,S)-4-(2,3-dichlorophenyl)-1,4-dihydro-2,6-dimethyl-3,5-pyridinedicarboxylic acid ethyl methyl ester)] displays an intermediate $t_{1/2}$ of 7 to 16 hours in humans with less than 5% of a dose excreted unchanged after oral or intravenous dosing (27,28). Intravenous clearance of felodipine varies between 50 and 65 L/h, and systemic availability, between 10% and 20% after an oral dose (27,29,30). A comparable bioavailability was observed in patients with portacaval shunts, suggesting that extrahepatic sites make a significant contribution to first-pass metabolism (31). Felodipine is used therapeutically as a racemic mixture, but most of the pharmacologic activity resides in the S-enantiomer (32). The S-/R-enantiomer ratios were 2.39, 2.09, and 1.09 for AUC, C_{max}, and $t_{1/2}$, respectively, suggesting that availability rather than systemic clearance accounts for the enantioselectivity in plasma concentrations of felodipine (32). The primary pathway of felodipine metabolism is oxidation to the achiral and inactive pyridine, dehydrofelodipine (33). After both intravenous and oral administration of radiolabeled felodipine, approximately 80% was recovered in urine and feces as metabolites derived from the pyridine by methyl and ethyl ester cleavage and by hydroxylation of the methyl groups (28,29,34).

The oxidation of felodipine to the corresponding pyridine, dehydrofelodipine, in human liver microsomes was inhibited completely by anti-CYP3A antibody and gestodene (35). Furthermore, aromatization of felodipine was catalyzed by cDNA-expressed CYP3A4, and the rate of this reaction was highly correlated with the rate of nifedipine aromatization in a bank of human liver microsomes (35). CYP3A enzymes therefore appear to be the principal catalysts in the formation of the primary metabolite of felodipine, and metabolites with an intact dihydropyridine nucleus have not been detected (33). The identity of the enzymes responsible for the formation of secondary felodipine metabolites is unknown.

Drug Interactions In Vivo

Coadministration of established inhibitors of CYP3A enzymes result in significant elevations in felodipine plasma concentrations and exaggerated pharmacologic response due to increased availability and reduced systemic clearance. For example, oral administration of 200 mg itraconazole produced an eight-fold increase in oral AUC and a doubling of $t_{1/2}$ of felodipine (36). Similarly, oral cyclosporine A significantly elevated the felodipine oral AUC by 58%, and erythromycin elevated the oral AUC and half-life by 149% and 61%, respectively (37,38). Consistent with the dominant role of CYP3A enzymes in felodipine metabolism, there was a reduction in oral AUC to 7% of control in patients with epilepsy receiving phenytoin, carbamazepine, or phenobarbital, which are well-known inducers of CYP3A4 (39).

Grapefruit juice did not affect the pharmacokinetics of intravenously administered felodipine (40) but caused a 40% to 200% increase in the AUC of orally administered drug without a change in half-life (37,41–43). Thus as noted for other dihydropyridines, a single dose of grapefruit juice appears selectively to inhibit the CYP3A4 activity present in human small intestinal mucosa and thereby increase systemic availability of these drugs. The lack of effect of grapefruit juice on the hepatic N-demethylation of erythromycin is consistent with this hypothesis (44). Watkins et al. (44,45) have demonstrated that this inhibition is irreversible in nature and corresponds to loss of immunodetectable CYP3A4 in duodenal biopsies obtained from volunteers who had consumed grapefruit juice. This mechanism of inhibition is consistent with the observation that the AUC of felodipine is elevated for up to 24 hours after consumption of a single dose of grapefruit juice (41).

Isradipine

Isradipine [(R,S)-4-(4-benzofurazanyl)-1,4-dihydro-2,6-dimethyl-3,5-pyridinedicarboxylic acid methyl 1-methylethyl ester] is completely absorbed from the gastrointestinal tract, but because of a high degree of first-pass metabolism, has a systemic availability of approximately 17% (46). Isradipine has a $t_{1/2}$ of 3 to 6 hours and is eliminated completely by metabolism. The primary pathways of isradipine elimination involve the formation of the pyridine metabolite and deesterification at the 3 position of the dihydropyridine ring to form a carboxylate (47). The metabolites do not contribute to the cardiovascular effects of the drug (48). A rigorous evaluation of the enzymes that catalyze the biotransformation of isradipine is lacking, but in human lymphoblastoid cells that expressed CYP3A4, the only detectable derivative of isradipine was the pyridine metabolite (49).

Drug Interactions In Vivo

Consistent with the involvement of CYP3A enzymes in the elimination of isradipine, the manufacturers have noted a 50% increase in the AUC after a 7-day course of cimetidine. Similarly, a 6-day treatment with rifampin led to undetectable plasma concentrations of isradipine. Changes in the disposition of isradipine due to coadministration of other drugs have not been reported, but significant changes should be anticipated when potent inhibitors and inducers of CYP3A enzymes are encountered.

Lacidipine

Lacidipine [1,4-dihydro-2,6-dimethyl-4-(2-(1,2-propylene t-butyl ester)phenyl)-3,5-pyridinedicarboxylic acid diethyl ester] exhibits a $t_{1/2}$ of approximately 8 hours and an extremely low bioavailability of 2% to 9% because of extensive first-pass metabolism (50,51). After oral administration of radiolabeled lacidipine to volunteers, the clearance was entirely by metabolism to inactive metabolites, and no parent drug was detected in either the urine or feces. In humans lacidipine is eliminated primarily by oxidation to the pyridine and deesterification to a carboxylic acid (52).

Drug Interactions In Vivo

Drug interactions that significantly influence the pharmacokinetics of lacidipine have not been reported but should be expected when potent inhibitors or inducers of CYP3A are used concomitantly.

Nicardipine

Nicardipine [(R,S)-1,4-dihydro-2,6-dimethyl-4-(3-nitrophenyl)-3,5-pyridinedicarboxylic acid methyl 2-[methyl-(phenylmethyl) amino] ethyl ester] is used clinically as a racemic mixture of (+)- and (−)-enantiomers, which exhibit an activity ratio of 3:1 (53). The absorption of nicardipine from the gastrointestinal tract is essentially complete, but first-pass metabolism reduces the oral bioavailability to approximately 10% (54). Plasma concentrations of nicardipine decline with a terminal half-life of 2 to 7 hours and a (+)/(−) ratio of approximately 2.5 (54,55). The two major urinary metabolites (36% of dose) of nicardipine were the glucuronides of the pyridine metabolite dealkylated at the nitrogen of the side chain (S14) and the dihydropyridine metabolite dealkylated at the nitrogen of the side chain (S16) (56). Other significant urinary metabolites (37% of dose) were the carboxylic acid metabolite of S14 (M9), the carboxylic acid metabolite of S16 (S18), and a carboxylic acid (position 3) metabolite (M6). Major metabolites identified in plasma were the acid metabolites M6 and M9, composing about 20% and 15% of the total radioactivity, respectively, and S16, which accounted for an additional 15%. Nicardipine and metabolite M5 accounted for about 15% of total radioactivity in plasma. Metabolites, M6, M9, and S16 possessed less than 1/200 the potency compared with nicardipine (56). Thus the primary pathways of nicardipine elimination are aromatization to the pyridine and dealkylation of the side chain at position 3. The enzymes that catalyze these biotransformations have not been characterized.

Drug Interactions In Vivo

Based on an analogy with other dihydropyridines, it is reasonable to assume that CYP3A enzymes will catalyze the initial oxidation of nicardipine to the pyridine metabolite. This hypothesis is supported by the observation that grapefruit juice increases the AUC of (+)-nicardipine by approximately 30% and the (−)-enantiomer by 100% (57). Interactions with other potent inhibitors and inducers of CYP3A should be anticipated.

Nimodipine

Nimodipine [(R,S)-1,4-dihydro-2,6-dimethyl-4-(3-nitrophenyl)-3,5-pyridinedicarboxylic acid 2-methoxyethyl 1-methylethyl ester] is used as a racemic mixture primarily for the prevention of cerebral vasospasm in patients with subarachnoid hemorrhage and to improve cerebral function in some elderly populations. The half-life of nimodipine is 5 to 10 hours, and bioavailability is 5% to 13% of an oral dose, primarily because of extensive first-pass elimination (58). Plasma concentrations of nimodipine are enriched four- to six-fold in the less active R-enantiomer, primarily because of a less efficient first-pass elimination of this isomer (59). Excretion of unchanged nimodipine is insignificant, and the primary pathway of elimination is oxidation to the inactive pyridine, but O-demethylation of the 3-methoxy group also occurs to a lesser extent (58,60). The rate of oxidation to the pyridine metabolite by human liver microsomes was highly correlated with the rate of nifedipine and felodipine aromatization and could be catalyzed by CYP3A4 expressed in transfected yeast cells (35).

Drug Interactions In Vivo

Few effects of concomitant drugs on nimodipine disposition have been observed, but inhibitors and inducers of CYP3A enzymes do result in the expected interactions. For example, prolonged anticonvulsant therapy, including carbamazepine, phenobarbital, phenytoin, or combinations thereof, reduced the AUC of nimodipine seven-fold because of induction of CYP3A-mediated first-pass metabolism (61). In addition, cimetidine (100 mg/day for 7 days) results in a doubling of the AUC for nimodipine (62). Grapefruit juice also increases the AUC of nimodipine by approximately 150% (63). Valproic acid therapy resulted in a 50% increase in nimodipine plasma concentrations, but the metabolic basis of this effect is unclear (61).

Nisoldipine

Nisoldipine [(R,S)-1,4-dihydro-2,6-dimethyl-4(2-nitrophenyl)-3,5-pyridinecarboxylic acid methyl 2-methylpropyl ester] is available as a racemic mixture of the active (+)- and inactive (−)-isomers, and its terminal $t_{1/2}$ has been reported to vary between 2 and 12 hours (64). The excretion of radiolabeled nisoldipine after intravenous dosage was 82% in urine and 14% in feces after a 4-day collection. After oral administration of radiolabeled nisoldipine, the average excretion was 74% in urine and 12% in feces after a 6-day collection but excretion of unchanged drug was negligible (65). Thus nisoldipine is eliminated completely by metabolism, and at least 85% of an oral dose is absorbed from the gastrointestinal tract. However, first pass metabolism of nisoldipine is extensive and systemic availability is 3% to 8% of an oral dose (64,66). The primary metabolic pathways of nisoldipine are formation of the pyridine derivative and hydroxylation of the isobutyl ester group (65). Hydroxylation of the isobutyl side chain results in a metabolite that has about 10% of activity of the parent drug (66). The rate of formation of the pyridine metabolite of nisoldipine by human liver microsomes was highly correlated with the rates of aromatization of nifedipine and felodipine. Furthermore, in common with most other dihydropyridines, cDNA-expressed CYP3A4 in yeast cells efficiently catalyzed this oxidation of nisoldipine (35). CYP3A enzymes are expected to play a major role in the inactivation of nisoldipine by humans.

Drug Interactions In Vivo

As expected for a CYP3A substrate that undergoes substantial first pass metabolism, the plasma concentrations of nisoldipine were markedly affected by grapefruit juice consumption; maximal plasma concentrations after oral administration increased 400%, and AUC, by 200% (67). Cimetidine treatment resulted in a modest increase in the bioavailability of nisoldipine from 3.9% to 5.7% without affecting systemic clearance (68,69). In line with the effect of these CYP3A inhibitors on nisoldipine disposition, there was a highly significant interaction with the CYP3A4 inducer phenytoin. Patients with epilepsy receiving stable phenytoin therapy experienced AUC values that were ten-fold lower than those seen in matched controls (70). Interactions with other potent inhibitors or inducers of CYP3A should be anticipated.

Nitrendipine

Nitrendipine [(R,S)-1,4-dihydro-2,6-dimethyl-4-(3-nitrophenyl)-3,5-pyridinedicarboxylic acid ethyl methyl ester] is available as a racemic mixture, but the S-enantiomer is almost ten times more potent than its antipode (2,71). The systemic clearance and $t_{1/2}$ of nitrendipine are approximately 1.6 L/min and 5 to 10 hours, respectively, with little if any enantioselectivity (72,73). Approximately 85% of an orally administered dose of radiolabeled nitrendipine was recovered in urine and feces over a 96-hour period with negligible excretion of unchanged drug, indicating almost complete absorption (74). However, because of enantioselective first pass metabolism, the oral bioavailability of R- and S-nitrendipine were 8% and 13%, respectively (72). After an oral dose, the achiral pyridine metabolite of R- and S-nitrendipine is rapidly formed and is detectable in plasma along with the secondary carboxylic acids formed by methyl or ethyl ester hydrolysis and the tertiary methyl hydroxylated products (74). These secondary and tertiary metabolites constitute the major urinary metabolites in their conjugated forms (73,74). The major metabolites of nitrendipine metabolism are thought to be pharmacologically inactive (2,73). Thus oxidation to the pyridine appears to be the major primary pathway of nitrendipine elimination. This is consistent with the good correlation ($r \geq 0.88$) between the AUCs of nifedipine, nitrendipine, and felodipine in a group of 12 healthy volunteers (32). However, based on the administration of the individual enantiomers and *in vitro* studies, it has been suggested that ester hydrolysis of nitrendipine may occur to a minor extent before pyridine formation (2,75).

Drug Interactions In Vivo

Enzymes in the CYP3A subfamily catalyze primarily the formation of the pyridine metabolite of nitrendipine by human liver microsomes *in vitro*, and therefore inhibitors and inducers of these enzymes should be expected to alter the pharmacokinetics of nitrendipine (35). In accord with this expectation, both cimetidine and grapefruit juice administration resulted in 125% to 150% increases in the AUC for the individual enantiomers of nitrendipine (76).

DILTIAZEM

Diltiazem (R,S) is a benzothiazepine calcium channel blocker that is commonly used as intravenous or sustained-release oral preparations (Fig. 24-2). Estimates of systemic clearance for diltiazem after intravenous infusion range from 14 to 21 mL/min/kg with a $t_{1/2}$ of approximately 3 hours (77,78). Orally administered diltiazem is rapidly absorbed from the gastrointestinal tract, with a systemic bioavailability of 33% to 44% (79). The cumulative excretion of radioactivity during the 120 hours after a single intravenous dose, a single oral dose, or multiple oral doses constituted 88% of the dosage, of which 71% was recovered from urine, and 17% was recovered from feces (78,80,81). After oral administration, less than 5% of the parent compound was excreted unchanged in the 0- to 24-hour urine (82). These data illustrate that diltiazem is well absorbed from the gastrointestinal lumen, but first pass elimination accounts for more than half of the dose.

After intravenous infusion of radiolabeled diltiazem to humans, N-desmethyldiltiazem (MA), desacetyldiltiazem (M1), N-desmethyldesacetyldiltiazem (M2), and the parent compound have been quantified in plasma (see Fig. 24-2; 78). Similarly, for oral dosing of 1 week to healthy volunteers, the metabolite plasma concentrations relative to parent drug were MA, 41%; N,O-didesmethyldiltiazem (MB), 16%; O-desmethyldiltiazem (MX), 15%; and less than 10% for M2, M1, N,O-didesmethyldesacetyldiltiazem (M6) and diltiazem N-oxide (83,84). Thus the initial metabolic steps in the elimination of diltiazem are N-demethylation, O-demethylation, and deacetylation. Early studies of diltiazem disposition suggested that M1 was the most abundant metabolite, but this was an artifact due to poorly validated analytic systems and/or chemical degradation (84,85). As many as five acidic and nine basic metabolites have been detected in a 24-hour urine after diltiazem oral administration, of which MA and MB were the most abundant (86).

The rate of diltiazem N-demethylation in primary cultures of human hepatocytes or human liver microsomes correlated with erythromycin N-demethylation rates and was inhibited by anti-CYP3A7 antibody (87). In general agreement with these observations, Sutton et al. (88) demonstrated that the rate of MA formation correlated with testosterone 6β-hydroxylation ($r = 0.82$), a CYP3A-mediated reaction, and tolbutamide hydroxylation ($r = 0.59$), a CYP2C8/9-mediated reaction, in 17 human liver microsomal samples; ketoconazole and triacetyloleandomycin, known CYP3A inhibitors, inhibited diltiazem N-demethylation by approximately 90%, whereas tolbutamide had no effect on diltiazem N-demethylation. Similarly, cDNA-expressed CYP3A4 catalyzed MA formation, but CYP2C8 and CYP2C9 were relatively ineffective catalysts (88). Thus diltiazem N-demethylation is primarily catalyzed by CYP3A *in vitro*. Corresponding studies

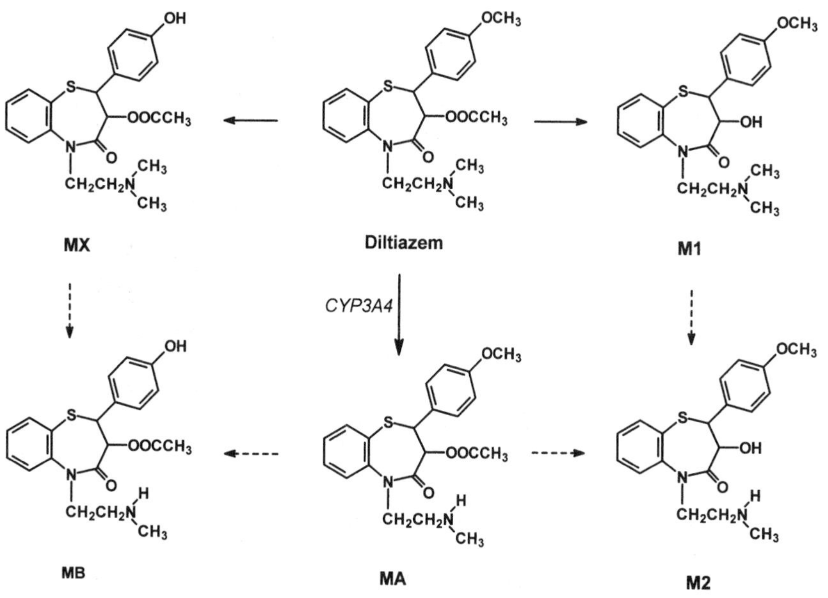

FIG. 24-2. Biotransformation of diltiazem in humans. MA (*N*-desmethyldiltiazem), M1 (desacetyldiltiazem), MX (*O*-desmethyldiltiazem), M2 (*N*-desmethyldesacetyldiltiazem), MB (*N,O*-didesmethyldiltiazem).

aimed at characterizing the other human biotransformations of diltiazem have not been reported.

A number of studies have addressed the pharmacodynamic activity of the significant metabolites of diltiazem. MA, M1, M2, *O*-desmethyldesacetyldiltiazem (M4), and M6 exhibited greater potency than diltiazem in adenosine diphosphate (ADP)-induced platelet-aggregation studies (89). Platelet aggregation may play a role in the cause or exacerbation of various cardiovascular diseases (89). The effects of MA, M1, M2, M4, and M6 on canine coronary blood flow, blood pressure, heart rate, and left ventricular pressure were qualitatively similar to those of diltiazem, which was the most potent (90). M4 and M1 were more potent than diltiazem in the inhibition of adenosine uptake by human erythrocytes, which may play a significant role in coronary circulation, but M2, M6, M1 *N*-oxide, and M4 *N*-oxide were inactive; MA exhibited some activity but was less potent than diltiazem (91). The vasorelaxant activities of diltiazem and metabolites on hamster aorta had the following rank order: diltiazem > M1 > MA > MX > M4 > MB > M9, but diltiazem was about 2.5 times as potent as M1 (92). Clearly the metabolites possess pharmacologic activity, but their role in therapeutic effects that stem from diltiazem administration is still unclear.

Drug Interactions *In Vivo*

Few studies have assessed the effect of concomitant drug therapy on diltiazem plasma concentrations in humans. The effect of CYP inducers on diltiazem disposition has not been reported. Nifedipine, a CYP3A substrate, had no effect on diltiazem pharmacokinetics (93).

In addition, grapefruit juice (200 mL) at 0, 2, 4, 8, and 12 hours after drug intake had no effect on the AUC or maximal plasma concentrations of diltiazem, but the half-life increased significantly (94). Quinidine, a known CYP3A substrate and CYP2D6 inhibitor, had no effect on the pharmacokinetics of diltiazem (95). Cimetidine (1,200 mg/day) dosing for 7 days resulted in a minor (less than 40%) but significant increase in the plasma AUC after a single dose of diltiazem (96).

The lack of effect of established inhibitors of CYP3A on the disposition of diltiazem is unexpected in view of the clear involvement of this enzyme in the formation of the major metabolite of diltiazem. However, it is clear that diltiazem is a potent inhibitor of CYP3A despite a relatively low capability for inhibition of this enzyme ($K_i \approx 50 \ \mu M$) by competitive inhibition *in vitro* (87,97). Furthermore, prolonged dosing results in an increase in diltiazem $t_{1/2}$ and bioavailability (81,98–100). These observations suggest that autoinhibition of CYP3A may readily occur after diltiazem administration, thus obviating inhibition by other CYP3A inhibitors and resulting in time-dependent nonlinear disposition. Possible mechanistic explanations for this nonlinearity include potent competitive enzyme inhibition and/or irreversible inhibition, by diltiazem and/or metabolites. Consistent with this hypothesis are the observations that MA ($K_i \approx 0.1 \ \mu M$) and *N,N*-didesmethyldiltiazem ($K_i \approx 0.1 \ \mu M$) were more potent than diltiazem as competitive inhibitors of CYP3A activity (88) and that intravenous infusion of diltiazem reduced diltiazem clearance in rabbits (101). Importantly, incubation of diltiazem with rat liver microsomes or administration to rats resulted in significant inactivation of cytochrome P450 by metabolic intermediate complex formation (102). We have confirmed that significant metabolic intermediate complex formation and inactivation of CYP3A4 and 3A5 occur with human liver microsomes and cDNA-expressed enzymes (D.R. Jones, unpublished observations). The combination of reversible and irreversible inhibition of CYP3A *in vivo* likely contributes to the nonlinear pharmacokinetics of diltiazem and the apparent resistance to interactions with concomitant medications.

MIBEFRADIL

Mibefradil is a calcium channel blocker in a distinct chemical class that contains a tetraline ring system linked by an aliphatic tertiary amine to a benzimidazole group (Fig. 24-3). After oral administration to steady state in humans, the major metabolite of mibefradil in plasma was Ro 40-5966, which is the alcohol metabolite resulting from deesterification (see Fig. 24-3; 103). This metabolite exhibited plasma AUC_{0-24hr} greater than that of mibefradil. The benzylic hydroxylation products and an aromatic hydroxylated form of Ro 40-5966 also were present in plasma (see Fig. 24-3; 103). The biotransformations that determine the intrinsic clearance of mibefradil, the enzymes that catalyze these steps, and the relative pharmacologic activities of the metabolites have not been reported. Mibefradil labeling indicated that it was an inhibitor of CYP1A2, CYP2D6, and CYP3A4. Its potential to participate in drug–drug interactions was fully

realized on its introduction and was so prevalent as to result in its withdrawal soon after.

VERAPAMIL

Verapamil is a phenylalkylamine and is most commonly administered as an equal mixture of R(d,+)- and S(l,-)-enantiomers in intravenous- and oral-dosage forms (Fig. 24-4). Approximately 70% of a radiolabeled dose of verapamil was excreted in the urine in 120 hours after intravenous or oral administration, and an additional 10% of the intravenous dose was excreted in the feces within 5 days (104). Thus absorption from the gastrointestinal tract is essentially complete.

When R- and S-verapamil were administered intravenously on separate occasions to humans, the plasma clearance of the S-enantiomer (1,411 mL/min) was about twice that of the R-enantiomer (797 mL/min), and a corresponding difference in half-life was noted, 4.8 hours for the S- and 4.1 hours for the R-enantiomer (105). However, after oral administration, the apparent clearance for S-verapamil of 2,400 mL/min was 3 to 4 times greater than that for the R-enantiomer (106,107). The S-enantiomer therefore exhibited a lower bioavailability of 18% compared with 39% for R-verapamil (106). The greater overall bioavailability of R-verapamil reflects hepatic and intestinal wall availability of approximately 0.6 for this enantiomer compared with estimates of approximately

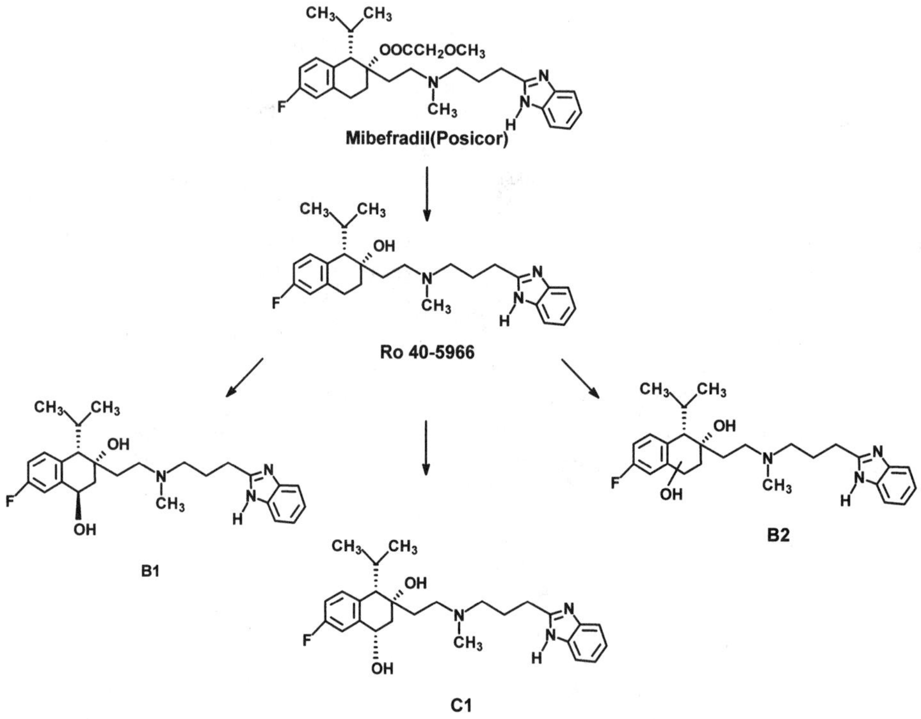

FIG. 24-3. Mibefradil metabolism in humans. Ro 40-5966 (alcohol metabolite of mibefradil), B1 (benzylic hydroxylated alcohol metabolite), C1 (benzylic hydroxylated alcohol metabolite), B2 (aromatic hydroxylated alcohol metabolite).

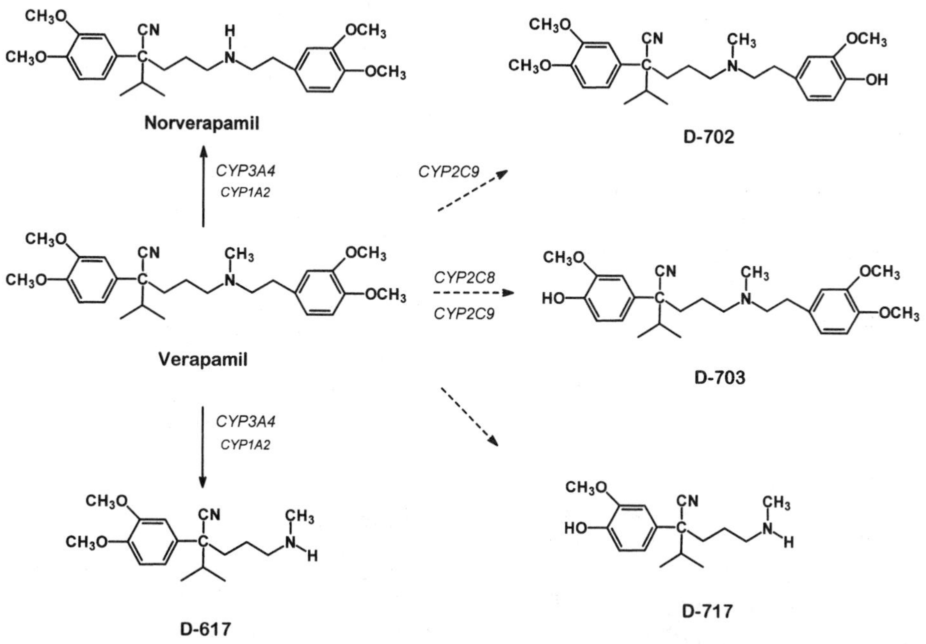

FIG. 24-4. Biotransformation of verapamil in humans. Cytochrome P450s responsible for each pathway are indicated. Norverapamil (*N*-desmethylverapamil), D-617 (*N*-desalkylverapamil), D-702 (*O*-desmethylverapamil), D-703 (*O*-desmethylverapamil), D-717 (*O*-desmethyl,*N*-desalkylverapamil).

0.4 for S-verapamil (108). Thus hepatic and intestinal wall sites contribute significantly to the first pass elimination of verapamil.

Many oxidative metabolites have been detected in urine after oral administration to humans, but excretion of unchanged verapamil has accounted for only 3% to 4% of the dose (109). An *N*-desalkylverapamil, D-617, was the most abundant metabolite in the 0- to 48-hour urine collection, with a percentage of the excreted dose of 22%, followed by the *O*-demethylated product, D-703 (7%), norverapamil (NVP; 6%), and the *O*-desmethyl *N*-desalkylverapamil, D-717 (6%; see Fig. 24-4) (109). A more recent study confirmed that D-617 is the major metabolite in urine, and NVP is the major metabolite in plasma (110). Although D-703 and *O*-desmethylverapamil are significant products of verapamil metabolism *in vitro*, they are not urinary metabolites *in vivo* (106,110). This discrepancy may be the result of preferred biliary excretion of the *O*-desmethylverapamil metabolite. D-617 and NVP have not exhibited any stereoselectivity with regard to $t_{1/2}$ and AUC after oral verapamil dosing (106).

The relative potency of verapamil and its major metabolites in vasodilation of coronary arteries has been studied after intracoronary administration to dogs. Verapamil exhibited the greatest vasodilatory potency, followed by NVP, with approximately five-fold lower activity, but D-617 and D-620 were essentially inactive (111). S-verapamil has been shown to exhibit approximately 10 times the dromotropic activity of the R-enantiomer in studies in humans (112).

Multiple enzymes are involved in the biotransformation of verapamil *in vitro*. On incubation of S- or R-verapamil with human liver microsomes, the intrinsic clearances of metabolite formation declined in the order D-617 > NVP > D-703 > D-702 and were always enantioselective in favor of the S-enantiomer (see Fig. 24-4) (106). D-617 formation from R-, S-, or racemic verapamil in 21 human liver microsomal samples was highly correlated with CYP3A catalytic activity ($r > 0.85$). For S-verapamil, D-617 formation significantly correlated with CYP1A2 catalytic activity ($r = 0.84$). For NVP formation from R-, S-, or racemic verapamil, significant correlations were seen with CYP3A and CYP1A2 activities. Furthermore, an anti-CYP3A antibody reduced the maximal formation of D-617 and NVP by 39% and 33% of control activity (110). cDNA-expressed CYP3A4 and CYP1A2 catalyzed the formation of D-617, whereas only CYP3A4 catalyzed NVP formation (110). These data illustrate that CYP3A and, to a lesser extent, CYP1A2 are the principal mediators of verapamil biotransformation in humans.

Anti-LKM2 antibodies (anti-CYP2C9 and anti-CYP2C19) inhibited the formation of the minor human metabolites, D-702 and D-703, by 82% and 53%, respectively, in four human liver microsomal samples (113). Additionally, sulfaphenazole inhibited D-702 and D-703 by 62% and 26%, respectively. cDNA-expressed CYP2C9 formed D-702 and expressed CYP2C8, and CYP2C9 formed D-703, with CYP2C8 displaying the highest V_{max} and the lowest K_m for the formation of D-703 (113). These *in vitro* results suggest that CYP2C8 and CYP2C9 may play a minor role in verapamil disposition.

Drug Interactions In Vivo

Very few reports of concomitant drug therapy influencing the plasma concentrations of verapamil have appeared. As expected from *in vitro* data, rifampin, a potent inducer of CYP3A, dramatically reduced the efficacy of oral verapamil, whereas no significant changes were observed after intravenous administration (108,114). This interaction coincided with a drastic reduction in verapamil oral bioavailability from 26% to 2% (114). A later study supported the conclusion that rifampin reduced verapamil oral bioavailability to less than 10% (110). By using simultaneous oral and intravenous administration of verapamil, Fromm et al. (108) estimated that rifampin reduced the hepatic availability of R-verapamil from 0.6 to 0.2 and the intestinal availability from 0.6 to 0.05. S-verapamil was similarly affected by rifampin, with hepatic availability changing from 0.3 to 0.15 and the intestinal availability changing from 0.45 to 0.05. As a result of these changes in availability, the apparent oral clearance increased by factors of 32 and 57 for S- and R-verapamil, respectively (108). The lack of effect of rifampin on the intravenous efficacy of verapamil corresponds to a modest 1.3-fold increase in hepatic clearance of S-verapamil. This, in turn, reflects the relative insensitivity of hepatic clearance to an increase in hepatic intrinsic clearance for this well-extracted drug. A similar effect by rifampin on verapamil disposition was observed in elderly volunteers (115). As expected from the response to rifampin, there was a doubling of the intravenous clearance and a five-fold increase in oral clearance of verapamil after daily treatment with phenobarbital (116). A case report suggests that induction of verapamil metabolism should also be expected with the CYP3A inducer, phenytoin (117).

As expected from the significant contribution of intestinal wall metabolism to verapamil bioavailability, grapefruit juice increased the oral bioavailability of verapamil by 1.4-fold (118). Similarly, cimetidine caused a significant increase in bioavailability of oral verapamil from 26% to 49%, but the pharmacokinetics of intravenous verapamil were not affected (119).

BEPRIDIL

Bepridil is a diarylaminopropylamine that is available as the racemate and differs from the other calcium channel blockers in structure as well as in pharmacokinetic characteristics. The half-life of bepridil approaches 2 days, and it is completely absorbed after oral administration (120,121). Oral bioavailability is approximately 60% and results in multiple metabolite formation (120). At least 25 metabolites of bepridil have been isolated and identified from plasma, urine, and fecal samples of humans receiving oral doses; less than 0.1% of the administered dosage of bepridil is recovered unchanged in urine. An aromatic hydroxy-metabolite has demonstrated cardiovascular activity similar to the parent compound but was less than 5% of the pooled 0- to 24-hour plasma total radioactivity compared with 16% for unchanged bepridil (120). In humans, the primary circulating metabolite is an N-dealkylated metabolite, and its conjugate constitutes the primary urinary metabolite (120–122). The metabolism of bepridil has not been characterized *in vitro*, and there is a general absence of controlled studies addressing the potential for bepridil to interact with other drugs *in vivo*.

OVERVIEW

In general, the calcium channel blockers are CYP3A substrates that display incomplete bioavailability because of intestinal wall and hepatic metabolism. Interactions at these first pass sites dominate the drug-interaction landscape for this class of drug. This feature provides a rational basis for anticipating potential drug interactions. However, many calcium channel blockers are also substrates for *p*-glycoprotein, the product of the multidrug resistance gene (MDR1). This protein is responsible for the secretion of some drugs into the intestinal lumen, the renal tubular fluid, and the biliary tract. Many inhibitors of CYP3A are also inhibitors of *p*-glycoprotein activity. Therefore it is theoretically possible that interactions with some calcium channel blockers could occur at the level of *p*-glycoprotein, and these would be clinically indistinguishable from interactions at the level of CYP3A. The relative contributions of these two mechanisms of interaction to drug interactions awaits full definition.

ACKNOWLEDGMENT

The support of the NIH through RO1 AG 13718 is gratefully acknowledged.

REFERENCES

1. Soons PA, Mulders TMT, Ucida E, Schoemaker HC, Cohen AF, Breimer DD. Stereoselective pharmacokinetics of oral felodipine and nitrendipine in healthy subjects: correlation with nifedipine pharmacokinetics. *Eur J Clin Pharmacol* 1993;44:163–169.
2. Mikus G, Mast V, Ratge D, Wisser H, Eichelbaum M. Stereoselectivity in cardiovascular and biochemical action of calcium antagonists: studies with the enantiomers of the dihydropyridine nitrendipine. *Clin Pharmacol Ther* 1995;57:52–61.
3. Raemsch KD, Sommer J. Pharmacokinetics and metabolism of nifedipine. *Hypertension* 1983;5(4 suppl):18–24.
4. Waller DG, Renwick AG, Gruchy BS, George CF. The first pass metabolism of nifedipine in man. *Br J Clin Pharmacol* 1984;18:951–954.
5. Challenor VF, Waller DG, Renwick AG, Gruchy BS, George CF. The trans-hepatic extraction of nifedipine. *Br J Clin Pharmacol* 1987;24:473–477.

6. Horster FA, Maul DW, Medenwald H, Patzschke K, Weger LA. Klinissche Untersuchungen zur Pharmackokinetik von radioaktiv markiertem 4-(2'-Nitrophenyl)-2,6-dimethyl-1,4-dihydropyridin-3,5-dicarbonsauredimethylester. *Arzneimittelforshung* 1972;22:330–334.

7. Kleinbloesem CH, van Brummelen P, van de Linde JA, Voogd PD, Breimer DD. Nifedipine: kinetics and dynamics in healthy subjects. *Clin Pharmacol Ther* 1984;35:742–749.

8. Guengerich FP, Margin MV, Beaune PH, Kremers P, Wolff T, Waxman DJ. Characterization of rat and human liver microsomal cytochrome P-450 forms involved in nifedipine oxidation, a prototype for genetic polymorphism in oxidative drug metabolism. *J Biol Chem* 1986;261: 5051–5060.

9. Böcker RH, Guengerich FP. Oxidation of 4-aryl- and 4-alkyl-substituted 2,6-dimethyl-3-5-bis (alkoxycarbonyl)-1,4,-dihydropyridines by human liver microsomes and immunochemical evidence for the involvement of a form of cytochrome P-450. *J Med Chem* 1986;29: 1596–1603.

10. Yamazake H, Nakano M, Imai Y, Yune-Fang U, Guengerich FP, Shimada T. Roles of cytochrome b5 in the oxidation of testosterone and nifedipine by recombinant cytochrome P450 3A4 and by human liver microsomes. *Arch Biochem Biophys* 1996;325:174–182.

11. Guengerich FP, Peterson LA, Böcker RH. Cytochrome P-450-catalyzed hydroxylation and carboxylic acid ester cleavage of Hantzsch pyridine esters. *J Biol Chem* 1988;263:8176–8183.

12. Funaki T, Soons PA, Guengerich FP, Breimer DD. In vivo oxidative cleavage of a pyridine-carboxylic acid ester metabolite of nifedipine. *Biochem Pharmacol* 1989;38:4213–4216.

13. Tateishi T, Ohashi K, Sudo T, et al. Dose dependent effect of diltiazem on the pharmacokinetics of nifedipine. *J Clin Pharmacol* 1989;29: 994–997.

14. Bowles SK, Reeves RA, Cardozo L, Edwards DJ. Evaluation of the pharmacokinetic pharmacodynamic interaction between quinidine and nifedipine. *J Clin Pharmacol* 1993;33:727–731.

15. Schellens JH, Ghabrial H, vander Wart HH, Bakker EN, Wilkinson GR, Breimer DD. Differential effects of quinidine on the disposition of nifedipine, sparteine, and mephenytoin in humans. *Clin Pharmacol Ther* 1991;50:520–528.

16. Khan A, Langley SJ, Mullins FG, Toon S. The pharmacokinetics and pharmacodynamics of nifedipine at steady state during concomitant administration of cimetidine or high dose ranitidine. *Br J Clin Pharmacol* 1991;32:519–522.

17. Tailor SA. Peripheral edema vasodilation due to nifedipine-itraconazole interaction: a case report. *Arch Dermatol* 1996;132:1374.

18. Sigusch H, Hippius M, Henschel L, Kaufmann K, Hoffmann A. Influence of grapefruit juice on the pharmacokinetics of a slow release nifedipine formulation. *Pharmazie* 1994;49:522–524.

19. Rashid TJ, Martin U, Clarke H, Waller DG, Renwick AG, George CF. Factors affecting the absolute bioavailability of nifedipine. *Br J Clin Pharmacol* 1995;40:51–58.

20. Holtbecker N, Fromm MF, Kromer HK, Ohnhaus EE, Heidemann H. The nifedipine-rifampin interaction: evidence for induction of gut wall metabolism. *Drug Metab Dispos* 1996;24:1121–1123.

21. Faulkner JK, McGibney D, Chasseaud LF, Perry JL. The pharmacokinetics of amlodipine in healthy volunteers after single intravenous and oral doses after 14 repeated oral doses given once daily. *Br J Clin Pharmacol* 1986;22:21–25.

22. Williams DM, Cubeddu LX. Amlodipine pharmacokinetics in healthy volunteers. *J Clin Pharmacol* 1988;28:990–994.

23. Abernethy DR, Gutkowska J, Lambert MD. Amlodipine in elderly hypertensive patients; pharmacokinetics and pharmacodynamics. *J Cardiovasc Pharmacol* 1988;12:S67–S71.

24. Stopher DA, Berefore AP, Macrae PV, Humphrey MJ. The metabolism and pharmacokinetics of amlodipine in humans and animals. *J Cardiovasc Pharmacol* 1988;12:S55–S59.

25. Laufen H, Leitold M. Enantioselective disposition of oral amlodipine in healthy volunteers. *Chirality* 1994;6:531–536.

26. Josefsson M, Zackrisson AL, Ahlner J. Effect of grapefruit juice on the pharmacokinetics of amlodipine in healthy volunteers. *Eur J Clin Pharmacol* 1996;51:189–193.

27. Dunselman PHJM, Edgar B, Scaf AHJ, Kunze CEE, Wesseling H. Pharmacokinetics of felodipine after intravenous and chronic oral administration in patients with congestive heart failure. *Br J Clin Pharmacol* 1989;66:45–52.

28. Weidolf L, Borg KO, Hoggman K-J. Urinary metabolites of felodipine: a new vasodilator drug, in man, dog, and mouse. *Xenobiotica* 1984;14:657–666.

29. Edgar B, Regardh CG, Johnsson G, et al. Felodipine kinetics in healthy men. *Clin Pharmacol Ther* 1985;38:205–211.

30. Saltiel E, Ellrodt AG, Monk JP, Langley MS. Felodipine: a review of its pharmacodynamic properties and therapeutic use in hypertension. *Drugs* 1988;36:387–428.

31. Lundahl J, Regardh CG, Edgar B, Johnsson G. Relationship between time of intake of grapefruit juice and its effect on pharmacokinetics and pharmacodynamics of felodipine in healthy subjects. *Eur J Clin Pharmacol* 1995;49:61–67.

32. Soons PA, Mulders TMT, Uchida E, Schoemaker HC, Cohen AF, Breimer DD. Stereoselective pharmacokinetics of oral felodipine and nitrendipine pharmacokinetics. *Eur J Clin Pharmacol* 1993;44: 163–169.

33. Bäärnhielm C, Backman A, Hoffmann KJ, Weidolf L. Biotransformation of felodipine in liver microsomes from rat, dog, and man. *Drug Metab Dispos* 1986;14:613–618.

34. Hoffmann KJ, Andersson L. Metabolism of [^{14}C]felodipine: a new vasodilating drug, in healthy volunteers. *Drugs* 1987;34(suppl 3): 43–52.

35. Guerngerich FP, Brian WR, Iwasake M, Sari M-A, Bäärnhielm C, Berntsson P. Oxidation of dihydropyridine calcium channel blockers and analogues by human liver cytochrome P-450 IIIA4. *J Med Chem* 1991;34:1838–1844.

36. Jalava KM, Olkkola KT, Neuvonen PJ. Itraconazole greatly increases plasma concentrations and effects of felodipine. *Clin Pharmacol Ther* 1997;61:410–415.

37. Bailey DG, Bend JR, Arnold JM, Tran LT, Spence JD. Erythromycin-felodipine interaction: magnitude, mechanism, and comparison with grapefruit juice. *Clin Pharmacol Ther* 1996;60:25–33.

38. Madsen JK, Jensen JD, Jensen LW, Pedersen EB. Pharmacokinetic interaction between cyclosporine and the dihydropyridine calcium antagonist felodipine. *Eur J Clin Pharmacol* 1997;52:161.

39. Capewell S, Freestone S, Critchley JA, Pottage A, Prescott LF. Reduced felodipine bioavailability in patients taking anticonvulsants. *Lancet* 1988;2:480–482.

40. Lundahl J, Regardh CG, Edgar B, Johnsson G. Effects of grapefruit juice ingestion: pharmacokinetics and haemodynamics of intravenously and orally administered felodipine in healthy men. *Eur J Clin Pharmacol* 1997;52:139–145.

41. Lundahl J, Regardh CG, Edgar B, Johnsson G. Relationship between time of intake of grapefruit and its effect on pharmacokinetic and pharmacodynamics of felodipine in healthy subjects. *Eur J Clin Pharmacol* 1995;49:61–67.

42. Bailey DG, Arnold JM, Munoz C, Spence JD. Grapefruit juice-felodipine interaction: mechanism, predictability, and effect of naringin. *Clin Pharmacol Ther* 1993;53:637–642.

43. Edgar B, Bailey D, Bergstrand R, Johnsson R, Regardh CG. Acute effects of drinking grapefruit juice on the pharmacokinetics and dynamics of felodipine and its potential clinical relevance. *Eur J Clin Pharmacol* 1992;42:313–317.

44. Lown KS, Bailey DG, Fontana RJ, et al. Grapefruit juice increases felodipine oral availability in humans by decreasing intestinal CYP3A protein expression. *J Clin Invest* 1997;99:2545–2553.

45. Schmieldin-Ren P, Edwards DJ, Fitzsimmons ME, et al. Mechanisms of enhanced oral availability of CYP3A4 substrates by grapefruit constituents: decreased enterocyte CYP3A4 concentration and mechanism-based inactivation by furanocoumarins. *Drug Metab Dispos* 1997;25:1228–1233.

46. Tse FLS, Jaffe JM. Pharmacokinetics of PN 200-110 (isradipine): a new calcium antagonist, after oral administration in man. *Eur J Clin Pharmacol* 1987;32:361–365.

47. Clifton GD, Blouin RA, Dilea C, et al. The pharmacokinetics of oral isradipine in normal volunteers. *J Clin Pharmacol* 1988;28:36–42.

48. Brogden RN, Sorkin EM. Isradipine: an update of its pharmacodynamic and pharmacokinetic properties and therapeutic efficacy in the treatment of mild to moderate hypertension. *Drugs* 1995;49:618–649.

49. Bidouil S, Dubois J, Hanocq M. Isocratic high-performance liquid chromatographic method for the separation of isradipine and its main metabolites: application to in vitro metabolization by h3A4/OR cells. *J Chromatogr B* 1997;693:359–366.

50. Hall ST, Harding SM, Evans GL, Pellegatti M, Rizzini P. Clinical pharmacology of lacidipine. *J Cardiovasc Pharmacol* 1991;17(suppl 4):S9–S13.

51. Squassante L, Caveggion E, Braggio S, Pellegatti M, Baroldi P. A study of plasma disposition kinetics of lacidipine after single oral ascending doses. *J Cardiovasc Pharmacol* 1994;23(suppl 5):S94–97.

52. Lee CR, Bryson HM. Lacidipine: a review of its pharmacodynamic and pharmacokinetic properties and therapeutic potential in the treatment of hypertension. *Drugs* 1994;48:274–296.

53. Takenaka T, Miyazaki I, Asano M, Higuchi S, Maeno H. Vasodilator and hypotensive effects of the optical isomers of nicardipine (YC-93): a new Ca^{2+} antagonist. *Jpn J Pharmacol* 1982;32:665–670.

54. Guerret M, Cheymol G, Hubert M, Julien-Larose C, Lavene D. Simultaneous study of the pharmacokinetics of intravenous and oral nicardipine using a stable isotope. *Eur J Clin Pharmacol* 1989;37: 381–385.

55. Inotsome N, Iwaoka T, Honda M, et al. Pharmacokinetics of nicardipine enantiomers in healthy young volunteers. *Eur J Clin Pharmacol* 1997;52:289–292.

56. Rush WR, Alexandar O, Hall DJ, Cairncross L, Dow RJ, Graham DJG. The metabolism of nicardipine hydrochloride in healthy male volunteers. *Xenobiotica* 1986;16:341–349.

57. Uno T, Ohkubo T, Sugawara K, Higashiyama A, Motomura S. Effect of grapefruit juice on the disposition of nicardipine after intravenous and oral doses. *Clin Pharmacol Ther* 1997;61:209.

58. Rämsch K-D, Graefe K-H, Scherling D, Sommer J, Ziegler R. Pharmacokinetics and metabolism of calcium-blocking agents nifedipine, nitrendipine and nimodipine. *Am J Nephrol* 1986;6:73–80.

59. Muck W, Tanaka T, Ahr G, Kuhlmann J. No interethnic differences in stereoselective disposition of oral nimodipine between Caucasian and Japanese subjects. *Int J Clin Pharmacol Ther* 1996;34:163–171.

60. Langley MS, Sorkin EM. Nimodipine: a review of its pharmacodynamic and pharmacokinetic properties, and therapeutic potential in cerebrovascular disease. *Drugs* 1989;37:669–699.

61. Tartara A, Galimberti CA, Manni R, et al. Differential effects of valproic acid and enzyme-inducing anticonvulsants on nimodipine pharmcokinetics in epileptic patients. *Br J Clin Pharmacol* 1991;32:335–340.

62. Muck W, Wingender W, Seiberling M, Woelke E, Ramsch KD, Kuhlmann J. Influence of the H_2-receptor antagonists cimetidine and ranitidine on the pharmacokinetics of nimodipine in healthy volunteers. *Eur J Clin Pharmacol* 1992;42:325–328.

63. Fuhr U, Maier A, Blume H, et al. Grapefruit juice increases oral nimodipine bioavailability. *Eur J Clin Pharmacol* 1994;47:A100.

64. Friedel HA, Sorkin EM. Nisoldipine: a preliminary review of its pharmacodynamic and pharmacokinetic properties, and therapeutic efficacy in the treatment of angina pectoris, hypertension and related cardiovascular disorders. *Drugs* 1988;36:682–731.

65. Scherling D, Karl W, Ahr G, Ahr HJ, Wehinger E. Pharmacokinetics of nisoldine. III. Biotransformation of nisoldine in rat, dog, monkey, and man. *Arzneimittelforschung* 1988;38:1105–1110.

66. Langtry HD, Spencer CM. Nisoldipine coat-core. *Drugs* 1997;53: 867–884.

67. Bailey DG, Arnold JMO, Strong HA, Munoz C, Spence JD. Effect of grapefruit juice and naringin on nisoldine pharmacokinetics. *Clin Pharmacol Ther* 1993;54:589–594.

68. van Harten J, van Brummelen P, Lodewijks MT, Danhof M, Breimer DD. Pharmacokinetics and hemodynamic effects of nisoldipine and its interaction with cimetidine. *Clin Pharmacol Ther* 1988;43:332–341.

69. Brendel E, Heinig R, Ahr G, et al. Influence of cimetidine and ranitidine on the pharmacokinetics of controlled-release formulations of the two calcium-antagonists nifedipine and nisoldipine. *Naunyn Schmiedebergs Arch Pharmacol* 1992;345(suppl):R3.

70. Michelucci R, Cipolla G, Passarelli D, et al. Reduced plasma nisoldipine concentrations in phenytoin-treated patients with epilepsy. *Epilepsia* 1995;37:1107–1110.

71. Eltze M, Boer R, Sanders KH, Boss K, Ulrich WR, Flockerzi D. Stereoselective inhibition of thromboxane-induced coronary vasoconstriction by 1,4-dihydropyridine calcium channel antagonist. *Chirality* 1990;2:233–240.

72. Soons PA, Breimer DD. Stereoselective pharmacokinetics of oral and intravenous nitrendipine healthy male subjects. *Br J Clin Pharmacol* 1991;32:11–16.

73. Mast V, Fischer C, Mikur G, Eichelbaum M. Use of pseudoracemic nitrendipine to elucidate the metabolic steps responsible for stereoselective disposition of nitrendipine enantiomers. *Br J Clin Pharmacol* 1992;33:51–59.

74. Krol GJ, Lettieri JT, Yeh SC, Burkholder DE, Birkett JP. Disposition and pharmacokinetics of ^{14}C-nitrendipine in healthy volunteers. *J Cardiovasc Pharmacol* 1987;9:S122–S128.

75. Böcker RH, Preuss E, Peter R. High-performance liquid chromatography of the metabolites of nitrendipine and investigation into the metabolic pathways of this dihydropyridine. *J Chromatogr B* 1990; 530:206–211.

76. Soons PA, Vogels BA, Roosemalen MC, et al. Grapefruit juice and cimetidine inhibit stereoselective metabolism of nitrendipine in humans. *Clin Pharmacol Ther* 1991;50:394–403.

77. Hermann P, Rodger SD, Remones G, Thenot JP, London DR, Morselli PL. Pharmacokinetics of diltiazem after intravenous and oral administration. *Eur J Clin Pharmacol* 1983;24:349–352.

78. Höglund P, Nilsson L-G. Physiological disposition of intravenously administered ^{14}C-labeled diltiazem in healthy volunteer. *Ther Drug Monit* 1988;1:401–409.

79. Ochs HR, Knüchel M. Pharmacokinetics and absolute bioavailability of diltiazem in humans. *Klin Wochenschr* 1984;62:303–306.

80. Höglund P, Nilsson L-G. Pharmacokinetics of diltiazem and its metabolites after repeated multiple-dose treatments in healthy volunteers. *Ther Drug Monit* 1989;11:543–550.

81. Höglund P, Nilsson L-G. Pharmacokinetics of diltiazem and its metabolites after single and multiple dosing in healthy volunteers. *Ther Drug Monit* 1989;11:558–566.

82. Sugihara J, Sugawara Y, Ando H, Harigaya S, Etoh A, Kohno K. Studies on the metabolism of diltiazem in man. *J Pharmacobiodyn* 1984; 7:24–32.

83. Yeung PKF, Buckley SJ, Hung OR, et al. Steady-state plasma concentrations of diltiazem and its metabolites in patients and healthy volunteers. *Ther Drug Monit* 1996;18:40–45.

84. Yeung PKF, Montague TJ, Tsui B, McGregor C. High-performance liquid chromatographic assay of diltiazem and six of its metabolites in plasma: application to a pharmacokinetic study in healthy volunteers. *J Pharmacol Sci* 1989;78:592–597.

85. Abernethy DR, Schwartz JB, Todd EL. Diltiazem and desacetyldiltiazem analysis in human plasma using high-performance liquid chromatography: improved sensitivity without derivatization. *J Chromatogr* 1985;342:216–220.

86. Sugawara Y, Nakamura S, Usuke S, et al. Metabolism of diltiazem II: metabolic profile in rat, dog and man. *J Pharmacobiodyn* 1988;11: 224–233.

87. Pichard L, Gillet G, Fabre I, et al. Identification of the rabbit and human cytochromes P-450IIIA as the major enzymes involved in the N-demethylation of diltiazem. *Drug Metab Dispos* 1990;18:711–719.

88. Sutton D, Butler AM, Nadin L, Murray M. Role of CYP3A4 in human hepatic diltiazem N-demethylation: inhibition of CYP3A4 activity by oxidized diltiazem metabolites. *J Pharmacol Exp Ther* 1997;282: 294–300.

89. Kiyomoto A, Sasaki Y, Odawara A, Morita T. Inhibition of platelet aggregation by diltiazem: comparison with verapamil and nifedipine and inhibitory potencies of diltiazem metabolites. *Circ Res* 1983;52: I115–I119.

90. Yabana H, Nagao T, Sato M. Cardiovascular effects of the metabolites of diltiazem in dogs. *Cardiovasc Pharmacol* 1985;7:152–157.

91. Yeung PKF, Mosher SJ, Macrae DA, Klassen GA. Effects of diltiazem and its metabolites on the uptake of adenosine in blood: an *in vitro* investigation. *J Pharm Pharmacol* 1991;43:685–689.

92. Li R, Farmer PS, Xie M, et al. Synthesis, characterization, and Ca^{2+} antagonistic activity of diltiazem metabolites. *Am Cancer Soc* 1992; 92:3246–3253.

93. Toyosaki N, Toyo-Oka T, Natsume T, et al. Combination therapy with diltiazem and nifedipine in patients with effort angina pectoris. *Circulation* 1988;77:1370–1375.

94. Sigusch H, Henschel S, Kraul H, Merkel U, Hoffmann A. Lack of effects of grapefruit juice on diltiazem bioavailability in normal subjects. *Pharmazie* 1994;49:675–679.

95. Laganiére S, Davies RF, Carignan G. Pharmacokinetic and pharmacodynamic interactions between diltiazem and quinidine. *Clin Pharmacol Ther* 1996;60:255–264.

96. Winship LC, McKenney JM, Wright JT, Wood JH Jr, Goodman RP. The effect of ranitidine and cimetidine on single-dose diltiazem pharmacokinetics. *Pharmacotherapy* 1985;5:16–19.

97. Pichard L, Fabre I, Fabre G, et al. Cyclosporin A drug interactions: screening for inducers and inhibitors of cytochrome P-450 (cyclosporin A oxidase) in primary cultures of human hepatocytes and in liver microsomes. *Drug Metab Dispos* 1990;18:595–606.

98. Caille G, Boucher S, Spenard J, et al. Diltiazem pharmacokinetics in elderly volunteers after single and multiple doses. *Eur J Drug Metab Pharmacokinet* 1991;16:75–80.

99. Montamat SC, Abernethy DR. *N*-Monodesmethyldiltiazem is the predominant metabolite of diltiazem in the plasma of young and elderly hypertensives. *Br J Clin Pharmacol* 1987;24:185–189.

100. Abernethy DR, Montamat SC. Acute and chronic studies of diltiazem in elderly versus young hypertensive patients. *Am J Cardiol* 1987;60: 116I–120I.

101. Lefebvre M, Caille G, Souich PD. Organ-specific pattern of inhibition of diltiazem metabolism at steady state in rabbits. *J Pharmacol Exp Ther* 1996;279:902–907.

102. Bensoussan C, Delaforge M, Mansuy D. Particular ability of cytochromes P450 3A to form inhibitory P450-iron-metabolite complexes upon metabolic oxidation of aminodrugs. *Biochem Pharmacol* 1995; 49:591–602.

103. Wiltshire HR, Sutton BM, Heeps G, et al. Metabolism of the calcium antagonist, mibefradil (POSICOR™, Ro 40-5967). Part III: comparative pharmacokinetics of mibefradil and its major metabolites in rat, marmoset, cynomolgus monkey and man. *Xenobiotica* 1997;27: 557–571.

104. Schomerus M, Spiegelhalder B, Stieren B, Eichelbaum M. Physiological disposition of verapamil in man. *Cardiovasc Res* 1976;10:605–612.

105. Eichelbaum M, Mikus G, Vogelgesang B. Pharmacokinetics of (+)-, (−)-, and (±)-verapamil after intravenous administration. *Br J Clin Pharmacol* 1984;17:453–458.

106. Kroemer HK, Echizen H, Heidemann H, Eichelbaum M. Predictability of the *in vivo* metabolism of verapamil from *in vitro* data: contribution of individual metabolic pathways and stereoselective aspects. *J Pharmacol Exp Ther* 1992;260:1052–1057.

107. Vogelgesang B, Echizen H, Schmidt E, Eichelbaum M. Stereoselective first-pass metabolism of highly cleared drugs: studies of the bioavailability of L- and D-verapamil examined with a stable isotope technique. *Br J Clin Pharmacol* 1984;18:733–740.

108. Fromm MF, Busse D, Kroemer HK, Eichelbaum M. Differential induction of prehepatic and hepatic metabolism of verapamil by rifampin. *Hepatology* 1996;24:796–801.

109. Eichelbaum M, Enge M, Remberg G, Schomerus M, Dengler HJ. The metabolism of DL-[^{14}C] verapamil in man. *Drug Metab Dispos* 1979;7:145–148.

110. Kroemer HK, Gautier JC, Beaune P, Henderson C, Wolf CR, Eichelbaum M. Identification of P450 enzymes involved in metabolism of verapamil in humans. *Naunyn Schmiedebergs Arch Pharmacol* 1993; 348:332–337.

111. Neugebauer G. Comparative cardiovascular actions of verapamil and its major metabolites in the anaesthetised dog. *Cardiovasc Res* 1978; 12:247–254.

112. Echizen H, Vogelgesang B, Eichelbaum M. Effects of d,l-verapamil on atrioventricular conduction in relation to its stereoselective first-pass metabolism. *Clin Pharmacol Ther* 1985;38:71–76.

113. Busse D, Cosme J, Beaune P, Kroemer HK, Eichelbaum M. Cytochromes of the P450 2C subfamily are the major enzymes involved in the *O*-demethylation of verapamil in humans. *Naunyn Schmiedebergs Arch Pharmacol* 1995;353:116–121.

114. Barbarash RA, Bauman JL, Fisher JL, Knodos GT, Batenhorst RL. Near-total reduction in verapamil bioavailability by rifampin electrocardiographic correlates. *Chest* 1988;94:964–995.

115. Fromm MF, Dilger K, Busse D, Kroemer HK, Eichelbaum M, Klots U. Gut wall metabolism of verapamil in older people: effects of rifampicin-mediated enzyme induction. *Br J Clin Pharmacol* 1998; 45:247–255.

116. Rutledge DR, Pieper JA, Mirvis DM. Effects of chronic phenobarbital on verapamil disposition in humans. *J Pharmacol Exp Ther* 1988; 246:7–13.

117. Woodcock BG, Kirsten R, Nelson K, Rietbrock S, Hopf R, Kaltenback M. A reduction in verapamil concentrations with phenytoin. *N Engl J Med* 1991;325:1179.

118. Fuhr U, Kroemer HK, Schymanski P. Effects of narigenen and naringin on verapamil metabolism in human liver microsomes. *Naunyn Schmiedebergs Arch Pharmacol* 1993;347:122.

119. Smith MS, Benyunes MC, Bjornsson TD, Shand DG, Pritchett EL. Influence of cimetidine on verapamil kinetics and dynamics. *Clin Pharmacol Ther* 1984;36:551–554.

120. Benet LZ. Pharmacokinetics and metabolism of bepridil. *Am J Cardiol* 1985;55:8C–13C.

121. Awni WM, Halstenston CE, Kayak RK, et al. Pharmacokinetics of bepridil and two of its metabolites in patients with end-stage renal disease. *J Clin Pharmacol* 1995;35:379–383.

122. Wu WN, Hills JF, Chang SY, Ng KT. Metabolism of bepridil in laboratory animals and humans. *Drug Metab Dispos* 1988;16:69–77.

CHAPTER 25

β-Adrenoceptor Antagonists

Martin S. Lennard

The β-adrenoceptor antagonists (β-blockers) remain a first-line therapy for hypertension in patients who do not have obstructive airway disease or cardiac failure and in the treatment of supraventricular arrhythmias. They also are a mainstay of treatment for angina and significantly reduce the incidence of a second myocardial infarction in patients who have had one previously. In addition they are used as an adjunct to therapy in the treatment of anxiety, thyrotoxicosis, and in the prophylaxis of migraine. Several β-blockers, particularly timolol, are also used topically in glaucoma. There were more than 14,000,000 prescriptions for β-blockers in England alone in 1996 (*Prescription Cost Analysis England 1996,* UK Government Department of Health). Accordingly, because many patients taking β-blockers are likely to be receiving combination drug therapy, the potential for drug–drug interactions is substantial.

More than 15 β-blockers are available worldwide for clinical use. They cover a wide range of lipophilicities. Atenolol, nadolol, and sotalol are very hydrophilic, resulting in their elimination from the body almost entirely by renal and fecal excretion of unchanged drug. In general, these drugs will not be subject to metabolically based pharmacokinetic interactions, although they do inhibit drug metabolism to a small degree. However, the more lipid-soluble compounds such as propranolol, metoprolol, and timolol undergo highly variable first pass metabolism, catalyzed mainly by cytochrome P450, with very little of the drug being excreted unchanged. Thus inhibition or induction of their metabolism by cytochrome P450 may have important clinical implications. The consequences of elevated plasma drug concentrations are excessive β-blockade, which may rarely be associated with heart failure, and bronchoconstriction. Less serious adverse effects, which

M. S. Lennard: Division of Clinical Sciences, Section of Molecular Pharmacology and Pharmacogenetics, University of Sheffield, Royal Hallamshire Hospital, Glossop Road, Sheffield S10 2JF, United Kingdom

may nevertheless substantially affect quality of life, include fatigue and lethargy, sleep disturbances, and gastrointestinal disturbances.

Some β-blockers, particularly propranolol, are also inhibitors of cytochrome P450 enzyme activities, which has clinical implications in patients taking other drugs with a narrow therapeutic range, and which are metabolized by cytochrome P450.

In this chapter, interactions involving β-blockers that are thought to occur through changes in metabolism are reviewed. It should be stressed that many of the pharmacokinetic data discussed were obtained from relatively small numbers of subjects. Thus many of the mean differences quoted will inevitably have large 95% confidence intervals and should be interpreted in this light.

THE METABOLISM OF THE MAIN LIPID-SOLUBLE β-BLOCKERS

Only the metabolism of those β-blockers for which significant numbers of clinically relevant metabolic interactions have been reported are discussed.

Propranolol

In humans propranolol is rapidly and completely absorbed, and undergoes high first pass metabolism, with very little of the dose being eliminated as unchanged drug (1). Although at least 13 metabolites have been identified, propranolol is metabolized through three primary routes: aromatic hydroxylation (mainly 4-hydroxylation), *N*-dealkylation followed by further side-chain oxidation, and direct glucuronidation (Fig. 25-1). It has been estimated that the percentage contributions of these routes to total metabolism are 42% (range, 27%—59%), 41% (range, 32%–50%), and 17% (10%–25%), respectively, but with considerable variability between individuals (2). The oral clearance of (R)-propranolol is significantly greater than that of the (S)-form (3), which appears largely due to

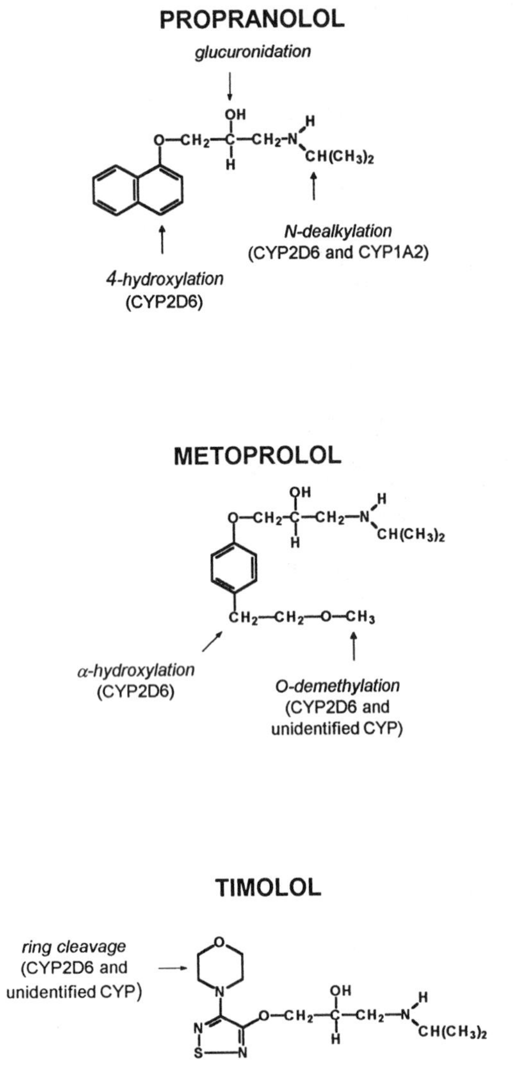

PROPRANOLOL

glucuronidation

N-dealkylation
(CYP2D6 and CYP1A2)

4-hydroxylation
(CYP2D6)

METOPROLOL

α-hydroxylation
(CYP2D6)

O-demethylation
(CYP2D6 and
unidentified CYP)

TIMOLOL

ring cleavage
(CYP2D6 and
unidentified CYP)

FIG. 25-1. The major routes of propranolol, metoprolol, and timolol metabolism in humans and the isoforms of cytochrome P450 catalyzing these reactions.

stereoselective aromatic ring hydroxylation (4). *In vitro* studies have indicated that the aromatic hydroxylation of propranolol is catalyzed mainly by polymorphic CYP2D6 (5,6). Both CYP2D6 and CYP1A2 catalyze side-chain oxidation, but their relative contributions show marked variation between individual livers (7). On average, the contribution of CYP2D6 to the overall elimination of propranolol is insufficient to cause differences in its pharmacokinetics between phenotypes (8,9).

Metoprolol

About 95% of a dose of metoprolol is metabolized in humans, and the major routes are shown in Fig. 25-1. α-Hydroxylation, which accounts for 10% or less of the dose (10,11), is entirely catalyzed by the polymorphically expressed enzyme, CYP2D6 (12). The major route of metoprolol metabolism is *O*-demethylation (65% of the

dose), which is partially catalyzed by CYP2D6, with a contribution from another unidentified isoform or isoforms of cytochrome P450. The *O*-demethylation but not the α-hydroxylation of metoprolol shows a modest degree of stereoselectivity favoring the (S)-enantiomer. *In vivo* CYP2D6 oxidation phenotype is a major determinant of the pharmacokinetics and pharmacodynamics of metoprolol, with poor metabolizers (8% of the white population) achieving, on average, 6 times higher plasma concentrations and experiencing a more intense and prolonged degree of β-blockade than do extensive metabolizers (13).

Timolol

At least 80% of an oral dose of timolol is thought to be metabolized in humans (14). The major urinary products, an ethanolamine and a glycine, arise through morpholino ring cleavage (see Fig. 25-1), but they account for only 26% of the dose. The metabolism of timolol is catalyzed by CYP2D6 (15) but not to the same extent as is metoprolol. Plasma concentrations of the clinically administered (S)-enantiomer of timolol in poor metabolizers are about double those in extensive metabolizers (15).

INHIBITION OF THE METABOLISM OF β-BLOCKERS BY OTHER DRUGS

Anesthetics

Anesthesia with *halothane* was shown to cause a large decrease (from 6.14 to 1.84 L/min) in the intrinsic clearance of propranolol in the dog (16). The intrinsic clearance of the (S)-enantiomer was affected to a greater extent than that of (R)-propranolol. Anesthesia with *propofol* also was associated with decreased intrinsic clearance of propranolol in the dog (17). Propofol was later found to inhibit the glucuronidation but not the oxidation of propranolol by dog and human liver microsomes (18) (Table 25-1).

Antiarrhythmic Agents

The class III antiarrhythmic drug *amiodarone* is a potent and relatively nonspecific inhibitor of cytochrome P450–mediated metabolism in humans (19). Its concurrent use with β-blockers is not uncommon, particularly in the treatment of refractory life-threatening arrhythmias and to prevent sudden death in patients with cardiac hypertrophy (19). It has not been established whether amiodarone causes elevations in the plasma concentrations of β-blockers, but two cases reports are compatible with this. In one case, two patients taking amiodarone had a cardiac arrest shortly after beginning propranolol therapy (19). In the other case, a patient receiving 1,200 mg of amiodarone daily complained of dizziness, weakness, and blurred vision shortly after taking 100 mg of metoprolol (20). The latter drug was discontinued, and

TABLE 25-1. *Interactions probably caused by inhibition of the metabolism of β-blockers by other drugs*

Other drug	β-Blocker	Type of study	Effect on PK	Effect on CYP or other enzyme activity	Effect on PD/response	Reference
Anesthetics						
Halothane	P	PK/dog	63% Decrease in intrinsic clearance			16
Propofol	P	PK/dog	40% Decrease in AUC	Glucuronyltransferase inhibited		17
Antiarrhythmic agents						
Amiodarone	P	Case report			1) Ventricular fibrillation, 2) Asystole	19,20
	M	Case report			Dizziness, weakness, blurred vision	21,22
Quinidine	P	PK	100% Increase in AUC	CYP2D6 inhibited	Increased β-blockade, prolongation of QT$_c$ and P	24
	T	Case report	100% Increase in Cp	CYP2D6 inhibited	Orthostatic hypotension	26
	M	PK	300% Increase in Cp	CYP2D6 inhibited	Small decrease in heart rate	28
Calcium channel antagonists						
Nifedipine	P,M,T, At,B	PK	Conflicting data on whether PK affected			33–36
Felodipine	M	PK	38% Increase in Cp			37
	M, P, Pi	PD			No changes in heart rate, PR interval, or blood pressure	38
Nicardipine	M	PK	28% Increase in Cp	CYP2D6 activity not affected		39
Isradipine	P	PK	30%–60% Increase in Cp			40
Lacidipine						41
Nisoldipine						42
Nimodipine	P	PK	PK unaffected			43
Verapamil	P	Case report	<50% Increase in Cp		Associated with cardiac failure	45
	M	PK	<50 Increase in Cp			44
Diltiazem	P	PK	48% Increase in Cp			47
	M	PK	33% Increase in Cp			47
Chlorpromazine	P	PK	30% Decrease in oral clearance			48
Opioid analgesics						
Dextropropoxyphene	P	PK	70% Increase in bioavailability	CYP2D6 inhibited		50
	M	PK	400% Increase in bioavailability	CYP2D6 inhibited		50
Dextromoramide	P	Case report			Bradycardia, severe hypotension	51
Oral contraceptives	P	PK	PK unaffected			53
	M	PK				52
Propafenone	M	PK	200%–500% increase in AUC	CYP2D6 inhibited	Nightmares in one patient, acute ventricular failure in another	31
	P	PK	100% increase in steady-state AUC		Modest increase in β-blocking effects	32
4-Quinolone antibacterials						
Ciprofloxacin	M	PK	42% Increase in AUC			57
SSRI antidepressants						
Fluoxetine	P	Case report		CYP2D6 inhibited?	Fatigue, bradycardia	60
	M	Case report		CYP2D6 inhibited?	Heart block	59
Ulcer-healing drugs						
Cimetidine	P	PK	100% Increase in AUC			62
	M	PK	60% Increase in AUC			63
	L	PK	80% Increase in bioavailability			64
Omeprazole	P	PK	No effect			66
	M	PK	No effect			67
Misoprostol	M	PK	40% increase in AUC			68

PK, pharmacokinetic; PD, pharmacodynamic; Cp, plasma concentration; AUC, area under the plasma concentration-time curve; At, atenolol; Al, alprenolol; B, betaxolol; L, labetalol; M, metoprolol; P, propranolol; Pi, pindolol; T, timolol.

the patient recovered within 24 hours. Although the basis of these reports requires further investigation, their findings emphasize the need for caution when using an extensively metabolized β-blocker in combination with amiodarone.

It has been shown that a subtherapeutic dose (50 mg) of *quinidine* increases the plasma concentration of propranolol (single 80-mg dose) through inhibition of CYP2D6 activity, leading to increased β-blockade and prolongation of the QT_c and PR intervals (21,22). The effect on the QT_c interval is almost certainly a direct action of quinidine. The increase in plasma drug concentration is stereoselective, quinidine having a greater effect on the clearance of inactive (R)-propranolol (21). However, it is not clear why quinidine has such a substantial effect on the elimination of propranolol, when no differences in the kinetics of the latter have been found between poor and extensive metabolizers with respect to CYP2D6 (8,9).

Combining quinidine with a β-blocker normally results in a beneficial interaction. Relatively small doses of quinidine and propranolol can effectively treat atrial defibrillation in patients resistant to high-dose quinidine alone (23). Adverse effects of this combination seem rare. An isolated report describes orthostatic hypotension in a patient taking quinidine and propranolol (24).

The systemic effects of timolol given topically for glaucoma are well recognized, and in some patients, the drug has caused life-threatening bronchoconstriction (25). Low-dose (50 mg) quinidine inhibits the CYP2D6-catalyzed metabolism of ophthalmic timolol, leading to increased plasma drug concentrations and a further modest decrease in heart rate (26). Thus the development of a bradycardia of 36 beats/min, in a patient being treated with eye drops when high-dose quinidine (500 mg/day) was introduced, may have been caused by inhibition of metabolism (27).

Quinidine (single 50-mg dose) also inhibits the CYP2D6-catalyzed metabolism of metoprolol (single 100-mg dose) (28), but there have been no reports of unwanted effects in patients taking this drug combination.

Propafenone

In patients being treated for ventricular arrhythmias, propafenone, which is a substrate and inhibitor of CYP2D6 (29,30) (150 mg, 3 times daily for 4 days), increased the area under the curve (AUC) of metoprolol (50 mg, 3 times daily, or 100 mg, twice daily for 1 to 4 weeks before the study) two- to five-fold (31) (Fig. 25-2). This was associated with severe adverse effects in two patients (distressing nightmares in one, acute ventricular failure in the other), which disappeared on reducing the dose of metoprolol in the former patient and discontinuing the drug in the latter.

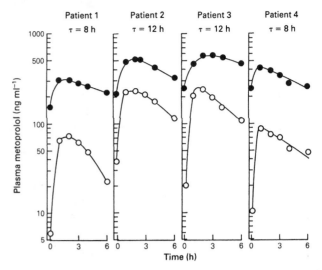

FIG. 25-2. Steady-state plasma concentrations of metoprolol in four patients with ventricular arrhythmias taking metoprolol (150–200 mg, daily) alone (open dots) or with propafenone (450 mg, daily for 4 days; closed dots). Reproduced from Wagner F, Kalushce D, Trenk D, Jahnchen E, Roskamm H. Drug interaction between propafenone and metoprolol. *Br J Clin Pharmacol* 1987;24:213–220, with permission).

When given daily, propafenone (225 mg) increased steady-state plasma propranolol (50 mg every 8 hours) concentrations by more than 100%, but caused only small changes in β-blockade (32).

Calcium Channel Antagonists

Calcium antagonists and β-blockers are often used together in patients with angina inadequately controlled by monotherapy.

There are conflicting data on whether *nifedipine* affects the pharmacokinetics of β-blockers (33–36). However, this drug combination is normally beneficial and safe in the treatment of hypertension. *Felodipine* (10 mg, twice daily) caused a small (38%) increase in the plasma concentration of metoprolol (100 mg, twice daily) when both drugs were given together over a 5-day period to healthy volunteers (37). In another study of healthy subjects given single therapeutic doses of felodipine (10 mg) with either propranolol (80 mg), metoprolol (100 mg), pindolol (5 mg), or timolol (10 mg), no clinically important changes in heart rate, PR interval, or blood pressure were observed (38). However, the majority reported some adverse reactions. Laurent-Kenesi et al. (39) reported that *nicardipine* (50 mg, twice daily) increases slightly the plasma concentrations of metoprolol (120 mg, twice daily) when both drugs are given together over a 5.5-day period to healthy volunteers. The impairment in metoprolol clearance occurred as a result of inhibition of a CYP2D6-independent route of elimination, because clearance to α-hydroxy-metoprolol was unaffected. Single-dose *isradipine* (10 mg) (40), *lacidipine* (4 mg) (41), and *nisoldipine* (20 mg) (42) increase plasma propranolol (80–160 mg) concentrations by 30% to 60%, whereas *nimodipine* (30 mg, thrice daily for 4 days) has no effect on propranolol (40 mg, thrice daily for 4 days) pharmacokinetics (43).

Verapamil (120 mg, thrice daily for 6 days) has been shown to cause modest increases (less than 50%) in the AUCs of metoprolol (100 mg, thrice daily for 1 week) (44) and propranolol (80 mg, thrice daily for 6 days) (45), which may contribute to the benefits of cotreatment. However, the combined use of verapamil, which has a negative inotropic effect on the heart, with a β-blocker has been associated with cardiac failure (46). Thus, close observation of patients is essential if this drug combination is used.

Although a number of adverse events during the concurrent use of *diltiazem* and β-blockers have been described, this drug combination is widely used and usually causes no major problems. Diltiazem (30 mg, daily for 3 days) increases the AUCs of single-dose propranolol (20 mg) and metoprolol (40 mg) by 48% and 33%, respectively (47), probably through inhibition of their metabolism, although there is no information about which isoform of cytochrome P450 might be affected.

Chlorpromazine

Although most antipsychotics are metabolized extensively by cytochrome P450 and, therefore, are potential inhibitors, only chlorpromazine has been studied with respect to its effect on the disposition of β-blockers. Vestal et al. (48) found that the steady-state plasma concentration of propranolol (80 mg, thrice daily for 4 days) was increased by 70% after 4 days of treatment with this drug (50 mg, thrice daily). However, there were no statistically significant effects on β-blockade.

Opioid Analgesics

Dextropropoxyphene is a potent inhibitor of CYP2D6 activity in human liver microsomes (49). Lundborg and Regard (50) showed that single doses of dextropropoxyphene (not stated) increase the bioavailability of single-dose metoprolol (100 mg) by about 400% and propranolol (40 mg) by 70%. Although there is no firm evidence that concurrent use of these drugs causes problems, excessive β-blockade could be experienced by patients taking dextropropoxyphene and metoprolol. The risk would seem less with propranolol.

Marked bradycardia and severe hypotension have reported in two patients given *dextromoramide* (1.25 and 4 mg) and propranolol (30 mg) by intravenous injection during general anesthesia, but the basis of this was not established (51).

Oral Contraceptives

Treatment with low-dose combined oral contraceptives increased the peak plasma concentration and AUC of metoprolol after a single 100-mg dose by 70% and 36%, respectively (52), but a similar regimen did not affect the pharmacokinetics of propranolol (53). The basis of the interaction with metoprolol is unclear, because oral contraceptive treatment has been shown not to affect CYP2D6 activity (54). The findings are probably not important clinically, and no special care is needed when it is given to women taking oral contraceptives.

4-Quinoline Antibacterials

The fluoroquinolone class of antibacterial drugs is known to inhibit cytochrome P450 activity (55), particularly that of CYP1A2 (56), but very little information is available on potential interactions between these drugs and β-blockers. Ciprofloxacin (five 12-hourly 500-mg doses) has been shown to cause a small increase (42%) in the AUC of metoprolol, which was thought not to be clinically important (57).

Selective Serotonin Reuptake Inhibitor Antidepressants

Although *fluoxetine* and *paroxetine* are both potent inhibitors of the activities of CYP2D6 and other cytochrome P450 isoforms (58), their effects on the pharmacokinetics of metoprolol and propranolol have not been studied. However, there have been two reports of patients taking metoprolol or propranolol having adverse effects 2 days after starting fluoxetine (20 mg daily). The patient taking metoprolol (100 mg daily) complained of profound fatigue and had a bradycardia of 36 beats/min (59). His heart rate returned to its previous value of 64 beats/min 5 days after discontinuation of fluoxetine. When metoprolol was replaced by sotalol, and fluoxetine treatment resumed, the patient had no further adverse effects. An alternative plan would have been to continue treatment with metoprolol and substitute fluoxetine with an antidepressant that does not inhibit CYP2D6 activity. The other patient, who had been taking propranolol (80 mg daily) for anxiety, had complete heart block after being started on fluoxetine (20 mg daily) 2 weeks previously (60). Propranolol and fluoxetine were stopped immediately, and the patient had a pacemaker inserted. He reverted to sinus rhythm within 2 days. Propranolol was then reintroduced with no subsequent adverse effects. Although fluoxetine alone can cause bradycardia and syncope (61), Walley et al. (59) suggested that inhibition of cytochrome P450–mediated metabolism may have been the cause of this interaction.

In view of the widespread use of both selective serotonin reuptake inhibitor (SSRI) antidepressants and β-blockers, their combined use will not be insignificant.

Unless there are compelling reasons not to do so, it is probably best to avoid giving a lipid-soluble β-blocker with an SSRI that inhibits cytochrome P450 activity.

Ulcer-Healing Drugs

The metabolism of orally administered metoprolol (100 mg, twice daily for 8 days), propranolol (160 mg daily, for 13 days) and labetalol (single 200-mg dose) is inhibited by *cimetidine* (1–1.2 g daily for 3–7 days), leading to increases in the AUC curve of 60% to 100% (62–64), but the clinical significance of these interactions was not evaluated. Cimetidine also decreases the clearance of intravenous propranolol, which is primarily dependent on liver blood flow (65). Ranitidine does not appear to affect the pharmacokinetics of metoprolol (63) or propranolol (62).

In a randomized double blind crossover study in healthy volunteers, it was shown that daily dosing with *omeprazole* (20 mg, daily for 8 days) had no effect on the pharmacokinetics or pharmacodynamics of propranolol (80 mg, twice daily for 8 days) (66). In a similar study, the pharmacokinetics of metoprolol (100 mg, daily for 8 days) enantiomers also were unaffected by omeprazole (40 mg, daily for 8 days) (67).

Bennett et al. (68) showed that 14 days of treatment with *misoprostol* (400 μg, twice daily for 2 weeks) causes about a 40% increase in the AUC of propranolol (80 mg, twice daily for 4 weeks) dosed to steady state.

INDUCTION OF THE METABOLISM OF β-BLOCKERS BY OTHER DRUGS

Barbiturates

Treatment with pentobarbitone (100 mg daily for 10 days; Table 25-2) or phenobarbitone (69) increases the clearance of single-dose metoprolol (100 mg) and timolol (70) in healthy volunteers by 32% and 24%, respectively. A much larger increase (up to 80%) in clearance has been observed for alprenolol (single 200-mg dose), with corresponding increases in heart rate and blood pressure (71,72). The latter interaction would be clinically significant, if this drug combination were not such a rarity.

Rifampicin

Rifampicin is a potent inducer of the metabolism of propranolol (120 mg, thrice daily for 5 weeks), the clearance of which increases three- to four-fold when rifampicin is given for 3 weeks at 600 mg daily (73,74) (Fig. 25-3). The clinical importance of this interaction has not been established, but a diminished clinical effect might be anticipated. The metabolism of single-dose metoprolol (100 mg) is less affected (40% decrease in AUC) by treatment with rifampicin (600 mg, daily for 17 days) (75), almost certainly because CYP2D6, which is primarily responsible for metabolizing metoprolol, is particularly resistant to induction (76).

Smoking

The induction of the CYP1A subfamily by constituents of tobacco smoke has led to a number of clinically significant drug interactions (77). With respect to β-blockers, serum concentrations of propranolol (80 mg, thrice daily for 2 days) are decreased up to two-fold in smokers (78). This is associated with a diminished pharmacologic effect (79,80). Smoking itself increases heart rate, blood pressure, and the severity of myocardial ischemia. Thus the effects of smoking on the actions of propranolol are

TABLE 25-2. *Interactions probably caused by induction of the metabolism of β-blockers by other drugs*

Other drug	β-Blocker	Type of study	Effect on PK	Effect on individual CYP or other enzyme activity	Effect on PD/response	Reference
Barbiturates						
Pentobarbitone	M	PK	32% increase in oral clearance			69
	Al	PK	80% increase in oral clearance		Increase in heart rate and blood pressure	71,72
Phenobarbitone	T	PK	24% increase in oral clearance			70
Rifampicin	P	PK	400% increase in oral clearance			73,74
	M	PK	40% decrease in AUC			75
Smoking	P	PK/PD	200% decrease in CP		Increase in heart rate and blood pressure	78–80
	M	PK	PK unaffected			81

PK, pharmacokinetic; PD, pharmacodynamic; Cp, plasma concentration; AUC, area under the plasma concentration–time curve; At, atenolol; Al, alprenolol; B, betaxolol; L, labetalol; M, metoprolol; P, propranolol; Pi, pindolol; T, timolol.

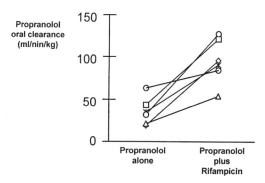

FIG. 25-3. Steady-state oral blood clearance of propranolol when given alone (120 mg, every 8 hours for 2 weeks) or with rifampicin (600 mg daily for 3 weeks) to six healthy subjects. Data redrawn from Herman RJ, Nakanura K, Wilkinson GR, Wood AJJ. Induction of propranolol metabolism by rifampicin. *Br J Clin Pharmacol* 1983;16:565–569, with permission.

probably a combination of pharmacokinetic and pharmacodynamic factors.

Smoking does not affect the clearance of single-dose metoprolol (100–200 mg) (81), which is in accordance with the low inducibility of CYP2D6.

EFFECT OF β-BLOCKERS ON THE ELIMINATION OF OTHER DRUGS

β-Blockers have been shown to alter the elimination of other drugs by affecting their cytochrome P450-mediated metabolism (Table 25-3). Significant correlations between their lipid solubility and inhibitory potency have been reported in liver microsomes (82–84) (Fig. 25-4). For example, propranolol, which has high lipid solubility, is a potent inhibitor of lignocaine and dextromethorphan metabolism, whereas atenolol, which is very hydrophilic, has little or no affect on the metabolism of these drugs. Although it is an important contributory factor, lipid solubility alone cannot account for the inhibition of the activity of individual isoforms of cytochrome P450, as there are large discrepancies between the inhibitory potencies of compounds possessing similar solubilities. This is exemplified by the 100 times greater potency of quinidine as an inhibitor of CYP2D6 compared with its diastereoisomer quinine (85), indicating the importance of structural factors. With respect to propranolol, inhibition of oxidative metabolism is not mediated solely by competition from unchanged drug, because there is strong *in vitro* evidence of a role for an irreversibly bound metabolic intermediate of propranolol, a product of 4-hydroxypropranolol, in the inhibition of cytochrome P450 activity (86). Furthermore, *in vivo* studies indicate that propranolol is a relatively selective inhibitor of CYPs 2D6 and 1A2, the major isoforms catalyzing its metabolism (see later).

Rowland et al. (86), examining the effect of propranolol on the CYP2D6 phenotype, showed that there was significant inhibition of the metabolism of debrisoquine to 4-hydroxydebrisoquine after 1 week of treatment with propranolol (80 mg, twice daily). However, the magnitude of the change was not sufficient to result in phenocopying: the conversion of the extensive-metabolizer phenotype to that of an apparent poor metabolizer (Fig. 25-5). The latter might have been anticipated from *in vitro* evidence suggesting the 4-hydroxypropranolol (formed by CYP2D6; see Fig. 25-1), is further metabolized to a reactive intermediate that covalently binds to and inactivates CYP2D6. However, it seems likely that the appearance of such a reactive metabolite might be decreased *in vivo* by parallel conjugation of 4-hydroxypropranolol and scavenging by glutathione and other nucleophiles.

Whatever the mechanism of inhibition of cytochrome P450 activity by β-blockers, it is apparent that propranolol and to a lesser extent metoprolol impair the elimination of a number of clinically used drugs *in vivo*. Peet et al. (87) reported that high-dose propranolol (8.1 mg/kg per day) increases plasma *chlorpromazine* (21 mg/kg per day) concentrations by 100% to 500% in schizophrenic patients, which may explain the increased efficacy of chlorpromazine when given with propranolol. In a single case report of a patient receiving both long-term chlorpromazine and thiothixine, administration of propranolol led to severe antipsychotic-induced adverse effects (delirium, grand mal seizure, photosensitivity), which disappeared rapidly on discontinuation of the β-blocker (88).

Several groups have shown that daily treatment with therapeutic doases of oral propranolol increases (19%–46%) the steady-state concentration of intravenously infused *lignocaine* (89–92), probably as a result of both inhibition of cytochrome P450 enzyme activity and a reduction in hepatic blood flow secondary to the decrease in cardiac output produced by β-blockade (93). There are several case reports of lignocaine toxicity during treatment with propranolol (94,95). Conflicting evidence on whether metoprolol affects the pharmacokinetics of lignocaine has been published. In one study, lignocaine clearance was decreased by 31% (92), but in two other studies, its elimination was unaltered (96,97). Because patients may receive β-blockers and lignocaine simultaneously, and increased lignocaine concentrations are associated with toxicity, the potential for interactions between these drugs should not be ignored.

Conrad and Nyman (98) and Miners et al. (99) reported a decrease (37%–52%) in the clearance of *theophylline* (375 mg, daily for 10 days or a single i.v. infusion of 5.7–6.4 mg/kg), which is metabolized mainly by CYP1A2 (100,101), during oral treatment with propranolol (120–720 mg, daily for up to 5 days) but not metoprolol (50 mg, every 6 hours for 54 hours). Because it is

TABLE 25-3. *Interactions probably caused by inhibition of the metabolism of other drugs by β-blockers*

β-Blocker	Other drug	Type of study	Effect on PK	Effect on individual CYP or other enzyme activity	Effect on PD/response	Reference
P	Debrisoquine (CYP2D6 probe)	PK		Small decrease in CYP2D6, activity, as reflected by a median change of 0.6 in the debrisoquine metabolic ratio	Not relevant	86
P	Chlorpromazine	PK	100%–500% Increase in Cp		Increased efficacy of chlorpromazine	87
P	Lignocaine (i.v. infusion)	PK/Case reports	19%–46% Increase in Cp		Lignocaine toxicity	89–92
M		PK	0–31% Decrease in clearance			92,96,97
P	Theophylline	PK	37%–52% Decrease in oral clearance; no effect on PK	CYP1A2 inhibited		98,99
M						98
P	Pravastatin	PK	Minor or no effect on AUC			102
P	Lovastatin	PK				102
P	Fluvastatin	PK				103
M	Diazepam	PK	25% increase in AUC			105
P	Diazepam	PK	Negligible effect on PK			105
P	Tolbutamide	PK	PK unaffected	No effect on CYP2C9 activity		97
P	Quinidine	PK	PK unaffected	No effect on CYP3A activity		108
P	Imipramine	Case report	>400 ng/ml plasma imipramine + desipramine Cp		No adverse effects reported	109
Pi	Fluoxetine	Clinical trial	Not investigated		Increased efficacy of fluoxetine	110
P,Pi	Thioridazine	PK	47% Increase in Cp	Possible inhibition of CYP2D6 activity		111,112
P,Pi	Haloperidol	PK	No effect on PK			111,112

PK, pharmacokinetic; PD, pharmacodynamic; Cp, plasma concentration; AUC, area under the plasma concentration–time curve; At, atenolol; Al, alprenolol; B, betaxolol; L, labetalol; M, metoprolol; P, propranolol; Pi, pindolol; T, timolol.

354

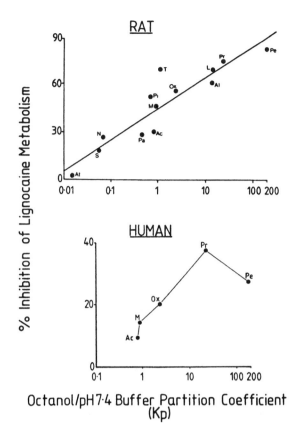

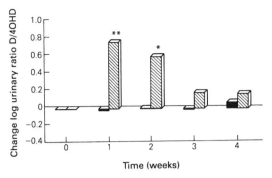

FIG. 25-5. Mean change from baseline in the log₁₀ 0- to 8-hour urinary debrisoquine/4-hydroxydebrisoquine ratio for nine patients treated with propranolol (80 mg, twice daily) for weeks 1 and 2, followed by a further 2 weeks (3 and 4) of atenolol treatment (hatched bars) and 10 patients continuing on atenolol 5 to 100 mg, daily for the entire 4 weeks (solid bars). *$p < 0.04$; **$p < 0.01$. From Rowland K, Yeo WW, Ellis SW, et al. Inhibition of CYP2D6 activity by treatment with propranolol and the role of 4-hydroxypropranolol. *Br J Clin Pharmacol* 1994;38:9–14, with permission.

FIG. 25-4. Relationship between percentage inhibition of lignocaine metabolism and octanol/buffer distribution coefficients (K_p) of a series of β-blockers (50 μM) in rat (lignocaine concentration, 4.27 μM) and human (lignocaine concentration, 42.7 μM) liver microsomes. At, atenolol; S, sotalol; N, nadolol; Pa, pamatolol; Ac, acebutolol; Pi, pindolol; T, timolol; Ox, oxprenolol; M, metoprolol; L, labetalol; Al, alprenolol; Pr, propranolol; Pe, penbutolol. Reproduced from Al-Asadi SAH, Black GL, Lennard MS, Tucker GT, Woods HF. Inhibition of lignocaine metabolism by β-adrenoceptor antagonists in rat and human liver microsomes. *Xenobiotica* 1989;19:929–944, with permission.

not considered safe to give noncardioselective β-blockers like propranolol to asthmatic patients, this drug combination is unlikely to be used widely in clinical practice.

Pharmacokinetic interactions have been studied between the 3-hydroxy-3-methylglutaryl coenzyme A (HMG-CoA) reductase inhibitors *pravastatin* (20 mg), *lovastatin* (20 mg) (102), and *fluvastatin* (40 mg) (103), all given as a single dose, and propranolol (40 mg, twice daily for 2–7 days), indicating no effect on or small decreases in the AUC of these lipid-lowering drugs.

Coadministration of propranolol (40–80 mg, twice daily for 5 days) or metoprolol (50–100 mg, twice daily for 5 days) with *diazepam* (10 mg, daily for 5 weeks), which is metabolized by CYPs 2C19 and 3A (104), produced small increases in the AUC of the benzodiazepine (105). Only the change caused by metoprolol reached statistical significance.

Propranolol (80 mg, twice or thrice daily for 3 days) has no effect on the elimination of intravenous *tolbutamide* (500 mg; metabolized mainly by CYP2C9) (97,106) or *quinidine* (200 mg, thrice daily for 3 days; CYP3A) (107,108).

Most tricyclic antidepressants and antipsychotics are substrates of CYP2D6 or CYP1A2. Gillette and Tannery (109) described two cases of children who achieved potentially toxic concentrations of *imipramine* and *desipramine* (more than 400 ng/ml total) when taking the former (40–75 mg daily) with propranolol (10–480 mg daily), although neither child reported any adverse effects. This is the only published example of apparent inhibition of tricyclic antidepressant metabolism by β-blockers, but the common use of this combination in patients with anxiety and depression or panic disorder raises the possibility that clinically significant interactions can be undetected.

Recent work has shown that augmentation of *fluoxetine* therapy with pindolol increases antidepressant efficacy (110). It has not been established whether such an effect is the result of increased plasma concentrations of fluoxetine, which is metabolized by CYP2D6. However, this seems unlikely because pindolol is a relatively weak inhibitor of CYP2D6 activity (82,83), and patients were receiving only small daily doses (2.5 mg) of the β-blocker. Furthermore, there is a relatively flat relationship between plasma SSRI concentration and response.

In schizophrenic patients, a β-blocker is sometimes added to existing antipsychotic therapy to treat anxiety. High doses of both propranolol (maximum, 520 mg/day) and pindolol (maximum, 40 mg/day) have been shown to increase serum concentrations of *thioridazine* but not *haloperidol* (doses not stated) (111,112). If β-blocker/antipsychotic therapy is indicated, the use of a nonphenathiazine agent has been recommended (113). However, interactions between β-blockers and other types of antipsychotic drugs cannot be ruled out.

CONCLUSIONS

β-Blockers are used in combination with many commonly prescribed drugs. A large number of pharmacokinetic interactions involving β-blockers have been reported, most of them occurring as a result of inhibition or induction of cytochrome P450–catalyzed metabolism. However, the majority of these interactions do not appear to result in serious toxicity. On the other hand, some of the anecdotal reports of clinically significant drug interactions involving β-blockers may well have arisen through changes in metabolism, but the basis of these observations has generally not been investigated further. Although β-blockers are generally well tolerated, elevated blood concentrations may be associated with effects that are not life threatening but that cause considerable discomfort to the patient. If a clinically significant pharmacokinetic interaction is suspected in a patient taking a β-blocker that is extensively metabolized, changing to a polar β-blocker such as atenolol should be considered. Indeed, there is a case that polar β-blockers should be preferred over their lipid-soluble counterparts when beginning treatment. However, prescriptions for propranolol, metoprolol, and timolol still represent about 20% of all prescriptions for β-blockers (*Prescription Cost Analysis England 1996,* UK Government Department of Health).

This review of pharmacokinetic interactions should be considered alongside the many reports of clinically significant pharmacodynamic interactions (84). In view of the widespread use of β-blockers and the likelihood that many patients taking tham will not receive monotherapy, it would seem desirable to gain as much knowledge as possible on potential interactions. A increasing number of novel drugs are introduced into clinical use each year, and the clinician should also be aware of the potential of new drugs to interact with β-blockers. Methods based on our increased knowledge of cytochrome P450 substrate specificity have been developed to allow prediction of pharmacokinetic interactions at an early stage of drug development. As an aid to better prescribing, such information is being added to the data sheets of many new drugs.

REFERENCES

1. Smith AJ, Tucker GT. Kinetics and biotransformation of adrenergic inhibitors. In: Szerkeres L, ed. *Adrenergic activators and inhibitors, handbook of experimental pharmacology.* 54/11. Berlin: Springer, 1981:417–501.
2. Walle T, Walle UK, Olanoff LS. Quantitative account of propranolol metabolism in urine of normal men. *Drug Metab Dispos* 1987;13:204–209.
3. Walle T, Webb JG, Bagwell EE, Walle UK, Daniell HB, Gaffney TE. Stereoselective delivery and action of beta-adrenoceptor antagonists. *Biochem Pharmacol* 1988;37:115–124.
4. Nelson WL, Shetty HU. Stereoselective oxidation of propranolol in microsomal fractions from rat and human liver: use of deuterium labelling and pseudoracemic mixtures. *Drug Metab Dispos* 1986;14:506–508.
5. Otton SV, Gillam EMJ, Lennard MS, Tucker GT, Woods HF. Propranolol oxidation by human liver microsomes: the use of cumene hydroperoxide to probe isoenzyme and regio- and stereoselectivity. *Br J Clin Pharmacol* 1990;30:751–760.
6. Yoshimoto K, Echizen H, Chiba K, Tani M, Ishizaki T. Identification of human CYP isoforms involved in the metabolism of propranolol enantiomers: N-deisopropylation is mediated mainly by CYP1A2. *Br J Clin Pharmacol* 1995;39:421–431.
7. Rowland K, Ellis SW, Lennard MS, Tucker GT. Variable contribution of CYP2D6 to the N-dealkylation of propranolol by human liver microsomes. *Br J Clin Pharmacol* 1996;42:390–393.
8. Lennard MS, Jackson PR, Freeston S, Tucker GT, Ramsay LE, Woods HF. The relationship between debrisoquine oxidation phenotype and the pharmacokinetics and pharmacodynamics of propranolol. *Br J Clin Pharmacol* 1984;17:679–685.
9. Raghuram TC, Koshakji RP, Wilkinson GR, Wood AJJ. Polymorphic ability to metabolise propranolol alters 4-hydroxypropranolol levels but not beta-blockade. *Clin Pharmacol Ther* 1984;36:51–56.
10. Borg KO, Carlsson E, Hoffman K-J, Johnsson TE, Thorin H, Wallin B. Metabolism of metoprolol-(-H³) in man, the dog and the rat. *Acta Pharmacol Toxicol* 1975;35(suppl V):125–135.
11. McGourty JC, Silas JS, Lennard MS, Tucker GT, Woods HF. Metoprolol metabolism and debrisoquine oxidation polymorphism: population and family studies. *Br J Clin Pharmacol* 1985;20:555–566.
12. Otton SV, Crewe HK, Lennard MS, Tucker GT, Woods HF. Use of quinidine to define the role of the sparteine/debrisoquine cytochrome P450 in metoprolol oxidation by human liver microsomes. *J Pharmacol Exp Ther* 1988;247:242.
13. Lennard MS, Silas JH, Freestone S, Ramsay LE, Tucker GT, Woods HF. Oxidation phenotype: major determinant of metoprolol metabolism and response. *N Engl J Med* 1982;307:1558–1560.
14. Tocco DJ, Duncan AEW, de Luna FA, Hucker HB, Gruber VF, Vanden Heuval WJA. Physiological disposition and metabolism of timolol in man and laboratory animals. *Drug Metab Dispos* 1975;3:361–370.
15. Lewis RV, Lennard MS, Jackson PR, Tucker GT, Ramsay LE, Woods HF. Timolol and atenolol: relationship between oxidation phenotype, pharmacokinetics and pharmacodynamics. *Br J Clin Pharmacol* 1985;19:329–333.
16. Whelan E, Wood AJJ, Koshakji R, Shay S, Wood M. Halothane inhibition of propranolol metabolism is stereoselective. *Anesthesiology* 1989;71:561–564.
17. Perry SM, Whelan EE, Shay S, Wood AJJ, Wood M. Effect of iv anesthesia with propofol on drug distribution and metabolism in the dog. *Br J Anaesth* 1991;66:66–72.
18. Whalley PM, Tucker GT, Reilly CS. Effect of propofol on propranolol metabolism by human liver microsomes. *Br J Anaesth* 1993;71:P306–P307.
19. Lesko LJ. Pharmacokinetic drug interactions with amiodarone. *Clin Pharmacokinet* 1989;17:130–140.
19a. Derrida JP, Ollagnier J, Benaim R, Haiat R, Chiche P. Amiodarone et propranolol; une association dangereuse? *Nouv Presse Med* 1979;8:1429.
20. Leor J, Levartowsky D, Sharon C, Farfel Z. Amiodarone and beta-adrenergic blockers: an interaction with metoprolol but not with atenolol. *Am Heart J* 1988;116:206–207.
21. Zhou H-H, Anthony LB, Roden DM, Wood AJJ. Quinidine reduces clearance of (+)-propranolol more than (−)-propranolol through marked reduction in 4-hydroxylation. *Clin Pharmacol Ther* 1990;47:686–693.
22. Yasuhara M, Yatsuzuka A, Yamada K, et al. Alteration of propranolol pharmacokinetics and pharmacodynamics by quinidine in man. *J Pharmacobiodyn* 1990:13:681–687.
23. Fors Wj, Vanderark CR, Reynolds JW. Evaluation of propranolol and quinidine in the treatment of quinidine-resistant arrhythmias. *Am J Cardiol* 1971;27:190.
24. Loon NR, Wilcox CS, Folger W. Orthostatic hypotension due to quinidine and propranolol. *Am J Med* 1986;81:1101–1104.

25. Fraunfelder FT. Ocular β-blockers and systemic effects. *Arch Intern Med* 1986;146:1073–1074.

26. Edeki TI, Huabing H, Wood AJJ. Pharmacogenetic explanation for excessive β-blockade following timolol eyedrops. *JAMA* 1995;274:1611–1613.

27. Dinai Y, Mordechar S, Haveh N, Halkin H. Bradycardia induced by interaction between quinidine and ophthalmic timolol. *Arch Intern Med* 1985;103:890–891.

28. Leemann T, Dayer P, Meyer UA. Single dose quinidine treatment inhibits metoprolol oxidation in extensive metabolisers. *Eur J Clin Pharmacol* 1986;29:739–741.

29. Buchert E, Woosley RE. Clinical implications of variable antiarrhythmic drug metabolism. *Pharmacogenetics* 1992;2:2–11.

30. Siddoway LA, McCallister CB, Thompson KA, et al. Inhibition of debrisoquine metabolism by propafenone. *Clin Res* 1985;33:A288.

31. Wagner F, Kalushce D, Trenk D, Jahnchen E, Roskamm H. Drug interaction between propafenone and metoprolol. *Br J Clin Pharmacol* 1987;24:213–220.

32. Kowey PR, Kirsen EB, Fu C-HJ, Mason WD. Interaction between propranolol and propafenone in healthy volunteers. *J Clin Pharmacol* 1989;29:512–517.

33. Gangji D, Juvent M, Niset G, Wathieu M, Degreve M, Bellens R. Study of the influence of nifedipine on the pharmacokinetics and pharmacodynamics of propranolol metoprolol and atenolol. *Br J Clin Pharmacol* 1984;17:29S–35S.

34. Kendall MJ, Jack DB, Laugher SJ, Lobo J, Smith R. Lack of a pharmacokinetic interaction between nifedipine and the beta-adrenoceptor blockers metoprolol and timolol. *Br J Clin Pharmacol* 1984;18:331–335.

35. Vincenaux P, Canal M, Domart Y, et al. Pharmacokinetic and pharmacodynamic interactions between nifedipine and propranolol or betaxolol. *Int J Clin Pharmacol Ther Toxicol* 1986;24:153–158.

36. Rosenkrantz B, Ledermann H, Frolich JC. Interaction between nifedipine and atenolol: pharmacokinetics and pharmacodynamics in normotensive volunteers. *J Cardiovasc Pharmacol* 1986;8:943–949.

37. Smith SR, Wilkins MR, Jack DB, Kendall MJ, Laugher S. Pharmacokinetic interactions between felodipine and metoprolol. *Eur J Clin Pharmacol* 1987;31:575–578.

38. Carruthers SG, Bailey DG. Tolerance and cardiovascular effects of single dose felodipine/beta-blocker combinations in healthy subjects. *J Cardiovasc Pharmacol* 1987;10(suppl 1):S169–S177.

39. Laurent-Kenesi M-A, Funck-Brentano C, Poirier J-M, Decolin D, Jaillon P. Influence of CYP2D6-dependent metabolism on the steady-state pharmacokinetics and pharmacodynamics of metoprolol and nicardipine, alone and in combination. *Br J Clin Pharmacol* 1993;36:531–538.

40. Shepherd AMM, Brodie CL, Carrillo DW, Kwan CM. Pharmacokinetic interactions between isradipine and propranolol. *Clin Pharmacol Ther* 1988;43:194.

41. Hall ST, Harding SM, Hassant H, Keene ON, Pellegatti M. The pharmacokinetic and pharmacodynamic interaction between lacidipine and propranolol in healthy volunteers. *J Cardiovasc Pharmacol* 1991;18(suppl 11):S13–S17.

42. Elliott HL, Meredith PA, McNally C, Reid JL. The interactions between nisoldipine and two beta-adrenoceptor antagonists: atenolol and propranolol. *Br J Clin Pharmacol* 1991;32:379–385.

43. Horstman R, Weber H, Wingender W, Ramsch K-O, Kuhlmann J. Does nimodipine interact with beta-adrenergic blocking agents? *Eur J Clin Pharmacol* 1989;36:A258.

44. Keech AC, Harper RW, Harrison PM, Pitt A, McLean AJ. Pharmacokinetic interaction between oral metoprolol and verapamil for angina pectoris. *Am J Cardiol* 1985;55:1628–1629.

45. Hung BA, Bottorff MB, Herring VL, Self TH, Lalonde RL. Effects of calcium channel blockers on the pharmacokinetics of propranolol stereoisomers. *Clin Pharmacol Ther* 1990;47:584–591.

46. McGourty JC, Silas JH. Beta-blockers and verapamil: a cautionary tale. *Br Med J* 1984;289:1624.

47. Tateisha T, Nakashima, Shitou T, et al. Effect of diltiazem on the pharmacokinetics of propranolol, metoprolol and atenolol. *Eur J Clin Pharmacol* 1989;6:67–70.

48. Vestal RE, Kornhauser DM, Hollifield DW, Shand DG. Inhibition of propranolol metabolism by chlorpromazine. *Clin Pharmacol Ther* 1979;25:19–24.

49. Henthorn TK, Spina E, Dumont E, von Bahr C. In vitro inhibition of a polymorphic human liver P-450 isozyme by narcotic analgesics. *Anesthesiology* 1989;70:339–342.

50. Lunborg P, Regard CG. The effect of propoxyphene pretreatment on the disposition of metoprolol and propranolol. *Clin Pharmacol Ther* 1981;29:263–264.

51. Cabanne F, Wilkening M, Caillard B, Foissac JC, Aepecle P. Interferences medicamenteuses induites par l'association propranolol-dextromoramide. *Anesth Analg (Paris)* 1973;30:369–375.

52. Kendall MJ, Quarterman CP, Jack DB, Beeley L. Metoprolol pharmacokinetics and the oral contraceptive pill. *Br J Clin Pharmacol* 1982;14:120–122.

53. Fagan TC, Walle T, Walle UK, Topmiller MJ. Ethynyl oestradiol alters propranolol metabolism pathway-specifically. *Clin Pharmacol Ther* 1993;53:241.

54. Bock KW, Schrenk D, Forster A, et al. The influence of environmental and genetic factors on CYP2D6, CY1A2 and UDP-glucuronyltransferases in man using sparteine, caffeine and paracetamol as probes. *Pharmacogenetics* 1994;4:209–218.

55. McLellan RA, Drobitch RK, Monshouwer M, Renton KW. Fluoroquinolone antibiotics inhibit cytochrome P450-mediated microsomal drug-metabolism in rat and human. *Drug Metab Dispos* 1996;24:1134–1138.

56. Fuhr U, Strobl G, Manaut F, et al. Quinoline antibacterial agents: relationship between structure and *in vitro* inhibition of the human cytochrome P450 isoform CYP1A2. *Mol Pharmacol* 1993;43:191–199.

57. Waite NM, Rutledge DR, Warbasse LH, Edwards DJ. Disposition of the (+)- and (−)-isomers of metoprolol following ciprofloxacin treatment. *Pharmacotherapy* 1990;10:236.

58. Crewe HK, Lennard MS, Tucker GT, Woods FR, Haddock RE. The effect of serotonin re-uptake inhibitors on cytochrome P450 2D6 (CYP2D6) activity in human liver microsomes. *Br J Clin Pharmacol* 1992;34:262–265.

59. Walley T, Pirmohamed M, Proudlove C, Maxwell D. Interaction of metoprolol and fluoxetine. *Lancet* 1993;341;967–968.

60. Drake WM, Gordon GD. Heart block in a patient on propranolol and fluoxetine. *Lancet* 1994;343:425.

61. Ellison JM, Milofsky JE, Ely E. Fluoxetine-induced bradycardia and syncope in two patients. *J Clin Psychiatry* 1990;51:385–386.

62. Reinmann IW, Klotz U, Frohlich JC. Cimetidine increases steady-state plasma levels of propranolol. *Br J Clin Pharmacol* 1981;12:785–790.

63. Toon S, Davison EM, Garstang FM, Batra H, Bowers RJ, Rowland M. The racemic metoprolol H₂-antagonist interaction. *Clin Pharmacol Ther* 1988;43:283–289.

64. Daneshmend TK, Roberts CJC. The effects of enzyme induction and enzyme inhibition on labetalol pharmacokinetics. *Br J Clin Pharmacol* 1984;18:393–400.

65. Feely J, Wilkinson GR, Wood AJJ. Reduction in liver blood flow and propranolol metabolism by cimetidine. *N Engl J Med* 1981;304:692–695.

66. Henry D, Brent P, Whyte I, Mihaly G, Devenish-Meares S. Propranolol steady-state pharmacokinetics are unaltered by omeprazole. *Eur J Clin Pharmacol* 1987;33:369–373.

67. Andersson T, Lundborg P, Regardh CG. Lack of effect of omeprazole treatment on steady-state plasma levels of metoprolol. *Eur J Clin Pharmacol* 1991;40:61–65.

68. Bennett PN, Fenn GC, Notarianni LJ. Potential drug interactions with misoprostol: on the pharmacokinetics of antipyrine and propranolol. *Postgrad Med J* 1988;64(suppl 1):21–24.

69. Haglund K, Seidemann P, Collste P, Borg K-O, von Bahr C. Influence of pentobarbitone on metoprolol plasma levels. *Clin Pharmacol Ther* 1979;26:326.

70. Mantyla R, Mannisto P, Nykanen S, Kopenen A, Lamminisivu U. Pharmacokinetic interactions of timolol with vasodilating drugs, food and phenobarbital in healthy volunteers. *Eur J Clin Pharmacol* 1983;24:227–230.

71. Alvan G, Piafsky K, Lind M, von Bahr C. Effect of pentobarbital on the disposition of alprenolol. *Clin Pharmacol Ther* 1977;22:316.

72. Seidemann P, Borg K-O, Haglund K, von Bahr C. Decreased plasma concentrations and clinical effects of alprenolol during combined treatment with pentobarbitone in hypertension. *Br J Clin Pharmacol* 1987;23:267–271.

73. Herman RJ, Nakanura K, Wilkinson GR, Wood AJJ. Induction of propranolol metabolism by rifampicin. *Br J Clin Pharmacol* 1983;16:565–569.

74. Shaheen O, Biollaz J, Koshakji RP, Wilkinson GR, Wood AJJ. Influence of debrisoquine phenotype on the inducibility of propranolol metabolism. *Clin Pharmacol Ther* 1989;45:439–443.

75. Bennett PN, John VA, Whitmarsh VB. Effects of rifampicin on metoprolol and antipyrine kinetics. *Br J Clin Pharmacol* 1982;13:387.

76. Eichelbaum M, Mineshita A, Ohnhaus EE, Zekorn C. The influence of enzyme induction on polymorphic sparteine induction. *Br J Clin Pharmacol* 1986;22:49–53.

77. Stockley IH. *Drug interactions*. 4th ed. London: Pharmaceutical Press, 1996.

78. Vestal RE, Wood AJJ, Branch RA, Shand DG, Wilkinson GR. Effects of age and cigarette smoking on propranolol disposition. *Clin Pharmacol Ther* 1979;26:8–15.

79. Fox KM, Jonathan A, Williams H, Selwyn A. Interaction between cigarettes and propranolol in the treatment of angina pectoris. *Br Med J* 1980;3:191–193.

80. Fox K, Deanfield J, Krikler S, Ribeiro P, Wright C. The interaction of cigarette smoking and beta-adrenoceptor blockade. *Br J Clin Pharmacol* 1984;17:92S–93S.

81. Schaaf LJ, Campbell SC, Mayersohn MB, Vagedes T, Perrier DG. Influence of smoking on the disposition kinetics of metoprolol. *Eur J Clin Pharmacol* 1987;33:355–361.

82. Deacon CS, Lennard MS, Bax NDS, Woods HF, Tucker GT. Inhibition of oxidative drug metabolism by β-adrenoceptor antagonists is related to their lipid solubility. *Br J Clin Pharmacol* 1981;12:429–432.

83. Ferrari S, Leemann T, Dayer P. The role of lipophilicity in the inhibition of polymorphic cytochrome P450IID6 oxidation by beta-blocking agents in vitro. *Life Sci* 1991;48:2259–2265.

84. Blauford I, Pfeifer TM, Frishman WH. β-Blockers: drug interactions of clinical significance. *Drug Safety* 1995;13:359–370.

85. Otton SV, Inaba T, Kalow. Competitive inhibition of sparteine oxidation in human liver by beta-adrenoceptor antagonists and other cardiovascular drugs. *Life Sci* 1984;34:73–80.

86. Rowland K, Yeo WW, Ellis SW, et al. Inhibition of CYP2D6 activity by treatment with propranolol and the role of 4-hydroxypropranolol. *Br J Clin Pharmacol* 1994;38:9–14.

87. Peet M, Middlemiss DN, Yates RA. Propranolol in schizophrenia, II: clinical and biochemical aspects of combining propranolol with chlorpromazine. *Br J Psychiatry* 1981;138:112.

88. Miller FA, Rampling D. Adverse effects of combined propranolol and chlorpromazine therapy. *Am J Psychiatry* 1982;139:1198–1199.

89. Schneck DW, Luderer JR, Davis D, Vary J. Effects of nadolol and propranolol lidocaine clearance. *Clin Pharmacol Ther* 1984;36:584–587.

90. Ochs HR, Carstens G, Greenblatt DJ. Reduction of lidocaine clearance during continuous infusion and by co-administration of propranolol. *N Engl J Med* 1980;303:373.

91. Svendsen TL, Tango M, Waldorff S, Steiness E, Trap-Jensen J. Effects of propranolol and pindolol on plasma lignocaine clearance. *Br J Clin Pharmacol* 1982;13:223S–226S.

92. Conrad KA, Byers JM, Finley PR, Burnham L. Lidocaine elimination: effects of metoprolol and propranolol. *Clin Pharmacol Ther* 1983;33:133–138.

93. Tucker GT, Bax NDS, Lennard, Al-Asady S, Bharaj HS, Woods. Effects of β-adrenoceptor antagonist on the pharmacokinetics of lignocaine. *Br J Clin Pharmacol* 1984;17:21S–28S.

94. Wyse DG, Kellen J, Tam Y, Rademaker AW. Increased efficacy and toxicity of lignocaine in patients on beta-blockers. *Int J Cardiol* 1988:21:59–70.

95. Graham CF, Turner WM, Jones JK. Lidocaine-propranolol interactions. *N Engl J Med* 1981;304:1301.

96. Jordo L, Johnsson G, Lundborg P, Regardh CG. Pharmacokinetics of lidocaine in healthy individuals pretreated with multiple doses of metoprolol. *Int J Clin Pharmacol Ther Toxicol* 1984;22:312–315.

97. Miners JO, Wing LMH, Lillywhite KJ, Smith KJ. Failure of "therapeutic" doses of beta-adrenoceptor antagonists to alter the disposition of tolbutamide and lignocaine. *Br J Clin Pharmacol* 1984;18:853–860.

98. Conrad KA, Nyman DW. Effects of metoprolol and propranolol on theophylline elimination. *Clin Pharmacol Ther* 1980;28:463.

99. Miners JO, Wing LMH, Lillywhite KJ, Robson RA. Selectivity and dose-dependency of the inhibitory effect of propranolol on theophylline metabolism in man. *Br J Clin Pharmacol* 1985;20:219–223.

100. Robson RA, Miners JO, Matthews AP, et al. Characterisation of theophylline metabolism by human liver microsomes. *Biochem Pharmacol* 1988;37:1651–1657.

101. Rasmussen BB, Maenpaa J, Pelkonen O, et al. Selective serotonin reuptake inhibitors and theophylline metabolism in human liver microsomes: potent inhibition by fluvoxamine. *Br J Clin Pharmacol* 1995;39:151–159.

102. Pan HY, Triscari J, DeVault AR, et al. Pharmacokinetic interaction between propranolol and the HMG-CoA reductase inhibitors pravastatin and lovastatin. *Br J Clin Pharmacol* 1991;32:665–670.

103. Smith HT, Jokubaitis LA, Troendle AJ, Hwang DS, Robinson WT. Pharmacokinetics of fluvastatin and specific drug interactions. *Am J Hypertens* 1993;6:375S–382S.

104. Andersson T, Miners JO, Veronese ME, Birkett DJ. Diazepam metabolism by human liver microsomes is mediated by both S-mephenytoin hydroxylase and CYP3A isoforms. *Br J Clin Pharmacol* 1994;38:131–137.

105. Hawkesworth G, Betts T, Crowe A, et al. Diazepam/β-adrenoceptor antagonist interactions. *Br J Clin Pharmacol* 1984;17:69S–76S.

106. Relling MV, Toshifumi A, Gonzalez F, Meyer UA. Tolbutamide and mephenytoin hydroxylation by human cytochrome P450s in the CYP2C subfamily. *J Pharmacol Exp Ther* 1990;252:442–447.

107. Guengerich FP, Muller-Enoch D, Blair IA. Oxidation of quinidine by human liver cytochrome P450. *Mol Pharmacol* 1986;30:287–295.

108. Fenster P, Perrier P, Mayorsohn M, Marku FI. Kinetic evaluation of the propranolol-quinidine interaction. *Clin Pharmacol Ther* 1980;27:450–453.

109. Gillette DW, Tannery LP. Beta-blockers inhibit tricyclic metabolism. *J Am Acad Child Adolesc Psychiatry* 1993;33:223–224.

110. Perez V, Gilaberte I, Fairies D, Alvarez E, Artigas F. Randomised, double blind, placebo controlled trial of pindolol in combination with fluoxetine antidepressant treatment. *Lancet* 1997;349:1594–1597.

111. Greendyke RM, Kanter DR. Plasma propranolol levels and their effect on plasma thioridazine and haloperidol concentrations. *J Clin Psychopharmacol* 1987;7:178–182.

112. Greendyke RM, Gulya A. Effect of pindolol administration on serum levels of thioridazine, haloperidol, phenytoin and phenobarbital. *J Clin Psychiatry* 1988;49:105–107.

113. Markowitz JS, Wells BG, Carson WH. Interactions between antipsychotic and antihypertensive drugs. *Ann Pharmacother* 1995;29:603–609.

114. Al-Asadi SAH, Black GL, Lennard MS, Tucker GT, Woods HF. Inhibition of lignocaine metabolism by β-adrenoceptor antagonists in rat and human liver microsomes. *Xenobiotica* 1989;19:929–944.

CHAPTER 26

Angiotensin II Antagonists, ACE Inhibitors, and Diuretics

Michael Goldberg

The potential for significant drug interactions is high in patients undergoing treatment for chronic cardiovascular diseases. Hypertensive patients, in particular, often require long-term treatment with multiple pharmacologic agents to achieve optimal blood pressure control and they frequently take a variety of additional prescription and over-the-counter medications for associated medical conditions (1). In these circumstances, clinically significant pharmacodynamic or pharmacokinetic drug–drug interactions can occur because one drug may enhance or inhibit the pharmacologic effects, absorption, distribution, excretion, or metabolism of another. Since the early 1990s, significant advances have been made in modern understanding of enzymatic processes involved in drug metabolism, particularly with respect to the cytochrome P450 isoenzymes. Indeed, it has become theoretically possible to estimate the likelihood of metabolic drug–drug interactions in the early stages of drug development once specific metabolizing enzymes and pathways have been characterized in *in vitro* systems.

This chapter specifically reviews the metabolic pathways of three major classes of drugs used to treat cardiovascular diseases: the angiotensin II (AII) antagonists, angiotensin-converting enzyme (ACE) inhibitors, and diuretics. The review focuses on the involvement of specific metabolic enzymes such as isoenzymes of the P450 family and glucuronyltransferases in the disposition of each drug, the pharmacologic activity of any metabolites generated, and, where applicable, an assessment of whether metabolic enzyme induction or inhibition by spe-

cific drugs can explain drug–drug interactions observed clinically. When possible, the principal routes of metabolism and disposition of a particular drug in humans are described. However, when metabolic data in humans are unavailable, *in vitro* or *in vivo* animal studies are reviewed. Angiotensin II receptor antagonists, representing a new and growing class of agents, are emphasized over other classes of drugs in this chapter.

ANGIOTENSIN II ANTAGONISTS

AII antagonists represent the newest class of cardiovascular drugs available to treat hypertension, heart fail-

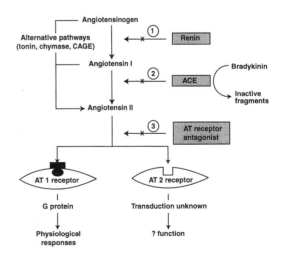

FIG. 26-1. Renin angiotensin system bioenzymatic cascade and potential steps to block the system. Angiotensin II antagonists block the action of AII generated by ACE and alternative pathways. Reproduced from Johnson CI. Angiotensin receptor antagonists: focus on losartan. *Lancet* 1995;346: 1403–1407, with permission.

M. Goldberg: Department of Clinical Pharmacology, Thomas Jefferson University School of Medicine, 132 South 10th Street, Philadelphia, Pennsylvania 19107-5244 and Department of Clinical Pharmacology, Merck Research Laboratories, 10 Sentry Parkway, Blue Bell, Pennsylvania 19422

ure, and potentially other cardiovascular diseases such as left ventricular hypertrophy and renal impairment (2–7). The therapeutic actions of AII antagonists result from their ability to selectively block the interaction of AII with its receptor present on target tissues such as vascular smooth muscle, zona glomerulosa of the adrenal gland, and afferent and efferent arterioles of the kidney (8,9). In contrast to the ACE inhibitors, AII antagonists block the action of AII formed by both ACE and non-ACE routes (Fig. 26-1) and do not produce alterations in the metabolism of other endogenous peptides (e.g., bradykinin), implicated in adverse reactions to ACE inhibitors (10).

AII, the principal effector of the renin-angiotensin cascade, interacts with at least two classes of receptors on target tissues (11). The principal AII receptors have been designated AT_1 and AT_2 and are typical polypeptide (360 amino acids) receptors with seven transmembrane domains (5). Most of the physiologic actions of AII, such as vasoconstriction, aldosterone stimulation, and salt and water homeostasis, are mediated by AT_1.

The sequence of events that ultimately led to the development of a specific, selective, and therapeutically useful AT_1 antagonist began in the early 1970s with pharmacologic studies of several peptide analogues of AII, including saralasin, 1-sarcosine,8-isoleucine angiotensin II, and other

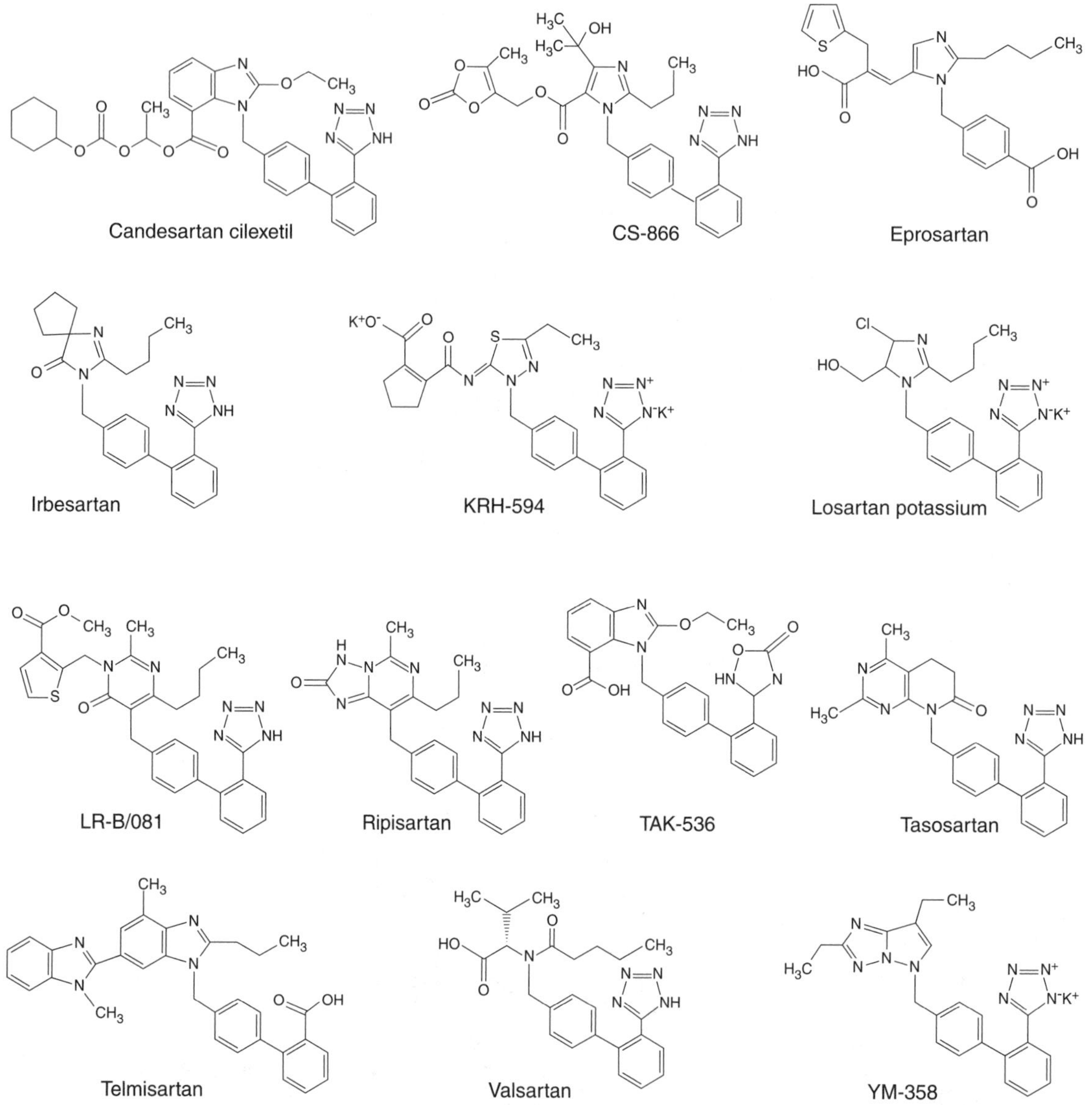

FIG. 26-2. Chemical structures of angiotensin II receptor antagonists launched or in clinical development. Adapted from Casas A, Merios M, Castaner J. Irbesartan. *Drugs Fut* 1997;22:481–491, with permission.

8-substituted angiotensins (12). These compounds were all found to be potent AII antagonists but unsuitable for clinical use because they retained significant partial agonist activity and had to be administered by constant intravenous infusion (13). These early observations prompted medicinal chemists to synthesize a series of nonpeptide AII antagonists based on the imidazole and imidazole-5-acetic acid structures (14). Two of these derivatives, referred to simply as S-8307 and S-8308, were capable of specifically blocking the actions of AII but displayed only weak blood pressure–lowering effects. In a sequence of elegant chemical modifications of these lead molecules, Timmermans and colleagues developed losartan, the first orally active, selective, and potent nonpeptide AT_1 antagonist (15).

The development of losartan prompted chemists to synthesize a plethora of nonpeptide AII antagonists using losartan or its intermediates as a molecular model (Fig. 26-2), and many of these are currently in various stages of clinical development (Table 26-1). This section reviews the metabolism of the most actively studied compounds to date: losartan, candesartan, irbesartan, eprosartan, and valsartan.

AII antagonists are principally metabolized by the liver to active or inactive metabolites. This biotransformation appears to involve several isoenzymes of the P450 family and UDP-glucuronyltransferases.

Losartan

Several investigators have evaluated the major pathways and enzymes of losartan metabolism using liver microsomes or hepatic tissue from humans and other species (16–18). Incubation of losartan with human liver slices revealed three principal metabolic pathways: (a) oxidation of the alcohol to the carboxylic acid, (b) monohydroxylation of the butyl side chain, and (c) glu-

curonidation of the tetrazole moiety. These pathways gave rise to a total of six losartan metabolites: M1, M2, M4, M5, M6, and M7 (Fig. 26-3) (18). The in vitro metabolism of losartan was not dominated by a single metabolite and both oxidized and glucuronidated metabolites were present. When tested in vitro for their ability to bind to the AII receptor, the C1- and C3-hydroxybutyl metabolites (M5 and M2), the hemiaminal decomposition products (M1′ and M1′′), and both the O- and tetrazole-N2-glucuronic acid conjugates possessed much lower activity than the parent compound. Only the carboxylic acid metabolite (M6), E3174, was found to be more potent in binding to the AII receptor than losartan.

Analysis of the mechanism of the biotransformation of losartan to E3174 in human liver microsomes revealed the involvement of CYP3A and CYP2C isoforms (17). These isoenzymes generated the active carboxylic acid metabolite by way of formation of an aldehyde intermediate (E3179) (Fig. 26-4). The biotransformation of losartan in vitro could be blocked by gestodene and ketoconazole (inhibitors of CYP3A4/5) and by sulfaphenazole (inhibitor of CYP2C9/10), supporting the potential involvement of these isoforms. Based on the low level of inhibition observed with quinidine and 4-methylpyrazole, it appeared that CYP2D6 and CYP2E1 were not involved in the metabolism of losartan or E3174. These observations are consistent with the findings of Sandwall and colleagues who evaluated losartan pharmacokinetics in subjects who were extensive or poor metabolizers of debrisoquine or mephenytoin (19). These pharmacokinetic studies also showed that CYP2D6 or CYP2C19 do not appear to play a role in the metabolism of losartan to E3174.

In vivo studies of losartan disposition in healthy male subjects revealed that approximately 14% of an oral or intravenous dose is converted to E3174 and that both presystemic and systemic mechanisms appear to contribute to this transformation (20). Losartan is eliminated primarily by nonrenal mechanisms, but E3174 elimination occurs by both renal and nonrenal routes. As summarized in Table 26-2, peak concentrations of losartan were attained approximately 1 hour after oral administration, whereas peak E3174 concentrations occurred later (4.1 hours).

Even though the metabolite E3174 is pharmacologically active, losartan is not a prodrug because losartan itself is a potent AII antagonist (20). However, the active metabolite E3174 likely contributes to the antihypertensive effect of losartan and likely accounts for the once-a-day efficacy observed with this agent (20,21).

Pharmacokinetic parameters are based on the following doses (20,22–24):

Losartan oral 50 mg, intravenous 20 mg
Candesartan oral 5 mg
Irbesartan oral 150 to 600 mg
Valsartan 160 mg

TABLE 26-1. *Angiotensin II receptor antagonists launched or in clinical development*

Compound	Company
Losartan	DuPont Merck
Candesartan cilexetil	Takeda/Astra
Irbesartan	Elf Sanofi/Bristol-Myers Squibb/Shionogi
Eprosartan	SmithKline Beecham
Telmisartan	Boehringer-Ingelheim
Valsartan	Novartis
Tasosartan	American Home Products
Ripisartan	Bristol-Myers Squibb (UPSA)
CS-866	Sankyo/Recordati
DA-727	Daiichi/Kotobuki
KRH-594	Wakunaga/Kissei
LR-B/081	Lusofarmaco/Menarini
TAK-536	Takeda
YM-358	Yamanouchi

Adapted from Casas A, Merios M, Castaner J. Irbesartan *Drugs Fut* 1997;22:481–491.

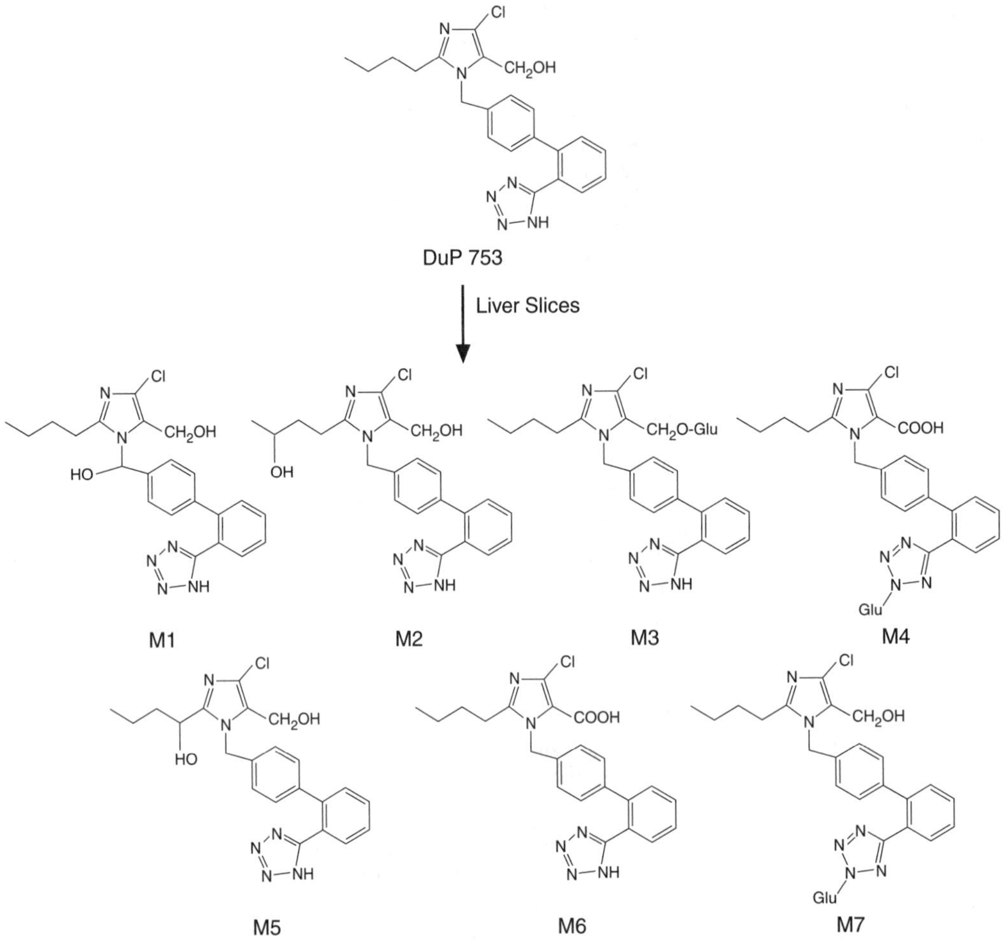

FIG. 26-3. Summary of metabolites formed by incubating losartan with human liver slices. Metabolite M3 has been isolated only in monkey and rat liver slices. Glu = 2β-glucuronic acid. From Stearns RA, Miller RR, Doss GA, et al. The metabolism of DuP 753, a nonpeptide angiotensin II receptor antagonist, by rat, monkey, and human liver slices. *Drug Metab Dispos* 1992;20:281–287, with permission.

Interestingly, recent reports by McCrea, Spielberg, and colleagues have described two healthy subjects with an amino acid substitution in CYP2C9 that resulted in a marked decrease in the metabolism of losartan to its active metabolite (25,26). Less than 1% of an oral losartan dose was metabolized to E3174. When the coding regions of the CYP2C9 gene were sequenced, these investigators found that both subjects were homozygous for a mutation causing an ILE for LEU substitution of residue 359, exon 7.

These subjects showed an extended half-life for losartan. Further studies are needed to assess the incidence of this infrequent variant enzyme and how this mutation influences the enzymatic function of CYP2C9 and the clinical efficacy of losartan. However, because the variant is infrequent, minimal impact is expected on the overall efficacy and safety profile of losartan.

Because losartan is metabolized to its active metabolite E3174 *in vitro* by several P450 isoforms, it is theoreti-

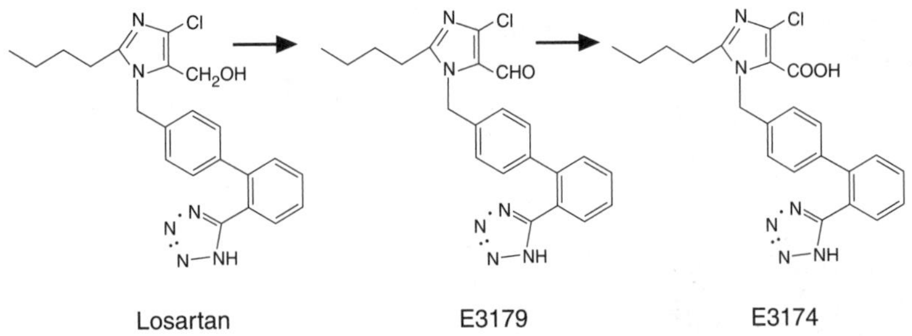

FIG. 26-4. Schema for the oxidative biotransformation of losartan to its active carboxylic acid metabolite. From Stearns RA, Chakravarty PK, Chen R, et al. Biotransformation of losartan to its active carboxylic acid metabolite in human liver microsomes. *Drug Metab Dispos* 1995;23:207–215, with permission.

TABLE 26-2. *Pharmacokinetic parameters for losartan and other angiotensin II receptor antagonists*

Pharmacokinetic parameter	Losartan	E3174 (active losartan metabolite)	CV-11974/M-1 (active candesartan metabolite)	Irbesartan	Valsartan
AUC (ng · hr/mL)	476	1915	681	—	16940
T_{max} (hr)	1.0	4.1	3.3	1.5–2	2[a]
C_{max} (ng/mL)	296	249	79	—	3130
$T_{1/2}$ (hr)	2.1	6.4	2.0	11–15	5.9[a]
V_{ss} IV admin (L)	28.4	10.3	—	—	—
Oral bioavailability (%)	32.6[b]	—	—	—	—
CL IV admin (mL/min)	636	46.9	—	—	—
CL_R IV admin (mL/min)	72.1	25.9	—	—	—

[a]Median value
[b]Geometric mean
AUC, area under the plasma-concentration curve; C_{max}, peak plasma concentration, T_{max}, time to reach C_{max}; $T_{1/2}$, half life; V_{ss}, volume of distribution at steady-state after IV administration; CL, plasma clearance after IV administration; CL_R, renal clearance after IV administration.

cally possible for the metabolism of this agent to be altered *in vivo* by drugs that either inhibit these enzymatic pathways (e.g., cimetidine) or induce P450 activity (e.g., phenobarbital). However, pharmacokinetic studies in healthy males showed that no clinically meaningful interaction occurred between losartan and either cimetidine or ketoconazole, two drugs that inhibit CYP3A4 (27,28). Cimetidine, a widely used H_2-antagonist, has been shown to inhibit the metabolism of several drugs metabolized by CYP3A4, including nifedipine, nisolodipine, and dapsone (29–31). However, when administered to healthy male subjects, multiple-dose cimetidine did not alter the pharmacokinetics or pharmacodynamics of losartan to a clinically significant degree. Cimetidine increased the AUC for losartan by 18% but had no effect on the AUC for E3174. Similarly, administration of ketoconazole over a 6-day period to healthy subjects produced little or no effect on either the systemic conversion of losartan to E3174 or the plasma clearances of losartan and E3174 (28). In addition, oral administration of losartan concomitantly with the CYP3A4 inhibitor, erythromycin, did not alter plasma concentrations of E3174 (32).

As indicated earlier, CYP2C9 appears to play a major role in the conversion of losartan to E3174. Few drugs in widespread clinical use are known to inhibit this pathway. In a recent study by Meadowcroft and colleagues, concomitant administration of fluvastatin (a specific CYP2C9 inhibitor) with losartan in healthy volunteers failed to significantly alter the steady-state pharmacokinetics of losartan or its metabolite E3174 (33). In contrast, the antimycotic fluconazole (an inhibitor of CYP2C9 and, to a lesser extent CYP3A4), appears to inhibit the conversion of losartan to E3174 (34,35).

Induction of CYP450 activity using phenobarbital as a nonspecific inducer also produced no clinically meaningful effect on losartan pharmacokinetics in healthy male subjects (36). Administration of phenobarbital produced no change in the plasma half-life of losartan or E3174

and produced minor, clinically unimportant reductions (about 20%) in the AUC for these compounds. However, phenobarbital administration resulted in a two-fold increase in the ratio of 6-β-hydroxycortisol to 17-hydroxycorticosteroids, indicating that induction of P450 drug-metabolizing enzymes had occurred. Similar effects of rifampin have been reported (32).

Losartan, like many antihypertensive agents, is often administered in combination with a diuretic, particularly hydrochlorothiazide. Hydrochlorothiazide is not metabolized *in vivo* and the kidney clears the majority of this diuretic—more than 95% of an oral dose appears in the urine unchanged. Because losartan is cleared mainly by nonrenal mechanisms, no clinically significant interaction between losartan and hydrochlorothiazide would be expected to occur in humans. The predicted absence of a significant pharmacokinetic interaction between these antihypertensive agents was recently confirmed in a randomized, crossover study in hypertensive patients (37).

In summary, the critical conversion of losartan to its active metabolite, E3174, would appear to be susceptible to inhibition by drugs such as fluconazole, which reduce the activity of CYP2C9. However, few clinically useful drugs inhibit this pathway at relevant concentrations, and those that do, like fluconazole, are prescribed infrequently and for only short treatment intervals so that an effect on the clinical profile of losartan would appear to be unlikely. Although CPY3A4 can catalyze the reaction *in vitro*, specific inhibitors of this pathway have not been shown to alter the conversion *in vivo* in humans. Thus, in contrast to drugs such as terfenadine, clinically significant interactions between inhibition of this pathway and losartan have not been demonstrated thus far. In patients undergoing long-term therapy with inducers of cytochrome P450 (e.g., phenobarbital), a minimal interaction might occur and the patient's antihypertensive response should be monitored if these agents are added or discontinued during prolonged losartan therapy.

Candesartan

Candesartan (TCV-116), a biphenyltetrazole imidazole, is an inactive prodrug that must be converted to its active carboxylic acid metabolite (CV11974) to achieve pharmacologic activity (38). In isolated rabbit aortic strips, candesartan is approximately 30 times less active than CV11974 in antagonizing AII-induced contraction (38).

Recent studies by Kondo and colleagues in rats and dogs showed that oral administration of candesartan cilexetil generated several key metabolites (Fig. 26-5) (39,40). These investigators found that candesartan was rapidly absorbed from the small intestine and hydrolyzed completely to a pharmacologically active metabolite (CV11974, or M-1). Subsequent metabolism of M-1 either by glucuronidation of the carboxylic acid side chain or tetrazole ring generated two additional metabolites (M-1-AG and M-1-NG, respectively). In addition, M-1 was also metabolized to M-II by way of

elimination of the ethyl group from the benzimidazole moiety (40).

Drug disposition studies in healthy males have also shown that the majority of orally administered candesartan (20 mg) is metabolized to the active metabolite M-1 or M-II (Fig. 26-6) (41). Levels of unchanged candesartan were low in both serum and urine.

Approximately 10% of the administered dose of candesartan appears in the urine during the first 24 hours after single or repeated dosing (22). This suggests that absorption from the gastrointestinal tract may be poor, with most of the drug being excreted in the feces. Pharmacokinetic parameters for the active metabolite M-1 are summarized in Table 26-2.

A recent randomized study in healthy volunteers by Jonkman and colleagues investigated potential pharmacokinetic drug interactions between candesartan cilexetil and hydrochlorothiazide, nifedipine, glibenclamide, warfarin, digoxin, or an oral contraceptive (42). Concomitant administration of hydrochlorothiazide and candesartan cilexetil resulted in a slight but significant decrease in the AUC of hydrochlorothiazide and a significant increase in the bioavailability and C_{max} values for candesartan (18% and 25%, respectively). Candesartan coadministration with warfarin also produced a 7% decrease in the trough plasma warfarin concentration. In contrast, coadministration of candesartan with nifedipine, glibenclamide, digoxin, or oral contraceptive did not influence the pharmacokinetic parameters of candesartan.

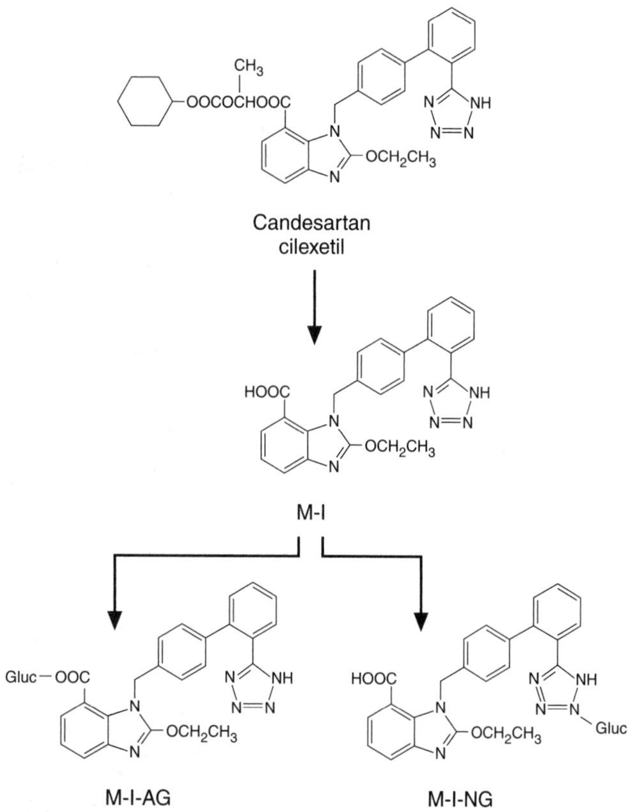

FIG. 26-5. Proposed metabolic pathway of candesartan cilexetil (TCV-116). From Kondo T, Yoshida K, Yoshimura Y, et al. Characterization of conjugated metabolites of a new angiotensin II receptor antagonist, candesartan cilexetil, in rats by liquid chromatography/electrospray tandem mass spectrometry following chemical derivativization. *J Mass Spect* 1996;31:873–878, with permission.

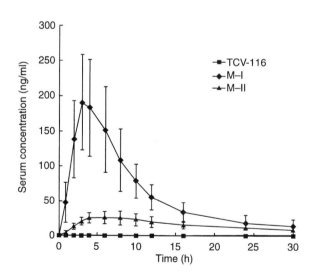

FIG. 26-6. Serum concentrations of candesartan, M-I, or M-II after a single oral dose of candesartan (20 mg) to 6 healthy males. From Miyabayashi T, Okuda T, Motohashi M, et al. Quantitation of a new potent angiotensin II receptor antagonist, TCV-116, and its metabolites in human serum and urine. *J Chromatogr* 1996;677:123–132, with permission.

Irbesartan

Irbesartan, a biphenyltetrazole imidazole AII antagonist (also known as SR-47436, BMS-186295), is extensively metabolized in humans. Administration of (C^{14})-irbesartan resulted in formation of seven metabolites (M1–M7), which were identified in urine, feces, and plasma samples by high-pressure liquid chromatography (Fig. 26-7) (43). In urine and feces, irbesartan itself and irbesartan glucuronide accounted for greater than 90% of the radioactivity (44).

Perrier and colleagues extensively studied the glucuronidation of irbesartan by UDP-glucuronosyltransferase in human, rat, and monkey hepatic microsomes (45). These investigators demonstrated that irbesartan undergoes N-glucuronidation on the tetrazole moiety. The reaction followed Michaelis-Menten kinetics and was optimal at pH 5.0 (K$_m$ 0.1 mM, V$_{max}$ 1.28 nmol/min/mg). Irbesartan glucuronide does not appear to contribute to the biologic activity of the parent compound (46). Additional

experiments using specific inhibitors of glucuronosyltransferase isoforms (Table 26-3) revealed that the irbesartan serves as a substrate for a dexamethazone-inducible UDP-glucuronosyltransferase molecular species. This isoform appeared to be different from that involved in the glucuronidation of monodigitoxigenin-monodigitoxoside.

The role, if any, of a specific isoform of cytochrome P450 in the formation of oxidative metabolites of irbesartan (e.g., M1–M7) has not been reported. However, because these metabolites contributed to a substantive fraction of total radioactivity after administration of 14$_C$-irbesartan (43), it is hard to predict which potential drug interaction may occur.

Preliminary pharmacokinetic data from a placebo-controlled, double-blind ascending dose study (150, 300, 600, and 900 mg) showed that steady-state irbesartan concentrations occurred after 3 days (47). Values for T$_{max}$ (1.5–2 hours), half-life (11–15 hours), and percent urinary excretion (0.7%–1.2%) appeared to be constant over the range of irbesartan doses studied. In a recent study by

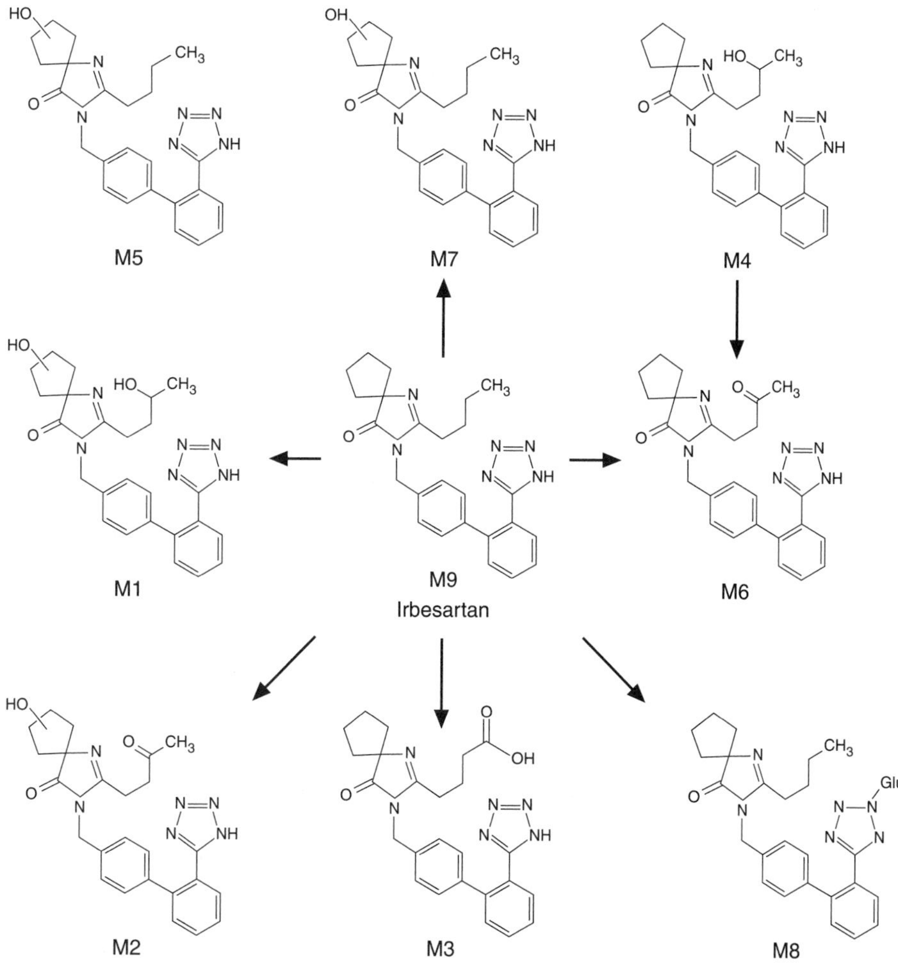

FIG. 26-7. Biotransformation of irbesartan in humans. From Casas A, Merios M, Castaner J. Irbesartan. *Drugs Fut* 1997;22:481–491, with permission.

TABLE 26-3. *Inhibitory effect of various compounds on the glucuronidation of irbesartan in human hepatic microsomal fractions*

Compounds	% of Inhibition	Type of inhibition
Phenols		
ρ-Nitrophenol	>10	
α-Naphthol	>10	
β-Naphthol	>10	
Estrone	>45.9	Noncompetitive
Methylumbelliferone	>10	
Paracetamol	>10	
Phenolphthaleine	>10	
Morphine	>10	
Harmol	>10	
Alcohol		
Chloramphenicol	>10	
Norethindrone	>33.8	Noncompetitive
Testosterone	>36.8	Noncompetitive
Carboxylic acid		
DT1	>28.1	Noncompetitive
7,7,7-Triphenylheptanoic acid	>34.6	Noncompetitive
Valproic acid	>10	
Probenecid	>10	
Naproxen	>34.1	Noncompetitive
Flurbiprofen	>46.3	Noncompetitive
Bilirubin	>14.1	
Tertiary amines		
Amitryptilline	>10	
Carbamazepine	>10	
Imipramine	>10	
Chlorpromazine	>10	

Human hepatic microsomes (HTL-27 preparation; 2 mg/mL) were incubated for 30 min with 100 μM SR 47436 (BMS 186295) in pH 5.0 Tris HCl (0.1 M)-MgCl$_2$ (5 mM) buffer with 0.2 mg of Brij 58 per mg of microsomal protein and 3 mM UDPGA in the absence or the presence of an equimolar concentration of different drugs known to be metabolized by various UDP-glucuronosyltransferase isoforms. When inhibition occurred, this later was investigated further by determining the type of inhibition (based on Lineweaver-Burk plots).

From Perrier L, Bourrie M, Marti E, et al. In vitro N-glucuronidation of SR47436 (BMS 186295), a new AT1 nonpeptide angiotensin II receptor antagonist, by rat, monkey and human hepatic microsomal fractions. *J Pharmacol Exp Ther* 1994;271:91–99.

Marino and colleagues, addition of hydrochlorothiazide to irbesartan monotherapy in mild-to-moderate hypertensive patients did not alter the pharmacokinetics of irbesartan, including C_{max}, T_{max}, and AUC (47).

Eprosartan

Limited data are available on the metabolism of eprosartan. This nonbiphenyltetrazole imidazole AII antagonist (SKF 108566) appears to be primarily eliminated in feces as unchanged drug and does not appear to be metabolized by the cytochrome P450 system (48). Renal clearance of eprosartan constitutes approximately 30% of the total clearance (49). More than 97% of plasma eprosartan is protein bound (50), raising the possibility of drug interactions with other protein-bound drugs. However, a recent pharmacodynamic study indicated that eprosartan did not significantly influence the 24-hour plasma glucose profiles of patients with type II diabetes stabilized on the highly protein-bound hypoglycemic drug glyburide (51). Eprosartan also produced no effect on the pharmacokinetics of oral digoxin in healthy males (49).

Valsartan

Valsartan (CGP 48933), a nonheterocyclic nonpeptide AII antagonist, is structurally related to losartan—the heterocyclic imidazole of losartan has been replaced with a nonplanar, acylated amino acid (46,52). Few studies have been published on the metabolism of valsartan in humans. Absorption and disposition of ^{14}C-labeled valsartan in rats and marmosets revealed that the majority of valsartan is excreted unchanged in the urine and feces (53). Oxidative *in vivo* biotransformation of valsartan in these species was found to be minimal; one minor metabolite occurred in marmosets and accounted for approximately 10% of the total plasma AUC for valsartan (53). This unidentified metabolite had a 200-fold lower affinity for the AT_1 receptor than the parent compound.

After oral administration in human subjects, valsartan is rapidly absorbed, with a time to peak plasma concentrations of approximately 2 hours (see Table 26-2) (24,53). Absorption of orally administered valsartan is reduced by more than 45% when administered with food (53). A recent randomized, open-label, crossover study in healthy volunteers showed that the single-dose pharmacokinetics of valsartan were essentially unchanged by coadministration of cimetidine, except for an increase in C_{max}, which was judged by the authors to be of little or no clinical relevance (54).

ANGIOTENSIN CONVERTING ENZYME INHIBITORS

The introduction of ACE inhibitors has markedly improved the management of a variety of cardiovascular diseases. Initially introduced as antihypertensive agents and representing one of the most efficacious and gener-

ally well-tolerated classes of drugs, ACE inhibitors have also revolutionized the treatment of congestive heart failure. A number of large multicenter clinical studies, including CONSENSUS, SOLVD, and V-HeFT II, have demonstrated that ACE inhibitors produce clinical improvement, slow the progression of symptoms, reduce total mortality rate, and reduce cardiovascular mortality rate in patients with heart failure or postmyocardial left ventricular dysfunction (55–57). ACE inhibitors also have clinical applications in treating progressive renal impairment and sclerodermal renal crisis (58).

ACE inhibitors arose as a result of research in the 1960s that showed that components of venom isolated from the Brazilian arrowhead viper *Bothrops jararaca* inhibited the enzyme responsible for degrading bradykinin–kinase II (59). Subsequent research established that kininase II and ACE (an enzyme generating angiotensin II) were, in fact, the same enzyme. A synthetic version of the nonapeptide fraction of snake venom

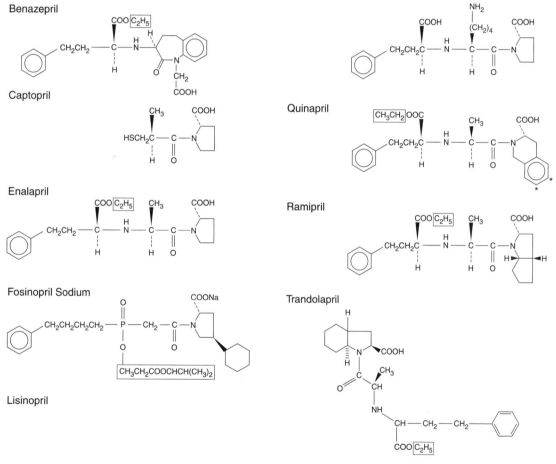

FIG. 26-8. Chemical structure of angiotensin-converting enzyme inhibitors approved for clinical use in the United States. The structures enclosed in boxes are removed by esterases and replaced with a hydrogen atom to form the active molecule *in vivo* (e.g., enalapril to enalaprilat). The asterisks (*) indicate the dimethoxy substitution (positions 6 and 7). From Jackson EK, Garrison JC. Renin and angiotensin. In: Hardman JG, Limbird LE, eds. *Goodman and Gilman's the pharmacological basis of therapeutics,* 9th ed. New York: McGraw-Hill, 1996:733–758, with permission.

(teprotide) produced a decrease in blood pressure when injected intravenously into patients with essential hypertension and also produced beneficial effects in heart failure patients (60). Cushman and colleagues at Squibb in the late 1970s further investigated the mechanism of action of teprotide and found that ACE inhibition could be achieved by succinyl amino acids such as carboxy alkanoyl and mercapto alkanoyl derivatives (61). This research ultimately led to the discovery of captopril—the first orally active, competitive inhibitor of ACE (62).

Since the development of captopril, a plethora of ACE inhibitors have been synthesized and developed—as of 1997, nine ACE inhibitors had been approved for clinical use in the United States (Fig. 26-8). ACE inhibitors share a common chemical moiety that is capable of interacting with the zinc ion located at the active site of ACE (63). Indeed, the chemical nature of this moiety is fundamental to the way in which ACE inhibitors are categorized—sulfhydryl-containing ACE inhibitors (e.g., captopril), dicarboxyl-containing inhibitors (e.g., enalapril, lisinopril, benzapril, quinapril, ramipril), and the phosphorus-containing inhibitors (e.g., fosinopril).

As discussed in this section, many ACE inhibitors including enalapril, quinapril, moexipril, benazepril, fosinopril, ramipril, and spirapril must be converted *in vivo* by esterases in liver or plasma to their corresponding diacids for maximal pharmacologic activity. Others such as captopril and lisonopril are themselves active molecules and do not require conversion. Many of the newer types of ACE inhibitors (e.g., benazepril, ramipril, lisinopril) are eliminated from the body renally and typically undergo minimal hepatic metabolism by CYP450 isoenzymes (59). As a result, these agents should be expected to present little or no risk for metabolic drug interactions.

Captopril

The metabolism of captopril, a potent ACE inhibitor containing a sulfhydryl moiety, has been extensively studied in animal models, normal subjects, and patients with heart failure, hypertension, and chronic renal failure (64). The principal pathways of captopril metabolism are summarized in Fig. 26-9. The presence of a free sulfhydryl group results in rapid binding of captopril to albumin and other plasma proteins and the formation of mixed disulfides with endogenous thiol-containing compounds (e.g., cysteine, glutathione) (64). This binding is reversible and may produce a reservoir of captopril in blood.

Studies in normal subjects using ^{35}S-labeled captopril (100 mg) showed that the primary route of captopril elimination is the kidney (65). The majority of orally administered captopril was eliminated in the urine (68%), with approximately 38% of the oral dose appearing as captopril and the rest as captopril disulfide (1.5%) and polar metabolites (26%). Peak plasma concentrations of captopril occur 1 hour after oral administration, and the drug is cleared rapidly with a half-life of approximately 2 hours

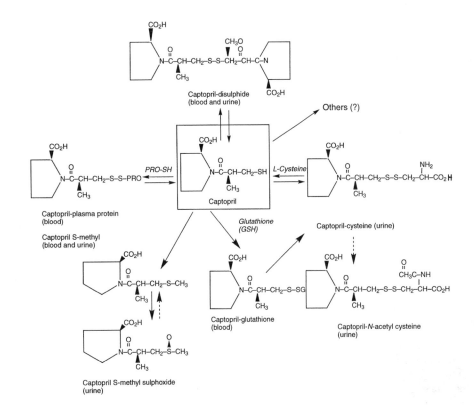

FIG. 26-9. Summary of biotransformation of captopril in blood and urine. Proposed metabolic pathways are indicated by the dotted arrows. From Migdalof BH, Antonaccio MJ, McKinstry DN, et al. Captopril: pharmacology, metabolism, and disposition. *Drug Metab Disp* 1984; 841–869, with permission.

(66). The oral bioavailability of captopril is roughly 62% (66). S-Methyl-captopril has also been identified in urine, accounting for about 1% of the oral dose (67). In dogs and monkeys but not humans, a sulfoxide metabolite may be present in urine.

Although captopril bioavailability may be reduced by coadministration of probenecid or antacids (64), these drug interactions are unlikely to be the result of alterations in captopril metabolism.

Enalapril

Enalapril, the second ACE inhibitor approved in the United States, is a prodrug that must be converted by hydrolysis *in vivo* to its bioactive form, enalaprilat (68).

In humans, the liver appears to be the principal site of conversion of enalapril to enalaprilat (69). Enalapril is rapidly absorbed from the gastrointestinal tract after oral administration, with peak serum concentrations of unchanged enalapril occurring after approximately 1 hour (Fig. 26-10). In contrast, peak enalaprilat concentrations are not achieved until 3 to 4 hours after enalapril dosing, but detectable levels may still be present after 72 to 96 hours, reflecting tight binding to plasma ACE, a phenomenon common to all ACE inhibitors (70,71). Renal excretion represents the primary route of excretion of enalapril. After a 10-mg dose of enalapril in healthy subjects, the majority of the drug can be recovered in urine (18% enalapril, 43% enalaprilat), with small amounts in the feces (6% enalapril, 27% enalaprilat) (72). Enalapril and enalaprilat are not metabolized further in humans (69) and no clinically significant drug interactions resulting from changes in their metabolism have yet been described.

Benazepril

The nonsulfhydryl ACE inhibitor benazepril is a prodrug that requires biotransformation *in vivo* to the free acid benazeprilat for maximal biological activity (59). Benazeprilat is approximately 200 times more potent than the parent compound in inhibiting ACE (59). Activation of benazepril involves cleavage of the ethoxycarbonyl group by hepatic esterases (73).

After oral administration, peak plasma concentrations of benazepril and benazeprilat occur within 0.5 hour and 1 to 1.5 hours, respectively (74). Benazepril is extensively metabolized with less than 1% of the dose excreted in the urine as unchanged benazepril (75). The primary urinary metabolites of benazepril were benazeprilat, accounting for 17% of the oral dose, and glucuronide conjugates of benazepril and benazeprilat, accounting for 4% and 8% of the dose, respectively. The main route of elimination of benazeprilat is by way of the kidneys, although biliary excretion may also occur (74). No clinically significant metabolic drug interactions with benazepril have yet been described.

Quinapril

Quinapril, a nonsulfhydryl, monoethyl ester ACE inhibitor, is a prodrug that is converted to the more active diacid metabolite, quinaprilat, *in vivo* by esterases present in the liver, gastrointestinal tract, and extravascular tissue (76). As illustrated in Fig. 26-11, quinapril is rapidly metabolized after absorption from the gastrointestinal tract primarily to quinaprilat but also to a limited extent to two diketopiperazine analogues of quinapril (PD109488 and PD113413), neither of which possesses ACE inhibitor activity (76,77).

Orally administered quinapril is rapidly absorbed in healthy male subjects, with peak plasma concentrations of quinapril and quinaprilat occurring after 1 and 2 hours, respectively. After a 40-mg dose, peak concentrations of quinaprilat in plasma were roughly four-fold higher than quinapril (77). Urinary excretion of quinaprilat and quinapril respectively account for approximately 30% and 3% of the administered quinapril dose. Excretion of

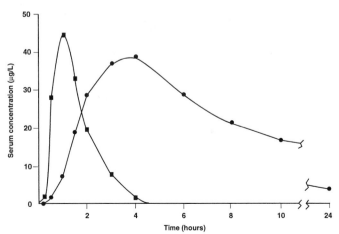

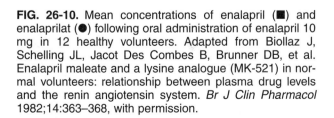

FIG. 26-10. Mean concentrations of enalapril (■) and enalaprilat (●) following oral administration of enalapril 10 mg in 12 healthy volunteers. Adapted from Biollaz J, Schelling JL, Jacot Des Combes B, Brunner DB, et al. Enalapril maleate and a lysine analogue (MK-521) in normal volunteers: relationship between plasma drug levels and the renin angiotensin system. *Br J Clin Pharmacol* 1982;14:363–368, with permission.

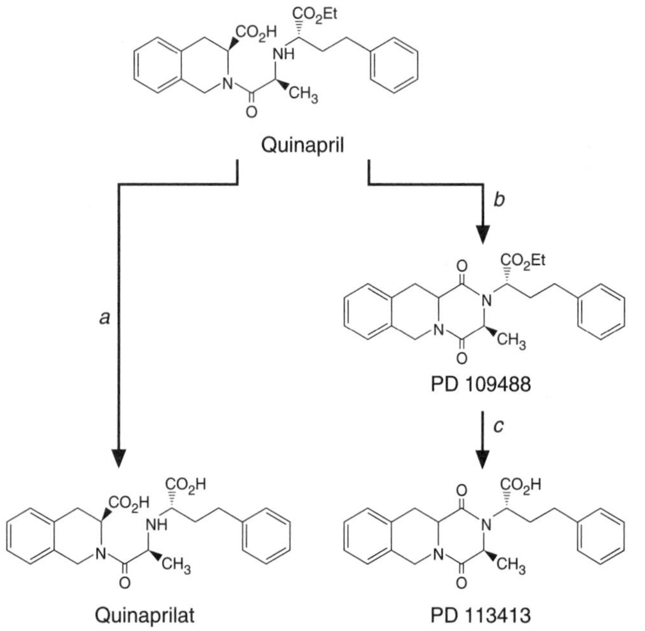

FIG. 26-11. Proposed metabolic pathways of quinapril in humans. From Olson SC, Horvath AM, Michniewicz BM, et al. The clinical pharmacokinetics of quinapril. *Angiology* 1989; 40:351–359, with permission.

each of the two diketopiperazine metabolites accounts for 6% of the dose. No clinically significant metabolic drug interactions with quinapril have yet been described.

Ramipril

The prodrug ramipril (HOE-698) is a dicarboxylic acid monoethyl ester derivative, which must be metabolized to the corresponding dicarboxylic acid (ramiprilat) to become effective as an ACE inhibitor (78). Based on urinary recovery studies in healthy subjects, approximately 56% of an orally administered dose (10 mg) is absorbed (78). After absorption in humans, ramipril is rapidly converted to ramiprilat in the liver and possibly the intestinal wall by saponification of the ester (78). Peak serum concentrations of the active metabolite ramiprilat and unchanged ramipril are achieved in approximately 3 hours and 1 hour, respectively (71). The pharmacokinetics of ramiprilat follows a triphasic elimination pattern, with an initial half-life (2–4 hours) resulting from extensive tissue distribution, an intermediate half-life (9–18 hours) resulting from plasma clearance of free ramiprilat, and terminal half-life (>50 hours) resulting from dissociation of ramiprilat from tissue ACE (73).

Ramipril is metabolized not only to ramiprilat but also to inactive metabolites, including glucuronides of ramipril and ramiprilat and diketopiperazine derivatives (79). No clinically significant drug interactions resulting from changes in ramipril metabolism have yet been described.

Lisinopril

Lisinopril (MK-521) is a pharmacologically active diacid, similar in structure to enalapril except that the methyl group is replaced with a butylamino group—in other words, lisinopril is a lysine analogue of enalaprilat (59,80). Unlike many ACE inhibitors, lisinopril is not a prodrug and requires no metabolic conversion for activity. Absorption of lisinopril after an oral dose of 10 mg is relatively slow, with peak levels occurring in roughly 6 to 7 hours (69,81). In healthy subjects, the majority of a 10-mg oral dose (97%) appeared unchanged in urine and feces, indicating the absence of significant metabolism of lisinopril either systemically or in the gastrointestinal tract (72). As a result, it is unlikely that clinically significant drug metabolic interactions would occur between lisinopril and drugs metabolized by CYP450 isoenzymes.

Fosinopril

Fosinopril is a phosphorus-containing ACE inhibitor prodrug (82). Following ingestion, fosinopril is rapidly hydrolyzed to its active diacid metabolite, fosinoprilat, by hepatic and gastrointestinal esterases (83). In healthy subjects, approximately 70% to 80% of an orally administered dose (10 mg) was hydrolyzed to fosinoprilat within 1 day after ingestion, and less than 1% remained as fosinopril. Acyl β-glucuronide conjugate was found to comprise the remainder (83). No clinically significant drug interactions resulting from interference with fosinopril metabolism have yet been described.

Moexipril

Moexipril (RS-10085) is a non-sulfhydryl-containing precursor of the active ACE inhibitor moexiprilat (84). Moexipril belongs to the carboxyl-containing class of ACE inhibitors and is chemically related to enalapril (84). The antihypertensive effect of moexipril can be almost entirely attributed to the effects of moexiprilat, the deesterified metabolite of moexiprilat (85).

Absorption of moexipril is incomplete with a bioavailability of approximately 13% after oral dosing (85). Moexipril is rapidly converted to moexiprilat—peak plasma concentrations of the active metabolite occur after approximately 1.5 hours. The half-life of moexipril and moexiprilat in plasma are estimated to be 1.3 and 9.8 hours, respectively (85). Approximately 7% of an orally administered dose appears in the urine as moexiprilat and 1% appears as moexipril. Small amounts (roughly 5% of an oral dose) of diketopiperazine derivatives and unidentified metabolites of moexipril and moexiprilat have also been identified in urine. The greatest proportion of an orally administered dose appears in feces as either moexiprilat (52%) or moexipril (1%). No clinically significant drug interactions resulting from changes in ramipril metabolism have yet been described. However, food has been shown to markedly impair the bioavailability of an orally administered dose.

Trandolapril

Like many of the ACE inhibitors discussed, trandolapril is a nonsulfhydryl prodrug that must be converted by non-specific hydrolysis in the liver to its pharmacologically active diacid, trandolaprilat (86). To a limited extent, both the parent drug and trandolaprilat are metabolized to conjugates of glucuronide. In addition, aromatization pathways lead to generation of minor amounts of diketopiperazine derivatives of both trandolapril and trandolaprilat (86). Trandolaprilat and its glucuronide conjugate represent the primary urinary excretion products (87). No clinically significant drug interactions resulting from changes in trandolaprilat metabolism have yet been described.

DIURETICS

Diuretics are extensively used to treat a variety of diseases, including hypertension, acute and chronic heart failure, acute and chronic renal failure, nephrotic syndrome, and cirrhosis (73). These agents are capable of changing the volume and composition of body fluids by increasing the renal excretion of sodium, chloride, and water (73,88). Diuretic-induced renal sodium and water excretion results from the ability of diuretic agents to inhibit sodium reabsorption in various regions of the tubular portion of the nephron (88).

A seminal observation in 1949 was that sulfanilamide, an antibiotic and inhibitor of carbonic anhydrase, possessed a diuretic effect in patients with congestive heart failure (89). Shortly afterward in 1950, investigators synthesized acetazolamide and other heterocyclic sulfonamides with increased specificity and activity against carbonic anhydrase (89). Acetazolamide became available for clinical use in the United States in 1953 (90). Several years later, a major breakthrough in diuretic development occurred with the synthesis of chlorothiazide, an orally active benzothiadiazine diuretic.

Since the late 1950s, numerous diuretics have been synthesized, developed, and marketed. Currently, diuretics are classified into four basic groups according to their mechanism of action: loop diuretics (e.g., ethacrynic acid, furosemide, torsemide), potassium-sparing diuretics (e.g., spironolactone, amiloride), thiazides and related diuretics (e.g., chlorothiazide, hydrochlorothiazide, hydroflumethiazide, and metolazone), and carbonic anhydrase inhibitors (e.g., acetazolamide). This latter group is not used in the treatment of cardiovascular diseases and is not reviewed further here.

In general, the potential for drug interactions with diuretics is high. For example, loop diuretics may interact with several types of drugs, including the following (73):

- Aminoglycosides (synergism of ototoxicity)
- Anticoagulants (increased anticoagulant activity)
- Digitalis glycosides (increased digitalis-induced arrhythmias)
- Lithium (increased plasma lithium levels)
- Propranolol (increased plasma propranolol levels)
- Sulfonylureas (hyperglycemia)
- Cisplatin (increased risk of diuretic-induced ototoxicity)
- Nonsteroidal anti-inflammatory drugs (blunted diuretic response)
- Probenecid (blunted diuretic response)
- Thiazide diuretics (synergistic diuretic effect, leading to profound diuresis)

Many diuretics, such as hydrochlorothiazide, amiloride, and chlorothiazide, are excreted in the urine or bile with little if any metabolic transformation and, therefore, the potential for metabolic drug interactions with these agents is minimal. However, several diuretics such as torsemide and spironolactone are extensively metabolized by the hepatic CYP450 system and the possibility exists for interactions with other drugs capable of inhibiting or inducing the enzymes of this microsomal system.

Furosemide

Furosemide (frusemide), an anthranilic acid derivative, is a potent loop diuretic. In healthy subjects, the bioavailability of orally administered furosemide ranges from 50% to 69% and peak plasma drug concentrations occur between 60 and 90 minutes (91,92). This diuretic is eliminated by both renal and nonrenal mechanisms (92). Furosemide is eliminated in the urine as unchanged drug and several metabolites, including furosemide glucuronide, 2-amino-4-chloro-5-sulfamoylanthranilic acid (CSA), and anthranilic acid (93–95). The enzymes involved in the hepatic metabolism of furosemide have not been clearly delineated. However, furosemide has been shown to stimulate hepatic microsomal enzyme activity, as evidenced by increased excretion of glucaric acid in the urine (96).

Ethacrynic Acid

Ethacrynic acid, an alpha, beta unsaturated ketone derivative of aryloxyacetic acid (97) is metabolized in humans, with only 30% to 40% of an oral dose excreted unchanged in the urine (98). Studies in dogs and rats show that ethacrynic acid is metabolized to three metabolites: ethacrynic acid glutathione (EA-GSH), ethacrynic acid mercapturate, and ethacrynic acid cysteine (Fig. 26-12) (97).

Several investigators have proposed that one or more metabolites of ethacrynic acid are biologically active (99,100). Indeed, based on the studies on the thick

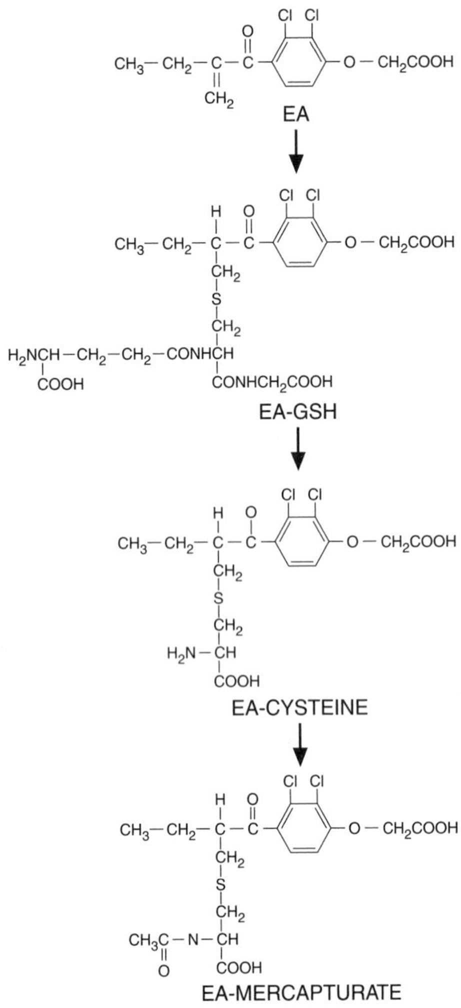

FIG. 26-12. Proposed pathways for metabolism of ethacrynic acid in dog and rat. From Klaassen CD, Fitzgerald TJ. Metabolism and biliary excretion of ethacrynic acid. *J Pharmacol Exp Ther* 1974;191:548–556, with permission.

ascending limb of Henle's loop in the rabbit, Burg and Green suggested that the ethacrynic acid–cysteine complex is not only the major urinary excretion product but also the major active species of the drug *in vivo* (99).

Limited clinical data are available on the metabolism and pharmacokinetics of ethacrynic acid in humans. Recently, however, Lacreta and colleagues reported the pharmacokinetics and bioavailability of ethacrynic acid in patients with cancer (100). These investigators studied cancer patients because ethacrynic acid may modulate resistance to several anticancer drugs by inhibiting glutathione S-transferases. After oral administration, ethacrynic acid rapidly appeared in plasma (peak concentration between 40 and 92 minutes) but had a low bioavailability (9.8%).

Torsemide

Torsemide (torasemide) is a loop diuretic belonging to the anilinopyridine sulfonylurea class (101). Orally admin-

istered torsemide is rapidly absorbed, with plasma concentrations peaking after 1 hour (102). This diuretic has an oral bioavailability approaching 90% (103). Torsemide is extensively metabolized (Fig. 26-13) and only 20% of the drug is excreted unchanged in the urine—the remaining 80% is metabolized by the liver (104).

Hepatic metabolism of torsemide is believed to occur predominantly, if not solely, from CYP450 2C9 activity (101,105). Metabolites M1 (resulting from hydroxylation of the methyl group), M3 (resulting from *para*-hydroxylation), and M5 (formed by oxidation of M1 at the carboxylic acid group) are the only metabolic products found in humans (101). M1 and M3 are both biologically active and likely contribute to the diuretic effect of torsemide (103); M1 possesses approximately one-tenth the activity of torsemide and M3 is approximately equivalent in potency to the parent compound. M5, the major metabolite in humans, is biologically inactive. Following a single oral dose, the cumulative total amount of torsemide and metabolites recovered in the urine was 83% (25% torsemide, 11% M1, 3% M3, and 44% M%) (103).

Because torsemide is metabolized via CYP2C9, the possibility exists for interactions with other drugs capable of inhibiting or inducing this enzyme such as diclofenac, phenytoin, piroxicam, tenoxicam, ticrynafen, tolbutamide, (S)-warfarin, carbamazepine, phenobarbital, rifampin, dicumarol, chloramphenicol, cotrimoxazole, azole antifungals, phenylbutazone, sulfaphenazole, and sulfinpyrazone (105). However, recent clinical data suggest that administration of cimetidine had no effect on the pharmacokinetics and pharmacodynamics of torsemide (106).

Spironolactone

Spironolactone is a steroid derivative that indirectly antagonizes the action of aldosterone (92). After oral administration in healthy subjects, this diuretic is rapidly absorbed (maximum plasma levels occur within 30 to 60 minutes) and undergoes extensive metabolism to a complex array of products, including canrenone, 6β-hydroxy-thiomethyl spironolactone, 7α-sulfoxidized spironolactone, and 6β-hydroxy 7α-sulfoxidized spironolactone (Fig. 26-14) (107). These metabolites are excreted in urine and bile (92).

Spironolactone initially undergoes esterolysis to a thiol intermediate followed by hydrolysis to canrenone or methylation to thiomethylspironolactone (92). Canrenone may be hydroxylated to 15α-hydroxycanrenone or converted to canrenoate and conjugated with glucuronic acid. In addition, thiomethylspironolactone may undergo a number of chemical modifications including hydroxylation, sulfoxidation, peroxidation, and conjugation (92). Canrenone and possibly some sulfur-containing metabolites are believed to be biologically active in humans (92). Spironolactone initially undergoes esterolysis to a thiol

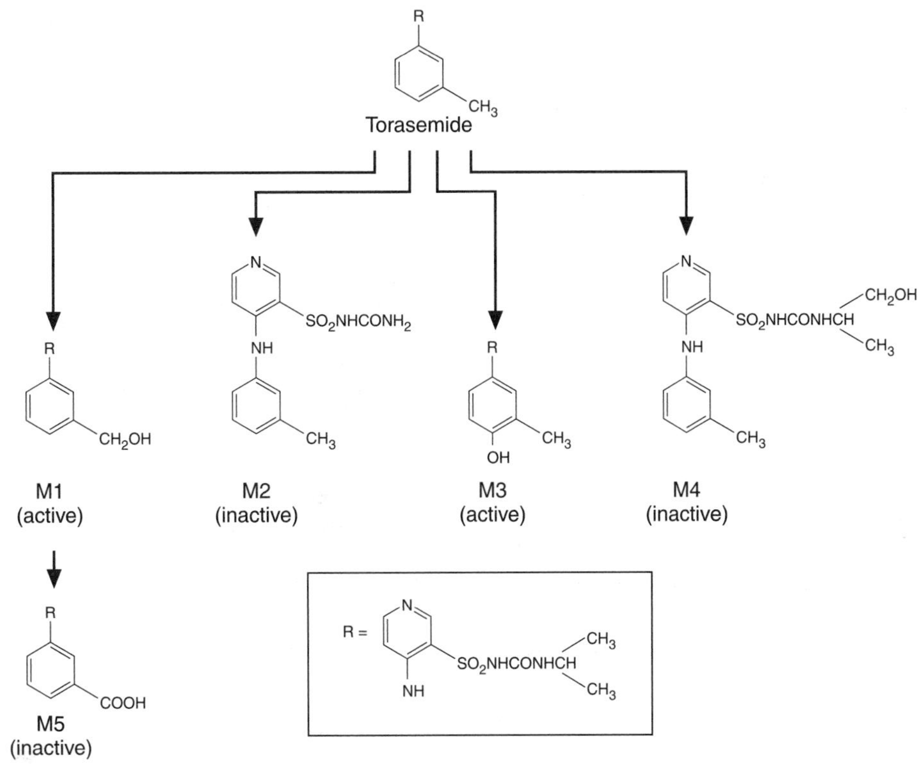

FIG. 26-13. Metabolism of torsemide to two active and three inactive metabolites; only M1, M3, and M5 are found in humans, with M5 being the major metabolite. Adapted from Karnes HT, Farthing D, Besenfelder E. Solid phase extraction with automated elution and HPLC of torsemide and metabolites from plasma. *J Liq Chromatogr* 1989;12:1809–1818, with permission.

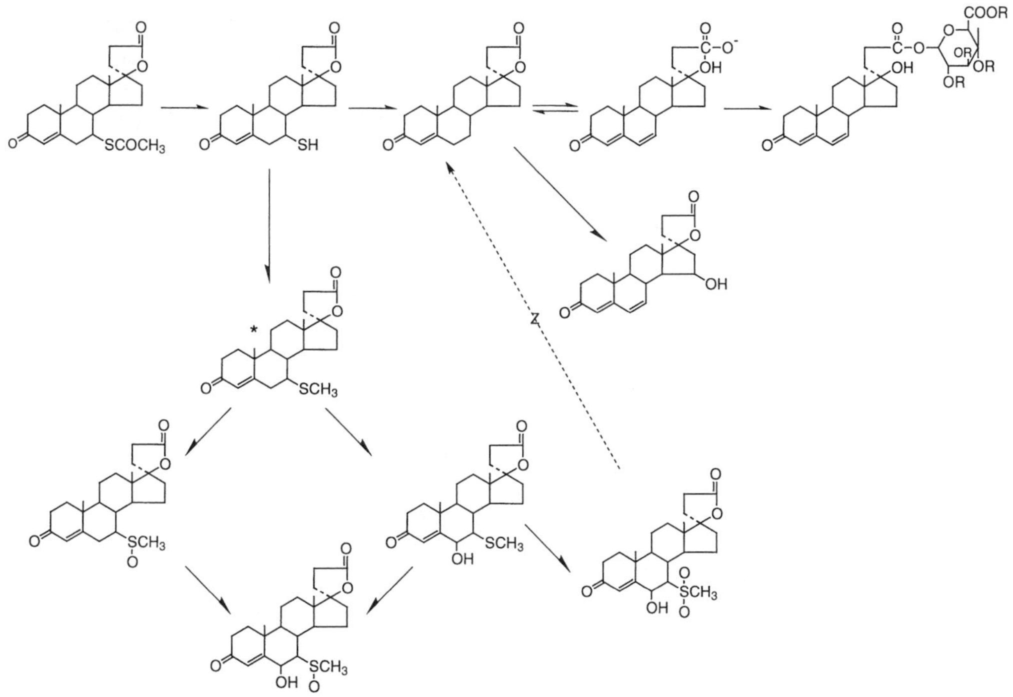

FIG. 26-14. Proposed scheme of metabolic degradation of spironolactone in man. *, postulated intermediate. From Abshagen U, Rennekamp H, Luszpinski G. Pharmacokinetics of spironolactone in man. *Naunyn-Schmiedeberg's Arch Pharmacol* 1976;296:37–45, with permission.

intermediate followed by hydrolysis to canrenone or methylation to thiomethylspironolactone (92). Canrenone may be hydroxylated to 15α-hydroxycanrenone or converted to canrenoate and conjugated with glucuronic acid. In addition, thiomethylspironolactone may undergo a number of chemical modifications including hydroxylation, sulfoxidation, peroxidation, and conjugation (92). Canrenone and possibly some sulfur-containing metabolites are believed to be biologically active in humans (92).

Spironolactone has been shown to induce hepatic enzymes involved in microsomal hydroxylation in humans and to increase CYP450 and cytochrome c reductase activity in *in vitro* animal models (108–110). Administration of spironolactone to nine healthy subjects was associated with a reduction in the half-life of antipyrine, increased excretion of 4-hydroxy-antipyrine, and 6β-hydroxy cortisol (108). Spironolactone, however, does not induce its own metabolism (111). Because spironolactone is capable of inducing hepatic microsomal enzyme hydroxylation, the potential exists for metabolic drug interactions with other drugs metabolized in this way (e.g., warfarin and dicoumarol) (92).

Amiloride

Amiloride, a pyrazine-carbonyl guanidine, is an antikaliuretic diuretic agent. There is no evidence of metabolic transformation of this diuretic in humans (112). Following oral administration of ^{14}C-labeled amiloride to healthy volunteers, peak drugs levels occurred at 3 to 4 hours (half-life 6 hours) and approximately 50% of the dose appeared unchanged in the urine (112,113). Renal clearance of amiloride occurs primarily by renal tubular excretion (112).

Chlorothiazide

Chlorothiazide is a nonmercurial diuretic agent that is not appreciably metabolized in humans (114). Intravenously administered ^{14}C-chlorothiazide is completely recovered in the urine within 24 hours; urinary recovery of an orally administered chlorothiazide is a much lower (33% to 58%). The plasma half-life of chlorothiazide after oral administration is relatively short, averaging 1.5 hours (73).

Hydrochlorothiazide

Hydrochlorothiazide, a member of the thiazide class of diuretics, is not metabolized in humans and is eliminated mainly by the kidneys (115). In normal subjects and patients with hypertension, greater than 95% of orally or intravenously administered ^{14}C-labeled hydrochlorothiazide dose is excreted unchanged in the urine (115). Hydrochlorothiazide was rapidly absorbed from the duodenum and upper jejunum and maximal plasma levels occurred between 1.5 and 5 hours following oral doses ranging from 12.5 mg to 75 mg (116). The plasma half-life of a 12.5-mg oral dose of hydrochlorothiazide averaged 2.6 hours (116).

Hydroflumethiazide

Hydroflumethiazide, an oral thiazide (benzothiadiazide) diuretic, is incompletely absorbed following oral administration. In adult, healthy male subjects, an oral dose of 100 mg hydroflumethiazide produced peak plasma concentrations after 2.6 hours. The plasma half-life of hydroflumethiazide averaged 2 hours and approximately 47% of the dose appeared in the urine over a 24-hour period (117). Hydroflumethiazide is partially metabolized in the body (approximately 2% to 3% of an oral dose) to 2,4-disulfamyl-5-trifluoromethylaniline (DTA) and both parent compound and metabolite are excreted in the urine (118). DTA has a longer half-life in the body compared to hydroflumethiazide but its biologic activity is unknown.

Metolazone

Metolazone, a derivative of quinethazone, is a thiazide diuretic. Studies in dogs and monkeys show that metolazone is metabolized (119). In humans, metolazone is primarily excreted unchanged in the urine (80%), with smaller amounts of intact drug either secreted in bile (10%) or metabolized (10%) (73). After administration of a single oral 5-mg dose to heart failure patients, metolazone first appeared in the urine between 1 and 1.5 hours and peak excretion rate occurred between 11 and 14 hours (120). The plasma half-life of metolazone is between 4 and 5 hours and approximately 65% of an oral dose is absorbed (73).

SUMMARY

This chapter summarizes available information on the potential for metabolic drug interactions relating to the cytochrome P450 system for AII receptor antagonists, ACE inhibitors, and diuretics. The latter two classes of drugs are commonly used in the treatment of hypertension and congestive heart failure. Based on available information to date, these two drug classes would appear to be generally unsusceptible to clinically important drug interactions based on inhibition or induction of cytochrome P450. Conjugation and excretion in the urine are the primary routes of elimination for these drugs. As a result, few studies on the effects of cytochrome P450 inhibitors or inducers on the elimination of these agents appear to have been carried out. Indeed, these types of studies would be of limited clinical relevance unless subsequent observations *in vitro* or *in vivo* indicate the potential for such interactions. However, the clinical profile of

ACE inhibitors and diuretics is not ideal. ACE inhibitors often result in cough, and less frequently, angioedema, both of which have been postulated to result from interaction of ACE inhibitors with the metabolism of other biologically active peptides (e.g., bradykinin). Diuretics have pronounced dose-related effects on urinary electrolyte excretion, which negatively impacts the benefit-risk profile of these agents. Thus, the recent development of selective inhibitors of the AT_1 receptor (e.g., losartan) has provided another therapeutic option for patients with cardiovascular disorders, especially with respect to the treatment of hypertension. The efficacy and general tolerability profile of this new class of agent suggests their potential to be a clear therapeutic advance over ACE inhibitors and diuretics.

While the clinical advantages of the angiotensin II antagonists are becoming accepted, their full clinical profile continues to be elucidated. In particular, the potential for metabolic interactions has only been well described for one of the AT_1 receptor antagonists. The generation of the active metabolite of losartan by CYP2C9 indicates the potential for inhibition of this pathway by specific drugs such as fluconazole. However, the clinical consequences of such inhibition remains to be investigated in that inhibition of this conversion does result in increased concentrations of the active parent drug. Published data on other angiotensin II antagonists are incomplete.

REFERENCES

1. Lam YWF, Shepherd AMM. Drug interactions in hypertensive patients. Pharmacologic, pharmacodynamic, and genetic considerations. *Clin Pharmacokinet* 1990;18:295–317.
2. Crozier I, Ikram H, Awan N, et al. Losartan in heart failure. Hemodynamic effects and tolerability. *Circulation* 1995;91:691–697.
3. Carr AA, Prisant LM. Losartan: first of a new class of angiotensin antagonists for the management of hypertension. *J Clin Pharmacol* 1996;36:3–12.
4. Gottlieb SS, Dickstein K, Fleck E, et al. Hemodynamic and neurohormonal effects of the angiotensin II antagonist losartan in patients with congestive heart failure. *Circulation* 1993;88:1602–1609.
5. Goodfriend TL, Elliott ME, Catt KJ. Angiotensin receptors and their antagonists. *N Engl J Med* 1996;334:1649–1654.
6. Gansevoort RT, deZeeüw D, Shahinfar S, et al. Effects of the angiotensin II antagonist losartan in hypertensive patients with renal disease. *J Hypertens* 1994;12[Suppl 2]:S37–S42.
7. Pitt B, Segal R, Martinez FA, et al. Randomized trial of losartan versus captopril in patients over 65 with heart failure (Evaluation of Losartan in the Elderly Study, ELITE). *Lancet* 1997;349:747–752.
8. Smith RD, Chiu AT, Wong PC, et al. Pharmacology of nonpeptide angiotensin II receptor antagonists. *Annu Rev Pharmacol Toxicol* 1992;32:135–165.
9. Messerli FH, Weber MA, Brunner HR. Angiotensin II receptor inhibition. A new therapeutic principle. *Arch Intern Med* 1996;156:1957–1965.
10. Johnson CI. Angiotensin receptor antagonists: focus on losartan. *Lancet* 1995;346:1403–1407.
11. de Gasparo M, Husain A, Alexander W, et al. Proposed update of angiotensin receptor nomenclature. *Hypertension* 1995.25;924–927.
12. Regoli D, Park WK, Rioux F. Pharmacology of angiotensin. *Pharmacol Rev* 1974;26:69–123.
13. Smith RD, Sweet CS, Goldberg A, Timmermans, PBMWM. Losartan potassium (COZAAR): a nonpeptide antagonist of angiotensin II. *Drugs Today* 1996;32[Suppl F]:1–42.
14. Furakawa Y, Kishimoto S, Nishikawa K. Hypotensive imidazole derivatives and hypotensive imidazole-5-acetic acid derivatives. Patents issued to Takeda Chemical Industries, Ltd, on July 20, 1982, and October 19, 1982, respectively. US Patents 4,340,598 and 4,355,040, Osaka, Japan, 1982.
15. Timmermans PBMWM, Wong PC, Chiu AT, et al. Angiotensin II receptors and angiotensin II receptor antagonists. *Pharmacol Rev* 1993;45:205–251.
16. Yun CH, Lee HS, Lee H, et al. Oxidation of the angiotensin II receptor antagonist losartan (DuP 753) in human liver microsomes. Role of cytochrome P450 3A(4) in formation of the active metabolite EXP 3174. *Drug Metab Dispos* 1995;23:285–289.
17. Stearns RA, Chakravarty PK, Chen R, et al. Biotransformation of losartan to its active carboxylic acid metabolite in human liver microsomes. *Drug Metab Dispos* 1995;23:207–215.
18. Stearns RA, Miller RR, Doss GA, et al. The metabolism of DuP 753, a nonpeptide angiotensin II receptor antagonist, by rat, monkey, and human liver slices. *Drug Metab Dispos* 1992;20:281–287.
19. Sandwall P, Lo MW, Dahlen P, et al. The metabolism of losartan to the active metabolite E3174 in subjects who are extensive and poor metabolizers of debrisoquine (CYP2D6) or mephenytoin (CYP2C19). *Br J Clin Pharmacol* 1997;43:215(abstr).
20. Lo MW, Goldberg MR, McCrea JB, et al. Pharmacokinetics of losartan, an angiotensin II receptor antagonist and its active metabolite EXP3174 in humans. *Clin Pharmacol Ther* 1995;58:641–649.
21. Wong PC, Price WA, Chiu AT, et al. Nonpeptide angiotensin II receptor antagonists. XI. Pharmacology of EXP3174: an active metabolite of DuP 753, and orally active antihypertensive agent. *J Pharmacol Exp Ther* 1990;255:211–217.
22. Ogihara T, Nagano M, Mikami H, et al. Effects of the angiotensin II antagonist, TCV-116, on blood pressure and the renin-angiotensin system in healthy subjects. *Clin Ther* 1994;16:74–86.
23. Marino MP, Langenbacher KM, Ford NF, et al. Safety, tolerability, pharmacokinetics of irbesartan after single and multiple doses in healthy male subjects. *Clin Pharmacol Ther* 1997;62(2):PIII-53 (abstr).
24. Czendlik CH, Sioufi A, Preiswerk G, et al. Pharmacokinetic and pharmacodynamic interaction of single doses of valsartan and atenolol. *Eur J Clin Pharmacol* 1997;52:451–459.
25. McCrea JB, Lo MW, Kong T, et al. A rare deficiency of the conversion of losartan to its active metabolite E3174. *Clin Pharmacol Ther* 1995;57:154(abstr PI-76).
26. Spielberg S, McCrea J, Cribb A, et al. A mutation in CYP2C9 is responsible for decreased metabolism of losartan. *Clin Pharmacol Ther* 1996;59:215(abstr).
27. Goldberg MR, Lo MW, Bradstreet TE, et al. Effects of cimetidine on pharmacokinetics and pharmacodynamics of losartan, an AT1-selective non-peptide angiotensin II receptor antagonist. *Eur J Clin Pharmacol* 1995;49:115–119.
28. McCrea JB, Lo MW, Furtek CI, et al. Ketoconazole does not affect the systemic conversion of losartan to E3174. *Clin Pharmacol Ther* 1996;59:169(abstr).
29. van Harten J, van Brummelen P, Lodewijks MTM, et al. Pharmacokinetics and hemodynamic effects of nisoldipine and its interaction with cimetidine. *Clin Pharmacol Ther* 1988;43:332–341.
30. Schwartz JB, Upton RA, Lin ET, et al. Effect of cimetidine or ranitidine administration on nifedipine pharmacokinetics and pharmacodynamics. *Clin Pharmacol Ther* 1988;43:673–680.
31. Coleman MD, Scott AK, Breckenridge AM, et al. The use of cimetidine as a selective inhibitor of dapsone N-hydroxylation in man. *Br J Clin Pharmacol* 1990;30:761–767.
32. Williamson KM, Patterson JH, Pieper JA, et al. Effects of erythromycin or rifampin on steady-state losartan pharmacokinetics in healthy volunteers. *Clin Pharmacol Ther* 1997;61:202(abstr PIII-31).
33. Meadowcroft AM, Williamson KM, Patterson JH, et al. The effects of fluvastatin, a CYP2C9 inhibitor, on losartan pharmacokinetics in health volunteers. *Clin Pharmacol Ther* 1998;63:213(abstr PIII-23).
34. Kazierad DJ, Martin DE, Tenero D, et al. Fluconazole (F) significantly alters the pharmacokinetics (PK) of losartan (L) but not eprosartan (E). *Clin Pharmacol Ther* 1997;61:203(abstr).
35. Kaukonen KM, Olkkola KT, Neuvonen PJ. Fluconazole but not itraconazole decreases the metabolism of losartan. *Eur J Clin Pharmacol* 1998;53:445–449.
36. Goldberg MR, Lo MW, Deutsch PJ, et al. Phenobarbital minimally alters plasma concentrations of losartan and its active metabolite E-3174. *Clin Pharmacol Ther* 1996;59:268–274.

37. McCrea JB, Lo MW, Tomasko L, et al. Absence of a pharmacokinetic interaction between losartan and hydrochlorothiazide. *J Clin Pharmacol* 1995;35:1200–1206.

38. Shibouta Y, Inada Y, Ojima M, et al. Pharmacological profile of a highly potent and long-acting angiotensin II receptor antagonist, 2-ethoxy-1-[[2′-(1H-tetrazol-5-yl)biphenyl-4-yl]methyl]-1H-benzimidazole-7-carboxylic acid (CV-11974) and its prodrug, (±)-1-(cyclohexyloxycarbonyloxy)-ethyl 2-ethoxy-1-[[2′-1H-tetrazol-5-yl-biphenyl-4-yl]methyl]-1H-benzimidazole-7-carboxylatge (TCV-116). *J Pharmacol Exp Ther* 1993;266:114–120.

39. Kondo T, Yoshida K, Yoshimura Y, et al. Disposition of the new angiotensin II receptor antagonist candesartan cilexetil in rats and dogs. *Arzneim Forsch Drug Res* 1996;46:594–600.

40. Kondo T, Yoshida K, Yoshimura Y, et al. Characterization of conjugated metabolites of a new angiotensin II receptor antagonist, candesartan cilexetil, in rats by liquid chromatography/electrospray tandem mass spectrometry following chemical derivativization. *J Mass Spect* 1996;31:873–878.

41. Miyabayashi T, Okuda T. Motohashi M, et al. Quantitation of a new potent angiotensin II receptor antagonist, TCV-116, and its metabolites in human serum and urine. *J Chromatogr* 1996;677:123–132.

42. Jonkman JH, van Lier JJ, van Heiningen PN, et al. Pharmacokinetic drug interaction studies with candesartan cilexetil. *J Hum Hypertens* 1997;11[Suppl 2]:S31–S35.

43. Casas A, Merios M, Castaner J. Irbesartan. *Drugs Fut* 1997;22: 481–491.

44. Chando TJ, Everett DW, Kahle AD, et al. Biotransformation of irbesartan (SR 47436/BMS 186295) in man. 7th North American ISSX Meeting Oct. 20–24, San Diego, 1996, Abstract 322.

45. Perrier L, Bourrie M, Marti E, et al. In vitro N-glucuronidation of SR47436 (BMS 186295), a new AT1 nonpeptide angiotensin II receptor antagonist, by rat, monkey and human hepatic microsomal fractions. *J Pharmacol Exp Ther* 1994;271:91–99.

46. Csajka C, Buclin T, Brunner HR, et al. Pharmacokinetic-pharmacodynamic profile of angiotensin II receptor antagonists. *Clin Pharmacokinet* 1997;32:1–29.

47. Marino MP, Langenbacher KM, Ford NF, et al. Effect of hydrochlorothiazide on the pharmacokinetics and pharmacodynamics of the angiotensin II blocker irbesartan. *Clin Drug Invest* 1997;14: 383–391.

48. Merlos M, Casas A, Graul A, Castaner J. Eprosartan. *Drugs Fut* 1997; 22:1079–1085.

49. Martin DE, Tompson D, Boike SC, et al. Lack of effect of eprosartan on the single dose pharmacokinetics of orally administered digoxin in healthy male volunteers. *Br J Clin Pharmacol* 1997;43:661–664.

50. Weinstock J, Keenan RM, Samanen J, et al. 1-(carboxy-benzyl)imidazole-5-acrylic acids: potent and selective angiotensin II antagonists. *J Med Chem* 1991;34:1514–1517.

51. Martin DE, DeCherney S, Ilson BE, et al. Eprosartan, an angiotensin II receptor antagonist, does not affect the pharmacodynamics of glyburide in patients with type II diabetes mellitus. *J Clin Pharmacol* 1997;37:155–159.

52. Criscione L, de Gasparo M, Buhlmayer P, et al. Pharmacological profile of valsartan: a potent, orally active, nonpeptide antagonist of the angiotensin II AT1-receptor subtype. *Br J Pharmacol* 1993;110: 761–771.

53. Criscione L, Bradley WA, Buhlmayer P, et al. Valsartan: preclinical and clinical profile of an antihypertensive angiotensin-II antagonist. *Cardiovasc Drug Rev* 1995;13:230–250.

54. Schmidt EK, Antonin KH, Flesch G, Racine-Poon A. An interaction study with cimetidine and the new angiotensin II antagonist valsartan. *Eur J Clin Pharmacol* 1998;53:451–458.

55. The CONSENSUS Trial Study Group. Effects of enalapril on mortality in severe congestive heart failure. Results of the Cooperative North Scandinavian Enalapril Survival Study (CONSENSUS). *N Engl J Med* 1987;316:1429–1435.

56. The SOLVD Investigators. Effect of enalapril on survival in patients with reduced left ventricular ejection fractions and congestive heart failure. *N Engl J Med* 1991;325:293–302.

57. Cohn JN, Johnson G, Ziesche S, et al. A comparison of enalapril with hydralazine-isosorbide dinitrate in the treatment of chronic congestive heart failure. *N Engl J Med* 1991;325:303–310.

58. Oates JA. Antihypertensive agents and the drug therapy of hypertension. In: Hardman JG, Limbird LE, eds. *Goodman and Gilman's the pharmacological basis of therapeutics,* 9th ed. New York: McGraw-Hill, 1996:780–808.

59. Kelly JG, O'Malley K. Clinical pharmacokinetics of the newer ACE inhibitors. *Clin Pharmacokinet* 1990;19:177–196.

60. Jackson EK, Garrison JC. Renin and angiotensin. In: Hardman JG, Limbird LE, eds. *Goodman and Gilman's the pharmacological basis of therapeutics,* 9th ed. New York: McGraw-Hill, 1996:733–758.

61. Cushman DW, Cheung HS, Sabo EF, et al. Design of potent competitive inhibitors of angiotensin converting enzyme. Carboxylalkanoyl and mercaptoalkanoyl amino acids. *Biochemistry* 1977;16:5484–5491.

62. Petrillo EW Jr, Ondetti MA. Angiotensin-converting enzyme inhibitors: medicinal chemistry and biological actions. *Med Res Rev* 1982;2:1–41.

63. Ondetti MA. Structural relationships of angiotensin converting enzyme inhibitors to pharmacologic activity. *Circulation* 1988;77 [Suppl 1]:I74–I78.

64. Duchin KL, McKinstry DN, Cohen AI, et al. Pharmacokinetics of captopril in healthy subjects and in patients with cardiovascular diseases. *Clin Pharmacokinet* 1988;14:241–259.

65. Kripalani KJ, McKinstry DN, Singhvi SM, et al. Disposition of captopril in normal subjects. *Clin Pharmacol Ther* 1980;27:636–641.

66. Duchin KL, Singhvi SM, Willard DA, et al. Captopril kinetics. *Clin Pharmacol Ther* 1982;31:452–458.

67. Drummer OH, Workman BS, Miach PJ, et al. The pharmacokinetics of captopril and captopril disulfide conjugates in uraemic patients on maintenance dialysis: comparison with patients with normal renal function. *Eur J Clin Pharmacol* 1987;32:267–271.

68. Gomez HJ, Cirillo VJ, Irvin JD. Enalapril: a review of human pharmacology. *Drugs* 1985;30[Suppl 1]:13–24.

69. Ulm EH. Enalapril maleate (MK-421), a potent, nonsulfhydryl angiotensin-converting enzyme inhibitor: absorption, disposition, and metabolism in man. *Drug Metab Rev* 1983;14:99–110.

70. Till AE, Gomez HJ, Hichens M, et al. Pharmacokinetics of repeated oral doses of enalapril (MK-421) in normal volunteers. *Biopharm Drug Dispos* 1984;5:273–280.

71. Todd PA, Heel RC. Enalapril: a review of its pharmacodynamic and pharmacokinetic properties, and therapeutic use in hypertension and congestive heart failure. *Drugs* 1986;31:198–248.

72. Ulm EH, Hichens M, Gomez HJ, et al. Enalpril maleate and a lysine analogue (MK-521): disposition in man. *Br J Clin Pharmacol* 1982; 14:357–362.

73. Jackson EK. Diuretics. In: Hardman JG, Limbird LE, eds. *Goodman and Gilman's the pharmacological basis of therapeutics,* 9th ed. New York: McGraw-Hill, 1996:685–713.

74. Balfour JA, Goa KL. Benazepril. A review of its pharmacodynamic and pharmacokinetic properties, and therapeutic efficacy in hypertension and congestive heart failure. *Drugs* 1991;42:511–539.

75. Waldmeier F, Kaiser G, Ackermann R, et al. The disposition of [14C]-labelled benazepril HCl in normal adult volunteers after single and repeated oral dose. *Xenobiotica* 1991;21:251–261.

76. Wadworth AN, Brogden RN. Quinapril. A review of its pharmacological properties, and therapeutic efficacy in cardiovascular disorders. *Drugs* 1991;41:378–399.

77. Olson SC, Horvath AM, Michniewicz BM, et al. The clinical pharmacokinetics of quinapril. *Angiology* 1989;40:351–359.

78. Eckert HG, Badian MJ, Gantz D, et al. Pharmacokinetics and biotransformation of 2-(N-((S)-1-ethoxycarboxyl-3-phenylpropyl)-L-alanyl)-(1S,3S, 5S)-2-azabicyclo (3.3.0) octane-3-carboxylic acid (HOE 498) in rat, dog, and man. *Arzneimittel-Forschung* 1984;34:1435–1447.

79. Todd PA, Benfield P. Ramipril: a review of its pharmacological properties and therapeutic efficacy in cardiovascular disorders. *Drugs* 1990;39:110–135.

80. Lancaster SG, Todd PA. Lisinopril. A preliminary review of its pharmacodynamic and pharmacokinetic properties, and therapeutic use in hypertension and congestive heart failure. *Drugs* 1988;35:646–669.

81. Biollaz J, Schelling JL, Jacot Des Combes B, Brunner DB, et al. Enalapril maleate and a lysine analogue (MK-521) in normal volunteers: relationship between plasma drug levels and the renin angiotensin system. *Br J Clin Pharmacol* 1982;14:363–368.

82. Wagstaff AJ, Davis R, McTavish D. Fosinopril. A reappraisal of its pharmacology and therapeutic efficacy in essential hypertension. *Drugs* 1996;51:777–791.

83. Singhvi SM, Duchin KL, Morrison RA, et al. Disposition of fosinopril sodium in healthy subjects. *Br J Clin Pharmacol* 1988;25:9–15.

84. Edling O, Bao G, Feelisch, et al. Moexipril, a new angiotensin-converting enzyme (ACE) inhibitor: pharmacological characterization and comparison with enalapril. *J Pharmacol Exp Ther* 1995;275:854–863.

85. Univasc (moexipril hydrochloride tablets) Prescribing Information. Schwartz Pharma, Milwaukee, Wisconsin 53201, 1996.

86. Wiseman LR, McTavish D. Trandolapril. A review of its pharmacodynamic and pharmacokinetic properties, and therapeutic use in essential hypertension. *Drugs* 1994;48:71–90.

87. Conen H, Brunner HR. Pharmacologic profile of trandolapril, a new angiotensin-converting enzyme inhibitor. *Am Heart J* 1993;125:1525–1531.

88. Rahn KH. Clinical pharmacology of diuretics. *Clin Exp Hypertens* 1983;A5:157–166.

89. Maren TH, Meyer E, Wadsworth BC. Carbonic anhydrase inhibition. I. The pharmacology of Diamox 2-acetylamino-1,3,4-thiadiazole-5-sulfonamide. *Bull Johns Hopkins Hosp* 1954;95:199–243.

90. Brest AN, Moyer JH. Clinical pharmacology of diuretic drugs. *Am J Cardiol* 1966;17:626–630.

91. Cutler RE, Blair AD. Clinical pharmacokinetics of frusemide. *Clin Pharmacokinet* 1979;4:279–296.

92. Beermann B, Groschinsky-Grind M. Clinical pharmacokinetics of diuretics. *Clin Pharmacokinet* 1980;5:221–245.

93. Andreasen F, Mikkelsen E. Distribution, elimination, and effect of furosemide in normal subjects and in patients with heart failure. *Eur J Clin Pharmacol* 1977;12:15–22.

94. Beermann B, Dalen E, Lindstrom B, Rosen A. On the fate of furosemide in man. *Eur J Clin Pharmacol* 1975;9:57–61.

95. Andreasen F, Hansen HE, Mikkelsen E. Pharmacokinetics of furosemide in anephric patients and in normal subjects. *Eur J Clin Pharmacol* 1978;13:41–48.

96. Herzberg M, Fishel B, Wiener MH. Hepatic microsomal enzyme induction and its evaluation in a clinical laboratory. *Isr J Med Sci* 1977;13:471–476.

97. Klaassen CD, Fitzgerald TJ. Metabolism and biliary excretion of ethacrynic acid. *J Pharmacol Exp Ther* 1974;191:548–556.

98. Peters G, Roch-Ramel F, Peters-Haefeli L. Pharmacology of diuretics: a progress report, 1968–1971. *Adv Nephrol Necker Hosp* 1972;2:191–230.

99. Burg M, Green N. Effect of ethacrynic acid on the thick ascending limb of Henle's loop. *Kidney Int* 1973;4:301–308.

100. Lacreta FP, Brennan JM, Nash SL, et al. Pharmacokinetics and bioavailability study of ethacrynic acid as a modulator of drug resistance in patients with cancer. *J Pharmacol Exp Ther* 1994;270:1186–1191.

101. Friedel HA, Buckley MMT. Torasemide: a review of its pharmacological properties and therapeutic potential. *Drugs* 1991;41:81–103.

102. Blose JS, Adams KF, Patterson JH. Torsemide: a pyridine-sulfonylurea loop diuretic. *Ann Pharmacother* 1995;29:396–402.

103. Neugebauer G, Besenfelder E, Mollendorff EV. Pharmacokinetics and metabolism of torasemide in man. *Arzneim Forsch Drug Res* 1988;38:164–166.

104. Brater C. Pharmacokinetics and pharmacodynamics of torasemide in health and disease. *J Cardiovascular Pharmacol* 1993;22[Suppl 3]:S24–S31.

105. Miners JO, Rees DLP, Valente L, et al. Human hepatic cytochrome P450 2C9 catalyzes the rate-limiting pathway of torsemide metabolism. *J Pharmacol Exp Ther* 1995;272:1076–1081.

106. Kramer WG. Lack of effect of cimetidine on torsemide pharmacokinetics and pharmacodynamics in healthy subjects. In: Puschett JB, ed. *Diuretics IV: chemistry, pharmacology, and clinical applications.* Amsterdam: Elsevier 1993:361–364.

107. Abshagen U, Rennekamp H, Luszpinski G. Pharmacokinetics of spironolactone in man. *Naunyn-Schmiedeberg's Arch Pharmacol* 1976;296:37–45.

108. Taylor SA, Rawlins MD, Smith SE. Spironolactone—a weak enzyme inducer in man. *J Pharm Pharmacol* 1972;24:578–579.

109. Gerald MC, Feller DR. Stimulation of barbiturate metabolism by spironolactone in mice. *Arch Int Pharmacodyn Ther* 1970;187:120–124.

110. Huffman DH, Shoeman DW, Pentikainen P, et al. The effect of spironolactone on antipyrine metabolism in man. *Pharmacology* 1973;10:338–344.

111. Sadee W, Schroder R, Leitner E, et al. Multiple dose kinetics of spironolactone and canrenoate-potassium in cardiac and hepatic failure. *Eur J Clin Pharmacol* 1974;7:195–200.

112. Weiss P, Hersey RM, Dujovne CA, et al. The metabolism of amiloride hydrochloride in man. *Clin Pharmacol Ther* 1969;10:401–406.

113. Smith AJ, Smith RN. Kinetics and bioavailability of two formulations of amiloride in man. *Br J Pharmacol* 1973;48:646–649.

114. Brettell HR, Aikawa JK, Gordon GS. Studies with chlorothiazide tagged with radioactive carbon (C14) in human beings. *Arch Intern Med* 1960;106:57–63.

115. Beermann B, Groschinsky-Grind M, Rosen A. Absorption, metabolism, and excretion of hydrochlorothiazide. *Clin Pharmacol Ther* 1976;19:531–537.

116. Beermann B, Groschinsky-Grind M. Pharmacokinetics of hydrochlorothiazide in man. *Eur J Clin Pharmacol* 1977;12:297–303.

117. Yakatan GJ, Smith RB, Frome EL, et al. Pharmacokinetics of orally administered hydroflumethiazide in man. *J Clin Pharmacol* 1977;17:37–47.

118. Brors O, Jacobsen S, Arnesen E. Pharmacokinetics of a single oral dose of hydroflumethiazide in health and in cardiac failure. *Eur J Clin Pharmacol* 1978;14:29–37.

119. Cohen AI, Hinsvark ON, Sullivan DJ. Metabolism of 14C-metolazone, a new diuretic, in naïve and chronically treated dogs and monkeys. *Tox Appl Pharmacol* 1970;17:285(abstr).

120. Farthing D, Fakhry I, Gehr TWB, et al. Quantitation of metolazone in urine by high-performance liquid chromatography with fluorescence detection. *J Chromatogr* 1990;534:228–232.

CHAPTER 27

Cholesterol-Lowering Agents and Cardiac Glycosides

Yves Horsmans

Cholesterol-lowering agents and cardiac glycosides are widely used and are commonly prescribed on a long-term basis. Their potential interactions with other drugs deserve particular attention. For both groups, each class of drugs is reviewed and the potential mechanisms responsible for such interactions are highlighted.

CHOLESTEROL-LOWERING AGENTS

A variety of cholesterol lowering agents are used, including hydroxymethylglutaryl-coenzyme A (HMG-CoA) reductase inhibitors, bile acid–binding resins, nicotinic acid, fibric acid derivatives, probucol, and guar gum.

HMG-CoA Reductase Inhibitors

These drugs are specific competitive inhibitors of HMG-CoA reductase, which catalyzes the rate-limiting step in cholesterol biosynthesis (1). Their efficacy and their high level of patient acceptance and safety is greatly responsible for their success (2,3). However, such compounds may produce various side effects (e.g., myopathy), mostly occurring through drug–drug interaction.

The six HMG-CoA reductase inhibitors currently available include lovastatin, simvastatin, pravastatin, fluvastatin, atorvastatin, and cerivastatin. Drug interactions may occur through different mechanisms:

1. *At the level of digestive absorption:* The absorption of all HMG-CoA reductase inhibitors is reduced by the coadministration of a bile acid–binding resin or an antacid (4–6). This pharmacokinetic interaction

induces a 10% to 50% reduction in plasma concentration of the HMG-CoA reductase inhibitor (7). However, in case of antacid coadministration, such pharmacokinetic effect does not affect the impact of HMG-CoA reductase inhibitor on the plasma level of cholesterol-low density lipoproteins (c-LDL) (7–9). More importantly, the pharmacokinetic effect observed with the coadministration of a bile acid–binding resin on HMG-CoA reductase inhibitors is associated with a greater lowering effect on plasma c-LDL linked to the intrinsic properties of both drugs. This pharmacokinetic effect may be avoided by temporal dispersion of drug administration.

2. *At the level of hepatic blood flow:* Coadministration of propranolol reduced to 20% the area under the curve (AUC) of lovastatin (10,11) and pravastatin (11), whereas no effect was observed on simvastatin (12), fluvastatin (13), or atorvastatin (14) pharmacokinetic parameters. It has been suggested that such a phenomenon is linked to the lowering effect of propranolol on the hepatic blood flow, thereby increasing first pass extraction of these drugs. Such an effect is surprising, however, in view of the high hepatic extraction ratio of all HMG-CoA reductase inhibitors, except pravastatin. This illustrates the difficulties of the studies devoted to the effects on hepatic blood flow in absence of its direct determination. Nevertheless, this type of interaction does not lead to clinically important modification in the cholesterol-lowering effect of these HMG-CoA reductase inhibitors.

   Theoretically, all drugs that lower hepatic blood flow might exert a similar effect, that is, the capability to decrease oral bioavailability of lovastatin and pravastatin by increasing their first pass extraction.

Y. Horsmans: Department of Gastroenterology, Catholic University of Louvain and Cliniques Universitaires St. Luc, 10 Avenue Hippocrate, Brussels 1200 Belgium

3. *At the level of first pass metabolism:* Diclofenac and fluvastatin coadministration induces a transient change in pharmacokinetic parameters of both drugs (15). The oral clearance of diclofenac is reduced by ±15% but no data are given for fluvastatin. This interaction is thought to be related to the high clearance of both drugs, which could be responsible for an inhibition of the first pass metabolism of both drugs. However, these two drugs are also substrates of the same cytochrome P450 enzyme (CYP2C9), suggesting that a competitive inhibition between these drugs could also be responsible for this pharmacokinetic effect. Similarly, simvastatin and fluvastatin increase the bioavailability of glibenclamide by 20% when coadministered and this effect probably derives from an inhibition of the first pass metabolism of glibenclamide (15). This phenomenon does not, however, induce any clinically significant pharmacodynamic effect.

The importance of this mechanism deserves attention, but no other similar interaction between HMG-CoA reductase inhibitors and other drugs characterized by a high clearance has been described.

4. *At the level of plasma protein binding:* HMG-CoA reductase inhibitors exhibit a relatively high plasma protein binding (>95%), of which albumin is the most important, with the exception of pravastatin

TABLE 27-1. *Substrates, inducers, and inhibitors of CYP3A*

Main drugs metabolized by CYP3A family
Nifedipine, felodipine, nisoldipine, nimodipine, verapamil
Lovastatin, simvastatin, atorvastatin, cerivastatin
Cyclosporine, FK506 (tacrolimus)
Midazolam, triazolam, diazepam
Ethynyloestradiol
Erythromycin, clarithromycin, roxithromycin
Alfentanil
Digitoxin
Quinidine
Tamoxifen, taxol
Lidocaine
(R)-warfarin
Terfenadine, astemizole, loratidine
Cisapride
Indinavir, ritonavir, saquinavir
Carbamazepine
Dapsone
Omeprazole, lansoprazole
Amiodarone
Main CYP3A-inducing drugs
Phenylbutazone, rifampicin, carbamazepine
Barbiturates, phenytoin
Main CYP3A-inhibiting drugs
Cimetidine, quinidine, erythromycin, triacetyloleandomycin
Ketoconazole, itraconazole, miconazole
Propoxyphene

TABLE 27-2. *Substrates, inducers, and inhibitors of CYP2C9*

Main drugs metabolized by CYP2C9 enzyme
Diclofenac
Phenytoin
Piroxicam, tenoxicam
Tolbutamide
(S)-warfarin
Fluvastatin
Main CYP2C9-inducing drug
Rifampicin
Main CYP2C9-inhibiting drug
Sulfaphenazole

(±50%) (11,16). Theoretically, interactions could occur at this pharmacokinetic level, but no systematic study has been conducted to document this phenomenon. Nevertheless, this type of drug interaction is rarely of clinical significance because the displaced drug distributes rapidly in the tissues and a higher amount of free drug can be metabolized and eliminated.

5. *At the level of metabolism:* All HMG-CoA reductase inhibitors except pravastatin are metabolized by the CYP system. Lovastatin, simvastatin, atorvastatin, and cerivastatin are mainly metabolized by the CYP3A family, whereas fluvastatin is mainly metabolized by the CYP2C9 enzyme (8,16–18). Cerivastatin is also metabolized by the CYP2C8 enzyme (6). Pravastatin is mainly eliminated unchanged and phase II reactions are most important for pravastatin elimination (19) even though it has been hypothesized that pravastatin might also be a CYP3A substrate (20).

Theoretically, all CYP3A substrates and modulators (Table 27-1) may thus interact with lovastatin, simvastatin, atorvastatin, and cerivastatin metabolism, whereas all CYP2C9 substrates or modulators (Table 27-2) may interact with fluvastatin metabolism.

Role of P-glycoprotein

HMG-CoA reductase inhibitors are P-glycoprotein (P-gp) substrates (21,22). P-gp acts as a drug efflux pump and is expressed in high levels in several normal tissues (23). P-gp seems to reduce drug absorption in the small intestinal tissue and in hepatic canalicular membranes, and to enhance drug elimination in proximal renal tubules. This way, P-gp influences at least partially the degree of oral bioavailability of HMG-CoA reductase inhibitors. P-gp and CYP3A proteins are colocalized in enterocytes and hepatocytes, acting together to reduce the intracellular concentrations of their substrates. Moreover, the spectrum of drugs and substrates interacting with these two proteins is similar (24). Until recently, it was difficult to determine the relative influence of CYP3A or P-gp on any substrate and vice versa.

The existence of interactions between HMG-CoA reductase inhibitors and CYP or P-gp has been confirmed in *in vitro* studies (18,20). The *in vivo* interaction of HMG-CoA reductase inhibitors with cyclosporine, a potent CYP3A/P-gp substrate may lead to the most severe side effect of these drugs, that is, myopathy and rhabdomyolysis (12,16). This side effect may rarely occur without the coadministration of other drugs and its incidence is dose dependent (25–27).

Cyclosporine

Coadministration of lovastatin and simvastatin with cyclosporine not only changes the pharmacokinetic parameters of both drugs but is also responsible for a major increase in risk of myopathy and rhabdomyolysis (25,28–31). A three- to 20-fold increase in AUC values for lovastatin and simvastatin has been observed in such circumstances. Because lovastatin, simvastatin, and cyclosporine are CYP3A and P-gp substrates, this pharmacokinetic drug interaction might occur at these levels. Because atorvastatin and cerivastatin are also CYP3A substrates, clinically significant drug interactions can be anticipated when one of these two drugs is combined with cyclosporine. Consequently, patients given cyclosporine should receive markedly lower doses of HMG-CoA reductase inhibitors whose metabolism is CYP3A dependent and they should undergo close blood cyclosporine monitoring. In contrast, pravastatin and fluvastatin metabolism is not CYP3A dependent, even though they are P-gp substrates. As expected, pravastatin or fluvastatin and cyclosporine interaction is milder, inducing only a two- to five-fold increase in cyclosporine bioavailability (32–35). No case of myopathy has been described in the case of pravastatin or fluvastatin and cyclosporine coadministration.

Other CYP3A Substrates and Inhibitors

Among other substrates of CYP3A, some macrolide antibiotics and antifungal agents are known to be metabolized by these enzymes but they are also potent CYP3A inhibitors (see Table 27-1). They greatly increase plasma concentrations of lovastatin, simvastatin, and atorvastatin (16,25,36–38). Moreover, such interactions may be responsible for the occurrence of rhabdomyolysis (29,31). With regard to atorvastatin, the coadministration of erythromycin increases the steady-state concentration of the drug by 40% (8). Imidazole agents are also potent CYP3A inhibitors and exert major effects on pharmacokinetic parameters of lovastatin, simvastatin, cerivastatin, and atorvastatin as those observed with macrolides (6,36,37). Similarly, administration of grapefruit juice, a potent CYP3A inhibitor at the small intestinal level,

greatly increases serum concentrations of lovastatin and simvastatin (39).

With regard to other CYP3A substrates and the potential occurrence of drug interaction, no exhaustive *in vivo* study has been conducted (38). Packages of several HMG-CoA reductase inhibitors include a warning about the potential of these drugs to enhance plasma norethindrone and ethinylestradiol concentrations but the clinical impact of such effect seems limited.

The influence of long-term CYP3A inducer therapy (see Table 27-1) on the pharmacokinetics of HMG-CoA reductase inhibitors remains poorly studied. It has been demonstrated that the bioavailability of these HMG-CoA reductase inhibitors is greatly reduced during rifampicin administration (7,16). However, the potential pharmacodynamic impact of this interaction has not been studied.

In contrast, coadministration of cimetidine, the most powerful aspecific CYP inhibitor in clinical practice, only exerts a small effect on the pharmacokinetics of HMG-CoA reductase inhibitors (9,15).

Interactions With Warfarin

Interactions between warfarin (whose metabolism is stereoselective: (R)-warfarin being metabolized by CYP3A enzymes and (S)-warfarin by CYP2C9 enzyme) and lovastatin, simvastatin, or atorvastatin has been observed. Hypoprothrombinemia or bleeding as a result of these combinations has been observed during clinical trials (25,40–42) and in healthy subjects (12,43). The mechanism of this interaction remains unknown. Some authors favor the possibility of an interaction at the level of warfarin metabolism that enhances its hypoprothrombinemic activity (40,42). Interaction between pravastatin and warfarin is responsible for an increase in the AUC and C_{max} of warfarin without any effect on pravastatin pharmacokinetic parameters. However, this effect does not alter the hypoprothrombinemic activity of warfarin (44,45). Caution must be advocated with regard to this last affirmation in that Trenque and colleagues (46) have recently reported one case of interaction between pravastatin and warfarin being responsible for the occurrence of hematuria in a 64-year-old woman.

Fluvastatin

As previously described, fluvastatin metabolism differs from that of other HMG-CoA reductase inhibitors. *In vitro* studies have demonstrated possible interactions with CYP2C9 substrates (20). *In vivo* drug interactions may thus occur with other CYP2C9 substrates such as nonsteroidal antiinflammatory drugs (NSAIDs), phenytoin, tolbutamide, omeprazole, and (S)-warfarin (see Table 27-2). *In vivo* coadministration studies conducted with diclofenac, tolbutamide, omeprazole, and (S)-warfarin have demonstrated significant interactions (15) only with diclofenac and omeprazole. Appel and Dingemanse showed a mutual transient change in pharmacokinetic parameters of both fluvastatin and diclofenac when given together (15). In the case on fluvastatin and omeprazole coadministration (47), a significant increase in the C_{max} (50%) and AUC (33%) for fluvastatin was observed, with a 23% decrease in the plasma clearance of fluvastatin. All these studies emphasize the need for corroborating *in vitro* data with *in vivo* studies before drawing any definitive conclusions for clinical practice. It must also be emphasized that even *in vivo* studies performed on small groups of healthy subjects deserve attention. With regard to warfarin and fluvastatin coadministration, three cases of interaction between these drugs have recently been reported (48).

The influence of long-term CYP2C9 inducer therapy on the pharmacokinetics of fluvastatin remains poorly studied. The bioavailability of fluvastatin is significantly reduced with rifampicin administration (47). Once again, the potential pharmacodynamic impact of this interaction has not been studied.

Coadministration of cimetidine induces an 18% decrease in the plasma clearance of fluvastatin (15).

Digoxin

An interaction between HMG-CoA reductase inhibitors and digoxin has also been reported. Simvastatin (49) and atorvastatin (13) increase plasma digoxin concentrations by 20%, necessitating frequent therapeutic drug monitoring for digoxin. In contrast, lovastatin (50), pravastatin (51), cerivastatin (6), and fluvastatin (15) do not seem to exert any significant effect on plasma digoxin concentrations even when a slight increase in the C_{max} of digoxin is observed after fluvastatin administration (52). Conversely, pravastatin AUC is increased by digoxin administration (38) without inducing any significant clinical effect. The mechanism of this interaction remains unknown. It is, however, tempting to speculate that interaction between digoxin and several HMG-CoA reductase inhibitors might occur at the P-gp level.

Lipid-Lowering Agents

Besides these pharmacokinetic phenomena, potential interactions of HMG-CoA reductase inhibitors with other lipid-lowering agents must be emphasized. Such coadministration may be responsible for an increased risk of myopathy or rhabdomyolysis through an unknown mechanism. Myopathy is one of the most serious side effects observed at an incidence of ±0.1% when an HMG-CoA reductase inhibitor is administrated alone (5,53). Coadministration of lovastatin with nicotinic acid (54,55) or fibric acid derivatives (particularly, gemfibrozil) (56,57) has been associated with an increased occurrence of myopathy. The side effect has also been reported with the

coadministration of pravastatin and clofibrate (52). No case of myopathy using other combinations has been reported. Pravastatin and gemfibrozil coadministration results in an elevation in serum creatinine phosphokinase level, but no clinically significant adverse effects (58,59). Caution is needed when prescribing combination therapy because there are limited data.

Several hypotheses have been postulated to explain the interaction between cholesterol-lowering agents (60). First, nicotinic acid and fibric acid derivatives could modify the pharmacokinetic parameters of HMG-CoA reductase inhibitors as described previously in case of their coadministration with erythromycin or cyclosporine. However, this hypothesis has never been validated. Second, a drug-induced membrane-destabilizing effect has been postulated (61–63). Third, in cell culture, HMG-CoA reductase inhibitor–induced myotoxicity has been recently shown to be likely related to reduced posttranslational modification of specific regulatory proteins by geranylgeraniol, an intermediate metabolite in cholesterol biosynthesis pathway (64). Other phenomena, such as preexisting mild renal impairment, which may decrease fibrate elimination, could also be evoked.

Summary

HMG-CoA reductase inhibitors may interact with numerous drugs (Table 27-3). However, most of these interactions do not have a significant clinical impact on the efficacy of HMG-CoA reductase inhibitors to reduce c-LDL. In contrast, despite pharmacokinetic interactions with other cholesterol-lowering agents, these combinations are associated with a greater reducing effect on plasma c-LDL linked to the intrinsic properties of these agents. However, coadministration of HMG-CoA reductase inhibitor and fibrate or nicotinic acid increases the risk of myopathy or rhabdomyolysis. Such a risk may also occur through a modulation of CYP3A activity by CYP3A inhibitors or other CYP3A substrates (see Table 27-1) for lovastatin, simvastatin, atorvastatin, and cerivastatin.

Other clinically significant interactions are those observed with warfarin and digoxin. Concerning digoxin, this potential effect seems to be only observed with simvastatin and atorvastatin. Monitoring of prothrombin time or digoxin levels are thus necessary in these situations.

Bile Acid–Binding Resins

Cholestyramine and colestipol are anion-exchange resins that are not absorbed by the gut. They are thus nonsystemic agents and they only produce drug interactions by binding any negatively charged drugs or compounds present in the gut at the time of their administration.

The bioavailability of acidic drugs is reduced when they are administered concomitantly to resins. In con-

TABLE 27-3. *Drug–drug interactions with HMG-CoA reductase inhibitors*

Drug	Effect	Prevention
Interactions shown of clinical significance		
Nicotinic acid	Enhanced risk of myopathy	Avoid concomitant administration with lovastatin and simvastatin; caution is needed with other HMG-CoA reductase inhibitors.
Fibrates	Enhanced risk of myopathy	Avoid concomitant administration. If needed, monitor plasma CPK level.
Cyclosporine	Enhanced risk of myopathy	Avoid concomitant administration. Fluvastatin or pravastatin should be preferred. Serum cyclosporine and CPK levels must be regularly determined.
Erythromycin	Enhanced risk of myopathy	Avoid concomitant administration with lovastatin and simvastatin; caution is needed with atorvastatin and cerivastatin.
Grapefruit juice	Enhanced risk of myopathy	Avoid concomitant administration with lovastatin and simvastatin; caution is needed with other CYP3A-dependent HMG-CoA reductase inhibitors.
Warfarin	Risk of hypoprothrombinemia or bleeding	Monitor prothrombin time.
Digoxin	Increased serum digoxin concentrations	With simvastatin, and atorvastatin, decrease dose of digoxin by 20%. Monitor serum digoxin levels.
Interactions of minimal or unknown clinical significance		
Propranolol	Reduction of lovastatin and pravastatin AUC by ±20%	None.
Glibenclamide	Fluvastatin increases by ±20% glibenclamide bioavailability	Monitor blood glucose levels but such a potential effect seems weak.
Potential interactions, concern for the future		
Substrates of CYP3A and lovastatin, simvastatin, atorvastatin, or cerivastatin: interaction similar to that observed with cyclosporine should be assessed for all these drugs (see Table 27-1).		
Substrates of CYP2C9 and fluvastatin: potential interaction similar to those observed with glibenclamide.		

trast, differential timing of drug administration minimizes or avoids such problems. Therefore, such drugs should be administered 1 hour before or 4 hours after taking the resin.

Systematic studies about the possibility of binding of acidic drug to resin have not been performed. It has been reported that resin decreases the absorption of thyroxine (65), digitalis glycosides (66,67), coumarin anticoagulants, paracetamol (68), some thiazides (69), propranolol, tetracyclines (70), furosemide, nicotinic acid, clofibrate, gemfibrozil (71), and HMG-CoA reductase inhibitors (72,73).

Nicotinic Acid

Few drug interactions have been reported with nicotinic acid. Clonidine coadministration may inhibit skin vasodilation induced by nicotinic acid (74); similar observation was made when acetylsalicylic acid was given shortly before nicotinic acid ingestion (75). No interactions have been described with resins or other lipid-lowering agents.

Fibric Acid Derivatives

Fibric acid is the parent compound of clofibrate, gemfibrozil, bezafibrate, ciprofibrate, and fenofibrate. They are commonly used in primary or secondary dyslipidemia, which is mainly characterized by a high serum level of triglycerides.

Except for gemfibrozil, they are characterized by a high degree of gut absorption, a very high binding affinity to plasma albumin, an extensive hepatic metabolism, and a urinary excretion as glucuronide conjugates.

Clofibrate

Because of its high binding affinity to plasma proteins, especially albumin (96%), clofibrate may produce a displacement of drugs from albumin. This has been demonstrated with coumarin anticoagulants (76,77) and sulphonylurea compounds given in the treatment of diabetes mellitus (78,79). Such enhancement in hypoprothrombinemic and hypoglycemic effects has been observed in case reports. However, no study has been devoted specifically to these problems. Moreover, several authors have suggested that the potentiation of action of warfarin by clofibrate is not due to an effect at the albumin level but rather is linked to an increased receptor sensitivity (80,81). Similarly, clofibrate may exert other effects on glucose metabolism. It has been suggested that clofibrate might reduce insulin resistance by mechanisms unrelated to pharmacokinetic interaction (82).

Displacement from albumin by clofibrate has also been demonstrated with metformin (83), furosemide (84), and clometacin (85).

Theoretically, all drugs characterized by a high degree of albumin-bound affinity might be displaced by clofibrate coadministration, resulting in an increase in the unbound fraction of the drug and, potentially, in an enhanced clinical effect of such a drug. Practically, a close monitoring of prothrombin time and serum glucose level should be advocated in patients given these drugs and in whom a treatment with clofibrate is initiated. This monitoring must be performed until plasma concentrations of both drugs have attained a new steady-state.

In rats, clofibrate has been reported to produce endoplasmic reticulum hyperplasia and induction of CYP4A with potential changes in drug and endogenous metabolism (86). Such an effect has not been observed in humans.

In contrast, rifampicin and other inducing cytochrome P450 drugs increase the metabolism of clofibrate, reducing its serum concentration and, therefore, decreasing its therapeutic efficacy (87).

An intriguing interaction between clofibrate and probucol is characterized by a profound reduction (60%–70%) in serum cholesterol–high density lipoproteins (c-HDL), whereas clofibrate alone produces an increase in serum c-HDL. The mechanism of this paradoxical interaction remains poorly determined (88).

Glucuronidation is the main step of clofibric acid metabolism. This step is enhanced by oral contraceptives. It has been suggested that this induction may be of clinical significance in terms of dosing schedule and duration of action (89).

The hepatic conjugation of clofibric acid with glucuronide is reduced by probenecid use (90). Because probenecid also inhibits the renal tubular secretion of the glucuronides of clofibric acid, an increase in serum clofibrate concentrations is observed in case of coadministration of these drugs.

Gemfibrozil

As observed with clofibrate, gemfibrozil may be involved in the displacement of drug–protein binding. Such an effect has been demonstrated with coumarin anticoagulants (91,92). Moreover, the metabolism of warfarin might be inhibited by gemfibrozil, thus producing higher warfarin concentrations and leading to an increased risk of bleeding (93).

With regard to other highly albumin-bound drugs, it seems that the displacement produced by gemfibrozil is absent or minimal (94). Concerning antidiabetic drugs and in contrast to clofibrate, gemfibrozil may induce per se a hyperglycemic effect (95), which could necessitate an adjustment in the dosage of oral hypoglycemics or insulin. This could explain why only one case of hypo-

glycemia resulting from an interaction between gemfibrozil and an oral hypoglycemic drug (glyburide) has been observed (96).

The most important interaction with gemfibrozil is discussed in the section on HMG-CoA reductase inhibitors and the occurrence of myopathy. As observed with clofibrate, coadministration of gemfibrozil and probucol may induce a paradoxical decrease in c-HDL (88,97).

Fenofibrate, Bezafibrate, Ciprofibrate

Interaction between these three fibrates and other drugs has only been reported in small clinical studies or case reports.

Fenofibrate potentiates the effect of oral anticoagulants, and the dosage of these agents should be reduced by about one-third at the initiation of fenofibrate (98). However, only one case of adverse interaction between fenofibrate and oral anticoagulant has been reported; a reduction of one-third of fenofibrate dose was needed to return to the previous prothrombin-time values (99).

One study has been devoted to the interaction between bezafibrate and racemic phenprocoumon, showing that bezafibrate administration requires a reduction in the phenprocoumon dose (100). This phenomenon has been attributed to an enhanced response to the anticoagulant drug by increasing the affinity of the receptor site for coumarin or to the rate of degradation of the vitamin K–dependent clotting factors.

Studies in patients with diabetes have suggested that coadministration of fenofibrate or bezafibrate and oral antidiabetic drugs does not necessitate dose adjustment for both drugs (99–103).

No published data are available on the interaction of ciprofibrate with oral hypoglycemics.

Probucol

No adverse drug interactions have been reported with probucol. However, because probucol increases the QTc interval (104), it is advisable to avoid coadministration of probucol with other drugs susceptible to induce similar prolongation in QT interval, such as class I or III antiarrhythmic agents, tricyclic antidepressants, terfenadine, or astemizole.

A favorable influence of the interaction between probucol and resins has been demonstrated. This combination indeed reduces gastrointestinal symptoms (e.g., diarrhea, flatulence) observed when they are given alone.

Guar Gum

Guar gum is a dietary fiber that may slightly reduce serum total cholesterol. Its mechanism of action is thought to be similar to that of the bile acid–binding resins. Similarly to resins, it is not absorbed by the gut and it may affect the absorption of various drugs. Such an effect is related to the prolonged gastric time of transit induced by guar gum and to a reduced diffusion of drugs through guar gum. By these mechanisms, guar gum decreases the rate but not the extent of absorption of paracetamol (105), digoxin (106,107), and bumetanide (108). Not only the rate but also the extent of absorption of metformin is reduced (109). Nevertheless, all these interactions do not seem to induce a significant clinical effect.

CARDIAC GLYCOSIDES

Cardiac glycosides have been administered in the treatment of heart failure for more than 200 years. Their use remains particularly difficult with regard to their narrow therapeutic-toxic ratio. The difficulty is compounded by the potential drug interactions that may modify the pharmacokinetic parameters of glycosides.

The clinician must be aware of the pharmacokinetic parameters of cardiac glycosides to understand and to prevent potential drug interactions with these agents (110). The clinician must also be aware of potential drug interactions at the pharmacodynamic level.

Digoxin, the most prescribed cardiac glycoside, is absorbed in the gastrointestinal tract, is bound to proteins (±25%) and tissues, and is mainly excreted by glomerular filtration and filtration in the kidneys without being metabolized (111). Nevertheless, bacterial transformation of digoxin (=10%) may occur in the gut lumen by the action of *Eubacterium lentum* (112).

With regard to these pharmacokinetic parameters, drug interaction mainly occurs in the absorption phase, on the digoxin volume of distribution, and in the kidneys by modifying digoxin excretion. Recently, it was demonstrated that P-gp plays a key role in digoxin absorption and excretion (113,114). P-gp is a member of the adenosine triphosphate–binding cassette family of transporter proteins. It is found in the apical membranes of mucosal cells in the intestine, the bile canalicular membranes of hepatocytes, and the brush-border membranes of proximal tubules of the kidney (23). Inhibitors of P-gp function thus profoundly modify digoxin pharmacokinetic parameters by interacting with P-gp at different levels:

1. *At the absorption level:* Several drugs may increase or reduce digoxin absorption. Resins (115), neomycin (116), sulfasalazine (117), sucralfate (118), and antacids containing aluminum or magnesium compounds (119,120) decrease digoxin absorption and require a temporal dispersion of digoxin doses. For resins, this is a binding effect, but the mechanism of this interaction for the other agents remains poorly defined. A similar effect has been recently reported between digoxin and acarbose (121).

In contrast, erythromycin (122,123), roxithromycin (124), clarithromycin (125–127), omeprazole (128), lansoprazole (129), tetracyclines (122), rifampicin (130), and quinidine (131) increase digoxin absorption, and their concurrent administration necessitates a careful monitoring of serum digoxin levels. With regard to macrolides and tetracyclines, such an effect is at least partly linked to the modification in intestinal microorganisms induced by these antibiotics that reduce the transformation of digoxin into its inactive metabolite (122). Recently, it was shown that the effect of rifampicin and quinidine at this level is partially due to an action of these drugs on intestinal P-gp facilitating digoxin absorption (113,114,132,133). The same mechanism may account for the drug interaction of digoxin with other multiple drug resistance agents, such as verapamil and nifedipine. Such a possibility requires further investigation.

2. *At the volume of distribution level:* Several drugs may increase or reduce digoxin volume of distribution. Propafenone (134), quinidine (135,136), verapamil (137,138), amiodarone (139), captopril (140), diltiazem (141,142), nifedipine, and nitrendipine (143) may decrease digoxin volume of distribution. However, concerning captopril and dihydropyridine calcium antagonists, opposite results (i.e., an absence of effect) have been observed (144–147). Digoxin volume of distribution may be increased by thyroxine and albuterol (148) administration.

3. *At the excretion level:* Renal clearance of digoxin may be increased by concomitant administration of thyroxine and, conversely, renal clearance of digoxin may be reduced by concomitant administration of clarithromycin (149), propafenone (150), quinidine (151), verapamil (137,143), amiodarone (139), diltiazem (152), spironolactone (153), nifedipine, and nitrendipine (147,154).

Again, with diltiazem and dihydropyridine calcium antagonists, opposite results (i.e., an absence of effect) have been observed (155). The inhibiting effect of clarithromycin, quinidine, and verapamil on renal P-gp may be partly responsible for this phenomenon (156,157). It has also been suggested that captopril may induce similar effects on renal clearance of digoxin (140). However, there are contrary data on pharmacokinetic interactions between captopril and digoxin (144).

This effect is also indirectly observed when there is concomitant administration of digoxin and drugs that may alter renal function (i.e., aminoglycoside antibiotics, cyclosporine) (158). Such alteration would indirectly reduce digoxin clearance. With regard to cyclosporine, an effect on renal P-gp is also at least in part responsible for an interaction with digoxin (156,157). The same phenomenon could also be partly responsible for the interaction observed between digoxin and propafenone (159).

Itraconazole has also been shown to elevate serum digoxin levels in several case reports (160–162). Interaction at the level of P-gp or digoxin liver metabolism has been postulated (162).

An interaction between two HMG-CoA reductase inhibitors and digoxin has also been reported. Simvastatin (49) and atorvastatin (13) slightly increase plasma digoxin concentration.

In comparison to digoxin, digitoxin is nearly completely absorbed by the gut, is extensively bound to proteins (±97%), is metabolized by enzymes of the CYP3A family into several inactive and active substances, and is excreted in urine and bile. Pharmacokinetic interactions may thus also occur at the protein-binding level (e.g., with warfarin) and at the metabolism level. In contrast, the impact of renal function is less important than that produced on digoxin pharmacokinetic parameters. Cytochrome P450-inducing drugs such as rifampicin (163), barbiturates (164), phenytoin (165), and phenylbutazone (165) have been shown to greatly enhance digitoxin metabolism. Interaction with other CYP3A substrates has been demonstrated with verapamil, diltiazem, and amiodarone (137,166).

Interactions may also be observed at the pharmacodynamic level. Cardiac glycosides exert different actions,

TABLE 27-4. *Interactions of digoxin with other drugs classified by class, type of drug–drug interaction, and potential prevention*

Drug	Mechanisms	Prevention
Interactions shown of clinical significance		
Cardiovascular drugs		
Amiodarone	PK(1): Reduction in volume of distribution Reduction in elimination	Decrease dose of digoxin by 50% before amiodarone administration.
Propafenone	PK: Reduction in volume of distribution Reduction in renal excretion	Decrease dose of digoxin by 25% before propafenone administration.
Quinidine	PK: Increase in absorption Reduction in volume of distribution Reduction in renal excretion	Decrease dose of digoxin by 50%. Monitor serum digoxin level and ECG.
Flecanaide	PD(2): Electrophysiologic effects	Monitor ECG.
Disopyramide	PD: Electrophysiologic effects	Monitor ECG.
Verapamil	PK: Reduction in renal excretion Reduction in volume of distribution PD: Electrophysiologic effects	Decrease dose of digoxin by 50%.
Bepridil	PD: Electrophysiologic effects	Monitor ECG
β-blockers	PD: Reduction of cardiac contractile state Electrophysiologic effects	Monitor serum digoxin level and ECG
Reserpine	PD: Electrophysiologic effects	Monitor ECG
Catecholamines	PD: Increased automaticity	Monitor ECG
Antacids	PK: Decrease absorption by ±25%	Space drugs at least 2 hours apart
Resins	PK: Decrease absorption by ±25%	Space drugs at least 2 hours apart
Sulfasalazine	PK: Decrease absorption by ±25%	Space drugs at least 2 hours apart
Antimicrobial agents		
Rifampicin	PK: Reduction in absorption	Temporal dispersion of doses.
Neomycin	PK: Reduction in absorption	Temporal dispersion of doses.
Macrolides	PK: Enhancement in absorption	Monitor serum digoxin levels.
Tetracyclines	PK: Enhancement in absorption	Monitor serum digoxin levels.
Amphotericin B	PK: Reduction in renal excretion	Monitor serum digoxin levels.
Thyroxine	PK: Enhancement in volume of distribution Enhancement in renal excretion	Monitor serum digoxin levels.
Albuterol	PK: Enhancement in volume of distribution	Monitor serum digoxin levels.
HMG-CoA reductase inhibitors		
Simvastatin and atorvastatin	PK: Unknown	Decrease dose of digoxin by 20%. Monitor serum digoxin level.
Interactions of minimal or unknown clinical significance		
Diltiazem	Contradictory data (see text)	
Dihydropyridine drugs	Contradictory data (see text)	
Captopril	Contradictory data (see text)	
Spironolactone	PK: Reduction in renal excretion	Monitor serum digoxin level.
Itraconazole	Unknown	Monitor serum digoxin level.
Acarbose	PK: Decrease absorption	Temporal dispersion of doses.
Proton pump inhibitors		
Omeprazole and lansoprazole	PK: Increase absorption	Monitor serum digoxin level.

PK, pharmacokinetic mechanism; PD, pharmacodynamic mechanism; ECG, electrocardiogram.
Modification of serum potassium or calcium level increases the risk of digoxin toxicity.

among which an inhibition of NA+,K+-ATPase enzyme of cell membranes, a positive inotropic effect, a regulation of sympathetic nervous system activity, and various electrophysiologic actions. Pharmacodynamic drug interactions may be observed with drugs also possessing similar mechanisms of action.

Coadministration of β-adrenergic receptor antagonists (167), verapamil (137,138,143,146), diltiazem (137,141, 142), flecainide (168, 169), reserpine (170), disopyramide (171), or bepridil (172) may induce bradycardia by decreasing sinoatrial or atrioventricular junctional conduction or automaticity.

Drugs that provoke a hypokalemia, such as kaliuretic diuretics, corticosteroids, or amphotericin B (173,174), may increase automaticity, promote inhibition of NA+,K+-ATPase enzyme, and facilitate the development of digitalis toxicity. Modification of calcium stores by administration of parenteral calcium or diuretics may also provoke arrhythmias in patients with digitalis toxicity.

Both sympathomimetic drugs and cardiac glycosides may increase automaticity and cause ectopic pacemaker activity. Their concomitant use could thus increase the possible occurrence of cardiac arrhythmias. Sympathomimetics with β-receptor stimulant activity such as epinephrine and isoproterenol would be the most likely to produce this effect (175). Electrocardiogram monitoring must be performed to avoid the side effects.

Verapamil (176) and β-adrenergic receptor antagonists (167) might counteract the inotropic effect produced by cardiac glycosides. To avoid these interactions, the administration of calcium channel blocker or β-adrenergic receptor antagonists must be discontinued or their doses must be drastically reduced.

The pharmacokinetic parameters of digoxin and ditoxin and the risk of interaction between these drugs and other ones must be kept in mind to avoid manifestations of cardiac glycoside toxicity (Table 27-4). Such phenomena can be serious or fatal because these drugs may enhance cardiac automaticity and cause ventricular tachycardia or fibrillation. With regard to this potential toxicity linked to a narrow therapeutic-toxic ratio, it is imperative to monitor serum digoxin concentration.

REFERENCES

1. Endo A. The discovery and development of HMG-CoA reductase inhibitors. *J Lipid Res* 1992;33:1569–1582.
2. Expert Panel on Detection, Evaluation, and Treatment of High Blood Cholesterol in Adults. Summary of the second report of the National Cholesterol Education Program (NCEP). *JAMA* 1993;269:3015–3023.
3. Steiner A, Weisser B, Vetter W. A comparative review of the adverse effects of treatments for hyperlipidemia. *Drug Saf* 1991;6:118–130.
4. Pan HY, De Vault AR, Swites BJ, et al. Pharmacokinetics and pharmacodynamics of pravastatin alone and with cholestyramine in hypercholesterolemia. *Clin Pharmacol Ther* 1990;48:201–207.
5. Henwood JM, Heel RC. Lovastatin: a preliminary review of its pharmacodynamic properties and therapeutic use in hyperlipidemia. *Drugs* 1988;36:429–454.
6. Mück W. Rational assessment of the interaction profile of cerivastatin

7. supports its low propensity for drug interactions. *Drugs* 1998;56 [Suppl 1]:15–23.
7. Jokubaitis LA. Updated clinical safety experience with fluvastatin. *Am J Cardiol* 1994;2:18D–24D.
8. Lea AP, McTavish D. Atorvastatin: a review of its pharmacologically and therapeutic potential in the management of hyperlipidemias. *Drugs* 1997;53:828–847.
9. Mück W, Ritter W, Dietrich H, Frey R, Kuhlmann J. Influence of the antacid Maalox and the H2 antagonist cimetidine on the pharmacokinetics of cerivastatin. *Int J Clin Pharmacol Ther* 1997;35:261–264.
10. McKenney JM. Lovastatin: a new cholesterol-lowering agent. *Clin Pharm* 1988;7:21–36.
11. Pan HY, Triscari J, De Vault AR, et al. Pharmacokinetic interaction between propranolol and the HMG-CoA reductase inhibitors pravastatin and lovastatin. *Br J Clin Pharmacol* 1991;31:665–670.
12. Todd PA, Goa KL. Simvastatin: a review of its pharmacological properties and therapeutic potential in hypercholesterolemia. *Drugs* 1990; 40:583–607.
13. Blum CB. Comparison of properties of four inhibitors of 3-hydroxy-3-methyl-glutaryl-coenzyme A reductase. *Am J Cardiol* 1994;73: 3D–11D.
14. Warner-Lambert/Parke-Davis. Atorvastatin clinical product monograph, October 1996.
15. Appel S, Dingemanse J. Pharmacokinetic and pharmacodynamic interactions of fluvastatin and their therapeutic implications. *Rev Contemp Pharmacother* 1996;7:167–182.
16. Desager JP, Horsmans Y. Clinical pharmacokinetics of 3-hydroxy-3-methylglutaryl-coenzyme A reductase inhibitors. *Clin Pharmacokinet* 1996;5:348–371.
17. Wang RW, Kari PH, Lu AYH, Thomas PE, Guengerich FP, Vyas KP. Biotransformation of lovastatin-IV. Identification of cytochrome P450 3A proteins as the major enzymes responsible for the oxidative metabolism of lovastatin in rat and human liver microsomes. *Arch Biochem Biophys* 1991;290:355–361.
18. Boberg M, Angerbauer R, Fey P, et al. Metabolism of cerivastatin by human liver microsomes in vitro: characterization of primary metabolic pathways and of cytochrome P450 isozymes involved. *Drug Metab Dispos* 1997;25:321–331.
19. Everett DW, Chando TJ, Didonato GC, Singhvi SM, Pan HY, Weinstein SH. Biotransformation of pravastatin sodium in humans. *Drug Metab Dispos* 1991;19:740–748.
20. Transon C, Leemann T, Dayer P. In vitro comparative inhibition profiles of major human drug metabolising cytochrome P450 isozymes (CYP2C9, CYP2D6 and CYP3A4) by HMG-CoA reductase inhibitors. *Eur J Clin Pharmacol* 1996;50:209–215.
21. Dimitrakoulos J, Yeger H. HMG-CoA reductase mediates the biologic effects of retinoic acid on human neuroblastoma cells: lovastatin specifically targets p-glycoprotein expressing cells. *Nature Med* 1996;2:326–333.
22. Yamazaki M, Suzuki H, Sugiyama Y. Recent advances in carrier-mediated hepatic uptake and biliary excretion of xenobiotics. *Pharm Res* 1996;13:497–513.
23. Gottesman MM, Pastan I. Biochemistry of multidrug resistance mediated by the multidrug transporter. *Annu Rev Biochem* 1993;62: 385–427.
24. Wacher VJ, Wu CY, Benet LZ. Overlapping substrate specificities and tissue distribution of cytochrome P450 3A and P-glycoprotein:implications for drug delivery and activity in cancer chemotherapy. *Mol Carcinogen* 1995;13:129–134.
25. Tobert JA. Efficacy and long-term adverse effect pattern of lovastatin. *Am J Cardiol* 1988;62:28J–34J.
26. Berland Y, Vacher-Coponat H, Durand C, Baz M, Laugier R, Musso JL. Rhabdomyolysis with simvastatin use. *Nephron* 1991;57:365–366.
27. Rosenberg AD, Neuwirth MG, Kagen LJ, Singh K, Fischer HD, Bernstein RL. Intraoperative rhabdomyolysis in a patient receiving pravastatin, a 3-hydroxy-3-methylglutaryl coenzyme A (HMG CoA) reductase inhibitor. *Anesth Analg* 1995;81:1089–1091.
28. Arnadottir M, Eriksson L-O, Thyssell H, Karkas JB. Plasma concentration profiles of simvastatin 3-hydroxy-3-methyl-glutaryl-coenzyme A reductase inhibitory activity in kidney transplant recipients with and without ciclosporin. *Nephron* 1993;65:410–413.
29. Grunden JW, Fisher KA. Lovastatin-induced rhabdomyolysis possibly associated with clarithromycin and azithromycin. *Ann Pharmacother* 1997;31:859–863.

30. East C, Alivizatos PA, Grundy SM, Jones PH, Farmer JA. Rhabdomyolysis in patients receiving lovastatin after cardiac transplantation. *N Engl J Med* 1988;318:47–48(letter).

31. Meier C, Stey C, Brack T, Maggiorini M, Ritsi B, Krahenbuhl S. Rhabdomyolysis in patients treated with simvastatin and ciclosporin: role of hepatic cytochrome P450 system activity. *Schweiz Med Wochenschr* 1995;125:1342–1346.

32. Regazzi MB, Iacona I, Campana C, Gavazzi A, Vigano M, Perani G. Altered disposition of pravastatin following concomitant drug therapy with cyclosporin A in transplant recipients. *Transplant Proc* 1993;25: 2732–2734.

33. Goldberg RB, Roth D. A preliminary report of the safety and efficacy of fluvastatin for hypercholesterolemia in renal transplant recipients receiving cyclosporine. *Am J Cardiol* 1995;76:107A–109A.

34. Li PKT, Mak TWL, Wang AYM, et al. The interaction of fluvastatin and cyclosporin A in renal transplant patients. *Int J Clin Pharmacol Ther* 1995;33:246–248.

35. Olbricht C, Wanner C, Eisenhauer T, et al. Accumulation of lovastatin, but not pravastatin, in the blood of cyclosporine-treated kidney graft patients after multiple doses. *Clin Pharmacol Ther* 1997;62: 311–321.

36. Neuvonen PJ, Kantola T, Kivistö KT. Simvastatin but not pravastatin is very susceptible to interaction with the CYP3A4 inhibitor itraconazole. *Clin Pharmacol Ther* 1998;63:332–341.

37. Kantola T, Kivistö KT, Neuvonen P. Effect of itraconazole on the pharmacokinetics of atorvastatin. *Clin Pharmacol Ther* 1998;64:58–65.

38. Garnett W R. Interactions with hydroxymethylglutaryl-coenzyme A reductase inhibitors. *Am J Health Syst Pharm* 1995;52:1639–1645.

39. Lilja JJ, Kivistö KT, Neuvonen P. Grapefruit juice-simvastatin interaction: effect on serum concentrations of simvastatin, simvastatin acid, and HMG-CoA reductase inhibitors. *Clin Pharmacol Ther* 1998; 64:477–483.

40. Ahmad S. Lovastatin: warfarin interaction. *Arch Intern Med* 1990; 150:2407.

41. Tobert JA, Shear CL, Chremos AN, Mantell GE. Clinical experience with lovastatin. *Am J Cardiol* 1990;65:23F–26F.

42. Hoffman HS. The interaction of lovastatin and warfarin. *Conn Med* 1992;56:107(letter).

43. Pan HY. Clinical pharmacology of pravastatin, a selective inhibitor of HMG-CoA reductase. *Eur J Clin Pharmacol* 1991;40[Suppl I]: S15–S18.

44. Walker JF. Simvastatin: the clinical profile. *Am J Med* 1989;87[Suppl 4A]:44–46.

45. Catalano P. Pravastatin safety: an overview. In: Wood C, ed. *Lipid management:pravastatin and the differential pharmacology of HMG-CoA reductase inhibitors.* Royal Society of Medicine Round Table Series No 16. Oxford: Alden Press 1990;16:26–31.

46. Trenque T, Choisy H, Germain M-L. Pravastatin: interaction with oral anticoagulant? *BMJ* 1996;312:886.

47. Sandoz Pharmaceuticals. Lescol package insert. East Hanover, NJ, 1994.

48. Kline SS, Harrell CC. Potential warfarin–fluvastatin interaction. *Ann Pharmacother* 1997;31:790.

49. Merck. Zocor package insert. West Point, PA, July 1993.

50. Merck. Mevacor package insert. West Point, PA, November 1992.

51. Bristol-Myers Squibb. Pravachol package insert. Princeton, NJ, 1993.

52. Garnett WR, Venitz J, Wilkens R, Dimenna G. Pharmacokinetic effects of fluvastatin in patients chronically receiving digoxin. *Am J Med* 1994;96[Suppl 6A]:84–86.

53. Haria M, McTavish D. Pravastatin: a reappraisal of its pharmacological properties and therapeutic use in the management of coronary heart disease. *Drugs* 1997;53:299–336.

54. Reaven P, Witztum JL. Lovastatin, nicotinic acid, and rhabdomyolysis. *Ann Intern Med* 1988;109:597–598.

55. Norman DJ, Illingworth DR, Munson J, Hosenpud J. Myolysis and acute renal failure in heart-tranplant recipient receiving lovastatin. *N Engl J Med* 1988;318:46–47.

56. Pierce LR, Wysowski DK, Gross TP. Myopathy and rhabdomyolysis associated with lovastatin-gemfibrozil combination therapy. *JAMA* 1990;264:71–75.

57. Marais GE, Larson KK. Rhabdomyolysis and acute renal failure induced by combination lovastatin and gemfibrozil therapy. *Ann Intern Med* 1990;112:228–230.

58. Newman TJ, Kassler-Taub KB, Gelarden RT, et al. Safety of pravastatin in long-term clinical trials conducted in the United States. *J Drug Dev* 1990;3[Suppl 2]:275–281.

59. Wiklund O, Angelin B, Bergman M, et al. Pravastatin and gemfibrozil alone and in combination for the treatment of hypercholesterolemia. *Am J Med* 1993;94:13–20.

60. Smith PF, Eydelloth RS, Grossman SJ, et al. HMG-CoA reductase inhibitor-induced myopathy in the rat: cyclosporine A interaction and mechanism studies. *J Pharmacol Exp Ther* 1991;257:1225–1235.

61. Mastaglia FL. Adverse effects of drugs on muscles. *Drugs* 1982;24: 304–321.

62. Corpier CL, Jones PH, Suki WN, et al. Rhabdomyolysis and renal injury with lovastatin use: report of two cases in cardiac transplant recipients. *JAMA* 1988;260:239–241.

63. Masters BA, Palmoski MJ, Flint OP, Gregg RE, Wang-Iverson D, Durham SK. In vitro myotoxicity of the 3-hydroxy-3-methylglutaryl Coenzyme A reductase inhibitors, pravastatin, lovastatin, and simvastatin, using neonatal rat skeletal myocytes. *Toxicol Appl Pharmacol* 1995;131:163–174.

64. Flint OP, Masters BA, Gregg RE, Durham SK. HMG CoA reductase inhibitor induced myotoxicity: pravastatin and lovastatin inhibit the geranylgeranylation of low molecular weight proteins in neonatal rat muscle cell culture. *Toxicol Appl Pharmacol* 1997;145:99–110.

65. Northcutt RC, Stiel JN, Hollifield JW, Stant EG Jr. The influence of cholestyramine on thyroxin absorption. *JAMA* 1969;208:1857–1861.

66. Bazzano G, Bazzano GD. Digitalis intoxication: treatment with a new steroid-binding resin. *JAMA* 1972;220:828–830.

67. Caldwell JH, Bush CA, Greenberger NJ. Interruption of the enterohepatic circulation of digoxin by cholestyramine. *J Clin Invest* 1971; 50:2638–2644.

68. Dordoni B, Wilson RA, Thompson RPH, Williams R. Reduction of absorption of paracetamol by activated charcoal and cholestyramine: a possible therapeutic measure. *BMJ* 1973;3:86–87.

69. Hunninghake DB, King S, La Croix K. The effect of cholestyramine and colestipol on the absorption of hydrochlorothiazide. *Int J Clin Pharmacol, Ther Toxicol* 1982;20:151–154.

70. Kaufffman RE, Azarnoff DL. Effect of colestipol on gastrointestinal absorption of chlorothiazide in man. *Clin Pharmacol Ther* 1973;14: 886–890.

71. Forland SC, Feng Y, Cutler RE. Apparent reduced absorption of gemfibrozil when given with colestipol. *J Clin Pharmacol* 1990;30:29–32.

72. Richter WO, Jacob BG, Schwandt P. Interaction between fibre and lovastatin. *Lancet* 1991;338:706(letter).

73. Smith HT, Jokubaitis LA, Troendle A. Pharmacokinetics of fluvastatin and specific drug interactions. *Am J Hypertens* 1993;6: 375S–382S.

74. Sigroth K. Effect of clonidine on nicotinic acid flushing. *Lancet* 1974;2:58.

75. Olsson AG, Carlson LA, Anggard E, Ciabattioni G. Prostaglandin production augmented in the short term by nicotinic acid. *Lancet* 1983;2: 565–567.

76. Eastment R.D. Warfarin dosage influenced by clofibrate plus age. *Lancet* 1973;1:1450.

77. Solomon RB, Rosner F. Massive hemorrhage and death during treatment with clofibrate and warafarin. *N Y State J Med* 1973;73: 2002–2003.

78. Daubresse JC, Luyckx AS, Lefebvre PJ. Potentiation of hypoglycemic effect of sulfonylureas by clofibrate. Correspondence. *N Engl J Med* 1976;294:613.

79. Jain AK, Ryan JR, McMahon FG. Potentiation of hypoglycemic effect of sulfonylureas by clofibrate. Correspondence. *N Engl J Med* 1976;294:613.

80. Bjornsson TD, Meffin PJ, Swezey S, Blaschke TF. Clofibrate displaces warfarin from plasma proteins in man: an example of a pure displacement interaction. *J Pharmacol Exp Ther* 1979;210:316–321.

81. O'Reilly RA, Sahud MA, Robinson AJ. Studies on the interaction of warfarin and clofibrate in man. *Thromb Diath Haemorrh* 1972;37: 309–318.

82. Ferrari C, Romussu M, Bertazzone A, Testori GP, Grimaldi MG. Effect of short-term clofibrate on glucose metabolism and insulin secretion in patients with mild maturity-onset diabetes mellitus. *Biomedicine* 1978;29:133–136.

83. DeSilva SR, Betteridge DJ, Shawe JE, Cudworth AG, Alberti KG. Metformin and clofibrate in maturity-onset diabetes mellitus: advantages of combined treatment. *Diabetes Metab* 1979;5:223–229.

84. Odegaard OR. Drugs affecting lipid metabolism. In: *Meyler's side effects of drugs*, 11th ed. Amsterdam: Elsevier.

85. Zini R, Barre J, D'Athis P, Tillement JP. Bindings of clometacin to human serum albumin. Interactions with clofibrate, indomethacin, salicylic acid and warfarin. *Biochem Pharmacol* 1983;32:2909–2914.

86. Aoyama T, Hardwick JP, Imoka S, Funae Y, Gelboin HV, Gonzalez FJ. Clofibrate-inducible rat hepatic P450s IVA1 and IVA3 catalyze the w- and (w-1) hydroxylation of fatty acids and the w-hydroxylation of prostaglandins E1 and F2ol. *J Lipid Res* 1990;31:1477–1482.

87. Houin G, Tillement JP. Clofibrate and enzymatic induction in man. *Int J Clin Pharmacol Biopharm* 1978;16:150–154.

88. Yokoyama S, Yamamoto A, Kurasawa T. A little more information about aggravation of probucol-induced HDL-reduction by clofibrate. *Atherosclerosis* 1988;70:179–181(erratum 72, 240).

89. Miners JO, Robson RA, Birkett DJ. Gender and oral contraceptive steroids as determinants of drug glucuronidation: effects on clofibric acid elimination. *Br J Clin Pharmacol* 1984;18:240–243.

90. Veenendaal JR, Brooks PM, Meffin PJ, Ahmad S. Probenecid-clofibrate interaction. *Clin Pharmacol Ther* 1981;29:351–358.

91. McEvoy GK, McQuarrie GM (eds). Drug information 1986;86:472, American Society of Hospital Pharmacists, Bethesda, 1986.

92. Todd PA, Ward A. Gemfibrozil: a review of its pharmacodynamic and pharmacokinetic properties, and therapeutic use in dyslipidaemia. *Drugs* 1988;36:314–339.

93. Ahmad S. Gemfibrozil interaction with warfarin sodium (Coumadin). *Chest* 1990;98:1041–1042.

94. Hamberger C, Barre J, Zini R, Taiclet A, Houin, Tillement JP. In vitro binding study of gemfibrozil to human serum proteins and erythrocytes: interactions with other drugs. *Int J Clin Pharmacol Res* 1986;6:441–449.

95. Brown MS, Goldstein JL. Drugs used in the treatment of hyperlipoproteinemias. In: Gilman AG (ed). *Goodman and Gilman's the pharmacological basis of therapeutics*, 8th ed. New York: Pergamon, 1990:886–889.

96. Ahmad S. Gemfibrozil: interaction with glyburide. *South Med J* 1991;84:102(letter).

97. Klosiewitz-Latoszek L, Szostak WB. Comparative studies on the influence of different fibrates on serum lipoproteins endogenous hyperlipoproteinaemia. *Eur J Clin Pharmacol* 1991;40:33–41.

98. Harvengt C, Heller F, Desager JP. Hypolipidemic and hypouricemic action of fenofibrate in various types of hyperlipoproteinemias. *Artery* 1980;7:459–463.

99. Roberts WC. Safety of fenofibrate—US and worldwide experience. *Cardiology* 1989;76:169–179.

100. Zimmermann R, Ehlers W, Walter E, et al. The effect of bezafibrate on the fibrinolytic enzyme system and the drug interaction with racemic phenprocoumon. *Atherosclerosis* 1978;29:477–485.

101. Blane GF. Comparative toxicity and safety profile of fenofibrate and other fibric acid derivatives. *Am J Med* 1987;83[Suppl 5B]:26–36.

102. Brown WV, Dujovne CA, Farquhar JW, et al. Effects of fenofibrate on plasma lipids. Double-blind, multicenter study in patients with type IIA or IIB hyperlipidemia. *Arteriosclerosis* 1986;6:670–678.

103. Monk JP, Todd PA. Bezafibrate. A review of its pharmacodynamic and pharmacokinetic properties, and therapeutic use in hyperlipidemia. *Drugs* 1987;33:539–576.

104. Browne KF, Prystowsky EN, Heger JJ, Cerimele BJ, Fineberg N, Zipes DP. Prolongation of the QT interval induced by probucol: demonstration of a method for determining QT interval change induced by a drug. *Am Heart J* 1984;107:680–684.

105. Holt S, Heading RC, Carter DC, Prescott LF, Tothill P. Effect of gel fibre on gastric emptying and absorption of glucose and paracetamol. *Lancet* 1979;1:636–639.

106. Huupponen R, Seppala P, Iisalo E. Effects of guar gum, a fibre preparation on digoxin and penicillin absorption in man. *Eur J Clin Pharmacol* 1984;26:279–281.

107. Lembcke B, Hasler K, Kramer P, Caspary WF, Creutzfeldt W. Plasma digoxin concentrations during administration of dietary fibre (guar gum) in man. *Z Gastroenterol* 1982;20:164–167.

108. Lowe CH, Daneshmend TK, Hunter KR. The effect of guar on bumetanide-induced diuresis. *Br J Clin Pharmacol* 1985;20:544–545.

109. Gin H, Orgerie MB, Aubertin J. The influence of guar gum on absorption of metormin from the gut in healthy volunteers. *Horm Metab Res* 1989;21:81–83.

110. Magnani B, Malini PL. Cardiac glycosides. Drug interactions of clinical significance. *Drug Saf* 1995;12:97–109.

111. Koren G. Clinical pharmacokinetic significance of the renal tubular secretion of drugs. *Clin Pharmacokinet* 1988;15:165–179.

112. Saha J, Butler VP, Neu HC, Lindenbaum J. Digoxin-inactivating bacteria: identification in human gut flora. *Science* 1983;220:325–327.

113. Schinkel AH, Mayer U, Wagenaar E, et al. Normal viability and altered pharmacokinetics in mice lacking MDR1 type (drug transporting) P glycoproteins. *Proc Natl Acad Sci* 1997;94:4028–4033.

114. Schinkel AH, Wagenaar E, Vandeemter L, Mol-Caam, Borst P. Absence of the MDR1A P glycoprotein in mice affects tissue distribution and pharmacokinetics of dexamethasone, digoxin and cyclosporin A. *J Clin Invest* 1995;96:1698–1705.

115. Hall WH, Shapell SD, Doherty JE. Effect of cholestyramine on digoxin absorption and excretion in man. *Am J Cardiol* 1977;39:213–216.

116. Lindenbaum J, Maulitz RM, Butler VP Jr. Inhibition of digoxin absorption by neomycin. *Gastroenterology* 1976;71:399–404.

117. Juhl RP, Summers RW, Guillory JK, Blaug SM, Cheng FH, Brown DD. Effect of sulphasalazine on digoxin bioavailability. *Clin Pharmacol Ther* 1976;20:387–394.

118. Rey AM, Gums JG. Altered absorption of digoxin, sustained-release quinidine, and warfarin with sucralfate administration. *Ann Pharmacother* 1991;25:745–746.

119. Allen MD, Greenblatt DJ, Harmartz JS, Smith TW. Effect of magnesium-aluminum hydroxyde and kaolin-pectin on absorption of digoxin from tablets and capsules. *J Clin Pharmacol* 1981;21:26–30.

120. Gugler R, Allgayer H. Effects of antacids on the clinical pharmacokinetics of drugs. An update. *Clin Pharmacokinet* 1990;18:210–219.

121. Serrano JS, Jimenez CM, Serrano MI, Balboa B. A possible interaction of potential clinical interest between digoxin and acarbose. *Clin Pharmacol Ther* 1996;60:589–592.

122. Lindenbaum J, Rund DG, Butler VP Jr, Tse-Eng D, Saha JR. Inactivation of digoxin by the gut flora: reversal by antibiotic therapy. *N Engl J Med* 1981;305:789–794.

123. Maxwell DL, Gilmour-White SK, Hall MR. Digoxin toxicity due to interaction of digoxin with erythromycin. *BMJ* 1989;298:572.

124. Corallo CE, Rogers IR. Roxithromycin induced digoxin toxicity. *Med J Aust* 1996;165:433–434.

125. Midoneck SR, Etingin OR. Clarithromycin related toxic effects of digoxin. *N Engl J Med* 1995;333:1505(letter).

126. Guerriero SE, Ehrenpreis E, Gallagher KL. Two cases of clarithromycin induced digoxin toxicity. *Pharmacotherapy* 1997;17:1035–1037.

127. Nawarskas JJ, McCarthy DM, Spinler SA. Digoxin toxicity secondary to clarithromycin therapy. *Ann Pharmacother* 1997;31:864–866.

128. Oosterhuis B, Jonkman JH, Andersson T, Zuiderwijk PB, Jedena JN. Minor effect of omeprazole on the pharmacokinetics of digoxin after a single oral dose. *Br J Clin Pharmacol* 1991;32:569–572.

129. Andersson T. Pharmacokinetics, metabolism and interactions of acid pump inhibitors. Focus on omeprazole, lansoprazole and pantoprazole. *Clin Pharmacokinet* 1996;31:9–28.

130. Gault H, Longerich L, Dawe M, et al. Digoxin-rifampicin interaction. *Clin Pharmacol Ther* 1984;35:750–754.

131. Bigger JT, Strauss HC. Digitalis toxicity: drug interactions promoting toxicity and the management of toxicity. *Semin Drug Treat* 1972;2:147–177.

132. Su SF, Huang JD. Inhibition of the intestinal digoxin absorption and exsorption by quinidine. *Drug Metab Dispos* 1996;24:142–147.

133. Greiner B, von Richter O, Fritz P, et al. Pharmacokinetic interaction between digoxin and rifampin—the role of P-glycoprotein. *Arch Pharmacol* 1998;358[Suppl 2]:abstract 47.29.

134. Nolan PE Jr, Marcus FI, Erstad BL, Hoyer GL, Furman C, Kirsten EB. Effects of coadministration of propafenone on the pharmacokinetics of digoxin in healthy volunteer subjects. *J Clin Pharmacol* 1989;29:46–52.

135. Bigger JT, Leahey EB. Quinidine and digoxin: an important interaction. *Drugs* 1982;24:229–239.

136. Kuhlmann J, Dorhmann R, Marcin S. Effects of quinidine on pharmacokinetics and pharmacodynamics of digitoxin achieving steady-state conditions. *Clin Pharmacol Ther* 1986;39:288–294.

137. Kuhlmann J. Effects of verapamil, diltiazem and nifedine on plasma levels and renal excretion of digitoxin. *Clin Pharmacol Ther* 1985;38:667–673.

138. Klein OH, Lang R, Weiss E, et al. The influence of verapamil on serum digoxin concentration. *Circulation* 1982;65:998–1003.

139. Fenster PE, White Jr NW, Hanson CD. Pharmacokinetic evaluation of the digoxin-amiodarone interaction. *J Am Coll Cardiol* 1985;5:108–112.

140. Cleland JG, Dargie HJ, Pettigrow A, Gillen G, Robertson JI. The effects of captopril on serum digoxin and urinary urea and digoxin clearances in patients with congestive heart failure. *Am Heart J* 1986; 112:130–135.

141. Andrejak M, Hary L, Andrejak MT, Lesbre JP. Diltiazem increases steady-state digoxin levels in patients with cardiac disease. *J Clin Pharmacol* 1987;27:967–970.

142. Rameis H, Magometschnigg D, Ganzinger U. The diltiazem-digoxin interaction. *Clin Pharmacol Ther* 1984;36:183–189.

143. Belz GG, Doering W, Munkes R, Matthews J. Interaction between digoxin and calcium antagonists and antiarrhythmic drugs. *Clin Pharmacol Ther* 1983;33:410–417.

144. Miyakawa T, Shionoiri H, Takasaki I, Kobayashi K, Ishii M. The effect of captopril on pharmacokinetics of digoxin in patients with mild congestive heart failure. *J Cardiovasc Pharmacol* 1991;17:576–580.

145. Jones WM, Kern K, Rindone J, Mayersohn M, Bliss M, Goldman S. Digoxin-diltiazem interactions: a pharmacokinetic evaluation. *Eur J Clin Pharmacol* 1986;31:351–353.

146. Rodin S, Johnson BF, Wilson J, Ritchie P, Johnson J. Comparative effects of verapamil and isradipine upon steady-state digoxin kinetics. *Clin Pharmacol Ther* 1988;43:668–672.

147. Kirch W, Hutt HJ, Dylewicz P, Graf KJ, Ohnhaus EE. Dose dependence of nifedipine-digoxin interaction? *Clin Pharmacol Ther* 1986;39:35–39.

148. Edner M, Jogestrand T. Oral salbutamol decreases serum digoxin concentration. *Eur J Clin Pharmacol* 1990;38:195–197.

149. Wakasugi H, Yano I, Ito T, et al. Effect of clarithromycin on renal excretion of digoxin: interaction with P-glycoprotein. *Clin Pharmacol Ther* 1998;64:123–128.

150. Calvo MV, Martin-Suarez A, Martin-Luengo C, Avila C, Cascon M, Dominguez-Gil-Hurle A. Interaction between digoxin and propafenone. *Ther Drug Monit* 1989;11:10–15.

151. Fichtl B, Doering W. The quinidine-digoxin interaction in perspective. *Clin Pharmacokinet* 1983;8:137–154.

152. Yoshida A, Fujita M, Kurosawa N, et al. Effects of diltiazem on plasma level and urinary excretion of digoxin in healthy subjects. *Clin Pharmacol Ther* 1984;35:681–686.

153. Waldorff S, Andersen JD, Heeboll-Nielsen N, et al. Spironolactone-induced changes in digoxin kinetics. *Clin Pharmacol Ther* 1978;24:162–167.

154. Belz GG, Aust PE, Munkes R. Digoxin plasma concentrations and nifedipine. *Lancet* 1984;1:844.

155. Kuhlmann J. Effects of nifedipine and diltiazem on plasma levels and renal excretion of beta-acetyldigoxin. *Clin Pharmacol Ther* 1985;37:150–156.

156. Okamura N, Hirai M, Tanigawara Y, et al. Digoxin-cyclosporine A interaction: modulation of multidrug transporter P-glycoprotein in the kidney. *J Pharmacol Exp Ther* 1993;266:1614–1619.

157. de Lannoy IAM, Koren G, Klein J, Charuk J, Silverman M. Cyclosporin and quinidine inhibition of renal digoxin excretion: evidence for luminal secretion of digoxin. *Am J Physiol* 1992;263: F613–F622.

158. Dorian P, Strauss M, Cardella C, David T, East S, Ogilvie R. Digoxin-cyclosporine interaction: severe digitalis toxicity after cyclosporine treatment. *Clin Invest Med* 1988;11:108–112.

159. Woodland C, Verjee Z, Giesbrecht E, Koren G, Ito S. The digoxin propafenone interaction: characterization of a mechanism using renal tubular cell monolayers. *J Pharmacol Exp Ther* 1997;283:39–45.

160. Rex J. Itraconazole-digoxin interaction. *Ann Intern Med* 1992;116: 525(letter).

161. Kauffman CA, Bagnasco FA. Digoxin toxicity associated with itraconazole therapy. *Clin Infect Dis* 1992;15:886–887(letter).

162. Jalava KM, Partanen J, Neuvonen PJ. Itraconazole decreases renal clearance of digoxin. *Ther Drug Monit* 1997;19:609–613.

163. Poor DM, Self TH, Davis HL. Interaction of rifampin and digitoxin. *Arch Intern Med* 1983;143:599.

164. Jelliffe RW, Blankenhorn DH. Effect of phenobarbital on digitoxin metabolism. *Clin Res* 1966;14:160–164.

165. Solomon HM, Abrahams WB. Interactions between digitoxin and other drugs in man. *Am Heart J* 1971;83:277–280.

166. Läer S, Scholz H, Buschmann I, Thoenes M, Meinertz T. Digitoxin intoxication during concomitant use of amiodarone. *Eur J Clin Pharmacol* 1998;54:95–96.

167. Cruickshank JM, Prichard BNC, eds. *Beta-blockers in clinical practice*. New York: Churchill Livingstone, 1987.

168. Tjandramaga TB, Verbesselt A, Van Hecken A, Mullie A, De Schepper PJ. Oral digoxin pharmacokinetics during multiple-dose flecainide treatment. *Arch Int Pharmacodyn Ther* 1982;260:302–303.

169. Lewis GP, Holtzman JL. Interaction of flecainide with digoxin and propranolol. *Am J Cardiol* 1984;53:52B–57B.

170. Dick H. Reserpine-digitalis toxicity. *Arch Intern Med* 1962;109: 503–505.

171. Kelly RA, Smith TW. Pharmacological treatment of heart failure. In: *Goodman & Gilman's the pharmacological basis of therapeutics*, 9th ed. New York: McGraw-Hill, 1996:809–838.

172. Belz GG, Wistuba S, Matthews JH. Digoxin and bepridil: pharmacokinetic and pharmacodynamic interactions. *Clin Pharmacol Ther* 1986;39:65–71.

173. Miller RP, Bates JH. Amphotericin B toxicity. A follow-up report of 53 patients. *Ann Intern Med* 1969;71:1089–1093.

174. Fenster PE, Hager WD, Goodman MM. Digoxin-quinidine-spironolactone interaction. *Clin Pharmacol Ther* 1984;36:70–73.

175. Becker DJ, Nonkin PM, Bennet LD. Effects of isoproterenol on digitalis cardiotoxicity. *Am J Cardiol* 1962;10:242–247.

176. Schwartz JB, Keefe D, Kates RE, Kirsten E, Harrison DC. Acute and chronic pharmacodynamic interaction of verapamil and digoxin in atrial fibrillation. *Circulation* 1982;65:1163–1170.

CHAPTER 28

Antiarrhythmics

Martin F. Fromm and Michel Eichelbaum

Antiarrhythmic drugs are an excellent example of how detailed knowledge of metabolism and pharmacodynamic properties of parent compound and metabolites may help explain interindividual differences in pharmacokinetics and drug effects. Several factors influencing antiarrhythmic therapy must be considered for each individual antiarrhythmic drug. First, is the antiarrhythmic effect caused by the parent compound? If there are pharmacologically active metabolites, what is their antiarrhythmic potency relative to the parent compound and are plasma concentrations of the metabolites in a range to contribute significantly to the therapeutic efficacy in humans? Second, is the major route of elimination primarily renal or by metabolism? Third, are polymorphic enzymes (e.g., CYP2D6, CYP2C19) involved to a major extent in the metabolism of an antiarrhythmic and what are the consequences of the polymorphism for the pharmacokinetics and drug effects (see Chapter 8 and ref. 1)? Fourth, are cytochrome P450 enzymes involved in metabolism of the antiarrhythmic, which can be induced or inhibited by comedications (e.g., rifampin-mediated induction of CYP3A4)? Finally, is the antiarrhythmic administered as a racemate with the enantiomers differing in their pharmacokinetic and pharmacodynamic properties? All these determinants of disposition and effect of antiarrhythmic drugs have been studied and are discussed for each individual drug within this chapter.

AMIODARONE

Amiodarone is a lipophilic drug, which accumulates in adipose tissue, liver, and heart (2). Its pharmacokinetics are characterized by considerable interindividual variability and a very long terminal half-life (weeks to months). N-desethylamiodarone, which has been reported to be equipotent as a sodium channel blocker and less potent as a calcium channel antagonist (2), is the main metabolite of amiodarone in plasma and may therefore contribute to the antiarrhythmic effect of amiodarone. During long-term therapy, the plasma concentration ratio of amiodarone and N-desethylamiodarone is approximately 1:1 (3). Excretion of amiodarone occurs mainly in the bile, whereas urinary excretion of amiodarone and N-desethylamiodarone is negligible (4–7). In vitro experiments with human liver microsomes indicate that CYP3A is the major enzyme metabolizing amiodarone to N-desethylamiodarone (8,9). These in vitro findings are in agreement with results from a study in healthy volunteers. Phenytoin, which has been shown to induce CYP3A in cultures of human hepatocytes (10), decreased amiodarone serum concentrations and increased serum concentrations of N-desethylamiodarone (11), suggesting induction of CYP3A-mediated formation of N-desethylamiodarone by phenytoin.

APRINDINE

After a single oral dose of aprindine, 65% of the administered dose is excreted in urine and 35% is found in feces (12). N-desethylaprindine was the major metabolite found in plasma (13,14). It has been reported to have antiarrhythmic activity similar to that of the parent compound (13). Two hydroxylated metabolites of aprindine (HA$_1$, HA$_2$) are the major metabolites in urine (40% and 20% of an oral dose, respectively, mainly excreted as glucuronides), whereas only a small amount of the administered dose is found as parent compound (12). In vitro experiments showed that these hydroxylated metabolites are formed by the polymorphic CYP2D6 in human liver microsomes from extensive metabolizers, but not in

M. F. Fromm and M. Eichelbaum: Dr. Margarete Fischer-Bosch-Institute of Clinical Pharmacology, Auerbachstrasse 112, D-70376 Stuttgart, Germany

human liver microsomes from a poor metabolizer of sparteine/debrisoquine (15). The role of CYP2D6 in formation of the hydroxylated metabolites was confirmed *in vivo*. After administration of a single oral dose of aprindine to one extensive and one poor metabolizer of sparteine/debrisoquine, these metabolites were only detectable in urine of the extensive metabolizer (15). Because CYP2D6 plays a major role for elimination of aprindine, considerable differences in pharmacokinetics of this antiarrhythmic can be expected between extensive and poor metabolizers of sparteine/debrisoquine, which, however, have not been investigated in *in vivo* studies. Aprindine is no longer used in clinical practice because of its severe side effects. It can be speculated that the occurrence of side effects might be related to the patient's CYP2D6 genotype.

BRETYLIUM

More than 85% of intravenously administered bretylium is excreted unchanged in urine, indicating that this drug does not undergo significant hepatic metabolism (16). Thus, clearance of bretylium primarily depends on the patient's kidney function (17). There are no reports that metabolic drug interactions contribute to variable pharmacokinetics and pharmacodynamics of this antiarrhythmic.

DISOPYRAMIDE

Disopyramide, which is administered as a racemate, with S-disopyramide having the greater electrophysiologic potency compared to the R-enantiomer, is predominantly excreted unchanged in urine. Twenty percent of a given dose is eliminated by the kidneys as its active mono-*N*-dealkylated metabolite (18,19). Mono-*N*-dealkylated disopyramide has 20% to 25% of the potency in prolonging the refractory period in guinea pig atria compared to racemic disopyramide (20). Striking anticholinergic activity of this metabolite has been reported in comparison to the parent compound, suggesting that the anticholinergic side effects of disopyramide are mainly due to its metabolite (21,22). Ratios of plasma mono-*N*-dealkylated disopyramide and total (S- plus R-enantiomer) parent compound are between 0.34 and 1.21 and depend on kidney function and comedication (enzyme inducing drugs) (23). Enantioselective disopyramide mono-*N*-dealkylation has been characterized using human liver microsomes (24). Because the mono-*N*-dealkylation of disopyramide showed biphasic kinetics, probably two enzymes are involved in this reaction. Mean intrinsic clearance for the high-affinity site was about 30 times greater than that for the low-affinity site (25). The mean intrinsic clearance of the high-affinity component of S-disopyramide mono-*N*-dealkylation was signifi-

cantly greater than that for R-disopyramide, which is consistent with *in vivo* pharmacokinetic observations. Data point to a contribution of CYP3A4 to disopyramide mono-*N*-dealkylation, in that the CYP3A4-inhibitor erythromycin inhibited the high-affinity site of disopyramide mono-*N*-dealkylation with a K_i of 19.5 μM (25).

Potentially fatal interactions have been reported in patients undergoing treatment with disopyramide; these interactions included prolonged QTc intervals, ventricular tachycardias, and elevated disopyramide concentrations after coadministration of erythromycin or clarithromycin (26,27). Moreover, rifampin, phenytoin, and phenobarbital, which are inducers of CYP3A4, caused a marked decrease in disopyramide plasma concentrations in patients and healthy volunteers (28–30).

DOFETILIDE

Dofetilide is one of the newer class III antiarrhythmics. This drug has a bioavailability of about 80%. After oral and intravenous administration of ^{14}C-dofetilide, 75% of total radioactivity in plasma is represented by the parent compound. The major proportion of dofetilide is excreted unchanged in urine (about 60% of the administered dose with the total urinary excretion of radioactivity after oral and intravenous administration of ^{14}C-dofetilide being about 85% of the dose within 96 hours) (31). In urine, several metabolites, which were formed by *N*-oxidation or *N*-dealkylation of the tertiary nitrogen atom, were found after intravenous administration. None of these metabolites accounted for more than 3% of total radioactivity in urine. The metabolites of dofetilide are unlikely to contribute significantly to its pharmacologic activity, because their class III activity is 20-fold less than that of the parent compound, only dofetilide *N*-oxide has marginal class I activity (32), and plasma concentrations of the metabolite are small in comparison to the parent compound. Formation of one of the major metabolites (*N*-desmethyldofetilide) is catalyzed by CYP3A4 (32). Because of the pharmacokinetic characteristics of the parent compound and its metabolite, it is unlikely that metabolic drug interactions resulting from induction or inhibition of CYP3A4 will have profound influence on the pharmacokinetics of dofetilide.

ENCAINIDE

Although the sodium channel blocker encainide is no longer marketed, it is an excellent example of a racemate (with its enantiomers having similar electrophysiologic properties) whose biotransformation to multiple potent metabolites is dependent on the CYP2D6 polymorphism. After oral administration, its bioavailability is low (30%) in extensive metabolizers of sparteine/debrisoquine as a result of presystemic elimination. In contrast, poor metabolizers have an almost complete bioavailability (83%) (33). Formation of the major metabolites of encainide in plasma and urine, O-desmethylencainide (ODE), and its subsequent metabolite 3-methoxy-O-desmethylencainide (MODE) is catalyzed by CYP2D6 (33–35). Urinary excretion of ODE and MODE was considerably reduced in poor metabolizers in comparison to extensive metabolizers (ODE: 3% versus 11% after intravenous administration; MODE: not detectable versus 4%), whereas poor metabolizers excreted significantly more unchanged encainide and N-desmethylencainide in urine (encainide: 39% versus 5%; and N-desmethylencainide: 2% versus not detectable) (33). In extensive metabolizers, serum concentrations of ODE and MODE are about four-fold higher during steady-state conditions than serum concentrations of encainide (33). In contrast, area under the serum-concentration time curve (AUC) of encainide is at least 20-fold larger than AUC of ODE and MODE in poor metabolizers. The sodium channel blocking activity of encainide is less than that of ODE (about one-tenth) and similar to that of MODE (36,37). Because formation of ODE and MODE is catalyzed by CYP2D6 (33–35), QRS interval prolongation is more pronounced in extensive metabolizers in comparison to poor metabolizers (33,38). Consequences of these differences for therapeutic effects and side effects remain unclear, although some data indicate an increased risk of proarrhythmic events in extensive metabolizers with equal therapeutic efficacy in both phenotypes (39). As might be anticipated, the CYP2D6 inhibitor quinidine exerts a striking effect on pharmacokinetics of encainide. Coadministration of quinidine considerably reduces nonrenal clearance of encainide in extensive metabolizers of sparteine/debrisoquine, whereas no alterations were found in poor metabolizers (40,41).

FLECAINIDE

Flecainide is marketed as a racemic mixture of S- and R-flecainide. Both enantiomers have similar electrophysiologic properties (42,43). During steady-state, a considerable fraction (CYP2D6 extensive metabolizers: 36%; CYP2D6 poor metabolizers: 46%) of the administered dose is excreted as unchanged flecainide (44). In addition to renal excretion of the parent compound, which depends on urine flow and pH, CYP2D6 genotype influences the pharmacokinetics of flecainide after administration of a single oral dose. The two major metabolites found in urine are meta-O-dealkylated flecainide (MODF) and its lactam (MODLF), which have little pharmacologic activity (45,46). After administration of a single oral dose, poor metabolizers had a higher AUC of flecainide and excreted significantly more unchanged flecainide in the urine in comparison to extensive metabolizers (55% versus 32%) (47–49). Moreover, urinary excretion of MODF and MODLF was lower in poor metabolizers compared to

extensive metabolizers (MODF: 11% versus 17% of the administered dose; MODLF: 8% versus 15%) (47,48). These data indicate that CYP2D6 activity influences the pharmacokinetics of flecainide after administration of a single dose. The lower recovery, but not the total absence of flecainide metabolites indicates the involvement of enzymes other than CYP2D6 in formation of MODF and MODLF.

During steady-state conditions, the differences in flecainide plasma pharmacokinetics between extensive and poor metabolizers had a similar trend as reported in the single dose studies, but were statistically not significant (44). Mean steady-state concentrations and QRS interval prolongation were not different between both phenotypes, but nonlinear pharmacokinetics and a shortened half-life were observed in extensive metabolizers. However, poor metabolizers with renal failure are likely to be of greater risk attaining higher flecainide concentrations and hence adverse reactions (50,51). Similar to the observations with encainide, coadministration of quinidine and flecainide resulted in a reduced oral clearance of R-flecainide and a decreased formation of the two major metabolites in extensive metabolizers of sparteine/debrisoquine on chronic flecainide therapy, but had no effect in one poor metabolizer (52).

The use of antiarrhythmics in therapy of cardiac arrhythmias has considerably changed since the publication of the results of the Cardiac Arrhythmia Suppression Trial (CAST) (53). As a result of the increased mortality rate in patients given encainide or flecainide after a myocardial infarction in comparison to placebo, there has been speculation whether CYP2D6 phenotype might be a factor predisposing to therapeutic outcome. Although this question could not be clearly answered, data indicate no excess of drug effect (determined by QRS or QT intervals) in patients who died during therapy (39,53,54). Moreover, the continuous increase in mortality rate during the course of the study argues against a major role of reduced drug metabolism in poor metabolizers, because higher drug concentrations and an increased risk of toxicity would be expected primarily in the early phase of the trial. Rather, a pharmacodynamic explanation seems more likely, for example, presence of a drug in combination with other factors such as transient coronary ischemia, which may have caused fatal arrhythmias in susceptible patients.

LIDOCAINE

Lidocaine is a local anaesthetic that is also used for acute intravenous treatment of ventricular arrhythmias. After oral administration, it undergoes extensive and variable first pass metabolism. Its major metabolites in plasma are mono- and di-N-desethylated compounds. The plasma ratios of monoethylglycinexylidide (MEGX) and lidocaine and of glycinexylidide (GX) and lidocaine are approximately 0.3 and 0.1, respectively (55,56). In different arrhythmia models, antiarrhythmic potency of MEGX was 0.8 to 1.0 of the parent compound (57–59). The relative potency of GX in relation to lidocaine was 0.10 to 0.26 (22,57,58). Moreover, GX actually reversed the sodium channel block produced by lidocaine under certain *in vitro* conditions (60). Formation of MEGX from lidocaine, which is the first step of the major metabolic pathway of lidocaine elimination (ultimately resulting in formation of conjugated 4-hydroxy-2,6-dimethylaniline, which is the major metabolite in urine) (61), is catalyzed primarily by CYP3A4 (62,63). This was shown with human liver microsomes using inhibitory CYP3A antibodies (Fig. 28-1), correlation of CYP3A content and lidocaine-*N*-deethylation activity, and expression of CYP3A4 cDNA in HepG2 cells (62,63). Little is known about the influence of inducers or inhibitors of CYP3A on pharmacokinetics of lidocaine in humans. Rifampin, the potent inducer of intestinal and hepatic CYP3A4, caused a considerable increase in the CYP3A-mediated formation of MEGX in cultured human hepatocytes (64). However, this interaction has limited clinical relevance, because lidocaine is a high clearance drug and is only intravenously administered. A moderate decrease in systemic clearance of lidocaine (−20%) with a decrease in plasma concentrations of its metabolite MEGX was observed when amiodarone was coadministered (65). According to *in vitro* experiments with human liver microsomes, this interaction was attributed, at least in part, to inhibition of CYP3A4-mediated formation of

MEGX by amiodarone and possibly by its metabolite *N*-desethylamiodarone (65). Reduction in the systemic lidocaine clearance is also expected with concomitant administration of potent CYP3A4 inhibitors such as ketoconazole, erythromycin, and ritonavir.

MEXILETINE

Mexiletine is used as a racemate with the enantiomers of mexiletine differing about two-fold in their affinities for sodium channels and exhibiting different antiarrhythmic properties in an animal model (66,67). Minor stereoselectivity in the disposition of mexiletine is observed with preferential metabolism of the R-enantiomer (68,69). Mexiletine is extensively metabolized in humans, with about 10% of a given dose excreted unchanged in urine (70,71). The major metabolites found in urine of extensive metabolizers of sparteine/debrisoquine are *N*-hydroxymexiletine (14% of the administered dose), hydroxymethylmexiletine (9%), *p*-hydroxymexiletine (5%), and *m*-hydroxymexiletine (2%) (70), none of which have relevant pharmacologic activities (71). *In vitro* experiments with human liver microsomes using either quinidine or substrates of CYP2D6 as inhibitors of CYP2D6 and the use of inhibitory CYP2D6 antibodies (anti-LKM1) showed that CYP2D6 plays an important role in formation of hydroxymethylmexiletine and *p*-hydroxymexiletine (72,73). These findings were confirmed by *in vivo* studies. First, clearance of mexiletine is about two-fold higher in extensive metabolizers of sparteine/debrisoquine in comparison to poor metabolizers (69,70,74). A higher incidence of adverse reactions such as nausea and light headedness has been reported for poor metabolizers compared to extensive metabolizers (74). Second, metabolic clearance to hydroxymethylmexiletine, *p*-hydroxymexiletine (in accordance with the *in vitro* findings described above), and *m*-hydroxymexiletine is significantly lower in poor metabolizers in comparison to extensive metabolizers (70). Finally, coadministration of the CYP2D6 inhibitor quinidine and mexiletine significantly decreased the oral clearance of mexiletine in extensive metabolizers, but did not have any effect on mexiletine pharmacokinetics in poor metabolizers (Fig. 28-2). In addition, urinary excretion of three metabolites (hydroxymethylmexiletine, *p*-hydroxymexiletine, *m*-hydroxymexiletine) was reduced by quinidine in extensive metabolizers of sparteine/debrisoquine (70,75). Several studies suggest that a combination therapy of mexiletine and quinidine is a very effective antiarrhythmic combination (76,77). A part of the increased therapeutic efficacy in comparison to monotherapy could be due to the pharmacokinetic interaction described earlier, which results in increased mexiletine plasma concentrations.

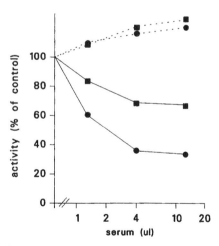

FIG. 28-1. Dose-dependent inhibition of lidocaine deethylation in human liver microsomes with polyclonal rabbit antiserum against human CYP3A4 (*solid lines*) or a preimmune serum (*broken lines*) using two different liver preparations (*squares, circles*). From Bargetzi MJ, Aoyama T, Gonzalez FJ, Meyer UA. Lidocaine metabolism in human liver microsomes by cytochrome P450IIIA4. *Clin Pharmacol Ther* 1989;46:521–527, with permission.

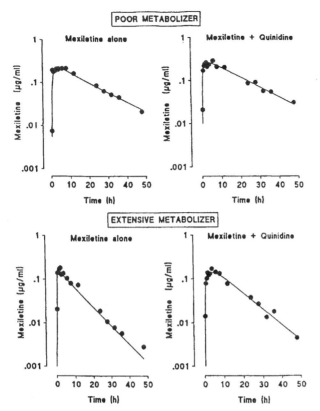

FIG. 28-2. Plasma concentration–time curves after administration of a single oral dose of mexiletine to one poor metabolizer (PM) (*upper panels*) and one extensive metabolizer (EM) of sparteine/debrisoquine without (*left panels*) and with (*right panels*) coadministration of quinidine. Mean apparent oral clearance of mexiletine of all subjects: PM (no quinidine)— 315 mL/min; PM (with quinidine)—314 mL/min; EM (no quinidine)—621 mL/min; EM (with quinidine)—471 mL/min. From Turgeon J, Fiset C, Giguere R, et al. Influence of debrisoquine phenotype and of quinidine on mexiletine disposition in man. *J Pharmacol Exp Ther* 1991;259:789–798, with permission.

N-PROPYLAJMALINE

Another substrate of CYP2D6 is *N*-propylajmaline (NPAB) (78). Mean apparent oral clearance and terminal half-life showed eight-fold and six-fold differences between extensive and poor metabolizers. Thus, it is not surprising that 30-fold differences in plasma concentrations were observed in patients given a fixed dose of 60 mg/day (79). After intravenous administration of ^{14}C-labeled *N*-propylajmaline, about 66% of the radioactivity in plasma results from the parent compound (80). In extensive metabolizers, about one-third of an oral dose is excreted as unchanged parent compound and another 30% as its monohydroxylated metabolite M1 (80). In contrast, poor metabolizers excrete 70% of an oral dose as parent compound, whereas only a very small amount (2%) of M1 is detectable in urine.

In a prospective study, the metabolic ratio of sparteine was used to select the appropriate dose to reach steady-state concentrations, which are required for effective antiarrhythmic treatment. One poor metabolizer required only a daily dose of 7 mg, in contrast to an extensive metabolizer, who was given 110 mg daily (51,81). Moreover, sufficient arrhythmia suppression was clearly correlated to *N*-propylajmaline steady-state plasma concentrations (81).

PROCAINAMIDE

Between 50% and 70% of procainamide is eliminated unchanged in urine (16). The major metabolite of procainamide in plasma and urine is the pharmacologically active *N*-acetylprocainamide. The formation of this metabolite is catalyzed by the polymorphic *N*-acetyltransferase (NAT 2). The ratio of plasma concentrations of *N*-acetylprocainamide and procainamide depends on the acetylator phenotype; means are 1.8 and 0.6 in rapid and slow metabolizers, respectively (82). This difference is of clinical interest, because procainamide and *N*-acetylprocainamide have different antiarrhythmic, electrophysiologic, and toxic properties (1,39). Whereas procainamide is primarily a sodium channel blocker, *N*-acetylprocainamide has no effect on sodium channels, but markedly prolongs action potential duration (83). This is in accordance with the fact that *N*-acetylprocainamide is primarily responsible for most of the QT interval prolongation observed after therapy with procainamide (84). Moreover, torsades de pointes in patients given procainamide is likely to occur mainly by elevated plasma concentrations of *N*-acetylprocainamide resulting from rapid acetylator phenotype or renal insufficiency (85).

The development of antinuclear antibodies and the procainamide-induced lupus erythematosus syndrome occurs more rapidly in slow acetylators compared to fast acetylators (86,87). It has recently been shown by *in vitro* studies that formation of another metabolite of procainamide (*N*-hydroxyprocainamide) is primarily catalyzed by CYP2D6 (88). Because this is the metabolite implicated in immunotoxicity after administration of procainamide and because this metabolite would not be formed in poor metabolizers of sparteine/debrisoquine, this finding could explain why procainamide-induced lupus erythematosus syndrome does not develop in all slow acetylators.

PROPAFENONE

Propafenone, which is marketed as a racemic mixture of S- and R-propafenone, is extensively metabolized in humans, and formation of major active metabolite 5-hydroxypropafenone is catalyzed by CYP2D6 (89–91).

Substantially higher drug concentrations of the parent compound are observed in poor metabolizers and are associated with a considerably higher risk of central nervous side effects in poor metabolizers (67% versus 14%) (89). Several aspects have to be considered in patients undergoing treatment with propafenone. First, in extensive metabolizers, nonlinear pharmacokinetics of propafenone have been observed with increased dosage, which has been attributed to saturation of CYP2D6-mediated first pass metabolism (89). Second, like several other antiarrhythmics, propafenone is administered as a racemate with its enantiomers differing in their pharmacokinetic and pharmacodynamic properties (92). Whereas both enantiomers of propafenone have the same potency as a sodium channel blocker, the S-enantiomer is a β-adrenoceptor antagonist, which on a molecular basis has 2% to 5% of the β-blocking activity of propranolol. Indeed, β-blockade after administration of propafenone was observed in both phenotypes, but it was more pronounced in the poor metabolizers (93). Because much higher plasma concentrations of S-propafenone are observed in poor metabolizers, the increased rate of central nervous side effects in this subset of patients might be due to a considerable β-blockade caused by S-propafenone. Finally, *in vitro* and *in vivo* data clearly showed that first pass metabolism of propafenone is altered as a result of an enantiomer–enantiomer interaction, thereby modifying β-blocking effects of racemic propafenone (94,95).

As mentioned earlier, *in vivo* and *in vitro* data obtained from human liver microsomes clearly indicate that CYP2D6 catalyzes the formation of 5-hydroxypropa-

fenone (Fig. 28-3) (89,90). The formation of *N*-desalkylpropafenone, which is a minor metabolite, is catalyzed by CYP3A4 and CYP1A2 (96). *In vitro*, 5-hydroxypropafenone is as potent a sodium channel blocker as propafenone, whereas *N*-desalkylpropafenone is less potent (91). Because these metabolites are very weak β-adrenoceptor antagonists, they do not contribute to *in vivo* β-blockade (91). In extensive metabolizers, the mean steady-state plasma concentration of 5-hydroxypropafenone (dose of propafenone: 150 mg 3x/day) was about 50% of the parent compound. Poor metabolizers had no detectable 5-hydroxypropafenone in plasma (93). In contrast, no major differences were found in the plasma concentration ratio of *N*-desalkylpropafenone and propafenone between extensive and poor metabolizers (0.13 versus 0.08) (93). In addition, diastereomeric R- and S-propafenone glucuronides, which are not pharmacologically active, can be detected in plasma in concentrations being equal to unconjugated R/S-propafenone (in extensive metabolizers) (97). The major metabolites found in urine of extensive metabolizers are conjugated 5-hydroxypropafenone (14% of an oral dose) (98) and (R + S)-propafenone glucuronides (15%) (99). Minor fractions are excreted as conjugated and unconjugated *N*-desalkylpropafenone and as unchanged parent compound (98,100). Because of the inability of poor metabolizers to form 5-hydroxypropafenone, the major fraction of a dose of propafenone is excreted as (R + S)-propafenone glucuronides (50%) (99).

In view of the major role of CYP2D6 for elimination of propafenone, drug interactions resulting from inhibition of CYP2D6 are likely to have a major impact on

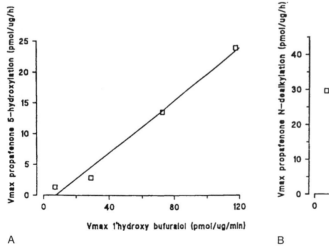

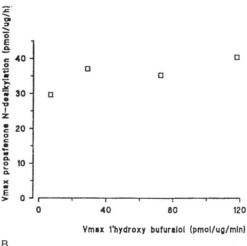

A   B

FIG. 28-3. Relationship between cumene hydroperoxide-mediated bufuralol 1′-hydroxylation, a CYP2D6-mediated reaction, and NADPH-mediated propafenone metabolite formation in liver microsomes of four human livers. (**A**) 5-hydroxylation. (**B**) *N*-dealkylation. From Kroemer HK, Mikus G, Kronbach T, Meyer UA, Eichelbaum M. In vitro characterization of the human cytochrome P450 involved in polymorphic oxidation of propafenone. *Clin Pharmacol Ther* 1989;45:28–33, with permission.

CHAPTER 28. ANTIARRHYTHMICS / 397

pharmacokinetics in extensive metabolizers only. Coadministration of the potent inhibitor of CYP2D6, quinidine, resulted in increased (two-fold) plasma concentrations of propafenone and decreased concentrations of 5-hydroxy-propafenone in extensive metabolizers, whereas no alterations were observed in poor metabolizers (100). The pharmacodynamic consequences of this drug interaction were investigated in a subsequent study (101). Quinidine increased the β-blockade, which is caused by the parent compound, during administration of propafenone in extensive metabolizers, but did not have any additional effect in poor metabolizers. The involvement of CYP3A4 in propafenone N-dealkylation provides an explanation for some observed drug interactions. For example, decreased propafenone plasma concentrations during concomitant therapy with rifampin could be explained, at least in part, by induction of CYP3A4-mediated propafenone N-dealkylation (102).

QUINIDINE

Quinidine has an oral bioavailability of about 70%, and approximately 20% to 37% of a dose is excreted unchanged by the kidneys (103,104). Several metabolites have been detected in plasma and urine. Marked interindividual variability has been observed for plasma concentrations of 3-hydroxyquinidine and 2'-oxoquinidinone. The mean ratios 3-hydroxyquinidine/quinidine, quinidine-N-oxide/quinidine, and 2'-oxoquinidinone/quinidine in serum of patients with normal kidney function were 0.36, 0.18, and 0.04, respectively (105,106). In a considerable percentage of patients, plasma concentrations of 3-hydroxyquinidine were even higher than those of quinidine when the unbound fraction was determined (107,108). Metabolites of quinidine in urine are 3-hydroxyquinidine (5%–21%), O-desmethylquinidine (1%–2%), quinidine-N-oxide (0.1%), and 2'-oxoquinidinone (traces) (104,105,109). The major metabolite 3-hydroxyquinidine is nearly as potent as the parent compound in blocking cardiac sodium channels and prolonging cardiac action potentials (103) and therefore is likely to contribute to the antiarrhythmic properties of quinidine. Moreover, the other aforementioned metabolites have also electrophysiologic properties in canine Purkinje fibers that are qualitatively similar to those of quinidine (110). They are, however, less potent and have lower plasma concentrations than quinidine, and thus are unlikely to contribute to the antiarrhythmic and proarrhythmic effects of quinidine (103).

In vitro studies using human liver microsomes clearly indicate that formation of the two major quinidine metabolites in plasma—3-hydroxyquinidine and quinidine-N-oxide—is catalyzed by CYP3A4 (111). The considerable decrease (two- to six-fold) in AUC of quinidine as a result of coadministration of rifampin, phenytoin, and phenobarbital can be explained, at least in part, by

induction of intestinal and hepatic CYP3A4 by these drugs (112,113). Although quinidine is a potent inhibitor of CYP2D6-mediated reactions (see Chapter 45), *in vitro* and *in vivo* data clearly indicate that quinidine itself is not metabolized by CYP2D6 (109,111).

Recent evidence has shown that quinidine is a substrate of the drug efflux pump P-glycoprotein (114,115), which is located in tissues with excretory function, such as liver, kidney, and small intestine. Thus, serum and tissue concentrations of quinidine might be influenced by individual expression and function of P-glycoprotein. The observation of a reduced quinidine clearance by coadministration of the CYP3A- and P-glycoprotein inhibitor verapamil in humans (116), for example, might be due to a metabolic drug interaction or inhibition of P-glycoprotein mediated drug transport.

SPARTEINE

The potent antiarrhythmic sparteine shows a wide range of plasma concentrations resulting from CYP2D6 catalyzing formation of 2- and 5-dehydrosparteine (117, 118). It has been speculated that this is why sparteine never gained any importance in treatment of arrhythmias. It appears that, with the recommended dose of 300 to 400 mg daily, only poor metabolizers will reach plasma concentrations in a range required for arrhythmia suppression (51). The remaining 90% of the population will only have subtherapeutic levels and no sufficient antiarrhythmic response. The role of sparteine for the discovery of the CYP2D6 polymorphism (sparteine/debrisoquine polymorphism) is described in detail in Chapter 8.

TOCAINIDE

Approximately 40% to 50% of a dose of the racemic drug tocainide is excreted as unchanged parent compound (119,120). Another 23% of a tocainide dose is excreted by the kidneys as tocainide carbamoyl O-β-D-glucuronide (120). Elimination of tocainide is stereoselective, resulting in an S-/R-tocainide plasma concentration ratio between 1.3 and 4.0 (121). Moreover, R-tocainide has been shown to be three times more potent than the S-enantiomer as an antiarrhythmic agent in a mouse model, and smaller differences have been reported for coronary-ligated dogs (122). Tocainide does not appear to have pharmacologically active metabolites (123). According to these data, significant alteration in the pharmacokinetics of tocainide resulting from metabolic drug interactions is unlikely. Dosage adjustments, however, appear necessary in patients with impaired kidney function.

IBUTILIDE

Ibutilide is one of the newer class III antiarrhythmics, which was approved in 1995 by the US Food and Drug

Administration for rapid conversion of recent-onset atrial fibrillation and atrial flutter (124). It is administered as a racemate with both enantiomers having similar pharmacokinetic properties. Intravenous administration of (+)-ibutilide to healthy volunteers resulted in a greater QT interval prolongation in comparison to (−)-ibutilide (125). The majority of an ibutilide dose (82%) is excreted in the urine as metabolites and parent compound. Unchanged drug contributes only 7% to the overall urinary elimination (124). *In vitro* experiments indicate that only the A-hydroxyl metabolite has class III antiarrhythmic activity equal to the parent compound. Because its plasma concentrations are only 10% of ibutilide, a major contribution of this metabolite to the overall drug effect appears unlikely (124). The enzymes catalyzing biotransformation of ibutilide have not yet been identified, but it has been reported that CYP3A4 and CYP2D6 do not seem to be involved (124).

MORICIZINE

Similar to encainide and flecainide in the CAST study, treatment of asymptomatic or mildly symptomatic ventricular premature depolarizations in survivors of myocardial infarction with moricizine (CAST-II study) resulted in an excess mortality rate compared to placebo (126). Moricizine is extensively metabolized in humans. Approximately 40 metabolites have been isolated, and the antiarrhythmic potency is unknown for most of them (127). So far, enzymes catalyzing the biotransformation of moricizine have not been identified.

CONCLUSION

Increased knowledge about drug-metabolizing enzymes involved in biotransformation of antiarrhythmics, interindividual differences in expression and function of these enzymes (e.g., resulting from genetic polymorphisms), pharmacologic properties of parent compound and its metabolites, and altered drug disposition by diseases (e.g., renal failure) provides a sound basis for a safer antiarrhythmic drug therapy. Moreover, studying the metabolic profile of a compound has come to play a very important part in drug development. There are current *in vitro* data and results from animal studies about the importance of the drug efflux pump P-glycoprotein for serum and tissue concentrations of some cardiovascular active drugs (e.g., quinidine, digoxin). It appears that some of the observed drug interactions could be due to both modification of the function of drug-metabolizing enzymes and modification of the function of P-glycoprotein. Further studies are necessary to clarify the latter issue.

ACKNOWLEDGMENT

Our own work cited in this review was supported by the Robert Bosch Foundation (Stuttgart, Germany). The work of Dr. Fromm in Nashville was supported by the Deutsche Forschungsgemeinschaft (Bonn, Germany; grant Fr 1298/1-1).

REFERENCES

1. Fromm MF, Kroemer HK, Eichelbaum M. Impact of P450 genetic polymorphism on first-pass extraction of cardiovascular and neuroactive drugs. *Adv Drug Del Rev* 1997;27:171–199.
2. Roden DM. Pharmacokinetics of amiodarone: implications for drug therapy. *Am J Cardiol* 1993;72:45F–50F.
3. Harris L, McKenna WJ, Rowland E, et al. Plasma amiodarone and desethyl amiodarone levels in chronic oral therapy. *Circulation* 1981;64[Suppl IV]:263(abstr).
4. Andreasen F, Agerbaek H, Bjerregaard P, Gotzsche H. Pharmacokinetics of amiodarone after intravenous and oral administration. *Eur J Clin Pharmacol* 1981;19:293–299.
5. Riva E, Gerna M, Latini R, Giani P, Volpi A, Maggioni A. Pharmacokinetics of amiodarone in man. *J Cardiovasc Pharmacol* 1982;4:264–269.
6. Harris L, Hind CR, McKenna WJ, et al. Renal elimination of amiodarone and its desethyl metabolite. *Postgrad Med J* 1983;59:440–442.
7. Gill J, Heel RC, Fitton A. Amiodarone. An overview of its pharmacological properties, and review of its therapeutic use in cardiac arrhythmias. *Drugs* 1992;43:69–110.
8. Trivier JM, Libersa C, Belloc C, Lhermitte M. Amiodarone N-deethylation in human liver microsomes: involvement of cytochrome P450 3A enzymes (first report). *Life Sci* 1993;52:PL91–PL96.
9. Fabre G, Julian B, Saint-Aubert B, Joyeux H, Berger Y. Evidence for CYP3A-mediated N-deethylation of amiodarone in human liver microsomal fractions. *Drug Metab Dispos* 1993;21:978–985.
10. Pichard L, Fabre I, Fabre G, et al. Cyclosporin A drug interactions. Screening for inducers and inhibitors of cytochrome P-450 (cyclosporin A oxidase) in primary cultures of human hepatocytes and in liver microsomes. *Drug Metab Dispos* 1990;18:595–606.
11. Nolan PE Jr, Marcus FI, Karol MD, Hoyer GL, Gear K. Effect of phenytoin on the clinical pharmacokinetics of amiodarone. *J Clin Pharmacol* 1990;30:1112–1119.
12. Fasola AF, Carmichael R. The pharmacology and clinical evaluation of aprindine a new antiarrhythmic agent. *Acta Cardiol* 1974;Suppl 18:317–333.
13. Murphy PJ. Metabolic pathways of aprindine. *Acta Cardiol* 1974;Suppl 18:131–142.
14. Wirth KE, Breithardt G, Michaelis L. Detection of aprindine and its metabolites in plasma and urine. *Herz* 1983;8:302–308.
15. Ebner T, Eichelbaum M. The metabolism of aprindine in relation to the sparteine/debrisoquine polymorphism. *Br J Clin Pharmacol* 1993;35:426–430.
16. Siddoway LA, Roden DM, Woosley RL. Clinical pharmacology of old and new antiarrhythmic drugs. *Cardiovasc Clin* 1985;15:199–248.
17. Rapeport WG. Clinical pharmacokinetics of bretylium. *Clin Pharmacokinet* 1985;10:248–256.
18. Rangno RE, Warnica W, Ogilvie RI, Kreeft J, Bridger E. Correlation of disopyramide pharmacokinetics with efficacy in ventricular tachyarrhythmia. *J Int Med Res* 1976;4:54–58.
19. Woosley RL, Funck-Brentano C. Overview of the clinical pharmacology of antiarrhythmic drugs. *Am J Cardiol* 1988;61:61A–69A.
20. Grant AM, Marshall RJ, Ankier SI. Some effects of disopyramide and its N-dealkylated metabolite on isolated nerve and cardiac muscle. *Eur J Pharmacol* 1978;49:389–394.
21. Baines MW, Davies JE, Kellett DN, Munt PL. Some pharmacological effects of disopyramide and a metabolite. *J Int Med Res* 1976;4:5–7.
22. Kates RE. Metabolites of cardiac antiarrhythmic drugs: their clinical role. *Ann NY Acad Sci* 1984;432:75–89.
23. Aitio ML. Plasma concentrations and protein binding of disopyramide and mono-N-dealkyldisopyramide during chronic oral disopyramide therapy. *Br J Clin Pharmacol* 1981;11:369–375.
24. Echizen H, Mochizuki K, Tani M, Ishizaki T. Interspecies differences in enantioselective mono-N-dealkylation of disopyramide by human and mouse liver microsomes. *J Pharmacol Exp Ther* 1994;268:1518–1525.
25. Echizen H, Kawasaki H, Chiba K, Tani M, Ishizaki T. A potent

inhibitory effect of erythromycin and other macrolide antibiotics on the mono-N-dealkylation metabolism of disopyramide with human liver microsomes. *J Pharmacol Exp Ther* 1993;264:1425–1431.

26. Ragosta M, Weihl AC, Rosenfeld LE. Potentially fatal interaction between erythromycin and disopyramide. *Am J Med* 1989;86:465–466.

27. Paar D, Terjung B, Sauerbruch T. Life-threatening interaction between clarithromycin and disopyramide. *Lancet* 1997;349:326–327.

28. Aitio ML, Mansury L, Tala E, Haataja M, Aitio A. The effect of enzyme induction on the metabolism of disopyramide in man. *Br J Clin Pharmacol* 1981;11:279–285.

29. Aitio ML, Vuorenmaa T. Enhanced metabolism and diminished efficacy of disopyramide by enzyme induction? *Br J Clin Pharmacol* 1980;9:149–152.

30. Kapil RP, Axelson JE, Mansfield IL, et al. Disopyramide pharmacokinetics and metabolism: effect of inducers. *Br J Clin Pharmacol* 1987;24:781–791.

31. Smith DA, Rasmussen HS, Stopher DA, Walker DK. Pharmacokinetics and metabolism of dofetilide in mouse, rat, dog and man. *Xenobiotica* 1992;22:709–719.

32. Walker DK, Alabaster CT, Congrave GS, et al. Significance of metabolism in the disposition and action of the antidysrhythmic drug, dofetilide. In vitro studies and correlation with in vivo data. *Drug Metab Dispos* 1996;24:447–455.

33. Wang T, Roden DM, Wolfenden HT, Woosley RL, Wood AJ, Wilkinson GR. Influence of genetic polymorphism on the metabolism and disposition of encainide in man. *J Pharmacol Exp Ther* 1984;228:605–611.

34. Woosley RL, Wood AJ, Roden DM. Drug therapy. Encainide. *N Engl J Med* 1988;318:1107–1115.

35. Woosley RL, Roden DM, Dai GH, et al. Co-inheritance of the polymorphic metabolism of encainide and debrisoquin. *Clin Pharmacol Ther* 1986;39:282–287.

36. Roden DM, Duff HJ, Altenbern D, Woosley RL. Antiarrhythmic activity of the O-demethyl metabolite of encainide. *J Pharmacol Exp Ther* 1982;221:552–557.

37. Davy JM, Dorian P, Kantelip JP, Harrison DC, Kates RE. Qualitative and quantitative comparison of the cardiac effects of encainide and its three major metabolites in the dog. *J Pharmacol Exp Ther* 1986;237:907–911.

38. Funck-Brentano C, Thomas G, Jacqz-Aigrain E, et al. Polymorphism of dextromethorphan metabolism: relationships between phenotype, genotype and response to the administration of encainide in humans. *J Pharmacol Exp Ther* 1992;263:780–786.

39. Buchert E, Woosley RL. Clinical implications of variable antiarrhythmic drug metabolism. *Pharmacogenetics* 1992;2:2–11.

40. Turgeon J, Pavlou HN, Wong W, Funck-Brentano C, Roden DM. Genetically determined steady-state interaction between encainide and quinidine in patients with arrhythmias. *J Pharmacol Exp Ther* 1990;255:642–649.

41. Funck-Brentano C, Turgeon J, Woosley RL, Roden DM. Effect of low dose quinidine on encainide pharmacokinetics and pharmacodynamics. Influence of genetic polymorphism. *J Pharmacol Exp Ther* 1989;249:134–142.

42. Kroemer HK, Turgeon J, Parker RA, Roden DM. Flecainide enantiomers: disposition in human subjects and electrophysiologic actions in vitro. *Clin Pharmacol Ther* 1989;46:584–590.

43. Smallwood JK, Robertson DW, Steinberg MI. Electrophysiological effects of flecainide enantiomers in canine Purkinje fibres. *Naunyn Schmiedebergs Arch Pharmacol* 1989;339:625–629.

44. Funck-Brentano C, Becquemont L, Kroemer HK, et al. Variable disposition kinetics and electrocardiographic effects of flecainide during repeated dosing in humans: contribution of genetic factors, dose-dependent clearance, and interaction with amiodarone. *Clin Pharmacol Ther* 1994;55:256–269.

45. Roden DM, Woosley RL. Drug therapy. Flecainide. *N Engl J Med* 1986;315:36–41.

46. Conard GJ, Ober RE. Metabolism of flecainide. *Am J Cardiol* 1984;53:41B–51B.

47. Gross AS, Mikus G, Fischer C, Eichelbaum M. Polymorphic flecainide disposition under conditions of uncontrolled urine flow and pH. *Eur J Clin Pharmacol* 1991;40:155–162.

48. Gross AS, Mikus G, Fischer C, et al. Stereoselective disposition of flecainide in relation to the sparteine/debrisoquine metaboliser phenotype. *Br J Clin Pharmacol* 1989;28:555–566.

49. Mikus G, Gross AS, Beckmann J, Hertrampf R, Gundert-Remy U, Eichelbaum M. The influence of the sparteine/debrisoquin phenotype on the disposition of flecainide. *Clin Pharmacol Ther* 1989;45:562–567.

50. Evers J, Eichelbaum M, Kroemer HK. Unpredictability of flecainide plasma concentrations in patients with renal failure: relationship to side effects and sudden death? *Ther Drug Monit* 1994;16:349–351.

51. Eichelbaum M, Gross AS. The genetic polymorphism of debrisoquine/sparteine metabolism—clinical aspects. *Pharmacol Ther* 1990;46:377–394.

52. Birgersdotter UM, Wong W, Turgeon J, Roden DM. Stereoselective genetically-determined interaction between chronic flecainide and quinidine in patients with arrhythmias. *Br J Clin Pharmacol* 1992;33:275–280.

53. Echt DS, Liebson PR, Mitchell LB, et al. Mortality and morbidity in patients receiving encainide, flecainide, or placebo. The Cardiac Arrhythmia Suppression Trial. *N Engl J Med* 1991;324:781–788.

54. The Cardiac Arrhythmia Suppression Trial (CAST) Investigators. Preliminary report: effect of encainide and flecainide on mortality in a randomized trial of arrhythmia suppression after myocardial infarction. The Cardiac Arrhythmia Suppression Trial (CAST) Investigators. *N Engl J Med* 1989;321:406–412.

55. Halkin H, Meffin P, Melmon KL, Rowland M. Influence of congestive heart failure on blood vessels of lidocaine and its active monodeethylated metabolite. *Clin Pharmacol Ther* 1975;17:669–676.

56. Drayer DE, Lorenzo B, Werns S, Reidenberg MM. Plasma levels, protein binding, and elimination data of lidocaine and active metabolites in cardiac patients of various ages. *Clin Pharmacol Ther* 1983;34:14–22.

57. Burney RG, DiFazio CA, Peach MJ, Petrie KA, Silvester MJ. Antiarrhythmic effects of lidocaine metabolites. *Am Heart J* 1974;88:765–769.

58. Strong JM, Mayfield DE, Atkinson AJ Jr, et al. Pharmacological activity, metabolism, and pharmacokinetics of glycinexylidide. *Clin Pharmacol Ther* 1975;17:184–194.

59. Freedman MD, Gal J, Freed CR. Decreased toxicity and equipotent antiarrhythmic potency of monoethylglycine xylidide compared to lidocaine. *Clin Res* 1982;327:87A(abstr).

60. Bennett PB, Woosley RL, Hondeghem LM. Competition between lidocaine and one of its metabolites, glycylxylidide, for cardiac sodium channels. *Circulation* 1988;78:692–700.

61. Keenaghan JB, Boyes RN. The tissue distribution, metabolism and excretion of lidocaine in rats, guinea pigs, dogs and man. *J Pharmacol Exp Ther* 1972;180:454–463.

62. Bargetzi MJ, Aoyama T, Gonzalez FJ, Meyer UA. Lidocaine metabolism in human liver microsomes by cytochrome P450IIIA4. *Clin Pharmacol Ther* 1989;46:521–527.

63. Imaoka S, Enomoto K, Oda Y, et al. Lidocaine metabolism by human cytochrome P-450s purified from hepatic microsomes: comparison of those with rat hepatic cytochrome P-450s. *J Pharmacol Exp Ther* 1990;255:1385–1391.

64. Li AP, Rasmussen A, Xu L, Kaminski DL. Rifampicin induction of lidocaine metabolism in cultured human hepatocytes. *J Pharmacol Exp Ther* 1995;274:673–677.

65. Ha HR, Candinas R, Stieger B, Meyer UA, Follath F. Interaction between amiodarone and lidocaine. *J Cardiovasc Pharmacol* 1996;28:533–539.

66. Hill RJ, Duff HJ, Sheldon RS. Determinants of stereospecific binding of type I antiarrhythmic drugs to cardiac sodium channels. *Mol Pharmacol* 1988;34:659–663.

67. Turgeon J, Uprichard AC, Belanger PM, Harron DW, Grech-Belanger O. Resolution and electrophysiological effects of mexiletine enantiomers. *J Pharm Pharmacol* 1991;43:630–635.

68. Grech-Belanger O, Turgeon J, Gilbert M. Stereoselective disposition of mexiletine in man. *Br J Clin Pharmacol* 1986;21:481–487.

69. Abolfathi Z, Fiset C, Gilbert M, Moerike K, Belanger PM, Turgeon J. Role of polymorphic debrisoquin 4-hydroxylase activity in the stereoselective disposition of mexiletine in humans. *J Pharmacol Exp Ther* 1993;266:1196–1201.

70. Turgeon J, Fiset C, Giguere R, et al. Influence of debrisoquine phenotype and of quinidine on mexiletine disposition in man. *J Pharmacol Exp Ther* 1991;259:789–798.

71. Gillis AM, Kates RE. Clinical pharmacokinetics of the newer antiarrhythmic agents. *Clin Pharmacokinet* 1984;9:375–403.

72. Broly F, Libersa C, Lhermitte M, Dupuis B. Inhibitory studies of mexiletine and dextromethorphan oxidation in human liver microsomes. *Biochem Pharmacol* 1990;39:1045–1053.

73. Broly F, Libersa C, Lhermitte M. Mexiletine metabolism in vitro by human liver. *Drug Metab Dispos* 1990;18:362–368.

74. Lledo P, Abrams SM, Johnston A, Patel M, Pearson RM, Turner P. Influence of debrisoquine hydroxylation phenotype on the pharmacokinetics of mexiletine. *Eur J Clin Pharmacol* 1993;44:63–67.

75. Broly F, Vandamme N, Libersa C, Lhermitte M. The metabolism of mexiletine in relation to the debrisoquine/sparteine-type polymorphism of drug oxidation. *Br J Clin Pharmacol* 1991;32:459–466.

76. Duff HJ, Mitchell LB, Manyari D, Wyse DG. Mexiletine-quinidine combination: electrophysiologic correlates of a favorable antiarrhythmic interaction in humans. *J Am Coll Cardiol* 1987;10:1149–1156.

77. Duff HJ, Roden D, Primm RK, Oates JA, Woosley RL. Mexiletine in the treatment of resistant ventricular arrhythmias: enhancement of efficacy and reduction of dose-related side effects by combination with quinidine. *Circulation* 1983;67:1124–1128.

78. Zekorn C, Achtert G, Hausleiter HJ, Moon CH, Eichelbaum M. Pharmacokinetics of N-propylajmaline in relation to polymorphic sparteine oxidation. *Klin Wochenschr* 1985;63:1180–1186.

79. Schwartzkopff B, Schilling G, Simon H. Comparison of tocainide and prajmalium bitartrate for the treatment of ventricular arrhythmias. *Arzneimittelforschung* 1983;33:153–158.

80. Hausleiter HJ, Achtert G, Khan MA, Kukovetz WR, Beubler E. Pharmacokinetics and biotransformation of N-propylajmaline hydrogen tartrate in man. *Eur J Drug Metab Pharmacokinet* 1982;7:329–339.

81. Mörike K, Hardtmann E, Heimburg P, Eichelbaum M. The impact of polymorphic N-propylajmaline metabolism on dose requirement and antiarrhythmic efficacy of the drug. *Eur J Pharmacol* 1990;183:628–629.

82. Reidenberg MM, Drayer DE, Levy M, Warner H. Polymorphic acetylation procainamide in man. *Clin Pharmacol Ther* 1975;17:722–730.

83. Jaillon P, Rubenson D, Peters F, Mason JW, Winkle RA. Electrophysiologic effects of N-acetylprocainamide in human beings. *Am J Cardiol* 1981;47:1134–1140.

84. Funck-Brentano C, Light RT, Lineberry MD, Wright GM, Roden DM, Woosley RL. Pharmacokinetic and pharmacodynamic interaction of N-acetyl procainamide and procainamide in humans. *J Cardiovasc Pharmacol* 1989;14:364–373.

85. Woosley RL, Roden DM. Pharmacologic causes of arrhythmogenic actions of antiarrhythmic drugs. *Am J Cardiol* 1987;59:19E–25E.

86. Woosley RL, Drayer DE, Reidenberg MM, Nies AS, Carr K, Oates JA. Effect of acetylator phenotype on the rate at which procainamide induces antinuclear antibodies and the lupus syndrome. *N Engl J Med* 1978;298:1157–1159.

87. Henningsen NC, Cederberg A, Hanson A, Johansson BW. Effects of long-term treatment with procaine amide. A prospective study with special regard to ANF and SLE in fast and slow acetylators. *Acta Med Scand* 1975;198:475–482.

88. Lessard E, Fortin A, Belanger PM, Beaune P, Hamelin BA, Turgeon J. Role of CYP2D6 in the N-hydroxylation of procainamide. *Pharmacogenetics* 1997;7:381–390.

89. Siddoway LA, Thompson KA, McAllister CB, et al. Polymorphism of propafenone metabolism and disposition in man: clinical and pharmacokinetic consequences. *Circulation* 1987;75:785–791.

90. Kroemer HK, Mikus G, Kronbach T, Meyer UA, Eichelbaum M. In vitro characterization of the human cytochrome P-450 involved in polymorphic oxidation of propafenone. *Clin Pharmacol Ther* 1989;45:28–33.

91. Funck-Brentano C, Kroemer HK, Lee JT, Roden DM. Propafenone. *N Engl J Med* 1990;322:518–525.

92. Kroemer HK, Funck-Brentano C, Silberstein DJ, et al. Stereoselective disposition and pharmacologic activity of propafenone enantiomers. *Circulation* 1989;79:1068–1076.

93. Lee JT, Kroemer HK, Silberstein DJ, et al. The role of genetically determined polymorphic drug metabolism in the beta-blockade produced by propafenone. *N Engl J Med* 1990;322:1764–1768.

94. Kroemer HK, Fischer C, Meese CO, Eichelbaum M. Enantiomer/enantiomer interaction of (S)- and (R)-propafenone for cytochrome P450IID6-catalyzed 5-hydroxylation: in vitro evaluation of the mechanism. *Mol Pharmacol* 1991;40:135–142.

95. Kroemer HK, Fromm MF, Buhl K, Terefe H, Blaschke G, Eichelbaum M. An enantiomer-enantiomer interaction of (S)- and (R)-propafenone modifies the effect of racemic drug therapy. *Circulation* 1994;89:2396–2400.

96. Botsch S, Gautier JC, Beaune P, Eichelbaum M, Kroemer HK. Identification and characterization of the cytochrome P450 enzymes involved in N-dealkylation of propafenone: molecular base for interaction potential and variable disposition of active metabolites. *Mol Pharmacol* 1993;43:120–126.

97. Fromm MF, Botsch S, Heinkele G, Evers J, Kroemer HK. Influence of renal function on the steady-state pharmacokinetics of the antiarrhythmic propafenone and its phase I and phase II metabolites. *Eur J Clin Pharmacol* 1995;48:279–283.

98. Vozeh S, Haefeli W, Ha HR, Vlcek J, Follath F. Nonlinear kinetics of propafenone metabolites in healthy man. *Eur J Clin Pharmacol* 1990;38:509–513.

99. Botsch S, Heinkele G, Meese CO, Eichelbaum M, Kroemer HK. Rapid determination of CYP2D6 phenotype during propafenone therapy by analysing urinary excretion of propafenone glucuronides. *Eur J Clin Pharmacol* 1994;46:133–135.

100. Funck-Brentano C, Kroemer HK, Pavlou H, Woosley RL, Roden DM. Genetically-determined interaction between propafenone and low dose quinidine: role of active metabolites in modulating net drug effect. *Br J Clin Pharmacol* 1989;27:435–444.

101. Mörike KE, Roden DM. Quinidine-enhanced beta-blockade during treatment with propafenone in extensive metabolizer human subjects. *Clin Pharmacol Ther* 1994;55:28–34.

102. Castel JM, Cappiello E, Leopaldi D, Latini R. Rifampicin lowers plasma concentrations of propafenone and its antiarrhythmic effect. *Br J Clin Pharmacol* 1990;30:155–156.

103. Roden DM. Antiarrhythmic drugs. Hardman JG, Limbird LE, eds. *Goodman & Gilman's. The pharmacological basis of therapeutics.* New York: McGraw-Hill, 1996:839–874.

104. Brosen K, Davidsen F, Gram LF. Quinidine kinetics after a single oral dose in relation to the sparteine oxidation polymorphism in man. *Br J Clin Pharmacol* 1990;29:248–253.

105. Drayer DE, Lowenthal DT, Restivo KM et al. Steady-state serum levels of quinidine and active metabolites in cardiac patients with varying degrees of renal function. *Clin Pharmacol Ther* 1978;24:31–39.

106. Kewitz G, Ha HR, Ganzinger U, Follath F. Serumkonzentration des Chinidins und seiner Metabolite nach repetierter Dosierung. *Schweiz Med Wochenschr* 1980;110:1706.

107. Drayer DE, Hughes M, Lorenzo B, Reidenberg MM. Prevalence of high (3S)-3-hydroxyquinidine/quinidine ratios in serum, and clearance of quinidine in cardiac patients with age. *Clin Pharmacol Ther* 1980;27:72–75.

108. Wooding-Scott RA, Visco J, Slaughter RL. Total and unbound concentrations of quinidine and 3-hydroxyquinidine at steady state. *Am Heart J* 1987;113:302–306.

109. Mikus G, Ha HR, Vozeh S, Zekorn C, Follath F, Eichelbaum M. Pharmacokinetics and metabolism of quinidine in extensive and poor metabolisers of sparteine. *Eur J Clin Pharmacol* 1986;31:69–72.

110. Thompson KA, Blair IA, Woosley RL, Roden DM. Comparative in vitro electrophysiology of quinidine, its major metabolites and dihydroquinidine. *J Pharmacol Exp Ther* 1987;241:84–90.

111. Guengerich FP, Muller-Enoch D, Blair IA. Oxidation of quinidine by human liver cytochrome P-450. *Mol Pharmacol* 1986;30:287–295.

112. Data JL, Wilkinson GR, Nies AS. Interaction of quinidine with anticonvulsant drugs. *N Engl J Med* 1976;294:699–702.

113. Twum-Barima Y, Carruthers SG. Quinidine-rifampin interaction. *N Engl J Med* 1981;304:1466–1469.

114. Kusuhara H, Suzuki H, Terasaki T, Kakee A, Lemaire M, Sugiyama Y. P-glycoprotein mediates the efflux of quinidine across the blood-brain barrier. *J Pharmacol Exp Ther* 1997;283:574–580.

115. Fromm MF, Kim RB, Stein CM, Wilkinson GR, Roden DM. Inhibition of P-glycoprotein-mediated drug transport: a unifying mechanism to explain the interaction between digoxin and quinidine. *Circulation* 1999;99:552–557.

116. Edwards DJ, Lavoie R, Beckman H, Blevins R, Rubenfire M. The effect of coadministration of verapamil on the pharmacokinetics and metabolism of quinidine. *Clin Pharmacol Ther* 1987;41:68–73.

117. Eichelbaum M, Spannbrucker N, Dengler HJ. Influence of the defective metabolism of sparteine on its pharmacokinetics. *Eur J Clin Pharmacol* 1979;16:189–194.

118. Eichelbaum M, Reetz KP, Schmidt EK, Zekorn C. The genetic polymorphism of sparteine metabolism. *Xenobiotica* 1986;16:465–481.

119. Lalka D, Meyer MB, Duce BR, Elvin AT. Kinetics of the oral antiarrhythmic lidocaine congener, tocainide. *Clin Pharmacol Ther* 1976; 19:757–766.

120. Elvin AT, Keenaghan JB, Byrnes EW, et al. Tocainide conjugation in humans: novel biotransformation pathway for a primary amine. *J Pharm Sci* 1980;69:47–49.

121. Sedman AJ, Gal J, Mastropaolo W, Johnson P, Maloney JD, Moyer TP. Serum tocainide enantiomer concentrations in human subjects. *Br J Clin Pharmacol* 1984;17:113–115.

122. Byrnes EW, McMaster PD, Smith ER, et al. New antiarrhythmic agents. 1. Primary alpha-amino anilides. *J Med Chem* 1979;22: 1171–1176.

123. Roden DM, Woosley RL. Drug therapy. Tocainide. *N Engl J Med* 1986; 315:41–45.

124. Cropp JS, Antal EG, Talbert RL. Ibutilide: a new class III antiarrhythmic agent. *Pharmacotherapy* 1997;17:1–9.

125. Jungbluth GL, Della-Coletta AA, VanderLugt JT. Evaluation of the pharmacokinetics and pharmacodynamics of ibutilide fumarate and its enantiomers in healthy male volunteers. *Pharmazeutical Research* 1991;8[Suppl 9]:S249(abstr).

126. The Cardiac Arrhythmia Suppression Trial II Investigators. Effect of the antiarrhythmic agent moricizine on survival after myocardial infarction. The Cardiac Arrhythmia Suppression Trial II Investigators. *N Engl J Med* 1992;327:227–233.

127. Clyne CA, Estes NA 3d, Wang PJ. Moricizine. *N Engl J Med* 1992; 327:255–260.

CHAPTER 29

Oral Anticoagulants

William F. Trager

BACKGROUND AND HISTORY

Like most drugs in the clinical armamentarium of medicine, the oral anticoagulants are derived from a bioactive plant substance that causes some profound pharmacologic effect. In this case, the drugs were discovered during the hemorrhagic plague of the 1920s and 1930s that first appeared in the prairies of North Dakota and in Alberta, Canada, and decimated livestock, particularly cattle, that had been fed on improperly cured sweet clover hay. Dicumarol (methylene bis-4,4'-hydroxycoumarin) (Fig. 29-1), the active agent present in the hay, was first isolated in the 1930s and its structure was established shortly thereafter by Karl P. Link and his research group at the University of Wisconsin (1). This group also recognized that a substance that had the ability to suppress blood clot formation had the potential to be of significant value to clinical medicine. While dicumarol was shown to be effective in humans, the anticoagulant response it produced tended to be highly variable, presumably because of its erratic absorption characteristics (2). Not long after the discovery of dicumarol, a synthetic program was initiated to find active dicumarol analogues with favorable pharmacokinetic properties. Warfarin (Fig. 29-2) was one of the early, very potent, compounds to emerge from this synthetic program. In contrast to dicumarol, warfarin is well absorbed (3). Because it is so potent, it was believed initially to be too toxic for use in humans; thus, it found extensive use as a rodenticide. Indeed, the name warfarin was coined in recognition of the Wisconsin Alumni Foundation that supplied support for its development as a rodenticide (1). In 1952, a report appeared in the literature of an individual who attempted

suicide by repeatedly ingesting large amounts of warfarin (4). The attempt was unsuccessful. Shortly thereafter, the safety of the drug was established for human use and it was introduced into clinical medicine (5). Five decades later, warfarin remains the oral anticoagulant of choice in North America. Of the hundreds of potential oral anticoagulants that have been synthesized, only two others—phenprocoumon (Fig. 29-3) and acenocoumarol (Fig. 29-4)—have found prominent clinical use, and that primarily in Europe. This chapter focuses on these three major oral anticoagulants.

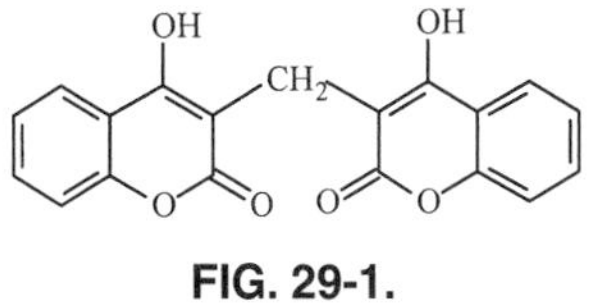

FIG. 29-1.

FIG. 29-2.

FIG. 29-3.

FIG. 29-4.

W. F. Trager: Department of Medicinal Chemistry, University of Washington, Box 357610, H172 Health Sciences Building, Seattle, Washington, 98195

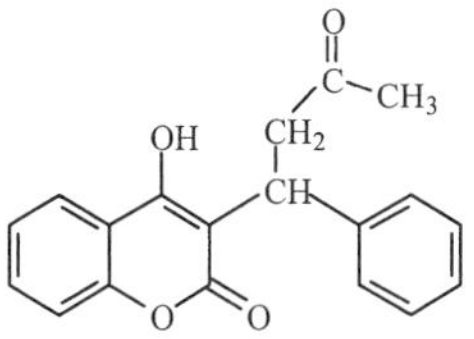

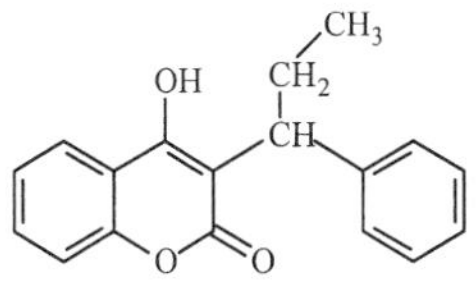

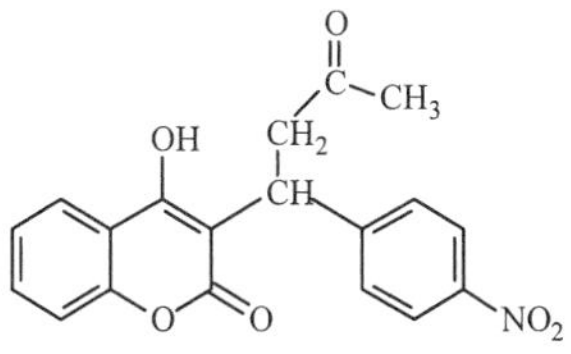

MODE OF ACTION

The coumarin-based oral anticoagulants like warfarin work by interfering with the synthesis of the vitamin K–dependent protein clotting factors, factors II (prothrombin), VII, IX, X, protein C, and protein S (6). Vitamin K is a cofactor of a carboxylation enzyme that catalyzes the incorporation of carbon dioxide into the methylene group immediately adjacent to the side chain carboxyl groups of a number (9–12) of glutamic acid residues (Glu) located near the N-terminus of the preclotting factors to form γ-carboxyglutamate residues (Gla) and generate the active clotting factors, which effectively bind Ca^{2+} (6,7). The ability of the protein factors to bind Ca^{2+} is essential to the process of clot formation (Fig 29-5). The active form of the vitamin is the reduced form, the hydroquinone or dihydro vitamin K, whereas the storage, or inactive form of the vitamin, is the oxidized form, vitamin K epoxide. Conversion of dihydro vitamin K back to vitamin K epoxide is coupled to the conversion of the Glu to Gla residues (Fig. 29-6) (6). The regeneration of dihydro vitamin K from vitamin K epoxide by a reductase is the specific process that is inhibited by the coumarin-based oral anticoagulants and is the basis for their anticoagulant activity (6,8,9).

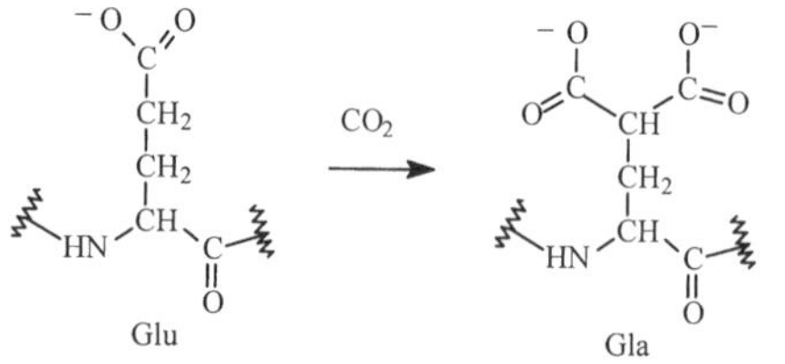

FIG. 29-5.

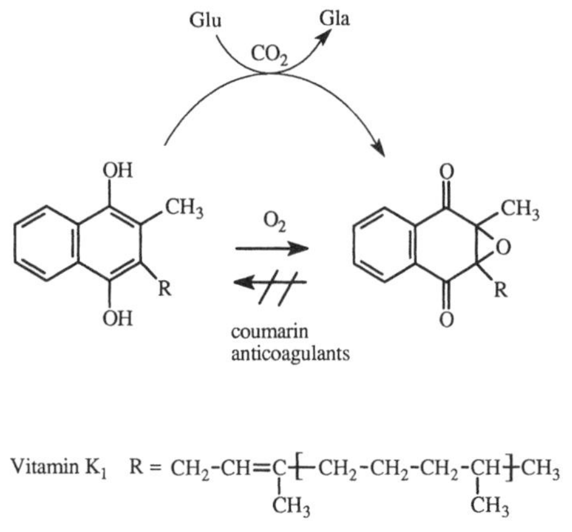

FIG. 29-6.

THERAPEUTIC MONITORING

Because the oral anticoagulants have a rather narrow therapeutic index and are frequently administered on a long-term basis, it is necessary to monitor pharmacologic activity, both to establish a maintenance dose and to periodically determine that the desired level of anticoagulation is maintained within defined limits. For many years this was achieved with a prothrombin time (PT) test. In this test, thromboplastin (a saline brain extract, generally obtained from the rabbit, which contains tissue factor, a nonenzymatic lipoprotein cofactor, and phospholipids) is added to a recalcified citrated plasma sample. The time for a clot to form is then measured and compared to a standard. In the absence of an anticoagulant, a normal clotting time (prothrombin time) under these conditions is 12 to 14 seconds.

Because there is inherent variability in the PT test resulting from a variety of factors, including the thromboplastin reagent itself, an international normalized ratio (INR) method of reporting anticoagulant activity has been adopted to standardize reporting between laboratories (10). In this method, the PT for the patient, PT_{pt}, is determined by a standard method using commercial thromboplastin and then compared (as a ratio) to the PT_{ref}, which would have been obtained by this method if the primary standard of human thromboplastin from the World Health Organization had been used. The INR is then calculated from the following equation:

$$INR = (PT_{pt}/PT_{ref})^{ISI}$$

where ISI = the international sensitivity index. A typical goal for an INR is 2 to 3, but this often depends on the specific condition being treated (11–13).

At therapeutic doses, the oral anticoagulants are pharmacologically clean, that is, they have few side effects. Their only significant biologic effect, in most circumstances, is their inhibitory effect on the synthesis of the vitamin K–dependent clotting factors. Although these agents are usually free of serious side effects, they are contraindicated in pregnancy and can induce full-thickness skin necrosis (14). Of more general therapeutic concern are the frequent drug–drug interactions that have been encountered when anticoagulants are coadministered with other medications. The potential causes of such drug–drug interactions include effects on the synthesis, function, or clearance of any factor, whether it is vitamin K, the anticoagulant, or the biochemical machinery involved in the blood clotting process. If the interaction operates at the level of vitamin K or some aspect of the biochemical machinery, then the chemical identity of the oral anticoagulant that is used is irrelevant and the observed effects will only be a function of the properties of the coadministered medication. Conversely, if the interactant effects are a function of the specific oral anticoagulant that is used, they are likely to be metabolically based, that is, the coadministered medication directly affects the absorption, distribution, or clearance of the anticoagulant. This chapter focuses on oral anticoagulant drug interactions that fall into the latter category—those that are based specifically in metabolism and have enzyme inhibition as their root cause. Interactions involving induction of anticoagulant clearance are relatively rare. Inducers and are discussed in Chapters 51–53. A major mechanism by which such interactions are likely to occur is by altering the clearance of the parent drug, so detailed knowledge of the metabolism of the parent drug in the human is crucial to understanding the cause of a drug interaction at the molecular level.

PHARMACOKINETICS, STEREOCHEMISTRY, AND METABOLISM

Warfarin

Warfarin, a weak organic acid (pKa approximately 6), is administered as the sodium salt. It is well absorbed (93% ± 8%) and reaches a maximum plasma concentration, Cp, within 2 hours; it is highly plasma protein bound (99% ± 1%). It has a whole body clearance, CL, of 0.045 ± 0.024 mL·min^{-1}·kg^{-1}, a volume of distribution, Vd, of 5.0 ± 2.1 L/kg, a half-life, t$_{1/2}$, of 37 ± 15 hours, and an effective plasma concentration of 2.2 ± 0.4 µg/mL (15). Because the molecule has a single asymmetric center, it exists in two enantiomeric forms—(R)- and (S)-warfarin—but it is only available clinically as the racemic mixture. The potency of (S)-warfarin as an anticoagulant is approximately 5 to 6 times greater than that of (R)-warfarin (16–18) and has a shorter t$_{1/2}$, 32 ± 12 hours versus 43 ± 14 hours (15). Thus, any process that specifically alters the clearance of (S)-warfarin would be expected to have a coupled, but opposite, effect on anticoagulation. If the clearance of (S)-warfarin decreases, anticoagulant response should increase, whereas if the clearance increases, anticoagulant response should decrease. This fact was the key that clarified the paradoxical *in vivo* results associated with the warfarin–phenylbutazone interaction.

An earlier study (19) had indicated that, when phenylbutazone was present, an enhanced anticoagulant response was observed along with an increase in the rate of elimination of warfarin. That is, there appeared to be no dose-response relationship between warfarin plasma concentration and the anticoagulant response elicited. In subsequent single-dose studies in which the individual (R)- and (S)-warfarin isomers were administered separately (20) or as a pseudoracemate (13C-(S)-warfarin/12C-(R)-warfarin) (21), the clearance of (S)-warfarin was suppressed in the presence of phenylbutazone, relative to its absence. Conversely, the clearance of the

(R)-isomer was accelerated. These results resolve the dilemma of the lack of correlation between plasma warfarin concentration and anticoagulant response. Depending on which effect is greater, suppression of the clearance of (S)-warfarin or acceleration of the clearance of (R)-warfarin determines whether the plasma concentration of total warfarin [mixture of (R)- and (S)-warfarin] in the presence of phenylbutazone will be greater, less, or unchanged relative to what it would be in the absence of phenylbutazone. Regardless of what the plasma concentration of total warfarin is in the presence of phenylbutazone, the concentration of (S)-warfarin in the presence of phenylbutazone will always be greater than what it would be in its absence. An enhanced anticoagulant response can always be expected when racemic warfarin is coadministered with phenylbutazone or indeed any drug that inhibits the clearance of (S)-warfarin.

A likely mechanism by which the clearance of (S)-warfarin could be reduced is through inhibition of its metabolism. Thus, if a drug interaction is to be understood, it becomes particularly important to define the metabolic profile of the drug that is subject to the interaction. Initial work to investigate the metabolism of warfarin was done in the rat by Link's group at the University of Wisconsin. These investigators were able to identify 6-, 7-, 8-, and 4'-hydroxywarfarin as primary metabolites (22). Subsequently, studies from other laboratories with rat liver microsomes and rat liver supernatant confirmed the identity of the reported metabolites along with several new metabolites (Fig. 29-7). The new metabolites were 9-hydroxywarfarin (23), dehydrowarfarin, 10-hydroxywarfarin (24), and the two diastereoisomeric "warfarin alcohols" resulting from reduction of the side chain carbonyl group (23).

The first human metabolites to be identified were 6- and 7-hydroxywarfarin along with the two warfarin alco-

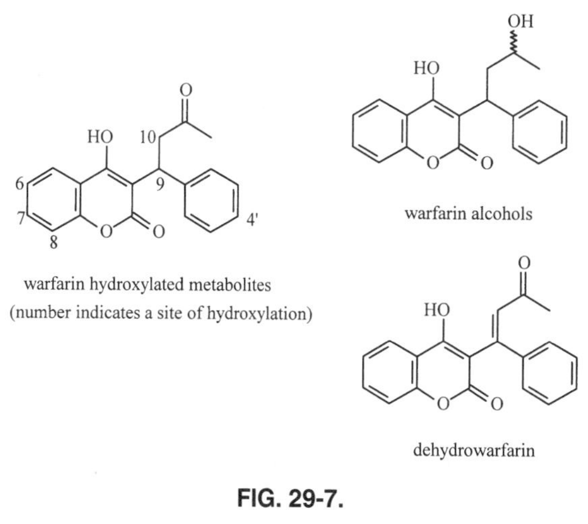

warfarin hydroxylated metabolites
(number indicates a site of hydroxylation)

warfarin alcohols

dehydrowarfarin

FIG. 29-7.

hols (25,26). The 7-hydroxy metabolite was found to originate almost exclusively from (S)-warfarin, whereas the 6-hydroxy metabolite was formed from both (R)- and (S)-warfarin (20). Warfarin alcohol 1, the major reductive metabolite, was formed from (R)-warfarin (20) and had the (9R,11S) absolute configuration (27), whereas warfarin alcohol 2 was formed from (S)-warfarin (20) and had the (9S,11S) absolute configuration (27). Later, the 8-hydroxy- and 4'-hydroxywarfarin metabolites were also found in humans. In humans, the formation of 8-hydroxywarfarin is stereoselective for (R)-warfarin (28), whereas the formation of 4'-hydroxywarfarin is stereoselective for (S)-warfarin (29). However, (S)-4'-hydroxywarfarin is such a minor metabolite that it is normally only seen under conditions of enzyme induction, such as with rifampin treatment (29).

Preliminary evidence for 9-hydroxywarfarin as a human metabolite was gained from mass spectral analysis of the urinary extract of a volunteer who had received an oral dose of 9-deuteriowarfarin (23), but its presence as a normal metabolite lacks confirmation. Structurally, it is likely to be relatively unstable and prone to dehydrate to dehydrowarfarin. Indeed, it has been suggested that metabolic formation of dehydrowarfarin occurs via cytochrome P450-catalyzed 9-hydroxylation followed by spontaneous dehydration (24).

Dehydrowarfarin and 10-hydroxywarfarin were first identified as human metabolites of warfarin after incubation with human liver microsomes (30). Later, dehydrowarfarin was confirmed as a urinary warfarin metabolite in a drug interaction study with diltiazem (31).

10-Hydroxywarfarin was synthesized and chemically characterized, and the absolute configurations of the four possible isomers were determined (32). Once synthetic standards were available, (9R,10S)-10-hydroxywarfarin was found to be a significant (10%–20%) metabolite of (R)-warfarin in humans (33). Virtually all of an oral dose of racemic warfarin can be accounted for by recovered parent drug and the summed contribution of the primary metabolites listed earlier. There are no major human metabolites of either (R)- or (S)-warfarin left to be discovered. Furthermore, in the human, secondary metabolism in the form of conjugation of the primary metabolites does not appear to be quantitatively important. Moreover, any sulfated or glucuronidated species that might be present in urine can be enzymatically hydrolyzed back to primary metabolites before analysis.

The increasing availability of human liver microsomes and cDNA-expressed forms of the various P450s produced a major breakthrough in the metabolic arena by allowing the specific P450s associated with a given metabolic transformation to be identified. Specific human P450s that contribute to the metabolism of (R)- and (S)-warfarin are listed in Table 29-1.

Phenprocoumon

Like warfarin, phenprocoumon is a weak organic acid with a pKa of approximately 5. It is well absorbed (43) and at least 98% plasma protein bound (44). It has a whole body clearance, CL, of about 0.01 mL·min^{-1}·kg^{-1}, a volume of distribution, Vd, of 0.11 to 0.18 L/kg, and a

TABLE 29-1. *Relative* in vivo *quantitative importance of human metabolites of (R)- and (S)-warfarin and the enzymes responsible for their formation*

Warfarin metabolite	Enzyme[a] that forms metabolite		In vivo[b] relative importance	
	(R)-metabolite	(S)-metabolite	(R)-metabolite	(S)-metabolite
4'-Hydroxy	3A4 (34,35); 1A2 (35); 2C18, 2C19 (38)	3A4 (35); 1A2 (35); 2C8, 2C18, 2C19 (38)	Trace (29[c],31)	Minor (29[c],31)
6-Hydroxy	**1A2**[d] (35,39); 3A4 (34); 2C19 (38)	**2C9** (35,38); 1A2 (35); 3A4 (35,39)	Moderate (28, 29,33,40–42)	Moderate (28,29,33,40–42)
7-Hydroxy	1A2 (35,39); 3A4 (35); 2C8 (38)	**2C9** (35,38); 1A2, 3A4 (35)	Minor (28,29,33, 40–42)	Major (28,29,33,40–42)
8-Hydroxy	**2C19** (36,38); 1A2 (35,37,39); 1A1 (37)	1A2 (35); 3A4 (35)	Moderate (28, 29,33,41,42)	Trace (28,33,41,42) Minor (29)
9-Hydroxy			Trace (23)	Trace (23)
Dehydro	3A4 (34)	3A4 (34)	Minor (31)	Minor (31)
10-Hydroxy	**3A4** (34,35,39)	3A4 (35)	Moderate (33)	
Alcohol 1 (R,S)	Ketoreductase		Moderate (28,29, 33,40–42)	Trace (29,41)
Alcohol 2 (S,S)		Ketoreductase	Trace (29,41)	Minor (28,29,33, 40–42)

[a]All enzymes are cytochrome P450s except for the ketoreductase.
[b]Trace <2%, minor <10%, moderate <35%, major >35%.
[c]Rifampin induction.
[d]Bold letters identify the major contributing isoform at therapeutic concentrations.

half-life, $t_{1/2}$, of 5.4 to 5.5 days (45,46). Also like warfarin, the benzylic carbon atom (C9) of phenprocoumon is chiral. The (S)-enantiomer is the more potent (1.5–2.5) anticoagulant (45), but the drug is only available clinically as the racemic mixture.

Metabolites of phenprocoumon were first identified from the rat and were found to be the 6-, 7-, 8-, and 4'-hydroxylated analogues (47–49). Unlike warfarin, phenprocoumon and its metabolites are extensively conjugated in the human. The elimination products of two-thirds of an administered dose are found in urine whereas one-third is found in feces. After enzymatic hydrolysis (glusulase), 6-, 7-, and 4'-hydroxyphenprocoumon were identified as metabolites. Together with parent drug (one-third of the dose), these metabolites accounted for virtually 100% of the administered dose (43). Evidence for the formation of 8-hydroxyphenprocoumon was noticeably absent (43). Similar to the quantitative metabolism of warfarin, the dominant metabolic pathway was formation of (S)-7-hydroxyphenprocoumon, followed by formation of (R)- and (S)-6-hydroxyphenprocoumon in almost equal amounts. In contrast to warfarin metabolism, 4'-hydroxylation [stereoselective for (S)-phenprocoumon], but not 8-hydroxylation, is a significant metabolic pathway for phenprocoumon (43). Unexpectedly, human liver microsomal metabolism of phenprocoumon did not mirror its metabolism *in vivo. In vitro*, the major metabolite formed was 4'-hydroxyphenprocoumon, not 7-hydroxyphenprocoumon. In addition, 8-hydroxyphenprocoumon is definitely formed, albeit as a minor product, and all four metabolites—4'-hydroxy, 6-hydroxy, 7-hydroxy, and 8-hydroxy—are formed with little apparent stereoselective preference (50). The reasons for the apparent differences in human *in vivo* and *in vitro* metabolism of phenprocoumon could be caused by a number of factors: (a) different levels of expression of the various P450s in the livers in the two experiments, (b) extrahepatic contributions to the metabolite pool, or (c) the extensive formation of a conjugate of phenprocoumon and its subsequent hydroxylation.

Expressed P450 2C9–catalyzed turnover of phenprocoumon is stereoselective for (S)-phenprocoumon, but the enzyme shows little regioselectivity, that is, all four metabolites are produced by P450 2C9 at roughly comparable levels except there is a much lower production of 8-hydroxyphenprocoumon (50). The identities of additional specific human P450s that contribute to phenprocoumon metabolism have not yet been published.

Acenocoumarol

Acenocoumarol, the *p*-nitrophenyl analogue of warfarin, is well absorbed and highly (98%) plasma protein bound (51,52). It has a whole body clearance, CL, of about 3.5 L/hour and a half-life, $t_{1/2}$, of approximately 9

hours (52–54). In contrast to warfarin and phenprocoumon, (R)-acenocoumarol rather than (S)-acenocoumarol has been reported to be responsible for most of the anticoagulant activity of a racemic dose of the drug (54,55). Because all three drugs—warfarin, phenprocoumon, and acenocoumarol—are closely related structurally and elicit their anticoagulant effects by the same mechanism (inhibition of vitamin K epoxide reductase), one would expect stereochemically related enantiomers for each drug to be the most potent. (S)-warfarin and (S)-phenprocoumon are more active than their respective (R) counterparts, but the opposite was reported to be true for acenocoumarol (54). The possibility of this seeming anomaly being due to a misassignment of absolute configurations has been eliminated by the definitive determinations of the absolute configurations of all three drugs (56–60). Rather than (R)-acenocoumarol being intrinsically more potent than (S)-acenocoumarol, the clinical effect appears to be attributable to the much higher plasma concentration of (R)-acenocoumarol that develops because of the much more rapid clearance of (S)-acenocoumarol (54).

Dieterle and co-workers (51) were the first to study the metabolism of acenocoumarol in humans. They identified two oxidized and four reduced metabolites. The two oxidized metabolites—6- and 7-hydroxyacenocoumarol—accounted for 20% to 40% of the administered dose. Of the four reduced metabolites, the two diastereomeric alcohols, resulting from reduction of the side chain carbonyl group, accounted for 6% to 13% of the dose, whereas 4'-aminoacenocoumarol, resulting from reduction of the 4'-nitro group, and its *N*-acetylated conjugate, accounted for 19% to 31% of the dose. Subsequently, Thijssen and colleagues (52,61,62) demonstrated that 4'-aminoacenocoumarol and its *N*-acetylated conjugate were formed primarily by intestinal microflora and therefore the amount formed was highly dependent on the formulation of acenocoumarol used for oral administration. Administration of tablets (Sintrom) leads to rapid absorption and virtually no formation of the amino metabolite and its derivative. More prolonged adsorption, the result of encapsulated acenocoumarol administration, leads to significant formation of both metabolites. In an extensive *in vitro* study with human liver microsomes, Hermans and Thijssen (63) demonstrated that the metabolism of both (R)- and (S)-acenocoumarol correspond qualitatively to the metabolism of (R)- and (S)-warfarin, respectively. For both drugs, the 6- and 7-hydroxy metabolites are quantitatively the most important. However, clearance to these two metabolites is much more rapid for acenocoumarol, particularly (S)-acenocoumarol. The microsomal results are consistent with an earlier *in vivo* study in which the half-lives of (S)- and (R)-acenocoumarol were found to be 0.5 to 1.0 and 8 to 10 hours, respectively, whereas those for (S)- and (R)-warfarin were found to be

24 to 33 and 35 to 58 hours, respectively (64). Extensive inhibition of the 6- and 7-hydroxylation of both (R)- and (S)-acenocoumarol by 25 μM of the selective P450 2C9 inhibitor sulfaphenazole, indicates that this specific enzyme is a major contributor to the metabolism of acenocoumarol. A similar, but less extensive, inhibitory profile with 100 μM omeprazole indicates that P450 2C19 also contributes to the formation of these two metabolites, again from both enantiomers (63). These results, although compelling, remain to be confirmed with expressed P450 2C9 and P450 2C19. Metabolic studies with acenocoumarol and expressed human P450s have yet to be published.

DRUG INTERACTIONS

The oral anticoagulants are classic in terms of a drug group that is susceptible to drug interactions. There is extensive published material, particularly for warfarin, listing the drugs and foods with which it is believed to interact [see numerous pharmacological texts, compendia, and reviews (65–70)]. A discussion follows on those interactions that are metabolic in origin, specifically those that are caused by inhibition of the enzymes (primarily P450s) responsible for the metabolic transformation and deactivation of the active anticoagulant. For the 4-hydroxycoumarin oral anticoagulants, this would mean interactions resulting from a significantly decreased clearance of the S-enantiomer of the anticoagulant, because it is inherently the most pharmacologically active.

To begin to understand such interactions, one first needs to know which enzymes are the main contributors to the metabolism of the drug. Ultimately, such knowledge can only be gained from *in vitro* experiments using isolated purified P450s or cDNA-expressed P450s. However, with the availability of expressed P450s, human liver microsomes, and a well-established database of selective inhibitors, the task has become considerably easier. Once the P450s responsible for the metabolism of a drug are known, some means of relating their *in vitro* to their *in vivo* catalytic activity toward the drug must be used. One approach is to determine the kinetic parameters associated with the formation of the metabolites of the drug that is catalyzed by a specific P450. The *in vitro* V_{max}/K_m value for metabolite formation that is catalyzed by a single P450 should be comparable to the formation clearance, CL_f, for that metabolite *in vivo*, as long as no other P450s are significant contributors to that metabolite at the concentration of drug that prevails *in vivo*. The determination of V_{max}/K_m provides a necessary, albeit not perfect, linkage for correlating *in vitro* with *in vivo* metabolic behavior. If the fraction of parent drug that is converted to a specific metabolite by a specific P450 is known, the goodness of the correlation depends primarily on two factors: (a) the relative concentration of that specific P450 in human liver preparations versus its *in vivo* concentration in the liver and (b) the fidelity of P450 behavior across the *in vitro* and *in vivo* environments. The potential power of the correlation is highlighted by the rank-order correlation that was achieved for warfarin metabolism at a time when its complete metabolism and the relative contributions of specific P450s were unknown (71) (Table 29-2).

Because the K_i value of a competitive inhibitor toward an enzyme is independent of both inhibitor and enzyme concentration, it is a parameter that (theoretically) should provide an even better correlation of *in vitro* and *in vivo* metabolic behavior (see Chapter 1). Assuming that the fidelity of P450 behavior across the *in vitro* and *in vivo* environments is maintained, then equal concentrations of the inhibitor at the enzyme either *in vitro* or *in vivo* should produce the same degree of inhibition. Thus, if a drug attains an *in vivo* plasma concentration that approximates or exceeds its K_i for the inhibition of some P450 that dominates the clearance of a second drug, a significant interaction would be expected between the two drugs if they were coadministered. As the extrapolation of *in*

TABLE 29-2. *Comparison of normalized warfarin metabolite clearances from human liver microsomes versus normalized metabolite formation clearances from human subjects*

Warfarin metabolites	*In vitro* Metabolite clearance, V_{max}/K_m % of total metabolism; N = 3	*In vivo* Human subjects, Cl_f % of total Cl
(S)-4′-hydroxy	1.3–5.6	0
(S)-6-hydroxy (high K_m)	1.2–2.8	—
(S)-6-hydroxy (low K_m)	18.9–25.6	16.3
(S)-7-hydoxy	43.3–63.9	63.1
(S)-8-hydoxy	0–0.4	0.3
(R)-4′-hydroxy	0.5–2.5	0
(R)-6-hydroxy	4.7–16.5	9.2
(R)-7-hydroxy	0.9–3.5	4.7
(R)-8-hydroxy	1.5–4.9	6.4

Data from Rettie AE, Eddy AC, Heimark LD, Gibaldi M, Trager WR. Characteristics of warfarin hydroxylation catalyzed by human liver microsomes. *Drug Metab Dispos* 1989;17:265–270.

vitro K_i to identify possible *in vivo* interactions has gained wide acceptance, factors that confound the correlation (mechanism-based or time-dependent inhibitors, inhibitory properties of metabolites, possible differences in unbound inhibitor plasma concentration, and inhibitor concentration at the active site of the enzyme) are being recognized and are receiving considerable attention (72). Considerations of this sort have led to the formulation of an *in vivo* K_i (73), which together with the *in vitro* K_i, is being explored as an approach to quantitative *in vitro/in vivo* comparisons as a means of circumventing some of the problems discussed in Chapter 1.

The following discussion involves specific drug interactions for warfarin, phenprocoumon, and acenocoumarol that have enzyme inhibition as the basis for the interaction. Because the metabolic contributions of the various P450s to the elimination of the three anticoagulants being considered are quantitatively and, to some extent, qualitatively different, the susceptibility of the individual anticoagulants to the inhibitory effects of a comedication should differ, and this, indeed, appears to be the case.

Warfarin

The metabolic inactivation of (S)-warfarin, the pharmacologically more potent enantiomer, is controlled by a single enzyme, P450 (CYP) 2C9 (35). The formation of (S)-6- and (S)-7-hydroxywarfarin by 2C9 accounts for at least 80% of the systemic clearance of (S)-warfarin (28). Because this single enzyme controls such a large fraction of the clearance of (S)-warfarin, inhibition of 2C9 is expected to have a major impact on (S)-warfarin clearance and result in an enhanced anticoagulant response. In contrast, no single enzyme dominates the metabolism of (R)-warfarin. P450s 3A4, 2C19, and 1A2 are the major contributors together with a ketoreductase that forms warfarin alcohol 1 (28,36,71). Thus, even extensive inhibition of any one of these enzymes would not be expected to have a major impact on (R)-warfarin clearance and anticoagulant response. In general, this is what is found.

Phenylbutazone

Coadministration of warfarin as a racemate (20) or as separate individual (R)- and (S)-enantiomers (21) with phenylbutazone results in a substantial increase in hypothrombinemic effect, which is accompanied by a decrease in the clearance of (S)-warfarin and an increase in the clearance of (R)-warfarin. When protein binding was taken into account, the unbound clearance of (S)-warfarin was then shown to decrease by four-fold relative to its unbound clearance in the absence of phenylbutazone, whereas the unbound clearance of (R)-was relatively unchanged (40). Consistent with the dramatic decrease in the unbound clearance of (S)-warfarin was the 90% and

93% reductions in the intrinsic formation clearances of (S)-6- and (S)-7-hydroxywarfarin, respectively.

Sulfinpyrazone

The sulfinpyrazone-warfarin interaction is similar to the phenylbutazone-warfarin interaction in that the increase in anticoagulant effect is accompanied by a significant decrease in the unbound clearance of (S)-warfarin and little change in the unbound clearance of (R)-warfarin (28,74). Again, the decrease in unbound (S)-warfarin clearance was associated with significant decreases in the intrinsic formation clearances for (S)-6- and (S)-7-hydroxywarfarin, 42% and 65%, respectively. Subsequently, it became known that P450 2C9 was responsible for the formation of virtually all (S)-7-hydroxywarfarin as well as most of (S)-6-hydroxywarfarin. Work was then initiated to determine whether the *in vitro* K_i for sulfinpyrazone inhibition of P450 2C9 in human liver microsomes would have predicted the interaction that was observed *in vivo*. The results revealed that sulfinpyrazone itself was probably not the primary inhibitory species, but rather it was the sulfide metabolite of sulfinpyrazone that was responsible for the interaction (75).

Amiodarone

Amiodarone inhibits the whole body clearance of both (R)- and (S)-warfarin when warfarin is present as either the racemic mixture or the individual enantiomers. The hypothrombinemic response is enhanced in all cases (76). In a subsequent investigation, the formation clearances of all metabolic pathways were depressed by amiodarone, although the metabolites of (S)-warfarin were affected to a greater extent than the metabolites of (R)-warfarin (77). The *in vivo* depression of warfarin clearances and metabolite formation was much greater than their depression *in vitro* (77). Even though the reason for the discrepancy is unknown, two possibilities seem likely. First, amiodarone is known to accumulate in liver such that liver concentrations can be orders of magnitude higher than plasma concentration (78). Second, the *N*-desethyl metabolite of amiodarone could make a significant contribution to the inhibitory profile because it is a secondary amine that could complex with heme and it achieves plasma concentrations that are as high as parent drug (79).

Miconazole

Miconazole markedly augments the anticoagulant effect and inhibits the whole body clearance of both (R)- and (S)-warfarin, but (S)-warfarin clearance is inhibited to the greatest extent. A 125-mg daily dose of miconazole inhibits the formation clearance of (S)-6-hydroxywarfarin by about 87% and that of (S)-7-hydroxywarfarin by about 94%. These results are consistent with the almost total blockade of P450 2C9 activity. The inhibitory effect of miconazole on (S)- and (R)-warfarin metabolism was qualitatively but not quantitatively predicted by *in vitro* kinetic data. The inhibitory potency of miconazole was found to be much greater *in vivo* than *in vitro*. The reason for the discrepancy is unknown (80).

Fluconazole

The ability of fluconazole to inhibit the oxidative pathways of (R)- and (S)-warfarin metabolism was first studied and K_i determined *in vitro* with human liver microsomes and expressed enzymes (39). P450 2C9 was found to be inhibited with a K_i of 7 to 8 μM, suggesting that, because the normal therapeutic plasma levels of fluconazole *in vivo* are 15 to 400 μM, a significant interaction should be expected. This was indeed found to be the case because fluconazole greatly increased anticoagulant effect and inhibited the (S)-warfarin formation clearances to (S)-6- and (S)-7-hydroxywarfarin by about 70% (33). The determination of an *in vivo* K_i for inhibition of (S)-7-hydroxywarfarin formation by fluconazole of 22 μM is in reasonable agreement with the K_i of 7 to 8 μM determined *in vitro*, indicating that, at least for fluconazole, *in vitro* data are highly predictive of *in vivo* behavior (73).

Cimetidine

Cimetidine inhibits the clearance of (R)-warfarin but has no effect on the clearance of (S)-warfarin (81–83). Whereas one study found an increased anticoagulant response with cimetidine (81), another did not (83). A dose of 1200 mg/day of cimetidine was used in the study that found the interaction, whereas a dose of 800 mg/day was used in the study that did not find an interaction, suggesting an effect that is dose dependent and marginal. It was later determined, based on apparent formation clearance values, that significant inhibition of metabolic pathways by cimetidine was restricted to the formation of (R)-6- and (R)-7-hydroxywarfarin, that is, it selectively affects the least potent warfarin enantiomer (84).

Enoxacin

The fluoroquinolone enoxacin does not enhance the anticoagulant effect of warfarin. It does significantly inhibit the P450 1A2–dependent 6-hydroxylation of (R)-warfarin while leaving the clearance of (S)-warfarin unaffected (85).

Diltiazem

The anticoagulant effect of warfarin is not potentiated by diltiazem. Diltiazem does inhibit the P450 1A2–cat-

alyzed inhibition of (R)-6-hydroxywarfarin and the P450 2C19–catalyzed inhibition of (R)-8-hydroxywarfarin without affecting the clearance of (S)-warfarin (31).

Phenprocoumon

The long half-life of phenprocoumon (approximately 5.5 days) coupled with the fact that approximately one-third of a dose is eliminated unchanged suggests that phenprocoumon should be less susceptible to metabolically based drug interactions than warfarin. Rodman and co-workers reported these clinically based findings in 1964 (86). In addition, the relative lack of established phenprocoumon drug interactions in the literature tend to support this assessment.

Phenylbutazone

Phenylbutazone has been reported to markedly increase racemic phenprocoumon plasma levels and prothrombin times, but that is the extent of knowledge of the interaction (87).

Sulfinpyrazone

In contrast to its effect on warfarin, sulfinpyrazone does not potentiate the anticoagulant activity of phenprocoumon nor decrease its clearance (87). A more extensive study on the fate of the individual enantiomers confirmed the findings of the earlier study and indicated that sulfinpyrazone inhibits the formation clearance of the oxidative metabolites derived from (S)-phenprocoumon by 40% to 60% (88). Presumably, the overall lower level of oxidative metabolism of (S)-phenprocoumon, relative to (S)-warfarin, coupled to its slower turnover rate, translates into a percent increase in parent drug concentration that is insufficient to cause a statistically distinct increase in prothrombin time.

Cimetidine

Cimetidine is reported to have no effect on either the clearance or the anticoagulant effect of phenprocoumon (89,90).

Acenocoumarol

The half-lives of (R)- and (S)-acenocoumarol—8 to 10 and 0.5 hours, respectively (64)—are the opposite extreme to those of (R)- and (S)-phenprocoumon, both of which are about 5.5 days (45,46). 6- and 7-Hydroxylation of both enantiomers of acenocoumarol are the major routes of elimination; P450 2C9 appears to be the major catalyst for the formation of all four metabolites (63). These data suggest that acenocoumarol should not only be subject to all of the P450-inhibitory drug interactions that warfarin is susceptible to, but also, for a given inhibitor, the effects should be more severe. Overall, this analysis suggests that, of the three anticoagulants, acenocoumarol should be the most susceptible to drug interactions. Even though more acenocoumarol than phenprocoumon drug interactions are documented in the literature, this is not true for warfarin, possibly because acenocoumarol has not been used as extensively as warfarin, nor has it been studied as extensively.

Sulfinpyrazone

Sulfinpyrazone was found to significantly augment the prothrombin time in a study of 22 patients taking acenocoumarol, but the pharmacokinetic parameters of parent drug or metabolites were not examined (91).

Amiodarone

Concomitant administration of amiodarone and acenocoumarol to 36 patients resulted in an augmented anticoagulant effect in 36 patients; in 7 of these patients, severe bleeding diathesis developed (92). Although blood levels of acenocoumarol or its metabolites were not determined, it was suggested in an earlier patient study that the basis of the interaction was inhibition of acenocoumarol metabolism (93).

Miconazole

Miconazole was found to lead to a marked increase in the anticoagulant activity elicited by acenocoumarol, but the interaction was not characterized further (94).

Cimetidine

A potential cimetidine-acenocoumarol interaction was studied in five subjects and the plasma concentrations of (R)- and (S)-acenocoumarol were determined. Cimetidine inhibited the clearance of (R)-acenocoumarol but not that of (S)-acenocoumarol. Despite a consistent pharmacokinetic effect on (R)-acenocoumarol clearance, an increased anticoagulant response was only produced in some of the subjects (95).

REFERENCES

1. Link KP. The discovery of dicumarol and its sequels. *Circulation* 1959; 19:97–107.
2. Weiner M, Shapiro S, Axelrod J, Cooper JR, Brodie BB. Physiological disposition of dicumarol in man. *J Pharmacol Exp Ther* 1950;99:409–420.
3. O'Reilly RA, Aggeler PM, Leong LS. Studies on the coumarin anticoagulant drugs: comparison of the pharmacodynamics of dicumarol and warfarin in man. *Thromb Diath Haemorrh* 1964;11:1–22.
4. Holmes RW, Love J. Suicide attempt with warfarin, a bishydroxycoumarin-like rodenticide. *JAMA* 1952;148:935–937.
5. Pollock BE. Clinical experience with warfarin (Coumadin) sodium, a new anticoagulant. *JAMA* 1955;159:1094–1097.
6. Suttie JW. Vitamin K-dependent carboxylation of glutamyl residues in proteins. *Biofactors* 1988;1:55–60.
7. Morris DP, Soute BAM, Vermeers C, Stafford DW. Characterization of the purified vitamin K-dependent τ-glutamyl carboxylase. *J Biol Chem* 1993;268:8735–8742.
8. Matschiner JR, Zimmerman A, Bell RG. The influence of warfarin on vitamin K epoxide reductase. *Thromb Diath Haemorrh Suppl* 1973;57:45–52.
9. Cain D, Hutson SM, Wallin R. Assembly of the warfarin-sensitive vitamin K 2,3-epoxide reductase enzyme complex in the endoplasmic reticulum membrane. *J Biol Chem* 1997;272:29068–29075.
10. WHO Expert Committee on Biological Standardization. 33rd Report, Geneva, Switzerland: World Health Organization; 1983. Technical Report Series No. 687.
11. Oertel LB. International normalized ratio (INR): an improved way to monitor oral anticoagulant therapy. *Nurse Pract* 1995;20(9):15–16, 21–22.
12. Hirsh J, Poller L. The international normalized ratio: a guide to understanding and correcting its problems. *Arch Intern Med* 1994;154:282–288.
13. Hirsh J, Dalen JE, Anderson DR, et al. Oral anticoagulants: mechanism of action, clinical effectiveness, and optimal therapeutic range. *Chest* 1998;114:445S–469S.
14. Pineo G, Hull RD. Adverse effects of coumarin anticoagulants. *Drug Saf* 1993;9(4):263–271.
15. Chan E, McLachlan AJ, Pegg M, MacKay AD, Cole RB, Rowland M. Disposition of warfarin enantiomers and metabolites in patients during multiple dosing with *rac*-warfarin. *Br J Clin Pharmacol* 1994;37:563–569.
16. Hewick DS, McEwen J. Plasma half-lives, plasma metabolite and the anticoagulant efficacies of the enantiomers of warfarin in man. *J Pharm Pharmacol* 1973;25:458–465.
17. Breckenridge A, Orme M, Wessling H, Lewis RJ, Gibbons R. Pharmacokinetics and pharmacodynamics of the enantiomers of warfarin in man. *Clin Pharmacol Ther* 1974;15:424–430.
18. O'Reilly RA. Studies on the optical enantiomorphs of warfarin in man. *Clin Pharmacol Ther* 1974;16:348–354.
19. Aggeler PM, O'Reilly RA, Leong L, Kowitz PE. Potentiation of anticoagulant effect of warfarin by phenylbutazone. *N Engl J Med* 1967;67:496–501.
20. Lewis RJ, Trager WF, Chan KK, et al. Warfarin: stereochemical aspects of it metabolism and the interaction with phenylbutazone. *J Clin Invest* 1974;53:1607–1617.
21. O'Reilly RA, Trager WF, Motley CH, Howald W. Stereoselective interaction of phenylbutazone with (^{12}C/^{13}C)warfarin pseudoracemates in man. *J Clin Invest* 1980;65:746–753.
22. Barker WM, Hermodson MA, Link KP. The metabolism of 4-^{14}C-warfarin sodium by the rat. *J Pharmacol Exp Ther* 1970;171:307–313.
23. Pohl LR, Garland WA, Nelson SD, Trager WF. The rapid identification of a new metabolite of warfarin via a chemical ionization mass spectrometry ion doublet technique. *Biomed Mass Spect* 1975;2:23–30.
24. Fasco MJ, Dymerski PP, Dos JD, Kaminsky LS. A new warfarin metabolite: structure and function. *J Med Chem* 1978;21:1054–1059.
25. Lewis RJ, Trager WF. Warfarin metabolism in man; identification of metabolites in urine. *J Clin Invest* 1970;49:907–913.
26. Trager WF, Lewis RJ, Garland WA. Mass spectral analysis in the identification of human metabolites of warfarin. *J Med Chem* 1970;13:1196–1204.
27. Chan KK, Lewis RJ, Trager WF. The absolute configuration of the four warfarin alcohols. *J Med Chem* 1972;15:1265–1270.
28. Toon S, Low LK, Gibaldi M, et al. The warfarin-sulfinpyrazone interaction: stereochemical considerations. *Clin Pharmacol Ther* 1986;39:15–25.
29. Heimark LD, Gibaldi M, Trager WF, O'Reilly RA, Goulart DA. The mechanism of the warfarin-rifampin drug interaction in humans. *Clin Pharmacol Ther* 1987;42:388–394.
30. Kaminsky LS, Dunbar DA, Wang PP, et al. Human hepatic cytochrome P-450 composition as probed by in vitro microsomal metabolism of warfarin. *Drug Metab Dispos* 1984;12:470–477.
31. Abernethy DL, Kaminsky LS, Dickinson DS. Selective inhibition of warfarin metabolism by diltiazem in humans. *J Pharmacol Exp Ther* 1991;257:411–415.

32. Lawrence RF, Rettie AE, Eddy AC, Trager WF. Chemical synthesis, absolute configuration, and stereochemistry of formation of 10-hydroxywarfarin: a major oxidative metabolite of (+)-(R)-warfarin from hepatic microsomal preparations. *Chirality* 1990;2:96–105.

33. Black DJ, Kunze KL, Wienkers LC, et al. Warfarin-fluconazole II: a metabolically based drug interaction: in vivo studies. *Drug Metab Dispos* 1996;24:422–428.

34. Brian WR, Sari M, Iwasaki M, Shimada T, Kaminsky LS, Guengerich FP. Catalytic activities of human liver cytochrome P-IIIA4 expressed in *Saccaromyces cerevisiae*. *Biochemistry* 1990;29:11280–11292.

35. Rettie AR, Korzekwa KR, Kunze KL, et al. Hydroxylation of warfarin by human cDNA expressed cytochrome P-450: a role for proteins encoded by CYP2C9 in the etiology of anticoagulant drug interactions. *Chem Res Toxicol* 1992;5:54–59.

36. Wienkers LC, Wurden CJ, Storch E, et al. Formation of (R)-8-hydroxywarfarin in human liver microsomes: a new metabolic marker for the (S)-mephenytoin hydroxylase, P4502C19. *Drug Metab Dispos* 1996;24:610–614.

37. Zhang Z, Fasco MJ, Huang Z, Guengerich FP, Kaminsky LS. Human cytochromes P450 1A1 and 1A2: R-warfarin metabolism as a probe. *Drug Metab Dispos* 1995;23:1339–1345.

38. Kaminsky LS, de Morais SM, Faletto MB, Dunbar DA, Goldstein JA. Correlation of human cytochrome P4502C substrates specificities with primary structure: warfarin as a probe. *Mol Pharmacol* 1993;43:234–239.

39. Kunze KL, Wienkers LC, Thummel KE, Trager WF. Warfarin-fluconazole I: inhibition of the human cytochrome P450-dependent metabolism of warfarin by fluconazole: in vitro studies. *Drug Metab Dispos* 1996;24:414–421.

40. Banfield C, O'Reilly R, Chan E, Rowland M. Phenybutazone-warfarin interaction in man: further stereochemical and metabolic considerations. *Br J Clin Pharmacol* 1983;16:669–675.

41. O'Reilly RA, Goulart DA, Kunze KL, et al. Mechanisms of the stereoselective interaction between miconazole and racemic warfarin in human subjects. *Clin Pharmacol Ther* 1992;51:656–667.

42. Heimark LD, Wienkers L, Kunze K, et al. The mechanism of the interaction between amiodarone and warfarin in humans. *Clin Pharmacol Ther* 1992;51:398–407.

43. Toon S, Heimark LD, Trager WF, O'Reilly RA. Metabolic fate of phenprocoumon in humans. *J Pharm Sci* 1985;74:1037–1040.

44. Husted S, Andreasen F. Individual variation in the response to phenprocoumon. *Eur J Clin Pharmacol* 1977;11:351–358.

45. Jänchen E, Meinertz T, Gilfrich H-J, Groth U, Martini A. The enantiomers of phenprocoumon: pharmacodynamic and pharmacokinetic studies. *Clin Pharmacol Ther* 1976;20:342–349.

46. Heimark LD, Toon S, Gibaldi M, Trager WF, O'Reilly RA, Goulart DA. The effect of sulfinpyrazone on the disposition of pseudoracemic phenprocoumon in humans. *Clin Pharmacol Ther* 1987;42:312–319.

47. Pohl LR, Haddock R, Trager WF. Synthesis, TLC, UV and MS properties of the anticoagulant phenprocoumon and its monohydroxylated derivatives. *J Med Chem* 1975;18:513–519.

48. Haddock R, Pohl LR, Trager WF. Biotransformation of phenprocoumon in the rat. *J Med Chem* 1975;18:519–523.

49. Wheeler C, Trager WF, Porter WR. Stereochemical aspects of the metabolism of phenprocoumon in rat liver microsomes. *Biochem Pharmacol* 1981;30:1785–1790.

50. He M. Catalytic characteristics of cytochrome P-450 2C9 and their relationship to the metabolism of coumarin anticoagulants and associated drug interactions. Ph.D. thesis, University of Washington, Seattle, Washington, 1995.

51. Dieterle W, Faigle JW, Montigel C, Sulc M, Theobald W. Biotransformation and pharmacokinetics of acenocoumarol (Sintrom) in man. *Eur J Clin Pharmacol* 1977;11:367–375.

52. Thijssen HHW, Baars LG. Active metabolites of acenocoumarol: do they contribute to the therapeutic effect? *Br J Clin Pharmacol* 1983;16:491–496.

53. Popovic J, Mikov M, Jakovljevic V. Pharmacokinetic analysis of a new acenocoumarol tablet formulation during a bioequivalence study. *Eur J Drug Metab Pharmacokinet* 1994;2:85–89.

54. Godbillon J, Richard J, Gerardin A, Meinertz T, Kasper W, Jähnchen E. Pharmacokinetics of the enantiomers of acenocoumarol in man. *Br J Clin Pharmacol* 1981;12:621–629.

55. Meinertz T, Kasper W, Kahl C, Jähnchen E. Anticoagulant activity of the enantiomers of acenocoumarol. *Br J Clin Pharmacol* 1978;5: 187–188.

56. West BD, Preis S, Schroeder CH, Link CP. Studies on the 4-hydroxycoumarins XVII: resolution and absolute configuration of warfarin. *J Am Chem Soc* 1961;83:2676–2679.

57. Valente EJ, Trager WF, Jensen LH. The crystal and molecular structure and absolute configuration of (−)(S)-warfarin. *Acta Cryst* 1975;B31:954–960.

58. West BD, Link KP. The resolution and absolute configuration of "marcumar" (1). *J Hetero Chem* 1965;2:93–94.

59. Valente EJ, Trager WF, Lingafelter EC. (−)-3-(1-Phenylpropyl)-4-hydroxycoumarin. *Acta Cryst* 1976;B32:277–279.

60. Wheeler CR, Trager WF. Absolute configuration of acenocoumarin. *J Med Chem* 1979;22:1122–1124.

61. Thijssen HH, Baars LG, Reijnders MJ. Analysis of acenocoumarin and its amino and acetamido metabolites in body fluids by high-performance liquid chromatography. *J Chromatogr* 1983;274:231–238.

62. Thijssen HH, Baars LG, Hazen MJ, Van den Bogaard AE. The role of intestinal microflora in the reductive metabolism of acenocoumarol in man. *Br J Clin Pharmacol* 1984;18:247–249.

63. Hermans JJ, Thijssen HH. Human liver microsomal metabolism of the enantiomers of warfarin and acenocoumarol: P450 isozyme diversity determines the differences in their pharmacokinetics. *Br J Pharmacol* 1993;110:482–490.

64. Thijssen HHW, Jansen GMJ, Baars LGM. Lack of effect of cimetidine on pharmacodynamics and kinetics of single oral doses of R- and S-acenocoumarol. *Eur J Pharmacol* 1986;30:619–623.

65. Drug interactions with anticoagulants and fibrinolytic agents. In: Griffin JP, D'Arcy PF, eds. *A manual of adverse drug interactions.* New York: Elsevier, 1997:177–208.

66. Anticoagulants. In: Burnham T, ed. *Drug facts and comparisons.* St. Louis: Michael R. Riley, 1999;88f–88g.

67. American Medical Association. *Drug evaluations annual 1995.* American Medical Association. Chicago: 1995:773.

68. Freedman MD, Olatidoye AG. Clinically significant drug interactions with the oral anticoagulants. *Drug Saf* 1994;10:381–394.

69. Wells PS, Holbrook AM, Crowther NR, Hirsh J. Interactions of warfarin with drugs and food. *Ann Intern Med* 1994;121:676–683.

70. Hirsh J, Dalen JE, Anderson DR, et al. Oral anticoagulants: mechanisms of action, clinical effectiveness, and optimal therapeutic range. *Chest* 1998;114[Suppl]:445S–469S.

71. Rettie AE, Eddy AC, Heimark LD, Gibaldi M, Trager WR. Characteristics of warfarin hydroxylation catalyzed by human liver microsomes. *Drug Metab Dispos* 1989;17:265–270.

72. Bertz RJ, Granneman GR. Use of in vitro and in vivo data to estimate the likelihood of metabolic pharmacokinetic interactions. *Clin Pharmacokinet* 1997;32:210–258.

73. Kunze KL, Trager WF. Warfarin-fluconazole III: a rational approach to management of a metabolically based drug interaction. *Drug Metab Dispos* 1996;24:429–435.

74. Toon S, Trager WF. Pharmacokinetic implications of stereoselective changes in plasma-protein binding: warfarin/sulfinpyrazone. *J Pharm Sci* 1984;73:1671–1673.

75. He M, Kunze KL, Trager WF. Inhibition of (S)-warfarin metabolism by sulfinpyrazone and its metabolites. *Drug Metab Dispos* 1995;23:659–663.

76. O'Reilly RA, Trager WF, Rettie AE, Goulart DA. Interaction of amiodarone with racemic warfarin and its separated enantiomorphs in humans. *Clin Pharmacol Ther* 1987;42:290–294.

77. Heimark LD, Wienkers L, Kunze K, et al. The mechanism of the interaction between amiodarone and warfarin in humans. *Clin Pharmacol Ther* 1992;51:398–407.

78. Adams PC, Holt DW, Storey GCA, Morley AR, Callaghan A, Campbell RWF. Amiodarone and its desethyl metabolite: tissue distribution and morphologic changes during long-term therapy. *Circulation* 1985;72:1064–1075.

79. Staubli M, Troendle A, Schmid B, et al. Pharmacokinetics of amiodarone, desethylamiodarone and other iodine-containing amiodarone metabolites. *Eur J Clin Pharmacol* 1985;29:417–423.

80. O'Reilly RA, Goulart DA, Kunze KL, et al. Mechanisms of the stereoselective interaction between miconazole and racemic warfarin in human subjects. *Clin Pharmacol Ther* 1992;51:656–667.

81. O'Reilly RA. Comparative interaction of cimetidine and ranitidine with racemic warfarin in man. *Arch Intern Med* 1984;144:989–991.

82. Choonara IA, Cholerton S, Haynes BP, Breckenridge AM, Park BK.

Stereoselective interaction between the R enantiomer of warfarin and cimetidine. *Br J Clin Pharmacol* 1986;21:271–277.

83. Toon S, Hopkins KJ, Garstang FM, Rowland M. Comparative effects of ranitidine and cimetidine on the pharmacokinetics and pharmacodynamics of warfarin in man. *Eur J Clin Pharmacol* 1987;32:165–172.

84. Niopas I, Toon S, Rowland M. Further insight into the stereoselective interaction between warfarin and cimetidine in man. *Br J Clin Pharmacol* 1991;32:508–511.

85. Toon S, Hopkins KJ, Garstang FM, et al. Enoxacin-warfarin interaction: pharmacokinetic and stereochemical aspects. *Clin Pharmacol Ther* 1987;42:33–41.

86. Rodman T, Pator BH, Resnick ME. Phenprocoumon, diphenadione, warfarin and bishydroxycoumarin: a comparative study. *Am J Med Sci* 1964;247:655–660.

87. O'Reilly RA. Phenylbutazone and sulfinpyrazone interaction with oral anticoagulant phenprocoumon. *Arch Intern Med* 1982;142:1634–1637.

88. Heimark LD, Toon S, Gibaldi M, Trager WF, O'Reilly RA, Goulart DA. The effect of sulfinpyrazone on the disposition of pseudoracemic phenprocoumon in humans. *Clin Pharmacol Ther* 1987;42:312–319.

89. Harenberg J, Staiger CH, de Vries JX, Walter E, Weber E, Zimmerman R. Cimetidine does not increase the anticoagulant effect of phenprocoumon. *Br J Clin Pharmacol* 1982;14:292–293.

90. Harenberg J, Zimmerman R, Staiger CH, de Vries JX, Walter E, Weber E. Lack of effect of cimetidine on action of phenprocoumon. *Eur J Clin Pharmacol* 1982;23:365–367.

91. Michot F, Holt NF, Fontailles F. The effect of sulfinpyrazone on the coagulation-inhibiting action of acenocoumarol. *Schweiz Med Wochenschr* 1981;111:255–260.

92. Caraco Y, Chajek-Shaul T. The incidence and clinical significance of amiodarone and acenocoumarol interaction. *Thromb Haemost* 1989;62:906–908.

93. Richard C, Riou B, Berdeaux A, et al. Prospective study of the potentiation of acenocoumarol by amiodarone. *Eur J Clin Pharmacol* 1985;28:625–629.

94. Ortin M, Olalla JI, Muruzabal MJ, Peralta FG, Gutierrez MA. Miconazole oral gel enhances acenocoumarol anticoagulant activity: a report of three cases. *Ann Pharmacother* 1999;33:175–177.

95. Gill TS, Hopkins KJ, Bottomley J, Gupta SK, Rowland M. Cimetidine-nicoumalone interaction in man: stereochemical considerations. *Br J Clin Pharmacol* 1989;27:469–474.

CHAPTER 30

Oral Antifungals

David J. Edwards

Since 1985, a substantial increase has occurred in the number of patients at risk for the development of systemic fungal infections. Most of these individuals are immunocompromised because they have been infected with diseases such as acquired immunodeficiency syndrome (AIDS) or they have undergone treatment of cancer or have used immunosuppressant drugs to prevent graft rejection following transplantation. Historically, amphotericin B was the only drug available for the treatment of such infections, but it was an unattractive choice because it must be administered intravenously and there is high risk of nephrotoxicity. However, a number of drugs have been developed in recent years that are effective against systemic fungal infections when administered orally and have an acceptable safety profile. This review focuses on the metabolism of ketoconazole, fluconazole, itraconazole, and terbinafine.

The chemical structures of these compounds are illustrated in Fig. 30-1. Ketoconazole, fluconazole, and itraconazole are chemically related, belonging to the class of drugs known as azoles. Ketoconazole contains the classic imidazole ring structure, whereas the latter two drugs are triazoles, having three nitrogen atoms in the azole ring. Terbinafine represents a different type of structure and is classified as an allylamine compound. Differences in chemical structure between the azoles and the allylamines are important determinants of the mechanism by which the drugs interfere with fungal cell growth. The azoles act primarily by blocking the synthesis of ergosterol, an important component of the fungal cell membrane (1). Inhibition of the cytochrome P450 enzyme C14 alpha demethylase by azoles reduces the conversion of lanosterol to ergosterol. Terbinafine also interferes with the production of ergosterol but at an earlier stage in the synthetic process by inhibiting squalene epoxidase, resulting in reduced conversion of squalene to squalene-2,3-epoxide (2).

Because all of these compounds act by inhibiting some aspect of oxidative metabolism in fungi with the azoles specifically interacting with cytochrome P450, it is not surprising that these drugs are substrates for and inhibitors of mammalian P450 enzymes. This review focuses on ketoconazole, fluconazole, itraconazole, and terbinafine as substrates for cytochrome P450, although there is a surprising lack of detailed published information concerning the metabolism of these drugs in humans and the specific cytochrome P450 enzymes involved. Ketoconazole, itraconazole, and fluconazole are among the most potent inhibitors of cytochrome P450 in clinical use. This subject is reviewed in detail in Chapter 47. Some of the data discussed in this chapter provide indirect evidence of the likely involvement of individual P450 enzymes in the metabolism of these compounds. The effect of other drugs on the metabolism of the antifungals is also reviewed with a focus on enzyme-inducing agents that have the potential to substantially reduce the clinical usefulness of antifungal drugs.

FLUCONAZOLE

Fluconazole is unique among the currently available antifungal drugs in that it is primarily eliminated by renal mechanisms with 65% to 90% of a dose excreted unchanged in the urine (3). There is no published information on the nature of the metabolites formed, although, according to data on file with the manufacturer, 11.4% of a dose was recovered in urine as metabolites in three healthy volunteers. Reported metabolites include a 1,2,4-triazole, an N-oxide compound, and a glucuronidated product, with no single metabolite accounting for more than 4% of the administered dose (4,5). There are no known active metabolites.

D. J. Edwards: Pharmacy Practice, College of Pharmacy and Allied Health Professions, Wayne State University, 1400 Chrysler Drive, Detroit, Michigan 48202

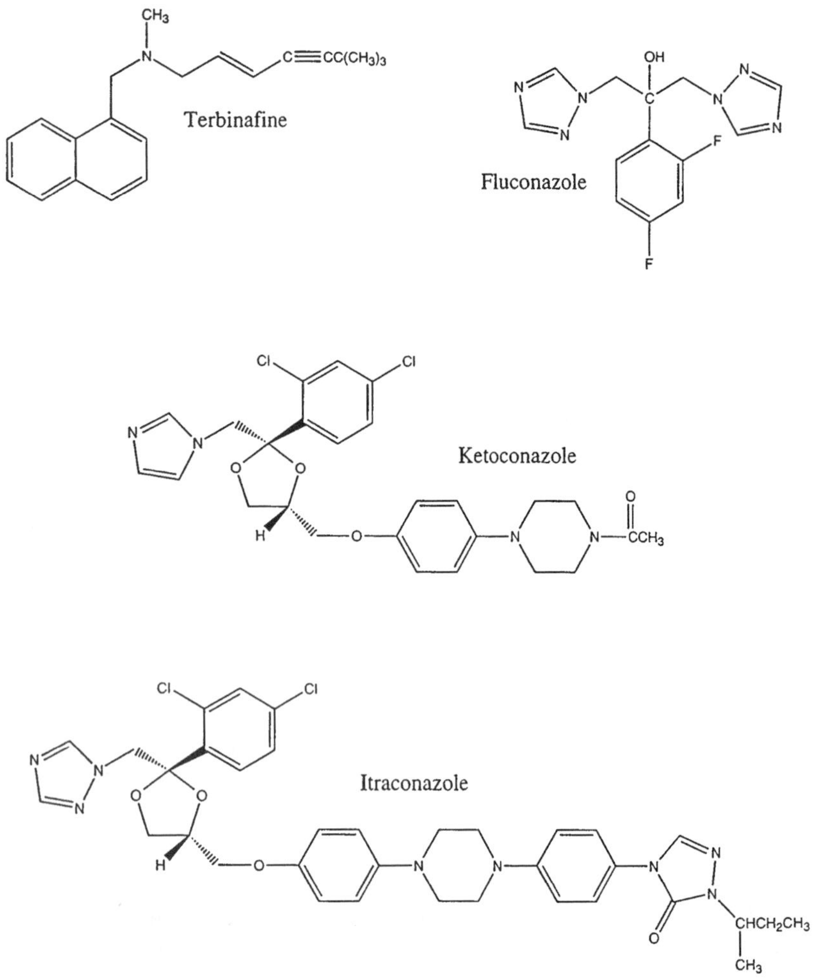

FIG. 30-1. Chemical structures of ketoconazole, fluconazole, itraconazole, and terbinafine.

Although the cytochrome P450 enzymes involved in the metabolism of fluconazole have not been reported in the literature, both *in vitro* and *in vivo* studies indicate that the drug interacts with the CYP2C9 and CYP3A4 enzymes. In comparison with ketoconazole, fluconazole was found to be a more potent inhibitor of the formation of 4-hydroxydiclofenac, a metabolite of diclofenac formed by CYP2C9, in human liver microsomes (6). Fluconazole also inhibited the hydroxylation of midazolam by CYP3A4 but was much less potent than either ketoconazole or itraconazole. Kunze and co-workers (7) reported that fluconazole was a potent inhibitor of the metabolism of (S)-warfarin by CYP2C9 (K_i = 7–8 µM) but also inhibited the 10-hydroxylation of (R)-warfarin mediated by CYP3A4 (K_i = 15–18 µM). Fluconazole had little effect on the activity of cDNA-expressed CYP1A2 with a K_i of greater than 800 µM. These studies are consistent with clinical studies that indicate that fluconazole decreases the clearance of (S)-warfarin (8), phenytoin (9), and tolbutamide (10), all of which are primarily cleared through CYP2C9-mediated metabolism. Studies with the CYP3A4 substrates triazolam (11) and cyclosporine (12) have suggested that fluconazole

impairs the elimination of these compounds in patients but generally appears to be a much weaker inhibitor of CYP3A4 than other azole antifungal drugs (6,7,13). The observation that fluconazole inhibits the metabolism of substrates for CYP2C9 and CYP3A4 suggests that fluconazole itself may be metabolized by these enzymes.

Drug Interactions Affecting Fluconazole

There are no reports of clinically significant inhibition of the metabolism of fluconazole in humans. However, this is not unexpected given the high proportion of the drug that is eliminated renally. Cimetidine, well known for its ability to inhibit cytochrome P450-mediated metabolism, lowered peak plasma concentrations of fluconazole by 20%, presumably by reducing absorption (10).

The effect of enzyme inducers on fluconazole disposition is of clinical interest and could potentially provide further insight into the enzymes involved in fluconazole metabolism. Although several studies have examined the effect of fluconazole on phenytoin disposition, the reverse interaction has not been examined in detail.

Coker and colleagues (14) reported that three patients treated concomitantly with rifampin and fluconazole appeared to suffer a relapse of their fungal infection. Apseloff and co-workers (15) administered 600 mg of rifampin orally to 16 healthy subjects and found that the area under the plasma concentration-time curve (AUC) for fluconazole decreased from 160.5 μg × hr/mL to 124 μg × hr/mL after 2 weeks of rifampin treatment. Although a decrease in plasma concentrations of this magnitude (23%) would not be expected to be clinically significant in most patients, larger changes are possible in individual patients. This study, along with the case reports, indicates that, even though the combination of rifampin should not usually render fluconazole ineffective, careful monitoring is required in patients receiving the combination.

Rifampin is an inducer of many cytochrome P450 enzymes. The metabolism of cyclosporine (16) and tolbutamide (17), substrates for CYP3A4 and CYP2C9, respectively, are both stimulated by rifampin, although the effect on CYP3A4 appears to be much stronger. Because rifampin is capable of inducing both CYP3A4 and CYP2C9, induction of fluconazole metabolism by rifampin does not allow one to draw any firm conclusions about the specific enzymes responsible for fluconazole metabolism. Rifabutin, a rifamycin derivative that is structurally related to rifampin, also induces CYP3A4 and other cytochrome P450 enzymes although to a lesser extent than rifampin. Fluconazole disposition was not significantly altered when given after 2 weeks of rifabutin pretreatment (18).

ITRACONAZOLE

Itraconazole is extensively metabolized in humans. Following administration of tritiated itraconazole to three healthy subjects, no unchanged itraconazole was recovered in the urine and less than 20% of the dose was recovered as parent compound in the feces (19). The major pathways for metabolism are oxidative scission of the dioxolane ring, oxidation of the piperazine ring, and both aliphatic oxidation and N-dealkylation at the 1-methylpropyl group. Although no single metabolite accounts for more than 5% of the total recovery of drug, oxidation of the 1-methylpropyl substituent produces hydroxyitraconazole. Peak hydroxyitraconazole concentrations in plasma after oral administration of itraconazole are typically 50% to 100% higher than those of the parent compound, while the hydroxyitraconazole AUC may be more than twice that of itraconazole (19–21). Itraconazole has incomplete oral bioavailability and appears to undergo substantial first pass metabolism to hydroxyitraconazole in the gut or liver. As a result, hydroxyitraconazole concentrations are much higher after oral administration of itraconazole than after intravenous administration (19). The first pass metabolism of itraconazole appears to be a saturable process and may account in part for the greater than proportional increases

in itraconazole concentrations with increasing dose. Van Peer and associates (22) reported that the AUC of itraconazole after a 200-mg oral dose was approximately tenfold higher than after a 50-mg dose.

Hydroxyitraconazole is a significant metabolite not only because of the high concentrations obtained in serum but also because it has antifungal activity. The in vitro antifungal effects of hydroxyitraconazole appear to be comparable to those of itraconazole although studies in animals have indicated that itraconazole is more active (19). The contribution of hydroxyitraconazole to the overall antifungal activity of itraconazole in humans is difficult to estimate. Hydroxyitraconazole is considerably more polar than itraconazole, such that concentrations at the site of infection could be lower than the parent compound despite higher concentrations in serum. The presence of hydroxyitraconazole in serum appears to account for a large discrepancy between serum concentrations of itraconazole measured by high performance liquid chromatography (HPLC) and those measured using a bioassay (23). Although equally active against fungal pathogens, hydroxyitraconazole was found to be more potent than itraconazole against the fungus commonly used in bioassays. Concentrations measured by bioassay are highly influenced by the amount of hydroxyitraconazole in the sample and may overestimate the itraconazole concentration by more than five-fold.

There are no published studies describing the in vitro metabolism of itraconazole by specific cytochrome P450 enzymes. Data on file with the manufacturer (Janssen Pharmaceutica, Belgium) indicate that the CYP3A4 enzyme is important in the metabolism of this compound (21). This is consistent with in vitro data showing that itraconazole inhibits the metabolism of substrates for CYP3A4. Although less potent than ketoconazole, itraconazole was a much more potent inhibitor than fluconazole of the CYP3A4-mediated metabolism of midazolam and cyclosporine (5,13). Studies in humans have demonstrated that itraconazole produces striking increases in the plasma concentrations of midazolam (ten- to 15-fold increase in AUC), triazolam (27-fold increase in AUC), felodipine (six-fold increase in AUC), terfenadine, and cyclosporine (24–28). All of these compounds are highly metabolized by CYP3A4 on first pass through the gut and liver with inhibition at both sites by itraconazole, contributing to the large increase in AUC. However, these interactions may not be solely due to the effect of itraconazole on CYP3A4 activity because many of these compounds are also substrates for P-glycoprotein (P-gp), the multidrug transporter present in the intestinal endothelium. Itraconazole has also been shown to inhibit the activity of P-gp (29).

Drug Interactions Affecting Itraconazole

There are few studies examining the effect of inhibitors of drug metabolism on itraconazole disposition. Cimetidine was found to increase the half-life of itraconazole by about 40%, although no significant difference in AUC was observed. The interpretation of this interaction is complicated by the fact that cimetidine raises gastric pH whereas itraconazole requires an acidic pH for maximal absorption. Inhibitors of CYP3A4 such as erythromycin and some of the recently developed protease inhibitors for the treatment of human immunodeficiency virus (HIV) infection (30) might be expected to inhibit itraconazole metabolism but detailed studies have not yet been reported.

The effect of enzyme inducers such as rifampin and phenytoin on itraconazole disposition is a significant clinical concern. Rifampin may be used in patients with fungal infections for either synergistic antifungal activity or for treatment of concomitant mycobacterial infection (e.g., tuberculosis). Phenytoin is useful for the prevention of seizures in patients whose fungal infections have spread to the central nervous system. Tucker and colleagues (31) described a series of patients receiving itraconazole with either phenytoin or rifampin. Three patients receiving the combination of rifampin and itraconazole and four patients receiving phenytoin and itraconazole failed to respond to the antifungal treatment or suffered a relapse. Drayton and associates (32) described a patient with AIDS receiving treatment with rifampin for pulmonary tuberculosis and itraconazole for infection with *Histoplasma capsulatum*. The patient failed to respond to itraconazole and serum levels of itraconazole were unmeasurable. After discontinuation of rifampin, measurable serum concentrations of itraconazole were achieved and the patient responded to therapy. This interaction has been studied in Yucatan miniature pigs (33). Rifampin reduced peak concentrations of itraconazole by 18-fold whereas the AUC was reduced 22-fold.

The effect of phenytoin on itraconazole disposition has been examined in healthy human volunteers (21). A single 200-mg dose of itraconazole was administered before and after treatment with phenytoin 300 mg daily for 15 days. Phenytoin decreased peak concentrations of itraconazole from 215 to 37 ng/mL whereas AUC was reduced by approximately 15-fold. Similar changes were observed in the peak concentration and AUC of hydroxyitraconazole, suggesting that phenytoin may also induce the metabolism of the metabolite. The dramatic decrease in itraconazole concentration with phenytoin is likely due to the combination of inducing the metabolism of CYP3A4 coupled with a reduction in the degree of saturable metabolism normally exhibited by the drug. Clearly, an interaction of this magnitude is almost certain to make itraconazole ineffective. Unless itraconazole concentrations can be routinely monitored to ensure therapeutic concentrations are present, the combination of itraconazole with enzyme-inducing agents such as phenytoin and rifampin should be avoided if possible.

KETOCONAZOLE

Ketoconazole is widely used in drug research for its ability to inhibit the activity of CYP3A4 *in vitro*. Testing the effect of ketoconazole on the metabolism of a new compound has become part of standard protocols for identifying the cytochrome P450 enzymes responsible. Although ketoconazole, like itraconazole, is extensively metabolized, detailed studies of the metabolic pathways and P450 enzymes involved in humans have not been published. In three male subjects given radiolabeled ketoconazole, unchanged drug accounted for only a small portion of the recovered radioactivity (34,35). The primary metabolic pathways are reported to involve oxidative degradation of the imidazole and piperazine rings, aromatic hydroxylation, and *O*-dealkylation. The metabolites produced by humans have not been specifically identified in the literature. Whitehouse and associates (36) have isolated and identified seven metabolites after incubation of ketoconazole with liver homogenates from mice. The primary metabolites were formed through metabolism of the 1-acetyl piperazine moiety. Removal of the acetyl group forms *N*-deacetyl ketoconazole, a product that has also been identified in rat hepatic microsomes (37). None of the metabolites of ketoconazole are reported to have antifungal activity. However, *N*-deacetyl ketoconazole has been reported to be cytotoxic in cultured rat hepatocytes, suggesting that it may play a role in ketoconazole-induced hepatitis (38).

There are no published reports documenting metabolism of ketoconazole by specific cytochrome P450 enzymes, although CYP3A4 would appear to be a likely candidate given the *in vitro* and *in vivo* effects of ketoconazole on substrates for this enzyme. Ketoconazole inhibits cyclosporine oxidase and testosterone 6β-hydroxylation *in vitro*. Although capable of inhibiting other forms of cytochrome P450, ketoconazole is a much more potent inhibitor of CYP3A4 activity (39,40). This is consistent with studies demonstrating dramatic increases in plasma concentrations of the CYP3A4 substrates cyclosporine, midazolam, triazolam, and terfenadine when given with ketoconazole (15,24,25,41) with minimal effects on theophylline (CYP1A2), phenytoin (CYP2C9), and prednisolone (9,42,43).

Drug Interactions Affecting Ketoconazole

Induction of the metabolism of ketoconazole is a significant concern with respect to the antifungal activity of the drug. Similar to the situation with itraconazole, interactions with rifampin and phenytoin have been reported. Rifampin has been implicated in several case reports of therapeutic failures with ketoconazole. Significant decreases in ketoconazole concentration have been documented (44–47). In a single patient, the AUC of ketoconazole was reduced from 9.15 to 2.02 µg × hr/mL after 5 months of treatment with rifampin (47). This interaction has been studied in six healthy subjects (48). The AUC following a single 200-mg dose of ketoconazole was reduced from 8.91 under control conditions to 1.79 mg × hr/L when given after several days of treatment with rifampin 600 mg. Peak ketoconazole concentrations were also significantly decreased.

Phenytoin has also been reported to reduce ketoconazole concentrations (31,47), although there are no detailed pharmacokinetic studies of this interaction. Clinically significant inhibition of the metabolism of ketoconazole has not been reported.

TERBINAFINE

Terbinafine is the only systemically active oral antifungal agent currently available that does not act by inhibiting a cytochrome P450 enzyme in fungi. It is, however, extensively metabolized and the metabolic pathways have been well described. Following administration of ^{14}C-terbinafine to human subjects, most of the radioactivity was recovered in the urine as metabolites with little unchanged drug (49,50). The major metabolites that have been detected in human plasma are produced from either N-demethylation or hydroxylation of the allyl side chain of the drug, with further metabolism of these compounds producing 15 identified metabolites (49,50). Carboxybutylterbinafine is present in plasma in significant concentrations with the AUC being about 13-fold higher than for terbinafine, while at least two other metabolites (demethyl terbinafine and demethyl carboxy terbinafine) are present in concentrations exceeding those of the parent compound (50). None of the metabolites are believed to possess antifungal activity.

Although the metabolic pathways for terbinafine have been well delineated, metabolism of the drug by specific cytochrome P450 enzymes has not been reported. No inferences as to the enzymes involved can be made on the basis of the inhibition of the metabolism of other P450 substrates because terbinafine is not a significant inhibitor of cytochrome P450 activity *in vitro* or *in vivo*. Negligible inhibition of substrates such as cyclosporine, tolbutamide, and ethoxycoumarin has been observed in human liver microsomes (13,39). Administration of terbinafine to healthy human subjects has not resulted in significant inhibition of the metabolism of antipyrine, midazolam, warfarin, or triazolam (11,51,53,54).

Drug Interactions Affecting Terbinafine

Cimetidine and terfenadine reduce the clearance of terbinafine by 33% and 16%, respectively, according to the *Physician's Desk Reference* (55). Of more concern clinically is the fact that rifampin increases the clearance

of terbinafine by 100%. A detailed description of this interaction has not been published. The apparent induction by rifampin suggests that CYP3A4 may play some role in the metabolism of terbinafine and that interactions with inducers such as phenytoin should be suspected.

CONCLUSION

The involvement of specific cytochrome P450 enzymes in the metabolism of the orally active systemic antifungal agents remains largely unreported to date. Inferences can be drawn on the basis of the ability of some of these compounds to inhibit specific forms of cytochrome P450. CYP3A4 is likely involved in the metabolism of itraconazole and ketoconazole with CYP2C9 playing a role in the metabolism of fluconazole. Induction of metabolism by rifampin and phenytoin leading to clinical failure has been reported for itraconazole and ketoconazole. A similar interaction may also occur with terbinafine. Because fluconazole is primarily eliminated by renal excretion of unchanged drug, it is much less susceptible to this type of interaction.

REFERENCES

1. Como JA, Dismukes WE. Oral azole drugs as systemic antifungal therapy. *N Engl J Med* 1994;530:263–272.
2. Ryder NS. Specific inhibition of fungal sterol biosynthesis by SF 86-327, a new allylamine antimycotic agent. *Antimicrob Agents Chemother* 1985;27:252–256.
3. Shiba K, Saito A, Miyahara T. Safety and pharmacokinetics of single oral and intravenous doses of fluconazole in healthy subjects. *Clin Ther* 1990;12:206–215.
4. Debruyne D, Ryckelynck J-P. Clinical pharmacokinetics of fluconazole. *Clin Pharmacokinet* 1993;24:10–27.
5. Dudley MN. Clinical pharmacology of fluconazole. *Pharmacotherapy* 1990; 10(Suppl):141S–145S.
6. Hargreaves JA, Jezequel S, Houston JB. Effect of azole antifungals on human microsomal metabolism of diclofenac and midazolam. *Br J Clin Pharmacol* 1994;38:175P.
7. Kunze KL, Wienkers LC, Thummel KE, Trager WF. Warfarin-fluconazole I. Inhibition of the human cytochrome P450-dependent metabolism of warfarin by fluconazole: in vitro studies. *Drug Metab Dispos* 1996;24:414–421.
8. Black DJ, Kunze KL, Wienkers LC, et al. Warfarin-fluconazole II. A metabolically based drug interaction: in vivo studies. *Drug Metab Dispos* 1996;24:422–428.
9. Touchette MA, Chandrasekar PH, Milad MA, Edwards DJ. Contrasting effects of fluconazole and ketoconazole on phenytoin and testosterone disposition in man. *Br J Clin Pharmacol* 1992;34:75–78.
10. Lazar JD, Wilner JD. Drug interactions with fluconazole. *Rev Infect Dis* 1990;12:S327–S333.
11. Varhe A, Olkkola KT, Neuvonen PJ. Fluconazole, but not terbinafine, enhances the effects of triazolam by inhibiting its metabolism. *Br J Clin Pharmacol* 1996;41:319–323.
12. Canafax DM, Graves NM, Hilligoss DM, Carleton BC, Gardner MJ, Matas AJ. Interaction between cyclosporine and fluconazole in renal allograft recipients. *Transplantation* 1991;51:1014–1018.
13. Back DJ, Tjia JF, Abel SM. Azoles, allylamines and drug metabolism. *Br J Dermatol* 1992;126(Suppl 39):14–18.
14. Coker RJ, Tomlinson DR, Parkin J, Harris JRW, Pinching AJ. Interaction between fluconazole and rifampicin. *BMJ* 1991;301:818.
15. Apseloff G, Hilligoss DM, Gardner MJ, et al. Induction of fluconazole metabolism by rifampin: in vivo study in humans. *J Clin Pharmacol* 1991;31:358–361.

16. Gomez DY, Wacher VJ, Tomlanovich SJ, Hebert MF, Benet LZ. The effects of ketoconazole on the intestinal metabolism and bioavailability of cyclosporine. *Clin Pharmacol Ther* 1995;58:15–19.

17. Zilly W, Breimer DD, Richter E. Stimulation of drug metabolism by rifampicin in patients with cirrhosis or cholestasis measured by increased hexobarbital and tolbutamide clearance. *Eur J Clin Pharmacol* 1977;11:287–293.

18. Trapnell CB, Lavelle JP, O'Leary CR, et al. Rifabutin does not alter fluconazole pharmacokinetics. *Clin Pharmacol Ther* 1993;53:196.

19. Heykants J, Van Peer A, Van de Velde V, et al. The clinical pharmacokinetics of itraconazole: an overview. *Mycoses* 1989;32(Suppl 1):67–87.

20. Barone JA, Koh JG, Bierman RH, et al. Food interaction and steady-state pharmacokinetics of itraconazole capsules in healthy male volunteers. *Antimicrob Agents Chemother* 1993;37:778–784.

21. Ducharme MP, Slaughter RL, Warbasse LH, et al. Itraconazole and hydroxyitraconazole serum concentrations are reduced more than tenfold by phenytoin. *Clin Pharmacol Ther* 1995;58:617–624.

22. Van Peer A, Woestenborghs R, Heykants J, Gasparini R, Gauwenbergh G. The effects of food and dose on the oral systemic availability of itraconazole in healthy subjects. *Eur J Clin Pharmacol* 1989;36:423–426.

23. Hostetler JS, Heykants J, Clemons KV, Woestenborghs R, HansonLH, Stevens DA. Discrepancies in bioassay and chromatography determinations explained by metabolism of itraconazole to hydroxyitraconazole: Studies of interpatient variations in concentrations. *Antimicrob Agents Chemother* 1993;37:2224–2227.

24. Olkkola KT, Backman JT, Neuvonen PJ. Midazolam should be avoided in patients receiving the systemic antimycotics ketoconazole or itraconazole. *Clin Pharmacol Ther* 1994;55:481–485.

25. Varhe A, Olkkola KT, Neuvonen PJ. Oral triazolam is potentially hazardous to patients receiving systemic antimycotics ketoconazole or itraconazole. *Clin Pharmacol Ther* 1994;56:601–607.

26. Jalava K-M, Olkkola KT, Neuvonen PJ. Itraconazole greatly increases plasma concentrations and effects of felodipine. *Clin Pharmacol Ther* 1997;61:410–415.

27. Honig PK, Wortham DC, Hull R, Zamani K, Smith JE, Cantilena LR. Itraconazole affects single-dose terfenadine pharmacokinetics and cardiac repolarization pharmacodynamics. *J Clin Pharmacol* 1993;33:1201–1206.

28. Kramer MR, Marshall SE, Denning DW, et al. Cyclosporine and itraconazole interaction in heart and lung transplant recipients. *Ann Intern Med* 1990;113:327–329.

29. Guan L, Benet LZ. Inhibitory effects of four azole antifungal agents (itraconazole, ketoconazole, miconazole and fluconazole) on digoxin transport across MDR1-MDCK cell monolayers. Proceedings of the 8th North American ISSX meeting, 1997:137.

30. Van Cleef GF, Fisher EJ, Polk RE. Drug interaction potential with inhibitors of HIV protease. *Pharmacotherapy* 1997;17:774–778.

31. Tucker RM, Denning DW, Hanson LH, et al. Interaction of azoles with rifampin, phenytoin, and carbamazepine: in vitro and clinical observations. *Clin Infect Dis* 1992;14:165–174.

32. Drayton J, Dickinson G, Rinaldi MG. Coadministration of rifampin and itraconazole leads to undetectable levels of serum itraconazole. *Clin Infect Dis* 1994;18:266.

33. Kaltenbach G, Leveque D, Peter J-D, et al. Pharmacokinetic interaction between itraconazole and rifampin in Yucatan miniature pigs. *Antimicrob Agents Chemother* 1996;40:2043–2046.

34. Daneshmend TK, Warnock DW. Clinical pharmacokinetics of ketoconazole. *Clin Pharmacokinet* 1988;14:13–34.

35. Heel RC, Brogden RN, Carmine A, Morley PA, Speight TM, Avery GS.

Ketoconazole: a review of its therapeutic efficacy in superficial and systemic fungal infections. *Drugs* 1982;23:1–36.

36. Whitehouse LW, Menzies A, Dawson B, et al. Mouse hepatic metabolites of ketoconazole: isolation and structure elucidation. *J Pharm Biomed Anal* 1994;12:1425–1441.

37. Rodriguez RJ, Acosta D. Metabolism of ketoconazole and deacetylated ketoconazole by rat hepatic microsomes and flavin-containing monooxygenases. *Drug Metab Dispos* 1997;25:772–777.

38. Rodriguez RJ, Acosta D. N-deacetyl ketoconazole-induced hepatotoxicity in a primary culture system of rat hepatocytes. *Toxicology* 1997;117:123–131.

39. Back DJ, Stevenson P, Tjia JF. Comparative effects of two antimycotic agents, ketoconazole and terbinafine on the metabolism of tolbutamide, ethinylestradiol, cyclosporin and ethoxycoumarin by human liver microsomes *in vitro*. *Br J Clin Pharmacol* 1989;28:166–170.

40. Baldwin SJ, Bloomer JC, Smith GJ, Ayrton AD, Clarke SE, Chenery RJ. Ketoconazole and sulphaphenazole as the respective selective inhibitors of P450 3A and 2C9. *Xenobiotica* 1995;25:261–270.

41. Honig PK, Wortham DC, Zamani K, Conner DP, Mullin JC, Cantilena LR. Terfenadine-ketoconazole interaction. Pharmacokinetic and electrocardiographic consequences. *JAMA* 1993;269:1513–1518.

42. Heusner JJ, Dukes GE, Rollins DE, Tolman KG, Galinsky RE. Effect of chronically administered ketoconazole on the elimination of theophylline in man. *DICP* 1987;21:514–517.

43. Yamashita SK, Ludwig EA, Middleton E, Jusko WJ. Lack of pharmacokinetic and pharmacodynamic interactions between ketoconazole and prednisolone. *Clin Pharmacol Ther* 1991;49:558–570.

44. Abadie-Kemmerly S, Pankey GA, Dalvisio JR. Failure of ketoconazole treatment of *Blastomyces dermatidis* due to interaction of isoniazid and rifampin. *Ann Intern Med* 1988;109:844–845.

45. Doble N, Hykin P, Shaw R, Keal EE. Pulmonary *Mycobacterium* tuberculosis in acquired immune deficiency syndrome. *BMJ* 1985;291:849–850.

46. Meunier F. Serum fungicidal activity in volunteers receiving antifungal agents. *Eur J Clin Microbiol* 1986;5:103–109.

47. Brass C, Galgiani JN, Blaschke TF, Defelice R, O'Reilly RA, Stevens DA. Disposition of ketoconazole, an oral antifungal, in humans. *Antimicrob Agents Chemother* 1982;21:151–158.

48. Doble N, Shaw R, Rowland-Hill C, Lush M, Warnock DW, Keal EE. Pharmacokinetic study of the interaction between rifampicin and ketoconazole. *J Antimicrob Chemother* 1988;21:633–635.

49. Jensen JC. Clinical pharmacokinetics of terbinafine (Lamisil). *Clin Exp Dermatol* 1989;14:110–113.

50. Humbert H, Cabiac MD, Denouel J, Kirkesseli S. Pharmacokinetics of terfinafine and of its five main metabolites in plasma and urine, following a single oral dose in healthy subjects. *Biopharm Drug Dispos* 1995;16:685–694.

51. Ahounen J, Olkkola KT, Neuvonen PJ. Effect of itraconazole and terbinafine on the pharmacokinetics and pharmacodynamics of midazolam in healthy volunteers. *Br J Clin Pharmacol* 1995;40:270–272.

52. Seyffer R, Eichelbaum M, Jensen JC, Klotz U. Antipyrine metabolism is not affected by terbinafine. *Eur J Clin Pharmacol* 1989;37:231–233.

53. Guerret M, Francheteau P, Hubert M. Evaluation of effects of terbinafine on single oral dose pharmacokinetic and anticoagulant actions of warfarin in healthy volunteers. *Pharmacotherapy* 1997;17:767–773.

54. Abdel-Rahman SM, Nahata MC. Oral terbinafine: a new antifungal agent. *Ann Pharmacother* 1997;31:445–456.

55. *Physician's Desk Reference*, 51st ed. Montvale, NJ: Medical Economics Company, 1997:2394.

CHAPTER 31

Antivirals

Jashvant D. Unadkat and Yi Wang

INTRODUCTION

Viruses are classified as DNA or RNA viruses. Typically, DNA viruses propagate in host cells by synthesizing viral mRNA by using the mRNA polymerase of the host cell. This viral mRNA is then translated into virus-specific proteins. Hepatitis and herpes are examples of diseases caused by DNA viruses. In contrast, RNA viruses propagate in host cells by synthesizing viral mRNA by using viral enzymes or by using the viral RNA as its own source of mRNA. Retroviruses, a special type of RNA virus, use viral reverse transcriptase to synthesize viral DNA. The viral DNA is then incorporated into the host genome where it uses the host cellular machinery to synthesize additional virus particles. An enzyme important in this synthetic pathway is the viral protease. The causative agent for acquired immunodeficiency syndrome (AIDS), human immunodeficiency virus-1 (HIV-1), is an example of a retrovirus. Anti-HIV drugs currently approved for use in the clinic target either the HIV-1–specific reverse transcriptase (e.g., nonnucleoside or nucleoside reverse transcriptase inhibitors such as nevirapine or azidothymidine) or the protease (e.g., protease inhibitors such as indinavir).

Among all viral diseases, AIDS is unique in that the treatment of this syndrome requires therapy with multiple anti-HIV and antiopportunistic infection (anti-OI) drugs. Because many of these anti-HIV and anti-OI drugs are inhibitors and/or substrates of cytochrome P450 (CYP) enzymes, the potential for drug interactions is high. The number of drugs approved for the treatment of viral diseases other than AIDS has increased considerably in the recent years. Of these, a majority are polar and therefore largely excreted by the kidneys. For the purposes of discussion of metabolic interactions of drugs in this chapter, we have categorized the drugs into two major categories: anti-HIV drugs and other antiviral agents.

METABOLISM OF ANTIVIRAL DRUGS

Anti-HIV drugs

Protease Inhibitors

This category of drugs has been highly effective in treating people with AIDS when used in combination with nucleoside reverse transcriptase inhibitors (RTIs) (1,2). The target of these drugs is the viral protease that is a key enzyme in the synthesis of new viral particles (3). Currently the protease inhibitors (PIs) approved for use in the clinic are amprenavir (Agenerase), indinavir sulfate (Crixivan), nelfinavir mesylate (Viracept), ritonavir (Norvir), and saquinavir mesylate [Invirase (hard-gel capsule) and Fortovase (soft-gel capsule)] (Fig. 31-1). All the members of this class of drugs are large, with molecular weights greater than 500 (from 506 to 766); they are hydrophobic and, except for indinavir, highly protein-bound to plasma proteins (more than 90%; predominantly to α-acid glycoprotein; Table 31-1) (4). These drugs are predominantly eliminated in the feces as metabolites (about 80% of the dose) (4). *In vitro* studies have shown that the formation of the majority of the identified metabolites of these PIs is catalyzed by CYP3A4/5 enzymes (5–9). Thus, as detailed later, clinically significant interactions of these PIs with CYP3A4/5 inhibitors are to be expected. A complicating factor in the interpretation of these interactions is that the PIs also are substrates of the efflux pump, *P*-glycoprotein (10–13). Thus drugs that are inhibitors of the CYP3A4/5 and *P*-glycoprotein may interact with the protease inhibitors by a dual mechanism, inhibition of metabolism by CYP3A4/5 and

J. D. Unadkat and Y. Wang: Department of Pharmaceutics, University of Washington, Box 357610, H272 Health Sciences Building, Seattle, Washington 98195-7610

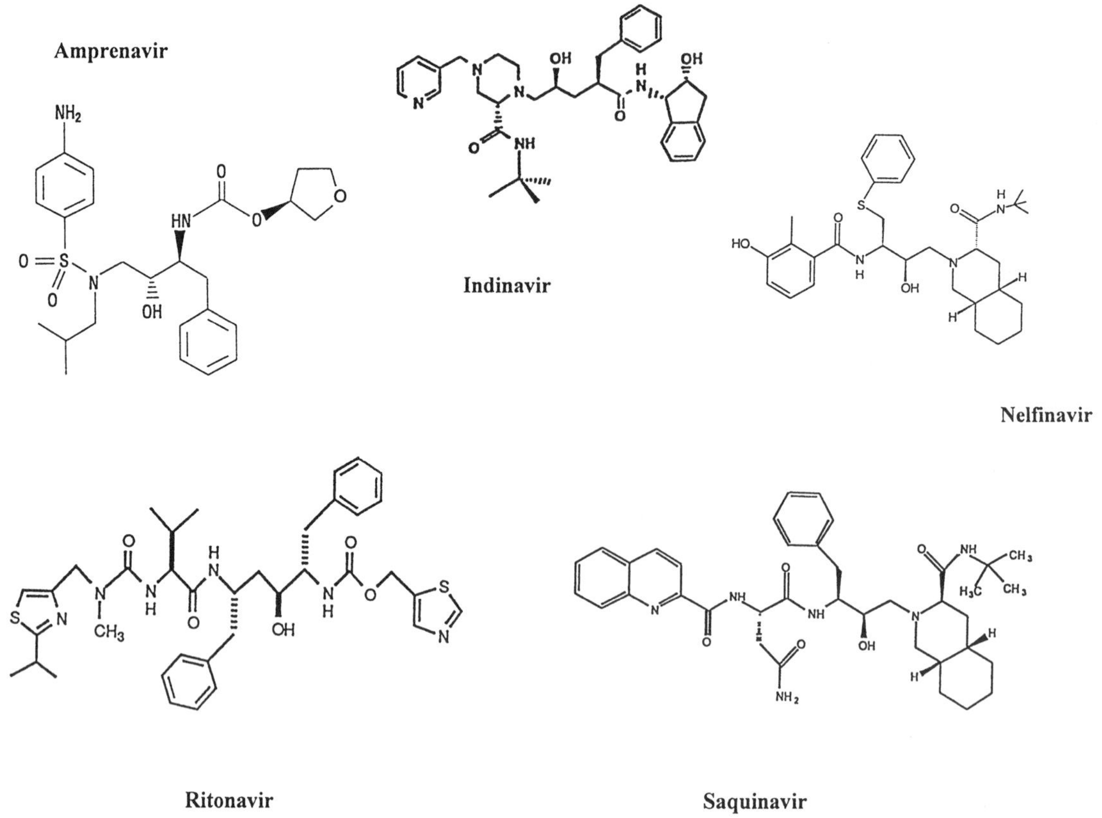

Amprenavir

Indinavir

Nelfinavir

Ritonavir

Saquinavir

FIG. 31-1. Chemical structures of the protease inhibitors: amprenavir, indinavir, nelfinavir, ritonavir, saquinavir.

inhibition of efflux into the intestinal lumen or bile by the P-glycoprotein (see Chapter 11).

Amprenavir

Amprenavir (14) is the most recent protease inhibitor approved by the Food and Drug Administration (FDA; April 1999). The multiple-dose and single-dose pharmacokinetics of amprenavir are dose independent over the dose range from 300 to 1,200 mg, b.i.d. The terminal plasma half-life of amprenavir ranges from 7.1 to 10.6 hours. The oral clearance of amprenavir at the dose used clinically (1,200 mg, b.i.d.) is 1,081 mL/min (manufacturer's data). Amprenavir is excreted primarily in the feces as metabolites (74% of the dose). Two oxidative metabolites (oxidation of the tetrahydrofuran and aniline moieties), formed in part by CYP3A4/5 (5), account for more than 90% of the [^{14}C]amprenavir found in the feces.

Indinavir

After single-dose administration, indinavir displays nonlinear pharmacokinetics over the dose range from 40 to 1,000 mg (15). The oral clearance of indinavir at the dose used in the clinic (800 mg q8h) is 711 mL/min (manufacturer's data). Indinavir is rapidly eliminated,

with a terminal plasma half-life of 1.8 ± 0.4 hours, and is extensively metabolized *in vivo*. Approximately 83% and 19% of total radioactivity is found in the feces and urine, respectively, after administration of a 400-mg dose of [^{14}C]indinavir (16). Of these fractions, only 20% and 9%, respectively, of the radioactivity is attributable to the unchanged drug. The metabolites identified in the urine and the feces are quaternary pyridine N-glucuronide (M1); 2', 3'-*trans*-dihydroxyindanylpyridine N-oxide (M2); 2', 3'-*trans*-dihydroxyindan (M3); and pyridine N-oxide (M4a) analog, and despyridylmethyl analogs of M3 (M5); and indinavir (M6) (16). In the feces, the radioactivity is predominantly due to M3 (21%), M5 (14%), M6 (13%), and the parent compound (19%) (16). M5 and M6 are the major metabolites in urine (17). Besides glucuronosyltransferases, CYP3A4 (K_m, 0.04 μM) (18) and 3A5 (K_m, 0.21 μM) (18) are the major enzymes found to form indinavir metabolites *in vitro* (6). In the fetal liver, which expresses only CYP3A7, the qualitative pattern of metabolism of indinavir and the K_m for its metabolism are similar to those in the adult liver (19).

Nelfinavir

The single-dose pharmacokinetics of nelfinavir are nonlinear. The oral clearance of nelfinavir at the dose used

TABLE 31-1. *Doses used in the clinic, steady-state maximum plasma concentration (C_{max}), plasma protein binding and major metabolizing enzymes of various antiviral drugs*

Generic name (Other names)	Trade name	Dose (P.O.)	Plasma concentration C_{max} (μg/ml) [μM]	Plasma protein binding (%)	Metabolizing enzyme
Anti-HIV agents					
Abacavir sulfate	Ziagen	300 mg/b.i.d.	3.0 ± 0.89 [4.5 ± 1.3]	50	Alcohol dehydrogenase, UGT
Didanosine (Dideoxyinosine, ddI)	Videx	200 mg/b.i.d.	1.3 [5.5]	<5	Adenylate kinase
Lamivudine (3TC)	Epivir	150 mg/b.i.d.	1.5 ± 0.5 [6.6 ± 2.1]	<36	Deoxycytidine kinase
Stavudine (d4T)	Zerit	40 mg/b.i.d.	603 ± 160 [2.6 ± 0.7]	Negligible	Thymidine kinase, thymidylate kinase
Zalcitabine (Dideoxycytidine, ddC)	Hivid	0.75 mg/q.i.d.	0.016–0.0375 [0.08–0.2]	<4	Deoxycytidine kinase
Zidovudine (Azidothymidine, AZT)	Retrovir	600 mg/q.d.	1.06 [4.0]	34–38	UGT, thymidine kinase, thymidylate kinase
Amprenavir	Agenerase	1200 mg/b.i.d.	5.36 [10.6]	90	CYP3A4/5
Indinavir sulfate	Crixivan	800 mg/q.i.d.	7.7 ± 2.5 [12.6 ± 4.1]	60	CYP3A4/5/7, UGT
Nelfinavir mesylate	Viracept	750 mg/t.i.d.	3–4 [5.3–7.0]	>98	CYP3A4/5, CYP2C19
Ritonavir	Norvir	600 mg/q.i.d.	11.2 ± 3.6 [15.5 ± 5.0]	>98	CYP3A4/5, CYP2D6
Saquinavir Mesylate	Fortovase	1200 mg/t.i.d.	2.2 [3.3]	98	CYP3A4/5
Delavirdine Mesylate	Rescriptor	400 mg/t.i.d.	19.3 ± 11 [35 ± 20]	98	CYP3A4/5, CYP2D6
Efavirenz	Sustiv	600 mg/q.d.	4.0 ± 1.1 [15.0 ± 4.1]	99.5	CYP3A4/5, CYP2B6
Nevirapine	Viramune	200 mg/q.d.	2 ± 0.4 [8.8 ± 1.5]	60	CYP3A4/5, UGT
Other antiviral agents					
Famciclovir	Famvir	500 mg/q.i.d.	3.3 [10.2]	<20	Aldehyde oxidase
Ribavirin	Rebetol	600 mg/b.i.d.	2.2 [9.0]	–	Adenosine kinase
Rimantadine HCl	Flumadine	100 mg/b.i.d.	0.05–0.1 0.2 ± 0.6	40	–

–: Data not available; UGT: uridine diphosphate glucuronosyltransferase.

in the clinic (750 mg, t.i.d.) is about 534 mL/min (20). After a 750-mg dose of [^{14}C]nelfinavir given orally, the majority (87%) of radioactivity was found in the feces. Of this, 78% was associated with oxidative metabolites, and 22% as the parent drug (manufacturer's data). In human liver microsomes, nelfinavir is metabolized to five metabolites: hydroxylation of the perhydroisoquinoline group, hydroxylation of the banzamide group; *S*-oxidation, and hydroxylation of the thiophenyl ring, and hydroxylation of the *t*-butylamide group (M8) (21). The formation of the first four metabolites is dominated by CYP3A, whereas the last metabolite listed, which is also the major active (equipotent to nelfinavir) circulating metabolite in the plasma [about one third of plasma nelfinavir concentration (22)], is formed by 2C19 (23,24).

Ritonavir

Multiple-dose pharmacokinetics of ritonavir are reported as both dose and time dependent (25). On single-dose administration of ritonavir, the oral clearance of ritonavir decreased from 218 to 110 mL/min over the dose range from 200 to 500 mg. Because ritonavir has been shown to be a substrate and a potent inhibitor of CYP3A enzymes (8), the most likely explanation for this dose-dependency is saturation of metabolism by CYP3A. The *in vivo* K_m of this saturable pathway was estimated as 3.4 μg/mL. Based on these data, the steady-state area under the curve (AUC) of 500 mg ritonavir administered q12h should theoretically be three-fold higher than that of a single 500-mg dose. However, the AUC after multiple-dose administration of ritonavir at 500 mg, q12h, was found to be not significantly different from that obtained after a single 500-mg dose. The authors of this study concluded that autoinduction is the most likely explanation for these observations (25). The hypothesis that ritonavir may be an enzyme inducer appears to be supported by the observation that ritonavir increases the oral clearance of ethinyl estradiol (26), azidothymidine (27), and theophylline (28).

After a 600-mg dose of [^{14}C]ritonavir solution given orally, 11.3% and 86.3% of the dose was excreted in the urine and feces, respectively. Of these fractions, the majority of the radioactivity was associated with metabolites, whereas 30.5% and 33.8%, respectively, was the parent drug. The isopropylthiazole oxidation metabolite (M2) was the only circulating (at about 1/30 the concentration of the parent drug) and active (equipotent to ritonavir) metabolite found in the plasma; it is also the predominant metabolite found in the feces (24% total radioactivity) and the urine (57% of total radioactivity). CYP3A4 is a significant contributor to the formation of three other metabolites (M1, M2, and M11) formed in human liver microsomes, whereas both CYP3A4/5 and CYP2D6 contribute to the formation of M2 (8). K_m values for the turnover of ritonavir by lymphoblast-expressed CYP3A4 and 3A5 range from 0.05 to 0.07 μM (29). Ritonavir is highly bound to plasma proteins (98% to 99%) (30). However, this binding is not saturable within the clinical concentration range of the drug and is not affected by other highly bound drugs such as warfarin (30).

Saquinavir

Saquinavir is available in two formulations, a hard-gel capsule (HGC; Invirase) which has an absolute bioavailability of 4%, and a soft-gel capsule (SGC; Fortovase), which has a bioavailability of 331% relative to that of the HGC (manufacturer's data). Because the active ingredient is identical in the two formulations, the following summary (except for bioavailability and therefore oral clearance values) should apply to both formulations. The pharmacokinetics of both Invirase (75–600 mg, t.i.d.) (31) and Fortovase (400–1,200 mg, t.i.d.) are dose dependent after single and multiple doses (32,33). The oral clearances of these drugs at the clinically recommended doses (600 mg, t.i.d., and 1,200 mg, b.i.d., respectively) are 27,855 and 275 mL/min (manufacturer's data). The terminal plasma half-life of saquinavir is 1.38 hours (34). After oral administration of 600 mg [^{14}C]saquinavir mesylate, about 88% and 1% of the total radioactivity was recovered in feces and urine, respectively. In human liver microsomes, the metabolism of saquinavir is primarily (about 90%) mediated by CYP3A4 (9,35). Human intestine and liver microsomes metabolize saquinavir to numerous inactive mono- and dihydroxylated species (36,37). Of these, the major metabolites are M-2 and

M-7, formed by monohydroxylations of the octahydro-2-(1H)-isoquinolinyl and (1,1-dimethylethyl) amino groups, respectively (9). The K_m for the formation of these metabolites in human intestinal microsomes ranges from 0.3 to 0.5 μM. Saquinavir is also a highly bound drug to plasma proteins (more than 98%) (4).

Collectively, all the protease inhibitors are highly bound to plasma proteins (except indinavir), are substrates of CYP3A, and are extensively metabolized (after oral administration) to inactive metabolites that are largely excreted in the feces. Thus as detailed later, the pharmacokinetics of all the protease inhibitors have the potential to be clinically significantly affected by coadministration of drugs that are inhibitors or inducers of CYP3A.

Nucleoside Analogs

Except for abacavir, which is a synthetic carbocyclic nucleoside, all other approved anti-HIV nucleoside analogs, didanosine (ddI), stavudine (d4T), zalcitabine (ddC), zidovudine (AZT), and lamivudine (3TC) are 2′,3′ dideoxynucleosides (Fig. 31-2). The pharmacokinetics of these nucleoside RTIs are dose independent (38,39). The percentage of the dose excreted in the urine and feces as the unchanged drug and metabolites after oral administration is provided in Table 31-2. Only nucleoside drugs that are extensively metabolized and for which the metabolic enzymes have been identified are discussed.

AZT can be metabolized *in vivo* to an inactive but hematologically toxic metabolite, 3′-amino-3′-deoxy thymidine (AMT), whose concentration in the circulation achieves an AUC about one fifth that of AZT (40). It is not clear whether AMT contributes to the overall *in vivo* hematologic toxicity of AZT. *In vitro* studies, by using human liver microsomes, indicated that the reduction of AZT to AMT involves cytochrome b5 and P450 enzymes plus their corresponding reductases (41). The *in vitro* formation of this metabolite is significantly inhibited by the CYP3A4 inhibitors ketoconazole, fluconazole, indinavir, and ritonavir (42). However, because an extremely high concentration of the inhibitors (1 mM) was used in this study, the clinical relevance of these *in vitro* interactions cannot be assessed.

Both abacavir and AZT are metabolized primarily to their glucuronides (43; manufacturer's data). Although the glucuronosyl transferase isoform(s) responsible for mediating metabolism of abacavir is not known, AZT appears to be metabolized by a form of uridine diphosphate glucuronosyl transferase (UDPGT$_2$; UGT2B) with a K_m of about 5 mM (44). In addition, abacavir is significantly metabolized to 5′-carboxylic acid by alcohol dehydrogenase (manufacturer's data).

All nucleoside RTIs are prodrugs; they must be activated intracellularly by host-cell enzymes to form their triphosphates to produce anti-HIV activity (45). This acti-

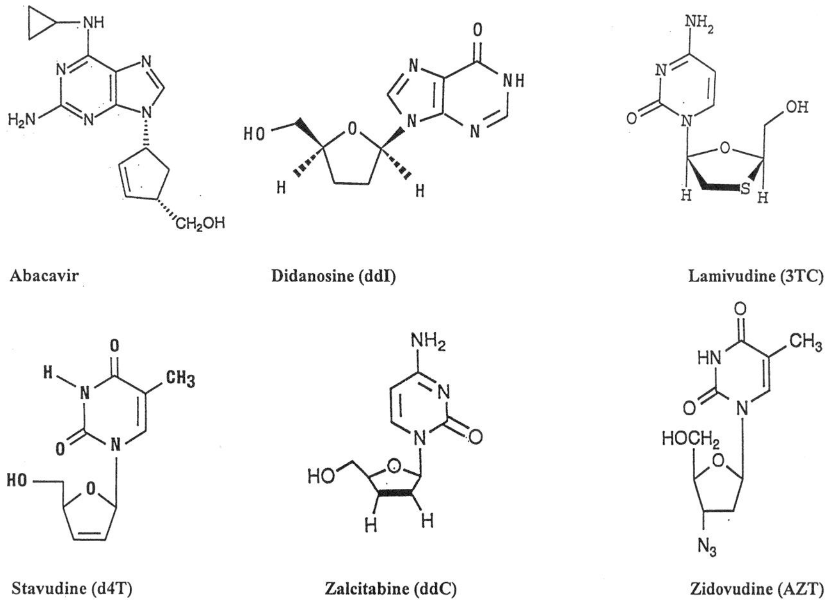

FIG. 31-2. Chemical structures of the nucleoside reverse transcriptase inhibitors: abacavir, didanosine, lamivudine, stavudine, zalcitabine, zidovudine.

vation occurs in multiple steps by various nucleoside phosphorylase enzymes, depending on the nucleoside involved. Therefore even though the fraction of the dose of each of these drugs that is intracellularly phosphorylated is low, interactions that affect these phosphorylation pathways will have a substantial impact on the efficacy of these drugs. However, such interactions are unlikely to result in a significant effect on the systemic pharmacokinetic parameters of the drugs. Intracellular drug interactions can be discerned only by measuring the concentration of the intracellular triphosphate metabolites of the drugs. Unfortunately, because of the low concentrations of these intracellular metabolites, development of detection methods with sufficient sensitivity to measure the *in vivo* intracellular concentrations of the triphosphates of the RTIs are arduous and fraught with difficulties (46–48).

AZT and d4T are both activated intracellularly by the same enzymes. Thymidine kinase phosphorylates these thymidine analogues to the monophosphate, thymidylate kinase phosphorylates the monophosphate to the diphosphate, and nucleoside diphosphate kinase phosphorylates the diphosphate to the triphosphate (49). Because both AZT and d4T are phosphorylated by the same enzymatic pathway, they are expected to compete for metabolism, especially because the affinity of the two compounds for thymidine kinase differs markedly. AZT has a much higher affinity for this enzyme (K_m, 14 μM) than does d4T (K_m, 142 μM) (50). At equimolar concentrations of the two drugs, d4T phosphorylation in cell cultures was reduced to less than 35% of that found in the absence of AZT (51). If these drugs are coadministered in the clinic, AZT would be preferentially phosphorylated intracellularly. Likewise, both ddC and 3TC are intracellularly

TABLE 31-2. *Excretory and metabolic profile of orally administered anti-HIV nucleoside reverse transcriptase inhibitors*

	Percent dose excreted in the urine		Percent dose excreted in the feces
Drug	Parent drug	Metabolite(s)	Parent drug + metabolites
Abacavir*	1.0%	5-carboxylic acid (25%) 5-glucuronide (30%) unidentified (13%)	16%
Didanosine[87] (ddl)	25%	dihydro-5-hydroxymethyl-2(3H)-furanone (–)	–
Lamivudine[88] (3TC)	70%	Trans-sulfoxide (5.2%)	–
Stavudine[89] (d4T)	39 ± 23%	unidentified	–
Zalcitabine** (ddC)	60%	dideoxyuridine (15%)	10%
Zidovudine[90] (AZT)	13%	5-O-glucuronide (68%)	10%

–: Data not available.
*Ziagan. From package insert, Glaxo Wellcome, 1998.
**Hivid. From package insert, Roche, 1998.

activated by deoxycytidine kinase (52). Not surprisingly, ddC significantly inhibited 3TC phosphorylation *in vitro,* in both peripheral blood mononuclear cells (PBMCs) and U937 cells (53). Based on these data, the combinations AZT and d4T or ddC and 3TC should not be used in the clinic. Indeed, data from clinical trials (as detailed later) support this conclusion.

Nonnucleoside analogs

There are currently three nonnucleoside RTIs (NNR-TIs) approved in the United States: efavirenz, delavirdine, and nevirapine (Fig. 31-3). These compounds are a heterogeneous group of drugs that are not nucleoside analogues. They inhibit HIV-1 reverse transcriptase at nanomolar concentrations in a noncompetitive manner, and unlike nucleoside RTIs, do not need to undergo intracellular activation for efficacy. Like the protease inhibitors, all three NNRTIs are hydrophobic, are substrates of CYP3A, and are clinically recommended to be used in combination with other anti-HIV drugs.

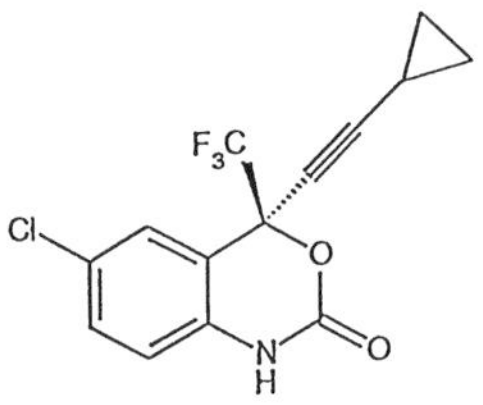

Efavirenz

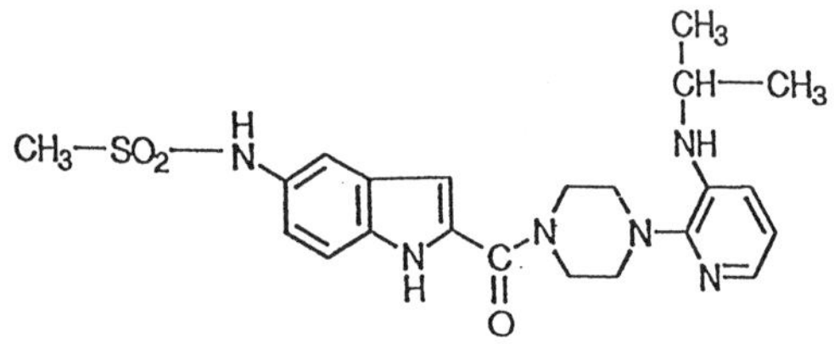

Delavirdine

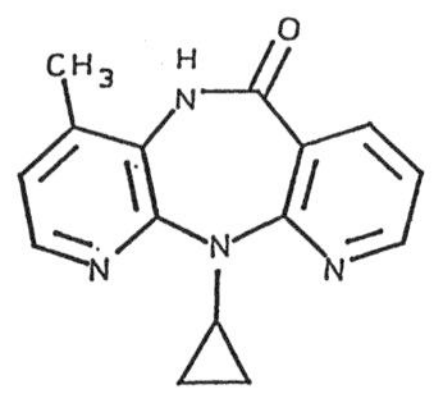

Nevirapine

FIG. 31-3. Chemical structures of the non-nucleoside reverse transcriptase inhibitors: efavirenz, delavirdine, nevirapine.

Efavirenz

At steady state, the pharmacokinetics of efavirenz are dose proportional in the dose range 200 to 600 mg, qd (manufacturer's data). However, the accumulation of the drug after multiple dosing is less than that predicted from the single-dose data. In addition, the terminal plasma half-life is shorter after multiple dosing than after a single dose (40–55 hours vs. 52–76 hours). Efavirenz is an inducer of its own metabolism. The oral plasma clearance of efavirenz at its clinically recommended dose (600 mg, qd) is 152 mL/min. On administration of [^{14}C]efavirenz (400 mg) on day 8 of a 1-month mass–balance study, approximately 14% to 34% of the radiolabeled drug was recovered in the urine, and 16% to 61% was recovered in feces. The majority of the radioactivity in the urine was associated with metabolites, whereas that in the feces was predominantly the unchanged drug. Human liver microsomal studies have demonstrated that efavirenz is principally metabolized by CYP3A4 and 2B6 to hydroxylated metabolites, with subsequent glucuronidation of these inactive hydroxylated metabolites. Efavirenz is highly bound to plasma proteins (99.5%–99.75%) (manufacturer's data).

Delavirdine

Delavirdine exhibits dose-dependent pharmacokinetics on multiple dosing (t.i.d.) in the dose range from 400 to 1,200 mg/day (54,55). The oral clearance of the drug decreased from 183 mL/min at 400 mg/day to 80 mL/min at 1,200 mg/day, and the terminal plasma half-life increased from 2.8 hours to 7.3 hours. Equal amounts of radioactivity were found in urine (51%) and feces (44%) when [^{14}C]delavirdine was administered orally to subjects who received multiple doses of delavirdine (300 mg, t.i.d.). Less than 5% of the delavirdine dose was recovered unchanged in the urine. In human liver microsomes, delavirdine is metabolized to three inactive metabolites, desalkyl delavirdine, and two as yet incompletely identified pyridine hydroxylated metabolites (MET-7 and MET-7a) (56). Desalkyl delavirdine was formed in human liver microsomes with a K_m of 6.8 µM. Only expressed human CYP3A4 (5.4 µM) and CYP2D6 (10.9 µM) catalyzed the formation of desalkyl delavirdine, whereas only expressed CYP3A4 mediated the formation of MET-7 and MET-7a. By using both human liver microsomes and expressed CYP3A4, delavirdine was found to be a mechanism-based inactivator of CYP3A4 (57). Delavirdine is highly bound to plasma proteins (about 98%).

Nevirapine

On multiple-dose administration (200–400 mg, qd), the pharmacokinetics of nevirapine are linear. However,

CHAPTER 31. ANTIVIRALS / **427**

the oral clearance of nevirapine at steady state (200–400 mg, qd) is 1.5- to two-fold higher [44 ± 12 mL/kg/h (58)] than that observed after a single dose, which suggests autoinduction of nevirapine metabolism (59; manufacturer's data). After administration of a single, 50-mg oral dose of [^{14}C]nevirapine to volunteers dosed to steady state (200 mg, b.i.d.), almost 81% of radioactivity is recovered in the urine, with 80% of this radioactivity consisting of glucuronide conjugates of hydroxylated metabolites. The major hydroxylated metabolites were 2-, 3-, and 12-hydroxy nevirapine. Minor metabolites were 8-hydroxy and 4-carboxy nevirapine (60). In human liver microsomes, nevirapine is metabolized by CYPs to 2-, 3-, 8-, and 12-hydroxy nevirapine. 2-Hydroxy and 12-hydroxy metabolites are formed by CYP3A, whereas 3-hydroxy nevirapine is formed by CYP2B6 (61). The anti-HIV activity of these metabolites is not known. To determine whether nevirapine induces CYP3A, 2B6, or both, Lamson et al. (59) determined nevirapine pharmacokinetics and the erythromycin breath test (ERMBT) in HIV-infected patients on four occasions: at baseline, after 14 and 28 days of nevirapine therapy, and at 2 weeks after discontinuing nevirapine. Fourteen days of 200-mg nevirapine, qd, increased the mean ERMBT by 22%. Increasing the dose to 200 mg, b.i.d., did not further increase the mean ERMBT. However, the formation clearance of the CYP2B6 metabolite (3-hydroxy nevirapine) was substantially increased, suggesting induction of CYP2B6. The plasma protein binding of nevirapine is 60%.

Other Antiviral Agents

Although a number of other antiviral agents are used in the clinic to treat a variety of other viral diseases such as cytomegalovirus infection and hepatitis (see Table 31-1), the majority of the drugs used are polar compounds and therefore are mostly excreted unchanged in the urine. Where the drugs are extensively metabolized, they are described later.

Famciclovir, a 9-substituted guanine derivative, is a prodrug that undergoes rapid and complete oxidation in humans to yield the active antiherpes agent, penciclovir (62,63), although small amounts of 8-oxo and 6,8-dioxometabolites also are formed. The majority of penciclovir formed (more than 80%) is excreted unchanged in the urine (64). Studies with cytosol from human liver and intestine and expressed enzyme have indicated that famciclovir is metabolized to penciclovir (by an intermediate) by aldehyde oxidase with a K_m of 115 ± 23 μM (65). Therefore any drug that inhibits aldehyde oxidase, a major metabolizing enzyme for famciclovir, will likely reduce the production of penciclovir.

Rimantadine is used for the treatment of influenza A. Rimantadine is extensively metabolized after an oral dose, with less than 25% of the dose excreted unchanged in the urine. Three hydroxylated metabolites and a glu-

curonide conjugate are reported to be excreted in the urine (66–69). However, the enzymes mediating these metabolic pathways have not been identified.

Ribavirin must be activated by cellular phosphorylation, probably adenosine kinase. Ribavirin inhibits d4T phosphorylation in both PBMCs and U937 cells (51), suggesting that thymidine kinase may be involved in the phosphorylation of ribavirin. After oral administration (800 mg), approximately 29% and 4% are recovered in the urine as the 1,2,4-triazole-3-carboxamide metabolite and the parent drug, respectively (70). The enzyme(s) responsible for the formation of the major metabolite have not been identified.

METABOLIC DRUG INTERACTIONS OF ANTIVIRAL DRUGS

Based on the earlier information, clinically significant metabolic interactions with most of these antiviral agents are likely to be mediated by inhibitors or inducers of CYP3A, glucuronosyltransferases, and phosphorylation kinases. The degree to which these interactions occur will depend on many factors, such as the contribution of these enzymes to the overall clearance of the drugs, the concentration of the inhibitor or inducer at the site of metabolism, and the *in vivo* inhibitory capacity of the inhibitor (*in vivo* K_i) (71). Because the latter two values are generally not available, the average unbound concentration of the inhibitor in the plasma (fu·[I]) is generally assumed to reflect the concentration of the inhibitor at the site of metabolism, and the *in vitro* K_i value is assumed to reflect the *in vivo* K_i. In the presence of a competitive or a noncompetitive inhibitor, assuming that the concentration of the substrate is less than the K_m, the degree of inhibition of the *in vivo* clearance of a drug by an inhibitor may be estimated from the formula

$$AUC_i/AUC = 1 + fu \cdot [I]/K_i \tag{1}$$

where AUC_i and AUC are the area under the plasma concentration–time profile of a drug in the presence and absence of the inhibitor (see Chapter 1) (72). Thus a ratio of fu · [I]/K_i that is much greater than unity would predict a clinically significant drug interaction with the inhibitor.

CYP3A Inhibitors and Inducers

CYP3A Inhibitors

Because most PIs are extensively metabolized by CYP 3A4/5, inducers and inhibitors of these enzymes result in clinically significant interactions with these drugs (see Chapter 10). Table 31-3 lists drugs that are either CYP3A4/5 inhibitors or inducers and their effect on the area under the plasma concentration–time profiles of PIs and NNRTIs when coadministered in the clinic. The [I]/K_i values of the CYP3A4 inhibitors (where available)

TABLE 31-3. *Effect of inhibitors or inducers of CYP3A (dose in parentheses) on the pharmacokinetics (% changes in AUC[a]) of antiviral drugs that are CYP3A4/5 substrates*

CYP3A inhibitor or inducer	K_i (μM)[e]	fu-[I]/K_i	[I]/K_i[f]	Protease inhibitor					Nonnucleoside reverse transcriptase inhibitor		
				Amprenavir	Indinavir	Nelfinavir	Ritonavir	Saquinavir	Efavirenz	Delavirdine	Nevirapine
Inhibitor											
Clarithromycin	48[d91]	0.008	0.06	18↑(300 mg/b.i.d.)[g]	29↑(500 mg/b.i.d.)[92]	—	12.5↑(500 mg/b.i.d.)[92]	300↑(500 mg/b.i.d.)	0↔(500 mg/b.i.d.)[93]	—	—
Fluconazole	1.3–25.1[c94,95]	0.8–16.4	0.9–18.4	—	19↓(400 mg/q.d.)[96]	—	15↑(200 mg/q.d.)[97]	—	16↑(200 mg/q.d.)	0↔[b]	—
Ketoconazole	0.015–0.13[c95,98]	0.2–1.9	22.3–193.2	31↑(400 mg)	68↑(400 mg)	35↑(400 mg/q.d.)[99]	18↑(200 mg/q.d.)[100]	300↑(200 mg/q.d.)	—	—	15–30↑(200 mg/q.d.)[101]
Amprenavir	0.5[5]	0.6	6.1	—	38↓(800 mg)	15↑(800 mg)	—	18↓(800 mg)	16↑(1200 mg)	—	—
Indinavir	0.2–0.9[d102,103]	1.7–7.6	4.2–19	33↑(800 mg/t.i.d.)	—	83↑(1000 mg/b.i.d.)	—	620↑(800 mg/t.i.d.*)[33]	0↔(800 mg/t.i.d.)	0↔(800 mg)[104]	0↔(800 mg/t.i.d.)
Nelfinavir	0.31–4.8[d7,103]	0.02–0.3	0.8	0↔(750 mg/t.i.d.)	51↑(750 mg/b.i.d.)	—	152↑(500 mg/b.i.d.)	500↑(750 mg/b.i.d.*)[105]	0↔(750 mg/t.i.d.)[106]	58↓(750 mg/t.i.d.)[106]	0↔(750 mg/b.i.d.)[107]
Ritonavir	0.019–0.46[c102,103]	0.2–5.3	10.9–262.8	—	475↑(400 mg/q.d.)[108]	152↑(500 mg/b.i.d.)	0↔(600 mg)[110]	>5000↑(600 mg)[109,110]	21↑(600 mg/b.i.d.)[111]	0↔(300 mg/b.i.d.)[112]	0↔(600 mg/b.i.d.)
Saquinavir	0.7–4.4[d9,103]	0.006–0.4	0.3–1.9	32↓(800 mg/t.i.d.)	—	18↑(1200 mg/t.i.d.*)	163↑(400 mg/t.i.d.)[113]	—	12↓(1200 mg/t.i.d.*)	0↔(600 mg/t.i.d.)[113]	0↔(600 mg/t.i.d.)[114]
Delavirdine	21.6[57,103]	0.02	1.0	—	44↑(400 mg/t.i.d.)[106]	192↑(400 mg/t.i.d.)[115]		500↑(400 mg/t.i.d.)		—	—
Inducer											
Efavirenz				—	31↓(200 mg/q.d.)	20↑(600 mg/q.d.)[116]	18↑(600 mg/q.d.)[111]	62↓(600 mg/t.i.d.)	—	—	—
Nevirapine				—	28↓(200 mg/b.i.d.)[116]	50↓(200/q.d.)[20]	11↓(200 mg/b.i.d.)	25↓[b]	—	—	—
Rifampin				82↓(300 mg/q.d.)	89↓(600 mg/q.d.)	566↓(600 mg/q.d.)[118]	35↓(600 mg/q.d.)	84↓(600 mg/q.d.)	26↓(600 mg/q.d.)[119]	2700↓(600 mg/q.d.)[120]	58↓(600 mg/q.d.)[123]
Rifabutin				15↓(150 mg/q.d.)	34↓(150 mg/q.d.)[121]	32↓(150 mg/q.d.)	—	40↓[b]	0↔(450 mg/q.d.)	500↓(300 mg/q.d.)[122]	—

[a]Data without citation are from pharmaceutical company's package inserts.
[b]Data are from the Guidelines for the Use of Antiretroviral Agents in HIV-Infected Adults and Adolescents at the web site of HIV/AIDS Treatment Information Service (ATIS) (www.hivatis.org).
[c]Noncompetitive inhibition.
[d]Competitive inhibition.
[e]The lowest and highest K_i values found in the literature.
[g]Dose of the inhibitor used in the study.
[I]: Average steady-state plasma concentration of the inhibitor; K_i: Apparent *in vitro* inhibitory constant in human liver microsomes; –: Data not available; *: Soft-gel saquinavir (Fortovase) was used in the study.

also are included in Table 31-3. Because several estimates of *in vitro* K_i values are available in the literature for most of the drugs listed, we have provided a range (lowest to the highest) of K_i values and therefore a range of $[I]/K_i$ values. Based on these values, except for delavirdine, the rank order of potency of the inhibitors based on *in vitro* K_i values ($[I]/K_i$ ratio) correlates relatively well with that observed *in vivo*. Ritonavir and ketoconazole are predicted to be the most potent CYP3A4 inhibitors and indeed decrease the clearance of the protease inhibitors to the largest extent. Next in potency and clustered together are fluconazole, indinavir, nelfinavir, and amprenavir. The inhibitors predicted to be the least potent are saquinavir, clarithromycin, and delavirdine. Delavirdine is more potent *in vivo* than would be predicted from its $[I]/K_i$ ratio, most likely because it is a mechanism-based inhibitor of CYP3A4 (57). Interestingly, this correlation of rank order of potency is poor if the free drug concentration is used (i.e., fu · $[I]/K_i$) to predict *in vivo* inhibitory capacity. In this case, fluconazole is predicted to be the most potent inhibitor of the *in vivo* clearance of the protease inhibitors, which it clearly is not. Although there is a rank-order correlation between the *in vivo* data and the predicted potency of CYP3A4 inhibitors, this correlation is not quantitative. For example, based on the $[I]/K_i$ ratio, amprenavir, indinavir, and nelfinavir are predicted to decrease significantly and substantially the *in vivo* clearance of other PIs. However, they either do not affect the clearance of other PIs or affect it only marginally. There are several possible explanations for this lack of quantitative correlation with the *in vivo* data. The formula ($[I]/K_i$ ratio) assumes that the substrate is present at a concentration below the K_m of the enzyme, CYP3A4. However, at the doses used in the clinic, the pharmacokinetics of many of the PIs are nonlinear, indicating saturation of their metabolism, presumably by CYP3A4. Second, the assumption that metabolism by CYP3A4 is the predominant elimination pathway may not be correct for all the PIs. Third, most of these protease inhibitors are substrates of the *P*-glycoprotein efflux pump (10,13,73), which is expressed in the intestine and in the bile canalicular membrane (74). Thus many of these interactions are likely to be taking place at the level of inhibition of both CYP3A4 and *P*-glycoprotein efflux. For example, the inhibition of CYP3A4-mediated metabolism of saquinavir in both the intestine and the liver and inhibition of *P*-glycoprotein efflux in the intestine are the most likely explanations for the observation that interaction of CYP3A4 inhibitors with saquinavir is quantitatively the largest among all the PIs (9). The role of *P*-glycoprotein efflux in the absorption of saquinavir is supported by the observation that cyclosporine, a poor inhibitor of CYP3A4 but a potent inhibitor of *P*-glycoprotein, increases the AUC of saquinavir by 430% (75).

Because CYP2D6 is thought to play a role in the metabolism of ritonavir, it is interesting to note that flu-

oxetine, a potent CYP2D6 inhibitor, only modestly increases the AUC of ritonavir (19%; $p < 0.05$) (76). This observation supports the conclusion that CYP2D6 is a minor contributor to the overall *in vivo* clearance of ritonavir. The CYP3A4 inhibitors do not appear to affect the clearance of the NNRTIs. The reason for this lack of interaction is clear if the metabolic profiles of these drugs are examined. None of these drugs is exclusively or primarily metabolized by CYP3A4/5.

CYP3A4 Inducers

The rifamycins, rifampin and rifabutin, are frequently used to treat *Mycobacterium tuberculosis* or *Mycobacterium avium-intracellulare*, two opportunistic infections that afflict people with AIDS. Rifampin and rifabutin are both inducers of CYP3A4 (77–80). The *in vitro* induction potency of rifabutin of CYP3A4 activity has previously been documented to be weaker than that of rifampin (78). Consistent with these *in vitro* data, the induction of clearance (as reflected by a decrease in the AUC) of both PIs and the NNRTIs decreases in the order rifampin > rifabutin = nevirapine > efavirenz. At first glance, the large inductive effect of rifampin on NNRTI clearances appears inconsistent with the data on the lack of effect of CYP3A4 inhibitors on the AUC of these drugs. However, it should be noted here that CYP3A4 may be a minor contributor to the overall clearance of the NNRTIs in the noninduced subject but a major contributor (because of induction) in the induced subject.

Intracellular Phosphorylation

A clinical trial of AZT plus d4T versus d4T alone in AZT-experienced subjects (ACTG 290) found that patients receiving both drugs experienced a decline in CD4 cell counts, whereas those taking d4T alone did not. This observation is predictable based on the *in vitro* data (see earlier) that AZT inhibits the intracellular phosphorylation of d4T (51). Therefore this combination is equivalent to administering AZT alone. Because AZT-experienced patients usually harbor AZT-resistant virus, administration of AZT alone to this group of patients will result, as observed, in a decline in CD4 cell count. Consequently this combination is no longer recommended for use in the clinic (81).

Glucuronosyltransferases

A number of drugs, when coadministered with AZT, significantly increase the AUC of AZT by inhibiting its metabolism to the glucuronide. Valproic acid (VPA), an anticonvulsant drug, is eliminated from the body by metabolism to the glucuronide by glucuronosyltransferases. Thus an interaction between VPA and AZT is theoretically possible. Indeed, Lertora et al. (82) reported that VPA (250 mg, t.i.d.) increases the AUC of AZT by 44% and decreases the AZT glucuronide/AZT concentration ratio in the urine by about 50%. Atovaquone (750 mg, b.i.d.), an antibiotic, when coadministered with AZT increases the AUC of AZT by 31% and decreases the AZT-glucuronide/AZT plasma AUC ratio by 30% (83). Likewise, fluconazole (400 mg, qd) increases the AUC of AZT by 74% and decreases the apparent formation clearance to the glucuronide by 48% (84). Although the therapeutic concentrations of AZT are not well defined, changes of more than 30% in AZT plasma concentrations are likely to warrant a modification in the dose of AZT because of the potential of high AZT plasma concentrations to produce hematologic toxicity. In human liver microsomes, the median inhibitory concentration (IC_{50}) values for the inhibition of formation of AZT glucuronide by atovaquone, fluconazole, and VPA were found to be more than 100, 50, and 100 μg/ml, respectively. The IC_{50} values of fluconazole and VPA are within the range of plasma concentrations of these drugs, whereas the IC_{50} value of atovaquone is ten-fold higher than its clinical plasma concentration. Thus the *in vitro* data in human liver microsomes are not consistently predictable of *in vivo* interactions with AZT (85). Besides inducing CYP enzymes, rifampin also induces glucuronosyltransferases. Burger et al. (86) found that rifampin (600 mg, qd) increases the clearance of AZT by about 58%. Such a magnitude of change in exposure of the patient to the drug is likely to call for an upward adjustment of the AZT dose.

CONCLUSIONS

CYP3A4/5, glucuronosyltransferases, and intracellular kinases are the major enzymes involved in the activation and/or metabolic clearance of antiviral drugs. Coadministration of potent inhibitors or inducers of these enzymes is likely to result in clinically significant interactions with antiviral drugs.

Supported in part by NIH AI38698.

REFERENCES

1. Vittinghoff E, Scheer S, O'Malley P, Colfax G, Holmberg SD, Buchbinder SP. Combination antiretroviral therapy and recent declines in AIDS incidence and mortality. *J Infect Dis* 1999;179:717–720.
2. Palella FJ Jr, Delaney KM, Moorman AC, et al. Declining morbidity and mortality among patients with advanced human immunodeficiency virus infection: HIV Outpatient Study Investigators [Comments]. *N Engl J Med* 1998;338:853–860.
3. Robins T, Plattner J. HIV protease inhibitors: their anti-HIV activity and potential role in treatment. *J Acquir Immune Defic Syndr* 1993;6:162–170.
4. Barry M, Gibbons S, Back D, Mulcahy F. Protease inhibitors in patients with HIV disease: clinically important pharmacokinetic considerations. *Clin Pharmacokinet* 1997;32:194–209.
5. Decker CJ, Laitinen LM, Bridson GW, Raybuck SA, Tung RD, Chaturvedi PR. Metabolism of amprenavir in liver microsomes: role of CYP3A4 inhibition for drug interactions. *J Pharmacol Sci* 1998;87:803–807.
6. Chiba M, Hensleigh M, Nishime JA, Balani SK, Lin JH. Role of cytochrome P450 3A4 in human metabolism of MK-639: a potent human immunodeficiency virus protease inhibitor. *Drug Metab Dispos* 1996;24:307–314.
7. Lillibridge JH, Liang BH, Kerr BM, et al. Characterization of the selectivity and mechanism of human cytochrome P450 inhibition by the human immunodeficiency virus-protease inhibitor nelfinavir mesylate. *Drug Metab Dispos* 1998;26:609–616.
8. Kumar GN, Rodrigues AD, Buko AM, Denissen JF. Cytochrome P450-mediated metabolism of the HIV-1 protease inhibitor ritonavir (ABT-538) in human liver microsomes [published erratum appears in *J Pharmacol Exp Ther* 1997;281:1506]. *J Pharmacol Exp Ther* 1996;277:423–431.
9. Fitzsimmons ME, Collins JM. Selective biotransformation of the human immunodeficiency virus protease inhibitor saquinavir by human small-intestinal cytochrome P4503A4: potential contribution to high first-pass metabolism. *Drug Metab Dispos* 1997;25:256–266.
10. Alsenz J, Steffen H, Alex R. Active apical secretory efflux of the HIV protease inhibitors saquinavir and ritonavir in Caco-2 cell monolayers [published erratum appears in *Pharmacol Res* 1998;15:958]. *Pharmacol Res* 1998;15:423–428.
11. Kim RB, Fromm MF, Wandel C, et al. The drug transporter *P*-glycoprotein limits oral absorption and brain entry of HIV-1 protease inhibitors. *J Clin Invest* 1998;101:289–289.
12. Srinivas RV, Middlemas D, Flynn P, Fridland A. Human immunodeficiency virus protease inhibitors serve as substrates for multidrug transporter proteins MDR1 and MRP1 but retain antiviral efficacy in cell lines expressing these transporters. *Antimicrob Agents Chemother* 1998;42:3157–3162.
13. Washington CB, Duran GE, Man MC, Sikic BI, Blaschke TF. Interaction of anti-HIV protease inhibitors with the multidrug transporter *P*-glycoprotein (P-gp) in human cultured cells. *J Acquir Immune Defic Syndr Hum Retrovirol* 1998;19:203–209.
14. Adkins JC, Faulds D. Amprenavir. *Drugs* 1998;55:837–842; discussion 843–844.
15. Yeh KC, Deutsch PJ, Haddix H, et al. Single-dose pharmacokinetics of indinavir and the effect of food [published erratum appears in *Antimicrob Agents Chemother* 1998;42:1308]. *Antimicrob Agents Chemother* 1998;42:332–338.
16. Balani SK, Woolf EJ, Hoagland VL, et al. Disposition of indinavir: a potent HIV-1 protease inhibitor, after an oral dose in humans. *Drug Metab Dispos* 1996;24:1389–1394.
17. Balani SK, Arison BH, Mathai L, et al. Metabolites of L-735,524: a potent HIV-1 protease inhibitor in human urine. *Drug Metab Dispos* 1995;23:266–270.
18. Chiba M, Hensleigh M, Lin JH. Hepatic and intestinal metabolism of indinavir: an HIV protease inhibitor, in rat and human microsomes: major role of CYP3A. *Biochem Pharmacol* 1997;53:1187–1195.
19. Chiba M, Nshime JA, Lin JH. In vitro metabolism of indinavir in the human fetal liver microsomes. *Drug Metab Dispos* 1997;25:1219–1222.
20. Merry C, Barry MG, Mulcahy F, et al. The pharmacokinetics of combination therapy with nelfinavir plus nevirapine [Comments]. *AIDS* 1998;12:1163–1167.
21. Sandoval T, Grettenberger H, Zhang K, et al. Metabolism of nefilnavir mesylate, an HIV-1 protease inhibitor, by human liver microsomes and recombinant human isoforms. *Pharmacol Sci* 1998;1:1096.
22. Lillibridge J, Lee C, Pithavala Y, et al. The role of polymorphic CYP2C19 in the metabolism of nelfinavir mesylate. *Pharmacol Sci* 1998;1:1156.
23. Webber S, Shetty B, Wu E. In vitro and in vivo metabolism and cytochrome P450 induction studies with HIV-1 protease inhibitor, Viracept 9Rm (AG1343). 3rd Conference on Retroviruses and Opportunistic Infections 1996; Washington, DC:79.
24. Perry CM, Benfield P. Nelfinavir. *Drugs* 1997;54:81–87, discussion 88.
25. Hsu A, Granneman GR, Witt G, et al. Multiple-dose pharmacokinetics of ritonavir in human immunodeficiency virus-infected subjects. *Antimicrob Agents Chemother* 1997;41:898–905.
26. Ouellet D, Hsu A, Qian J, et al. Effect of ritonavir on the pharmacokinetics of ethinyl oestradiol in healthy female volunteers. *Br J Clin Pharmacol* 1998;46:111–116.
27. Cato A III, Qian J, Hsu A, Levy B, Leonard J, Granneman R. Multidose pharmacokinetics of ritonavir and zidovudine in human immuno-

deficiency virus-infected patients. *Antimicrob Agents Chemother* 1998;42:1788–1793.

28. Hsu A, Granneman G, Witt G, Cavanaugh J, Leonard J. Assessment of multiple doses of ritonavir on the pharmacokinetics of theophylline. *Int Conf AIDS* 1996;11:89.

29. Koudriakova T, Iatsimirskaia E, Utkin I, et al. Metabolism of the human immunodeficiency virus protease inhibitors indinavir and ritonavir by human intestinal microsomes and expressed cytochrome P4503A4/3A5: mechanism-based inactivation of cytochrome P4503A by ritonavir. *Drug Metab Dispos* 1998;26:552–561.

30. Hsu A, Granneman GR, Bertz RJ. Ritonavir: clinical pharmacokinetics and interactions with other anti-HIV agents [published erratum appears in *Clin Pharmacokinet* 1998;35:473]. *Clin Pharmacokinet* 1998;35:275–291.

31. Perry CM, Noble S. Saquinavir soft-gel capsule formulation: a review of its use in patients with HIV infection. *Drugs* 1998;55:461–486.

32. Muirhead G, Shaw T, Williams P. Pharmacokinetics of the HIV-protease inhibitor, RO31-8959, after a single dose and multiple doses in healthy volunteers. *Br J Pharmacol* 1992;34:170P–17IP.

33. Buss N. Saquinavir soft gel capsule (Fortovase): pharmacokinetics and drug interactions. 5th Conf Retrovir Oppor Infect February 1–5, 1998:145.

34. Vanhove GF, Kastrissios H, Gries JM, et al. Pharmacokinetics of saquinavir, zidovudine, and zalcitabine in combination therapy. *Antimicrob Agents Chemother* 1997;41:2428–2432.

35. Farrar G, Mitchell A, Marsh K. Prediction of potential drug interactions of saquinavir (Ro 31-8959) from in vitro data. *Br J Clin Pharmacol* 1994;38:162p.

36. Moyle G. Saquinavir: a review of its development, pharmacological properties and clinical use. *Expert Opin Invest Drugs* 1996;5:155–167.

37. Noble S, Faulds D. Saquinavir: a review of its pharmacology and clinical potential in the management of HIV infection. *Drugs* 1996;52:93–112.

38. Morse GD, Shelton MJ, O'Donnell AM. Comparative pharmacokinetics of antiviral nucleoside analogues. *Clin Pharmacokinet* 1993;24:101–123.

39. Dudley MN. Clinical pharmacokinetics of nucleoside antiretroviral agents. *J Infect Dis* 1995;171(suppl 2):S99–S112.

40. Stagg MP, Cretton EM, Kidd L, Diasio RB, Sommadossi JP. Clinical pharmacokinetics of 3′-azido-3′-deoxythymidine (zidovudine) and catabolites with formation of a toxic catabolite, 3′-amino-3′-deoxythymidine. *Clin Pharmacol Ther* 1992;51:668–676.

41. Pan-Zhou XR, Cretton-Scott E, Zhou XJ, Yang MX, Lasker JM, Sommadossi JP. Role of human liver P450s and cytochrome b5 in the reductive metabolism of 3′-azido-3′-deoxythymidine (AZT) to 3′-amino-3′-deoxythymidine. *Biochem Pharmacol* 1998;55:757–766.

42. Fayz S, Inaba T. Zidovudine azido-reductase in human liver microsomes: activation by ethacrynic acid, dipyridamole, and indomethacin and inhibition by human immunodeficiency virus protease inhibitors. *Antimicrob Agents Chemother* 1998;42:1654–1658.

43. Veal GJ, Back DJ. Metabolism of zidovudine. *Gen Pharmacol* 1995;26:1469–1475.

44. Rajaonarison JF, Lacarelle B, De Sousa G, Catalin J, Rahmani R. In vitro glucuronidation of 3′-azido-3′-deoxythymidine by human liver: role of UDP-glucuronosyltransferase 2 form. *Drug Metab Dispos* 1991;19:809–815.

45. Peter K, Gambertoglio JG. Intracellular phosphorylation of zidovudine (ZDV) and other nucleoside reverse transcriptase inhibitors (RTI) used for human immunodeficiency virus (HIV) infection. *Pharmacol Res* 1998;15:819–825.

46. Peter K, Lalezari JP, Gambertoglio JG. Quantification of zidovudine and individual zidovudine phosphates in peripheral blood mononuclear cells by a combined isocratic high performance liquid chromatography radioimmunoassay method. *J Pharm Biomed Anal* 1996;14:491–499.

47. Robbins BL, Rodman J, McDonald C, Srinivas RV, Flynn PM, Fridland A. Enzymatic assay for measurement of zidovudine triphosphate in peripheral blood mononuclear cells. *Antimicrob Agents Chemother* 1994;38:115–121.

48. Robbins BL, Tran TT, Pinkerton FH Jr, et al. Development of a new cartridge radioimmunoassay for determination of intracellular levels of lamivudine triphosphate in the peripheral blood mononuclear cells of human immunodeficiency virus-infected patients. *Antimicrob Agents Chemother* 1998;42:2656–2660.

49. Qian M, Chandrasena G, Ho RJ, Unadkat JD. Comparison of rates of intracellular metabolism of zidovudine in human and primate peripheral blood mononuclear cells. *Antimicrob Agents Chemother* 1994;38:2398–2403.

50. Balzarini J, Herdewijn P, De Clercq E. Differential patterns of intracellular metabolism of 2′,3′-didehydro-2′,3′-dideoxythymidine and 3′-azido-2′,3′-dideoxythymidine, two potent anti-human immunodeficiency virus compounds. *J Biol Chem* 1989;264:6127–6133.

51. Hoggard PG, Kewn S, Barry MG, Khoo SH, Back DJ. Effects of drugs on 2′,3′-dideoxy-2′,3′-didehydrothymidine phosphorylation in vitro. *Antimicrob Agents Chemother* 1997;41:1231–1236.

52. Veal GJ, Barry MG, Khoo SH, Back DJ. In vitro screening of nucleoside analog combinations for potential use in anti-HIV therapy. *AIDS Res Hum Retroviruses* 1997;13:481–484.

53. Kewn S, Veal GJ, Hoggard PG, Barry MG, Back DJ. Lamivudine (3TC) phosphorylation and drug interactions in vitro. *Biochem Pharmacol* 1997;54:589–595.

54. Cheng CL, Smith DE, Carver PL, et al. Steady-state pharmacokinetics of delavirdine in HIV-positive patients: effect on erythromycin breath test [Comments]. *Clin Pharmacol Ther* 1997;61:531–543.

55. Freimuth WW. Delavirdine mesylate: a potent non-nucleoside HIV-1 reverse transcriptase inhibitor. *Adv Exp Med Biol* 1996;394:279–289.

56. Voorman RL, Maio SM, Hauer MJ, Sanders PE, Payne NA, Ackland MJ. Metabolism of delavirdine: a human immunodeficiency virus type-1 reverse transcriptase inhibitor, by microsomal cytochrome P450 in humans, rats, and other species: probable involvement of CYP2D6 and CYP3A. *Drug Metab Dispos* 1998;26:631–639.

57. Voorman RL, Maio SM, Payne NA, Zhao Z, Koeplinger KA, Wang X. Microsomal metabolism of delavirdine: evidence for mechanism-based inactivation of human cytochrome P450 3A. *J Pharmacol Exp Ther* 1998;287:381–388.

58. Havlir D, Cheeseman SH, McLaughlin M, et al. High-dose nevirapine: safety, pharmacokinetics, and antiviral effect in patients with human immunodeficiency virus infection. *J Infect Dis* 1995;171:537–545.

59. Lamson M, Macgregor T, Riska P, et al. Nevirapine induces both CYP3A4 and CYP2B6 metabolic pathways. *Clin Pharmacol Ther* 1996;65:PI–79.

60. Riska P, Erickson D, Joseph D, Dinallo R, Hattox S. Nevirapine, a nonnucleoside reverse transcriptase inhibitor: metabolism in man, mouse, rat, dog, cynomolgus monkey and chimpanzee. *Int Conf AIDS* 1996;11:321.

61. Erickson D, Riska P, Hattox S, et al. Nevirapine hydroxylation, an in vitro probe for the simultaneous determination of CYP3A and CYP2B6 activity in human liver microsomes. ISSX-U.S.A. regional meeting, 1997:98.

62. Harrell AW, Wheeler SM, Pennick M, Clarke SE, Chenery RJ. Evidence that famciclovir (BRL 42810) and its associated metabolites do not inhibit the 6 beta-hydroxylation of testosterone in human liver microsomes. *Drug Metab Dispos* 1993;21:18–23.

63. Gill KS, Wood MJ. The clinical pharmacokinetics of famciclovir. *Clin Pharmacokinet* 1996;31:1–8.

64. Filer CW, Allen GD, Brown TA, et al. Metabolic and pharmacokinetic studies following oral administration of ^{14}C-famciclovir to healthy subjects. *Xenobiotica* 1994;24:357–368.

65. Rashidi MR, Smith JA, Clarke SE, Beedham C. In vitro oxidation of famciclovir and 6-deoxypenciclovir by aldehyde oxidase from human, guinea pig, rabbit, and rat liver. *Drug Metab Dispos* 1997;25:805–813.

66. Rubio FR, Fukuda EK, Garland WA. Urinary metabolites of rimantadine in humans. *Drug Metab Dispos* 1988;16:773–777.

67. Wills RJ, Farolino DA, Choma N, Keigher N. Rimantadine pharmacokinetics after single and multiple doses. *Antimicrob Agents Chemother* 1987;31:826–828.

68. Choma N, Davis PP, Edom RW, Fukuda EK. Quantitation of the enantiomers of rimantadine and its hydroxylated metabolites in human plasma by gas chromatography/mass spectrometry. *Biomed Chromatogr* 1992;6:12–15.

69. Brown SY, Garland WA, Fukuda EK. Isolation and characterization of an unusual glucuronide conjugate of rimantadine. *Drug Metab Dispos* 1990;18:546–547.

70. Paroni R, Del Puppo M, Borghi C, Sirtori CR, Galli Kienle M. Pharmacokinetics of ribavirin and urinary excretion of the major metabolite 1,2,4-triazole-3-carboxamide in normal volunteers. *Int J Clin Pharmacol Ther Toxicol* 1989;27:302–307.

71. Bertz RJ, Granneman GR. Use of in vitro and in vivo data to estimate the likelihood of metabolic pharmacokinetic interactions. *Clin Pharmacokinet* 1997;32:210–258.

72. Shaw PN, Houston JB. Kinetics of drug metabolism inhibition: use of metabolite concentration-time profiles. *J Pharmacokinet Biopharmacol* 1987;15:497–510.

73. Kim AE, Dintaman JM, Waddell DS, Silverman JA. Saquinavir, an HIV protease inhibitor, is transported by *P*-glycoprotein. *J Pharmacol Exp Ther* 1998;286:1439–1445.

74. Pavelic ZP, Reising J, Pavelic L, Kelley DJ, Stambrook PJ, Gluckman JL. Detection of *P*-glycoprotein with four monoclonal antibodies in normal and tumor tissues. *Arch Otolaryngol Head Neck Surg* 1993; 119:753–757.

75. Brinkman K, Huysmans F, Burger DM. Pharmacokinetic interaction between saquinavir and cyclosporine [Letter]. *Ann Intern Med* 1998;129:914–915.

76. Ouellet D, Hsu A, Qian J, et al. Effect of fluoxetine on pharmacokinetics of ritonavir. *Antimicrob Agents Chemother* 1998;42: 3107–3112.

77. Lake BG, Ball SE, Renwick AB, et al. Induction of CYP3A isoforms in cultured precision-cut human liver slices. *Xenobiotica* 1997;27: 1165–1173.

78. Li AP, Reith MK, Rasmussen A, et al. Primary human hepatocytes as a tool for the evaluation of structure-activity relationship in cytochrome P450 induction potential of xenobiotics: evaluation of rifampin, rifapentine and rifabutin. *Chem Biol Interact* 1997;107: 17–30.

79. Oesch F, Arand M, Benedetti MS, Castelli MG, Dostert P. Inducing properties of rifampicin and rifabutin for selected enzyme activities of the cytochrome P-450 and UDP-glucuronosyltransferase superfamilies in female rat liver. *J Antimicrob Chemother* 1996;37:1111–1119.

80. Gillum JG, Israel DS, Polk RE. Pharmacokinetic drug interactions with antimicrobial agents. *Clin Pharmacokinet* 1993;25:450–482.

81. Havlir D, Friedland G, Pollard R, et al. Combination of zidovudine (ZDV) and stavudine (d4T) therapy versus other nucleosides: report of two randomized trials (ACTG290 and 298). 5th Conference on Retroviruses and Opportunistic Infections, 1998:79.

82. Lertora JJ, Rege AB, Greenspan DL, et al. Pharmacokinetic interaction between zidovudine and valproic acid in patients infected with human immunodeficiency virus. *Clin Pharmacol Ther* 1994;56: 272–278.

83. Lee BL, Tauber MG, Sadler B, Goldstein D, Chambers HF. Atovaquone inhibits the glucuronidation and increases the plasma concentrations of zidovudine. *Clin Pharmacol Ther* 1996;59:14–21.

84. Sahai J, Gallicano K, Pakuts A, Cameron DW. Effect of fluconazole on zidovudine pharmacokinetics in patients infected with human immunodeficiency virus [Comments]. *J Infect Dis* 1994;169:1103–1107.

85. Trapnell CB, Klecker RW, Jamis-Dow C, Collins JM. Glucuronidation of 3′-azido-3′-deoxythymidine (zidovudine) by human liver microsomes: relevance to clinical pharmacokinetic interactions with atovaquone, fluconazole, methadone, and valproic acid. *Antimicrob Agents Chemother* 1998;42:1592–1596.

86. Burger DM, Meenhorst PL, Koks CH, Beijnen JH. Pharmacokinetic interaction between rifampin and zidovudine. *Antimicrob Agents Chemother* 1993;37:1426–1431.

87. Knupp CA, Shyu WC, Dolin R, et al. Pharmacokinetics of didanosine in patients with acquired immunodeficiency syndrome or acquired immunodeficiency syndrome-related complex. *Clin Pharmacol Ther* 1991;49:523–535.

88. van Leeuwen R, Lange JM, Hussey EK, et al. The safety and pharmacokinetics of a reverse transcriptase inhibitor, 3TC, in patients with HIV infection: a phase I study. *AIDS* 1992;6:1471–1475.

89. Dudley MN, Graham KK, Kaul S, et al. Pharmacokinetics of stavudine in patients with AIDS or AIDS-related complex. *J Infect Dis* 1992;166:480–485.

90. Blum MR, Liao SH, Good SS, de Miranda P. Pharmacokinetics and bioavailability of zidovudine in humans. *Am J Med* 1988;85:189–194.

91. Rodrigues AD, Roberts EM, Mulford DJ, Yao Y, Ouellet D. Oxidative metabolism of clarithromycin in the presence of human liver microsomes: major role for the cytochrome P4503A (CYP3A) subfamily. *Drug Metab Dispos* 1997;25:623–630.

92. Ouellet D, Hsu A, Granneman GR, et al. Pharmacokinetic interaction between ritonavir and clarithromycin. *Clin Pharmacol Ther* 1998;64: 355–362.

93. Benedek IH, Joshi A, Fiske WD, et al. Pharmacokinetic (PK) interaction studies in healthy volunteers with efavirenz (EFV) and the macrolide antibiotics, azithromycin (AZM) and clarithromycin (CLR). 5th Conf Retrovir Oppor Infect 1998:144 [Abstract].

94. von Moltke LL, Greenblatt DJ, Schmider J, et al. Midazolam hydroxylation by human liver microsomes in vitro: inhibition by fluoxetine, norfluoxetine, and by azole antifungal agents. *J Clin Pharmacol* 1996; 36:783–791.

95. Omar G, Whiting PH, Hawksworth GM, Humphrey MJ, Burke MD. Ketoconazole and fluconazole inhibition of the metabolism of cyclosporin A by human liver in vitro. *Ther Drug Monit* 1997;19: 436–445.

96. De Wit S, Debier M, De Smet M, et al. Effect of fluconazole on indinavir pharmacokinetics in human immunodeficiency virus-infected patients. *Antimicrob Agents Chemother* 1998;42:223–227.

97. Cato A III, Cao G, Hsu A, Cavanaugh J, Leonard J, Granneman R. Evaluation of the effect of fluconazole on the pharmacokinetics of ritonavir. *Drug Metab Dispos* 1997;25:1104–1106.

98. Gibbs MA, Thummel KE, Shen DD, Kunze KL. Inhibition of cytochrome P-450 3A (CYP3A) in human intestinal and liver microsomes: comparison of K_i values and impact of CYP3A5 expression. *Drug Metab Dispos* 1999;27:180–187.

99. Kerr B, Yuen G, Daniels R, Quart B, Anderson R. Strategic approach to nelfinavir mesylate (NFV) drug interactions involving CYP3A metabolism. 4th Conf Retro and Opportun Infect 1997.

100. Bertz R, Wong C, Carother L, Il L, Dennis S, Valdes J. Evaluation of the pharmacokinetics of multiple dose ritonavir and ketoconazole in combination. *Clin Pharmacol Ther* 1998;63:230.

101. Lamson M, Robinson P, Gigliotti M, Myers MW. The pharmacokinetic interactions of nevirapine and ketoconazole (Keto). Int Conf AIDS 1998;12:55 [Abstract].

102. Eagling VA, Back DJ, Barry MG. Differential inhibition of cytochrome P450 isoforms by the protease inhibitors, ritonavir, saquinavir and indinavir. *Br J Clin Pharmacol* 1997;44:190–194.

103. Wang Y, Unadkat J. Differential inhibitory capacities of indinavir (IND) and ritonavir (RIT) towards cytochrome P450 (CYP) enzymes 3A4 and 3A5. *Pharmacol Sci* 1998;1:1128.

104. Ferry JJ, Herman BD, Carel BJ, Carlson GF, Batts DH. Pharmacokinetic drug-drug interaction study of delavirdine and indinavir in healthy volunteers. *J Acquir Immune Defic Syndr Hum Retrovirol* 1998;18:252–259.

105. Merry C, Barry MG, Mulcahy F, Halifax KL, Back DJ. Saquinavir pharmacokinetics alone and in combination with nelfinavir in HIV-infected patients. *AIDS* 1997;11:F117–120.

106. Cox S, Schneck D, Herman B, et al. Delavirdine (DLV) and nelfinavir (NFV): a pharmacokinetic (PK) drug-drug interaction study in healthy adult volunteers. 5th Conf Retrovir Oppor Infect 1998:144 (abstract no. 345).

107. Skowron G, Leoung G, Kerr B, et al. Lack of pharmacokinetic interaction between nelfinavir and nevirapine [Editorial; comment]. *AIDS* 1998;12:1243–1244.

108. Hsu A, Granneman GR, Cao G, et al. Pharmacokinetic interaction between ritonavir and indinavir in healthy volunteers. *Antimicrob Agents Chemother* 1998;42:2784–2791.

109. Hsu A, Granneman GR, Cao G, et al. Pharmacokinetic interactions between two human immunodeficiency virus protease inhibitors, ritonavir and saquinavir. *Clin Pharmacol Ther* 1998;63:453–464.

110. Merry C, Barry MG, Mulcahy F, et al. Saquinavir pharmacokinetics alone and in combination with ritonavir in HIV-infected patients. *AIDS* 1997;11:F29–F33.

111. Fiske W, Benedek I, Joseph J, et al. Pharmacokinetics of efavirenz (EFV) and ritonavir (RIT) after multiple oral doses in healthy volunteers. Int Conf AIDS 1998;12:827 (abstract no. 42269).

112. Ferry J, Schneck D, Carlson G, et al. Evaluation of the pharmacokinetic (PK) interaction between ritonavir (RIT) and delavirdine (DLV) in healthy volunteers. 4th Conf Retrovir Opportun Infect 1997;Jan 22–26.

113. Cox S, Batts D, Stewart F, et al. Evaluation of the pharmacokinetic (PK) interaction between saquinavir (SQV) and delavirdine (DLV) in healthy volunteers. 4th Conf Retrovir Opportun Infect 1997;Jan 22–26.

114. Sahai J, Cameron W, Salgo M, et al. Drug interaction study between saquinavir (SQV) and nevirapine (NVP). 4th Conf Retrovir Opportun Infect 1997;Jan 22–26:178 (abstract no. 614).

115. Morse G, Shelton M, Hewitt R, et al. Ritonavir (RIT) pharmacoki-

netics (PK) during combination therapy with delavirdine (DLV). 5th Conf Retrovir Opportun Infect 1998, February 1–5 (abstract no. 343).

116. Fiske W, Benedek I, White S, Pepperess K, Joseph J, Kornhauser D. Pharmacokinetic interaction between efavirenz (EFV) and nelfinavir mesylate (NFV) in healthy volunteers. 5th Conf Retrovir Oppor Infect 1998, February 1–5:144 (abstract no. 349).

117. Murphy R, Gagnier P, Lamson M, Dusek A, Ju W, Hsu A. Effect of nevirapine (NVP) on pharmacokinetics (PK) of indinavir (IDV) and ritonavir (RTV) in HIV-1 patients. 4th Conf Retrovir Opportun Infect 1997:133 (abstract).

118. Yuen G, Anderson R, Sandoval T, Wu E, Shetty B, Kerr B. The pharmacokinetics (PK) of nelfinavir (NVR) administered alone and with rifampin (RIF) in healthy volunteers [Abstract]. *Clin Pharmacol Ther* 1997;61:147.

119. Benedek I, Joshi A, Fiske W, et al. Pharmacokinetic interaction between efavirenz (EFV) and rifampin (RIF) in healthy volunteers. Int Conf AIDS 1998;12:829 (abstract no. 42280).

120. Borin M, Cox S, Chambers J, Freimuth W, Gagnon S. Effect of rifampin (RIF) on delavirdine (DLV) pharmacokinetics in HIV+ patients. In: Program of abstracts from the Interscience Conference. Bethesda, MD: American Society for Microbiology, 1994, p. 82.

121. Winchell G, McCrea J, Carides A, et al. Pharmacokinetic interaction between indinavir and rifabutin [Abstract PI-66]. *Clin Pharmacol Ther* 1997;61:153.

122. Borin MT, Chambers JH, Carel BJ, Freimuth WW, Aksentijevich S, Piergies AA. Pharmacokinetic study of the interaction between rifabutin and delavirdine mesylate in HIV-1 infected patients. *Antiviral Res* 1997;35:53–63.

123. Robinson P, Lamson M, Gigliotti M, Myers M. Pharmacokinetic (PK) interaction between nevirapine (NVP) and rifampin (RMP). Int Conf AIDS 1998;12:1115 (abstract no. 60623).

CHAPTER 32

H₁-Receptor Antagonists

Danny D. Shen, Soraya Madani, Christopher Banfield, and Robert P. Clement

INTRODUCTION

The available H₁-receptor antagonists—antihistamines—are divided into two classes. The first-generation antihistamines, including diphenhydramine, chlorpheniramine, tripelennamine, and hydroxyzine, are capable of penetrating the blood–brain barrier, interacting with the central H₁ receptor, and causing drowsiness and impairment of cognitive function. These older antihistamines also interact with cholinergic receptors to elicit anticholinergic side effects. Despite these drawbacks, the first-generation antihistamines have been used widely for many years without any safety problems.

The second-generation antihistamines are much more selective toward the peripheral H₁ receptors, and distribute into the brain poorly. As a result, they are remarkably free from central and peripheral nervous system side effects and are considered nonsedating. Introduction of the first two second-generation antihistamines, terfenadine and astemizole, in the early 1980s, heralded a new era in the treatment of seasonal allergies and was a huge commercial success. However, case reports of serious and occasionally fatal ventricular arrhythmia (viz., torsades de pointes) associated with terfenadine overdose, as well as combined use of terfenadine with some antifungals and macrolide antibiotics, began to appear by 1990 (1,2). Soon afterward, the adverse drug interactions with terfenadine were shown to be the result of profound inhibition of CYP3A-mediated terfenadine metabolism. Similar occur-

rence of cardiotoxicity was observed later with astemizole. These reported incidents of adverse drug interactions with terfenadine were the first of many significant metabolic drug interactions involving the CYP3A enzymes that were to follow throughout the 1990s. The discovery of such a potentially fatal metabolic drug interaction also attracted the attention of the US Food and Drug Administration (FDA), which led to the demand for prospective in vitro and in vivo studies of metabolic drug interactions during new drug development.

This chapter reviews the available literature on metabolic interactions with the nonsedating antihistamines with a focus on the role of CYP3A. Detailed information is available on drug interactions involving terfenadine, whereas much fewer data exist in the open literature for the other nonsedating antihistamines. Therefore the emphasis of our presentation is on terfenadine.

TERFENADINE

Metabolism and Disposition

Terfenadine is eliminated entirely by oxidative metabolism. Detailed studies on the metabolic fate of terfenadine have been conducted in vitro by using human liver microsomes (3,4). Two primary pathways have been identified: C-hydroxylation of the tert-butyl side chain to yield the alcohol metabolite (TOH), and N-dealkylation to form azacyclonol (AZ) and 4-(4-t-butylphenyl)-4-hydroxybutyraldehyde (see Fig. 32-1). Terfenadine alcohol undergoes rapid, successive oxidative steps to form the carboxylic acid metabolite, terfenadine acid (TCOOH). Terfenadine acid is the major circulating metabolite and is responsible for the antihistaminic effects of terfenadine. The alcohol metabolite also undergoes a minor amount of N-dealkylation to AZ.

Yun et al. (3) were the first investigators to establish that CYP3A4 is the main enzyme responsible for the two primary pathways of terfenadine through activity correlation

D. D. Shen: Department of Pharmaceutics, School of Pharmacy, University of Washington, Box 357610, Room H272 Health Sciences Building, Seattle, Washington 98195-7610

S. Madani: Center for Drug Evaluation and Research, Food and Drug Administration, 5600 Fishers Lane, HFD 870, Rockville, Maryland 20857

C. Banfield and R. P. Clement: Department of Drug Metabolism and Pharmacokinetics, Schering-Plough Research Institute, 2015 Galloping HIll Road, Kenilworth, New Jersey 07033-0539

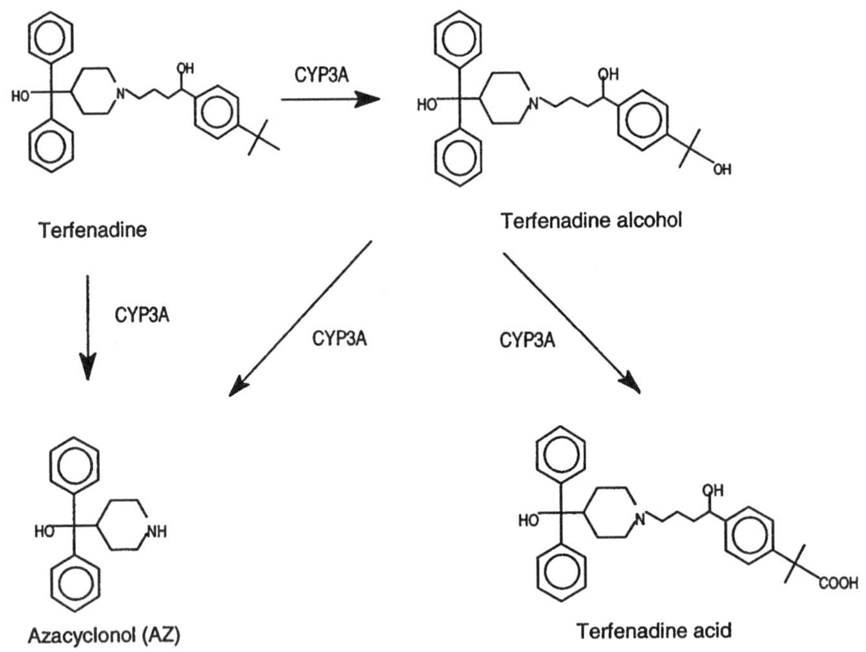

FIG. 32-1. Metabolic pathways for terfenadine oxidation.

in a liver bank with a CYP3A catalytic probe and chemical and immuno-inhibition studies. Jones et al. (4) recently showed that terfenadine can be oxidized to its alcohol metabolite by microsomes derived from B-lymphoblastoid cells expressing CYP2D6. However, the V_{max} (per picomole P450) of terfenadine oxidation with cDNA-expressed CYP2D6 was one sixth of that observed for CYP3A4. Given the relatively low constitutive level of CYP2D6 in human liver, the contribution of CYP2D6 is estimated to be well less than 5% that of CYP3A4 in the hepatic metabolism of terfenadine. In fact, Jones et al. (4) reported that quinidine at a concentration of 1 μM, which selectively inhibits CYP2D6, did not affect the rate of terfenadine oxidation in pooled human liver microsomes.

In a follow-up to the study of Yun et al., Ling et al. (5) examined the secondary oxidation of alcohol to the acid, and concluded that CYP3A4 is also the rate-determining enzyme. They further showed that, at a relatively high substrate concentration of 30 μM, C-oxidation accounted for 75% and N-dealkylation 25% of primary oxidation. Formation of acid metabolite accounts for 90% of terfenadine alcohol oxidation, whereas N-dealkylation of TOH to AZ accounts for the remaining 10%. Thus most of terfenadine is eventually converted to the acid metabolite (about 68%) in vitro.

Investigations into the bioavailability and pharmacokinetics of terfenadine have been hampered by the lack of an intravenous formulation. An early study by Okerholm et al. (6) compared the disposition kinetics of ^{14}C-labeled with unlabeled terfenadine at an oral dose of 60 mg in healthy human volunteers. Plasma terfenadine was analyzed by a radioimmunoassay. After the unlabeled dose, very low

plasma concentrations of intact terfenadine were observed. A mean peak plasma concentration of 1.54 ± 0.73 ng/mL was achieved in 0.79 ± 0.43 hours. In comparison, a mean peak plasma radioactivity corresponding to 351 ± 43 ng/mL equivalent of terfenadine was attained in 1.67 ± 0.41 hours after ^{14}C-terfenadine administration. A recent study by Lalonde et al. (7), which collected single-dose pharmacokinetic data in 132 healthy, nonsmoking, male volunteers by using a sensitive liquid chromatography–mass spectrometry (LC–MS) assay, confirmed the low circulating concentrations of terfenadine. They observed a geometric mean, peak plasma concentration of 1.54 ng/mL (60% coefficient of variation) after 120 mg, twice the terfenadine dose used in the Okerholm study. Okerholm et al. (6) estimated the oral bioavailability of terfenadine at 0.5%, based on the ratio of the area under the plasma concentration–time curve (AUC) of unlabeled terfenadine to that of radiolabeled terfenadine. A later study by Gartiez et al. (8) showed that 45% to 63% of a 60-mg oral dose of terfenadine was recovered as its carboxylic acid metabolite; 15% to 20% was excreted in urine, and 30% to 50% in feces. An additional 20% of the dose was recovered as AZ in urine only. Therefore between 65% and 85% of the terfenadine oral dose is accounted for in the form of metabolites. These observations have led to the conclusion that the gastrointestinal absorption of terfenadine is nearly complete, and the estimated more than 99% loss in oral dose is due to extensive first pass metabolism.

It should be noted that the often-quoted first pass estimate of 99.5% relied on the implicit (and rather unconventional) assumption that the clearance of terfenadine and that of its circulating metabolites are comparable.

The exact sites of first pass metabolism (i.e., intestines, liver, and the lungs) have not been defined, an issue that is important in our understanding of the kinetics of drug interactions. A recent report of an inhibition of terfenadine metabolism by grapefruit juice (see later section), which selectively inhibits and inactivates gut CYP3A enzymes (9), does point to the involvement of terfenadine first pass metabolism at the intestinal epithelium.

In Vitro Metabolic Kinetics

The metabolic kinetics of terfenadine in human liver microsomes have been characterized by a number of investigators (10–14), often as part of a study to elucidate *in vivo* drug interactions with terfenadine. Only two recent studies from Raeissi et al. (13) and our laboratory (14) have investigated terfenadine metabolism *in vitro* in both the liver and intestinal mucosa. Raeissi et al. (13) compared terfenadine metabolism in microsomes prepared from one human liver and one human intestinal mucosa, and from a subclone of Caco-2 cells (TC7) in culture that expresses CYP3A5. Our study was performed on microsomes prepared from separate panels of human livers and intestinal mucosa ($n = 4$ each) (14).

Table 32-1 lists the published enzyme kinetic parameters and the relevant conditions of the metabolic experiments. The reported K_m and V_{max} values vary widely and are accompanied by notable differences in the microsomal incubation condition between studies. For the human liver, K_m ranges from well less than 1 μM as observed in our laboratory (14) to as high as 60 μM reported by Jurima-Romet et al. (10). Two of the studies could not report V_{max} because of the lack of metabolite standards

for assay calibration. The V_{max} for formation of varied TOH from the other three studies varies by about two-fold. The largest variation is observed with the reported values of V_{max}/K_m or intrinsic clearance for TOH formation, ranging from more than 1,300 μL/min/mg protein in our study (14) to as low as 24 μL/min/mg in the study of Rodrigues et al. (12). The same sort of difference appears to exist for the intestinal data between the study of Raessi et al. (13) and Madani (14). We observed K_m values for terfenadine oxidation to either TOH or AZ to be less than 0.7 μM, whereas Raessi et al. reported slightly higher values (more than 1.4 μM). Our V_{max} values for both pathways were markedly greater than the estimates of Raessi et al. (13). These differences translate into many-fold differences between intrinsic clearance estimates for the intestine, more than 700 μL/min/mg from our study (14) versus less than 24 μL/min/mg from Raessi et al. (13).

Deviation from an initial velocity condition, nonspecific microsomal protein binding of terfenadine, and lack of measurements at appropriately low substrate concentrations (at or below K_m) probably account for much of the variation between studies. By using a sensitive LC–MS method for the assay of terfenadine metabolites, we found that initial velocity conditions could be achieved only by keeping the microsomal protein concentrations below 0.2 mg/mL and incubation time less than 10 minutes at substrate concentrations around the K_m (less than 1 μM) (13). The alcohol metabolite is rapidly lost by further oxidation to terfenadine acid. Moreover, at terfenadine concentrations exceeding 10 μM, substrate inhibition kinetics were observed. The high protein concentration and long incubation times adopted by several of the earlier studies were probably necessitated by

TABLE 32-1. *Summary of literature data on the kinetics of microsomal terfenadine oxidation in vitro*

Tissue/Study	Terfenadine (μM)	Incubation time (min)	Protein conc. (mg/mL)	Species assayed	K_M (μM)	V_{max} (pmol/ min/mg)	$Cl_{int,mic}$ (μL/min/mg)
Liver							
Jurima-Romet et al. (10), N = 3	10–400	30	2.0	TOH	60 ± 8	NA	NA
				AZ	27 ± 8		
von Moltke et al. (11), N = 3	5–150	20	0.25	TOH	15.2 ± 2.3	NA	NA
				AZ	4.6 ± 0.3		
Rodrigues et al. (12), N = 3	1–200	60	2.0	T	9.6 ± 2.8	234 ± 63	24
	1–200	10	2.0	TOH	12.9 ± 3.7	188 ± 51	15
Raessi et al. (13), N = 1	1–42	5	0.125	TOH	1.8	370	205
				AZ	0.8	60	75
Madani et al. (14), N = 4	0.05–30	6	0.075	TOH	0.23 ± 0.15[a]	253 ± 237	1,367 ± 791
				AZ	3.3 ± 3.0	132 ± 89	120 ± 156
Intestine							
Raessi et al. (13), N = 1	1–42	30	0.25	TOH	2.5	61	24
				AZ	1.4	14	10
Madani et al. (14), N = 4	0.05–30	6	0.10	TOH	0.22 ± 0.09	243 ± 46	1,295 ± 599
				AZ	0.38–036	179 ± 73	765 ± 426
Caco-2 (CYP3A5) Raessi et al (13)	1–42	45	1.0	TOH	1.9	2.1	1.1

NA, not available.

[a]Based on unbound terfenadine concentration in microsomal suspension.

limited metabolite assay sensitivity. In view of these technical limitations with the earlier studies, only the data from the recent studies of Raessi et al. (13) and Madani (14) represent reasonably accurate parameter estimates for the Michaelis–Menten kinetics of terfenadine oxidation in human liver and intestinal microsomes. Moreover, those incubation protocols that resulted in non–initial velocity conditions will also lead to an overestimation of median inhibitory concentration (IC_{50}) or K_i from in vitro inhibition studies (see later section). Nevertheless, rank order in vitro/in vivo correlation of K_i data for a given set of incubation conditions may still be feasible.

In vitro/in vivo scaling of terfenadine metabolism was performed on the estimates of hepatic and intestinal microsomal intrinsic clearance for primary oxidation obtained from our study (i.e., 1,495 ± 697 μL/min/mg and 2,060 ± 629 μL/min/mg, respectively). A satisfactory prediction of the oral clearance of terfenadine reported by Lalonde et al. (7) was obtained. More important, the average first pass extraction of terfenadine by intestinal and hepatic CYP3As was predicted to be 96% and 27% with a well-stirred organ extraction model and accounting for plasma protein binding in estimating the hepatic intrinsic clearance. These theoretical predictions suggest that gut wall metabolism may be a major contributor to the extensive first pass effect of this antihistamine. The presence of mucosal CYP3A-mediated metabolism may explain the profound inhibition of terfenadine first pass during simultaneous dosing with CYP3A inhibitors, because the local concentration of inhibitor at the luminal surface could be very high.

Cardiotoxicity

Woosley et al. (15) were the first investigators to show that terfenadine, but not the major circulating carboxylic acid metabolite, inhibits delayed-rectifier potassium current in isolated cat ventricular myocytes in a manner much like quinidine. Subsequent studies in human and rodent ventricular myocytes (16,17) showed that terfenadine blocks multiple potassium currents: the inward-rectifier (I_K1), the delayed rectifier (I_K), and the transient outward (I_{to}) currents. Together these actions lead to delayed repolarization, QT-interval prolongation, and enhanced susceptibility to premature ventricular depolarizations, which trigger polymorphic ventricular arrhythmia or torsades de pointes. Near-complete inhibition of the various cardiac potassium currents was generally noted at terfenadine concentrations between 1 and 10 μM (0.5–5 μg/mL).

The normally low circulating concentrations (about 1 ng/mL or less) of terfenadine at therapeutic doses of the antihistamine, primarily a result of extensive first pass metabolism, do not elicit significant effects on cardiac potassium channels. However, after overdose or when terfenadine metabolism is impaired, such as in liver disease or through drug interactions, plasma terfenadine can be elevated to concentrations that are associated with signif-

icant blockade of cardiac potassium currents and increased risk of ventricular arrhythmia.

In Vivo Interactions

This section summarizes the reported pharmacokinetic studies investigating drug interactions with terfenadine, most of which were performed in healthy volunteers. The studies concentrated on azole antifungals, macrolide antibiotics, and antidepressants, three classes of drugs that were identified in adverse drug reaction reports to the FDA and considered to have a high frequency of combined use with terfenadine.

Azole Antifungals

Ketoconazole was the first drug that was implicated in adverse drug interactions with terfenadine in the landmark report by Monahan et al. in 1990 (2). Shortly afterward, the same investigative group reported a pharmacokinetic and electrocardiographic (ECG) study in six healthy volunteers (18). The volunteers received 60 mg of terfenadine twice daily for 8 days, and then 200 mg ketoconazole given twice a day was added to the subjects' regimen and continued for another 7 days. Pharmacokinetic profiling of terfenadine was performed on day 8, and again after 6 days of concomitant administration of ketoconazole and terfenadine. ECG recordings were obtained at baseline, at the time of predose after 1 week taking terfenadine alone, and after the addition of ketoconazole to the regimen.

Plasma terfenadine concentrations were below the high-performance liquid chromatography (HPLC) assay detection limit (about 5 ng/mL) in all but a single subject after 1 week of terfenadine treatment. After combined treatment with ketoconazole, plasma terfenadine concentration became readily measurable. Peak terfenadine concentration ranged from 25 to 80 ng/mL, and trough concentration varied from 15 to 50 ng/mL. Because baseline plasma terfenadine could not be measured, the exact magnitude of increase in apparent oral clearance of terfenadine could not be ascertained. If we were to compare the observed range of C_{max} after addition of ketoconazole to the population-average C_{max} of 0.75 ng/mL for a 60-mg dose, as reported by Lalonde at el. (7), we estimate a remarkable 32- to 100-fold increase in peak concentration.

Although the acid metabolite of terfenadine did not show changes in peak concentration (177–488 ng/mL) and time to peak (about 2 hours) on addition of ketoconazole, a prolongation in the terminal half-life was observed. There was a 57% increase in metabolite AUC. This suggests that ketoconazole inhibited the elimination clearance of terfenadine acid in a significant fashion.

A slight increase in mean QT interval was observed at the time of predose after 1 week of terfenadine treatment compared with baseline (416 ± 6 ms vs. 408 ± 8 ms). All six subjects exhibited prolongation of QT_c to a mean of 490 ± 16 ms after the addition of ketoconazole. There was an excellent correlation between the increase in QT$_c$ and plasma terfenadine concentration.

Honig et al. (19) also investigated the interaction between itraconazole and terfenadine after case reports of torsades de pointes in patients receiving the two drugs in combination (20), and in view of the ability of itraconazole to inhibit cyclosporine clearance. Terfenadine pharmacokinetics and QT intervals were studied after a 120-mg dose in six healthy volunteers, before and after 7 days of oral itraconazole at 200 mg daily. As was observed in the ketoconazole study, plasma terfenadine concentration increased from a barely or less than detectable level to readily quantifiable levels after ketoconazole treatment. Itraconazole did not elevate the peak terfenadine concentrations to a level as high as those observed in the ketoconazole study (10–20 ng/mL vs. 25–80 ng/mL). This is consistent with the fact that itraconazole is a slightly weaker inhibitor of hepatic microsomal CYP3A metabolism in vitro (21), although the difference in terfenadine treatment (single vs. steady state) may also be a factor in determining the magnitude of terfenadine interaction between the two antifungal drugs. A rough estimate of the magnitude of increase in terfenadine C_{max} based on a population baseline value of 0.75 ng/mL would yield a 12- to 26-fold increment. A modest increase in the QT$_c$ (425 ± 9 ms to 432 ± 12 ms) was associated with the less dramatic increase in plasma terfenadine after itraconazole.

Honig et al. (22) also observed itraconazole-induced changes in the acid metabolite pharmacokinetics that differed from those with ketoconazole: a significant delay in time to peak (2–3 to 4–6 hours), a lowering of C_{max} (469 ± 136 ng/mL to 272 ± 37 ng/mL), and a modest 30%

decrease in AUC. These data suggest that itraconazole did not inhibit the elimination clearance of the acid metabolite significantly, and most of the observed changes reflected the delay and slight reduction in formation of the acid metabolite.

Further studies on the pharmacokinetics of terfenadine interaction have been reported for fluconazole and terbinafine (22,23). Fluconazole treatment (200 mg, once daily) did not lead to an increase in plasma terfenadine above detectable levels in a group of healthy volunteers; neither was there a significant change in QT$_c$ interval on their ECG recordings. Fluconazole did cause a small increase in the acid metabolite C_{max} and AUC, suggesting an interfering effect on terfenadine acid disposition. In the case of terbinafine, no significant differences in terfenadine or acid metabolite pharmacokinetics were observed when comparing the addition of terfenadine with an ongoing regimen of terbinafine (250 mg, once daily) versus placebo. No ECG changes were noted during combined terbinafine and terfenadine treatment. The lack of an interaction between terfenadine and terbinafine is not unexpected, because its known K_i for CYP3A-mediated metabolism is more than 100 µM (see Chapter 47, Neuvonen), which is well above terbinafine therapeutic plasma, and presumably intestinal enterocyte, concentrations. The absence of a significant interaction between fluconazole and terfenadine is more curious because fluconazole will inhibit the oral clearance of midazolam (24), another selective CYP3A substrate. The apparent K_i for inhibition of midazolam 1'-hydroxylation is approximately 10 µM (25). However, the K_i of fluconazole for inhibition of terfenadine metabolism is apparently greater than 100 µM (Table 32-2) and above circulating flucona-

TABLE 32-2. *Summary of in vitro K_i against C-oxidation of terfenadine in human liver microsomes for azole antifungals and selective serotonin reuptake inhibitors*

Inhibitor	Competitive K_i (µM)		Therapeutic plasma concentration of inhibitor (µM)
	Von moltke et al.[a] (Ref. 11)	Shen et al.[b] (unpublished data)	
Azole antifungals			
Ketoconazole	0.34	0.30	1–10
Clotrimazole	—	0.08	1.9 ± 4.5 (oral) 0.015 (troche)
Miconazole	—	0.71	16 (i.v.) 0.42 (oral) 0.011–0.033 (vaginal)
Itraconazole	2.1	0.70	3.2
Fluconazole	>20	133	3.9–30
SSRIs			
Fluoxetine	66	47	0.5–1.5
Norfluoxetine	13	17	0.5–1.5
Paroxetine	56	53	0.1–0.4
Sertraline	30	77	0.1–0.3
Desmethylsertraline	7.5	—	0.1–0.3
Fluvoxamine	51	—	0.5–1.5

[a]Incubation condition: 0.25 mg/mL microsomal protein, 20-min incubation time, NADPH-generating system.
[b]Incubation condition: 0.5 mg/mL microsomal protein, 10-min incubation time, NADPH-generating system, 1 mM NAD.

zole concentrations, suggesting that the effect of a CYP3A inhibitor is substrate dependent.

Macrolide Antibiotics

Erythromycin is the macrolide antibiotic that has most frequently been associated with clinical reports of terfenadine cardiotoxicity. Honig et al. (26) investigated the effects of concomitant erythromycin treatment on terfenadine pharmacokinetics and ECG pharmacodynamics in nine healthy volunteers. The subjects received 60 mg terfenadine b.i.d. for 7 days before the addition of oral erythromycin at 500 mg every 8 hours. The combined treatment continued for another 6 days. Serial blood collection and electrocardiographic recordings were performed after the morning dose on the last day of treatment with terfenadine alone, and after 6 days of combined treatment.

Three of the nine subjects had detectable accumulation of intact terfenadine in plasma (peak concentrations of 11–34 ng/mL). The mean QT_c interval increased by 18 ms between baseline (predrug) and after 1 week of terfenadine treatment. A further increase in mean QT_c by 19 ms was observed after addition of erythromycin to the terfenadine regimen. Although neither increase was statistically significant, Honig et al. commented that the increase in mean QT_c (64 ms) for the subgroup of subjects with a measurable increase in plasma terfenadine during terfenadine and erythromycin combination treatment did attain statistical significance.

An approximate two-fold increase in C_{max} and AUC of terfenadine acid metabolite, along with a delay in time to peak (2.2 ± 0.2 hours to 4.0 ± 0.3 hours) also were observed. It appears that erythromycin has a remarkable inhibitory effect on elimination of the carboxylic acid metabolite, at a magnitude that is greater than that observed with ketoconazole or itraconazole.

Overall, the data of Honig et al. (26) support the hypothesis that erythromycin inhibits terfenadine first pass metabolism and presents a risk for cardiotoxicity. However, the inhibitory effect is less predictable among individuals, and of a lesser magnitude than that observed with ketoconazole.

In a follow-up study (27), Honig et al. compared the effects of 1-week treatment with erythromycin (500 mg, t.i.d.), clarithromycin (500 mg, b.i.d.), and azithromycin (500 mg load, 250 mg, once daily) on the steady-state pharmacokinetics and ECG effects of terfenadine (60 mg, b.i.d.; $n = 6$ in each group). The results for the erythromycin treatment group replicated those observed in the earlier study. The effects with clarithromycin treatment resembled those observed with erythromycin [i.e., variable (detectable levels in three of the six subjects) and modest elevations in plasma terfenadine (peak concentration from 6 to 12 ng/mL), and small but definite increases in QT_c, particularly in those subjects with a measurable

increase in plasma terfenadine]. Azithromycin treatment did not alter the pharmacokinetics or the cardiac effects of terfenadine. The absence of an interaction between azithromycin and terfenadine was confirmed later in a study by Harris et al. (28).

It should be noted that both erythromycin and clarithromycin are mechanism-based inhibitors *in vitro* and may exert some of their *in vivo* inhibitory effects through their metabolites (see Chapter 46, Polk). Therefore, inhibitory interactions with these drugs are likely to depend on the duration and schedule of antibiotic treatment. It may also explain the intersubject variability in their inhibitory effect.

Antidepressants

The possible involvement of selective serotonin reuptake inhibitors (SSRIs) in adverse drug interactions with terfenadine was first raised in the literature by two isolated case reports of a possible interaction between fluoxetine and terfenadine (29,30). Whereas fluoxetine and its metabolite, norfluoxetine, are known to be weak inhibitors of CYP3A (i.e., their therapeutic concentrations are less than one tenth of the reported K_i values; see Table 32-2), the possibility of a metabolic or pharmacodynamic interaction under exceptional circumstances, such as with unusually high doses of fluoxetine, cannot be ruled out. Recently Bergstrom et al. (31) conducted a human volunteer study to compare the pharmacokinetics and QT response of a single 60-mg test dose of terfenadine before and after treatment with a loading regimen of fluoxetine at 60 mg daily for 9 days. This loading regimen yielded plasma levels of fluoxetine and norfluoxetine that are close to the steady-state levels observed during regular administration of a 20-mg antidepressant dose of fluoxetine. By using a sensitive LC–MS method for the assay of plasma terfenadine, they were able to characterize the plasma concentration time course of intact terfenadine after a single 60-mg dose of terfenadine. Fluoxetine treatment resulted in an unexpected decrease in plasma terfenadine: a 30% decrease in C_{max} and a 42% decrease in AUC. The fluoxetine loading regimen did not alter the time course of the terfenadine acid metabolite. A comparison of serial QT-interval measurements over a 12-hour period after the two single test doses of terfenadine did not reveal a significant increase after the 9-day regimen of fluoxetine.

Interaction studies with two other monoamine reuptake inhibitors, paroxetine (32) and venlafaxine (33), have been reported. Terfenadine AUC was determined during steady-state dosing with either terfenadine alone (60 mg, b.i.d.) or after addition of terfenadine to a paroxetine regimen (20 mg, daily). The venlafaxine–terfenadine study examined a single test dose (120 mg) of terfenadine before and after an escalating regimen of venlafaxine (37.5 mg, b.i.d., for 3 days followed by 75 mg, b.i.d., for

5 days). In both studies, concomitant treatment or pretreatment with the antidepressant did not alter plasma terfenadine kinetics as measured by LC-MS. QT_c was monitored in the paroxetine study and did not show any measurable increase as a result of coadministration of paroxetine and terfenadine over terfenadine alone. In both studies, small but measurable decreases in the C_{max} and AUC of terfenadine acid metabolite in plasma were noted.

Miscellaneous Drugs

Recently Ng et al. (34) reported a single case of torsades de pointes during concomitant use of terfenadine and cimetidine in a 21-year-old Chinese woman. However, Honig et al. (35) showed earlier that neither the addition of cimetidine at 600 mg every 12 hours nor ranitidine at 150 mg every 12 hours to a 60-mg/day regimen of terfenadine resulted in measurable accumulation of plasma terfenadine, change in acid metabolite pharmacokinetics, or increase in QT interval. The negative finding is consistent with the fact that cimetidine inhibits terfenadine metabolism in human liver microsomes only at concentrations more than 500 μM (unpublished data).

Stern et al. (36) recently reported on a volunteer study to examine the potential effect of atorvastatin, a CYP3A4 substrate, on the pharmacokinetics of a single 120-mg test dose of terfenadine. One-week pretreatment with a high 80-mg daily dose of atorvastatin lowered the mean C_{max} slightly, but increased the mean AUC of plasma terfenadine by 35%. There was a slight decrease in both the mean C_{max} and AUC of the acid metabolite. However, none of these changes was statistically significant. These investigators concluded that atorvastatin does not pose a risk when combined with terfenadine; however, no ECG assessment was performed to confirm the lack of pharmacodynamic effects.

Negative findings also were reported from a recent terfenadine interaction study with a new antipsychotic sertindole, which is a substrate of CYP2D6 and CYP3A4 (37).

Grapefruit Juice

Grapefruit juice is known to inhibit the first pass metabolism of a number of high first pass CYP3A substrates, most notably dihydropyridine calcium channel blockers and cyclosporine (9). Recent studies showed that grapefruit juice constituents, in addition to being competitive inhibitors of CYP3A4, are capable of inactivating mucosal CYP3A4. This suggests that the inhibitory effect of grapefruit juice may be localized at the intestinal mucosa. As mentioned earlier, we have demonstrated a high rate of terfenadine oxidation in microsomes prepared from the mucosa of human small intestine. Therefore any inhibitory effects of grapefruit juice on terfena-

dine pharmacokinetics may be indicative of intestinal first pass metabolism of terfenadine.

Since 1996, four separate studies have investigated the effects of grapefruit juice on terfenadine pharmacokinetics and effects on QT interval (38–41). The first two studies by Honig et al. (38) and Benton et al. (39) involved a two-phase, repetitive terfenadine dosing protocol. In phase I, the two daily doses of terfenadine (60 mg each) were taken with 240 mL of water. Throughout phase II, terfenadine was taken along with 240 mL of double-strength grapefruit juice prepared from frozen concentrate. Each phase lasted 1 week. The study of Honig et al. was performed in six healthy volunteers who were slow metabolizers of terfenadine. The second study by Benton et al. was conducted in an unselected group of 12 volunteers. In addition, during phase II, half of the subjects (n = 6) received the double-strength grapefruit juice simultaneous with terfenadine (simultaneous group); the other subjects received grapefruit juice 2 hours after terfenadine (delayed group). In both studies, modest but consistent elevation in plasma terfenadine was observed during simultaneous dosing of terfenadine with grapefruit juice compared with terfenadine with water. Peak plasma concentrations of terfenadine observed during phase II were mostly around or less than 10 ng/mL and did not exceed 20 ng/mL. Only two of the six subjects who delayed taking grapefruit juice 2 hours after terfenadine had a measurable increase in plasma terfenadine. Consistent increase (22%–55%) in plasma concentration of terfenadine acid metabolite was observed, the effect being greater in the "simultaneous" group. In both studies, a small and statistically significant increase in mean QT_c interval was observed in the grapefruit juice phase compared with the control phase; individual increases were especially noted in those subjects who had a detectable increase in plasma terfenadine concentration.

The more recent studies from Clifford et al. (40) and Rau et al. (41) were single-dose, grapefruit juice–terfenadine interaction studies. By using a sensitive LC-MS assay, Clifford et al. documented a roughly three-fold increase in the C_{max} and AUC of plasma terfenadine when terfenadine was taken with 300 mL of freshly squeezed grapefruit juice as compared with when it was taken with water. However, they were not able to discern a significant lengthening in the mean QT_c. On the other hand, Rau et al. (41) compared the effects of regular and double-strength grapefruit juice and found no difference in their ability to elevate plasma terfenadine. Similar to the study by Clifford et al. (40), but in contrast to the earlier long-term dosing studies, QT interval was not altered.

The clinical significance of grapefruit juice–terfenadine interaction remains uncertain. There is, however, no dispute that terfenadine metabolism is inhibited to a lesser degree than that induced by ketoconazole or erythromycin, and most likely reflects a selective inhibition of gut CYP3A-mediated first pass.

In Vitro Interactions

Several groups of investigators, including our laboratory, have studied the interaction of terfenadine with known CYP3A inhibitors or substrates in human liver microsomes to support a metabolic mechanism for *in vivo* findings of terfenadine–drug interactions, and to explore *in vitro/in vivo* kinetic correlations. The earliest study by Jurima-Romet et al. (10) reported K_i values for a series of azole antifungals, macrolide antibiotics, and other known CYP3A substrates. In contrast to *in vivo* findings, little distinction in their *in vitro* K_i was observed across the antifungals or macrolide antibiotics. For example, both ketoconazole and fluconazole had K_i values around 10 μM. These K_i estimates may be confounded by inappropriate incubation conditions (see Table 32-1), as mentioned earlier; for example, exceptionally high microsomal protein concentration (2 mg/mL) and long incubation time (30 minutes) were used.

A later study by von Moltke et al. (11) reported *in vitro* K_i for azole antifungals and SSRIs that appear to be much more in line qualitatively with *in vivo* interaction data. Table 32-2 presents their K_i data for terfenadine *C*-oxidation, along with unpublished data collected in our laboratory by using a similar incubation protocol. Several comments are in order. First, there is a good agreement in the K_i values between the two laboratories. Second, *in vitro* inhibitory potency can be ranked by comparing the therapeutic plasma concentration of the inhibitor with its K_i value (i.e., I/K_i ratio). Accordingly, there appears to be an excellent rank-order correlation between the *in vitro* and *in vivo* inhibitory potency of the azole antifungals (i.e., ketoconazole > itraconazole > fluconazole). The K_i values of SSRIs were uniformly high relative to their known therapeutic plasma concentrations, suggesting that they are very weak inhibitors *in vivo*.

Von Moltke et al. (11) attempted a quantitative prediction of *in vivo* inhibition through *in vitro/in vivo* scaling based on their *in vitro* K_i values and accounting for partitioning of the inhibitor between liver tissue and plasma. These investigators assumed that intrahepatic inhibitor concentration (as opposed to total or unbound plasma concentration) is a more appropriate measure of the inhibitor concentration at the site of enzyme. Their predicted range of AUC increments [i.e., nine to 37 for ketoconazole and two to ten for itraconazole, and around one for fluconazole (negligible inhibition)], were somewhat below the increment observed *in vivo* as described in the previous section. The cause of the slight underprediction is not known, and may be related to the neglect of intestinal first pass metabolism in the scaling approach.

The same *in vitro/in vivo* scaling when applied to the SSRIs yielded a respective prediction of two- to five-fold and 1.2- to 1.4-fold increment in terfenadine AUC for fluoxetine and paroxetine. The prediction for fluoxetine clearly does not agree with the *in vivo* findings of a decrease in plasma terfenadine (31). The metabolic interaction between fluoxetine and terfenadine probably involves a mechanism other than enzyme inhibition. The inhibitory effect of paroxetine appears to be overpredicted when compared with that in the human volunteer study of Martin et al. (32). It is possible that the assumption of intrahepatic concentration as the effective inhibitory concentration of SSRIs may not be appropriate. If total or free plasma concentration was used, a negligible interaction would have been predicted, which is more consistent with actual observation.

Jurima-Romet et al. (42) have reported the use of human hepatocytes in short-term, primary culture for the study of terfenadine drug interactions. They reported K_i values for several antifungals and macrolide antibiotics that were comparable to what has been determined in human liver microsomes.

As already mentioned, the *in vitro/in vivo* scaling described earlier did not account for the full possibility of sequential first pass metabolism of terfenadine at the intestine and the liver. Unfortunately, we have very little data on the inhibition kinetics of terfenadine metabolism in human intestinal microsomes. Raeissi et al. (13) have reported data on inhibition of terfenadine *C*-oxidation in human jejunal microsomes by ketoconazole and troleandomycin. The apparent IC_{50} values at 20 μM terfenadine appear to be consistent with those observed in human liver microsomes.

This discussion illustrates the challenges of *in vitro/in vivo* scaling of metabolic inhibition, even in the case of terfenadine and CYP3A, for which a great deal of data have been amassed. Further presentation of this topic is found in Chapter 1.

FEXOFENADINE

Fexofenadine, the carboxylic acid metabolite of terfenadine, was introduced as an alternative to terfenadine in late 1997. This eventually led to the withdrawal of terfenadine from the US market. Clinical trials have shown that clinically effective dosages of fexofenadine, 120 or 180 mg daily, do not produce prolongation of the cardiac QT interval and should be free of the cardiotoxic effects of its precursor (43). This is consistent with the minimal effects of fexofenadine on repolarizing potassium currents in the myocardium (16) and cloned human cardiac potassium channels (44–46,49).

In human volunteers, 92% of a 60-mg dose of [^{14}C]fexofenadine was recovered, 80% from feces and 12% from the urine. More than 85% of the recovered radioactivity was in the form of unchanged drug, indicating minimal metabolism (43). Potential interactions with ketoconazole or erythromycin have been investigated by the manufacturer, Hoechst Marion Roussel (47). When erythromycin (500 mg, q8h) or ketoconazole (400 mg, once daily) was added to a high-dose regimen of fexofenadine (120 mg, twice daily), nearly 100% to 150% increases in steady-state C_{max} and AUC of fexofenadine were observed. This is reminiscent of the previously reported increase in plasma acid metabolite concentration after terfenadine when erythromycin or ketoconazole was coadministered (18,24,25). Very recently, Soldner et al. (48) showed that fexofenadine is subject to efflux transport by P-glycoprotein (MDR1) or other multidrug resistance–associated proteins (MRPs) in Caco-2 cells. Because ketoconazole is known to be an inhibitor of P-glycoprotein and erythromycin a substrate (see Chapter 11), the elevation in plasma concentration during combined administration of fexofenadine with these two antimicrobial agents may reflect a blockade of its excretion in the bile or efflux at the gastrointestinal epithelium.

ASTEMIZOLE

Astemizole is known to cause torsades de pointes in overdose situations and when combined with azole antifungals and erythromycin (47). Although the adverse drug interactions with astemizole have repeatedly been attributed to inhibition of CYP enzymes (putatively CYP3A4) in literature reviews, few, if any, reported studies have documented details of the metabolic mechanism.

In humans, astemizole is known to undergo oxidative metabolism to yield three major metabolites, desmethylastemizole, norastemizole (N-dealkylation at the piperidine nitrogen), and 6-hydroxydesmethylastemizole (50). Unlike the situation with terfenadine, both the O- and N-dealkyl-metabolites as well as astemizole possess antihistaminic effect (51), and have been shown to block delayed-rectifier potassium currents in isolated myocytes and perfused cat hearts (47). Astemizole and its desmethyl-metabolite were equally potent, and norastemizole was slightly less potent in prolonging QT interval in perfused feline hearts.

Like terfenadine, orally administered astemizole is subject to extensive first pass metabolism (about 90% of dose) (52). Therefore, circulating concentrations of astemizole are very low (less than 1 ng/mL). Desmethylastemizole is thought to be a major metabolite (about 50%) formed during first pass. Desmethylastemizole has a very long terminal half-life, ranging from 10 days after a single dose to 20 days after steady-state dosing; this compares with a half-life of 1 to 2 days for the parent drug. Therefore desmethylastemizole and with its hydroxylated metabolite accumulate over 4 to 8 weeks of continuous dosing, and reach concentrations well exceeding that of unchanged astemizole.

In its product literature (53), the manufacturer (Janssen Pharmaceutica) reports in vitro studies with human liver microsomes that show CYP3A4 to be the principal enzyme responsible for the formation of desmethylastemizole. It also states that CYP1A2 and CYP2D6 are involved in the "minor pathways"; however, the identity of these minor pathways (possibly including formation of norastemizole) was not revealed. Moreover, the enzyme(s) responsible for the 6-hydroxylation of desmethylastemizole was not mentioned. Layrijsen et al. (54) reported that ketoconazole, itraconazole, and erythromycin all inhibited O-desmethylation of astemizole with IC_{50} values that were higher than those observed with terfenadine hydroxylation. N-dealkylation of astemizole also was inhibitable by erythromycin.

There is only one published report on the pharmacokinetic interaction between itraconazole and astemizole in 12 male healthy volunteers (55). A 10-mg test dose of astemizole was administered on two separate occasions, once during steady state (daily administration of 200 mg itraconazole) and once during placebo administration. Itraconazole treatment prolonged the mean terminal half-life of astemizole from 2.1 to 3.6 days and increased its AUC by nearly three-fold. The C_{max} of astemizole did not change (0.74 vs. 0.81 ng/mL). The time to peak concentration of desmethylastemizole was delayed significantly (28 to 195 hours), and there was a two-fold increase in metabolite AUC. These data suggest inhibition of elimination clearance of both the parent drug and the O-desmethyl-metabolite; the secondary metabolism of desmethylastemizole also may involve CYP3A. There was, however, no statistically significant difference in the mean QT_c interval between the itraconazole- and placebo-treatment phase of the single-dose astemizole study. In the product literature (53), the manufacturer stated that interactions with other inhibitors of CYP3A (particular highlighting of ketoconazole, miconazole, metronidazole, fluconazole, erythromycin, clarithromycin, troleandomycin, and mibefradil) also result in markedly elevated plasma concentrations of astemizole and desmethylastemizole. In view of these findings, coadministration of any of these inhibitors with astemizole should be avoided.

LORATADINE

Loratadine is mainly eliminated by CYP-mediated oxidation to an important circulating active metabolite, descarboethoxyloratadine (DCL), which is in turn hydroxylated and excreted in urine and feces as conjugates. The CYP isoenzymes involved in loratadine metabolism were identified by using liver bank correlation, chemical and immunoinhibition studies, microsomes containing cDNA-expressed human CYPs, and molecular modeling (56). These in vitro methods showed that DCL formation is predominantly mediated by CYP3A4 and to a lesser extent by CYP2D6. At relatively high substrate concentrations (more than 1 μM or 400 ng/mL), CYP3A4 accounts for 75%, and CYP2D6, 25% of primary oxidation.

Separate human volunteer studies have been conducted to investigate the effects of concurrent administration of two prototypic CYP3A inhibitors, erythromycin (57) and ketoconazole (58), and a modest inhibitor of CYP2D6 and CYP3A4, cimetidine (57), on loratadine and DCL pharmacokinetics to assess the clinical relevance of the CYP enzyme profile observed *in vitro*. All three studies followed the same randomized, three-way crossover design ($N = 24$ in each study) with the inhibitors dosed at their clinically recommended dose and frequency. Once admitted into the protocol, subjects were randomly assigned to one of the following treatments: (a) one loratadine 10-mg tablet early in the morning for 10 days with concurrent administration of the inhibitor, (b) one loratadine 10-mg tablet daily in the morning for 10 days with concurrent administration of placebo, or (c) one placebo tablet daily in the morning for 10 days with concurrent administration of the inhibitor. A 14-day washout period separated each phase of the crossover periods. A "third party" assigned subjects to the various treatment groups because of differences in the dosage forms.

Safety and tolerability of the treatments were evaluated by physical examination and routine clinical laboratory tests. In addition, ECGs were performed at specified times before initiation of treatment, daily during treatment periods, and on day 10 of each treatment period. On day 10 of each period, blood samples were collected at specified times for the determination of plasma concentrations of loratadine, DCL, and the inhibitor drug. No subject was withdrawn from any of the studies for any ECG-related reason. The inhibitory effects of erythromycin, cimetidine, and ketoconazole on the plasma AUCs of loratadine and DCL are summarized in Table 32-3.

The importance of CYP3A in the clearance of loratadine was confirmed by the impairment of the loratadine metabolism during concurrent administration with the two CYP3A inhibitors. Erythromycin cotreatment resulted in a modest increase in loratadine AUC, whereas a remarkable three-fold increase in AUC was observed with ketoconazole cotreatment. This is consistent with the relative potency of the two inhibitors toward CYP3A activity.

If the loratadine dose were completely converted to DCL, no change in the primary metabolite AUC would

TABLE 32-3. *Percentage change in AUC (0–24h) of loratadine and DCL after 10 days of coadministration of loratadine with erythromycin, cimetidine, or ketoconazole*

Inhibitor	Loratadine	DCL
Erythromycin (500 mg, q8h)	+40%	+46%
Ketoconazole (200 mg, q12h)	+307%	+73%
Cimetidine (300 mg, q.i.d.)	+103%	+6%

have been expected. However, for both CYP3A inhibitors, DCL AUC was increased significantly, suggesting that CYP3A also is important in the clearance of DCL.

Cimetidine coadministration led to a significant increase in loratadine AUC, which probably reflects mostly inhibition of the CYP2D6 component of loratadine oxidation, although a small contribution from CYP3A inhibition cannot be ruled out because cimetidine does have a weak inhibitory effect on CYP3A. The absence of a significant change in the DCL AUC in the presence of cimetidine suggests a minor role for CYP2D6 in the clearance of DCL.

In all three studies, no prolongation in QT_c interval was observed. The lack of any cardiac effect is consistent with the absence of reports that clearly associate loratadine treatment with incidents of torsades de pointes (49). In addition, a 3-month study in 50 healthy volunteers given a daily dose of loratadine at four times the recommended level (40 mg) did not reveal any evidence of QT_c prolongation (58). Therefore metabolic interactions with CYP3A inhibitors do not appear to have adverse consequences.

CETIRIZINE

Cetirizine was formerly identified as a metabolite of hydroxyzine, a first-generation antihistamine. Cetirizine is eliminated largely as unchanged drug in urine, and to a smaller extent in feces, in total accounting for more than 65% of the dose (61). A small amount of *O*-dealkylated metabolite has been detected in blood or urine. Given its limited metabolism, significant metabolic interactions are not expected. Indeed, one interaction study with cimetidine yielded negative findings (62).

CONCLUSION

Our experience with the adverse drug interactions involving CYP3A-mediated metabolism of the nonsedating antihistamines over this past decade has given us rich insights into the pharmacokinetics of CYP3A inhibition. It is clear that dramatic metabolic interaction and possibly serious adverse events can result when a high–first pass drug (e.g., terfenadine) is combined with a number of marketed drugs that are potent CYP3A inhibitors (e.g., ketoconazole). We are also beginning to appreciate the critical role of intestinal CYP3A in determining the magnitude of the metabolic interaction. As a result, metabolic profiling of candidate molecules has become an essential part of high-throughput screening during the early stage of new drug development. It has also become an important consideration in drug selection and therapeutic substitution.

REFERENCES

1. Davies AJ, Harindra V, McEwan A, Ghose RR. Cardiotoxic effect with convulsions in terfenadine overdose. *Br Med J* 1989;298:325.

2. Monahan BP, Ferguson CL, Killeavy ES, Lloyd BK, Troy J, Cantilena LR Jr. Torsades de pointes occurring in association with terfenadine use. *JAMA* 1990;264:2788–2790.

3. Yun C, Okerholm RA, Guengerich FP. Oxidation of the antihistaminic drug terfenadine in human liver microsomes: role of cytochrome P-450 3A(4) in *N*-dealkylation and *C*-hydroxylation. *Drug Metab Disp* 1992; 21:403–409.

4. Jones BC, Hyland R, Ackland M, Tyman CA, Smith DA. Interaction of terfenadine and its primary metabolites with cytochrome P450 2D6. *Drug Metab Disp* 1998;26:875–882.

5. Ling HJ, Leeson GA, Burmaster SD, Hook RH, Reith MK, Cheng LK. Metabolism of terfenadine associated with CYP3A(4) activity in human hepatic microsomes. *Drug Metab Disp* 1995;23:631–636.

6. Okerholm RA, Weiner DL, Hook RH, et al. Bioavailability of terfenadine in man. *Biopharm Drug Dispos* 1981;2:185–190.

7. Lalonde RL, Lessard D, Gaudreault J. Population pharmacokinetics of terfenadine. *Pharm Res* 1996;13:832–838.

8. Garteiz DA, Hook RH, Walker BJ, Okerholm RA. Pharmacokinetics and biotransformation studies of terfenadine in man. *Arzneimittelforschung* 1982;32:1185–1190.

9. Bailey DG, Malcolm J, Arnold O, Spence JD. Grapefruit juice-drug interactions. *Br J Clin Pharmacol* 1998;46:101–110.

10. Jurima-Romet M, Crawford K, Cyr T, Inaba T. Terfenadine metabolism in human liver: in vitro inhibition by macrolide antibiotics and azole antifungals. *Drug Metab Dispos* 1994;22:849–857.

11. von Moltke L, Greenblatt DJ, Duan SX, Harmatz JS, Wright CE, Shader RI. Inhibition of terfenadine metabolism in vitro by azole antifungal agents and by selective serotonin reuptake inhibitor antidepressants: relation to pharmacokinetic interactions in vitro. *J Clin Psychopharmacol* 1996;16:104–112.

12. Rodrigues AD, Mulford DJ, Lee RD, et al. In vitro metabolism of terfenadine by a purified recombinant fusion protein containing cytochrome P4502A4 and NADPH-P450 reductase: comparison to human liver microsomes and precision-cut tissue slices. *Drug Metab Dispos* 1995;23:765–775.

13. Raeissi SD, Guo Z, Dobson GL, Artursson P, Hidalgo IJ. Comparison of CYP3A activities in a subclone of Caco-2 cells (TC9) and human intestine. *Pharm Res* 1997;14:1019–1025.

14. Madani S. The role of CYP2D6 and CYP3A4 in first-pass intestinal drug metabolism. Ph.D. thesis, University of Washington, 1998.

15. Woolsey RL, Chen Y, Freiman JP, Gillis RA. Mechanism of the cardiotoxic actions of terfenadine. *JAMA* 1993;269:1532–1536.

16. Crumb WJ, Wible B, Arnold DJ, Payne JP, Brown AM. Blockade of multiple human cardiac potassium currents by the antihistamine terfenadine: possible mechanism for terfenadine-associated cardiotoxicity. *Mol Pharmacol* 1995;47:181–190.

17. Berul CI, Morad M. Regulation of potassium channels by nonsedating antihistamines. *Circulation* 1995;91:2220–2225.

18. Honig PK, Wortham DC, Zamani K, Conner DP, Mullin JC, Cantilena LR Jr. Terfenadine-ketoconazole interaction: pharmacokinetic and electrocardiographic consequences. *JAMA* 1993;269:113–1518.

19. Honig PK, Wortham DC, Hull R, Zamani K, Smith JE, Cantilena LR. Itraconazole affects single-dose terfenadine pharmacokinetics and cardiac repolarization pharmacodynamics. *J Clin Pharmacol* 1993;33: 1201–1206.

20. Pohjola-Sintonen S, Viitasalo M, Toivonen L, Neuvonen P. Torsades de pointes after terfenadine-itraconazole interaction. *Br Med J* 1993;306: 186.

21. Back DJ, Tjia JF. Comparative effects of the antimycotic drugs ketoconazole, fluconazole, itraconazole and terbinafine on the metabolism of cyclosporin by human liver microsomes. *Br J Clin Pharmacol* 1991; 32:624–626.

22. Honig PK, Wortham DC, Zamani K, Mullin JC, Conner DP, Cantilena LR. The effect of fluconazole on the steady-state pharmacokinetics and electrocardiographic pharmacodynamics of terfenadine in humans. *Clin Pharmacol Ther* 1993;53:630–636.

23. Robbins B, Chang CT, Cramer JA, et al. Safe administration of terbinafine and terfenadine: a placebo-controlled crossover study of pharmacokinetic and pharmacodynamic interactions in healthy volunteers. *Clin Pharmacol Ther* 1996;59:275–283.

24. Ahonen J, Olkkola KT, Takala A, Neuvonen PJ. Interaction between fluconazole and midazolam in intensive care patients. *Acta Anaesthesiol Scand* 1999;43:509–514.

25. Gibbs MA, Thummel KE, Shen DD, Kunze KL. Inhibition of

cytochrome P-450 3A (CYP3A) in human intestinal and liver microsomes: comparison of Ki values and impact of CYP3A5 expression. *Drug Metab Dispos* 1999;27:180–187.

26. Honig PK, Woosley RL, Zamani K, Conner DP, Cantilena LR Jr. Changes in the pharmacokinetics and electrocardiographic pharmacodynamics of terfenadine with concomitant administration of erythromycin. *Clin Pharmacol Ther* 1992;52:231–218.

27. Honig PK, Wortham DC, Zamani K, Cantilena LR. Comparison of the effect of the macrolide antibiotics erythromycin, clarithromycin and azithromycin on terfenadine steady-state pharmacokinetics and electrocardiographic parameters. *Drug Invest* 1994;7:148–156.

28. Harris S, Hilligoss DM, Colangelo PM, Eller M, Okerholm R. Azithromycin and terfenadine: lack of drug interaction. *Clin Pharmacol Ther* 1995;58:310–315.

29. Swims MP. Potential terfenadine-fluoxetine interaction. *Ann Pharmacother* 1993;27:1404–1405.

30. Marchiando RJ, Cook MD, Jue SG. Probable terfenadine-fluoxetine-associated cardiac toxicity. *Ann Pharmacother* 1995;29:937–938.

31. Bergstrom RF, Goldberg MJ, Cerimele BJ, Hatcher BL. Assessment of the potential for a pharmacokinetic interaction between fluoxetine and terfenadine. *Clin Pharmacol Ther* 1997;62:643–650.

32. Martin DE, Zussman BD,Everett D, Benincosa LJ, Etheredge RC, Jorkasky DK. Paroxetine does not affect the cardiac safety and pharmacokinetics of terfenadine in healthy adult men. *J Clin Psychopharmacol* 1997;17:451–459.

33. Amchin J, Zarycranski W, Taylor KP, Albano D, Klockowski PM. Effect of venlafaxine on the pharmacokinetics of terfenadine. *Psychopharmacol Bull* 1998;34:383–389.

34. Ng PW, Chan WK, Chan TYK. Torsades de pointes during the concomitant use of terfenadine and cimetidine. *Aust NZ J Med* 1998;26:120–121.

35. Honig PK, Wortham DC, Zamani K, Conner DP, Mullin JC, Cantilena LR. Effect of concomitant administration of cimetidine and ranitidine on the pharmacokinetics and electrocardiographic effects of terfenadine. *Eur J Clin Pharmacol* 1993;45:41–46.

36. Stern RH, Smithers JA, Olson SC. Atorvastatin does not produce a clinically significant effect on the pharmacokinetics of terfenadine. *J Clin Pharmacol* 1998;38:753–757.

37. Wong SL, Cao G, Mack R, Granneman GR. Lack of CYP3A inhibition effects of sertindole on terfenadine in healthy volunteers. *Int J Clin Pharmacol Ther* 1998;36:146–151.

38. Honig PK, Wortham DC, Lazarev A, Cantilena LR. Grapefruit juice alters the systemic bioavailability and cardiac repolarization of terfenadine in poor metabolizers of terfenadine. *J Clin Pharmacol* 1996;36:345–351.

39. Benton RE, Honig PK, Zamani K, Cantilena LR, Woosley RL. Grapefruit juice alters terfenadine pharmacokinetics, resulting in prolongation of repolarization on the electrocardiogram. *Clin Pharmacol Ther* 1996;59:383–388.

40. Clifford CP, Adams DA, Murray S, et al. The cardiac effects of terfenadine after inhibition of its metabolism by grapefruit juice. *Eur J Clin Pharmacol* 1997;52:311–315.

41. Rau SE, Bend JR, Arnold MO, Tran LT, Spence JD, Bailey DG. Grapefruit juice-terfenadine single-dose interaction: magnitude, mechanism, and relevance. *Clin Pharmacol Ther* 1997;61:401–409.

42. Jurima-Romet M, Huang HS, Beck DJ, Li AP. Evaluation of drug interactions in intact hepatocytes: inhibitors of terfenadine metabolism. *Toxicol In Vitro* 1996;10:655–663.

43. Markham A, Wagstaff AJ. Fexofenadine. *Drugs* 1998;55:269–274.

44. Rampe D, Wile B, Brown AM, Dage RC. Effects of terfenadine and its metabolites on a delayed rectifier K⁺ channel cloned from human heart. *Mol Pharmacol* 1993;44:1240–1245.

45. Yang T, Prakash C, Roden DM, Snyders DJ. Mechanism of block of a human cardiac potassium channel by terfenadine racemate and enantiomers. *Br J Pharmacol* 1995;115:267–274.

46. Roy ML, Dumaine R, Brown AM. *HERG*: a primary human ventricular target of nonsedating antihistamine terfenadine. *Circulation* 1996; 94:817–823.

47. Woosley RL. Cardiac actions of antihistamines. *Annu Rev Pharmacol Toxicol* 1996;36:233–252.

48. *Physicians' Desk Reference*. Montvale, NJ: Medical Economics Company, 1999:1289–1291.

49. Soldner A, Christians U, Susanto M, Wacher VJ, Silverman JA, Benet LZ. Grapefruit juice activates P-glycoprotein-mediated drug transport. *Pharmacol Res* 1999;16:478–485.

50. Meuldermans W, Hendrickx J, Lauwers W, Hurkmans R, Swysen E,

Heykants J. Excretion and biotransformation of astemizole in rats, guinea pigs, dogs, and man. *Drug Dev Res* 1986;8:37–51.

51. Kamei C, Mio M, Izushi K, et al. Antiallergic effects of major metabolites of astemizole in rats and guinea pigs. *Arzneimittelforschung* 1991; 41:932–936.

52. Heykants J, van Peer A, Woestenborghs R, Jageneau A, Vanden Bussche G. Dose-proportionality, bioavailability, and steady-state kinetics of astemizole in man. *Drug Dev Res* 1986;8:71–78.

53. *Physicians' Desk Reference*. Montvale, NJ: Medical Economics Company, 1999:1423–1426.

54. Layrijsen K, van Houdt J, Thijs D, Meuldermans W, Janssens M, Heykants J. The interaction of ketoconazole, itraconazole and erythromycin with the in vitro metabolism of antihistamines in human liver microsomes [Abstract]. *Allergy* 1993;48(suppl 16):34.

55. Lefebvre RA, van Peer A, Woestenborghs R. Influence of itraconazole on the pharmacokinetics and electrocardiographic effects of astemizole. *Br J Clin Pharmacol* 1997;43:319–322.

56. Yumibe N, Huie K, Chen K-J, Snow M, Clement RP, Cayen MN. Identification of human liver cytochrome P450 enzymes that metabolize the nonsedating antihistamine loratadine. *Biochem Pharmacol* 1996;51: 165–172.

57. Brannan MD, Reidenberg P, Radwanski E, et al. Loratadine administered concomitantly with erythromycin: pharmacokinetic and electrographic evaluations. *Clin Pharmacol Ther* 1995;58:269–278.

58. Brannan MD, Reidenberg P, Radwanski E, Shneyer L, Lin C, Affrime MB. Evaluation of pharmacokinetic and electrocardiographic parameters following 10 days of concomitant administration of loratadine with ketoconazole [Abstract]. *J Clin Pharmacol* 1994;34:1016.

59. Brannan MD, Affrime MB, Reidenberg P, Radwanski E, Lin CC. Evaluation of the pharmacokinetics and electrocardiographic pharmacodynamics of loratadine with concomitant administration of cimetidine [Abstract]. *Pharmacotherapy* 1994;14:347.

60. Affrime MB, Lorber R, Danzig M, Cuss F, Brannan MD. Three month evaluation of electrocardiographic effects of loratadine in humans [Abstract]. *Allergy* 1993;48(suppl 16):29.

61. Spencer CM, Faulds D, Peters DH. Cetirizine: a reappraisal of its pharmacological properties and therapeutic use in selected allergic disorders. *Drugs* 1993;46:1055–1080.

62. Simons FE, Sussman GL, Simon KJ. Effect of the H_2-antagonist cimetidine on the pharmacokinetics and pharmacodynamics of the H_1-antagonist hydroxyzine and cetirizine in patients with chronic urticaria. *J Allergy Clin Immunol* 1994;95:685–693.

CHAPTER 33

Analgesics–Antipyretics

Sidney D. Nelson

INTRODUCTION

This chapter describes the known pathways of metabolism of acetaminophen and tramadol, and then highlights drug interactions observed for each drug, particularly in humans. Most of the discussion focuses on those interactions observed in humans that appear to modulate toxic effects of the drugs. Although an attempt is made to classify drug interactions of acetaminophen based on metabolic pathways, the reader should keep in mind that more than one pathway may be affected by the same agent. Acetaminophen is by far the most widely used analgesic–antipyretic agent, and several instances of drug interactions have been reported (1). However, despite the frequency with which this drug is used (and abused), in only a few instances have therapeutic consequences resulted from drug interactions.

ACETAMINOPHEN

Pathways of Drug Metabolism

Documented pathways of metabolism of acetaminophen are shown in Fig. 33-1 [refer to Chapter 6, ref. 1, for a review of pathways and their relative importance]. Although metabolic routes appear to be the same in all species, including humans, formation rates for each pathway vary considerably among species and may vary significantly within a species, depending on a variety of genetic and epigenetic factors. The following discussion of these pathways relates primarily relates to humans.

Glucuronidation and sulfation are the major pathways of elimination of acetaminophen in all animals and account for approximately 50% and 30%, respectively, of therapeutic doses of the drug in humans. Of the human

S. D. Nelson: Department of Medicinal Chemistry, School of Pharmacy, University of Washington, Box 357631, H375 Health Sciences Building, Seattle, Washington 98195-7631

uridine diphosphate (UDP)-glucuronosyltransferases (UGTs) tested, UGT1*6 has the highest affinity (K_m, about 2 mM), although several isoforms could catalyze the reaction (K_m, more than 12 mM) (2,3). Of the human sulfotransferases (SULTs), members of phenol sulfotransferase *SULT1* gene subfamily are active in acetaminophen sulfation (4,5), but kinetic parameters for the various isoforms have not been reported.

Hydrolysis of acetaminophen to p-aminophenol, and its subsequent reacetylation back to acetaminophen, has been shown to occur in rats (6,7). Approximately 10% of a dose of acetaminophen was determined to undergo this so-called "futile cycling" by stable-isotope labeling of the drug and nuclear magnetic resonance (NMR) spectroscopic analysis of urine (7). These same reactions are assumed to occur in humans because both species have homologous carboxylesterases of the *CES1* gene subfamily (8) and homologous N-acetyltransferases of the *NAT1* and *NAT2* gene subfamilies (9).

Oxidation of acetaminophen to N-acetyl-p-benzoquinone imine (NAPQI) by cytochromes P450 (CYPs) is considered to be the major pathway involved in hepatotoxicity caused by acetaminophen in overdose and some other situations (1,10,11). After taking normal therapeutic doses of acetaminophen, humans excrete into urine approximately 5% to 10% as thiol ether metabolites derived from reaction of glutathione (GSH) with NAPQI (1,12–14). This is likely an underestimation of the extent of oxidation of acetaminophen to NAPQI because it is known that this highly reactive quinone imine is subject to reduction back to acetaminophen by reduced nicotinamide adenine dinucleotide phosphate (NADPH), NADH, NADPH–cytochrome P450 reductase, and DT-diaphorase (11,15,16), as well as through *ipso* adduct decomposition reactions (17,18).

CYPs also oxidize acetaminophen to a catechol, 3-hydroxyacetaminophen (see Fig. 33-1), which is considered nontoxic based on studies in mice (19). The catechol

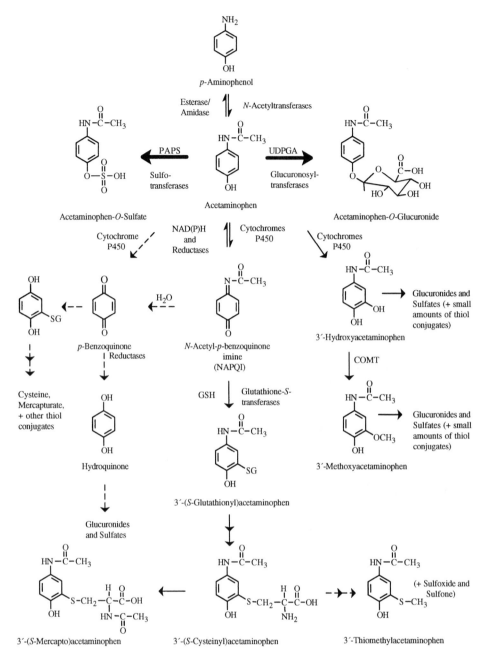

FIG. 33-1. Pathways of metabolism for acetaminophen. Bold arrows, major pathways in humans at therapeutic doses of acetaminophen (more than 20% of administered dose); regular arrows, intermediate pathways (more than 5%, less than 20%); and dashed arrows, minor pathways (less than 5%, many of which have been quantified only in laboratory animals).

plus its secondary metabolites account for about 4% to 8% of therapeutic doses of acetaminophen in humans (12–14). Whereas several human CYPs have been shown to oxidize acetaminophen to NAPQI (20–23), only a few have been found to form the catechol at detectable levels (Table 33-1) (23). Based on kinetic data obtained with purified enzymes, CYP1A2 and CYP3A4 should be the most efficient P450 isoforms in the oxidation of acetaminophen to NAPQI at therapeutic concentrations (about 0.1 mM) of the drug, whereas CYP1A1, CYP1A2, and

CYP2E1 should be most efficient at moderately high concentrations (0.5–2 mM). At concentrations of more than 2 mM, CYP2A6 and CYP2D6 contribute significantly to acetaminophen oxidation (20–23 and unpublished data). In contrast, only CYP2A6 and CYP2E1 contribute significantly to formation of the catechol metabolite.

However, these results with purified CYP isoforms should be interpreted cautiously because they do not take into consideration relative amounts of the different iso-

TABLE 33-1. *Activity of human cytochromes P450 (CYPs) in the oxidation of acetaminophen (1 Mm) to NAPQI, measured as its glutathione conjugate, 3′-(S-glutathionyl) acetaminophen, and the catechol, 3′-hydroxyacetaminophen*

Human isoform	3′-(S-glutathionyl) acetaminophen	3′-hydroxy-acetaminophen
CYP1A1[a]	6.7	ND[c]
CYP1A2[b]	10.0	0.1
CYP1B1[a]	ND[c]	ND[c]
CYP2A6[b]	1.7	6.6
CYP2B6[b]	ND[c]	ND[c]
CYP2C8[b]	0.2	0.1
CYP2C9[b]	0.1	ND[c]
CYP2C19[a]	ND[c]	ND[c]
CYP2D6[b]	1.6	ND[c]
CYP2E1[b]	4.6	0.6
CYP3A4[b]	1.2	0.1

Values expressed as nmol/min/nmol P450.
[a]Baculovirus-expressed Supersomes from Gentest Corp.
[b]Purified from baculovirus-expressed enzymes.
[c]Not detectable at the limits of the HPLC/EC assay used.

forms in the intestine and liver, nor do they consider competition of the isoforms for factors involved in reduction of the different CYPs. For example, based on the kinetic data, CYP1A1 and CYP1A2 should be significant contributors to NAPQI formation. However, CYP1A1 is almost absent in most human intestinal and liver tissue, and CYP1A2 appears to play little role in the bioactivation of acetaminophen in mice (24,25). Even on induction, neither CYP1A1 nor CYP1A2 appears to play a significant role in the metabolism of acetaminophen in humans (12,26,27).

Addition of GSH to NAPQI occurs rapidly and spontaneously with little contribution of glutathione S-transferases (GSTs) unless concentrations of GSH and NAPQI are very low, as would occur when GSH is depleted from liver cells after overdoses of acetaminophen (17). Human GSTs of the π gene family are most active in the conjugation reaction (17).

No studies have been reported on the enzymes involved in formation of other metabolites depicted in Fig. 33-1. Metabolites of the *p*-benzoquinone pathway have so far been detected only in mice (28) and represent less than 3% of toxic doses. Of mechanistic interest is that *p*-benzoquinone can arise by two pathways: oxidation of acetaminophen by P450 and hydrolysis of NAPQI (unpublished data). Products of further oxidation of 3-hydroxyacetaminophen and 3-methoxy-acetaminophen have also been identified only as minor metabolites of acetaminophen when mice are administered toxic doses (28). The remainder of the chapter focuses on drug interactions occurring only with primary pathways of metabolism.

Drug Interactions with the Glucuronidation Pathway

Although several drugs can alter the extent of glucuronidation of acetaminophen in laboratory animals and in humans (see Table 7.4 in ref. 1), in only a few cases has the extent of glucuronidation apparently decreased enough to augment hepatotoxicity. Congenic rats with a hereditary deficiency in bilirubin UDP-glucuronosyltransferase have significantly reduced glucuronidation activity toward acetaminophen with a concomitant two- to three-fold increase in the fraction of the acetaminophen dose converted to thioether conjugates (a measure of bioactivation to the toxic metabolite, NAPQI), and these rats are much more susceptible to hepatotoxicity caused by acetaminophen (29). The results show that severe impairment of glucuronidation can increase the risk for hepatotoxicity. Studies in limited numbers of patients with Gilbert's disease indicate that those with the greatest deficiency in glucuronidation activity toward acetaminophen may also be at higher risk for hepatotoxicity because of substantial two- to four-fold increases in acetaminophen thioether conjugate formation (30,31).

The drugs probenecid (32,33), salicylamide (34), and zidovudine (35) have been shown to inhibit competitively the glucuronidation of acetaminophen, and are known to decrease the extent of its glucuronidation in humans. However, there is only one case report of hepatotoxicity in an acquired immunodeficiency syndrome (AIDS) patient receiving zidovudine and acetaminophen that implicates this as a mechanism of increased risk of toxicity from acetaminophen (36). Conversely, a report associated acetaminophen with a higher frequency of hematologic toxicity in AIDS patients taking zidovudine (37). However, this is apparently unrelated to an effect of acetaminophen on glucuronidation of zidovudine, inasmuch as acetaminophen does not significantly inhibit this conjugation pathway (35,38). Acetaminophen has been observed to decrease significantly the elimination rate of chloramphenicol as its glucuronide, thereby putting patients at risk of chloramphenicol toxicity, but this occurred only when the drugs were given intravenously (39).

Several drugs (ascorbic acid, diphenylhydantoin, oral contraceptives, phenobarbital, rifampin, and sulfinpyrazone) and other factors (cigarette smoking, diets rich in cruciferous vegetables) can increase the extent of glucuronidation of acetaminophen in laboratory animals and humans; however, many of these also decrease extents of sulfation and/or increase the extent of formation of the major toxic metabolite of acetaminophen, so it is unclear in many cases what the overall effect on toxicity will be (see Table 7.4 in ref. 1).

Drug Interactions with the Sulfation Pathway

There are no reports of drug interactions with the sulfation pathway whereby the risk of toxicity caused by acetaminophen has increased. Sulfation is a detoxification pathway for acetaminophen, and decreases in the extent of metabolism of acetaminophen through this pathway in humans appear to be accompanied by an increase in detoxification through the glucuronidation pathway (see Table 7.4 in ref. 1).

N-Acetyl-L-cysteine, a widely used and effective treatment for acetaminophen overdose (40), significantly increases the fraction of a dose of acetaminophen that is cleared through the sulfation pathway (13,41). However, the primary mechanism of protection from hepatotoxicity by N-acetyl-L-cysteine appears to be enhanced GSH synthesis (see Drug Interactions with Cytochrome P450 Pathways).

Acetaminophen has been found to decrease the formation of sulfate conjugates of the oral contraceptive estrogen, ethinyl estradiol (42), of the renal vasodilator, fenoldepam (43), and of the active sulfate metabolite of the antihypertensive and hair-growth stimulatory drug, minoxidil (44), in humans. No changes in therapeutic efficacy of any of these drugs were noted.

Drug Interactions with Cytochrome P450 Pathways

Hundreds of chemicals are known to induce and/or activate cytochromes P450, and because the major toxic metabolite of acetaminophen, NAPQI, is formed by cytochrome P450 oxidation, it is not surprising that many of these chemicals have been found to increase the extent of toxicity caused by acetaminophen in laboratory animals (see Table 14.1 in ref. 1). However, most of these chemicals, including drugs used in humans, exert their effects only at supraphysiologic or supratherapeutic concentrations such that only a few drugs apparently increase risk of acetaminophen toxicity in humans. Even in some situations in which induction of cytochrome P450 isoforms would be anticipated to increase the rate of formation of NAPQI (e.g., induction of CYP1A family P450s by polycyclic aromatic hydrocarbons found in cigarette smoke and charcoal-broiled meat, and by the drug

omeprazole), no such increase has been observed in humans (12,26,27,45).

Several anticonvulsant drugs that induce more than one *CYP* gene family, such as phenobarbital, phenytoin, and carbamazepine, have been found to increase the formation of thioether conjugates as a marker of the oxidation of acetaminophen to NAPQI in humans (26,45,46). These drugs also increase the extent of glucuronidation of acetaminophen (26,45,47,48), which is a detoxification pathway, and may be the reason that only a few cases have been reported that link the ingestion of anticonvulsants with increased risk of hepatotoxicity caused by acetaminophen (49–51). This same argument may hold for other inducers of the metabolism of acetaminophen, such as rifampin (45,47) and sulfinpyrazone (26).

Just as many chemicals induce and/or activate cytochromes P450, many also repress and/or inhibit these enzymes and should protect against acetaminophen toxicity. Studies in laboratory animals demonstrate such protection for several chemicals (see Table 14.1 in ref. 1), but only a few drugs have been shown to decrease the oxidative metabolism of acetaminophen in humans.

Interferons may repress some cytochromes P450, and induction of interferon synthesis in mice can prevent acetaminophen-mediated hepatotoxicity (52), apparently by decreasing the rate of oxidation of acetaminophen by cytochromes P450 (53). However, induction of interferons by influenza vaccine has no effect on the metabolism of acetaminophen in humans (54), although one case has been reported of a cancer patient treated with interferons plus vinblastine who sustained hepatotoxicity after receiving therapeutic doses of acetaminophen (55).

There is one report that the relatively nonspecific inhibitor of human liver CYPs, ketoconazole, decreases the elimination rate of acetaminophen in humans (56), and one report that methoxsalen, a relatively specific inhibitor of CYP2A6, decreases the formation of thioether conjugates of acetaminophen in humans (57). Methoxsalen has been shown to decrease hepatotoxicity caused by acetaminophen in mice (58).

Propoxyphene is an analgesic that is used in combination with acetaminophen, and when given acutely, it is a potent inhibitor of cytochromes P450 by formation of a tight-binding metabolite complex with P450 heme (59). One case report suggested that propoxyphene protected against hepatotoxicity that would normally have been observed after human ingestion of a very large dose of acetaminophen (60). Other reports suggest that deaths associated with combinations of propoxyphene and acetaminophen are caused either by propoxyphene itself or by an induction effect of propoxyphene on acetaminophen metabolism to toxic metabolites (61).

Paradoxic inhibition and induction of cytochromes P450 are believed to be the basis for the complex drug interactions between some CYP2E1 inhibitors/inducers, such as ethanol and isoniazid, and acetaminophen

(14,62,63). These interactions are consistent with a time-dependent model of induction of CYP2E1 by ligand stabilization, a mechanism that results in the inhibition of CYP2E1 activity while the inducer is present and the enhancement of activity after the inducer is removed (64) (see Chapter 53, Slattery). For example, isoniazid is known to inhibit the oxidation of acetaminophen to NAPQI in humans for nearly 24 hours after coadministration (14,65), but from 24 to nearly 48 hours after administration, significant increases in its formation were observed (14). This increase may, in part, be responsible for some cases of hepatotoxicity and nephrotoxicity reported in patients receiving acetaminophen and isoniazid (66–68).

It also is known that ethanol is both an inhibitor and inducer of CYP2E1, at least in part by the same mechanism of protein stabilization as is isoniazid (69–71). Ethanol, given acutely, is known to inhibit the metabolism of acetaminophen and to protect against acetaminophen toxicity in laboratory animals (72–74), and may do so in humans as well (75). In contrast, prolonged ethanol administration potentiates liver injury caused by acetaminophen. This finding was first reported almost 20 years ago (76), and has been observed in several studies in laboratory animals and case reports and studies in humans since then (see Table 7.4 in ref. 1 and refs. 77–80). Although induction of CYP2E1 is likely to play a role in the potentiation of acetaminophen toxicity, because it is a major isoform involved in acetaminophen oxidation (20–24), selective induction of other P450 isoforms (such as CYP3A4) (81) and poor nutrition (82–84) are likely to play important roles in alcoholics as well.

Drug Interactions with the Glutathione Pathway

Glutathione is an important scavenger of reactive metabolites of acetaminophen, as was determined more than 25 years ago in pioneering studies by Mitchell et al. (85). In fact, the international standard treatment for acetaminophen poisoning is treatment with *N*-acetylcysteine (40), which appears to provide *L*-cysteine to replenish depleted glutathione stores in hepatocytes (86). Several other thiol-containing compounds and/or pro-drugs of *L*-cysteine have been found to protect against toxicity caused by acetaminophen in laboratory animals, apparently by a similar mechanism, although other mechanisms (e.g., antioxidant mechanisms) also may be involved (see Table 14.1 in ref. 1).

Ethanol is the only drug that has been demonstrated to decrease glutathione stores in hepatocytes and to potentiate hepatotoxicity caused by acetaminophen (82,87). Although it might be anticipated that some alkylating agents used in high-dose chemotherapy regimens could deplete glutathione to an extent that would potentiate acetaminophen toxicity, no studies of these possible drug–drug interactions have been reported.

Summary

Metabolic drug–drug interactions with acetaminophen are expected to be common because acetaminophen is a widely used drug taken in relatively high doses and is metabolized by several phase I and phase II pathways. Surprisingly, few of these drug interactions have been reported, and only a very small number have apparent therapeutic or toxicologic consequences. On the other hand, because of its widespread use and potential to cause life-threatening liver and kidney injury, awareness of the metabolic pathways of acetaminophen that may be affected to an extent that could cause increased risk of injury is important.

A recent example is that of a potential interaction with the new antidiabetic drug, acarbose (88–90). This drug exerts its pharmacologic effect in the gastrointestinal (GI) tract by competitively inhibiting some α-glucosidases, thereby decreasing postprandial blood glucose concentrations (91). Although only about 1% of a dose of acarbose reaches the systemic circulation, several cases of hepatotoxicity and allergic reactions have been associated with the drug (92). Apparently as a result of the effect on glucose concentrations, CYP2E1 was induced in rats by acarbose treatment, an effect that is augmented by ethanol treatment, and these rats became very susceptible to acetaminophen hepatotoxicity (88). However, as suggested in an editorial (89), acarbose may also decrease rates of glucuronidation of acetaminophen by decreasing glucose concentrations, and ethanol can have several effects on glutathione and other pathways. Whether some of the cases of hepatotoxicity reported after acarbose therapy in humans are related to coingestion of acetaminophen, or whether acarbose even potentiates acetaminophen toxicity in humans is not known.

The potential interaction between acetaminophen and warfarin received a great deal of attention recently (93). Results of a retrospective study suggested that acetaminophen was an underrecognized cause of overcoagulation, especially in elderly patients receiving warfarin therapy. Considering the large number of patients who have used acetaminophen as an analgesic-antipyretic when taking warfarin over the last 50 years, very few case reports have suggested that acetaminophen increased the anticoagulant effect of warfarin (94–97). Results of a recent case-controlled study indicate that acetaminophen does not significantly alter either the pharmacokinetics or pharmacodynamics of warfarin (98), and another study showed that acetaminophen did not significantly inhibit the metabolism of the therapeutically active *S*-warfarin to its inactive 7-hydroxy metabolite by CYP2C9 (99), the major route of elimination of *S*-warfarin in humans. Thus it seems unlikely that a metabolic drug–drug interaction occurs in the vast majority of patients, although some unusual genetic or environmental/nutritional/social factors may play a role in a small number of individuals.

Ingestion of alcohol is the most likely factor that could be involved in a metabolic drug–drug interaction with acetaminophen, and patients discontinuing therapy with isoniazid could be at risk as well. The number of cases involving other drug–drug interactions with acetaminophen is too small to suggest that they present a risk to most patients.

TRAMADOL

Pathways of Drug Metabolism

Tramadol (Ultram) is an analgesic with a unique mechanism of action introduced in the United States only recently, although it has been used in Europe since 1977 (100). Tramadol is *O*-demethylated to a therapeutically active phenolic metabolite by CYP2D6 and *N*-demethylated to an inactive metabolite by CYP3A4 (101). Secondary metabolites arise by further *N*- and *O*-demethylation and glucuronidation and sulfation of the phenolic hydroxy group (Fig. 33-2). Tramadol is administered as the racemate of the geometric isomer shown in Fig. 33-2, and *O*-demethylation occurs approximately twice as

rapidly with the (−)-enantiomer, whereas *N*-demethylation is stereoselective for the (+)-enantiomer (101,102).

Studies in humans indicate that both *O*-demethylation and mono-*N*-demethylation are major routes of metabolism in humans; unchanged tramadol accounts for approximately 25% to 75% of the administered dose in the urine, and the sum of *O*-demethyltramadol, *N*-demethyltramadol, and *N*,*O*-didemethyltramadol plus conjugates accounts for most of the rest, whereas the *N*,*N*-didemethyl metabolites account for less than 3% of the dose (102,103). The formation rates of *N*- versus *O*-demethylated metabolites show wide interindividual variation, as might be expected because of CYP2D6 genetic polymorphisms and interindividual variation in CYP3A4/3A5 levels.

Drug Interactions with Tramadol

The only drug interaction reported to date in the clinical literature is a case report of increased anticoagulant effect of phenprocoumon, presumably as a result of tramadol treatment (104), although this has been disputed (105). It is anticipated that the CYP2D6 poor-metabolizer

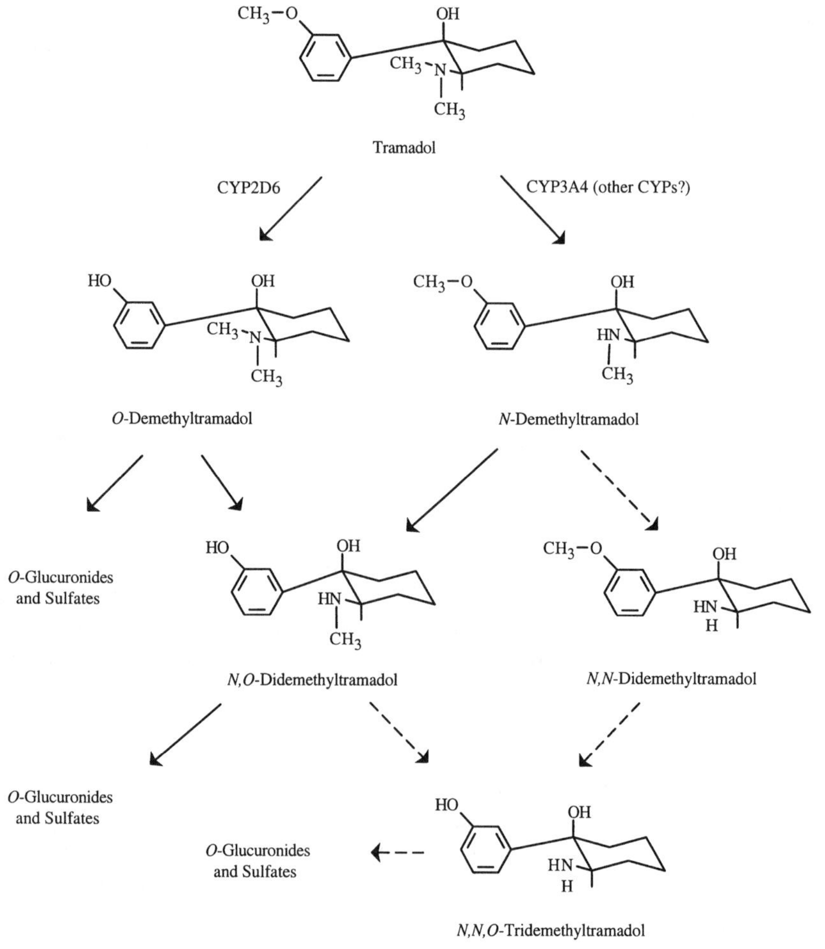

FIG. 33-2. Pathways of tramadol metabolism. Regular arrows, major pathways in humans; dashed arrows, minor pathways.

phenotype may derive less therapeutic effect from tramadol if the *O*-demethylated metabolite is significantly more active than tramadol itself, and this same reasoning applies to possible inhibition of CYP2D6 by quinidine and other inhibitors of this isoform (106). Moreover, drugs that induce CYP3A4, such as carbamazepine, are expected to increase the fraction of a tramadol dose that is eliminated by *N*-demethylation and to decrease the therapeutic effect of tramadol (106). Alternatively, inhibitors of CYP3A4 may increase the intrinsic therapeutic activity and/or prolong the activity of the drug, although no such effects have been reported or investigated. Tramadol itself does not inhibit the metabolism of probe substrates of several human liver CYPs (106 and unpublished data).

REFERENCES

1. Prescott LF. *Paracetamol (acetaminophen): a critical bibliographic review*. London: Taylor & Francis, 1996.
2. Bock KW, Forster A, Gschaidmeier H, et al. Paracetamol glucuronidation by recombinant rat and human phenol UDP-glucuronosyltransferases. *Biochem Pharmacol* 1993;45:1809–1814.
3. Burchell B, Brierley CH, Rance D. Specificity of human UDP-glucuronosyltransferases and xenobiotic glucuronidation. *Life Sci* 1995;57:1819–1831.
4. Duffel MW. Sulfotransferases. In: Guengerich FP, ed. *Comprehensive toxicology. Vol 3, biotransformation*. Oxford: Elsevier, 1997:365–383.
5. Weinshilboum RM, Otterness DM, Aksoy IA, Wood TC, Her C, Raftogianis RB. Sulfation and sulfotransferases 1: sulfotransferase molecular biology: cDNAs and genes. *FASEB J* 1997;11:3–14.
6. Newton JF, Kuo C-H, DeShone GM, Hoefle D, Bernstein J, Hook JB. The role of *p*-aminophenol in acetaminophen-induced nephrotoxicity: effect of bis(*p*-nitrophenyl) phosphate on acetaminophen and *p*-aminophenol nephrotoxicity and metabolism in Fischer 344 rats. *Toxicol Appl Pharmacol* 1985;81:416–430.
7. Nicholls AW, Caddick S, Wilson ID, Farrant RD, Lindon JC, Nicholson JK. The use of isotopic labelling and high field NMR to investigate the nephrotoxic effects of paracetamol in the rat [Abstract]. *ISSX Proc* 1994;6:276.
8. Satoh T, Hosokawa M. The mammalian carboxylesterases: from molecules to functions. *Annu Rev Pharmacol Toxicol* 1998;38:257–288.
9. Vatsis KP, Weber WW, Bell DA, et al. Nomenclature for *N*-acetyltransferases. *Pharmacogenetics* 1995;5:1–17.
10. Jollow DJ, Thorgeirsson SS, Potter WZ, Hashimoto M, Mitchell JR. Acetaminophen-induced hepatic necrosis VI: metabolic disposition of toxic and nontoxic doses of acetaminophen. *Pharmacology* 1974;12:251–271.
11. Dahlin DC, Miwa GT, Lu AYH, Nelson SD. *N*-Acetyl-*p*-benzoquinone imine: a cytochrome P450-mediated oxidation product of acetaminophen. *Proc Natl Acad Sci USA* 1984;81:1327–1331.
12. Anderson KE, Schneider J, Pantuck EJ, et al. Acetaminophen metabolism in subjects fed charcoal-broiled beef. *Clin Pharmacol Ther* 1983;34:369–374.
13. Slattery JT, Wilson JM, Kalhorn TF, Nelson SD. Dose-dependent pharmacokinetics of acetaminophen: evidence of glutathione depletion in humans. *Clin Pharmacol Ther* 1987;41:413–418.
14. Zand R, Nelson SD, Slattery JT, et al. Inhibition and induction of cytochrome P450-2E1-catalyzed oxidation by isoniazid in humans. *Clin Pharmacol Ther* 1993;54:142–149.
15. Powis G, Svingen BA, Dahlin DC, Nelson SD. Enzymatic and nonenzymatic reduction of *N*-acetyl-*p*-benzoquinone imine. *Biochem Pharmacol* 1984;33:2367–2370.
16. Powis G, See KL, Santone KS, Melder DC, Hodnett EM. Quinone imines as substrates for quinone reductase (NAD(P)H: (quinone-acceptor) oxidoreductase) and the effect of dicoumarol on their cytotoxicity. *Biochem Pharmacol* 1987;36:2473–2479.
17. Coles B, Wilson I, Wardman P, Hinson JA, Nelson SD, Ketterer B. The

18. Chen W, Shockor JP, Tonge R, Hunter A, Gartner C, Nelson SD. Protein and nonprotein cysteinyl thiol modification by *N*-acetyl-*p*-benzoquinone imine via a novel *ipso* adduct. *Biochemistry* 1999;38:8159–8166.
19. Forte AJ, Wilson JM, Slattery JT, Nelson SD. The formation and toxicity of catechol metabolites of acetaminophen in mice. *Drug Metab Dispos* 1984;12:484–491.
20. Raucy JL, Lasker JM, Lieber CS, Black M. Acetaminophen activation by human liver cytochromes P450IIE1 and P450IA2. *Arch Biochem Biophys* 1989;271:270–283.
21. Patten CJ, Thomas PE, Guy RL, et al. Cytochrome P450 enzymes involved in acetaminophen activation by rat and human liver microsomes and their kinetics. *Chem Res Toxicol* 1993;6:511–518.
22. Thummel KE, Lee CA, Kunze KL, Nelson SD, Slattery JT. Oxidation of acetaminophen to *N*-acetyl-*p*-benzoquinone imine by human CYP3A4. *Biochem Pharmacol* 1993;45:1563–1569.
23. Chen W, Koenigs LL, Thompson SJ, et al. Oxidation of acetaminophen to its toxic quinone imine and nontoxic catechol metabolites by baculovirus-expressed and purified human cytochromes P450 2E1 and 2A6. *Chem Res Toxicol* 1998;11:295–301.
24. Zaher H, Buters JTM, Ward JM, et al. Protection against acetaminophen toxicity in CYP1A2 and CYP2E1 double-null mice. *Toxicol Appl Pharmacol* 1998;152:193–199.
25. Tonge RP, Kelly EJ, Bruschi SA, et al. Role of CYP1A2 in the hepatotoxicity of acetaminophen: investigations using *Cyp1a2* null mice. *Toxicol Appl Pharmacol* 1998;153:102–108.
26. Miners JO, Attwood J, Birkett DJ. Determinants of acetaminophen metabolism: effects of inducers and inhibitors of drug metabolism on acetaminophen's metabolic pathways. *Clin Pharmacol Ther* 1984;35:480–486.
27. Sarich T, Kalhorn T, Magee S, et al. The effect of omeprazole pretreatment on acetaminophen metabolism in rapid and slow metabolizers of *S*-mephenytoin. *Clin Pharmacol Ther* 1997;62:21–28.
28. Rashed MS, Myers TG, Nelson SD. Hepatic protein arylation, glutathione depletion, and metabolite profiles of acetaminophen and a non-hepatotoxic regioisomer, 3'-hydroxyacetanilide, in the mouse. *Drug Metab Dispos* 1990;18:765–770.
29. deMorais SMF, Chow SYM, Wells PG. Biotransformation and toxicity of acetaminophen in congenic RHA rats with or without a hereditary deficiency in bilirubin UDP-glucuronosyltransferase. *Toxicol Appl Pharmacol* 1992;117:81–87.
30. deMorais SMF, Uetrecht JP, Wells PG. Decreased glucuronidation and increased bioactivation of acetaminophen in Gilbert's syndrome. *Gastroenterology* 1992;102:577–586.
31. Esteban A, Pérez-Mateo M. Gilbert's disease: a risk factor for paracetamol overdosage? *J Hepatol* 1993;18:257–258.
32. Abernathy DR, Greenblatt DJ, Ameer B, Shader RI. Probenecid impairment of acetaminophen and lorazepam clearance: direct inhibition of ether glucuronide formation. *J Pharmacol Exp Ther* 1985;234:345–349.
33. Kamali F. The effect of probenecid on paracetamol metabolism and pharmacokinetics. *Eur J Clin Pharmacol* 1993;45:551–553.
34. Levy G, Yamada H. Drug biotransformation interactions in man III: acetaminophen and salicylamide. *J Pharmacol Sci* 1971;60:215–227.
35. Kamali F, Rawlins MD. Influence of probenecid and paracetamol (acetaminophen) on zidovudine glucuronidation in human liver *in vitro*. *Biopharm Drug Dispos* 1992;13:403–409.
36. Shiner K, Goetz MB. Severe hepatotoxicity in a patient receiving both acetaminophen and zidovudine. *Am J Med* 1992;93:94–96.
37. Richman DD, Fischi MA, Grieco MH, et al. AZT Collaborative Working Group: the toxicity of azidothymine (AZT) in the treatment of patients with AIDS and AIDS-related complex. *N Engl J Med* 1987;317:192–197.
38. Sattler FR, Ko R, Atoniskis D, et al. Acetaminophen does not impair clearance of zidovudine. *Ann Intern Med* 1991;114:937–940.
39. Stein CM, Thornhill DP, Neill P, Nyazema NZ. Lack of effect of paracetamol on the pharmacokinetics of chloramphenicol. *Br J Clin Pharmacol* 1989;27:262–264.
40. Smilkstein MJ, Knapp GL, Kulig KW, Rumack BH. Efficacy of oral *N*-acetylcysteine in the treatment of acetaminophen overdose. *N Engl J Med* 1988;319:1557–1562.

41. Prescott LF. Kinetics and metabolism of paracetamol and phenacetin. *Br J Clin Pharmacol* 1980;10(suppl 2):291S–298S.

42. Rogers SM, Back DJ, Stevenson PJ, Grimmer SFM, Orme ML'E. Paracetamol interaction with oral contraceptive steroids: increased plasma concentrations of ethinylestradiol. *Br J Clin Pharmacol* 1987; 23:721–726.

43. Zemniak JA, Allison N, Boppana VK, Dubb J, Stote R. The effect of acetaminophen on the disposition of fenoldepam: competition for sulfation. *Clin Pharmacol Ther* 1987;41:275–281.

44. Buhl AE, Waldon DJ, Baker CA, Johnson GA. Minoxidil sulfate is the active metabolite that stimulates hair follicles. *J Invest Dermatol* 1990;95:553–557.

45. Bock KW, Wiltfang J, Blume R, Ullrich D, Bircher J. Paracetamol as a test drug to determine glucuronide formation in man: effects of inducers and of smoking. *Eur J Clin Pharmacol* 1987;31:677–683.

46. Mitchell JR, Thorgeirsson SS, Potter WZ, Jollow DJ, Keiser H. Acetaminophen-induced hepatic injury: protective role of glutathione in man and rationale for therapy. *Clin Pharmacol Ther* 1974;16:676–684.

47. Prescott LF, Critchley JAJH, Bulali-Mood M, Pentland B. Effects of microsomal enzyme induction on paracetamol metabolism in man. *Br J Clin Pharmacol* 1981;12:149–153.

48. Dolara P, Lodovici M, Salvadori M, Zaccara G, Muscas GC. Urinary 6-beta-OH-cortisol and paracetamol metabolites as a probe for assessing oxidation and conjugation of chemicals in humans. *Pharmacol Res Commun* 1987;19:261–273.

49. Wright JN, Prescott LF. Potentiation by previous drug therapy of hepatotoxicity following paracetamol overdosage. *Scott Med J* 1973;18: 56–58.

50. Wilson JT, Kasantikul V, Harbison R, Martin D. Death in an adolescent following an overdose of acetaminophen and phenobarbital. *Am J Dis Child* 1978;132:466–473.

51. Minton NA, Henry JA, Frankel RJ. Fatal paracetamol poisoning in an epileptic. *Hum Toxicol* 1988;7:33–34.

52. Renton KW, Dickson G. The prevention of acetaminophen-induced hepatotoxicity by the interferon inducer poly (rI:rC). *Toxicol Appl Pharmacol* 1984;72:40–45.

53. Dolphin CT, Caldwell J, Smith RL. Effect of poly rI:rC treatment upon the metabolism of [^{14}C]-paracetamol in the BALB/cJ mouse. *Biochem Pharmacol* 1987;36:3835–3840.

54. Scavone JM, Blyden GT, Greenblatt DJ. Lack of effect of influenza vaccine on the pharmacokinetics of antipyrine, alprazolam, paracetamol (acetaminophen) and lorazepam. *Clin Pharmacokinet* 1989;16:180–185.

55. Kellokumpu-Lehtinen P, Iiasolo E, Nordman E. Hepatotoxicity of paracetamol in combination with interferon and vinblastine. *Lancet* 1989;1:1143.

56. Seddon CE, Boobis AR, Davies DS. Comparative activation of paracetamol in the rat, mouse and man. *Arch Toxicol* 1987;suppl 11: 305–309.

57. Amoual G, Larrey D, Letteron P, et al. Effects of methoxsalen on the metabolism of acetaminophen in humans. *Biochem Pharmacol* 1987; 36:2349–2352.

58. Letteron P, Descutoire V, Larrey D, et al. Pre- or post-treatment with methoxsalen prevents the hepatotoxicity of acetaminophen in mice. *J Pharmacol Exp Ther* 1986;239:559–567.

59. Peterson GR, Hostetler RM, Lehman T, Covault HP. Acute inhibition of oxidative drug metabolism by propoxyphene. *Biochem Pharmacol* 1979;28:1783–1789.

60. Pond SM, Tong TG, Kaysen GA, et al. Massive intoxication with acetaminophen and propoxyphene: unexplained survival and unusual pharmacokinetics of acetaminophen. *J Toxicol Clin Toxicol* 1982;19:1–16.

61. Robinson AE, Sattar H, McDowall RD, Holder AT, Powell R. Forensic toxicology of some deaths associated with the combined use of propoxyphene and acetaminophen (paracetamol). *J Forensic Sci* 1977; 22:708–717.

62. Chien JY, Peter RM, Nolan CM, et al. Influence of polymorphic N-acetyltransferase phenotype on the inhibition and induction of acetaminophen bioactivation with long-term isoniazid. *Clin Pharmacol Ther* 1997;61:24–34.

63. Slattery JT, Nelson SD, Thummel KE. The complex interaction between ethanol and acetaminophen. *Clin Pharmacol Ther* 1996;60:241–246.

64. Chien JY, Thummel KE, Slattery JT. Pharmacokinetic consequences of induction of CYP2E1 by ligand stabilization. *Drug Metab Dispos* 1997;25:1165–1174.

65. Epstein MM, Nelson SD, Slattery JT, Kalhorn TF, Wall RA, Wright JM. Inhibition of the metabolism of paracetamol by isoniazid. *Br J Clin Pharmacol* 1991;31:139–142.

66. Murphy R, Scartz R, Watkins PB. Severe acetaminophen toxicity in a patient receiving isoniazid. *Ann Intern Med* 1990;113:799–800.

67. Moulding TS, Redeker AG, Kanel GC. Acetaminophen, isoniazid, and hepatic toxicity. *Ann Intern Med* 1991;114:431.

68. Nolan CM, Sandblom RE, Thummel KE, Slattery JT, Nelson SD. Hepatotoxicity associated with acetaminophen usage in patients receiving multiple drug therapy for tuberculosis. *Chest* 1994;105: 408–411.

69. Eliasson E, Johansson I, Ingelman-Sundberg M. Ligand-dependent maintenance of ethanol-inducible cytochrome P-450 in primary hepatocyte cultures. *Biochem Biophys Res Commun* 1988;150:436–443.

70. Roberts BJ, Song B-J, Soh Y, Park SS, Shoat SE. Ethanol induces CYP2E1 by protein stabilization. *J Biol Chem* 1995;50:29632–29635.

71. Lieber CS. Cytochrome P4502E1: its physiological and pathological role. *Physiol Rev* 1997;77:517–544.

72. Wong LT, Whitehouse LW, Solomonraj G, Paul CJ. Effect of a concomitant single dose of ethanol on the hepatotoxicity and metabolism of acetaminophen in mice. *Toxicology* 1980;17:297–309.

73. Sato H, Nakano M, Lieber CS. Prevention of acetaminophen hepatotoxicity by acute ethanol administration in the rat: comparison with carbon tetrachloride-induced hepatotoxicity. *J Pharmacol Exp Ther* 1981;218:805–810.

74. Banda PW, Quart BD. The effect of alcohol on the toxicity of acetaminophen in mice. *Res Commun Chem Pathol Pharmacol* 1984;43: 127–138.

75. Critchley JAJH, Dyson EH, Scott AW, Jarvie DR, Prescott LF. Is there a place for cimetidine or ethanol in the treatment of paracetamol poisoning? *Lancet* 1983;1:1375–1376.

76. McClain CJ, Kromhaut JP, Peterson FJ, Holtzman JL. Potentiation of acetaminophen hepatotoxicity by alcohol. *JAMA* 1980;244:251–253.

77. Seeff LB, Cuccherini BA, Zimmerman HJ, Adler E, Benjamin SB. Acetaminophen toxicity in the alcoholic: a therapeutic misadventure. *Ann Intern Med* 1986;104:399–404.

78. Nelson SD. Molecular mechanisms of the hepatotoxicity caused by acetaminophen. *Semin Liver Dis* 1990;10:267–278.

79. Zimmerman HJ, Maddrey WC. Acetaminophen (paracetamol) hepatotoxicity with regular intake of alcohol: analysis of instances of therapeutic misadventure. *Hepatology* 1995;22:762–777.

80. Johnston SC, Pelletier LL. Enhanced hepatotoxicity of acetaminophen in the alcoholic patient: two case reports and a review of the literature. *Medicine* 1997;76:185–191.

81. Sinclair J, Jeffery E, Wrighton S, et al. Alcohol-mediated increases in acetaminophen hepatotoxicity. *Biochem Pharmacol* 1998;55: 1557–1565.

82. Lauterburg BH, Velez ME. Glutathione deficiency in alcoholics: risk factor for paracetamol hepatotoxicity. *Gut* 1988;29:1153–1157.

83. Whitcomb DC, Block GD. Association of acetaminophen hepatotoxicity with fasting and ethanol use. *JAMA* 1994;272:1845–1850.

84. Hu Y, Ingelman-Sundberg M, Lindros KO. Induction mechanisms of cytochrome P450 2E1 in liver: interplay between ethanol treatment and starvation. *Biochem Pharmacol* 1995;50:155–161.

85. Mitchell JR, Jollow DJ, Potter WZ, Gillette JR, Brodie BB. Acetaminophen-induced hepatic necrosis IV: protective role of glutathione. *J Pharmacol Exp Ther* 1973;187:211–217.

86. Corcoran GB, Wong BK. Role of glutathione in prevention of acetaminophen-induced hepatotoxicity by N-acetyl-L-cysteine *in vivo*: studies with N-acetyl-D-cysteine in mice. *J Pharmacol Exp Ther* 1986; 238:54–61.

87. Lauterburg BH, Davies S, Mitchell JR. Ethanol suppresses hepatic glutathione synthesis in rats *in vivo*. *J Pharmacol Exp Ther* 1984;230: 7–11.

88. Wang P-Y, Kaneko T, Wang Y, Sato A. Acarbose alone or in combination with ethanol potentiates the hepatotoxicity of carbon tetrachloride and acetaminophen in rats. *Hepatology* 1999;29:161–165.

89. Krähenbül S. Acarbose and acetaminophen: a dangerous combination? *Hepatology* 1999;29:285–287.

90. Sato A. Acarbose and acetaminophen: a dangerous combination? [Letter]. *Hepatology* 1999;29:1914.

91. Balfour JA, McTavish D. Acarbose: an update of its pharmacology and therapeutic use in diabetes mellitus. *Drugs* 1993;46:1024–1054.

92. Kono T, Hayami M, Kobayashi H, Ishii M, Taniguchi S. Acarbose-induced generalised erythema multiforme. *Lancet* 1999;354:396–397.

93. Hylek EM, Heiman H, Skates SJ, Sheehan MA, Singer DE. Acetaminophen and other risk factors for excessive warfarin anticoagulation. *JAMA* 1998;279:657–662.
94. Autlitz AM, Mead JA, Tolentino MA. Potentiation of oral anticoagulant therapy by acetaminophen. *Curr Ther Res* 1968;10:501–507.
95. Boejings JJ, Boerstra EE, Ris P. Interaction between paracetamol and coumarin anticoagulants. *Lancet* 1982;1:506.
96. Rubin RN, Mentzner RL, Budzynski AZ. Potentiation of anticoagulant effect of warfarin by acetaminophen: Tylenol. *Clin Res* 1984;32:698a.
97. Bartle WR, Blakely JA. Potentiation of warfarin anticoagulation by acetaminophen. *JAMA* 1991;265:1260.
98. Kwan D, Bartle WR, Walker SE. The effects of acetaminophen on pharmacokinetics and pharmacodynamics of warfarin. *J Clin Pharmacol* 1999;39:68–75.
99. Takigawa T, Tainaka H, Mihara K, Ogata H. Inhibition of *S*-warfarin metabolism by nonsteroidal antiinflammatory drugs in human liver microsomes *in vitro*. *Biol Pharmacol Bull* 1998;21:541–543.
100. Raffa RB, Friderichs E, Reimann W, Shank RP, Codd EE, Vaught JL. Opioid and nonopioid components independently contribute to the mechanism of action of tramadol an "atypical" opioid analgesic. *J Pharmacol Exp Ther* 1992;260:275–285.
101. Paar WD, Frankus P, Dengler HJ. The metabolism of tramadol by human liver microsomes. *Clin Invest* 1992;70:708–710.
102. Elsing B, Blaschke G. Achiral and chiral high-performance liquid chromatographic determination of tramadol and its major metabolites in urine after oral administration of racemic tramadol. *J Chromatogr* 1993;612:223–230.
103. Lintz VW, Evlain S, Frankus E, Uragg H. Metabolismus von Tramadol bei Mensch and Tier. *Arzneimittelforschung/Drug Res* 1981;31:1932–1943.
104. Madsen H, Møller-Rasmussen J, Brøsen K. Interaction between tramadol and phenprocoumon. *Lancet* 1997;350:637.
105. Boeijinga JK, van Meegen E, van den Ende R, Schook CE, Cohen AF. Is there interaction between tramadol and phenprocoumon? *Lancet* 1997;350:1552–1553.
106. *Physicians Desk Reference*. Montvale, NJ: Medical Economics Co., 1999:2554–2557.

CHAPTER 34

Nonsteroidal Antiinflammatory Drugs

Timothy S. Tracy

INTRODUCTION

Nonsteroidal antiinflammatory drugs (NSAIDs) are used in the treatment of various conditions involving pain and/or inflammation. These conditions may include such maladies as arthritis (both rheumatoid and osteoarthritis), musculoskeletal pain, dysmenorrhea, headaches, and other conditions. The NSAIDs exert their action by inhibiting cyclooxygenase (1). Cyclooxygenase exists in at least two isoforms (cyclooxygenase-1 and cyclooxygenase-2), which appear to have different actions within the body (2). The drugs mentioned in this chapter inhibit both isoforms, although some have slightly greater specificity for cyclooxygenase-2. It is thought that cyclooxygenase-1 is the isoform most ubiquitous in the body and responsible for the ulcerogenic properties of the NSAIDs. New drugs have just been approved (celocoxib and rofecoxib) by the Food and Drug Administration (FDA) that are selective for cyclo-oxygenase-2 and thus may have fewer adverse effects, such as gastrointestinal (GI) ulceration.

The NSAIDs (Fig. 34-1) are generally well absorbed and usually reach maximal levels in 30 to 90 minutes. The liver is the primary organ of metabolism, and the compounds are subject to both phase I and phase II metabolism (although a few are eliminated exclusively by phase II metabolism). Of the phase II metabolizing enzymes, glucuronosyl transferase is the predominant enzyme acting on the NSAIDs. An interesting feature of this glucuronidation is that these compounds form acyl glucuronides by conjugation at their carboxyl moiety, and subsequent to this conjugation, they can undergo acyl migration of the glucuronide moiety (3). That is, initially the glucuronide is formed at the β-position of the glu-

T. S. Tracy: Department of Basic Pharmaceutical Sciences, West Virginia University, P.O. Box 9530, Morgantown, West Virginia 26506

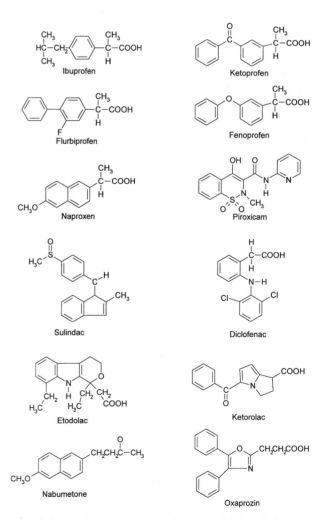

FIG. 34-1. Most commonly used nonsteroidal antiinflammatory drugs (NSAIDs) currently available in the United States.

curonic acid, but the bond can migrate around the glucuronic acid, producing a mixture of glucuronide conjugate isomers. This becomes particularly important when performing chemical analysis of these conjugates in that the acyl migration isomers are resistant to cleavage by β-glucuronidase. Thus to perform high-performance liquid chromatography (HPLC) analysis of the parent compound, the glucuronides must be subjected to either strong acid or base hydrolysis, generally under elevated temperatures, to achieve complete hydrolysis. Furthermore, the glucuronide conjugates of several NSAIDs eliminated all or in part by this route can irreversibly bind to albumin. This process has been implicated in immunogenic responses to the NSAIDs (3).

Finally, the parent NSAIDs are highly protein bound, usually greater than 99%, to plasma proteins, especially albumin. This protein binding can be stereoselective, in the case of chiral compounds, with differences in the unbound fraction of the two enantiomers being quite substantial. This becomes of particular relevance because for the chiral NSAIDs, cyclooxygenase inhibition is thought to reside in only one of the two enantiomers. Thus stereoselective binding can influence the free fraction of pharmacologically active drug.

ACETYLSALICYLIC ACID

Although aspirin was originally synthesized in 1853, the Bayer Company first commercially developed acetylsalicylic acid (ASA) in 1899. Interestingly, it was synthesized and commercialized in an attempt to avoid the untoward side effects, such as GI irritation, of sodium salicylate, which was used in the treatment of rheumatoid arthritis. Although now it is known that ASA is in fact more irritating to the GI tract than is sodium salicylate. ASA is metabolized by a number of pathways (Fig. 34-2) that are in part responsible for the variety of pharmacologic actions of ASA.

Both ASA and the released salicylate are absorbed relatively rapidly from the stomach, with peak plasma levels of aspirin occurring in 10 to 20 minutes and peak levels of salicylate occurring in 20 to 120 minutes (4). ASA is rapidly hydrolyzed by both nonenzymatic hydrolysis and plasma esterases, resulting in a plasma half-life ($t_{1/2}$) of approximately 10 to 20 minutes (4,5). It is this deacetylation of ASA (and subsequent binding to proteins) that is thought to result in its pharmacologic actions of irreversibly inhibiting blood platelet aggregation. Plasma protein binding of salicylic acid is approximately 80% to 90%, and the binding of ASA is thought to be similar (6).

Metabolism

After the conversion of ASA to salicylate by nonenzymatic or esterase hydrolysis, several enzymatic conversions can occur to the salicylate molecule (see Fig. 34-2). Salicylate can undergo cytochrome P450–mediated hydroxylation to form gentisic acid (GA) (7). It is also proposed that this process may occur to a small extent nonenzymatically through attack by hydroxyl radicals (7).

Glucuronidation of the phenolic or carboxylate moieties of salicylic acid also occur and are catalyzed by uridine diphosphate (UDP)-glucuronosyltransferases (8).

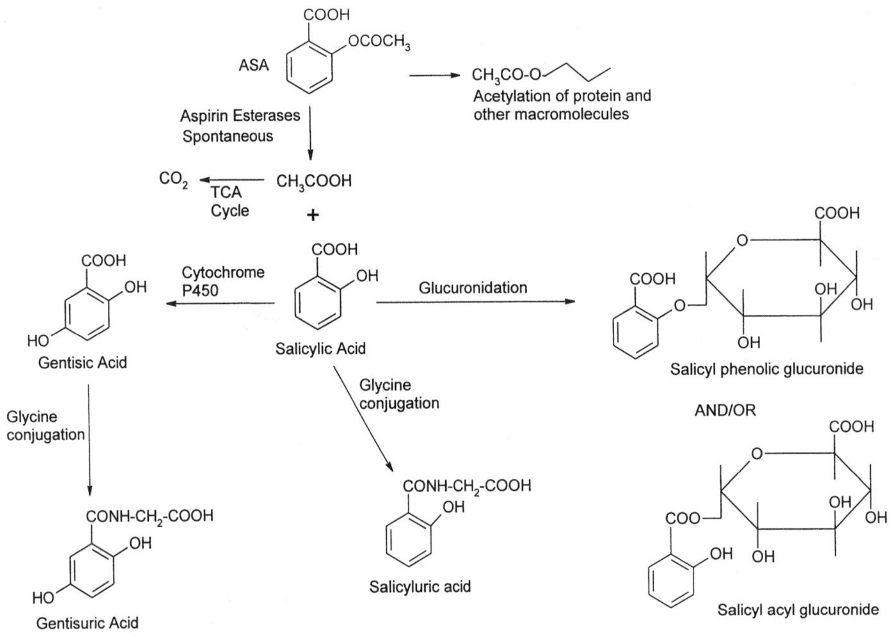

FIG. 34-2. Aspirin metabolism.

The phenolic moiety is glucuronidated to form salicyl phenolic glucuronide, and the carboxyl moiety is likewise glucuronidated to form salicylacyl glucuronide.

Finally, through formation of a salicyl-S coenzyme A (CoA) intermediate, either salicylic or gentisic acids form salicylurate or gentisurate, respectively. These reactions occur in the mitochondria, and after the reaction of the carboxylate groups of these molecules with CoA, the conjugate is then linked with glycine by a glycine N-acyl-transferase (9).

PROFEN NSAIDS

The "profen" NSAIDs have a common phenylpropionic acid structure with minor modifications. The first of these compounds to become commercially available was ibuprofen, and it offered the advantage of lower incidence of GI ulceration and toxicity than did aspirin. Interestingly, several of the profen NSAIDs are chiral compounds and as such exhibit stereoselective pharmacokinetics and pharmacodynamics. For example, as mentioned earlier, only the S-enantiomer of these compounds inhibits cyclooxygenase and as such is the active moiety, with the R-enantiomer being either inactive or converted to the active enantiomer by chiral inversion (see later). All of the profen NSAIDs undergo glucuronidation as one of their elimination pathways, but some also undergo cytochrome P450–mediated oxidative metabolism, which can also be followed by glucuronidation.

Ibuprofen

After oral administration, the bioavailability of ibuprofen [±2-(p-isobutylphenyl)propionic acid] is essentially complete (more than 90%) (10). Studies have shown the half-life of both R- and S-ibuprofen to be about 2 to 4 hours, and the volume of distribution limited to the plasma volume (10,11). The total urinary recovery of ibuprofen and its metabolites was approximately 70% after administration of either R- or racemic-ibuprofen but

was slightly greater than 80% when only S-ibuprofen was given (12).

Metabolism

Two different oxidative metabolites of ibuprofen have been observed in human urine, a 2-hydroxy metabolite and a carboxy-metabolite (Fig. 34-3). Because ibuprofen is administered as a racemic mixture, and formation of the carboxy metabolite results in the introduction of a second chiral center into the molecule, six metabolites are formed, including S-2-hydroxyibuprofen, R-2-hydroxyibuprofen, S,S-carboxyibuprofen, S,R-carboxyibuprofen, R,R-carboxyibuprofen, and R,S-carboxyibuprofen. It is of note that these carboxyibuprofen metabolites are actually a secondary product (resulting from nonmicrosomal dehydrogenation) of 3-hydroxyibuprofen originally formed by microsomal cytochrome P450. The 2-hydroxyibuprofen metabolites recovered represent about 22% of the administered dose, whereas the carboxyibuprofen metabolites represent about 36% of the administered dose of ibuprofen (12).

Studies have been undertaken to determine the cytochrome P450 isoforms responsible for the oxidative metabolism of R- and S-ibuprofen. By using microsomes from B-lymphoblastoid cell lines expressing various cytochrome P450 isoforms, Hamman et al. (13) found that CYPs 2C9 and 2C8 produced significant ibuprofen hydroxylation. CYP2C9 exhibited the greatest intrinsic clearance, with selectivity toward S-3-hydroxyibuprofen formation. In contrast, CYP2C8 demonstrated selectivity toward formation of 2-hydroxyibuprofen. These processes were readily inhibited by sulfaphenazole and correlated significantly with tolbutamide methylhydroxylation (CYP2C9) and taxol 6α-hydroxylation (CYP2C8), measured in a bank of human liver microsomes. These same authors found that the CYP2C9*2 (Arg144Cys) variant also metabolized ibuprofen but to a lesser extent than CYP2C9*1 (wild type). More recently, studies with chimeric 2C9/2C19 enzymes demonstrated that residues at positions 286 and 289 of the CYP2C9 enzyme are crit-

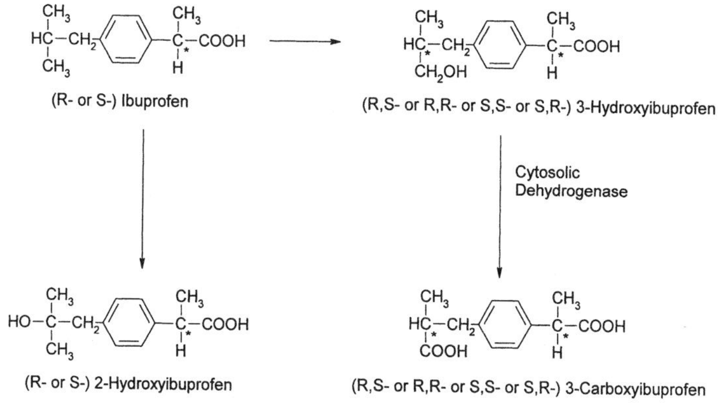

FIG. 34-3. Ibuprofen oxidative metabolism. *Chiral center.

ical for the binding of ibuprofen and its subsequent hydroxylation (14).

Aside from oxidative metabolism, ibuprofen and its metabolites can also undergo glucuronidation, generally thought to occur on the carboxylate moiety of the phenylpropionic acid structure. In fact, a very small portion (less than 2%) of parent ibuprofen is excreted unchanged. Glucuronide conjugates of ibuprofen, hydroxyibuprofen and carboxyibuprofen, are recovered in the urine of patients given ibuprofen (12). As implied earlier, the glucuronide conjugates can undergo acyl migration, producing a number of glucuronide isomers. These glucuronide conjugates can bind covalently to albumin with unknown effects. Interestingly, studies with UDP-glucuronosyltransferase expressed in COS-7 cells showed that ibuprofen was stereoselectively glucuronidated by this enzyme with an S/R ratio of 1.6 (15).

Chiral Inversion

Early investigators of ibuprofen metabolism conducted *in vivo* studies on the disposition of each enantiomer administered individually, because the enantiomers were already known to differ *in vitro* with respect to their pharmacologic activity (16). From these studies, it was noted that when R-ibuprofen was given to humans, both R- and S-ibuprofen and their metabolites were excreted in the urine, and roughly equivalent pharmacologic activity was noted regardless of the enantiomer administered (16,17). One of the first studies attempting to quantitate the degree of this inversion was conducted by Lee et al. (11). By using plasma data from patients given racemic-ibuprofen, R-ibuprofen, or S-ibuprofen on separate occasions, these investigators calculated the mean fraction of R-ibuprofen inverted to S-ibuprofen as 63%. This estimation of the fraction of R-ibuprofen inverted to S-ibuprofen *in vivo* has been confirmed by other investigators with either plasma or urine data (12).

After the *in vivo* confirmation in humans, several laboratories undertook a series of *in vitro* investigations to determine the mechanism of this chiral inversion. In an abstract, it was suggested that the formation of a CoA thioester with ibuprofen might be an intermediate in this inversion process, but no data to substantiate this claim were given (18). Several investigators were able to show, by using indirect methods, that if CoA and tissue were allowed to incubate and then the products hydrolyzed before assay for ibuprofen, that chiral inversion could be observed (19–21). However, because the CoA thioester of ibuprofen was not directly measured, it could only be surmised to be present. Shortly thereafter, R-ibuprofenyl CoA and S-ibuprofenyl CoA were chemically synthesized and an assay developed by using a chiral α1-acid glycoprotein column to measure both species in a reaction directly without acid hydrolysis (22). This advancement then allowed experiments to determine the rate of

ibuprofenyl-CoA formation (23), the epimerization of these thioesters, and their rate of hydrolysis (24) in human liver tissue, and subsequently, led to the reaction scheme presented in Fig. 34-4. It was later confirmed that this inversion process occurs essentially exclusively in the liver and not in the gut (10). It is interesting to note that flurbiprofen, another NSAID that does not undergo chiral inversion, can be made to invert if the CoA thioester is formed chemically and then allowed to react with tissue (25). Later studies have focused on the exact mechanism by which the atoms around the chiral center become inverted (26–28), and identification of the exact nature of the formation, epimerization, and hydrolysis enzymes. Because this formation of an ibuprofenyl-CoA thioester is analogous to the activation of fatty acids before certain steps of their metabolism, investigators have searched for and found evidence in rats and humans that, like fatty acids, ibuprofen can become incorporated into triglycerides and phospholipids (29,30). Thus it has become clear that formation of a CoA thioester is obligatory for ibuprofen chiral inversion and plays a role in its distribution throughout the body.

Ketoprofen

Ketoprofen [±2-(3-benzoylphenyl)propionic acid] is rapidly absorbed after oral administration and reaches peak plasma concentrations in about 1 to 2 hours (31,32). Interestingly, the half-life of the R-enantiomer has been reported to be about two-fold greater (3.3 vs. 1.4 hours) than that of S-ketoprofen (31), but other studies have not confirmed this difference (32). Approximately 50% to 70% of an oral dose is recovered in the urine in 24 hours with an equal proportion of both enantiomers being excreted (31,32). Interestingly, two studies have reported that approximately 10% of the R-ketoprofen dose undergoes chiral inversion to the S-enantiomer (32,33). Even though it is thought that only the S-enantiomer inhibits cyclooxygenase, this minimal R- to S- inversion is probably of little clinical consequence. Like other NSAIDs,

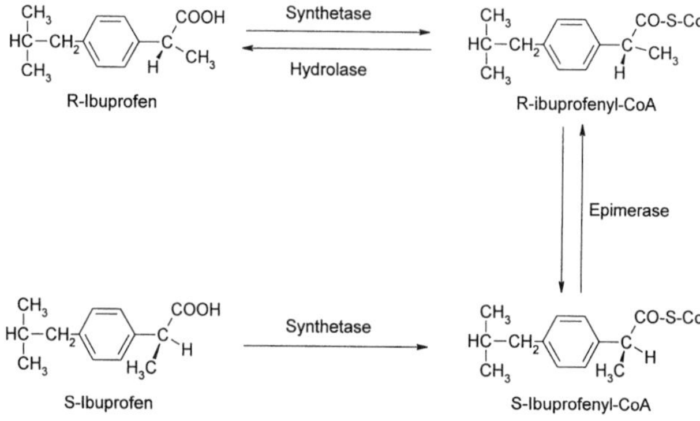

FIG. 34-4. Ibuprofen chiral inversion.

ketoprofen is highly bound to plasma proteins (i.e., albumin), and the percentage binding estimated to be 99.2%, with no difference between the enantiomers (34). Furthermore, ketoprofen glucuronide can irreversibly bind to human serum albumin, as can other NSAIDs (35).

Metabolism

As stated previously, 50% to 70% of an oral dose is recovered in the urine. Of this amount recovered, at least 90% is eliminated as the ketoprofen acyl glucuronide metabolite (32,36). *In vitro* studies have suggested that ketoprofen, along with several other NSAIDs, is conjugated with glucuronic acid by the UDP-glucuronosyltransferase UGT2B7 (15). Although it has been suggested that a minor pathway of ketoprofen elimination might be through oxidative hydroxylation, scant evidence exists to substantiate this hypothesis. However, *in vitro* at concentrations as low as 25 μM, ketoprofen can inhibit cytochrome P450 2C9–mediated flurbiprofen metabolism (T.S. Tracy and J.M. Hutzler, unpublished data, 1999), suggesting that ketoprofen may be a substrate for the CYP2C9 enzyme with a slow rate of turnover.

Flurbiprofen

Flurbiprofen [±2-(2-fluoro-4-biphenyl) propionic acid] is similar to the other profen NSAIDs in most characteristics. Flurbiprofen is eliminated from the body by both oxidative and conjugative processes and has a plasma half-life of 5.1 hours for R-flurbiprofen and 6.0 hours for S-flurbiprofen. Likewise, the areas under the curve (AUCs), oral clearances, and volumes of distribution appear to be equal for the two enantiomers, suggesting a lack of stereoselectivity in flurbiprofen elimination (37). Flurbiprofen has one of the highest degrees of protein binding of the NSAIDs, with binding being approximately equal for the S- and R-enantiomers (about 99.95% for both enantiomers) (37).

Metabolism

Flurbiprofen enantiomers are metabolized by the cytochrome P450 system to produce 4′-hydroxyflurbiprofen as the primary oxidative metabolite, which accounts for as much as 86% of the oxidative metabolites recovered. The production of hydroxyflurbiprofen is carried out essentially exclusively by cytochrome P450 2C9, and again, there does not appear to be any significant stereoselectivity in the formation of this metabolite by P450 2C9 (38,39). *In vitro* studies have demonstrated that CYP2C9*1 is the predominant variant of the isoform involved in this reaction, but that CYP2C9*2 also carries out this hydroxylation, albeit at levels approximately one-third those seen with CYP2C9*1 (39). CYP2C9*3 also will hydroxylate flurbiprofen, but at substantially reduced

turnover numbers compared with CYP2C9*1 (40). Furthermore, the K_m for this process increases substantially for the CYP2C9*3 variant as compared with the other two variants. The lack of stereoselectivity in flurbiprofen hydroxylation measured *in vitro* confirms results seen *in vivo* that demonstrate only modest stereoselectivity (R/S ratio, 0.8) (41). Flurbiprofen also forms a 3′,4′-dihydroxyflurbiprofen metabolite, and this compound can be methylated to form 3′-hydroxy-4′-methoxyflurbiprofen. It is this methylated form of the dihydroxy product that is detectable in urine.

Approximately 25% of the dose is excreted as either flurbiprofen or its glucuronide conjugate (37). However, only about 2% of the dose is excreted as unchanged flurbiprofen. The metabolites of flurbiprofen are also extensively glucuronidated, with these glucuronide conjugates composing the primary form found in the urine.

Fenoprofen

Fenoprofen [±2-(3-phenoxyphenyl) propionic acid] is structurally very similar to ketoprofen, except that the carbonyl function linking the two phenyl rings in ketoprofen is replaced in fenoprofen by an oxygen ether linkage. Like the other profen NSAIDs, it is readily absorbed, highly bound to plasma proteins (42), and can covalently bind to plasma proteins (43). It appears to be eliminated with a 2- to 3-hour half-life, and its volume of distribution approximates the vascular compartment (44).

Metabolism

Fenoprofen is oxidatively metabolized to 4′-hydroxyfenoprofen, and this metabolite accounts for about 34% of the administered dose (42). No other oxidative metabolites have been detected, and the enzymes (presumably P450 isoforms) that catalyze this hydroxylation have not been identified. The S/R ratio of 4′-hydroxyfenoprofen appears to be approximately unity in plasma despite the extensive chiral inversion (see later) (45).

Fenoprofen is readily glucuronidated, with less than 1% each of fenoprofen or its 4′-hydroxy metabolite excreted as the unconjugated compound (42). Approximately 65% of the fenoprofen dose is excreted as the glucuronide conjugate. Interestingly, as early as 1972, Rubin et al. (42) described an "acid-labile" conjugate of both fenoprofen and 4′-hydroxyfenoprofen that was resistant to β-glucuronidase. In light of current knowledge, it now seems justified to assume that this acid-labile conjugate was in fact the positional isomers of fenoprofen and 4′-hydroxyfenoprofen glucuronide resulting from the acyl-migration phenomenon. Although it is difficult to measure *in vivo* because of chiral inversion, *in vitro* studies have suggested that glucuronidation of the R-enantiomer occurs more rapidly (46).

Chiral inversion

Fenoprofen undergoes even more extensive chiral inversion than does ibuprofen, with virtually all of the R-enantiomer being converted to the S-enantiomer (47). This chiral inversion appears to occur by the same mechanism as does ibuprofen chiral inversion. Thus most of the inactive R-enantiomer is converted to the active S-form after administration. Although conducted in animals, studies have suggested that fenoprofen can be incorporated into triglycerides and phospholipids, presumably by formation of the CoA thioester and involvement in fatty acid metabolism pathways (48,49).

NAPROXEN

Naproxen [(+)-2-(6-methoxy-2-naphthyl)propionic acid] is closely related to the profen NSAIDs, except that it contains a naphthalene ring system instead of a phenyl ring. Naproxen is unique in that even though it is a chiral compound, it is marketed only as the S-(+)- enantiomer. This becomes important in that only the active compound is administered, and the issue of chiral inversion is avoided (animal studies suggest that R-naproxen is inverted to the S-enantiomer). Again, naproxen is highly bound to plasma proteins (50), but little work has been done to assess the degree of covalent binding to plasma proteins. The elimination half-life of naproxen is longer than that of most NSAIDs and has been reported to be approximately 14 hours in humans (50).

Metabolism

Approximately 5% of a naproxen dose is excreted as desmethylnaproxen, resulting from demethylation of the naphthalene methoxy substituent (51). In addition, another 23% of the dose is recovered as conjugates of desmethylnaproxen. The cytochrome P450 isoforms responsible for this demethylation have been identified. Cytochrome P450 2C9 provides the greatest contribution to naproxen demethylation, although cytochrome P450 1A2 also may contribute substantially to naproxen metabolism (52–54). Cytochrome P450 2C8 may also play a minor role in naproxen demethylation (54). The involvement of cytochrome P450 1A2 is notable in that it has not been implicated to play a substantial role in the metabolism of other NSAIDs. Of the CYP2C9 variants, CYP2C9*1 is the most active in demethylating naproxen, whereas CYP2C9*2 is less active, and CYP2C9*3 is very weakly active in carrying out this reaction (54).

Only 10% of a naproxen dose is excreted as unchanged drug, with the remainder being excreted as either oxidative or conjugated metabolites (51). Forty percent of the recovered dose has been reported to be naproxen glucuronide, with an additional 20% being an unknown conjugate of naproxen. Approximately 12% of the dose is recovered as the glucuronide of desmethylnaproxen. More recently, Kiang et al. (55) identified 6-desmethyl-naproxen sulfate as a metabolite of naproxen, which may account for the remainder of the excreted desmethyl-naproxen conjugate.

PIROXICAM

Piroxicam [4-hydroxy-2-methyl-N-2-pyridinyl-2H,1,2-benzothiazine-3-carboxamide 1,1-dioxide] is the only member of the oxicam class of NSAIDs available on the US market. Piroxicam has several unique properties, including its long half-life (about 55 hours) as compared with the other NSAIDs (56). Furthermore, the hydroxy metabolite (see later) has an even longer half-life (about 70 hours) and is less water soluble than the parent compound. This lessened water solubility of the hydroxyl metabolite is thought to be due to hydrogen bonding between the hydroxyl hydrogen and the proximal nitrogen of another piroxicam molecule, making the compound more attracted to itself than to water. The protein binding of piroxicam is quite high, as expected, being approximately 99% bound to albumin. Interestingly, meloxicam, an analogue of piroxicam, is currently under US FDA review, with the purported advantage of being more selective for cyclooxygenase-2 and thus presumably producing fewer adverse reactions than earlier NSAIDs.

Metabolism

As mentioned earlier, piroxicam is primarily oxidatively metabolized to 5'-hydroxypiroxicam (57). It has been speculated that this reaction is carried out by CYP2C9, based on reciprocal inhibition studies with tenoxicam (which was inhibited by the CYP2C9 inhibitor sulfaphenazole) (58). Unpublished studies in our laboratory with purified enzymes suggest that CYP2C19 may be as active as CYP2C9 in hydroxylating piroxicam and that liver concentrations of the individual isoforms may control the relative contribution of each (T. S. Tracy et al., unpublished data, 1999).

Piroxicam appears to be excreted in the urine almost exclusively as the glucuronide conjugate, with negligible amounts excreted as unchanged piroxicam (56). It has been reported that 25% to 60% of the excreted dose is recovered as 5'-hydroxypiroxicam, and of this amount, two thirds is eliminated as the glucuronide conjugate (56,59).

SULINDAC

Sulindac {(Z)-5-fluoro-2-methyl-1-[4-methylsulfinyl)phenylmethylene]-1H-indene-3-acetic acid} is a prodrug and thus its biotransformation is important to pharmacologic activity. Sulindac (sulfoxide) undergoes oxidation of the sulfinyl substituent to form a sulfone, and reduction of this same substituent to form a sulfide (60,61). This sulfide metabolite is thought to confer the primary pharmacologic activity, with sulindac having less antiinflammatory activity, and the sulfone being essentially devoid of activity (60). Sulindac is well absorbed after oral administration, and the sulfide metabolite exhibits a plasma half-life of 18 hours (62). The plasma protein binding is slightly less than that of other NSAIDs, ranging from 93% to 98%, depending on the species (parent, sulfide, or sulfone) (61).

Metabolism

The oxidation of sulindac sulfoxide to form the sulfone is an irreversible process that results in a pharmacologically inactive species. However, the reduction of sulindac sulfoxide is reversible, and thus the two molecules interconvert during time in the body (61). The conversion of the sulindac sulfide back to sulindac sulfoxide appears to occur through the flavin monooxygenase system (63). Approximately 75% of a dose of sulindac is recovered in the urine and feces within 5 days. However, although all three compounds (sulindac sulfoxide, sulindac sulfide, and sulindac sulfone) are found in the plasma, only the sulfoxide and sulfone compounds are excreted in the urine (61). Both the sulfoxide and sulfone compounds can be conjugated with glucuronic acid, and as such, they are excreted both as free and conjugated compound, with the glucuronide conjugate of sulindac sulfone being the metabolite found in the largest quantities in the urine (61)

DICLOFENAC

Diclofenac [{2-[2,6-dichlorophenyl)amino]benzene acetic acid} is rapidly absorbed after oral administration, reaching a maximal concentration in 10 to 40 minutes for the conventional dosage form and approximately 2 hours for the sustained-release product (64). The elimination half-life has been reported to be 1 to 2 hours (65). Plasma protein binding of diclofenac is approximately 99.7%, and it appears also to penetrate well into synovial fluid, where it can also be bound to plasma proteins (66).

Metabolism

Diclofenac is primarily oxidatively metabolized to form the 4'-hydroxy metabolite in humans, with its urinary excretion accounting for 30% of the dose and its biliary excretion accounting for another 10% to 20% of the dose (67). Smaller amounts of 3'-hydroxy, 5-hydroxy, 4',5-dihydroxy, and 3'-hydroxy-4'-methoxy metabolites have also been detected in either plasma or urine (67–69). Diclofenac 4'-hydroxylation appears to be predominantly catalyzed by cytochrome P450 2C9 (70). Diclofenac hydroxylation is not diminished substantially by the CYP2C9*2 variant, and the K_m is approximately equal to

that seen with wild type (2C9*1) enzyme (40). However, with the CYP2C9*3 variant, there is a reduction in V_{max} and an increase in K_m for diclofenac 4'-hydroxylation, resulting in a lower turnover. It appears that the metabolites as well as parent drug of diclofenac are excreted predominantly as the glucuronide conjugate in urine (67,69).

ETODOLAC

Etodolac [±1,8-diethyl-1,3,4,9-tetrahydropyrano-(3,4-b)indole-1-acetic acid], like several other NSAIDs, is marketed as a racemic mixture with antiinflammatory activity residing in the S-enantiomer. It has been suggested that an advantage of etodolac is that it has less propensity to cause gastric ulceration than do most other NSAIDs (71,72). Etodolac exhibits a plasma half-life of about 6 hours, and 99% of the drug is bound to plasma proteins (73,74). Like several of the other NSAIDs, etodolac has been found to bind irreversibly to albumin *in vitro* (75).

Metabolism

Etodolac undergoes a variety of biotransformations with less than 5% of the dose being excreted unchanged in the urine (74). Etodolac is hydroxylated at three different positions to form 6-hydroxyetodolac, 7-hydroxyetodolac, and 8-(1-hydroxyethyl)etodolac. These metabolites each compose 10% to 20% of the excreted dose and are excreted mainly as glucuronide conjugates. Less than 5% of the dose of etodolac is excreted as unchanged drug, with approximately 20% of the urinary recovery due to etodolac glucuronide. Altogether, 10% to 15% of the excreted dose is recovered as unchanged etodolac and its hydroxylated metabolites. The enzyme responsible for the hydroxylation of etodolac is unknown at this time.

KETOROLAC

Ketorolac [±5-benzoyl-2,3-dihydro-1H-pyrrolizine-1-carboxylic acid] is administered as the tromethamine salt and is a potent analgesic with cyclooxygenase inhibitory activity. Although primarily used for pain, it is structurally related to the other NSAIDs mentioned herein and also possesses antiinflammatory activity. Ketorolac is readily absorbed orally but also can be given by intravenous or intramuscular administration (which differentiates it from most other NSAIDs). The half-life appears to be approximately 5 hours, and the volume of distribution about 15 L, suggesting distribution in the vascular compartment (76). Ketorolac is about 99% bound to plasma proteins. Like many of the profen NSAIDs, ketorolac is chiral, with the cyclooxygenase inhibition and analgesic activity residing in the S-enantiomer (77). However, ketorolac does not undergo appreciable chiral inversion of the enantiomers in humans, with no R- to S-inversion occurring and only 6% of S-ketorolac being inverted to R-ketorolac (77).

Metabolism

Ketorolac is excreted into urine primarily as parent drug, ketorolac glucuronide, or as the *p*-hydroxyketorolac metabolite. It has been reported that approximately 60% of a dose of ketorolac is excreted as unchanged drug, with another 30% being excreted as the glucuronide conjugate, and the remaining 10% as the *p*-hydroxy metabolite (76,78). The enzyme producing this *p*-hydroxy metabolite is unknown as of this time, but because this metabolite only composes 10% of an excreted dose, its formation is probably of little consequence in drug interactions.

NABUMETONE

Nabumetone [4-(6-methoxy-2-naphthyl)-butan-2-one] is a prodrug with virtually no antiinflammatory activity; it must be converted to the 6-methoxy-2-naphthyl-acetic acid (6-MNA) metabolite to become active. The prodrug undergoes extensive first pass metabolism to 6-MNA, which has a half-life of about 28 hours in normal subjects (79). Nabumetone has been reported to be approximately 99% bound to plasma proteins (80) and exhibits a volume of distribution of approximately 30 L (79).

Metabolism

Nabumetone is readily converted in the body to the active metabolite 6-MNA by oxidative removal of two carbons (81). Approximately 15% of the dose is recovered as 6-MNA or its glucuronide conjugate, with less than 1% being found as free 6-MNA. 6-MNA can be further demethylated to metabolite M-I (6-hydroxy-2-naphthylacetic acid), which accounts for about 16% of the urinary metabolite recovery, with it being divided approximately equally between the glucuronidated and free forms of M-I. Parent nabumetone can also be demethylated to produce 4-(6-methoxy-2-naphthyl)-butan-2-one, known as metabolite M-IV. Metabolite M-IV is also readily detected in urine and accounts for approximately 10% of the dose, with it being essentially exclusively eliminated as the glucuronide conjugate. Finally, the carbonyl function of M-IV can be reduced to form the alcohol known as M-III, the glucuronide conjugate of which accounts for about 13% of the dose recovered in urine.

OXAPROZIN

Oxaprozin [4,5-diphenyl-2-oxazole propionic acid] differs somewhat from other NSAIDs in that peak plasma concentrations are not reached until 2 to 4 hours, and the terminal half-life of about 60 hours is substantially longer than that of most other agents of this class (82). Oxaprozin is extensively bound to plasma proteins, with binding greater than 99% (83). Furthermore, oxaprozin can covalently bind to serum albumin, as can several other NSAIDs (84,85). Approximately 60% of an oxaprozin dose is excreted in the urine as parent drug and metabolites, whereas another 30% is excreted in the feces (82).

Metabolism

Very little oxaprozin is eliminated as unchanged drug, with the primary metabolite being the ester glucuronide conjugate of parent oxaprozin, accounting for almost 50% of the recovered dose (82). The primary oxidative metabolite of oxaprozin is the 4-(*p*-hydroxyphenyl) metabolite, with traces of the 5-(*p*-hydroxyphenyl) metabolite being found. These hydroxyl metabolites are almost exclusively eliminated as the glucuronide conjugate, with less than 10% of the dose being eliminated as the unconjugated hydroxyl metabolites. However, approximately one third of the hydroxyl metabolites eliminated are the ether glucuronides, with the remainder being the ester glucuronides. To date, the enzyme responsible for the hydroxylation of oxaprozin has not been reported.

DIFLUNISAL

Diflunisal [2′4′-difluoro-4-hydroxy-3-biphenylcarboxylic acid] is an NSAID structurally related to aspirin. The plasma half-life of diflunisal is approximately 8 hours (86), and it has been reported to be 99.8% bound to plasma proteins (87). Because diflunisal lacks the acetyl group found in aspirin, it appears to have less effect on platelet function, and effects that do occur are reversible, as opposed to those seen with aspirin (88). Its primary route of elimination is through the kidneys, but some biliary elimination also occurs.

Metabolism

The primary elimination of diflunisal is through conjugation with either glucuronic acid or sulfate, but a small portion of the dose is eliminated as 3-hydroxydiflunisal (89). Diflunisal phenolic glucuronide composes approximately 30% of the dose recovered in the urine, whereas diflunisal acyl glucuronide makes up about 50% of the dose recovered in the urine (90). A sulfate conjugate of diflunisal also has been identified (91). After a single dose, this sulfate conjugate is only a very small portion (less than 10%) of the recovered dose, but upon repeated administration, it can become as much as 20% to 40% of the recovered dose (91). Interestingly, the partial metabolic clearances of diflunisal by acyl and phenolic glucuronide formation are reduced significantly after multiple dose administration (92). Very little diflunisal is excreted as unchanged drug.

In a study of the effects of gender, oral contraceptive use, and smoking on diflunisal elimination (93), it was discovered that the plasma clearance of diflunisal was higher in men and women taking oral contraceptives than in control women. Statistically significant changes, however, were noted between men and women only in the partial metabolic clearance of diflunisal by phenolic glucuronidation and between oral contraceptive users and control women for the acyl glucuronidation of diflunisal. Smoking resulted in a 35% increase in diflunisal clearance with a reduction in the urinary recovery of the glucuronide and sulfate conjugates. These authors postulated that smoking may have induced the hydroxylation of diflunisal, which is normally a minor pathway.

IN VIVO INTERACTIONS INVOLVING THE NSAIDS

Given their widespread use, it is fortunate that the NSAIDs are involved in very few clinically significant drug interactions. However, it is this safety profile that has probably led to wider use and availability of some agents (e.g., ibuprofen, naproxen, and ketoprofen) as over-the-counter (nonprescription) drugs. All of the interactions listed later are of either minor clinical significance or, if of more clinical significance, were generally reported as a case report in an individual patient and involved mitigating circumstances.

Case reports involving a fatal interaction of ketoprofen (94) or naproxen (95) in patients receiving high-dose methotrexate for treatment of cancer elicited great concern because the combination of NSAIDs and low-dose methotrexate was increasingly being used together for the treatment of rheumatoid arthritis. However, the clinical significance of this potential interaction has not been borne out. Several studies have shown that ibuprofen and the salicylates can decrease the renal clearance of methotrexate (96,97). Conflicting results have been obtained concerning the systemic clearance of methotrexate with the NSAIDs. For example, one study found that ibuprofen, naproxen, and a salicylate all produced statistically significant reductions in methotrexate systemic clearance (97); however, this was not confirmed by other studies (98–100). It is universally agreed that piroxicam, ketoprofen, and flurbiprofen have no effect on low-dose methotrexate pharmacokinetics (100,101). Regardless, because low-dose methotrexate is given only once a week for the treatment of rheumatoid arthritis, any interaction is probably of little clinical significance. It should be remembered that at high doses of methotrexate, such as those used in the treatment of cancer, the NSAIDs may have profound clinical implications.

The metabolic drug interaction involving the NSAIDs most likely to produce a change in NSAID kinetics is the interaction with probenecid. Studies have shown that probenecid can cause a 2.5-fold increase in naproxen half-life and a 66% reduction in naproxen conjugates excreted in the urine (102). Conversely, an eight-fold increase in the desmethylnaproxen metabolite excretion was noted. These authors hypothesized that the interaction was due to probenecid decreasing naproxen renal clearance and inhibiting naproxen glucuronide formation. Similar results have been noted for ketoprofen, which is predominantly eliminated by glucuronidation pathways. Coadministration of probenecid resulted in a 67% decrease in ketoprofen total clearance and a 93% reduction in the renal clearance of ketoprofen glucuronide conjugates (103). However, because of the wide therapeutic index of the NSAIDs, this interaction is probably of minor clinical significance.

Several studies have looked at the interaction of aspirin with various NSAIDs. In each study, no changes were noted in salicylate levels after NSAID coadministration (104–106). Aspirin did lower ibuprofen levels by 60%, but no change in $t_{1/2}$ was noted (104). Fenoprofen AUC was reduced 30% with aspirin coadministration, and a 15% increase in 4′-hydroxyfenoprofen excretion was noted (105). Aspirin had very little effect on naproxen levels but did cause a modest increase in naproxen renal clearance (106). Changes in protein binding of the NSAIDs have been postulated as the mechanism of these interactions.

Because the NSAIDs can affect renal function, it seems plausible that interactions at this level might occur. For example, case reports have suggested that either ibuprofen (107) or piroxicam (108) may cause development of lithium toxicity. However, clinical trials with ibuprofen (109), diclofenac (110), naproxen, or sulindac (111) have demonstrated only modest (20% or less) reduction in lithium clearance. It should be noted that in clinical trials, patients had normal renal function, but in case reports, the patients had developed acute renal dysfunction, which may have predisposed them to the toxicity.

Finally, one study attempted to discern whether ibuprofen might alter the pharmacokinetics of phenytoin, a plausible question, given the dependence of both on cytochrome P450 2C9 for metabolism. However, this single-dose phenytoin study demonstrated that ibuprofen, 1,600 mg/day, had no effect on any parameters of phenytoin pharmacokinetics (112). This finding fits well with the lack of documented interaction of NSAIDs with other CYP2C9 substrates. However, it has been noted that coadministration of phenobarbital reduced the fenoprofen AUC and increased the excretion of metabolites (113).

REFERENCES

1. Vane JR. Inhibition of prostaglandin synthesis as a mechanism of action for aspirin-like drugs. *Nature* 1971;231:232–235.

2. Vane JR, Bakhle YS, Botting RM. Cyclooxygenases 1 and 2. *Annu Rev Pharmacol Toxicol* 1998;120:3897–3120.
3. Spahn-Langguth H, Benet LZ. Acyl glucuronides revisited: is the glucuronidation process a toxification as well as detoxification mechanism? *Drug Metab Rev* 1992;24:5–48.
4. Rowland M, Riegelman S, Harris PA, Sholkoff SD. Absorption kinetics of aspirin in man following oral administratino of an aqueous solution. *J Pharm Sci* 1972;61:379–385.
5. Rowland M, Riegelman S. Pharmacokinetics of acetylsalicylic acid and salicylic acid after intravenous administration in man. *J Pharm Sci* 1968;57:1313–1319.
6. Wanwimolruk S, Birkett DJ, Brooks PM. Protein binding of some non-steroidal anti-inflammatory drugs in rheumatoid arthritis. *Clin Pharmacokinet* 1982;7:85–92.
7. Ingelman-Sundberg M, Kaur H, Terelius Y, Persson JO, Halliwell B. Hydroxylation of salicylate by microsomal fractions and cytochrome P-450: lack of production of 2,3-dihydroxybenzoate unless hydroxyl radical formation is permitted. *Biochem J* 1991;276:753–757.
8. Smith PK. The pharmacology of salicylates and related compounds. *Ann N Y Acad Sci* 1960;86:38–63.
9. Forman WB, Davidson ED, Webster LT. Enzymatic conversion of salicylate to salicylurate. *Mol Pharmacol* 1971;7:247–259.
10. Hall SD, Rudy AC, Knight PM, Brater DC. Lack of presystemic inversion of (R)- to (S)-ibuprofen in humans. *Clin Pharmacol Ther* 1993;53:393–400.
11. Lee EJ, Williams K, Day R, Graham G, Champion D. Stereoselective disposition of ibuprofen enantiomers in man. *Br J Clin Pharmacol* 1985;19:669–674.
12. Rudy AC, Knight PM, Brater DC, Hall SD. Stereoselective metabolism of ibuprofen in humans: administration of R-, S- and racemic ibuprofen [published erratum appears in *J Pharmacol Exp Ther* 1992;260:1456]. *J Pharmacol Exp Ther* 1991;259:1133–1139.
13. Hamman MA, Thompson GA, Hall SD. Regioselective and stereoselective metabolism of ibuprofen by human cytochrome P450 2C. *Biochem Pharmacol* 1997;54:33–41.
14. Klose TS, Ibeanu GC, Ghanayem BI, et al. Identification of residues 286 and 289 as critical for conferring substrate specificity of human CYP2C9 for diclofenac and ibuprofen. *Arch Biochem Biophys* 1998;357:240–248.
15. Jin C, Miners JO, Lillywhite KJ, Mackenzie PI. Complementary deoxyribonucleic acid cloning and expression of a human liver uridine diphosphate-glucuronosyltransferase glucuronidating carboxylic acid-containing drugs. *J Pharmacol Exp Ther* 1993;264:475–479.
16. Wechter WJ, Loughhead DG, Reischer RJ, VanGiessen GJ, Kaiser DG. Enzymatic inversion at saturated carbon: nature and mechanism of the inversion of R(−)p-iso-butyl hydratropic acid. *Biochem Biophys Res Commun* 1974;61:833–837.
17. Kaiser DG, Vangiessen GJ, Reischer RJ, Wechter WJ. Isomeric inversion of ibuprofen (R)-enantiomer in humans. *J Pharm Sci* 1976;65:269–273.
18. Nakamura Y, Yamaguchi S, Takahashi S, Hashimoto K, Iwatani K, Nakagawa Y. Optical isomerization mechanism of R(-)hydratropic acid derivatives. *J Pharmacobiodyn* 1981;4:S–1.
19. Knights KM, Drew R, Meffin PJ. Enantiospecific formation of fenoprofen coenzyme A thioester in vitro. *Biochem Pharmacol* 1988;37:3539–3542.
20. Knihinicki RD, Williams KM, Day RO. Chiral inversion of 2-arylpropionic acid non-steroidal anti-inflammatory drugs. I: In vitro studies of ibuprofen and flurbiprofen. *Biochem Pharmacol* 1989;38:4389–4395.
21. Knadler MP, Hall SD. Stereoselective arylpropionyl-CoA thioester formation in vitro. *Chirality* 1990;2:67–73.
22. Tracy TS, Hall SD. Determination of the epimeric composition of ibuprofenyl-CoA. *Anal Biochem* 1991;195:24–29.
23. Tracy TS, Wirthwein DP, Hall SD. Metabolic inversion of (R)-ibuprofen: formation of ibuprofenyl-coenzyme A. *Drug Metab Dispos* 1993;21:114–120.
24. Tracy TS, Hall SD. Metabolic inversion of (R)-ibuprofen: epimerization and hydrolysis of ibuprofenyl-coenzyme A. *Drug Metab Dispos* 1992;20:322–327.
25. Porubek DJ, Sanins SM, Stephens JR, et al. Metabolic chiral inversion of flurbiprofen-CoA in vitro. *Biochem Pharmacol* 1991;42:R1–R4.
26. Baillie TA, Adams WJ, Kaiser DG, et al. Mechanistic studies of the metabolic chiral inversion of (R)-ibuprofen in humans. *J Pharmacol Exp Ther* 1989;249:517–523.
27. Sanins SM, Adams WJ, Kaiser DG, et al. Mechanistic studies on the metabolic chiral inversion of R-ibuprofen in the rat. *Drug Metab Dispos* 1991;19:405–410.
28. Chen CS, Chen T, Shieh WR. Metabolic stereoisomeric inversion of 2-arylpropionic acids: on the mechanism of ibuprofen epimerization in rats. *Biochim Biophys Acta* 1990;1033:1–6.
29. Williams K, Day R, Knihinicki R, Duffield A. The stereoselective uptake of ibuprofen enantiomers into adipose tissue. *Biochem Pharmacol* 1986;35:3403–3405.
30. Johnson JL, Brater DC, Hall SD. Formation of "hybrid" glycerolipids in normal volunteers. *Clin Pharmacol Ther* 1995;57:213.
31. Foster RT, Jamali F, Russell AS, Alballa SR. Pharmacokinetics of ketoprofen enantiomers in healthy subjects following single and multiple doses. *J Pharmacol Sci* 1988;77:70–73.
32. Rudy AC, Liu YX, Brater DC, Hall SD. Stereoselective pharmacokinetics and inversion of (R)-ketoprofen in healthy volunteers. *J Clin Pharmacol* 1998;38(suppl):S10.
33. Jamali F, Russell AS, Foster RT, Lemko G. Ketoprofen pharmacokinetics in humans: evidence of enantiomeric inversion and lack of interaction. *J Pharm Sci* 1990;79:460–461.
34. Hayball PJ, Nation RL, Bochner F, Newton JL, Massy-Westropp RA, Hamon DP. Plasma protein binding of ketoprofen enantiomers in man: method development and application. *Chirality* 1991;3:460–466.
35. Presle N, Lapicque F, Fournel-Gigleux S, Magdalou J, Netter P. Stereoselective irreversible binding of ketoprofen glucuronides to albumin: characterization of the site and the mechanism. *Drug Metab Dispos* 1996;24:1050–1057.
36. Upton RA, Buskin JN, Williams RL, Riegelman S. Negligible excretion of unchanged ketoprofen, naproxen, and probenecid in urine. *J Pharm Sci* 1980;69:1254–1257.
37. Knadler MP, Brater DC, Hall SD. Stereoselective disposition of flurbiprofen in normal volunteers. *Br J Clin Pharmacol* 1992;33:369–375.
38. Tracy TS, Marra C, Wrighton SA, Gonzalez FJ, Korzekwa KR. Studies of flurbiprofen 4'-hydroxylation: additional evidence suggesting the sole involvement of cytochrome P450 2C9. *Biochem Pharmacol* 1996;52:1305–1309.
39. Tracy TS, Rosenbluth BW, Wrighton SA, Gonzalez FJ, Korzekwa KR. Role of cytochrome P450 2C9 and an allelic variant in the 4'-hydroxylation of (R)- and (S)-flurbiprofen. *Biochem Pharmacol* 1995;49:1269–1275.
40. Yamazaki H, Inoue K, Chiba K, et al. Comparative studies on the catalytic roles of cytochrome P450 2C9 and its cys- and leu-variants in the oxidation of warfarin, flurbiprofen, and diclofenac by human liver microsomes. *Biochem Pharmacol* 1998;56:243–251.
41. Knadler MP, Hall SD. High-performance liquid chromatographic analysis of the enantiomers of flurbiprofen and its metabolites in plasma and urine. *J Chromatogr* 1989;494:173–182.
42. Rubin A, Warrick P, Wolen RL, Chernish SM, Ridolfo AS, Gruber CM. Physiological disposition of fenoprofen in man. 3: Metabolism and protein binding of fenoprofen. *J Pharmacol Exp Ther* 1972;183:449–457.
43. Volland C, Sun H, Dammeyer J, Benet LZ. Stereoselective degradation of the fenoprofen acyl glucuronide enantiomers and irreversible binding to plasma protein. *Drug Metab Dispos* 1991;19:1080–1086.
44. Rubin A, Rodda BE, Warrick P, Ridolfo AS, Gruber CM. Physiological disposition of fenoprofen in man. II: Plasma and urine pharmacokinetics after oral and intravenous administration. *J Pharm Sci* 1972;61:739–745.
45. Volland C, Sun H, Benet LZ. Stereoselective analysis of fenoprofen and its metabolites. *J Chromatogr* 1990;534:127–138.
46. Volland C, Benet LZ. In vitro enantioselective glucuronidation of fenoprofen. *Pharmacology* 1991;43:53–60.
47. Rubin A, Knadler MP, Ho PP, Bechtol LD, Wolen RL. Stereoselective inversion of (R)-fenoprofen to (S)-fenoprofen in humans. *J Pharm Sci* 1985;74:82–84.
48. Sallustio BC, Knights KM, Meffin PJ. The stereospecific inhibition of endogenous triacylglycerol synthesis by fenoprofen in rat isolated adipocytes and hepatocytes. *Biochem Pharmacol* 1990;40:1414–1417.
49. Sallustio BC, Meffin PJ, Knights KM. The stereospecific incorpora-

tion of fenoprofen into rat hepatocyte and adipocyte triacylglycerols. *Biochem Pharmacol* 1988;37:1919–1923.

50. Runkel R, Forchielli E, Boost G, et al. Naproxen: metabolism, excretion and comparative pharmacokinetics. *Scand J Rheumatol* 1973;2:29–36.

51. Thompson GF, Collins J. Urinary metabolic profiles for choosing test animals for chronic toxicity studies: application to naproxen. *J Pharm Sci* 1973;62:937–941.

52. Rodrigues AD, Kukulka MJ, Roberts EM, Ouellet D, Rodgers TR. [O-methyl C-14]naproxen O-demethylase activity in human liver microsomes: evidence for the involvement of cytochrome P4501A2 and P4502C9/10. *Drug Metab Dispos* 1996;24:126–136.

53. Miners JO, Coulter S, Tukey RH, Veronese ME, Birkett DJ. Cytochromes P450, 1A2, and 2C9 are responsible for the human hepatic O-demethylation of R- and S-naproxen. *Biochem Pharmacol* 1996;51:1003–1008.

54. Tracy TS, Marra C, Wrighton SA, Gonzalez FJ, Korzekwa KR. Involvement of multiple cytochrome P450 isoforms in naproxen O-demethylation. *Eur J Clin Pharmacol* 1997;52:293–298.

55. Kiang CH, Lee C, Kushinsky S. Isolation and identification of 6-desmethylnaproxen sulfate as a new metabolite of naproxen in human plasma. *Drug Metab Dispos* 1989;17:43–48.

56. Richardson CJ, Blocka K, Ross SG, Verbeeck RK. Piroxicam and 5′-hydroxypiroxicam kinetics following multiple dose administration of piroxicam. *Eur J Clin Pharmacol* 1987;32:89–91.

57. Twomey TM, Hobbs DC. Biotransformation of piroxicam by man. *Fed Proc* 1978;37:271.

58. Zhao J, Leemann T, Dayer P. In vitro oxidation of oxicam NSAIDs by a human liver cytochrome P450. *Life Sci* 1992;51:575–581.

59. Wiseman EH, Boyle JA. Piroxicam (Feldene). *Clin Rheum Dis* 1980;6:583–613.

60. Duggan DE, Hooke KF, Risley EA, Shen TY, Arman CG. Identification of the biologically active form of sulindac. *J Pharmacol Exp Ther* 1977;201:8–13.

61. Hucker HB, Stauffer SC, White SD, et al. Physiologic disposition and metabolic fate of a new anti-inflammatory agent, cis-5-fluoro-2-methyl-1-[p-(methylsulfinyl)-benzylidenyl]-indene-3-acetic acid in the rat, dog, rhesus monkey and man. *Drug Metab Dispos* 1973;1:736.

62. Duggan DE, Hare LE, Ditzler CA, Lei BW, Kwan KC. The disposition of sulindac. *Clin Pharmacol Ther* 1977;21:326–335.

63. Light DR, Waxman DJ, Walsh C. Studies on the chirality of sulfoxidation catalyzed by bacterial flavoenzyme cyclohexanone monooxygenase and hog liver flavin adenine dinucleotide containing monooxygenase. *Biochemistry* 1982;21:2490–2498.

64. John VA. The pharmacokinetics and metabolism of diclofenac sodium (VoltarolR) in animals and man. *Rheumatol Rehabil* 1979;2:22–37.

65. Kendall MJ, Thornhill DP, Willis JV. Factors affecting the pharmacokinetics of diclofenac sodium (VoltarolR). *Rheumatol Rehabil* 1979;2:38–46.

66. Chan KKH, Vyas KH, Brandt KD. In vitro protein binding of diclofenac sodium in plasma and synovial fluid. *J Pharm Sci* 1987;76:105–108.

67. Stierlin H, Faigle JW. Biotransformation of diclofenac sodium (Voltaren) in animals and in man. II: quantitative determination of the unchanged drug and principal phenolic metabolites, in urine and bile. *Xenobiotica* 1979;9:611–621.

68. Faigle JW, Bottcher I, Godbillon J, et al. A new metabolite of diclofenac sodium in human plasma. *Xenobiotica* 1988;18:1191–1197.

69. Stierlin H, Faigle JW, Sallmann A, et al. Biotransformation of diclofenac sodium (Voltaren) in animals and in man. I: Isolation and identification of principal metabolites. *Xenobiotica* 1979;9:601–610.

70. Leemann T, Transon C, Dayer P. Cytochrome P450TB (CYP2C): a major monooxygenase catalyzing diclofenac 4′-hydroxylation in human liver. *Life Sci* 1993;52:29–34.

71. Laine L, Sloane R, Ferretti M, Cominelli F. A randomized double-blind comparison of placebo, etodolac, and naproxen on gastrointestinal injury and prostaglandin production. *Gastrointest Endosc* 1995;42:428–433.

72. Dvornik DM. Tissue selective inhibition of prostaglandin biosynthesis by etodolac. *J Rheumatol* 1997;47:40–47.

73. Cayen MN, Kraml M, Ferdinandi ES, Greselin E, Dvornik D. The metabolic disposition of etodolac in rats, dogs, and man. *Drug Metab Rev* 1981;12:339–362.

74. Ferdinandi ES, Sehgal SN, Demerson CA, et al. Disposition and biotransformation of ^{14}C-etodolac in man. *Xenobiotica* 1986;16:153–166.

75. Smith PC, Song WQ, Rodriguez RJ. Covalent binding of etodolac acyl glucuronide to albumin in vitro. *Drug Metab Dispos* 1992;20:962–965.

76. Mroszczak EJ, Jung D, Yee J, Bynum L, Sevelius H, Massey I. Ketorolac tromethamine pharmacokinetics and metabolism after intravenous, intramuscular, and oral administration in humans and animals. *Pharmacotherapy* 1990;10:33S–39S.

77. Mroszczak E, Combs D, Chaplin M, et al. Chiral kinetics and dynamics of ketorolac. *J Clin Pharmacol* 1996;36:521–539.

78. Mroszczak EJ, Lee FW, Combs D, et al. Ketorolac tromethamine absorption, distribution, metabolism, excretion, and pharmacokinetics in animals and humans. *Drug Metab Dispos* 1987;15:618–626.

79. Brier ME, Sloan RS, Aronoff GR. Population pharmacokinetics of the active metabolite of nabumetone in renal dysfunction. *Clin Pharmacol Ther* 1995;57:622–627.

80. Hyneck M, Audet P, Nichols A, et al. Steady-state pharmacokinetics and ex vivo protein binding of nabumetone. *Clin Pharmacol Ther* 1993;53:212.

81. Haddock RE, Jeffery DJ, Lloyd JA, Thawley AR. Metabolism of nabumetone (BRL 14777) by various species including man. *Xenobiotica* 1984;14:327–337.

82. Janssen FW, Jusko WJ, Chiang ST, et al. Metabolism and kinetics of oxaprozin in normal subjects. *Clin Pharmacol Ther* 1980;27:352–362.

83. Aubry A-F, Markoglou N, Adams MH, Longstreth J, Wainer IW. The effect of co-administered drugs on oxaprozin binding to human serum albumin. *J Pharm Pharmacol* 1995;47:937–944.

84. Ruelius HW, Kirkman SK, Young EM, Janssen FW. Reactions of oxaprozin-1-O-acyl glucuronide in solutions of human plasma and albumin. *Adv Exp Med Biol* 1986;197:431–441.

85. Wells DS, Janssen FW, Ruelius HW. Interactions between oxaprozin glucuronide and human serum albumin. *Xenobiotica* 1987;17:1437–1449.

86. Tempero KF, Cirillo VJ, Steelman SL. Diflunisal: a review of pharmacokinetic and pharmacodynamic properties, drug interactions, and special tolerability studies in humans. *Br J Clin Pharmacol* 1977;4:31S–36S.

87. Verbeeck RK, Boel A, Buntinx A, DeSchepper PJ. Plasma protein binding and interaction studies with diflunisal: a new salicylate analgesic. *Biochem Pharmacol* 1980;29:571–576.

88. Green D, Davies RO, Holmes GI, et al. Effects of diflunisal on platelet function and fecal blood loss. *Pharmacotherapy* 1983;3:65S–69S.

89. Macdonald JI, Dickinson RG, Reid RS, Edom RW, King AR, Verbeeck RK. Identification of a hydroxy metabolite of diflunisal in rat and human urine. *Xenobiotica* 1991;21:1521–1533.

90. Loewen GR, Herman RJ, Ross SG, Verbeeck RK. Effect of dose on the glucuronidation and sulphation kinetics of diflunisal in man: single dose studies. *Br J Clin Pharmacol* 1988;26:31–39.

91. Loewen GR, McKay G, Verbeeck RK. Isolation and identification of a new major metabolite of diflunisal in man: the sulfate conjugate. *Drug Metab Dispos* 1986;14:127–131.

92. Verbeeck RK, Loewen GR, Macdonald JI, Herman RJ. The effect of multiple dosage on the kinetics of glucuronidation and sulphation of diflunisal in man. *Br J Clin Pharmacol* 1990;29:381–389.

93. Macdonald JI, Herman RJ, Verbeeck RK. Sex-difference and the effects of smoking and oral contraceptive steroids on the kinetics of diflunisal. *Eur J Clin Pharmacol* 1990;38:175–179.

94. Thyss A, Milano G, Kubar J, Namer M, Schneider M. Clinical and pharmacokinetic evidence of a life-threatening interaction between methotrexate and ketoprofen. *Lancet* 1986;I:256–258.

95. Singh RR, Malaviya AN, Pandey JN, Guleria JS. Fatal interaction between methotrexate and naproxen. *Lancet* 1986;I:1390.

96. Liegler DG, Henderson ES, Hahn MA, Oliverio VT. The effect of organic acids on renal clearance of methotrexate in man. *Clin Pharmacol Ther* 1969;10:849–857.

97. Tracy TS, Krohn K, Jones DR, Bradley JD, Hall SD, Brater DC. The effects of a salicylate, ibuprofen, and naproxen on the disposition of methotrexate in patients with rheumatoid arthritis. *Eur J Clin Pharmacol* 1992;42:121–125.

98. Stewart CF, Fleming RA, Arkin C, Evans WE. Coadministration of naproxen and low-dose methotrexate in patients with rheumatoid arthritis. *Clin Pharmacol Ther* 1990;47:540–546.

99. Furst D, Herman R, Koehnke R, et al. The effect of aspirin and sulindac on methotrexate clearance. *J Pharm Sci* 1990;79:782–786.

100. Skeith KJ, Russell AS, Jamali F, Coates J. Lack of significant interaction between low-dose methotrexate and ibuprofen or flurbiprofen in patients with arthritis. *J Rheumatol* 1990;17:1008–1010.

101. Tracy TS, Worster T, Bradley JD, Greene PK, Brater DC. Methotrexate disposition following concomitant administration of ketoprofen, piroxicam and flurbiprofen in patients with rheumatoid arthritis. *Br J Clin Pharmacol* 1994;37:453–456.

102. Runkel R, Mroszczak E, Chaplin M, Sevelius H, Segre E. Naproxen-probenecid interaction. *Clin Pharmacol Ther* 1978;24:706–713.

103. Upton RA, Williams RL, Buskin JN, Jones RM. Effects of probenecid on ketoprofen kinetics. *Clin Pharmacol Ther* 1982;31:705–712.

104. Grennan DM, Ferry DG, Ashworth ME, Kenny RE, Mackinnon M. The aspirin-ibuprofen interaction in rheumatoid arthritis. *Br J Clin Pharmacol* 1979;8:497–503.

105. Rubin A, Rodda BE, Warrick P, Gruber CM, Ridolfo AS. Interactions of aspirin with nonsteroidal antiinflammatory drugs in man. *Arthritis Rheum* 1973;16:635–645.

106. Segre EJ, Chaplin M, Forchielli E, Runkel R, Sevelius H. Naproxen-aspirin interactions in man. *Clin Pharmacol Ther* 1974;15:375–379.

107. Khan IH. Lithium and non-steroidal anti-inflammatory drugs. *Br Med J* 1991;302:1537–1538.

108. Nadarajah J, Stein GS. Piroxicam induced lithium toxicity. *Ann Rheum Dis* 1985;44:502.

109. Kristoff CA, Hayes PE, Barr WH, Small RE, Townsend RJ, Ettigi PG. Effect of ibuprofen on lithium plasma and red blood cell concentrations. *Clin Pharmacol* 1986;5:51–55.

110. Reimann IW, Frolich JC. Effects of diclofenac on lithium kinetics. *Clin Pharmacol Ther* 1981;30:348–352.

111. Ragheb M, Powell AL. Lithium interaction with sulindac and naproxen. *J Clin Psychopharmacol* 1986;6:150–154.

112. Bachmann KA, Schwartz JI, Forney RB, Jauregui L, Sullivan TJ. Inability of ibuprofen to alter single dose phenytoin disposition. *Br J Clin Pharmacol* 1986;21:165–169.

113. Rubin A, Chernish SM, Crabtree R, et al. A profile of the physiological disposition and gastro-intestinal effects of fenoprofen in man. *Curr Med Res Opin* 1974;2:529–544.

CHAPTER 35

Methylxanthines

Donald J. Birkett and John O. Miners

INTRODUCTION

The methylxanthines comprise caffeine (CA; 1,3,7-trimethylxanthine) and its demethylated metabolites theophylline (TP), theobromine (TB), and paraxanthine (PX). Caffeine and TP are widely consumed in beverages such as coffee and tea, whereas TB is the major methylxanthine in chocolate. Theophylline has been extensively used in the treatment of obstructive airways disease and, because it has a narrow therapeutic window and severe dose-related toxicity, its pharmacokinetics and metabolism have been intensively studied. Caffeine has been used as a metabolic probe for cytochrome P450 (CYP) isoforms, N-acetyltransferase and xanthine oxidase. Its role as an *in vivo* metabolic probe for CYP1A2 is dealt with in Chapter 6. In this chapter, TP is discussed first because of its role as a therapeutic agent. Theobromine, PX, and CA are then discussed, and finally reference is made to some other methylxanthine analogues that have been developed as drugs.

THEOPHYLLINE

In Vivo Metabolism

Theophylline (TP; 1,3-dimethylxanthine) is extensively metabolized *in vivo* with only about 5% to 15% of the dose being excreted unchanged. The *in vivo* clearance is about 0.05 L/h/kg, so that TP is classified as a low-hepatic-extraction-ratio drug. Bioavailability is essentially complete from immediate-release and most controlled-release dosage forms. The intravenous dosage form most used is aminophylline, which is the ethylenediamine salt of TP and contains about 80% TP.

Like the other methylxanthines, TP is metabolized by demethylation to 1-methylxanthine (1-MX) and 3-methylxanthine (3-MX), and by 8-oxidation to 1,3-dimethyluric acid (1,3-DMU) (Fig. 35-1). 1-MX is further metabolized almost completely to 1-methyluric acid (1-MU), but 3-MX is excreted without further metabolism.

There have been numerous studies of TP metabolism *in vivo*, the first of which was in 1957 by Cornish and Christman (1) in two subjects. The results of a number of these studies are shown in Table 35-1. The results have been remarkably consistent, with the metabolite excretion as a percentage of total metabolites plus TP in urine being 17% to 27% for 1-MU, 10% to 18% for 3-MX, 44% to 55% for 1,3-DMU, and 2% to 17% for unchanged TP. Only trace amounts of 1-MX and 3-MU have been detected.

The formation of 1-MU could occur through either 1-MX or 1,3-DMU as intermediates. This was clarified by Grygiel et al. (7), who administered TP in the presence and absence of the xanthine oxidase inhibitor allopurinol. Allopurinol resulted in an increase in excretion of 1-MX, an approximately stoichiometric decrease in excretion of 1-MU, and no change in the excretion of 1,3-DMU (see Table 35-1). This was confirmed by Birkett et al. (11), who administered 1-MX and 1,3-DMU intravenously to healthy subjects. 1,3-DMU was excreted unchanged, whereas 1-MX was recovered in urine largely as 1-MU. When 1-MX was administered with allopurinol, the major part of the dose was recovered unchanged as 1-MX. This confirmed that 1-MU derived from TP is formed from the intermediate metabolite, 1-MX.

As TP is used to prevent neonatal apnea, there have been a number of studies of its metabolism in premature neonates. All pathways of metabolism are reduced in premature neonates, with 40% to 60% of the dose being excreted as unchanged TP (12–14). In addition, TP is methylated at the 7-position to form CA (1,3,7-trimethylxanthine), with CA accounting for about 10% of

D. J. Birkett and J. O. Miners: Department of Clinical Pharmacology, Flinders University and Flinders Medical Center, Bedford Park, South Australia 5042, Australia

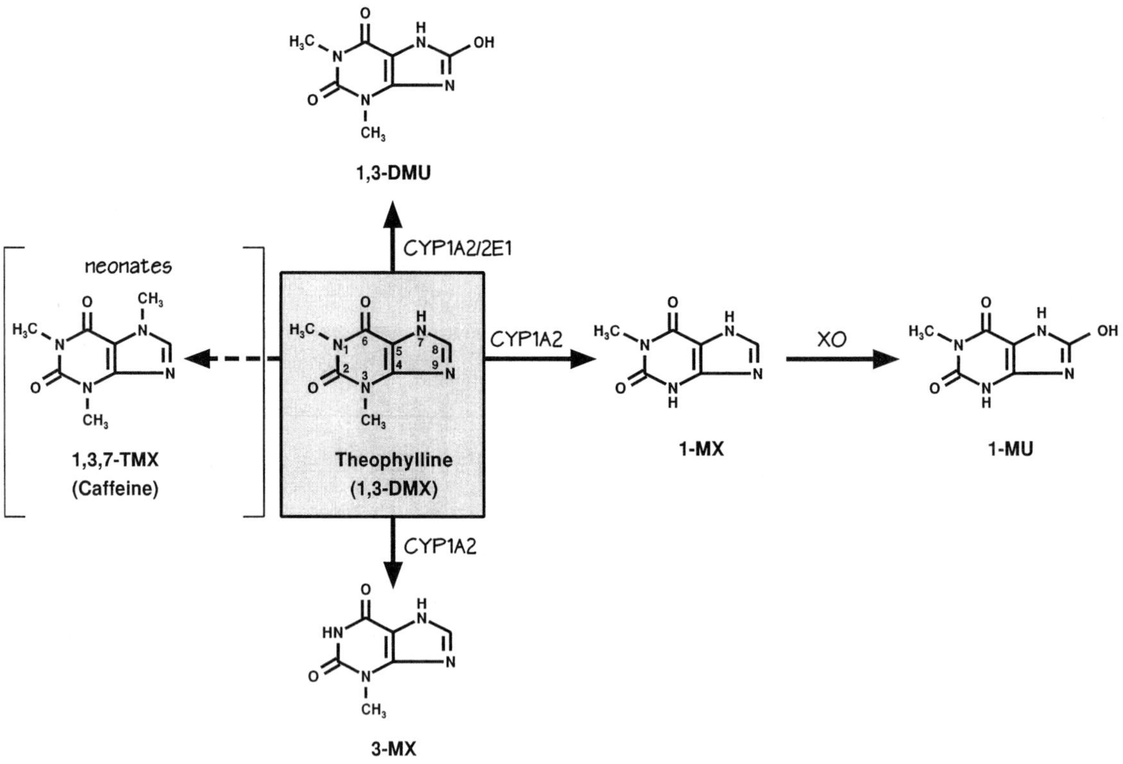

FIG. 35-1. Pathways of theophylline metabolism in humans.

TP and its metabolites excreted in urine (12–15). It is not clear whether this pathway is apparent only in neonates because of the immaturity of the other metabolic pathways, or whether the 7-methylation enzyme is not expressed in adults. It is difficult in adults to exclude a minor 7-methylation pathway because of the ubiquity of dietary CA intake.

TP metabolic pathways mature to reach adult levels at about age 55 weeks after conception (12). Compared with adults, 3-MX excretion is low relative to the other metabolites in premature neonates. Differences in cytochrome P450 (CYP) isoform maturation rates may mean that different enzymes are responsible for the metabolism of TP in this age group compared with adults. Kraus et al. (12) concluded that maturation of TP clearance in premature neonates was related to the development of the 1-demethylation pathway to 3-MX, whereas Tserng et al. (13) concluded that maturation of 8-oxidation to 1,3-DMU was the main factor. Jager-Roman et al. (16) found that prenatal treatment with betamethasone

TABLE 35-1. *Theophylline metabolite excretion in humans*

No. of subjects	Percentage of total excreted as[a]					Subjects	Reference
	1-MX	1-MU	3-MX	1,3-DMU	Theophylline		
2		27.5	19.5	51.5	1.5	Adults	1
	2.0	26.0	11.0	42.0	19.0	Adults	2
12		32.0	17.6	41.0	9.1	Adults	3
21	4.1	19.4	17.2	41.4	18.1	Adults	4
8		24.7	14.9	54.6	5.6	Adult smokers	5
9		20.6	11.7	54.1	13.1	Adult nonsmokers	5
16		23.5	16.2	52.8	7.1	Children 2–12 yr	6
14		20.0	13.5	55.4	10.5	Adult nonsmokers	6
10		20.2	13.1	53.2	12.5	Adults	7
10	13.5	5.4	13.2	54.5	13.4	With allopurinol	7
8		21.1	14.4	47.4	17.0	Nonsmokers	8
2		19.0	10.0	69.5	1.5	Aduls	9
15		16.5	36.2	39.6	7.7	Adults	10

[a]Expressed as percentage of total theophylline and metabolites recovered in urine.

resulted in increased TP metabolism in the neonate and suggested that this was due to prenatal maturation of CYP isoforms induced by the corticosteroid.

In children, TP clearance is increased compared with adults, and the half-life is shorter. The profile of metabolite excretion in children is similar to that in adults (6), indicating that all metabolic pathways are increased to a similar extent. Part, but not all, of the increased clearance is due to a larger liver weight/body weight ratio in children compared with adults (17).

There have been several studies on the linearity of TP metabolism *in vivo* in humans. Tang-Liu et al. (18) found K_m values for the conversion of TP to 1-MU, 3-MX, and 1,3-DMU of 2.7 mg/L, 9.3 mg/L, and 14.2 mg/L, respectively. Dahlqvist et al. (19) found somewhat higher K_m values for the same pathways: 16 mg/L, 16 mg/L, and 32 mg/L, respectively. The V_{max} values reported were 5 mg/h, 13 mg/h, and 34 mg/h, respectively, for 1-MU, 3-MX, and 1,3-DMU by Tang-Liu et al. (18), and 20 mg/h, 14 mg/h, and 65 mg/h, respectively, by Dahlqvist et al. (19).

The renal clearances of TP metabolites are high. Tang-Liu et al. (18) reported the renal clearances of 1-MU, 3-MX, and 1,3-DMU to be 22.5 L/h, 12 L/h, and 22.6 L/h, respectively. These values are well above the clearance by glomerular filtration, indicating substantial renal tubular secretion of all three metabolites. The elimination of the metabolites was rate limited by the elimination of TP. A similar order of relative renal clearances of the three metabolites can be inferred from the data in Rodopoulos et al. (2). The renal clearance of TP itself is dependent on urine flow, with TP being reabsorbed in the renal tubule to approximate equilibrium with the unbound concentration in plasma (20). After single doses to nontolerant

individuals, TP renal clearance is initially increased because of the diuresis produced by the drug (7,20). Plasma concentrations of the metabolites are low because of their high renal clearance, being less than 10% of the TP plasma concentration in each case (2,18,21,22).

Structure–activity studies of xanthine analogues suggest that a methyl group in the 1-position is essential for adenosine antagonism and that substituents of increasing length in the 3-position confer increasing bronchodilator activity. Thus a xanthine analogue enprofylline, 3-propylxanthine, was more potent than TP as a bronchodilator but lacked central nervous stimulant and other activities associated with adenosine antagonism (23,24). In agreement with this, 3-MX was found to produce similar effects to TP in a variety of pharmacologic models (25), but was less potent than TP. The low concentrations of the metabolites after dosing with TP indicate that they add very little to the overall therapeutic effects, although the extent to which they accumulate in renal dysfunction has not been investigated.

In Vitro Metabolism Studies

The two main approaches to defining the CYP isoforms responsible for the metabolism of a drug substrate are human liver microsomal studies and studies with recombinant P450s. Both of these approaches have been used with TP.

Studies with human liver microsomes (HLMs) have given reasonably consistent results (Table 35-2). Two studies have found biphasic kinetic plots (Eadie–Hofstee plots), and one, linear kinetics. The first study by Robson et al. (26), which reported linear kinetics, used a TP concentration range of 0.025 mM to 0.5 mM, lower than

TABLE 35-2. *Kinetics of theophylline metabolism in vitro in human liver microsomes and with recombinant CYP isoforms*

Preparation	Apparent K_m			V_{max}			Cl_{int}			% Total			Ref
	1-MX	3-MX	1,3-DMU	1-MX	3-MX	1,3-DMU	1-MX	3-MX	1,3-DMU	1-MX	3-MX	1,3-DMU	
Human liver microsomes													
High affinity	0.64	0.55	0.79	2.8	2.6	11.2	4.5	4.9	14.3	189	20.6	60.4	26
High affinity	0.6	0.6	8.5	31.7	51.7	466	52.8	86.2	54.8	27.2	44.4	28.3	28
High affinity	0.29	0.28	0.31	5.9	3.3	43.3	20.4	11.9	140	11.8	6.9	81.2	27
Low affinity	25.8	36	31	14.8	14.2	478	0.6	0.4	15.4	3.5	2.4	94.1	
Isoforms													
CYP1A2			0.6			0.9			1.5				31
CYP2D6			14.4			1.4			0.1				
CYP2E1			19.9			12.9			0.6				
CYP3A4			24.1			0.4			0.2				
CYP1A1	0.31			0.2			0.64						33
CYP1A2	0.38	1.1	0.23	6	2.5	7.3	15.8	2.2	31.8	31.7	4.4	63.9	
CYP2D6	7		8.1	1.8		8	0.3		1				
CYP2E1			15.3			68.7			4.5				

Units: K_m, mM; V_{max} (HLM), pmol/min/mg microsomal protein; V_{max} (recombinant isoforms), pmol/min/pmol CYP; Cl_{int} (HLM), μL/min/mg microsomal protein; CL_{int} (recombinant isoforms), μL/min/pmol CYP.

those of the other two studies, in which substrate ranges of 0.05 mM to 20 mM (27) and 0.2 mM to 18 mM (28)) were used. Absence of activity without a reduced nicotinamide adenine dinucleotide phosphate (NADPH) generating system (26) and essentially complete inhibition of metabolism by an anti-human NADPH-cytochrome P450 reductase antibody (29) confirmed that TP is metabolized in HLMs by CYP isoforms.

K_m and V_{max} values for TP metabolic pathways in HLM and with cDNA-expressed CYP isoforms are shown in Table 35-2. The results of the various microsomal studies are reasonably consistent, with K_m values in the range 0.3 mM to 0.8 mM, except for the value of 8.5 mM for 1,3-DMU formation reported by Rasmussen et al. (28). In this latter case, the lowest substrate concentration used was 0.2 mM, so the high-affinity K_m may not have been well defined. Tjia et al. (27) reported low-affinity K_m values of the order of 25 mM to 36 mM for the three pathways. The similarity of the high-affinity K_m values for the three pathways suggests that the reactions are carried out by the one CYP isoform, but does not exclude the involvement of multiple isoforms with similar K_m values. Both Tjia et al. (27) and Rasmussen et al. (28) indicated that, at therapeutic concentrations of TP, the majority of the metabolism would be carried out by the high-affinity forms. When the kinetic constants are used to calculate Cl_{int} values for the three pathways, the order of activity is similar to that seen *in vivo* (see Table 35-2).

Robson et al. (29) found no inhibition by tolbutamide or sulfaphenazole (CYP2C9), mephenytoin (CYP2C19), or debrisoquine (CYP2D6). 7,8-Benzoflavone (CYP1A2) at a low concentration was a potent inhibitor of all three pathways, but at a high concentration (0.1 mM) activated the 8-oxidation to 1,3-DMU. Nifedipine also inhibited the demethylation pathways but activated 8-oxidation. Inhibition also was observed with the less-selective inhibitors verapamil, dextropropoxyphene, cimetidine, and propranolol.

Tjia et al. (27) found potent inhibition of all three pathways by the CYP1A2-selective inhibitors furafylline, elliptocine, and 7,8-benzoflavone. Selective inhibitors for CYP3A (ketoconazole, troleandomycin, and gestodene), CYP2C9 (tolbutamide and sulfaphenazole), and CYP2D6 (quinidine) had no effect. The CYP2E1 inhibitor, diethyldithiocarbamate, inhibited all pathways but is known to be not completely selective for CYP2E1. The selective CYP2E1 substrate, 4-nitrophenol, inhibited the 8-oxidation by 30% but had little effect on the demethylations. They also found marked stimulation of 8-oxidation but not the demethylations by 7,8-benzoflavone at high concentrations. A similar activating effect of 7,8-benzoflavone on 8-oxidation had previously been reported by Robson et al. (29), who found that nifedipine also stimulated the 8-oxidation but not the demethylations. *In vitro* activation by 7,8-benzoflavone has been considered to be characteristic of CYP3A4

activities. However, Tassaneeyakul et al. (30) have reported that at high concentrations (more than 0.015 mM), 7,8-benzoflavone activated both 4-nitrophenol hydroxylation and chlorzoxazone 6-hydroxylation, activities selective for human CYP2E1. Thus the observed effects may not be inconsistent with a role of CYP2E1 in the formation of 1,3-DMU.

Rasmussen et al. (28) investigated the effects of a range of selective serotonin reuptake inhibitors (SSRIs) and a selection of CYP isoform–selective inhibitors on TP metabolism in HLMs. The CYP3A4 inhibitor, ketoconazole, and the CYP2D6 inhibitor, quinidine, had essentially no effect. Fluvoxamine, a potent inhibitor of CYP1A2, inhibited all three pathways of TP metabolism, but the K_i was somewhat higher for the 8-oxidation than for the demethylations. Of the other SSRIs tested, paroxetine, sertraline, litoxetin, and norfluoxetine inhibited TP metabolism, and in all cases the effect was less marked for the 8-oxidation than for the demethylations. Fluoxetine, which is a potent CYP2D6 inhibitor, citalopram. and desmethylcitalopram were not inhibitors. These investigators also studied the effect of ethanol at concentrations from 0.17 mM to 86 mM, which do not exhibit nonspecific inhibition of P450s. At a concentration of 86 mM, ethanol decreased the formation of 1,3-DMU by 42% but did not affect the demethylation pathways. Ethanol and fluvoxamine in combination essentially abolished 1,3-DMU formation. Zhang and Kaminsky (31) found a strong correlation of TP 8-oxidation with CYP1A2 form-specific activities at low TP concentration (5 mM), and with CYP2E1 activities at a high TP concentration (40 mM). Weaker correlations with CYP3A4 activities were observed at both TP concentrations.

Taken together, the inhibition and correlation studies of TP metabolism suggest a predominant role for CYP1A2 in formation of the demethylated metabolites 1-MX and 3-MX. CYP1A2 also is important in the formation of 1,3-DMU, but a number of findings strongly suggest that a second isoform, probably CYP2E1, also is involved in this pathway.

A number of studies have investigated TP metabolism by cDNA-expressed CYP isoforms. The qualitative activities found are shown in Table 35-3. CYP2A6 and CYP2B6 have consistently been found not to metabolize TP. CYP2C9 was found by Shimada et al. (32) to have some activity, but not by Zhang et al. (31). CYP1A1, CYP1A2, CYP1B1, CYP2D6, CYP2E1, and CYP3A4 have all been found to have activity in the production of one or more of the TP metabolites. CYP1A2 has consistently been found to have higher activity than the other CYP isoforms. Two of the studies included formal kinetic characterization of the activities, and the K_m and V_{max} values found are shown in Table 35-2. CYP1A2 is the only isoform to show K_m values for all three metabolic pathways less than 1 mM (31,33), similar to those found with HLMs. The V_{max} for CYP2E1-mediated formation of 1,3-

TABLE 35-3. *Metabolism of theophylline by recombinant CYP isoforms*

Reference	Metabolites detected with									
	1A1	1A2	1B1	2A6	2B6	2C9	2D6	2E1	3A4	3A5
33	1MX	1MX 3MX DMU		Nil	Nil		1MX DMU	DMu	Nil	
27		1MX 3MX DMU							DMU	Nil
32	1MX 3MX DMU	1-MX 3MX DMU	1MX 3MX DMU			1MX DMU	1M DMU	1MX DMU	1MX DMU	
89		1-MX 3-MX DMU		Nil	Nil			DMU	DMU	Nil
31[a]	Nil	DMU		Nil	Nil	Nil	DMU	DMU	DMU	

Blank spaces not tested; nil, below the limit of detection for all three metabolites.
[a]Only DMU was investigated.

DMU was 14-fold (31), and 9.4-fold (33) higher than that for CYP1A2, indicating that CYP2E1 has a high capacity for TP 8-oxidation. However, the K_m for CYP2E1 was much higher than that for CYP1A2. When expressed as an intrinsic clearance (V_{max}/K_m), CYP1A2 is two-fold (31) or seven-fold (33) more active than CYP2E1. Both CYP2D6 and CYP3A4 have a high K_m and relatively low V_{max} (see Table 35-2), making it unlikely that these isoforms contribute substantially to TP metabolism *in vivo*. If the data of Ha et al. (33) with CYP1A2 are expressed as percentage of total metabolism based on the intrinsic clearance values, the results (1-MX, 31.7%; 3-MX, 4.5%; 1,3-DMU, 63.8%) are similar to the relative formation of the metabolites *in vivo* and in HLMs.

The results of studies with HLMs and with cDNA-expressed CYP isoforms are therefore consistent, and indicate that 1-MX and 3-MX are formed by CYP1A2, whereas both CYP1A2 and CYP2E1 are likely to be involved in the 8-oxidation to 1,3-DMU.

Krenitsky et al. (34) studied the metabolism of a series of methylated xanthines by xanthine oxidase. 1-MX was actively converted to 1-MU, but 3-MX was a poor substrate for this enzyme. This is consistent with the *in vivo* findings of essentially complete conversion of 1-MX to 1-MU, which is blocked by the xanthine oxidase inhibitor allopurinol, whereas 3-MX is excreted without further biotransformation.

In Vivo Interaction Studies

TP is a metabolized drug with a low therapeutic index and as such has become a "standard" for drug-interaction studies. The many studies prior to 1991 have been exhaustively reviewed by Upton (35,36). Taken as a whole, the *in vivo* interaction studies are reasonably consistent with the isoform assignments on the basis of *in vitro* data.

Cigarette smoking, a classic inducer of CYP1A2, has been shown to increase TP clearance (5). In agreement with this, fluvoxamine, a potent inhibitor of CYP1A2, has been shown to reduce TP CL by 75%, confirming the dominant role of CYP1A2 in the *in vivo* metabolism of TP (3). Disulfiram, the *in vivo* precursor of the CYP2E1 inhibitor diethyldithiocarbamate, has been shown to reduce TP CL by about 20% (37).

Interactions with TP of a number of inhibitors or substrates of CYP3A4 have been investigated *in vivo*. The prototype CYP3A4 inhibitors ketoconazole (38,39) and grapefruit juice (40) were shown to have essentially no effect on TP CL. There have been a number of studies with diltiazem with variable results. These have included no change in TP CL (41–44), or small decreases in CL by 22% (45), 9% (46), 12% (47), and 21% (48). Diltiazem has much larger effects on substrates such as cyclosporine, which are metabolized predominantly by CYP3A4. Verapamil has been found in various studies to cause a small decrease of 14% to 23% in TP clearance (42,47,49,50). Nifedipine, also a CYP3A4 substrate, has essentially no effect on TP clearance (43,47,49,51–53).

The macrolide antibiotics are mechanism-based inhibitors of CYP3A4. Although the *in vitro* data and the *in vivo* interaction data discussed earlier do not suggest a role for this isoform in the metabolism of TP, inhibitory interactions have been found *in vivo*. Troleandomycin, the most potent CYP3A4 inhibitor of the macrolides, has been shown to reduce TP clearance by 50% (54). Naline et al. (38) also found that troleandomycin caused a 50% decrease in TP clearance and further showed that all three TP metabolic pathways were affected to about the same extent. Numerous studies with erythromycin found either no change or decreases of up to 35% in TP CL (for a detailed discussion, see reference 35). A small effect (14%) has also been found with roxithromycin (55). The macrolides are known to become nonspecific CYP inhibitors at higher concentrations *in vitro*. The inhibitory effects observed *in vivo* may therefore be the result of nonspecific mechanism-based CYP inhibition occurring with prolonged (days to weeks) exposure.

A number of the quinolone antibiotics are potent inhibitors of TP clearance. In particular, enoxacin decreases TP CL by up to 74% (56,57), and ciprofloxacin by up to 55% (58–62). Perfloxacin reduces TP clearance by about 30% (58). The quinolones are known inhibitors of CYP1A2 (63,64), but the specificity of their inhibition of other CYP isoforms has not been studied systematically.

Other drugs that inhibit TP metabolism *in vivo* include cimetidine (65), a general CYP inhibitor; propranolol (66); acyclovir (67); and mexiletine (68,69). Sulfinpyrazone, which inhibits the CYP2C9 substrate tolbutamide (70), induces the metabolism of TP (71). Other drugs that induce TP metabolism are rifampicin (72), phenytoin (73), and moricizine (74). These drugs are nonselective CYP inhibitors or inducers, or their CYP isoform selectivity has not been investigated.

A number of the studies that have determined partial clearances along the three metabolic pathways for TP have found differential effects on the demethylations compared with the 8-oxidation. Greater effects on the demethylations than on the 8-oxidation have been found for fluvoxamine (3), ciprofloxacin (75–77), enoxacin (78,79), mexiletine (68,69), cimetidine (38,65), propranolol (66), and tocainide (80). By contrast, the *in vivo* effect of disulfiram, a CYP2E1 inhibitor, was due to inhibition of the formation CL of 1,3-DMU, with no effect on the demethylation pathways (37). These differential *in vivo* effects on the demethylation and 8-oxidation pathways strongly support a significant role for CYP2E1 in the 8-oxidation, as has been inferred from the *in vitro* studies.

Overall, therefore, the *in vivo* interaction results are reasonably consistent with the *in vitro* results, with both indicating that 1-MX and 3-MX are formed by CYP1A2, whereas 1,3-DMU is formed by both CYP1A2 and CYP2E1.

THEOBROMINE

Early studies identified 3-MX, 7-methylxanthine (7-MX), and 7-methyluric acid (7-MU) as the major urinary metabolites of TB in humans (1). Subsequently, 3,7-dimethyluric acid (3,7-DMU) and 6-amino-5-(*N*-methylformylamino)-1-methyluracil (3,7-DAU; a **dia**minouracil) were also detected in the urine of subjects administered TB in the form of cocoa (81).

Quantitative studies of TB disposition in humans indicate that 3-demethylation to give 7-MX and 7-MU is the major metabolic pathway (82–84). 7-MX and 7-MU, which are formed in the approximate ratio of 4:1, have been reported to account for 48.0% to 60.8% of TB-derived products excreted in urine. Excretion of 3-MX,

3,7-DAU, and unchanged TB ranged from 16.6% to 22.3%, 8.1% to 13.2%, and 10.9% to 15.8% of the dose administered, respectively. Formation of 3,7-DMU generally accounts for less than 2% of TB metabolism *in vivo* and, like TP, 3-MU is not detected as a biotransformation product of TB. Studies in a rat model demonstrated that 3,7-DAU and 3,7-DMU were derived from a common oxidized intermediate of TB (Fig. 35-2) (85). In the presence of glutathione, or some other cellular thiol, the intermediate is converted to 3,7-DAU. 3,7-DMU formation predominates after depletion of reducing thiols. *C*8–*N*9 bond scission to form a di- (or tri-) aminouracil also occurs with PX and CA (see later), but not TP. Thus the presence of an *N*7-methyl group appears to be obligatory for this pathway.

TB is well absorbed after oral administration; recovery of TB-derived products in urine is greater than 90% (82–84). Reported mean total plasma TB clearances for nonsmoking men from five studies, which used doses ranging from approximately 3 to 10 mg/kg, ranged from 0.045 to 0.075 L/h/kg (82–84,86,87). There is no evidence of dose-dependent elimination from these studies, although this point was not addressed specifically in any of the investigations. Comparative pharmacokinetic stud-

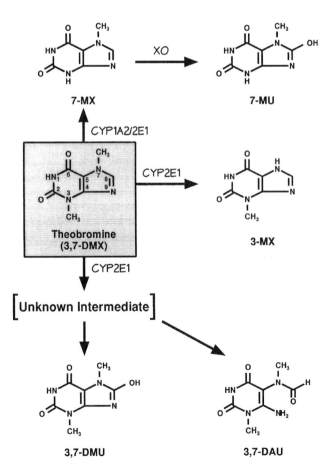

FIG. 35-2. Pathways of theobromine metabolism in humans.

ies undertaken in the same subjects have shown that the total plasma clearance of TB is higher than that of TP (by 30% to 45%), but unbound plasma clearances are almost identical (83,87). The unbound fraction of TB (0.86) is significantly higher than the mean unbound fractions of TP (0.58), PX (0.54), and CA (0.68) (87).

Evidence for the involvement of xanthine oxidase and CYP in TB metabolism in humans was provided initially by interaction studies *in vivo* (82,86). Allopurinol treatment abolished the formation of 7-MU and increased the excretion of 7-MX, but the partial metabolic clearance to 7-MX plus 7-MU was not different with and without allopurinol. Thus xanthine oxidase catalyzes the conversion of 7-MX to 7-MU (see Fig. 35-2). Plasma TB clearance was decreased by the concomitant administration of cimetidine, whereas pretreatment with sulfinpyrazone, a known inducer of TP metabolism, increased all metabolic clearances of TB. A modest increase in TB clearance was noted in cigarette smokers. These observations suggested a contribution of CYP, possibly the polycyclic aromatic hydrocarbon–inducible CYP1A2, to the primary metabolic pathways of TB.

Kinetic and inhibitor studies with HLMs and recombinant P450s subsequently confirmed a contribution of both CYP2E1 and CYP1A2 to human hepatic TB metabolism (88,89). Diethyldithiocarbamate and 4-nitrophenol, probes for CYP2E1, inhibited the microsomal formation of 3-MX, 7-MX, and 3,7-DMU by 55% to 60%, 35% to 55% and 85%, respectively. The CYP1A2 inhibitor furafylline variably inhibited (0 to 65%) 7-MX formation, but had no effect on other pathways. Consistent with the microsomal inhibition data, recombinant CYP1A2 and CYP2E1 exhibited similar apparent K_m values for 7-MX formation, and CYP2E1 was further shown to have the capacity to convert TB to both 3-MX and 3,7-DMU (89). Collectively, these results indicate that CYP2E1 and CYP1A2 together are responsible for 7-MX formation, whereas CYP2E1 is essentially solely responsible for 3,7-DMU (and, by inference, 3,7-DAU) formation. CYP2E1 and an unidentified isoform(s) catalyze the conversion of TB to 3-MX.

PARAXANTHINE

PX is the major biotransformation product of CA (see Caffeine) and consumers of CA-containing beverages are continuously exposed to this compound (90,91). Despite this widespread exposure, PX disposition and toxicity have not been studied widely. 1-MX, 1-MU, 7-MX, 7-MU, 1,7-dimethyluric acid (1,7-DMU), 6-amino-5-(N-formylmethylamino)-3-methyluracil (1,7-DAU), 5-acetylamino-6-formylamino-3-methyluracil (AFMU), and 5-acetylamino-6-amino-3-methyluracil (AAMU) have been identified in the urine of subjects administered PX (Fig. 35-3) (92,93). AAMU is a decomposition product of AFMU, which undergoes spontaneous deformylation in

urine (94). Excretion in urine of 1-MX, 1-MU, AFMU, 7-MX, 1,7-DMU, and unchanged PX have been reported to account, on average, for 17.8%, 34.8%, 14.2%, 5.2%, 7.7%, and 9.0%, respectively, of a PX dose administered orally to humans (93). Other potential metabolites, including 1,7-DAU and 7-MU, were not measured. Thus formation of the N7-demethylated metabolites 1-MX, 1-MU, and AFMU account for two thirds of PX biotransformation.

By analogy with the other N7-methylated xanthines TB and CA, it is assumed that 1,7-DAU and 1,7-DMU are derived from a common oxidized intermediate (see Fig. 35-3). There is also some evidence demonstrating that the N7-demethylated metabolites 1-MX, 1-MU, and AFMU arise from a common intermediate (93). Treatments that affect the conversion of PX to 1-MX *in vivo* (for example, cimetidine) influence AFMU formation similarly. It has therefore been proposed that N7-demethylation of PX proceeds by way of an unstable ring-opened intermediate that undergoes either acetylation or internal rearrangement to give AFMU and 1-MX, respectively (see Fig. 35-3) (93).

Two studies have reported pharmacokinetic parameters for PX in nonsmoking adult men (87,93). Mean total plasma clearances were 0.132 and 0.103 L/h/kg. Total and unbound plasma clearances of PX (*viz.*, 0.132 and 0.248 L/h/kg, respectively) determined in one of the studies were almost two-fold higher than those of TP and TB measured in the same group of subjects, but similar to values determined for CA (87).

Like the monodemethylations of TP and TB, CYP is responsible for PX N3- and N7-demethylation. Clearances to 7-MX and the N7-demethylated metabolites (i.e., 1-MX + 1-MU + AFMU) are both decreased by cimetidine treatment *in vivo* (93). *In vitro*, rates of PX N1- and N7-demethylation correlated significantly with the microsomal ethoxyresorufin O-deethylase and CA N3-demethylase activities of a panel of human livers (95). Moreover, mutual competitive inhibition was observed for ethoxyresorufin and PX (N1- and N3-demethylation and 1,7-DMU formation). Because ethoxyresorufin O-deethylation and CA N3-demethylation are both catalyzed by hepatic CYP1A2 (see following section and Chapter 6, CYP1A), these data are suggestive of a contribution of CYP1A2 to each of the primary PX metabolic pathways. An involvement of CYP1A2 in PX metabolism was subsequently demonstrated by using recombinant enzymes (89). Recombinant CYP1A2, but not CYP 2A6, 2B6, 2E1, 3A4, or 3A5, catalyzed the N1- and N7-demethylations of PX. In contrast, both CYP1A2 and CYP2A6 were able to convert PX to 1,7-DMU (and presumably also 1,7-DAU).

Once formed, 1-MX and 7-MX are converted partially to 1-MU and 7-MU, respectively (see Fig. 35-3) (92,93). Interestingly, the 1-MU to 1-MX ratio in urine after administration of PX, CA, or 1-MX itself ranges from

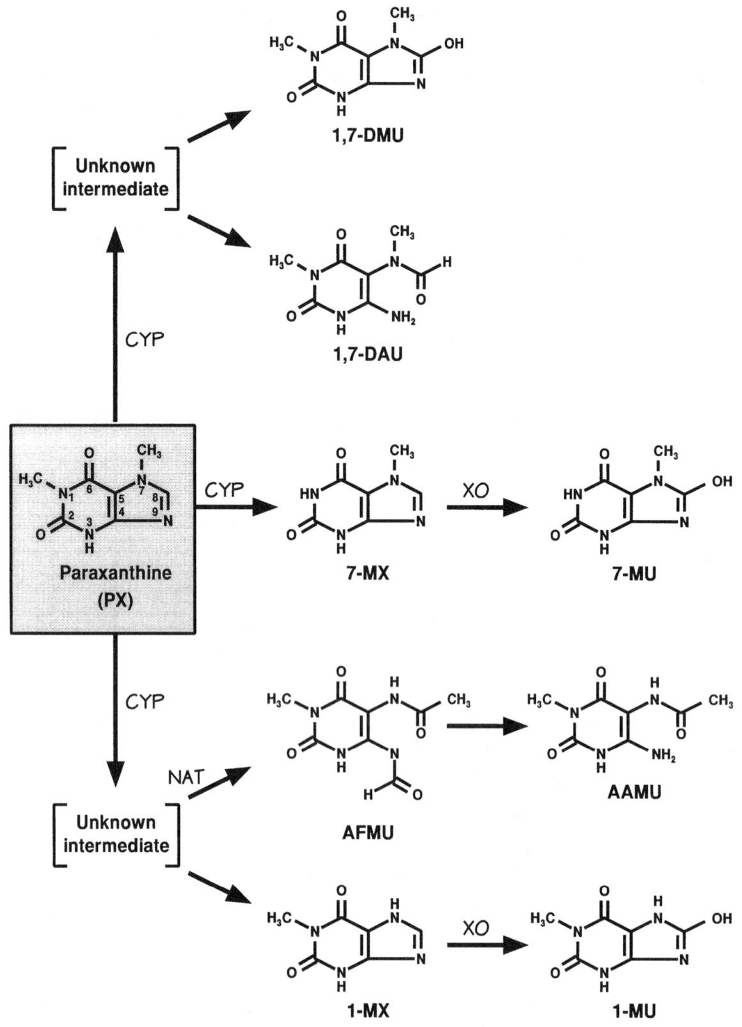

FIG. 35-3. Pathways of paraxanthine metabolism in humans.

approximately one to three, whereas it is more than ten when these compounds are derived from TP (7,93). Coadministration of PX and allopurinol increased the ratio of 1-MX to 1-MU in urine, consistent with the involvement of xanthine oxidase in this reaction (93). Allopurinol has also been shown to inhibit the 8-oxidation of PX-derived 1-MX after CA administration (see following section) in a dose-dependent manner (96). Furthermore, the relation between the plasma oxypurinol (the active metabolite of allopurinol) concentration and the decrement in the urinary 1-MX to 1-MU ratio fitted well by using a sigmoid E_{max} model (97). Collectively, these data suggest that the 1-MX to 1-MU ratio after CA administration provides an *in vivo* index of xanthine oxidase activity and a simple method for monitoring the allopurinol effect in patients with gouty arthritis.

Acetylation of the putative intermediate arising from PX *N*7-demethylation, which results in formation of AFMU (see Fig. 35-3), is catalyzed by the polymorphic *N*-acetyltransferase, NAT2. The urinary ratios of PX-derived AFMU to 1-MX and of AFMU to (AFMU + 1-MX + 1-MU) after CA administration show concordance with both dapsone and sulfamethazine *N*-acetylation in population studies (98,99). Theoretically, use of (AFMU + 1-MX + 1-MU) as the denominator is preferable for NAT2 phenotyping because it precludes xanthine oxidase activity as a variable.

CAFFEINE

CA metabolism in humans is complex, with at least 17 biotransformation products being excreted in urine. Primary metabolic pathways, inferred initially from urine excretion data (92,100), are *N*1-demethylation to form TB, *N*3-demethylation to form PX, *N*7-demethylation to form TP, and production of 1,3,7-trimethyluric acid (1,3,7-TMU) and 6-amino-5-(*N*-formylmethylamino)-1,3-diaminouracil (1,3,7-TAU; a triaminouracil) (Fig. 35-4). Like TB, there is direct evidence in a rodent model that 1,3,7-TMU and 1,3,7-TAU are derived from a common oxidized intermediate (101).

By using areas under the plasma concentration–time curves for each of the dimethylxanthines in subjects administered CA to steady state and plasma clearances of PX, TB, and TP determined in the same individuals, it has

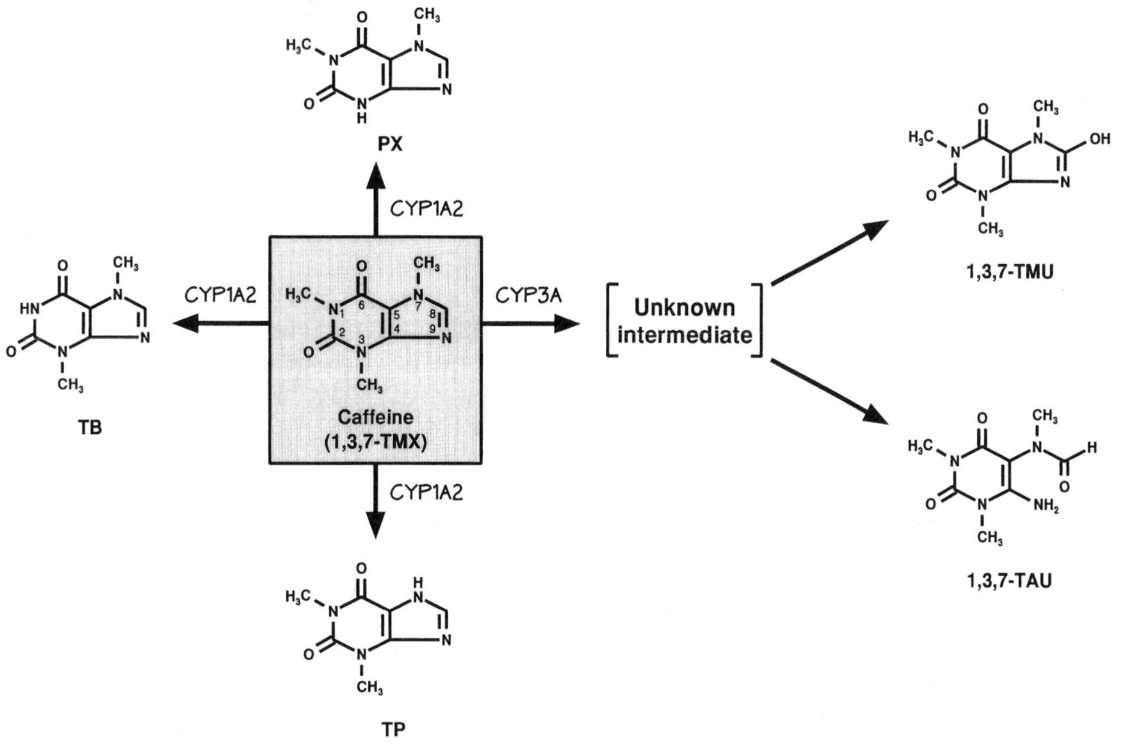

FIG. 35-4. Primary metabolic pathways of caffeine in humans.

been demonstrated that the *N*-demethylations account, on average, for 95% of CA clearance (91). Mean fractional conversions of CA to PX, TB, and TP were approximately 80%, 11%, and 4%, respectively. 3,7-DMU and 3,7-TAU formation and excretion of unchanged CA account for the remainder of CA elimination. Thus 3-demethylation to form PX is the major determinant of plasma CA clearance in humans.

As described in preceding sections, once formed PX, TB, and TP are subject to extensive biotransformation, giving rise to the characteristic pattern of urine metabolites observed after CA administration (see Fig. 6-2, Chapter 6). Because *N*3-demethylation is the dominant pathway of CA clearance, the most abundant urinary metabolites are those derived from PX (92,100,102–104). AFMU, 1-MX, and 1-MU together account for about 60% of the CA-derived products in urine. Caution is necessary, however, in the interpretation of urine excretion data because each of the monomethylxanthines and monomethylurates may be derived from two precursor dimethylxanthines (see Fig. 6-2, Chapter 6).

CA is essentially completely absorbed after oral administration (105). Total plasma clearances in healthy nonsmoking subjects from representative, well-controlled pharmacokinetic studies with CA doses 5 mg/kg or less range from 0.091 to 0.158 L/h/kg (87,106–109). An unbound plasma clearance of 0.187 L/h/kg has been reported for CA (87) and, as noted previously, unbound and total clearances

of CA and PX are similar but higher than those of TP and TB. Area under the plasma concentration–time curve has been reported to increase linearly for short-term administration of CA over the dose range 50 to 750 mg (approximately 0.75–10 mg/kg) (110). However, there is evidence that, under prolonged dosing conditions, plasma CA clearance may be dose dependent. Plasma clearance was 22% lower in subjects administered 12 mg/kg/day of CA compared with a group receiving 4.2 mg/kg/day (111). Like TP, and probably the other dimethylxanthines, CA renal clearance is dependent on urine flow, and CA is reabsorbed from the renal tubule to equilibrium with the unbound compound in blood (112,113).

As noted previously, TP metabolism is impaired in premature neonates, and a similar phenomenon is observed for CA in this age group. Mean total CA plasma clearance in 32 premature infants with apnea was 0.009 L/h/kg (114), approximately ten-fold lower than values reported for adult nonsmokers (see earlier). With the exception of 7-MU (a lower-abundance metabolite even in older age groups), all CA biotransformation products identified in adults have been detected in the urine of premature and term neonates (115–117). CA has been reported to account for more than 85% of urinary products soon after birth (115). Rates of maturation of the *N*-demethylation pathways with postnatal age estimated from both *in vivo* and *in vitro* studies vary, and range from 4 to 9 months (115,116,118).

It is now accepted that CYP1A2 is the enzyme that is essentially solely responsible for human hepatic CA $N3$-monodemethylation (i.e., PX formation) at plasma concentrations associated with normal dietary intake (see CYP1A, Chapter 6). Biphasic kinetics are observed for each of the CA N-demethylations in human liver microsomes, with high-affinity (K_m less than 0.5 mM) and low-affinity (K_m more than 19 mM) components (see Fig. 6-3 of Chapter 6) (95,119). The high-affinity reactions are inhibited selectively by prototypic CYP1A inhibitors (95,119,120). In particular, HLM CA $N3$-demethylation is inhibited more than 95% by furafylline. In microsomes from panels of human liver, rates of the high-affinity CA $N3$-demethylase activity correlate significantly with immunoreactive CYP1A2 content and a range of CYP1A2 activities, including phenacetin O-deethylation, ethoxyresorufin O-deethylation, 4-aminobiphenyl N-oxidation, and 2-acetylaminofluorene N-hydroxylation (95,120–122). Moreover, purified and recombinant human CYP1A2 have the capacity to convert CA to PX (119–123), and reported apparent K_m values for the recombinant enzyme match that for the high-affinity component of CA $N3$-demethylation. Like most CYP1A2 substrates, CA also is metabolized by CYP1A1 (119,124). However, given the negligible expression of CYP1A1 in uninduced liver and apparent low intrinsic clearance for CA $N3$-demethylation, this enzyme would not be expected to contribute significantly to CA elimination *in vivo*.

CYP1A2 also appears to be the major enzyme responsible for the high-affinity components of HLM CA $N1$- and $N7$-demethylation. Each of these reactions is inhibited by prototypic CYP1A inhibitors (95,119). Correlations between the high-affinity activities of all CA N-demethylations were highly significant in microsomes from a panel of livers, and the high-affinity components of TB and TP formation correlated with other CYP1A2 activities (122). Furthermore, apparent K_m values for CA $N1$- and $N7$-demethylation catalyzed by recombinant CYP1A2 were in agreement with the values reported for the high-affinity HLM reactions (122). Although recombinant CYP2E1 and CYP3A4 have also been reported to convert CA to TB and TP (89), these enzymes probably contribute to the low-affinity reactions. Apparent K_m values for CA $N1$- and $N7$-demethylation by cDNA-expressed CYP2E1 were 28 mM and 43 mM, respectively (122).

Microsomal kinetic studies are generally consistent with a major role of CYP3A in 1,3,7-TMU (and by inference, 1,3,7-TAU) formation. Typical of numerous CYP3A-catalyzed pathways, 1,3,7-TAU formation in HLMs exhibits substrate activation and is stimulated by 7,8-benzoflavone (119). In addition, the reaction is inhibited by a specific CYP3A antibody, and rates of 1,3,7-TMU formation correlate significantly with immunoreactive CYP3A content and activities (e.g., omeprazole

sulfoxidation) in microsomes from a panel of human livers (119,122). 1,3,7-DMU formation is the dominant pathway of CA metabolism in fetal liver *in vitro* (118). This is consistent with the expression of a CYP3A subfamily isoform (*viz.*, CYP3A7), but not CYP1A, in fetal liver.

Interaction data *in vivo* are consistent with an involvement of CYP1A2 in CA elimination (104). In particular, CA plasma clearance is enhanced in cigarette smokers and decreased by furafylline coadministration. CA plasma clearance and elimination rate may be almost doubled in cigarette smokers (107,125), whereas pretreatment with the CYP1A2 inhibitor furafylline essentially abolishes CA metabolic clearance (126). Consistent with induction of CA metabolism by cigarette smoking, plasma CA concentration increases significantly on cessation of smoking (127).

Other interactions involving CA are broadly similar to the pattern of metabolic drug interactions reported for TP (see previous discussion). Enoxacin, ciprofloxacin, and pipemidic acid have been shown to be potent inhibitors (K_i values less than 0.2 mM) of HLM CA $N3$-demethylation, whereas lomefloxacin and ofloxacin were weak inhibitors of this pathway (128). *In vivo*, therapeutic doses of enoxacin and pipemidic acid reduce plasma CA clearance by 60% or more (129,130). Lesser inhibition was observed with ciprofloxacin, whereas either marginal or nonsignificant effects on plasma CA clearance were reported after norfloxacin or ofloxacin administration. Coadministration of fluvoxamine, a very potent but probably nonselective CYP1A2 inhibitor, reduced plasma CA clearance on average by 80% (131). Cimetidine has been reported to affect CA elimination variably; the reduction of clearance ranged from 0 to approximately 50% in five subjects (132). There is a modest reduction (about 20%–30%) in plasma CA clearance in both normal subjects and recovering alcoholics treated with disulfiram (133). Whether this reflects a contribution of CYP2E1, which exhibits low affinity for CA, or nonspecific inhibition by disulfiram (and/or its active metabolite, diethyldithiocarbamate) is not clear. Consistent with the minor contribution of CYP3A to CA biotransformation *in vitro*, ketoconazole administration has little or no effect on plasma CA clearance (134).

Plasma CA clearance has been reported to be more than two-fold higher in patients with epilepsy receiving phenytoin compared with a nonmedicated control group (135). In contrast, CA elimination was apparently unaffected by carbamazepine and valproic acid. As noted in Chapter 6, the possible induction of CYP1A by omeprazole and other gastric proton-pump inhibitors has been the subject of considerable attention. Available evidence, however, indicates that therapeutic doses of omeprazole, lansoprazole, and pantoprazole have little or no effect on plasma CA clearance (136). Higher doses of omeprazole may have a modest effect on CA clearance, especially in CYP2C19 poor metabolizers (137).

OTHER METHYLXANTHINES

A number of synthetic substituted xanthines have been developed for clinical use as bronchodilators (e.g., doxophylline, dyphylline, enprofylline, isbufylline, pimefylline, proxyphylline), but relatively few found widespread clinical acceptance, and compared with theophylline, their therapeutic importance is minimal. Substituted xanthines used for other disorders include pentoxifylline, indicated primarily for the treatment of intermittent claudication, and lisofylline, an antiinflammatory that inhibits stress-activated lipid metabolic pathways. Pentoxifylline and lisofylline are structurally related (Fig. 35-5), and relations between metabolic pathways have been investigated recently.

Lisofylline contains a chiral carbon atom in its side chain, and the R-enantiomer has been developed as an antiinflammatory. Pentoxifylline is reduced entirely in human liver cytosol to the S-enantiomer of lisofylline, and this pathway also predominates in microsomes (138). Intrinsic clearance by cytosolic reduction is 4 times greater than microsomal reduction. The S-enantiomer of lisofylline is reoxidized to pentoxifylline, but less than 50% of the oxidation of lisofylline itself (i.e., the R-antipode) occurs by this route (138). Other oxidation pathways comprise the formation of aliphatic diols.

Although carbonyl reductases are assumed to be responsible for pentoxifylline reduction, CYP has been implicated in the oxidation of lisofylline to pentoxifylline. HLM lisofylline oxidation exhibits biphasic kinetics (139). The low-affinity oxidase is not a P450, but CYP1A2 is a major contributor to the high-affinity pathway. The high-affinity reaction is inhibited by furafylline and correlates with warfarin 6-hydroxylation, a

CYP1A2-catalyzed reaction (139). In addition, recombinant CYP1A2 was shown to catalyze the conversion of lisofylline to pentoxifylline. Furafylline, 1,8-dimethyl-3-(2′-furfuryl)methylxanthine, is known to be a mechanism-based inhibitor of CYP1A2 (see Chapter 6) (140,141). Taken together with the lisofylline data, this suggests that CYP1A2 has the capacity to accept as substrates xanthines N-alkylated with substituents that are larger and more polar than the methyl group.

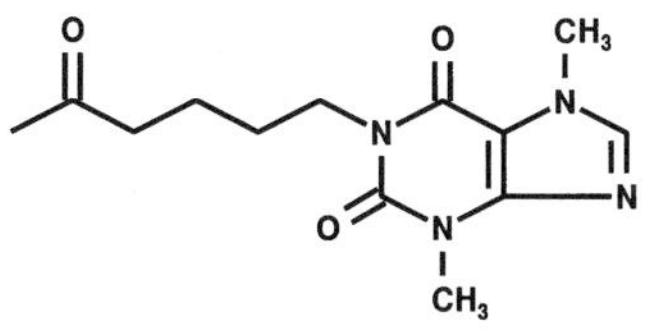

FIG. 35-5. Structures of pentoxifylline and lisofylline.

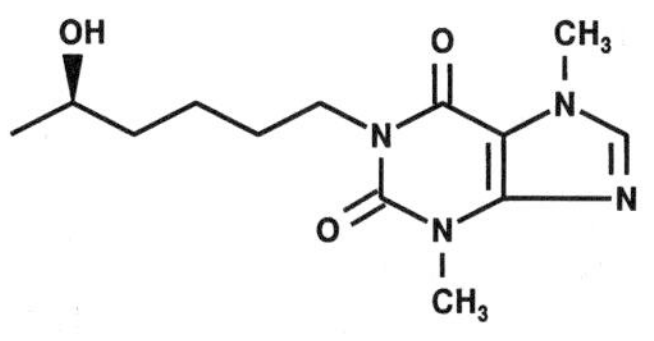

REFERENCES

1. Cornish HH, Christman AA. A study of the metabolism of theobromine, theophylline and caffeine in man. *J Biol Chem* 1957;228:315–323.
2. Rodopoulos N, Norman A. Elimination of theophylline metabolites in healthy adults. *Scand J Clin Lab Invest* 1997;57:233–240.
3. Rasmussen BB, Jeppesen U, Gaist D, Brosen K. Griseofulvin and fluvoxamine interactions with the metabolism of theophylline. *Ther Drug Monit* 1997;19:56–62.
4. Kamali F, Edwards C, Rawlins MD. Lack of effect of flosequinan on the pharmacokinetics of theophylline. *Br J Clin Pharmacol* 1991;32:124–126.
5. Grygiel JJ, Birkett DJ. Cigarette smoking and theophylline clearance and metabolism. *Clin Pharmacol Ther* 1981;30:491–496.
6. Grygiel JJ, Birkett DJ. Effect of age on patterns of theophylline metabolism. *Clin Pharmacol Ther* 1980;28:456–462.
7. Grygiel JJ, Wing LM, Farkas J, Birkett DJ. Effects of allopurinol on theophylline metabolism and clearance. *Clin Pharmacol Ther* 1979;26:660–667.
8. St. Pierre MV, Spino M, Isles AF, Tesoro A, MacLeod SM. Temporal variation in the disposition of theophylline and its metabolites. *Clin Pharmacol Ther* 1985;38:89–95.
9. Thompson RD, Nagasawa HT, Jenne JW. Determination of theophylline and its metabolites in human urine and serum by high-pressure liquid chromatography. *J Lab Clin Med* 1974;84:584–593.
10. Jenne JW, Nagasawa HT, Thompson RD. Relationship of urinary metabolites of theophylline to serum theophylline levels. *Clin Pharmacol Ther* 1976;19:375–381.
11. Birkett DJ, Miners JO, Attwood J. Secondary metabolism of theophylline biotransformation products in man—route of formation of 1-methyluric acid. *Br J Clin Pharmacol* 1983;15:117–119.
12. Kraus DM, Fischer JH, Reitz SJ, et al. Alterations in theophylline metabolism during the first year of life. *Clin Pharmacol Ther* 1993;54:351–359.
13. Tserng KY, Takieddine FN, King KC. Developmental aspects of theophylline metabolism in premature infants. *Clin Pharmacol Ther* 1983;33:522–528.
14. Tserng KY, King KC, Takieddine FN. Theophylline metabolism in premature infants. *Clin Pharmacol Ther* 1981;29:594–600.
15. Boutroy MJ, Vert P, Royer RJ, Monin P, Royer-Morrot MJ. Caffeine, a metabolite of theophylline during the treatment of apnea in the premature infant. *J Pediatr* 1979;94:996–998.
16. Jager-Roman E, Doyle PE, Thomas D, Baird-Lambert J, Cvejic M, Buchanan N. Increased theophylline metabolism in premature infants after prenatal betamethasone administration. *Dev Pharmacol Ther* 1982;5:127–135.
17. Grygiel JJ, Ward H, Ogborne M, Goldin A, Birkett DJ. Relationships between plasma theophylline clearance, liver volume and body weight in children and adults. *Eur J Clin Pharmacol* 1983;24:529–532.
18. Tang-Liu DD, Williams RL, Riegelman S. Nonlinear theophylline elimination. *Clin Pharmacol Ther* 1982;31:358–369.
19. Dahlqvist R, Billing B, Miners JO, Birkett DJ. Nonlinear metabolic disposition of theophylline. *Ther Drug Monit* 1984;6:290–297.
20. Tang-Liu DD, Tozer TN, Riegelman S. Urine flow-dependence of theophylline renal clearance in man. *J Pharmacokinet Biopharmacol* 1982;10:351–364.
21. Rasmussen BB, Brosen K. Theophylline has no advantages over caf-

feine as a putative model drug for assessing CYP1A2 activity in humans. *Br J Clin Pharmacol* 1997;43:253–258.

22. Reinhardt D, Berdel D, Heimann G, et al. Steady state pharmacokinetics, metabolism and pharmacodynamics of theophylline in children after unequal twice-daily dosing of a new sustained-release formulation. *Chronobiol Int* 1987;4:369–380.

23. Persson CG, Karlsson JA, Erjefalt I. Differentiation between bronchodilation and universal adenosine antagonism among xanthine derivatives. *Life Sci* 1982;30:2181–2189.

24. Persson CG. Development of safer xanthine drugs for treatment of obstructive airways disease. *J Allergy Clin Immunol* 1986;78:817–824.

25. Persson CG, Andersson KE. Respiratory and cardiovascular effects of 3-methylxanthine, a metabolite of theophylline. *Acta Pharmacol Toxicol (Copenh)* 1977;40:529–536.

26. Robson RA, Matthews AP, Miners JO, et al. Characterisation of theophylline metabolism in human liver microsomes. *Br J Clin Pharmacol* 1987;24:293–300.

27. Tjia JF, Colbert J, Back DJ. Theophylline metabolism in human liver microsomes: inhibition studies. *J Pharmacol Exp Ther* 1996;276:912–917.

28. Rasmussen BB, Maenpaa J, Pelkonen O, et al. Selective serotonin reuptake inhibitors and theophylline metabolism in human liver microsomes: potent inhibition by fluvoxamine. *Br J Clin Pharmacol* 1995;39:151–159.

29. Robson RA, Miners JO, Matthews AP, et al. Characterisation of theophylline metabolism in human liver microsomes inhibition and immunochemical studies. *Biochem Pharmacol* 1988;37:1651–1659.

30. Tassaneeyakul W, Veronese ME, Birkett DJ, Gonzalez FJ, Miners JO. Validation of 4-nitrophenol as an in vitro substrate probe for human liver CYP2E1 using cDNA expression and microsomal kinetic techniques. *Biochem Pharmacol* 1993;46:1975–1981.

31. Zhang ZY, Kaminsky LS. Characterization of human cytochromes P450 involved in theophylline 8-hydroxylation. *Biochem Pharmacol* 1995;50:205–211.

32. Shimada T, Gillam EM, Sutter TR, Strickland PT, Guengerich FP, Yamazaki H. Oxidation of xenobiotics by recombinant human cytochrome P450 1B1. *Drug Metab Dispos* 1997;25:617–622.

33. Ha HR, Chen J, Freiburghaus AU, Follath F. Metabolism of theophylline by cDNA-expressed human cytochromes P-450. *Br J Clin Pharmacol* 1995;39:321–326.

34. Krenitsky TA, Neil SM, Elion GB, Hitchings GH. A comparison of the specificities of xanthine oxidase and aldehyde oxidase. *Arch Biochem Biophys* 1972;150:585–599.

35. Upton RA. Pharmacokinetic interactions between theophylline and other medication (Part I). *Clin Pharmacokinet* 1991;20:66–80.

36. Upton RA. Pharmacokinetic interactions between theophylline and other medication (Part II). *Clin Pharmacokinet* 1991;20:135–150.

37. Loi CM, Day JD, Jue SG, et al. Dose-dependent inhibition of theophylline metabolism by disulfiram in recovering alcoholics. *Clin Pharmacol Ther* 1989;45:476–486.

38. Naline E, Sanceaume M, Pays M, Advenier C. Application of theophylline metabolite assays to the exploration of liver microsome oxidative function in man. *Fund Clin Pharmacol* 1988;2:341–351.

39. Brown MW, Maldonado AL, Meredith CG, Speeg KV Jr. Effect of ketoconazole on hepatic oxidative drug metabolism. *Clin Pharmacol Ther* 1985;37:290–297.

40. Fuhr U, Maier A, Keller A, Steinijans VW, Sauter R, Staib AH. Lacking effect of grapefruit juice on theophylline pharmacokinetics. *Int J Clin Pharmacol Ther* 1995;33:311–314.

41. Adebayo GI, Akintonwa A, Mabadeje AF. Attenuation of rifampicin-induced theophylline metabolism by diltiazem/rifampicin coadministration in healthy volunteers. *Eur J Clin Pharmacol* 1989;37:127–131.

42. Abernethy DR, Egan JM, Dickinson TH, Carrum G. Substrate-selective inhibition by verapamil and diltiazem: differential disposition of antipyrine and theophylline in humans. *J Pharmacol Exp Ther* 1988;244:994–999.

43. Smith SR, Haffner CA, Kendall MJ. The influence of nifedipine and diltiazem on serum theophylline concentration-time profiles. *J Clin Pharmacol Ther* 1989;14:403–408.

44. Christopher MA, Harman E, Hendeles L. Clinical relevance of the interaction of theophylline with diltiazem or nifedipine. *Chest* 1989;95:309–313.

45. Soto J, Sacristan JA, Alsar MJ. Diltiazem treatment impairs theophylline elimination in patients with bronchospastic airway disease. *Ther Drug Monit* 1994;16:49–52.

46. Ohashi K, Sakamoto K, Sudo T, et al. Effects of diltiazem and cimetidine on theophylline oxidative metabolism. *J Clin Pharmacol* 1993;33:1233–1237.

47. Sirmans SM, Pieper JA, Lalonde RL, Smith DG, Self TH. Effect of calcium channel blockers on theophylline disposition. *Clin Pharmacol Ther* 1988;44:29–34.

48. Nafziger AN, May JJ, Bertino JS Jr. Inhibition of theophylline elimination by diltiazem therapy. *J Clin Pharmacol* 1987;27:862–865.

49. Robson RA, Miners JO, Birkett DJ. Selective inhibitory effects of nifedipine and verapamil on oxidative metabolism: effects on theophylline. *Br J Clin Pharmacol* 1988;25:397–400.

50. Nielsen-Kudsk JE, Buhl JS, Johannessen AC. Verapamil-induced inhibition of theophylline elimination in healthy humans. *Pharmacol Toxicol* 1990;66:101–103.

51. Jackson SH, Shah K, Debbas NM, et al. The interaction between i.v. theophylline and chronic oral dosing with slow release nifedipine in volunteers. *Br J Clin Pharmacol* 1986;21:389–392.

52. Garty M, Cohen E, Mazar A, Ilfeld DN, Spitzer S, Rosenfeld JB. Effect of nifedipine and theophylline in asthma. *Clin Pharmacol Ther* 1986;40:195–198.

53. Adebayo GI, Mabadeje AF. Effect of nifedipine on antipyrine and theophylline disposition. *Biopharmacol Drug Dispos* 1990;11:157–164.

54. Weinberger M, Hudgel D, Spector S, Chidsey C. Inhibition of theophylline clearance by troleandomycin. *J Allergy Clin Immunol* 1977;59:228–231.

55. Saint-Salvi B, Tremblay D, Surjus A, Lefebvre MA. A study of the interaction of roxithromycin with theophylline and carbamazepine. *J Antimicrob Chemother* 1987;20:121–129.

56. Rogge MC, Solomon WR, Sedman AJ, Welling PG, Koup JR, Wagner JG. The theophylline-enoxacin interaction. II: Changes in the disposition of theophylline and its metabolites during intermittent administration of enoxacin. *Clin Pharmacol Ther* 1989;46:420–428.

57. Rogge MC, Solomon WR, Sedman AJ, Welling PG, Toothaker RD, Wagner JG. The theophylline-enoxacin interaction. I: Effect of enoxacin dose size on theophylline disposition. *Clin Pharmacol Ther* 1988;44:579–587.

58. Wijnands WJ, Vree TB, Baars AM, van Herwaarden CL. The influence of the 4-quinolones ciprofloxacin, pefloxacin and ofloxacin on the elimination of theophylline. *Pharmacol Weekbl Sci* 1987;9(suppl):S72–S75.

59. Wijnands WJ, Vree TB, van Herwaarden CL. The influence of quinolone derivatives on theophylline clearance. *Br J Clin Pharmacol* 1986;22:677–683.

60. Niki Y, Soejima R, Kawane H, Sumi M, Umeki S. New synthetic quinolone antibacterial agents and serum concentration of theophylline. *Chest* 1987;92:663–669.

61. Bachmann KA, Schwartz JI, Jauregui L. Predicting the ciprofloxacin-theophylline interaction from single plasma theophylline measurements. *Br J Clin Pharmacol* 1988;26:191–194.

62. Schwartz J, Jauregui L, Lettieri J, Bachmann K. Impact of ciprofloxacin on theophylline clearance and steady-state concentrations in serum. *Antimicrob Agents Chemother* 1988;32:75–77.

63. Harder S, Fuhr U, Staib AH, Wolff T. Ciprofloxacin-caffeine: a drug interaction established using in vivo and in vitro investigations. *Am J Med* 1989;87:89S–91S.

64. Fuhr U, Strobl G, Manaut F, et al. Quinolone antibacterial agents: relationship between structure and in vitro inhibition of the human cytochrome P450 isoform CYP1A2. *Mol Pharmacol* 1993;43:191–199.

65. Grygiel JJ, Miners JO, Drew R, Birkett DJ. Differential effects of cimetidine on theophylline metabolic pathways. *Eur J Clin Pharmacol* 1984;26:335–340.

66. Miners JO, Wing LM, Lillywhite KJ, Robson RA. Selectivity and dose-dependency of the inhibitory effect of propranolol on theophylline metabolism in man. *Br J Clin Pharmacol* 1985;20:219–223.

67. Maeda Y, Konishi T, Omoda K, et al. Inhibition of theophylline metabolism by aciclovir. *Biol Pharm Bull* 1996;19:1591–1595.

68. Loi CM, Wei XX, Vestal RE. Inhibition of theophylline metabolism by mexiletine in young male and female nonsmokers. *Clin Pharmacol Ther* 1991;49:571–580.

69. Hurwitz A, Vacek JL, Botteron GW, Sztern MI, Hughes EM, Jayaraj

A. Mexiletine effects on theophylline disposition. *Clin Pharmacol Ther* 1991;50:299–307.

70. Miners JO, Foenander T, Wanwimolruk S, Gallus AS, Birkett DJ. The effect of sulphinpyrazone on oxidative drug metabolism in man: inhibition of tolbutamide elimination. *Eur J Clin Pharmacol* 1982;22:321–326.

71. Birkett DJ, Miners JO, Attwood J. Evidence for a dual action of sulphinpyrazone on drug metabolism in man: theophylline-sulphinpyrazone interaction. *Br J Clin Pharmacol* 1983;15:567–569.

72. Robson RA, Miners JO, Wing LM, Birkett DJ. Theophylline-rifampicin interaction: non-selective induction of theophylline metabolic pathways. *Br J Clin Pharmacol* 1984;18:445–448.

73. Adebayo GI. Interaction between phenytoin and theophylline in healthy volunteers. *Clin Exp Pharmacol Physiol* 1988;15:883–887.

74. Pieniaszek HJ Jr, Davidson AF, Benedek IH. Effect of moricizine on the pharmacokinetics of single-dose theophylline in healthy subjects. *Ther Drug Monit* 1993;15:199–203.

75. Loi CM, Parker BM, Cusack BJ, Vestal RE. Aging and drug interactions. III: Individual and combined effects of cimetidine and cimetidine and ciprofloxacin on theophylline metabolism in healthy male and female nonsmokers. *J Pharmacol Exp Ther* 1997;280:627–637.

76. Batty KT, Davis TM, Ilett KF, Dusci LJ, Langton SR. The effect of ciprofloxacin on theophylline pharmacokinetics in healthy subjects. *Br J Clin Pharmacol* 1995;39:305–311.

77. Loi CM, Parker BM, Cusack BJ, Vestal R. Individual and combined effects of cimetidine and ciprofloxacin on theophylline metabolism in male nonsmokers. *Br J Clin Pharmacol* 1993;36:195–200.

78. Konishi H, Morita K, Yamaji A. Effect of fluconazole on theophylline disposition in humans. *Eur J Clin Pharmacol* 1994;46:309–312.

79. Sano M, Kawakatsu K, Ohkita C, et al. Effects of enoxacin, ofloxacin and norfloxacin on theophylline disposition in humans. *Eur J Clin Pharmacol* 1988;35:161–165.

80. Loi CM, Wei X, Parker BM, Korrapati MR, Vestal RE. The effect of tocainide on theophylline metabolism. *Br J Clin Pharmacol* 1993;35:437–440.

81. Arnaud MJ, Welsch C. Metabolic pathway of theobromine in the rat and identification of two new metabolites in human urine. *J Agric Food Chem* 1979;27:524–527.

82. Miners JO, Attwood J, Birkett DJ. Theobromine metabolism in man. *Drug Metab Dispos* 1982;10:672–675.

83. Birkett DJ, Dahlqvist R, Miners JO, Lelo A, Billing B. Comparison of theophylline and theobromine metabolism in man. *Drug Metab Dispos* 1985;13:725–728.

84. Tarka SM Jr, Arnaud MJ, Dvorchik BH, Vesell ES. Theobromine kinetics and metabolic disposition. *Clin Pharmacol Ther* 1983;34:546–555.

85. Lelo A, Birkett DJ, Miners JO. Mechanism of formation of 6-amino-5-(N-methylformylamino)-1-methyluracil and 3,7-dimethyluric acid from theobromine in the rat in vitro: involvement of cytochrome P-450 and a cellular thiol. *Xenobiotica* 1990;20:823–833.

86. Miners JO, Attwood J, Wing LM, Birkett DJ. Influence of cimetidine, sulfinpyrazone, and cigarette smoking on theobromine metabolism in man. *Drug Metab Dispos* 1985;13:598–601.

87. Lelo A, Birkett DJ, Robson RA, Miners JO. Comparative pharmacokinetics of caffeine and its primary demethylated metabolites paraxanthine, theobromine and theophylline in man. *Br J Clin Pharmacol* 1986;22:177–182.

88. Gates S, Miners JO. Cytochrome P450 isoform selectivity in human hepatic theobromine metabolism. *Br J Clin Pharmacol* 1999;47:299–305..

89. Gu L, Gonzalez FJ, Kalow W, Tang BK. Biotransformation of caffeine, paraxanthine, theobromine and theophylline by cDNA-expressed human CYP1A2 and CYP2E1. *Pharmacogenetics* 1992;2:73–77.

90. Lelo A, Miners JO, Robson R, Birkett DJ. Assessment of caffeine exposure: caffeine content of beverages, caffeine intake, and plasma concentrations of methylxanthines. *Clin Pharmacol Ther* 1986;39:54–59.

91. Lelo A, Miners JO, Robson RA, Birkett DJ. Quantitative assessment of caffeine partial clearances in man. *Br J Clin Pharmacol* 1986;22:183–186.

92. Arnaud MJ, Welsch C. Caffeine metabolism in human subjects. *IX International Colloquium on science and technology of coffee.* London: Association Scientific Internationale du Cafe, 1980:385–395.

93. Lelo A, Kjellen G, Birkett DJ, Miners JO. Paraxanthine metabolism in

humans: determination of metabolic partial clearances and effects of allopurinol and cimetidine. *J Pharmacol Exp Ther* 1989;248:315–319.

94. Tang BK, Grant DM, Kalow W. Isolation and identification of 5-acetylamino-6-formylamino-3-methyluracil as a major metabolite of caffeine in man. *Drug Metab Dispos* 1983;11:218–220.

95. Campbell ME, Grant DM, Inaba T, Kalow W. Biotransformation of caffeine, paraxanthine, theophylline, and theobromine by polycyclic aromatic hydrocarbon-inducible cytochrome P-450 in human liver microsomes. *Drug Metab Dispos* 1987;15:237–249.

96. Grant DM, Tang BK, Campbell ME, Kalow W. Effect of allopurinol on caffeine disposition in man. *Br J Clin Pharmacol* 1986;21:454–48.

97. Birkett DJ, Miners JO, Valente L, Lillywhite KJ, Day RO. 1-Methylxanthine derived from caffeine as a pharmacodynamic probe of oxypurinol effect. *Br J Clin Pharmacol* 1997;43:197–200.

98. Kilbane AJ, Silbart LK, Manis M, Beitins IZ, Weber WW. Human N-acetylation genotype determination with urinary caffeine metabolites *Clin Pharmacol Ther* 1990;47:470–477.

99. Tang BK, Kadar D, Qian L, Iriah J, Yip J, Kalow W. Caffeine as a metabolic probe: validation of its use for acetylator phenotyping. *Clin Pharmacol Ther* 1991;49:648–657.

100. Callahan MM, Robertson RS, Arnaud MJ, Branfman AR, McComish MF, Yesair DW. Human metabolism of (1-methyl-^{14}C)- and (2-^{14}C)caffeine after oral administration. *Drug Metab Dispos* 1982;10:417–423.

101. Ferrero JL, Neims AH. Metabolism of caffeine by mouse liver microsomes: GSH or cytosol causes a shift in products from 1,3,7-trimethylurate to a substituted diaminouracil. *Life Sci* 1983;33:1173–1178.

102. Callahan MM, Robertson RS, Branfman AR, McComish MF, Yesair DW. Comparison of caffeine metabolism in three nonsmoking populations after oral administration of radiolabeled caffeine. *Drug Metab Dispos* 1983;11:211–217.

103. Miners JO, Birkett DJ. The use of caffeine as a metabolic probe for human drug metabolizing enzymes. *Gen Pharmacol* 1996;27:245–249.

104. Kalow W, Tang BK. The use of caffeine for enzyme assays: a critical appraisal. *Clin Pharmacol Ther* 1993;53:503–514.

105. Blanchard J, Sawers SJ. The absolute bioavailability of caffeine in man. *Eur J Clin Pharmacol* 1983;24:93–98.

106. Blanchard J, Sawers SJ. Comparative pharmacokinetics of caffeine in young and elderly men. *J Pharmacokinet Biopharm* 1983;11:109–126.

107. Parsons WD, Neims AH. Effect of smoking on caffeine clearance. *Clin Pharmacol Ther* 1978;24:40–45.

108. Cheng WSC, Murphy TL, Smith MT, Cooksley WGE, Halliday JW, Powell LW. Dose-dependent pharmacokinetics of caffeine in humans: relevance as a test of quantitative liver function. *Clin Pharmacol Ther* 1990;47:516–524.

109. Denaro CP, Jacob P 3rd, Benowitz NL. Evaluation of pharmacokinetic methods used to estimate caffeine clearance and comparison with a bayesian forecasting method. *Ther Drug Monit* 1998;20:78–87.

110. Newton R, Broughton LJ, Lind MJ, Morrison PJ, Rogers HJ, Bradbrook ID. Plasma and salivary pharmacokinetics of caffeine in man. *Eur J Clin Pharmacol* 1981;21:45–52.

111. Denaro CP, Brown CR, Wilson M, Jacob P 3d, Benowitz NL. Dose-dependency of caffeine metabolism with repeated dosing. *Clin Pharmacol Ther* 1990;48:277–285.

112. Birkett DJ, Miners JO. Caffeine renal clearance and urine caffeine concentrations during steady state dosing: implications for monitoring caffeine intake during sports events. *Br J Clin Pharmacol* 1991;31:405–408.

113. Blanchard J, Sawers SJ. Relationship between urine flow rate and renal clearance of caffeine in man. *J Clin Pharmacol* 1983;23:134–138.

114. Aranda JV, Cook CE, Gorman W, et al. Pharmacokinetic profile of caffeine in the premature newborn infant with apnea. *J Pediatr* 1979;94:663–668.

115. Aldridge A, Aranda JV, Neims AH. Caffeine metabolism in the newborn. *Clin Pharmacol Ther* 1979;25:447–453.

116. Carrier O, Pons G, Rey E, et al. Maturation of caffeine metabolic pathways in infancy. *Clin Pharmacol Ther* 1988;44:145–151.

117. Gorodischer R, Zmora E, Ben Zvi Z, et al. Urinary metabolites of caffeine in the premature infant. *Eur J Clin Pharmacol* 1986;31:497–499.

118. Cazeneuve C, Pons G, Rey E, et al. Biotransformation of caffeine in human liver microsomes from foetuses, neonates, infants and adults. *Br J Clin Pharmacol* 1994;37:405–412.

119. Tassaneeyakul W, Mohamed Z, Birkett DJ, et al. Caffeine as a probe for human cytochromes P450: validation using cDNA-expression,

immunoinhibition and microsomal kinetic and inhibitor techniques. *Pharmacogenetics* 1992;2:173–183.

120. Bloomer JC, Clarke SE, Chenery RJ. Determination of P4501A2 activity in human liver microsomes using (3-^{14}C-methyl)caffeine. *Xenobiotica* 1995;25:917–927.

121. Butler MA, Iwasaki M, Guengerich FP, Kadlubar FF. Human cytochrome P-450PA (P-4501A2), the phenacetin *O*-deethylase, is primarily responsible for the hepatic 3-demethylation of caffeine and *N*-oxidation of carcinogenic arylamines. *Proc Natl Acad Sci USA* 1989;86:7696–7700.

122. Tassaneeyakul W, Birkett DJ, McManus ME, et al. Caffeine metabolism by human hepatic cytochromes P450: contributions of 1A2, 2E1 and 3A isoforms. *Biochem Pharmacol* 1994;47:1767–1776.

123. Fuhr U, Doehmer J, Battula N, et al. Biotransformation of caffeine and theophylline in mammalian cell lines genetically engineered for expression of single cytochrome P450 isoforms. *Biochem Pharmacol* 1992;43:225–235.

124. Tassaneeyakul W, Birkett DJ, Veronese ME, et al. Specificity of substrate and inhibitor probes for human cytochromes P450 1A1 and 1A2. *J Pharmacol Exp Ther* 1993;265:401–407.

125. Kotake AN, Schoeller DA, Lambert GH, Baker AL, Schaffer DD, Josephs H. The caffeine CO$_2$ breath test: dose response and route of *N*-demethylation in smokers and nonsmokers. *Clin Pharmacol Ther* 1982;32:261–269.

126. Tarrus E, Cami J, Roberts DJ, Spickett RG, Celdran E, Segura J. Accumulation of caffeine in healthy volunteers treated with furafylline. *Br J Clin Pharmacol* 1987;23:9–18.

127. Benowitz NL, Hall SM, Modin G. Persistent increase in caffeine concentrations in people who stop smoking. *Br Med J* 1989;298:1075–1076.

128. Fuhr U, Wolff T, Harder S, Schymanski P, Staib AH. Quinolone inhibition of cytochrome P450 dependent caffeine metabolism in human liver microsomes. *Drug Metab Dispos* 1990;18:1005–1010.

129. Harder S, Fuhr U, Staib AH, Wolff T. Ciprofloxacin-caffeine: a drug interaction established using in vivo and in vitro investigations. *Am J Med* 1989;87(suppl 5A):89S–91S.

130. Carbo M, Segura J, de la Torre R, Badenas JM, Cami J. Effect of quinolones on caffeine disposition. *Clin Pharmacol Ther* 1989;45:234–240.

131. Jeppesen U, Loft S, Poulson HE, Brosen K. A fluvoxamine-caffeine interaction study. *Pharmacogenetics* 1996;6:213–222.

132. Broughton LJ, Rogers HJ. Decreased systemic clearance of caffeine due to cimetidine. *Br J Clin Pharmacol* 1981;12:155–159.

133. Beach CA, Mays DC, Guiler RC, Jacober CH, Gerber N. Inhibition of elimination of caffeine by disulfiram in normal subjects and recovering alcoholics. *Clin Pharmacol Ther* 1986;39:265–270.

134. Wahllander A, Paumgartner G. Effect of ketoconazole and terbinafine on the pharmacokinetics of caffeine in healthy volunteers. *Eur J Clin Pharmacol* 1989;37:279–283.

135. Weitholtz H, Zysset TH, Kreiten K, Kohl D, Buchsel R, Matern S. Effect of phenytoin, carbamazepine and valproic acid on caffeine metabolism. *Eur J Clin Pharmacol* 1989;36:401–406.

136. Andersson T, Holmberg J, Walan A. Pharmacokinetics and effect on caffeine metabolism of the proton pump inhibitors omeprazole, lansoprazole and pantoprazole. *Br J Clin Pharmacol* 1998;45:369–375.

137. Rost LK, Brosicke H, Heinemeyer G, Roots I. Specific and dose-dependent enzyme induction by omeprazole in human beings. *Hepatology* 1994;20:1204–1212.

138. Lillibridge JA, Kalhorn TF, Slattery JT. Metabolism of lisofylline and pentoxifylline in human liver microsomes and cytosol. *Drug Metab Dispos* 1996;24:1174–1179.

139. Lee SH, Slattery JT. Cytochrome P450 isozymes involved in lisofylline metabolism to pentoxifylline in human liver microsomes. *Drug Metab Dispos* 1997;25:1354–1358.

140. Kunze KL, Trager WF. Isoform-selective mechanism-based inhibition of human cytochrome P450 1A2 by furafylline. *Chem Res Toxicol* 1993;6:649–656.

141. Tassaneeyakul W, Birkett DJ, Veronese ME, McManus ME, Tukey RH, Miners JO. Direct characterization of the selectivity of furafylline as an inhibitor of human cytochromes P450 1A1 and 1A2. *Pharmacogenetics* 1994;4:281–284.

CHAPTER 36

H₂-Antagonists, Proton-Pump Inhibitors, and Antiemetics

Ronald M. Laethem and Cosette J. Serabjit-Singh

INTRODUCTION

The three classes of drugs covered in this chapter, H₂-antagonists, the substituted benzimidazole proton-pump inhibitors, and the 5-HT₃ antagonists, represent gastrointestinal therapies prescribed to very large proportions of the population. With ranitidine hydrochloride alone, more than 209 million patient treatments have been dispensed in more that 120 countries since 1981 (1). Overall, the aforementioned drug classes represent some of the safest drugs on the market today. However, with the staggering numbers of people taking these drugs under countless different conditions, metabolic drug interactions can occur. For the most part, these interactions appear to not have clinically significant pharmacodynamic manifestations. The last 10 years have seen many important advances in our mechanistic understanding of drug–drug interactions. The advances seen in the field of metabolic enzymes, specifically cytochromes P450, have led to the ability to predict some drug interactions. A limitation to this approach is the array of genetic and environmental factors that contribute to an individual's drug-metabolizing capability. This chapter is intended to provide information on the metabolic characteristics of these classes of drugs for the interpretation of known interactions and prediction of drug interactions with drugs for which no specific interaction data are available.

H₂ ANTAGONISTS

Histamine is a signaling molecule that causes acid secretion by binding to H₁ and H₂ receptors present on acid-secreting cells in the gastric mucosa. H₂-receptor antagonists competitively inhibit the receptor, thus suppressing acid secretion, causing an increase in gastric pH. The H₂-antagonists are a diverse group of drugs based on the structure of histamine. The first drugs in this class contained an imidazole moiety, but later it was found that other five-membered rings could substitute for the imidazole group and give superior drug characteristics.

Cimetidine

Cimetidine (Table 36-1) was approved for use in 1977 and is the first widely prescribed H₂ antagonist. It is a modification of histamine that retains the imidazole moiety of histamine. The major route of elimination for cimetidine is renal excretion. The renal clearance of cimetidine ranges from 23 to 36 L/h (2), which is much greater than the glomerular filtration rate of 6 to 7 L/h, indicating that active renal tubular secretion of cimetidine plays a major role in its renal clearance. Cimetidine undergoes some hepatic metabolism, with less than 20% of a given dose of cimetidine metabolized in the liver (3). Oral dosing of cimetidine in humans results in 70% of the dose recovered in the urine by 24 hours (4). In the same period, 5% of the dose is recovered in the feces through biliary excretion (5). Unchanged cimetidine accounts for 64% of the recovered urinary dose, with the main phase I metabolite, cimetidine S-oxide (6), accounting for 8% (4). The major metabolite recovered in the urine is cimetidine N-glucuronide, which makes up 22% of the dose (4,7). Other minor metabolites found in the urine are the 5-hydroxymethyl metabolite (4% of the dose), cimetidine

R. M. Laethem: Department of Bioanalysis and Drug Metabolism, Glaxo Wellcome Inc., 3030 Cornwallis Road, Research Triangle Park, North Carolina 27709

C. J. Serabjit-Singh: Departments of Science Development and Bioanalysis and Drug Metabolism, Glaxo Wellcome Inc., 5 Moore Drive, Research Triangle Park, North Carolina 27709

TABLE 36-1. *Summary of currently available H₂-antagonists*

	Oral bioavailability (%)	Elimination route	Renal clearance (L/h)	Parent excreted (%)[a]	Relative potency[b]	Metabolism	Metabolites	Structure
Cimetidine	63–78	Renal	24–36	75	1	FMO3	Sulfoxide hydroxymethyl	
Famotidine	37–45	Renal	14–26	70	40	?	S-oxide	
Nizatidine	98	Renal	27–36	63[b]	10	?	N2-monodesmethyl N2-oxide	
Ranitidine	52	Renal Biliary	24–32	70	6	FMO; P450	N-oxide N-desmethyl sulfoxide	

[a]Urinary excretion in 24 h after i.v. dose.
[b]Equimolar basis for comparison.
[c]In decreasing order of abundance.
[d]Single 150-mg oral dose.

484

guanylurea (2% of the dose), and cimetidine guanidine (4). Cimetidine is believed to be the only pharmacologically active agent after oral dosing, as cimetidine *S*-oxide has no H$_2$-antagonist activity in rodents (8).

Early work indicated that formation of cimetidine *S*-oxide could potentially be mediated by either cytochrome P450 or flavin-containing monooxygenase (FMO) (9,10). Studies with animal tissues established the stereopreference of cytochrome P450 and FMO1 to form sulfoxides with (*S*) and (*R*) absolute stereochemistry, respectively (11,12). Cashman et al. (13,14) reported that in humans, FMO3 (originally designated FMO2) was the enzyme responsible for the *S*-oxidation of cimetidine. This group demonstrated that even though cimetidine could interact with pig liver FMO1 (10) and cytochrome P450 could oxidize cimetidine (9), these reactions could not account for the stereoselective ratio of urinary (+) and (−)-cimetidine formed in humans (13). This group also reported that selective conditions and agents for inhibition of FMO or cytochrome P450 supported the role of FMO3 in cimetidine oxidation, as did experiments using Western blots to assess the relative levels of various cytochromes P450 and FMO1 and FMO3 in human liver microsomes.

Interactions between cimetidine and other drugs metabolized by FMO3 have not been described. At present, our knowledge of the role of FMO3 in drug metabolism is rather limited, and consequently this aspect of cimetidine metabolism is not well explored. However, based on the relatively minor role that FMO3 appears to play in the metabolism of cimetidine, one would not expect drug interactions of major clinical consequence from this mechanism. Cimetidine undergoes secondary metabolism by glucuronidation (4,7); however, it does not interact with drugs primarily cleared by glucuronidation such as lorazepam or oxazepam (15,16), indicating that cimetidine does not interact with this enzyme system. Cimetidine is a well-known inhibitor of cytochrome P450 monooxygenases (17), and some drug interactions arise through this mechanism (covered in Chapter 49 of this volume). Because no CYP isoforms play a role in cimetidine clearance, no drug interaction with this enzyme system through competitive, noncompetitive, or mixed inhibition–type mechanisms is possible.

Famotidine

Famotidine (see Table 36-1) has a guanidinothiazole moiety replacing the imidazole found in histamine and is the most potent H$_2$ antagonist, being 40 times more potent than cimetidine (2). As with cimetidine, famotidine undergoes little first pass metabolism and is largely cleared by renal excretion. The renal-clearance rate of famotidine exceeds that of the glomerular filtration rate of creatinine by three-fold, indicating that active secretion of the drug by the kidney plays a significant role in the renal clearance of famotidine (18). Hepatic metabolism

of famotidine results in a single major metabolite, famotidine *S*-oxide (19). After an oral dose of famotidine, 65% to 70% is excreted in the urine (20), although one report with four individuals demonstrated that after a single oral dose of famotidine, 38% was excreted in the urine and 51% in the feces within 96 hours (21). Biliary excretion of famotidine is reported to be negligible (22). Parent drug excreted in the urine accounts for 30% of the administered dose (21,23), but the recovery of the dose in the urine has a wide range (19), indicating that metabolism may vary considerably. Famotidine *S*-oxide is recovered in the urine as approximately 5% of an i.v. dose (24) and has been shown to have no pharmacologic activity (25).

The enzymes responsible for the small amount of famotidine metabolism have not yet been identified. The package insert for famotidine indicates that no significant drug interactions have yet been found (26); therefore it seems that the importance of identifying these enzymes is mitigated. It is apparent that drug interactions with CYP isoforms either do not occur or are undetectable. The possibility exists that FMO may be involved in the *S*-oxidation of famotidine; however, the lack of drug interactions indicates that there is no adverse interaction between famotidine and this enzyme system. No glucuronidated metabolites of famotidine have been identified, and *in vitro* it does not interfere with the microsomal glucuronidation of 7-hydroxy-4-methylcoumarin (27), indicating no interaction with this phase II enzyme system. It has been shown *in vitro* that famotidine has no affinity for CYP isoforms, as evidenced by spectral changes (28), and it does not significantly inhibit cytochrome P450–mediated *O*-deethylation of 7-ethoxycoumarin or the *N*-demethylation of benzphetamine (28). Nearly 20 million patients have been treated with famotidine since its introduction in 1985, and in that time, this drug has proven to be very safe, with an excellent drug-interaction profile (29).

Nizatidine

Nizatidine (see Table 36-1) has a thiazole ring nucleus similar to famotidine and the side chains of ranitidine. Nizatidine is rapidly cleared by renal filtration and tubular secretion and undergoes minimal first pass metabolism in the liver (30). Up to 60% of an oral dose in the plasma can be attributed to parent drug, and more than 90% of an oral dose is recovered in the urine by 16 hours, with 65% to 75% of the excreted drug being unchanged parent. Approximately 6% to 7% of an oral dose of nizatidine is excreted in the feces (30). The main metabolites of nizatidine are *N*2-monodesmethylnizatidine, which accounts for approximately 8% of an oral dose, and nizatidine *N*2-oxide, composing 6% of the dose (31). *N*2-monodesmethylnizatidine has 60% of the H$_2$-antagonist activity of nizatidine (32); nizatidine sulfoxide is devoid of H$_2$-antagonist activity; and the biologic activity of the *N*2-oxide is unknown (33).

Nizatidine appears to behave much like famotidine with respect to interactions with drug-metabolizing enzymes. The enzymes responsible for the minor amount of nizatidine metabolism have not yet been identified. Nizatidine does not interact with CYP isoforms (34) and does not affect the pharmacokinetics of lorazepam, indicating that it does not interfere with glucuronidation of drugs (35). There has been only one report of a drug interaction with nizatidine (26). Nizatidine given concurrently with high doses of aspirin may cause increased blood salicylate levels, probably through inhibition of renal secretion of salicylate. This interaction was not clinically significant in that bleeding time was not altered; aspirin-induced gastric mucosal irritation and fecal blood loss was reduced in the subjects receiving nizatidine (36). From all the available data, it appears that nizatidine, like famotidine, is a safe drug devoid of any clinically significant drug interactions.

Ranitidine

Ranitidine (see Table 36-1) has a furan ring rather than the imidazole found in histamine. Ranitidine was the first marketed H_2-antagonist without the imidazole moiety found in cimetidine and is approximately four- to six-fold more potent than this drug (25). Ranitidine clearance is primarily accomplished by renal excretion, with both glomerular filtration and extensive tubular secretion playing a role (3,37). Renal clearance is responsible for 70% of the total clearance of ranitidine, and in the urine, approximately 30% of the dose is unchanged parent (38). Hepatic metabolism of ranitidine appears to contribute little to the overall clearance of this drug. Three metabolites of ranitidine are found in humans: ranitidine N-oxide, desmethyl ranitidine, and ranitidine S-oxide (39). Within the first 24 hours of an oral dose of ranitidine, ranitidine N-oxide is the major urinary metabolite, accounting for 3% to 6% of the dose, followed by the desmethyl and S-oxide metabolites, each composing approximately 1% of the dose (38).

The minor amount of ranitidine metabolism is carried out primarily by FMO3. *In vitro* studies with recombinant human FMO3 and FMO5 demonstrated that both enzymes yielded the N- and S-oxides of ranitidine (40). The oxidation rates with FMO5 were 100-fold less than those with FMO3, indicating that *in vivo*, FMO3 is probably the most relevant enzyme. Neither FMO carried out the N-demethylation of ranitidine, suggesting that an unidentified CYP isoform or isoforms is responsible for this reaction. Similar to the other H_2 antagonists, ranitidine is not metabolized significantly by these enzyme systems; therefore at the recommended doses of ranitidine, drug interactions through competition for enzyme active sites will not occur. Ranitidine inhibition of CYP isoforms has been reported; however, it does not interact as strongly with CYP isoforms as does cimetidine (20). This lower affinity, coupled with the lower doses of ranitidine necessary to achieve therapeutic results, ensures that the significant concentration-dependent P450 inhibition observed with cimetidine will not occur with ranitidine.

No clinically significant drug interactions are reported in the package insert for ranitidine; however, there is a warning that interactions of high-dose ranitidine (more than 400 mg/day) with warfarin have not been studied (26). The evidence that ranitidine can interfere with warfarin metabolism is scant, concerning a single study with five subjects, in which warfarin clearance was decreased, but no change in elimination half-life was detected (41). One anecdotal report of a 65-year-old woman was published (42). The case for a lack of interaction between ranitidine and warfarin is more persuasive (1). In a situation in which high-dose ranitidine is to be given with warfarin, care should be exercised by the prescribing physician to avoid a potentially toxic interaction, or a different course of therapy may be sought. Ranitidine treatment concomitant with a plethora of other drugs has resulted in few adverse drug interactions since its introduction in 1981, thus establishing the excellent safety profile of ranitidine (1).

PROTON-PUMP INHIBITORS

The major proton-pump inhibitors are a group of antisecretory drugs comprising substituted benzimidazole derivatives of timoprazole. This class of agents binds covalently to the H^+/K^+-adenosine triphosphatase (ATPase) in the parietal cells of the stomach, thus blocking the final step in acid production. The substituted benzimidazoles are actually prodrugs, with the active form being the sulfenamide derivatives formed at acidic pH. The drugs are absorbed from the small intestine and reach the parietal cells through the bloodstream, where the acidic environment of the secretory canaliculus results in activation of the prodrug with subsequent binding to and inhibition of the H^+/K^+-ATPase. Inactivation of the H^+/K^+-ATPase is essentially irreversible, leading to very long pharmacodynamic effects relative to plasma areas under the concentration–time curve (AUCs).

Lansoprazole

Lansoprazole (Table 36-2) is the second of the substituted benzimidazole class of proton-pump inhibitors and is a modification of omeprazole. Lansoprazole is extensively metabolized by the liver, with two major metabolites, lansoprazole sulfone and 5-hydroxylansoprazole, found in the serum (43). After a single oral dose of lansoprazole, approximately 20% of the dose is recovered in the urine as conjugated and unconjugated metabolites (44), with the remainder of the dose excreted in the feces (45). No parent compound has been found in the urine of patients in clinical trials (45).

TABLE 36-2. *Summary of currently prescribed proton-pump inhibitors*

	Oral bioavailability (%)	Elimination route	Parent excreted (% in urine)	Relative potency[a]	Metabolism	Metabolites[b]	Structure
Lansoprazole	81	Hepatic	0	1.5	CYP2C19, CYP3A	Hydroxy Sulfone	
Omeprazole	40	Hepatic	0	2	CYP2C19, CYP3A	5-hydroxy sulfone 5-O-desmethyl 3-hydroxy	
Pantoprazole	75	Hepatic	0	1	CYP2C19, CYP3A	4-Desmethyl sulfone	

[a]Daily recommended dose used for comparison.
[b]In decreasing order of abundance.

The major primary metabolite of lansoprazole found in the serum is lansoprazole sulfone, resulting from oxidation of the sulfoxide radical in lansoprazole. It appears that this reaction is catalyzed predominantly by P450 3A4/5 (46,47), which also can oxidize carbon 5 of the benzimidazole moiety, forming 5-hydroxylansoprazole. This reaction was catalyzed by CYP2C18 and 3A4/5 when 10 μM lansoprazole was used in vitro (46). However, at the more physiologically relevant concentration of 1 μM, it was demonstrated that CYP2C19 is the predominant isoform catalyzing the sulfoxidation (47). Neither lansoprazole sulfone nor 5-hydroxylansoprazole has any pharmacologic activity (48).

In contrast to imidazole-containing drugs such as cimetidine, the benzimidazole moiety in lansoprazole does not appear to be a nonspecific inhibitor of CYP isoforms (49). In human liver microsomes, lansoprazole is a potent competitive inhibitor of CYP2C19 (K_i, 3.4 μM), a moderate competitive inhibitor of CYP2C9, a moderate mixed inhibitor of CYP2D6, a weak noncompetitive inhibitor of CYP3A, and without effect on CYP1A2 or CYP2E1 (50). Lansoprazole does not significantly interfere with substrates of CYP2C isoforms, and as indicated in Table 36-3, drug interactions with lansoprazole are very few, with no clinically significant interactions reported (51), although many interactions remain to be characterized. Because CYP2C19 plays a relatively minor role in the metabolism of drugs, lansoprazole inhibition of this isoform should result in the decreased clearance of few if any drugs. No interaction has been observed with S-warfarin (52), diazepam (53), or phenytoin (54), all substrates for CYP2C9, and to a lesser extent, for CYP2C19. These findings are consistent with the in vitro results in which lansoprazole was found to be a moderate competitive inhibitor of CYP2C19 with a K_i of 50 μM.

It appears that CYP3A4 plays a secondary, but not minor, role in lansoprazole metabolism (55,51), suggesting that interactions with substrates of this CYP isoform may not predominate. Interaction studies with some of the prototypical CYP3A4 substrates such as nifedipine, cyclosporine, lidocaine, and quinidine have not been reported. In vitro, lansoprazole was found to be a weak noncompetitive inhibitor of CYP3A4 with a K_i of 165 μM for dextromethorphan N-demethylation (50). Based on this in vitro inhibition potency, it is predicted that any drug interaction with CYP3A4 substrates is likely to be weak and not clinically significant. However, many CYP3A4 substrates remain to be tested for interaction with lansoprazole, and this prediction may not be valid for all CYP3A substrates in all situations.

One of the two major enzymes involved in the metabolism of lansoprazole, CYP2C19, is polymorphically expressed (56). Approximately 2% to 5% of whites (57), 15% to 20% of Asians (58), and 2% of African Americans (59) would be expected to metabolize lansoprazole more slowly than the remaining population, leading to

TABLE 36-3. *Interactions of proton-pump inhibitors with other drugs*

Drug tested	Major P450	Lansoprazole	Omeprazole	Pantoprazole
Theophylline	CYP1A2	(↑Cl)	No IA	No IA
Caffeine	CYP1A2	NT	↑Cl[a]	No IA
Phenytoin	CYP2C9	No IA	↓Cl	No IA
Warfarin	CYP2C9	No IA	(↓Cl)	No IA
Tolbutamide	CYP2C9	(↓Cl)	NT	NT
Carbamazepine	CYP2C8	DC NT	↓Cl	No IA
Diclofenac	CYP2C9	NT	NT	No IA
Phenprocoumon	?	NT	NT	No IA
Mephenytoin	CYP2C19	NT	↓M	No IA
Diazepam	CYP2C19	No IA	↓Cl	No IA
Debrisoquine	CYP2D6	NT	No IA	No IA
Propranolol	CYP2D6 + others	No IA	No IA	NT
Metoprolol	CYP2D6	NT	No IA	NT
Nifedipine	CYP3A4	NT	(↓Cl?)	No IA
Cyclosporine	CYP3A4	NT	No IA	NT
Lidocaine	CYP3A4	NT	No IA	NT
Quinidine	CYP3A4	NT	No IA	NT
Contraceptives	CYP3A4	Eff. on ovul.?	NT	No IA
Alcohol	CYP2E1	NT	NT	No IA
Antipyrene	CYP3A/2C/1A2	(↑Cl)	(↓Cl)	No IA

IA, interaction; Cl, clearance; M, metabolism; NT, not tested; (), of questionable significance.
[a]Observed in poor metabolizers.
Modified from Meyer UA. Interaction of proton pump inhibitors with cytochromes P450: consequences for drug interactions. *Yale J Biol Med* 1996;69:203–209, with permission.

significant increases in plasma concentration. It has been shown that poor *S*-mephenytoin metabolizers are poor lansoprazole metabolizers as well (60). The major role of CYP2C19 in lansoprazole metabolism *in vivo* is further validated in studies with poor metabolizers of *S*-mephenytoin, in which increases in the AUCs for lansoprazole, omeprazole, and pantoprazole were of similar magnitude, indicating major metabolism carried out by the same CYP isoform (55). It should be noted, however, that in light of 24-hour dosing regimens, even the 4-hour elimination half-life in poor lansoprazole metabolizers is still relatively short compared with that of extensive metabolizers (1.5 hours). An increased plasma AUC of lansoprazole in poor metabolizers will probably not result in clinically significant interactions because the number of drugs cleared by CYP2C19 is rather limited. However, more studies are necessary to evaluate the clinical significance of CYP2C19 polymorphism and the safety of lansoprazole therapy with coadministered drugs.

Lansoprazole has been shown to induce to CYP1A1/2 and 3A4 activity in cultured human hepatocytes (61) and CYP1A1/2 activity and protein levels in rats (62). The induction of CYP1A2 also can be observed *in vivo*, as lansoprazole causes a slight, but significant decrease in the AUC of theophylline (63,64). This approximately 10% decrease in the AUC of theophylline is the only drug interaction (other than absorption effects) mentioned in the package insert for lansoprazole; however, it is noted that this small change is not clinically relevant (26). The clinical significance of CYP1A2 induction has not been determined; therefore drug monitoring of theophylline and other drugs metabolized primarily by CYP1A2 is prudent when they are used in combination with lansoprazole.

Omeprazole

Omeprazole (see Table 36-2) is the first substituted benzimidazole proton-pump inhibitor based on the structure of timoprazole. It is completely metabolized by the liver, with no parent compound detectable in the urine or feces after oral and i.v. doses (65). Approximately 80% of a given dose of omeprazole is excreted in the urine (65), with the remainder found in the feces as a result of biliary excretion (66). The two major plasma metabolites of omeprazole are 5-hydroxyomeprazole and omeprazole sulfone (67), neither of which is pharmacologically active (57). Both primary metabolites undergo secondary metabolism to the hydroxysulfone (68). The 5-hydroxyomeprazole metabolite is further metabolized to the corresponding carboxylic acid, and these two metabolites compose 50% of the recovered dose in the urine at 0 to 2 hours (47% of total dose), with the

remainder composed of at least four other metabolites of omeprazole (69,70).

The same CYP isoforms that metabolize lansoprazole also carry out most of the primary metabolism of omeprazole; however, the abundance of the two major metabolites is reversed for the two drugs. The major plasma metabolite of omeprazole is 5-hydroxyomeprazole, whereas the major metabolite for lansoprazole is the sulfone. Hydroxylation of both lansoprazole and omeprazole is carried out by CYP2C19, but on opposite sides of the molecules (71). The 5-hydroxylation of omeprazole occurs on the pyridinyl methyl group, but takes place on the 5 carbon of the benzimidazole moiety of lansoprazole. Formation of omeprazole sulfone is analogous to that of lansoprazole, being catalyzed by CYP3A4/5 on the sulfoxide group in the middle of both molecules. A minor metabolite of omeprazole is 5-*O*-desmethylomeprazole, which is catalyzed primarily by CYP2C19 (and to a smaller extent by P450 2D6), indicating that the analogous position in both lansoprazole and omeprazole can be metabolized by this isoform (71).

Omeprazole sulfone and 5-hydroxyomeprazole are further metabolized to form several secondary metabolites (71). The hydroxysulfone derivative of omeprazole is the major secondary metabolite from both omeprazole sulfone and 5-hydroxyomeprazole (68). It was shown *in vitro* that formation of the hydroxysulfone metabolite from 5-hydroxyomeprazole was catalyzed by CYP3A4/5, and conversion from omeprazole sulfone was catalyzed by CYP2C19 (68). CYP3A4/5 was also shown to catalyze the formation of pyridine-*N*-oxide omeprazole sulfone from omeprazole sulfone (68). These *in vitro* studies confirmed earlier *in vivo* studies, indicating that secondary metabolism of omeprazole sulfone was mediated by CYP2C19, but that of 5-hydroxyomeprazole was not (65).

Polymorphically expressed CYP2C19 is the major enzyme responsible for omeprazole metabolism (71). Like lansoprazole, omeprazole is a potent competitive inhibitor of CYP2C19 in human liver microsomes, with a K_i between 1 and 4 μM (50,72). Omeprazole also was found to be a moderate competitive inhibitor of CYP2C9, a very weak competitive inhibitor of CYP2D6, a weak noncompetitive inhibitor of CYP3A, and without effect on CYP1A2 or CYP2E1 (50). The affinity of omeprazole and CYP3A4 is ten-fold less than that with CYP2C19 (73), indicating the potential for significant drug interactions with CYP2C19 substrates. Omeprazole inhibits the clearance of diazepam by approximately 25% to 50% and shows dependence on the extensive mephenytoin hydroxylator phenotype (74–76); however, this interaction appears not to have serious clinical consequences. Omeprazole inhibition of diazepam clearance contrasts with results for lansoprazole, with which no inhibition was observed, suggesting that lansoprazole has less affinity for CYP2C19 than does omeprazole. However, this explanation is at odds with the determination that omeprazole and lansoprazole have similar K_i values for CYP2C19 in vitro (50). This result is also in contrast to similar studies carried out in rats, in which lansoprazole was found to inhibit the metabolism of diazepam (77), highlighting the potential pitfalls of extrapolating animal data to humans.

The effects of omeprazole on CYP2C9 are demonstrated in studies with phenytoin (74) and S-warfarin (78), which are metabolized primarily by CYP2C9, and to a smaller extent by CYP2C19. Omeprazole has been shown to cause no effect (79,80) or to cause a modest increase in the plasma phenytoin AUC (74,81). Omeprazole appears to cause a slight (12%) increase in the plasma AUC of R-warfarin, but not S-warfarin, the pharmacologically more active enantiomer (82). The effects on CYP2C9 substrates can readily be explained by omeprazole inhibition of minor CYP2C19 metabolism of these drugs (55). The rapid clearance of omeprazole and its metabolites ensures that low effective concentrations of the drug are maintained, thereby reducing the magnitude of any competitive interactions with the CYP2C family. Thus drugs with narrow therapeutic margins coadministered with omeprazole should be monitored; however, the probability of significant toxic interactions appears to be quite low.

The affinity of omeprazole for CYP3A4 is ten-fold less than that for CYP2C19 (73); however, because CYP2C19 represents less than 10% of total P450 in the liver (83), conditions in which omeprazole saturates this isoform could lead to significant CYP3A4 interactions. It has been reported that omeprazole and its sulfone and cimetidine were equipotent inhibitors of midazolam metabolism in human liver microsomes (84); however, this observation has not been validated in vivo. There are also reports that omeprazole interferes with cyclosporine clearance (26); however, there is also evidence against such an interaction (85). No significant interactions of omeprazole with CYP3A4 substrates have been reported, indicating that at standard therapeutic doses, plasma concentrations of omeprazole are not high enough to interfere with CYP3A4 (49). This was further established in a study reporting that omeprazole does not inhibit CYP3A4 activity in vivo when measured with the erythromycin breath test (86).

It has recently been shown that omeprazole has the capacity to interfere with the activation of proguanil to cycloguanil by CYP2C19 and 3A4 (87). It was previously determined in vivo that omeprazole caused a 2.5-fold increase in the proguanil-to-cycloguanil urinary ratio (88). This preliminary finding was confirmed by determining that omeprazole caused a 32% decrease in the apparent oral clearance of proguanil and a 65% decrease

in the metabolism of proguanil to cycloguanil in humans (87). The clinical significance of the decreased cycloguanil formation has yet to be determined, but it is conceivable that this may have important implications for protection against malaria in patients receiving both omeprazole and proguanil.

CYP2D6 may be involved in the metabolism of omeprazole, albeit at a low level (68). Metoprolol is metabolized by CYP2D6, and propranolol is partially metabolized by this CYP isoform; the pharmacokinetic parameters of both drugs are not significantly altered by omeprazole (89,90). Because of the minor role of CYP2D6 in omeprazole metabolism, it would be expected that drug interactions of omeprazole with drugs metabolized predominantly by CYP2D6 should be of no clinical consequence.

Omeprazole has been shown to be an aryl hydrocarbon–like inducer of CYP1A2 in cultures of human hepatocytes and in hepatic and gut biopsies of patients receiving repeated doses of omeprazole (91,92). Omeprazole was also shown to induce CYP1A1 in both the Caco-2 cell line (93) and the HepG2 cell line (94). Omeprazole and its sulfone metabolite were shown to induce CYP3A in primary cultures of human hepatocytes (61). This was further confirmed in vivo by demonstrating increased metabolism of caffeine after omeprazole treatment (95). Clearly, omeprazole is qualitatively an inducer of CYP1A; however, the quantitative significance of the induction is questionable. CYP1A can be induced by many environmental factors such as diet, exercise, and smoking (96), and the clinical consequences of elevated CYP1A levels due to omeprazole versus elevated levels resulting from environmental factors is unknown. Indeed, in the study with biopsies from the human gastrointestinal tract, the authors concluded that the induction of CYP1A in response to omeprazole was less than that attributable to inducers found in the diet (92). More studies will be necessary in this area to determine the probability of clinically significant drug interactions resulting from elevated CYP1A levels during omeprazole therapy.

Pantoprazole

Pantoprazole (see Table 36-2) is the latest substituted benzimidazole and is considered the safest from a drug-interaction standpoint. Pantoprazole is rapidly cleared from serum and extensively metabolized by the liver, yielding 4-desmethyl pantoprazole as the major plasma metabolite. Nearly 80% of an intravenous dose is converted to metabolites (mostly 4-desmethyl pantoprazole) and excreted in the urine, with the remaining dose found as metabolites in the feces resulting from biliary excretion. In contrast to lansoprazole and omeprazole, phase II metabolism is significant for 4-hydroxypantoprazole, which is rapidly conjugated with sulfate (97). This rapid conjugation and elimination of pantoprazole may in part explain the lack of interactions observed with this drug. Pantoprazole metabolism is complete, as no parent compound was found to be excreted in the urine (97). None of the metabolites of pantoprazole have any pharmacologic activity (98).

The major site of metabolism on pantoprazole is *O*-demethylation at the 4 position of the pyridine ring, yielding the corresponding hydroxy metabolite (98). This reaction was found to be catalyzed by CYP2C19 in human liver microsomes (72). A minor route of metabolism is formation of pantoprazole sulfone, which is carried out by CYP3A (72), and it has been suggested that CYP2C9 and 2D6 may play a minor role in pantoprazole metabolism; however, details are not available (51). Pantoprazole does not interfere with the clearance of nifedipine (99), a CYP3A4 substrate, or with metoprolol (100), a CYP2D6 substrate, indicating that significant interactions with drugs oxidized by these isoforms will probably not be clinically relevant.

Pantoprazole appears to be remarkably free from any type of drug interactions with the substances thus far analyzed as summarized in Table 36-1 (51,101). Studies done *in vitro* with rat liver microsomes indicated that pantoprazole has a greatly reduced capacity to interact with CYP isoforms when compared with omeprazole and lansoprazole (102,103). Pantoprazole does not appear to interact with CYP2C isoforms. Pantoprazole has no effect the pharmacokinetics of phenytoin (104) or *S*-warfarin (105), both substrates of CYP2C9. It also does not affect the disposition of diazepam (106) or *R*-warfarin (105), which are largely metabolized by CYP2C19. One caveat of these studies is that pantoprazole was only administered i.v. in the diazepam study, which results in lower exposure of the liver than in the case of oral dosing. However, the lack of interaction with diazepam was also demonstrated in an *in vivo* rat study in which it took three-fold more pantoprazole to produce the same prolongation of diazepam effect as it did omeprazole (76).

In contrast to the other substituted benzimidazoles, pantoprazole does not induce CYP1A isoforms. Pantoprazole has been found to have no effect on the pharmacokinetics of theophylline (107) or caffeine (101), it seems that pantoprazole does not have any interaction with CYP1A2 (108). These data, together with evidence that pantoprazole does not interfere with antipyrene clearance (109), also suggest that pantoprazole does not induce CYP1A2 *in vivo*. This lack of CYP isoform induction coupled with a notable lack of CYP isoform interaction make pantoprazole a very safe drug with the least risk of drug interaction compared with omeprazole or lansoprazole.

ANTIEMETICS

Serotonin is a signaling molecule involved in the vomiting reflex. It is released from enterochromaffin cells in the gut and binds to serotonin$_3$ (5-HT$_3$) receptors on vagal afferent neurons, which when stimulated, induce vomiting. The vomiting reflex can be prevented by 5-HT$_3$–receptor antagonists. One widely used group of antiemetics is based on the structure of serotonin, and these drugs competitively inhibit the stimulation of 5-HT$_3$ receptors by serotonin.

Granisetron

Granisetron (Table 36-4) is the second member of the 5-HT$_3$–receptor antagonist group of drugs and is 5 to 10 times more potent than ondansetron (110) and tropisetron (111). The primary route of granisetron clearance is through hepatic oxidation primarily to 7-hydroxygranisetron (112), with renal clearance playing a less important role (113). Route of administration has little effect on the pharmacokinetic disposition of granisetron dosages (112). 7-Hydroxygranisetron and its conjugates make up the majority of the dose found in plasma, urine, and feces; approximately 25% of a dose of granisetron is excreted in the urine as 7-hydroxygranisetron and its conjugates. Generally less than 20% of a given dose is excreted unchanged in the urine (113), with less than 1% excreted unchanged in the feces (112). Other minor metabolites of granisetron include *N*9′-desmethylgranisetron and the secondary metabolites, 6,7-dihydrodiolgranisetron and *N*9′-desmethyl-7-hydroxygranisetron, in addition to glucuronide and sulfate conjugates of these metabolites (112). Because most of these metabolites circulate as conjugates, their impact on pharmacologic activity of granisetron is expected to be minimal.

The CYP isoform responsible for granisetron metabolism is still an active area of research, with only one study reporting the CYP isoforms involved in granisetron 7-hydroxylation and *N*9′-desmethylation (114). *In vitro*, CYP3A3/4 is responsible for the *N*9′-desmethylation of granisetron; however, the 7-hydroxylation of granisetron is carried out by a CYP3A isoform that has not been positively identified. The formation of 7-hydroxygranisetron is potently inhibited by 0.6 µ*M* ketoconazole; however, the 7-hydroxylation reaction did not correlate with two prototypical CYP3A activities, testosterone 6β-hydroxylation, or cyclosporine oxidation. The authors speculated that either CYP3A5 or 3A7 is responsible for formation of 7-hydroxygranisetron.

Drug-interaction studies with granisetron are scant at this time. Because granisetron is metabolized by CYP3A3/4, there exists the potential for interactions with drugs metabolized by this pathway. Granisetron does not

TABLE 36-4. Summary of currently prescribed 5-HT$_3$-receptor antagonists

	Oral bioavailability (%)	Elimination route	Renal clearance (L/h)	Parent excreted (% in urine)	Relative potency[a]	Metabolism	Metabolites[b]	Structure
Granisetron	60	Hepatic	4–5	8–17	5–10	CYP3A	7-Hydroxy N9′-desmethyl	
Ondansetron	60	Hepatic	<1	<5	1	CYP1A2, CYP3A, CYP2D6	5-Hydroxy sulfone 5-O-Desmethyl 3-hydroxy	
Tropisetron	60[c]; 100[d]	Hepatic Renal	5[c,d]	0[c], 10[d]	1	CYP2D6	4-Desmethyl sulfone	

[a]*In vitro* pharmacologic activity used for comparison.
[b]In decreasing order of abundance.
[c]Extensive debrisoquine metabolizers.
[d]Poor debrisoquine metabolizers.

492

interact with emetogenic cancer therapies so far tested and does not induce or inhibit CYP isoforms (26).

Ondansetron

Ondansetron (see Table 36-4) is a carbazole and is the prototypical 5-HT$_3$–receptor antagonist. It is extensively metabolized in the liver, with more than 95% of a given dose cleared by this route. The major oxidative metabolite is 8-hydroxyondansetron, followed by 7-hydroxyondansetron; however, these metabolites are very difficult to detect in the plasma because they are rapidly conjugated to glucuronide and sulfate by phase II enzymes before leaving the liver to be excreted in the urine (115). Less than 5% of a given dose of ondansetron is excreted unchanged in the urine or feces (116).

Four metabolites of ondansetron are formed in humans as a result of oxidation at the indole moiety. The major metabolites of ondansetron are 8-hydroxyondansetron, which accounts for 40% of a given dose, and 7- hydroxyondansetron, representing 20% of the dose. There is also a minor amount of oxidation forming 6-hydroxyondansetron, accounting for less than 5% of the dose and a very minor amount of N-dealkylation yielding N-desmethylondansetron (115). Multiple forms of cytochrome P450 are involved in the oxidative metabolism of ondansetron in the liver (117,118). CYP2D6 was found to be involved in the hydroxylation of ondansetron; as determined with an inhibitor of CYP2D6 (quinidine), cDNA expressed CYP2D6 and inhibition of CYP2D6-dependent O-demethylation of dextromethorphan (117). This study also showed that CYP3A was involved, as evidenced by inhibition of CYP3A-specific metabolism of cyclosporine by ondansetron (117). These results were later confirmed and expanded to include CYP1A1 and 1A2 (118). In lymphoblastoid cells expressing CYP isoforms, CYP1A1 and 1A2 were found to metabolize ondansetron to products consistent with the *in vivo* metabolic profile and at a rate similar to CYP2D6. Inhibitors were used to determine that CYP1A1 and 1A2 play the most important role for ondansetron hydroxylation, whereas CYP2D6 plays a relatively minor role. The involvement of CYP3A seems important only at relatively high concentrations of ondansetron (118).

The major metabolite of ondansetron, 8-hydroxyondansetron, is as potent as the parent, with the remaining hydroxy metabolites also being active, but at reduced potency relative to ondansetron. These metabolites are rapidly conjugated to inactive compounds that do not accumulate in the plasma. As a consequence of this lack of systemic exposure, the metabolites of ondansetron do not contribute pharmacologically to the action of ondansetron (115).

Multiple CYP isoforms are involved in the metabolism of ondansetron. This redundancy of pathways predicts minimal clinically significant drug interactions. This seems to be the case in practice, as there are no clinically significant drug interactions of ondansetron and any other drug, and no dosage adjustments are required (26). Because polymorphically expressed CYP2D6 is involved in the clearance of ondansetron, a study with poor and extensive debrisoquine metabolizers was conducted to determine if differences in ondansetron clearance could occur (119). It was found that the status of CYP2D6 had no effect on the clearance, AUC, C_{max}, or half-life of ondansetron. Despite the involvement of the CYP2D6 polymorphism, ondansetron appears to be a safe drug, with an absence of clinically significant drug interactions.

Tropisetron

Tropisetron (see Table 36-4) is the latest member of the substituted benzimidazole antiemetic family of drugs. It is metabolized in the liver; however, there is a minimal first pass effect (120). Tropisetron is metabolized through oxidation at the 5, 6, or 7 positions of the indole moiety, and these metabolites are conjugated to sulfate and glucuronide before excretion (121). Minor pathways of metabolism result in N-demethylation and N-oxygenation at the tropinyl nitrogen of tropisetron (121). The predominant metabolites excreted in the urine are 6-hydroxytropisetron and its sulfated conjugate, accounting for approximately 46% of a given dose, whereas 5-hydroxytropisetron and its sulfated and glucuronidated metabolites are approximately 12% of the dose (121). Only 9% of a dose is excreted unchanged in the urine, and approximately 15% is found in the feces, almost entirely as metabolites (122). In the plasma, the major metabolites are the glucuronide conjugates of 5-hydroxytropisetron, followed by lesser amounts of 6-hydroxytropisetron and its sulfate conjugates (121).

Polymorphically expressed CYP2D6 is involved in the hydroxylation of tropisetron, as determined with several methods. Quinidine, a CYP2D6 inhibitor, reduced tropisetron hydroxylation by 67% when used at 1 μM in human liver microsomes; cDNA-expressed CYP2D6 was able to hydroxylate tropisetron, and tropisetron was a competitive inhibitor of CYP2D6-dependent O-demethylation of dextromethorphan (117). This study also demonstrated that CYP3A may play a minor role in the metabolism of tropisetron, and this was subsequently confirmed in a later report (123). Firkusny et al. (123) showed that the formation of 5- and 6-hydroxytropisetron in the presence of CYP2D6 inhibitory antibodies correlated to the content of CYP3A4, and addition of ketoconazole abolished this hydroxylation. It was further suggested that CYP3A4 was the isoform responsible for the formation of *N*-desmethyltropisetron, although detailed study of this reaction was not possible because of technical limitations (123). The contribution of CYP3A4 may become significant in CYP2D6 poor metabolizers. Because the plasma concentration of tropisetron reaches 50 n*M* only after a single 5-mg oral dose, no competitive inhibition of CYP2D6 or 3A4 would be expected, as this is well below the effective K_i for both CYP isoforms (124).

As with the other antiemetics, there is a paucity of definitive drug-interaction studies. The major involvement of CYP2D6 in tropisetron metabolism can potentially be a source of adverse drug interactions. The metabolic clearance of tropisetron is decreased in poor metabolizers relative to extensive metabolizers, leading to a five-fold increase in the elimination half-life (122). The current perception is that the risk of tropisetron accumulation in poor metabolizers is low, considering the recommended dosage levels and short-term treatment regimen necessary to achieve antiemetic action (120).

FUTURE PERSPECTIVES

It is now possible to address many questions about drug interactions preclinically by using *in vitro* techniques. Determination of the metabolic pathway specific for a particular drug and the contribution of metabolism to total drug clearance are important in anticipating adverse interactions with coadministered drugs. These predictions can help in the proper design of clinical trials and aid the physician in prescribing drug combinations not previously examined for interactions. The challenge for the prescriber is weighing the many factors that also contribute to the potential for interactions to occur and the clinical significance of those interactions that are manifest.

The incidence of clinically relevant drug interactions with the H_2 antagonists, substituted benzimidazole proton-pump inhibitors, and 5-HT$_3$ antagonists currently on the market is quite low. In general, these drugs appear to be safe; however, drug interactions can still occur in small subsets of the general population. The H_2 antagonists have been given to millions of patients with little incidence of clinically significant drug interactions, but continued diligence with coadministered drugs with a narrow therapeutic ratio is appropriate. The H_2 antagonists do not appear to interact with renally cleared drugs, but the potential for drug interaction with a drug cleared by the same mechanism may exist in an as-yet-undiscovered entity. The substituted benzimidazole proton-pump inhibitors appear safe, but as a class, are not so mature as some of the H_2 antagonists, and drug interactions may well remain to be uncovered. The recent interest in the potential danger of omeprazole inhibition of proguanil-to-cycloguanil activation in the treatment of malaria is a case in point (87). The 5-HT$_3$–receptor antagonists are the newest class of drugs covered in this chapter, and the paucity of drug-interaction studies in this area is sure to spur active research for some time. Although this class of drugs appears to have an excellent safety profile, optimization of dosing regimens is incomplete. The relation between dosage and pharmacodynamic effects in relieving nausea together with emesis must be defined to ensure that patients receive the appropriate amount of drug.

REFERENCES

1. Mills JG, Koch KM, Webster C, Sirgo MA, Fitzgerald K, Wood JR. The safety of ranitidine in over a decade of use. *Aliment Pharmacol Ther* 1997;11:129–137.
2. Lin JH. Pharmacokinetic and pharmacodynamic properties of histamine H$_2$-receptor antagonists: relationship between intrinsic potency and effective plasma concentrations. *Clin Pharmacokinet* 1991;20:218–236.
3. Louis WJ, Mihaly GW, Hanson RG, et al. Pharmacokinetic and gastric secretory studies of ranitidine in man. *Scand J Gastroenterol* 1981;16 (suppl 69):11–15.
4. Mitchell SC, Idle JR, Smith RL. The metabolism of [^{14}C] cimetidine in man. *Xenobiotica* 1982;12:283–292.
5. Schentag JJ, Cerra FB, Calleri GM, Leising ME, French MA, Bernhard H. Age, disease, and cimetidine disposition in healthy subjects and chronically ill patients. *Clin Pharmacol Ther* 1981;29:737–743.
6. Taylor DC, Cresswell PR, Bartlett DC. The metabolism and elimination of cimetidine: a histamine H$_2$-receptor antagonist, in the rat, dog, and man. *Drug Metab Dispos* 1978;6:21–30.
7. Mitchell SC, Ritchie JC, Idle JR, Smith RL. Nature of the polar urinary metabolites of metiamide and cimetidine in man. *Biochem Soc Trans* 1982;10:123–124.
8. Speeg KV Jr, Patwardhan RV, Avant GR, Mitchell MC, Schenker S Jr. Inhibition of microsomal drug metabolism by histamine H$_2$-receptor antagonists *in vivo* and *in vitro* in rodents. *Gastroenterology* 1982;82:89–96.
9. Schulz M, Schmoldt A. On the sulphoxidation of cimetidine and etintidine by rat and human liver microsomes. *Xenobiotica* 1988;18:983–989.
10. Oldham HG, Chenery RJ. Interaction of cimetidine and ranitidine with the FAD monooxygenase in pig liver microsomes. *Biochem Pharmacol* 1985;34:2398–2401.
11. Cashman JR, Olsen LD, Bornheim LM. Enantioselective S-oxygenation by flavin-containing and cytochrome P-450 monooxygenases. *Chem Res Toxicol* 1990;3:344–349.
12. Rettie AE, Bogucki BD, Lim I, Meier GP. Stereoselective sulfoxidation of a series of alkyl *p*-tolyl sulfides by microsomal and purified flavin-containing monooxygenases. *Mol Pharmacol* 1990;37:643–651.
13. Cashman JR, Park SB, Yang Z-C, et al. Chemical, enzymatic, and human enantioselective S-oxygenation of cimetidine. *Drug Metab Dispos* 1993;21:587–597.
14. Cashman JR, Park SB, Berkman CE, Cashman LE. Role of hepatic flavin-containing monooxygenase 3 in drug and chemical metabolism in adult humans. *Chem Biol Interact* 1995;96:33–46.
15. Patwardhan RV, Yarborough GW, Desmond PV, Johnson RF, Schenker S, Speeg KV Jr. Cimetidine spares the glucuronidation of lorazepam and oxazepam. *Gastroenterology* 1980;79:912–916.
16. Greenblatt DJ, Abernethy DR, Koepke HH, Shader RI. Interaction of cimetidine with oxazepam, lorazepam, and flurazepam. *J Clin Pharmacol* 1984;24:187–193.
17. Knodell RG, Browne DG, Gwozdz GP, Brian WR, Guengerich FP. Differential inhibition of individual human liver cytochromes P-450 by cimetidine. *Gastroenterology* 1991;101:1680–1691.
18. Takabatake T, Ohta H, Maekawa M, et al. Pharmacokinetics of famotidine: a new H$_2$-receptor antagonist, in relation to renal function. *Eur J Clin Pharmacol* 1985;28:327–332.
19. Hucker HB, Hutt JE, Chremos AN, Rotmensch H. Disposition and metabolism of famotidine: a potent H$_2$-receptor blocker [Abstract]. *Fed Proc* 1984;43:655.

20. Schunack W. Pharmacology of H₂-receptor antagonists: an overview. *J Intern Med Res* 1989;17:9A–16A.
21. Yeh KC, Chremos AN, Lin JH, et al. Single-dose pharmacokinetics and bioavailability of famotidine in man: results of multicenter collaborative studies. *Biopharm Drug Dispos* 1987;8:549–560.
22. Klotz U, Walker S. Biliary excretion of H₂-receptor antagonists. *Eur J Clin Pharmacol* 1990;39:91–92.
23. Kawai R, Yamada S, Kawanyra S, Miwa T, Miwa M. Metabolic fate of famotidine (YM-11170), a new potent H₂-receptor agonist: absorption and excretion in dogs and humans. *Pharmacometrics* 1984;27:73–77.
24. Kroemer H, Klotz U. Pharmacokinetics of famotidine in man. *Int J Clin Pharmacol Ther Toxicol* 1987;25:458–463.
25. Schunack W. What are the differences between the H₂-receptor antagonists? *Aliment Pharmacol Ther* 1987;1:493S–503S.
26. *Physicians Desk Reference.* 47th ed. Montvale, NJ: Medical Economics Company, 1997.
27. Irshaid Y, Abu-Khalaf M. Lack of effect of certain histamine H₂-receptor blockers on the glucuronidation of 7-hydroxy-4-methylcoumarin by human liver microsomes. *Pharmacol Toxicol* 1992;71:294–296.
28. Wang RW, Miwa GT, Argenbright LS, Lu AYH. *In vitro* studies on the interaction of famotidine with liver microsomal cytochrome P-450. *Biochem Pharmacol* 1988;37:3049–3053.
29. Howden CW, Tytgat GN. The tolerability and safety profile of famotidine. *Clin Ther* 1996;18:36–54.
30. Knadler MP, Bergstrom RF, Callaghan JT, Rubin A. Nizatidine, an H₂-blocker: its metabolism and disposition in man. *Drug Metab Dispos* 1986;14:175–182.
31. Callaghan JT, Bergstrom RF, Rubin A, et al. A pharmacokinetic profile of nizatidine in man. *Scand J Gastroenterol* 1987;22(suppl 136):9–17.
32. Gladziwa U, Klotz U. Pharmacokinetics and pharmacodynamics of H₂-receptor antagonists in patients with renal insufficiency. *Clin Pharmacokinet* 1993;24:319–332.
33. Price AH, Brogden RN. Nizatidine: a preliminary review of its pharmacodynamic and pharmacokinetic properties, and its therapeutic use in peptic ulcer disease. *Drugs* 1988;36:521–539.
34. Klotz U. Lack of effect of nizatidine on drug metabolism. *Scand J Gastroenterol* 1987;22(suppl 136):18–23.
35. Secor JW, Speeg KV Jr, Meredith CG, Johnson RF, Snowdy P, Schenker S. Lack of effect of nizatidine on hepatic drug metabolism in man. *Br J Clin Pharmacol* 1985;20:710–713.
36. Callaghan JT, Ridolfo AS, Crabtree RE, Obermeyer BD, Offen WW, DeSante KA. Nizatidine: effect on aspirin-induced gastrointestinal red blood cell loss [Abstract]. *Gastroenterology* 1987;92:1336.
37. Carey PF, Martin LE, Owen PE. Determination of ranitidine and its metabolites in human urine by reversed-phase ion-pair high-performance liquid chromatography. *J Chromatogr* 1981;225:161–168.
38. Garg DC, Weidler DJ, Eshelman FN. Ranitidine bioavailability and kinetics in normal male subjects. *Clin Pharmacol Ther* 1983;33:445–452.
39. Bell JA, Dallas FAA, Jenner WN, Martin LE. The metabolism of ranitidine in animals and man. *Biochem Soc Trans* 1980;8:93.
40. Overby LH, Carver GC, Philpot RM. Quantitation and kinetic properties of hepatic microsomal and recombinant flavin-containing monooxygenases 3 and 5 from humans. *Chem Biol Interact* 1997;106:29–45.
41. Desmond PV, Mashford ML, Harman PJ, Morphett BJ, Breen KJ, Wang YM. Decreased oral warfarin clearance after ranitidine and cimetidine. *Clin Pharmacol Ther* 1984;35:338–341.
42. Baciewicz AM, Morgan PJ. Ranitidine-warfarin interaction. *Ann Intern Med* 1990;112:76–77.
43. Tateno M, Nakamura N. Phase I study of lansoprazole (AG-1749) antiulcer agent: capsule form. *Rinsho Iyaku* 1991;7:51–62.
44. Hongo M, Ohara S, Hirasawa Y, Abe S, Asaki S, Toyota T. Effect of lansoprazole on intragastric pH: comparison between morning and evening dosing. *Dig Dis Sci* 1992;37:882–890.
45. Barradell LB, Faulds D, McTavish D. Lansoprazole: a review of its pharmacodynamic and pharmacokinetic properties and its therapeutic efficacy in acid-related disorders. *Drugs* 1992;44:225–250.
46. Pichard L, Curi-Pedrosa R, Bonfils C, et al. Oxidative metabolism of lansoprazole by human liver cytochromes P450. *Mol Pharmacol* 1995;47:410–418.
47. Pearce RE, Rodrigues AD, Goldstein JA, Parkinson A. Identification of the human P450 enzymes involved in lansoprazole metabolism. *J Pharmacol Exp Ther* 1996;277:805–816.
48. Zimmermann AE, Katona BG. Lansoprazole: a comprehensive review. *Pharmacotherapy* 1997;17:308–326.
49. Tucker GT. The interaction of proton pump inhibitors with cytochromes P450. *Aliment Pharmacol Ther* 1994;8(suppl 1):33–38.
50. Ko JW, Sukova N, Thacker D, Chen P, Flockhart DA. Evaluation of omeprazole and lansoprazole as inhibitors of cytochrome P450 isoforms. *Drug Metab Dispos* 1997;25:853–862.
51. Meyer UA. Interaction of proton pump inhibitors with cytochromes P450: consequences for drug interactions. *Yale J Biol Med* 1996;69:203–209.
52. Cavanaugh JH, Winters EP, Cohen A, Braeckman R. Lack of effect of lansoprazole on steady state warfarin metabolism [Abstract]. *Gastroenterology* 1991;100:A40.
53. Lefebre RA, Flouvat B, Karolac-Tamisier S, Moerman E, van Ganse E. Influence of lansoprazole treatment on diazepam plasma concentrations. *Clin Pharmacol Ther* 1992;52:458–463.
54. Karol MD, Mukherji D, Cavanaugh JH. Lack of effect of concomitant multidose lansoprazole on single-dose phenytoin pharmacokinetics in subjects [Abstract]. *Gastroenterology* 1994;106:A103.
55. Andersson T. Pharmacokinetics, metabolism and interactions of acid pump inhibitors: focus on omeprazole, lansoprazole and pantoprazole. *Clin Pharmacol* 1996;31:9–28.
56. Küpfer A, Preisig R. Pharmacogenetics of mephenytoin: a new drug hydroxylation polymorphism in man. *Eur J Clin Pharmacol* 1984;26:753–759.
57. Andersson T, Regårdh CG, Dahl-Puustinen ML, Bertilsson L. Slow omeprazole metabolizers are also poor S-mephenytoin hydroxylators. *Ther Drug Monit* 1990;12:415–416.
58. Sohn D-R, Kobayashi K, Chiba K, Lee K-H, Shin S-G, Ishizaki T. Disposition kinetics and metabolism of omeprazole in extensive and poor metabolizers of S-mephenytoin 4′-hydroxylation recruited from an Oriental population. *J Pharmacol Exp Ther* 1992;262:1195–1202.
59. Marinac JS, Balian JD, Foxworth JW, et al. Determination of CYP2C19 phenotype in black Americans with omeprazole: correlation with genotype. *Clin Pharmacol Ther* 1996;60:138–144.
60. Katsuki H, Nakamura C, Arimori K, Fujiyama S, Nakano M. Genetic polymorphism of CYP2C19 and lansoprazole pharmacokinetics in Japanese subjects. *Eur J Clin Pharmacol* 1997;52:391–396.
61. Curi-Pedrosa R, Daujat M, Pichard L, et al. Omeprazole and lansoprazole are mixed inducers of CYP1A and CYP3A in human hepatocytes in primary culture. *J Pharmacol Exp Ther* 1994;269:384–392.
62. Masubuchi N, Hakusui H, Okazaki O. Effects of pantoprazole on xenobiotic metabolizing enzymes in rat liver microsomes: a comparison with other proton pump inhibitors. *Drug Metab Dispos* 1997;25:584–589.
63. Granneman GR, Karol MD, Locke CS, Cavanaugh JH. Pharmacokinetic interaction between lansoprazole and theophylline. *Ther Drug Monit* 1995;17:460–464.
64. Kokufu T, Ihara N, Sugioka N, et al. Effects of lansoprazole on pharmacokinetics and metabolism of theophylline. *Eur J Clin Pharmacol* 1995;48:391–395.
65. Regårdh CG, Andersson T, Lagerström PO, Lundborg P, Skånberg I. The pharmacokinetics of omeprazole in humans: a study of single intravenous and oral doses. *Ther Drug Monit* 1990;12:163–172.
66. Lind T, Andersson T, Skånberg I, Olbe L. Biliary excretion of intravenous [¹⁴C] omeprazole in humans. *Clin Pharmacol Ther* 1987;42:504–508.
67. Cederberg C, Andersson T, Skånberg I. Omeprazole: pharmacokinetics and metabolism in man. *Scand J Gastroenterol* 1989;24(suppl 166):33–40.
68. Andersson T, Miners JO, Veronese ME, Birkett DJ. Identification of human liver cytochrome P450 isoforms mediating secondary omeprazole metabolism. *Br J Clin Pharmacol* 1994;37:597–604.
69. Renberg L, Simonsson R, Hoffmann KJ. Identification of two main urinary metabolites of [¹⁴C]omeprazole in humans. *Drug Metab Dispos* 1989;17:69–76.
70. Regårdh CG. Pharmacokinetics and metabolism of omeprazole in man. *Scand J Gastroenterol* 1986;21(suppl 118):99–104.
71. Andersson T, Miners J-O, Tassaneeyakul W, Veronese ME, Meyer UA, Birkett DJ. Identification of human liver cytochrome P450 isoforms mediating omeprazole metabolism. *Br J Clin Pharmacol* 1993;36:521–530.

72. VandenBranden M, Ring BJ, Binkley SN, Wrighton SA. Interaction of human liver cytochromes P450 *in vitro* with LY307640: a gastric proton pump inhibitor. *Pharmacogenetics* 1996;6:81–91.

73. Chiba K, Kobayashi K, Manabe K, Tani M, Kamataki T, Ishizaki T. Oxidative metabolism of omeprazole in human liver microsomes: cosegregation with *S*-mephenytoin 4′-hydroxylation. *J Pharmacol Exp Ther* 1993;266:52–59.

74. Gugler R, Jensen JC. Omeprazole inhibits oxidative drug metabolism: studies with diazepam and phenytoin in vivo and 7-ethoxycoumarin *in vitro*. *Gastroenterology* 1985;89:1235–1241.

75. Andersson T, Cederberg C, Edvardsson G, Heggelund A, Lundborg P. Effect of omeprazole treatment on diazepam plasma levels in slow versus normal rapid metabolizers of omeprazole. *Clin Pharmacol Ther* 1990;47:79–85.

76. Caraco Y, Tateishi T, Wood AJJ. Interethnic difference in omeprazole's inhibition of diazepam metabolism. *Clin Pharmacol Ther* 1995; 58:62–72.

77. Hanauer G, Graf U, Meissner T. *In vivo* cytochrome P 450 interactions of the newly developed H+/K(+)-ATPase inhibitor pantoprazole (BY 1023/SK&F 96022) compared to other antiulcer drugs. *Methods Find Exp Clin Pharmacol* 1991;13:63–67.

78. Rettie AE, Korzekwa KR, Kunze KL, et al. Hydroxylation of warfarin by human cDNA-expressed cytochrome P-450: a role for P-4502C9 in the etiology of (*S*)-warfarin-drug interactions. *Chem Res Toxicol* 1992; 5:54–59.

79. Andersson T, Lagerström PO, Unge P. A study of the interaction between omeprazole and phenytoin in epileptic patients. *Ther Drug Monit* 1990;12:329–333.

80. Bachmann KA, Sullivan TJ, Lauregut L, Reese JH, Miller K, Levine L. Absence of an inhibitory effect of omeprazole and nizatidine in phenytoin disposition: a marker of CYP2C activity. *Br J Clin Pharmacol* 1993;36:380–382.

81. Prichard PJ, Walt RP, Kitchingman GK, et al. Oral phenytoin pharmacokinetics during omeprazole therapy. *Br J Clin Pharmacol* 1987;24: 543–545.

82. Sutfin T, Balmer K, Bostrom H, Eriksson S, Hoglund P, Paulsen O. Stereoselective interaction of omeprazole with warfarin in healthy men. *Ther Drug Monit* 1989;11:176–184.

83. Jung F, Richardson TH, Raucy JL, Johnson EF. Diazepam metabolism by cDNA-expressed human 2C P450s: identification of P4502C18 and P4502C19 as low K_m diazepam *N*-demethylases. *Drug Metab Dispos* 1997;25:133–139.

84. Li G, Klotz U. Inhibitory effect of omeprazole on the metabolism of midazolam *in vitro*. *Arzneimittelforschung* 1990;40:1105–1107.

85. Blohme I, Idstrom JP, Andersson T. A study of the interaction between omeprazole and cyclosporine in renal transplant patients. *Br J Clin Pharmacol* 1993;35:156–160.

86. Tateishi T, Graham SG, Krivoruk Y, Wood AJ. Omeprazole does not affect measured CYP3A4 activity using the erythromycin breath test. *Br J Clin Pharmacol* 1995;40:411–412.

87. Funck-Brentano C, Becquemont L, Lenevu A, Roux A, Jaillon P, Beaune P. Inhibition by omeprazole of proguanil metabolism: mechanism of the interaction *in vitro* and prediction of *in vivo* results from the *in vitro* experiments. *J Pharmacol Exp Ther* 1997;280: 730–738.

88. Partovian C, Jacqz-Aigrain E, Keundjian A, Jaillon P, Funck-Brentano C. Comparison of chloroguanide and mephenytoin for the in vivo assessment of genetically determined CYP2C19 activity in humans. *Clin Pharmacol Ther* 1995;58:257–263.

89. Andersson T, Lundborg P, Regårdh CG. Lack of effect of omeprazole treatment on steady-state plasma levels of metoprolol. *Eur J Clin Pharmacol* 1991;40:61–65.

90. Henry D, Brent P, Whyte I, Mihaly G, Devenish-Meares S. Propranolol steady-state pharmacokinetics are unaltered by omeprazole. *Eur J Clin Pharmacol* 1987;33:369–373.

91. Diaz D, Fabre I, Daujat M, et al. Omeprazole is an aryl hydrocarbon-like inducer of human hepatic cytochrome P450. *Gastroenterology* 1990;99:737–747.

92. McDonnell WM, Scheiman JM, Traber PG. Induction of cytochrome P4501A genes (CYP1A) by omeprazole in the human alimentary tract. *Gastroenterology* 1992;103:1509–1516.

93. Daujat M, Charrasse S, Fabre I, et al. Induction of CYP1A1 gene by benzimidazole derivatives during Caco-2 cell differentiation: evidence

94. for an aryl-hydrocarbon receptor-mediated mechanism. *Eur J Biochem* 1996;237:642–652.

94. Krusekopf S, Kleeberg U, Hildebrandt AG, Ruckpaul K. Effects of benzimidazole derivatives on cytochrome P450 1A1 expression in a human hepatoma cell line. *Xenobiotica* 1997;27:1–9.

95. Rost KL, Brösicke H, Brockmöller J, Scheffler M, Helge H, Roots I. Increase of cytochrome P450IA2 activity by omeprazole: evidence by the 13C-(*N*-3-methyl)-caffeine breath test in poor and extensive metabolizers of *S*-mephenytoin. *Clin Pharmacol Ther* 1992;52: 170–180.

96. Vistisen K, Loft S, Poulsen HE. Cytochrome P450IA2 activity in man measured by caffeine metabolism: effect of smoking, broccoli and exercise. *Adv Exp Med Biol* 1991;283:407–411.

97. Steinijans VW, Huber R, Hartmann M, et al. Lack of pantoprazole drug interactions in man. *Int J Clin Pharmacol Ther* 1994;32:385–399.

98. Huber R, Kohl B, Sachs G, et al. Review article: the continuing development of proton pump inhibitors with particular reference to pantoprazole. *Aliment Pharmacol Ther* 1995;9:363–378.

99. Bliesath H, Huber R, Hartmann M, Kunz K, Koch HJ, Wurst W. Pantoprazole does not influence the steady state pharmacokinetics of nifedipine [Abstract]. *Gastroenterology* 1994;106:A55.

100. Koch HJ, Hartmann M, Bliesath H, et al. Pantoprazole does not influence metoprolol pharmacokinetics in man [Abstract]. *Gastroenterology* 1996;110:A158.

101. Steinijans VW, Huber R, Hartmann M, et al. Lack of pantoprazole drug interactions in man: an updated review. *Int J Clin Pharmacol Ther* 1996;34:S31–S50.

102. Kromer W, Postius S, Riedel R, et al. BY 1023/SK &F 96022INN pantoprazole: a novel gastric proton pump inhibitor, potently inhibits acid secretion but lacks relevant cytochrome P450 interactions. *J Pharmacol Exp Ther* 1990;254:129–135.

103. Simon WA, Büdingen C, Fahr S, Kinder B, Koske M. The H+, K(+)-ATPase inhibitor pantoprazole (BY1023/SK&F96022) interacts less with cytochrome P450 than omeprazole and lansoprazole. *Biochem Pharmacol* 1991;42:347–355.

104. Middle MV, Muller FO, Schall R, et al. No influence of pantoprazole on the pharmacokinetics of phenytoin. *Int J Clin Pharmacol Ther* 1996;34(1 suppl):S72–S75.

105. Duursema L, Muller FO, Schall R, et al. Lack of effect of pantoprazole on the pharmacodynamics and pharmacokinetics of warfarin. *Br J Clin Pharmacol* 1995;39:700–703.

106. Gugler R, Hartmann M, Rudi J, et al. Lack of effect of pantoprazole and diazepam in man [Abstract]. *Gastroenterology* 1992;102:A77.

107. Schulz HU, Hartmann M, Steinijans VW, et al. Lack of influence of pantoprazole on the disposition kinetics of theophylline in man. *Int J Clin Pharmacol Ther Toxicol* 1991;29:369–375.

108. Hartmann M, Bliesath H, Zeck K, et al. Pantoprazole does not influence CYP1A2 activity in man [Abstract]. *Gastroenterology* 1995;108 (suppl 4):A109.

109. De Mey C, Meineke I, Steinijans VW, et al. Pantoprazole lacks interaction with antipyrine in man, either by inhibition or induction. *Int J Clin Pharmacol Ther* 1996;34:S58–S66.

110. Andrews PL, Bhandari P, Davey PT, Bingham S, Marr HE, Blower PR. Are all 5-HT3 receptor antagonists the same? *Eur J Cancer* 1992; 28A:S2–S6.

111. Diehl V, Marty M. Efficacy and safety of antiemetics. *Cancer Treat Rev* 1994;20:379–392.

112. Clarke SE, Austin NE, Bloomer JC, et al. Metabolism and disposition of 14C-granisetron in rat, dog and man after intravenous and oral dosing. *Xenobiotica* 1994;24:1119–1131.

113. Allen A, Asgill CC, Pierce DM, Upward J, Zussman BD. Pharmacokinetics and tolerability of ascending intravenous doses of granisetron: a novel 5-HT3 antagonist, in healthy human subjects. *Eur J Clin Pharmacol* 1994;46:159–162.

114. Bloomer JC, Baldwin SJ, Smith GJ, Ayrton AD, Clarke SE, Chenery RJ. Characterisation of the cytochrome P450 enzymes involved in the *in vitro* metabolism of granisetron. *Br J Clin Pharmacol* 1994;38: 557–566.

115. Pritchard JF. Ondansetron metabolism and pharmacokinetics. *Semin Oncol* 1992;19:9–15.

116. Saynor DA, Dixon CM. The metabolism of ondansetron. *Eur J Cancer Clin Oncol* 1989;25:S75–S77.

117. Fischer V, Vickers AE, Heitz F, et al. The polymorphic cytochrome P-

4502D6 is involved in the metabolism of both 5-hydroxytryptamine antagonists, tropisetron and ondansetron. *Drug Metab Dispos* 1994; 22:269–274.

118. Dixon CM, Colthup PV, Serabjit-Singh CJ, et al. Multiple forms of cytochrome P450 are involved in the metabolism of ondansetron in humans. *Drug Metab Dispos* 1995;23:1225–1230.

119. Ashforth EIL, Palmer JL, Bye A, Bedding A. The pharmacokinetics of ondansetron after intravenous injection in healthy volunteers phenotyped as poor or extensive metabolisers of debrisoquine. *Br J Clin Pharmacol* 1994;37:389–391.

120. Kutz K. Pharmacology, toxicology and human pharmacokinetics of tropisetron. *Ann Oncol* 1993;4:15–18.

121. Fischer V, Baldeck JP, Tse FL. Pharmacokinetics and metabolism of the 5-hydroxytryptamine antagonist tropisetron after single oral doses in humans. *Drug Metab Dispos* 1992;20:603–607.

122. de Bruijn KM. Tropisetron: a review of the clinical experience. *Drugs* 1992;43:11–22.

123. Firkusny L, Kroemer HK, Eichelbaum M. *In vitro* characterization of cytochrome P450 catalyzed metabolism of the antiemetic tropisetron. *Biochem Pharmacol* 1995;49:1777–1784.

124. Vickers AEM, Fischer V, Connors MS, et al. Biotransformation of the antiemetic 5-HT₃ antagonist tropisetron in liver and kidney slices of human, rat and dog with a comparison to in vivo. *Eur J Drug Metab Pharmacokinet* 1996;21:43–50.

CHAPTER 37

Immunosuppressive Agents

Mary F. Hebert

The currently available immunosuppressive agents have been used for the management of patients with a wide range of medical issues, such as organ transplantation, autoimmune diseases, asthma, and rheumatoid arthritis, among others. All of the agents have relatively narrow therapeutic ranges, with significant dose-limiting toxicities. This chapter discusses the following immunosuppressive agents: azathioprine, cyclosporine, glucocorticoids, mycophenolate mofetil, and tacrolimus. For each, this chapter reviews the major metabolic pathways, the enzymes involved in metabolism, the metabolite activity, and the drug interactions. Even for the agents whose use has been established for a while, such as azathioprine and glucocorticoids, modern understanding is still incomplete.

AZATHIOPRINE

Major Metabolic Pathways *In Vivo*

Azathioprine, a chemical analogue of the purines, is a compound that undergoes significant metabolism. It is rapidly converted *in vivo* to 6-mercaptopurine (1–5). Subsequently, the metabolism of 6-mercaptopurine proceeds by way of three pathways, including degradation to thiouric acid (4,6), conversion to thiopurine nucleotides (3–5,7,8), and methylation of the thiol group (9,10). As is discussed later, many of these metabolites have immunosuppressive properties.

Specific Enzymes

There are several enzymes involved in the metabolism of azathioprine and the subsequent metabolism of 6-mer-

captopurine. Azathioprine is converted to 6-mercaptopurine by glutathione-S-transferase (11–13). The three separate pathways by which 6-mercaptopurine is metabolized involves three distinct enzymes. The metabolism of 6-mercaptopurine to thiouric acid occurs via xanthine oxidase (6). This is an essential pathway in the detoxification of this compound. Inhibition of this pathway can lead to life-threatening bone marrow suppression. The metabolism of 6-mercaptopurine to the thiopurine nucleotides occurs by way of hypoxanthine guanine phosphoribosyltransferase. Elevated levels of the 6-thioguanine nucleotides have been associated with the myelotoxicity of azathioprine and 6-mercaptopurine. Thiol methylation of 6-mercaptopurine occurs via thiopurine methyltransferase (9,10). Thiopurine methyltransferase is controlled by a common genetic polymorphism, with one in 300 subjects being homozygous for low activity, approximately 11% with intermediate activity, and 89% high enzyme activity (14,15). The clinical significance of this polymorphism with respect to azathioprine is not well understood.

Metabolite Activity

The immunosuppressive effects of azathioprine and its metabolites are multifaceted. Several of the metabolites (including 6-mercaptopurine, 6-thioguanine nucleotides, thioinosinic acid, and the S-methylated thiopurines) exhibit immunosuppressive effects. Thioinosinic acid competitively inhibits hypoxanthine-guanine phosphoribosyltransferase, resulting in inhibition of nucleic acid and protein synthesis. Several metabolites of 6-mercaptopurine reduce endogenous purines, such as the 6-thioguanine nucleotides and S-methylated thiopurines. The 6-thioguanine nucleotides can also incorporate into RNA and DNA (16–19). In addition, elevated levels of 6-thioguanine nucleotides have been associated with azathioprine myelotoxicity (3,8,20,21). On the other hand,

M. F. Hebert: Department of Pharmacy, University of Washington, Box 357630, H375 Health Sciences Center, Seattle, Washington 98195-7610

499

not all metabolites of 6-mercaptopurine are active, such as 6-thiouric acid (22). The formation of 6-thiouric acid is a detoxifying pathway for 6-mercaptopurine.

Drug Interactions, Enzyme Inhibitors

Allopurinol, a known inhibitor of xanthine oxidase (23), has been found to dramatically decrease the metabolism of 6-mercaptopurine. Allopurinol pretreatment has been shown to increase the peak plasma concentration and the area under the concentration time curve (AUC) of oral 6-mercaptopurine by 500% (24). The decreased metabolism of 6-mercaptopurine associated with concomitant administration of allopurinol and azathioprine, has resulted in clinically significant bone marrow suppression. In some cases, the myelosuppression has been severe or even fatal (25–28). Anticipatory azathioprine dose reduction, with the initiation of allopurinol, appears to decrease the risk of myelosuppression, but does not always eliminate it (25). In general, avoiding this combination is wise.

CYCLOSPORINE

Major Metabolic Pathways *In Vivo*

Cyclosporine is a lipophilic, cyclic polypeptide containing 11 amino acids. Its molecular weight is 1202.63 Da. More than 30 metabolites of cyclosporine have been identified (29–31). After much confusion regarding the identification of the various metabolites, standardization of the nomenclature for the metabolites was developed and described in the 1990 consensus document (32). Both primary and secondary metabolism of cyclosporine occurs. Hydroxylation, *N*-demethylation, cyclization, and oxidation to the aldehyde or acid, all take place in the metabolism process.

Some metabolites, such as AM1, AM9, AM1c, AM19, and AM4N, can usually be measured in the blood of patients with normal hepatic function (33,34). Following cyclosporine administration, AM1 has the highest concentration in humans not receiving interacting agents (33). The major metabolites in bile include AM19, AM1c9, AM4N9, AM1A, AM1, and AM1c. The dominant metabolite in bile is AM1A (35–41). Only a small amount of cyclosporine is excreted unchanged by the kidney (33) or in feces (30).

Specific Enzymes

Cyclosporine is metabolized by cytochrome P450 3A4 (CYP3A4) and to a lesser extent cytochrome P450 3A5 (CYP3A5) (42–44). Both CYP3A4 and CYP3A5 exist in human liver (45,46) and intestine (42). It is clear that hepatic metabolism is a major site of elimination for cyclosporine. However, Wu and colleagues (47), through

the analysis of three drug interaction studies (48–50), showed the clinical importance of the intestinal metabolism of cyclosporine as well. Kolars and co-workers (51) measured the metabolites of cyclosporine (AM9 and AM4N) in the portal veins of patients during the anhepatic phase of liver transplantation. An interfering substance prevented AM1 from being measured. If the rate of formation of AM1 and AM9 were the same in these patients as was seen in enterocyte microsomal preparations, then as much as 50% of orally administered cyclosporine may be metabolized in the intestine.

Another factor that appears to play a significant role in the metabolism of cyclosporine is P-glycoprotein (P-gp). P-gp is a membrane efflux pump that, when overly expressed, has been associated with multidrug resistance in tumor cells (52). P-gp works by pumping drugs out of the cell, thereby keeping intracellular concentrations low (53). P-gp is also expressed on the surface of normal cells, such as small and large intestinal epithelium, bile canaliculi, and kidney proximal tubules (54). Lown and colleagues (55) conducted the first study documenting the clinical importance of intestinal P-gp. In 19 kidney transplant patients who underwent the erythromycin breath test (to estimate hepatic CYP3A4 activity), small intestinal biopsies (to measure intestinal CYP3A4 and P-gp), and steady-state oral cyclosporine pharmacokinetics, it was found that 56% of the variability in the apparent oral cyclosporine clearance could be explained by hepatic CYP3A4 activity and 17% of the variability could be explained by intestinal P-gp content. The variability of oral cyclosporine pharmacokinetics did not appear to be influenced by intestinal CYP3A4 content. Therefore, although intestinal metabolism appears to be important for the pharmacokinetics of cyclosporine, it may be enzyme exposure (regulated by P-gp), rather than content, that dictates overall intestinal impact.

Metabolite Activity

Limited information is available on the immunosuppressive or toxic effects of the metabolites of cyclosporine. One problem in obtaining this information is a direct result of the difficulty in obtaining sufficient quantities of purified metabolites to conduct the studies. Another problem is that animal studies have questionable application to humans. Animal immune response as well as tolerance of nephrotoxicity can be quite different than human responses. *In vitro* studies have similar limitations. *In vitro* immunosuppressive studies have found that AM1 and AM9 have much lower immunosuppressive effects than cyclosporine. AM1 has been found to cause approximately 10% (56,57) of the immunosuppressive effects as cyclosporine and AM9 about 3% (56). Attempting to evaluate the nephrotoxicity of the metabolites, Donatsch and co-workers (58) found that subcutaneous administration of AM1, AM9, and AM4N did not cause nephrotoxicity in rats. Sewing and associates (59) conducted an *in vivo* study in liver transplant patients to evaluate the nephrotoxicity of the metabolites. They reported that liver transplant patients with renal dysfunction had elevated levels of AM1c9. It is unclear whether the elevated levels of AM1c9 is a cause of the renal impairment or a result of impaired clearance of the metabolite in patients with renal dysfunction.

Drug Interactions

Many agents have been shown to interact with cyclosporine. Interactions can be used intentionally to assist clinicians in maintaining therapeutic cyclosporine levels and, in some cases, decreasing drug costs. The addition of a known enzyme inhibitor can decrease cyclosporine dosing requirements, thereby decreasing drug costs (60). This benefit can be obtained if the inhibitor is less costly than the cyclosporine. An unexpected or unintentional interaction with cyclosporine can lead to significant problems. For example, the addition of an enzyme inhibitor (e.g., ketoconazole or erythromycin) to a patient's drug therapy when the patient has been stabilized on cyclosporine can result in substantial renal impairment as a result of elevated cyclosporine levels. On the other hand, the addition of an enzyme inducer (e.g., rifampin or phenytoin) can lead to a decrease in cyclosporine concentrations and lack of efficacy.

Although drug interactions are becoming better understood, they are not completely understood. Cyclosporine is metabolized by CYP3A4 and CYP3A5 in the liver and intestine. In addition, cyclosporine is a substrate for P-gp. Any agent given concomitantly with cyclosporine, which induces or inhibits CYP3A4, CYP3A5, or P-gp, will potentially alter the concentration of cyclosporine. The data currently available for assessing the mechanisms of drug interactions, are incomplete and potentially limited in their applicability to the clinical situation. The evaluation of drug-induced changes in CYP3A has usually been done *in vitro* in animal or human microsomal systems. In other cases, a probe compound has been used to assess the effects of various drugs on the enzymes of interest. Assessments of the impact of various agents on P-gp have been done *in vitro* with animals or on multidrug-resistant tumor cell lines. The *in vitro* data may or may not correlate with what is actually taking place *in vivo* in humans.

Drug Interactions, Enzyme Inhibitors

Many agents have been shown to increase cyclosporine concentrations and potentially lead to cyclosporine-induced toxicity (Table 37-1). Because of the immunosuppressive and hypertensive effects of cyclosporine, the antifungal azoles, macrolide antibiotics, and some of the calcium channel blockers are of particular clinical interest because they potentially would be added to the drug therapy of a patient who has been stabilized on cyclosporine. It appears that the drug interactions may affect both intestinal as well as hepatic metabolism (47–49). When coadministered, the antifungal azoles can increase cyclosporine concentrations. It appears that ketoconazole has the greatest effect, followed by itraconazole and then fluconazole. Gomez and associates (49) found that ketoconazole decreased the clearance of cyclosporine in healthy volunteers (0.32 ± 0.09 L/hr/kg versus 0.18 ± 0.05 L/hr/kg) and increased its bioavailability ($22.4\% \pm 4.8\%$ versus $56.4\% \pm 11.7\%$). The large increase in bioavailability was greater than could be explained by the decrease in hepatic clearance alone. This finding is consistent with ketoconazole having an effect on intestinal P-gp and/or intestinal CYP3A4 as well as hepatic metabolism. In this case, the *in vitro* data (i.e., ketoconazole inhibits CYP3A and P-gp activity) are consistent with the clinical results (i.e., ketoconazole results in increased cyclosporine levels) (see Table 37-1).

The macrolide antibiotics seem to have complex effects on CYP3A (see Table 37-1). First, they appear to increase CYP3A content (45). In addition, they inhibit CYP3A activity (69,88,89). This inhibition, in part, occurs through metabolism of the macrolide antibiotics. The metabolites tightly bind to the heme moiety of CYP3A, forming an inactive stable complex (115). Gant and colleagues (90)

TABLE 37-1. *Agents that increase cyclosporine levels in vivo and their effects on CYP3A and P-glycoprotein*

Agent (ref.)	CYP3A effect (ref.)	P-glycoprotein effect (ref.)
Amiodarone (61–63)		Inhibits (64–66)
Clarithromycin (67,68)	Inhibits (69)	
Diltiazem (70–74)	Inhibits (110)	Inhibits (75,76)
Erythromycin (50,77–87)	Increases content, Inhibits (69,88,89)	Increases expression (90)
Fluconazole (91–94)	Inhibits (69)	
Grapefruit juice (95)	Inhibits (96,97)	
Itraconazole (98–100)	Inhibits (69)	Inhibits (101)
Ketoconazole (49,102–106)	Inhibits (69,107)	Inhibits (108)
Nicardipine (109)	Inhibits (110)	Inhibits (111)
Verapamil (74,112,113)	Inhibits (110)	Inhibits Decreases expression (64,65,75,114)

found that erythromycin increases *mdr2* mRNA. The expression of *mdr2*, should increase biliary P-gp content. Whether or not erythromycin would also increase intestinal P-gp has yet to be determined. Nonetheless, the dominant effect of erythromycin on the metabolism of CYP3A substrates, such as cyclosporine, is inhibition. Gupta and colleagues (50) demonstrated this effect by showing that erythromycin slightly decreased the clearance of cyclosporine (0.31 ± 0.16 L/hr/kg versus 0.27 ± 0.15 L/hr/kg). At the same time, erythromycin dramatically increased the bioavailability of cyclosporine ($36 \pm 12\%$ versus $60 \pm 20\%$). As with the antifungal azoles, erythromycin appears to have a greater effect on intestinal metabolism than hepatic CYP3A.

When evaluating the calcium channel blockers, it is important to evaluate each agent individually. That is, it is not possible to look at the class of drugs as a whole with respect to drug interaction potential. Some agents, such as verapamil (74,112,113), diltiazem (70–74), and nicardipine (109), when given concomitantly with cyclosporine, lead to elevated cyclosporine concentrations. Other calcium channel blockers, such as nifedipine (113) and isradipine (116), do not appear to alter cyclosporine levels.

Drug Interactions, Enzyme Inducers

Other agents, primarily the antituberculosis agent rifampin and some of the antiseizure medications (Table 37-2), have been shown to lower cyclosporine levels. Although rifampin may have a complex interaction affecting both CYP3A and P-gp, the ultimate result is a decrease in cyclosporine levels. Hebert and associates have shown (48) that rifampin clearly increases cyclosporine clearance in healthy volunteers (0.30 ± 0.05 L/hr/kg versus 0.42 ± 0.10 L/hr/kg) through induction of hepatic metabolism. In addition, rifampin markedly decreased cyclosporine bioavailability ($27 \pm 9\%$ versus $10 \pm 3\%$). The large decrease in bioavailability can be explained by rifampin inducing intestinal CYP3A and/or P-gp as well as hepatic metabolism.

TABLE 37-2. *Agents that decrease cyclosporine levels in vivo and their effects on CYP3A and P-glycoprotein*

Agent (ref.)	CYP3A effect (ref.)	P-glycoprotein effect (ref.)
Carbamazepine (117)	Induces (110,118)	
Phenobarbital (119)	Induces (45,120–125)	Induces (126)
Phenytoin (127,128)	Induces (110,118)	Induces (126)
Rifampin (48,129–134)	Induces (135,136)	Induces
		Inhibits (126,137)

GLUCOCORTICOIDS

Major Metabolic Pathways *In Vivo*

Many systemic glucocorticoids are available (e.g., cortisol, cortisone, prednisone, prednisolone, dexamethasone, methylprednisolone). In general, steroid metabolism involves sequential hydroxylation, followed by conjugation to water-soluble metabolites. Cortisol (11β, 17, 21-trihydrxoypregn-4-ene-3,20-dione) and cortisone (17, 21-dihydroxypregn-4-ene-3,11,20-trione) are endogenously produced corticosteroids. They can also be administered exogenously. Cortisol, also known as hydrocortisone, has been found to be metabolized to many metabolites, with the dominant route being A-ring reduction and subsequent conjugation (138,139). A-ring reduction can occur with both cortisol and cortisone, leading to tetrahydrocortisol and tetrahydrocortisone (140). Relatively smaller quantities of unconjugated polar metabolites (e.g., 6β-hydroxycortisol, 6β-hydroxycortisone, 2α-hydroxycortisone, 6α-hydroxycortisol, as well as 11-keto and 11-hydroxy metabolites of cortisol) have also been recovered in urine (138). Canalis and co-workers (141) found that 6β-hydroxycortisol is the major unconjugated urinary metabolite of cortisol, making up approximately 1% of the total cortisol secretion. Kornel and colleagues (142) measured cortisol and its metabolites in human plasma. Glucuronide conjugates, including steroids reduced at the A-ring and those not reduced at the A-ring but hydroxylated in C-6 position or reduced at C-20, were present in the highest concentrations ($47.4\% \pm 2.8\%$ of total). The next highest concentrations in plasma were the free steroids, primarily cortisol and cortisone ($45.1\% \pm 4.7\%$ of total). Sulfate conjugates ($3.6\% \pm 1.0\%$ of total) followed a similar pattern as the glucuronide conjugates. Very polar metabolites of cortisol, those hydroxylated at C-6 and reduced at C-20 and bound to nucleosides, made up $3.9\% \pm 1.0\%$ of the total metabolites.

Prednisone (17α, 21-dihydroxypregna-1,4-diene-3,11,20-trione) and prednisolone (11β, 17α, 21-trihydroxypregna-1,4-diene-3, 20-dione) are synthetic analogues of cortisol. Like cortisol, prednisolone can be hydroxylated at the 6β position. Urinary elimination of 6β-hydroxyprednisolone makes up 8% to 10% of the dose when either prednisone or prednisolone is administered (143,144). Following oral administration of prednisone, prednisolone concentrations are four- to ten-fold greater than prednisone concentrations (145–147). The pharmacokinetics of prednisone and prednisolone have been shown to be nonlinear (145,148–152). This may in part be related to the concentration-dependent binding of prednisolone to plasma proteins (150,153). Conversion of prednisone to prednisolone can be followed by partial reconversion back to prednisone (154,155). The interconversion appears to favor prednisolone, in that the concentrations of prednisolone are 4 to 10 times higher than prednisone when either prednisone or prednisolone is administered (154).

The nonlinear relationship of the AUC ratio for prednisone and prednisolone may be due to dose-dependent interconversion between the two or different degrees of nonlinearity in disposition. Both prednisone and prednisolone can also undergo reduction of the 20-ketone group (155). The interconversion of prednisone and prednisolone is thought to be rapid and efficient. Equal doses of prednisolone and prednisone produce similar prednisone concentration time profiles (156). Both prednisone and prednisolone are primarily metabolized. When either prednisone (143–145, 154) or prednisolone (143,144,154,157) is administered, only a small amount is excreted in the urine as prednisone (2%–5%) or prednisolone (7%–24%). The major pathway of elimination of both agents is biotransformation to a variety of oxidative products.

Specific Enzymes

The enzymes involved in the interconversion of cortisol and cortisone, as well as prednisone and prednisolone, have not been determined. Although a relatively minor pathway, cortisol is thought to be metabolized to 6β-hydroxycortisol by CYP3A (158). Both CYP3A4 and CYP3A5 catalyze the 6β-hydroxylation of cortisol. CYP3A5 catalyzes the reaction at about one-half the rate of CYP3A4 *in vitro* (159). The urinary excretion of 6β-hydroxycortisol, or its ratio to cortisol, initially was suggested to be a marker of CYP3A activity. However, Hunt and colleagues (160) found no correlation between the urinary ratio of 6β-hydroxycortisol/cortisol and erythromycin *N*-demethylation, as measured by the erythromycin breath test. Although the ratio of 6β-hydroxycortisol/cortisol may be a good marker of enzyme induction (161–163), it may not correlate well with hepatic CYP3A activity ($r = 0.59$, as measured by the erythromycin breath test) (164), because of the many other factors that may affect the ratio, such as extrahepatic CYP3A activity as well as potential contributions by more than one CYP3A isozyme.

Metabolite Activity

Even though cortisol, cortisone, prednisone, and prednisolone can be administered exogenously for their glucocorticoid effects, only cortisol and prednisolone are active. The metabolic interconversion of the agents to the active forms allows for agents such as prednisone and cortisone to be therapeutically effective. Cortisone and prednisone have low binding affinities for the glucocorticoid receptor as compared with hydrocortisone and prednisolone (165). Cortisone and prednisone presumably also have no antiinflammatory activity (166).

Drug Interactions, Enzyme Inhibitors

One clinical difficulty with drug interactions that alter glucocorticoid levels is that therapeutic monitoring of blood or plasma concentrations for these agents is not routinely done. Ketoconazole and oral contraceptives have been shown to decrease the clearance of prednisolone (143,167–169). Zurcher and colleagues (143) reported that ketoconazole significantly reduced prednisolone clearance (2.37 ± 0.30 mL/min/kg versus 1.72 ± 0.20 mL/min/kg) with no change in the ratio of AUCs for prednisolone/prednisone in healthy volunteers. Boekenoogen and co-workers (167) reported that oral contraceptive users had a much lower clearance of prednisolone (96 ± 89 mL/min/1.73 m²) than female controls (187 ± 22 mL/min/1.73 m²). Legler and Benet (168) found that, although dose-dependent prednisolone kinetics were maintained, women on oral contraceptives had a substantial decrease in prednisolone clearance.

Drug Interactions, Enzyme Inducers

As with cyclosporine, rifampin and some of the antiseizure medications can induce the metabolism of the glucocorticoids. Concomitant administration of rifampin with the corticosteroids has resulted in an increase in prednisolone clearance and exacerbation of underlying disease (170,171). In addition, the metabolism of endogenous corticosteroids appears to be induced by rifampin (158,172). Buffington and associates (170) reported three cases of renal transplant patients in whom renal allograft dysfunction appeared to develop as a result of rifampin inducing the metabolism of the glucocorticoids. The hydroxylation of the 3-keto-Δ^4 steroids at the 6β position is usually a minor pathway, but it can be induced by rifampin (158,172). Mean urinary excretion of 6β-hydroxycortisol increased 268% to 416% with rifampin (172). Similar results were found by others (158, 173). Roots and colleagues (161) reported a four-fold increase in urinary excretion of 6β-hydroxycortisol and no change in 17-hydroxy corticosteroids with rifampin as compared with controls.

Phenobarbital has been shown to induce the metabolism of endogenous as well as exogenously administered glucocorticoids. Hydroxylation of 3-keto-Δ^4 steroids at the 6β position can be induced by phenobarbital (158,172). This induction has been associated with 105% increase in the mean urinary 6β-hydroxycortisol excretion (172). Saenger and colleagues (174) found that phenobarbital increased 6β-hydroxycortisol levels in random urine samples four- to five-fold. Brooks and associates (175) found that phenobarbital increased the urinary excretion of 6-hydroxycortisol from a mean of 0.17 mg/day to 0.32 mg/day in seven patients with asthma. In addition, three prednisone-dependent patients with asthma underwent clinical worsening with the initiation of phenobarbital. Brooks and colleagues (176) found that phenobarbital was associated with a shorter prednisolone half-life, leading to the clinical worsening of disease in nine patients with rheumatoid arthritis.

Phenytoin has been associated with an increase in clearance of prednisolone (177) and cortisol (178). Werk and associates (163) have also shown that phenytoin alters the metabolism of cortisol, increasing the proportion excreted as polar unconjugated metabolites, such as 6-hydroxycortisol, and a decrease in the proportion undergoing A-ring reduction and glucuronide conjugation. They also found an increase in conversion of tetrahydrocortisol to tetrahydrocortisone and other tetrahydro metabolites. Phenytoin was also found to slightly decrease the urinary excretion of 17-hydroxycorticosteroids and 17-ketosteroids. However, earlier work showed that plasma levels of 17-hydroxycorticosteroids are normal during phenytoin therapy (179,180). Roots and associates (161) found an average nine-fold increase in urinary excretion of 6β-hydroxycortisol with phenytoin alone or phenytoin in combination with primidone, diazepam, clonazepam, or carbamazepine. Moreland and co-workers (162) found that carbamazepine tripled the urinary excretion of 6β-hydroxycortisol.

MYCOPHENOLATE MOFETIL

Major Metabolic Pathways *In Vivo*

Mycophenolate mofetil (2-morpholinoethyl ester of mycophenolic acid) appears to be rapidly and completely metabolized to mycophenolic acid. Following oral administration of mycophenolate mofetil, parent compound has not been quantifiable in plasma (181, 182). With intravenous administration of mycophenolate mofetil, parent compound is only detectable in plasma during the infusion. After discontinuation of the infusion, mycophenolate mofetil is no longer measurable in plasma (183). Mycophenolic acid concentrations were found to peak at the end of the infusion (183). Mycophenolic acid is subsequently conjugated to mycophenolic acid glucuronide, which is the primary urinary excretion product (182,183). Following a single intravenous dose of mycophenolate mofetil, more than 80% of the administered dose was excreted in urine as mycophenolic acid glucuronide, and less than 1% as mycophenolic acid (183). Following long-term dosing of oral mycophenolate mofetil, the AUC for mycophenolic acid glucuronide is 24 to 65 times that of mycophenolic acid in liver transplant patients (181). Following a single intravenous dose of mycophenolate mofetil, the AUC for mycophenolic acid glucuronide is approximately three-fold higher than for mycophenolic acid (183). Mycophenolic acid appears to undergo enterohepatic recirculation as a result of biliary excretion of mycophenolic acid glucuronide and reconversion to mycophenolic acid in the intestine. This results in a second peak in the plasma concentration time curve for mycophenolic acid (184). Three other metabolites have been recovered in the urine following oral administra-

tion of mycophenolate mofetil (N-(2-carboxymethyl)-morpholine, N-(2-hydroxyethyl)-morpholine, and N-oxide of N-(2-hydroxyethyl)-morpholine) (185).

Specific Enzymes

The ethyl ester is cleaved off of mycophenolate mofetil, producing mycophenolic acid by esterases. Mycophenolic acid is then conjugated to mycophenolic acid glucuronide by glucuronyl transferase (185). This reaction can also be reversed, removing the glucuronide and producing free mycophenolic acid, most likely by intestinal bacteria glucuronidases.

Metabolite Activity

The *in vitro* antiproliferative effects of mycophenolate mofetil and mycophenolic acid are approximately the same. They have similar concentration response curves for human peripheral blood cells simulated by phytohemagglutinin (PHA, a T-cell mitogen) (186). Mycophenolate mofetil has also been shown to inhibit mixed lymphocyte culture (187), tetanus-specific IgG memory (187), and pokeweed mitogen (PWM, T-dependent B-cell mitogen) (188) and IgG (188) responses *in vitro*.

Mycophenolic acid inhibits inosine monophosphate dehydrogenase, thereby decreasing guanine nucleotide levels (189–194). Inhibition of inosine monophosphate dehydrogenase results in inhibition of *de novo* purine synthesis and lymphocyte proliferation (190,194–197). The type II isoform of inosine monophosphate dehydrogenase is five times more susceptible than the type I isoform to mycophenolic acid inhibition (193,195). Mycophenolic acid has also been shown to inhibit the attachment of monocytes to endothelial cells and laminin (198), thus inhibiting adhesion. Mycophenolic acid concentrations between 2.0 and 5.0 mg/L have been shown *in vitro* to inhibit inosine monophosphate dehydrogenase by approximately 50% (192). Mycophenolic acid glucuronide has much less effect on inosine monophosphate dehydrogenase than mycophenolic acid (192). Concentrations of mycophenolic acid glucuronide of 100 mg/L inhibit inosine monophosphate dehydrogenase activity by approximately 26% (192). Concentrations higher than that were not studied.

Drug Interactions

There are currently no known metabolic drug interactions with mycophenolate mofetil. However, there are two agents known to substantially alter the AUC of mycophenolic acid. Antacids (aluminum and magnesium hydroxide), when given concomitantly with mycophenolate mofetil, reduce the maximum concentration achieved by 15% and the 24-hour AUC by 37% for both mycophenolic acid and mycophenolic acid glucuronide.

The decrease in absorption seen may be a result of chelation (199). The coadministration of cholestyramine and mycophenolate mofetil has also been associated with a decrease in the AUC for mycophenolic acid by approximately 40% (185).

TACROLIMUS

Major Metabolic Pathways *In Vivo*

Tacrolimus is a 23-member macrolide lactone, with a molecular weight of 803.5 Da. At least nine metabolites have been identified (200–202). Tacrolimus appears to undergo demethylation or hydroxylation. Christians and colleagues (201) studied tacrolimus and its metabolites in liver transplant patients. They found tacrolimus and a demethylated metabolite in the blood. In urine, they found tacrolimus, a didemethylated and hydroxylated metabolite, and two didemethylated metabolites. When analyzing bile, they found a dihydroxylated metabolite, a didemethylated metabolite, a didemethylated and hydroxylated metabolite, and a didemethylated and dihydroxylated metabolite.

Specific Enzymes

Tacrolimus metabolism and transport by P-gp is similar to that of cyclosporine. Tacrolimus is metabolized primarily by CYP3A4 (203). Lampen and co-workers (204) have shown that tacrolimus is metabolized *in vitro* by both liver and intestinal microsomes. Formation of tacrolimus metabolites was similar in human liver and intestinal microsomes. Saeki and colleagues (205) reported that tacrolimus is transported by P-gp as well.

Metabolite Activity

Christians and co-workers (200) purified two tacrolimus metabolites. They found that the demethylated metabolite retained 10% of the immunosuppressive activity of tacrolimus [as determined by phytohemagglutinin (PHA) stimulation of human lymphocytes] and the double demethylated metabolite 7% of the parent compound immunosuppressive activity. Iwasaki and colleagues (202) evaluated the immunosuppressive effects of tacrolimus metabolites produced in phenobarbital-treated rat liver microsomes. Four metabolites were identified and tested for immunosuppressive effects. Two of the metabolites had negligible immunosuppressive effects (*O*-demethylated at position 15 and monohydroxylated at position 12 with a tetrahydrofuran ring configuration). One of the metabolites had comparable immunosuppressive activity to tacrolimus (*O*-demethylated at position 31). The fourth metabolite had less than one-tenth the activity of tacrolimus (*O*-demethylated at position 13 and tetrahydrofuran ring arrangement).

TABLE 37-3. *Agents that increase tacrolimus levels in vivo and their effects on CYP3A and P-glycoprotein*

Agent (ref.)	CYP3A effect (ref.)	P-glycoprotein effect (ref.)
Erythromycin (206,207)	Increases content Inhibits (69,88,89)	Increases expression (90)
Fluconazole (208)	Inhibits (69)	
Ketoconazole (209)	Inhibits (69,107)	Inhibits (108)

Drug Interactions

Available information on drug interactions is much more limited with tacrolimus than with cyclosporine. This is most likely a result of the shorter time that tacrolimus has been available. Until data are available to the contrary, it should be assumed that those agents that interact with cyclosporine will also interact with tacrolimus.

Drug Interactions, Enzyme Inhibitors

As with cyclosporine, agents such as the macrolide antibiotics (i.e., erythromycin) and the azole antifungal agents (i.e., ketoconazole and fluconazole) have been associated with increased tacrolimus levels (Table 37-3). Floren and colleagues (209) conducted a study in healthy volunteers that showed a significant increase in tacrolimus bioavailability (14% ± 5% versus 30% ± 8%) with ketoconazole. At the same time, there was no consistent change in clearance or volume of distribution. The change in bioavailability can be explained by a local inhibitory effect of ketoconazole on tacrolimus intestinal metabolism or P-gp transport.

Drug Interactions, Enzyme Inducers

There is a published case report documenting decreased tacrolimus levels with rifampin (210). This interaction is expected, because rifampin is known to induce CYP3A activity (135,136). The P-gp effect of rifampin appears mixed, with both induction and inhibition having been reported (126,137). In addition, the interaction between rifampin and cyclosporine has been well described, with rifampin increasing cyclosporine clearance and dramatically decreasing bioavailability (48).

SUMMARY

The metabolism of the immunosuppressive agents (azathioprine, cyclosporine, glucocorticoids, mycophenolate mofetil, and tacrolimus) is complex. Each agent undergoes primary, secondary, and in some cases tertiary metabolism to multiple metabolites. Some of the metabolites are active and others are not. Several enzymes are involved in the metabolism of these compounds. In addition, P-gp plays a significant role in the intestinal metabolism of cyclosporine and tacrolimus. All of the immunosuppressive agents have relatively narrow therapeutic ranges, significant dose-limiting toxicities, and undergo clinically important drug interactions. The concomitant administration of enzyme inducers can lead to decreased concentrations of the immunosuppressive agents and impair effectiveness. The concomitant administration of enzyme inhibitors can lead to elevated concentrations and increased toxicity. Caution is warranted when using combination therapy involving the immunosuppressive agents and potentially interacting compounds.

REFERENCES

1. Lin S-N, Jessup K, Ployd M, et al. Quantitation of plasma azathioprine and 6-mercaptopurine levels in renal transplant patients. *Transplantation* 1980;29:290–294.
2. Odlind B, Hartvig P, Lindstrom B, Lonnerholm G, Tufveson G, Grefberg N. Serum azathioprine and 6-mercaptopurine levels and immunosuppressive activity after azathioprine in uremic patients. *Int J Immunopharmacol* 1986;8:1–11.
3. Lennard L, Brown CB, Fox M, Maddocks JL. Azathioprine metabolism in kidney transplant recipients. *Br J Clin Pharmacol* 1984;18:693–700.
4. Chan GLC, Erdmann GR, Gruber SA, Matas AJ, Canafax DM. Azathioprine metabolism: pharmacokinetics of 6-mercaptopurine, 6-thiouric acid and 6-thioguanine nucleotides in renal transplant patients. *J Clin Pharmacol* 1990;30:358–363.
5. Lennard L, Maddocks JL. Assay of 6-thioguanine nucleotide, a major metabolite of azathioprine, 6-mercaptopurine and 6-thioguanine in human red blood cells. *J Pharm Pharmacol* 1983;35:15–18.
6. Elion GB, Callahan S, Nathan H, Bieber S, Rundles RW, Hitchings GH. Potentiation by inhibition of drug degradation: 6-substituted purines and xanthine oxidase. *Biochem Pharmacol* 1963;12:85–93.
7. Bergan S, Rugstad HE, Bentadal O, Stokke O. Monitoring of azathioprine treatment by determination of 6-thioguanine nucleotide concentrations in erythrocytes. *Transplantation* 1994;58:803–808.
8. Lennard L, Harrington CI, Wood M, Maddocks JL. Metabolism of azathioprine to 6-thioguanine nucleotides in patients with pemphigus vulgaris. *Br J Clin Pharmacol* 1987;23:229–233.
9. Remy CN. Metabolism of thiopyrimidines and thiopurines: S-methylation with S-adenosylmethionine transmethylase and catabolism in mammalian tissue. *J Biol Chem* 1963;238:1078–1084.
10. Woodson LC, Weinshilboum RM. Human kidney thiopurine methyltransferase: purification and biochemical properties. *Biochem Pharmacol* 1983;32:819–826.
11. Kaplowitz N, Kuhlenkamp J. Inhibition of hepatic metabolism of azathioprine in vivo. *Gastroenterology* 1978;74:90–92.
12. Watanabe A, Hobara N, Nagashima H. Demonstration of enzymatic activity converting azathioprine to 6-mercaptopurine. *Acta Med Okayama* 1978;32:173–179.
13. Hobara N, Watanabe A. Impaired metabolism of azathioprine in carbon tetrachloride-injured rats. *Hepato Gastroenterol* 1981;28:192–194.
14. Weinshilboum RM, Sludek SL. Mercaptopurine pharmacogenetics: monogenic inheritance of erythrocyte thiopurine methyltransferase activity. *Am J Hum Genet* 1980;32:651–662.
15. Szumlanski CL, Honchel R, Scott MC, Weinshilboum RM. Human liver thiopurine methyltransferase pharmacogenetics: biochemical properties, liver-erythrocyte correlation and presence of isozymes. *Pharmacogenetics* 1992;2:148–159.
16. Scannell JP, Hitchings GH. Thioguanine in deoxyribonucleic acid from tumors of 6-mercaptopurine–treated mice. *Proc Soc Exp Biol Med* 1966;122:627–629.
17. Bieber S, Dietrich LS, Elion GB, Hitchings GH, Martin DS. The incorporation of 6-mercaptopurine-S^{35} into the nucleic acids of sensitive and nonsensitive transplantable mouse tumors. *Cancer Res* 1961;21:228–231.
18. Tidd DM, Paterson ARP. A biochemical mechanism for the delayed cytotoxic reaction of 6-mercaptopurine. *Cancer Res* 1974;34:738–746.
19. Tay BS, Lilley RM, Murray AW, Atkinson MR. Inhibition of phosphoribosyl pyrophosphate amidotransferase from Ehrlich ascites—tumor cells by thiopurine nucleotides. *Biochem Pharmacol* 1969;18:936–938.
20. Schutz E, Gummert J, Mohr FW, Armstrong VW, Oellerich M. Azathioprine myelotoxicity related to elevated 6-thioguanine nucleotides in heart transplantation. *Transplant Proc* 1995;27:1298–1300.
21. Lennard L, Van Loon JA, Weinshilboum RM. Pharmacogenetics of acute azathioprine toxicity: relationship to thiopurine methyltransferase genetic polymorphism. *Clin Pharmacol Ther* 1989;46:149–154.
22. Elion GB, Callahan S, Rundles RW, Hitchings GH. Relationships between metabolic fates and antitumour activities of thiopurines. *Cancer Res* 1963;23:1207–1217.
23. Watts RWE, Watts JEM, Seegmiller JE. Xanthine oxidase activity in human tissues and its inhibition by allopurinol. *J Lab Clin Med* 1965;66:688–697.
24. Zimm S, Collins JM, O'Neill D, Chabner BA, Poplack DG. Inhibition of first-pass metabolism in cancer chemotherapy: interaction of 6-mercaptopurine and allopurinol. *Clin Pharmacol Ther* 1983;34:810–816.
25. Cummins D, Sekar M, Halil O, Banner N. Myelosuppression associated with azathioprine–allopurinol interaction after heart and lung transplantation. *Transplantation* 1996;61:1661–1662.
26. Schutz E, Gummert J, Mohr FW, Armstrong VW, Oellerich M. Should 6-thioguanine nucleotides be monitored in heart transplant recipients given azathioprine? *Ther Drug Monit* 1996;18:228–233.
27. Venkat Raman G, Sharman VL, Lee HA. Azathioprine and allopurinol: a potentially dangerous combination. *J Intern Med* 1990;228:69–71.
28. Kennedy DT, Hayney MS, Lake KD. Azathioprine and allopurinol: the price of an avoidable drug interaction. *Ann Pharmacother* 1996;30:951–954.
29. Maurer G, Loosli HR, Schreier E, Keller B. Disposition of cyclosporin in several animal species and man. I. Structural elucidation of its metabolites. *Drug Metab Dispos* 1984;12:120–126.
30. Maurer G, Lemaire M. Biotransformation and distribution in blood of cyclosporin and its metabolites. *Transplant Proc* 1986;18:25–34.
31. Christians U, Schlitt HJ, Bleck JS, et al. Measurement of cyclosporine and 18 metabolites in blood, bile and urine by high-performance liquid chromatography (HPLC). *Transplant Proc* 1988;20:609–613.
32. Kahan BD, Shaw LM, Holt D, Grevel J, Johnston A. Consensus document: Hawk's Cay meeting on therapeutic drug monitoring of cyclosporine. *Clin Chem* 1990;36:1510–1516.
33. Bleck JS, Schlitt HJ, Christians U, et al. Urinary excretion of cyclosporin and 17 of its metabolites in renal allograft recipients. *Pharmacology* 1989;39:160–164.
34. Awni WM, Kasiske BL, Heim-Duthoy K, Rao KV. Long-term cyclosporin pharmacokinetic changes in renal transplant recipients; effect of binding and metabolism. *Clin Pharmacol Ther* 1989;45:41–48.
35. Sewing KF, Christians U, Bleck JS, Schottmann R, Strohmeyer SS. Measurement and disposition of cyclosporin and its metabolites. *Bibliotheca Cardiol* 1988;43:63–72.
36. Christians U, Strohmeyers, Kownatzki R, et al. Investigations on the metabolic pathways of cyclosporin: II. Elucidation of the metabolic pathways in vitro by human liver microsomes. *Xenobiotica* 1991;21:1199–1210.
37. Cheung F, Wong PY, Loo J, Cole EH, Levy GA. Identification of cyclosporine metabolites in human blood, bile, and urine by high-performance liquid chromatography/radioimmunoassay/fast atomic bombardment mass spectroscopy. *Transplant Proc* 1988;20:602–608.
38. Wallemacq PE, Lhoest G, Latinne D, DeBruyere M. Isolation, characterization and in vitro activity of human cyclosporin A metabolite. *Transplant Proc* 1989;21:906–910.
39. Hartmann NR, Jardine I. The in vitro activity, radioimmunoassay, and molecular weight of thirteen rabbit cyclosporine metabolites. *Drug Metab Dispos* 1987;15:661–664.
40. Wang PC, Hartmann NR, Venkataramanan R, et al. Isolation of 10 cyclosporine metabolites from human bile. *Drug Metab Dispos* 1989;17:292–296.

41. Hartmann NR, Trimble LA, Vederas JC, Jardine I. An acid metabolite of cyclosporine. *Biochem Biophys Res Commun* 1985;133:964–971.
42. Lown KS, Kolars JC, Thummel KE, et al. Interpatient heterogeneity in expression of CYP3A4 and CYP3A5 in small bowel. Lack of prediction by the erythromycin breath test. *Drug Metab Dispos* 1994;22:947–955.
43. Watkins PB. Drug metabolism by cytochromes P450 in the liver and small bowel. *Gastroenterol Pharmacol* 1992;21:511–526.
44. Aoyama T, Yamano S, Waxman DJ, et al. Cytochrome P-450 hPCN3, a novel cytochrome P-450 IIIA gene product that is differentially expressed in adult human liver. *J Biol Chem* 1989;264:10388–10395.
45. Watkins PB, Wrighton SA, Maurel P, et al. Identification of an inducible form of cytochrome P-450 in human liver. *Proc Natl Acad Sci USA* 1985;82:6310–6314.
46. Wrighton SA, Ring BJ, Watkins PB, Vandenbranden M. Identification of a polymorphically expressed member of the human cytochrome P-450III family. *Mol Pharmacol* 1989;36:97–105.
47. Wu CY, Benet LZ, Hebert MF, Gupta SK, Rowland M, Gomez DY, Wacher VJ. Differentiation of absorption and first-pass gut and hepatic metabolism in humans: studies with cyclosporine. *Clin Pharmacol Ther* 1995;58:492–497.
48. Hebert MF, Roberts JP, Prueksaritanont T, Benet LZ. Bioavailability of cyclosporine with concomitant rifampin administration is markedly less than predicted by hepatic enzyme induction. *Clin Pharmacol Ther* 1992;52:453–457.
49. Gomez DY, Wacher VJ, Tomlanovich SJ, Hebert MF, Benet LZ. The effects of ketoconazole on the intestinal metabolism and bioavailability of cyclosporine. *Clin Pharmacol Ther* 1995;58:15–19.
50. Gupta SK, Bakran A, Johnson RWG, Rowland M. Cyclosporin-erythromycin interaction in renal transplant patients. *Br J Clin Pharmacol* 1989;27:475–481.
51. Kolars JC, Merion R, Awni WM, Watkins PB. First pass metabolism of cyclosporin by the gut. *Lancet* 1991;338:1488–1490.
52. Roninson IB, Chin JE, Choi K, et al. Isolation of human mdr DNA sequences amplified in multidrug-resistant KB carcinoma cells. *Proc Natl Acad Sci USA* 1986;83:4538–4542.
53. Kartner N, Riordan JR, Ling V. Cell surface p-glycoprotein is associated with multidrug resistance in mammalian cell lines. *Science* 1983;221:1285–1288.
54. Pavelic ZP, Reising J, Pavelic L, Kelley DJ, Stambrook PJ, Gluckman JL. Detection of p-glycoprotein with four monoclonal antibodies in normal and tumor tissues. *Arch Otolaryngol Head Neck Surg* 1993;119:753–757.
55. Lown KS, Mayo RR, Leichtman AB, et al. Role of intestinal p-glycoprotein (mdr1) in interpatient variation in the oral bioavailability of cyclosporine. *Clin Pharmacol Ther* 1997;62:1–13.
56. Rosano TG, Brooks CA, Dybas MT, Cramer SM, Stevens C, Freed BM. Selection of an optimal assay method for monitoring cyclosporine therapy. *Transplant Proc* 1990;22:1125–1128.
57. Fahr A, Hiestand P, Ryffel B. Studies on the biological activities of Sandimmun metabolites in humans and in animal models: review and original experiments. *Transplant Proc* 1990;22:1116–1124.
58. Donatsch P, Rickenbacher U, Ryffel B, Brouillard JF. Sandimmun metabolites—their potential to cause adverse reactions in the rat. *Transplant Proc* 1990;22:1137–1140.
59. Sewing K-Fr, Christians U, Kohlhaw K, et al. Biologic activity of cyclosporine metabolites. *Transplant Proc* 1990;22:1129–1134.
60. First MR, Schroeder TJ, Weiskittel P, Myre SA, Alexander JW, Pesce AJ. Concomitant administration of cyclosporin and ketoconazole in renal transplant recipients. *Lancet* 1989;2:1198–1201.
61. Nicolau DP, Uber WE, Crumbley AJ, Strange C. Amiodarone-cyclosporine interaction in heart transplant patient. *J Heart Lung Transplant* 1992;11:564–568.
62. Chitwood KK, Abdul-Haqq AJ, Heim-Duthoy KL. Cyclosporine-amiodarone interaction. *Ann Pharmacother* 1993;27:569–571.
63. Mamprin F, Mullins P, Graham T, et al. Amiodarone-cyclosporine interaction in cardiac transplantation. *Am Heart J* 1992;123:1725–1726.
64. Dodic N, Dumaitre B, Daugan A, Pianetti P. Synthesis and activity against multidrug resistance in Chinese hamster ovary cells of new acridone-4-carboxamides. *J Med Chem* 1995;38:2418–2426.
65. Shapiro AB, Ling V. Reconstitution of drug transport purified p-glycoprotein. *J Biol Chem* 1995;270:16167–16175.
66. Wigler PW, Patterson FK. Reversal agent inhibition of the multidrug resistance pump in human leukemic lymphoblasts. *Biochim Biophys Acta* 1994;1189:1–6.
67. Gersema LM, Porter CB, Russell EH. Suspected drug interaction between cyclosporine and clarithromycin. *J Heart Lung Transplant* 1994;13:343–345.
68. Ferrari SL, Goffin E, Mourad M, Wallemacq P, Squifflet JP, Pirson Y. The interaction between clarithromycin and cyclosporine in kidney transplant recipients. *Transplantation* 1994;58:725–727.
69. Jurima-Romet M, Crawford K, Cyr T, Inaba T. Terfenadine metabolism in human liver. In vitro inhibition by macrolide antibiotics and azole antifungals. *Drug Metab Dispos* 1994;22:849–857.
70. Neumayer HH, Wagner K. Diltiazem and economic use of cyclosporin. *Lancet* 1986;2:523.
71. Grino JM, Sabate I, Castelao AM, Alsina J. Influence of diltiazem on cyclosporin clearance. *Lancet* 1986;1:1387.
72. Pochet JM, Pirson Y. Cyclosporin-diltiazem interaction. *Lancet* 1986;1:979.
73. Valantine H, Keogh A, McIntosh N, Hunt S, Oyer P, Schroeder J. Cost containment: coadministration of diltiazem with cyclosporine after heart transplantation. *J Heart Lung Transplant* 1992;11:1–8.
74. Sketris IS, Methot ME, Nicol D, Belitsky P, Knox MG. Effect of calcium-channel blockers on cyclosporine clearance and use in renal transplant patients. *Ann Pharmacother* 1994;28:1227–1231.
75. Horio M, Lovelace E, Pastan I, Gottesman MM. Agents which reverse multidrug-resistance are inhibitors of (³H)vinblastine transport by isolated vesicles. *Biochim Biophys Acta* 1991;1061:106–110.
76. Barancik M, Polekovà L, Mràzovà T, Breier A, Stankovicovs T, Slezàk J. Reversal effects of several Ca(2+)-entry blockers, neuroleptics and local anaesthetics on p-glycoprotein–mediated vincristine resistance of L1210/VCR mouse leukaemic cell line. *Drugs Exp Clin Res* 1994;20:13–18.
77. Hourmant M, LeBigot JF, Vernillet L, Sagniez G, Remi JP, Soulillou JP. Coadministration of erythromycin results in an increase of blood cyclosporine to toxic levels. *Transplant Proc* 1985;17:2723–2727.
78. Ptachinski RJ, Carpenter BJ, Burckart GJ, Venkataramanan R, Rosenthal JT. Effect of erythromycin on cyclosporine levels. *N Engl J Med* 1985;313:1416–1417.
79. Grino JM, Sabate I, Castelao AM, Guardia M, Seron D, Alsina J. Erythromycin and cyclosporine. *Ann Intern Med* 1986;105:467–468.
80. Godin JRP, Sketris IS, Belitsky P. Erythromycin-cyclosporine interaction. *Drug Intell Clin Pharm* 1986;20:504–505.
81. Kessler M, Louis J, Renoult E, Vigneron B, Netter P. Interaction between cyclosporin and erythromycin in a kidney transplant patient. *Eur J Clin Pharmacol* 1986;30:633–634.
82. Kohan DE. Possible interaction between cyclosporine and erythromycin. *N Engl J Med* 1986;314:448.
83. Freeman DJ, Martell R, Carruthers SG, Heinrich SD, Keown PA, Stiller CR. Cyclosporin-erythromycin interaction in normal subjects. *Br J Clin Pharmacol* 1987;23:776–778.
84. Wadhwa NK, Schroeder TJ, O'Flaherty E, et al. Interaction between erythromycin and cyclosporine in a kidney and pancreas allograft recipient. *Ther Drug Monit* 1987;9:123–125.
85. Jensen CWB, Flechner SM, Van Buren CT, et al. Exacerbation of cyclosporine toxicity by concomitant administration of erythromycin. *Transplantation* 1987;43:263–270.
86. Harnett JD, Parfrey PS, Paul MD, Gault MH. Erythromycin-cyclosporine interaction in renal transplant recipients. *Transplantation* 1987;43:316–318.
87. Zylber-Katz E. Multiple drug interactions with cyclosporine in a heart transplant patient. *Ann Pharmacother* 1995;29:127–131.
88. Miura T, Iwasaki M, Komori M, et al. Decrease in a constitutive form of cytochrome P-450 by macrolide antibiotics. *J Antimicrob Chemother* 1989;24:551–559.
89. Wrighton SA, Ring BJ. Inhibition of human CYP3A catalyzed 1'-hydroxy midazolam formation by ketoconazole, nifedipine, erythromycin, cimetidine, and nizatidine. *Pharm Res* 1994;11:921–924.
90. Gant TW, O'Connor CK, Corbitt R, Thorgeirsson U, Thorgeirsson SS. In vivo induction of liver p-glycoprotein expression by xenobiotics in monkeys. *Toxicol Appl Pharmacol* 1995;133:269–276.
91. Lopez-Gil JA. Fluconazole-cyclosporine interaction: a dose-dependent effect? *Ann Pharmacother* 1993;27:427–430.
92. Sugar AM, Saunders C, Idelson BA, Bernard DB. Interaction of fluconazole and cyclosporine. *Ann Intern Med* 1989;110:844.

93. Graves NM, Matas AJ, Hilligoss DM, Canafax DM. Fluconazole/cyclosporine interaction. *Clin Pharmacol Ther* 1990;43:208.

94. Collignon P, Hurley B, Mitchell D. Interaction of fluconazole with cyclosporin. *Lancet* 1989;1:1262.

95. Ducharme MP, Warbasse LH, Edwards DJ. Disposition of intravenous and oral cyclosporine after administration with grapefruit juice. *Clin Pharmacol Ther* 1995;57:485–491.

96. Edwards DJ, Bernier SM. Naringin and naringenin are not the primary CYP3A inhibitors in grapefruit juice. *Life Sci* 1996;59:1025–1030.

97. Miniscalco A, Lundahl J, Regardh CG, Edgar B, Eriksson UG. Inhibition of dihydropyridine metabolism in rat and human liver microsomes by flavonoids found in grapefruit juice. *J Pharmacol Exp Ther* 1992;261:1195–1199.

98. Trenk D, Brett W, Jahnchen E, Birnbaum D. Time course of cyclosporin/itraconazole interaction. *Lancet* 1987;2:1335–1336.

99. Kwan JTC, Foxall PJD, Davidson DGC, Bending MR, Eisinger AJ. Interaction of cyclosporin and itraconazole. *Lancet* 1987;2:282.

100. Kramer MR, Marshall SE, Denning DW, et al. Cyclosporine and itraconazole interaction in heart and lung transplant recipients. *Ann Intern Med* 1990;113:327–329.

101. Kurosawa M, Okabe M, Hara N, et al. Reversal effect of itraconazole on adriamycin and etoposide resistance in human leukemia cells. *Ann Hematol* 1996;72:17–21.

102. Morgenstern GR, Powles R, Robinson B, McElwain TJ. Cyclosporine interaction with ketoconazole and melphalan. *Lancet* 1982;2:1342.

103. Ferguson RM, Sutherland DER, Simmons RL, Najarian JS. Ketoconazole, cyclosporin metabolism and renal transplantation. *Lancet* 1982;2:882–883.

104. Sorenson AL, Lovdahl M, Hewitt JM, et al. The effect of ketoconazole on cyclosporine metabolism in renal allograft recipients. *Transplant Proc* 1994;26:2822.

105. First MR, Schroeder TJ, Michael A, Hariharan S, Weiskettel P, Alexander JW. Cyclosporine-ketoconazole interaction. *Transplantation* 1993;55:1000–1004.

106. First MR, Schroeder TJ, Alexander JW, et al. Cyclosporine dose reduction by ketoconazole administration in renal transplant recipients. *Transplantation* 1991;51:365–370.

107. Labroo RB, Thummel KE, Kunze KL, Podoll T, Trager WF, Kharasch ED. Catalytic role of cytochrome p450 3A4 in multiple pathways of alfentanil metabolism. *Drug Metab Dispos* 1995;23:490–496.

108. Siegsmund MJ, Cardarelli C, Aksentijevich I, Sugimoto Y, Pastan I, Gottesman MM. Ketoconazole effectively reverses multi-drug resistance in highly resistant KB cells. *J Urol* 1994;151:485–491.

109. Bourbigot B, Guiserix J, Airiau J, Bressollette L, Morin JF, Cledes J. Nicardipine increases cyclosporin blood levels. *Lancet* 1986;1:1447.

110. Pichard L, Fabre I, Fabre G, et al. Cyclosporine A drug interactions. Screening for inducers and inhibitors of cytochrome P-450 (cyclosporin A oxidase) in primary culture of human hepatocytes and in liver microsomes. *Drug Metab Dispos* 1990;18:595–606.

111. Kobayashi Y, Yamashiro T, Nagatake H, et al. Expression and function of multidrug resistance p-glycoprotein in a cultured natural killer cell-rich population revealed by MRK16 monoclonal antibody and AHC-52. *Biochem Pharmacol* 1994;48:1641–1646.

112. Lindholm A, Henricsson S. Verapamil inhibits cyclosporin metabolism. *Lancet* 1987;1:1262–1263.

113. Tortorice KL, Heim-Duthoy KL, Awni WM, Rao KL, Kasiske BL. The effect of calcium channel blockers on cyclosporine and its metabolites in renal transplant recipients. *Ther Drug Monit* 1990;12:321–328.

114. Muller C, Bailly JD, Goubin F, et al. Verapamil decreases p-glycoprotein expression in multidrug-resistant human leukemic cell lines. *Int J Cancer* 1994;56:749–754.

115. Wrighton SA, Maurel P, Schuetz EG, Watkins PB, Young B, Guzelian PS. Identification of the cytochrome p-450 induced by macrolide antibiotics in rat liver as the glucocorticoid responsive cytochrome p-450p. *Biochemistry* 1985;24:2171–2178.

116. Endresen L, Bergan S, Holdaas H, Pran T, Sinding-Larsen B, Berg KJ. Lack of effect of the calcium antagonist isradipine on cyclosporine pharmacokinetics in renal transplant patients. *Ther Drug Monit* 1991;13:490–495.

117. Cooney GF, Mochon M, Kaiser B, Dunn SP, Goldsmith B. Effects of carbamazepine on cyclosporine metabolism in pediatric renal transplant recipients. *Pharmacotherapy* 1995;15:353–356.

118. Backman JT, Olkkola KT, Ojala M, Laaksovirta H, Neuvonen PJ. Concentrations and effects of oral midazolam are greatly reduced in patients treated with carbamazepine or phenytoin. *Epilepsia* 1996;37:253–257.

119. Carstensen H, Jacobsen N, Dieperink H. Interaction between cyclosporin A and phenobarbitone. *Br J Clin Pharmacol* 1986;21:550–551.

120. Thummel KE, Shen DD, Podoll TD, et al. Use of midazolam as a human cytochrome P450 3A probe: II. Characterization of inter- and intraindividual hepatic CYP3A variability after liver transplantation. *J Pharmacol Exp Ther* 1994;271:557–566.

121. Shaw PM, Barnes TS, Cameron D, et al. Purification and characterization of an anticonvulsant-induced human cytochrome P-450 catalyzing cyclosporin metabolism. *Biochem J* 1989;263:653–663.

122. Donato MT, Castell JV, Gomez-Lechon MJ. Effect of model inducers on cytochrome P450 activities of human hepatocytes in primary culture. *Drug Metab Dispos* 1995;23:553–558.

123. Schuetz EG, Schuetz JD, Strom SC, et al. Regulation of human liver cytochromes P-450 in family 3A in primary and continuous culture of human hepatocytes. *Hepatology* 1993;18:1254–1262.

124. Manke A, Roos PH, Hanstein WG, Chabot GG. In vivo induction of cytochrome P450 CYP3A expression in rat leukocytes using various inducers. *Biochem Pharmacol* 1996;51:1579–1582.

125. Murayama N, Shimada M, Yamazoe Y, et al. Distinct effects of phenobarbital and its N-methylated derivative on liver cytochrome p450 induction. *Arch Biochem Biophys* 1996;328:184–192.

126. Schuetz EG, Beck WT, Schuetz JD. Modulators and substrates of p-glycoprotein and cytochrome P4503A coordinately up-regulate these proteins in human colon carcinoma cells. *Mol Pharmacol* 1996;49:311–318.

127. Freeman DJ, Laupacis A, Keown PA, Stiller CR, Carruthers SG. Evaluation of cyclosporin-phenytoin interaction with observations on cyclosporin metabolites. *Br J Clin Pharmacol* 1984;18:887–893.

128. Keown PA, Laupacis A, Carruthers G, et al. Interaction between phenytoin and cyclosporine following organ transplantation. *Transplantation* 1984;38:304–306.

129. Van Buren D, Wideman CA, Ried M, et al. The antagonistic effect of rifampin upon cyclosporine bioavailability. *Transplant Proc* 1984;16:1642–1645.

130. Modry DL, Stinson EB, Oyer PE, Jamieson SW, Baldwin JC, Shumway NE. Acute rejection and massive cyclosporine requirements in heart transplant recipients treated with rifampin. *Transplantation* 1985;39:313–314.

131. Offermann G, Keller F, Molzahn M. Low cyclosporin A blood levels and acute graft rejection in a renal transplant recipient during rifampin treatment. *Am J Nephrol* 1985;5:385–387.

132. Vandevelde C, Chang A, Andrews D, Riggs W, Jewesson P. Rifampin and ansamycin interactions with cyclosporine after renal transplantation. *Pharmacotherapy* 1991;11:88–89.

133. Cassidy MJD, Van Zyl-Smit R, Pascoe MD, Swanepoel CR, Jacobson JE. Effect of rifampicin on cyclosporin A blood levels in a renal transplant recipient. *Nephron* 1985;41:207–208.

134. Langhoff E, Madsen S. Rapid metabolism of cyclosporin and prednisone in kidney transplant patient receiving tuberculostatic treatment. *Lancet* 1983;2:1031.

135. Kolars JC, Schmiedlin-Ren P, Schuetz J, Ghosh M, Dobbins WO, Watkins PB. Expression of P450IIIA4 in duodenal mucosa: interpatient variability and regulation in cultured explants. *Gastroenterology* 1991;100:A221.

136. Kolars JC, Schmiedlin-Ren P, Schuetz JD, Fang C, Watkins PB. Identification of rifampin-inducible P450IIIA4 (CYP3A4) in human small bowel enterocytes. *J Clin Invest* 1992;90:1871–1878.

137. Fardel O, Lecureur V, Loyer P, Guillouzo A. Rifampicin enhances anticancer drug accumulation and activity in multidrug-resistant cells. *Biochem Pharmacol* 1995;49:1255–1260.

138. Frantz AG, Katz FH, Jailer JW. 6β-hydroxycortisol and other polar corticosteroids: measurement and significance in human urine. *J Clin Endocrinol Metab* 1961;21:1290–1330.

139. Kornel L, Moore JT, Noyes I. Corticosteroids in human blood: IV. Distribution of cortisol and its metabolites between plasma and erythrocytes in vivo. *J Clin Endocrinol* 1970;30:40–50.

140. Jenkins JS, Sampson PA. Conversion of cortisone to cortisol and prednisone to prednisolone. *BMJ* 1967;2:205–207.

141. Canalis E, Reardon GE, Caldarella AM. A more specific liquid-chromatographic method for free cortisol in urine. *Clin Chem* 1982;28:2418–2420.

142. Kornel L, Miyabo S, Saito Z, Cha R-W, Wu F-T. Corticosteroids in human blood. VIII. Cortisol metabolites in plasma of normotensive subjects and patients with essential hypertension. *J Clin Endocrinol Metab* 1975;40:949–958.

143. Zurcher RM, Frey BM, Frey FJ. Impact of ketoconazole on metabolism of prednisolone. *Clin Pharmacol Ther* 1989;45:366–372.

144. Frey FJ, Schnetzer A, Horber FF, Frey BM. Evidence that cyclosporine does not affect the metabolism of prednisolone after renal transplantation. *Transplantation* 1987;43:494–498.

145. Rose JQ, Yurchak AM, Jusko WJ. Dose dependent pharmacokinetics of prednisone and prednisolone in man. *J Pharmacokin Biopharm* 1981;9:389–417.

146. Uribe M, Summerskill WhJ, Go VLW. Comparative serum prednisone and prednisolone concentrations following administration to patients with chronic active liver disease. *Clin Pharmacokin* 1982;7:452–459.

147. Sullivan TJ, Hallmark MR, Sakmar E, Weidler DJ, Earhart RH, Wagner JG. Comparative bioavailability: eight commercial prednisone tablets. *J Pharmacokin Biopharm* 1976;4:157–172.

148. Lewis GP, Jusko WJ, Burke CW, Graves L. Prednisone side-effects and serum protein levels. *Lancet* 1971;2:778–781.

149. Meikle AW, Weed JA, Tyler FH. Kinetics and interconversion of prednisolone and prednisone studied with new radioimmunoassays. *J Clin Endocrinol Metab* 1975;41:717–721.

150. Pickup ME, Lose JR, Leatham PA, Rhind VM, Wright V, Downie WW. Dose dependent pharmacokinetics of prednisolone. *Eur J Clin Pharmacol* 1977;12:213–219.

151. Loo JCK, McGilveray IJ, Jordan N, Moffat J, Brien R. Dose dependent pharmacokinetics of prednisone and prednisolone in man. *J Pharm Pharmacol* 1978;30:736.

152. Tanner A, Bochner F, Caffin J, Halliday J, Powell L. Dose dependent prednisolone kinetics. *Clin Pharmacol Ther* 1979;25:571–578.

153. Chen PS, Mills IH, Barttler FC. Ultrafiltration studies of steroid-protein binding. *J Endocrinol* 1961;23:129–137.

154. Rose JQ, Yurchak AM, Jusko WJ, Powell D. Bioavailability and disposition of prednisone and prednisolone from prednisone tablets. *Biopharm Drug Dispos* 1980;1:247–258.

155. Gray CH, Green MAS, Holness NJ, Lunnon JB. Urinary metabolic products of prednisone and prednisolone. *J Endocrinol* 1956;14:146–154.

156. Powell LW, Axelsen E. Corticosteroids in liver disease: studies on the biological conversion of prednisone to prednisolone and plasma protein binding. *Gut* 1972;13:690–696.

157. English J, Chakraborty J, Marks V, Trigger DJ, Thomson AG. Prednisolone levels in the plasma and urine. A study of two preparations in man. *Br J Clin Pharmacol* 1975;2:327–332.

158. Ged C, Rouillon JM, Pichard L, et al. The increase in urinary excretion of 6β-hydroxycortisol as a marker of human hepatic cytochrome P450IIIA induction. *Br J Clin Pharmacol* 1989;28:373–387.

159. Wrighton SA, Brian WR, Sari M-A, et al. Studies on the expression and metabolic capabilities of human liver cytochrome P450IIIA5 (HLp3). *Mol Pharmacol* 1990;38:207–213.

160. Hunt CM, Watkins PB, Saenger P, et al. Heterogeneity of CYP3A isoforms metabolizing erythromycin and cortisol. *Clin Pharmacol Ther* 1992;51:18–23.

161. Roots I, Holbe R, Hovermann W, Nigam S, Heinemeyer G, Hildebrandt AG. Quantitative determination by HPLC of urinary 6β-hydroxycortisol, an indicator of enzyme induction by rifampicin and antiepileptic drugs. *Eur J Clin Pharmacol* 1979;16:63–71.

162. Moreland TA, Park BK, Rylance GW. Drug metabolising enzyme induction in children. *Br J Clin Pharmacol* 1981;11:420p–421p.

163. Werk EE, MacGee J, Sholiton LJ. Effect of diphenylhydantoin on cortisol metabolism in man. *J Clin Invest* 1964;43:1824–1835.

164. Watkins PB, Turgeon K, Saenger P, et al. Comparison of urinary 6-β-cortisol and the erythromycin breath test as measures of hepatic P450IIIA (CYP3A) activity. *Clin Pharmacol Ther* 1992;52:265–273.

165. Ponec M, Kempenaar J, Shroot B, Caron J-C. Glucocorticoids: binding affinity and lipophilicity. *J Pharm Sci* 1986;75:973–975.

166. Hollander JL, Brown EM, Jessar RA, et al. Hydrocortisone and cortisone injected into arthritic joints: comparative effects of and use of hydrocortisone as a local antiarthritic agent. *JAMA* 1951;147:1629–1635.

167. Boekenoogen SJ, Szefler SJ, Jusko WJ. Prednisolone disposition and protein binding in oral contraceptive users. *J Clin Endocrinol Metab* 1983;56:702–709.

168. Legler UF, Benet LZ. Marked alterations in dose-dependent prednisolone kinetics in women taking oral contraceptives. *Clin Pharmacol Ther* 1986;39:425–429.

169. Kozower M, Veatch L, Kaplan MM. Decreased clearance of prednisolone, a factor in the development of corticosteroid side effects. *J Clin Endocrinol Metab* 1974;38:407–412.

170. Buffington GA, Dominguez JH, Piering WF, Hebert LA, Kauffman HM, Lemann J. Interaction of rifampin and glucocorticoids. *JAMA* 1976;236:1958–1960.

171. Hendrickse W, McKiernan J, Pickup M, Lowe J. Rifampicin-induced non-responsiveness to corticosteroid treatment in nephrotic syndrome. *BMJ* 1979;1:306.

172. Ohnhaus EE, Park BK. Measurement of urinary 6-β-hydroxycortisol excretion as an in vivo parameter in the clinical assessment of the microsomal enzyme-inducing capacity of antipyrine, phenobarbitone and rifampicin. *Eur J Clin Pharmacol* 1979;15:139–145.

173. Desager JP, Dumont E, Harvengt C. The urinary 6β-hydroxycortisol excretion in man on inducers and inhibitors of the hepatic mixed function oxidase. *Pharmacol Ther* 1987;33:197–199.

174. Saenger P. 6β-hydroxycortisol in random urine samples as an indicator of enzyme induction. *Clin Pharmacol Ther* 1983;34:818–821.

175. Brooks SM, Werk EE, Ackerman S, Sullivan I, Thrasher K. Adverse effects of phenobarbital on corticosteroid metabolism in patients with bronchial asthma. *N Engl J Med* 1972;286:1125–1128.

176. Brooks PM, Buchanan WW, Grove M, Downie WW. Effects of enzyme induction on metabolism of prednisolone. *Ann Rheum Dis* 1976;35:339–343.

177. Petereit LB, Meikle AW. Effectiveness of prednisolone during phenytoin therapy. *Clin Pharmacol Ther* 1977;22:912–916.

178. Choi Y, Thrasher K, Werk EE, Sholiton LJ, Olinger C. Effect of diphenylhydantoin on cortisol kinetics in humans. *J Pharmacol Exp Ther* 1971;176:27–34.

179. Bray PF, Ely RS, Zapata G, Kelley VC. Adrenocortical function in epilepsy. I. The role of cortisol (hydrocortisone) in the mechanism and management of seizures. *Neurology* 1960;10:842–846.

180. Christy NP, Hofmann AD. Effects of diphenylhydantoin upon adrenal cortical function in man. *Neurology* 1959;9:245–250.

181. Hebert MF, Benet LZ, Gomez D, et al. Pharmacokinetics of oral mycophenolate mofetil in liver transplant patients. *Clin Pharmacol Ther* 1994;55:164.

182. Shah J, Bullingham R, Rice P, Tsina I, Swan S, Halstenson C. Pharmacokinetics of oral mycophenolate mofetil (MMF) and metabolites in renally impaired patients. *Clin Pharmacol Ther* 1995;57:149.

183. Shah J, Linna J, Tsina I. Pharmacokinetics of mycophenolate mofetil in healthy male volunteers after single intravenous ascending doses. *Pharm Res* 1993;10:S-339.

184. Shaw LM, Sollinger HW, Halloran P, et al. Mycophenolate mofetil: a report of the consensus panel. *Ther Drug Monit* 1995;17:690–699.

185. Roche Laboratories Inc. CellCept (mycophenolate mofetil capsules) package insert. Nutley, NJ: June 1997.

186. Allison AC, Almquist SJ, Muller CD, Eugui EM. In vitro immunosuppressive effects of mycophenolic acid and an ester pro-drug, RS61443. *Transplant Proc* 1991;23:10–14.

187. Burlingham WJ, Grailer AP, Hullett DA, Sollinger HW. Inhibition of both MLC and an in vitro IgG memory response to tetanus toxoid by RS-61443. *Transplantation* 1991;51:545–547.

188. Grailer A, Nichols J, Hullett D, Sollinger HW, Burlingham WJ. Inhibition of human B cell responses in vitro by RS-61443, cyclosporine A and DAB486 IL-2. *Transplant Proc* 1991;23:314–315.

189. Carter SB, Franklin TJ, Jones DF, et al. Mycophenolic acid: an anticancer compound with unusual properties. *Nature* 1969;223:848–850.

190. Franklin TJ, Cook JM. The inhibition of nucleic acid synthesis by mycophenolic acid. *Biochem J* 1969;113:515–524.

191. Franklin TJ, Morris WP. Pharmacodynamics of inhibition of GTP synthesis in vivo by mycophenolic acid. *Adv Enzym Regul* 1994;34:107–117.

192. Langman LJ, LeGatt DF, Yatscoff RW. Pharmacodynamic assessment of mycophenolic acid-induced immunosuppression by measuring IMP dehydrogenase activity. *Clin Chem* 1995;41:295–299.

193. Makara GM, Keseru GM, Kajtar-Peredy M, Anderson WK. Nuclear magnetic resonance and molecular modeling study on mycophenolic acid: implications for binding inosine monophosphate dehydrogenase. *J Med Chem* 1996;39:1236–1242.

194. Eugui EM, Almquist SJ, Muller CD, Allison AC. Lymphocyte-selec-

tive cytostatic immunosuppressive effects of mycophenolic acid in vitro: role of deoxyguanosine nucleotide depletion. *Scand J Immunol* 1991;33:161–173.

195. Carr SF, Papp E, Wu JC, Natsumeda Y. Characterization of human type I and II IMP dehydrogenases. *J Biol Chem* 1993;268:27286–27290.

196. Wu JC. Mycophenolate mofetil: molecular mechanisms of action. *Perspect Drug Discov Design* 1994;2:185–204.

197. Nowak I, Shaw LM. Mycophenolic acid binding to human serum albumin: characterization and relation to pharmacodynamics. *Clin Chem* 1995;41:1011–1017.

198. Laurent AF, Dumont S, Poindron P, Muller CD. Mycophenolic acid suppresses protein N-linked glycosylation in human monocytes and their adhesion to endothelial cells and to some substrates. *Exp Hematol* 1996;24:59–67.

199. Bullingham R, Shah J, Goldblum R, Schiff M. Effects of food and antacid on the pharmacokinetics of single doses of mycophenolate mofetil in rheumatoid arthritis patients. *Br J Clin Pharmacol* 1996;41:513–516.

200. Christians U, Druse C, Kownatzki R, et al. Measurement of FK 506 by HPLC and isolation and characterization of metabolites. *Transplant Proc* 1991;23:940–941.

201. Christians U, Braun F, Kosian N, et al. High performance liquid chromatography/mass spectrometry of FK506 and its metabolites in blood, bile, and urine of liver grafted patients. *Transplant Proc* 1991;23:2741–2744.

202. Iwasaki K, Shiraga T, Nagase K, et al. Isolation, identification, and biological activities of oxidative metabolites of FK506, a potent immunosuppressive macrolide lactone. *Drug Metab Dispos* 1993;21:971–977.

203. Sattler M, Guengerich FP, Yun C-H, Christians U, Sewing K-F. Cytochrome p-4503A enzymes are responsible for biotransformation of FK506 and rapamycin in man and rat. *Drug Metab Dispos* 1992;20:753–761.

204. Lampen A, Christians U, Guengerich FP, et al. Metabolism of the immunosuppressant tacrolimus in the small intestine: cytochrome P450, drug interactions, and interindividual variability. *Drug Metab Dispos* 1995;23:1315–1324.

205. Saeki T, Ueda K, Tanigawara Y, Hori R, Komano T. Human p-glycoprotein transports cyclosporin A and FK506. *J Biol Chem* 1993;268:6077–6080.

206. Shaeffer MS, Collier D, Sorrell MF. Interaction between FK506 and erythromycin. *Ann Pharmacother* 1994;28:280–281.

207. Jensen C, Jordan M, Shapiro R, et al. Interaction between tacrolimus and erythromycin. *Lancet* 1994;344:825.

208. Osowski CL, Dix SP, Lin LS, Mullins RE, Geller RB, Wingard JR. Evaluation of the drug interaction between intravenous high-dose fluconazole and cyclosporine or tacrolimus in bone marrow transplant patients. *Transplantation* 1996;61:1268–1272.

209. Floren LC, Bekersky I, Benet LZ, Mekki Q, Dressler D, Lee JW, Roberts JP, Hebert MF. Tacrolimus oral bioavailability doubles with coadministration of ketoconazole. *Clin Pharmacol Ther* 1997;62:41–49.

210. Furlan V, Perello L, Jacquemin E, Debray D, Taburet AM. Interactions between FK506 and rifampicin or erythromycin in pediatric liver recipients. *Transplantation* 1995;59:1217–1218.

CHAPTER 38

Estrogens and Progestins

Maurice G. Emery

The steroid hormone compounds in this review were some of the earliest marketed pharmaceutical products to be used for endocrine disorders; some have been in use for more than 40 years. These compounds have been used to treat endocrine disorders and malignancies, to provide effective contraception, and to treat endogenous estrogen deficiency occurring with the menopause.

The first breakthrough that made these products inexpensive and readily available came with the discovery of naturally occurring precursors for synthesis of a wide variety of steroids. Organic chemists have continued to modify two plant steroid precursors—diosgenin from the Mexican yam and stigmasterol from soybeans—to produce many of the so-called "newer generation" steroid hormones currently in use.

The other major obstacle to be overcome was to improve the oral bioavailability of these compounds. One such modification of interest to drug metabolism was the introduction of alkynl groups. Although this particular strategy led to acceptable oral absorption, it has become widely recognized as one that may produce mechanism-based inhibition of some cytochrome P450 isoforms.

With additional understanding of endogenous steroid hormone action and roles in modifying disorders associated with their perturbation, newer steroid and nonsteroid compounds have been developed. Some of the more recent advances include the identification of estrogen receptor subsets (1) with the development of selective estrogen receptor modulators (SERMs), the evolution of androgen inhibitors, and continued refinement of currently used steroids to maximize benefits and minimize the adverse event profile. Soon, continued progress in steroid hormone action will no doubt be accompanied by a number of clinically useful agents.

M. G. Emery: Abbott Laboratories, Department of Metabolism, Radiochemistry, and Cellular Toxicity, Building AP9-LL, 100 Abbott Park Road, Abbott Park, Illinois 60064

ESTROGENS

The metabolic fate of estrogen compounds is exceedingly complex for three main reasons. First, endogenous and exogenous estrogenic compounds undergo extensive metabolism by cytochrome P450 and these pathways usually represent the major route of elimination for these compounds. Adding to the complexity of their metabolism, orally administered estrogens are also subject to extensive first pass sulfate and glucuronide conjugation. Second, because they are directly conjugated in the liver and gut wall, these metabolites can then undergo enterohepatic recirculation whereby they are excreted in the bile, and then reabsorbed (Fig. 38-1). In the gut, normal flora can affect the biologic activity through reduction reactions to form more potent steroids (e.g., estrone to estradiol). Furthermore, these bacteria can affect the degree of reabsorption through glucuronide, sulfate, and methyl deconjugation reactions (2). Third, the interconversion and conjugation of the major endogenous estrogens serve to provide a large stable pool of circulating estrogen, principally as sulfoconju-

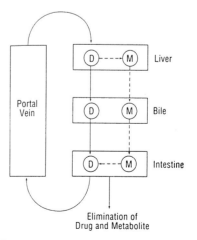

FIG. 38-1. Enterohepatic recirculation of steroid metabolites.

gates. These processes add to the complexity of interpreting the effect of metabolism on the overall clinical effect of a drug interaction in that these forms may act as a source of continuing drug action and absorption.

Endogenous Estrogens (Estradiol and Estrone)

Metabolic Disposition

The metabolic scheme of the principal endogenous estrogens is shown in Fig. 38-2. The quantitative aspects of 17β-estradiol exhibit route dependency resulting from extensive first pass metabolism. When administered by the oral route to reproductive-age women, only about 10% of the dose was absorbed as unchanged estradiol (3). The oral administration of 17β-estradiol results in 65% of the dose being converted to the biologically less active metabolite estrone through interconversion by steroid 17β-dehydrogenase. Following a 2-mg oral dose of micronized 17β-estradiol, average peak plasma concentrations of estrone and estradiol are 0.9 nM and 0.2 nM, respectively.

Significant conjugation of estradiol and estrone also occurs. By comparing fractional clearances, approximately 15% of the dose is converted to estrone, 25% to estrone sulfate, 25% to estrone glucuronide, and 25% to estradiol glucuronide. When administered by non-oral routes (i.e., transdermal, vaginal, intravenous), relatively larger amounts of estradiol and hydroxylated estrogens and less estrone and estrone glucuronide are formed (4,5). Therefore, routes of estradiol administration that bypass the portal circulation may affect the disposition of 17β-estradiol and relative importance of oxidative metabolic pathways.

The oxidative metabolism of 17β-estradiol in humans occurs principally in two major locations—aromatic hydroxylations at the 2 and 4 positions to form catecholestrogens and D-ring 16α-hydroxylation. The 2-hydroxylation is the predominant pathway, being responsible for approximately 30% of 17β-estradiol metabolism (6). Hydroxylation at the 16 position to form either 16α-OH estrone or estriol accounts for about 10% of an intravenous 17β-estradiol dose (3).

Enzyme Identification of Metabolite Formation

The 17β-estradiol 2- and 4-hydroxylations have been studied extensively in human liver microsomes and expressed enzymes. Correlation of these products with typical substrates and immunoreactive protein as well as

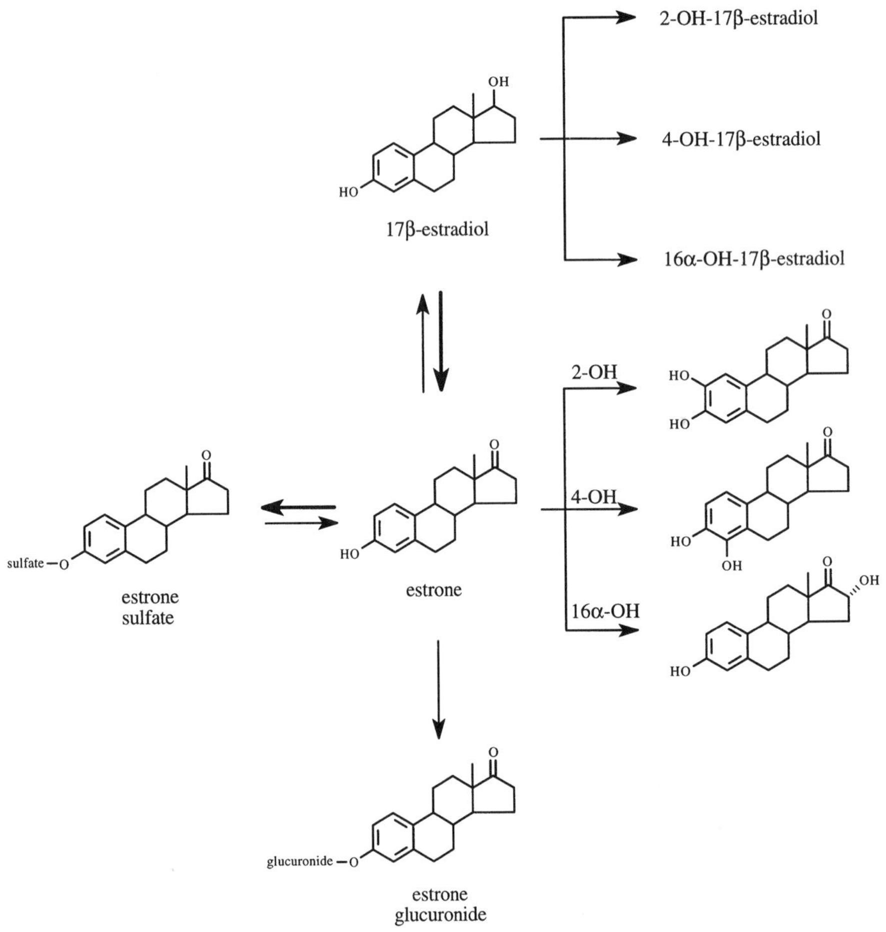

FIG. 38-2. Biotransformation pathways for principal endogenous estrogens.

antibody and substrate inhibition studies has identified CYP3A as the major isoform responsible for these oxidations (7,8). Typical to CYP3A substrates, *in vitro* α-naphthflavone, testosterone, and progesterone increased the 2-hydroxylation activity, suggesting an activation mechanism. The *in vitro* K_m of the 2- and 4-hydroxylation reactions was approximately 10 μM. After ablation of CYP3A activity by preincubation with gestodene, a CYP3A mechanism-based inhibitor, the remaining activity attributable to other CYP isoforms was 20%.

In vitro, CYP1A1 and CYP1A2 cDNA–expressed enzyme demonstrates 2-hydroxylase activity with a turnover rate similar to that of CYP3A (9,10), and heavy cigarette smoking, a known inducer of CYP1A in women increases the *in vivo* estradiol 2-hydroxylation (11). This evidence collectively suggests that the remaining activity may be due to CYP1A and may be an important pathway under induced conditions.

Like the other estrogen hydroxylation reactions, CYP3A was recently identified to catalyze the 16α-hydroxylation of estrone (12,13). The *in vitro* K_m for hepatic microsomes was 150 μM and was in good agreement with cDNA-expressed enzyme. Of interest, the metabolic rates of estrone 16α-hydroxylation in the presence of human microsomal sulfatases were significantly increased when estrone sulfate was used as the substrate compared to estrone.

17α-Ethinyl Estradiol/Mestranol

Ethinyl estradiol (EE2) and its 3-methyl ether—mestranol—are the principal estrogens used in combined oral contraceptives and have been in use for nearly 40 years.

The estrogen component of oral contraceptives has been associated with both beneficial and adverse effects. Older formulations with higher estrogen doses (100–150 μg EE2) were associated with thromboembolic disease. This risk has been minimized by newer formulations that reduced overall estrogen exposure. The newest formulations, containing 15 to 20 μg EE2, are likely the lowest combination doses possible that still maintain contraceptive efficacy. Alterations in the disposition of contraceptive estrogens could, therefore, be associated with either lack of efficacy or adverse effects.

Metabolic Disposition

EE2 is well absorbed but subject to extensive first pass elimination upon oral administration with an average bioavailability of approximately 40% (14). In addition, there is a wide variation of systemic bioavailability ranging from 20% to 65%. Further studies revealed that the principal site of this presystemic elimination was the gut mucosa, which was responsible for the loss of approximately 44% of the EE2 dose (15). Sulfation is the principal route of presystemic elimination but appears to only account for about 60% of the first pass metabolism.

Mestranol is a prodrug of EE2 and is also rapidly absorbed. Average peak plasma mestranol concentrations occur within 1 to 2 hours, followed by a peak in the EE2 concentration. Approximately 50% of a mestranol dose is converted to EE2 (16,17).

The metabolic scheme for mestranol and EE2 is shown in Figure 38-3. Once absorbed, the principal route of elimination is by oxidation at the 2 position. The 2-OH

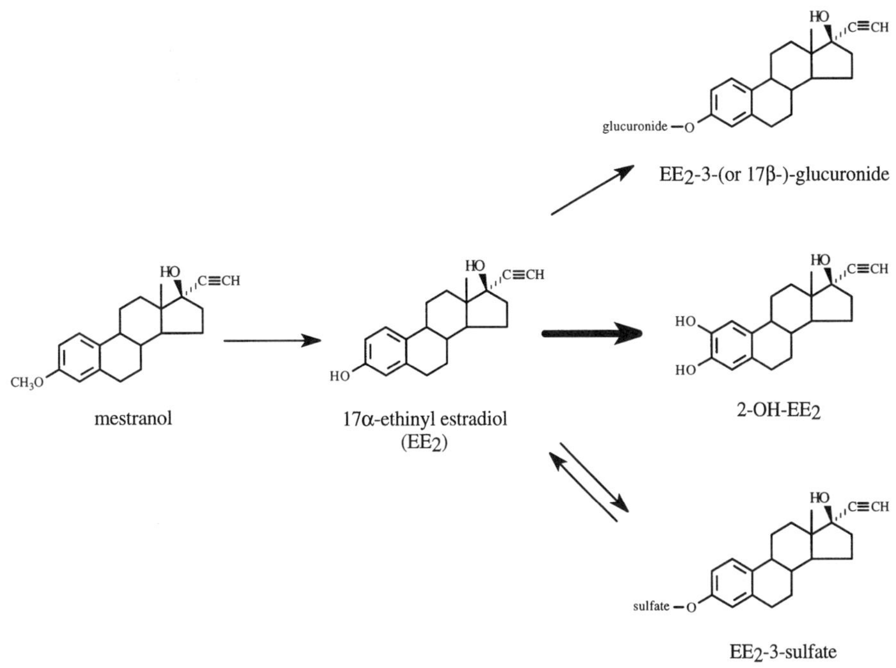

FIG. 38-3. Biotransformation pathways for mestranol and 17α-ethinyl estradiol.

metabolite accounts for an average 30% but has been reported to be as great as 60% of an EE_2 dose (18,19). Hydroxylations also occur at the 4 and 16 positions.

EE_2 also undergoes enterohepatic recirculation following glucuronide conjugation. Eventually, approximately 30% of EE_2 can be recovered in feces. The direct 3- or 17-O-glucuronides have been identified (20). This pathway appears to be minor, although it may be more important if oxidative metabolism is not available (21).

Enzyme Identification of Metabolite Formation

Mestranol owes its activity to ethinyl estradiol and must undergo 3-O-demethylation. *In vitro* human liver microsomal studies demonstrate a role for CYP2C9 in the O-demethylation of mestranol (22). Although complete characterization of inhibition has not been performed, at a mestranol concentration of 3 µM, significant inhibition was observed with sulfaphenazole (IC_{50} 3.6 µM) and miconazole (IC_{50} 1.5 µM). No inhibition was observed with either quinidine or troleandomycin (10 µM). The clinical significance of CYP2C9 inhibition on mestranol conversion has not been studied but such an interaction could conceivably result in loss of contraceptive efficacy.

Ethinyl estradiol 2-hydroxylation is catalyzed by CYP3A and has been well characterized (23). EE_2 2-hydroxylase activity correlated with nifedipine oxidation ($r = 0.95$), immunoreactive CYP3A ($r = 0.98$), and was inhibited by either troleandomycin or anti-CYP3A antibody. Of interest in this study was the finding that preincubation with EE_2 resulted in loss of nifedipine, its own oxidation, and spectrally determined microsomal CYP P450. Further evidence of CYP3A involvement was observed in human liver microsomes prepared from biopsies obtained from subjects taking rifampin. Although a distinction between 2 and 4 hydroxylation could not be made, a five-fold increase in A-ring oxidation was observed when compared to historical control microsomes (24).

In vitro evidence of CYP3A is supported by *in vivo* interactions involving EE_2. In the early 1970s, a number of episodes of breakthrough bleeding and pregnancies were reported, indicating loss of efficacy; these were associated with the concomitant use of rifampin. Consequently, an increase the clearance of EE_2 by rifampin was noted (18). The effect of grapefruit juice, which contains CYP3A inhibitors, on the relative bioavailability of EE_2, has also been studied (25). Although this study did not characterize metabolite formation and administered the grapefruit juice within one-half hour of EE_2 administration, a significant increase (37%) in the mean C_{max} was observed. Because 40% of the first pass metabolism is unaccounted for, this suggests a possible role for intestinal hydroxylation by CYP3A as possibly influencing the bioavailability of EE_2 and warrants further study.

Conjugated Equine Estrogens

Conjugated equine estrogen (CEE) is the most widely used product for menopausal estrogen replacement. The CEE currently in clinical use consists of a mixture containing ten different sulfate esters of estrogens, all with significant estrogenic activity. These include estrogens found in humans (estrone, estradiol) as well as those unique to equine species, the major difference between human and equine estrogen being B-ring unsaturation. The largest component of the currently available combination (Premarin) is estrone sulfate (45%), followed by equilin sulfate (25%), 17α-dihydroequilin sulfate (15%), 17β-dihydroequilin sulfate (4%), and delta-8-estrone sulfate (3.5%). Small amounts of 17α-estradiol, 17β-estradiol, equilenin, 17α-dihydroequilenin, and 17β-dihydroequilenin have also been isolated from this mixture.

This degree of complexity makes the prediction of drug interactions difficult. Nonetheless, it is possible that unique profiles of effect may be produced as a result of differential interactions with some or all of these estrogens. For example, differences in a number of biologic effects were observed following the administration of this combination or of estrone sulfate alone to women despite the attainment of similar plasma estrone and estradiol concentrations (26). This activity can be attributed to the effect of the equine estrogens. See Endogenous Estrogens (p. 512) for information on those estrogens present in humans.

Metabolic Disposition

Following oral administration of a 10-mg dose, equilin attained an average peak plasma concentration of 2.7 nM (27). The major circulating form, equilin sulfate, like other estrogen sulfoconjugates serves as a highly plasma protein–bound, low-clearance source of equilin through the action of sulfatase. Information regarding the quantitative aspects of equilin disposition is incomplete, with only 50% of the dose being accounted for in urine.

The known metabolic fate of equilin sulfate is shown in Figure 38-4. Equilin sulfate undergoes 17β-reduction, deconjugation to form equilin and B-ring reduction in humans. 17β-dihydroequilin sulfate, equilin, and 17β-equilenin formation accounts for approximately 30%, 19%, and 10% of equilin sulfate disposition, respectively (28).

Oxidation at the 16 position to form hydroxyl metabolites has been identified (29). These metabolites of 17β-dihydroequilin and 17β-dihydroequilenin, however, probably represent significant elimination pathways because, following the administration of 17β-dihydroequilin sulfate, a large number of unknown radioactive polar metabolites were identified. Even though 2- and 4-hydroxy metabolites have yet to be identified as for other estrogens, these probably are formed as well. Quantita-

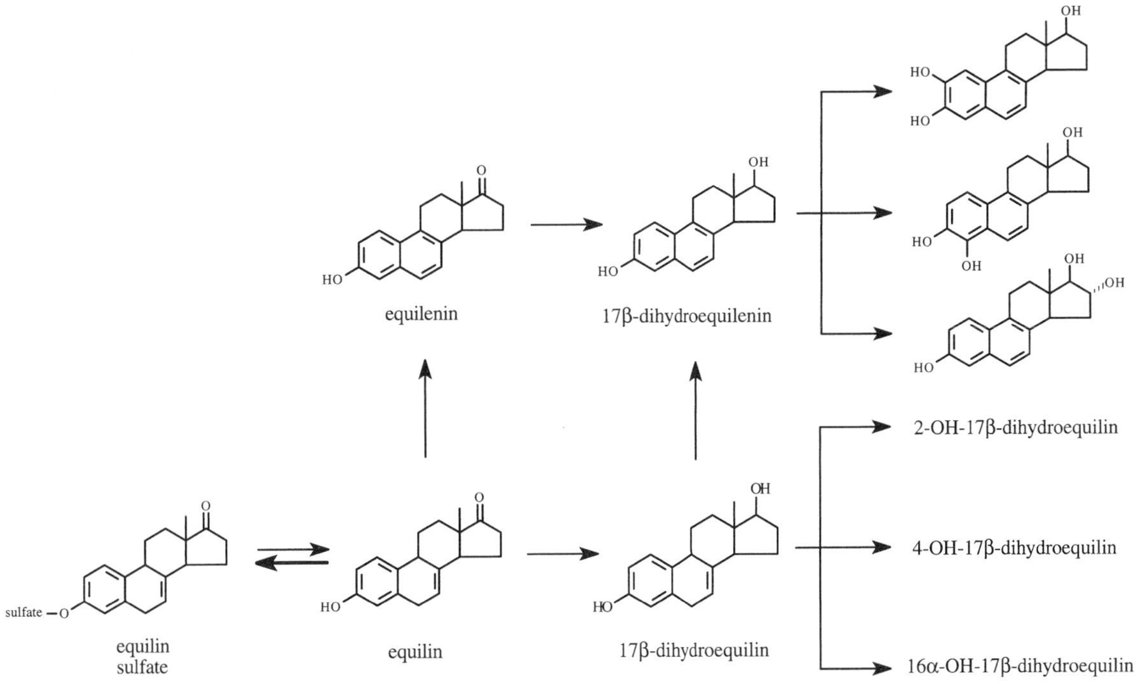

FIG. 38-4. Biotransformation pathways for equilin sulfate.

tively, these polar metabolites accounted for greater than 60% of the dose. The quantitative aspect of these metabolites to the overall metabolic fate is unknown.

Enzyme Identification of Metabolite Formation

The enzymes responsible for the 17β reduction are probably those belonging to a family of steroid dehydrogenases and are responsible for the generation of potent steroids. These conversions are important because they probably are responsible for generating the active estrogen species similar to the relationship between the naturally occurring human estrogens, estrone, and 17β-estradiol. *In vitro* human receptor binding studies and *in vivo* studies following oral administration indicate that these metabolites are indeed more potent than their oxidized forms (29,30). Multiple forms of steroid dehydrogenase have been reported; however, the specific steroid dehydrogenase isoform responsible for the interconversion of equine estrogens in humans is unknown. Furthermore, although this conversion has been shown to occur in human endometrium, the major site of equine estrogen metabolic conversion is unknown (31). Early studies identified tissue supplied by splanchnic circulation, including the liver, as the primary source of endogenous estrogen conversion and, therefore, it is likely that the same occurs for the B-ring unsaturated estrogens.

Further B-ring reduction to form corresponding derivatives from equilin and 17β-equilin is evidence for 6, 8(9) steroid dehydrogenase-isomerase activity in humans (32).

This metabolic conversion also leads to considerably more potent estrogens. The enzyme responsible for this activity has yet to be identified as well. Identification of enzymes responsible for the formation of B-ring oxidative metabolites (2-, 4-, and 16-hydroxylated estrogens) have not yet been identified.

Tamoxifen/Toremifene

Tamoxifen and a chlorinated derivative, toremifene, are nonsteroidal estrogen receptor modulators with both agonist and antagonist activity. They are indicated for the treatment of breast cancer, and recent tamoxifen clinical studies have focused on its use in preventing breast cancer in high-risk subjects (33).

Metabolic Disposition

Tamoxifen metabolism has been well studied in humans. Five major metabolites, mainly involving the dimethylaminoethoxy side chain, have been identified and are shown in Fig. 38-5. Quantitatively, *N*-desmethyltamoxifen (DMT) is the major metabolic product, accounting for 50% of the dose. Smaller amounts of *N*-desdimethyltamoxifen (DDMT), the primary ethoxy alcohol, 4-OH hydroxyltamoxifen (4-OHT), and the side chain *N*-oxide have also been identified in humans (34,35). Glucuronide conjugates of tamoxifen metabolites are excreted in the bile and participate in enterohepatic recirculation of tamoxifen (36). The average

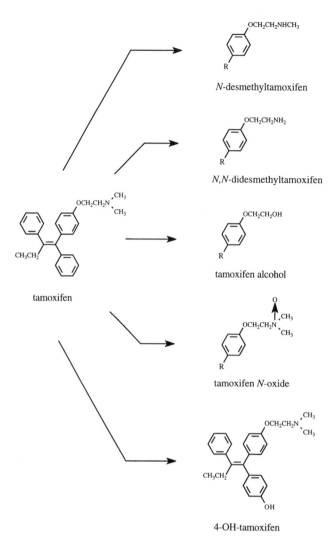

FIG. 38-5. Biotransformation pathways of tamoxifen.

steady-state plasma concentration of tamoxifen is approximately 250 nM. In adults younger than 50 years of age, the DMT, DDMT, 4-OHT, and primary alcohol steady-state concentration average is 400, 55, 10, and 30 nM, respectively. All steady-state plasma concentrations increase with advancing age, although the ratio of the various metabolites remains constant (34). All metabolites have been shown to possess estrogen receptor activity and probably contribute to the effect of tamoxifen (37).

The metabolic fate of toremifene is similar to that of tamoxifen. The major metabolites identified are *N*-desmethyltoremifene and the deaminohydroxy (primary alcohol) metabolite. After a single 120-mg oral dose, the peak plasma concentrations of the toremifene and desmethylmetabolite are 1.2 μM and 0.45 μM, respectively (38). Following multiple dosing, the concentrations of the desmethyl metabolite are two to four times greater than the parent compound, with steady-state concentrations of toremifene and desmethyl metabolite being reached in about 4 weeks. The predominant route of elimination is

fecal; only 10% of the toremifene dose is recovered in the urine. As with tamoxifen, toremifene undergoes extensive enterohepatic recirculation.

Enzyme Identification of Metabolite Formation

N-demethylation of tamoxifen has been well characterized and has been attributed to CYP3A (39,40). Inhibition of DMT formation in human liver microsomes is nearly complete with erythromycin, cyclosporine, and nifedipine. In addition, tamoxifen demethylase activity correlated with testosterone 6β-hydroxylation ($r = 0.90$) and immunoreactive CYP3A content ($r = 0.87$), and anti-CYP3A antibody was able to inhibit more than 70% of this activity. The *in vitro* K_m of this reaction was 98 μM. Toremifene demethylation has also been identified in human liver microsomes and is attributed to CYP3A (41).

As predicted, *in vivo* studies of tamoxifen and toremifene following rifampin administration demonstrated an 85% reduction in the oral tamoxifen area under the plasma concentration time curve (AUC) when compared to baseline. The C_{max} was reduced by 45% and the elimination half-life was reduced by 50% of control values. The reduction in the C_{max} suggests an increase in presystemic clearance. The AUC metabolite to parent ratio increased from 2.1 to 5.6, probably as the result of a marked increase in the formation clearance of metabolite. This interaction may have clinical significance because residence and peak concentrations of both parent compound and the major metabolite are reduced.

Although the 4-OH pathway accounts for a very small fraction of metabolism (approximately 2%), there is interest in identifying its metabolic pathway. The 4-OH metabolite binds to estrogen receptor as an antagonist with 100 times more affinity than the parent compound and, therefore, may contribute to the overall effect of tamoxifen (42). 4-OH tamoxifen also appears to undergo metabolic isomerization from the *trans* to *cis* isomer, rendering it inactive (43). Finally, 4-OH metabolite may be a bioactivated form that forms DNA adducts *in vitro* and *in vivo* (44,45).

Some controversy exists surrounding the identification of human CYP isoforms catalyzing the 4-hydroxylation of tamoxifen. Using statistical correlation of content and activity in human liver microsomes, the strongest correlations were observed with CYP2C8, CYP2C9, and CYP2D6 (46). Later work attempting to better characterize the 4-hydroxylase activity used human microsomes and recombinant enzyme. The suggestion that 4-OH tamoxifen formation could be catalyzed by CYP2D6, 2C9, and 3A4 was supported by the use of quinidine (1 μM), sulfaphenazole (20 μM), and ketoconazole (2 μM) as inhibitors. In microsomal studies, this resulted in inhibition ranging from 0% to 80%, 0% to 80%, and 12% to 57%, respectively (47). A previous study that suggested no involvement for CYP2D6 may have demonstrated the lack of CYP2D6 because of the variability of expression of various CYP isoforms in the small number of livers studied (48).

Dehal and Kupfer using *Escherichia coli*–expressed human P450 systems suggested that only CYP2D6 participates in the 4-hydroxylation of tamoxifen (44). However, in their human liver microsomal experiments, only 30% inhibition of 4-hydroxylation was observed using 20 μM quinidine or a polyclonal CYP2D6 antibody. Therefore, it seems likely that CYP2D6 and 2C9 are principally involved in tamoxifen 4-hydroxylation. Estimation of the kinetic parameters has not been possible because (a) the behavior of the *in vitro* system is unusual, (b) protein and drug concentration dependencies have been demonstrated, and (c) there have been no *in vivo* studies that have definitively identified the clinically important CYP enzymes in 4-hydroxylation of tamoxifen.

The *N*-oxide metabolite of tamoxifen has also been studied. The use of purified mouse enzyme and methimazole as well as temperature-dependent studies in human liver microsomes suggests a role for flavin monooxygenases (FMO) in the oxidation at the tertiary amine (40).

Finally, tamoxifen has produced a significant and serious interaction with warfarin, causing hypothrombinemia probably through inhibition of its metabolism (49). It appears that, at least *in vivo*, tamoxifen may inhibit CYP2C9.

Raloxifene

Raloxifene is an estrogen from a class of benzothiophene estrogenic compounds referred to as SERM. These compounds appear to act as both agonists and antagonists at differing receptors. In this regard, raloxifene appears to act as an agonist on bone and lipoprotein, whereas antagonistic activity is displayed in uterus and breast.

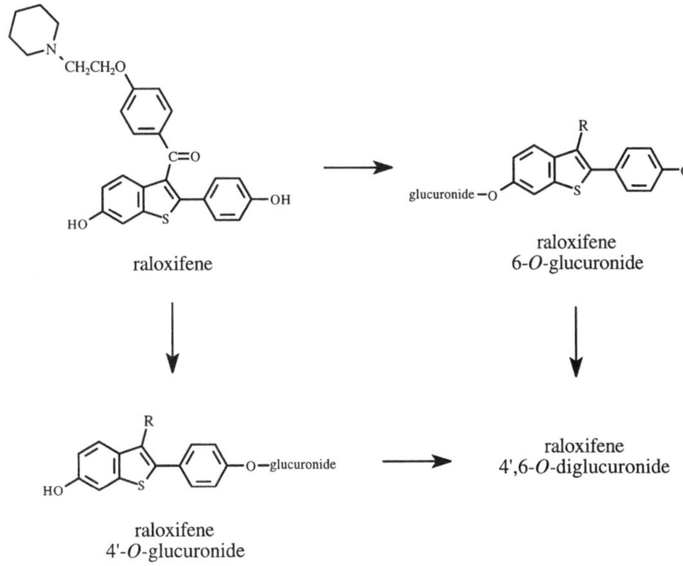

FIG. 38-6. Biotransformation pathways for raloxifene.

Metabolic Disposition

The metabolic scheme for raloxifene is shown in Fig. 38-6. Raloxifene undergoes extensive first pass metabolism and, although 60% of the dose is absorbed, the overall bioavailability is only 2%. The major metabolites identified are the 6- and 4'-glucuronide conjugates and the 4',6-diglucuronide. The major route of elimination is fecal, and there is substantial evidence that raloxifene undergoes extensive enterohepatic recirculation (50).

Enzyme Identification of Metabolite Formation

There is no evidence that CYP enzymes are involved in the metabolism of this compound because no other metabolites have been identified. Furthermore, no significant drug–drug interactions with known inhibitors of CYP enzymes are known.

The isoform of human UDP-glucuronyltransferase that catalyzes raloxifene metabolism has not yet been reported. Raloxifene glucuronides have little affinity for estrogen receptors and appear to be significantly less active than the parent compound in human breast cancer cell line studies (51).

PROGESTINS

Progestins are compounds that bind to progesterone receptor and exhibit some progesterone-like activity, most often defined on a particular *in vivo* or *in vitro* parameter (e.g., endometrial histology). In general, progestins antagonize the effect of estrogens.

Progestins and the endogenous steroid progesterone have been classified based on their structural backbone; they can be divided into two broad groups: (a) the C-21 (pregnane) progestins and (b) those derived from androgens—the 19-nortestosterone analogues. These compounds have found use as oral contraceptives and in many conditions including endometrial hyperplasia and carcinoma, and cachexia associated with cancer and acquired immunodeficiency syndrome. Recently, progesterone has been marketed to prevent endometrial hyperplasia secondary to postmenopausal estrogen therapy.

Progesterone

Progesterone is the naturally occurring C-21 steroid. Significant progesterone production occurs during the reproductive years in women and is present primarily following ovulation and during pregnancy. Maximum physiologic progesterone plasma concentrations of approximately 80 and 450 nM are produced from synthesis by the postovulatory follicle and the placenta, respectively.

Poor oral bioavailability prevented its use but the impact on hepatic protein synthesis made progesterone an attractive therapy when compared with 19-nortestosterone derivatives. The development of micronized particles has sufficiently increased the availability, making oral progesterone useful in treating secondary amenorrhea and as part of menopausal hormone replacement therapy.

Metabolic Disposition

The metabolic fate of progesterone, like other endogenous steroids, is complicated. Early studies of progesterone metabolic fate suffered from problems of nonspecific immunoquantitation. Furthermore, significant enterohepatic recirculation and multiple reductive metabolic pathways are known to occur (52). The use of mass spectroscopy technology has assisted in the identification of metabolic fate but the story is not complete. In addition, route-dependent metabolism of progesterone occurs and there are large interspecies differences in progesterone disposition. Therefore, in the interest of current therapeutic importance, this section addresses what is known about the disposition of exogenously administered oral progesterone.

The average absolute bioavailability of orally administered micronized progesterone is 8.6% (53). Following oral administration, dose proportionality is observed, and a 300-mg dose produces average peak concentrations of approximately 100 nM. The precise nature of poor bioavailability is unclear; however, evidence suggests that in humans both first pass and luminal escape may be important.

Differences in metabolic profiles of major metabolites have been observed following absorption by portal (oral) and nonportal routes (vaginal, intravenous). In humans, oral administration resulted in much greater plasma of 5α- and 5β-pregnane-3, 20-dione, and 11-deoxycorticosterone (4-pregnen-21-ol-3, 20-dione), suggesting greater first pass metabolism (54). These data and biliary secretion data from previous studies suggest that rapid reductive metabolism must contribute significantly to the first pass effect (52).

A significant fraction of administered progesterone undergoes enterohepatic recirculation. Following intravenous administration, approximately 30% of the progesterone dose is secreted in bile (55). It is likely that progesterone metabolites secreted in bile undergo many cycles of secretion and reabsorption (57). The systemic entrance of hydroxylated progesterone analogues is inversely correlated with oral absorption of progesterone, suggesting that metabolic hydroxylation is likely to result in less reabsorption (56).

The known metabolic scheme for orally administered progesterone is shown in Fig. 38-7. Following administration of radiolabeled progesterone, approximately 70% of the dose can be recovered, 60% percent as urinary metabolites and 10% as fecal metabolites (58). The metabolic fate of the remainder (30%) remains unknown, and hepatic metabolism accounts for only about half of all metabolic pathways (59). Progesterone undergoes both reductive and oxidative metabolism, the major metabolite

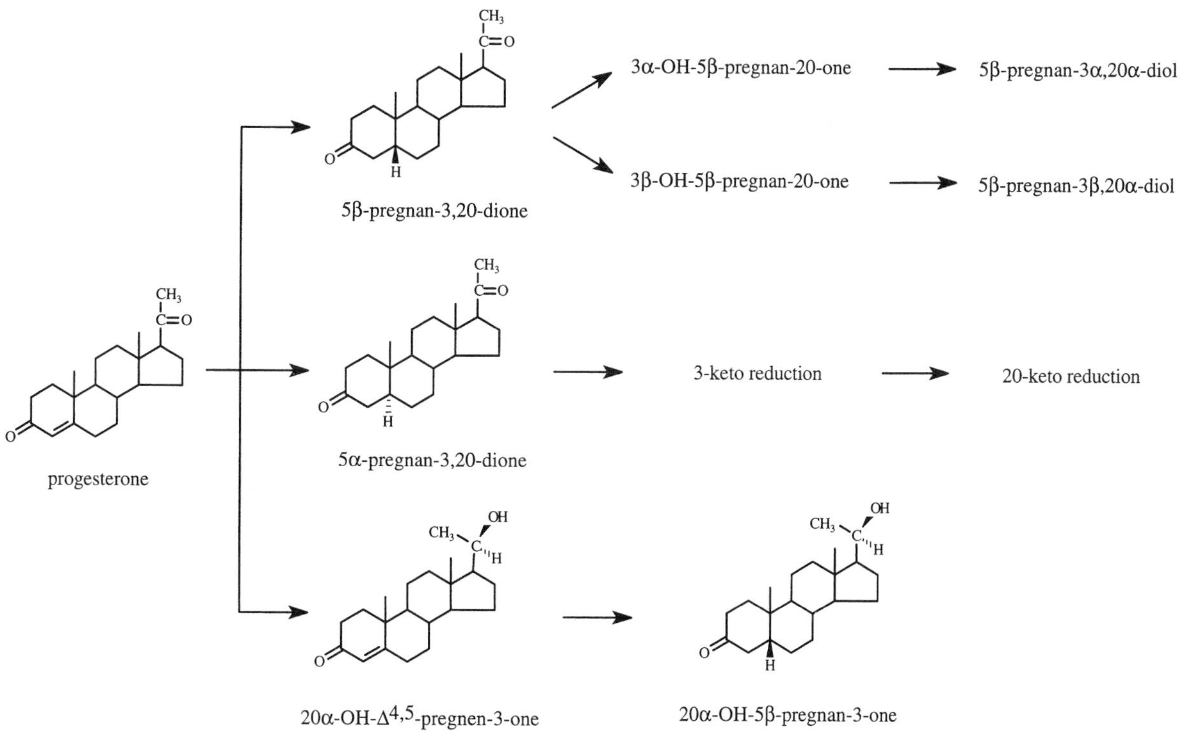

FIG. 38-7. Biotransformation pathways for progesterone.

(approximately 25%) being 5β-pregnane-3α, 20α diol (pregnanediol) glucuronide. Besides 5α- and β-reduction and 3- and 20-α hydroxyl formation, there is some *in vivo* and *in vitro* evidence for oxidation at the 6, 16, 17, and 21 positions as well (60–62).

Administration of 5α-dihydroprogesterone (5α-DHP) to women allowed the quantitation of its major metabolites (63). In this study, only 37% of the administered intravenous dose was recovered. The major metabolites were identified as the 3α- or 3β-6α-dihydroxy-5α-pregnan-20-one glucuronides, accounting for 16% and 6% of the 5α-DHP dose, respectively.

Some metabolites of progesterone have activity and may be responsible for some side effects observed with oral progesterone treatment. It has long been recognized that a number of compounds derived from progesterone possess sedative effects (64). Four such compounds were identified in the plasma of women who were administered oral progesterone (65). One subject experienced a severe hypnotic state that persisted for 2 hours following a 400-mg oral dose.

Enzyme Identification of Metabolite Formation

The identification of the 5-position reductive metabolism remains unclear. The *in vivo* 5β-reduction of progesterone appears to be confined to the liver. 3β-oxidation is likely to occur by a member of the steroid hydrogenase family but neither of the enzymes responsible for their formation has been described. 5α-reduction appears to be mainly extrahepatic and evidence suggests that the 6-hydroxylation of 5α-steroids does not appear to be CYP mediated (66–67).

Recently, the 6β-hydroxylation of progesterone was identified as the major *in vitro* hepatic oxidative pathway in human liver (68). This activity was attributed to CYP3A from substrate and antibody inhibition, and correlation with other known CYP3A substrate oxidation rates and immunoreactive protein content. Whether this pathway contributes *in vivo* as a major route of progesterone elimination in humans is unknown. The concentration of progesterone used in this study was 25 μM. These concentrations exceed the *in vivo* concentrations by more than two log concentrations; therefore, it is unclear what role, if any, CYP3A has in the disposition of progesterone. Yamazaki and Shimada determined the K_m for progesterone 6β-hydroxylation from recombinant human CYP3A enzyme to be 80 μM (69). Interestingly, they found evidence for CYP2C19 involvement in 16- and 21-hydroxylation. Given that only a small fraction of progesterone disposition has been accounted for, it seems plausible that metabolic pathways similar to other endogenous and synthetic neutral steroids may involve hepatic CYP enzymes. Further studies are needed to define the significance of hepatic CYP isoforms on the disposition of progesterone in humans, especially under conditions of induction or inhibition.

Norethindrone

Metabolic Disposition

Norethindrone (norethisterone, NET) appears to be well absorbed. Peak plasma NET concentrations following a 1-mg oral dose are approximately 20 nM (70). The absolute bioavailability after a single dose averages 64%, indicating the presence of significant first pass metabolism. Two other progestins—norethindrone acetate (17β-acetyl NET) and ethynodiol diacetate (3, 17β-diacetyl NET)—are prodrugs of NET and therefore are not considered separately.

Following administration of radiolabeled NET, more than 50% of the dose can be recovered in urine and up to 40% of the dose can be recovered in feces. Most of the radiolabeled compounds were recovered as glucuronide conjugates (71).

The biotransformation scheme of NET is shown in Fig. 38-8. The major metabolites identified are those similar to other neutral steroids and include 5α- and β-reduction and 3α- and β-hydroxylation (72). The major metabolite recovered in the glucuronide fraction was the 3α-OH, 5β-norethindrone, accounting for approximately 15% of the dose. Other hydroxylation pathways have been known for some time and include 10β-hydroxylation (73). Other unidentified highly polar, water-soluble, polyhydroxylated metabolites have been seen; however, little other informa-tion is known about the quantitative aspect of NET disposition despite its use for more than 30 years (74).

Enzyme Identification of Metabolite Formation

To predict oral bioavailability of various 19-nor testosterone compounds, such as NET, intrinsic clearance was estimated from NADPH-dependent disappearance of NET in human liver microsomes (75). From the *in vitro* data, a scaled *in vivo* Cl_{int} of 81 L/hour was estimated. These data suggest a potentially significant role for CYP enzymes in the elimination of NET. However, specific metabolites and the enzymes catalyzing a particular metabolic pathway have yet to be studied.

Evidence for a significant CYP3A role in the overall metabolism of NET is suggested by *in vivo* interaction studies. Concomitant administration of NET-containing combination oral contraceptives with CYP3A-inducing agents results in significant changes in the NET oral clearance (76). Ten days of either rifampin or rifabutin (300 mg/day) increased the NET oral clearance by 60% or 20%, respectively. Furthermore, the NET C_{max} was reduced by approximately the same amount (30%) with each drug. However, rifampin reduced the terminal half-life of NET 58%, whereas rifabutin had less of an effect (35% decrease). These data suggest that when CYP3A is induced, it affects the first pass of NET similarly but that

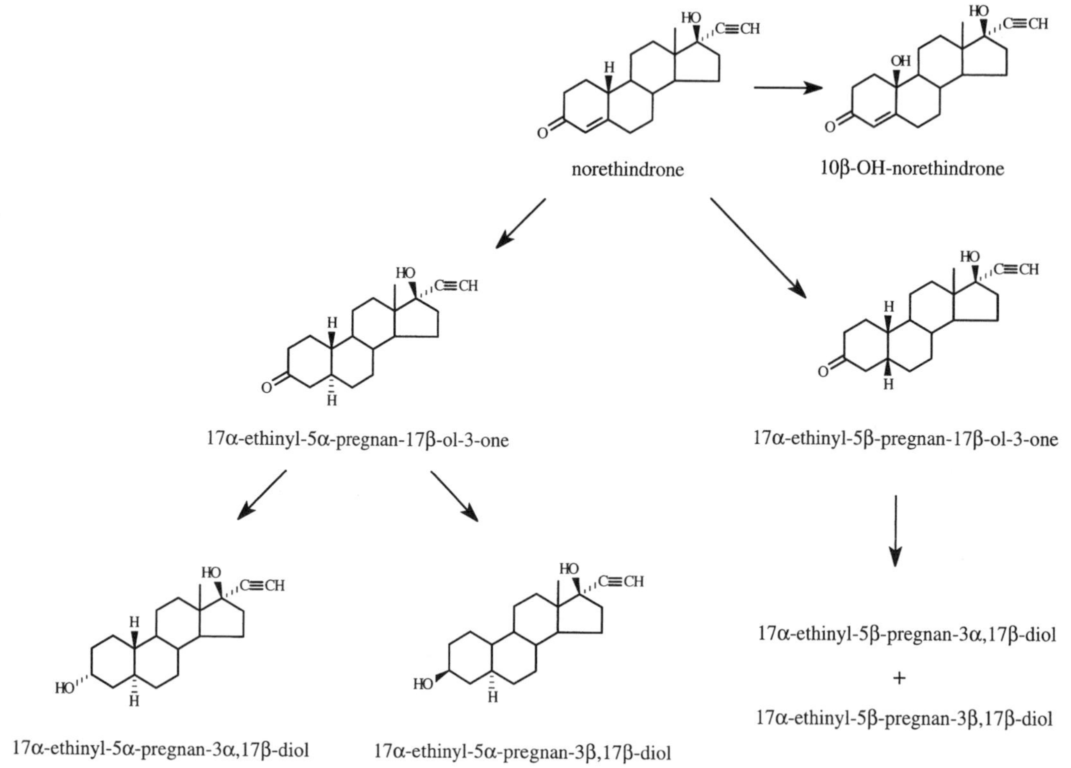

FIG. 38-8. Biotransformation pathways for norethindrone.

rifabutin has less of an effect on systemic clearance of NET and that CYP3A contributes significantly to the overall metabolic fate of NET.

Levonorgestrel

Metabolic Fate

Unlike norethindrone, levonorgestrel (LNG) is not subject to a large first pass effect but is primarily metabolized, less than 1% recovered in the urine unchanged. Sisenwine reported that approximately 45% and 30% of a radiolabeled dose was recovered in the urine and feces, respectively (78). In urine, the majority of these compounds were predominantly glucuronide conjugates. The major metabolite in the urine was 3α, 5β-tetrahydrolevonorgestrel; however, this accounted for only 11% of the dose. Urinary hydroxylated metabolites (2 and 16 position) have also been isolated, corresponding to approximately 3% of the dose. Unknown urinary metabolites were seen that have yet to be identified. As with norethindrone, there is a significant gap in both the qualitative and quantitative aspects of its metabolic fate despite its widespread use as a contraceptive.

Enzyme Identification

There is no information on the identification of enzymes responsible for the metabolic disposition of LNG.

Norgestimate

Norgestimate is one of three recently developed gonanes characterized by 3-keto and 13-ethyl groups on the 19-nortestosterone backbone, constituting the third generation progestins. These compounds appear to have a beneficial effect on lipoproteins.

Metabolic Fate

Following oral administration of norgestimate, peak plasma concentrations of norgestimate and its primary circulating metabolite, 17-desacetyl norgestimate, are quickly observed in the plasma (79). Mean peak plasma concentrations of the parent and deacetylated compound are 12.3 nM and 10.9 nM, respectively.

Only one study has been published reporting the metabolic fate of norgestimate (80). Overall, slightly greater than 80% of a radioactive dose was recovered where aver-

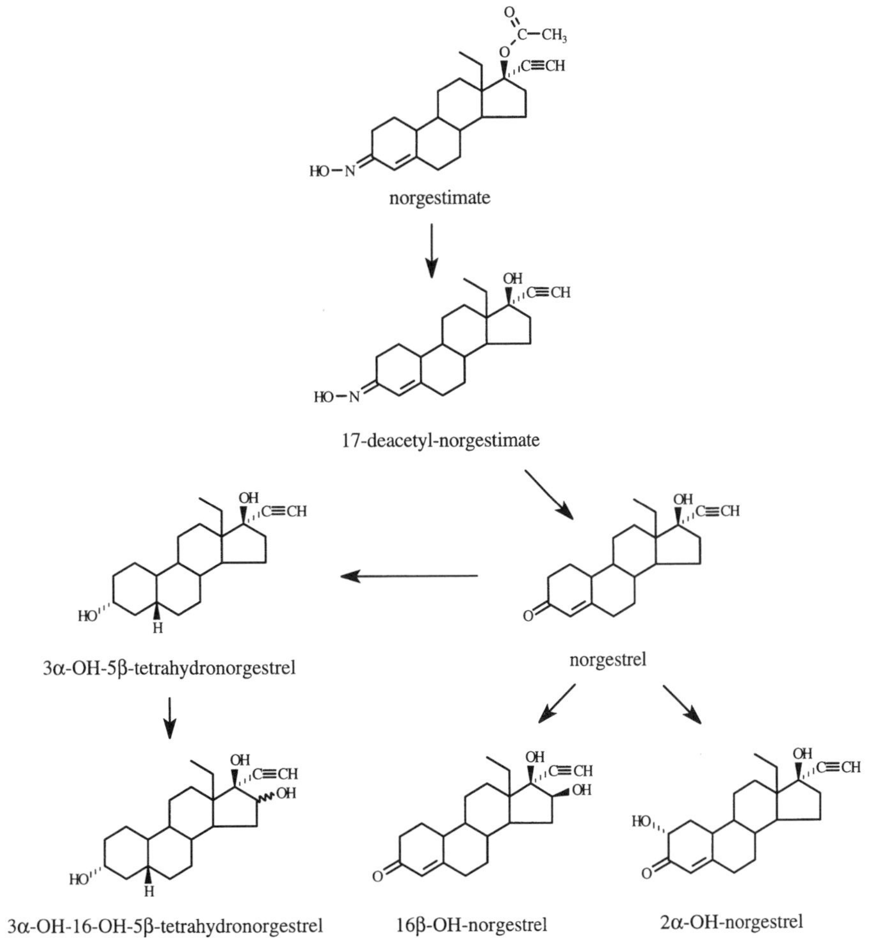

FIG. 38-9. Biotransformation pathways for norgestimate.

ages of 47% and 37% were found in the urine and feces, respectively. Five metabolites were isolated from the urine and are shown in Fig. 38-9. These metabolites indicate that there is deacetylation at the 17-position and loss of the 3-oxime to form a 3-keto group. The predominant metabolite was 3α, 5β-tetrahydronorgestrel (approximately 8% of the dose), followed by norgestrel (approximately 5%). Other metabolites included 2- and 16-hydroxylated metabolites of norgestrel and triols. Additional hydroxylated metabolites were observed but not identified.

Because administration of norgestimate leads to formation of norgestrel, it has been suggested that norgestimate is a prodrug. By comparing levonorgestrel AUC following levonorgestrel and norgestimate, it has been estimated that approximately 21% of a norgestimate dose is converted to levonorgestrel and, therefore, may contribute to its *in vivo* activity (77).

The pharmacologic profile of the 17-desacetyl norgestimate is similar to the parent compound and is about equally active in various *in vitro* and *in vivo* activity assays (81). Although a reasonable amount of levonorgestrel and its metabolites appear to be formed, the effect of norgestimate containing combined oral contraceptives on lipoproteins suggests that levonorgestrel does not contribute to the major progestin action *in vivo*.

Enzyme Identification

Studies done in human intestinal mucosa and liver microsomes demonstrate that 17-deacetylation did not require NADPH and that it accounted for about 40% of hepatic activity and probably is catalyzed by microsomal esterases. Incubation in hepatic microsomes identified a number of metabolites. Less than 2% was identified as 3-keto norgestimate, but norgestrel and other unidentified metabolites accounted for 10% and 15% of microsomal metabolism (82). The specific enzymes responsible for the NADPH-dependent oxidation pathways remain unknown.

Desogestrel

Metabolic Fate

Desogestrel (DSG) is considered to be a prodrug in that, following oral administration, DSG is rapidly and completely converted to the active metabolite, 3-keodesogestrel (3-KDSG). Following a 2.5-mg oral DSG dose, peak DSG and 3-KDSG plasma concentrations were reported to be 2 nM and 30 nM, respectively. Little circulating DSG can be detected following oral administration of DSG and the 3-KDSG AUC is the same when nearly equimolar oral doses of DSG or 3-KDSG were administered (84,85). Furthermore, an *in vivo* study demonstrated that 3-KDSG exerts progestational activity much greater than the parent compound (85).

DSG is fairly well absorbed although there is a great deal of intersubject variability. The absolute bioavailability was determined to be 76% (range, 40%–113%) and, in subsequent study by the same investigators, 62% (range, 51%–78%) (86,87). The possibility for both incomplete

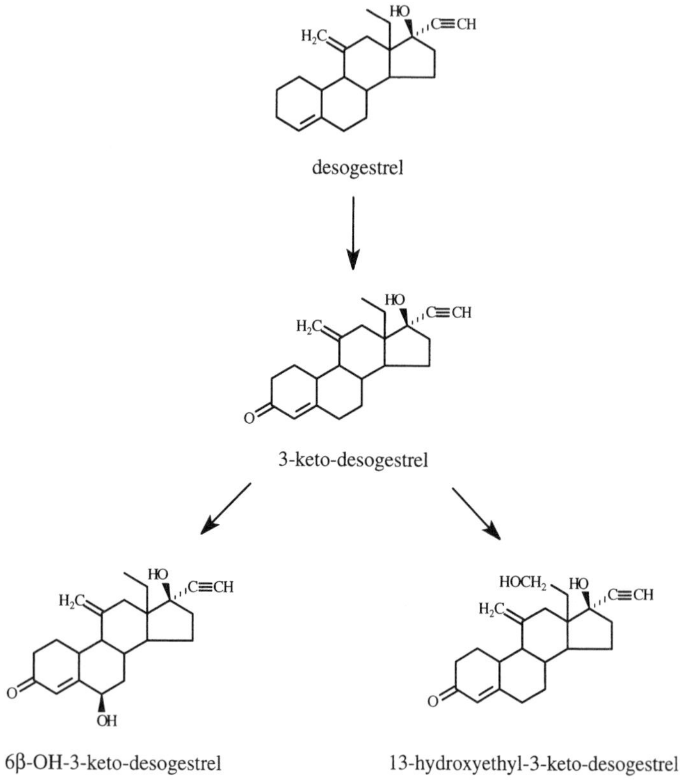

FIG. 38-10. Biotransformation pathways for desogestrel.

absorption and first pass intestinal metabolism exists for this compound because phase I and II intestinal metabolism has been demonstrated *in vitro* (88).

Figure 38-10 depicts the putative metabolic pathway for DSG. Following oral administration, conversion of DSG to 3α- or β-OH DSG is seen in human liver microsomal studies, and this oxidation is thought to represent the intermediate step to formation of the 3-keto metabolite (89). *In vitro* evidence from human liver microsomal studies suggests that 3-KDSG can undergo further oxidation to form 6β- and 13-ethyl hydroxyl metabolites (90). Besides oxidation, there is *in vitro* evidence for reduction of the Δ^4 double bond similar to other progestational compounds. This metabolism occurs in human liver homogenate and in the cytosolic fraction (91,92). The relative contribution of this metabolic pathway is unknown.

Enzyme Identification

The enzymes responsible for oxidation at the 3 position were recently investigated (89). Using NADPH reductase antibody, the role of CYP in the oxidation of DSG was established. From this study, it appears that CYP2C9 and 2C19 contribute to the oxidation of DSG at the 3 position similar to mestranol biotransformation. Only sulfaphenazole produced significant inhibition using selective CYP enzyme inhibitors for 3A4, 2E1, 2D6, 2A6, and 1A2. Maximum inhibition (65%) was observed after combining sulfaphenazole and mephenytoin (10 μM and 100 μM, respectively). In an expressed CYP2C9 lymphoblast system, a K_m of 6.5 μM for DSG 3α-hydroxylation and a K_i of 0.91 μM for sulfaphenazole were observed.

Human liver microsomal studies demonstrated the formation of 3α- and 3β-OH DSG metabolites after a 5-minute incubation, and longer incubation (30 minutes) resulted in the formation of 3-keto DSG. Because of the role of CYP3A in steroid metabolism, extensive work was done to characterize CYP3A involvement in DSG metabolism. There was no correlation with CYP3A4 content and an anti-CYP3A antibody or incubation with ketoconazole did not inhibit 3-KDSG formation. In fact, incubation with ketoconazole markedly increased the amount of 3-keto DSG. Because the intestine has a role in oxidative metabolism of DSG, this suggests that further DSG oxidative metabolism (6β- and 13-ethyl hydroxylation) may be the result of CYP3A or CYP1A activity (90,93).

The reduction of the 3-OH DSG is probably the result of activity of 3α-hydroxysteroid dehydrogenase enzyme that has been isolated from human liver (94). The cytosolic 5α- or 5β-reductase may catalyze Δ^{4-5} reduction. The enzyme pathways responsible for DSG phase I metabolism and *in vivo* disposition require further investigation.

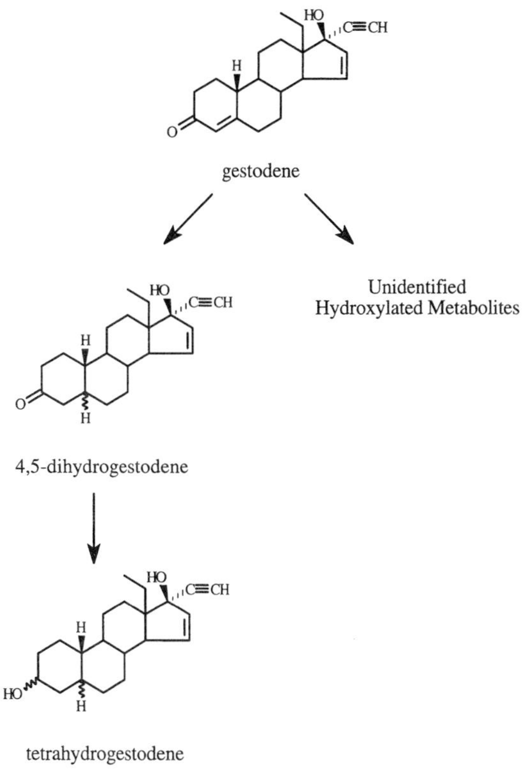

FIG. 38-11. Biotransformation pathways for gestodene.

Gestodene

Metabolic Fate

Gestodene is well absorbed after oral administration. The absolute bioavailability has been estimated to be about 90% (87,95). The major metabolic pathways identified for gestodene are shown in Fig. 38-11. *In vivo* metabolism studies demonstrate that the major urinary metabolites include Δ^{4-5} reduction and various hydroxyl metabolites.

Enzyme Identification

Little is known about the precise nature of enzymes that catalyze the various metabolites of gestodene. Ward and Back examined the role of various hepatic subcellular fractions in gestodene metabolism (96). Hepatic cytosol was efficient at A-ring reduction, producing 5-dihydrogestodene and 3-keto reduction (tetrahydrogestodene), although the latter was produced in lesser amounts. The techniques employed did not allow for determination of the axial hydrogen (5α or 5β) arrangement. Enzyme kinetic parameters of Δ^{4-5} reduction yielded an apparent K_m of (5.0 μM) and inhibition studies demonstrated that androstenedione and cortisol both inhibited this metabolite formation in a noncompetitive fashion (K_i values 2.9 and 24.1 μM, respectively). The enzymes responsible may be the mammalian cytosolic Δ^4-reductase and the cytosolic and microsomal 3-ketoreductase enzymes. Microsomal metabolism demonstrated an NADPH-dependent hydroxyl metabolite of gestodene. Preliminary evidence suggested that the enzyme involved is CYP3A in that ketoconazole markedly inhibited the formation of this metabolite ($IC_{50} < 100$ nM).

Gestodene at concentrations of 100 μM appear to be mechanism-based inhibitors of CYP3A (97). In this study, inhibition EE_2 2-hydroxylation, a CYP3A-mediated metabolic step, was demonstrated, raising the possibility of a drug interaction because these compounds are administered in combination. However, multiple pharmacokinetic studies comparing DSG and gestodene in combination with EE_2 were not able to demonstrate differences in EE_2 clearance after single or multiple dosing. Because the concentration used in vitro is three orders of magnitude than those obtained in vivo, it is likely that an effect may not be observed. It might be possible that local concentrations at the intestinal surface may be greater and, if inhibition did occur, first pass might not be observed because there are other metabolic pathways. Studies that examine the metabolic disposition of EE_2 with and without gestodene may help determine whether differential first pass occurs. It is unlikely, however, to be of clinical significance.

C-21 Pregnane Progestins (Medroxyprogesterone Acetate, Megestrol)

Medroxyprogesterone (MPA) is widely used in hormone replacement and contraceptive regimens. Megesterol (MEG) has been used in the treatment of breast cancer and, recently, as adjunct therapy in cachexia resulting from chronic diseases. Despite the widespread use, little is known about the metabolic fate of these compounds.

Metabolic Fate

The precise MPA fraction absorbed is unknown because no studies have compared oral and intravenous doses. However, when compared to intramuscular and intraperitoneal administration, the estimated bioavailability is low—17.4% and 0.2%, respectively. MEG appears to be better absorbed, in that, following oral administration of labeled drug, urinary recovery ranged between 55% and 80% (98). However, whether first pass metabolism occurs is unknown. Single oral doses of MPA (1200 mg) and MEG (160 mg) produce peak concentrations of approximately 150 nM; however, MPA doses employed clinically may be as low as 2.5 mg per day. The depot form of MPA (1200 mg) produces much lower concentrations, approximately 20 nM (99).

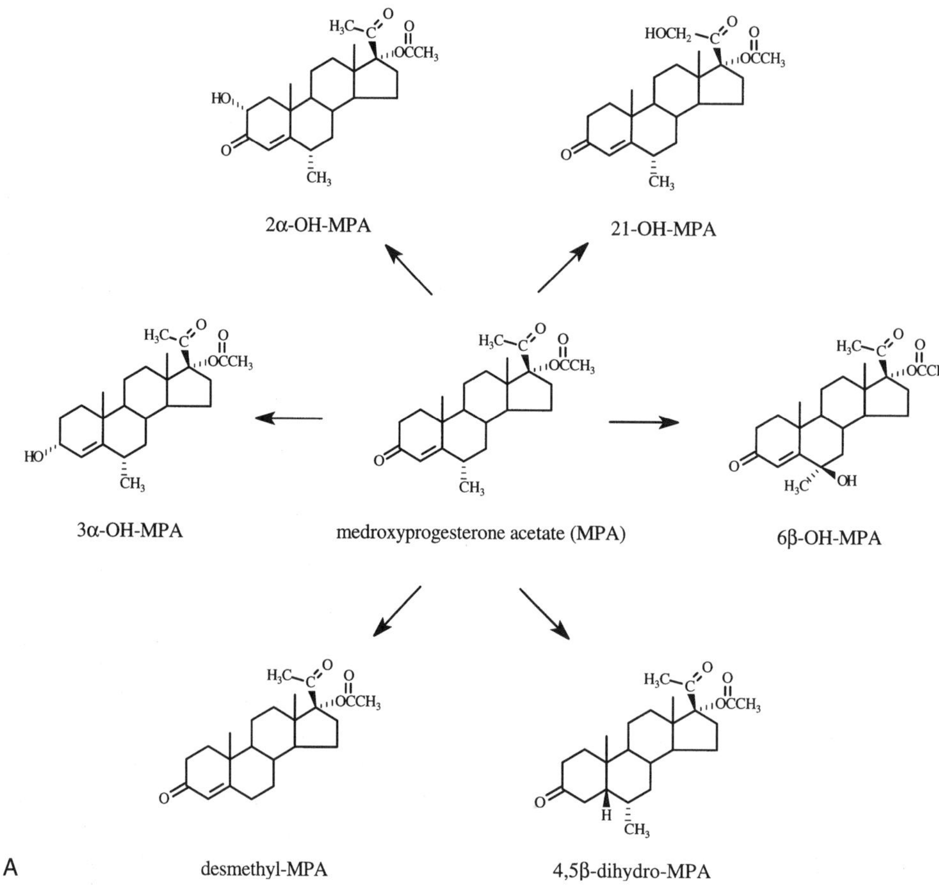

FIG. 38-12. (A) Biotransformation pathways of medroxyprogesterone acetate.

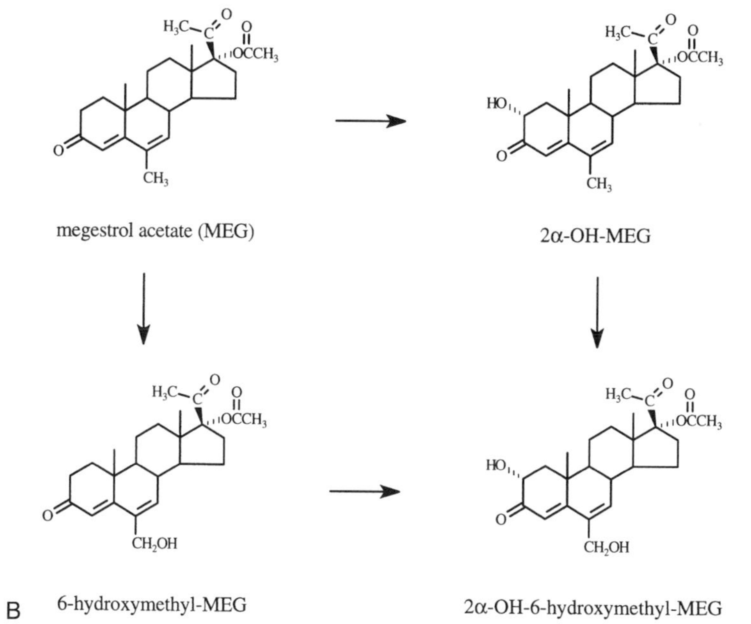

megestrol acetate (MEG) 2α-OH-MEG

6-hydroxymethyl-MEG 2α-OH-6-hydroxymethyl-MEG

B

FIG. 38-12. (B) Biotransformation pathways of megestrol acetate.

Following an intravenous dose, almost all of MPA undergoes metabolism; less than 3% of a dose is recovered as unchanged drug in urine. However, only about 50% of a dose can be accounted for. Single-dose radiolabel studies of MPA can account for approximately 60% of the administered dose: 25% to 50% appears in urine and approximately 5% to 10% can be recovered in feces (100,101). For MEG, total recovery of label ranged from 83% to 95%, with the remainder between total radioactivity and urinary excretion (55–80%) found in the feces.

The proposed metabolic scheme for MPA and MEG is shown in Figure 38-12. The major metabolite of MPA is a glucuronide conjugate, presumably at the 3-oxo position. Nonetheless, 15 metabolites have been recovered in the urine, representing 2-, 6-, and 21-hydroxylation, reduction, demethylation, and sequential metabolic products of these pathways (100,102). MEG has three hydroxyl metabolites (2-OH, 6-methyl-OH, and the 2-OH, 6-methyl-OH dihydroxy) recovered as the corresponding glucuronides from urine. These metabolites, however, only account for approximately 8% of the total radioactivity.

Enzyme Identification of Metabolite Formation

No information exists regarding the enzymes that catalyze the various metabolites of either MPA or MEG. Of note, MEG appears to be an efficient inhibitor of MDR transport protein in several human cell culture lines (103). Given the relationship between MDR and CYP3A, it is possible that MEG is also a substrate or inhibitor of CYP3A.

Mifepristone

Mifepristone is an 11-substituted (dimethylaminopropyl) steroid in a relatively new class of drugs with antiprogestin activity; therefore, this class of compounds has utility in the management of reproductive system disorders. In addition to its action at the progesterone receptor, mifepristone also has affinity for the glucocorticoid receptor with relatively higher affinity than dexamethasone, an action associated with its use in the treatment of Cushing's syndrome (104,105).

Metabolic Fate

Mifepristone is administered orally and exhibits marked variability in its bioavailability, ranging from 30% to 56% following a 100-mg dose. Peak plasma concentrations are approximately 2 to 4 μM and do not increase further in proportion to the dose. This nonlinear behavior occurs with doses greater than 100 mg and is probably related to saturable plasma binding of α-1 acid glycoprotein. Although parent compound plasma AUC does not increase proportionally, metabolite AUC following mifepristone administration suggests that this phenomenon is not the result of changes in metabolic clearance or bioavailability changes from a first pass effect (106).

Metabolism of mifepristone is extensive and only a small fraction of the dose appears unchanged in urine. The primary metabolites identified are the 17-propynl hydroxymetabolite and at the tertiary amine, where sequential demethylation occurs (Fig. 38-13) (105,106). These metabolites undergo further biotransformation and are excreted into the bile (107).

Compared to the parent drug, the metabolites display less than 20% of *in vitro* human progesterone receptor binding activity but still retain approximately 50% of their potency to the glucocorticoid receptor, suggesting that the metabolites might contribute to antiglucocorticoid effect but probably will not contribute much to its antiprogesterone action (104).

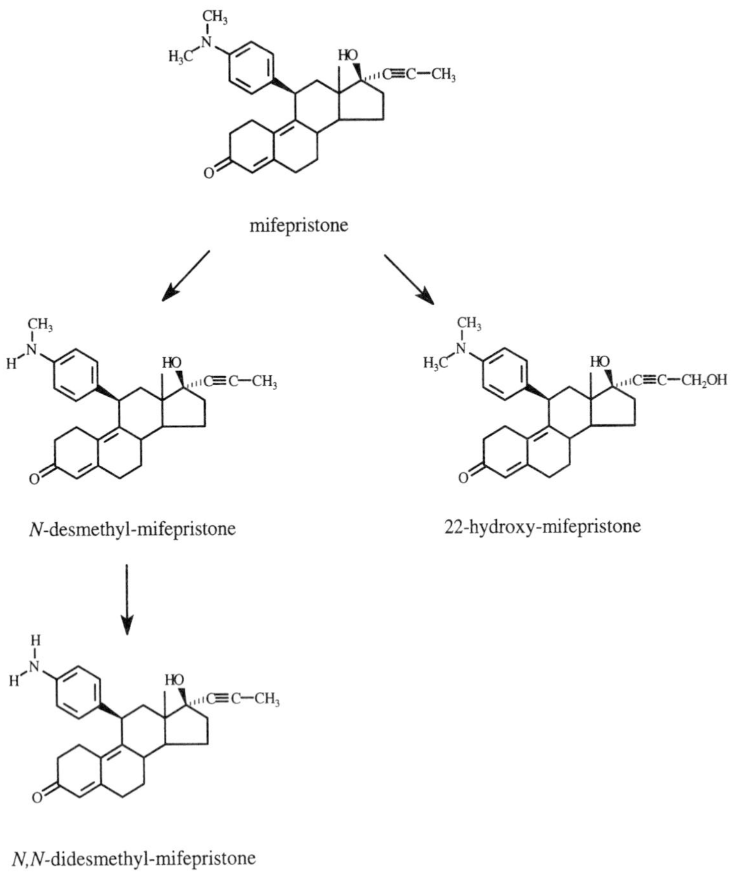

mifepristone

N-desmethyl-mifepristone

22-hydroxy-mifepristone

N,N-didesmethyl-mifepristone

FIG. 38-13. Biotransformation pathways of mifeprostone.

Enzyme Identification of Metabolite Formation

Substantial evidence points to CYP3A as the major isoform responsible for the formation of the oxidative metabolites of mifepristone (108). Mifepristone oxidation rates significantly correlate with CYP3A protein content, and activities and are inhibited by CYP3A antibodies and inhibitors. Consistent with the *in vivo* observations, the monodesmethyl metabolite was the major metabolite formed in human liver microsomal studies. The hydroxylation and demethylation apparent K_m values were 9.9 and 10.6 µM, respectively.

Mifepristone also demonstrates time-dependent and NADPH-dependent inactivation of CYP3A in human liver microsomes (109). Possible mechanisms involving the regions of metabolism include activation of a propynl group and the formation of metabolic intermediate complexation. He and co-workers estimated the hepatic microsomal K_i and K_{inact} to be 4.7 µM and 0.089 min^{-1}, respectively (110). Therefore, mifepristone is one of the more potent CYP3A inactivating drugs identified to date. Evidence for heme adduct formation was not found, although binding to CYP3A protein was identified in a ratio of 1:1 with mifepristone. Finally, mifepristone demonstrates *in vitro* CYP3A induction in rat, rabbit, and human hepatocyte culture (111). This may be due to stabilization of protein from MI complexation or by transcriptional activation. It is possible that mifepristone may interact with other

CYP3A substrates at either the level of intestinal first pass or clearance. There are no known studies to date that confirm these observations with *in vivo* interactions in humans.

REFERENCES

1. Mosselman S, Pohlman J, Dijekma R. ER beta: identification and characterization of a novel human estrogen receptor. *FEBS Lett* 1996;392: 49–53.
2. Jarvenpaa P. In vitro metabolism of catechol estrogens by human fecal microflora. *J Steroid Biochem* 1990;35:289–292.
3. Longcope C, Gorbach S, Goldin B, Woods M, Dwyer J, Warram J. The metabolism of estradiol; oral compared to intravenous administration. *J Steroid Biochem* 1985;23:1065–1070.
4. O'Connell M. Pharmacokinetic and pharmacologic variation between different estrogen products. *J Clin Pharmacol* 1995;35:18S–24S.
5. Lobo R, Cassidenti D. Pharmacokinetics of oral 17β-estradiol. *J Reprod Med* 1992;37:77–84.
6. Ball P, Knuppen R. Formation, metabolism, and physiologic importance of catecholestrogens. *Am J Obstet Gynecol* 1990;163:2163–2170.
7. Kerlan V, Dreano Y, Bercovici J, Beaune P, Floch H, Berthou F. Nature of cytochromes P450 involved in the 2/4-hydroxylations of estradiol in human liver microsomes. *Biochem Pharmacol* 1992;44:1745–1756.
8. Aoyama T, Korzekwa K, Nagata K, Gillette J, Gelboin H, Gonzalez F. Estradiol metabolism by complementary deoxyribonucleic acid-expressed human cytochrome P450s. *Endocrinology* 1990;126: 3101–3106.
9. Spink D, Eugster H, Lincoln D 2nd, et al. 17β-estradiol hydroxylation catalyzed by human cytochrome P450 1A1: a comparison of the activities induced by 2,3,7,8-tetrachlorodibenzo-p-dioxin in MCF-7 cells with those from heterologous expression of the cDNA. *Arch Biochem Biophys* 1992;293:342–348.
10. Fisher CW, Caudle DL, Martin-Wixtrom C, et al. High-level expression of functional human cytochrome P450 1A2 in *Escherichia coli*. *FASEB J* 1992;6:759–764.

11. Michnovicz J, Hershcopf R, Nagnuma H, Bradlow H, Fishman J. Increased 2-hydroxylation of estradiol as a possible mechanism for the anti-estrogenic effect of cigarette smoking. *N Engl J Med* 1986;20: 1305–1309.

12. Shou M, Korzekwa K, Brooks E, Krausz K, Gonzalez F, Gelboin H. Role of human hepatic cytochrome P450 1A2 and 3A4 in the metabolic activation of estrone. *Carcinogenesis* 1997;18:207–214.

13. Huang Z, Guengerich F, Kaminsky L. 16 alpha-hydroxylation of estrone by human cytochrome P4503A4/5. *Carcinogenesis* 1998;19:867–872.

14. Back DJ, Breckenridge A, Crawford F, et al. An investigation of the pharmacokinetics of ethinylestradiol in women using radioimmuno-assay. *Contraception* 1979;20:263–273.

15. Back D, Breckenridge A, MacIver M, et al. The gut wall metabolism of ethinyloestradiol and its contribution to the pre-systemic metabolism of ethinyloestradiol in humans. *Br J Clin Pharmacol* 1982;13:325–330.

16. Bird C, Clark A. Metabolic clearance rates and metabolism of mestranol and ethinylestradiol in normal young women. *J Clin Endocrinol Metab* 1973;36:296–302.

17. Bolt H, Bolt W. Pharmacokinetics of mestranol in man in relation to its oestrogenic activity. *Eur J Clin Pharmacol* 1974;7:295–305.

18. Bolt H, Bolt M, Kappus H. Interaction of rifampicin treatment with pharmacokinetics and metabolism of ethinyloestradiol in man. *Acta Endocrinol (Copenh)* 1977;85:189–197.

19. Williams M, Helton E, Goldzieher J. The urinary metabolites of 17 alpha-ethinylestradiol-9 alpha, 11xi-3H in women. Chromatographic profiling and identification of ethynl and non-ethynl compounds. *Steroids* 1975;25:229–246.

20. Sahlberg B, Axelson M, Collins D, Sjovall J. Analysis of isomeric ethynylestradiol glucuronides in urine. *J Chromatogr* 1981;6:453–461.

21. Maggs J, Grimmer S, Orme M, Breckenridge A, Park B, Gilmore I. The biliary and urinary metabolites of [3H]17 alpha-ethynylestradiol in women. *Xenobiotica* 1983;13:421–431.

22. Schmider J, Greenblatt D, von Moltke L, et al. Biotransformation of mestranol to ethinyl estradiol *in vitro*: the role of cytochrome P-450 2C9 and metabolic inhibitors. *J Clin Pharmacol* 1997;37:193–200.

23. Guengerich F. Oxidation of 17 alpha-ethynylestradiol by human liver cytochrome P-450. *Mol Pharmacol* 1988;33:500–508.

24. Bolt H, Kappus H, Bolt M. Effect of rifampin treatment on metabolism of oestradiol and 17 alpha-ethynylestradiol by human liver microsomes. *Eur J Clin Pharmacol* 1975;8:301–307.

25. Weber A, Jager R, Borner A, et al. Can grapefruit juice influence ethinylestradiol bioavailability? *Contraception* 1996;53:41–47.

26. Mashchak C, Lobo R, Dozono-Takano R, et al. Comparisons of pharmacodynamic properties of various estrogen formulations. *Am J Obstet Gynecol* 1982;144:511–518.

27. Bhavnani B, Sarda I, Woolever C. Radioimmunoassay of plasma equilin and estrone in postmenopausal women after the administration of Premarin. *J Clin Endocrinol Metab* 1981;52:741–747.

28. Bhavnani, Cecutti A. Metabolic clearance rate of equilin sulfate and its conversion to plasma equilin, conjugated and unconjugated equilenin, 17β-dihydroequilin and 17β-dihydroequilenin in normal postmeno-pausal women and men under steady state conditions. *J Clin Endo-crinol Metab* 1993;77:1269–1274.

29. Bhavnani B. Pharmacokinetics and pharmacodynamics of conjugated equine estrogens: chemistry and metabolism. *Proc Soc Exp Biol Med* 1998;217:6–16.

30. Bhavnani B, Woolever C. Interaction of ring B unsaturated estrogens with estrogen receptors of human endometrium and rat uterus. *Steroids* 1991;56:201–210.

31. Bhavnani B, Gerulath A. Metabolism of [3H]equilin in normal and malignant human endometrium and in endometrial adenocarcinoma transplanted into nude mice. *J Steroid Biochem Mol Biol* 1991;38: 433–439.

32. Bhavnani B, Cecutti A, Wallace D. Metabolism of [3H] 17β-dihydroe-quilin and [3H] 17β-dihydroequilin sulfate in normal postmenopausal women. *Steroids* 1994;59:389–394.

33. Jordan V. Alternate antiestrogens and approaches to the prevention of breast cancer. *J Cell Biochem Suppl* 1995;22:51–57.

34. Peyrade F, Frenay M, Etienne M, et al. Age-related difference in tamoxifen disposition. *Clin Pharmacol Ther* 1996;59:401–410.

35. Lien E, Solheim, Lea O, Lundgren S, Kvinnsland S, Ueland P. Distri-bution of 4-hydroxy-N-desmethyltamoxifen and other tamoxifen metabolites in human biological fluids during tamoxifen treatment. *Cancer Res* 1989;49:2175–2183.

36. Buckley M, Goa K. Tamoxifen. A reappraisal of its pharmacodynamic and pharmacokinetic properties, and therapeutic use. *Drugs* 1989;37: 451–490.

37. Borgna JL, Rochefort H. Hydroxylated metabolites of tamoxifen are formed in vivo and bound to estrogen receptor in target tissues. *J Biol Chem* 1981;256:859–868.

38. Kivisto K, Villika K, Nyman L, Anttila M, Neuvonen P. Tamoxifen and toremifene concentrations in plasma are greatly decreased by rifampin. *Clin Pharmacol Ther* 1998;64:648–654.

39. Jacolot F, Simon I, Dreano Y, Beaune P, Riche C, Berthou F. Identifi-cation of the cytochrome P450 IIIA family as the enzymes involved in the N-demethylation of tamoxifen in human liver. *Biochem Pharmacol* 1991;41:1911–1919.

40. Mani C, Hodgson E, Kupfer D. Metabolism of the antimammary can-cer antiestrogenic agent tamoxifen. II Flavin-containing monooxyge-nase-mediated N-oxidation. *Drug Metab Dispos* 1993;21:657–661.

41. Berthou F, Dreano Y, Belloc C, Kangas L, Gautier J, Beaune P. Involve-ment of cytochrome P450 3A enzyme family in the major metabolic pathways of toremifene in human liver microsomes. *Biochem Pharma-col* 1994;47:1883–1895.

42. Jordan V, Collins M, Rowsby L, Prestwich G. A monohydroxylated metabolite of tamoxifen with potent antiestrogenic activity. *J Endo-crinol* 1977;75:305–316.

43. Williams M, Lennard M, Martin I, Tucker G. Interindividual variation in the isomerization of 4-hydroxytamoxifen by human liver micro-somes: involvement of cytochromes P450. *Carcinogenesis* 1994;15: 2733–2738.

44. Dehal SS, Kupfer D. CYP2D6 catalyzes tamoxifen 4-hydroxylation in human liver. *Cancer Res* 1997;57:3402–3406.

45. Moorthy B, Sriram P, Pathak D, Bodell W, Randerath K. Tamoxifen metabolic activation: comparison of DNA adducts formed by micro-somal and chemical activation of tamoxifen and 4-hydroxytamoxifen with DNA adducts formed in vivo. *Cancer Res* 1996;56:53–57.

46. White I, De Matteis F, Gibbs A, et al. Species differences in the cova-lent binding of [14C] tamoxifen to liver microsomes and the forms of cytochrome P450 involved. *Biochem Pharmacol* 1995;49:1035–1042.

47. Crewe H, Ellis S, Lennard M, Tucker G. Variable contribution of cyto-chromes P450 2D6, 2C9 and 3A4 to the 4-hydroxylation of tamoxifen by human liver microsomes. *Biochem Pharmacol* 1997;53:171–178.

48. Blankson E, Ellis S, Lennard M, Tucker G, Rogers K. The metabolism of tamoxifen by human liver microsomes is not mediated by cyto-chrome P450IID6. *Biochem Pharmacol* 1991;42[Suppl]:S209–S212.

49. Lodwick R, McConkey B, Brown A. Life threatening interaction between tamoxifen and warfarin. *BMJ (Clin Res Ed)* 1987;295:1141.

50. Ni L, Allerheiligen S, Basson R. Pharmacokinetics of raloxifene in men and psotmenopausal women volunteers. *Pharm Res* 1996;13 [Suppl]:S430.

51. Dodge J, Lugar C, Cho S, et al. Evaluation of the major metabolites of raloxifene as modulators of tissue selectivity. *J Steroid Biochem Mol Biol* 1997;61:97–106.

52. Adlercreutz H, Martin F. Biliary excretion and intestinal metabolism of progesterone and estrogens in man. *J Steroid Biochem* 1980;13: 231–244.

53. Simon J, Robinson D, Andrews M, et al. The absorption of oral micron-ized progesterone: the effect of food, dose proportionality, and com-parison with intramuscular progesterone. *Fertil Steril* 1993;60:26–33.

54. De Lignieres B, Dennerstein L, Backstrom T. Influence of route of administration on progesterone metabolism. *Maturitas* 1995;21: 251–257.

55. Sandberg A, Slaunwhite W. The metabolic fate of 14C progesterone in human subjects. *J Clin Endocrinol Metab* 1958;18:253–265.

56. Schedl H. Absorption of steroid hormones from the human small intestine. *J Clin Endocrinol Metab* 1965;25:1309–1316.

57. Eriksson H. Absorption and enterohepatic recirculation of neutral steroids in the rat. *Eur J Biochem* 1971;19:416–423.

58. Aufrere M, Benson H. Progesterone: an overview and recent advances. *J Pharm Sci* 1976;65:783–800.

59. MacDonald P, Dombrooski R, Casey M. Recurrent secretion of proges-terone in large amounts: an endocrine/metabolic disorder unique to young women? *Endocr Rev* 1991;12:372–401.

60. Laatikainen T, Karjalainen O. Excretion of conjugates of neutral ster-oids in human bile during late pregnancy. *Acta Endocrinol (Copenh)* 1972;69:775–788.

61. Whitehead M, Townsend P, Gill D, Collins W, Campbell S. Absorption and metabolism of oral progesterone. *BMJ* 1980;280:825–827.

62. Niwa T, Yabusaki Y, Honma K, et al. Contribution of human hepatic

cytochrome P450 isoforms to regioselective hydroxylation of steroid hormones. *Xenobiotica* 1998;28:539–547.

63. Chantilis S, Dombroski R, Shakleton C, Casey M, MacDonald P. Metabolism of 5α-dihydroprogesterone in women and men: 3β- and 3α-, 6α-dihydroxy-5α-pregnan-20-ones are major urinary metabolites. *J Clin Endocrinol Metab* 1996;81:3644–3649.

64. Heuser G. Induction of anesthesia, seizures and sleep by steroid hormones. *Anesthesiology* 1967;28:173–183.

65. Arafat E, Hargrove J, Maxson W, Desiderio D, Wentz A, Andersen R. Sedative and hypnotic effects of oral administration of micronized progesterone may be mediated through its metabolites. *Am J Obstet Gynecol* 1988;159:1203–1209.

66. Gemzik B, Parkinson A. Hydroxylation of 5α-androstane-3β, 17β-diol by rat prostate microsomes: potent inhibition by imidazole-type antimycotic drugs and lack of inhibition by steroid 5α-reductase inhibitors. *Arch Biochem Biophys* 1992;296:366–373.

67. Haarparanta T, Glaumann H, Gustafsson J. Characterization and endocrine regulation of the cytochrome P-450 dependent microsomal hydroxylation of 5α-androstane-3β, 17β-diol in the rat ventral prostate. *Endocrinology* 1984;114:2293–1300.

68. Waxman D, Attisano C, Guengerich F, Lapenson D. Human liver microsomal steroid metabolism: identification of the major microsomal steroid hormone 6β hydroxylase cytochrome P-450 enzyme. *Arch Biochem Biophys* 1988;263:424–436.

69. Yamazaki H, Shimada T. Progesterone and testosterone hydroxylation by cytochromes P450 2C19, 2C9, and 3A4 in human liver microsomes. *Arch Biochem Biophys* 1996;346:161–169.

70. Back D, Breckenridge A, Crawford F, et al. Kinetics of norethindrone in women. *Clin Pharmacol Ther* 1978;24:439–447.

71. Kamyab S, Fotherby K, Klopper A. Metabolism of [4-14C] norethisterone in women. *J Endocrinol* 1968;41:263–272.

72. Gerhards E, Hecker W, Hitze H, Nieuweboer B, Bellmann O. The metabolism of norethisterone (17-ethinyl-4-estrene-17-ol-3-one) and of DL- and D-norgestrel (18-methyl-17-ethinyl-4-estrene-17-ol-3-one) in man. *Acta Endocrinol (Copenh)* 1971;68:219–248.

73. Layne D, Golab T, Arai K, Pincus G. The metabolic fate of orally administered 3H-noretynodrl and 3H-norethindrone in humans. *Biochem Pharmacol* 1963;12:905–913.

74. Stanczyk F, Roy S. Metabolism of levonorgestrel, norethindrone, and structurally related contraceptive steroids. *Contraception* 1990;42:67–96.

75. Kuhnz W, Gleschen H. Predicting the oral bioavailability of 19-nortestosterone progestins in vivo from their metabolic stability in human liver microsomal preparations in vitro. *Drug Metab Dispos* 1998;26:1120–1127.

76. LeBel M, Masson E, Guilbert E, et al. Effects of rifabutin and rifampicin on the pharmacokinetics of ethinylestradiol and norethindrone. *J Clin Pharmacol* 1998;38:1042–1050.

77. Kuhnz W, Blode H, Mahler M. Systemic availability of levonorgestrel after single oral administration of a norgestimate-containing combination oral contraceptive to 12 young women. *Contraception* 1994;49:255–263.

78. Sisenwine S, Kimmel H, Liu A, Ruelius H. Excretion and stereoselective biotransformation of dl-, d- and l-norgestrel in women. *Drug Metab Dispos* 1975;3:180–188.

79. McGuire J, Phillips A, Hahn D, Tolman E, Flor S, Kafrissen M. Pharmacologic and pharmacokinetic characteristics of norgestimate and its metabolites. *Am J Obstet Gynecol* 1990;163:2127–2131.

80. Alton K, Hetyei N, Shaw C, Patrick J. Biotransformation of norgestimate in women. *Contraception* 1984;29:19–29.

81. Phillips A, Demarest K, Hahn D, Wong F, McGuire J. Progestational and androgenic receptor binding affinities and in vivo activities of norgestimate and other progestins. *Contraception* 1990;41:399–410.

82. Madden S, Back D. Metabolism of norgestimate by human gastrointestinal mucosa and liver microsomes in vitro. *J Steroid Biochem Mol Biol* 1991;38:497–503.

83. Viinikka L. Radioimmunoassay of a new progestagen, Org 2969, and its metabolite. *J Steroid Biochem* 1978;9:979–982.

84. Hasenack H, Bosch A, Kaar K. Serum levels of 3-keto-desogestrel after oral administration of desogestrel and 3-keto-desogestrel. *Contraception* 1986;33:591–596.

85. Viinikka L, Ylikorkala O, Nummi S, et al. Biological effects of a new and potent progestagen. A clinical study. *Acta Endocrinol (Copenh)* 1976;83:429–438.

86. Back D, Grimmer S, Shenoy N, Orme M. Plasma concentration of 3-keto-desogestrel after oral administration of desogestrel and intravenous administration of 3-keto-desogestrel. *Contraception* 1987;35:619–626.

87. Orme M, Back D, Ward S, Green S. The pharmacokinetics of ethynylestradiol in the presence and absence of gestodene and desogestrel. *Contraception* 1991;43:305–316.

88. Madden S, Back D, Martin C, Orme M. Metabolism of the contraceptive steroid desogestrel by the intestinal mucosa. *Br J Clin Pharmacol* 1989;27:295–299.

89. Gentile D, Verhoeven C, Shimada T, Back D. The role of CYP2C in the in vitro bioactivation of the contraceptive desogestrel. *J Pharmacol Exp Ther* 1998;287:975–982.

90. Verhoeven C, Krebbers S, Wagenaars G, Vos R. In vitro and in vivo metabolism of desogestrel in several species. *Drug Metab Dispos* 1998;26:927–936.

91. Viinikka L. Metabolism of a new synthetic progestagen, Org 2969, by human liver in vitro. *J Steroid Biochem* 1979;10:353–357.

92. Viinikka L, Ylikorkala O, Vihko R, Wijnand H, Booij M, van der Veen F. Metabolism of a new synthetic progestagen, Org 2969, in female volunteers. Pharmacokinetics after an oral dose. *Eur J Clin Pharmacol* 1979;15:349–355.

93. Paine M, Schmiedlin-Ren P, Watkins P. Cytochrome p-450 1A expression in human small bowel: interindividual variation and inhibition by ketoconazole. *Drug Metab Dispos* 1999;27:360–364.

94. Iyer RB, Binstock J, Schwartz I, Gordon G, Weinstein B, Southren A. Purification and properties of human hepatic 3 alpha-hydroxysteroid dehydrogenase. *J Steroid Biochem Mol Biol* 1992;43:343–349.

95. Tauber U, Tack J, Matthes H. Single dose pharmacokinetics of gestodene in women after intravenous and oral administration. *Contraception* 1989;40:461–479.

96. Ward S, Back D. Metabolism of gestodene in human liver cytosol and microsomes in vitro. *J Steroid Biochem Mol Biol* 1993;46:235–243.

97. Guengerich F. Mechanism-based inactivation of human liver microsomal cyochrome P-450 IIIA4 by gestodene. *Chem Res Toxicol* 1990;3:363–371.

98. Cooper J, Kellie A. The metabolism of megestrol acetate (17-alpha-acetoxy-6-methylpregna-4,6-diene-3,20-dione) in women. *Steroids* 1968;11:133–149.

99. Lober J, Mouridsen H, Salimtschik M, Johanson E. Pharmacokinetics of medroxyprogesterone acetate administered by oral and intramuscular route. *Acta Obstet Scand Suppl* 1981;101:71–74.

100. Fukushima DK, Levin J, Liang J, Smulowitz M. Isolation and partial synthesis of a new metabolite of medroxyprogesterone acetate. *Steroids* 1979;34:57–72.

101. Utaaker E, Lundgren S, Kvinnsland S, Aakvaag A. Pharmacokinetics and metabolism of medroxyprogesterone acetate in patients with advanced breast cancer. *J Steroid Biochem* 1988;31:437–441.

102. Sturm G, Haberlein H, Bauer T, Plaum T, Stalker D. Mass spectrometric and high-performance liquid chromatographic studies of medroxyprogesterone acetate metabolites in human plasma. *J Chromatogr* 1991;562:351–362.

103. Fleming GF, Amato J, Agresti M, Safa A. Megestrol acetate reverses multidrug resistance and interacts with P-glycoprotein. *Cancer Chemother Pharmacol* 1992;29:445–449.

104. Heikinheimo O, Kontula K, Croxatto H, Spitz I, Luukkainen T, Lahteenmaki P. Plasma concentrations and receptor binding of RU486 and its metabolites in humans. *J Steroid Biochem* 1987;26:279–284.

105. Nieman L, Chrousos G, Kellner C, et al. Successful treatment of Cushing's syndrome with the glucocorticoid antagonist RU486. *J Clin Endocrinol Metab* 1985;61:536–540.

106. Lahteenmaki P, Heikinheimo O, Croxatto H, et al. Pharmacokinetics and metabolism of RU486. *J Steroid Biochem* 1987;27:859–863.

107. Deraedt R, Bonnat C, Busigny M, et al. Pharmacokinetics of RU486. In: Baulieu E, Segal S, eds. *The antiprogestin steroid RU486 and human fertility control.* New York: Raven Press, 1985:103–122.

108. Jang GR, Wrighton SA, Benet LZ. Identification of CYP3A4 as the principle enzyme catalyzing mifepristone (RU486) oxidation in human liver microsomes. *Biochem Pharmacol* 1996;52:753–761.

109. Jang JR, Benet LZ. Antiprogestin-mediated inactivation of cytochrome P450 3A4. *Pharmacology* 1998;56:150–157.

110. He K, Woolf T, Hollenberg P. Mechanism-based inactivation of cytochrome P-450-3A4 by mifepristone (RU486). *J Pharmacol Exp Ther* 1999;288:791–797.

111. Kocarek T, Schuetz E, Strom S, Fisher R, Guzelian P. Comparative analysis of cytochrome P4503A induction in primary cultures of rat, rabbit and human hepatocytes. *Drug Metab Dispos* 1995;23:415–421.

CHAPTER 39

Hypoglycemic Agents

William R. Brian

DIABETES MELLITUS

Diabetes mellitus is best characterized by consistently elevated blood glucose levels, resulting from inadequate or no production of the hormone insulin or lack of responsiveness of tissues to insulin. Diabetes is clinically characterized by altered metabolism of carbohydrates, lipids, and proteins, and by certain types of vascular and neural pathologies. In healthy humans, insulin produced in the β cells of the pancreas controls blood glucose concentrations and other metabolic processes. Increases in blood glucose concentration signals release of insulin from the β cells through a cyclic guanosine monophosphate-mediated mechanism. Insulin then interacts with receptors on liver, adipose, and peripheral muscle cells to direct the uptake of blood glucose. Blood glucose concentrations are usually kept within a fairly narrow range in healthy people (70–120 mg/dL).

If left untreated or poorly controlled, diabetes leads to lifestyle-changing and life-threatening peripheral pathologies. Some of the major microvascular and macrovascular pathologies include degradation and loss of vision caused by retinopathy, nephropathy leading to end-stage renal disease, coronary artery disease resulting from changes in cholesterol and triglyceride status, and decreased vascularization of the extremities, often resulting in hypertension and infection, sometimes with surgical loss of extremities. For more detail on diabetes mellitus, refer to References 1 and 2.

Two general classes of diabetes mellitus have been described. Insulin-dependent diabetes, referred to as type I or juvenile-onset diabetes, results from the lack of insulin production by the pancreatic β cells. Approximately 10% of all diabetes cases are type I. Current thinking is that this form of diabetes results from an autoimmune

response, with loss of β cell function. Without endogenous insulin production, type I diabetes requires the use of exogenous insulin to control blood glucose levels. Recombinant human insulin administered subcutaneously is used successfully in these patients.

Non–insulin-dependent diabetes is referred to as type II or adult-onset diabetes. It results from decreased production and release of insulin from the pancreatic β cells or from decreased sensitivity of liver, adipose, or muscle cells to insulin. Decreased insulin sensitivity is thought to be due to decreased numbers of insulin receptors on the cell surface. Approximately 90% of patients with diabetes have this form of the disease.

Initially, type II diabetes may be treated using a combination of diet and exercise. Obesity plays a major role in decreasing insulin sensitivity in type II diabetes. Generally, as the obese person loses weight, insulin sensitivity increases. If drug treatment is required, insulin can be used or, more likely, one of several oral medications may be used. These drugs are typically called hypoglycemic agents, although the goal in their use is to maintain normal blood glucose concentrations. There are several chemical classes of these drugs, which cause release of insulin from the pancreatic β cells or increase the sensitivity of adipose, liver, and muscle cells to insulin. Alternatively, the alpha-glucosidase inhibitors are drugs that structurally mimic saccharides and function by inhibiting the intestinal degradation of saccharides to glucose, reducing absorption of glucose and minimizing postprandial elevations in blood glucose concentrations.

DRUG INTERACTIONS

Because management of diabetes usually involves treatment of concurrent pathologies, drug–drug interactions must be considered with the hypoglycemic drugs. In this chapter, drug–drug interactions based on drug metabolism mechanisms (i.e., the effect of one drug on the metabolism of another drug) are considered, resulting

W. R. Brian: Departments of Clinical Metabolism and Pharmacokinetics, Sanofi-Synthelabo Research, 9 Great Valley Parkway, Malvern, Pennsylvania 19355

in pharmacokinetic changes for a drug. An extensive literature search indicated that most of the published interactions describe the effect of a concomitant drug on the hypoglycemic drug.

Several issues were identified in reviewing the drug interaction literature for the hypoglycemic drugs. Many reported interactions are based on small but statistically significant changes in drug pharmacokinetics, but blood glucose concentrations were not altered or were not determined. Therefore, the clinical significance of these findings is questionable. Relationships between plasma drug and blood glucose concentrations are not always direct. Small to moderate decreases in blood glucose concentrations do not always result in clinically significant hypoglycemia, which is typically characterized by sweating, shaking, sudden onset of fatigue, and, if severe, loss of consciousness. Designs of interaction trials differed between studies. Variables included dosage amounts, times and routes of drug administration relative to each other, and the use of single versus multiple doses. The majority of the interaction reports based on clinical presentations of hypoglycemia occurred after multiple doses of both drugs. However, many of the clinical trials designed to directly investigate drug interactions used only single doses of the hypoglycemic drug or coadministered drug. Finally, many of the sulfonylurea hypoglycemic drugs were developed years ago when knowledge of drug metabolism and mechanisms of drug interactions were not well defined. Where possible, underlying mechanisms based on current knowledge are described or proposed. With these caveats, some drug interactions or lack of interactions are obvious, based on well designed studies or years of clinical practice. Some of the drugs for which interactions have been described have been largely replaced by newer drugs, but they are included for historical reasons. By understanding the mechanisms for drug interactions with the older drugs, predictions of clinically significant interactions can be made for some of the currently prescribed drugs.

Other drug–drug interactions with the hypoglycemic drugs based on pharmacodynamic mechanisms have been reported. Some of the more notable interactions are with the sulfonylurea drugs (see later text) in combination with salicylic acid, ethanol, some β-adrenergic receptor antagonists, or monoamine oxidase inhibitors. These drugs have some inherent hypoglycemic activity alone, which gives an additive effect with the sulfonylurea drugs. Refer to recent reviews in References 3 through 5.

There are apparently no metabolism-based drug interactions with the alpha-glucosidase inhibitors. Hypoglycemia has been described to be a result of the combined pharmacodynamic effects of insulin and acarbose, an alpha-glucosidase inhibitor (6).

Because insulin is a protein, it is not expected to have any pharmacokinetic interactions with the oral hypoglycemic drugs and, indeed, no reports were found in an extensive literature search. In some clinical protocols, insulin is coadministered with oral hypoglycemic agents to improve control of blood glucose in type II diabetes (2).

SULFONYLUREA DRUGS

Development of the sulfonylurea drugs for diabetes treatment resulted from an observation in the 1940s that a sulfonamide antibiotic caused hypoglycemia in some patients (7–9). This observation eventually led to the introduction of chlorpropamide and tolbutamide for the clinical management of diabetes in the 1950s.

The mechanism by which the sulfonylurea drugs work to lower blood glucose is somewhat controversial (reviewed in Ref. 10). Initially, the sulfonylurea drugs bind to pancreatic β cells to cause release of insulin. These drugs do not work in patients without at least some functional β cells. However, over time, insulin release from the β cells in response to these drugs returns to predrug levels, although the drugs remain effective at keeping blood glucose concentrations at or near normal levels. Some researchers propose that long-term administration of a sulfonylurea drug increases the number of insulin receptors on adipose, liver, and muscle cells, increasing the sensitivity of these tissues to insulin. In many patients, these drugs eventually lose their effectiveness as the ability of the β cells to produce insulin is reduced or lost. The sulfonylurea drugs are truly hypoglycemic agents because they can decrease blood glucose below normal levels.

Sulfonylurea drugs are typically classified as first or second generation, based on their potency for reducing blood glucose concentrations. The first generation sulfonylurea drugs include chlorpropamide, tolbutamide, and acetohexamide. They are still prescribed, although in a relatively low number of patients who have had long-term success with them. Smaller doses of the second generation drugs are required to achieve the same effect as the first generation drugs. Most type II patients are routinely started on a second generation sulfonylurea or newer oral drug, at least in the United States and western Europe. Structures of these drugs are shown in Fig. 39-1.

In general, the sulfonylurea drugs are extensively metabolized, increasing the potential for metabolism-based drug–drug interactions. One of the sulfonylurea drugs, tolbutamide, has been widely used as a general noninvasive probe of drug metabolism, because it is essentially completely cleared by oxidation. The initial hydroxylation step is catalyzed by the cytochrome P450 2C9 isoform (CYP2C9) (11,12). Although the other sulfonylurea drugs are structurally similar to tolbutamide, the role of CYP2C9 or other enzymes in their metabolism has not been clearly established.

Most of the sulfonylurea drugs are highly bound to plasma proteins and the first generation drugs, in particular, have low clearance rates. Drug–drug interactions

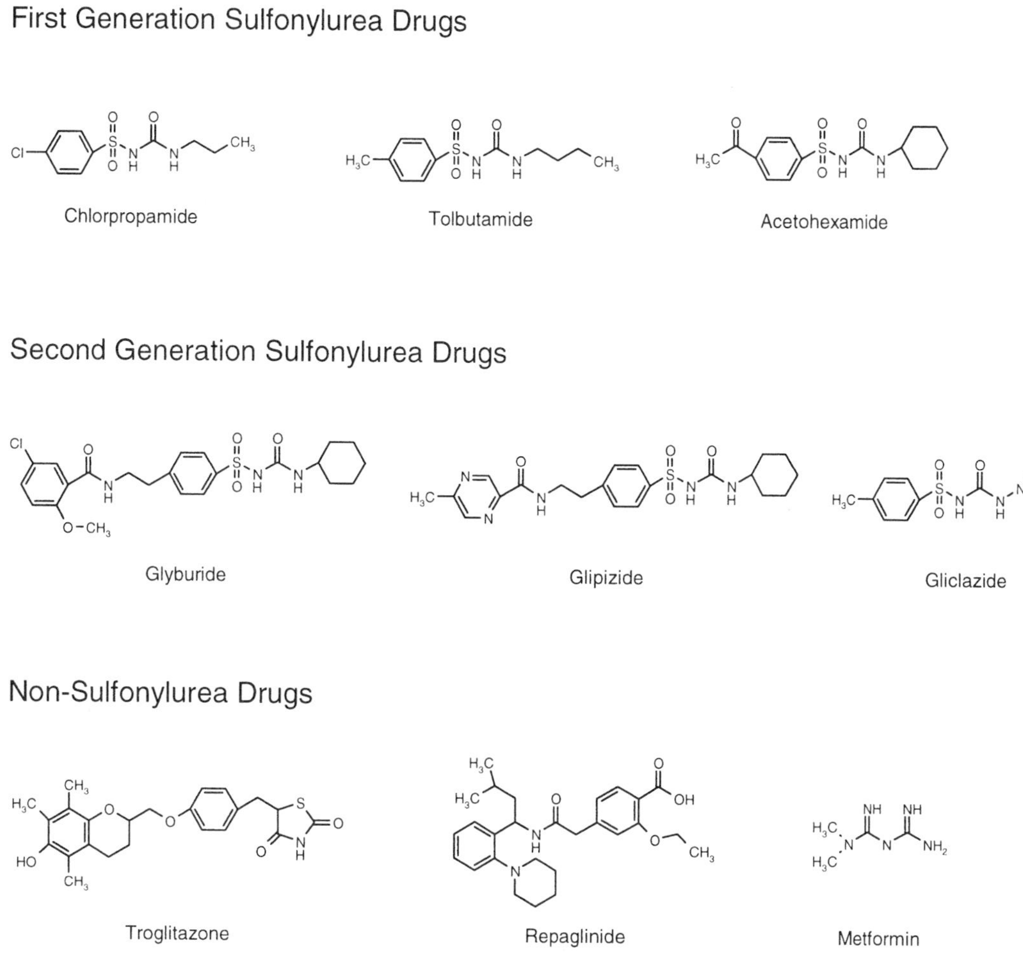

First Generation Sulfonylurea Drugs

Chlorpropamide

Tolbutamide

Acetohexamide

Second Generation Sulfonylurea Drugs

Glyburide

Glipizide

Gliclazide

Non-Sulfonylurea Drugs

Troglitazone

Repaglinide

Metformin

FIG. 39-1. Structures of oral hypoglycemic drugs.

were initially observed for some of these drugs 30 to 40 years ago, and they were commonly assumed to be due to displacement of the sulfonylurea drug from plasma proteins by the coadministered drug. Based on pharmacokinetic models of tolbutamide interactions, however, displacement from plasma proteins should have a small and only transient effect, if any, on insulin release from the pancreas (described for tolbutamide and sulfaphenazole in Refs. 13 and 14). With further analysis and clinical studies, many of the drug interactions originally ascribed to changes in plasma protein binding are considered to result from inhibition of the enzymes responsible for metabolic clearance of the sulfonylurea drug.

FIRST GENERATION SULFONYLUREA DRUGS

Chlorpropamide

Chlorpropamide was one of the first successful sulfonylurea drugs marketed for type II diabetes mellitus. A typical oral dose of chlorpropamide is 250 mg daily, resulting in maximum plasma concentrations (C_{max}) of approximately 30 μg/mL (15). The dose can vary from 100 to 750 mg daily depending on the patient's response. The plasma elimination half-life in healthy subjects and patients with diabetes is approximately 36 hours but there is high variability (8,16). The drug is approximately 90% protein bound in plasma, primarily to albumin (17).

Chlorpropamide is extensively metabolized, with approximately 20% of a single-250 mg dose excreted unchanged in the urine of male patients with diabetes (15). Major metabolites identified in urine were 2-hydroxychlorpropamide and p-chlorobenzenesulfonylurea (a breakdown product of p-chlorobenzenesulfonamide), representing approximately 55% and 23% of a single dose, respectively. Approximately 2% to 3% of the dose was recovered as 3-hydroxychlorpropamide. The 2- and 3-hydroxylated metabolites have weak pharmacologic activity. Although assumed to be CYP mediated, the isoforms catalyzing these reactions have not been identified. Because some chlorpropamide is cleared by renal excretion, hypoglycemia has been reported in renally compromised patients (16).

Chloramphenicol

Chloramphenicol is an antibiotic used primarily as a last resort to treat serious microbial infections that are resistant to safer antibiotics. Chloramphenicol (1–2 g daily) increased the mean plasma half-life of a single 1-g dose of chlorpropamide from approximately 36 hours to 91 hours in healthy subjects (16). The authors hypothesized that the interaction was due to decreased renal excretion of chlorpropamide. However, chloramphenicol is a known inhibitor of drug metabolism (18), acting as a cytochrome P450 inhibitor (19). Thus, the interaction could also be due to inhibition of chlorpropamide metabolism.

Vitamin K Antagonists

Severe hypoglycemia was observed in an elderly male patient stabilized on chlorpropamide (250 mg daily) after initiation of anticoagulant therapy with dicoumarol (bishydroxycoumarin) (20). This reaction was studied further in four patients with diabetes given daily doses of 250 mg of chlorpropamide. Repeated administration of dicoumarol, at dosages sufficient to reduce blood clotting times to 40% of normal, approximately doubled the plasma concentration and elimination half-life of chlorpropamide. A similar effect was observed in two healthy subjects receiving a single dose of 450 mg of chlorpropamide. Acenecoumarol, another vitamin K antagonist, more than doubled the plasma half-life of chlorpropamide in a woman with diabetes (16). The mechanisms for these interactions were not studied but it can be speculated that the interaction involved inhibition of CYP2C9, the isoform primarily responsible for the metabolism of the vitamin K antagonist (S)-warfarin (21). Whether dicoumarol or acenecoumarol, which are structurally related to warfarin, are substrates or inhibitors of CYP2C9 has not been determined.

Sulfonamides

Single incidences of hypoglycemia have been reported as resulting from coadministration of chlorpropamide with some sulfonamide antibiotics, such as sulfamethazine (also known as sulfadimidine) (22), sulfisoxazole (23), or cotrimoxazole (a combination of the sulfonamide drug sulfamethoxazole and trimethoprim) (24).

Phenylbutazone

Phenybutazone is a nonsteroidal antiinflammatory drug (NSAID) that is rarely used to treat rheumatoid arthritis. Daily administration of phenylbutazone (300 mg) and chlorpropamide (125 to 250 mg) resulted in a small but statistically significant reduction in fasting blood glucose levels in nine patients with diabetes (25). Approximately 3 weeks were required for the effect to become significantly different from placebo and clinical hypoglycemia

did not occur. The authors proposed that the interaction could be due to changes in protein binding, changes in metabolism, or interference with renal excretion. It was proposed, but not tested, that clinically significant hypoglycemia may occur in patients taking larger doses of chlorpropamide.

Phenylbutazone is structurally related to sulfaphenazole (see later text), a known selective inhibitor of CYP2C9. It can be speculated that the interaction between phenylbutazone and chlorpropamide is due, at least in part, to inhibition of CYP2C9 by phenylbutazone.

Rifampin

In a single case study in an elderly man with diabetes stabilized on chlorpropamide, initiation of rifampin treatment for tuberculosis (600 mg daily) decreased serum chlorpropamide concentrations to approximately 30% of those observed before rifampin (26). The daily chlorpropamide dosage was increased from 250 to 400 mg to maintain control of blood glucose. After discontinuing rifampin, without adjusting the chlorpropamide dose, serum chlorpropamide concentrations increased approximately four-fold. The patient did not experience hypoglycemia with this large increase. This effect can be attributed to the well-characterized induction of CYP2C9 and CYP3A4 by rifampin.

Halofenate

Halofenate was in development as an antilipemic drug. Long-term administration of halofenate decreased the plasma glucose levels in patients with diabetes taking chlorpropamide alone or in combination with phenformin (a biguanide drug used to treat diabetes; see later text) (27,28). A reduction in chlorpropamide dose was required in some patients receiving this combination. The authors proposed that this effect was due to displacement of chlorpropamide from plasma proteins by halofenate, resulting in higher plasma chlorpropamide concentrations. However, in the study by Jain and co-workers (27), the full effect of this interaction was observed only after 1 month of daily administration. The potential of slow inactivation of an enzyme (possibly CYP2C9) responsible for chlorpropamide metabolism must also be considered.

Other Drugs

Petitpierre and colleagues (16) anecdotally reported that chlorpropamide plasma half-life was not altered with coadministration of diphenylhydantoin, diazepam, demethylchlortetracycline, doxycycline, gentamicin, penicillin, digoxin, bromhexine, or papaverine. However, details were not provided.

Coadministration of the NSAID ibuprofen with chlorpropamide did not change fasting blood glucose levels relative to chlorpropamide alone (25). Coadministration of salicylate and chlorpropamide resulted in significantly lower blood glucose concentrations than was observed with either agent alone (29). This is apparently due to the well-described blood glucose–lowering property of salicylate rather than to the alteration in chlorpropamide pharmacokinetics.

Significant interactions resulting in elevated plasma chlorpropamide concentrations resulting from inhibition of renal excretion, rather than metabolism, are reported for probenecid, allopurinol, and clofibrate (summarized in Ref. 5).

Tolbutamide

Typical oral and intravenous (IV) dosages of tolbutamide are 500 mg to 2 g daily. Plasma half-life values for tolbutamide administered orally or intravenously are in the range of 4 to 8 hours (14,30,31). The drug is approximately 95% protein bound in plasma, primarily to albumin (32).

Tolbutamide is almost quantitatively cleared by hydroxylation of the methyl group, followed by further oxidation to carboxytolbutamide and then excretion in the urine (33). Methyl hydroxylation was shown to be catalyzed by the cytochrome P450 isoform that is currently known as CYP2C9 (11,12). Hydroxytolbutamide has some hypoglycemic activity, although it does not contribute to the pharmacologic activity of the drug because it circulates at very low concentrations in blood (34). Carboxytolbutamide is not inherently active as a hypoglycemic agent. Tolbutamide hydroxylation is routinely used to measure the activity of CYP2C9 in microsomes from human liver and heterologous expression systems (35,36).

The hydroxylation of tolbutamide by CYP2C9 was initially thought to be polymorphically expressed (37). However, it appears that rather than a true polymorphism, there are some rare variants of the human CYP2C9 gene producing an enzyme with reduced catalytic activity (38).

Chloramphenicol

As with chlorpropamide, the disposition of tolbutamide is affected by coadministration of the antibiotic chloramphenicol. This interaction was first observed in an elderly subject receiving tolbutamide for Parkinson's disease (39). The subject began treatment for a urinary tract infection with 2 g daily of chloramphenicol while continuing to receive 2 g daily of tolbutamide. After 3 days, the subject experienced hypoglycemia. In a clinical study to examine this interaction, patients with diabetes receiving oral dosages of 1500 mg of tolbutamide daily (3 divided doses of 500 mg) were given 2 g daily of chloramphenicol (18). After several days, this regimen doubled serum concentrations and half-lives of tolbutamide without significant hypoglycemia. These results are consistent with chloramphenicol acting as a CYP inhibitor.

Similar results were observed in another study in which eight women with diabetes, stabilized on tolbutamide (1.5 g/day), were given chloramphenicol (2 g/day) (40). Blood glucose levels in five of the eight patients decreased by an average of approximately 30% after 9 days of concomitant administration. In a second study with a similar dosing schedule, serum tolbutamide concentrations approximately doubled in seven of eight patients and blood glucose levels decreased by about 24% in all patients. None of these patients experienced clinical hypoglycemia, and the authors suggested that significant hypoglycemia resulting from this interaction would be rare.

Vitamin K Antagonists

Perhaps the first indication of an interaction with tolbutamide and a vitamin K antagonist was contained in an anecdotal report in 1957. Prothrombin times increased in two patients stabilized on dicoumarol (bishydroxycoumarin) within 24 to 48 hours of starting tolbutamide therapy to treat their diabetes (41). However, this was not observed in three other patients receiving the same treatment.

Hypoglycemia and a prolonged elimination half-life of tolbutamide were reported within days of initiating dicoumarol treatment in an elderly patient with diabetes stabilized on tolbutamide (42). Similar findings were reported in an elderly patient with diabetes on long-term treatment with dicoumarol 2 hours after a single 1-g oral dose of tolbutamide (43). This was then tested in four patients with diabetes who were stabilized on a 500-mg daily dose of tolbutamide. After receiving dicoumarol for at least 3 days, there was an approximate two- to threefold increase in plasma tolbutamide concentrations, which correlated with decreased blood glucose levels in these patients. When dicoumarol administration was stopped, plasma tolbutamide levels returned to normal. This effect was repeated in eight additional healthy subjects following 1-week administration of dicoumarol. In the first four patients receiving tolbutamide and dicoumarol, concentrations of carboxytolbutamide in plasma were undetectable, whereas it can usually be detected when tolbutamide is given alone. This led the authors to suggest that this interaction was due to dicoumarol decreasing the metabolism of tolbutamide.

A similar effect of elevated plasma concentrations and prolonged half-life of tolbutamide was observed in three healthy subjects receiving 1 g of tolbutamide intravenously and either dicoumarol (50 mg daily, orally for 7 days) or phenyramidol (400 mg daily, orally for 4 days) (44). Dicoumarol (600-mg single oral dose) was again reported to increase the plasma concentrations of tolbutamide (1 g daily dose) in four healthy subjects (45). Again, it could be speculated that the interactions with tolbutamide and dicoumarol or phenyramidol involved inhibition of CYP2C9.

Interestingly, tolbutamide increased the elimination rate of dicoumarol in two of the four subjects tested (45), but without significant impact on anticoagulant activity. Administration of tolbutamide (0.5–2 g daily) did not change the plasma concentration or half-life of phenprocoumon following a single oral dose of 12 mg in ten patients with diabetes on long-term treatment with tolbutamide (46).

Sulfonamides

Two patients with diabetes receiving tolbutamide (oral dosages of 0.5 or 2 g daily) developed severe hypoglycemia after beginning treatment with the sulfonamide sulfisoxazole (oral dosages of 2 or 4 g daily) (47). One of these subjects died, even after intensive glucose administration.

Administration of the antibacterial combination agent cotrimoxazole, which contains sulfamethoxazole (1600 mg) and trimethoprim (320 mg), for 7 days before administration of tolbutamide (500 mg IV) in healthy subjects resulted in a statistically significant 25% decrease in unbound tolbutamide clearance and 30% increase in plasma half-life of tolbutamide (48). Tolbutamide plasma protein binding was reduced by 6% and steady-state volume of distribution increased by 10%. These changes are consistent with inhibition of tolbutamide metabolism by cotrimoxazole. In general, the effect was additive for the two components of cotrimoxazole, with each component alone causing smaller, but still statistically significant, changes in tolbutamide disposition. However, blood glucose concentrations did not change during the study and the authors concluded that there was only a minor risk of hypoglycemia with coadministration of cotrimoxazole and tolbutamide.

Administration of sulfamethizole (4 g daily) to six healthy subjects for 7 days resulted in a 61% increase in tolbutamide half-life and a 38% decrease in plasma clearance after a single 750 mg IV dose of tolbutamide (49). Blood glucose concentrations were not measured. Sulfamethizole also caused similar pharmacokinetic effects with diphenylhydantoin and warfarin. These drugs are substrates of CYP2C9, suggesting that sulfamethizole is acting by inhibition of this isoform (21,50).

There was no significant hypoglycemia or elevation in serum tolbutamide concentrations when the sulfonamides sulfafurazole, sulfadimethoxine, sulfamethoxypyridazine, or sulfadiazine were coadministered with tolbutamide in subjects with diabetes (51).

Sulfaphenazole

Sulfaphenazole is a potent and selective inhibitor of CYP2C9 in human liver microsomes and is routinely used in this capacity (35,36). A clinical interaction between sulfaphenazole and tolbutamide was first described in 1963 (51). The authors reported that three

elderly patients with diabetes experienced severe hypoglycemia within days of receiving tolbutamide (0.5–1 g daily) and sulfaphenazole (1–2 g daily). This was reproduced in a clinical study with another five patients with diabetes receiving daily dosages of 1.5 g of tolbutamide and 2 g of sulfaphenazole. In these subjects, decreased blood glucose and elevated plasma tolbutamide concentrations (approximately three- to five-fold above normal) were observed within a few days of beginning sulfaphenazole treatment. After sulfaphenazole administration was stopped, blood glucose levels returned to normal after 24 to 48 hours. In a parallel study, three patients with diabetes received sulfaphenazole alone (without tolbutamide) without any effect on blood glucose, indicating that sulfaphenazole had no hypoglycemic effect by itself. When a healthy subject was given sulfaphenazole for 9 days (apparently 2 g/day), the plasma elimination half-life of tolbutamide (1 g IV) increased to approximately 18.5 hours, compared to 4.5 hours before sulfaphenazole administration.

In another study, the plasma half-life of tolbutamide was increased two- to five-fold in two healthy male subjects receiving a single 500-mg oral dose of tolbutamide after 7 days of treatment with oral sulfaphenazole (2 g/day) (52). A similar result was observed in two subjects following a single oral dose of 1 g of sulfaphenazole. Sulfaphenazole treatment reduced the urinary elimination of tolbutamide metabolites. Others have reported similar interactions with coadministration of tolbutamide and sulfaphenazole (53,54).

Sulfaphenazole was shown to approximately double the concentration of unbound tolbutamide in plasma (51), suggesting that a decrease in protein binding of tolbutamide may contribute to the hypoglycemia and change in tolbutamide pharmacokinetics. However, sulfadimethoxine, another sulfonamide drug, had a similar effect on protein binding of tolbutamide without changing total plasma tolbutamide concentrations or inducing hypoglycemia. Therefore, with knowledge that sulfaphenazole is a potent inhibitor of tolbutamide hydroxylation in human liver microsomes, it appears that the clinical effect of sulfaphenazole on tolbutamide kinetics is primarily due to its inhibition of CYP2C9.

Phenylbutazone

Phenylbutazone is structurally related to sulfaphenazole. The first clinical indication of an interaction between phenylbutazone and tolbutamide was in patients with diabetes, after coadministration of these drugs restored normal blood glucose concentrations when tolbutamide alone was insufficient (55; reported in Ref. 56).

Following 8 days of treatment with 600 mg of phenylbutazone, the serum tolbutamide concentration and half-life in a patient was significantly increased (51). In another study with nine patients with diabetes, administration of phenylbutazone for 7 days reduced tolbutamide clearance by 51% and increased tolbutamide plasma half-life by 125% following a single 3 g oral dose of tolbutamide (56). Blood glucose concentrations were not monitored in either of these studies. In the latter study, the plasma half-life of phenylbutazone was reduced and the clearance increased following daily oral administration of tolbutamide, suggesting that tolbutamide acted as an inducer of phenylbutazone metabolism.

Other authors have also reported interactions with phenylbutazone, resulting in changes in tolbutamide pharmacokinetics (52,57,58). Pond and colleagues (52) observed that single doses of phenylbutazone did not affect the plasma pharmacokinetics of tolbutamide and that multiple doses were required.

The mechanism of the phenylbutazone–tolbutamide interaction is complex. Phenylbutazone displaces tolbutamide from plasma proteins (59). However, as discussed earlier, this probably contributes very little, if at all, to changes in tolbutamide clearance with chronic administration. Phenylbutazone decreases renal excretion of some drugs by competitive inhibition of anionic secretion transporters, but this is unlikely to affect the disposition of tolbutamide because it is cleared by metabolism. Others proposed that, in addition to these mechanisms, phenylbutazone decreased the oxidative metabolism of tolbutamide (51,60). In support of this, phenylbutazone, and its oxidative metabolite oxyphenbutazone, inhibited tolbutamide hydroxylation (CYP2C9) in human liver microsomes *in vitro* (52,61). Also, phenylbutazone decreased the clearance of (S)-warfarin, which is consistent with an inhibitory effect on CYP2C9 (21,62). Thus, the major effect of phenylbutazone on tolbutamide clearance is probably due to CYP2C9 inhibition.

Azapropazone

Azapropazone is a nonsteroidal antirheumatic drug that is structurally similar to phenylbutazone. Two reports indicate that severe hypoglycemia developed in elderly patients with diabetes who were stabilized on tolbutamide (500 mg twice daily) after starting on azapropazone (900–1200 mg daily) for treatment of bone pain (63,64). This interaction was confirmed in three healthy subjects who were given 900 mg of azapropazone daily for 4 days before IV administration of 500 mg of tolbutamide (63). Concomitant administration increased the tolbutamide plasma half-life two- to five-fold and decreased tolbutamide clearance by the same magnitude.

Rifampin

Tolbutamide was used as a model substrate to noninvasively monitor the effect of rifampin on oxidative drug metabolism (31). Tolbutamide (20 mg/kg) labeled with 35S was administered intravenously to five healthy sub-

jects before and after 8 days of oral treatment with 1.2 g/day of rifampin. The plasma half-life of tolbutamide was reduced from 418 to 183 minutes by rifampin and tolbutamide plasma clearance increased approximately two-fold, from 0.21 mL/min/kg to 0.47 mL/min/kg, without a significant change in the volume of distribution. The excretion of 35S in the urine within the first 6 hours after receiving tolbutamide increased from 45% of the administered dose before rifampin administration to 71% after rifampin treatment. These results indicate that rifampin increased the metabolism of tolbutamide, which has come to be attributed to induction of CYP2C9. Blood glucose concentrations were not monitored in this study and projections were not made of the clinical significance of rifampin treatment on control of blood glucose in patients with diabetes using tolbutamide. In a similar study conducted by these authors, rifampin also induced the metabolism of hexobarbital, another selective substrate of CYP2C9 (12).

This finding was repeated in 16 patients with tuberculosis who received 45 to 65 mg of rifampin daily for 4 weeks (65,66). In these patients, the serum half-life of tolbutamide decreased by 43% and the serum concentrations of tolbutamide decreased by 30% to 49% between 180 and 360 minutes after a single 1 g IV dose. Serum insulin and glucose concentrations before and after rifampin treatment were not significantly different, even with the change in tolbutamide pharmacokinetics.

H₂-antagonists

Many clinically significant drug interactions have been reported with coadministration of cimetidine and, to a lesser extent, ranitidine. Interactions with cimetidine appear to be due predominantly to inhibition of CYP isoforms, with potential contribution from inhibition of renal excretion (summarized in Ref. 67). Interactions with cimetidine caused by decreases in liver blood flow or changes in gastric pH are considered rare. Using purified and heterologously expressed CYP isoforms, cimetidine was found to be a relatively poor inhibitor of CYP2C9, especially when compared to its inhibition of CYP2D6 and CYP3A4 (68).

The effect of cimetidine or ranitidine on tolbutamide metabolism and clearance has been studied several times. Typically, little or no clinically significant effects on tolbutamide half-life or clearance were observed with either cimetidine or ranitidine (less than 20% change in mean values for either parameter) (69–71). In these studies, cimetidine was usually given at daily dosages of 1200 mg or less. Dosages of ranitidine were typically 300 mg or less. However, in one study, cimetidine at a daily dosage of 1600 mg caused a significant increase in tolbutamide plasma half-life and decreased tolbutamide clearance (72). This suggests a dose-dependent effect of cimetidine on tolbutamide pharmacokinetics.

Alcohol

Some of the first studies to examine the effect of alcohol on the drug metabolism system used tolbutamide as a probe. Tolbutamide clearance was studied in subjects who chronically ingested at least 250 g of alcohol daily for 2 or more years, with no evidence of liver damage. Results were compared to control subjects who abstained from alcohol or drank less than 10 g daily. Following IV administration of 1 g of tolbutamide, the plasma half-life of tolbutamide was reduced to approximately 165 minutes in alcoholics, compared to approximately 350 minutes in the nonalcoholics (73,74). In addition, chronic alcohol ingestion decreased the plasma half-lives of diphenylhydantoin and warfarin, which are selectively metabolized by CYP2C9, as is tolbutamide.

A similar finding was reported for 10 chronic alcoholics (with normal liver function) who received 1 g of tolbutamide intravenously at least several days after the last drink of alcohol (75). The clearance of tolbutamide was significantly elevated, and the plasma half-life significantly reduced (approximately two-fold) in these subjects relative to a control group that ingested little or no ethanol before or during the study.

Conversely, healthy subjects received an IV infusion of ethanol before and after a 1-g IV dose of tolbutamide (75). The clearance of tolbutamide in these subjects was greatly reduced relative to the same subjects given tolbutamide without concomitant ethanol infusion. The changes in tolbutamide clearance observed with concomitant alcohol injection are consistent with the paradoxical induction and inhibitory effects of ethanol on CYP2E1 activity (see Chapter 9). Although a similar mechanism has never been described for human CYP2C9, it is interesting to speculate on the possibility as an explanation for the clinical interaction.

Fluconazole

The effect of the antifungal agent fluconazole on tolbutamide pharmacokinetics was tested in 19 healthy subjects (76). When 500 mg of tolbutamide was administered orally 2 hours after a single oral 150 mg dose of fluconazole, statistically significant increases in tolbutamide maximal plasma concentrations (C_{max}) and area under the plasma concentration–time curve (AUC) values were observed. The plasma elimination half-life approximately doubled. The pharmacokinetic changes were maintained and did not increase with continuation of daily dosages of 100 mg of fluconazole for 6 additional days. Blood glucose concentrations did not change with either dosage protocol, but the authors suggested that blood glucose levels should be monitored if tolbutamide and fluconazole were coadministered in patients with diabetes. The interaction between fluconazole and tolbutamide is consistent with the inhibition of CYP2C9 by fluconazole as reported previously (77).

Other Drugs

No or very small changes in tolbutamide pharmacokinetics were observed in clinical trials with propranolol, metoprolol or atenolol (78), sulindac (79), dextropropoxyphene (80), primaquine (72), and sertraline (81). Interactions between these drugs and tolbutamide that result in hypoglycemia are not expected.

Acetohexamide

Acetohexamide differs from the other sulfonylurea drugs because it undergoes reductive metabolism rather than oxidation. The metabolite, hydroxyhexamide, is actually the active agent, with approximately 1.5- to 2-fold more pharmacologic activity than the parent drug (8). The plasma elimination half-life of hydroxyhexamide is approximately 5 hours, whereas the half-life of acetohexamide is approximately 1.5 hours. Hydroxyhexamide is cleared primarily by renal excretion. A literature search did not reveal any drug–drug interactions resulting from inhibition of the reduction of acetohexamide, probably because of the large capacity of carbonyl reductases in the body. Also, interactions resulting from interference with hydroxyhexamide excretion have not been reported.

Phenylbutazone

One interaction that has been described involved the coadministration of acetohexamide with phenylbutazone (82). In eight subjects, phenylbutazone decreased blood glucose concentrations in subjects receiving acetohexamide. Through careful pharmacokinetic analysis, it was determined that phenylbutazone was not inhibiting the reduction of acetohexamide, but rather was inhibiting the renal excretion of hydroxyhexamide, resulting in prolonged exposure and hypoglycemia.

SECOND GENERATION SULFONYLUREA DRUGS

Several oral hypoglycemic drugs with greater potency were introduced after the first generation agents. These second generation drugs contain a sulfonylurea pharmacophore and apparently function by the same mechanisms as the first generation drugs. The increased potency allows administration of lower dosages but does not result in increased release of insulin or better control of blood glucose levels when compared with the first generation drugs. A greater possibility of hypoglycemia resulting from their increased potency has been suggested but has not been clinically evident. The same pharmacodynamic interactions described for the first generation sulfonylureas have been documented with the second generation drugs.

Glybenclamide (Glyburide)

The most studied of the second generation sulfonylurea drugs is glybenclamide, which is used extensively. Typical oral dosages are 5 to 15 mg daily. Glybenclamide is extensively metabolized, with the 4-hydroxy metabolite being predominant and there being lesser amounts of the 3-hydroxy metabolite and a small amount (<2% of dose) of an unidentified metabolite (83). Approximately equal amounts of drug-related material are excreted in urine and feces, contrasting with first generation agents and their metabolites, which are primarily excreted in urine (84). The metabolites have minimal hypoglycemic activity in rabbits and, presumably, humans (85). The plasma half-life of glybenclamide following a single oral dose is approximately 5 hours.

Evidence from our laboratory indicates that the 3- and 4-hydroxy metabolites are produced primarily by CYP2C9 in human liver microsomes (*unpublished data*, 1998). Thus, coadministered drugs that inhibit CYP2C9 might be expected to decrease the clearance of glybenclamide. Another predominant metabolite observed in NADPH-supplemented human liver microsomes is ethylhydroxyglybenclamide, which is produced by CYP3A4 (*unpublished data*, 1998). This does not appear to be a major metabolite in humans *in vivo*, so interactions with CYP3A-specific inhibitors are not expected.

Glybenclamide is highly bound (approximately 99%) to plasma proteins (86). Unlike the first generation sulfonylureas, which bind to albumin through ionic interactions, glybenclamide binds to albumin via hydrophobic interactions.

Vitamin K Antagonists

Vitamin K antagonists do not appear to be potent inhibitors of glybenclamide metabolism, in that no reports have been found in a literature search. There was a report of prolonged warfarin clearance when coadministered with glybenclamide in an elderly patient who had been stabilized on warfarin for many years. After initiating glybenclamide treatment (10 mg daily), the patient's prothrombin times more than tripled within 48 hours and she experienced severe internal bleeding that ultimately led to her death (87). This suggests an interaction resulting from glybenclamide competitively inhibiting CYP2C9, although this has not been studied. However, glybenclamide (2.5–6 mg daily for at least 8 days) was reported to have no effect on plasma concentrations or half-life of phenprocoumon following a single oral dose of 12.7 mg in patients with diabetes (46). This is consistent with the absence of a pharmacokinetic interaction observed between tolbutamide and phenprocoumon (46).

Cotrimoxazole

In a retrospective analysis, seven of 57 patients with diabetes taking glybenclamide experienced severe hypoglycemia during simultaneous treatment with cotrimoxazole (trimethoprim and sulfamethoxazole) (88). In a study to specifically examine whether the concomitant administration of these drugs resulted in hypoglycemia, eight patients with diabetes who were stabilized on glybenclamide (5–15 mg daily) received cotrimoxazole for 4 to 6 days (dose not given) to treat bacterial infections (89). In contrast to observations from the retrospective analysis, the plasma AUC of glybenclamide was not significantly changed during this study, nor were concentrations of insulin or glucose.

Rifampin

Rifampin (600 mg daily) increased the plasma clearance of glybenclamide in a 67-year-old woman on stable glybenclamide therapy (5 mg daily) (90). She required an increased dosage of glybenclamide (15 mg daily) after beginning rifampin treatment for tuberculosis. Even with this increase in glybenclamide dosage, insulin therapy also had to be added to control blood glucose levels. After the rifampin treatment was discontinued, serum glybenclamide concentrations increased dramatically and her glybenclamide dosage was reduced to the 5-mg daily dose used before initiation of rifampin. Although her plasma glybenclamide concentrations increased approximately five-fold within 20 days of stopping rifampin treatment, there was no appreciable change in her blood glucose levels. The authors suggested a potential risk of hypoglycemia for some patients when glybenclamide is coadministered with rifampin, although other incidences were not found in the literature. This interaction is consistent with the known CYP-inducing effect of rifampin.

H2 Antagonists

Cimetidine (1200 mg daily for 4 days) increased the plasma AUC of glybenclamide in healthy male subjects receiving a single 5 mg dose of glybenclamide during a glucose tolerance test (91). In the same study, coadministration of ranitidine (300 mg daily for 4 days) and glybenclamide did not significantly change the AUC of glybenclamide. Plasma glucose concentrations were elevated, however, in these studies. The mechanism of this effect has not been elucidated.

A single incidence of an interaction with glybenclamide and ranitidine in an elderly man with diabetes was reported (92). This man, stabilized on glybenclamide (5 mg daily), had severe hypoglycemia 6 days after initiation of ranitidine treatment (300 mg daily). Treatment required constant infusion of glucose for approximately 16 hours.

Miconazole

A significant decrease in blood glucose was observed after a single 375-mg oral dose of miconazole in an elderly woman with diabetes, stabilized on a daily oral dose of 15 mg of glybenclamide (93). A reduction in the miconazole dose to 250 mg daily was required to return her blood glucose to the premiconazole concentration. The authors proposed that this interaction was due to inhibition of oxidative metabolism by the imidazole-containing miconazole.

Miconazole is an antifungicide, which is currently primarily used topically (suppositories). When used topically, little of the drug is absorbed systemically, so risk of the interaction described is very small. This effect of miconazole is consistent with inhibition of CYP enzymes by imidazole-containing drugs.

Verapamil

Single-dose administration of glybenclamide and verapamil in nine healthy subjects resulted in statistically significant increases in peak plasma glybenclamide concentrations and AUC values compared to the same subjects receiving glybenclamide with placebo (94). Concentrations of blood glucose or other biochemical markers for diabetes were not significantly different from placebo values. The authors suggested that this interaction resulted from inhibition of glybenclamide metabolism by verapamil but clinically significant changes in blood glucose concentrations were not expected.

Other Drugs

In other studies to investigate specific drug–drug interactions, glybenclamide pharmacokinetics or plasma glucose levels were not affected by diclofenac (95), propranolol (96), acebutolol (96) (acebutolol and propranolol did have a pharmacodynamic effect), fluconazole (97), clotrimazole (97), or fluvastatin (98).

Glipizide

Glipizide is another second generation sulfonylurea, with typical daily oral dosages of 5 to 15 mg. It is essentially completely absorbed and is extensively metabolized, with only approximately 2% to 9% of a single oral dose excreted as glipizide in urine (99). In another study, glipizide in urine and feces accounted for approximately 2% to 3% of the administered dose (100). The two major metabolites observed in urine were 4-*trans*-hydroxyglipizide and 3-*cis*-hydroxyglipizide, with the former present in three- to five-fold excess over the latter. Glipizide is approximately 98% protein bound in plasma.

Because glipizide is structurally similar to glybenclamide and other second generation sulfonylureas, similar metabolism-based drug–drug interactions would be expected but very few have been reported. Small changes in pharmacokinetic parameters (C_{max}, AUC, or half-life) of glipizide were reported following a single 400-mg dose of cimetidine (101), a single 150-mg dose of ranitidine (102), indubofen (200 mg for 5 days) (103), and a

single 20 mg dose of nifedipine (104). Blood glucose concentrations were unaffected and hypoglycemia did not occur in these clinical studies.

Gliclazide

Typical oral dosages of gliclazide range from 40 to 320 mg/day. Following a single dose of ^{14}C-gliclazide, 60% to 70% of the dose was excreted in urine, with another 10% to 20% excreted in feces (105,106). The drug is extensively metabolized, with less than 20% of the administered dose recovered as gliclazide. The major metabolites are the carboxylic acid and hydroxymethyl derivatives, with five other minor metabolites detected but not structurally characterized.

Some drug–drug interactions with gliclazide were tabulated without supporting references in a recent review, but a literature search did not confirm these (107). The drugs reported to decrease gliclazide clearance were similar to those reported for other sulfonylurea drugs, such as sulfonamides, vitamin K antagonists, and phenylbutazone. Increased clearance of gliclazide by enzyme-inducing drugs, such as rifampin, phenytoin, and barbiturates was also noted.

A few interaction reports were found in literature searches. Cimetidine administration (800 mg/day) initiated in an elderly subject stabilized on gliclazide (160 mg/day) resulted in severe hypoglycemia (108). In an elderly woman stabilized in gliclazide (40 mg/day), hypoglycemia developed 5 days after a single IV dose of 400 mg miconazole. The hypoglycemia was prolonged and resistant to glucose infusion, even after discontinuing gliclazide (109). Gliclazide plasma concentrations were elevated approximately 20-fold over premiconazole levels. Two additional incidences were reported in elderly patients with diabetes following IV miconazole administration (93). As discussed for glibenclamide, these interactions were probably due to inhibition of gliclazide metabolism by miconazole. Coadministration of gliclazide (dose not reported) with fluconazole (50 mg/day orally for 14 days) or clotrimazole (100 mg/day intravaginally for 14 days) in women with diabetes did not cause hypoglycemia or alter blood glucose (97).

NONSULFONYLUREA DRUGS

In addition to the sulfonylurea drugs, other drugs are available for the treatment of type II diabetes. In contrast to the sulfonylurea drugs, these drugs are truly antihyperglycemic, meaning that they reduce blood glucose levels to typical ranges but do not cause hypoglycemia. Structures of these drugs are shown in Figure 39-1.

Repaglinide

Repaglinide is an oral drug recently approved for the US market for treating type II diabetes. It functions by causing release of insulin from the pancreatic β cells, like the sulfonylurea drugs. However, it is structurally different, belonging to the meglitinide class of drugs. Unlike the sulfonylurea drugs, stimulation of insulin release by repaglinide is dependent on the presence of glucose in the blood. Hypoglycemia is then less of a risk, compared to the risk with sulfonylureas. Typical dosages are 0.5 to 4 mg daily, divided into portions taken prior to meals.

Repaglinide is rapidly absorbed and has a plasma half-life of approximately 1 hour (110). After a single oral dose of radiolabeled repaglinide, approximately 90% and 8% of the dose was excreted in the feces and urine, respectively. Less than 2% of the dose was excreted as parent drug. Repaglinide is extensively metabolized by direct glucuronidation and oxidation, predominantly by CYP3A4. The metabolites are not pharmacologically active. Repaglinide is highly bound (98%) to plasma proteins.

Drug–drug interactions with warfarin, digoxin or theophylline are not expected, based on clinical trials with healthy volunteers (111). Coadministration of cimetidine (800 mg/day for 5 days) with repaglinide (2 mg three times daily for 4 days) did not change repaglinide pharmacokinetics from control values or result in hypoglycemia (112). Coadministration of repaglinide with digoxin (0.25 mg daily for 9 days) did not affect repaglinide or digoxin pharmacokinetics in a similar study design (113). Combination therapy with repaglinide and metformin was well tolerated. Treatment of 83 patients with diabetes with metformin (1–3 g/day) and repaglinide (0.5–4 mg daily) for many months improved control of blood glucose levels without any incidences of hypoglycemia (114). The clinical effects of potent CYP3A inhibitors or CYP3A inducers on repaglinide pharmacokinetics have apparently not been tested. Therefore, drug interactions with these agents cannot be ruled out (109).

Metformin

The biguanides used for treatment of type II diabetes were introduced in the 1950s. Three drugs—metformin (glucophage), phenformin, and buformin—were initially marketed but only metformin is still available. Several comprehensive reviews have been published on metformin (10,115–118).

Use of the biguanide drugs has been controversial because they can produce lactic acidosis, which may be fatal. However, this is very rare with metformin, usually occurring only in patients with compromised renal function. Lactic acidosis was much more common with phenformin and buformin, which are no longer marketed because of this toxicity.

Metformin improves glucose control by increasing insulin-mediated glucose uptake by hepatocytes, muscle, and adipose tissue, by inhibiting hepatic gluconeogensis, and perhaps by delaying glucose absorption in the gastrointestinal tract. The increased glucose uptake appears to be the result of increasing the number of glucose transporters on cellular plasma membranes. Metformin does not increase insulin secretion from the pancreatic β cells as is done by the sulfonylurea drugs or repaglinide, so it will not cause hypoglycemia. Metformin requires some insulin production to control blood glucose concentrations.

Metformin is not metabolized in humans after oral or IV administration (119–122). Recoveries of 80% to 100% of the metformin dose in urine as unchanged drug have been reported in humans after IV administration. After oral administration, approximately 60% to 65% of the dose was recovered in urine. No oxidative or conjugated metabolites of metformin have been observed in plasma, urine, or feces. The drug is eliminated by renal excretion by way of active tubular secretion, hence the increased risk of lactic acidosis in renally compromised patients. Metformin is contraindicated in these patients.

Conversely, phenformin was extensively metabolized, primarily to the 4-hydroxy metabolite (123). CYP2D6 is the primary isoform responsible for 4-hydroxylation (124). Many of the cases of lactic acidosis observed with this drug may have been the result of reduced metabolism in patients lacking functional CYP2D6. Buformin was the least used of the biguanide drugs. It was primarily cleared via renal excretion.

Because metformin is not metabolized, metabolism based drug–drug interactions resulting in metformin pharmacokinetic changes are not expected. The effect of metformin on regulation of some drug metabolism activities was tested *ex vivo* using hepatic microsomes from rats dosed orally with metformin (50 mg daily) for 10 days (125). Metformin did not change the rates of aminopyrine N-demethylation, benzo(a)pyrene hydroxylation, or epoxide hydrolase (tested with styrene 7,8-oxide), relative to controls. In a clinical study, 850 mg of metformin administered orally twice daily for 4 weeks did not alter the plasma clearance or half-life of antipyrene, or the urinary excretion of glucaric acid or 6β-hydroxycortisol. This information, although not specific by current standards, is consistent with current clinical practice that metabolism-based drug interactions with metformin do not occur.

The use of metformin with sulfonylurea drugs to achieve better control of type II diabetes is common. Drug–drug interactions between these classes of drugs do not occur, beyond the combined effect on blood glucose (3). Combination therapy with repaglinide and metformin is also practiced (126). Caution must be taken when the second drug is added to the diabetes treatment, because metformin increases insulin sensitivity and sulfonylurea drugs or repaglinide increase circulating insulin concentrations. Hypoglycemia is possible under this scenario. Dosage adjustments may be necessary to reduce the risk of hypoglycemia.

Troglitazone (Rezulin)

Troglitazone is an orally active antihyperglycemic drug in the novel thiazolidinedione class. It is the first marketed compound in this class, although related compounds are in development. It functions as an insulin sensitizer in peripheral tissues, increasing the ability of cells to take up glucose and reducing the concentrations of insulin required to keep blood glucose at normal levels (127,128). The drug may also have some effect in increasing glycolysis and reducing gluconeogenesis in liver cells.

Typical dosages of troglitazone are 200 to 600 mg daily. Plasma half-life values are in the range of 16 to 34 hours (129). After 14 days of daily dosages of 400 mg, approximately 85% of the parent and metabolites are excreted in the feces, with another 3% excreted in the urine (130). Troglitazone is extensively metabolized, primarily via sulfation (131). Minor amounts of a glucuronide conjugate and a quinone metabolite have been identified. The drug is extensively (>99%) bound to plasma albumin (127). Troglitazone has been reported to cause liver damage in a small number of patients (132). Therefore, monitoring of liver function tests is required.

Troglitazone was reported to inhibit CYP3A4 by 60% in human liver microsomes, although troglitazone concentrations and reaction conditions were not described, so the clinical relevance of this is unclear (133). According to the package insert, troglitazone tested *in vitro* at clinically relevant concentrations did not inhibit any of the major hepatic CYP isoforms, using heterologously expressed isoforms (134). Therefore, drug interactions caused by inhibition of CYP isoforms by troglitazone are unexpected.

Potential clinical drug–drug interactions with troglitazone and other drugs have been tested. Interactions were not observed following concomitant administration of troglitazone and glybenclamide (135), digoxin (136), acetaminophen, warfarin, or a single dose of alcohol (137).

Results of other clinical studies suggest that troglitazone is an inducer of CYP3A4. Daily troglitazone treatment in healthy subjects (600 mg) for 14 days resulted in decreased AUC values for terfenadine and its acid metabolite of approximately 62% and 34%, respectively, apparently as a result of CYP3A4 induction (133,138). Plasma cyclosporine concentrations in a heart transplant recipient decreased to below detectable levels within 1 month of initiating troglitazone treatment (400 mg daily). The cyclosporine dosage was increased (to 400 mg daily) and troglitazone stopped, resulting in a four-fold increase in typical plasma cyclosporine concentrations 1 week later. After returning to the initial cyclosporine dosage, plasma cyclosporine concentrations stabilized as before troglitazone treatment (139). Plasma concentrations of ethinyl estradiol and norethindrone, in an oral contraceptive formulation, were reduced by approximately 30% when coadministered with troglitazone (137).

CONCLUSION

Several classes of oral drugs are used to treat type II diabetes mellitus. These include the sulfonylurea drugs, which share some common structural elements, metformin, repaglinide, and troglitazone. The sulfonylurea drugs have generally been available longer than the other drugs, but the first generation drugs are no longer extensively used. Metabolism-based drug interactions are described or anticipated with all but metformin.

After reviewing more than 40 years of clinical literature on drug interactions with the sulfonylurea drugs, it appears that metabolism-based interactions are limited to a small number of concomitant drugs. These include vitamin K antagonists, chloramphenicol, sulfonamides, some older NSAIDS, some azole-containing drugs, and rifampin. Acetohexamide is an exception because of its unique reductive metabolism. CYP2C9 has only been reported to catalyze tolbutamide hydroxylation, but drug interactions with the other sulfonylurea drugs are generally consistent with inhibition of CYP2C9. However, renal excretion, hepatic insufficiency and plasma protein binding may also be involved in the disposition of some of these drugs. Many of the spontaneous interactions involved elderly patients, suggesting a greater possibility of interactions with reduced liver or kidney function or compromised nutritional status.

With the exception of glybenclamide, in general, the use of the sulfonylurea drugs is declining, as is the use of many of the identified inhibitor drugs. Therefore, the incidence of drug interactions with the sulfonylurea drugs should decline also. The sulfonylurea drugs provide an interesting story, in that they were the first significant oral treatment for type II diabetes and drug interactions were clinically evident long before the underlying mechanisms were elucidated.

Metabolic drug interactions with troglitazone, caused by inhibition, are unexpected because sulfation is the primary route of troglitazone metabolism. However, because of the action of troglitazone as a CYP inducer, significant drug interactions must be considered, primarily with drugs metabolized by CYP3A.

Significant metabolic drug interactions have not been reported for the relatively new drug repaglinide. Since CYP3A predominates in the metabolism of the drug, interactions with inhibitors or inducers of CYP3A may be anticipated.

There are no metabolic drug interactions with metformin, because it is not metabolized and does not inhibit the metabolism of other drugs.

Pharmacodynamic interactions are also reported for these drugs, especially those resulting in hypoglycemia, but they were not discussed in this chapter. The pharmacodynamic interactions are well understood and are easily managed clinically.

Based on general clinical practice with the oral hypoglycemic drugs, metabolic drug interactions are reserved for a small number of well-defined drugs and are typically not a concern. Many patients have safely taken these drugs with great benefit and minor risk of drug interactions, if prescribed and taken correctly.

REFERENCES

1. Hardman JG, Gilman AG, Limbird LE, eds. *The pharmacological basis of therapeutics*, Vol. 9. New York: McGraw-Hill, 1996.
2. Lebovitz HE, ed. *Therapy for diabetes mellitus and related disorders.* Alexandria, VA: American Diabetes Association, 1991.
3. Scheen AJ, Lefebvre PJ. Antihyperglycaemic agents: drug interactions of clinical importance. *Drug Safety* 1995;12:32–45.
4. Hansten PD, Horn JR. Antidiabetic drug interactions. In: Hansten PD, Horn JR, eds. *Drug interactions: clinical significance of drug–drug interactions,* 6th ed. Philadelphia: Lea & Febiger, 1989:161–176.
5. Stockley IH. Hypoglycaemic agent drug interactions. In: Stockley IH, ed. *Drug interactions. A source book of adverse interactions: their mechanisms, clinical importance and management,* 3rd ed. Oxford: Blackwell Scientific, 1994:538–576.
6. Campbell LK, White JR, Campbell RK. Acarbose: its role in the treatment of diabetes mellitus. *Ann Pharmacother* 1996;30:1255–1262.
7. Feldman J. Glyburide: a second-generation sulfonylurea hypoglycemic agent. History, chemistry, metabolism, pharmacokinetics, clinical use and adverse effects. *Pharmacotherapy* 1985;5:43–62.
8. Jackson JE, Bressler R. Clinical pharmacology of sulphonylurea hypoglycemic agents: Part 1. *Drugs* 1981;22:211–245.
9. Gerich JE. Oral hypoglycemic agents. *N Engl J Med* 1989;321:1231–1245.
10. Krentz AJ, Ferner RE, Bailey CJ. Comparative tolerability profiles of oral antidiabetic agents. *Drug Saf* 1994;11:223–241.
11. Knodell RG, Hall SD, Wilkinson GR, Guengerich FP. Hepatic metabolism of tolbutamide: characterization of the form of cytochrome P-450 involved in methyl hydroxylation and relationship to in vivo disposition. *J Pharmacol Exp Ther* 1987;241:1112–1118.
12. Brian WR, Srivastava PK, Umbenhauer DR, Lloyd RS, Guengerich FP. Expression of a human liver cytochrome P-450 protein with tolbutamide hydroxylase activity in *Saccharomyces cerevisiae*. *Biochemistry* 1989;28:4993–4999.
13. Rowland M, Tozer TN. *Clinical pharmacokinetics: concepts and applications*, 2nd ed. Philadelphia: Lea & Febiger, 1989.
14. Rowland M, Matin SB, Thiessen J, Karam J. Kinetics of tolbutamide interactions. In: Morselli PL, Garattini S, Cohen SN, eds. *Drug interactions.* New York: Raven Press, 1974:199–211.
15. Taylor JA. Pharmacokinetics and biotransformation of chlorpropamide in man. *Clin Pharmacol Ther* 1972;13:710–718.
16. Petitpierre B, Perrin L, Rudhardt M, Herrera A, Fabre J. Behaviour of chlorpropamide in renal insufficiency and under the effect of associated drug therapy. *Int J Clin Pharmacol* 1972;6:120–124.
17. Balant L. Clinical pharmacokinetics of sulphonylurea hypoglycemic drugs. *Clin Pharmacokin* 1982;6:215–241.
18. Christensen LK, Skovsted L. Inhibition of drug metabolism by chloramphenicol. *Lancet* 1969;2:1397–1399.
19. Halpert J, Naslund B, Betner I. Suicide inactivation of rat liver cytochrome P-450 by chloramphenicol *in vivo* and *in vitro*. *Mol Pharmacol* 1983;23:445–452.
20. Kristensen M, Hansen JM. Accumulation of chlorpropamide caused by dicoumarol. *Acta Med Scand* 1968;183:83–86.
21. Rettie AE, Korzekwa KR, Kunze KL, et al. Hydroxylation of warfarin by human cDNA-expressed cytochrome P-450: A role for P-4502C9 in the etiology of (S)-warfarin drug interactions. *Chem Res Toxicol* 1992;5:54–59.
22. Dall JLC, Conway H, McAlpine SG. Hypoglycaemia resulting from chlorpropamide. *Scot Med J* 1967;12:403–404.

23. Tucker HSG, Hirsch JI. Sulfonamide-sulfonylurea interaction. *N Engl J Med* 1972;286:110–111.
24. Baciewicz AM, Swafford WB. Hypoglycemia induced by the interaction of chlorpropamide and cotrimoxazole. *Drug Intelligence and Clinical Pharmacy* 1984;18:309–310.
25. Shah SJ, Bhandarkar SD, Satoskar RS. Drug interaction between chlorpropamide and non-steroidal anti-inflammatory drugs, ibuprofen and phenylbutazone. *Int J Clin Pharmacol Ther Toxicol* 1984;22:470–472.
26. Self TH, Morris T. Interaction of rifampin and chlorpropamide. *Chest* 1980;77:800–801.
27. Jain AK, Ryan JR, McMahon FG. Potentiation of hypoglycemic effect of sulfonylureas by halofenate. *N Engl J Med* 1975;293:1283–1286.
28. Kudzma DJ, Friedberg SJ. Potentiation of hypoglycemic effect of chlorpropamide and phenformin by halofenate. *Diabetes* 1976;26:291–295.
29. Richardson T, Foster J, Mawer GE. Enhancement by sodium salicylate of the blood glucose lowering effect of chlorpropamide—drug interactions or summation of similar effects? *Br J Clin Pharmacol* 1986;22:43–48.
30. Sotaniemi EA, Huhti E. Half life of intravenous tolbutamide in the serum of patients in medical wards. *Ann Clin Res* 1974;6:146–154.
31. Zilly W, Breimer DD, Richter E. Induction of drug metabolism in man after rifampicin treatment measured by increased hexobarbital and tolbutamide clearance. *Europ J Clin Pharmacol* 1975;9:219–227.
32. Wishinsky H, Glaser EJ, Perkal S. Protein interactions of sulfonylurea compounds. *Diabetes* 1962;11:18–25.
33. Thomas RC, Ikeda GJ. The metabolic fate of tolbutamide in man and the rat. *J Med Chem* 1966;9:507–510.
34. Schulz E, Schmidt FH. Abbauhemmung von tolbutamid durch sulfaphenazol beim menschen. *Pharmacol Clin* 1970;2:150–154.
35. Newton DJ, Wang RW, Lu AYH. Cytochrome P450 inhibitors: evaluation of specificities in the in vitro metabolism of therapeutic agents by human liver microsomes. *Drug Metab Dispos* 1995;23:154–158.
36. Bournie M, Meunier V, Berger Y, Fabre G. Cytochrome P450 isoform inhibitors as a tool for the investigation of metabolic reactions catalyzed by human liver microsomes. *J Pharmacol Exp Ther* 1996;277:321–332.
37. Scott J, Poffenbarger PL. Pharmacogenetics of tolbutamide metabolism in humans. *Diabetes* 1979;28:41–51.
38. Miners JO, Birkett DJ. Cytochrome P4502C9: an enzyme of major importance in human drug metabolism. *Br J Clin Pharmacol* 1998;45:525–538.
39. Hansen JM, Kristensen M. Tolbutamide in the treatment of Parkinson's disease: a double blind trial. *Dan Med Bull* 1965;12:181–184.
40. Brunova E, Slabochova Z, Platilova H, Pavlik F, Grafnetterova J, Dvoracek K. Interaction of tolbutamide and chloramphenicol in diabetic patients. *Int J Clin Pharmacol* 1977;15:7–12.
41. Chaplin H, Cassell M. Studies on the possible relationship of tolbutamide to dicoumarol in anticoagulant therapy. *Am J Med Sci* 1958;235:706–715.
42. Spurny OM, Wolf JW, Devins GS. Protracted tolbutamide-induced hypoglycemia. *Arch Intern Med* 1965;115:53–56.
43. Kristensen M, Hansen JM. Potentiation of the tolbutamide effect by dicoumarol. *Diabetes* 1967;16:211–214.
44. Solomon HM, Schrogie JJ. Effect of phenyramidol and bishydroxycoumarin on the metabolism of tolbutamide in human subjects. *Metabolism* 1967;16:1029–1033.
45. Jahnchen E, Meinerts T, Gilfrich H-J, Groth U. Pharmacokinetic analysis of the interaction between dicoumarol and tolbutamide in man. *Eur J Clin Pharmacol* 1976;10:349–356.
46. Heine P, Kewitz H, Wiegboldt KA. The influence of hypoglycaemic sulphonylureas on elimination and efficacy of phenprocoumon following a single oral dose in diabetic patients. *Eur J Clin Pharmacol* 1976;10:31–36.
47. Soeldner JS, Steinke J. Hypoglycemia in tolbutamide-treated diabetes. *JAMA* 1965;193:148–149.
48. Wing LMH, Miners JO. Cotrimoxazole as an inhibitor of oxidative drug metabolism: effects of trimethoprim and sulphamethoxazole separately and combined on tolbutamide disposition. *Br J Clin Pharmacol* 1985;20:482–485.
49. Lumholtz B, Siersbaek-Nielsen K, Skovsted L, Kampmann J, Hansen JM. Sulfamethizole-induced inhibition of diphenylhydantoin, tolbutamide, and warfarin metabolism. *Clin Pharmacol Ther* 1975;17:731–734.

50. Doecke CJ, Veronese ME, Pond SM, et al. Relationship between phenytoin and tolbutamide hydroxylations in human liver microsomes. *Br J Clin Pharmacol* 1991;31:125–130.
51. Christensen LK, Hansen JM, Kristensen M. Sulphaphenazole-induced hypoglycemic attacks in tolbutamide-treated diabetics. *Lancet* 1963;2: 1298–1301.
52. Pond SM, Birkett DJ, Wade DN. Mechanisms of inhibition of tolbutamide metabolism: phenylbutazone, oxyphenbutazone, sulfaphenazole. *Clin Pharmacol Ther* 1977;22:573–579.
53. Rowlands M, Matin SB. Kinetics of drug-drug interactions. *J Pharmacokin Biopharm* 1973;1:553–567.
54. Schulz E, Schmidt FH. Abbauhemmung von tolbutamide durch sulfaphenazol beim menschen. *Pharmacologia Clinica* 1970;2:150–154.
55. Gulbrandsen R. Okt tolbutamid–effect. Ved Hjelp au fenylbutazon? *T Norske Haegeforen* 1959;79:1127–1128.
56. Szita M, Gachalyi B, Tornyossy M, Kaldor A. Interaction of phenylbutazone and tolbutamide in man. *Int J Clin Pharmacol Ther Toxicol* 1980;18:378–380.
57. Dent LA, Jue SG. Tolbutamide-phenylbutazone interaction. *Drug Intelligence and Clinical Pharmacy* 1976;10:711.
58. Tannebaum H, Anderson LG, Soeldner JS. Phenylbutazone-tolbutamide drug interaction. *N Engl J Med* 1974;290:344.
59. Stowers JM, Borthwick LJ. Oral hypoglycemic drugs: clinical pharmacology and therapeutic use. *Drugs* 1977;14:41–56.
60. Ober KF. Mechanism of interaction of tolbutamide and phenylbutazone in diabetic patients. *Eur J Clin Pharmacol* 1974;7:291–294.
61. Miners JO, Smith KJ, Robson RA, McManus ME, Veronese ME, Birkett DJ. Tolbutamide hydroxylation by human liver microsomes. *Biochem Pharmacol* 1988;37:1137–1144.
62. O'Reilly RA. Studies on the optical enantiomorphs of warfarin in man. *Clin Pharmacol Ther* 1974;16:348–354.
63. Andreasen PB, Simonsen K, Brocks K, Dimo B, Bouchelouche P. Hypoglycaemia induced by azapropazone-tolbutamide interaction. *Br J Clin Pharmacol* 1981;12:581–583.
64. Waller DG, Waller D. Hypoglycaemia due to azapropazone-tolbutamide interaction. *Br J Rheumatol* 1984;23:24–25.
65. Syvalahti E, Pihlajamaki KK, Iisalo EJ. Rifampin and drug metabolism. *Lancet* 1974;2:232–233.
66. Syvalahti E, Pihlajamaki K, Iisalo E. Effect of tuberculostatic agents on the response of serum growth hormone and immunoreactive insulin to intravenous tolbutamide, and on the half-life of tolbutamide. *Int J Clin Pharmacol* 1976;13:83–89.
67. Shinn AF. Clinical relevance of cimetidine drug interactions. *Drug Saf* 1992;7:245–267.
68. Knodell RG, Browne DG, Gwozdz GP, Brian WR, Guengerich FP. Differential inhibition of individual human liver cytochromes P-450 by cimetidine. *Gastroenterology* 1991;101:1680–1691.
69. Cate EW, Rogers JF, Powell JR. Inhibition of tolbutamide elimination by cimetidine but not ranitidine. *J Clin Pharmacol* 1986;26:372–377.
70. Adebayo GI, Coker HAB. Lack of efficacy of cimetidine and ranitidine as inhibitors of tolbutamide metabolism. *Eur J Clin Pharmacol* 1988;34:653–656.
71. Toon S, Holt BL, Mullins FGP, Khan A. Effects of cimetidine, ranitidine and omeprazole on tolbutamide pharmacokinetics. *J Pharm Pharmacol* 1995;47:85–88.
72. Back DJ, Tjia J, Moenig H, Ohnhaus EE, Park BK. Selective inhibition of drug oxidation after simultaneous administration of two probe drugs, antipyrine and tolbutamide. *Eur J Clin Pharmacol* 1988;34:157–163.
73. Kater RMH, Roggin G, Tobon F, Zieve P, Iber FL. Increased rate of clearance of drugs from the circulation of alcoholics. *Am J Med Sci* 1969;258:35–39.
74. Kater RMH, Tobon F, Iber FL. Increased rate of tolbutamide metabolism in alcoholic patients. *JAMA* 1969;207:363–365.
75. Carulli N, Manenti F, Gallo M, Salvioli GF. Alcohol-drugs interaction in man: alcohol and tolbutamide. *Eur J Clin Invest* 1971;1:421–424.
76. Lazar JD, Wilner KD. Drug interactions with fluconazole. *Rev Infect Dis* 1990;12:S327–S333.
77. Kunze KL, Wienkers LC, Thummel KE, Trager WF. Warfarin-fluconazole: inhibition of the human cytochrome P450-dependent metabolism of warfarin by fluconazole. *Drug Metab Disp* 1996;24(4):414–421.
78. Miners JO, Wing LMH, Lillywhite KJ, Smith KJ. Failure of "therapeutic" doses of β-adrenoceptor antagonists to alter the disposition of tolbutamide and lignocaine. *Br J Clin Pharmacol* 1984;18:853–860.
79. Ryan JR, Jain AK, McMahon FG, Vargas R. On the question of an interaction between sulindac and tolbutamide in the control of diabetes. *Clin Pharmacol Ther* 1977;21:231–233.
80. Robson RA, Miners JO, Whitehead AG, Birkett DJ. Specificity of the inhibitory effect of dextropropoxyphene on oxidative drug metabolism in man: effects on theophylline and tolbutamide disposition. *Br J Clin Pharmacol* 1987;23:772–775.
81. Tremaine LM, Wilner KD, Preskorn SH. A study of the potential effect of sertraline on the pharmacokinetics and protein binding of tolbutamide. *Clin Pharmacokinet* 1997;32:31–36.
82. Field JB, Ohta M, Boyle C, Remer A. Potentiation of acetohexamide hypoglycemia by phenylbutazone. *N Engl J Med* 1967;277:889–894.
83. Rupp W, Christ O, Heptner W. Resorption, ausscheidung und metabolismus nach intravenoser und oraler gabe von HB 419-14C an menschen. *Arzneim Forsch* 1969;19:1428–1434.
84. Rupp W, Christ O, Fulberth W. Untersuchungen zur bioavailability von glibenclamid. *Arzneim Forsch* 1972;22:471–473.
85. Heptner W, Kellner H-M, Christ O, Weihrauch D. Metabolismus von HB 419 am tier. *Arzneim Forsch* 1969;19:1400–1404.
86. Christ O, Heptner W, Rupp W. Investigations on absorption, excretion and metabolism in man after administration of ^{14}C-labelled HB 419. *Horm Metab Res* 1969;1:51–54.
87. Jassel SV. Drug points. *BMJ* 1991;303:789.
88. Asplund K, Wiholm BE, Lithner F. Glibenclamide-associated hypoglycaemia: a report on 57 cases. *Diabetologia* 1983;24:412–417.
89. Sjoberg S, Wiholm BE, Gunnarsson R, et al. Lack of pharmacokinetic interaction between glibenclamide and trimethoprim-sulphamethoxazole. *Diabetic Med* 1987;4:245–247.
90. Self TH, Tsiu SJ, Fowler JW. Interaction of rifampin and glyburide. *Chest* 1989;96:1443–1444.
91. Kubacka RT, Antal EJ, Juhl RP. The paradoxical effect of cimetidine and ranitidine on glibenclamide pharmacokinetics and pharmacodynamics. *Br J Clin Pharmacol* 1987;23:743–751.
92. Lee K, Mize R, Lowenstein SR. Glyburide-induced hypoglycemia and ranitidine. *Ann Intern Med* 1987;107:261–262.
93. Loupi E, Descotes J, Lery N, Evreux JC. Interactions medicamenteuses et miconazole. *Therapie* 1982;37:437–441.
94. Semple CG, Omile C, Buchanan KD, Beastall GH, Paterson KR. Effect of oral verapamil on glibenclamide stimulated insulin secretion. *Br J Clin Pharmacol* 1986;22:187–190.
95. Chlud K. Untersuchungen zur wechselwirkung von diclofenac and glibenclamid. *Zeit Rheum* 1976;35:377–382.
96. Zaman R, Kendall MJ. The effect of acebutolol and propranolol on the hypoglycaemic action of glibenclamide. *Br J Clin Pharmacol* 1982; 13:507–512.
97. Rowe BR, Thorpe J, Barnett A. Safety of fluconazole in women taking oral hypoglycaemic agents. *Lancet* 1992;39:255–256.
98. Appel S, Rufenacht T, Kalafsky G, et al. Lack of interaction between fluvastatin and oral hypoglycemic agents in healthy subjects and in patients with non-insulin-dependent diabetes mellitus. *Am J Cardiol* 1995;76:29A–32A.
99. Schmidt HAE, Schoog M, Schweer KH, Winkler E. Pharmacokinetics and pharmacodynamics as well as metabolism following orally and intravenously administered ^{14}C-glipizide, a new antidiabetic. *Diabetologia* 1973;9:320–330.
100. Fuccella LM, Tamassia V, Valzelli G. Metabolism and kinetics of the hypoglycemic agent glipizide in man—comparison with glybenclamide. *J Clin Pharmacol* 1973;13:68–75.
101. Feely J, Peden NR. Enhanced sulphonylurea-induced hypoglycaemia with cimetidine. *Br J Clin Pharmacol* 1983;16:607P.
102. MacWalter RS, Debani AH, Feely J, Stevenson IH. Potentiation by ranitidine of the hypoglycaemic response to glipizide in diabetic patients. *Br J Clin Pharmacol* 1985;19:121–124.
103. Elvander-Stahl E, Melander A, Wahlin-Boll E. Indobufen interacts with the sulphonylurea, glipizide, but not with the β-adrenergic receptor antagonists, propranolol and atenolol. *J Clin Pharmacol* 1984;18: 773–778.
104. Connacher AA, El Debani EH, Isles TE, Stevenson IH. Disposition and hypoglycaemic action of glipizide in diabetic patients given a single dose of nifedipine. *Eur J Clin Pharmacol* 1987;33:81–83.
105. Campbell DB, Adrianessens P, Hopkins YW, Gordon B, Williams JRB. Pharmacokinetics and metabolism of gliclazide: a review. In: *Gliclazide and the treatment of diabetes*. International congress and symposium series no. 20. London: Academic Press and Royal Society of Medicine 1980;71–82.

106. Oida T, Yoshida K, Kagemoto A, Sekine Y. The metabolism of gliclazide in man. *Xenobiotica* 1985;15:87–96.

107. Palmer KJ, Brogden RN. Gliclazide: an update of its pharmacological properties and therapeutic efficacy in non-insulin-dependent diabetes mellitus. *Drugs* 1993;46:92–125.

108. Archambeaud-Mouveroux F, Nouaille Y, Nadalon S, Treves R, Merle L. Interaction between gliclazide and cimetidine. *Eur J Clin Pharmacol* 1987;31:631.

109. Tanabashi S, Mihara M. A case of non-insulin-dependent diabetes mellitus with hypoglycemia induced by miconazole during treatment with gliclazide. *J Japan Diab Soc* 1995;38:389–394.

110. Brodows R. Prandin: a new therapy for type 2 diabetes. *Practical Diabetology* 1998;17:1–4.

111. *Physicians' desk reference*, 53rd ed. Montvale, NJ: Medical Economics, 1999:2108.

112. Schwietert R, Wemer J, Jonkman JHG, Hatorp V, Thomsen MS. No change in repaglinide pharmacokinetics with cimetidine co-administration. *Eur J Clin Pharmacol* 1997;52:A140.

113. Schwietert R, Wemer J, Jonkman JHG, Thomsen MS, Hatorp V. Co-administration of repaglinide does not affect digoxin pharmacokinetics. *Eur J Clin Pharmacol* 1997;52:A140.

114. Moses R, Slobodniuk R, Boyages S, et al. Additional treatment with repaglinide provides significant improvement in glycaemic control in NIIDM patients poorly controlled on metformin. *Diabetologia* 1997; 40:A322.

115. Sirtori CR, Pasik C. Re-evaluation of a biguanide, metformin: mechanism of action and tolerability. *Pharmacol Res* 1994;30:187–228.

116. Dunn CJ, Peters DH. Metformin: a review of its pharmacological properties and therapeutic use in non-insulin-dependent diabetes mellitus. *Drugs* 1995;49:721–749.

117. Hermann LS, Melander A. Biguanides: basic aspects and clinical uses. In: Alberti KGMM, DeFronzo RA, Keen H, Zimmet P, eds. *International textbook of diabetes mellitus,* Vol 28. New York: John Wiley and Sons, 1992:774–795.

118. Wildasin EM, Skaar DJ, Kirchain WR, Hulse M. Metformin, a promising oral antihyperglycemic for the treatment of noninsulin-dependent diabetes mellitus. *Pharmacotherapy* 1997;17:62–73.

119. Beckmann R. Resorption, verteilung im organismus und ausscheidung von metformin. *Diabetologia* 1969;5:318–324.

120. Pentikaiinen PJ, Neuvonen PJ, Penttila A. Pharmacokinetics of metformin after intravenous and oral administration to man. *Eur J Clin Pharmacol* 1979;16:195–202.

121. Tucker GT, Casey C, Phillips PJ, Connor H, Ward JD, Woods HF. Metformin kinetics in healthy subjects and in patients with diabetes mellitus. *Br J Clin Pharmacol* 1981;12:235–246.

122. Sirtoris CR, Franceschini G, Galli-Kienle M, et al. Disposition of metformin (N,N-demethylbiguanide) in man. *Clin Pharmacol Ther* 1978;24:683–693.

123. Bisisio E, Galli-Kienle M, Galli G, et al. Defective hydroxylation of phenformin as a determinant of drug toxicity. *Diabetes* 1981;30: 644–649.

124. Shah RR, Evans DA, Oates NS, Idle JR, Smith RL. The genetic control of phenformin 4-hydroxylation. *J Med Genet* 1985;22:361–366.

125. Ohnhaus EE, Berger W, Duckert F, Oesch F. The influence of dimethylbiguanide on phenprocoumon elimination and its mode of action. *Klin Wochenschr* 1983;61:851–858.

126. *Physicians' desk reference*, 53rd ed. Montvale, NJ: Medical Economics, 1999:2109.

127. Chen C. Troglitazone: an antidiabetic agent. *Am J Health Syst Pharm* 1998;55:905–925.

128. Johnson MD, Campbell LK, Campbell RK. Troglitazone: review and assessment of its role in the treatment of patients with impaired glucose tolerance and diabetes mellitus. *Ann Pharmacother* 1998;32:337–348.

129. Sparano N, Seaton TL. Troglitazone in type II diabetes mellitus. *Pharmacotherapy* 1998;18:539–548.

130. Shibata H, Nii S, Kobayashi M, et al. Phase I study of a new hypoglycemic agent CS-045 in healthy volunteers: safety and pharmacokinetics in single administration. *Rinsho Iyaku* 1993;9:1503–1518.

131. Young MA, Robinson CE, Devoy MAB, Minton NA. The influence of food on the pharmacokinetics of GR92132X, a thiazolidinedione, in healthy subjects. *Br J Clin Pharmacol* 1994;37:482P.

132. *Physicians' desk reference*, 53rd ed. Montvale, NJ: Medical Economics, 1999:2310.

133. Loi CM, Stern, R, Vassos AB, Koup JR, Sedman A. Effect of troglitazone on terfenadine pharmacokinetics. *Clin Pharmacol Ther* 1998; 63:228.

134. *Physicians' desk reference*, 53rd ed. Montvale, NJ: Medical Economics, 1999:2311.

135. Puchler K, Sasahara K, Witte PU, Wasserhess P. Lack of pharmacokinetic interaction between troglitazone and glibenclamide in NIDDM patients. *Diabetologia* 1996;39:A232.

136. Loi C-M, Knowlton PW, Stern R, et al. Effect of troglitazone on steady-state pharmacokinetics of digoxin. *J Clin Pharmacol* 1998; 38:178–183.

137. *Physicians' desk reference*, 53rd ed. Montvale, NJ: Medical Economics, 1999:2313.

138. Loi CM, Knowlton P, Stern R, Koup JR, Vassos AB, Sedman AJ. Effect of troglitazone on terfenadine pharmacokinetics when dosed 4-hours apart. *Clin Pharmacol Ther* 1998;63:229.

139. Frantz, RP, Nguyen TT. Rezulin (troglitazone) greatly increases cyclosporine metabolism. *J Heart Lung Transplant* 1998;17: 1037–1038.

CHAPTER 40

Antineoplastic Agents

James B. Mangold and Volker Fischer

Anticancer agents are frequently administered as a combination therapy as well as with supporting comedications, such as antiemetics, to reduce unwanted side effects. The therapeutic window for the anticancer agent is typically narrow and drug interactions could lead to exaggerated toxicity of the anticancer drug or reduced efficacy. The study of interactions involving anticancer agents typically cannot be conducted in healthy volunteers for ethical reasons. In patients, characterization of these interactions is hindered not only by the complexity of the clinical drug regimens used but also by factors relating to the variability in the patient populations and many factors that limit or preclude a comprehensive study of the interaction. Despite these limitations, drug interactions in this area are of considerable clinical importance and are the subject of several recent reviews (1–5).

In many cases, particularly when drug resistance has developed as a result of the efflux of the anticancer agent from the tumor cell by P-glycoprotein (P-gp), a pharmacokinetic interaction in which P-gp is inhibited is actually desirable to maintain adequate intracellular concentrations. Toward this end, several multidrug resistance (MDR)-modifying agents such as valspodar (PSC 833) are being developed. Inhibition of P-gp, however, is not selective for tumor cells; it is also an important factor in controlling absorption as well as renal and hepatic clearance of unchanged drug. The pivotal role of this transporter system in the disposition of a variety of drugs is discussed in this chapter in the context of anticancer agents.

Also of importance are pharmacokinetic interactions involving metabolic reactions. Many substrates of P-gp also appear to be substrates for cytochrome P450 (CYP) enzymes, in particular CYP3A (6). This fact can make it difficult to determine the relative contributions of P-gp and CYP to the observed effect. Additional information

such as the amount absorbed and the amount excreted unchanged may help to distinguish these processes. The increasing availability of the molecular tools (e.g., recombinant CYP isoforms) necessary to delineate the kinetics of these competing processes has greatly improved modern understanding of these complex interactions, but much additional research is needed.

This chapter provides an overview of several pharmacokinetic drug interactions involving anticancer agents and discusses the relevant pharmacokinetic and mechanistic information involved. This information may help guide further study of the specific interactions discussed and help predict potential interactions for compounds not specifically investigated. An overview is given in Table 40-1.

5-FLUOROURACIL

5-Fluorouracil (5-FU) is a highly toxic antineoplastic antimetabolite with a narrow therapeutic index. It exerts its antineoplastic effects by inhibiting the formation of thymidylic acid by way of blocking the methylation of uridylic acid. This results in a decrease in DNA and, to some extent, RNA, thereby interfering with cell growth, particularly rapidly growing cells. After intravenous administration, 5-FU exhibits a relatively short plasma elimination half-life of approximately 16 minutes and up to 20% of the dose is excreted unchanged in the urine within 6 hours, mostly during the first hour (7). The catabolism of 5-FU involves a multistep pathway in which the enzyme, dihydropyrimidine dehydrogenase (DPD), catalyzes the first rate-limiting step (8,9). The ultimate degradation products, CO_2, urea, and α-fluoro-β-alanine, are not biologically active.

Although catabolism of 5-FU by DPD is thought to occur largely in the liver, enzyme activity has also been measured in the blood. The importance of this enzyme in governing 5-FU catabolism and therefore toxicity is illustrated by the severe toxicity seen in a small population of

J. B. Mangold and V. Fischer: Department of Drug Metabolism and Pharmacokinetics, Novartis Institute for Biomedical Research, 59 Route 10, East Hanover, New Jersey 07936-1080

TABLE 40-1. *Overview of observed drug interactions, potentially relevant pharmacokinetic parameters, and proposed mechanisms*

Compound	Relevant enzyme	K_m (μM)	Pathway	P-gp substrate	% Absorbed	Excreted unchanged	AUC change with coadministration	Proposed mechanism	Reference for interaction
5-FU	Dihydropyrimidine dehydrogenase (DPD)	3.3	Dihydro-5-FU	NK	IV	20% (urine)	Sorivudine↑	DPD inhibitor	13–15
							Metronidazole↑	NK	19
							Cimetidine↑	NK	20
Paclitaxel	CYP2C8	16.0	6α-OH	Yes	IV	10%	Valspodar 50%↑	CYP/P-gp inhibitor	36
	CYP3A	34.8	p-phenyl-OH						
Docetaxel	CYP3A4	0.9/1.1	All	Yes	IV	Mainly metabolites	Barbiturates↓	CYP inducer	45
Doxorubicin	CYP3A5	9.3	Doxorubicinol	Yes	IV	50%	Doxorubicin↑	CYP/Pgp inhibitor	47
	Aldoketoreductase	NK					Valspodar↑	P-gp inhibitor	36
							Paclitaxel 30%↑	P-gp inhibitor	51–53
Vincristine	CYP3A	NK	NK	Yes	IV	NK	Nifedipine↑	CYP/P-gp inhibitor	67
							Itraconazole↑	CYP/P-gp inhibitor	59,63
Vinblastine	CYP3A	6.8	NK	Yes	IV	NK	Tamoxifen↑	CYP/P-gp inhibitor	121
Etoposide	CYP3A	53.9	3'-desmethyl	Yes	PO ~50% BA	20%–35%	Cyclosporine↑	CYP/P-gp inhibitor	36,77
		42–115							
Teniposide	CYP3A	19.7–43.5	3'-desmethyl	Yes	IV	~5%	Phenobarbitone↓	CYP inducer	75
							Phenytoin↓	CYP inducer	75
							Cyclosporine↑	CYP-P-gp inhibitor	78
							Fluconazole↑	CYP/P-gp inhibitor	104
Cyclosphosphamide	CYP2C9	49/95	4-OH	NK	IV	Up to 50% (urine)			
	CYP3A4/2B6	~5000	4-OH		PO >75%		Dexamethasone↓	CYP inducer	105
	CYP3A4/2B6	~8000	Deschloroethyl				Phenytoin↓	CYP inducer	106
6-Mercaptopurine	Xanthine oxidase (XO)	NK	8-OH	NK	~50%	NK	Methotrexate↑	XO inhibitor	85,86
Tamoxifen	CYP3A4	98	N-desmethyl	Yes	NK	<30%	Allopurinol↑	XO inhibitor	109,110
	CYP2C9	NK	4-OH				Rifampin↓	CYP inducer	125
	CYP2D6	NK	4-OH				Aminoglutethimide↓	CYP inducer	126
	FMO	NK	N-Oxide				Phenobarbital↓	CYP inducer	7
							Bromocriptine↑	CYP inhibitor	7

IV, intravenous; NK, not known; PO, by mouth; BA, bioavailability; AUC, area under plasma concentration versus time curve; P-gp, P-glycoprotein.

patients deficient in this enzyme (8,10–12). Agents that inhibit DPD, such as certain antiviral agents [e.g., sorivudine and its metabolite, (E)-5-(2-bromovinyl)uracil], have been reported to increase 5-FU exposure and accompanying toxicity in several instances (13–15).

In contrast, there are a number of reports of apparent interactions related to 5-FU therapy that remain unexplained. The ability of interferon-α to influence the pharmacokinetics of 5-FU is still somewhat controversial. Interferon-α has been reported to increase 5-FU levels in some studies (16), but not in others (17). The reasons for these conflicting reports are unclear.

In a related situation, the apparent enhancement in 5-FU activity when combined with either interferon-α or leukovorin, led to the investigation of the feasibility of combining all three medications (18). During this study, an interaction was noted in which concomitant interferon-α and leukovorin treatment resulted in significantly higher serum levels of leukovorin and its metabolite 5-methyltetrahydrofolate. Again, the underlying mechanism is unclear for this effect.

Prior metronidazole treatment has been reported to significantly reduce 5-FU clearance (19), as can chronic cimetidine administration (20), but the mechanisms underlying these apparent interactions are also unknown. 5-FU is not a known P-gp substrate and the effect of metronidazole and cimetidine on the 5-FU-metabolizing dihydropyrimidine dehydrogenase has not been investigated.

PACLITAXEL

Paclitaxel is a semisynthetic natural product derived from the Pacific yew, *Taxus baccata*. Antitumor effects of paclitaxel are due to its interference with the normal microtubule reorganization processes that are critical for interphase and mitotic functions in the cell, and thereby cell division (21). Paclitaxel exhibits biphasic plasma elimination after intravenous administration (7,22,23). A rapid decline in the early phase is attributed to both elimination and distribution to the periphery and is followed by a second phase, suggesting the slow release of the drug from the periphery back to the central compartment. The extensive distribution of paclitaxel to the tissues is supported with the high mean steady-state volume of distribution values (227–688 L/m^2) observed after a 24-hour infusion. Plasma protein binding ranges from 89% to 98% based on *in vitro* studies with human serum proteins.

After intravenous administration, paclitaxel clearance occurs largely in the liver, with an average of approximately 70% of a radioactive dose found in the feces and 14% in urine within 120 hours (7). Only approximately 10% of the dose is eliminated as parent drug in urine and feces and the major metabolite in feces is 6α-hydroxypaclitaxel (24). Paclitaxel is a substrate for P-gp, which prevents its application as an orally administered drug (25) and may also contribute to its elimination as unchanged

drug. Metabolism to the two primary metabolites 6α-hydroxypaclitaxel and 3-*p*-hydroxypaclitaxel is by way of CYP2C8 and CYP3A4, respectively (26,27). The K$_m$ values are 16 and 35 µM for CYP2C8 and CYP3A4, respectively (28,29). In 75% of human liver microsomal preparations, 6α-hydroxypaclitaxel is the major metabolite, but in 25%, 3-*p*-hydroxypaclitaxel is more important (30).

Because metabolism appears to play an important role in the elimination of paclitaxel, agents that could compete with or inhibit the involved enzymes would be expected to result in increased paclitaxel serum levels. For example, an interaction with ketoconazole might be initially anticipated because of the ability of ketoconazole to inhibit several CYP isoforms, especially CYP3A [K$_i$ = 0.01–0.04 µM, (28,31)], and P-gp (32,33). But when paclitaxel is given to patients concomitantly with ketoconazole, no pharmacokinetic interaction is observed, apparently because insufficient concentrations of ketoconazole are achieved after typical clinical doses (34). *In vitro* experiments have suggested that a ketoconazole concentration of about 37µM is necessary to inhibit CYP2C8-mediated paclitaxel 6α-hydroxylation by 50% (35). However, a 50% dose reduction of paclitaxel is required upon coadministration with the MDR modifier valspodar (36). Valspodar is a potent inhibitor of P-gp and CYP3A, but not CYP2C8 (28,37–39). Similarly, (R)-verapamil, which also inhibits both P-gp (40) and CYP3A (41), significantly increases the toxicity and reduces the clearance of paclitaxel (42). Other reports of putative interactions with paclitaxel have appeared (see Doxorubicin and Platinum complexes).

DOCETAXEL

Docetaxel is another semisynthetic natural product, obtained from yew plant needles. Like paclitaxel, its mechanism of antineoplastic action centers around microtubule network disruption and resulting interference with interface and mitotic processes. After intravenous dosing, the pharmacokinetics of docetaxel in plasma are triphasic, including an initial rapid distribution phase to the peripheral compartment (mean steady-state volume of distribution of 113L/kg) and a late terminal phase slow efflux from that compartment (7,43,44). Plasma protein binding of docetaxel is approximately 94% based on *in vitro* studies and involves α$_1$-acid glycoprotein, albumin, and lipoproteins. Somewhat higher protein binding, approximately 97%, is observed *in vivo* in cancer patients.

Docetaxel elimination occurs primarily in the feces (approximately 75%) and to a lesser extent (approximately 6%) in urine (7). Of the fecal elimination, unchanged docetaxel accounts for less than 8%, whereas the remainder consists of one major and several minor metabolites. The major metabolite is monohydroxylated docetaxel, resulting from hydroxylation of the *tert*-butyl ester group. *In vitro* studies have implicated the CYP3A subfamily as the major catalyst of docetaxel metabolism (45,46). Accordingly, use of docetaxel in patients also receiving medications known to induce or inhibit CYP3A poses the potential for an interaction. Consistent with this prediction, patients pretreated with barbiturates, inducers of CYP3A, showed enhanced hydroxylation of docetaxel (45). Additionally, the role of P-gp in docetaxel elimination is implicated in the interaction in which prior treatment with doxorubicin results in significant increases in docetaxel AUC (area under the plasma-time curve) values (47) (see Doxorubicin). Doxorubicin inhibits CYP3A-catalyzed reactions at concentrations (IC_{50} approximately 20 μM), which are at least 100-fold higher than therapeutic concentrations (<0.2μM) (28,48).

DOXORUBICIN

The anthracycline antibiotic, doxorubicin, a product of *Streptomyces peucetius* var. *caesius* cultures, is believed to exert its cytotoxic effects by binding to nucleic acids mainly through intercalation. This intercalation interferes with DNA synthesis by inhibiting DNA and RNA polymerases and replication. In addition, the ability of doxorubicin to interact with topoisomerase II, yielding DNA-cleavable complexes, contributes to its overall cytotoxic action (49,50). The pharmacokinetics of plasma after intravenous administration show a rapid distribution phase (approximately 5 minutes) to the tissues, followed by slow terminal half-life of 20 to 48 hours (7). Considerable tissue distribution was indicated by high steady-state volume of distribution values of greater than 20 to 30 L/kg. Binding of doxorubicin and its major metabolite, doxorubicinol, to plasma proteins is moderate (approximately 75%). Doxorubicin clearance involves mainly metabolism and biliary excretion with approximately 40% of the dose eliminated in the bile and 5% to 12% in urine within 120 hours (7). Doxorubicinol, which is formed by reduction at the 7-position and loss of the amino sugar, has similar pharmacokinetic properties to doxorubicin.

When doxorubicin treatment is combined with paclitaxel, the sequence of administration has been shown to be important in limiting the apparent interaction between the two agents (51–53). When doxorubicin treatment immediately follows paclitaxel, plasma levels of doxorubicin are approximately 70% higher and its clearance is reduced by about 30%. This effect and the accompanying dose-limiting toxicity was proposed to be due to the ability of paclitaxel to slow doxorubicin metabolism (51), although the mechanistic basis for this is unclear. As mentioned earlier, doxorubicin metabolism involves primarily reduction and loss of the amino sugar to yield the major metabolite, doxorubicinol, and the ability of paclitaxel to interfere with these reactions has not been documented. An alternative possibility was that the interaction involved the competition for biliary clearance of these agents, possibly involving P-gp (54). Additionally, Cremophor EL used in the paclitaxel clinical formulation was proposed to contribute to this putative P-gp–related interaction (54). More research is necessary to clarify these possibilities. Nevertheless, it has been recommended that the administration of doxorubicin should precede that of paclitaxel to avoid this interaction (51,52).

A similar interaction has been reported when the MDR-modifying agent valspodar was given concomitantly with doxorubicin (36). Valspodar coadministration resulted in significant increases in doxorubicin and doxorubicinol serum AUC values. The mechanism underlying this interaction is likely an inhibition of P-gp in that valspodar did not inhibit doxorubicin metabolism in human liver microsomes (28). The inhibition of P-gp and corresponding decrease in doxorubicin and doxorubicinol clearance is consistent with the previously described paclitaxel interaction mechanism, as well as with an earlier report of the ability of verapamil to interact with doxorubicin, presumably through effects on P-gp (55).

VINCA ALKALOIDS

The vinca alkaloid family of antineoplastic agents includes vinblastine, vincristine, and vinorelbine (56). All three of these vinca alkaloids share similar mechanisms of action, which include inhibition of microtubule assembly, thereby arresting the dividing cell at the metaphase. Other contributing actions differentiate these compounds in terms of their overall biologic effects. All display triphasic plasma pharmacokinetics, characterized by relatively rapid uptake into tissues with a later slow efflux back to the central compartment. For vincristine, intravenous administration results in plasma half-lives of 5 minutes, 2.3 hours, and 85 hours with considerable intersubject variability in the terminal half-life value ranging from 19 to 155 hours (7). The corresponding half-lives for vinblastine are 3.7 minutes, 1.6 hours, and 24 hours. The terminal plasma half-lives of vinorelbine range from 28 to 44 hours.

The metabolism of the vinca alkaloids in general appears to be mediated primarily by the CYP3A subfamily (57,58) and excretion occurs mainly in bile. For most vinca alkaloids, it is not known whether they are excreted mainly as metabolites or unchanged. In the case of vinorelbine, however, considerable unchanged drug was found in the feces after intravenous administration. This is consistent with the reporting of several vinca alkaloids as substrates for P-gp. Therefore, the potential for CYP or P-gp inhibition to contribute to clinical interactions involving the vinca alkaloids has been proposed (59–61) and a number of case reports supportive of such interactions have appeared (62). Enhanced neurotoxicity of vincristine has been reported when it was given with the antifungal agent itraconazole (59,63). Itraconazole has the potential to inhibit both CYP3A (64) and P-gp (6,65).

Coadministration of vincristine with nifedipine, which also can inhibit CYP3A (64) and P-gp (66), leads to a decreased vincristine clearance from the body (67).

ETOPOSIDE AND TENIPOSIDE

Etoposide (VP-16) and teniposide (VM-26) are semi-synthetic derivatives of podophyllotoxin, which act through inhibition of topoisomerase II. Topoisomerase II plays an essential role in the proliferation of eukaryotic cells. The cytotoxic effects of these agents are mainly due to their ability to trap the DNA–topoisomerase II complex and inhibit DNA synthesis (68–70). After intravenous doses, etoposide exhibits biphasic plasma pharmacokinetics with a distribution half-life of 1.5 hours and terminal half-life of 4 to 11 hours (7). Teniposide pharmacokinetics in plasma are also biphasic with a terminal half-life of 5 hours (7). The steady-state volume of distribution ranges from 7 to 17 L/m^2 for etoposide and 8 to 44 L/m^2 for teniposide. Both are highly protein bound (97% for etoposide and >99% for teniposide) based on *in vitro* studies. Elimination of a radiolabeled intravenous etoposide dose involves both urinary and fecal elimination routes, with recoveries in urine and feces of 42% to 67% and 0% to 16%, respectively. Less than half the urinary excretion was unchanged etoposide. The majority of the biliary–fecal elimination is due to metabolism, with less than 6% unchanged etoposide in bile after an intravenous dose. The major urinary metabolite is the hydroxy acid derivative, in which the etoposide lactone has been opened. Other metabolites in urine include sulfate and glucuronide conjugates of etoposide. When given orally, bioavailability is about 50% with no first-pass effect observed. For teniposide, intravenous administration of radiolabeled teniposide results in approximately 44% of the dose being eliminated in urine, including 4% to 12% of the dose as parent drug. The excretion of radioactivity in feces by 72 hours was 0% to 10% of the dose.

Interactions in which systemic exposure to etoposide or teniposide is altered may arise from CYP or P-gp interaction (71). CYP involvement in etoposide and teniposide metabolism has been investigated (72–74) and the major metabolic pathway of 3′-demethylation is catalyzed by CYP3A4. Induction of CYP metabolism observed with concomitant phenobarbitone or phenytoin therapy decreased the systemic clearance of teniposide two- to three-fold (75). Also consistent with CYP involvement in etoposide and teniposide metabolism is the reported increase in systemic exposure when other CYP3A4 substrates (e.g., cyclosporine analogues such as valspodar) are coadministered (28,36,76–78); however, the likely contribution of P-gp inhibition to the observed increase in exposure must also be considered.

The ability of etoposide to function as an inhibitor of other CYP reactions *in vitro* has also been reported. Etoposide was found to inhibit paclitaxel 6α- and 3′-p-hydroxylation *in vitro* (79), reactions attributed to CYP isoforms 2C8 and 3A4, respectively (26,27,30). Other reports have pointed to the inhibitory effects of etoposide on CYP2C19 (80,81). The clinical significance, in light of the possible contribution of P-gp effects, is difficult to assess, but nonetheless cannot be discounted.

METHOTREXATE

Methotrexate (MTX) is an antimetabolite that exerts its antineoplastic effects through the inhibition of tetrahydrofolate reductase (TFR) and, therefore, DNA synthesis. This inhibition of TFR leads to a decrease in available tetrahydrofolates that are needed as one-carbon carriers in the synthesis of purine nucleotides and thymidylate. MTX may be given either orally or intravenously (82–84). When administered orally, dose-dependent absorption is observed. At lower doses (30 mg/m^2 or less), MTX is well absorbed with a bioavailability of approximately 60%, but at higher doses (80 mg/m^2 or greater), absorption is less (7). After lower doses, the terminal plasma half-life ranges from 3 to 10 hours and, after high doses, from 8 to 15 hours. After intravenous administration, the steady-state volume of distribution ranges from 0.4 to 0.8 L/kg and MTX protein binding in serum is approximately 50% (7). Upon absorption, MTX is converted to polyglutamated metabolites, which also act as TFR and thymidylate synthetase inhibitors. These metabolites may also be converted back to free MTX by cellular hydrolases. Some oxidative metabolism occurs as well to form 7-hydroxy-MTX. Elimination of MTX is primarily renal, with 80% to 90% of an intravenous dose being excreted unchanged in urine. The renal excretion involves both glomerular filtration and active tubular secretion.

Because MTX disposition is predominantly influenced by renal function, drug interactions generally involve renal impairment either by the drug itself or a concomitant medication. However, MTX has other actions that lead to potential pharmacokinetic interactions with other drugs. One such case stems from the ability of MTX to inhibit xanthine oxidase (XO), an enzyme system important in the metabolism of 6-mercaptopurine (6-MP). This inhibition may not be of great clinical significance except in high MTX dose situations because of the high interpatient variability in 6-MP pharmacokinetics. With high dose MTX, substantial increases in 6-MP bioavailability are seen with increases in both C_{max} and AUC (85,86). Another inhibitor of XO, allopurinol, can also inhibit first pass metabolism of 6-MP (see 6-Mercaptopurine) and lead to a similar pharmacokinetic drug interaction.

PLATINUM COMPLEXES

Carboplatin and cisplatin are platinum-containing complexes that produce interstrand cross-links in DNA. Both agents have as part of their structure two ammonia molecules complexed to the platinum. For activity, these agents must be converted to their active "aquated" form in which the ammonia molecules are replaced by two water molecules. The rate at which this aquation occurs appears to determine potency (87,88). Carboplatin is primarily eliminated by the renal route, with about 71% of the dose eliminated in urine within 24 hours in patients with normal renal function (7,89–91). All of the platinum in the 24-hour urine was present as carboplatin. After intravenous infusion, biphasic kinetics are observed in plasma with half-lives ranging from 1.1 to 2.0 hours and 2.6 to 5.9 hours (7). The apparent volume of distribution is about 16 L and carboplatin in not bound to plasma proteins. Cisplatin after intravenous injection (either bolus or infusion) displays monophasic plasma kinetics with a half-life of approximately 30 minutes (7). Although cisplatin does not exhibit typical reversible plasma protein–binding behavior, approximately 90% of the platinum after a 3-hour infusion is tightly bound to plasma protein. This bound platinum remains associated with the protein for extended periods (half-life > 5 days). Elimination of cisplatin is mainly in urine, involving both glomerular filtration and active secretion processes. The urinary platinum is present as unchanged cisplatin, free (ultrafiltrable) platinum, and other platinum-containing compounds.

Most concern for interactions with platinum agents relate to renal function. Agents that influence renal function or that have nephrotoxic effects could pose serious problems if used concomitantly with platinum complexes. The use of paclitaxel concomitantly with carboplatin has been reported to result in an apparent reduction in the anticipated carboplatin AUC value, suggestive of a pharmacokinetic interaction. However, it was subsequently concluded that the lower than anticipated AUC values were most likely due to an inadequate assessment of glomerular filtration rate used to establish the carboplatin dose (92,93).

CYCLOPHOSPHAMIDE AND IFOSFAMIDE

Cyclophosphamide and ifosfamide are biotransformed by CYP and the reactive metabolites formed produce DNA cross-links, preferentially targeting rapidly growing cells. Cyclophosphamide is administered both orally and intravenously (94), and ifosfamide is only given intravenously (95,96). After oral dosing, cyclophosphamide is well absorbed, with a bioavailability of approximately 75% and elimination half-lives of 3 to 12 hours (7). Although most cyclophosphamide elimination involves metabolism, up to 25% of the dose may be excreted in urine unchanged. Plasma protein binding of cyclophosphamide is low. Ifosfamide (94) shows dose-dependent pharmacokinetics with terminal plasma half-lives ranging from up to 15 hours after high doses (3.8–5 g/m²/d) to 7 hours after lower doses (1.6–2.4 g/m²/d) and sat-

urable metabolism is observed (7). The proportion of unchanged drug excreted in urine is also dose dependent, ranging from 61% after the high dose to 12% to 18% after the lower dose. Because activity of these agents resides in their metabolites, the relationship of parent drug pharmacokinetics to pharmacodynamics is not always meaningful. In fact, enhanced metabolism is typically associated with increased therapeutic effect.

Metabolic activation of cyclophosphamide and ifosfamide occurs by way of 4-hydroxylation, primarily catalyzed by CYP2B6 in the case of cyclophosphamide and CYP3A4 for ifosfamide (97). Additionally, recent reports suggest that members of the CYP2C family, in particular 2C19 and 2C9, may also contribute to the activation of both agents (98,99). A second metabolic reaction of importance appears to be side chain oxidation. This N-dechloroethylation pathway, catalyzed primarily by CYP3A4 (99–101), produces chloroacetaldehyde, a potential neurotoxin, and is therefore implicated in the neurotoxicity associated with these agents. Because different CYP isoforms catalyze the pathways associated with cyclophosphamide activation and toxicity, modulation of the reactions that could improve the therapeutic profile of the drug have been proposed (97). The potential of this approach was recently demonstrated in an animal model in which troleandomycin, a known CYP3A inhibitor, was used to reduce the formation of toxic metabolites without apparent adverse effect on antitumor activity (102). For ifosfamide, however, the involvement of CYP3A4 in both activation and toxification reactions makes such a strategy nonviable.

The role of CYP3A4 in cyclophosphamide biotransformation has posed the potential for interactions with other agents metabolized by this isoform (101). Ifosfamide and cyclophosphamide were found to competitively inhibit CYP3A-catalyzed testosterone 6β-hydroxylation in human liver microsomes, but with relatively high K_i values of 510 μM and 490 μM, respectively (103). Known inhibitors of CYP3A4 would be expected to hinder the activation reaction. This possibility was supported by a retrospective study of cyclophosphamide with and without concomitant fluconazole therapy (104). Fluconazole, a known CYP3A4 and CYP2C9 inhibitor, was observed to reduce cyclophosphamide clearance by approximately 50% (2.4 versus 4.2 L/h/m²). The in vitro inhibition of cyclophosphamide 4-hydroxylation by fluconazole in human liver microsomes was associated with IC_{50} values ranging from 9 to 80 μM (104). Although the clinical significance of this is not clear, the potential for a reduction in therapeutic effect must be considered.

Cyclophosphamide and ifosfamide pharmacokinetics and metabolism are also influenced by enzyme induction (94,95). Prior treatment with dexamethasone resulted in an increase in cyclophosphamide clearance in children, which was attributed to induction of CYP enzymes (105). The administration of busulfan together with phenytoin was also found to increase cyclophosphamide clearance in cancer patients (106). The ability of typical CYP inducers—phenobarbital, dexamethasone, and rifampin—to enhance activation of cyclophosphamide and ifosfamide has been demonstrated *in vitro* using primary human hepatocyte cultures (107). A 200% to 400% increase in 4-hydroxylation activity relative to controls was observed, accompanied by increases in CYP2B6, CYP2C8, CYP2C9, and CYP3A4 immunoreactive protein. Autoinduction was also observed in this system with either ifosfamide or cyclophosphamide, and resulted in increases in CYP3A4, CYP2C8, and CYP2C9 protein levels (107). However, for ifosfamide in the clinic, a significant pharmacokinetic interaction involving dexamethasone was not observed (108), but an apparent alteration in metabolism attributed to differential induction of CYP isoforms by phenytoin has been reported (109). Evidence of autoinduction has also been seen in the clinical setting (110).

6-MERCAPTOPURINE

The antimetabolite 6-MP interferes with nucleic acid biosynthesis and has demonstrated activity in the treatment of human leukemias (111). After oral administration, 6-MP absorption is variable and averages approximately 50%. Elimination half-life in plasma after intravenous dosing is approximately 22 minutes in children and 45 minutes in adults (7). 6-MP rapidly enters into endogenous pathways for purine metabolism and is converted to a variety of active metabolites within the cells. Consequently, the biologic activity of 6-MP persists for much longer than the measurable plasma drug levels. Overall, the metabolism of 6-MP is relatively complex. Among the enzymes involved in 6-MP metabolism, xanthine oxidase (XO) appears to play an important role, as does thiopurine methyltransferase. The importance of the former with regard to drug interaction potential is evidenced by the significant increases in systemic exposure to 6-MP when it is administered concomitantly with the xanthine oxidase inhibitor allopurinol (112,113) (see Methotrexate). Under these circumstances, substantial dosage adjustment is necessary to avoid unacceptable toxicity.

TAMOXIFEN

Tamoxifen is a nonsteroidal agent that exhibits antiestrogenic properties, probably because of its ability to compete with estrogen for its binding sites in target tissues. It is often used in the treatment of metastatic breast cancer in patients with estrogen receptor–positive tumors.

Tamoxifen is extensively metabolized after oral administration to numerous metabolites, with *N*-desmethyl-hydroxytamoxifen, 4-hydroxytamoxifen, and tamoxifen-*N*-oxide being the major ones (114). *N*-desmethyltamoxifen has equal antiestrogenic activity and

4-hydroxytamoxifen is 100 times more active than parent tamoxifen (115,116). The *N*-oxide metabolite may be considered as a depot form of tamoxifen in that it can easily be reduced to tamoxifen *in vivo*. CYP3A and flavin-containing monooxygenase have been identified to be the enzymes responsible for *N*-demethylation and *N*-oxide formation, respectively (117–119), and CYP2D6, CYP2C9, and CYP3A are involved in 4-hydroxylation of tamoxifen (120,121). Further *ortho*-hydroxylation of 4-hydroxytamoxifen to the corresponding catechol metabolite was found to be catalyzed primarily by CYP3A with lesser involvement of CYP2D6 (122).

Elimination of tamoxifen and its metabolites may also be mediated by P-gp because all three—tamoxifen, *N*-desmethyltamoxifen, and 4-hydroxy tamoxifen—have been reported to be substrates for P-gp, based on ATPase stimulation (123). Approximately 65% of the administered dose is excreted from the body primarily in feces. The drug is excreted mainly as polar conjugates, with unchanged drug and unconjugated metabolites accounting for less than 30% of the total fecal radioactivity. Drug interactions can thus be expected when P-gp or CYP3A is inhibited by concomitant medications, or when tamoxifen or its metabolites inhibit the activity of these proteins, thereby slowing the elimination of other drugs.

Although the effect of tamoxifen on the metabolism and excretion of other antineoplastic drugs, such as cyclophosphamide and other drugs that require CYP activation, is not known, high-dose oral tamoxifen was shown to inhibit vinblastine elimination (124). Also, when tamoxifen was used in combination with coumarin-type anticoagulants, a significant increase in anticoagulant effect was observed (125–127). This could indicate that tamoxifen is able to inhibit CYP2C9, but no confirming data are available.

Conversely, coadministration of the CYP3A substrate bromocriptine elevates serum tamoxifen and *N*-desmethyl-tamoxifen concentrations (7), whereas the effects of enzyme inducers such as phenobarbital or aminoglutethimide lower plasma concentrations of tamoxifen (7,128,129).

CONCLUSION

Considerable progress has been made in recent years in characterizing the mechanisms of drug disposition for anticancer agents, and this knowledge has improved understanding of the processes underlying clinically significant drug interactions. Recognition of P-gp as a key factor in drug absorption and elimination has provided new insight into factors that can be perturbed and thereby alter systemic exposure. However, the relative importance of this transporter for many anticancer agents is often unclear because basic information on extent of absorption and the amount of drug excreted unchanged is incomplete or lacking. In the future, the availability of new *in vitro* tools and model systems may enhance one's ability to quantify the contribution of P-gps.

Interindividual variability is also a factor that complicates the characterization of drug interactions. For metabolic reactions, much is known about the extent to which important enzyme systems (e.g., CYP enzymes) can vary across the population and be influenced by either inhibitors or inducers. This knowledge of CYP-mediated reactions can be exploited for therapeutic advantage as highlighted in the case of cyclophosphamide (see cyclophosphamide). However, comparable information on the interindividual variability in P-gp expression remains poorly understood, as do factors that modulate P-gp.

REFERENCES

1. McLeod HL. Clinically relevant drug–drug interactions in oncology. *Br J Clin Pharmacol* 1998;45:539–544.
2. Kivisto KT, Kroemer HK, Eichelbaum M. The role of human cytochrome P450 enzymes in the metabolism of anticancer agents: implications for drug interactions. *Br J Clin Pharmacol* 1995;40: 523–530.
3. van Meerten E, Verweij J, Schellens JH. Antineoplastic agents. Drug interactions of clinical significance. *Drug Saf* 1995;12:168–182.
4. Loadman PM, Bibby MC. Pharmacokinetic drug interactions with anticancer drugs. *Clin Pharmacokinet* 1994;26:486–500.
5. Balis FM. Pharmacokinetic drug interactions of commonly used anticancer drugs. *Clin Pharmacokinet* 1986;11:223–235.
6. Wacher VJ, Wu CY, Benet LZ. Overlapping substrate specificities and tissue distribution of cytochrome P450 3A and P-glycoprotein: implications for drug delivery and activity in cancer chemotherapy. *Mol Carcinog* 1995;13:129–134.
7. *Physicians desk reference*, 53rd ed. Montvale, NJ: Medical Economics, 1999.
8. Lu Z, Zhang R, Diasio RB. Population characteristics of hepatic dihydropyrimidine dehydrogenase activity, a key metabolic enzyme in 5-fluorouracil chemotherapy. *Clin Pharmacol Ther* 1995;58:512–522.
9. Lu Z-H, Zhang R, Diasio RB. Purification and characterization of dihydropyrimidine dehydrogenase from human liver. *J Biol Chem* 1992;267:17102–17109.
10. Lu Z, Zhang R, Diasio RB. Dihydropyrimidine dehydrogenase activity in human peripheral blood mononuclear cells and liver: population characteristics, newly identified deficient patients, and clinical implications in 5-fluorouracil chemotherapy. *Cancer Res* 1993;53:5433–5438.
11. Harris BE, Carpenter JT, Diasio RB. Severe 5-fluorouracil toxicity secondary to dihydropyrimidine dehydrogenase deficiency. A potentially more common pharmacogenetic syndrome. *Cancer* 1991;68: 499–501.
12. Diasio RB. Sorivudine and 5-fluorouracil; a clinically significant drug–drug interaction due to inhibition of dihydropyrimidine dehydrogenase. *Br J Clin Pharmacol* 1998;46:1–4.
13. Watabe T, Okuda R, Ogura K. Lethal drug interactions of the new antiviral, sorvudine, with anticancer prodrugs of 5-fluorouracil. *Yakaguku Zasshi* 1997;117:910–21.
14. Ogura K, Nishiyama T, Takubo H, et al. Suicidal inactivation of human dehydrogenase by (E)-5-(2-bromovinyl)uracil derived from the antiviral, sorivudine. *Cancer Lett* 1998;122:107–113.
15. Peck R, Wiggs R, Callaghan J, et al. Inhibition of dihydropyrimidine dehydrogenase by 5-propynyluracil, a metabolite of the anti-varicella zoster virus agent, netvudine. *Clin Pharmacol Ther* 1996;59:22–31.
16. Schuller J, Czejka M. Pharmacokinetic interaction of 5-fluorouracil and interferon alpha-2b with or without folinic acid. *Med Oncol* 1995;12:47–53.
17. Seymour MT, Patel N, Johnston A, Joel SP, Slevin ML. Lack of effect of interferon alpha-2a upon fluorouracil pharmacokinetics. *Br J Cancer* 1994;70:724–728.
18. Sinnege HA, Buter J, de Vries EG, Uges DR, Roenhorst HW, Verschueren RC, Sleijfer DT, Willemse PH, Mulder NH. Phase I-II study

19. of the addition of alpha-2a interferon to 5-fluorouracil/leukovorin. Pharmacokinetic interaction of alpha-2a interferon and leukovorin. *Eur J Cancer* 1993;29A:1715–1720.
19. Bardakji Z, Jolivet J, Besner JB, Ayoub J. 5-Fluorouracil-metronidazole combination therapy in metastatic colorectal cancer. Clinical, pharmacokinetic and *in vitro* cytotoxicity studies. *Cancer Chemother Pharmacol* 1986;18:140–144.
20. Harvey VJ, Slevin ML, Dilloway MR, Clark PI, Johnston A, Lant AF. The influence of cimetidine on the pharmacokinetics of 5-fluorouracil. *Br J Clin Pharmacol* 1984;18:421–430.
21. Eisenhauer EA, Vermorken JB. The taxoids. Comparative clinical pharmacology and therapeutic potential. *Drugs* 1998;55:5–30.
22. Kearns CM. Pharmacokinetics of the taxanes. *Pharmacotherapy* 1997;17(5 Pt 2):105S –109S.
23. Sonnichsen DS, Relling MV. Clinical pharmacokinetics of paclitaxel. *Clin Pharmacokinet* 1994;27:256–269.
24. Walle T, Walle UK, Kumar GN, Bhalla KN. Taxol metabolism and disposition in cancer patients. *Drug Metab Dispos* 1995;23:506–512.
25. van Asperen J, van Tellingen O, Sparreboom A, et al. Enhanced oral bioavailability of paclitaxel in mice treated with the P-glycoprotein blocker SDZ PSC 833. *Br J Cancer* 1997;76:1181–1183.
26. Harris JW, Rahman A, Kim BR, Guengerich FP, Collins JM. Metabolism of taxol by human hepatic microsomes and liver slices: participation of cytochrome P450 3A4 and an unknown P450 enzyme. *Cancer Res* 1994;54:4026–4035.
27. Rahman A, Korzekwa KR, Grogan J, Gonzalez FJ, Harris JW. Selective biotransformation of taxol to 6-alpha-hydroxytaxol by human cytochrome P450 2C8. *Cancer Res* 1994;54:5543–5546.
28. Fischer V, Rodriguez-Gascon A, Heitz F, Tynes R, Hauck C, Cohen D. The multidrug resistance modulator valspodar (PSC 833) is metabolized by human cytochrome P450 3A: implications for drug–drug interactions and pharmacological activity of the main metabolite. *Drug Metab Dispos* 1998;26:802–811.
29. Cresteil T, Monsarrat B, Alvinerie P, Treluyer JM, Vieira I, Wright M. Taxol metabolism by human liver microsomes: identification of cytochrome P450 isozymes involved in its biotransformation. *Cancer Res* 1994;54:386–392.
30. Sonnichsen DS, Liu Q, Schuetz EG, Schuetz JD, Pappo A, Relling MV. Variability in human cytochrome P450 paclitaxel metabolism. *J Pharmacol Exp Ther* 1995;275:566–575.
31. Gibbs MA, Thummel KE, Shen DD, Kunze KL. Inhibition of cytochrome P-450 3A (CYP3A) in human intestinal and liver microsomes: comparison of K_i values and impact of CYP3A5 expression. *Drug Metab Dispos* 1999;27:180–187.
32. Takano M, Hasegawa R, Fukuda T, Yumoto R, Nagai J, Murakami T. Interaction with P-glycoprotein and transport of erythromycin, midazolam and ketoconazole in Caco-2 cells. *Eur J Pharmacol* 1998;358: 289–294.
33. Salphati L, Benet LZ. Effects of ketoconazole on digoxin absorption and disposition in rat. *Pharmacology* 1998;56:308–313.
34. Jamis-Dow CA, Pearl ML, Watkins PB, Blake DS, Klecker RW, Collins JM. Predicting drug interactions *in vivo* from experiments *in vitro*. Human studies with paclitaxel and ketoconazole. *Am J Clin Oncol* 1997;20:592–599.
35. Jamis-Dow CA, Klecker RW, Katki AG, Collins JM. Metabolism of taxol by human and rat *in vitro*: a screen for drug interactions and interspecies differences. *Cancer Chemother Pharmacol* 1995;36: 107–114.
36. Fisher GA, Sikic BI. Clinical studies with modulators of multidrug resistance. *Drug Resist Clin Oncol Haematol* 1995;9:363–382.
37. Boesch D, Muller K, Pourtier-Manzanedo A, Loor F. Restoration of daunomycin retention in multidrug-resistant P388 cells by submicromolar concentrations of SDZ PSC 833, a nonimmunosuppressive cyclosporin derivative. *Exp Cell Res* 1991;196:26–32.
38. Twentyman PR, Bleehen NM. Resistance modification by PSC-833, a novel non-immunosuppressive cyclosporin. *Eur J Cancer* 1991;27: 1639–1642.
39. te Boekhorst PA, van Kapel J, Schoester M, Sonneveld P. Reversal of typical multidrug resistance by cyclosporin and its non-immunosuppressive analogue SDZ PSC 833 in Chinese hamster ovary cells expressing the mdr1 phenotype. *Cancer Chemother Pharmacol* 1992;30:238–242.
40. Beck WT, Qian XD. Photoaffinity substrates for P-glycoprotein. *Biochem Pharmacol* 1992;43:89–93.

41. Kroemer HK, Gautier J-C, Beaume P, Henderson C, Wolf CR, Eichelbaum M. Identification of P450 enzymes involved in the metabolism of verapamil in humans. *Naunyn-Schmiedeberg Arch Pharmacol* 1993;348:332–337.

42. Tolcher AW, Cowan KH, Solomon D, et al. Phase I crossover study of paclitaxel with r-verapamil in patients with metastatic breast cancer. *J Clin Oncol* 1996;14:1173–1184.

43. Bruno R, Riva A, Hille D, Lebecq A, Thomas L. Pharmacokinetic and pharmacodynamic properties of docetaxel: results of phase I and phase II trials. *Am J Health Syst Pharm* 1997;54[24 Suppl 2]:S16–S19.

44. Fulton B, Spencer CM. Docetaxel. A review of its pharmacodynamic and pharmacokinetic properties and therapeutic efficacy in the management of metastatic breast cancer. *Drugs* 1996;51:1075–1092.

45. Royer I, Monsarrat B, Sonnier M, Wright M, Cresteil T. Metabolism of docetaxel by human cytochromes P450: interactions with paclitaxel and other neoplastic drugs. *Cancer Res* 1996;56:58–65.

46. Marre F, Sanderink GJ, de Sousa G, Gaillard C, Martinet M, Rahmani R. Hepatic biotransformation of docetaxel (Taxotere) *in vitro*: involvement of the CYP3A subfamily in humans. *Cancer Res* 1996;56:1296–1302.

47. D'Incalci M, Schuller J, Colombo T, Zucchetti M, Riva A. Taxoids in combination with anthracyclines and other agents: pharmacokinetic considerations. *Semin Oncol* 1998;25[6 Suppl 13]:16–20.

48. Meyer FP. Indicative therapeutic and toxic drug concentrations in plasma: a tabulation. *Int J Clin Pharmacol Ther* 1994;32:71–81.

49. Hortobagyi GN. Anthracyclines in the treatment of cancer. An overview. *Drugs* 1997;54[Suppl 4]:1–7.

50. Robert J, Gianni L. Pharmacokinetics and metabolism of anthracyclines. *Cancer Surv* 1993;17:219–252.

51. Holmes FA. Update: the M.D. Anderson Cancer experience with paclitaxel in the management of breast carcinoma. *Semin Oncol* 1995;22[4 Suppl 8]:9–15.

52. Holmes FA, Madden T, Newman RA, et al. Sequence dependent alteration of doxorubicin pharmacokinetics by paclitaxel in a phase I study of paclitaxel and doxorubicin in patients with metastatic breast cancer. *J Clin Oncol* 1996;14:2713–2721.

53. Baker SD. Drug interactions with the taxanes. *Pharmacotherapy* 1997;17[5 Part 2]:126S–132S.

54. Gianni L, Vigano L, Locatelli A, et al. Human pharmacokinetic characterization and *in vitro* study of the interaction between doxorubicin and paclitaxel in patients with breast cancer. *J Clin Oncol* 1997;15:1906–1915.

55. Kerr DJ, Graham J, Cummings J, et al. The effect of verapamil on the pharmacokinetics of adriamycin. *Cancer Chemother Pharmacol* 1986;18:239–242.

56. Zhou XJ, Rahmani R. Preclinical and clinical pharmacology of vinca alkaloids. *Drugs* 1992;44[Suppl 4]:1–16; discussion 66–69.

57. Zhou XJ, Zhou-Pan XR, Gauthier T, Placidi M, Maurel P, Rahmani R. Human liver microsomal cytochrome P450 3A isozymes mediated vindesine biotransformation. *Biochem Pharmacol* 1993;45:853–861.

58. Zhou-Pan XR, Seree E, Zhou XJ, et al. Involvement of human liver P450 3A in vinblastine metabolism: drug interactions. *Cancer Res* 1993;53:5121–5126.

59. Böhme A, Ganser A, Hoelzer D. Aggravation of vincristine-induced neurotoxicity by itraconazole in the treatment of adult ALL. *Ann Hematol* 1995;71:311–312.

60. Crom WR, de Graff SS, Synold T, et al. Pharmacokinetics of vincristine in children and adolescents with acute lymphocytic leukemia. *J Pediatr* 1994;125:642–649.

61. Watanabe T, Iwasaki M, Todaka T, Morikawa H, Ohtawa M. Effect of SDZ PSC 833 ([3'-keto-Bmt1]-[Val2]-cyclosporin) on serum protein binding and distribution to blood cells of doxorubicin, vincristine and etoposide *in vitro*. *Anticancer Drugs* 1997;8:400–404.

62. Chan JD. Pharmacokinetic drug interactions of vinca alkaloids: summary of case reports. *Pharmacotherapy* 1998;18:1304–1307.

63. Gillies J, Hung KA, Fitzsimons E, Soutar R. Severe vincristine toxicity in combination with itraconazole. *Clin Lab Haematol* 1998;20:123–124.

64. Gascon MP, Dayer P. *In vitro* forecasting of drugs which may interfere with the biotransformation of midazolam. *Eur J Clin Pharmacol* 1991;41:573–578.

65. Miyama T, Takanaga H, Matsuo H, et al. P-glycoprotein-mediated transport of itraconazole across the blood-brain barrier. *Antimicrob Agents Chemother* 1998;42:1738–1744.

66. Rebbeor JF, Senior AE. Effects of cardiovascular drugs on ATPase activity of P-glycoprotein in plasma membranes and in purified reconstituted form. *Biochim Biophys Acta* 1998;1369:85–93.

67. Fedeli L, Colozza M, Boschetti E, et al. Pharmacokinetics of vincristine in cancer patients treated with nifedipine. *Cancer* 1989;64:1805–1811.

68. Clark PI, Slevin ML. The clinical pharmacology of etoposide and teniposide. *Clin Pharmacokinet* 1987;12:223–242.

69. Stewart CF. Use of etoposide in patients with organ dysfunction: pharmacokinetic and pharmacodynamic considerations. *Cancer Chemother Pharmacol* 1994;34[Suppl]:S76–S83.

70. McLeod HL, Evans WE. Clinical pharmacokinetics and pharmacodynamics of epipodophyllotoxins. *Cancer Surv* 1993;17:253–268.

71. Böhme M, Büchler M, Müller M, Keppler D. Differential inhibition by cyclosporins of primary active ATP-dependent transporters in the hepatocyte canalicular membrane. *FEBS Lett* 1993;333:193–196.

72. Relling MV, Evans R, Dass C, Desiderio DM, Memec J. Human cytochrome P450 metabolism of teniposide and etoposide. *J Pharmacol Exp Ther* 1992;261:491–496.

73. Relling MV, Memec J, Schuetz EG, Schuetz JD, Gonzalez FJ, Korzekwa KR. O-Demethylation of epipodophyllotoxins is catalyzed by human cytochrome P450 3A4. *Mol Pharmacol* 1993;45:352–358.

74. Kawashiro T, Yamashita K, Zhao XJ, et al. A study on the metabolism of etoposide and possible interactions with antitumor or supporting agents by human liver microsomes. *J Pharmacol Exp Ther* 1998;286:1294–1300.

75. Baker DK, Relling MV, Pui CH, Christensen ML, Evans WE, Rodman JH. Increased teniposide clearance with concomitant anticonvulsant therapy. *J Clin Oncol* 1992;10:311–315.

76. Kronbach T, Fischer V, Meyer UA. Cyclosporin metabolism in human liver: identification of a cytochrome P-450III gene family as the major cyclosporin-metabolizing enzyme explains interactions of cyclosporin with other drugs. *Clin Pharmacol Ther* 1988;43:630–635.

77. Lum BL, Kaubisch S, Yahanda AM, et al. Alteration of etoposide pharmacokinetics and pharmacodynamics by cyclosporin in a phase I trial to modulate multidrug resistance. *J Clin Oncol* 1992;10:1635–1642.

78. Gigante M, Sorio R, Colussi AM, et al. Effect of cyclosporine on teniposide pharmacokinetics and pharmacodynamics in patients with renal cell cancer. *Anticancer Drugs* 1995;6:479–482.

79. Desai PB, Duan JZ, Zhu YW, Kouzi S. Human liver microsomal metabolism of paclitaxel and drug interactions. *Eur J Drug Metab Pharmacokinet* 1998;23:417–424.

80. Wrighton SA, Stevens JC. The human hepatic cytochromes P450 involved in drug metabolism. *Crit Rev Toxicol* 1992;22:1–21.

81. Goldstein JA, de Morais SM. Biochemistry and molecular biology of the human CYP2C subfamily. *Pharmacogenetics* 1994;4:285–299.

82. Pignon T, Lacarelle B, Duffaud F, et al. Pharmacokinetics of high-dose methotrexate in adult osteogenic sarcoma. *Cancer Chemother Pharmacol* 1994;33:420–424.

83. Peters GJ, Schornagel JH, Milano GA. Clinical pharmacokinetics of anti-metabolites. *Cancer Surv* 1993;17:123–156.

84. Hudes GR, LaCreta F, Walczak J, et al. Pharmacokinetic study of trimetrexate in combination with cisplatin. *Cancer Res* 1991;51:3080–3087.

85. Innocenti F, Danesi R, DiPaulo A, et al. Clinical and experimental pharmacokinetic interaction between 6 mercaptopurine and methotrexate. *Cancer Chemother Pharmacol* 1996;37:409–414.

86. Balis FM, Holcenberg JS, Zimm S, et al. The effect of methotrexate on the bioavailability of oral 6 mercaptopurine. *Clin Pharmacol Ther* 1987;41:384–387.

87. Murry DJ. Comparative clinical pharmacology of cisplatin and carboplatin. *Pharmacotherapy* 1997;17[5 Pt 2]:140S–145S.

88. Long DF, Repta AJ. Cisplatin: chemistry, distribution and biotransformation. *Biopharm Drug Dispos* 1981;2:1–16.

89. Duffull SB, Robinson BA. Clinical pharmacokinetics and dose optimisation of carboplatin. *Clin Pharmacokinet* 1997;33:161–183.

90. van der Vijgh WJ. Clinical pharmacokinetics of carboplatin. *Clin Pharmacokinet* 1991;21:242–261.

91. Ribaud P, Gouveia J, Bonnay M, Mathe G. Clinical pharmacology and pharmacokinetics of cis-platinum and analogs. *Cancer Treat Rep* 1981;65[Suppl 3]:97–105.

92. Calvert AH, Boddy A, Bailey NP, et al. Carboplatin in combination with paclitaxel in advanced ovarian cancer: dose determination and pharmacokinetic and pharmacodynamic interactions. *Semin Oncol* 1995;22[5 Suppl 12]:91–98.

93. Kearns CM, Belani CP, Erkmen K, et al. Pharmacokinetics of pacli-taxel and carboplatin in combination. *Semin Oncol* 1995;22[5 Suppl 12]:1–4.

94. Moore MJ. Clinical pharmacokinetics of cyclophosphamide. *Clin Pharmacokinet* 1991;20:194–208.

95. Wagner T. Ifosfamide clinical pharmacokinetics. *Clin Pharmacokinet* 1994;26:439–456.

96. Kaijser GP, Beijnen JH, Bult A, Underberg WJ. Ifosfamide metabolism and pharmacokinetics (review). *Anticancer Res* 1994;14:517–531.

97. Chang TK, Weber GF, Crespi CL, Waxman DJ. Differential activation of cyclophosphamide and ifosfamide by cytochromes P-450 2B and 3A in human liver microsomes. *Cancer Res* 1993;53:5629–5637.

98. Chang TK, Yu L, Goldstein JA, Waxman DJ. Identification of the polymorphically expressed CYP2C19 and the wild-type CYP2C9-ILE359 allele as low-Km catalysts of cyclophosphamide and ifos-famide activation. *Pharmacogenetics* 1997;7:211–221.

99. Ren S, Yang JS, Kalhorn TF, Slattery JT. Oxidation of cyclophos-phamide to 4-hydroxycyclophosphamide and deschloroethylcy-clophosphamide in human liver microsomes. *Cancer Res* 1997;57:4229–4235.

100. Walker D, Flinois JP, Monkman SC, et al. Identification of the major human hepatic cytochrome P450 involved in activation and N-dechloroethylation of ifosfamide. *Biochem Pharmacol* 1994;47:1157–1163.

101. Bohnenstengel F, Hofmann U, Eichelbaum M, Kroemer HK. Charac-terization of the cytochrome P450 involved in side-chain oxidation of cyclophosphamide in humans. *Eur J Clin Pharmacol* 1996;51:297–301.

102. Yu LJ, Drewes P, Gustafsson K, Brain EG, Hecht JE, Waxman DJ. *In vivo* modulation of alternative pathways of P-450–catalyzed cyclophosphamide metabolism: impact on pharmacokinetics and anti-tumor activity. *J Pharmacol Exp Ther* 1999;288:928–937.

103. Murray M, Butler AM, Stupans I. Competitive inhibition of human liver microsomal cytochrome P450 3A-dependent steroid 6 beta-hydroxylation activity by cyclophosphamide and ifosfamide *in vitro*. *J Pharmacol Exp Ther* 1994;270:645–649.

104. Yule SM, Walker D, Cole M, et al. The effect of fluconazole on cyclophosphamide metabolism in children. *Drug Metab Dispos* 1999;27:417–421.

105. Yule SM, Boddy AV, Cole M, et al. Cyclophosphamide pharmacoki-netics in children. *Br J Clin Pharmacol* 1996;41:13–19.

106. Slattery JT, Kalhorn TF, McDonald GB, et al. Conditioning regimen-dependent disposition of cyclophosphamide and hydroxycyclophos-phamide in human marrow transplantation patients. *J Clin Oncol* 1996;14:1484–1494.

107. Chang TK, Yu L, Maurel P, Waxman DJ. Enhanced cyclophosphamide and ifosfamide activation in primary human hepatocyte cultures: response to cytochrome P-450 inducers and autoinduction by oxaza-phosphorines. *Cancer Res* 1997;57:1946–1954.

108. Singer JM, Hartley JM, Brennan C, Nicholson PW, Souhami RL. The pharmacokinetics and metabolism of ifosfamide during bolus and infusional administration: a randomized cross-over study. *Br J Cancer* 1998;77:978–984.

109. Ducharme MP, Bernstein ML, Granvil CP, Gehrcke B, Wainer IW. Phenytoin-induced alteration in the N-dechloroethylation of ifosfamide stereoisomers. *Cancer Chemother Pharmacol* 1997;40:531–533.

110. Kaijser GP, Keizer HJ, Beijnen JH, Bult A, Underberg WJ. Pharmaco-kinetics of ifosfamide, 2- and 3-dechloroethylifosfamide in plasma

and urine of cancer patients treated with a 10-day continuous infusion of ifosfamide. *Anticancer Res* 1996;16:3247–3257.

111. Lennard L. The clinical pharmacology of 6-mercaptopurine. *Eur J Clin Pharmacol* 1992;43:329–339.

112. Kennedy DT, Hayney MS, Lake KD. Azathioprine and allopurinol: the price of an avoidable drug-interaction. *Ann Pharmacother* 1996;30:951–954.

113. Poplack DG, Balis FM, Zimm S. The pharmacology of orally admin-istered chemotherapy. A reappraisal. *Cancer* 1986;58:473–480.

114. Poon GK, Chui YC, McCague R, et al. Analysis of phase I and phase II metabolites of tamoxifen in breast cancer patients. *Drug Metab Dis-pos* 1993;21:1119–1124.

115. Buckley MM, Goa KL. Tamoxifen. A reappraisal of its pharmacody-namic and pharmacokinetic properties, and therapeutic use. *Drugs* 1989;37:451–490.

116. Jordan VC, Collins MM, Rowsby L, Prestwich G. A monohydroxy-lated metabolite of tamoxifen with potent antioestrogenic activity. *J Endocrinol* 1977;75:305–316.

117. Jacolot F, Simon I, Dreano Y, Beaune P, Riche C, Berthou F. Identifi-cation of the cytochrome P450 IIIA family as the enzymes involved in the N-demethylation of tamoxifen in human liver microsomes. *Biochem Pharmacol* 1991;41:1911–1919.

118. Mani C, Gelboin HV, Park SS, Pearce R, Parkinson A, Kupfer D. Metabolism of the antimammary cancer antiestrogenic agent tamox-ifen. I. Cytochrome P-450-catalyzed N-demethylation and 4-hydroxy-lation. *Drug Metab Dispos* 1993;21:645–656.

119. Mani C, Hodgson E, Kupfer D. Metabolism of the antimammary can-cer antiestrogenic agent tamoxifen. II. Flavin-containing monooxyge-nase-mediated N-oxidation. *Drug Metab Dispos* 1993;21:657–661.

120. Crewe HK, Ellis SW, Lennard MS, Tucker GT. Variable contribution of cytochromes P450 2D6, 2C9 and 3A4 to the 4-hydroxylation of tamoxifen by human liver microsomes. *Biochem Pharmacol* 1997;53:171–178.

121. Dehal SS, Kupfer D. CYP2D6 catalyzes tamoxifen 4-hydroxylation in human liver. *Cancer Res* 1997;57:3402–3406.

122. Dehal SS, Kupfer D. Cytochrome P450 3A and 2D6 catalyze *ortho*-hydroxylation of 4-hydroxytamoxifen and 3-hydroxytamoxifen (droloxifene) yielding tamoxifen catechol: involvement of catechols in covalent binding to hepatic proteins. *Drug Metab Dispos* 1999;27:681–688.

123. Rao US, Fine RL, Scarborough GA. Antiestrogens and steroid hor-mones: substrates of the human P-glycoprotein. *Biochem Pharmacol* 1994;48:287–292.

124. Trump DL, Smith DC, Ellis PG, et al. High-dose oral tamoxifen, a potential multidrug-resistance-reversal agent: phase I trial in combi-nation with vinblastine. *J Natl Cancer Inst* 1992;84:1811–1816.

125. Lodwick R, McConkey B, Brown AM. Life threatening interaction between tamoxifen and warfarin. *BMJ (Clin Res Ed)* 1987;295:1141.

126. Tenni P, Lalich DL, Byrne MJ. Life threatening interaction between tamoxifen and warfarin. *BMJ* 1989;298:93.

127. Ritchie LD, Grant SM. Tamoxifen-warfarin interaction: the Aberdeen hospital's drug file. *BMJ* 1989;298:1253.

128. Kivisto KT, Villikka K, Nyman L, Anttila M, Neuvonen PJ. Tamoxifen and toremifene concentrations in plasma are greatly decreased by rifampin. *Clin Pharmacol Ther* 1998;64:648–654.

129. Lien EA, Anker G, Lonning PE, Solheim E, Ueland PM. Decreased serum concentrations of tamoxifen and its metabolites induced by aminoglutethimide. *Cancer Res* 1990;50:5851–5857.

SECTION IV

Drugs as Inhibitors of Metabolic Enzymes

CHAPTER 41

Anticonvulsants

René H. Levy, Gary G. Mather, and Gail D. Anderson

In the process of drug development, initial studies with antiepileptic drugs (AEDs) are generally conducted in patients with refractory seizures in which one drug is added to a regimen of established drugs (add-on trials). In addition to providing information regarding the anticonvulsant potential of the new drug, these studies also evaluate pharmacokinetic interactions between the two (or more) drugs used in the study. Thus, reports of interactions among drugs within this therapeutic class are common. Typically, the effects of AEDs on the metabolism of drugs used for other therapeutic purposes are reported only after the new AED has been introduced during clinical use. Because carbamazepine (CBZ), phenytoin (PHT), and phenobarbitol (PB) are among the most potent enzyme-inducing drugs known, the clinical literature is replete with publications regarding the inductive effects of AEDs. However, some evidence of inhibition by AEDs also exists. Evidence in recently developed drugs is in the form of *in vitro* testing conducted before release of the drug into clinical practice. This information often details the specific isozymes that may be affected. For the older, more established drugs, evidence comes in the form of reports of clinical interactions and the involvement of specific enzymes can only be inferred based on a knowledge of the metabolic fate of the affected drug. In this chapter, the evidence regarding the potential for metabolic inhibition by AEDs is reviewed. When available, both *in vitro* and *in vivo* data are presented and the degree of correlation is assessed.

CARBAMAZEPINE

In Vivo

Although numerous studies report drug interactions caused by metabolic induction resulting from administration of CBZ, few studies have investigated the inhibitory capacity of CBZ and its metabolites. However, some evidence of inhibition by CBZ exists. The effect of CBZ comedication on PHT plasma concentrations was evaluated by making intrapatient comparisons at a constant PHT dose (1). Significant increases in steady-state PHT plasma concentrations were observed in half of the patients after CBZ was added to the treatment regimen compared to PHT monotherapy. In a subset of patients in whom signs of drug toxicity developed, the mean concentration of PHT increased from 12.54 µg/mL to 22.7 µg/mL when CBZ was added. Patients with higher initial PHT concentrations appeared to be at higher risk of PHT toxicity as a result of the addition of CBZ. This evidence suggests that administration of CBZ inhibits the metabolic clearance of PHT *in vivo*. Although the inhibition spectra for CBZ and carbamazepine epoxide (CBZE) have not been characterized, this evidence suggests that administration of CBZ may inhibit the metabolic clearance of PHT *in vivo* and that a likely mechanism for this interaction is inhibition of CYP2C19. Thus, it appears that the effects of CBZ on PHT metabolism are dependent not only on CBZ dose but also on initial PHT dose and plasma concentration. These complex interactions may be explained by a balance of CBZ induction and inhibition, probably mediated through CYP2C19.

FELBAMATE

In Vitro Inhibition Studies

The inhibitory effects of felbamate toward seven P450 isoforms were investigated *in vitro* by incubating probes specific for each isoform in human liver microsomes. The

R.H. Levy: Departments of Pharmaceutics and Neurological Surgery, University of Washington, Box 357610, H272 Health Sciences Building, Seattle, Washington 98195

G.G. Mather: CEDRA Corporation, 8609 Cross Park Drive, Austin, Texas 78754

G.D. Anderson: Department of Pharmacy, University of Washington, Box 357630, H375 Health Sciences Building, Seattle, Washington 98195

formation rate of each specific metabolite was monitored in the presence or absence of felbamate to determine the potential for inhibition by felbamate. No significant inhibition was observed when felbamate was added (up to 1000 μM) to incubations with probes for CYP2A6, CYP2C9, CYP2E1, CYP2D6, or CYP3A4 (2). The formation rate of 6-hydroxy-(R)-warfarin was slightly decreased when felbamate 1000 μM was included. Because this metabolite is formed by both CYP1A2 and CYP2C19, felbamate was incubated with theophylline or (S)-mephenytoin as additional measures of CYP1A2 or CYP2C19 activity, respectively. The formation of 1,3-dimethyluric acid was decreased only 13% when felbamate was added at a concentration of 1500 μM, suggesting little or no inhibition of CYP1A2. However, the formation rate of 4′-OH-(S)-mephenytoin was decreased substantially. The inhibition constant describing felbamate inhibition of CYP2C19 was 225 μM, a concentration within the therapeutic range.

In Vivo

In early add-on studies, increases in PHT plasma concentrations were observed when felbamate was coadministered with PHT, and reductions in PHT dose were required (3,4). In a subsequent study, ten patients stabilized on PHT were closely monitored as felbamate was added incrementally in doses up to 3600 mg/day (5). Phenytoin dose reductions were required in all patients beyond felbamate doses of 1200 mg/day or 1800 mg/day. Felbamate inhibited the hydroxylation of PHT and the ratio of pHPPH AUC$_\tau$ to PHT AUC$_\tau$ was reduced in a dose-dependent manner. These findings are consistent with inhibition of CYP2C19 in that this enzyme catalyzes the formation of p-hydroxyphenytoin (pHPPH) in addition to CYP2C9. Two studies demonstrated 20% to 30% increases in phenobarbital plasma concentrations when it was coadministered with felbamate (6,7). An approximate 55% reduction of phenobarbital hydroxylation in these studies is consistent with a role for CYP2C19 in the formation of this metabolite. A similar interaction has been reported in three patients given felbamate and methsuximide. All patients had increased normethsuximide concentrations after initiation of felbamate and methsuximide dose reductions were required. This interaction may result either from induction of normethsuximide formation or from inhibition of normethsuximide clearance by felbamate.

The effect of felbamate on the disposition kinetics of valproic acid (VPA) has been studied in adult and pediatric patients with epilepsy and mechanistically in healthy volunteers. In a group of adult patients, coadministration of 1200 or 2400 mg/day felbamate increased the mean VPA peak concentrations from 86.1 to 115 and 133 mg/mL, respectively (8). No changes were observed in the extent of VPA protein binding. Delgado (9) observed 15% to 38% increases in VPA plasma concentrations in children when felbamate was added (average dose 18.5 mg/kg/day) even in the face of a concomitant 30% reduction in VPA dose. In a group of 18 healthy volunteers given VPA 400 mg/day for a total of 21 days, felbamate was coadministered 1200 to 3600 mg/day on days 8 to 21 (10). VPA kinetics were measured in the control period (day 7) and in the combination treatment phase (day 21). VPA plasma concentrations were approximately 40% higher and the excretion of 3-oxo-VPA in urine was significantly reduced in the presence of felbamate. The effects were dose dependent and were maximal at a felbamate dose of approximately 2400 mg/day. These findings may be due to inhibition of β-oxidation by felbamate because 3-oxo-VPA is a product of this mitochondrial pathway.

LAMOTRIGINE

In Vivo

Early add-on trials with lamotrigine (LTG) suggested an interaction between LTG and CBZE, resulting in increased CBZE levels and an increased CBZE to CBZ ratio. Warner and colleagues (11) reported an increase of 45% in the mean plasma concentration of CBZE following introduction of LTG in a study of nine patients. Although these data suggest reduction of CBZE clearance, two placebo-controlled studies have failed to verify the existence of this interaction. In a study of 11 patients, CBZ levels were 8.3 and 8.7 μg/mL in the placebo and LTG treatment phases, and CBZE concentrations were 2.1 and 2.0 μg/mL, respectively (12). Similarly, no significant changes in CBZ or CBZE concentrations resulting from coadministration of LTG were reported in a second crossover add-on trial in 22 patients (13).

PHENYTOIN

In Vitro Inhibition Studies

The saturable kinetics of PHT in clinical use are widely known and the effects of other drugs on the metabolism of PHT have been studied extensively. Although the effects of PHT on the metabolism of other drugs are less well known, the effects of PHT specifically on CYP2C9 and CYP2C19 have recently been clarified. Doecke and co-workers (14), in the discovery of the role of CYP2C9 in the metabolism of PHT, determined an inhibition constant (K_i) of 22.6 μM for PHT inhibition of tolbutamide hydroxylation in human liver microsomes. Other studies by the same group demonstrated a K_i of 19.1 μM when the experiment was conducted in expressed CYP2C9 (15). Subsequently, the role of CYP2C19 was elucidated and K_ms for the formation of (R)-pHPPH and (S)-pHPPH were determined in expressed CYP2C9 and CYP2C19 (16). As expected, the K_ms for formation of either product by a single enzyme were equal to the K_m for CYP2C9 formation of (R)- or (S)-pHPPH (approximately 5.5 μM) and the K_m for CYP2C19 formation of these metabolites (approximately 70 μM). Using a model of competitive inhibition, K_m is equal to K_i. Because the therapeutic range of PHT is 20 to 80 μM, these studies suggest that PHT will inhibit CYP2C9 *in vivo* and may have some inhibitory effects on CYP2C19 at the higher concentrations as well.

In Vivo

Two case reports suggest inhibition of CYP2C9 by PHT *in vivo*. In one patient previously stabilized on warfarin therapy, the prothrombin time increased from 21 to 32 seconds when PHT was added, even though the warfarin dose was reduced (17). In a second case report, the interaction between warfarin and PHT resulted in hemorrhage and cardiac arrest. Although warfarin had been used previously for 5 months without adversity, the international normalized ratio for warfarin increased from 2.87 to 10.41 (therapeutic range 2.5–4.0) when PHT was administered concomitantly (18). Based on the fact that the clearance of the active S-enantiomer of warfarin is dependent on CYP2C9 (19) and that therapeutic levels of PHT are higher than its K_m, these interactions can be attributed to inhibition of CYP2C9, although additional inhibition of CYP2C19 cannot be excluded.

TOPIRAMATE

In Vitro Inhibition Studies

Topiramate was incubated with probe substrates for seven major P450 isoforms in order to characterize its spectrum of P450 inhibition. Significant inhibition of CYP2C19 catalyzed formation of 1″ R-OH,1′(R)-bufuralol and 4′-OH-(S)-mephenytoin reached 29% inhibition at 900 μM (20). Topiramate did not inhibit any other of the isoforms tested at similar concentrations.

In Vivo

Consistent with slight inhibition of CYP2C19, 6 of 12 patients given PHT had increased PHT plasma concentrations after the addition of topiramate. Plasma concentrations in the remaining six subjects were unchanged in the cotreatment period (21). The inhibitory effects of topiramate toward PHT are more evident at higher initial concentrations of PHT (i.e., in patients in whom CYP2C19 is likely to play a more prominent role in PHT clearance). In a similar study with CBZ, no significant changes were observed in total or unbound CBZ or CBZE pharmacokintecs during topiramate administration (22).

VALPROATE

Valproate is a broad-spectrum inhibitor that has been reported to decrease the metabolic clearance of drugs metabolized by cytochrome P450, uridine diphosphate (UDP) glycosylstransferases (UGTs), and microsomal epoxide hydrolase (mEH). Valproate undergoes extensive hepatic metabolism to at least 15 different metabolites. However, circulating plasma concentrations of the metabolites are 100- to 1000-fold less than the parent compound (23).

In Vitro Inhibition Studies

The *in vitro* inhibition profile of valproate for cytochrome P450 isozymes was determined in human liver microsomes using model substrates (24). Valproate significantly inhibited CYP2C9 with an average K_i of 1209 μM. At the highest valproate concentration (3000 μM), CYP1A2, CYP2C19, and CYP3A4 were only slightly inhibited (8%–17%). Valproate had little or no effect on CYP2D6 or CYP2E1.

In vitro human liver microsomal studies evaluating the effect of valproate on epoxide hydrolase have yielded conflicting results. Using CBZE and styrene oxide as substrates, Kerr and colleagues (25) determined that valproate inhibited epoxide hydrolase with an average K_i of 550 μM. In contrast, other investigators found only a slight inhibition (16%) at significantly higher valproate concentrations (10 mM) (26) or no inhibition (27).

There are no data demonstrating the *in vitro* inhibitor profile of valproate for UGT substrates in human liver microsomes. In rat liver microsomal preparations, valproate inhibits the glucuronidation of parahydroxyphenobarbital, the major oxidative metabolite of phenobarbital (28), 4-hydroxyandrostenedione, a synthetic steroid (29), and SN-38, the active metabolite of irinotecan (30). Using stable expressed human UDP glucuronosyltransferases, valproate competitively inhibited the glucuronidation of dihydrotestosterone and propofol, substrates for UGT2B15 and UGT1A8, respectively (31). Valproate is a substrate for UGT1A6 (9,32), UGT1A8 (31), and possibly UGT2B7 (33); however, it is not a substrate for UGT2B15 (31).

In Vivo Interactions

A summary of the reported clinical interactions attributed to valproate is given in Table 41-1. Valproate does not alter plasma concentrations of oral contraceptives (34) or cyclosporine (35), which are both CYP3A4 substrates. This suggests that, *in vivo*, the predominant substrates inhibited by valproate are of the CYP2C family. Clinically, CBZE plasma concentrations are elevated with concurrent valproate administration (36,37) and valproate inhibits the epoxide hydrolase catalyzed formation of carbamazepine transhydrodiol by 20% at average total valproate plasma concentrations of 113 μM.

The largest inhibitory effect of valproate is on drugs metabolized by the UGT family of enzymes including both

TABLE 41-1. *Drugs with metabolic clearances decreased by VPA*

Drugs	CYP isozymes	Other pathways	Extent of interaction	References
Amitriptyline	CYP2C19 CYP2D6 CYP3A4		++	48
Carbamazepine	CYP1A2 CYP2C8	UDPGT	+++	25,36,37,49
CBZ-epoxide	CYP3A4	Epoxide hydrolase		
Diazepam	CYP2C19 CYP3A4		++	50,51
Ethosuximide	Not known	Not known	−/+	52–54
Lamotrigine		UDPGT	++++	55
Lorazepam		UDPGT	+++	38
Nimodipine	CYP3A4		++	56
Phenobarbital	CYP2C9 CYP2C19	UDP glucosyltransferase	++++	43,44
Phenytoin	CYP2C9 CYP2C19		++	16
Zidovudine		UDPGT	++++	41

UDPGT, UDP glucuronosyltransferases; VPA, valproic acid.

UDP glucuronyltransferases and UDP glucosyltransferase. Valproate significantly decreases the formation clearance of lorazepam glucuronide (38,39), LTG *N*-glucuronide (40), zidovudine glucuronide (41,42), and phenobarbital *N*-glucoside (43,44). The identity of the UGT isozyme responsible for the conjugation of the aforementioned drugs is known only for LTG, which is metabolized by UGT1A4, an enzyme that predominantly metabolizes primary, tertiary, and quaternary amines substrates (45).

In Vitro Versus *In Vivo* Correlation

The *in vitro* spectrum of valproate on cytochrome P450 substrates underestimates the *in vivo* inhibition spectrum. The K_i describing valproate inhibition of CYP2C9 is in the range of total valproate plasma concentrations found clinically, but is 20-fold higher than unbound plasma concentrations of valproate. However, of the drugs with known clinical interactions with valproate, only phenobarbital and PHT are significantly metabolized by CYP2C9. The results of Kerr and colleagues (25) are consistent with the effect of valproate on the elimination of CBZE found clinically; however, the K_i is significantly higher than the unbound plasma study of valproate *in vivo*. At this time, there is too little information available to determine whether the *in vitro* inhibition of the UGTs estimates the *in vivo* inhibition spectrum of valproate.

ZONISAMIDE

In Vitro Inhibition Studies

The inhibition spectrum for zonisamide has been characterized for the major P450 isoforms (46). These *in vitro* studies demonstrated that zonisamide does not signifi-

cantly inhibit CYP1A2 and CYP2D6 up to concentrations of 1000 μM, a concentration substantially greater than therapeutic levels (up to 200 μM). Incubation of zonisamide with (S)-mephenytoin, a probe for CYP2C19, resulted in inhibition reaching approximately 50% when the zonisamide concentration was 1000 μM. Slightly less inhibition was observed in metabolism catalyzed by CYP2A6, CYP2C9, and CYP2E1 at the same zonisamide concentration. The K_i determined for inhibition of CYP3A4 (the enzyme that catalyzes the reductive metabolism of zonisamide) was 1076 μM. Thus, it appears that zonisamide should not inhibit these seven P450 isozymes if the plasma concentration is the same or nearly the same as the concentration at the enzyme site.

In Vivo

The only suggestion that administration of zonisamide may result in inhibition of P450 metabolism comes from a population pharmacokinetic study in which the K_m for PHT appeared to be increased 16% when coadministered with zonisamide (47). Although this observation was not explained by the authors, such an increase would be consistent with slight inhibition of CYP2C19.

REFERENCES

1. Zielinski JJ, Haidukewych D, Leheta BJ. Carbamazepine-phenytoin interaction: elevation of plasma phenytoin concentrations due to carbamazepine comedication. *Ther Drug Monit* 1985;7(1):51–53.
2. Glue P, Banfield CR, Perhach JL, Mather GG, Racha JK, Levy RH. Pharmacokinetic interactions with felbamate. In vitro-in vivo correlation. *Clin Pharmacokinet* 1997;33(3):214–224.
3. Fuerst RH, Graves NM, Leppik IE, Brundage RC, Holmes GB, Remmel RP. Felbamate increases phenytoin but decreases carbamazepine concentrations. *Epilepsia* 1988;29(4):488–491.
4. Wilensky AJ, Friel PN, Ojemann LM, Kupferberg HJ, Levy RH. Phar-

macokinetics of W-554 (ADD 03055) in epileptic patients. *Epilepsia* 1985;26(6):602–626.

5. Sachdeo R, Wagner M, Sachdeo S, Shumaker RC, Perhach JL, Ward DL. Steady-state pharmacokinetics of phenytoin when coadministered with felbamate (Felbatol). *Epilepsia* 1992;33[Suppl 3]:84.

6. Sachdeo RC, Padela MF. The effect of felbamate on phenobarbital serum concentrations. *Epilepsia* 1994;35[Suppl 8]:94.

7. Kerrick JM, Wolff DL, Risinger MW, Graves NM. Increased phenobarbital plasma concentrations after felbamate initiation. *Epilepsia* 1994;35[Suppl 8]:96.

8. Wagner ML, Graves NM, Leppik IE, Remmel RP, Shumaker RC, Ward DL, Perhach JL. The effect of felbamate on valproic acid disposition. *Clin Pharmacol Ther* 1994;56(5):494–502.

9. Delgado MR. Changes in valproic acid concentrations and dose/level ratios by felbamate coadministration in children. *Ann Neurol* 1994; 36(3):538.

10. Hooper WD, Franklin ME, Glue P, et al. Effect of felbamate on valproic acid disposition in healthy volunteers: inhibition of beta-oxidation. *Epilepsia* 1996;37(1):91–97.

11. Warner T, Patsalos PN, Prevett M, Elyas AA, Duncan JS. Lamotrigine-induced carbamazepine toxicity: an interaction with carbamazepine-10,11-epoxide. *Epilepsy Res* 1992;11(2):147–150.

12. Schapel GJ, Beran RG, Vajda FJ, et al. Double-blind, placebo controlled, crossover study of lamotrigine in treatment resistant partial seizures. *J Neurol Neurosurg Psychiatry* 1993;56(5):448–453.

13. Stolarek I, Blacklaw J, Thompson GG, Brodie MJ. Gamma vinyl GABA (Vigabatrin) and lamotrigine: synergism in refractory epilepsy? *Epilepsia* 1993;34[Suppl 2]:108–109.

14. Doecke CJ, Veronese ME, Pond SM, et al. Relationship between phenytoin and tolbutamide hydroxylations in human liver microsomes. *Br J Clin Pharmacol* 1991;31(2):125–130.

15. Veronese ME, Mackenzie PI, Doecke CJ, McManus ME, Miners JO, Birkett DJ. Tolbutamide and phenytoin hydroxylations by cDNA-expressed human liver cytochrome P4502C9 [published erratum appears in *Biochem Biophys Res Commun* 1991 Nov 14;180(3);1527]. *Biochem Biophys Res Commun* 1991;175(3):1112–1118.

16. Bajpai M, Roskos LK, Shen DD, Levy RH. Roles of cytochrome P4502C9 and cytochrome P4502C19 in the stereoselective metabolism of phenytoin to its major metabolite. *Drug Metab Dispos* 1996;24(12): 1401–1403.

17. Nappi JM. Warfarin and phenytoin interaction [letter]. *Ann Intern Med* 1979;90(5):852.

18. Panegyres PK, Rischbieth RH. Fatal phenytoin warfarin interaction [letter]. *Postgrad Med J* 1991;67(783):98.

19. Rettie AE, Eddy AC, Heimark LD, Gibaldi M, Trager WF. Characteristics of warfarin hydroxylation catalyzed by human liver microsomes. *Drug Metab Dispos* 1989;17(3):265–270.

20. Levy RH, Bishop F, Streeter AJ, et al. Explanation and prediction of drug interactions with topiramate using a CYP450 inhibition spectrum. *Epilepsia* 1995;36[Suppl 4]:47.

21. Gisclon LG, Curtin CR, Kramer LD. The steady-state (SS) pharmacokinetics (PK) of phenytoin (Dilantin) and topiramate (Topamax) in epileptic patients on monotherapy, and during combination therapy. *Epilepsia* 1994;35[Suppl 8]:54.

22. Sachdeo RC, Sachdeo SK, Walker SA, Kramer LD, Nayak RK, Doose DR. Steady-state pharmacokinetics of topiramate and carbamazepine in patients with epilepsy during monotherapy and concomitant therapy. *Epilepsia* 1996;37(8):774–780.

23. Levy RH, Rettenmeier AW, Anderson GD, et al. Effects of polytherapy with phenytoin, carbamazepine, and stiripentol on formation of 4-ene-valproate, a hepatotoxic metabolite of valproic acid. *Clin Pharmacol Ther* 1990;48(3):225–235.

24. Hurst S, Labroo R, Carlson S, Mather G, Levy R. In vitro inhibition profile of valproic acid for cytochrome P450. ISSX Proceedings: 8th North American ISSX Meeting, Hilton Head, SC, 1997:64.

25. Kerr BM, Thummel KE, Wurden CJ, et al. Human liver carbamazepine metabolism. Role of CYP3A4 and CYP2C8 in 10,11-epoxide formation. *Biochem Pharmacol* 1994;47(11):1969–1979.

26. Robbins DK, Wedlund PJ, Elsberg S, Oesch F, Thomas H. Interaction of valproic acid and some analogues with microsomal epoxide hydrolase. *Biochem Pharmacol* 1992;43(4):775–783.

27. Pacifici GM, Rane A. Valpromide but not sodium hydrogen divalproate inhibits epoxide hydrolase in human liver. *Pharmacol Toxicol* 1987; 60(3):237–238.

28. Taburet AM, Aymard P. Valproate glucuronidation by rat liver microsomes. Interaction with parahydroxyphenobarbital. *Biochem Pharmacol* 1983;32(24):3859–3861.

29. Parr IB, Rowlands MG, Houghton J, Jarman M. Inhibition of the formation of 4-hydroxyandrostenedione glucuronide by valproate. *Biochem Pharmacol* 1988;37(23):4581–4583.

30. Gupta E, Wang X, Ramirez J, Ratain MJ. Modulation of glucuronidation of SN-38, the active metabolite of irinotecan, by valproic acid and phenobarbital. *Cancer Chemother Pharmacol* 1997;39(5):440–444.

31. Anderson G, Ethell B, Burchell B. Effect of valproate on glucuronidation of endogenous steroids and model substrates in stably expressed human UDP glucuronosyltransferases (in press).

32. Ebner T, Burchell B. Substrate specificities of two stably expressed human liver UDP-glucuronosyltransferases of the UGT1 gene family. *Drug Metab Dispos* 1993;21(1):50–55.

33. Jin C, Miners JO, Lillywhite KJ, Mackenzie PI. Complementary deoxyribonucleic acid cloning and expression of a human liver uridine diphosphate-glucuronosyltransferase glucuronidating carboxylic acid-containing drugs. *J Pharmacol Exp Ther* 1993;264(1):475–479.

34. Crawford P, Chadwick D, Cleland P, et al. The lack of effect of sodium valproate on the pharmacokinetics of oral contraceptive steroids. *Contraception* 1986;33(1):23–29.

35. Hillebrand G, Castro LA, van Scheidt W, Beukelmann D, Land W, Schmidt D. Valproate for epilepsy in renal transplant recipients receiving cyclosporine [see comments]. *Transplantation* 1987;43(6):915–916.

36. McKee PJ, Blacklaw J, Butler E, Gillham RA, Brodie MJ. Variability and clinical relevance of the interaction between sodium valproate and carbamazepine in epileptic patients. *Epilepsy Res* 1992;11(3):193–198.

37. Bernus I, Dickinson RG, Hooper WD, Eadie MJ. The mechanism of the carbamazepine-valproate interaction in humans. *Br J Clin Pharmacol* 1997;44(1):21–27.

38. Anderson GD, Gidal BE, Kantor ED, Wilensky AJ. Lorazepam-valproate interaction: studies in normal subjects and isolated perfused rat liver. *Epilepsia* 1994;35(1):221–225.

39. Samara EE, Granneman RG, Witt GF, Cavanaugh JH. Effect of valproate on the pharmacokinetics and pharmacodynamics of lorazepam. *J Clin Pharmacol* 1997;37(5):442–450.

40. Yuen AW, Land G, Weatherley BC, Peck AW. Sodium valproate acutely inhibits lamotrigine metabolism. *Br J Clin Pharmacol* 1992;33(5): 511–513.

41. Lertora JJ, Rege AB, Greenspan DL, Akula S, George WJ, Hyslop NE Jr, Agrawal KC. Pharmacokinetic interaction between zidovudine and valproic acid in patients infected with human immunodeficiency virus. *Clin Pharmacol Ther* 1994;56(3):272–278.

42. Akula SK, Rege AB, Dreisbach AW, Dejace PM, Lertora JJ. Valproic acid increases cerebrospinal fluid zidovudine levels in a patient with AIDS. *Am J Med Sci* 1997;313(4):244–246.

43. Bernus I, Dickinson RG, Hooper WD, Eadie MJ. Inhibition of phenobarbitone N-glucosidation by valproate. *Br J Clin Pharmacol* 1994; 38(5):411–416.

44. Patel IH, Levy RH, Cutler RE. Phenobarbital—valporic acid interaction. *Clin Pharmacol Ther* 1980;27(4):515–521.

45. Green MD, Bishop WP, Tephly TR. Expressed human UGT1.4 protein catalyzes the formation of quaternary ammonium-linked glucuronides. *Drug Metab Dispos* 1995;23(3):299–302.

46. Mather GG, Carlson S, Trager WF, Buchanan RA, Levy RH. Prediction of zonisamide interactions based on metabolic isozymes. *Epilepsia* 1997;38[Suppl 8]:108.

47. Odani A, Hashimoto Y, Takayanagi K, et al. Population pharmacokinetics of phenytoin in Japanese patients with epilepsy: analysis with a dose-dependent clearance model. *Biol Pharm Bull* 1996;19(3):444–448.

48. Harvey AT, Preskorn SH. Cytochrome P450 enzymes: interpretation of their interactions with selective serotonin reuptake inhibitors. Part I. *J Clin Psychopharmacol* 1996;16(4):273–285.

49. Kerr BM, Rettie AE, Eddy AC, et al. Inhibition of human liver microsomal epoxide hydrolase by valproate and valpromide: in vitro/in vivo correlation [published erratum appears in *Clin Pharmacol Ther* 1989 Sep;46(3):343]. *Clin Pharmacol Ther* 1989;46(1):82–93.

50. Andersson T, Miners JO, Veronese ME, Birkett DJ. Diazepam metabolism by human liver microsomes is mediated by both S-mephenytoin hydroxylase and CYP3A isoforms. *Br J Clin Pharmacol* 1994;38(2): 131–137.

51. Dhillon S, Richens A. Valproic acid and diazepam interaction in vivo. *Br J Clin Pharmacol* 1982;13(4):553–560.

52. Bauer LA, Harris C, Wilensky AJ, Raisys VA, Levy RH. Ethosuximide kinetics: possible interaction with valproic acid. *Clin Pharmacol Ther* 1982;31(6):741–745.

53. Mattson RH, Cramer JA. Valproic acid and ethosuximide interaction. *Ann Neurol* 1980;7(6):583–584.

54. Pisani F, Narbone MC, Trunfio C, et al. Valproic acid-ethosuximide interaction: a pharmacokinetic study. *Epilepsia* 1984;25(2):229–233.

55. Cohen AF, Land GS, Breimer DD, Yuen WC, Winton C, Peck AW. Lamotrigine, a new anticonvulsant: pharmacokinetics in normal humans. *Clin Pharmacol Ther* 1987;42(5):535–541.

56. Guengerich FP, Brian WR, Iwasaki M, Sari MA, Baarnhielm C, Berntsson P. Oxidation of dihydropyridine calcium channel blockers and analogues by human liver cytochrome P-450 IIIA4. *J Med Chem* 1991; 34(6):1838–4184.

CHAPTER 42

Antidepressants

Mujeeb U. Shad and Sheldon H. Preskorn

INTRODUCTION

The importance of antidepressants as inhibitors of metabolic enzymes is underscored by the fact that the majority of patients taking an antidepressant are taking at least one other prescription drug, and from one third to two thirds are taking three or more drugs in addition to their antidepressant (1,2). As a result of this prevalence of polypharmacy, patients taking antidepressants are at risk for experiencing a drug–drug interaction. Knowledge of the material covered in this chapter can help the prescribing physician understand the potential drug–drug interactions, which can be caused by specific antidepressants when coprescribed with other drugs. This knowledge can aid the prescribing physician in managing pharmacotherapy to maximize the likelihood of an optimal treatment outcome.

The amount of research that has been done to assess the effects of antidepressants on metabolic enzymes ranges from minimal in the case of older antidepressants [e.g., tertiary amine tricyclic antidepressants (TCAs)] to substantial in the case of newer agents (e.g., selective serotonin reuptake inhibitors, SSRIs). Effects on metabolic enzymes have become important distinguishing characteristics among the newer antidepressants, particularly with regard to the various SSRIs. That is because the members of this class were designed to be quite similar in terms of their neuropsychopharmacology, their efficacy, their tolerability, and their safety. The research in this area was in part fueled by the finding that fluoxetine, which is the most widely prescribed antidepressant, inhibits several metabolic enzymes to a potentially clinically significant degree.

Clinical Pharmacology of Antidepressants

Although a full discussion of this topic and the relative efficacy of the various antidepressants are beyond the scope of this chapter, some comments are warranted as a frame of reference for interpreting the studies reviewed here. First, there are eight classes of antidepressants, based on the mechanism(s) of action as follows:

1. Multiple mechanisms of action agents: for example, tertiary amine TCAs;
2. Selective norepinephrine reuptake inhibitors: for example, secondary amine TCAs;
3. Monoamine oxidase (MAO-I; reversible/nonreversible and selective/nonselective);
4. Selective serotonin reuptake inhibitors (SSRIs);
5. Serotonin and norepinephrine reuptake inhibitors (SNRI): for example, venlafaxine;
6. Serotonin-2A (5HT2A) receptor blockers and serotonin reuptake inhibitors: for example, nefazodone;
7. Dopamine and norepinephrine reuptake inhibitors: for example, bupropion; and
8. α-2 Blocker and selective serotonin receptor blockers: for example, mirtazapine.

This classification system will be used as the outline for the review of *in vitro* and *in vivo* studies regarding inhibitory effects of the various antidepressants on metabolic enzymes. As this classification system implies, there are considerable differences in the clinical pharmacology of these eight classes of antidepressants, particularly with regard to their safety, their tolerability, and the types of pharmacodynamic drug–drug interactions they can cause. For example, the tertiary amine TCAs, by virtue of their multiple mechanisms of action, have a narrower therapeutic index, poorer tolerability profile, and more propensity for causing multiple types of pharmacodynamically mediated drug–drug interactions than do many of the other classes of antidepressants.

M. U. Shad and S. H. Preskorn: Department of Psychiatry and Behavioral Sciences, University of Kansas School of Medicine, 1010 N. Kansas, Wichita, Kansas 67214

A controversial topic is whether there is any difference among these classes in terms of their overall antidepressant efficacy. Based on the bulk of clinical trial data, monodrug therapy with any antidepressant from any class will produce a full remission in approximately 50% of outpatients with major depression. However, different patients are responsive to mechanistically different antidepressants, suggesting that there is more than one biochemical form of major depression.

From the standpoint of this discussion, the issue is, which dose of these various antidepressants is most clinically relevant? To answer that question, Table 42-1 presents the data from the fixed-dose clinical trials with the newer antidepressants. In these trials, researcher-administered rating scales such as the Hamilton Depression Rating Scale (HDRS) are typically used to quantitate the initial severity of the patient's depressive syndrome and then changes in that severity as a result of treatment. The reduction in HDRS scores, presented in Table 42-1, is specifically as a result of antidepressant therapy. As can be seen, effective antidepressants generally produce a 2.5- to 4.0-point decrease on the HDRS above and beyond that which is produced by placebo treatment. By using that as a standard, the roughly equivalent dosages of the newer antidepressants are as follows: 20 mg/day for fluoxetine and paroxetine, 400 mg/day for nefazodone, 50 mg/day for sertraline, and 75 mg/day for venlafaxine. From Table 42-1, it is evident that the SSRIs have a flat dose–antidepressant response relation, whereas nefazodone and venlafaxine have ascending dose–response relations. Thus there is no compelling reason to use higher than the minimal effective dosages of the SSRIs. In fact, nefazodone and venlafaxine are the only two antidepressants that have compelling data to support the use of higher doses in patients who did not benefit from their usually effective minimal dose, but higher doses of nefazodone and venlafaxine may well be helpful. These dose–antidepressant response data with the various antidepressants will be important later in this chapter when comparing the relative effects of these different antidepressants on metabolic enzymes. The ideal comparison studies would use dosages of the different antidepressants that are equivalent in terms of their antidepressant efficacy and would involve a dosing strategy that yields plasma concentrations of the different drugs closely approximating those that would occur in clinical practice.

TYPES OF STUDIES DONE ON THE EFFECT OF ANTIDEPRESSANTS ON METABOLIC ENZYMES

The effects of antidepressants have been examined *in vitro* primarily by using human hepatic microsome preparations and *in vivo* in formal pharmacokinetic drug–drug interaction studies primarily in normal volunteers, although some studies have been done in young patients and a few in elderly patients.

The *in vitro* studies permit determination of the potency of a drug to inhibit a specific metabolic enzyme. By using that information, *in vitro* modeling can be done to select which drugs and which effects to examine *in vivo*. That approach increases the efficiency of the *in vivo* studies, which is important because such studies involve some risks for the human subjects and hence are expensive and time-consuming. *In vitro* modeling involves estimating the hepatic concentration of the drug in question that would be expected under clinically relevant dosing conditions, based on the plasma concentration of the drug

TABLE 42-1. *Antidepressant effect[a] as a function of dose in fixed-dose, placebo-controlled studies*

	Daily dose (mg/day)					
Fluoxetine	5	20	40	60	—	—
Study 1 (32)						
ΔChange	—	4.1[b]	3.9[b]	1.5	—	—
Study 2 (32)						
Change	4.2[b]	3.0[b]	4.2[b]	—	—	—
Sertraline (78)	—	50	100	200	—	—
ΔChange	—	2.7[b]	2.8[b]	3.9[c]	—	—
Paroxetine (71)	10	20	30	40	—	—
ΔChange	−1.2	2.4[b]	1.5[b]	1.5[b]	—	—
Venlafaxine (86)	62.5	75	225	375	—	—
ΔChange	1.0	4.5[b]	6.0[b]	5.0[b]	—	—
Nefazodone[e]	200–250	300	400	500	600	—
ΔChange	1.7	2.0	2.7[b]	5.1[d]	0.6[d]	—

[a]Antidepressant effect [Δ Change in Hamilton Depression Rating Scale (HDRS)] = (baseline HDRS − final HDRS) on drug minus (baseline HDRS − final HDRS) on placebo.
[b]$p < 0.05$
[c]$p < 0.001$
[d]$p < 0.01$
[e]From Nefazodone presentation to the Food and Drug Administration Psychopharmacology Committee, Washington, DC, July 1993.

that typically occurs under such dosing conditions times the plasma/hepatic partition coefficient of the drug. The expected degree of metabolic enzyme inhibition that the drug would be expected to produce in clinical use is then predicted based on its *in vitro* inhibitory constant for that enzyme and its estimated hepatic concentration. For example, von Moltke et al. (3) have used such an *in vitro/in vivo* scaling approach to predict the inhibitory effects of SSRIs (fluoxetine, paroxetine, and sertraline) on desipramine (a model substrate for CYP2D6) clearance based on *in vitro* studies and the inhibitory effects of fluoxetine and fluvoxamine on alprazolam clearance (4,5). The predicted percentage inhibition in the clearance of desipramine by fluoxetine, paroxetine, and sertraline and of alprazolam by fluoxetine and fluvoxamine, respectively, correlated well with the observed *in vivo* inhibition (Tables 42-2 and 42-3). Thus *in vitro* modeling can be useful in predicting potential clinically important metabolic drug interactions. This topic is discussed further separately under each SSRI.

Several caveats are warranted when discussing *in vitro* modeling. First, efforts to date have been almost exclusively focused on estimating the degree of inhibition of the metabolic enzyme that we would expect to be produced in the liver. However, the liver is not necessarily the only site of interest. For example, the enzyme in the bowel wall is likely the critical site for interactions involving first pass metabolism, such as the one between terfenadine and CYP3A3/4 inhibitors. In this instance, the issue is what concentration of the inhibitor is achieved in the bowel at the time that the coprescribed drug is being absorbed. That concentration is dependent on a number of variables including the time of the administra-

tion of the two drugs and the rate and extent of the absorption of the inhibitor. That may well explain why *in vitro* modeling done with fluoxetine, paroxetine, and sertraline tended to overestimate their *in vivo* effects on the pharmacokinetics of terfenadine (Table 42-4). Second, the *in vitro* modeling has generally taken into account only the parent drug and perhaps its primary metabolite. Such modeling could underestimate the *in vivo* effect of a drug, which has a secondary metabolite with more potent inhibition of a metabolic enzyme than either the parent drug or its primary metabolite. Third, the *in vitro* approach does not take into account the fact that the drug *in vivo* may also induce the enzyme that it inhibits *in vivo*. For example, sertraline has modestly increased the rate of metabolism of antipyrine, which may reflect a weak inductive effect on CYP3A3/4. Such an offsetting inductive effect might further explain the discrepancy between the *in vitro* modeling, which predicted a mild inhibitory effect of sertraline on CYP3A substrates and the results of three *in vivo* studies, which showed no alteration in the pharmacokinetics of three different CYP3A substrates (i.e., alprazolam, carbamazepine, and terfenadine) when coadministered with sertraline (6,7).

In general, antidepressants competitively inhibit metabolic enzymes, so the magnitude of the inhibition is dependent on the concentration of the antidepressant, which in turn is determined by the dose and duration of drug administration. The *in vivo* studies that have been done with antidepressants can be divided into three types based on the dosing strategy used: single dose, loading dose, and steady-state dosing. The single-dose strategy is obviously the simplest and is prone to underestimate the magnitude of the effect that will occur in clinical practice,

TABLE 42-2. *Decrease in desipramine (a CYP 2D6 substrate) clearance as predicted by in vitro modeling, compared with the actual decrease observed as a result of coadministration of fluoxetine, paroxetine, and sertraline in humans*

	Fluoxetine (20 mg/day)	Paroxetine (20 mg/day)		Sertraline (dose for first and second studies, 50 mg/day and for third and fourth, 150 mg/day)			
		First study	Second study	First study	Second study	Third study	Fourth study
Predicted by model (3)	82%	50%	57%	18%	15%	37%	37%
Observed *in vivo*	79% (3)	80% (9)	81% (77)	17% (3)	29% (9)	43% (26)	35% (25)

TABLE 42-3. *Correlation between predicted and observed in vivo effects or SSRIs on CYP 3A3/4 substrates*

	Fluoxetine (20 mg/day)[a]		Fluvoxamine (100 mg/day)[a]	Fluoxetine (20 mg/day)[c]	Paroxetine (20 mg/day)[c]	Sertraline (200 mg/day)[c]
	First study	Second study				
Predicted by model (4)	26%	29%	43%[b]	45%	15%	60%
Observed *in vivo*	33% (38)	21% (39)	49% (55)	0 (51)	0 (76)	0 (6)

[a]Decrease in alprazolam (a CYP 3A3/4 substrate) clearance as predicted by *in vitro* modeling, compared with the actual decrease observed as a result of coadministration of fluoxetine and fluvoxamine in humans.
[b]From maximum Css
[c]Decrease in terfenadine (a CYP 3A3/4 substrates) clearance as predicted by *in vitro* modeling, compared with the actual decrease observed as a result of coadministration of fluoxetine, paroxetine, and sertraline in humans.

TABLE 42-4. *Decrease in terfenadine (a 3A3/4 substrate) clearance as predicted by in vitro modeling compared with the actual decreases in terfenadine, alprazolam, and carbamazepine (CYP 3A3/4 substrates) clearance observed as result of coadministration with fluoxetine, paroxetine, and sertraline*

Drug	In vitro (9)	In vivo		
		Terfenadine	Alprazolam	Carbamazepine
Fluoxetine (20 mg/day)	45%	0 (51)	26%–33% (39)	27% (40)
Paroxetine (20 mg/day)	15%	0 (76)	NA	0 (75)
Sertraline (dose)[a]	60%	0 (6)	0 (6)	0 (6)

[a]200 mg/day for terfenadine and carbamazepine and 50 mg/day for alprazolam study at steady state.

particularly for antidepressants having long half-lives and/or nonlinear pharmacokinetics such as fluoxetine, which requires 35 to 75 days to achieve steady state at its lowest recommended daily dose and longer at higher dosages. A second strategy uses a loading-dose approach to try to produce a plasma level of the antidepressant that will more closely approximate what would be expected under steady-state dosing conditions in clinical practice. For example, a common loading-dose strategy with fluoxetine to simulate 20 mg/day under steady state is to administer 60 mg/day of fluoxetine for 8 days (Table 42-7). Even this approach will somewhat underestimate the true steady-state condition, particularly for norfluoxetine, which is more potent than the parent drug at inhibiting several CYP enzymes. The best strategy is obviously to dose the drug for a sufficiently long interval to achieve a true steady-state condition, just as would occur under clinically relevant dosing conditions. That requires approximately 1 to 2 weeks of dosing for all commonly used antidepressants, with the exception of fluoxetine.

The *in vivo* studies typically assess the effect of the antidepressant on a metabolic enzyme by examining its effect on the pharmacokinetics of a coprescribed drug, which is principally dependent on a specific metabolic enzyme for its clearance. The bulk of these studies have been done by using drugs that are metabolized by the cytochrome P450 (CYP) enzyme system. Generally the outcome measures in these studies have been limited to changes in the pharmacokinetic parameters of the coprescribed drugs and perhaps the antidepressant as well. A few studies have also assessed whether the changes in the pharmacokinetics of the coprescribed drug resulted in measurable changes in its pharmacodynamics by including such measurements in the study. Without such measurements, one can only infer whether the change in the pharmacokinetics of the coprescribed drug are of sufficient magnitude that they are likely to result in clinically important changes in its pharmacodynamics. Such inferences are based on what effects would be expected to occur at a dose of the coprescribed drug that would be necessary to produce an equivalent accumulation of the drug as resulted from the antidepressant-induced change in its pharmacokinetics.

The importance of such *in vivo* studies extends beyond the relatively simple question of whether the antidepressant affects the pharmacokinetics of the specific drug used in the study. Because those changes reflect the effect of the antidepressant on a metabolic enzyme, the results extend to other drugs that are also metabolized by the same metabolic enzyme. A question has been, how well do changes in one substrate predict changes in another substrate? As reviewed latter in this chapter, accumulating data demonstrate good agreement between the relative effects of several antidepressants on different CYP2D6 substrates including desipramine, dextromethorphan, meta-chloropiperazine (mCPP), and perphenazine.

With this background, the research that has been done with antidepressants as inhibitors of metabolic enzymes will now be reviewed.

Multiple Mechanism of Action Agents: Tertiary Amine Tricyclic Antidepressants

This class of antidepressants comprises amitriptyline, clomipramine, doxepin, imipramine, and trimipramine. The *in vitro* study by Crewe et al. (8) observed that the inhibitory effects of clomipramine and amitriptyline are several-fold less than those of fluoxetine, paroxetine, or quinidine. No formal *in vivo* studies examined the inhibitory effects of tertiary amine TCAs on CYP enzymes. However, these medications show linear pharmacokinetics over their clinically relevant dosing range and are hydroxylated by CYP2D6 and demethylated by CYP1A2, -2C19, and -3A3/4, which means that these drugs may not saturate or inhibit these CYP enzymes at their usual therapeutic levels.

Selective Norepinephrine Reuptake Inhibitors: Secondary Amine Tricyclic Antidepressants

Few formal studies examined the inhibitory effects of secondary amine TCAs on CYP enzyme(s). Similar to tertiary amine TCAs, desipramine, a tertiary amine TCA, has weak *in vitro* inhibitory effects on CYP2D6 (8). This finding is supported by *in vivo* studies in which desipramine produced only modest increases in the plasma level of paroxetine (a substrate and an inhibitor of CYP2D6) (9). Similarly, coadministration of desipramine resulted in a modest increase in the plasma level of nefazodone under relevant steady-state dosing conditions (10).

Monoamine Oxidase Inhibitors (MAOIs)

These antidepressants are inhibitors of the metabolic enzymes, monoamine oxidase A and B. Conceivably they may inhibit other metabolic enzymes such as the CYP enzymes. However, there are no studies on this matter. There are also no reports of the MAOIs causing a change in the clearance of other drugs coadministered with them. However, that may be because of their limited use and the fact that physicians rarely used these agents in combination with other medications out of concern for causing a hypertensive crisis or a serotonin syndrome. Thus knowledge about the potential effects of MAOIs on the pharmacokinetics of other drugs is essentially an unaddressed but intriguing question.

Selective Serotonin Reuptake Inhibitors

Worldwide, five SSRIs are available for the treatment of depression:(a) citalopram, (b) fluoxetine, (c) fluvoxamine, (d) paroxetine, and (e) sertraline.

The inhibitory effects of different SSRIs on CYP enzymes have been extensively studied. For example, the relative effects of these drugs on CYP2D6 have been examined in 19 in vivo studies (9,11–28). The results of these and the other in vitro and in vivo studies are summarized in Tables 42-5, 42-6, and 42-7, and are discussed later in alphabetic order.

Citalopram

Citalopram is a weak inhibitor of CYP2D6 in vitro but has weak or no effects on CYP2C19, -1A2, and -3A3/4

(11,29). Effects on CYP2C9/10 have not been studied. As can be seen in Table 42-5, citalopram has much lower in vitro potency in comparison to other SSRIs in terms of inhibition of CYP1A2, CYP2C19, CYP2D6, and CYP3A3/4 (4,8,29–31). However, the potency of citalopram to inhibit CYP2D6 is relatively more than its potency to inhibit three other CYP enzymes.

Consistent with these in vitro findings, citalopram at 40 mg/day has been shown in vivo to produce a modest 47% increase in the plasma levels of desipramine (a CYP2D6 substrate; Tables 42-6 and 42-7) (11). In another study, Jeppesen et al. (28) studied the effect of a single dose of SSRIs on model substrates for three CYP enzymes: caffeine for CYP1A2, S-mephenytoin for CYP2C19, and sparteine for CYP2D6. However, the use of a single-dose approach significantly limits the interpretation of the results because the effect of the drugs is almost undoubtedly underestimated. Nevertheless, this study did compare the in vivo effects of citalopram with those of three other SSRIs (i.e., fluoxetine, fluvoxamine, and paroxetine) on these three CYP enzymes. This in vivo study confirmed the findings of the Gram et al. (11) study in terms of modest inhibitory effects of citalopram on CYP2D6 and found no effects of citalopram on CYP2C19 and -1A2. As can be seen from Tables 42-5 and 42-6, the in vitro findings are in accordance with the in vivo findings in terms of inhibitory effects of citalopram on CYP enzymes.

Fluoxetine

Fluoxetine has a flat dose–antidepressant response curve, meaning that the optimal response generally

TABLE 42-5. *Inhibitory potency of different SSRIs and their metabolites for specific CYP enzymes [expressed as the K_i (μm)], based on in vitro studies using human hepatic microsomes*

Reference	Substrate	Citalopram/ desmethylcitalopram	Fluvoxamine	Fluoxetine/ Norfluoxetine	Paroxetine/M2	Sertraline/ desmethylsertraline
CYP1A2[a]						
Brosen et al. (30)	Phenacetin	>100/>100	0.2	>100/>100	45/NA	70/NA
Rasmussen et al. (31)	Theophylline	>100/>100	0.2	>100/>100	50/NA	>100
von Moltke et al. (44)	Phenacetin	NA	0.24	4.4/5.9	5.5/NA	8.8/9.5
CYP2C9/10						
Schmider et al. (49)	Phenytoin	NA	6.0	19/17	35/NA	33/66
CYP2C19						
Kobayashi et al. (29)	S-mephenytoin	87.3/55.8	NA	5.2/1.1	7.7/NA	2.0/NA
CYP2D6[b]						
Crewe et al. (8)	Sparteine	5.1	8.2	0.60/0.45	0.15/0.50	0.70/NA
Skjelbo et al. (45)	Imipramine	19/1.3	3.9	0.92/0.33	0.36/NA	NA
von Moltke et al. (46)	Desipramine	NA	16.6	3.0/3.5	2.0/NA	22.7/16.0
Otton et al. (16)	Dextromethorphan	NA	NA	0.15/NA	0.065/NA	1.2/NA
Otton et al. (72)	Dextromethorphan	NA	NA	0.17/0.19	NA	1.5/NA
Belpaire et al. (73)	Metoprolol	44/23.7	13.5	1.3/1.2	1.2	16.5/23.7
CYP3A3/4[c]						
von Moltke et al. (46)	Alprazolam	NA	10.0	83.3/11.1	39.0/NA	23.8/20.4
Rasmussen et al. (31)	Cortisol	>100/>100	40	60/19	>70	90/NA
von Moltke et al. (7)	Terfenadine	NA	17.6	30.0/2.2	15.8/NA	4.7/1.4

K_i, inhibition constant (the smaller the value, the greater the potency on a molar basis); NA, data not available.
K_i, value for comparison: [a]fluvoxamine, 0.18 for ethoxyresorufin; [b]quinidine, 0.03 for sparteine; [c]ketoconazole, 0.04 for alprazolam.

TABLE 42-6. *In vivo change in the plasma levels of different CYP enzyme substrates by different SSRIs*

SSRIs	CYP1A2	CYP2C9/10		CYP2C19		CYP2D6	CYP3A3/4		
	CAF	TBA	PHT	DZ	MPT	DMI	APZ	CBZ	TERF
Citalopram	0[a]	NA	NA	NA	0[b]	47%[c]	NA	NA	NA
Fluoxetine	0[d]	4%[e]	161%[f]	50%[g]	NA	380%[h]–642%[i]	26%[j] 33%[k]	27%[l] 0–63%[m]	0[n]
Fluvoxamine	400%[o]	NA	NA	300%[p]	NA	14%[q]	100%[r]	30–70%[s]	NA
Paroxetine	0[t]	NA	0[u]	10%[v]	0[w]	327%[x]–421%[y]	NA	0[z]	0[aa]
Sertraline	0[bb]	18%[cc]	0[dd]	13%[ee]	NA	54%[ff]–70%[gg] 0–37%[hh]	0[ii]	0[jj]	0[kk]

CYP 1A2: CAF, caffeine; CYP 2C9/10: TBA, tolbutamide; PHT, phenytoin; CYP 2C19: DZ, diazepam; MPT, S-mephenytoin; CYP 2D6: DMI, desipramine; CYP 3A3/4: APZ, alprazolam; CBZ, carbamazepine; TERF, terfenadine; NA, data not available.

[a]Single-dose strategy up to 80 mg (28).
[b]Single-dose strategy up to 80 mg (28).
[c]40 mg × 10 days (11).
[d]Single-dose strategy up to 80 mg (28)
[e]30 mg/day × 8 days, an inadequate loading-dose strategy (50).
[f]Multiple case reports with dosages generally 20 mg/day (33–36).
[g]60 mg/day × 8 days (37).
[h]20 mg/day × 3 weeks (15).
[i]60 mg/day × 8 days (14).
[j]40 mg/day × 7 days (39).
[k]60 mg/day × 4 days (38).
[l]20 mg/day × 7 days (40).
[m]Multiple case reports with dose generally approximating 20 mg/day (41–43).
[n]60 mg/day × 9 days (51).
[o]50 mg/day × 4 days and 100 mg/day × 8 days (53).

[p]112 mg/day × 16 days (52).
[q]100 mg/day at steady state (18).
[r]100 mg/day × 10 days (55).
[s]Multiple case reports with dosages of 100–300 mg/day (54,56).
[t]Single-dose strategy up to 80 mg (28).
[u]Controlled-case series, 30 mg/day × 10–14 days (75,77)
[v]30 mg/day × 14 days (74).
[w]Single-dose strategy up to 80 mg (28).
[x]30 mg/day at steady state (20).
[y]20 mg/day × 9 days (9).
[z]Controlled-case series, 30 mg/day × 10 days (75).
[aa]20 mg/day × 15 days (76).
[bb]94 mg/day at steady state (23).
[cc]200 mg/day × 16 days (80).
[dd]200 mg/day × 16 days (81).
[ee]200 mg/day × 32 days (83).
[ff]150 mg/day × 8 days (25).
[gg]150 mg/day at steady state (26).
[hh]50 mg/day at steady state (9,22).
[ii]50 mg/day at steady state (67).
[jj]200 mg/day at steady state (6,79).
[kk]200 mg/day at steady state (6).

occurs with a dose of 20 mg/day, and further increase in the dose does not increase the average response rate in the patients treated in the clinical trials. Fluoxetine at 20 mg/day results in a 3- to 4-point decrease on HDRS (see Table 42-1) (32).

Fluoxetine, at 20 mg/day, inhibits CYP2D6 (12–17) and -2C9/10 (33–36) to a substantial degree, CYP2C19 moderately (29,37), and CYP3A3/4 mildly (31,38–43), but has no effects on CYP1A2 (28,30,31,44). The *in vitro* studies are summarized in Table 42-5. As can be seen, norfluoxetine, the primary metabolite of fluoxetine, is more potent than the parent drug in terms of the *in vitro* inhibition of several CYP enzymes: CYP2C19, -2D6, and -3A3/4 (8,29,31,45,46). Those facts are clinically relevant because the plasma concentrations of norfluoxetine exceed those of the parent drug under steady-state conditions, and its effect persists longer because of its extended half-life of 7 to 15 days (47,48). There is not a significant difference between *in vitro* inhibitory effects of fluoxetine and norfluoxetine on CYP2C9/10 (see Table 42-5) (49). Norfluoxetine, of all the SSRIs, is second only to paroxetine in terms of its *in vitro* potency for inhibiting CYP2D6 and is equipotent to fluvoxamine and more potent than the other SSRIs in terms of CYP3A3/4 inhi-

bition. Nevertheless, norfluoxetine and fluvoxamine are both several orders of magnitude less potent than ketoconazole as CYP3A3/4 inhibitors.

Consistent with the *in vitro* findings, fluoxetine, under dosing conditions that approximate steady-state conditions at 20 mg/day, has been shown in two *in vivo* studies to increase substantially the plasma levels of desipramine (a substrate for CYP2D6) by 380% to 640% (see Tables 42-6 and 42-7) (14,15). In another *in vivo* study, coadministration of fluoxetine with trazodone resulted in an average increase of 820% in the plasma level of mCPP (a substrate and a metabolite of trazodone), based on all the data. If the highest two increases are excluded, the average increase was 270% (17). Similarly, in two different *in vivo* studies, a 1,711% to 3,484% increase in dextromethorphan/dextrorphan (DM/DO) ratio was observed, when fluoxetine was coadministered with dextromethorphan (a model substrate for CYP2D6; see Table 42-7) (12,13). The results of these *in vivo* studies somewhat underestimated the full effect that would occur under steady-state conditions at 20 mg/day, given the loading-dosing strategy that was used. That is particularly true with regard to plasma levels of norfluoxetine, which takes, on average, 55 days of continuous dosing to reach

TABLE 42-7. *Sumary of in vivo effects of different SSRIs on substrates for CYP 2D6*

SSRI	Author	No	SSRI dose (mg/day)	Duration (days)	Substrate	Substrate dosing	Results AUC2–AUC1/AUC2	DM/DO	EMs to PMS
Citalopram	Gram (11)	8	40	10	DMI	Single dose	↑47%		
Fluoxetine	Lam (12)	8	60[a]	8	DM	Single dose		↑3,484%	62.5%
	Amchin (13)	12	20	28	DM	Single dose		↑1,711%	
	Bergstrom (14)	6	60[a]	8	DMI	Single dose	↑640%		
		6	60[a]	8	IMI	Single dose	IMI ↑235% DMI ↑430% Total ↑327%		
	Preskorn (15)	9	20	21	DMI	21 days	↑380%		
	Otton (16)	19	40	21	DM	Single dose			95%
	Maes (17)	11	20	28	mCPP	7 days	↑%820(↑270%)[b]		
Fluvoxamine	Lam (12)	8	100	8	DM	Single dose		↑6%	0
	Spina (18)	16	100	10	IMI	Single dose	↑263%		
		6	100	10	DMI	Single dose	↑14%		
Paroxetine	Alderman (9)	17	20	9	DMI	9 days	↑421%		
	Brosen (19)	9	20	8	DMI	Single dose	↑364%		78%
	Albers (20)	10	30	4	IMI	Single dose	↑IMI 74% ↑DMI 327% Total ↑223%		
	Lam (12)	8	20	8	DM	Single dose		↑3,943%	50%
Sertraline	Ozdemir (21)	8	20	10	PRZ	Single dose	↑595%		
	Preskorn (15)	9	50	21	DMI	21 days	↑23%		
	Jann (22)	4	50	7	DMI	7 days	↑0		
	Alderman (9)	17	50	9	DMI	9 days	↑37%		
	Ozdemir(23)	19	Mean, 94	?	DM	Single dose	↑0		0
	Sproule (24)	6	Mean, 108	21	DM	Single dose	↑5%	↑22%	0
	Lam (12)	7	100	8	DM	Single dose		↑28%	0
	Kurtz (25)	6	150	8	IMI	Single dose	↑68%		
		6	150	8	DMI	Single dose	↑54%		
	Zussman (26)	13	150	29	DMI	Single dose	↑70%		
	Solai(27)	7	100–150	≥5	NTP	Chronic dosing	↑70%		

AUC, area under the curve; DMI, desipramine; IMI, imipramine; DM, dextromethorphan; DO, dextrorphan; mCPP, *meta*-chlorophenypiperazine (a metabolite of trazodone); PRZ, perphenazine; NTP, nortriptyline.
[a]60 mg/day for 8 days is used to simulate a dose of 20 mg/day under steady state.
[b]820% is based on all the data. If the highest two increases are excluded, the average was 270%.

steady-state concentrations. Fluoxetine, at a dose that produced the plasma levels approximating those achieved at 20 mg/day, increased the plasma level of diazepam (which at the low doses used in this study is a CYP2C19 substrate) by 50% (37) and plasma levels of alprazolam and carbamazepine (both substrates for CYP3A3/4), by 33% and 0 to 63%, respectively (38,41–43). Fluoxetine increased the plasma concentration of phenytoin (a substrate for CYP2C9/10) *in vivo* by 161% (33–36). However, in another *in vivo* study, coadministration of fluoxetine at a dose of 30 mg/day for 8 days, which is an inadequate loading-dose strategy, resulted in a 4% increase in the plasma levels of tolbutamide (a CYP2C9/10 substrate) (50). A single dose of fluoxetine, up to 80 mg, did not have any *in vivo* inhibitory effects on CYP1A2 (28). Although the single-dose strategy would underestimate the effect of this drug, this finding is consistent with relatively weak *in vitro* potency of fluoxetine and norfluoxetine in terms of the inhibition of this enzyme. Unlike *in vitro* studies, in an *in vivo* study, a daily dose of 60 mg for 9 days of fluoxetine resulted in no increase in the plasma levels of coadministered terfena-

dine (a substrate for CYP3A3/4) (51). Based on an *in vitro/in vivo* scaling model proposed by von Moltke et al. (46), there is a great degree of *in vitro* and *in vivo* correlation in terms of percentage decrease in desipramine clearance by fluoxetine. As can be seen from Table 42-2, the observed and predicted percentage of decrease in desipramine clearance by fluoxetine was almost the same (i.e., 79% and 82%, respectively). Similarly, the observed versus predicted percentage decrease in the clearance of alprazolam by fluoxetine was 33% versus 26%, according to one study, and 21% versus 29%, according to another study, respectively (4).

Fluvoxamine

Although fluvoxamine has not been approved for the treatment of major depression in United States, it is an SSRI and therefore would be expected to have antidepressant efficacy. It is approved for the treatment of obsessive–compulsive disorder in the United States.

The *in vitro* studies are summarized under Table 42-5. As can be seen, fluvoxamine is the most potent *in vitro* inhibitor of CYP1A2, -2C9/10 and -3A3/4 in comparison to all of the other SSRIs. The results of *in vitro* studies in terms of inhibitory effects of fluvoxamine on CYP1A2 and -2C19 are consistent with *in vivo* findings. However, the potential inhibitory effects of fluvoxamine on CYP2C9/10 have not been formally tested *in vivo.*

Based on *in vivo* studies, fluvoxamine, at a dose of 100 mg/day and under steady-state conditions, inhibits CYP1A2 and -2C19 to a substantial degree (28,30,31,44, 52), CYP3A3/4 moderately (4), and has essentially no effects on CYP2D6 (8,18,45).

Fluvoxamine has been shown, *in vivo,* to increase the plasma level of caffeine (a substrate for CYP1A2) by 400% to 500% (53), diazepam (which at low levels is a substrate for CYP2C19) by 300% (52), and alprazolam and carbamazepine (substrates for CYP3A3/4) by 100% and 30% to 70%, respectively (54–56).

An *in vivo* study examined the inhibitory effects of fluvoxamine on racemic warfarin. Whereas (S)-warfarin is the active enantiomer, in terms of anticoagulant effect, and a substrate for CYP2C9/10 (57–59), (R)-warfarin is the inactive form and a substrate for CYP1A2. However, high levels of (R)-warfarin can competitively inhibit CYP 2C9/10 and thus increase plasma levels of (S)-warfarin, resulting in increased anticoagulation. Consistent with these facts, addition of fluvoxamine, for 14 days, to a stable regimen of racemic warfarin produced a 65% increase in the plasma levels of racemic warfarin and a resultant increase in prothrombin time (60). Given the complex interaction between R and S enantiomers of warfarin, results of this study do not rule out that fluvoxamine may have also increased the plasma levels of (S)-warfarin through a direct inhibitory effect on CYP2C9/10. Nevertheless, the known inhibitory effects of fluvoxamine on CYP1A2 and the subsequent inhibition of CYP2C9/10, resulting from the buildup of (R)-warfarin levels, can solely explain these results (61).

Consistent with these formal studies, a number of case reports indicated that coadministration of fluvoxamine can increase the plasma levels of coadministered drugs that are known substrates for CYP1A2 including clozapine, tertiary amine TCAs, and theophylline (62–70).

The inhibition in the clearance of alprazolam, observed during an *in vivo* study (55), correlated closely with the predicted decrease in the clearance of alprazolam by fluvoxamine by using von Moltke's *in vitro/in vivo* scaling model. The observed and predicted inhibition in the clearance of alprazolam by fluvoxamine was 49% and 43%, respectively (see Table 42-2) (5).

Paroxetine

Paroxetine has a flat dose–antidepressant response curve like all other SSRIs. The minimal effective dose of 20 mg/day produces a 2.4-point decrease in HDRS (see Table 42-1) (71).

Paroxetine is the most potent inhibitor of CYP2D6 (4, 8,16,45,72,73) of all antidepressants but is weak in terms of the inhibition of CYP1A2, CYP2C9/10, CYP2C19, and CYP3A3/4 (29–31,44,49,74,75). Based on *in vitro* studies, paroxetine is 2 to 4 times more potent than fluoxetine and an order of magnitude or more potent than citalopram, fluvoxamine, and sertraline in terms of CYP2D6 inhibition (see Table 42-5). In addition, the M2 metabolite of paroxetine, which does not inhibit serotonin uptake and therefore probably does not contribute to its antidepressant efficacy, is as potent as norfluoxetine in terms of *in vitro* inhibition of CYP2D6 (8).

Consistent with these *in vitro* findings, paroxetine, 20 mg/day, *in vivo* under near steady-state conditions increases the plasma levels of desipramine (a substrate for CYP2D6) by 327% to 421% (see Tables 42-6 and 42-7) (9,19,20). Consistence with these steady-state studies, Jeppesen et al. (28) showed that paroxetine, at a single dose of 40 mg, converted three of six extensive metabolizers into poor metabolizers of sparteine. Similarly, in another *in vivo* study, Ozdemir et al. (21) found a 595% increase in the plasma levels of perphenazine (a substrate for CYP2D6) when coadministered with paroxetine (see Table 42-7) (21). An *in vivo* study showed no increase in the plasma levels of terfenadine (a CYP3A3/4 substrate) when coadministered with paroxetine, 20 mg/day, under steady-state conditions (76). Consistent with an *in vitro* study (49), two *in vivo* studies have shown that coadministration of paroxetine at a dose of 30 mg/day for 10 to 14 days resulted in no change in the plasma levels of phenytoin (a CYP2C9/10 substrate) (75,77).

Based on von Moltke's *in vitro/in vivo* scaling model, the observed results of two *in vivo* studies have shown a high degree of correlation, with a predicted decrease in desipramine clearance by paroxetine, on the basis of its inhibition constants. As can be seen from Table 42-2, the observed versus the predicted inhibition of desipramine clearance was 80% versus 50% in one study and 81% versus 57% in the second study (3).

Sertraline

Like other SSRIs, sertraline has a flat dose–response curve and a decrease of 2.7 and 2.8 points is observed on HDRS at doses of either 50 or 100 mg/day, respectively (see Table 42-1) (78).

Sertraline, at its usually effective dose of 50 mg/day, has been found to have mild inhibitory effects on CYP2D6 (9,15,22) but no inhibitory effects on CYP1A2, CYP2C9/10, CYP2C19, and CYP3A3/4 (6,29–31,44).

As can be seen from Table 42-5, sertraline in three *in vitro* studies has been shown to be an order of magnitude less potent than fluoxetine and paroxetine in terms of CYP2D6 inhibition. The early study by Crewe et al. (8) is the only *in vitro* study to suggest that the potency of sertraline in terms of CYP2D6 inhibition is close to that of fluoxetine (see Table 42-5). Sertraline *in vitro* has been shown to have weak effects on CYP3A3/4 (46). An *in vitro* study showed that sertraline and its primary metabolite desmethylsertraline were about 2 and 4 times more potent in terms of inhibiting CYP3A3/4 than paroxetine and fluoxetine, respectively, but only half as potent as norfluoxetine and fluvoxamine (see Table 42-5) (46). However, another *in vitro* study with terfenadine (CYP3A3/4 substrate) found desmethylsertraline and sertraline more potent then any other SSRIs (see Table 42-5) (7).

Consistent with *in vitro* studies, sertraline was shown to have mild *in vivo* inhibitory effects on CYP2D6 (see Tables 42-6 and 42-7). Three formal *in vivo* pharmacokinetics studies showed that sertraline at its usually effective antidepressant dose (i.e., 50 mg/day) under steady-state dosing conditions, caused a modest 0 to 37% increase in the plasma levels of desipramine (a substrate for CYP2D6; see Table 42-7) (9,15,22). Sertraline is the only SSRI that has been studied at higher than its usually effective antidepressant dosages (i.e., 50–150 mg/day) in terms of its inhibitory effect on CYP2D6 (see Table 42-7). Because dextromethorphan is a model substrate for CYP2D6, the dextromethorphan/dextrorphan ratio has been used in three different *in vivo* studies to compare the inhibitory effects of sertraline on CYP2D6. In the first study, sertraline, at an average dose of 108 mg/day, caused a 5% prolongation in the clearance of dextromethorphan (a model substrate for CYP2D6) and a 22% increase in the DM/DO ratio (24). In the second study, coadministration of 100 mg/day of sertraline with DM under steady-state dosing conditions resulted in a 28% increase in the DM/DO ratio (12). Similarly, in the third study, Ozdemir et al. (23) found no change in the plasma levels of DM (a model substrate for CYP2D6) when coadministered with an average dose of 94 mg/day of sertraline under steady-state dosing conditions. Solai et al. (27) found an average 70% increase in the plasma level of nortriptyline (a substrate for CYP2D6) in elderly patients with a mean age of 72 years, with concomitantly prescribed sertraline at a daily dose of 100 to 150 mg under steady state (27). In two *in vivo* studies, coadministration of sertraline, at 150 mg/day, caused an average of 70% increase in desipramine levels (26).

One subject in one of the 150 mg/day studies experienced a 200% increase in desipramine plasma levels (25,26). This matter is important because the prescribing physician must be concerned about outliers such as this individual, as well as what happens to the usual patient. Thus it is of interest and importance to try to determine why this individual experienced more than a 3 times greater increase in desipramine plasma levels than

occurred in the average subject in this study. Examining the data revealed that this individual developed sertraline plasma levels 3 times higher than the average subject in this study, meaning that he was a slow metabolizer of sertraline. Thus the average subject in this study would have to take 450 mg/day of sertraline to achieve sertraline plasma levels comparable to those that occurred in this individual. Although the occurrence of this outlier is important as a "worst case scenario," he still developed only half the increase in desipramine plasma levels that occurs in the average subject taking fluoxetine and paroxetine at their lowest recommended dosages.

Contrary to the *in vitro* findings, in three formal *in vivo* pharmacokinetics studies done under steady-state dosing conditions, sertraline did not have detectable inhibitory effects on the metabolism of three different CYP3A substrates (see Table 42-6) (6). In one of these studies, sertraline, 50 mg/day, and steady state did not alter the plasma levels of alprazolam (a model substrate for CYP3A3/4). In two other *in vivo* studies, sertraline, at a dose of 200 mg/day, which is 4 times more than its usually effective antidepressant dose, did not increase the plasma levels of terfenadine and carbamazepine (also substrates for CYP3A3/4; see Table 42-6) (6). Another *in vivo* study showed no change in the plasma levels of carbamazepine coadministered with sertraline under relevant dosing conditions (79).

A formal, *in vivo,* pharmacokinetics study showed no changes in demethylation ratio of imipramine (imipramine level divided by desipramine level) when used concurrently with sertraline, 50 mg/day, under steady-state conditions (22). This pathway is mediated by three CYP enzymes: CYP1A2, -2C19, and -3A3/4. However, at a higher dose of 150 mg, which is 3 times its usual therapeutic dose, sertraline produced an average 68% increase in area under the curve (AUC) of imipramine, consistent with moderate inhibition of ring hydroxylation, which is mediated by CYP2D6 (25). In addition, there have been no case reports of interactions between sertraline and tertiary amine in which sertraline has increased the plasma levels of tertiary amine TCAs, *in vivo*, by inhibiting their biotransformation to secondary amine TCAs. The absence of such case reports is consistent with an absence of effect on CYP1A2, CYP2C19, and CYP3A3/4. In an *in vivo* study, coadministration of sertraline, at an average dose of 94 mg/day and under steady-state conditions, did not result in a change in the plasma levels of caffeine (see Table 42-6) (23).

The result of an *in vitro* study by Schmider et al. (49) is consistent with several pharmacokinetics studies, suggesting that sertraline produces minimal *in vivo* inhibition of CYP2C9/10. For example, at a dose of 200 mg/day, for 16 days, sertraline caused a modest 18% increase in the plasma levels of tolbutamide, which is a substrate for CYP2C9/10 (80). Two other *in vivo* studies were done with CYP2C9/10 substrates: phenytoin and warfarin. Sertraline, at a dose of 200 mg/day administered long enough to ensure steady-state conditions, did not alter the plasma levels of phenytoin, which is a substrate for CYP2C9/10 (81) and caused only a 9% increase in prothrombin AUC in 12 healthy volunteers taking warfarin (82). Because the last three studies were done at a dose of 200 mg/day of sertraline, it can be deduced that sertraline, at its usually effective antidepressant dose of 50 mg/day, should have minimal to no detectable effects in terms of CYP2C9/10 inhibition.

In terms of CYP2C19 inhibition, sertraline *in vivo* at a dose of 200 mg/day, under steady-state dosing conditions, showed a 13% decrease in the clearance of a single low dose of diazepam (a preferential substrate for CYP2C19 at low dosages) (83). Based on this result, sertraline, at its usually effective antidepressant dose of 50 mg/day, would have minimal to no detectable effects in terms of CYP2C19 inhibition.

In summary, to produce sufficient inhibition of CYP2D6 to be potentially clinically significant in the usual patient would require dosages well in excess of the maximal recommended daily dose, 200 mg/day. Because the principal metabolite of sertraline, desmethylsertraline, is as potent as the parent drug in inhibiting CYP enzymes and has a longer half-life (i.e., 62–104 hours), the period of potential drug–drug interaction may be prolonged. Fortunately, the duration of most studies with sertraline involved stable dosing for 14 to 16 days such that steady-state conditions were achieved for desmethylsertraline as well as for the parent drug.

von Moltke et al. (3) used four studies (9,25,26,84) to compare the predicted percentage inhibition of desipramine clearance by sertraline, based on *in vitro* studies with the actual decrease in the clearance observed *in vivo*. As can be seen from Table 42-2, the observed versus the predicted decrease in desipramine clearance during concomitant use of sertraline was 17% versus 18% in the first study, 29% versus 15% in the second study, 35% versus 37% in the third study, and 43% versus 37% in the fourth study. This high degree of *in vitro/in vivo* correlation observed with SSRIs suggests that *in vitro* data can

be used to predict the potential risk of metabolic drug interactions.

Selective Norepinephrine and Serotonin Reuptake Inhibitors: Venlafaxine

There is a convincing evidence that venlafaxine has an ascending dose–response curve with a decrease of 4.5 points on HDRS at an average dose of 75 mg/day and 6.0 at an average dose of 225 mg/day (see Table 42-1) (85).

Venlafaxine, at a dose of 150 mg/day, has modest inhibitory effects on CYP2D6 (72,86–93) and no significant effects on CYP1A2, CYP2C9/10, and CYP3A3/4 (86,94–98). In an *in vitro* study, venlafaxine had little effect on the metabolism of imipramine (a substrate for CYP1A2, -2C19, and -3A3/4 in terms of demethylation and CYP2D6 in terms of ring hydroxylation; Table 42-8) (99). Ball et al. (72) studied the *in vitro* inhibition of CYP2D6 by venlafaxine. In this study the *in vitro* potency of venlafaxine for inhibiting CYP2D6 was assessed in terms of inhibition of the biotransformation of DM to DO, which is mediated by CYP2D6. The apparent enzyme-inhibitor affinity constant (K_i) was 20 for venlafaxine versus 0.15 for fluoxetine, and 0.065 for paroxetine (see Table 42-8) (72). In the same study, *O*-desmethylvenlafaxine (ODV), the active metabolite of venlafaxine, had weak or no inhibitory effect, and *N*-desmethylvenlafaxine, a minor metabolite of venlafaxine, had the same inhibitory effects on CYP2D6 as the parent compound. Thus venlafaxine was more than two orders of magnitude less potent in terms of CYP2D6 inhibition than either paroxetine or fluoxetine and hence would need to achieve two orders of magnitude higher concentration, under clinically relevant dosing conditions, to achieve comparable CYP2D6 inhibition. The fact that such plasma levels are not achieved in routine clinical use predicts that venlafaxine should have a lower potential for affecting the clearance of concomitantly administered drugs, which are metabolized principally by CYP2D6.

In vivo, venlafaxine, under steady-state conditions, caused a modest 10% increase in the plasma level of

TABLE 42-8. *Inhibitory potency of mirtazapine, nefazodone, and venlafaxine, for specific CYP enzymes^a K_i^a (μM) based on in vitro studies using human hepatic microsomes*

Reference	Substrate	Mirtazapine	Nefazodone	Venlafaxine
CYP1A2[b]	Ethoxyresorufin	159 (112)	NA	>1,000 (86)
CYP2C9/10	Tolbutamide	NA	NA	>1,000 (86)
CYP2D6[c]	Dextromethorphan	NA	18–50 (108)	20.0 (72)
	Imipramine	NA	NA	41.0 (99)
	Bufuralol	41.1 (112)	NA	NA
CYP3A3/4[d]	Testosterone	210 (112)	NA	>1,000 (86)
	Triazolam	NA	0.6 (109)	NA

NA, data not available; ^{a}K_i, inhibition constant (the smaller the value, the greater the potency on a molar basis); K_i values for comparison: Expressed as the; [b]fluvoxamine, 0.18 for ethoxyresorufin; [c]quinidine, 0.03 for sparteine; [d]ketoconazole, 0.04 for alprazolam.

imipramine and a 50% increase in the plasma level of desipramine (a model substrate for CYP2D6; data presented by Dr. Preskorn at the Annual Meeting of Association of European Psychiatrists, 1996; Table 42-9). This result is consistent with the fact that imipramine is converted to desipramine by *N*-demethylation mediated by CYP1A2, -2C19, and -3A3/4, whereas desipramine is principally cleared by ring hydroxylation mediated by CYP2D6. The 50% increase in the plasma levels of desipramine is approximately the same degree of increase seen with sertraline at 150 mg/day, but is almost an order of magnitude less than that produced by fluoxetine and paroxetine at 20 mg/day (see Tables 42-7 and 42-9) (9,14, 15,19,20).

In another *in vivo* study, coadministration of venlafaxine, 150 mg/day for 4 weeks, with DM (a model substrate for CYP2D6) resulted in a 2 times increase in DM/DO ratio (13). In the same study, fluoxetine, 20 mg/day for 4 weeks, increased DM/DO ratio by 17 times. Because fluoxetine takes approximately 8 weeks, on average, to reach the steady-state concentration (C_{ss}), the increase in the DM/DO observed with fluoxetine would have been higher if fluoxetine had been used for longer than 4 weeks. A similar *in vivo* study showed a 33% increase in the DM/DO ratio when DM was coadministered with 150 mg/day of venlafaxine under steady-state conditions (100).

Although the precise mechanism remains uncertain, venlafaxine caused a 70% increase in the AUC of coadministered haloperidol (101). Because the metabolism of haloperidol is complex and the principal enzyme(s) involved in its metabolism have not been confirmed, this study does not shed light on which the metabolic enzyme is affected sufficiently by venlafaxine to produce this increase. It is clearly not due to CYP2D6 inhibition by venlafaxine. Nevertheless, the degree of *in vivo* CYP2D6 inhibition caused by venlafaxine in comparison to other antidepressants is higher than initially expected, given its weak

in vitro potency. The reason is most likely due to the higher total and free concentration of venlafaxine and its metabolite, ODV, in comparison to the concentration of other antidepressants at comparable antidepressant dosages.

In another *in vivo* study, a single dose of 10 mg of diazepam (a preferential substrate for CYP2C19 at such dosages) was coadministered with venlafaxine at a dose of 150 mg/day under steady-state conditions. The AUC for diazepam decreased 6%, with a 12% increase in its oral clearance (see Table 42-9) (94). This effect on CYP2C19 would be expected to be of little or no clinical significance for most drugs that are metabolized by these enzymes. Under the same dosing conditions as with diazepam, venlafaxine did not affect the pharmacokinetics (C_{max}, AUC, T_{max}) of a single 0.5-g/kg dose of ethanol (a substrate for CYP2E1) (102).

An *in vivo* study with alprazolam (a substrate for CYP3A3/4) showed that venlafaxine under steady-state and relevant dosing condition caused a 30% decrease in the plasma level of a single 2-mg dose of alprazolam (see Table 42-9) (95). The mechanism of this decrease in the plasma level of alprazolam is not completely understood at this time but would be consistent with a mild inductive effect on CYP3A3/4. A similar study with carbamazepine, another substrate for CYP3A3/4, showed that venlafaxine, 150 mg/day for 6 days, did not significantly alter the plasma level of carbamazepine or its major metabolite, carbamazepine-epoxide (98). These *in vivo* findings are consistent with *in vitro* findings that venlafaxine has a low or no potential to inhibit CYP3A3/4 and may even exert a mild inductive effect (86,95).

Selective Serotonin (5HT2a) Receptor Blockers and Serotonin Reuptake Inhibitors: Nefazodone

There is a preponderance of evidence that nefazodone, like venlafaxine, has an ascending dose–response curve

TABLE 42-9. *In vivo change in the plasma levels of different enzyme substrates by nefazodone and venlafaxine*

	CYP1A2		CYP2C9/10		CYP2C19		CYP2D6	CYP3A3/4		
	CAF	THY	PHT	TBA	DZ	MPT	DMI	TRF	TRZ	APZ
Nefazodone	NA	0[a]	0[a]	NA	NA	NA	↑8%[b]	NA	↑290%[c]	↑98%[c]
Venlafaxine	↓5%[d]	NA	NA	NA	↓6%[e]	NA	50%[f]	↑4%[g]	NA	↓30%[h]

CYP 1A2: CAF, caffeine; THY, theophylline; CYP 2C9/10: PHT, phenytoin; TBA, tolbutamide; CYP 2C19: DZ, diazepam; MPT, *S*-mephenytoin; CYP 2D6: DMI, desipramine; DM/DX, dextromethorphan/Dextrorphan ratio; CYP 3A3/4: APZ, alprazolam; TRZ, triazolam; TRF, terfenadine.

[a]Data on file, Medical Affairs Department, Bristol-Myers Squibb Company, Princeton, NJ.
[b]200 mg/day × 5 days and 300 mg/day × 14 days (104).
[c]400 mg/day × 7 days (105,106).
[d]75 mg/day × 2–4 days and 150 mg/day × 5–8 days (96).
[e]150 mg/day × 10 days (94).
[f]150 mg/day at steady state (Data presented by Dr. Preskorn at the Annual Meeting of Association of European Psychiatrists, 1996).
[g]75 mg/day × 5 days and 150 mg/day × 6–9 days (97).
[h]75 mg/day × 4–6 days and 150 mg/day × 7–12 days (95)

as suggested by only a 2.0-point decrease on HDRS at a dose of 300 mg/day in comparison to a 5.1-point decrease at 500 mg/day (see Table 42-1) (103). Nefazodone reaches plasma concentrations several-fold higher than the levels achieved by most other antidepressants. The peak steady-state levels of nefazodone and its active metabolite at a minimal effective dose of 300 mg/day average 1,450 ng/mL (104) versus 20 to 40 ng/mL for paroxetine and sertraline and versus 200 to 400 ng/mL for fluoxetine and venlafaxine at their minimal effective dosages (10,103). In addition, the plasma levels of nefazodone change substantially over a dosing interval ranging from 5,000 ng/mL at C_{max} to 500 ng/mL at C_{min} (10).

In vivo, nefazodone, at its minimal effective dosage of 300 mg/day, inhibits CYP3A3/4 substantially (105,106), CYP2D6 weakly (104,107), and does not inhibit CYP1A2 and CYP2C9/10 (data on file, Medical Affairs Department, Bristol Myers Squibb Company, Princeton, NJ, U.S.A.).

Nefazodone has been shown *in vitro* to be a potent inhibitor of CYP3A3/4 and a weak inhibitor of CYP2D6 (see Table 42-8) (108,109). In contrast to fluvoxamine, there was no *in vitro* inhibitory effect of nefazodone or its metabolites on CYP1A2 (Package insert for Serzone, Bristol-Myers Squibb, 1995). This was confirmed by an *in vivo* study in which nefazodone did not change the plasma levels of theophylline (a substrate for CYP1A2; see Table 42-9; data on file, Medical Affairs Department, Bristol-Myers Squibb Company). Similarly, no increase in the plasma levels of S-warfarin and phenytoin occurred with coadministered nefazodone, *in vivo*, suggesting that nefazodone does not have inhibitory effects on CYP2C9/10 (see Table 42-9; data on file, Medical Affairs Department, Bristol-Myers Squibb Company).

Consistent with *in vitro* studies, an *in vivo* study showed that nefazodone is more than 40 times less potent in terms of CYP2D6 inhibition than is fluoxetine (104). In this study, there was a modest increase of 8% and 10% in the AUC and C_{max} of desipramine (a model substrate for CYP2D6), respectively, when coadministered with nefazodone at a dose of 300 mg/day at steady state (see Table 42-9). This study also indicates that triazolodione and mCPP, the principal metabolites of nefazodone, do not inhibit CYP2D6.

Another *in vivo* study has shown a modest 35% increase in AUC of haloperidol when coadministered with nefazodone under relevant dosing conditions and steady state (107). As stated earlier, haloperidol has a complex metabolism and undoubtedly involves more than one metabolic enzyme. Thus studies with haloperidol, although clinically important, currently do not yield mechanistic information about metabolic enzymes involved in pharmacokinetic drug–drug interactions.

Multiple *in vivo* studies have confirmed that the potent *in vitro* inhibition of CYP3A3/4 by nefazodone translates to substantial *in vivo* inhibition, even at its minimally

effective dose of 300 mg/day. In two separate *in vivo* studies, coadministered nefazodone was shown to increase the plasma levels of triazolobenzodiazepines: alprazolam and triazolam (substrates for CYP3A3/4) by 98% and 290%, respectively (see Table 42-9) (105,106).

No studies have been published correlating the results from *in vitro* modeling with the results of formal *in vivo* studies with nefazodone. Nevertheless, the *in vitro* data on the inhibitory effects of nefazodone on CYP3A and CYP2D6 (in terms of the rank order and the magnitude of the difference in the inhibition constants for these two enzymes) is consistent with the findings of *in vivo* studies with triazolobenzodiazepines as CYP3A substrates and desipramine as a CYP2D6 substrate (see Tables 42-8 and 42-9).

Dopamine and Norepinephrine Reuptake Inhibitors: Bupropion

There have been no *in vitro* studies and no formal *in vivo* pharmacokinetics studies on the possible effects of bupropion on metabolic enzymes. In a study of the pharmacokinetics of bupropion in geriatric patients, the effect of bupropion on CYP2D6 was assessed in two CYP2D6 extensive metabolizers by using debrisoquine as the model substrate (110). In both patients, administration of bupropion resulted in a modest increase in the metabolic ratio of debrisoquine to its primary metabolite, suggesting that bupropion can inhibit CYP2D6. That conclusion is further supported by a case report documenting a four-fold increase in desipramine plasma levels as a result of bupropion coadministration (111).

α-2 Blockers and Selective Serotonin Receptor Inhibitors: Mirtazapine

Mirtazapine is the latest antidepressant approved by the Food and Drug Administration (FDA) to be used for the treatment of major depression. Based on preclinical *in vitro* studies, mirtazapine is a weak competitive inhibitor of CYP1A2, -2D6, and -3A3/4 (see Table 42-8) (112). In these *in vitro* studies, the inhibitory effects of mirtazapine on CYP1A2, -2D6, -3A3/4 were studied by using human hepatic microsomes with 7-ethoxyresorufin, bufuralol, and testosterone as model substrates for CYP1A2, -2D6, and -3A3/4, respectively. The inhibitory constants (K_i) of mirtazapine were compared with those of fluvoxamine for CYP1A2, fluoxetine for CYP2D6, and ketoconazole for CYP3A3/4. Table 42-8 shows that the inhibitory effects of mirtazapine on these CYP enzymes are one or more orders of magnitude less than fluvoxamine, fluoxetine, and ketoconazole.

In vitro modeling has been done and predicts that mirtazapine should not produce clinically meaningful inhibition of these three CYP enzymes (112). Although formal *in vivo* studies remain to be done, the pharmacokinetics of mirtazapine itself are consistent with this prediction as follows: Mirtazapine is metabolized by CYP1A2, -2D6, and -3A3/4 with each enzyme appearing to contribute approximately equally to its clearance (112). Mirtazapine has linear pharmacokinetics over its clinically relevant dosing range (i.e., 15–80 mg/day) (Package insert, Remeron tablets, Organon, 1997). These results are consistent with the prediction from *in vitro* modeling that mirtazapine should not cause clinically meaningful inhibition of CYP1A2, -2D6, and -3A3/4. Nevertheless, formal *in vivo* studies with model substrates are needed to provide a more definitive test of this hypothesis.

In conclusion, this chapter reviewed the existent knowledge about the eight different classes of antidepressants in terms of metabolic enzymes-mediated drug–drug interactions. This review considered first *in vitro* data and then predictions based on *in vitro* modeling, and finally the results of formal *in vivo* studies. A considerable range of data are available for different antidepressants, ranging from virtually none for many of the older agents as TCAs and MAOIs to an extensive amount for newer agents, particularly SSRIs. This information is important for optimal patient outcome because antidepressants are frequently prescribed to patients on other medications. There is tremendous expansion of knowledge in this area so that this chapter will likely be outdated shortly after publication, even though every effort has been made to be as complete and current as possible.

REFERENCES

1. Preskorn S. Do you feel lucky? *J Pract Psych Behav Health* 1998;4:37–40.
2. Shad MU, Carmichael CA, Preskorn S, Horst WD. Prevalence of polypharmacy in patients on antidepressants and its relation with drug-drug interactions. Am Psychiatric Assoc Annual Meeting New Research Program and Abstracts 1997;93 Abstract.
3. von Moltke LL, Greenblatt DJ, Shader RI. Predictable and modest inhibition of desipramine clearance by sertraline at low and high doses. New Research Program and Abstracts: The Annual Meeting of American Psychiatric Association, May, 1995, Miami, F 1995; Abstract.
4. von Moltke L, Greenblatt D, Cotreau-Bibbo M, Harmatz J, Shader R. Inhibitors of alprazolam metabolism in vitro: effect of serotonin-reuptake-inhibitor antidepressants, ketoconazole and quinidine. *Br J Clin Pharmacol* 1994;38:23–31.
5. von Moltke L, Greenblatt DJ, Court MH, Duan SX, Harmatz JS, Shader RI. Inhibition of alprazolam and desipramine hydroxylation in vitro by paroxetine and fluvoxamine: comparison with other selective serotonin reuptake inhibitor antidepressants. *J Clin Psychopharmacol* 1995;15:125–131.
6. Preskorn S, Alderman J, Greenblatt D, Horst W. Sertraline does not inhibit cytochrome P450 3A-mediated drug metabolism *in vivo. Psychopharmacol Bull* 1997;33:659–665.
7. von Moltke LL, Greenblatt DJ, Duan SX, Harmatz JS, Wright CE, Shader RI. Inhibition of terfenadine metabolism *in vitro* by azole antifungal agents and by selective serotonin reuptake inhibitor antidepressants: relation to pharmacokinetic interactions *in vivo. J Clin Psychopharmacol* 1996;16:104–112.
8. Crewe HK, Lennard MS, Tucker GT, Woods FR, Haddock RE. The effect of paroxetine and other specific serotonin re-uptake inhibitors on cytochrome P450IID6 activity in human liver microsomes. *Br J Clin Pharmacol* 1991;32:658P–659P.
9. Alderman J, Greenblatt DJ, Allison J, Preskorn S, Harrison W, Chung M. Desipramine pharmacokinetics with the selective serotonin reup-

10. take inhibitors (SSRIs), paroxetine or sertraline: poster presented at the American Psychiatric Association. Sesquicentennial Celebration, 1844–1994. Philadelphia: 1994.
10. Barbhaiya RH, Buch AB, Greene DS. A study of the effect of age and gender on the pharmacokinetics of nefazodone after single and multiple doses. *J Clin Psychopharmacol* 1996;16:19–25.
11. Gram LF, Hansen MGJ, Sindrup SH, Brosen K, Poulsen JH, Aaes-Jorgensen T, et al. Citalopram: interaction studies with levomepromazine, imipramine, and lithium. *Ther Drug Monit* 1993;15:18–24.
12. Lam YW, Ereshefsky L, Riesenman C, Simpson J. In vivo comparison of CYP 2D6 inhibition among SSRIs: implications for drug interactions. Abstract presented at the 1996 annual meeting of American Psychiatric Association, New York: 1996:Abstract.
13. Ereshefsky L, Amchin JD, Zarycranski WM, Heath G. Relationship of plasma concentrations of fluoxetine and venlafaxine with effects on CYP 2D6 in vivo. Presented at the 36th annual meeting of the New Clinical Drug Evaluation Unit of the NIMH, May 30th, 1996, Boca Raton, Florida: 1996:Abstract.
14. Bergstrom RF, Peyton AL, Lemberger L. Quantification and mechanism of the fluoxetine and tricyclic antidepressant interaction. *Clin Pharmacol Ther* 1992;51:239–248.
15. Preskorn S, Alderman J, Chung M, Harrison W, Messig M, Harris S. Pharmacokinetics of desipramine coadministered with sertraline or fluoxetine. *J Clin Psychopharmacol* 1994;14:90–8.
16. Otton SV, Wu D, Joffe RT, Cheung SW, Sellers EM. Inhibition by fluoxetine of cytochrome P450 2D6 activity. *Clin Pharmacol Ther* 1993;53:401–409.
17. Maes M, Westenberg H, Vandoolaeghe E, et al. Effects of trazodone and fluoxetine in the treatment of major depression: therapeutic pharmacokinetic and pharmacodynamic interactions through formation of metachlorophenylpiperazine. *J Clin Psychopharmacol* 1997;17:358–364.
18. Spina E, Pollicino AM, Avenoso A, Campo GM, Perucca E, Caputi AP. Effect of fluvoxamine on the pharmacokinetics of imipramine and desipramine in healthy subjects. *Ther Drug Monit* 1993;15:243–246.
19. Brosen K, Hansen JG, Neilsen KK, Sindrup SH, Gram LF. Inhibition by paroxetine of desipramine metabolism in extensive but not in poor metabolizers of sparteine. *Eur J Clin Pharmacol* 1993;44:349–355.
20. Albers LJ, Reist C, Helmeste D, Vu R, Tang SW. Paroxetine shifts imipramine metabolism. *Psychiatry Res* 1996;59:189–196.
21. Ozdemir V, Naranjo CA, Herrmann N, Reed K, Sellers E, Kalow W. Paroxetine potentiates the central nervous system side effects of perphenazine: contribution of cytochrome P4502D6 inhibition in vivo. *Clin Pharmacol Ther* 1997;62:334–47.
22. Jann M, Carson S, Grimsley S, Erikson S, Kumar A, Carter J. Effects of sertraline (SER) upon imipramine (IMI) pharmacodynamics [Abstract]. *Clin Pharmacol Ther* 1995;57:207.
23. Ozdemir V, Naranjo C, Herrmann N, Shulman R, Sellers E, Kalow W. Sertraline effects on CYP1A2 and CYP2D6 isozyme activities in younger adults and the elderly. Abstract presented at the Annual Meeting of the American Society of Clinical Pharmacology and Therapeutics, 1997 1997; 176 Abstract.
24. Sproule B, Otton S, Cheung S, Zhong X, Romach M, Sellers E. CYP2D6 inhibition in patients treated with sertraline. *J Clin Psychopharmacol* 1996;17:102–106.
25. Kurtz D, Bergstrom R, Goldberg M, Cerimale B. Drug interaction between sertraline and desipramine or imipramine [Abstract]. *J Clin Pharmacol* 1994;34:1030.
26. Zussman B, Davie C, Fowles S, et al. Sertraline, like other SSRIs, is a significant inhibitor of desipramine metabolism in vivo. *Br J Clin Pharmacol* 1995;39:550–551.
27. Solai E, Mulsant BH, Pollock BG, Sweet RA, Rosen J, Reynolds CF III. Effect of sertraline on nortriptyline plasma levels in elderly depressed patients. Presented at the 37th annual meeting of the New Clinical Drug Evaluation Unit of the NIMH, May 27–30, 1997, Boca Raton, Florida: 1997:Abstract.
28. Jeppesen U, Gram LF, Vistisen K, Loft S, Poulsen HE, Brosen K. Dose-dependent inhibition of CYP1A2, CYP2C19, and CYP2D6 by citalopram, fluoxetine, fluvoxamine and paroxetine. *Eur J Clin Pharmacol* 1996;51:73–78.
29. Kobayashi K, Yamumoto T, Chiba K, Tani M, Ishizaki T, Kuroiwa Y. The effects of selective serotonin reuptake inhibitors and their metabolites on S-mephenytoin 4′-hydroxylase activity in human liver microsomes. *Br J Clin Pharmacol* 1995;40:481–485.
30. Brosen K, Skjelbo E, Rasmussen BB, Poulsen HE, Loft S. Fluvoxam-

ine is a potent inhibitor of cytochrome P4501A2. *Biochem Pharmacol* 1993;45:1211–1214.

31. Rasmussen B, Maenpaa J, Loft S, Poulsen H, Lykkesfeldt J, Brosen K. Selective serotonin reuptake inhibitors and theophylline metabolism in human liver microsomes: potent inhibition by fluvoxamine. *Br J Clin Pharmacol* 1995;39:151–159.

32. Wernicke J, Dunlop S, Dornseif B, Zerbe R. Fixed dose fluoxetine therapy for depression. *Psychopharmacol Bull* 1987;23:164–168.

33. Darley J. Interaction between phenytoin and fluoxetine. *Seizure* 1994; 3:151–152.

34. Jalil P. Toxic reaction following the combined administration of fluoxetine and phenytoin: two case reports. *J Neurol Neurosurg Psychiatry* 1992;55:412–413.

35. Woods DJ, Coulter DM, Pillans P. Interaction of phenytoin and fluoxetine. *NZ Med J* 1994;107:19–19.

36. Shader RI, Greenblatt DJ, von Moltke LL. Fluoxetine inhibition of phenytoin metabolism [Editorial]. *J Clin Psychopharmacol* 1994;14: 375–376.

37. Lemberger L, Rowe H, Bosomworth JC, Tenbarge JB, Bergstrom RF. The effect of fluoxetine on the pharmacokinetics and psychomotor responses of diazepam. *Clin Pharmacol Ther* 1988;43:412–419.

38. Lasher TA, Fleishaker JC, Steenwyk RC, Antal EJ. Pharmacokinetic pharmacodynamic evaluation of the combined administration of alprazolam and fluoxetine. *Psychopharmacology* 1991;104:323–327.

39. Greenblatt DJ, Preskorn S, Cotreau MM, Horst WD, Harmatz JS. Fluoxetine impairs clearance of alprazolam but not of clonazepam. *Clin Pharmacol Ther* 1992;52:479–486.

40. Grimsley SR, Jann MW, Carter JG, D'Mello AP, D'Souza MJ. Increased carbamazepine plasma concentrations after fluoxetine coadministration. *Clin Pharmacol Ther* 1991;50:10–15.

41. Gernaat HBPE, Van De Woude J, Touw DJ. Fluoxetine and parkinsonism in patients taking carbamazepine. *Am J Psychiatry* 1991;148: 1604–1605.

42. Pearson HJ. Interaction of fluoxetine with carbamazepine. *J Clin Psychiatry* 1990;51:126.

43. Spina E, Avenoso A, Pollicino AM, Caputi AP, Fazio A, Pisani F. Carbamazepine coadministration with fluoxetine or fluvoxamine. *Ther Drug Monit* 1993;15:247–250.

44. von Moltke LL, Greenblatt DJ, Duan SX, Schmider J, Harmatz JS, Shader RI. In vitro biotransformation of phenacetin to acetaminophen: metabolic inhibition by antidepressants. *Am Soc Clin Pharmacol Ther* 1996;59:175–175(abst).

45. Skjelbo E, Brosen K. Inhibitors of imipramine metabolism by human liver microsomes. *Br J Clin Pharmacol* 1992;34:256–261.

46. von Moltke LL, Greenblatt DJ, Court MH, Duan SX, Harmatz JS, Shader RI. Inhibition of alprazolam and desipramine hydroxylation *in vitro* by paroxetine and fluvoxamine: comparison with other selective serotonin reuptake inhibitor antidepressants. *J Clin Psychopharmacol* 1995;15:125–131.

47. Preskorn S. Pharmacokinetics of antidepressants: why and how they are relevant to treatment. *J Clin Psychiatry* 1993;54(suppl 9):14–34.

48. Goodnick P. Pharmacokinetics a second generation of antidepressants: fluoxetine. *Psychopharmacol Bull* 1991;27:503–512.

49. Schmider J, Greenblatt DJ, von Moltke LL, Karsov D, Shader RI. Inhibition of CYP2C9 by selective serotonin reuptake inhibitors in vitro: studies of phenytoin para-hydroxylation. Poster presented at 36th Annual NCDEU meeting at Boca Raton, FL, May 28–31. 1996; Poster No. 122: Abstract.

50. Lemberger L, Bergstrom RF, Wolen RL, Farid NA, Enas GG, Aronoff GR. Fluoxetine: clinical pharmacology and physiologic disposition. *J Clin Psychiatry* 1985;46:14–19.

51. Bergstrom R, Goldberg M, Cerimele B, Hatcher B. Assessment of the potential for a pharmacokinetic interaction between fluoxetine and terfenadine. *Clin Pharmacol Ther* 1997;62:643–651.

52. Perucca E, Gatti G, Cipolla G, et al. Inhibition of diazepam metabolism by fluvoxamine: a pharmacokinetic study in normal volunteers. *Clin Pharmacol Ther* 1994;56:471–476.

53. Jeppesen U, Loft S, Poulsen H, Brosen K. A fluvoxamine-caffeine interaction study. *Pharmacogenetics* 1996;6:213–222.

54. Fritze J, Unsorg B, Lanczik M. Interaction between carbamazepine and fluvoxamine. *Acta Psychiatry Scand* 1991;84:583–584.

55. Fleishaker JC, Hulst LK. A pharmacokinetic and pharmacodynamic evaluation of the combined administration of alprazolam and fluvoxamine. *Eur J Clin Pharmacol* 1994;46:35–39.

56. Bonnet P, Vandel S, Nezelog S, Sechter D, Bizouard P. Carbamazepine, fluvoxamine: is there a pharmacokinetic interaction? *Therapie* 1992;47:165.

57. Rettie AE, Korzekwa KR, Kunze KL, et al. Hydroxylation of warfarin by human cDNA-expressed cytochrome P-450: a role for P-4502C9 in the etiology of (S)-warfarin-drug interactions. *Chem Res Toxicol* 1992; 5:54–59.

58. Lewis R, Trager W, Chan K, et al. Warfarin: stereochemical aspects of its metabolism and the interaction with phenylbutazone. *J Clin Invest* 1974;53:1607–1617.

59. Kunze K, Eddy AC, Gibaldi M, Trager W. Metabolic enantiomeric interactions: the inhibition of human (S)-warfarin-7-hydroxylase by (R)-warfarin. *Chirality* 1991;3:24–29.

60. Benfield P, Ward A. Fluvoxamine: a review of its pharmacodynamic and pharmacokinetic properties, and therapeutic efficacy in depressive illness. *Drugs* 1986;32:313–334.

61. Harvey A, Preskorn S. Cytochrome P450 enzymes: interpretation of their interactions with selective serotonin reuptake inhibitors: part II. *J Clin Psychopharmacol* 1996;16:345–355.

62. Baumann P, Bertschy G. Pharmacodynamic and pharmacokinetic interactions of selective serotonin re-uptake inhibiting antidepressants (SSRIs) with other psychotropic drugs. *Nord J Psychiatry* 1993;47 (suppl 30):13–19.

63. Bertschy G, Vandel S, Allers G, Volmat R. Fluvoxamine-tricyclic antidepressant interaction. *Eur J Clin Pharmacol* 1991;40:119–120.

64. Bertschy G, Vandel S, Francois T, et al. Metabolic interaction between tricyclic antidepressant and fluvoxamine and fluoxetine, a pharmacogenetic approach. *Clin Neuropharmacol* 1992;15(suppl 1, pt A): 78A–79A(abst).

65. Hartter S, Wetzel H, Hammes E, Hiemke C. Inhibition of antidepressant demethylation and hydroxylation by fluvoxamine in depressed patients. *Psychopharmacology* 1993;110:302–308.

66. Sperber AD. Toxic interaction between fluvoxamine and sustained release theophylline in an 11-year-old boy. *Drug Safety* 1991;6:460–462.

67. Jerling M, Lindstrom L, Bondesson U, Bertilsson L. Fluvoxamine inhibition and carbamazepine induction of the metabolism of clozapine: evidence from a therapeutic drug monitoring service. *Ther Drug Monit* 1994;16:368–374.

68. Thomson AH, McGovern EM, Bennie P, Caldwell G, Smith M. Interaction between fluvoxamine and theophylline. *Pharmaceut J* 1992;1: 137.

69. van Harten J. Clinical pharmacokinetics of selective serotonin reuptake inhibitors. *Clin Pharmacokinet* 1993;24:203–220.

70. Markowitz J, Gill H, Lavia M, DeVane C, Brewerton T. Fluvoxamine-clozapine dose dependent interaction. *Can J Psychiatry* 1996;41: 670–671.

71. Dunner DL, Dunbar GC. Optimal dose regimen for paroxetine. *J Clin Psychiatry* 1992;53(suppl 2):21–26.

72. Otton SV, Ball SE, Cheung SW, Inaba T, Sellers EM. Comparative inhibition of the polymorphic enzyme CYP2D6 by venlafaxine (VF) and other 5HT uptake inhibitors. *Clin Pharmacol Ther* 1994;55: 141–141(abst).

73. Belpaire F, Wijnant P, Temmerman A, Bogaert, Rasmussen B, Brosen K. Inhibition of the oxidative metabolism of metoprolol by the selective serotonin reuptake inhibitors in human liver microsomes. Abstract presented at the Annual Meeting of Belgian Society of Fundamentals of Physiology and Pharmacology, 1996; Abstract.

74. Bannister SJ, Houser VP, Hulse JD, Kisicki JC, Rasmussen JGC. Evaluation of the potential for interactions of paroxetine with diazepam, cimetidine, warfarin, and digoxin. *Acta Psychiatry Scand* 1989;80 (suppl 350):102–106.

75. Andersen BB, Mikkelsen M, Vesterager A, et al. No influence of the antidepressant paroxetine on carbamazepine, valproate and phenytoin. *Epilepsy Res* 1991;10:201–204.

76. Martin D, Zussman B, Everitt D, Benincosa L, Etheredge R, Jorkasky D. Paroxetine does not affect the cardiac safety and pharmacokinetics of terfenadine in healthy adult men. *J Clin Psychopharmacol* 1997;17: 451–459.

77. Kaye CM, Haddock RE, Langley PF, et al. A review of the metabolism and pharmacokinetics of paroxetine in man. *Acta Psychiatry Scand* 1989;80(suppl 350):60–75.

78. Preskorn S, Lane R. Sertraline 50 mg daily: the optimal dose in the treatment of depression. *Int J Clin Pharmacol* 1995;10:129–141.

79. Rapeport WG, Williams SA, Muirhead DC, Dewland PM, Tanner T,

Wesnes K. Absence of a sertraline-mediated effect on the pharmacokinetics and pharmacodynamics of carbamazepine. *J Clin Psychiatry* 1996;57(suppl 1):20–23.

80. Tremaine LM, Wilner KD, Preskorn S. A study of the potential effect of sertraline on the pharmacokinetics and protein binding of tolbutamide. *Clin Pharmacokinet* 1997;32:31–36.

81. Rapeport WG, Muirhead DC, Williams SA, Cross M, Wesnes K. Absence of effect of sertraline on the pharmacokinetics and pharmacodynamics of phenytoin. *J Clin Psychiatry* 1996;57(suppl 1):24–28.

82. Apseloff G, Wilner KD, Gerber N, Tremaine LM. Effect of sertraline on protein binding of warfarin. *Clin Pharmacokinet* 1997;32:37–42.

83. Gardner MJ, Baris BA, Wilner KD, Preskorn S. Absence of a clinically meaningful effect of sertraline on the pharmacokinetics and protein binding of diazepam in healthy volunteers. *Clin Pharmacokinet* 1997;32:43–49.

84. von Moltke LL, Greenblatt DJ, Cotreau-Bibbo MM, Duan SX, Harmatz JS, Shader RI. Inhibition of desipramine hydroxylation *in vitro* by serotonin-reuptake-inhibitor antidepressants, and by quinidine and ketoconazole: a model system to predict drug interactions *in vivo*. *J Pharmacol Exp Ther* 1994;268:1278–1283.

85. Preskorn S. Antidepressant drug selection: criteria and options. *J Clin Psychiatry* 1994;55(suppl A):6–24.

86. Ball SE, Ahern D, Scatina J, Kao J. Venlafaxine: in vitro inhibition of CYP 2D6 dependent imipramine and desipramine metabolism; comparative studies with selected SSRIs and effects on human hepatic CYP 3A4, CYP 2C9 and CYP 1A2. *Br J Pharmacol* 1997;43:619–626.

87. Ereshefsky L. Drug-drug interactions involving antidepressants: focus on venlafaxine. *J Clin Psychopharmacol* 1996;16(suppl 2):37–50.

88. Amchin J, Zarycranski W, Taylor KP, Albano D, Klockowski PM. Effect of venlafaxine on the pharmacokinetics of risperidone. *J Clin Pharmacol* 1999;39:297–309.

89. Amchin J, Zarycranski W. Effect of venlafaxine on the pharmacokinetics of alprazolam. *Psychopharmacol Bull* 1996;32:410.

90. Alfaro C, Ereshefsky L, Lam YW. Relationship of venlafaxine, fluoxetine, sertraline, and paroxetine plasma concentration with CYP 2D6 inhibition. Presented at the 37th annual meeting of the New Clinical Drug Evaluation Unit of the NIMH, May 27–30, 1997, Boca Raton, Florida 1997; Abstract.

91. Amchin JD, Albano D, Troy S. Venlafaxine's low drug interaction potential based on cytochrome P450: in vivo evidence confirming in vitro data of low CYP 2D6 and no CYP 3A4 inhibition. Presented at the annual meeting of Association of Medicine and Psychiatry, November 13, 1996, San Antonio, TX 1996; Abstract.

92. Amchin JD, Ereshefsky L, Zarycranski WM. Effect of venlafaxine versus fluoxetine on the metabolism of dextromethorphan, a CYP2D6 marker. American Psychiatric Association 1996 Annual Meeting New Research Program and Abstracts 1996; Abstract.

93. Otton SV, Ball SE, Cheung SW, Inaba T, Rudolph RL, Sellers EM. Venlafaxine oxidation in vitro is catalyzed by CYP2D6. *Br J Clin Pharmacol* 1996;41:149–156.

94. Troy S, Lucki I, Peirgies A, Parker V, Klockowski P, Chiang S. Pharmacokinetic and pharmacodynamic evaluation of the potential drug interaction between venlafaxine and diazepam. *J Clin Pharmacol* 1995;35:410–419.

95. Amchin JD, Zarycranski WM. Effect of venlafaxine on the pharmacokinetics of alprazolam. Presented at the 36th annual meeting of the New Clinical Drug Evaluation Unit of the NIMH, May 30th, 1996, Boca Raton, Florida; Abstract.

96. Amchin JD, Zarycranski WM, Taylor K. Evidence that venlafaxine does not inhibit CYP 1A2 as measured in vivo by the metabolism of caffeine. Abstract presented at the Annual Meeting of the American Society of Clinical Pharmacology and Therapeutics, 1997; Abstract.

97. Amchin JD, Zarycranski WM, Taylor K. Venlafaxine's lack of CYP 3A3/4 inhibition is further confirmed by an in vivo study with terfenadine. Abstract presented at the Annual Meeting of American College of Neuropsychopharmacology, 1996; Abstract.

98. Wiklander B, Danjou P, Tamin SK, Toon S. Evaluation of of the potential pharmacokinetic interaction of venlafaxine and carbamazepine. *Eur Neuropsychopharmacol* 1995;5:310–311(abst).

99. Ball SE, Ahern D, Kao J, Scatina J. Venlafaxine (VF): effects on CYP2D6 dependent imipramine (IMP) and desipramine (DMP) 2-hydroxylation; comparative studies with fluoxetine (FLU) and effects on CYP1A2, CYP3A4, and CYP2C9. *Clin Pharmacol Ther* 1996;59:170(abst).

100. Lam YW, Ereshefsky L, Riesenman C, Simpson RJ. In vivo comparison of CYP 2D6 inhibition among SSRIs: implications for drug interactions. Abstract presented at the 1996 annual meeting of American Psychiatric Association, May 7, 1996, New York 1996; Abstract.

101. Preskorn S, Nemeroff C. Debate: are CYP450 drug interactions really important, or is it all just marketing hype? *Prog Notes* 1997;8:57–63.

102. Effexor (venlafaxine hydrochloride) tablets. 1997; 51 ed. *Physician's desk reference* 51st ed. Montvale NJ: Prescribing information; Medical Economics Data, 1997:2664–2668.

103. Janicak P, Davis J, Preskorn S, Ayd F Jr. Treatment with antidepressants. In: Janicak P, ed. *Principles and practice pf psychopharmacotherapy.* 2nd ed. Baltimore: Williams & Wilkins, 1997:243–356.

104. Preskorn S, Magnus R, Horst W, Rosenblum J, Jody D, Ieni J. Pharmacokinetic and pharmacodynamic effects of co-administration of nefazodone and desipramine to normal volunteers. New Research Program and Abstracts (NR195): The Annual Meeting of American Psychiatric Association, May 4–9, 1996 New York, NY 1996; 120–121. Abstract.

105. Greene DS, Salazar DE, Dockens RC, Kroboth P, Barbhaiya RH. Coadministration of nefazodone and benzodiazepines. III: a pharmacokinetic interaction study with alprazolam. *J Clin Psychopharmacol* 1995;15:399–408.

106. Barbhaiya RH, Shukla U, Kroboth P, Greene DS. Coadministration of nefazodone and benzodiazepines. II: a pharmacokinetic interaction study with triazolam. *J Clin Psychopharmacol* 1995;15:320–326 (abst).

107. Barbhaiya RH, Shukla U, Greene DS, Breuel H, Midha K. Investigation of pharmacokinetic and pharmacodynamic interactions after coadministration of nefazodone and haloperidol. *J Clin Psychopharmacol* 1995;16:26–34(abst).

108. Schmider J, Greenblatt DJ, von Moltke LL, Harmatz JS, Shader RI. Inhibition of cytochrome P450 by nefazodone in vitro studies of dextromethorphan O- and N-demethylation. *Br J Clin Pharmacol* 1996;41:339–343.

109. von Moltke L, Greenblatt DJ, Harmatz JS, et al. Triazolam biotransformation by human liver microsomes in vitro: effects of metabolic inhibitors and clinical confirmation of a predicted interaction with ketoconazole. *J Pharmacol Exp Ther* 1996;276:370–379.

110. Pollock BG, Sweet RA, Kirshner M, Reynolds CF III. Bupropion plasma levels and CYP 2D6 phenotype. *Ther Drug Monit* 1996;18:581–585.

111. Shad MU, Preskorn S. A possible bupropion and imipramine interaction [Letter]. *J Clin Psychopharmacol* 1997;17:118–119.

112. Dahl ML, Voortman G., Alm C, et al. In vitro and in vivo studies on the disposition of mirtazapine in humans. *Clin Drug Invest* 1997;1:37–46(abst).

CHAPTER 43

Neuroleptics and Antipsychotics

Michael Murray

CHEMICAL CLASSES OF NEUROLEPTIC DRUGS

Neuroleptic drugs can be divided into several chemical classes. Well-established neuroleptics include the phenothiazines, thioxanthenes, butyrophenones, and diphenylbutylpiperidines. Benzamides have now been in use for almost two decades, but the indoles, dibenzodiazepines, and related heterocyclic agents are newer additions to the list of available antipsychotic drugs. Phenothiazines and butyrophenones remain the best known and most widely used neuroleptics, but side effects with phenothiazines and thioxanthenes are common and include sedation, antimuscarinic effects and α-adrenoreceptor antagonism. Extrapyramidal effects, such as ataxia and dystonia, are also relatively common. Butyrophenones and diphenylbutylpiperidines exhibit a high incidence of extrapyramidal problems, but other side effects are less common than with the phenothiazines. Some of the newer agents are often better tolerated, especially the benzamides and indoles, and this is a major reason for their increasing use (1). Dibenzodiazepines, such as clozapine and olanzapine, reportedly exhibit a moderately high incidence of side effects but have proven effective in cases in which the established neuroleptics have failed. This chapter outlines the pharmacokinetic interactions elicited by neuroleptics, but to interpret the significance of such interactions, it is necessary to appreciate the special features of antipsychotic therapy.

PHARMACOKINETIC PROPERTIES OF NEUROLEPTIC DRUGS

Individuals receiving antipsychotic medication often receive concurrent drug therapy, because of coexisting depression, anxiety, or other syndromes that necessitate

M. Murray: Heart Research Institute, Missenden Road, Campertown, New South Wales 2050, Australia

the inclusion of antidepressants, anxiolytics, or hypnotics into their therapeutic regimens. Thus the potential for pharmacokinetic drug interactions is considerable. However, in most clinical situations, the psychotic patient is stabilized with neuroleptic therapy, and further drugs are added as necessary. Accordingly, most pharmacokinetic drug interactions are documented in terms of impact on neuroleptic therapy.

Elimination half-lives for most neuroleptic agents are long, and volumes of distribution are usually large because of relatively high lipophilicity and extensive protein and tissue binding. Only the free concentration is relevant for interactions with CYPs or other enzymes. Effective serum concentrations for the more potent neuroleptics, such as haloperidol and perphenazine, are in the range of 1 to 25 ng/mL, whereas serum concentrations for the less-potent agents, like chlorpromazine and thioridazine, are five-fold to ten-fold higher (2). Intramuscular injection of oil-based depot dose forms allows the slow release of neuroleptic drugs into the circulation and ensures patient compliance, but also changes drug pharmacokinetics. Although some investigators favor routine monitoring of neuroleptic agents, others remain unconvinced that serum concentrations relate well to therapeutic control. Thus in cases of suspected pharmacokinetic drug interactions, the supporting serum data on drug concentrations are often unavailable. This complicates the optimal design of multiple-drug regimens and the identification of interacting drugs. Pharmacokinetic considerations are pertinent to the understanding of effects of neuroleptics on CYPs in the clinical setting.

Phenothiazines and Thioxanthenes

Chlorpromazine (Fig. 43-1) has a half-life of between 12 and 36 hours, is about 99% protein bound, has a large volume of distribution, and is metabolized along a variety of enzymatic pathways. Relatively high doses of

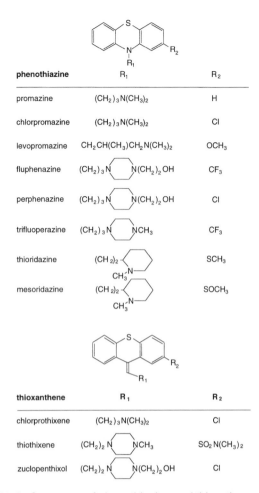

phenothiazine	R₁	R₂
promazine	$(CH_2)_3N(CH_3)_2$	H
chlorpromazine	$(CH_2)_3N(CH_3)_2$	Cl
levopromazine	$CH_2CH(CH_3)CH_2N(CH_3)_2$	OCH₃
fluphenazine	$(CH_2)_3N$ ⬡ $N(CH_2)_2OH$	CF₃
perphenazine	$(CH_2)_3N$ ⬡ $N(CH_2)_2OH$	Cl
trifluoperazine	$(CH_2)_3N$ ⬡ NCH_3	CF₃
thioridazine	$(CH_2)_2$	SCH₃
mesoridazine	$(CH_2)_2$	SOCH₃

thioxanthene	R₁	R₂
chlorprothixene	$(CH_2)_3N(CH_3)_2$	Cl
thiothixene	$(CH_2)_2N$ ⬡ NCH_3	$SO_2N(CH_3)_2$
zuclopenthixol	$(CH_2)_2N$ ⬡ $N(CH_2)_2OH$	Cl

FIG. 43-1. Structures of phenothiazine and thixanthene neuroleptics. Phenothiazines shown include those containing aliphatic side chains (e.g., chlorpromazine), piperidine-containing side chains (e.g., thioridazine), and piperazine-containing side chains (e.g., perphenazine).

chlorpromazine are used in therapy, and multiple doses lead to lower serum concentrations of drug (3). Thioridazine is probably the best known and most widely used piperidine-containing phenothiazine (see Fig. 43-1). Its pharmacokinetic behavior is similar to that of chlorpromazine. Deficient analytic methods precluded the accurate estimation of the pharmacokinetics of perphenazine (3), an important phenazine-containing phenothiazine (see Fig. 43-1). More recently, however, it has emerged that the drug also has a very long half-life (mean, about 13 hours) and undergoes extensive protein and tissue binding.

Three injectible forms of the thioxanthene zuclopenthixol exhibited different pharmacokinetic behavior (4). Maximal serum concentrations were obtained after 1 hour for the dihydrochloride, after 36 hours for the acetate (as an oily injection), and after about 7 days for the decanoate (also an oily injection). Slower release also led to longer periods over which the drug was detected (up to 14 days after a single dose of zuclopenthixol decanoate).

Butyrophenones and Diphenylpiperidines

The absorption rates of butyrophenones, such as haloperidol (Fig. 43-2), are extremely slow and constitute the rate-limiting step in drug elimination (giving rise to so-called "flip-flop'" kinetics) (5). Like the phenothiazines, the half-life of haloperidol is long (15 to 30 hours), and it is more than 90% bound to plasma proteins. Pimozide is a diphenylbutylpiperidine antipsychotic for which some pharmacokinetic parameters are available. This drug has an extremely long half-life of 30 to 150 hours, is about 97% bound to plasma proteins, and tissue binding is extensive (3).

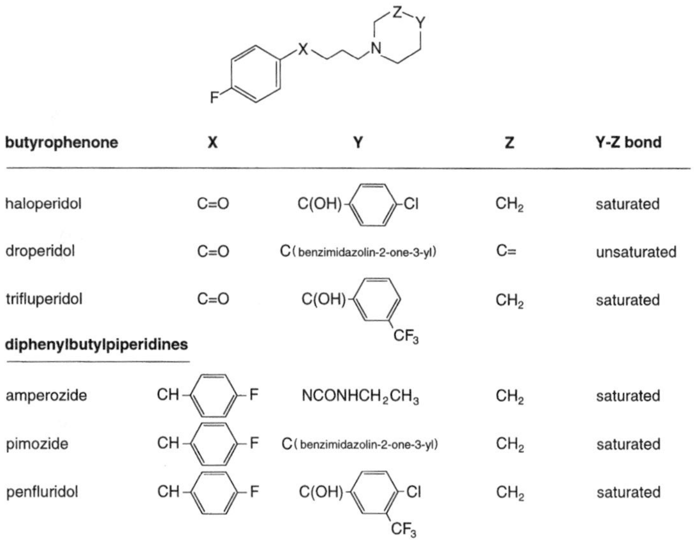

butyrophenone	X	Y	Z	Y-Z bond
haloperidol	C=O	C(OH)—⬡—Cl	CH₂	saturated
droperidol	C=O	C(benzimidazolin-2-one-3-yl)	C=	unsaturated
trifluperidol	C=O	C(OH)—⬡—CF₃	CH₂	saturated
diphenylbutylpiperidines				
amperozide	CH—⬡—F	NCONHCH₂CH₃	CH₂	saturated
pimozide	CH—⬡—F	C(benzimidazolin-2-one-3-yl)	CH₂	saturated
penfluridol	CH—⬡—F	C(OH)—⬡(Cl)(CF₃)	CH₂	saturated

FIG. 43-2. Structures of several butyrophenone and diphenylbutylpiperidine neuroleptics. Note the structural similarities between the two drug classes.

Benzamides

Like most benzamide neuroleptics, sulpiride is excreted unchanged, with a relatively long half-life around 7 to 15 hours (6). Its systemic availability is low (about 35%) (7), but this is due to poor absorption and not to extensive hepatic extraction (3). A half-life of 5 hours was documented for tiapride in six patients with Huntington's disease; most of the drug was eliminated unchanged (8,9). The clinical pharmacokinetics of remoxipride have been studied; a half-life of 4 to 7 hours has been reported for drug elimination, and at least 80% of the drug was protein bound (10,11); six minor oxidized metabolites were detected in urine (11).

Indoles

The indoles have not yet found widespread use in antipsychotic therapy. Molindone has a short half-life around 1.5 hours (12), but the half-life of sertindole (1) is extremely long (at least 24 hours). Sertindole is more than 99% bound to plasma proteins, and the volume of distribution is very high at 20 to 40 L/kg (13). Ziprasidone exhibits a half-life of about 10 hours (13). The drug is extensively bound to plasma proteins (more than 99%).

Dibenzodiazepines and Related Antipsychotics

The half-life of the dibenzodiazepine clozapine (Fig. 43-3) is 11 to 105 hours, and it is 92% to 95% plasma protein bound (13). The half-life of clozapine increases after a multiple-dosage regimen, suggesting that inhibitory metabolites may accumulate. The structurally similar olanzapine, which possesses a thiophene ring in place of one of the clozapine carbocyclic systems, also has a long half-life of 20 to 70 hours and is 93% bound to plasma proteins (13,14).

Risperidone

Risperidone is a substituted pyrimidinone and is one of several miscellaneous heterocyclic neuroleptics that are

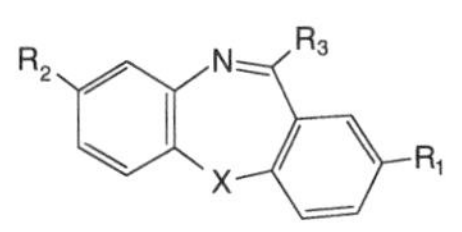

neuroleptic	X	R₁	R₂	R₃
clozapine	NH	H	Cl	N-piperazine-NCH₃
fluperlapine	CH₂	H	F	N-piperazine-NCH₃
lozapine	O	Cl	H	N-piperazine-NCH₃
zotepine	S	Cl	H	O(CH₂)₂N(CH₃)₂

FIG. 43-3. Structures of several neuroleptics related to the dibenzodiazepine clozapine.

in clinical use. The drug undergoes extensive presystemic elimination that decreases its bioavailability to about 70% (15). The half-life of the active moiety (risperidone and the major metabolite 9-hydroxyrisperidone) is around 20 hours. Plasma protein binding is 90% for the parent and 70% for the 9-hydroxy metabolite.

BIOTRANSFORMATION OF NEUROLEPTIC DRUGS

The biotransformation of most antipsychotic drugs is often complex and usually involves multiple enzymatic pathways. Some metabolites are pharmacologically active and may have a greater propensity than the parent drug to elicit pharmacokinetic drug interactions, but basic information on neuroleptic biotransformation is deficient. Extended dose regimens can influence the appearance of particular neuroleptic metabolites in serum, urine, or feces. There is also evidence of metabolite accumulation, which could arise because of impaired elimination, induction of biotransformation enzymes, or saturation of tissue sites that usually sequester the neuroleptic. Each of these possibilities may influence inhibitory interactions involving CYPs. To evaluate the available information on pharmacokinetic drug interactions, CYPs that mediate neuroleptic oxidation must be considered.

Phenothiazines and Thioxanthenes

Chlorpromazine sulfoxide was detected after oral dosing, but not after intramuscular injection, suggesting that it may be formed in the intestinal wall or by gut bacteria; a similar situation occurs with levopromazine (3). Because intestinal CYP3A4 contributes to extrahepatic biotransformation of some drugs (16), this enzyme may have a role in phenothiazine sulfoxidation. Indeed, oxidation of the heterocyclic sulfur atom of chlorpromazine is mediated by CYP3A4 in human hepatic microsomes (17). 7-Hydroxychlorpromazine has pharmacologic activity (13), and inhibition of its formation by quinidine implicates CYP2D6 in the pathway (18), but this has not been established unequivocally. It has also been demonstrated that formation of chlorpromazine N-oxide involves the flavin-containing monooxygenase and CYP2D6 (17). Thus several hepatic enzymes could well be targets for inhibition by chlorpromazine or its metabolites.

Thioridazine is probably the most common piperidine-containing phenothiazine. The carbon atom at position 2 of the piperidine nitrogen is a chiral center; the drug is administered as a racemate, and many metabolites are possible. The urinary elimination of thioridazine and its metabolites has been studied (19). Twelve metabolites were formed by oxidation at the side chain sulfur, further oxidation to the sulfone, N-oxidation, oxidation of the phenothiazine sulfur atom, and oxidation at the carbon adjacent to the piperidino nitrogen to produce the lactam. However, only 4% of the administered dose was recovered, suggesting that metabolism may be even more complex.

A role of CYP2D6 in thioridazine biotransformation appears likely from *in vivo* studies. Thus CYP2D6 has been implicated in thioridazine 2-sulfoxidation to mesoridazine and further oxidation to the sulfone sulforidazine (20,21); these are also neuroleptic drugs. Oxidation of the heterocyclic sulfur atom was not mediated by CYP2D6. Supportive evidence for a role for CYP2D6 in thioridazine thioether sulfoxidation was provided by experiments with the recombinant enzyme, but CYP3A4 did not support the pathway *in vitro* (22).

CYP2D6 status is also a major factor influencing perphenazine oxidation *in vivo* (23). The metabolic profiles of fluphenazine were different after oral ingestion and depot injection of the decanoate ester. Higher serum levels of the 7-hydroxy- and sulfoxide metabolites were observed after oral administration by comparison with depot injection of the decanoate ester (24).

Thioxanthene and flupenthixol metabolites include the sulfoxides, *N*-desmethylated analogues and the glucuronides (25,26). There is little information on the metabolic pathways of other thioxanthenes or the CYP enzymes that are involved, but first pass metabolism is extensive (3).

Butyrophenones and Diphenylbutylpiperidines

Pathways of haloperidol metabolism include oxidative cleavage to the fluorophenyl carbonic acid and piperidine-containing metabolites, as well as ketone reduction (25). Reduced haloperidol possesses pharmacologic activity, but this is lower than that of the parent drug (13). The formation of reduced haloperidol from haloperidol is mediated by a reduced nicotinamide adenine dinucleotide phosphate (NADPH)-dependent ketone reductase that is present in human liver cytosol (27,28).

The capacity of CYPs 3A4 and 2D6 to oxidize haloperidol and its reduced analogue in lymphoblastoid cell microsomes has been examined (29). Direct evidence was obtained for the conversion of haloperidol to haloperidol-1,2,3,4-tetrahydropyridine by CYP3A4, and its further oxidation to the corresponding pyridinium species by CYPs 3A4 and 2D6 (29,30). *N*-Dealkylation of haloperidol and reduced haloperidol was supported by CYPs 3A4/2D6 and CYP3A4, respectively. CYP3A4 also oxidized reduced haloperidol back to the parent. It would now be informative to determine whether other CYPs contribute to these pathways. Thus more cDNA-derived CYPs should be evaluated, and correlative studies with other CYP activities in human microsomal fractions would be valuable.

In regard to the potential involvement of CYP3A4 in haloperidol metabolism, it is noteworthy that plasma concentrations of the drug are decreased in patients receiving concurrent anticonvulsant therapy (31). This is consistent with CYP3A4 induction by the anticonvulsants but, more important, provides support for haloperidol oxidation by CYP3A4.

There is little information on the metabolism of the diphenylbutylpiperidines. Penfluridol undergoes *N*-dealkylation to the difluorophenylalkanoic acid and the phenylpiperidine metabolites (32). A similar metabolic profile has been observed for pimozide (33).

Benzamides

As indicated, benzamide antipsychotics are generally resistant to biotransformation. Metabolites of sulpiride have not been detected in urine or feces, and the drug is excreted largely unchanged by the kidney (34). Patients with renal impairment require dose reduction or extension of the dose interval (35). Biotransformation to the 4-oxo-derivative accounts for less than 10% of an administered dose of sultopride in humans (36).

Indoles

The indoles have not yet found widespread use in antipsychotic therapy (1). The metabolic ratio of dehydrosertindole to sertindole correlates well with the ratio of dextromethorphan to dextrorphan, thus supporting a role for CYP2D6 in dehydrosertindole formation (37). Other oxidized metabolites are pharmacologically inactive and CYPs 2D6 and 3A4 have been implicated in norsertindole formation. Excretion of sertindole into feces (after conjugation and biliary excretion) is significant.

Dibenzodiazepines and Related Drugs

Clozapine is metabolized extensively before elimination by *N*-demethylation, *N*-oxidation, sulfoxidation, and oxidation at the 3'-carbon and glucuronidation (3,38). Up to 90% of an administered dose was excreted in urine or feces (38,39). The *N*-desmethyl metabolite is reportedly active, but the *N*-oxide is not. Olanzapine metabolites include the *N*-glucuronide, 2-hydroxymethyl, the 4'-*N*-oxide, and 4'-*N*-desmethyl analogues. Loxapine metabolites detected in urine include those formed by aromatic hydroxylation, *N*-demethylation, and *N*-oxidation (40).

The role of CYPs in the metabolism of clozapine, fluperlapine, and olanzapine has been studied. Recombinant CYP2D6 oxidizes clozapine, but not to its principal metabolites (the *N*-oxide and *N*-desmethyl analogues), whereas fluperlapine is oxidized efficiently by CYP2D6 to its major metabolite 7-hydroxyfluperlapine (41). These observations suggest that fluperlapine, but not clozapine, may elicit drug interactions involving CYP2D6. Subsequent *in vitro* and *in vivo* studies have supported these findings.

The metabolism of clozapine and binding of a reactive clozapine metabolite to human liver microsomes *in vitro* has been described (42). Some evidence was obtained from inhibitor studies for the involvement of CYPs 1A2 and 3A4 in clozapine *N*-demethylation and for CYP3A4 and the flavin-containing monooxygenase in clozapine *N*-oxidation. Formation of the reactive metabolite was inhibited by chemicals that are known to interact with CYP3A4 and the flavin-containing monooxygenase. The nature of the reactive species was not investigated, but it is interesting that the same enzymes are implicated in the formation of the reactive and *N*-oxide metabolites.

The metabolism of olanzapine in human liver microsomes has also been studied *in vitro* (43). The 2-hydroxymethyl-, 7-hydroxy-, 4′-*N*-oxide-, and 4′-*N*-desmethyl metabolites were detected (K_m values of 30–75 μM). These values are larger than the free concentrations of drug in serum, so that biotransformation enzymes are unlikely to be saturated during therapy. The flavin-containing monooxygenase was implicated in *N*-oxide formation. CYP1A2 has a major role in formation of the *N*-desmethyl and 7-hydroxy metabolites, whereas CYP2D6 appears responsible for the 2-hydroxymethyl metabolite. This is in contrast with clozapine in which a role for CYP2D6 in formation of a major metabolite could not be established unequivocally (41).

Zotepine is structurally similar to the dibenzodiazepines and undergoes metabolism to the *N*-demethylated and hydroxylated analogues (44). Zotepine metabolism is inhibited by diazepam, but there appeared to be no association between *S*-mephenytoin hydroxylation and zotepine biotransformation (45). Thus it was suggested that the effect of diazepam is probably unrelated to CYP2C19 inhibition and that perhaps another CYP that mediates diazepam oxidation could be an alternate target (e.g., CYP3A4).

Risperidone

The pyrimidinone risperidone undergoes CYP2D6-mediated polymorphic hydroxylation to the 9-hydroxymetabolite, which is pharmacologically active. Other metabolites arise by *N*-dealkylation at the piperidine nitrogen and by 7-hydroxylation on the pyrimidinone ring system (15). Apart from risperidone, an increasing number of agents are structurally dissimilar from the major classes of neuroleptics. Because most of these agents are newly available or at the preclinical stage, information on their detailed biotransformation pathways is not readily accessible.

PHARMACOKINETIC DRUG INTERACTIONS INVOLVING NEUROLEPTICS

In Vitro Studies of CYP Inhibition by Phenothiazines Containing Aliphatic Side Chains

Chlorpromazine and levopromazine are probably the most widely used neuroleptic drugs in this category.

Chlorpromazine is a potent competitive inhibitor of the *p*-hydroxylation (K_i, 5.5 μM) and methylhydroxylation (K_i, 4.5 μM) of mexiletine, a type 1B antiarrhythmic agent (46). Because the hepatic *p*-hydroxylation of mexiletine is inducible by cigarette smoking, there may be a role for CYP1A in this pathway (47), which in turn suggests that chlorpromazine may be an inhibitor of CYP1A.

An association between mexiletine metabolism and CYP2D6 was also suggested (46). This is consistent with the competitive inhibition (K_i, 7 μM) by chlorpromazine of the *in vitro* metabolism of sparteine oxidation (48,49) and desipramine 2-hydroxylation (K_i, 6 μM) (50). Chlorpromazine also inhibited CYP2D6-mediated codeine *O*-demethylation in human liver microsomes by a competitive mechanism (K_i, 0.5 μM); levopromazine was similarly effective (51). Because the K_m for codeine *O*-demethylation was much larger (100–200 μM) than these K_i values, inhibition by chlorpromazine could be clinically significant. Indeed, inhibition of the *O*-demethylation of codeine to morphine may impair narcotic analgesia.

In Vivo Studies of CYP Inhibition by Phenothiazines Containing Aliphatic Side Chains

The toxicity of tricyclic antidepressants when serum concentrations exceed about 0.5 mg/mL underscores the importance attached to identification of pharmacokinetic interactions (2). Administration of chlorpromazine or levopromazine to patients who were stabilized with amitriptyline influenced the steady-state levels of the primary metabolite nortriptyline, but amitriptyline levels in serum were unchanged (52). In contrast, propiomazine exerted no discernible effects on the serum levels of amitriptyline or nortriptyline after dosage of patients with either drug.

These findings concur with several other reports that implicate chlorpromazine in CYP2D6 inhibition. Thus debrisoquine hydroxylation *in vivo* was inhibited by levopromazine and chlorpromazine (53), and chlorpromazine decreased the clearance of a pulse dose of [^{14}C]imipramine in patients whose antidepressant therapy had already attained steady state (54).

Chlorpromazine was found to impair moclobemide elimination *in vivo* in patients (55). Not previously suspected, this interaction suggests that chlorpromazine may be an inhibitor of CYP2C19, which has been associated with moclobemide oxidation (56). The interaction led to a median three-fold increase in moclobemide levels, achieving as much as a six-fold increase in some patients. It would now be useful to evaluate whether this putative interaction can be confirmed in human hepatic microsomes *in vitro*.

Chlorpromazine also has been linked to drug interactions with several antihypertensive agents, but it has proven difficult to account for these in terms of a pharmacokinetic mechanism. One of the most important interactions involves propranolol. Several case reports exist, but serum concentrations of the drugs have been measured in only a limited number of the studies. Thus an increase in plasma propranolol to about two-fold of starting levels was reported in five patients who were administered chlorpromazine; small decreases in blood pressure were noted in some of the patients (57). Despite this the elimination half-life of propranolol did not change markedly; the authors argued against an effect of chlorpromazine on the binding of propranolol to plasma proteins. The significance of these pharmacokinetic changes remains unclear because follow-up mechanistic studies do not appear to have been undertaken. Nevertheless, support for a pharmacokinetic interaction of potential significance was provided by Peet et al. (58), who reported an increase in serum chlorpromazine concentrations by propranolol. Indeed, the involvement of CYP2D6 in the 4-hydroxylation of propranolol has been established (59).

In Vitro Studies of CYP Inhibition by Piperidine-Containing Phenothiazines

Thioridazine inhibits CYP2D6-dependent desipramine 2-hydroxylation with a K_i of 0.75 μM in adult and fetal hepatic microsomes *in vitro* (50,60). Similarly, thioridazine inhibited codeine *O*-demethylation to morphine in human liver microsomes, and also appeared to be more potent than chlorpromazine and levopromazine (51). In contrast, a relatively weak effect of thioridazine on codeine *O*-demethylation *in vitro* was observed in two human livers (61). Apart from thioridazine, there is a deficiency of information on *in vitro* interactions involving CYPs and other piperidine-containing phenothiazines in human microsomal fractions.

In Vivo Studies of CYP Inhibition by Piperidine-containing Phenothiazines

The tricyclic antidepressants, amitriptyline and imipramine, undergo *N*-demethylation to nortriptyline and desipramine, respectively. One study demonstrated that levels of nortriptyline were significantly increased by thioridazine in patients who were receiving amitriptyline therapy (52). Similarly, nortriptyline concentrations in serum were elevated after coadministration of thioridazine and nortriptyline. This finding contrasts to some extent with the report that serum imipramine concentrations were increased by thioridazine to about 3 times those at steady state (62). This is because, as indicated earlier, imipramine is a structural analogue of amitriptyline, and serum amitriptyline concentrations were found not to be increased by concurrent thioridazine (52). A plausible explanation is that CYPs other than 2D6 may contribute more extensively

to the oxidation of amitriptyline than to that of imipramine. Consequently, CYP2D6 inhibition by thioridazine could have a greater impact on drugs whose metabolism relies on that enzyme.

A major effect of thioridazine on *in vivo* CYP2D6 activity emerges from several studies. Thus the inhibition of desipramine oxidation (63) and debrisoquine hydroxylation by thioridazine (53) has been noted. After administration at daily doses of 200 mg or 400 mg for 10 days, thioridazine decreased dextromethorphan oxidation in a population of extensive metabolizers to rates typical of those observed in poor metabolizers (64). It was concluded that thioridazine washout is warranted before commencement of therapy with agents that are metabolized extensively by CYP2D6. It also emerged from this study that thioridazine did not affect mephenytoin elimination, which implies that CYP2C19 is not a target for inhibition by this drug.

An interaction of potential interest has been documented in which serum phenytoin concentrations were increased from 11 to 56 mg/mL in a patient who also received thioridazine (65). CYPs 2C have been implicated in phenytoin metabolism (66), so it is possible that thioridazine can modulate the activity of these enzymes *in vivo*. However, caution must be exercised in the interpretation of this interaction because it is restricted to static measurements of drug concentrations in serum and not necessarily to changes in phenytoin elimination. Further, phenytoin is extensively bound to plasma proteins, and its displacement from these sites by thioridazine could have precipitated the adverse clinical interaction that occurred in this patient. Although actually the reverse of this discussion of neuroleptic effects on drug metabolism, it has been found that thioridazine levels in plasma were elevated by propranolol (67). As indicated previously, CYP2D6 participates in propranolol 4-hydroxylation (59). Thus two drugs with similar affinities for a CYP may elicit mutual inhibition of each other's metabolism, especially if that CYP has a dominant role in biotransformation.

In Vitro Studies of CYP Inhibition by Piperazine-containing Phenothiazines

This category of neuroleptics contains several agents in common use, notably perphenazine, fluphenazine, prochlorperazine, and trifluoperazine, but most of the available literature relates to perphenazine. Perphenazine was found to be a potent competitive inhibitor of bufuralol 1'-hydroxylation, a typical CYP2D6 reaction, in human liver microsomes *in vitro* (K_i, 1.9 μM) (68). However, the recommended therapeutic concentrations of potent neuroleptics are somewhat lower at 1 to 25 ng/mL, which corresponds to a maximal concentration of about 60 nM perphenazine. Thus it appears that CYP2D6 inhibition *in vivo* may not be clinically relevant, except where the substrate itself has a low affinity for the enzyme.

In Vivo Studies of CYP Inhibition by Piperazine-containing Phenothiazines

Perphenazine impairs the elimination of tricyclic antidepressants *in vivo*, including imipramine (52,54,69), desipramine (70), and nortriptyline (54,71). Indeed, subsequent administration of perphenazine (32–48 mg/day) decreased the excretion of imipramine and nortriptyline by up to 50% and 60%, respectively, and metabolites of nortriptyline accumulated in plasma. The study of Gram and Overϕ (54) encountered some criticism because it was thought that the doses of perphenazine used may have been excessive and not indicative of problems likely to be encountered during fluphenazine therapy (72). The alternate explanation that was provided was that the opposite inhibition process may have occurred: that the tricyclic antidepressant inhibited the elimination of the neuroleptic drug. The controversy surrounding this putative pharmacokinetic interaction emphasizes the need for systematic evaluation of interactions observed *in vivo* by using comparative experiments in microsomal fractions *in vitro*.

Serum concentrations of nortriptyline were found to be increased after perphenazine administration, but serum concentrations of amitriptyline were unchanged (52,71). This is compatible with the proposal that perphenazine may be oxidized relatively exclusively by CYP2D6. In this regard, perphenazine has been classified as a substrate for CYP2D6 (48), and another study related the disposition of perphenazine closely to polymorphic debrisoquine hydroxylation (73). Maximal serum concentrations of the parent drug were about three-fold higher in poor metabolizers of CYP2D6. At odds with these reports, it has been suggested that CYP2D6 may not be the sole catalyst of perphenazine biotransformation because interindividual variation in steady-state perphenazine serum concentrations appeared independent of the CYP2D6 metabolizer phenotype (74). Thus a definitive conclusion concerning the involvement of CYP2D6 in perphenazine oxidation has proven elusive.

In the study undertaken by Jerling et al. (52), dixyrazine, another piperazine-containing neuroleptic, had no effect on serum concentrations of amitriptyline or nortriptyline in amitriptyline-treated individuals.

There may be instances in which phenothiazines transiently influence serum concentrations of coadministered drugs. For example, a small increase in plasma concentration and decreased clearance of the anticonvulsant valproic acid has been attributed to chlorpromazine administration (75); normal valproate pharmacokinetics were restored by removal of chlorpromazine. Clinical consequences were not apparent, so the effect may not warrant modifications to therapy.

In Vitro and *In Vivo* Studies of CYP Inhibition by Thioxanthenes

Information on the *in vitro* effects of thioxanthene antipsychotics on CYP activities in human hepatic microsomes is deficient, but several *in vivo* studies have been conducted. Thus flupenthixol did not appear to influence serum levels of amitriptyline or nortriptyline in amitriptyline-treated subjects, or serum nortriptyline concentrations after administration of that drug (52). Unlike several phenothiazines, flupenthixol (3–6 mg/day) had no effect on the elimination of imipramine (54).

Zuclopenthixol did not affect serum levels of nortriptyline or amitriptyline in patients who received amitriptyline, even though zuclopenthixol is known to be partly dependent on CYP2D6 for its metabolism (71). By comparison, the piperazine-substituted phenothiazine perphenazine increased serum antidepressant concentrations during coadministration. Thus it was suggested that zuclopenthixol may have a lower affinity than perphenazine for CYP2D6. Considered together, it appears that thioxanthenes pose a smaller problem in terms of significant pharmacokinetic drug interactions. There is considerable structural similarity between these agents and the phenothiazines, but the thioxanthenes do contain an unsaturated bond between the thioxanthene nucleus and the side chain. Perhaps this structural feature confers a rigid conformation to the thioxanthenes that prevents their effective interaction with CYPs.

In Vitro Studies of CYP Inhibition by Butyrophenones and Diphenylbutylpiperidines

Several butyrophenones are inhibitors of CYP2D6-mediated bufuralol 1′-hydroxylation in human liver microsomes *in vitro* (68). Trifluperidol was a potent competitive inhibitor of the activity (K_i, 169 μM), and it may be anticipated that this drug could exert significant inhibition of CYP2D6 *in vivo*. Haloperidol was a order of magnitude less potent (K_i, 1.2 μM), although this would still be considered to be effective inhibition. Trifluperidol and haloperidol are structurally very similar and differ only in the nature of substitution of the phenyl ring in the 4-position of the piperidine ring (see Fig. 43-2). These substituents are 3′-trifluoromethyl- and 4′-chloro- in the respective drugs and possess similar hydrophobic, steric, and electronic properties (electron-withdrawing effect at the piperidine system). An interesting possibility is that the 3′-trifluoromethyl- substituent may coordinate efficiently with a region of the CYP2D6 active site that is crucial for catalysis. However, this possibility now requires extensive testing in microsomal fractions with similarly substituted butyrophenones.

A K_i of 1 μM also was determined for haloperidol against the CYP2D6-dependent oxidation of sparteine to 2-dehydrosparteine in human liver microsomes (49).

Three other butyrophenones (spiperone, droperidol, and benperidol) were less effective than haloperidol, and K_i values were not determined (68). The diphenylbutylpiperidine neuroleptic pimozide was not inhibitory toward CYP2D6 activity but was somewhat more effective against CYP2C19-dependent mephenytoin hydroxylation (49). However, the K_i was relatively large at 120 μM, which suggests that the likelihood of clinically significant pharmacokinetic interactions would probably be minimal.

In Vivo Studies of CYP Inhibition by Butyrophenones and Diphenylbutylpiperidines

As is the case with most other neuroleptic agents, considerable effort has been expended to evaluate whether haloperidol administration impairs CYP2D6 activity in vivo (76). Several reports support an association between CYP2D6 and haloperidol biotransformation. Thus haloperidol impaired debrisoquine elimination in vivo (64,70) and caused a marked increase in the metabolic ratio of sparteine (in favor of parent drug) (77). Another study demonstrated that the excretion of imipramine in patients is impaired by haloperidol and is consistent with a role for CYP2D6 in haloperidol metabolism (54). The butyrophenones haloperidol and melperone inhibited CYP2D6-mediated debrisoquine hydroxylation in vivo (53), so that these clinical findings are consistent with in vitro observations (28,29).

Several studies suggest that the association between haloperidol oxidation and CYP2D6 may be less clear than that for other neuroleptics. For example, it was noted that haloperidol did not convert extensive metabolizers to the poor-metabolizer phenotype (73). Further, haloperidol did not increase serum levels of amitriptyline or nortriptyline in patients who received these drugs (52), and no interaction between bromoperidol and desipramine was found in an in vivo study in schizophrenics (78).

It may be possible to reconcile these apparently disparate observations. Thus haloperidol administration increased serum levels of carbamazepine in patients by about 40% over steady-state levels (79). Indeed, the dose of carbamazepine was lower in those patients who also received haloperidol (about 75% of that in patients who received carbamazepine alone), so that the increase in serum carbamazepine may actually underestimate the interaction. The point of particular interest that emerges from this study is that carbamazepine is not considered to be a CYP2D6 substrate and is probably oxidized by CYP3A4. Therefore it is feasible that haloperidol has affinity for other CYPs, such as CYP3A4, which was also suggested from in vitro studies of CYP3A4 and haloperidol metabolism (29). It would now be informative to evaluate the effect of haloperidol on the elimination half-life of carbamazepine and for comparative in vitro information to be obtained from studies in microsomal incubations.

In Vitro and In Vivo Studies of CYP Inhibition by Benzamides

There is very little information on the capacity of benzamides to interact with the CYP-mediated metabolism of other drugs, but this is not surprising in view of the general unimportance of oxidation in benzamide biotransformation. This is supported by the observation that sulpiride has a minimal capacity to inhibit CYP2D6-mediated bufuralol 1'-hydroxylation in human liver microsomes (68). Pharmacokinetic interactions in vivo were not observed between remoxipride and either diazepam, ethanol, biperiden, or warfarin (11). These observations are readily understood in terms of the minor role that oxidative biotransformation plays in the elimination of benzamide drugs.

In Vitro and In Vivo Studies of CYP Inhibition by Indoles

Information on the capacity of indole neuroleptics to inhibit CYP activities also is limited. Median inhibitory concentration (IC_{50}) values have been presented for sertindole and dehydrosertindole against CYP2D6 and CYP3A4, but the substrates were not specified, and the range of inhibitor concentrations was not provided (13). Thus it was not possible to compare the potencies of sertindole against those of different CYPs. However, it is extremely interesting that the parent drug was more effective than its metabolite norsertindole against CYP2D6, whereas the metabolite was more effective than the parent against CYP3A4 activity. Thus it is possible that accumulation of the N-demethylated metabolite of sertindole could promote inhibition of CYP3A4. These preliminary observations require more thorough evaluation in further experiments and, ideally, corroboration in clinical studies.

In Vitro Studies of CYP Inhibition by Dibenzodiazepines and Related Neuroleptics

Olanzapine, which has recently entered clinical use (1), and clozapine are emerging as favored new-generation antipsychotic agents because they exhibit a lesser incidence of neurologic side effects (38) and because they may be effective in patients who are refractory to other neuroleptics (14). Considerably more information is available on the biotransformation and pharmacokinetic interactions associated with these neuroleptic drugs than for the indoles, benzamides, and diphenylbutylpiperidines.

The capacities of olanzapine and clozapine to inhibit the activities of four major CYPs in human liver were evaluated (80). The K_i values were determined in this study, which facilitates a clear interpretation of inhibitory effects. However, both drugs were essentially inactive as inhibitors of CYPs 2C9, 2C19, 2D6, and 3A4 activities, although clozapine was generally more potent than olanzapine. Thus K_i values were generally one or two orders of magnitude greater than those obtained for the reference inhibitors of these enzymes (phenytoin, omeprazole, quinidine, and ketoconazole, respectively). The structure of clozapine is shown in Fig. 43-3. Olanzapine is structurally similar but possesses a thiophene ring instead of one of the benzo systems; the other carbocyclic system is chlorinated in the case of clozapine (at position R_2; see Fig. 43-3) but is unsubstituted in olanzapine. It is well established that thiophene and benzene are bioisosteric (81), but the overall hydrophobicity of clozapine is about 1 log unit greater than that of olanzapine (calculated by the additivity principle) (82). This difference in hydrophobic character most probably accounts for the somewhat greater potency of clozapine, in that its movement out of the aqueous phase and to the active center of microsomal CYPs would be superior to that of olanzapine.

The significance of the inhibitory properties of clozapine and olanzapine was pursued, and it was argued that the serum free (non–protein bound) concentrations of the drugs that would likely be encountered during therapy would be below those necessary to elicit pharmacokinetic drug interactions. However, in view of the apparent association between CYP1A2 and clozapine biotransformation (see later), it would have been useful to determine the extent of CYP1A2 inhibition by the drugs.

In Vivo Studies of CYP Inhibition by Dibenzodiazepines and Related Neuroleptics

No association was found between CYP2D6 or CYP2C19 and clozapine elimination in vivo (39), but the involvement of CYP1A2 was found subsequently (83). This was established in studies of caffeine elimination [from area under the curve (AUC) measurements] and by using analysis of covariance. Supportive of a clinically relevant association between clozapine and CYP1A2 is a case report in which a patient who had been stabilized on clozapine suffered from adverse effects after ingestion of a high dose of caffeine (84). Serum levels of clozapine and norclozapine were about 2.5- and two-fold of those levels measured after a caffeine washout period of 7 days. Similarly, there have been other reports of acute psychotic episodes involving clozapine and coffee or caffeinated diet cola (85).

Erythromycin increased serum levels of clozapine to about two-fold of steady state (86). Although this may suggest a role for CYP3A4 in clozapine metabolism, it is unlikely that clozapine would elicit pharmacokinetic drug interactions involving CYP3A4 unless the drug in question had a lower affinity for the enzyme than did clozapine.

A potential pharmacokinetic interaction between clozapine and the angiotensin-converting enzyme inhibitor enalapril has emerged from a well-documented case report (87). Patients had been stabilized on the combination of enalapril and an antipsychotic but were then administered clozapine in place of the original neuroleptic agent. They became drowsy and hypotensive. After recovery they were rechallenged with lower doses of both enalapril and clozapine and had no ill effects. Thus close monitoring of dose is important with this drug combination.

It has been reported that a patient who was stabilized on clozapine and was then administered risperidone had adverse effects from a two-fold increase in serum clozapine concentrations after 2 weeks of concurrent therapy (88). Although this was accounted for in terms of a CYP2D6 interaction, the weight of evidence appears to be against a significant role for this enzyme in clozapine biotransformation, although it clearly participates in risperidone oxidation (15). It is possible that risperidone may also be a substrate for CYP1A2.

It has been suggested that serum levels of clozapine after single-dose administration are not predictive of effects seen after multiple dosage (89). Thus it is conceivable that clozapine metabolites inhibit biotransformation of the parent drug. Certainly a similar situation occurs with oxidized metabolites of the calcium channel blocker diltiazem both in vitro (90) and in vivo (91).

INTERPRETATION OF REPORTS OF CYP INHIBITION BY NEUROLEPTICS

The literature contains a number of reports of inhibitory effects of neuroleptics on the oxidative biotransformation of coadministered drugs. Several general observations can be made.

Much of the inhibition data has been obtained from in vivo studies in which neuroleptics have been found to impair the elimination of several classes of drugs, including tricyclic antidepressants and debrisoquine or other antihypertensives. Indeed, most of this literature has concentrated on inhibitory phenomena involving CYP2D6, the polymorphically distributed debrisoquine hydroxylase (52,53,63). Many neuroleptics have been found to inhibit CYP2D6 activity in extensive metabolizers. A notable exception is the atypical antipsychotic clozapine, which has been associated with pharmacokinetic drug interactions with substrates for CYP1A2 (83). Notwithstanding these important findings, the range of CYPs susceptible to inhibition by neuroleptic drugs remains underexplored. Fragments of information exist within the literature to associate, for example, haloperidol with CYP3A4 (29,30) and thioridazine with CYP2C9 (65). Unfortunately, demonstration that these enzymes are inhibited significantly by haloperidol or thioridazine requires extensive in vivo investigation, and ethical problems would arise immediately.

Difficulties also would be encountered because of the nature of the patient population. Inhibitory effects of neuroleptics on the elimination of coadministered psychoac-

588 / Drugs as Inhibitors of Metabolic Enzymes: CNS Diseases

tive drugs may not be readily apparent and may not be reported faithfully by the study subjects. Thus follow-up studies may not be undertaken by using serum drug monitoring because the potential drug interaction escapes initial detection. Perhaps this is a partial explanation for the concentration of studies in the context of CYP2D6, a well-established polymorphic enzyme whose metabolic function has been investigated thoroughly in many clinical studies.

Finally, it must be emphasized that neuroleptic drugs are used for the most part according to consistent drug regimens. Additional forms of therapy may be introduced to the patient who is stabilized on neuroleptic drugs, rather than the converse. For example, many reports of drug interactions with neuroleptics involve inhibitory processes on neuroleptic metabolism. Thus selective serotonin reuptake inhibitors and tricyclic antidepressants are well established for the capacity to impair the elimination of many important drugs, including neuroleptics (92). Such reports do not necessarily establish the significance of the reverse processes (inhibition of selective serotonin reuptake inhibitors or tricyclic antidepressant oxidation by neuroleptics). This consideration underscores the need for basic biochemical information obtained from studies in hepatic microsomes that would establish the relative inhibitory capacity of interacting drugs. That is, documentation of interactions between selective serotonin reuptake inhibitors and neuroleptics may be relevant in one or both directions. Until K_m and K_i data are obtained for mutual inhibition processes, firm conclusions cannot be reached.

The role of CYP2D6 in the oxidation of many neuroleptics and in pharmacokinetic drug interactions involving neuroleptics raises an interesting point in relation to CYP2D6 phenotype. Extensive metabolizers would be expected to be at greater risk from pharmacokinetic interactions than poor metabolizers. Thus it has been shown that administration of some drug substrates for CYP2D6 can "convert," at least temporarily, extensive metabolizers to the opposite phenotype (64). Serious pharmacokinetic interactions have been identified in extensive metabolizers, but poor metabolizers are already deficient in CYP2D6-mediated pathways. It may be for this reason that pharmacokinetic interactions with certain neuroleptics have been difficult to characterize in some studies.

It is noteworthy that most of the *in vivo* literature deals with studies on a limited number of neuroleptic agents, especially chlorpromazine, levopromazine, thioridazine, perphenazine, haloperidol, and clozapine, which are already used extensively. Information on the structural features of neuroleptics that contribute to inhibition is not currently available. Neither is appropriate information available from *in vitro* studies conducted in microsomal incubations, except from studies in microsomes from nonhuman species. Benzamides do not appear to repre-

sent risks from pharmacokinetic drug interactions because they are essentially refractory to oxidative metabolism (6), but information on other important neuroleptics is deficient.

The *in vitro* evidence of inhibition of CYP oxidation by neuroleptics is also relatively deficient. Very little information has been derived in human microsomal fractions concerning the capacity of neuroleptics to inhibit the activity of specific CYP enzymes. It is accepted that such studies would have to be interpreted carefully, especially when it is considered that the pharmacokinetic behavior of most neuroleptics is unusual. However, it would be extremely useful if the potential roles of neuroleptic metabolites in inhibition processes were evaluated systematically. Although it is not anticipated that these metabolites should form quasi-covalent complexes with CYPs, similar to those observed with macrolide antibiotics, or elicit autocatalytic inactivation of these enzymes (93), certain drug metabolites have been associated with potent reversible inhibition of CYP-mediated biotransformation. Thus *N*-desmethyldiltiazem was a more potent inhibitor than diltiazem of human hepatic microsomal CYP3A4 activity (90), and a similar finding was made with norfluoxetine compared with the parent drug fluoxetine (94). Reports from *in vivo* studies that multiple administrations of some neuroleptics decrease elimination rates of the parent drug suggest that drug metabolites may exert CYP inhibition (89). *In vitro* studies are now required to evaluate this possibility.

Although not directly applicable to the clinical situation, studies conducted in rat hepatic microsomes have indicated an order of potency for phenothiazines as inhibitors of several CYP activities. Thus thioridazine has emerged as a potent inhibitor of rat hepatic microsomal CYP2B1 (95). Indeed, of 12 phenothiazines that were tested, the potency of thioridazine was underpredicted by regression equations describing the relations between chemical structure and CYP inhibition (96). Apart from CYP2B1, it was also noted that CYP1A2 was effectively inhibited by some of the agents. These studies establish the paradigm that phenothiazines, and possibly other neuroleptic drugs, have the capacity to inhibit multiple CYPs. It is now important that analogous *in vitro* studies should be undertaken in human hepatic microsomes so that indications can be obtained on the true pharmacokinetic interaction potential of these important drugs.

REFERENCES

1. Citrome L. New antipsychotic medications: what advantages do they offer? *Postgrad Med* 1997;101:207–214.
2. Goff DC, Baldessarini RJ. Drug interactions with antipsychotic agents. *J Clin Psychopharmacol* 1990;13:57–67.
3. Balant-Gorgia AE, Balant LP, Andreoli A. Pharmacokinetic optimisation of the treatment of psychosis. *Clin Pharmacokinet* 1993;25:217–236.
4. Aaes-Jorgensen T. Pharmacokinetics of three different injectable zuclopenthixol preparations. *Prog Neuropsychopharmacol Biol Psychiatry* 1989;13:77–85.

5. Froemming JS, Lam YW, Jann MW, Davis CM. Pharmacokinetics of haloperidol. *Clin Pharmacokinet* 1989;17:396–423.
6. Bateman DN. Pharmacokinetics and metabolism of the benzamides. *Adv Biochem Psychopharmacol* 1982;35:143–162.
7. Caley CF, Weber SS. Sulpiride: an antipsychotic with selective dopaminergic antagonist properties. *Ann Pharmacother* 1995;29:152–160.
8. Norman T, Chiu E, James RH, Gregory MS. Single oral dose pharmacokinetics of tiapride in patients with Huntington's disease. *Eur J Clin Pharmacol* 1987;32:583–586.
9. Rey E, d'Athis P, Richard MO, de Lauture D, Olive G. Pharmacokinetics of tiapride and absolute bioavailability of three extravascular forms. *Int J Clin Pharmacol Ther Toxicol* 1982;20:62–67.
10. von Bahr C, Movin G, Yisak WA, Jostell KG, Widman M. Clinical pharmacokinetics of remoxipride. *Acta Psychiatry Scand* 1990;(suppl 358):41–44.
11. Wadsworth AN, Heel RC. Remoxipride: a review of its pharmacodynamic and pharmacokinetic properties, and therapeutic potential in schizophrenia. *Drugs* 1990;40:863–879.
12. Claghorn JL. Review of clinical and laboratory experiences with molidone hydrochloride. *J Clin Psychiatry* 1985;46:30–33.
13. Ereshefsky L. Pharmacokinetics and drug interactions: update for new antipsychotics. *J Clin Psychiatry* 1996;57(suppl 11):12–25.
14. Jann MW, Grimsley SR, Gray EC, Chang WH. Pharmacokinetics and pharmacodynamics of clozapine. *Clin Pharmacokinet* 1993;24:161–176.
15. DeVane CL. Brief comparison of the pharmacokinetics and pharmacodynamics of the traditional and newer antipsychotic drugs. *Am J Health Syst Pharmacol* 1995;52(suppl 1):S15–S18.
16. Kolars JC, Schmiedlin-Ren P, Schuetz JD, Fang C, Watkins PB. Identification of rifampicin-inducible P450IIIA4 (CYP3A4) in human small bowel enterocytes. *J Clin Invest* 1992;90:1871–1878.
17. Cashman JR, Yang Z, Yang L, Wrighton SA. Stereo- and regioselective *N*- and *S*-oxidation of tertiary amines and sulfides in the presence of adult human liver microsomes. *Drug Metab Dispos* 1993;21:492–501.
18. Muralidharan G, Cooper JK, Hawes EM, Korchinski ED, Midha KK. Quinidine inhibits the 7-hydroxylation of chlorpromazine in extensive metabolisers of debrisoquine. *Eur J Clin Pharmacol* 1996;50:121–128.
19. Lin G, Hawes EM, McKay G, Korchinski ED, Midha KK. Metabolism of piperidine-type phenothiazine antipsychotic agents IV: thioridazine in dog, man and rat. *Xenobiotica* 1993;23:1059–1074.
20. von Bahr C, Movin G, Nordin C, et al. Plasma levels of thioridazine and metabolites are influenced by the debrisoquin hydroxylation phenotype. *Clin Pharmacol Ther* 1991;49:234–240.
21. Eap CB, Guentert TW, Schaublin-Loidl M, et al. Plasma levels of the enantiomers of thioridazine, thioridazine 2-sulfoxide, thioridazine 2-sulfone, and thioridazine 5-sulfoxide in poor and extensive metabolizers of dextromethorphan and mephenytoin. *Clin Pharmacol Ther* 1996;59:322–331.
22. Blake BL, Rose RL, Mailman RB, Levi PE, Hodgson E. Metabolism of thioridazine by microsomal monooxygenases: relative roles of P450 and flavin-containing monooxygenase. *Xenobiotica* 1995;25:377–393.
23. Marder SR, Van Putten T, Avavagiri M, et al. Plasma parent drug and metabolites in patients receiving oral and depot fluphenazine. *Psychopharmacol Bull* 1989;25:479–482.
24. Midha KK, Hubbard JW, Marder SR, Marshall BD, Van Putten T. Impact of clinical pharmacokinetics on neuroleptic therapy in patients with schizophrenia. *J Psychiatry Neurosci* 1994;19:254–264.
25. Jann MW, Ereshefsky L, Saklad SR. Clinical pharmacokinetics of the depot antipsychotics. *Clin Pharmacokinet* 1985;10:315–333.
26. Ereshefsky L, Saklad SR, Watanabe MD, Davis CM, Jann MW. Thiothixene pharmacokinetic interactions: a study of hepatic enzyme inducers, clearance inhibitors, and demographic variables. *J Clin Psychopharmacol* 1991;11:296–301.
27. Inaba T, Kovacs J. Haloperidol reductase in human and guinea pig livers. *Drug Metab Dispos* 1989;17:330–333.
28. Tyndale RF, Kalow W, Inaba T. Oxidation of reduced haloperidol to haloperidol: involvement of human P450IID6 (sparteine/debrisoquine monooxygenase). *Br J Clin Pharmacol* 1991;31:655–660.
29. Fang J, Baker GB, Silverstone PH, Coutts RT. Involvement of CYP3A4 and CYP2D6 in the metabolism of haloperidol. *Cell Mol Neurobiol* 1997;17:227–233.
30. Usuki E, Pearce R, Parkinson A, Castagnoli N Jr. Studies on the conversion of haloperidol and its tetrahydropyridine dehydration product to potentially neurotoxic pyridinium metabolites by human liver microsomes. *Chem Res Toxicol* 1996;9:800–806.
31. Linnoila M, Viukari M, Vaisanen K, Auvinen J. Effect of anticonvulsants on plasma haloperidol and thioridazine levels. *Am J Psychiatry* 1980;137:819–821.
32. Migdalof BH, Grindel JM, Heykants JJP, Janssen PAJ. Penfluridol: a neuroleptic drug designed for long duration of action. *Drug Metab Rev* 1979;9:281–299.
33. McCreadie RG, Heykants JJP, Chalmers A, Anderson AM. Plasma pimozide profiles in chronic schizophrenics. *Br J Clin Pharmacol* 1979;7:533–534.
34. Bressolle F, Bres J, Faure-Jeantis A. Absolute bioavailability, rate of absorption, and dose proportionality of sulpiride in humans. *J Pharmacol Sci* 1992;81:26–32.
35. Bressolle F, Bres J, Mourad G. Pharmacokinetics of sulpiride after intravenous administration in patients with impaired renal function. *Clin Pharmacokinet* 1989;17:367–373.
36. Kobari T, Namekawa H, Kato Y, Yamada S. Biotransformation of sultopride in man and several animal species. *Xenobiotica* 1985;15:469–476.
37. Wong SL, Menacherry S, Mulford D, Schmitz PJ, Locke C, Granneman GR. Pharmacokinetics of sertindole and dehydrosertindole in volunteers with normal or impaired renal function. *Eur J Clin Pharmacol* 1997;52:223–227.
38. Dain JG, Nicoletti, Ballard F. Biotransformation of clozapine in humans. *Drug Metab Dispos* 1997;25:603–609.
39. Dahl ML, Llerena A, Bondesson U, Lindstrom L, Bertilsson L. Disposition of clozapine in man: lack of association with debrisoquine and S-mephenytoin hydroxylation polymorphisms. *Br J Clin Pharmacol* 1994;37:71–74.
40. Cooper SF, Dugal R, Bertrand MJ. Determination of loxapine in human plasma and urine and identification of three urinary metabolites. *Xenobiotica* 1979;9:405–414.
41. Fischer V, Vogels B, Maurer G, Tynes RE. The antipsychotic clozapine is metabolized by the polymorphic human microsomal and recombinant cytochrome P450 2D6. *J Pharmacol Exp Ther* 1992;260:1355–1360.
42. Pirmohamed M, Williams D, Madden S, Templeton E, Park BK. Metabolism and bioactivation of clozapine by human liver *in vitro*. *J Pharmacol Exp Ther* 1995;272:984–890.
43. Ring BJ, Catlow J, Lindsay TJ, et al. Identification of the human cytochromes P450 responsible for the *in vitro* formation of the major oxidative metabolites of the antipsychotic agent olanzapine. *J Pharmacol Exp Ther* 1996;276:658–666.
44. Noda K, Suzuki A, Okui H, Noguchi H, Nishiura M, Nishiura N. Pharmacokinetics and metabolism of 2-chloro-11-(2-dimethylaminoethoxy)-dibenzo[b,f]thiepine (Zotepine) in rat, mouse, dog and man. *Arzneimittelforschung* 1979;29:1595–1600.
45. Kondo T, Tanaka O, Otani K, et al. Possible inhibitory effect of diazepam on the metabolism of zotepine: an antipsychotic drug. *Psychopharmacology* 1996;127:311–314.
46. Broly F, Libersa C, Lhermitte M, Dupuis B. Inhibitory studies of mexiletine and dextromethorphan oxidation in human liver microsomes. *Biochem Pharmacol* 1990;39:1045–1053.
47. Grech-Belanger O, Gilbert M, Turgeon J, LeBlanc P. Effect of cigarette smoking on mexiletine kinetics. *Clin Pharmacol Ther* 1985;37:638–643.
48. Brøsen K, Gram LF. Clinical significance of the sparteine/debrisoquine oxidation polymorphism. *Eur J Clin Pharmacol* 1989;36:537–547.
49. Inaba T, Jurima M, Mahon WA, Kalow W. *In vitro* inhibition studies of two isozymes of human liver cytochrome P-450: mephenytoin *p*-hydroxylase and sparteine monooxygenase. *Drug Metab Dispos* 1985;13:443–448.
50. von Bahr C, Spina E, Birgersson C, et al. Inhibition of desmethylimipramine 2-hydroxylation by drugs in human liver microsomes. *Biochem Pharmacol* 1985;34:2501–2505.
51. Dayer P, Desmeules J, Striberni R. *In vitro* forecasting of drugs that may interfere with codeine bioactivation. *Eur J Drug Metab Pharmacokinet* 1992;17:115–120.
52. Jerling M, Dahl ML, Aberg-Wistedt A, et al. The CYP2D6 genotype predicts the oral clearance of the neuroleptic agents perphenazine and zuclopenthixol. *Clin Pharmacol Ther* 1996;59:423–428.
53. Syvahlahti EKG, Lindberg R, Kallio J, De Vocht M. Inhibitory effects of neuroleptics on debrisoquine oxidation in man. *Br J Clin Pharmacol* 1986;22:89–92.
54. Gram LF, Overø KF. Drug interaction: inhibitory effect of neuroleptics on metabolism of tricyclic antidepressants in man. *Br Med J* 1972;1:463–465.

55. Gex-Fabry M, Balant-Gorgia AE, Balant LP. Therapeutic drug monitoring databases for postmarketing surveillance of drug-drug interactions: evaluation of a paired approach for psychotropic medication. *Ther Drug Monit* 1997;19:1–10.

56. Gram LF, Guentert TW, Grange S, Vitisen K, Brøsen K. Moclobemide: a substrate of CYP2C19 and an inhibitor of CYP2C19, CYP2D6, and CYP1A2: a panel study. *Clin Pharmacol Ther* 1995;57:670–677.

57. Vestal RE, Kornhauser DM, Hollifield JW, Shand DG. Inhibition of propranolol metabolism by chlorpromazine. *Clin Pharmacol Ther* 1979;25:19–24.

58. Peet M, Middlemiss DN, Yates RA. Pharmacokinetic interaction between propranolol and chlorpromazine in schizophrenic patients. *Lancet* 1980;2:978.

59. Shaw L, Lennard MS, Tucker GT, Bax NDS, Woods HF. Irreversible binding and metabolism of propranolol by human liver microsomes: relationship to polymorphic oxidation. *Biochem Pharmacol* 1987;36:2283–2288.

60. Spina E, Pacifici GM, von Bahr C, Rane A. Characterization of desmethylimipramine 2-hydroxylation in human foetal and adult liver microsomes. *Acta Pharmacol Toxicol* 1986;58:277–281.

61. Yue QY, Sawe J. Different effects of inhibitors on the *O*- and *N*-demethylation of codeine in human liver microsomes. *Eur J Clin Pharmacol* 1997;52:41–47.

62. Maynard GL, Soni P. Thioridazine interferences with imipramine metabolism and measurement. *Ther Drug Monit* 1996;18:729–731.

63. Hirschowitz J, Bennet JA, Semian FP, Garber D. Thioridazine effect on desipramine plasma levels. *J Clin Psychopharmacol* 1983;3:376–379.

64. Baumann P, Meyer JW, Amey M, et al. Dextromethorphan and mephenytoin phenotyping of patients treated with thioridazine or amitriptyline. *Ther Drug Monit* 1992;14:1–8.

65. Vincent FM. Phenothiazine-induced phenytoin intoxication. *Ann Intern Med* 1980;93:56–57.

66. Veronese ME, Mackenzie PI, Doecke CJ, McManus ME, Miners JO, Birkett DJ. Tolbutamide and phenytoin hydroxylations by cDNA-expressed human liver cytochrome P4502C9. *Biochem Biophys Res Commun* 1991;175:1112–1118.

67. Silver JM, Yudofsky SC, Kogan M, Katz BL. Elevation of thioridazine plasma levels by propranolol. *Am J Psychiatry* 1986;143:1290–1292.

68. Fonne-Pfister R, Meyer UA. Xenobiotic and endobiotic inhibitors of cytochrome P-450db1 function: the target of the debrisoquine/sparteine type polymorphism. *Biochem Pharmacol* 1988;37:3829–3835.

69. Siris SG, Cooper TB, Rifkin AE, Brenner R, Lieberman JA. Plasma imipramine concentrations in patients receiving concomitant fluphenazine decanoate. *Am J Psychiatry* 1982;139:104–108.

70. Bock JL, Nelson JC, Gray S, Jatlow PI. Desipramine hydroxylation: variability and effect of antipsychotic drugs. *Clin Pharmacol Ther* 1983;33:322–328.

71. Linnet K. Comparison of the kinetic interactions of the neuroleptics perphenazine and zuclopenthixol with tricyclic antidepressives. *Ther Drug Monit* 1995;17:308–311.

72. Kragh-Sorensen P, Borga O, Garle M, et al. Effect of simultaneous treatment with low doses of perphenazine on plasma and urine concentrations of nortriptyline and 10-hydroxynortriptyline. *Eur J Clin Pharmacol* 1977;11:479–483.

73. Dahl-Puustinen ML, Liden A, Alm C, Nordin C, Bertilsson L. Disposition of perphenazine is related to polymorphic debrisoquin hydroxylation in human beings. *Clin Pharmacol Ther* 1989;46:78–81.

74. Linnet K, Wiborg O. Steady-state serum concentrations of the neuroleptic perphenazine in relation to CYP2D6 genetic polymorphism. *Clin Pharmacol Ther* 1996;60:41–47.

75. Ishizaki T, Chiba K, Saito M, Kobayashi K, Iizuka R. The effects of neuroleptics (haloperidol and chlorpromazine) on the pharmacokinetics of valproic acid in schizophrenic patients. *J Clin Psychopharmacol* 1984;4:254–261.

76. Llerena A, Dahl M-L, Ekqvist B, Bertilsson L. Haloperidol disposition is dependent on the debrisoquine hydroxylation phenotype: increased plasma levels of the reduced metabolite in poor metabolizers. *Ther Drug Monit* 1992;14:261–264.

77. Gram LF, Debruyne D, Caillard V, Boulenger JP, Lacotte J, Moulin M. Substantial rise in sparteine metabolic ratio during haloperidol treatment. *Br J Clin Pharmacol* 1989;27:272–275.

78. Suzuki A, Otani K, Ishida M, et al. No interaction between desipramine and bromoperidol. *Prog Neuropsychopharmacol Biol Psychiatry* 1996;20:1265–1271.

79. Iwahashi K, Miyatake R, Suwaki H, Hosokawa K, Ichikawa Y. The drug-drug interaction effects of haloperidol on plasma carbamazepine levels. *Clin Neuropharmacol* 1995;18:233–236.

80. Ring BJ, Binkley SN, Vandenbranden M, Wrighton SA. *In vitro* interaction of the antipsychotic agent olanzapine with human cytochromes P450 CYP2C9, CYP2C19, CYP2D6 and CYP3A. *Br J Clin Pharmacol* 1996;41:181–186.

81. Burger A. Isosterism and bioisosterism in drug design. *Prog Drug Res* 1991;37:287–371.

82. Hansch C, Leo A, Unger SH, Kim KH, Nikaitani D, Lien EJ. "Aromatic" substituent constants for structure-activity correlations. *J Med Chem* 1973;16:1207–1216.

83. Bertilsson L, Carrillo JA, Dahl ML, et al. Clozapine disposition covaries with CYP1A2 activity determined by a caffeine test. *Br J Clin Pharmacol* 1994;38:471–473.

84. Odom-White A, de Leon J. Clozapine levels and caffeine. *J Clin Psychiatry* 1996;57:175–176.

85. Vainer JL, Chouinard G. Interaction between caffeine and clozapine. *J Clin Psychopharmacol* 1994;14:284–285.

86. Funderburg LG, Vertrees JE, True JE, Miller AE. Seizure following addition of erythromycin to clozapine treatment. *Am J Psychiatry* 1994;151:1840–1841.

87. Aronowitz JS, Chakos MH, Safferman AZ, Liebman JA. Syncope associated with the combination of clozapine and enalapril. *J Clin Psychopharmacol* 1994;14:429–430.

88. Tyson SC, Devane CL, Risch SC. Pharmacokinetic interaction between risperidone and clozapine. *Am J Psychiatry* 1995;152:1401–1402.

89. Choc MG, Hsuan F, Honigfeld G, et al. Single- vs multiple-dose pharmacokinetics of clozapine in psychiatric patients. *Pharmaceut Res* 1990;7:347–351.

90. Sutton D, Butler AM, Nadin L, Murray M. Role of CYP3A4 in human hepatic diltiazem *N*-demethylation: inhibition of CYP3A4 activity by oxidized diltiazem metabolites. *J Pharmacol Exp Ther* 1997;282:294–300.

91. Abernethy DR, Montamat SC. Acute and chronic studies of diltiazem in elderly versus young hypertensive patients. *Am J Cardiol* 1987;60:116I–120I.

92. Baumann P. Pharmacokinetic-pharmacodynamic relationship of the selective serotonin reuptake inhibitors. *Clin Pharmacokinet* 1996;31:444–469.

93. Murray M, Reidy GF. Selectivity in the inhibition of mammalian cytochromes P-450 by chemical agents. *Pharmacol Rev* 1990;42:85–101.

94. Greenblatt DJ, von Moltke LL, Schmider J, Harmatz JS, Shader RI. Inhibition of human cytochrome P450-3A isoforms by fluoxetine and norfluoxetine: *in vitro* and *in vivo* studies. *J Clin Pharmacol* 1996;36:792–798.

95. Murray M, Reidy GF. *In vitro* inhibition of hepatic drug oxidation by thioridazine: kinetic analysis of the inhibition of cytochrome P-450 isoform-specific reactions. *Biochem Pharmacol* 1989;38:4359–4365.

96. Murray M. Inhibition of hepatic drug metabolism by phenothiazine tranquilizers: quantitative structure-activity relationships and selective inhibition of cytochrome P-450 isoform-specific activities. *Chem Res Toxicol* 1989;2:240–246.

CHAPTER 44

Calcium Channel Blockers

Dagmar Busse and Michel Eichelbaum

INTRODUCTION

Calcium channel blockers are widely prescribed in the treatment of angina pectoris, hypertension, and supraventricular arrhythmias. The frequent and increasing use provides a substantial potential for clinically relevant drug interaction with other coadministered drugs. In fact, drug interactions with calcium channel blockers have been reported in numerous *in vivo* and *in vitro* studies (1–4). The nature of the underlying mechanisms of most of the interactions, however, has not been elucidated in detail. Several mechanisms (concerning both pharmacokinetics and pharmacodynamics) have been identified to be potentially involved and should therefore be considered in the analysis of *in vivo* interaction studies.

This chapter focuses on inhibition of oxidative drug metabolism, which is one of the most frequent and clinically relevant mechanisms by which calcium channel blockers alter the disposition and elimination of coadministered drugs (5). Verapamil and diltiazem, for example, decrease the metabolism of phenazon, which is used as a general marker compound for hepatic oxidative metabolism, thereby indicating their potential to inhibit the cytochrome P450–mediated metabolism of other drugs. In addition, calcium channel blockers are extensively metabolized by the liver (6) and may therefore interfere with the hepatic metabolism of coprescribed drugs through competition for the same routes of biotransformation. In fact, many of the drugs that have been reported to interact are substrates of the same cytochrome P450 enzymes. Besides impairment of drug metabolism, calcium channel blockers have the potential to cause pharmacokinetic interactions by two further mechanisms. Verapamil and several dihydropyridines (e.g., nifedipine, nisoldipine) tend to increase liver blood flow (7,8), which could affect the elimination of drugs with a high hepatic-extraction ratio, resulting in increased bioavailability and enhanced systemic clearance (9). Furthermore, some of the calcium channel blockers (e.g., verapamil, nifedipine) are inhibitors of the P-glycoprotein efflux pump. They may therefore impair the P-glycoprotein–mediated intestinal, biliary, and/or renal secretion of coadministered drugs, thereby altering their disposition and elimination (10,11). This mechanism is likely to play a role in the pharmacokinetic interactions observed with P-glycoprotein substrates such as digoxin (12), paclitaxel (13), and doxorubicin (14). Finally, some of the drug interactions reported for calcium channel blockers can be attributed to additive pharmacologic effects (e.g., with other cardiovascular active drugs like β-blocking agents) or pharmacodynamic interactions caused by the calcium channel blocking activity, in particular at the neuromuscular and central nervous system (CNS) level (e.g., potentiation of the neuromuscular blockade produced by muscle relaxants (15,16)).

PHENYLALKYLAMINES

Verapamil

Numerous *in vitro* and *in vivo* reports indicate the potential of verapamil to inhibit cytochrome P450–dependent oxidative metabolism. In addition, some data suggest that its major plasma metabolite, norverapamil, may also inhibit cytochrome P450.

Verapamil undergoes extensive metabolism by several enzymes of the cytochrome P450 (CYP) family (including CYP3A4, CYP1A2, and CYP2C) to norverapamil and various other *N*- and *O*-dealkylated compounds (see Chapter 24). Serum concentrations of verapamil achieved *in vivo* vary considerably but usually are in the range between 100 and 500 ng/mL (i.e., less than 1 μ*M*) after standard oral medication (17). However, verapamil con-

D. Busse and M. Eichelbaum: Dr. Margarete Fischer-Bosch-Institute for Clinical Pharmacology, Auerbachstrasse 112, D-70376 Stuttgart, Germany

centrations reached at the enzyme active site in the liver may be much higher [in mouse liver, 1,000-fold higher than in plasma (18)], which should be considered when the results of *in vitro* inhibition studies are extrapolated to the clinical situation. In addition, after oral dosing, steady-state levels of norverapamil are of the same order of magnitude as verapamil concentrations and could therefore contribute to cytochrome P450 inhibition *in vivo* (19).

Inhibition of cytochrome P450–dependent drug bio-transformation by verapamil was first suggested by *in vitro* experiments, showing that verapamil was a potent inhibitor of aminopyrine *N*-demethylation in liver microsomes of the mouse (20,21). In the following, the general potential of verapamil and its metabolite norverapamil to influence cytochrome P450–mediated metabolism was demonstrated by their ability to inhibit the biotransformation of antipyrine, used as a marker compound for hepatic oxidative metabolism. *In vitro,* verapamil and norverapamil inhibited total microsomal cytochrome P450–mediated 4-hydroxylation and 3-hydroxylation of antipyrine (22). Accordingly, *in vivo,* verapamil pretreatment was found to reduce the oral clearance (range, 11%–34%) and to prolong the half-life (range, 14%–21%) of antipyrine significantly in a dose- and time-dependent manner, without affecting apparent volume of distribution (8,23–25). The changes in serum antipyrine pharmacokinetics were associated with a decrease in urinary recovery of the three major metabolites (24), which is consistent with impaired antipyrine metabolism. As at least two members of the CYP family are known to participate in the formation of each of the antipyrine metabolites (26,27), no information concerning an isozyme-selective inhibition by verapamil can be obtained from the antipyrine studies. However, inhibition of individual CYP isoforms has been demonstrated in human liver microsomes by the capacity of verapamil to inhibit typical metabolic reactions catalyzed by specific cytochrome P450 enzymes, including CYP3A4, CYP1A2, the CYP2C subfamily, and CYP2D6. Verapamil was a potent inhibitor of taxol 6α-hydroxylation (at 50 μ*M*, 60% inhibition) and of tacrolimus *O*-demethylation (K_i, 82 μ*M*), which are both known to be catalyzed by CYP3A4 (28–30). In addition, verapamil decreased the 3-demethylation of caffeine (at 500 μ*M*, 35% inhibition), thereby indicating its potential to inhibit CYP1A2 (31). Moreover, verapamil competitively inhibited tolbutamide hydroxylation (K_i, 115 μ*M*), which is catalyzed by enzymes of the CYP2C family (32,33). Finally, verapamil had an inhibitory effect on the α-hydroxylation of metoprolol, a pathway mediated by CYP2D6 (34). As the latter is not involved in verapamil metabolism, the inhibitory effect is not likely to result only from competition for the same routes of biotransformation. The ability of verapamil to act directly with cytochrome P450 was confirmed by spectral evidence, showing that verapamil caused a reverse type I change in the difference spectrum, which indicates the binding to be likely at a hydrophilic site of the heme iron (20,21,35).

Consistent with the *in vitro* data, several *in vivo* studies in both healthy volunteers and patients have demonstrated the potential of verapamil to cause drug interactions, probably involving inhibition of drug biotransformation. Verapamil decreases the clearance of a number of other compounds subject to oxidative metabolism in the liver, thereby leading to elevations in serum concentrations and, in some cases, increased toxicity. The most common and clinically relevant *in vivo* drug interactions are discussed in detail in the following and compared with *in vitro* data, if present.

β-Blocking Agents

Lipophilic β-blockers like metoprolol and propranolol undergo extensive hepatic metabolism by cytochrome P450 enzymes (see Chapter 25). In contrast, atenolol is a more hydrophilic compound and is excreted mainly unchanged by the kidneys. Coadministration of verapamil resulted in a significant increase in the plasma concentrations of metoprolol (36,37) and propranolol (38–40), but not of atenolol (41). In healthy volunteers, verapamil significantly reduced the oral clearance of propranolol by about 30%, whereas elimination half-life and systemic clearance were apparently not affected (39). As propranolol is a drug with a high extraction ratio [i.e., the systemic clearance and elimination half-life are both mainly dependent on liver blood flow (9)], these findings are consistent with a decrease in first pass metabolism based on impaired enzyme activity. A similar observation (i.e., a nearly complete reduction of first pass metabolism with coadministration of verapamil) has been reported for metoprolol in dogs (42). Consistent with the reported *in vivo* findings, verapamil significantly decreased the disappearance rate of propranolol in isolated rat hepatocytes (43) and inhibited both the α-hydroxylation and the *O*-demethylation of metoprolol in human liver microsomes, with K_i-estimates in the low micromolar range (34). In summary, the reported data indicate that the clinical and adverse effects observed during the combination therapy of verapamil with metoprolol or propranolol (44) do not exclusively result from additive pharmacologic effects, but may in part be attributed to pharmacokinetic interactions. Such alterations in the disposition may be important in patients particularly sensitive to additional β-blockade.

Carbamazepine

Coadministration of carbamazepine and verapamil resulted in increased carbamazepine levels and neurotoxicity (45–48). For example, Macphee et al. (45) report an increase in free and total carbamazepine levels of 33%

and 46%, respectively, with all patients exhibiting signs of neurotoxicity. Concurrently, the ratio of the principal metabolite (carbamazepine-10,11-epoxide) to parent compound was significantly reduced (−36%). Carbamazepine undergoes almost complete hepatic biotransformation by cytochrome P450 enzymes, predominantly involving CYP3A4 (see Chapter 17). Therefore impairment of carbamazepine metabolism by verapamil is a plausible mechanism for the observed *in vivo* interaction. The use of verapamil in combination with carbamazepine requires appropriate dosage adjustment of carbamazepine, based on clinical and laboratory monitoring.

Cyclosporine

Hypertension is common in renal transplant patients, and calcium channel blockers are effective antihypertensive agents in this situation. Cyclosporine is extensively metabolized by the cytochrome P450 enzyme system (predominantly CYP3A4) to more than 30 metabolites, the major primary metabolites being M1, M17, and M21 (see Chapter 37). In human liver microsomes, verapamil markedly decreased the disappearance rate of cyclosporine (49) and inhibited formation of M17 and M21 by approximately 30% and 28%, respectively, at a concentration of 50 μM (50). Accordingly, several studies and case reports indicated a clinically relevant interaction between verapamil and cyclosporine *in vivo*: coadministration of cyclosporine and verapamil has been shown to result in a two- to four-fold increase in cyclosporine blood levels (51–55) and in a significant decrease in apparent oral clearance (56) of cyclosporine. Systemic clearance of cyclosporine, however, was not significantly altered (57). These findings indicate that oral verapamil is likely to increase the bioavailability of cyclosporine by inhibiting its first pass metabolism, which is known to occur to a considerable extent in the liver and the gut-wall mucosa (58–60). Besides CYP3A4, a second component influencing intestinal disposition of cyclosporine is the activity of P-glycoprotein (61). The alterations in oral pharmacokinetics of cyclosporine may therefore additionally involve verapamil-induced modulation of intestinal P-glycoprotein. In the clinical setting, the combination of verapamil with cyclosporine requires careful dose adjustment of the latter, based on clinical and laboratory monitoring. As the oral dose of cyclosporine to maintain specific whole-blood concentrations is significantly lower during coadministration of verapamil (the dose may be reduced by one third), drug costs are significantly reduced (57).

Ethanol

In vitro experiments with human liver microsomes and liver cytosol, respectively, showed no effect of verapamil (50–1,000 μM) on either CYP2E1 or alcohol dehydrogenase (ADH) activity (62). Norverapamil, the main metabolite of verapamil, did not influence ADH activity as well, but had an inhibitory effect on CYP2E1 (at 1 mM, decrease in enzyme activity to 67% of control activity). Consistent with *in vitro* data, a single dose of verapamil failed to show any effect on ethanol pharmacokinetics (63,64). In contrast, a 5-day pretreatment with verapamil resulted in an increase in peak ethanol concentrations (+17%) and area under the curve (AUC; +30%) compared with placebo (65). After oral dosing of verapamil, steady-state levels of norverapamil have been found to be equal to or greater than verapamil levels (19). Although the serum concentrations of norverapamil reached *in vivo* are lower than those used in the *in vitro* experiments, a norverapamil-induced inhibition of CYP2E1 may be in part responsible for the increased ethanol levels observed during long-term treatment with verapamil.

Imipramine

Pretreatment with verapamil resulted in a significant increase of the imipramine AUC (+15%) and in a reduction of the apparent oral clearance (−25%) (66). Imipramine undergoes hepatic oxidative metabolism by the cytochrome P450 system, involving CYP2D6, CYP1A2, CYP2C19, and CYP3A4 (67) (see Chapter 18). As verapamil has demonstrated the potential to inhibit each of these CYP isoforms, the observed *in vivo* interaction may result from inhibition of imipramine metabolism. However, plasma concentrations and apparent renal clearance of the major imipramine metabolites (i.e., 2-hydroxy-imipramine, desipramine, and 2-hydroxydesipramine) were not altered with verapamil (66). The authors suggested that the increased bioavailability of imipramine may be due to impaired formation of additional, nonaccounted for metabolites (i.e., the *N*-oxide and didemethylated metabolite). The ultimate underlying mechanism for the observed *in vivo* interaction remains to be clarified.

Midazolam

Midazolam is a widely used short-acting hypnotic, which undergoes extensive hepatic metabolism primarily mediated by cytochromes of the CYP3A subfamily (68). Midazolam 1′-hydroxylation, a major metabolic pathway of midazolam biotransformation, was inhibited by verapamil in human liver microsomes (IC$_{50}$, 100 μM) (69). *In vivo*, coadministration of verapamil with midazolam resulted in a three-fold increase in the AUC of midazolam, a doubling of the peak concentrations, and a prolongation of the elimination half-life compared with placebo (70). The pharmacokinetic changes were associated with profound and prolonged sedative effects. According to the authors, the dosage of midazolam should be reduced up to 50% when used concurrently with verapamil.

Prazosin

An enhanced hypotensive effect has been observed during combination therapy of verapamil with the peripheral α_1-antagonist prazosin, more pronounced than when either drug was used alone. A pharmacologic investigation demonstrated that verapamil coadministration resulted in an increased peak concentration (55%–100%) and AUC (45%–80%) of prazosin (71,72), but did not significantly alter its elimination half-life. Prazosin is extensively metabolized in the liver (primarily by O-demethylation, which suggests involvement of cytochrome P450 enzymes) and has a high first pass effect (73). The mechanisms for the verapamil-induced increase in prazosin bioavailability remain unclear, but besides changes in liver blood flow, reduced first pass metabolism resulting from impaired enzyme activity may play a role.

Quinidine

In healthy volunteers, pretreatment with verapamil significantly reduced the oral clearance (−30%) and prolonged the half-life (+30%) of quinidine. In addition, coadministration of verapamil resulted in a marked decrease (60%–70%) in urinary recovery of 3-hydroxyquinidine, a major product of quinidine biotransformation (74). Quinidine undergoes extensive hepatic oxidative metabolism, mainly involving CYP3A4 (75) (see Chapter 28). The reported in vivo data suggest that verapamil could interfere with the CYP3A4-mediated oxidative metabolism of quinidine. As quinidine has recently been shown to be a substrate of P-glycoprotein in vitro, verapamil may additionally alter the disposition of quinidine by inhibiting possible P-glycoprotein–mediated absorption and/or elimination processes (see Chapter 28). The overall clinical significance of the verapamil/quinidine interaction is not clear. According to a case report, the verapamil-induced changes in quinidine concentrations could result in increased toxicity (76). Therefore patients should be closely monitored, and dose adjustments of quinidine may be required.

Theophylline

In vitro studies with human liver microsomes demonstrated that verapamil competitively inhibited all three major pathways of theophylline metabolism [i.e., the 1-demethylation, 3-demethylation, and 8-hydroxylation (77)], which is consistent with the documented potential of verapamil to interfere with CYP1A2 (31). In vivo, several case reports and pharmacokinetic studies have indicated that coadministration of verapamil increases theophylline plasma concentrations, reduces its systemic and apparent oral clearance (−11% to 20%), and increases its elimination half-life, without altering the volume of distribution (23,77–82). The effect varied considerably and appeared to be dose related (79). The pharmacokinetic

changes of serum theophylline were associated with a reduction in urinary recovery of theophylline metabolites (23,81) and an increase in renal excretion of unchanged parent compound (81), which is consistent with inhibition of metabolism. The extent of the verapamil/theophylline interaction is expected to be of minor clinical importance in the majority of the patients. However, theophylline concentrations should be monitored with coadministration of verapamil, especially in patients with theophylline concentrations in the upper end of the therapeutic range.

Others

In contrast to verapamil, there is little information concerning pharmacokinetic interactions of gallopamil and tiapamil with other drugs, and in particular, no relevant data regarding inhibition of oxidative metabolism have been reported.

BENZOTHIAZEPINES: DILTIAZEM

A reduction in hepatic oxidative enzyme activity during diltiazem treatment is well established, and most of the pharmacokinetic drug interactions involving diltiazem have been attributed to inhibition of cytochrome P450–mediated drug metabolism.

The capacity of diltiazem to inhibit microsomal drug oxidation was first reported by Renton (20), showing that diltiazem competitively inhibits aminopyrine N-demethylation in liver microsomes of the mouse. More recently, diltiazem metabolites have been implicated in P450 inhibition (84–86). Diltiazem is extensively metabolized in the liver into a host of metabolites, primarily by deacetylation and demethylation by CYP3A4 [(86); see Chapter 24]. In human liver microsomes, the N-demethylated metabolites N-desmethyl-diltiazem and N,N-didesmethyl-diltiazem (but not deacetyl-diltiazem) were inhibitors of CYP3A4-mediated testosterone 6β-hydroxylation and even more potent than diltiazem (at 50 μM, the IC$_{50}$ was 120, 11, and 0.6 μM for diltiazem, N-desmethyl-, and N,N-didesmethyl-diltiazem, respectively) (86). Multiple oral dosing results in a prolongation of the elimination half-life of diltiazem and in an increase of its bioavailability (87–89), which may be due to inhibition of diltiazem biotransformation by diltiazem itself or by accumulated metabolites. In fact, a significant accumulation of N-desmethyl-diltiazem has been reported to occur during prolonged diltiazem therapy [mean trough plasma level was approximately 50% that of the parent drug (87,88)], indicating that this metabolite may contribute to enzyme inhibition under a multiple-dose regimen in vivo. The capacity of diltiazem and N-desmethyl-diltiazem to generate a reversible binding interaction with ferric P450 was demonstrated by difference spectra: in liver microsomes of the rat/mouse, diltiazem caused a type I and N-desmethyl-diltiazem a type II spectral change (20,21,85).

Similar to verapamil, diltiazem inhibited metabolism of antipyrine, the most commonly used model drug to assess hepatic drug oxidation. *In vivo,* diltiazem significantly reduced the oral clearance (13%–33%) and prolonged the half-life (13%–47%) of antipyrine, without affecting apparent volume of distribution (8,23,90–93). In addition, urinary recovery of unchanged antipyrine was significantly increased (90,92), and the formation clearance of the three major metabolites reduced by 20% to 40% (23,90,91,93). Some authors reported a selective inhibitory effect on specific oxidative pathways (23,93), whereas others found a similar reduction in the formation rate constants of all three metabolites (90,91). In human liver microsomes, diltiazem and *N*-desmethyl-diltiazem selectively inhibited CYP3A4, but did not affect CYP1A2, CYP2C9, and CYP2E1 (as measured by testosterone 6β-hydroxylation, 7-ethylresorufin *O*-demethylation, tolbutamide methyl-hydroxylation, and aniline 4-hydroxylation, respectively) (86). In addition, diltiazem significantly increased the metabolic ratio of debrisoquine (urinary excretion of debrisoquine/4-hydroxydebrisoquine) (93), thereby indicating its potential to interfere with CYP2D6.

In the clinical setting, a number of pharmacokinetic interactions for diltiazem with other drugs, whose main route of elimination is P450-dependent oxidative metabolism, have been reported. The documented interactions mainly include CYP3A4 and CYP2D6 substrates, which is consistent with the preferential inhibition of these isozymes. As diltiazem seems to have no significant effect on liver blood flow (8,94), the induced changes in metabolism of high-extraction drugs observed *in vivo* can principally be attributed to alterations in enzyme activity.

β-Blocking Agents

Similar to verapamil, combined therapy with diltiazem significantly increased the AUC of metoprolol (about 30%) and propranolol (range, 30%–50%), but did not affect the pharmacokinetics of atenolol (39,95). In addition, oral clearance of propranolol was reduced by diltiazem (about 25%) (39), with no major changes in the elimination half-life (39,95). *In vitro,* diltiazem dose-dependently inhibited the disappearance rate of propranolol in isolated rat hepatocytes (43).

Carbamazepine

Concomitant administration of diltiazem has been reported to increase carbamazepine concentrations up to 40% to 50%, thereby resulting in enhanced neurotoxicity and necessitating a dose reduction up to 60% (48,96–98). Carbamazepine is a CYP3A4 substrate (see Chapter 17), and the most probable mechanism for this interaction is impairment of carbamazepine metabolism by diltiazem. It is recommended to monitor carbamazepine concentrations and clinical signs of carbamazepine toxicity carefully when this drug is combined with diltiazem.

Cyclosporine

Diltiazem is often coprescribed with cyclosporine in renal transplant patients to reduce transplant ischemia and to treat concomitant diseases such as hypertension and angina. Numerous case reports and clinical studies have reported a pharmacokinetic interaction between diltiazem and the CYP3A4 substrate cyclosporine, although a recent case report suggested that this interaction does not occur in all the patients (99). Diltiazem coadministration significantly increased cyclosporine blood levels (100–105) and reduced its systemic clearance (−27%) (57). In addition, a significant accumulation of M17, a major primary cyclosporine metabolite with immunosuppressive activity, has been observed during concomitant diltiazem therapy (104,106,107). It has been suggested that this may result from inhibition of succeeding metabolic steps, leading to formation of the secondary metabolites M8 and M18 (104). In contrast to multiple dosing, a single dose of diltiazem did not alter cyclosporine kinetics (108), which supports the findings that diltiazem metabolites contribute to the enzyme-inhibiting effect (84–86). Evaluation of cyclosporine metabolism in human liver microsomes by coincubation with diltiazem showed a decrease in the disappearance rate of cyclosporine (49) and a noncompetitive inhibition for the generation of M1 and M17, with K_i estimates of 70 and 100 μ*M*, respectively (50,104). However, diltiazem concentrations used for *in vitro* inhibition exceeded those usually reached in plasma [less than 1 μ*M* (88)]. The discrepancy could be due, for example, to hepatic tissue uptake, leading to higher diltiazem concentrations at the enzyme active site than in plasma or/and to the accumulation of enzyme-inhibiting metabolites of diltiazem during a multiple-dose regimen. Despite the pharmacokinetic interaction, only few case reports of increased nephrotoxicity have been reported during combined therapy of diltiazem with cyclosporine (101,109), which is possibly due to the apparent protective effect of diltiazem in renal transplant patients (110). However, cyclosporine concentrations should be monitored carefully, especially during initiation and discontinuation of concomitant diltiazem therapy. The interaction of diltiazem with cyclosporine decreases cyclosporine dosage requirements by approximately 30% (102,105,106,111–115), thereby leading to significant cost savings (102,116,117).

Imipramine and Nortriptyline

Diltiazem has been shown to increase the AUC (+30%) and to decrease the oral clearance (−35%) of the tricyclic antidepressant imipramine (66). Imipramine is highly metabolized by several CYP isozymes, including

CYP2D6 and CYP3A4, the two cytochromes that are preferentially inhibited by diltiazem and its metabolites [(67); see Chapter 18]. Therefore impairment of hepatic oxidative metabolism is a likely explanation for the observed increase in the bioavailability of imipramine when given concomitantly with diltiazem. A recent case report suggested that diltiazem also affects oral pharmacokinetics of the tricyclic antidepressant nortriptyline, which is as well a high-extraction drug that is metabolized mainly by CYP2D6 (see Chapter 18). Coadministration of diltiazem significantly increased the plasma concentrations of orally administered nortriptyline, suggesting decreased presystemic elimination (118). Caution is warranted when combining diltiazem with imipramine or nortriptyline.

Midazolam and Triazolam

A clinically relevant pharmacokinetic interaction of diltiazem has been reported with the short-acting hypnotic agents midazolam and triazolam, which are both substrates of CYP3A4. Diltiazem significantly increased the AUC (two- to three-fold) and the elimination half-life (two- to three-fold) of orally administered midazolam and triazolam, which was accompanied by increased and prolonged sedative effects (70,119,120). According to the authors' suggestion, care should be taken in the use of midazolam and triazolam in patients receiving diltiazem.

Nifedipine

Dual calcium channel blocker therapy is rarely used in clinical practice. However, combined therapy with diltiazem and the dihydropyridine nifedipine has been reported to be effective in variant angina (121) and in patients with effort angina pectoris (122). In healthy volunteers, marked changes in the pharmacokinetics of nifedipine were observed in relation to diltiazem pretreatment. Diltiazem caused a dose-dependent increase in the serum concentrations of nifedipine (two- to three-fold increase in the AUC), prolonged its elimination half-life (+30%–40%), and reduced its oral clearance (−60%), which resulted in an increased antihypertensive effect when compared with single treatment with either drug (96,123–125). Nifedipine is a CYP3A4 substrate (see Chapter 24), and impairment of nifedipine metabolism is the most likely explanation for this interaction. The assumption is further supported by the fact that diltiazem pretreatment decreased the AUC ratio of the primary nifedipine metabolite to parent compound (96).

Theophylline

CYP1A2, the major enzyme involved in theophylline metabolism, was not markedly inhibited by diltiazem and its N-demethylated metabolites in vitro (88). In agree-

ment, concurrent administration of theophylline and diltiazem has been reported to have no significant effect on the pharmacokinetics of single intravenous or multiple oral theophylline doses (23,126,127). However, other authors found that diltiazem modestly but significantly reduced total oral (−12%) and systemic clearance (−20%) of theophylline and increased its elimination half-life (+11%–24%) (84,128–130). The fractional clearances of the three major urinary theophylline metabolites indicated that diltiazem selectively decreased the metabolic clearance of 1,3-dimethyl uric acid (1,3-DMU), without affecting the formation rate of 1-methyl uric acid and 3-methylxanthine (23,129). According to recent in vitro results, in addition to CYP1A2, CYP2E1 plays a minor role for formation of 1,3-DMU but not for the other theophylline metabolites (131). However, in human liver microsomes, diltiazem and N-desmethyl-diltiazem did not affect CYP2E1 (88). Further studies are needed to clarify this issue.

Quinidine

Pretreatment with diltiazem has been reported to reduce the oral clearance significantly (−36%) and to prolong the elimination half-life (+27%) of the CYP3A4 substrate quinidine, resulting in significant pharmacodynamic changes (132). In contrast, other authors found no alteration in the kinetics of either drug during coadministration (133). More studies with these two agents are needed to confirm the extent of this interaction.

Additional pharmacokinetic interactions of diltiazem, possibly based on inhibition of metabolism, but of little clinical significance, have been reported with warfarin (134), encainide (135), and moricizine (136).

DIHYDROPYRIDINES

In contrast to diltiazem and verapamil, the dihydropyridines generally have a less-documented inhibitory effect on oxidative metabolism. Moreover, several dihydropyridines tend to increase liver blood flow (7,8,137), which complicates the analysis of in vivo pharmacokinetic interactions with high-extraction drugs.

In vitro inhibition of cytochrome P450-dependent metabolic pathways has been documented for some of the dihydropyridines: in rat liver microsomes, isradipine, nifedipine, and darodipine were inhibitors of the aminopyrine N-demethylation and produced a change in the difference spectrum, thereby indicating their ability to interact with P450 (21). Furthermore, amlodipine, isradipine, nicardipine, and nifedipine impaired metabolism of propranolol in isolated rat hepatocytes, with nicardipine and isradipine more potent than the other dihydropyridines and even more potent than verapamil and diltiazem (45). In human liver microsomes, nifedipine inhibited tolbutamide hydroxylation (K_i, 11 μM) (32) and theophylline demethylations (79), thereby indicating its ability to interfere with CYP2C9 and CYP1A2, respectively. In addition, nicardipine and nifedipine, which are both CYP3A4 substrates (see Chapter 24), competitively inhibited the CYP3A4-dependent metabolism of midazolam (71) and cyclosporine (138), with K_i estimates ranging between 5 and 10 μM. Henricsson et al. (51) found nifedipine to be as potent in inhibiting *in vitro* metabolism of cyclosporine as verapamil or diltiazem, whereas Brockmoeller et al. (104) reported that the effect was much less with nifedipine and from the competitive type (in contrast to noncompetitive inhibition by verapamil and diltiazem).

The inhibitory effect of nifedipine documented *in vitro* is not observed to any significant extent *in vivo*: the clearance of antipyrine was not altered by nifedipine (8,139, 140), and no relevant metabolic drug interactions with nifedipine have been reported in the clinical setting. The reason for this discrepancy remains unclear, but could possibly be attributed to differences in hepatic tissue uptake, leading to high concentrations at the enzyme active site in the liver for verapamil but not for nifedipine, for example (16). In contrast, the inhibitory *in vitro* effect of nicardipine on cyclosporine metabolism was confirmed by a clinically relevant interaction *in vivo* (141), suggesting that nicardipine may achieve sufficiently high concentrations in the liver to impair CYP3A4-dependent pathways competitively . No clinically important interactions involving oxidative drug metabolism have been reported for amlodipine, felodipine, isradipine, nimodipine, and nitrendipine (1–3,5,142).

β-Blocking Agents

Several dihydropyridines, including felodipine (143), isradipine (144), nisoldipine (145), nicardipine (146,147), and nifedipine (148,149), have been reported to increase the peak concentrations and the AUC of oral metoprolol or propranolol. In all cases, the interaction did not result in relevant pharmacodynamic changes. Apart from the study with felodipine, the investigations were carried out with single doses of the dihydropyridines, and the increased bioavailability was more attributed to a transient increase in liver blood flow rather than to inhibition of oxidative metabolism (147). In contrast to single-dose treatment, multiple-dose administration of nisoldipine did not alter the pharmacokinetics of oral propranolol (150).

Cyclosporine

In vitro experiments with human liver microsomes clearly indicated the potential of nifedipine and nicardipine to inhibit the metabolism of cyclosporine competitively, with K_i-estimates of 10 and 8 μM, respectively (51,52,138). Consistent with the *in vitro* results, nicardip-

ine led to a considerable increase in cyclosporine concentrations *in vivo* (141), resulting in a 30% reduction in daily dosage requirement and consequently in a significant cost containment (151). In contrast, nifedipine had no clinically relevant effect on the *in vivo* pharmacokinetics of cyclosporine in adults (1–5). However, a study in pediatric renal transplant patients suggested that nifedipine may impair cyclosporine elimination in children (152). Isradipine, nifedipine, nitrendipine, and felodipine had little, if any, effect on cyclosporine blood concentrations during concurrent therapy (1–5,153,154).

Tacrolimus

In human liver microsomes, nifedipine was found to inhibit competitively the CYP3A4-mediated metabolism of the immunosuppressant agent tacrolimus, with a K_i for tacrolimus *O*-demethylation of 12 μM (29). *In vivo*, a significant decrease (up to 30%) in the daily and cumulative dosage requirement of tacrolimus was reported in a recent retrospective study (155). According to the authors, blood concentrations of tacrolimus should be monitored during coadministration of nifedipine, as downward adjustment of dose may be required. Prospective pharmacokinetic studies are needed to confirm the extent of this interaction.

Theophylline

In vitro studies found that nifedipine was an inhibitor of theophylline 1- and 3-demethylation, but not of 8-hydroxylation (156). *In vivo* case reports suggest an increase in theophylline concentrations related to nifedipine dosage (157,158). However, minor or lacking effects of nifedipine on theophylline disposition have been reported in prospective studies (84,127,140,159,160). Only Robson et al. (156) were able to discern a modest decrease (9%) in mean total theophylline clearance due to decreased clearances by 1- and 3-demethylation. The equivocal findings suggest no clinically significant interaction between nifedipine and theophylline. Isradipine had no effect on theophylline pharmacokinetics (161), and felodipine was found to even decrease theophylline concentrations, probably by reducing the absorption (162).

Quinidine

Concurrent therapy with nifedipine or felodipine did not significantly alter the pharmacokinetics of the CYP3A4 substrate quinidine (163,164).

OTHERS

Little published work concerns inhibition of oxidative drug metabolism by the newer nondihydropyridine calcium channel blocker *bepridil,* a diarylaminopropylamine derivative (165).

In contrast, the tetralol derivative *mibefradil* was recently voluntarily withdrawn from the market almost exactly 1 year after the drug had been given marketing approval for Europe and the United States, as a result of several reports on potentially harmful drug interactions. Mibefradil is a selective T-type calcium channel antagonist and therefore pharmacologically represents a new molecule, which led to its classification as an additional category of calcium channel antagonist. The drug is virtually completely metabolized by esterase-catalyzed hydrolysis and CYP3A4-mediated oxidation (166). *In vitro* studies on human liver microsomes have shown that it is not only a substrate of CYP3A4, but also a potent inhibitor of CYP3A4 and CYP2D6 and hence likely to affect the pharmacokinetics of concomitant drugs *in vivo,* whose metabolism predominantly depends on these two isozymes (166,167). When mibefradil entered the market in the middle of 1997, *in vivo* drug interactions with several compounds were already described, among them the CYP3A4 substrates cyclosporine, terfenadine, and quinidine, as well as the CYP2D6 substrate metoprolol. After oral dosing, plasma concentrations of these drugs were considerably increased with concomitant mibefradil when compared with baseline values (166,167). These interactions did not result in major alterations of the pharmacodynamic effects of metoprolol and quinidine, but the increase in the plasma levels of cyclosporine and terfenadine is likely to be of clinical relevance because of the narrow therapeutic range of the immunosuppressant and the potentially dangerous QT_c interval prolongation with increased concentrations of terfenadine, respectively. Although there were no specific interaction studies with astemizole and cisapride, the labeling of mibefradil specifically stated that both compounds could also be expected to accumulate to dangerous levels if coadministered with this new calcium channel blocker, thereby (as with terfenadine) increasing the risk of QT_c interval prolongation as serious side effects. In the following, interactions with the 3-hydroxy-3-methylglutaryl–coenzyme A (HMG-CoA) reductase inhibitors simvastatin and lovastatin (which both depend on CYP3A4 for their metabolic clearance) were reported to result in a risk of potentially life-threatening muscle injury (rhabdomyolysis) (168). From spontaneous reports and ongoing trials, additional adverse reactions related to coadministration of mibefradil with several other drugs were continuously reported, finally resulting in a list of more than 25 drugs known to be potentially dangerous if used with mibefradil (169). The seriousness of the side effects and the complexity of the prescribing information needed in this case ultimately motivated the voluntary withdrawal of mibefradil from the market in June 1998.

CONCLUSION

The phenylalkylamine verapamil and the benzothiazepine diltiazem both inhibit oxidative drug metabolism catalyzed by cytochrome P450 enzymes, both *in vitro* and *in vivo*. Verapamil interacts with several CYP isozymes (including CYP1A2, CYP2C, CYP3A4, and CYP2D6), whereas diltiazem preferentially inhibits CYP3A4 and CYP2D6. The magnitude of the effect (particularly at high doses) is sufficient to warrant caution when administering these two calcium channel antagonists in combination with others drugs whose main route of elimination is P450-dependent oxidative metabolism. In particular, in drugs with a narrow therapeutic index, the increase in drug level can be of clinical relevance (e.g., with carbamazepine, quinidine, or cyclosporine). On the other hand, economic benefits arise from the decrease in the required dosage of cyclosporine, for example, when coadministered with diltiazem or verapamil. In the case of the tetralol-derivative mibefradil, a new selective T-type calcium channel antagonist that was approved in June 1997, the intensity of its inhibition of CYP3A4 and CYP2D6 resulted in so many clinically relevant drug interactions that mibefradil was finally voluntarily withdrawn from the market within 1 year after launch. The dihydropyridines (e.g., nifedipine, nicardipine, nisoldipine, nitrendipine, felodipine, amlodipine, and isradipine) generally have minor or negligible effects on oxidative metabolism of other drugs. They may therefore represent an alternative to verapamil and diltiazem when a calcium channel blocker is added to a given medication, and no interactions are desirable. No metabolic drug interactions have been documented so far for the second-generation phenylalkylamines (gallopamil, tiapamil) and the diarylaminopropylamine derivative bepridil.

REFERENCES

1. Schlanz KD, Myre SA, Bottorff MB. Pharmacokinetic interactions with calcium channel antagonists (Pt I). *Clin Pharmacokinet* 1991;21: 344–356.
2. Schlanz KD, Myre SA, Bottorff MB. Pharmacokinetic interactions with calcium channel antagonists (Pt II). *Clin Pharmacokinet* 1991; 21:448–460.
3. Rosenthal T, Ezra D. Calcium antagonists: drug interactions of clinical significance. *Drug Safety* 1995;13:157–187.
4. Hansten PD, Horn JR. *Drug interactions and updates quarterly.* Vancouver, WA: Lea & Febiger, Applied Therapeutics Inc., 1993.
5. Hung BA, Self TH, Lalonde RL, Bottorff MB. Calcium channel blockers as inhibitors of drug metabolism. *Chest* 1989;96:393–399.
6. Kelly JG, O'Malley K. Clinical pharmacokinetics of calcium antagonists. *Clin Pharmacokinet* 1992;22:416–433.
7. Meredith PA, Elliott HL, Pasanisi F, Kelman AW, Sumner DJ, Reid JL. Verapamil pharmacokinetics and apparent hepatic and renal blood flow. *Br J Clin Pharmacol* 1985;20:101–106.
8. Bauer LA, Stenwall M, Horn JR, Davis R, Opheim K, Greene L. Changes in antipyrine and indocyanine green kinetics during nifedipine, verapamil, and diltiazem therapy. *Clin Pharmacol Ther* 1986;40: 239–242.

9. Wilkinson GR, Shand DG. A physiological approach to hepatic drug clearance. *Clin Pharmacol Ther* 1975;18:377–390.

10. Fisher GA, Lum BL, Hausdorff J, Sikic BI. Pharmacological considerations in the modulation of multidrug resistance. *Eur J Cancer* 1996;32:1082–1088.

11. Relling MV. Are the major effects of P-glycoprotein modulators due to altered pharmacokinetics of anticancer drugs? *Ther Drug Monit* 1996;18:350–356.

12. Tanigawara Y, Okamura N, Hirai M, et al. Transport of digoxin by human P-glycoprotein in a porcine kidney epithelial cell line. *J Pharmacol Exp Ther* 1992;263:840–845.

13. Berg SL, Tocher A, O'Shaughnessy JA, et al. Effect of R-verapamil on the pharmacokinetics of paclitaxel in women with breast cancer. *J Clin Oncol* 1995;13:2039–2042.

14. Kerr DJ, Graham J, Cummings J, et al. The effect of verapamil on the pharmacokinetics of Adriamycin. *Cancer Chemother Pharmacol* 1986;18:239–242.

15. Jones RM, Cashman JN, Casson WR, Broadbent MP. Verapamil potentiation of neuromuscular blockade: failure of reversal with neostigmine but prompt reversal with edrophonium. *Anesth Analg* 1985;64:1021–1025.

16. Hamann SR, Todd GD, McAllister RG Jr. The pharmacology of verapamil. V: Tissue distribution of verapamil and norverapamil in rat and dog. *Pharmacology* 1983;27:1–8.

17. Echizen H, Eichelbaum M. Clinical pharmacokinetics of verapamil, nifedipine and diltiazem. *Clin Pharmacokinet* 1986;11:425–449.

18. Sekerci S, Tulunay M. Interactions of calcium channel blockers with non-depolarising muscle relaxants in vitro. *Anaesthesia* 1996;51:140–144.

19. Woodcock BG, Hopf R, Kaltenbach M. Verapamil and norverapamil plasma concentrations during long-term therapy in patients with hypertrophic obstructive cardiomyopathy. *J Cardiovasc Pharmacol* 1980;2:17–23.

20. Renton KW. Inhibition of hepatic microsomal drug metabolism by the calcium channel blockers diltiazem and verapamil. *Biochem Pharmacol* 1985;34:2549–2553.

21. Maenpaa J, Ruskoaho H, Pelkonen O. Inhibition of hepatic microsomal drug metabolism in rats by five calcium antagonists. *Pharmacol Toxicol* 1989;64:446–450.

22. Egan JM, Abernethy DR, Hughes H. Mechanisms of verapamil-mediated inhibition of drug oxidation. *Fed Proc* 1986;45:446.

23. Abernethy DR, Egan JM, Dickinson TH, Carrum G. Substrate-selective inhibition of verapamil and diltiazem: differential disposition of antipyrine and theophylline in humans. *J Pharmacol Exp Ther* 1988;244:994–999.

24. Bach D, Blevins R, Kerner N, Rubenfire M, Edwards DJ. The effect of verapamil on antipyrine pharmacokinetics and metabolism in man. *Br J Clin Pharmacol* 1986;21:655–659.

25. Rumiantsev DO, Piotrovskii VK, Riabokon OS, Slastnikova ID, Kokurina EV, Metelitsa VI. The effect of oral verapamil therapy on antipyrine clearance. *Br J Clin Pharmacol* 1986;22:606–609.

26. Engel G, Hofmann U, Heidemann H, Cosme J, Eichelbaum M. Antipyrine as a probe for human oxidative drug metabolism: identification of the cytochrome P450 enzymes catalyzing 4-hydroxyantipyrine, 3-hydroxymethylantipyrine, and norantipyrine formation. *Clin Pharmacol Ther* 1996;59:613–623.

27. Sharer JE, Wrighton SA. Identification of the human hepatic cytochromes P450 involved in the in vivo oxidation of antipyrine. *Drug Metab Dispos* 1996;24:487–494.

28. Kumar GN, Walle UK, Walle T. Cytochrome P450 3A-mediated human liver microsomal taxol 6 alpha-hydroxylation. *J Pharmacol Exp Ther* 1994;68:1160–1165.

29. Lampen A, Christians U, Guengerich FP, et al. Metabolism of the immunosuppressant tacrolimus in the small intestine: cytochrome P450, drug interactions, and interindividual variability. *Drug Metab Dispos* 1995;23:1315–1324.

30. Sattler M, Guengerich FP, Yun CY, Christians U, Sewing KF. Cytochrome P-450A4 is responsible for biotransformation of FK506 and rapamycin in man and rat. *Drug Metab Dispos* 1992;20:753–761.

31. Fuhr U, Woodcock BG, Siewert M. Verapamil and drug metabolism by the cytochrome P450 isoform CYP1A2. *Eur J Clin Pharmacol* 1992;42:463–464.

32. Miners JO, Smith KJ, Robson RA, McManus ME, Veronese ME, Birkett DJ. Tolbutamide hydroxylation by human liver microsomes: kinetic characterisation and relationship to other cytochrome P-450 dependent xenobiotic oxidations. *Biochem Pharmacol* 1988;37:1137–1144.

33. Veronese ME, Mackenzie PI, Doecke CJ, McManus ME, Miners JO, Birkett DJ. Tolbutamide and phenytoin hydroxylations by cDNA-expressed human liver cytochrome P4502C9. *Biochem Biophys Res Commun* 1991;175:1112–1118.

34. Kim M, Shen DD, Eddy AC, Nelson WL. Inhibition of the enantioselective oxidative metabolism of metoprolol by verapamil in human liver microsomes. *Drug Metab Dispos* 1993;21:309–317.

35. Kawahara M, Akita S, Fujii K, Morio M. Effect of the calcium channel blocking agents on the reductive metabolism of halothane. *J Appl Toxicol* 1991;11:29–31.

36. McLean AJ, Knight R, Harrison PM, Harper RW. Clearance-based oral drug interaction between verapamil and metoprolol and comparison with atenolol. *Am J Cardiol* 1985;55:1628–1629.

37. Keech AC, Harper RW, Harrison PM, Pitt A, McLean AJ. Pharmacokinetic interaction between oral metoprolol and verapamil for angina pectoris. *Am J Cardiol* 1986;58:551–552.

38. McCourty JC, Silas JH, Tucker GT, Lennard MS. The effect of combined therapy on the pharmacokinetics and pharmacodynamics of verapamil and propranolol in patients with angina pectoris. *Br J Clin Pharmacol* 1988;25:349–357.

39. Hunt BA, Bottorff MB, Herring VL, Self TH, Lalonde RL. Effects of calcium channel blockers on the pharmacokinetics of propranolol stereoisomers. *Clin Pharmacol Ther* 1990;47:584–591.

40. Murdoch DL, Thomson GD, Thompson GG, Murray GD, Brodie MJ, McInnes GT. Evaluation of potential pharmacodynamic and pharmacokinetic interactions between verapamil and propranolol in normal subjects. *Br J Clin Pharmacol* 1991;31:323–332.

41. Keech AC, Harper RW, Harrison PM, Pitt A, McLean AJ. Extent and pharmacokinetic mechanisms of oral atenolol-verapamil interaction in man. *Eur J Clin Pharmacol* 1988;35:363–366.

42. Murthy SS, Nelson WL, Shen DD, Power JM, Cahill CM, McLean AJ. Pharmacokinetic interactions between verapamil and metoprolol in the dog: stereochemical aspects. *Drug Metab Dispos* 1991;19:1093–1100.

43. Vercruysse I, Vermeulen AM, Belpaire FM, Massart DL, Dupont AG. The effect of different calcium antagonists and a calcium agonist on the metabolism of propranolol by isolated rat hepatocytes. *Fundam Clin Pharmacol* 1994;8:373–378.

44. Carruthers SG, Freeman DJ, Bailey DG. Synergistic adverse hemodynamic interactions between oral verapamil and propranolol. *Clin Pharmacol Ther* 1989;46:469–477.

45. Macphee GJA, Thompson GG, McInnes GT, Brodie MJ. Verapamil potentiates carbamazepine neurotoxicity: a clinically important inhibitory interaction. *Lancet* 1986;I:700–703.

46. Beattie B, Biller J, Melhaus B, Murray M. Verapamil-induced carbamazepine neurotoxicity. *Eur Neurol* 2988;28:104–105.

47. Price WA, Di Marzio LR. Verapamil-carbamazepine neurotoxicity. *J Clin Psychiatry* 1988;49:80.

48. Bahls FH, Ozuna J, Ritchie DE. Interaction between calcium channel blockers and the anticonvulsants carbamazepine and phenytoin. *Neurology* 1991;41:740–742.

49. Henricsson S, Lindholm A, Aravoglou M. Cyclosporine metabolism in human liver microsomes and its inhibition by other drugs. *Pharmacol Toxicol* 1990;66:49–52.

50. Tija JF, Back DJ, Breckenridge AM. Calcium channel antagonists and cyclosporine metabolism: in vitro studies with human liver microsomes. *Br J Clin Pharmacol* 1989;28:362–365.

51. Lindholm A, Henricsson S. Verapamil inhibits cyclosporine metabolism [Letter]. *Lancet* 1987;1:1262–1263.

52. Robson RA, Fraenkel M, Barratt LJ, Birkett DJ. Cyclosporine-verapamil interaction. *Br J Clin Pharmacol* 1988;25:402–403.

53. Maggio TG, Bartels DW. Increased cyclosporine blood concentrations due to verapamil interaction. *Drug Intell Clin Pharm* 1988;22:705–707.

54. Angermann CE, Spes CH, Anthuber M, Kemkes BM, Theisen K. Verapamil increases cyclosporin-A blood trough levels in cardiac transplant recipients. *J Am Coll Cardiol* 1988;11:206A.

55. Howard RL, Shapiro JI, Babcock S, Chan L. The effect of calcium channel blockers on the cyclosporine dose requirement in renal transplant recipients. *Ren Fail* 1990;12:89–92.

56. Sabaté I, Griño J, Castelao AM, Ortola J. Evaluation of cyclosporine-

verapamil interaction, with observation on parent cyclosporine and metabolites. *Clin Chem* 1988;34:2151–2152.

57. Sketris IS, Methot ME, Nicol D, Belitsky P, Knox MG. Effect of calcium-channel blockers on cyclosporine clearance and use in renal transplant patients. *Ann Pharmacother* 1994;28:1227–1231.

58. Kolars JC, Awni WM, Merion RM, Watkins PB. First-pass metabolism of cyclosporine by the gut. *Lancet* 1991;338:1488–1490.

59. Hebert MF, Roberts JP, Prueksaritanont T, Benet LZ. Bioavailability of cyclosporine with concomitant rifampin administration is markedly less than predicted by hepatic enzyme induction. *Clin Pharmacol Ther* 1992;52:453–457.

60. Gomez DY, Wacher VJ, Tomlanovich SJ, Hebert MF, Benet LZ. The effects of ketoconazole on the intestinal metabolism and bioavailability of cyclosporine. *Clin Pharmacol Ther* 1995;58:15–19.

61. Hebert MF. Contributions of hepatic and intestinal metabolism and P-glycoprotein to cyclosporine and tacrolimus oral drug delivery. *Adv Drug Deliver Rev* 1997;27:201–214.

62. Ammon E, Klotz U. In-vitro assessment of a possible verapamil/ethanol interaction. *Naunyn Schmiedebergs Arch Pharmacol* 1997;355:R123.

63. Perez-Reyes M, White WR, Hicks RE. Interaction between ethanol and calcium channel blockers in humans. *Alcohol Clin Exp Res* 1992;16:769–775.

64. Zacny JP, Yajnik S. Effects of calcium channel inhibitors on ethanol effects and pharmacokinetics in healthy volunteers. *Alcohol* 1993;10:505–509.

65. Bauer LA, Schumock G, Horn J, Opheim K. Verapamil inhibits ethanol elimination and prolongs the perception of intoxication. *Clin Pharmacol Ther* 1992;52:6–10.

66. Hermann DJ, Krol TF, Dukes GE, ET AL. Comparison of verapamil, diltiazem, and labetalol on the bioavailability and metabolism of imipramine. *J Clin Pharmacol* 1992;32:176–183.

67. Koyama E, Chiba K, Tani M, Ishizaki T. Reappraisal of human CYP isoforms involved in imipramine N-demethylation and 2-hydroxylation: a study using microsomes obtained from putative extensive and poor metabolizers of S-mephenytoin and eleven recombinant human CYPs. *J Pharmacol Exp Ther* 1997;281:1199–1210.

68. Kronbach T, Mathys D, Umeno M, Gonzales FJ, Meyer UA. Oxidation of midazolam and triazolam by human liver cytochrome P450IIIA4. *Mol Pharmacol* 1989;36:89–96.

69. Gascon M-P, Dayer P. In vitro forecasting of drugs which may interfere with the biotransformation of midazolam. *Eur J Clin Pharmacol* 1991;41:573–578.

70. Backman JT, Olkkola KT, Aranko K, Himberg JJ, Neuvonen PJ. Dose of midazolam should be reduced during diltiazem and verapamil treatments. *Br J Clin Pharmacol* 1994;37:221–225.

71. Pasanisi F, Elliott HL, Meredith PA, McSharry DR, Reid JL. Combined alpha adrenoceptor antagonism and calcium channel blockade in normal subjects. *Clin Pharmacol Ther* 1984;36:716–723.

72. Elliott HL, Meredith PA, Campbell L, Reid JL. The combination of prazosin and verapamil in the treatment of essential hypertension. *Clin Pharmacol Ther* 1988;43:554–560.

73. Jaillon P. Clinical pharmacokinetics of prazosin. *Clin Pharmacokinet* 1980;5:365–376.

74. Edwars DJ, Lavoie R, Beckman H, Belvins R, Rubenfire M. The effect of coadministration of verapamil on the pharmacokinetics and metabolism of quinidine. *Clin Pharmacol Ther* 1987;41:68–73.

75. Guengerich FP, Muller-Enoch D, Blair IA. Oxidation of quinidine by human liver cytochrome P-450. *Mol Pharmacol* 1986;30:287–295.

76. Trohman RG, Estes DM, Castellanos A, Palomo AR, Myerburg RJ, Kessler KM. Increased quinidine plasma concentrations during administration of verapamil: a new quinidine-verapamil interaction. *Am J Cardiol* 1986;57:706–707.

77. Robson RA, Miners JO, Matthew AP, et al. Characterisation of theophylline metabolism by human liver microsomes: inhibition and immunohistochemical studies. *Biochem Pharmacol* 1988;37:1651–1659.

78. Burnakis TG, Seldon M, Czaplicki AD. Increased serum theophylline concentrations secondary to oral verapamil. *Clin Pharm* 1983;2:458–461.

79. Stringer KA, Mallet J, Clarke M, Lindenfeld JA. The effect of three different oral doses of verapamil on the disposition of theophylline. *Eur J Clin Pharmacol* 1992;43:35–38.

80. Nielsen-Kudsk JE, Buhl JS, Johannessen AC. Verapamil-induced inhi-bition of theophylline elimination in healthy humans. *Pharmacol Toxicol* 1990;66:101–103.

81. Robson RA, Miners JO, Birkett DJ. Selective inhibitory effects of nifedipine and verapamil on oxidative metabolism: effects on theophylline. *Br J Clin Pharmacol* 1988;25:397–400.

82. Sirmans SM, Pieper JA, Lalonde RL, Smith DG, Self TH. Effect of calcium channel blockers on theophylline disposition. *Clin Pharmacol Ther* 1988;44:29–34.

83. Gin AS, Stringer KA, Welage LS, Wilton JH, Matthews GE. The effect of verapamil on the pharmacokinetic disposition of theophylline in cigarette smokers. *J Clin Pharmacol* 1989;29:728–732.

84. Tsao SC, Dickinson TH, Abernethy DR. Metabolite inhibition of parent drug biotransformation: studies of diltiazem. *Drug Metab Dispos* 1990;18:180–182.

85. Murray M, Butler AM. Enhanced inhibition of microsomal cytochrome P450 3A2 in rat liver during diltiazem biotransformation. *J Pharmacol Exp Ther* 1996;279:1447–1452.

86. Sutton D, Butler AM, Nadin L, Murray M. Role of CYP3A4 in human hepatic diltiazem N-demethylation: inhibition of CYP3A4 activity by oxidized diltiazem metabolites. *J Pharmacol Exp Ther* 1997;282:294–300.

87. Abernethy DR, Montamat SC. Acute and chronic studies of diltiazem in elderly versus young hypertensive patients. *Am J Cardiol* 1987;60:116I–120I.

88. Montamat SC, Abernethy DR. N-monodesmethyldiltiazem is the predominant metabolite of diltiazem in the plasma of young and elderly hypertensives. *Br J Clin Pharmacol* 1987;24:185189.

89. Hoglund P, Nilsson LG. Pharmacokinetics of diltiazem and its metabolites after single and multiple dosing in healthy volunteers. *Ther Drug Monit* 1989;11:558--566.

90. Carrum G, Egan JM, Abernethy DR. Diltiazem treatment impairs hepatic drug oxidation: studies of antipyrine. *Clin Pharmacol Ther* 1986;40:140–143.

91. Bottorff MB, Lalonde RL, Kazierad DJ, Hoon TJ, Tsiu SJ, Mirvis DM. The effects of encainide versus diltiazem on the oxidative metabolic pathways of antipyrine. *Pharmacotherapy* 1989;9:315--321.

92. Ohashi K, Sakamoto K, Sudo T, et al. The effect of diltiazem on hepatic drug oxidation assessed by antipyrine and trimethadione. *J Clin Pharmacol* 1991;31:1132–1136.

93. Sakai H, Kobayashi S, Hamada K, et al. The effects of diltiazem on hepatic drug metabolizing enzymes in man using antipyrine, trimethadione and debrisoquine as model substrates. *Br J Clin Pharmacol* 1991;31:353–355.

94. Tateishi T, Ohashi K, Sudo T, et al. Dose dependent effect of diltiazem on the pharmacokinetics of nifedipine. *J Clin Pharmacol* 1989;29:994–997.

95. Tateishi T, Nakashima H, Shitou T, et al. Effect of diltiazem on the pharmacokinetics of propranolol, metoprolol and atenolol. *Eur J Clin Pharmacol* 1989;36:67–70.

96. Brodie MJ, Macphee GJA. Carbamazepine neurotoxicity precipitated by diltiazem. *BMJ* 1986;292:1170–1171.

97. Eimer M, Carter BL. Elevated serum carbamazepine concentrations following diltiazem initiation. *Drug Intell Clin Pharm* 1987;21:340–342.

98. Maoz E, Grossman E, Thaler M, Rosenthal T. Carbamazepine neurotoxic reaction after administration of diltiazem. *Arch Intern Med* 1992;152:2503–2504.

99. Jones TE, Morris RG. Diltiazem does not always increase blood cyclosporin concentration. *Br J Clin Pharmacol* 1996;42:642–644.

100. Griño JM, Sabaté I, Castelao AM, Alsina J. Influence of diltiazem on cyclosporine clearance. *Lancet* 1986;1:1387.

101. Pochet JM, Pirson Y. Cyclosporine-diltiazem interaction. *Lancet* 1986;1:979.

102. McCauley J, Ptachcinski RJ, Shapiro R. The cyclosporine-sparing effects of diltiazem in renal transplantation. *Transplant Proc* 1989;21:3955–3957.

103. Sabaté I, Grino JM, Castelao AM, Huguet J, Serón D, Blanco A. Cyclosporin-diltiazem interaction: comparison of cyclosporin levels measured with two monoclonal antibodies. *Transplant Proc* 1989;21:1460–1461.

104. Brockmoller J, Neumayer HH, Wagner K, et al. Pharmacokinetic interaction between cyclosporine and diltiazem. *Eur J Clin Pharmacol* 1990;38:237–242.

105. Masri MA, Shakuntala V, Shanwaz M, et al. Pharmacokinetics of

cyclosporine in renal transplant patients on diltiazem. *Transplant Proc* 1994;26:1921.

106. Wagner K, Albrecht S, Neumayer HH. Prevention of posttransplant acute tubular necrosis by the calcium antagonist diltiazem: a prospective randomized study. *Am J Nephrol* 1987;7:287–291.

107. Kunzendorf U, Walz G, Brockmoeller J, et al. Effects of diltiazem upon metabolism and immunosuppressive action of cyclosporine in kidney graft recipients. *Transplantation* 1991;52:280–284.

108. Roy LF, East DS, Browning FM, et al. Short-term effects of calcium antagonists on hemodynamics and cyclosporine pharmacokinetics in heart-transplant and kidney-transplant patients. *Clin Pharmacol Ther* 1989;46:657–667.

109. Maddux MS, Jermis SA, Bauma YD, Pollak R. Significant drug interactions with cyclosporine. *Hosp Ther* 1987;12:56–70.

110. Wagner K, Henkel M, Heinemeyer G, Neumayer HH. Interaction of calcium blockers and cyclosporine. *Transplant Proc* 1988;20:561–568.

111. Kohlhaw K, Wonigeit K, Frei U, Oldhafer K, Neumann K, Pichlmayr R. Effect of the calcium channel blocker diltiazem on cyclosporine A blood levels and dose requirements. *Transplant Proc* 1988;20(suppl 2):572–574.

112. Campistol JM, Oppenheimer F, Vilardell J, et al. Interaction between ciclosporin and diltiazem in renal transplant patients. *Nephron* 1991;57:241–242.

113. Bourge RC, Kirklin JK, Naftel DC, Figg WD, White-Williams C, Ketchum C. Diltiazem-cyclosporine interaction in cardiac transplant recipients: impact on cyclosporine dose and medication costs. *Am J Med* 1991;90:402–404.

114. Tortorice KL, Heim-Duthoy KL, Awni WM, Rao KV, Kasiske BL. The effects of calcium channel blockers on cyclosporine and its metabolites in renal transplant recipients. *Ther Drug Monit* 1990;12:321–328.

115. Chrysostomou A, Walker RG, Russ GR, d'Apice AJ, Kincaid-Smith P, Mathew TH. Diltiazem in renal allograft recipients receiving cyclosporine. *Transplantation* 1993;55:300–304.

116. Neumayer HH, Wagner K. Diltiazem and economic use of cyclosporine [Letter]. *Lancet* 1986;2:523.

117. Jones TE. The use of other drugs to allow a lower dosage of cyclosporin to be used: therapeutic and pharmacoeconomic considerations. *Clin Pharmacokinet* 1997;32:357–367.

118. Krahenbuhl S, Smith-Gamble V, Hoppel CL. Pharmacokinetic interaction between diltiazem and nortriptyline. *Eur J Clin Pharmacol* 1996;49:417–419.

119. Varhe A, Olkkola KT, Neuvonen PJ. Diltiazem enhances the effects of triazolam by inhibiting its metabolism. *Clin Pharmacol Ther* 1996;59:369–375.

120. Kosuge K, Nishimoto M, Kimura M, Umemura K, Nakashima M, Ohashi K. Enhanced effect of triazolam with diltiazem. *Br J Clin Pharmacol* 1997;43:367–372.

121. Kimura E, Kishida H. Treatment of variant angina with drugs: a survey of 11 cardiology institutes in Japan. *Circulation* 1981;63:844–848.

122. Toyosaki N, Toyo-oka T, Natsume T, et al. Combination therapy with diltiazem and nifedipine in effort angina pectoris. *Circulation* 1988;77:1370–1375.

123. Ohashi K, Tateishi T, Sudo T, et al. Effects of diltiazem on the pharmacokinetics of nifedipine. *J Cardiovasc Pharmacol* 1990;15:96–101.

124. Ohashi K, Sudo T, Sakamoto K, et al. The influence of pretreatment periods with diltiazem on nifedipine kinetics. *J Clin Pharmacol* 1993;33:222–225.

125. Saseen JJ, Carter BL, Brown TE, Elliott WJ, Black HR. Comparison of nifedipine alone and with diltiazem or verapamil in hypertension. *Hypertension* 1996;28:109–114.

126. Smith SR, Haffner CA, Kendall MJ. The influence of nifedipine and diltiazem on serum theophylline concentration-time profiles. *J Clin Pharm Ther* 1989;14:403–408.

127. Christopher MA, Harman E, Hendeles L. Clinical relevance of the interaction of theophylline with diltiazem or nifedipine. *Chest* 1989;95:309–313.

128. Nafziger AN, May JJ, Bertino JS Jr. Inhibition of theophylline elimination by diltiazem therapy. *J Clin Pharmacol* 1987;27:862–865.

129. Ohashi K, Sakamoto K, Sudo T, et al. Effects of diltiazem and cimetidine on theophylline oxidative metabolism. *J Clin Pharmacol* 1993;33:1233–1237.

130. Soto J, Sacristan JA, Alsar MJ. Diltiazem treatment impairs theophylline elimination in patients with bronchospastic airway disease. *Ther Drug Monit* 1994;16:49–52.

131. Tjia JF, Colbert J, Back DJ. Theophylline metabolism in human liver microsomes: inhibition studies. *J Pharmacol Exp Ther* 1996;276:912–917.

132. Laganiere S, Davies RF, Carignan G, et al. Pharmacokinetic and pharmacodynamic interactions between diltiazem and quinidine. *Clin Pharmacol Ther* 1996;60:255–264.

133. Matera MG, De Santis D, Vacca C, et al. Quinidine-diltiazem: pharmacokinetic interaction in humans. *Curr Ther Res* 1986;40:653–656.

134. Stoysich AM, Lucas BD, Mohiuddin SM, Hilleman DE. Further elucidation of pharmacokinetic interaction between diltiazem and warfarin. *J Clin Pharm Ther* 1996;34:56–60.

135. Kazierad DJ, Lalonde RL, Hoon TJ, Mirvis DM, Bottorff MB. The effect of diltiazem on the disposition of encainide and its active metabolites. *Clin Pharmacol Ther* 1989;46:668–673.

136. Shum L, Pieniaszek HJ, Robinson CA, et al. Pharmacokinetic interactions of moricizine and diltiazem in healthy volunteers. *J Clin Pharmacol* 1996;36:1161–1168.

137. Klockowski PM, Lener ME, Sirgo MA, Rocci ML Jr. Comparative evaluation of the effects of isradipine and diltiazem on antipyrine and indocyanine green clearances in elderly volunteers. *Clin Pharmacol Ther* 1990;48:375–380.

138. Pichard L, Fabre I, Fabre G, et al. Cyclosporine A drug interactions: screening for inducers and inhibitors of cytochrome P-450 (cyclosporine A oxidase) in primary cultures of human hepatocytes and in liver microsomes. *Drug Metab Dispos* 1990;18:595–606.

139. Dickinson TH, Egan JM, Abernethy DR. Effects of nifedipine on hepatic drug oxidation. *Pharmacology* 1988;36:405–410.

140. Adebayo GI, Mabadeje AF. Effect of nifedipine on antipyrine and theophylline disposition. *Biopharm Drug Dispos* 1990;11:157–164.

141. Cantarovich M, Hiesse C, Lockiec F, Charpenter B, Fries D. Confirmation of the interaction between cyclosporine and the calcium channel blocker nicardipine in renal transplant patients. *Clin Nephrol* 1987;28:190–193.

142. Muck W, Ahr G, Kuhlmann J. Nimodipine: potential for drug-drug interactions in the elderly. *Drugs Aging* 1995;6:229–242.

143. Smith SR, Wilkins MR, Jack DB, Kendall MJ, Laugher S. Pharmacokinetic interactions between felodipine and metoprolol. *Eur J Clin Pharmacol* 1987;31:575–578.

144. Shepherd AMM, Brodie CL, Carrillo DW, Kwan CM. Pharmacokinetic interactions between isradipine and propranolol. *Clin Pharmacol Ther* 1988;43:194 (abst).

145. Levine MA, Ogilvie RI, Leenen FH. Pharmacokinetic and pharmacodynamic interactions between nisoldipine and propranolol. *Clin Pharmacol Ther* 1988;43:39–48.

146. Schoors DF, Vercruysse I, Musch G, Massart DL, Dupont AG. Influence of nicardipine on the pharmacokinetics and pharmacodynamics of propranolol in healthy volunteers. *Br J Clin Pharmacol* 1990;9:497–501.

147. Vercruysse I, Massart DL, Dupont AG. Increase in plasma propranolol caused by nicardipine is dependent on the delivery rate of propranolol. *Eur J Clin Pharmacol* 1995;49:121–125.

148. Vinceneux P, Canal M, Domart Y, et al. Pharmacokinetic and pharmacodynamic interactions between nifedipine and propranolol or betaxolol. *Int J Clin Pharmacol Ther Toxicol* 1986;24:153–158.

149. Bauer LA, Murray K, Horn JR, Opheim K, Olsen J. Influence of nifedipine therapy on indocyanine green and oral propranolol pharmacokinetics. *Eur J Clin Pharmacol* 1989;37:257–260.

150. Shaw-Stiffel TA, Walker SE, Ogilvie RI, Leenen FH. Pharmacokinetic and pharmacodynamic interactions during multiple-dose administration of nisoldipine and propranolol. *Clin Pharmacol Ther* 1994;55:661–669.

151. Duvoux C, Cherqui D, Di Martino V, et al. Nicardipine as antihypertensive therapy in liver transplant recipients: results of long-term use. *Hepatology* 1997;25:430–433.

152. Crocker JF, Renton KW, LeVatte TL, McLellan DH. The interaction of the calcium channel blockers verapamil and nifedipine with Cyclosporin A in pediatric renal transplant patients. *Pediatr Nephrol* 1994;8:408–411.

153. Copur MS, Tasdemir I, Turgan C, et al. Effects of nitrendipine on blood pressure and blood Cyclosporin A levels in patients with post transplant hypertension. *Nephron* 1989;52:227–230.

602 / Drugs as Inhibitors of Metabolic Enzymes: Cardiovascular Diseases

154. Madsen JK, Jensen JD, Jensen LW, Pedersen EB. Pharmacokinetic interaction between cyclosporine and the dihydropyridine calcium antagonist felodipine. Eur J Clin Pharmacol 1996;50:203–208.
155. Seifeldin RA, Marcos-Alvarez A, Gordon FD, Lewis WD, Jenkins RL. Nifedipine interaction with tacrolimus in liver transplant recipients. Ann Pharmacother 1997;31:571–575.
156. Robson RA, Miners JO, Matthews AP, et al. Characterisation of theophylline metabolism by human liver microsomes: inhibition and immunochemical studies. Biochem Pharmacol 1988;37:1651–1659.
157. Parillo SJ, Venditto M. Elevated theophylline blood levels from institution of nifedipine therapy. Ann Emerg Med 1984;13:216–217.
158. Harrod CS. Theophylline toxicity and nifedipine. Ann Intern Med 1987;106:480.
159. Garty M, Cohen E, Mazar A, Ilfeld DN, Spitzer S, Rosenfeld JB. Effect of nifedipine and theophylline in asthma. Clin Pharmacol Ther 1986;40:195–198.
160. Upton RA. Pharmacokinetic interactions between theophylline and other medication (Pt II). Clin Pharmacokinet 1991;20:135–150.
161. Perreault MM, Kazierad DJ, Wilton JH, Izzo JL Jr. The effect of isradipine on theophylline pharmacokinetics in healthy volunteers. Pharmacotherapy 1993;13:149–153.
162. Bratel T, Billing B, Dahlqvist R. Felodipine reduces the absorption of theophylline in man. Eur J Clin Pharmacol 1989;36:481–485.
163. Bailey DG, Freeman DJ, Melendez LJ, Kreeft JH, Edgar B, Carruthers SG. Quinidine interaction with nifedipine and felodipine: pharmacokinetic and pharmacodynamic evaluation. Clin Pharmacol Ther 1993;53:354–359.
164. Hippius M, Henschel L, Sigusch H, Tepper J, Brendel E, Hoffmann A. Pharmacokinetic interactions of nifedipine and quinidine. Pharmazie 1995;50:613–616.
165. Hollingshead LM, Faulds D, Fitton A. Bepridil: a review of its pharmacological properties and therapeutic use in stable angina pectoris. Drugs 1992;44:835–857.
166. Welker HA, Wiltshire H, Bullingham R. Clinical pharmacokinetics of mibefradil. Clin Pharmacokinet 1998;35:405–423.
167. Abernethy DR. Pharmacologic and pharmacokinetic profile of mibefradil, a T- and L-type calcium channel antagonist. Am J Cardiol 1997;80:4C–11C.
168. Ellison RH. Http:/www.dfa.gov/medwatch/safety/1997/posico.htm.
169. Li Wan Po A, Zhang WY. What lessons can be learnt from withdrawal of mibefradil from the market? [Commentary]. Lancet 1998;351:1829–1830.

CHAPTER 45

Antiarrhythmics

Kim Brøsen

QUINIDINE

Quinidine is one of the oldest antiarrhythmics still used in the prevention and treatment of atrial flutter and fibrillation, as well as for ventricular and supraventricular arrhythmias. After oral dosing, the bioavailability is only about 70%, and this may reflect the secretory effect of P-glycoprotein in the gut mucosa (1). Quinidine is 80% to 90% protein bound in plasma, and systemically available quinidine rapidly distributes to the heart, skeletal muscles, kidneys, and liver. The recommended therapeutic plasma concentration range is 5 to 15 μM. After oral intake, quinidine is almost undetectable in the cerebrospinal fluid of humans (2), and recent studies with a rat model showed that this may be due to the secretory action of P-glycoprotein in the blood–brain barrier (3).

About 10% to 20% of a quinidine dose is excreted unchanged in the urine through the kidneys. The total renal clearance ranged from 2.7 L/h to 8.3 L/h in a recent study of healthy subjects (4), and this greatly exceeds the estimated glomerular filtration clearance of about 0.8 to 1.6 L/h (estimated as the product between the non–protein bound fraction of 0.1–0.2 and the glomerular filtration rate of about 7.5 L/h). The discrepancy strongly suggests that quinidine undergoes active tubular secretion, and this may also be due to the secretory actions of P-glycoprotein (5). However, oxidation in the liver accounts for the majority of quinidine elimination, and in humans, the following metabolites have been identified: (3S)-3OH-quinidine, quinidine-N-oxide, quinidine-10,11-dihydrodiol, 2'-oxoquinidine, and O-desmethylquinidine (Fig. 45-1). The latter two are minor metabolites, and in practice, the only metabolites present in quantifiable amounts are (3S)-3hydroxy-quinidine and quinidine-N-oxide, both

K. Brøsen: Department of Clinical Pharmacology, Institute of Public Health, University of Southern Denmark—Odense University, Winslowparken 19 and Clinical Chemistry Department (KKA), Odense University Hospital, DK-5000 Odense, Denmark

of which possess antiarrhythmic effects. Quinidine still is derived from the bark of cinchona trees, and commercially available quinidine contains 5% to 20% of its dihydro analogue, dihydroquinidine deriving either from the extraction process of cinchona bark, or the epimerization process of quinine, the latter process being quantitatively the most important in the synthesis of quinidine. A third possibility, that dihydroquinidine is formed by biotransformation, was recently ruled out in a pharmacokinetic study (4) in which quinidine purified from dihydroquinidine was given to healthy subjects in a single oral dose. It was not possible to detect dihydroquinidine in either plasma or urine from any of the subjects.

In Vitro Studies

Assessment of sparteine metabolism by human liver microsomes or the 9,000 g supernatant was initially used as a method for identification of drugs subject to the sparteine oxidation polymorphism (6). Drugs that were identified as competitive inhibitors of sparteine metabolism were putative substrates of the enzyme cytochrome P450 2D6 (CYP2D6), and drugs that did not inhibit sparteine metabolism were not considered candidates for the sparteine oxidation polymorphism. Because quinidine and its diastereoisomer quinine, like sparteine, both are plant alkaloids, they were tested in the sparteine oxidation *in vitro* system and found to be very potent inhibitors (6). The inhibitor constants, K_i, for quinidine and quinine were 0.06 μM and 15 μM, respectively. Besides the discovery of quinidine as a very potent inhibitor of sparteine oxidation (alias CYP2D6), it was also the first proven example of stereoselective inhibition via CYP2D6: quinine was a less potent inhibitor than quinidine by two orders of magnitude. In a follow-up study, the same researchers found that this also applied when the other classic CYP2D6 substrate, debrisoquine, was used (7): the K_i values for inhibition

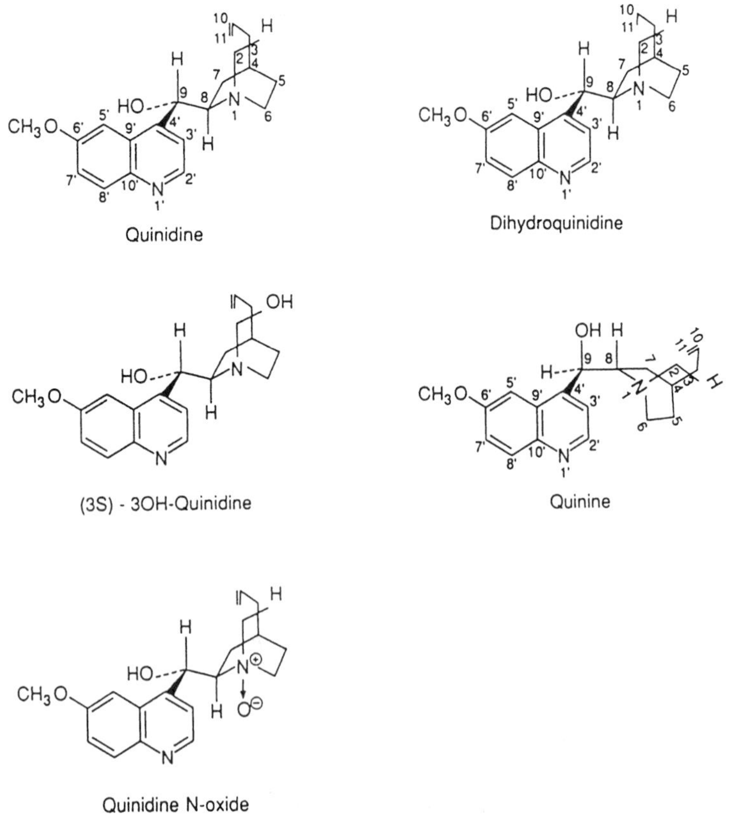

FIG. 45-1. The structural formulae of quinidine, its most important metabolites, dihydroquinidine and quinine.

of the 4-hydroxylation of debrisoquine were 0.030 μM and 10 μM for quinidine and quinine, respectively. The stereoselective inhibition of CYP2D6 also was confirmed by a radioreceptor assay technique by using ^{3}H-dihydroquinidine as a specific probe for the CYP2D6 site in human liver microsomes (7). Through the use of other substrates of CYP2D6, numerous subsequent *in vitro* studies have confirmed the potent inhibition by quinidine (Table 45-1): desipramine (8), bufuralol (9,10), dextromethorphan (11), mexiletine (12), imipramine (13,14), clomipramine, *N*-desmethylclomipramine (15), and metoprolol (16). Potent inhibition by quinidine has been reported for several other CYP2D6 substrates including

the (−)-*E*-10-hydroxylation of nortriptyline (17), the oxidation of reduced haloperidol to haloperidol (18), the demethylation of paroxetine (19), the *N*-dealkylation of *S*-(−)-propranolol (20), the *O*-demethylation of *p*-methoxy-amphetamine (21), and the 5-hydroxylation of tolterodine (22).

Ching et al. (23) expressed CYP2D6 in yeast microsomes and used the *O*-demethylation of dextromethorphan to probe the enzyme. Quinidine and dihydroquinidine were very potent inhibitors of CYP2D6 with K_i values in the nanomolar range, similar to values previously reported for quinidine (see Table 45-1). (3S)-3-hydroxyquinidine, quinidine-*N*-oxide, *O*-desmethylquini-

TABLE 45-1. *Quinidine inhibition of selected CYP2D6 marker reactions in vitro*

Drug	CYP2D6 marker reaction	Inhibitor constant (K_i) (μM)	Reference
Desipramine	2-hydroxylation	0.27	8
Bufuralol	1′-hydroxylation	0.01	9
	1′-hydroxylation	0.06	10
Dextromethorphan	*O*-demethylation	0.015	11
Mexiletine	Aliphatic hydroxylation	0.03	12
	Aromatic hydroxylation	0.03	12
Imipramine	2-hydroxylation	0.07	13
		0.009–0.092	14
Clomipramine	8-hydroxylation	0.010	15
N-desmethylclomipramine	8-hydroxylation	0.016	15
Metoprolol	α-hydroxylation	0.04–0.13	16
	O-demethylation	0.13–0.18	16

dine, and quinine were one or two orders of magnitude less potent inhibitors of CYP2D6.

A pharmacophore model was recently proposed for the structure–activity relation for the avid binding of quinidine (and other potent inhibitors) to CYP2D6 (24). According to the model, potent inhibitors of CYP2D6 have a positive nitrogen atom in their molecule and a flat hydrophobic region almost perpendicular to the N-H axis. The hydrophobic region should not extend more than 7.5 A from the nitrogen atom. The very potent inhibitors (including quinidine) have functional groups with negative electrostatic potential and hydrogen bond–acceptor properties on the opposite with distances of 4.8 to 5.5 A and 6.6 to 7.5 A, respectively, from the nitrogen atom (see Fig. 45-1). Similar structure–activity relation studies for the prediction of compounds that not only are bound, but actually also are oxidized by CYP2D6 have shown that the susceptible sites are 5 to 7 A from a basic nitrogen atom (original references are reviewed in 4). On the basis of a theoretic analysis of quinidine's molecular structure, it was concluded that it could not be ruled out that the formation of the two minor metabolites, 2'-oxoquinidine and O-desmethyl-quinidine, are catalyzed by CYP2D6, but that it is highly unlikely that this enzyme is involved in the formation of any of the other metabolites. Indeed, quinidine is not metabolized by CYP2D6 (4) but rather by CYP3A4 (25,26).

It was early suggested that quinidine could be used to distinguish those drugs metabolized by CYP2D6 from those metabolized by other enzymes (27). Quinidine, as expected, inhibited the 4-hydroxylation of debrisoquine and the 1'-hydroxylation of bufuralol in human liver microsomes but not the O-deethylation of phenacetin (27). The latter oxidation is catalyzed by CYP1A2, and hence quinidine does not inhibit this enzyme. In keeping with this, it was shown that the N-demethylation of imipramine catalyzed in combination by CYP1A2, CYP2C19, and CYP3A4 was not influenced by quinidine in vitro (13,14). Besides, the N1-, N3-, and N7-demethylations of caffeine, also catalyzed by CYP1A2, were not inhibited by quinidine in human liver microsomes (28). The lack of inhibition of imipramine's N-demethylation by quinidine makes it unlikely that CYP2C19 is influenced by quinidine. This notion was confirmed in a recent in vitro study by using proguanil as a model drug for CYP2C19 (29). Neither the formation of cycloguanil nor the formation of the pharmacologically inactive metabolite 4-chlorophenylbiguanide was inhibited by quinidine in human liver microsomes even at quinidine concentrations up to 100 μM (29). Bourrie et al. (30) recently screened quinidine for its ability to inhibit a number of important CYP-specific marker reactions in vitro: ethoxyresorufin O-deethylation (CYP1A1), phenacetin O-deethylation (CYP1A2), coumarin 7-hydroxylation (CYP2A6), tolbutamide 4-methylhydroxylation (CYP2C9), dextromethorphan O-demethylation (CYP2D6), aniline 4-hydroxylation (CYP2E1), and nifedipine dehydrogenation (CYP3A4). In keeping with the previous results, the K_i for inhibition of the CYP2D6 process was 0.4 μM, but even at quinidine concentrations 10 times higher than this value, no inhibition of the other marker reactions was observed. Indeed, this comprehensive study confirms and extends previous knowledge, and it seems fair to conclude that quinidine is both a potent and a selective inhibitor of CYP2D6. The finding of a K_i in the nanomolar range is a very specific and sensitive measure for the involvement of CYP2D6, and the finding of either lack of inhibition or much higher K_i values with great certainty rules out any role of CYP2D6 in the oxidation process under study.

In Vivo Studies

The *in vitro* studies regarding quinidine inhibition of CYP2D6 were followed up by a series of *in vivo* studies. The studies were apparently carried out more or less simultaneously, and they are briefly summarized here. Brinn et al. (31) carried out a sparteine test before and during daily treatment with quinidine 600 to 800 mg/day in eight patients aged 33 to 84 years with supraventricular tachyarrhythmias. The prequinidine sparteine metabolic ratio (sparteine/dehydrosparteines in the 12-hour urine) was 28 in one patient, phenotyped as a poor metabolizer, and it ranged from 0.34 to 6.4 in the remaining seven patients that were accordingly phenotyped as extensive metabolizers. With quinidine, the metabolic ratio was 160 in the poor metabolizer and increased to 21 to 490 in the extensive metabolizers. Hence, all patients were phenotypically poor metabolizers during therapeutic doses of quinidine, and the change was due to the increase in metabolic ratio in the extensive metabolizers. In another study (27), eight healthy extensive metabolizers were debrisoquine tested without and with concomitant oral intake of 50 mg quinidine. Their debrisoquine metabolic ratios (debrisoquine/4-hydroxydebrisoquine in the 6-hour urine) ranged from 0.3 to 5.6, well below the antimode of 12.6 for debrisoquine, and they all were classified as extensive metabolizers. With quinidine, the metabolic ratio increased by a factor of 5.5-fold to 66.7-fold, and all except two subjects had their phenotypes changed to poor metabolizer. In a follow-up study, a single oral dose of 50 mg of quinidine coadministered with debrisoquine converted four of six extensive metabolizers to poor metabolizers, and repetitive debrisoquine testing showed that this effect lasted for 3 days, but that the increase in debrisoquine metabolic ratio had disappeared after 1 week (32). The same duration of quinidine inhibition was reported after a single oral dose of 100 mg by using sparteine to probe CYP2D6 (33). Inaba et al. (34) gave 250 mg quinidine as a single oral dose to seven healthy extensive metabolizers and performed a sparteine test in each. There was a dramatic increase in the sparteine metabolic ratio in each subject, but it did not exceed the antimode of 20, so all remained extensive metabolizers. The sparteine metabolic ratio returned to the prequinidine level 7 days later, showing that the inhibition of CYP2D6 was reversible. Leemann et al. (9) gave racemic metoprolol as a single oral dose of 100 mg to five poor metabolizers and five extensive metabolizers. Then (+)- and (–)-metoprolol were assayed in serum after 3 hours before and after concomitant intake of quinidine, 50 mg. The ratio of the active (–) enantiomer to the lesser active (+) enantiomer was 1.68 ± 0.57 in the extensive metabolizers, and in the poor metabolizers, it was 1.05 ± 0.09, thereby confirming the well-known stereoselective preferential metabolism of (+)-metoprolol by CYP2D6. With quinidine, the (–)/(+) ratio decreased to 1.03 ± 0.07 in the extensive metabolizers, and it was unchanged in the poor metabolizers. Seven patients with supraventricular tachycardia were debrisoquine tested before and during quinidine treatment (600 to 800 mg/day) (35). The prequinidine metabolic ratio of debrisoquine ranged from 0.1 to 3.6, and all were therefore classified as extensive metabolizers. With quinidine, the debrisoquine metabolic ratio increased markedly in all patients, with a range from 15 to 51. Hence patients all became poor metabolizers with quinidine. The dose-dependency of quinidine inhibition was studied after the administration of single oral doses of 5, 10, 20, 40, and 80 mg of quinidine to 12 healthy extensive metabolizers with subsequent sparteine testing (33). In all subjects, there was a marked and dose-dependent increase in the sparteine metabolic ratio. After 80 mg of quinidine, eight of the 12 subjects became phenotypically poor metabolizers (metabolic ratio, more than 20).

For quinidine to become useful for assessment of the involvement of CYP2D6 *in vivo*, it is necessary that there exists a dose-window in which only CYP2D6 activity is abolished, without the involvement of other CYP enzymes. In a study (36), a cocktail consisting of mephenytoin (CYP2C19), sparteine (CYP2D6), and nifedipine (CYP3A4) was given alone and after 200 mg of quinidine. As expected, the formation of dehydrosparteines was abolished after quinidine, but there was no effect on the 4-hydroxylation of mephenytoin. The plasma concentration of nifedipine did not change during quinidine, but its mean elimination half-life increased from 1.9 to 2.8 hours, and the plasma level of the metabolite M-I decreased by approximately 40%. Both changes can be explained by quinidine and nifedipine being substrates for CYP3A4.

The differential inhibitory effect of quinidine on drug oxidation in poor and extensive metabolizers of debrisoquine was studied in three healthy subjects of the former phenotype and seven of the latter (37). The CYP2D6 substrate desipramine, 25 mg (corresponding to 82.5 μmol), was given to the volunteers, and urine was collected for 24 hours. In the extensive metabolizers, the mean recovery of 2-hydroxydesipramine was about 21 μmol in the extensive metabolizers, but only about 2 μmol in the poor metabolizers, and this confirmed that CYP2D6 is of paramount importance for the aromatic hydroxylation of desipramine. When the desipramine testing was repeated after 2 days of pretreatment with quinidine, the mean recovery of 2-hydroxydesipramine decreased to about 0.7 μmol in the extensive metabolizers and to about the same value in the poor metabolizers, yet another example of phenocopy caused by quinidine in relation to CYP2D6. In the third part of the experiment, the volunteers took quinine 750 mg/day for 2 days, and in both phenotypes, this had a much lesser impact on the 2-hydroxylation. Once again, the differential stereoselective inhibition of the two diastereomers was confirmed.

The impact of quinidine, 200 mg/day, on the plasma pharmacokinetics of imipramine and desipramine was studied in six healthy extensive metabolizers who took single oral doses of 100 mg of each of the two tricyclic antidepressants (38). With quinidine, the apparent total oral clearance of imipramine was reduced by 35% and that of desipramine by 85%. The clearance of imipramine through demethylation (desipramine formation) was not changed with quinidine, but its clearance by other pathways (largely 2-hydroxylation) was reduced 50%. 2-Hydroxyimipramine and 2-hydroxydesipramine were detected in plasma before quinidine but not with quinidine. The mean elimination half-life of imipramine increased by 50%, whereas that of desipramine increased almost 500% with quinidine. The study showed that quinidine, as expected, almost abolished the formation of 2-hydroxyimipramine and 2-hydroxydesipramine catalyzed by CYP2D6, but that it did not influence the N-demethylation of imipramine catalyzed by CYP1A2, CYP2C19, and CYP3A4. The results regarding imipramine were in full agreement with previous and subsequent *in vitro* studies (13). The pharmacokinetic parameters for both imipramine and desipramine obtained with quinidine were almost identical with those obtained in poor metabolizers who had not taken quinidine (38). The influence of quinidine on desipramine metabolism *in vivo* (37,38) also agreed with both earlier and later *in vitro* studies (8,39).

The antiarrhythmic drug encainide is sequentially oxidized by CYP2D6 to the two active metabolites, *O*-desmethyl encainide, and further to 3-methoxy-*O*-desmethyl encainide. In a panel study of seven extensive metabolizers of debrisoquine and four poor metabolizers (40), each subject took a single oral dose of 60 mg of encainide orally and was at the same time given a single intravenous bolus of [^{14}C]encainide. In a randomized crossover fashion, the encainide intake was carried out alone and together with the concomitant intake of quinidine, 200 mg/day in four divided doses every 6 hours. The mean systemic clearance of encainide in extensive metabolizers was 0.935 L/min before quinidine and decreased to 0.190 L/min with quinidine. The corresponding values were 0.128 and 0.119 L/min in the poor metabolizers. The mean of the elimination half-life increased from 1.8 hours before to 7.7 hours with quinidine. In the poor metabolizers, the corresponding values were 10.4 and 9.2 hours, respectively. *O*-Desmethyl encainide and 3-methoxy-*O*-desmethyl encainide achieved higher concentrations than the parent compound in the plasma in the extensive metabolizers without quinidine, but only the former metabolite could be detected with quinidine, although in a substantially lower concentration than without quinidine. In the extensive metabolizers, the QRS interval (an index for the blockade of the sodium channels) and PR interval increased approximately 10% with encainide, but only a minor increase was seen in the poor metabolizers, and the phenotype difference most likely was due to the high levels of the *O*-desmethyl encainide in the former. In further support of this, the electrocardiogram (ECG) changes disappeared in the extensive metabolizers with quinidine. The findings of the study with healthy volunteers could only partially be reproduced in a clinical follow-up study (41). Ten patients, eight extensive metabolizers and two poor metabolizers, who required treatment for ventricular arrhythmias, entered the open-label study. After a drug-free washout period, the patients entered the encainide phase in which the dose was titrated to achieve a 50% suppression of the ventricular ectopic beats. In that phase, the mean (±SD) encainide dose was 65 ± 34 mg/day. In the third phase, quinidine, 60 mg every 8 hours, was added, and in the fourth and last phase, while still taking quinidine, encainide treatment was temporarily stopped. With quinidine, the mean steady-state concentration of encainide was increased nearly 12-fold. The mean plasma concentration of 3-methoxy-*O*-desmethyl encainide decreased from a value of about 4 times the level of encainide before quinidine to a level that was barely detectable. Somewhat surprisingly, the steady-state level of *O*-desmethyl encainide was about 5 times higher than that of parent compound before quinidine but remained more or less unchanged during quinidine. This was a change compared with the results obtained in the healthy subjects after a single dose of encainide, and it may reflect that both the formation of *O*-desmethyl encainide and the further conversion of the metabolite to 3-methoxy-*O*-desmethyl encainide are catalyzed by CYP2D6 and hence inhibited by quinidine. In keeping with this, the QRS prolongation caused by encainide in the extensive metabolizers did not change with quinidine in contrast to the previous single dose study. There were no changes in the two poor metabolizers with quinidine, with regard to either the pharmacokinetics or the pharmacodynamics of encainide.

Renal excretion makes up a substantial part of the elimination of flecainide, up to 30% to 40%, but the residue is metabolized in the liver partially by CYP2D6. Six healthy subjects, one poor metabolizer of dextromethorphan and five extensive metabolizers, were given 150 mg of flecainide as a single intravenous dose

twice: alone and after a single oral dose of quinidine, 50 mg, taken the evening before (42). Without quinidine, the mean total clearance of flecainide was 10.5 mL/min/kg of body weight. After quinidine, the clearance decreased to 8.1 mL/min/kg, and the difference was statistically significant. The elimination half-life increased from 8.8 to 10.7 hours after quinidine. It may be concluded from the study that quinidine given in therapeutic doses would increase the flecainide plasma levels, especially in patients with renal impairment, and that this could lead to toxicity.

Mexiletine is eliminated in parallel by renal excretion and biotransformation, the former process accounting for about 10% of the total elimination. The main metabolic routes are aromatic hydroxylation to *p*-hydroxymexiletine, aliphatic hydroxylation to hydroxymethylmexiletine, and *N*-glucuronidation. In a preliminary study (43), six healthy extensive metabolizers of debrisoquine took a single oral dose of 200 mg of mexiletine followed by urine collection for 48 hours. This experiment was repeated with the addition of a single oral dose of 41.5 mg of quinidine base. The urinary content of unchanged mexiletine increased more than 50% with quinidine, whereas the recoveries of the two hydroxylated metabolites decreased by more than 50%, and that of the *N*-glucuronidated metabolite increased by approximately 20%. The results of the study are in keeping with CYP2D6 being an important, albeit not the only, enzyme catalyzing the two hydroxylations, thereby supporting previous *in vitro* work (12). The results also show that quinidine does not inhibit the *N*-glucuronyltransferases. In a parallel panel study performed by another research group (44), it was shown that quinidine reduced the total and nonrenal clearance of mexiletine as it reduced the partial formation clearances of the three primary hydroxylations leading to hydroxymethylmexiletine, *m*-hydroxymexiletine, and *p*-hydroxymexiletine. The reduction of clearance occurred in the extensive metabolizers only and not in the poor metabolizers. Mexiletine has in its molecular structure an asymmetric carbon atom; this gives rise to stereoisomers, and mexiletine is therefore administered as a racemic mixture that consists of R-(–)-mexiletine and S-(+)-mexiletine. In a follow-up study, the plasma and urine samples were reanalyzed by an enantioselective high-performance liquid chromatography (HPLC) method for its concentrations of the two enantiomers (45). There were 14 healthy subjects, 10 extensive and four poor metabolizers of debrisoquine/sparteine, and each had taken a single oral dose of 200 mg of racemic mexiletine before and during concomitant quinidine, 50 mg, every 6 hours. Before quinidine, the areas under the plasma concentration (AUC) curves were of equal size both for the R-(–) and the S-(+) enantiomers in both phenotypes. However, the AUC values were about 60% greater in the poor metabolizers than in the extensive metabolizers for both enantiomers. With quinidine, both AUC values increased in the extensive, but not in the poor metabolizers, and the phenotype differences were diminished, but not abolished. The R/S ratios were close to unity in both phenotypes with quinidine. A very large fraction, approximately 25% of the administered dose, was recovered in urine in the form of R-(−)-N-hydroxymexiletine glucuronide in both extensive and poor metabolizers, but the S-(+)-counterpart only made up a few percentages of the dose. This did not change with quinidine, and it may be concluded that the N-glucuronidation is highly stereoselective for the R-(−)-enantiomer and, as expected, independent of CYP2D6.

Propafenone is hydroxylated by CYP2D6 to its active metabolite, 5-hydroxypropafenone, and it is dealkylated by other enzymes (see Chapter 28) to desalkyl-propafenone. Nine patients treated with propafenone for symptomatic and frequent ventricular ectopic depolarization participated in a clinical study (46). Five patients were extensive metabolizers of debrisoquine, two were poor metabolizers, and two were not phenotyped. The mean propafenone dose was 825 mg/day (range, 450–900 mg/day), and subsequently, quinidine, 50 mg, was added to each propafenone dose. In the two poor metabolizers, there were no change in propafenone and 5-hydroxypropafenone concentrations before and with quinidine. In contrast, in the extensive metabolizers, the mean steady-state plasma concentration of propafenone increased from 408 to 1096 ng/mL with concomitant quinidine, but the concentration of 5-hydroxypropafenone decreased from 242 to 125 ng/mL. There were no changes in ECG intervals or in the frequency of arrhythmias in the extensive metabolizers with quinidine. One very plausible explanation for the lack of pharmacodynamic changes imposed by quinidine is that the lower 5-hydroxypropafenone concentrations outweigh the increase in parent compound concentration. Light and shade were introduced in a subsequent study regarding the clinical outcome of the propafenone–quinidine interaction (47). Nine healthy subjects, seven extensive metabolizers, and two poor metabolizer patients were included in a double-blind crossover study. The subjects received propafenone, 225 mg every 8 hours, plus quinidine, 60 mg every 8 hours, in one period of the study, and propafenone plus placebo in another period of the study. The steady-state concentration of each of the two enantiomers, R-propafenone and S-propafenone, as well as of the racemate, increased in the extensive metabolizers during quinidine albeit not to a level reaching statistical significance. The increase, however, was most pronounced in subjects with high CYP2D6 activity at baseline, as judged from their relatively low levels of propafenone before quinidine. In the extensive metabolizers, however, a statistically significant increase in the extent of propafenone-induced β-blockade was evident from a reduction in exercise-induced tachycardia and sensitivity to isoproterenol. One likely explanation for this is that propafenone both is a β-blocker and a blocker of sodium channels, but 5-hydroxypropafenone has only the latter pharmacodynamic property with very little β-blocking activity.

Topical administration of the nonselective β-blocker timolol in the eyes is widely used for the treatment of glaucoma. Adverse effects (e.g., in the form of bronchial constriction in patients with asthma) are well known and are due to the systemic absorption of timolol. Timolol is metabolized by CYP2D6 and therefore achieves higher plasma concentrations in poor metabolizers than in extensive metabolizers. In a single-blind randomized crossover study, timolol eyedrops or artificial eyedrops were administered with placebo or quinidine, 50 mg (48). The participants of the study were eight extensive metabolizers and five poor metabolizers. The plasma concentrations of timolol were statistically significantly higher in the poor metabolizers than in the extensive metabolizers. With quinidine, the timolol plasma concentration in the extensive metabolizers reached the same level as that in the poor metabolizers. The exercise heart rate was reduced in both phenotypes with timolol as compared with artificial tears, and the reduction was statistically significantly higher in the poor metabolizers compared with the extensive metabolizers.

Propranolol is a racemate administered as a mixture of (−) and (+)-propranolol. Concomitant intake of quinidine resulted in a doubling of the mean AUC of racemic propranolol (48) in six healthy subjects. The partial formation clearance of 4-hydroxypropranolol decreased more than 10-fold with quinidine. The metabolism of (+)-propranolol was more inhibited by quinidine than was the metabolism of (−)-propranolol. The AUC of the former increased by 177% and that of the latter by only 100%. There was a more pronounced reduction of exercise-induced tachycardia and in the QT_c and PR prolongations by propranolol combined with quinidine as compared with propranolol alone.

The metabolism of metoprolol was studied in 10 black and 10 white healthy extensive metabolizers (50) in a randomized crossover study. In both phases of the study, a single oral dose of 200 mg racemic metoprolol was administered. In one of the phases, the subjects took quinidine, 100 mg/day, starting 3 days before metoprolol. The means of the AUC of the active enantiomer, S-metoprolol, were 879 and 984 ng/mL/h in whites and blacks, respectively. With quinidine, the AUC increased to 2,515 and 2,719. Accordingly, the half-life of metoprolol was doubled with quinidine. The concentration of S-metoprolol was somewhat higher than that of R-metoprolol. Thus the S/R ratio without quinidine was 1.39 in both racial groups, but decreased to 0.89 and 1.03 in whites and blacks, respectively, with quinidine. The results of the study were in agreement with both previous (51) and later in vitro studies (16).

Several antipsychotic drugs are substrates for CYP2D6, but chlorpromazine had not previously been investigated in this regard. However, in a recent study (52), 10 healthy subjects, who were extensive metabolizers with regard to CYP2D6, took single oral doses of 100 mg of chlorpromazine without and with prior intake of quinidine, 250 mg. The urinary recovery of 7-hydroxychlorpromazine was reduced more than two-fold after quinidine. After quinidine, the AUC of chlorpromazine increased about 40%, and the AUC of 7-hydroxychlorpromazine decreased about 15%. Neither of the changes reached a level of statistical significance, but the data suggest that CYP2D6 is partially responsible for the biotransformation of chlorpromazine, especially through the 7-hydroxylation.

As outlined earlier, quinidine was a potent inhibitor of the oxidation of reduced haloperidol to haloperidol (18), suggesting a role of CYP2D6 for this oxidation. The interaction between haloperidol, reduced haloperidol, and quinidine has also been investigated *in vivo* (53). Eight healthy volunteers participated in a crossover study in which they took single oral doses of haloperidol, 5 mg, and reduced haloperidol, 5 mg, on separate occasions without and with intake of quinidine, 250 mg, 1 hour before. The AUCs of both parent compounds increased two- to three-fold after quinidine, but the study did not support that the interconversion between the two compounds is catalyzed by CYP2D6. A further discussion of this discrepancy between the results obtained with quinidine inhibition *in vitro* and *in vivo* is outside the scope of this chapter.

Codeine is predominantly eliminated by glucuronidation (80%) and to a much lesser extent by *O*-demethylation and *N*-demethylation (see Chapter 22). Codeine is a prodrug, and the active metabolite, morphine, is formed by *O*-demethylation catalyzed by CYP2D6 (54). Several studies have addressed the influence of quinidine on the pharmacokinetics and hypoalgesic effects of codeine. In a randomized double-blind study (55), eight healthy volunteers were included, seven of whom were extensive metabolizers, and one who was a poor metabolizer of dextromethorphan. Ten hours before intake of 100 mg of codeine, the volunteers took either placebo or quinidine, 50 mg. In both sessions, pain was elicited by electric stimulation. The pain threshold was determined by a visual analogue scale (VAS) as well as by means of electric stimulation of the sural nerve and recording of the so-called R-III reflex from the biceps femoris. The mean maximal morphine concentration after codeine preceded by placebo was 18 nM in the extensive metabolizers and less than 1 nM in the poor metabolizers. After codeine preceded by quinidine, the morphine level decreased to 1.5 nM in the extensive metabolizers, confirming the dominant role of CYP2D6 for the *O*-demethylation. In the extensive metabolizers, the combination of codeine and placebo resulted in a statistically significant increase in the pain thresholds measured both by the VAS scale and the R-III reflex as compared with the measurements after double placebo. No increase in pain thresholds was recorded when morphine formation

was abolished by quinidine. In a similar, but somewhat larger study (56), the analgesic effect of 100 mg codeine given orally with placebo was measured, and both drugs were given with and without pretreatment with a single oral dose of 200 mg of quinidine 3 hours before. The four different treatment sequences were placebo/placebo, quinidine/placebo, placebo/codeine, and quinidine/codeine. Pain was elicited by the output from an argon laser transmitted to the skin. This experimental pain model allowed determination of the pain threshold (pin-prick) and the pain tolerance. In agreement with a previous study (55), the median of the maximal concentration of morphine was 18 nM after codeine and placebo, and as expected, the value decreased to a level below the quantitation limit of the applied assay (less than 4 nM) after quinidine and codeine. The pin-prick pain thresholds were statistically significantly elevated after placebo/codeine but not after quinidine/codeine compared with placebo/placebo. However, both placebo/codeine and quinidine/codeine increased the pain tolerance thresholds compared with placebo/placebo. There were no statistically significant differences between quinidine/codeine and quinidine/placebo with regard to either pain thresholds or pain tolerance. The results regarding quinidine intake mimicking the poor metabolizer phenotype were clear regarding the pharmacokinetics of codeine but less clear with regard to the role of morphine in codeine hypoalgesia. The possible explanation for this could be either that quinidine in itself possesses analgesic effects that confounded the results or that quinidine does not traverse the blood–brain barrier and hence is unable to block the local CYP2D6-catalyzed morphine formation in the brain. In an attempt to support this hypothesis further, a study was undertaken (2). Seventeen patients, including 16 extensive metabolizers and one poor metabolizer of sparteine, undergoing spinal anesthesia for urinary tract surgery or examination, took either a single oral dose of 125 mg of codeine or the same dose of codeine preceded by quinidine, 200 mg, as a single oral dose. Two hours after codeine, a plasma and spinal fluid sample was drawn. The median protein binding of quinidine in plasma was 86%, and the median of the non–protein-bound concentration in plasma was 115 nM as compared with an unbound concentration of 10 nM in the cerebrospinal fluid. The total and the unbound concentration of quinidine were the same in the cerebrospinal fluid. The medians of the morphine concentrations in plasma were 10 and 1.5 nM, respectively, in the patients without and with quinidine, and the corresponding concentrations in the cerebrospinal fluid were 3.6 and 0.2 nM, respectively. The study confirmed that quinidine penetrates the blood–brain barrier poorly, but it did not show directly that morphine formation locally in the brain was not diminished by quinidine to a similar degree as that seen in the liver.

Sixteen healthy male subjects took 120 mg of codeine, 100 mg of quinidine, or placebo in a double-blind randomized experiment (57). There were 10 extensive and six poor metabolizers of debrisoquine, and the treatment combinations were codeine/placebo, codeine/quinidine, and placebo/quinidine. The formation clearance of morphine from codeine was on average 163 mL/min in extensive metabolizers and 0.86 mL/min in the poor metabolizers. After codeine, the average formation clearance dropped to 17 mL/min but was largely unchanged in the poor metabolizers. The near abolishment of morphine formation with quinidine in the extensive metabolizers reduced the respiratory, psychomotor, and pupillary effects.

There is evidence that both codeine and morphine are endogenous substances formed from two molecules of tyrosine (54) and that the O-demethylations of thebaine to oripavine and of codeine to morphine, two of the final steps in endogenous morphine formation, are catalyzed by CYP2D6. In a comparative study of the urinary excretion of codeine and morphine in 20 drug-free extensive metabolizers and 20 drug-free poor metabolizers (58), it was reported that mean recovery of the two compounds were 1,048 and 2,438 pmol/24 h, respectively, in the extensive metabolizers, and 588 and 2,124 pmol/24 h in the poor metabolizers, but neither of the differences between the phenotypes reached a level of statistical significance. The average codeine/morphine ratio was nearly 2 times higher in the poor metabolizers compared with extensive metabolizers, but the difference was not statistically significant. Four extensive metabolizers took a single oral dose of 50 mg of quinidine, but this apparently had no influence on the recovery of either codeine or morphine. The study did not support the role of CYP2D6 in the endogenous morphine formation, but this may have been due to a statistical type 2 error, due to the 1,000-fold interindividual differences in the excretion rate of codeine and morphine (51).

Hydrocodone is a structural analogue of codeine, the difference being that the hydroxy group in the 6-position of codeine is replaced by a ketone group in hydrocodone. Glucuronidation is therefore abolished, but like codeine, the drug is O-demethylated to an active metabolite, hydromorphone. The O-demethylation clearance of hydrocodone was on average 28 mL/h/kg in five extensive metabolizers compared with 3.4 mL/h/kg in six extensive metabolizers (59). Besides, pretreatment of the extensive metabolizers with 100 mg of quinidine resulted in a decrease of the O-demethylation clearance to 5 mL/h/kg, and this further supported the role of CYP2D6 in the formation of hydromorphone. In a follow-up study (60), 17 extensive metabolizers and eight poor metabolizers of dextromethorphan took single oral doses of hydrocodone in dosages of either 10 mg (one subject), 15 mg (10 subjects), or 22.5 mg (14 subjects). The hydrocodone intake was preceded 8 hours before by either placebo or quinidine, 100 mg. The ratio between the urinary recoveries of hydrocodone versus hydromorphone was higher in the extensive metabolizers than in the poor metabolizers during the placebo/hydrocodone

part of the study, but the phenotype difference was abolished in the quinidine/hydrocodone period. The subjects were tested with a battery of subjective and physiological experimental models for abuse liability. The conclusion on the pharmacodynamic investigation was that extensive and poor metabolizers were equally responsive to an oral dose of hydrocodone, even after quinidine.

The antitussive dextromethorphan is a widely used alternatively to sparteine and debrisoquine as a probe drug for CYP2D6 because the O-demethylation of dextromethorphan to form the metabolite dextrorphan is catalyzed by CYP2D6. Assessment of dextromethorphan and dextrorphan in urine after dextromethorphan intake and calculation of a metabolic ratio between the two may serve as a phenotype marker. Individuals with a dextromethorphan/dextrorphan ratio of less than 0.3 are classified as extensive metabolizers, and those with a ratio above 0.3 as poor metabolizers. Dextromethorphan is used as an antitussive, but its clinical use is somewhat hampered by its very low bioavailability. In a clinical study of seven patients with amyotrophic lateral sclerosis (61), repetitive dosing of 60 mg of dextromethorphan every 12 hours resulted in a mean steady-state concentration of 12 ng/mL. However, in the presence of quinidine, 75 mg, twice daily, this concentration increased to 241 ng/mL, illustrating that CYP2D6 is of paramount importance for the first pass metabolism of dextromethorphan. Similar results were obtained in a more recent study (62).

PROPAFENONE

Propafenone is hydroxylated to an active metabolite, 5-hydroxypropafenone, and dealkylated to N-desalkyl-propafenone. During repeated dosing, both metabolites accumulate to a degree that in part is determined by the patient's CYP2D6 phenotype. In a clinical study (46), five extensive metabolizers of debrisoquine, two presumed extensive metabolizers, and two phenotyped poor metabolizers were treated with propafenone, 150 mg, 3 times daily. The mean of their steady-state concentrations of propafenone, 5-hydroxypropafenone, and N-desalkyl-propafenone were 408, 242, and 91 ng/mL, respectively, in the extensive metabolizers. The corresponding values in the two poor metabolizers were 1,870 and 3,900, 15 and 25, and 202 and 192 ng/mL. Propafenone is administered as a racemate, and after oral administration, the plasma levels of S-propafenone are about 60% higher than the levels of R-propafenone (63), indicating that the R-enantiomer inhibits the biotransformation of the S-enantiomer.

In Vitro Studies

Racemic propafenone was a potent inhibitor of the 4-hydroxylation of debrisoquine in human liver microsomes with a K_i of 0.7 μM (64). In a separate study with human liver microsomes with bufuralol as a model drug

(65), R-propafenone proved to be a somewhat more potent inhibitor of the 1'-hydroxylation, having a K_i of 21 nM as compared with 56 nM for S-propafenone. The K_i for racemic propafenone in that study was an order of magnitude lower than that reported in the previous study (64), 50 nM. The corresponding values for racemic 5-hydroxypropafenone and racemic N-desalkylpropafenone were 855 and 1,530 nM, respectively. R-propafenone was an inhibitor of the 5-hydroxylation of S-[$^2H_4$]-propafenone, with a K_i of 2.9 μM (66), and the similar value for inhibition of the 5-hydroxylation of R-propafenone by S-[$^2H_4$]-propafenone was 5.2 μM. The study confirmed the earlier suspicion (63) that R-propafenone is a more potent inhibitor than S-propafenone of the CYP2D6-catalyzed 5-hydroxylation.

An *in vitro* study (67) showed that the N-dealkylation of propafenone is catalyzed in parallel by CYP1A2 and CYP3A4. This means that propafenone is a competitive inhibitor of both enzymes, and this was confirmed for the former in an *in vitro* study with the O-deethylation of phenacetin as a marker reaction for CYP1A2 (68). The median inhibitory concentration (IC_{50}) value of propafenone for the inhibition of the O-deethylation was 29 μM.

In Vivo Studies

Propafenone, as expected, also is a very potent inhibitor of CYP2D6 *in vivo*. Six extensive metabolizers and three poor metabolizers of debrisoquine (64) were debrisoquine tested before and during treatment with either 600 or 900 mg of propafenone per day. Before propafenone, the urinary recovery of 4-hydroxydebrisoquine made up more than 8% of the total recovery of 4-hydroxydebrisoquine and debrisoquine in the 8-hour urine, with a mean of 34%. With propafenone, the value dropped to 8%, and four of the six extensive metabolizers became poor metabolizers with propafenone. In the poor metabolizers, the recovery of the 4-hydroxylated metabolite was less than 8% both before and with propafenone. In another clinical study (69), the interaction between metoprolol and propafenone was studied. There were eight patients requiring treatment for ventricular arrhythmias and six healthy subjects in the study, but the CYP2D6 activity was not determined in any of the participants. The patients were divided in two groups, each consisting of four individuals. In one group, the patients were treated with metoprolol in doses of 150 to 200 mg/day, and the steady-state levels of metoprolol were determined before and after 4 days with concomitant intake of propafenone, 450 mg/day. The plasma levels of racemic metoprolol increased from nearly three-fold to more than five-fold with propafenone. The other group consisted of four patients treated concomitantly with propafenone, 450 mg/day, and metoprolol, 150 mg/day, for 1 week. The plasma levels of propafenone were deter-mined with metoprolol and 4 days after discontinuation of metoprolol. There were no consistent changes in the propafenone levels between the two periods. The six healthy subjects took single doses of metoprolol, 50 mg, and propafenone, 150 mg. It was an open-labeled three-fold crossover study in which either drug was given alone or in combination. The apparent oral clearance of metoprolol decreased from 2.32 L/min to 1.13 L/min with propafenone, and the difference was statistically significant. The median values for propafenone given alone and in combination with metoprolol were 2,908 L/min and 3,961 L/min in four subjects. The presumed inhibition of the metabolism of S-propafenone by R-propafenone (66) reported *in vitro* has also been investigated *in vivo* (70). In a single-blind, randomized study, propafenone in the form of the racemate, the R- and the S-enantiomers were administered on separate occasions. In each treatment session, the dosage was 150 mg every 6 hours for 4 days. The clearance of S-propafenone was on average 55% lower after the administration of racemic propafenone compared with the value obtained after S-propafenone alone, and this provided additional evidence that R-propafenone inhibits the biotransformation of S-propafenone. The maximal reduction of exercise heart rate was on average reduced by 8.8 and 4.3 beats/min after racemic and S-propafenone, respectively, and both changes were statistically significantly different from those with placebo. The change after R-propafenone was only 1.8 beats/min, but this was not statistically significantly different. The results of this part of the study were consistent with the S-enantiomer being responsible for the β-adrenoceptor blocking activity. All of the active-treatment periods were associated with a statistically significant increase in the QRS interval compared with placebo, and this is consistent with both of the enantiomers of propafenone being sodium channel blockers.

The inhibition of CYP1A2 reported *in vitro* (68) also was observed *in vivo*. Thus it has been reported (71,72) that the plasma levels of theophylline, a substrate of CYP1A2, increased during concomitant intake of propafenone, and that the increase was associated with serious toxicity. Warfarin is administered as a racemate; the anticoagulant properties are due mainly to S-warfarin, and CYP2C9 is the major enzyme responsible for the elimination of the active enantiomer. A pharmacokinetic and pharmacodynamic interaction study was performed between propafenone and warfarin (73). Eight healthy subjects took propafenone, 450 mg/day, alone for 1 week, racemic warfarin, 5 mg/day, alone for 1 week, and the combination of the two for yet another week. Warfarin did not change the steady-state plasma levels of propafenone, but the mean steady-state concentration of warfarin increased from 0.98 μg/mL to 1.36 μg/mL with propafenone. In agreement with this, the prothrombin time increased in all eight subjects during the combination of the two drugs compared with the measurement obtained on the last day of warfarin alone. The results of the study suggest that propafenone also inhibits CYP2C9.

AMIODARONE

Amiodarone is oxidized to the active metabolite *N*-desethylamiodarone. In 12 healthy male subjects, seven extensive metabolizers and five poor metabolizers of dextromethorphan treated with amiodarone, 200 mg, every 12 hours for 5 days (74), the mean amiodarone plasma concentration of amiodarone was 0.51 and 0.47 µg/mL in extensive and poor metabolizers, respectively, and the concentrations of *N*-desethylamiodarone were 0.25 and 0.24 µg/mL.

In Vitro Studies

S-warfarin is the more active enantiomer compared with R-warfarin, and the S-enantiomer is predominantly metabolized by CYP2C9 in the 6- and and the 7-positions. Amiodarone, in a final concentration of 50 µ*M*, was incubated with S-warfarin in a final concentration of 4.5 µ*M* in a human liver microsome preparation (75). With amiodarone, the rates of 6- and 7-hydroxylation were reduced by 17.3% and 30%, respectively, indicating that amiodarone is an inhibitor of CYP2C9. In another study, amiodarone was an inhibitor of dextromethorphan *O*-demethylation in human liver microsomes with a K_i of 30 µ*M* (76). In human liver microsomes, amiodarone was an inhibitor of the CYP3A4-catalyzed *N*-desethylation of lidocaine, with an inhibitor constant of 47 µ*M* (77)

In Vivo Studies

Seven healthy subjects were given a single intravenous bolus of phenytoin, 5 mg/kg (78), before and during concomitant intake of amiodarone, 200 mg/day, for 3 weeks. The mean AUC of phenytoin increased from 245 mg/h/L before amiodarone to 342 mg/h/L with amiodarone, and the mean elimination half-life of phenytoin increased from 16.1 to 22.6 hours with amiodarone. Both changes in phenytoin elimination kinetics are consistent with amiodarone being an inhibitor of CYP2C9.

Six healthy men on separate occasions (79) took single oral doses of racemic warfarin, 1.5 mg/kg, S-warfarin and R-warfarin, 0.75 mg/kg, twice on three separate occasions without and with concomitant amiodarone, 400 mg/day for 4 days. The AUC of racemic warfarin, S-warfarin, and R-warfarin were 624, 230, and 638 µg/h/mL without amiodarone, and the corresponding AUCs with amiodarone were 1,249, 485, and 1,036 µg/h/mL; all increases were statistically significant, and the same applied to the increases in hypothrombinemia with amiodarone compared with each of the three dose regimens of warfarin given alone.

In a follow-up study (75), five healthy subjects took single oral doses of pseudoracemic warfarin, 0.75 mg/kg, with and without concomitant amiodarone, 300 mg/day, and the study confirmed that amiodarone inhibited the biotransformation of both the enantiomers, although the difference in AUCs was not so pronounced as in the previous study.

The influence of amiodarone on three polymorphically expressed enzymes, *N*-acetyltransferase measured through the assessment of isoniazid metabolism, CYP2C19 assessed by mephenytoin 4-hydroxylation, and CYP2D6 measured by means of dextromethorphan (76), was investigated in eight patients with a maintenance dose of 200 to 400 mg amiodarone per day. Amiodarone inhibited the CYP2D6-catalyzed *O*-demethylation of dextromethorphan but not the metabolism of the two other marker reactions. An interaction between flecainide and amiodarone (74) was investigated by administering flecainide, 100 mg/day, without and with amiodarone, 400 mg/day, for 5 days. The mean flecainide plasma concentration increased from approximately 125 ng/mL without amiodarone to 192 ng/mL in the seven extensive metabolizers and from approximately 170 ng/mL to 282 ng/mL in the five poor metabolizers.

The interaction between amiodarone and lidocaine was investigated in six cardiac patients (77). Each patient was given a single intravenous dose of lidocaine, 1 mg/kg, on three occasions: alone and after accumulated doses of 3 and 13 grams, respectively, of amiodarone. The mean AUCs of lidocaine in the three sessions were 111,7, 135.3, and 131.7 µg/min/mL, thus confirming that amiodarone also inhibits lidocaine metabolism *in vivo*.

FLECAINIDE

Flecainide is predominantly excreted unchanged through the kidneys, and to a lesser extent, metabolized to its two inactive metabolites, meta-*O*-dealkylated flecainide and its lactam. In an *in vitro* study, flecainide was reported to have an inhibitor constant of 0.954 µ*M* for the 1'-hydroxylation of bufuralol in human liver microsomes (80). In eight extensive metabolizers of debrisoquine, the metabolic ratio of dextromethorphan was on an average 0.014, with a range from 0.003 to 0.04 before flecainide, but after 1 week of flecainide, 200 mg/day, it increased to 0.163, and one subject changed his phenotype to that of a poor metabolizer, having a metabolic ratio of 0.63.

REFERENCES

1. Emi Y, Tsunashima D, Ogawara K, Higaki K, Kimura T. Role of P-glycoprotein as a secretory mechanism in quinidine absorption from rat small intestine. *J Pharm Sci* 1998;87:295–299.
2. Sindrup SH, Hofmann U, Asmussen J, et al. Impact of quinidine on plasma and cerebrospinal fluid concentrations of codeine and morphine after codeine intake. *Eur J Clin Pharmacol* 1996;49:503–509.
3. Kusuhara H, Suzuki H, Terasaki T, Kakee A, Lemaire M, Sugiyama Y.

P-glycoprotein mediates the efflux of quinidine across the blood-brain barrier. *J Pharmacol Exp Ther* 1997;283:574–580.

4. Nielsen F, Rosholm J-U, Brøsen K. Lack of relationship between quinidine pharmacokinetics and the sparteine oxidation polymorphism. *Eur J Clin Pharmacol* 1995;48:501–504.

5. Woodland C, Ito S, Koren G. A model for the prediction of digoxin-drug interactions at the renal tubular cell level. *Ther Drug Monit* 1998; 20:134–138.

6. Otton SV, Inaba T, Kalow W. Competitive inhibition of sparteine oxidation in human liver by β-adrenoceptor antagonists and other cardiovascular drugs. *Life Sci* 1984;34:73–80.

7. Otton SV, Kalow W, Seeman P. High affinity of quinidine for a stereoselective microsomal binding site as determined by a radioreceptor assay. *Experientia* 1984;40:973–974.

8. von Bahr C, Spina E, Birgersson E, et al. Inhibition of desmethylimipramine 2-hydroxylation by drugs in human liver microsomes. *Biochem Pharmacol* 1985;34:2501–2505.

9. Leemann T, Dayer P, Meyer UA. Single-dose quinidine treatment inhibits metoprolol oxidation in extensive metabolizers. *Eur J Clin Pharmacol* 1986;29:739–741.

10. Gut J, Catin T, Dayer P, Kronbach T, Zanger U, Meyer UA. Debrisoquine/sparteine-type polymorphism of drug oxidation. *J Biol Chem* 1986;261:11734–11743.

11. Dayer P, Leemann T, Striberni R. Dextromethorphan *O*-demethylation in liver microsomes as a prototype reaction to monitor cytochrome P-450 db$_1$ activity. *Clin Pharmacol Ther* 1989;45:34–40.

12. Broly F, Libersa C, Lhermitte M, Dupuis B. Inhibitory studies of mexiletine and dextromethorphan oxidation in human liver microsomes. *Biochem Pharmacol* 1990;39:1045–1053.

13. Brøsen K, Zeugin T, Meyer UA. Role of P450IID6, the target of the sparteine-debrisoquin oxidation polymorphism, in the metabolism of imipramine. *Clin Pharmacol Ther* 1991;49:609–617.

14. Skjelbo E, Brøsen K. Inhibitors of imipramine metabolism by human liver microsomes. *Br J Clin Pharmacol* 1992;34:256–261.

15. Nielsen KK, Flinois JP, Beaune P, Brøsen K. The biotransformation of clomipramine *in vitro*, identification of the cytochrome P450s responsible for the separate metabolic pathways. *J Pharmacol Exp Ther* 1996; 277:1659–1664.

16. Belpaire FM, Wijnant P, Temmerman A, Rasmussen BB, Brøsen K. The oxidative metabolism of metoprolol in human liver microsomes: inhibition by the selective serotonin reuptake inhibitors. *Eur J Clin Pharmacol* 1998;54:261–264.

17. Dahl M-J, Nordin C, Bertilsson L. Enantioselective hydroxylation of nortriptyline in human liver microsomes, intestinal homogenate, and patients treated with nortriptyline. *Ther Drug Monit* 1991;13:189–194.

18. Tyndale RF, Kalow W, Inaba T. Oxidation of reduced haloperidol to haloperidol: involvement of human P450IID6 (sparteine/debrisoquine monooxygenase). *Br J Clin Pharmacol* 1991;31:655–660.

19. Bloomer JC, Woods FR, Haddock RE, Lennard MS, Tucker GT. The role of cytochrome P4502D6 in the metabolism of paroxetine by human liver microsomes. *Br J Clin Pharmacol* 1992;33:521–523.

20. Rowland K, Ellis SW, Lennard MS, Tucker GT. Variable contribution of CYP2D6 to the *N*-dealkylation of S-(–)-propranolol by human liver microsomes. *Br J Clin Pharmacol* 1996;42:390–393.

21. Wu D, Otton SV, Inaba T, Kalow W, Sellers EM. Interactions of amphetamine analogs with human liver CYP2D6. *Biochem Pharmacol* 1997; 53:1605–1612.

22. Postlind H, Danielson A, Lindgren A, Andersson SH. Tolterodine, a new muscarinic receptor antagonist, is metabolized by cytochromes P450 2D6 and 3A in human liver microsomes. *Drug Metab Dispos* 1998;26:289–293.

23. Ching MS, Blake CL, Ghabrial H, et al. Potent inhibition of yeast-expressed CYP2D6 by dihydroquinidine, quinidine, and its metabolites. *Biochem Pharmacol* 1995;50:833–837.

24. Strobl GR, von Kruedener S, Stöckigt J, Guengerich FP, Wolff T. Development of a pharmacophore for inhibition of human liver cytochrome P-450 2D6: molecular modeling and inhibition studies. *J Med Chem* 1993;36:1136–1145.

25. Guengerich FP, Muller-Enoch D, Blair IA. Oxidation of quinidine by human liver cytochrome P-450. *Mol Pharmacol* 1986;30:287–295.

26. Nielsen TL, Rasmussen BB, Flinoiss J-P, Beaune P, Brøsen K. In vitro metabolism of quinidine: the (3S)-3-hydroxylation of quinidine is a specific marker reaction for cytochrome P4503A4 activity in human liver microsomes. *J Pharmacol Exp Ther* 1998 (resubmitted).

27. Speirs CJ, Murray S, Boobis AR, Seddon CE, Davies DS. Quinidine and the identification of drugs whose elimination is impaired in subjects classified as poor metabolizers of debrisoquine. *Br J Clin Pharmacol* 1986;22:739–743.

28. Rasmussen BB, Nielsen TL, Brøsen K. Fluvoxamine is a potent inhibitor of the metabolism of caffeine in vitro. *Pharmacol Toxicol* 1998;83:240–245.

29. Rasmussen BB, Nielsen TL, Brøsen K. Fluvoxamine inhibits the CYP2C19-catalysed metabolism of proguanil in vitro. *Eur J Clin Pharmacol* 1998;54:735–740.

30. Bourrie M, Meunier V, Berger Y, Fabre G. Cytochrome P450 isoform inhibitors as a tool for the investigation of metabolic reactions catalyzed by human liver microsomes. *J Pharmacol Exp Ther* 1996;277: 321–332.

31. Brinn R, Brøsen K, Gram LF, Haghfelt T, Otton SV. Sparteine oxidation is practically abolished in quinidine-treated patients. *Br J Clin Pharmacol* 1986;22:194–197.

32. Ayesh R, Dawling S, Hayler A, et al. Comparative effects of the diastereoisomers, quinine and quinidine in producing phenocopy debrisoquine poor metabolisers (PMs) in healthy volunteers. *Chirality* 1991;3:14–18.

33. Nielsen MD, Brøsen K, Gram LF. A dose-effect study of the in vivo inhibitory effect of quinidine on sparteine oxidation in man. *Br J Clin Pharmacol* 1990;29:299–304.

34. Inaba T, Tyndale RE, Mahon WA. Quinidine: potent inhibition of sparteine and debrisoquine oxidation in vivo [Letter]. *Br J Clin Pharmacol* 1986;22:199–200.

35. Brøsen K, Gram LF, Haghfelt T, Bertilsson L. Extensive metabolizers of debrisoquine become poor metabolizers during quinidine treatment. *Pharmacol Toxicol* 1987;60:312–314.

36. Schellens JHM, Ghabrial H, van der Wart HHF, Bakker EN, Wilkinson GR, Breimer DD. Differential effects of quinidine on the disposition of nifedipine, sparteine, and mephenytoin in humans. *Clin Pharmacol Ther* 1991;50:520–528.

37. Steiner E, Dumont E, Spina E, Dahlqvist R. Inhibition of desipramine 2-hydroxylation by quinidine and quinine. *Clin Pharmacol Ther* 1988; 43:577–581.

38. Brøsen K, Gram LF. Quinidine inhibits the 2-hydroxylation of imipramine and desipramine but not the demethylation of imipramine. *Eur J Clin Pharmacol* 1989;37:155–160.

39. von Moltke LL, Greenblatt DJ, Cotreau-Bibbo MM, Duan SX, Harmatz JS, Shader RI. Inhibition of desipramine hydroxylation in vitro by serotonin reuptake-inhibitor antidepressants, and by quinidine and ketoconazole: a model system to predict drug interactions in vivo. *J Pharmacol Exp Ther* 1994;268:1278–1283.

40. Funck-Brentano C, Turgeon J, Woosley RL, Roden DM. Effect of low dose quinidine on encainide pharmacokinetics and pharmacodynamics: influence of genetic polymorphism. *J Pharmacol Exp Ther* 1989;249: 134–142.

41. Turgeon J, Pavlou HN, Wong W, Funck-Brentano C, Roden DM. Genetically determined steady-state interaction between encainide and quinidine in patients with arrhythmias. *J Pharmacol Exp Ther* 1990;255:642–649.

42. Munafo A, Buclin T, Tuto D, Biollaz J. The effect of a low dose of quinidine on the disposition of flecainide in healthy volunteers. *Eur J Clin Pharmacol* 1992;43:441–443.

43. Broly F, Vandamme N, Caron J, Libersa C, Lhermitte M. Single-dose quinidine treatment inhibits mexiletine oxidation in extensive metabolizers of debrisoquine. *Life Sci* 1991;48:PL-123–PL-128.

44. Turgeon J, Fiset C, Giguere R, et al. Influence of debrisoquine phenotype and of quinidine on mexiletine disposition in man. *J Pharmacol Exp Ther* 1991;259:789–798.

45. Abolfathi Z, Fiset C, Gilbert M, Moerike K, Bélanger PM, Turgeon J. Role of polymorphic debrisoquin 4-hydroxylase activity in the stereoselective disposition of mexiletine in humans. *J Pharmacol Exp Ther* 1993;266:1196–1201.

46. Funck-Brentano C, Kroemer HK, Pavlou H, Woosley RL, Roden DM. Genetically determined interaction between propafenone and low dose quinidine: role of active metabolites in modulating net drug effect. *Br J Clin Pharmacol* 1989;27:435–444.

47. Mörike KE, Roden DM. Quinidine-enhanced β-blockade during treatment with propafenone in extensive metabolizer human subjects. *Clin Pharmacol Ther* 1994;55:28–34.

48. Edeki TI, He H, Wood AJJ. Pharmacogenetic explanation for excessive β-blockade following timolol eye drops. *JAMA* 1995;274:1611–1613.

49. Zhou HH, Anthony LB, Roden DM, Wood AJ. Quinidine reduces clearance of (+)-propranolol more than (−)-propranolol through marked reduction in 4-hydroxylation. *Clin Pharmacol Ther* 1990;47:686–693.
50. Johnson JA, Burlew BS. Metoprolol metabolism via cytochrome P4502D6 in ethnic populations. *Drug Metab Disp* 1996;24:350–355.
51. Otton SV, Crewe HK, Lennard MS, Tucker GT, Woods HF. Use of quinidine inhibition to define the role of the sparteine/debrisoquine cytochrome P450 in metoprolol oxidation by human liver microsomes. *J Pharmacol Exp Ther* 1988;247:242–247.
52. Muralidharan G, Cooper JK, Hawes EM, Korchinski ED, Midha KK. Quinidine inhibits the 7-hydroxylation of chlorpromazine in extensive metabolisers of debrisoquine. *Eur J Clin Pharmacol* 1996;50:121–128.
53. Young D, Midha KK, Fossler MJ, et al. Effect of quinidine on the interconversion kinetics between haloperidol and reduced haloperidol in humans: implications for the involvement of cytochrome P450IID6. *Eur J Clin Pharmacol* 1993;44:433–438.
54. Sindrup SH, Brøsen K. The pharmacogenetics of codeine hypoalgesia. *Pharmacogenetics* 1995;5:335–346.
55. Desmeules J, Gascon M-P, Dayer P, Magistris M. Impact of environmental and genetic factors on codeine analgesia. *Eur J Clin Pharmacol* 1991;41:23–26.
56. Sindrup SH, Arendt-Nielsen L, Brøsen K, et al. The effect of quinidine on the analgesic effect of codeine. *Eur J Clin Pharmacol* 1992;42:587–592.
57. Caraco Y, Sheller J, Wood AJJ. Pharmacogenetic determination of the effects of codeine and prediction of drug interactions. *J Pharmacol Exp Ther* 1996;278:1165–1174.
58. Mikus G, Bochner F, Eichelbaum M, Horak P, Somogyi AA, Spector S. Endogenous codeine and morphine in poor and extensive metabolisers of the CYP2D6 (debrisoquine/sparteine) polymorphism. *J Pharmacol Exp Ther* 1994;268:546–551.
59. Otton SV, Schadel M, Cheung SW, Kaplan HL, Busto UE, Sellers EM. CYP2D6 phenotype determines the metabolic conversion of hydrocodone to hydromorphone. *Clin Pharmacol Ther* 1993;54:463–472.
60. Kaplan HL, Busto UE, Baylon GJ, Cheung SW, Otton SV, Somer G, Sellers EM. Inhibition of cytochrome P450 2D6 metabolism of hydrocodone to hydromorphone does not importantly affect abuse liability. *J Pharmacol Exp Ther* 1997;281:103–108.
61. Zhang Y, Britto MR, Valderhaug KL, Wedlund PJ, Smith RA. Dextromethorphan: enhancing its systemic availability by way of low-dose quinidine-mediated inhibition of cytochrome P4502D6. *Clin Pharmacol Ther* 1992;51:647–655.
62. Schadel M, Wu D, Otton SV, Kalow W, Sellers EM. Pharmacokinetics of dextromethorphan and metabolites in humans: influence of the CYP2D6 phenotype and quinidine inhibition. *J Clin Psychopharmacol* 1995;15:263–269.
63. Kroemer HK, Funck-Brentano C, Silberstein DJ, et al. Stereoselective disposition and pharmacologic activity of propafenone enantiomers. *Circulation* 1988;79:1068–1076.
64. Siddoway LA, Thompson KA, McAllister CB, et al. Polymorphism of propafenone metabolism and disposition in man: clinical and pharmacokinetic consequences. *Circulation* 1987;75:785–791.
65. Kroemer HK, Mikus G, Kronbach T, Meyer UA, Eichelbaum M. In vitro characterization of the human cytochrome P-450 involved in the polymorphic oxidation of propafenone. *Clin Pharmacol Ther* 1988;45:28–33.
66. Kroemer HK, Fischer C, Meese CO, Eichelbaum M. Enantiomer/enantiomer interaction of (S)- and (R)-propafenone for cytochrome P450IID6-catalyzed 5-hydroxylation: *in vitro* evaluation of the mechanism. *Mol Pharmacol* 1991;40:135–142.
67. Botsch S, Gautier JC, Beaune P, Eichelbaum M, Kroemer HK. Identification and characterization of the cytochrome P450 enzymes involved in *N*-dealkylation of propafenone: molecular base for interaction potential and variable disposition of active metabolites. *Mol Pharmacol* 1993;43:120–126.
68. Kobayashi K, Nakajima M, Chiba K, et al. Inhibitory effects of antiarrhythmic drugs on phenacetin *O*-deethylation catalyzed by CYP1A2. *Br J Clin Pharmacol* 1998;45:361–368.
69. Wagner F, Kalusche D, Trenk D, Jähnchen E, Roskamm H. Drug interaction between propafenone and metoprolol. *Br J Clin Pharmacol* 1987;24:213–220.
70. Kroemer HK, Fromm MF, Buhl K, Blaschke G, Eichelbaum M. An enantiomer-enantiomer interaction of (S)- and (R)-propafenone modifies the effect of racemic drug therapy. *Circulation* 1994;89:2396–2400.
71. Lee BL, Dohrmann ML. Theophylline toxicity after propafenone treatment: evidence for drug interaction. *Clin Pharmacol Ther* 1992;51:353–355.
72. Spinler SA, Gammaitoni A, Charland SL, Hurwitz J. Propafenone-theophylline interaction. *Pharmacotherapy* 1993;13:68–71.
73. Kates RE, Yee Y-G, Kirsten EB. Interaction between warfarin and propafenone in healthy volunteer subjects. *Clin Pharmacol Ther* 1987;42:305–311.
74. Funck-Brentano C, Becquemont L, Kroemer HK, et al. Variable disposition kinetics and electrocardiographic effects of flecainide during repeated dosing in humans: contribution of genetic factors, dose-dependent clearance, and interaction with amiodarone. *Clin Pharmacol Ther* 1994;55:256–269.
75. Heimark LD, Wienkers L, Kunze K, et al. The mechanism of the interaction between amiodarone and warfarin in humans. *Clin Pharmacol Ther* 1992;51:398–407.
76. Funck-Brentano C, Jacqz-Aigrain E, Leenhardt A, Roux A, Poirier J-M, Jaillon P. Influence of amiodarone on genetically determined drug metabolism in humans. *Clin Pharmacol Ther* 1991;50:259–266.
77. Ha HR, Stieger B, Meyer UA, Follath F. Interaction between amiodarone and lidocaine. *J Cardiovasc Pharmacol* 1996;28:533–539.
78. Nolan PE, Marcus FI, Hoyer GL, Bliss M, Gear K. Pharmacokinetic interaction between intravenous phenytoin and amiodarone in healthy volunteers. *Clin Pharmacol Ther* 1989;46:43–50.
79. O'Reilly RA, Trager WF, Rettie AE, Goulart DA. Interaction of amiodarone with racemic warfarin and its separated enantiomorphs in humans. *Clin Pharmacol Ther* 1987;42:290–294.
80. Haefeli WE, Bargetzi MJ, Follath F, Meyer UA. Potent inhibition of cytochrome P450IID6 (debrisoquin 4-hydroxylase) by flecainide in vitro and in vivo. *J Cardiovasc Pharmacol* 1990;15:776–779.

CHAPTER 46

Antimicrobials and Antiparasitics

Ronald E. Polk

Antimicrobial drugs are one of the most common causes of metabolic drug interactions (1–4). Since new drugs are being developed at an increasing rate because of the rapid rise in resistant organisms, the current prescribing guidelines must be consulted. This has become an important source, as many drug interaction investigations are conducted by the manufacturer and may not appear elsewhere.

FLUOROQUINOLONES

Background and Mechanisms

Some fluoroquinolone antibiotics are potent inhibitors of CYP1A2, and clinically important interactions have been described with theophylline, a substrate of this isoform. A metabolite was initially thought to be responsible for enzyme inhibition, but the metabolite does not inhibit P450s *in vitro* (5), whereas the parent compound does (6). It is unknown whether the fluoroquinolones that inhibit CYP1A2 also are metabolized by CYP1A2. Führ (7) evaluated the effects of 44 fluoroquinolones on *in vitro* inhibition of CYP1A2 and developed a model to predict quinolone inhibition of caffeine 3-demethylation from structure–activity relations. Presence of a nitrogen at position 4 or 7 reduces or increases inhibitory activity, respectively, and cleavage of the piperazine ring yields compounds that are more inhibitory than the parent compounds (8). The presence of a bulky substituent at position 8 may impair binding to CYP1A2, whereas a 4′-nitrogen atom in the 7-piperazinyl group may be required for inhibition, the latter possibly serving as the binding site to the enzymes (9).

The most clinically important metabolic interaction with fluoroquinolones is inhibition of drugs metabolized by CYP1A2, in particular, theophylline. Other substrates of CYP1A2, such as tacrine and clozapine, have not been thoroughly investigated.

Many of the older fluoroquinolones such as ciprofloxacin were developed when hepatic isoforms were not well characterized, and other important drug interactions were described as case reports, including cyclosporine (CsA) and warfarin (see later). Although fluoroquinolones can inhibit CYP3A4 *in vitro* (10), nearly all prospective clinical investigations with non-CYP1A2 substrates reported no inhibition (see later). It is probable that most case reports involving fluoroquinolones and non-CYP1A2 substrates do not reflect a causal relation, but are likely confounded by alternative explanations such as the suppression of metabolic enzyme activity by infection (see Chapters 11 and 12).

Methylxanthines

The inhibition of theophylline metabolism by certain fluoroquinolones is well known and thoroughly investigated (13–20). Evidence points to quinolone-induced inhibition of CYP1A2-mediated demethylations as the most important mechanism for this interaction (14,15), although the 8-hydroxylation step also is inhibited (6,15). It is now a routine preclinical investigation of a new fluoroquinolone to evaluate inhibition of CYP1A2, often by evaluating the effect of the quinolone on 1- and 3-demethylations or *O*-hydroxylation of theophylline *in vitro* (16). The magnitude of the interaction *in vivo* depends on the specific quinolone and dose; inhibition at clinically useful doses is greatest for enoxacin (approximately a 60% mean reduction in clearance), followed by clinafloxacin (50% decrease), ciprofloxacin and pefloxacin (approximately a 30% mean reduction in clearance for both) (17,18). There is little inhibition of theophylline metabolism, either *in vitro* or *in vivo,* for norfloxacin, ofloxacin, levofloxacin, sparfloxacin, fleroxacin, and lomefloxacin (17,19,20). Grepafloxacin inhibits theophylline metabolism to a similar extent as ciprofloxacin, whereas preliminary information for moxifloxacin, trovafloxacin, and gatifloxacin indicates that there is little clinically meaningful inhibition of CYP1A2 (20).

R. E. Polk: Department of Pharmacy, Virginia Commonwealth University, School of Pharmacy, 410 North 12th Street, Smith Building, Richmond, Virginia 23298-0533

The same fluoroquinolones that inhibit theophylline metabolism also inhibit caffeine metabolism (20–24). Enoxacin reduced caffeine clearance by approximately 80% and was associated with nausea and vomiting (20). Ciprofloxacin decreased caffeine clearance by 30% to 45%, and norfloxacin and ofloxacin had no significant effect. The clinical significance of these interactions is unclear, and there are no published reports of excessive central nervous system (CNS) stimulation from caffeine accumulation in patients treated with fluoroquinolones. In part this may reflect the fact that CNS stimulation is itself an adverse effect of fluoroquinolones, and any effect of caffeine accumulation would be difficult to discern (21).

Most drug–drug interaction investigations evaluate only the effect of one drug on the metabolism of another. Patients often receive multiple drugs, each of which may be an independent inhibitor (or inducer) of different P450 enzymes. The combination of cimetidine and ciprofloxacin resulted in a greater inhibition of theophylline metabolism than did either agent alone (25,26). However, a study in five subjects did not find the combination of clarithromycin (a CYP3A4 inhibitor) plus ciprofloxacin to result in additional inhibition of theophylline metabolism beyond that with ciprofloxacin alone (27).

Warfarin

Several case reports described prolongation of coagulation time, measured as prothrombin time (PT), or international normalized ratio (INR), in patients stabilized with warfarin therapy who received a quinolone (28–30). In contrast, a prospective trial by Toon (31) found that administration of enoxacin, 400 mg every 12 hours, for 14 days to six healthy volunteers, followed by single-dose warfarin, had no effect on the pharmacokinetics of the more pharmacologically active S-enantiomer of warfarin, although a 32% reduction in the renal clearance of the R-stereoisomer was noted. A prospective, placebo-controlled trial by Bianco (32) found that administration of ciprofloxacin, 500 mg every 12 hours for 10 days, had no significant effect on PT in 16 subjects receiving prolonged warfarin therapy (30). Similarly, a double-blind, placebo-controlled crossover trial in 36 patients receiving long-term warfarin found no statistically or clinically important effect on S-warfarin pharmacokinetics or anticoagulation response in patients who received a 12-day course of ciprofloxacin, 750 mg twice daily. Concentrations of the R-stereoisomer did increase significantly (33). Norfloxacin did not alter the pharmacokinetic disposition of warfarin in a prospective trial of 10 subjects (34), and levofloxacin did not alter warfarin pharmacokinetics (R- or L-stereoisomers) or anticoagulation response in 16 adults (35).

These clinical trials that report no important effect on the clinical response to warfarin can be explained. The pharmacologically active S-isomer is metabolized by CYP2C9 (see Chapter 29), an enzyme not inhibited by fluoroquinolones. The relatively inactive isomer, the R-enantio-mer, is metabolized by CYP1A2, consistent with the effects seen in the enoxacin, clinafloxacin, and ciprofloxacin investigations described earlier. Patients who are receiving warfarin in whom a quinolone is indicated (especially for clinafloxacin) can probably be treated safely, although it would be prudent to monitor prothrombin response.

Cyclosporine/Tacrolimus

Case reports suggest an interaction between fluoroquinolones and CsA, resulting in increases in serum creatinine and inconsistent changes in CsA concentrations (37). Retrospective investigations have reported that pediatric renal transplant patients required a lower dose of CsA to maintain therapeutic serum concentrations when norfloxacin was coadministered compared with a control group not receiving norfloxacin (38). However, prospective investigations have reported that fluoroquinolones have no effect on the pharmacokinetics of CsA. Renal transplant patients who received ciprofloxacin, 750 mg every 12 hours, for 2 weeks, or a similar regimen of pefloxacin had no alterations in CsA metabolism or serum creatinine (39). Pichard et al. (40) found that norfloxacin did not inhibit CsA metabolism in human liver microsomes in vitro, consistent with prospective clinical trials. These negative findings are consistent with observations that fluoroquinolones inhibit primarily CYP1A2, but not the rate-limiting cyclosporine-metabolizing enzyme, CYP3A4. Because of these findings, fluoroquinolones have been recommended to treat infections caused by Legionella pneumophila in transplant patients receiving CsA, instead of macrolides and rifampin, because of the well-known deleterious effects of the latter therapies on CsA concentrations (41). More recent investigations, however, have reported that ciprofloxacin increases production of interleukin-2 by human peripheral blood lymphocytes in vitro, and can antagonize the main pharmacologic effect of CsA and tacrolimus (42). A case control study in 42 patients found that ciprofloxacin was associated with a two-fold increase in rejection episodes among kidney transplant recipients (43). Recent reviews of antimicrobial drug interactions with CsA and tacrolimus concluded that the concentrations of ciprofloxacin and other fluoroquinolones are not likely to antagonize the effects of CsA and tacrolimus, but that some caution should be used until this issue is settled (44,45).

Miscellaneous

Both tacrine and clozapine are substrates for CYP1A2. In vitro studies have shown that enoxacin decreases conversion of tacrine to its hepatotoxic metabolite in vitro by inhibition of CYP1A2, an effect that could be of clinical importance (46). The clinical consequences of coadministration of an CYP1A2-inhibitory quinolone with tacrine is unknown. Limited clinical observations suggest that fluoroquinolones may decrease clearance of clozapine in humans (47).

In support of the selective inhibition of CYP1A2 by some fluoroquinolones, found that ciprofloxacin did not inhibit the metabolism of quinidine, a substrate for CYP3A4 (48) and gatifloxacin does not inhibit midazolam clearance (49).

MACROLIDES

Background and Mechanisms

Nearly all interactions with macrolide (14-member macrocyclic lactone rings) antibiotics result from dose-dependent inhibition of gastrointestinal and/or hepatic CYP3A4. The azalide (15-member rings) antibiotic, azithromycin, does not inhibit CYP3A4 (see later). Studies in human liver microsomes show differences in inhibitory activity between macrolides: troleandomycin is the most potent, followed by clarithromycin, erythromycin, roxithromycin, azithromycin, and spiramycin (50,51). Clinical studies have confirmed and extended these *in vitro* observations. At clinical doses, erythromycin and clarithromycin appear to be similar in inhibitory potency and in the spectrum of interacting drugs, whereas midecamycin, josamycin, and roxithromycin are much less inhibitory, and azithromycin, dirithromycin, rikamycin, and spiramycin have no important effect (52–55).

The proposed mechanism of enzyme inhibition is that macrolides such as erythromycin undergo *N*-demethylation by CYP3A4 to a nitrosoalkane, which forms a stable inactivating complex with the heme of P450 (51). These stable complexes are quasi-irreversible, and macrolides act as "mechanism-based" inhibitors of CYP3A4. Macrolides and azalides that do not form these stable complexes show little or no enzyme inhibition. This same *N*-demethylation step is the basis for the erythromycin breath test, reported to be a measure of hepatic CYP3A4 activity in humans (56). In addition to *N*-demethylation, clarithromycin is extensively metabolized by CYP3A4 to 14-hydroxyclarithromycin, a bioactive metabolite (57). Inhibition of CYP3A4 will decrease concentrations of 14-hydroxy-clarithromycin; the clinical significance is unknown. Induction of CYP3A4 increases clearance of clarithromycin (see later), but similar observations have not been made for erythromycin. It is possible that the poor bioavailability of erythromycin may in part reflect gastrointestinal metabolism of erythromycin by CYP3A4.

The clinically important drug interactions with the inhibitory macrolides, such as erythromycin and clarithromycin, are generally predictable and involve CYP3A4 substrates with a narrow therapeutic index: most commonly, CsA, tacrolimus, terfenadine, cisapride, midazolam, triazolam, and carbamazepine (see later). In addition, less well studied but important interacting drugs that appear to be CYP3A4 substrates include ergot and *Vinca* alkaloids (58), some hydroxymethylglutaryl–coenzyme A reductase inhibitors such as lovastatin (59), and pimozide. Two of the well-documented interactions with erythromycin, involving warfarin and theophylline, are not well explained because these are primarily CYP2C9 and CYP1A2 substrates, respectively, isoforms not known to be inhibited by erythromycin.

Theophylline

Of the 17 prospective clinical trials of the erythromycin–theophylline interaction reviewed by Periti et al. (60), 12 reported a statistically significant reduction in theophylline clearance after erythromycin. The inconsistent frequency of this interaction is used by Watkins (61) to illustrate the relation of between-subject variability in P450 activity and the unpredictable nature of some drug–drug interactions. Because erythromycin inhibits CYP3A4, but not CYP1A2 (62), an interaction is not expected when theophylline and erythromycin are coadministered. However, theophylline is also oxidized by 8-hydroxylation, which may be mediated by CYP3A4. A patient receiving erythromycin would be expected to "shunt" metabolism of theophylline away from 8-hydroxylation (CYP3A4) and toward *N*-demethylation (CYP1A2), with little net change in theophylline clearance. However, in patients with a relative deficiency in CYP1A2, CYP3A4 may be responsible for clearance of a greater proportion of the administered dose, and inhibition of CYP3A4 in these subjects by erythromycin may be sufficient to explain the increase in theophylline serum concentrations seen in some subjects. In addition, there may be an effect of downregulation of P450 activity by the infection that erythromycin is prescribed to treat.

Prospective trials that demonstrate a significant interaction reported that theophylline clearance is reduced by approximately 25%. The interaction is most likely to occur in subjects receiving higher erythromycin doses (more than 1.5 g/day), in those with higher serum concentrations, and in those given prolonged therapy (63). Because the frequency of this interaction is variable, and the contribution of "infection" is uncertain, patients receiving both drugs should have theophylline levels monitored.

Roxithromycin results in a small but statistically significant reduction in theophylline clearance, whereas the effects of josamycin on theophylline metabolism have been inconsistent (60). Clarithromycin (500 mg, b.i.d.) administered to 10 subjects reduced clearance of theophylline by 17% ($p < 0.05$) (64). In contrast, miocamycin, midecamycin and azithromycin do not alter theophylline clearance (53,54,60,65).

Cyclosporine/Tacrolimus

Cyclosporine and erythromycin both compete for metabolism by CYP3A4 (66), and CsA concentrations predictably increase in patients receiving concomitant erythromycin (67,68). All prospective trials in normal volunteers and transplant patients have found significant reductions in clearance of CsA with concomitant erythromycin. Azanza et al. (69) reported increased CsA concentrations in three transplant patients who received josamycin. A number of case reports of clarithromycin–CsA and tacrolimus interactions have been reported (70,71), and clarithromycin should not be administered with CsA or tacrolimus. Other macrolides, such as spiramycin, have no effect *in vitro* or *in vivo*. Azithromycin does not appear to interact with CsA (53).

The contribution of gastrointestinal versus hepatic CYP3A4 to CsA metabolism has been debated. It is not clear whether macrolides increase CsA concentrations through a gastrointestinal or hepatic effect on CYP3A4, or both (72). Drugs that appear to increase absorption of CsA may do so more through inhibition of P-glycoprotein (which normally pumps CsA back into the gut lumen), rather than through inhibition of gut CYP3A4 (73).

Oral Anticoagulants

Erythromycin may increase the hypoprothrombinemic effect of warfarin, probably by inhibition of warfarin metabolism. Case reports described bleeding in patients receiving warfarin after administration of erythromycin (74). Prospective studies have shown a modest but significant reduction in mean warfarin clearance (75,76). The pharmacologically active S-enantiomer of warfarin is metabolized by CYP2C9, and the interaction with erythromycin is not readily explained. Because it is not possible to predict those who will have an exaggerated response when erythromycin is taken by a patient receiving warfarin, patients should be monitored closely. Azithromycin has rarely been reported to affect PT in patients receiving warfarin (77), but most evidence indicates there is no interaction. There are similar case reports of clarithromycin increasing the response to warfarin (78).

Carbamazepine

Carbamazepine is metabolized by CYP3A4 to its epoxide, and there is a predictable and well-understood interaction with macrolides that inhibit CYP3A4 (79), resulting in classic signs of carbamazepine toxicity (dizziness, vomiting, ataxia, nystagmus). A study in healthy volunteers found a mean reduction in carbamazepine clearance of 17% when 250 mg of erythromycin was given every 6 hours for 8 days (80). This interaction also occurs with josamycin (81) and clarithromycin (82). Azithromycin is apparently free of this interaction (52).

Digoxin

An interaction with an unusual metabolic mechanism is found between some macrolides, most commonly erythromycin and clarithromycin, and digoxin. Approximately 10% of patients metabolize digoxin by a gastrointestinal tract bacterium, *Eubacterium lentum,* to "digoxin degradation products" (83). Erythromycin, clarithromycin, (and tetracycline) eradicate these bacteria, resulting in an increase in serum digoxin concentrations.

An alternative mechanism may be that clarithromycin can inhibit P-gp and interferes with digoxin transport in *in vitro* preparations (84). It is not clear which mechanism explains reports of digoxin toxicity in patients given these antibiotics. Because it is not possible to identify patients at risk *a priori,* digoxin concentrations should be monitored.

Terfenadine and Astemizole

The clinical observation that a patient taking terfenadine developed a severe arrhythmia when ketoconazole was coadministered initiated a series of investigations into this important interaction (85). Terfenadine is completely and extensively metabolized by CYP3A4 to the active antihistamine, terfenadine carboxylate (86,87). Accumulation of the parent compound resulting from inhibition of CYP3A4 can lead to fatal arrhythmias (torsades de pointes). Although macrolides are less potent inhibitors of CYP3A4 compared with ketoconazole, use of erythromycin and clarithromycin in the patient taking terfenadine and astemizole has resulted in life-threatening arrhythmias. Honig et al. (88) studied nine volunteers who received terfenadine, 60 mg every 12 hours, for 7 days, followed by erythromycin, 500 every 8 hours, for 7 days. Peak concentrations of terfenadine's active metabolite increased 107% after erythromycin administration, and three subjects had ECG changes. In a similar study, clarithromycin was found to be at least as potent an inhibitor of terfenadine metabolism as erythromycin; azithromycin had no effect (89,90). Despite extensive warnings of this interaction to professional and lay audiences, concomitant prescribing of inhibitors of CYP3A4 and terfenadine continued (91,92), resulting in removal of terfenadine from the US market on February 1, 1998. Astemizole has interactions and effects similar to those of terfenadine and was withdrawn in June 1999.

Triazolam/Midazolam/Alprazolam

Triazolam and midazolam are metabolized by CYP3A4 (93,94). Both erythromycin and troleandomycin reduce metabolic clearance of triazolam, which may result in psychomotor impairment and drowsiness. Studies in volunteers have shown 50% to 100% increases in peak plasma concentrations and a prolongation of triazolam half-life (95,96). Erythromycin and clarithromycin significantly impair metabolic clearance of midazolam, and azithromycin has no effect (97,98). Similar interactions are observed for alprazolam, although the clinical significance of the interactions may be less (99).

Cisapride

The interaction between cisapride and erythromycin or other inhibitors of CYP3A4 is very similar to that of terfenadine. Cisapride is extensively metabolized by CYP3A4 and can cause potentially fatal arrhythmias (torsades de pointes) when serum concentrations increase to toxic levels (100). A warning appears in the cisapride package insert of the dangers of coadministration of inhibitors of CYP3A4. Most of the interacting comedications given to patients receiving cisapride and reported to the Food and Drug Administration (FDA) were either macrolides or azoles. Clarithromycin causes effects similar to those of erythromycin, although patients with renal impairment or preexisting cardiac diseases may be most susceptible (101).

Miscellaneous Interactions

Interactions with the following drugs presumably reflect macrolide inhibition of CYP3A4, may result in severe clinical effects, but have not been extensively investigated: ergot alkaloids (102), methylprednisolone, *Vinca* alkaloids (103), valproate, alfentanil, clozapine (104), buspirone (105), lovastatin, simvastatin, and atorvastatin (106,107), pimozide (package insert, Orap), and disopyramide (108). Limited investigations reported that erythromycin does not alter the metabolism of glyburide (109), sufentanil (110), or phenytoin (111).

Quinupristine/Dalfopristine

Quinupristine/dalfopristine is a combination antimicrobial compound in the streptogramin class (112). It is available for intravenous use and is active for many gram-positive aerobic bacteria, including those that are often resistant to traditional agents such as vancomycin. Clinical investigations in the organ-transplant population revealed that it causes a doubling of the AUC of CsA in patients receiving both drugs, suggesting that quinupristine/dalfopristine is an inhibitor of CYP3A4 (112). Precautions are advised for combination therapy with other CYP3A4 substrates, similar to those for erythromycin and clarithromycin.

Rifabutin

There is a bidirectional drug–drug interaction with clarithromycin and rifabutin. Rifabutin, at a dose of 300 mg/day, induces the metabolism of clarithromycin to its 14-OH metabolite, resulting in a 50% reduction in the AUC of the parent clarithromycin. The clinical significance of this interaction is unknown (113). Likewise, clarithromycin inhibits the metabolism of rifabutin, either through inhibition of formation of its primary metabolite (25-desacetyl-rifabutin) (114) or the inhibition of subsequent metabolism of the main metabolite (115). An increase in serum concentrations of the parent compound (and/or its metabolite) can lead to uveitis, neutropenia and flu-like symptoms (116,117). Because of the toxicity of rifabutin in this setting and if azithromycin is effective prophylaxis for *Mycobacterium avium* complex (MAC) (118), rifabutin is rarely used. However, because rifampin cannot be used to treat infection with *M. tuberculosis* in patients receiving human immunodeficiency virus 1 (HIV-1) protease inhibitors (see Chapter 48), rifabutin is being reevaluated for this use in the HIV population.

Oral Contraceptives and "Antibiotics"

There are case reports of women who become pregnant while taking oral contraceptive agents and "antibiotics." Although rifampin (and to a lesser extent, rifabutin) clearly induces metabolism or ethinyl estradiol and norethindrone (119), there is little data that other antibiotics have any measurable effect (120–121). As a precaution patients who are receiving antibiotics are usually advised to use an alternative form of contraception.

ANTIPARASITIC DRUGS

Drugs that interact with antiparasitic drugs are included in Table 46-1. Although most of these drug are little used in developed countries, drug interactions with quinidine deserve special mention. Quinidine is effective in the treatment of acute malaria (122) and is primarily metabolized by CYP3A4. However, quinidine is a potent inhibitor of

TABLE 46-1. *Pharmacokinetic drug interactions with antiparasitic agents*

Anti-parasitic	Interacting drug	Clinical effect	References
Quinidine[Q]	Amiodarone[Q]	↑ quinidine concentrations; reports of torsades de pointes	126
	Astemizole	↑ quinidine concentrations; reports of torsades de pointes	127
Quinidine & Quinine[Q+Q]	Oral anticoagulants[Q+Q]	↑ anticoagulant effect	128, 129
	β-Blockers[Q]	↑ β-blocker concentrations	125
	Cimetidine[Q+Q]	↑ quinidine concentrations	130
	Diltiazem	↑ diltiazem concentrations	131
	Digitalis glycosides[Q+Q]	↓ digoxin clearance	132, 133
	Erythromycin	↑ quinidine concentrations; reports of torsades de pointes	134
	Itraconazole	↑ quinidine concentrations	135
	Ketoconazole[Q]	↑ quinidine concentrations	136
	Neuromuscular blocking agents[Q+Q]	↓ neuromuscular blocker metabolism	137
	Phenytoin[Q]	↓ quinidine concentrations	138
	Rifampin[Q]	↓ quinidine concentrations	139
Thiabendazole	Theophylline	↓ theophylline clearance	140
Praziquantel	Phenytoin	↓ praziquantel concentrations	141–143
	Cimetidine	↑ praziquantel concentration	

CYP2D6, and the metabolism of other drugs that are normally cleared by CYP2D6 will be suppressed (123,124). CYP2D6 is under genetic control, and 10% of the Northern European population is deficient in this enzyme. These individuals typically display an exaggerated response to drugs of which the metabolism is rate limited by this enzyme; the best-studied example is the antihypertensive, debrisoquine. Administration of quinidine converts an individual to a poor metabolizer of debrisoquine and other drugs that require this enzyme activity such as β-blockers, tricyclic antidepressants, and many antiarrhythmics (125).

REFERENCES

1. Gregg CR. Drug interactions and anti-infective therapies. *Am J Med* 1999;106:227–237.
2. Hersh EV. Adverse drug interactions in dental practice: interactions involving antibiotics. Part II of a series. *J Am Dent Assoc* 1999;130:236–251.
3. Horn JR, Hasten PD. Drug interactions with antibacterial agents. *J Fam Pract* 1995;41:81–90.
4. Griffin JP. Drug interactions with antimalarial agents. *Adverse Drug React Toxicol Rev* 1999;18:25–43.
5. Mulder GJ, Nagelkerke JF, Tudens RB, Wijnands WJ, Van der mark EJ. Inhibition of the oxidative metabolism of theophylline in isolated rat hepatocytes by the quinolone antibiotic enoxacin and its metabolite oxoenoxacin, but not by ofloxacin. *Biochem Pharmacol* 1988;37:2565–2568.
6. Sarkar M, Polk RE, Guzelian PS, Hunt C, Karnes HT. In vitro effect of fluoroquinolones on theophylline metabolism in human liver microsomes. *Antimicrob Agents Chemother* 1990;34:594–599.
7. Führ U, Strobl G, Manaut F, et al. Quinolone antibacterial agents: relationship between structure and in vitro inhibition of the human cytochrome P450 isoform CYP1A2. *Mol Pharmacol* 1993;43:191–199.
8. Sörgel F, Kinzig M. Pharmacokinetics of gyrase inhibitors, Part 2: renal and hepatic elimination pathways and drug interactions. *Am J Med* 1993;94:56S–69S.
9. Mizuki Y, Yamaguchi T, Fujiwara I. Pharmacokinetic interactions related to the chemical structures of fluoroquinolones. *J Antimicrob Chemother* 1996;37(suppl A):41–55.
10. McLellan RA, Renton KW, Monshouwer M, Drobitch RK. Fluoroquinolone antibiotics inhibit cytochrome P450-mediated microsomal drug metabolism in rat and human. *Drug Metab Dispos* 1996;24:1134–1138.
11. Shedlofsky SI, Israel BC, Tosheva R, Blouin RA. Endotoxin depresses hepatic cytochrome P450-mediated drug metabolism in women. *Br J Clin Pharmacol* 1997;43:627–632.
12. Shedlofsky SI, Israel BC, McClain CJ, Hill DB, Blouin RA. Endotoxin administration to humans inhibits hepatic cytochrome P450-mediated drug metabolism. *J Clin Invest* 1994;94:2209–2214.
13. Radandt JM, Marchbanks CR, Dudley MN. Interactions of fluoroquinolones with other drugs: mechanisms, variability, clinical significance, and management. *Clin Infect Dis* 1992;14:272–284.
14. Führ U, Anders EM, Mahr G, Sörgel F, Staib AH. Inhibitory potency of quinolone antibacterial agents against cytochrome P450IA2 activity in vivo and in vitro. *Antimicrob Agents Chemother* 1992;36:942–948.
15. Robson RA, Begg EJ, Atkinson HC, Saunders DA, Frampton CM. Competitive effects of ciprofloxacin and lomefloxacin on the oxidative metabolism of theophylline. *Br J Clin Pharmacol* 1990;29:491–493.
16. White RB, Stevens JC, Heyn H. The effect of RPR 102341 on theophylline metabolism and phenacetin O-deethylase activity in human liver microsomes. *Pharmacol Res* 1997;14:512–515.
17. Wijnands WJA, Vree TB, Van Herwaarden CLA. The influence of quinolone derivatives on theophylline clearance. *Br J Clin Pharmacol* 1986;22:677–683.
18. Randinitis EJ, Koup JR, Rausch G, Vassos AB. Effect of clinafloxacin administration on the single dose pharmacokinetics of theophylline and caffeine. In: *Proceedings and abstracts of the 38th Interscience Conference on Antimicrobial Agents and Chemotherapy*. Sept. 24–27, 1998. San Diego, CA: Sept. 24–27, 1998: Abstract A-019.
19. Parent M, LeBel M. Meta-analysis of quinolone-theophylline interactions. *Ann Pharmacother* 1991;25:191–194.
20. Stein GE. Pharmacokinetics and pharmacodynamics of newer fluoroquinolones. *Clin Infect Dis* 1996;23(suppl 1):S19–S24.
21. Harder S, Staib AH, Beer C, Papenberg A, Stille W, Shah PM. 4-Quinolones inhibit biotransformation of caffeine. *Eur J Clin Pharmacol* 1988; 35:651–656.
22. Healy DP, Polk RE, Kanawati L, Rock DT, Mooney ML. Interaction between oral ciprofloxacin and caffeine in normal volunteers. *Antimicrob Agents Chemother* 1989;33:474–478.
23. Barnett G, Segura J, De La Torre R, Carbo M. Pharmacokinetic determination of relative potency of quinolone inhibition of caffeine disposition. *Eur J Clin Pharmacol* 1990;39:63–69.
24. Peloquin CA, Nix DE, Sedman AJ, et al. Pharmacokinetics and clinical effects of caffeine alone and in combination with oral enoxacin. *Rev Infect Dis* 1989;11:S1095.
25. Loi CM, Parker B, Vestal RE. Combined effect of cimetidine and ciprofloxacin on theophylline disposition. *Clin Pharmacol Ther* 1991;49:130(abst).
26. Davis RL, Quenzer RW, Kelly HW, Powell JR. Effect of the addition of ciprofloxacin on theophylline pharmacokinetics in subjects inhibited by cimetidine. *Pharmacotherapy* 1992;26:11–13.
27. Gillum JG, Polk RE, Climo MW, Scott RB, Israel DS. Effect of combination therapy with ciprofloxacin and clarithromycin on theophylline pharmacokinetics in healthy volunteers. *Antimicrob Agents Chemother* 1996;40:1715–1716.
28. Linville T, Matanin D. Norfloxacin and warfarin [Letter]. *Ann Intern Med* 1989;110:751–752.
29. Leor J, Matetzki S. Ofloxacin and warfarin [letter]. *Ann Intern Med* 198;109:761.
30. Jolson HM, Tanner LA, Green L, Grasela TH. Adverse reaction reporting of interaction between warfarin and fluoroquinolones. *Arch Intern Med* 1991;151:1003–1004.
31. Toon S, Hopkins KJ, Garstang FM, et al. Enoxacin-warfarin interaction: pharmacokinetic and stereochemical aspects. *Clin Pharmacol Ther* 1987;42:33–41.
32. Bianco TM, Bussey HI, Farnett LE, et al. Potential warfarin-ciprofloxacin interaction in patients receiving long-term anticoagulation. *Pharmacotherapy* 1992;12:435–439.
33. Israel DS, Polk RE, Heller AH, et al. Effect of ciprofloxacin on the pharmacokinetics and pharmacodynamics of warfarin. *Clin Infect Dis* 1996;22:251–256.
34. Rocci ML Jr, Vlasses PH, Distlerath LM, et al. Norfloxacin does not alter warfarin's disposition or anticoagulant effect. *J Clin Pharmacol* 1990;30:728–732.
35. Liao S, Nayak RK, Fowler C, Palmer M. Absence of an effect of levofloxacin on warfarin pharmacokinetics and anticoagulation in male volunteers. *J Clin Pharmacol* 1996;36:1072–1077.
36. Randinitis EJ, Koup JR, Bron NJ, et al. Drug interactions studies with clinafloxacin and probenecid, cimetidine, phenytoin and warfarin. In: *Proceedings and abstracts of the 38th Interscience Conference on Antimicrobial Agents and Chemotherapy*. San Diego, CA: Sept. 24–27, 1998: Abstract A-020.
37. Avent CK, Krinsky D, Kirklin JK, Bourge RC, Figg WD. Synergistic nephrotoxicity due to ciprofloxacin and cyclosporine. *Am J Med* 1988;85:452–453.
38. McLellan RA, Renton KW, Monshouwer M, Drobitch RK. Fluoroquinolone antibiotics inhibit cytochrome P450-mediated microsomal drug metabolism in rat and human. *Drug Metab Dispos* 1996;24:1134–1138.
39. Lang J, Finaz de Villaine J, Garraffo R, Touraine JL. Cyclosporin (cyclosporin A) pharmacokinetics in renal transplant patients receiving ciprofloxacin. *Am J Med* 1989;87(suppl 5A):82s–85s.
40. Pichard L, Fabre I, Fabre G, et al. Screening for inducers and inhibitors of cytochrome P450 (cyclosporine A oxidase) in primary cultures of human hepatocytes and in liver microsomes. *Drug Metab Dispos* 1990;18:595–606.
41. Hooper TL, Gould FK, Swinburn CR, et al. Ciprofloxacin: a preferred treatment for *Legionella* infections in patients receiving cyclosporin A. *J Antimicrob Chemother* 1988;22:952–953.
42. Ho S, Crabtree GR, Nourse J, et al. The mechanism of action of cyclosporin A and FK506. *Clin Immunol Immunopathol* 1996;80(3 Pt 2):S40–S45.

43. Wrishko RE, Keown PA, Landsberg D, et al. Investigation of a possible interaction between ciprofloxacin and cyclosporine in renal transplant patients. *Transplantation* 1997;15:996–999.

44. Paterson D, Singh N. Interactions between tacrolimus and antimicrobial agents. *Clin Infect Dis* 1997;25:1430–1440.

45. Campana C, Molinaro M, Buggia I, Regazzi MB. Clinically significant drug interactions with cyclosporin: an update. *Clin Pharmacokinet* 1996;30:141–179.

46. Bezek S, Woolf TF, Pool WF, Kukan M. The effect of cytochromes P4501A induction and inhibition on the disposition of the cognition activator tacrine in rat hepatic preparations. *Xenobiotica* 1996;26:935–946.

47. Markowitz JS, Mintzer JE, Devane CL, Gill HS. Fluoroquinolone inhibition of clozapine metabolism [Letter]. *Am J Psychiatry* 1997;154:881.

48. Bleske BE, Carver PL, Annesley TM, Bleske JR, Morady F. The effect of ciprofloxacin on the pharmacokinetic and ECG parameters of quinidine. *J Clin Pharmacol* 1990;30:911–915.

49. Gajjar DA, Lacreta FP, Kollia GD, et al. Lack of effect of gatifloxacin on the pharmacokinetics of midazolam, a model substrate for cytochrome P450 3A (CYP3A4) activity in healthy adult volunteers. In: *Proceedings and abstracts of the 39th Interscience Conference on Antimicrobial Agents and Chemotherapy*. San Francisco, CA: Sept. 26–29, 1999: Abstract 197.

50. Gascon MP, Dayer P. Comparative effects of macrolide antibiotics on liver monooxygenases. *Clin Pharmacol Ther* 1991;49:158(abst).

51. Lindstrom TD, Hanssen BR, Wrighton SA. Cytochrome P-450 complex formation by dirithromycin and other macrolides in rat and human livers. *Antimicrob Agents Chemother* 1993;37:265–269.

52. McConnell SA, Amsden GW. Review and comparison of advanced-generation macrolides clarithromycin and dirithromycin. *Pharmacotherapy* 1999;19:404–415.

53. Nahata M. Drug interactions with azithromycin and the macrolides: an overview. *J Antimicrob Chemother* 1996;37(suppl C):133–142.

54. Amsden GW. Macrolides versus azalides: a drug interaction update. *Ann Pharmacother* 1995;29:906–917.

55. von Rosensteil NA, Adam D. Macrolide antibacterials: drug interactions of clinical significance. *Drug Safety* 1995;13:105–122.

56. Lown KS, Watkins PB, Berent S, et al. The erythromycin breath test predicts the clearance of midazolam. *Clin Pharmacol Ther* 1995;57:16–24.

57. Rodrigues AS, Roberts E, Mulford DJ, Yao Y, Ouellet D. Oxidative metabolism of clarithromycin in the presence of human liver microsomes: major role for the cytochrome P4503A (CYP3A) subfamily. *Drug Metab Dispos* 1997;25:623–630.

58. Tobe SW, Warner E, Murphy GF, Skorecki KL, Jamal SA, Siu LL. Vinblastine and erythromycin: an unrecognized serious drug interaction. *Cancer Chemother Pharmacol* 1995;35:188–190.

59. Garnett WR. Interactions with hydroxymethylglutaryl-coenzyme A reductase inhibitors. *Am J Health Syst Pharm* 1995;52:1639–1645.

60. Periti P, Mazzei T, Mini E, Novelli A. Pharmacokinetic drug interactions of macrolides. *Clin Pharmacokinet* 1992;23:106–131.

61. Watkins PB. Drug metabolism by cytochromes P450 in the liver and small bowel. *Gastroenterol Clin North Am* 1992;21:511–526.

62. Führ U, Staib AH, Kinzig M, Sörgel F. Lack of an effect of macrolides on cytochrome P4501A2 activity in human liver microsomes [abstract 206]. Program and abstracts, First international conference on the macrolides, azalides and streptogramins. Jan 22–25, Santa Fe, NM, 1992.

63. Prince RA, Wing DS, Weinberger MM, Hendles LS, Riegelman S. Effect of erythromycin on theophylline kinetics. *J Allergy Clin Immunol* 1981;68:427–431.

64. Ruff F, Chu S-Y, Sonders RC, Senello LT. Effects of multiple doses of clarithromycin on the pharmacokinetics of theophylline. In: *Abstracts of the 30th Interscience Conference on Antimicrobial Agents and Chemotherapy*. American Society for Microbiology; Atlanta: 1990: Abstract 761.

65. Felstead S. Azithromycin drug interactions. *Pathol Biol* 1995;436:512–514.

66. Pichard L, Fabre I, Fabre G, et al. Screening for inducers and inhibitors of cytochrome P450 (cyclosporine A oxidase) in primary cultures of human hepatocytes and in liver microsomes. *Drug Metab Dispos* 1990;18:595–606.

67. Jensen CWB, Flechner SM, Van Buren CT, et al. Exacerbation of cyclosporin toxicity by concomitant administration of erythromycin. *Transplantation* 1987;43:263–270.

68. Aoki FY, Yatscoff R, Jeffrey J, Rush D, Sitar D. Effects of erythromycin on cyclosporine A kinetics in renal transplant patients. *Clin Pharmacol Ther* 1987;41:221.

69. Azanza JR, Catalan M, Alvarez MP, et al. Possible interaction between cyclosporin and josamycin: a description of three cases. *Clin Pharmacol Ther* 1992;51:572–575.

70. Sketris IS, West ML, Wright MR. Possible role of the intestinal P-450 enzyme system in a cyclosporine-clarithromycin interaction. *Pharmacotherapy* 1996;16:301–305.

71. Gomez G, Alvarez ML, Errasti P, et al. Acute tacrolimus nephrotoxicity in renal transplant patients treated with clarithromycin. *Transplant Proc* 1999;31:2250–2251.

72. Gomez DY, Wacher VJ, Tomlanovich SJ, Hebert MF, Benet LZ. The effects of ketoconazole on the intestinal metabolism and bioavailability of cyclosporine. *Clin Pharmacol Ther* 1995;58:15–19.

73. Lown KS, Mayo RR, Leichtman AB, et al. Role of intestinal P-glycoprotein (mdr 1) in interpatient variation in the oral bioavailability of CsA. *Clin Pharmacol Ther* 1997;62:248–260.

74. Schwartz J, Bachmann K, Perrigo E. Interaction between warfarin and erythromycin. *South Med J* 1983;76:91–93.

75. Bachmann K, Schwartz JI, Fornay R Jr, Frogameni A, Jauregui LE. The effect of erythromycin on the disposition kinetics of warfarin. *Pharmacology* 1984;28:171–176.

76. Weibert RT, Lorentz SM, Townsend RJ, et al. Effect of erythromycin in patients receiving long-term warfarin therapy. *Clin Pharmacol* 1989;8:210–214.

77. Lane G. Increased hypoprothrombinemic effect of warfarin possibly induced by azithromycin [Letter]. *Ann Pharmacother* 1996;30:884–885.

78. Recker MW, Kier KL. Potential interaction between clarithromycin and warfarin. *Ann Pharmacother* 1997;31:996–998.

79. Stafstrom CE, DeLong GR, Boustany RM, Nahouraii R, Loganbill H, Nohria V. Erythromycin-induced carbamazepine toxicity: a continuing problem. *Arch Pediatr Adolesc Med* 1995;149:99–101.

80. Wong YY, Ludden TM, Bell RD. Effect of erythromycin on carbamazepine kinetics. *Clin Pharmacol Ther* 1983;33:460–464.

81. Vincon G, Albin H, Demotes-Mainard F, et al. Effects of josamycin on carbamazepine kinetics. *Eur J Clin Pharmacol* 1987;32:321–323.

82. O'Connor NK, Fris J. Clarithromycin-carbamazepine interaction in a clinical setting. *J Am Board Fam Pract* 1994;7:489–492.

83. Lindenbaum J, Rund DG, Butler VP, Tse-Eng D, Saha JN. Inactivation of digoxin by the gut flora: reversal by antibiotic therapy. *N Engl J Med* 1981;305:789–794.

84. Wakasugi H, Yano I, Ito T, et al. Effect of clarithromycin on renal excretion of digoxin: interaction with P-glycoprotein. *Clin Pharmacol Ther* 1998;64:123–128.

85. Mathews DR, McNutt B, Okerholm R, Flicker McBride G. Torsades de pointes occurring in association with terfenadine use [Letter]. *JAMA* 1991;266:2375–2376.

86. Jurima-Romet M, Inaba T, Cyr T, Crawford K. Terfenadine metabolism in human liver: in vitro inhibition by macrolide antibiotics and azole antifungals. *Drug Metab Dispos* 1994;22:849–857.

87. Monahan BP, Ferguson CL, Killeavy ES, et al. Torsades de pointes occurring in association with terfenadine use. *JAMA* 1990;264:2788–2790.

88. Honig PK, Woosley RL, Zamani K, Conner DP, Cantilena LR. Changes in the pharmacokinetics and electrocardiographic pharmacodynamics of terfenadine with concomitant administration of erythromycin. *Clin Pharmacol Ther* 1992;52:231–238.

89. Honig P, Wortham D, Zamani K, Conner D, Cantilena L. Effect of erythromycin, clarithromycin and azithromycin on the pharmacokinetics of terfenadine. *Clin Pharmacol Ther* 1993;53:161 (PI-106).

90. Harris S, Okerholm R, Eller M, Colangelo PM, Hilligoss DM. Azithromycin and terfenadine: lack of drug interaction. *Clin Pharmacol Ther* 1995;58:310–315.

91. Thompson D, Oster G. Use of terfenadine and contraindicated drugs. *JAMA* 1996;275:1339–1341.

92. Zechnich AD, Hedges JR. Use of terfenadine and contraindicated drugs [Letter]. *JAMA* 1996;276:953.

93. Kronbach T, Mathys D, Umeno M, Gonzales FJ, Meyer UA. Oxidation of midazolam and triazolam by human liver cytochrome CYP3A4. *Mol Pharmacol* 1989;36:89–96.

94. Gascon MP, Dayer P. In vitro forecasting of drugs which may interfere with the biotransformation of midazolam. *Eur J Clin Pharmacol* 1991;41:573–578.

95. Phillips JP, Antal EJ, Smith RB. A pharmacokinetic interaction between erythromycin and triazolam. *J Clin Psychopharmacol* 1986; 6:297–299.

96. Warot D, Bergougnan L, Lamiable D, et al. Troleandomycin-triazolam interaction in healthy volunteers: pharmacokinetic and psychometric evaluation. *Eur J Clin Pharmacol* 1987;32:389–393.

97. Zimmermann T, Wildfeuer A, Leitold M, Scharpf F, Laufen H, Yeates RA. Influence of the antibiotics erythromycin and azithromycin on the pharmacokinetics and pharmacodynamics of midazolam. *Arzneimittelforschung* 1996;46:213–217.

98. Yeates RA, Zimmermann T, Laufen H. Interaction between midazolam and clarithromycin: comparison with azithromycin. *Int J Clin Pharmacol Ther* 1996;34:400–405.

99. Yasui N, Ishizaki T, Chiba K, et al. Kinetic and dynamic study of oral alprazolam with and without erythromycin in humans: in vivo evidence for the involvement of CYP3A4 in alprazolam metabolism. *Clin Pharmacol Ther* 1996;59:514–519.

100. Wysowski DK, Bacsanyi J. Cisapride and fatal arrhythmia [Letter]. *N Engl J Med* 1996;335:290–291.

101. Sekkarie MA. Torsades de pointes in two chronic renal failure patients treated with cisapride and clarithromycin. *Am J Kidney Dis* 1997;30: 437–439.

102. Horowitz RS, Gomez HF, Dart RC. Clinical ergotism with lingual ischemia induced by clarithromycin-ergotamine interaction. *Arch Intern Med* 1996;156:456–458.

103. Tobe SW, Warner E, Murphy GF, Skorecki KL, Jamal SA, Siu LL. Vinblastine and erythromycin: an unrecognized serious drug interaction. *Cancer Chemother Pharmacol* 1995;35:188–190.

104. Cohen LG, Goff DC, Fisch J, Flood JG, Eugenio L, Chesley S. Erythromycin-induced clozapine toxic reaction. *Arch Intern Med* 1996;156:675–677.

105. Kivisto KT, Neuvonen PJ, Kantola T, Lamberg TS. Plasma buspirone concentrations are greatly increased by erythromycin and itraconazole. *Clin Pharmacol Ther* 1997;62:348–354.

106. Reference removed in proofs.

107. Grunden JW, Fisher KA. Lovastatin-induced rhabdomyolysis possibly associated with clarithromycin and azithromycin. *Ann Pharmacother* 1997;31:859–863.

108. Paar D, Sauerbruch T, Terjung B. Life-threatening interaction between clarithromycin and disopyramide. *Lancet* 1997;349:326–327.

109. Fleishaker JC, Phillips JP. Evaluation of a potential interaction between erythromycin and glyburide in diabetic volunteers. *J Clin Pharmacol* 1991;31:259–262.

110. Bartkowski RR, Goldberg ME, Huffnagle S, Epstein RH. Sufentanil disposition: is it affected by erythromycin administration? *Anesthesiology* 1993;78:260–265.

111. Milne RW, Coulthard K, Nation RL, Penna AC, Roberts G, Sansom LN. Lack of effect of erythromycin on the pharmacokinetics of single oral dose of phenytoin. *Br J Clin Pharmacol* 1988;26:330–333.

112. Rubinstein E, Prokocimer P, Talbot GH. Safety and tolerability of quinupristin/dalfopristin: administration guidelines. *J Antimicrob Chemother* 1999;44:37–46.

113. Wallace RJ Jr, Tanaka K, Girard W, Griffith DE, Brown BA. Reduced serum levels of clarithromycin in patients treated with multidrug regimens including rifampin or rifabutin for *Mycobacterium avium-M. intracellulare* infection. *J Infect Dis* 1995;171:747–750.

114. Trapnell CB, Collins JM, Klecker RW, Jamis-Dow C. Metabolism of rifabutin and its 25-desacetyl metabolite, LM565, by human liver microsomes and recombinant human cytochrome P-450 3A4: relevance to clinical interaction with fluconazole. *Antimicrob Agents Chemother* 1997;41:924–926.

115. Slatsimirskaia E, Koudriakova T, Gerber N, et al. Metabolism of rifabutin in human enterocyte and liver microsomes: kinetic parameters, identification of enzyme systems, and drug interactions with macrolides and antifungal agents. *Clin Pharmacol Ther* 1997;61:554–562.

116. Tseng AL, Walmsley SL. Rifabutin-associated uveitis. *Ann Pharmacother* 1995;29:1149–1155.

117. Griffith DE, Wallace RJ Jr, Girard WM, Brown BA. Adverse events associated with high-dose rifabutin in macrolide-containing regimens for the treatment of *Mycobacterium avium* complex lung disease. *Clin Infect Dis* 1995;21:594–598.

118. Benson CA. Disseminated *Mycobacterium avium* complex infection:

119. Barditch-Crovo P, Trapnell CB, Ette E, et al. The effects of rifampin and rifabutin on the pharmacokinetics and pharmacodynamics of a combination oral contraceptive. *Clin Pharmacol Ther* 1999;65: 428–438.

120. Weisberg E. Interactions between oral contraceptives and antifungals/antibacterials. Is contraceptive failure the result? *Clin Pharmacokinet* 1999;36:309–313.

121. Weaver K. Interaction between borad-spectrum antibiotics and the combined oral contraceptive pill. A literature review. *Contraception* 1999;59:71–78.

122. Miller KD, Greenberg AE, Campbell CC. Treatment of severe malaria in the United States with a continuous infusion of quinidine gluconate and exchange transfusion. *N Engl J Med* 1989;321:65–70.

123. Leemann T, Dayer P, Meyer UA. Single dose quinidine treatment inhibits metoprolol oxidation in extensive metabolizers. *Eur J Clin Pharmacol* 1986;29:739–741.

124. Brosen K, Gram LF. Clinical significance of the sparteine/debrisoquine oxidative polymorphism. *Eur J Clin Pharmacol* 1989;36: 537–547.

125. Caporoso NE, Shaw GL. Clinical implications of the competitive inhibition of the debrisoquine-metabolizing enzyme by quinidine. *Arch Intern Med* 1991;151:1985–1992.

126. Lesko LJ. Pharmacokinetic drug interactions with amiodarone. *Clin Pharmacokinet* 1989;17:130–140.

127. Martin ES, Black JN, Rogalski K. Quinine may trigger torsades de pointes during astemizole therapy. *Pacing Clin Electrophysiol* 1997; 20:2024–2025.

128. Koch-Weser J. Quinidine-induced hypoprothrombinemic hemorrhage in patients on chronic warfarin therapy. *Ann Intern Med* 1968;68: 511–517.

129. Gazzaniga AB, Stewart DR. Possible quinidine-induced hemorrhage in a patient on warfarin sodium. *N Engl J Med* 1969;280:711–712.

130. Penston J, Wormsley KG. Adverse reactions and interactions with H_2-receptor antagonists. *Med Toxicol* 1986;1:192–216.

131. Laganiere S, McGilveray I, Pereira C, et al. Pharmacokinetic and pharmacodynamic interactions between diltiazem and quinidine. *Clin Pharmacol Ther* 1996;60:255–264.

132. Rodin SM, Johnson BF. Pharmacokinetic interactions with digoxin. *Clin Pharmacokinet* 1988;15:227–244.

133. Pederson KE, Madsen JL, Klitgaard NA, Kjaer K, Hvidt S. Effect of quinine on plasma digoxin concentration and renal digoxin clearance. *Acta Med Scand* 1985;218:229–232.

134. Lin JC, Quasny HA. QT prolongation and development of torsades de pointes with the concomitant administration of oral erythromycin base and quinidine. *Pharmacotherapy* 1997;17:626–630.

135. Kaukonen KM, Neuvonen PJ, Olkkola KT. Itraconazole increases plasma concentrations of quinidine. *Clin Pharmacol Ther* 1997;62: 510–517.

136. McNulty RM, Lazor JA, Sketch M. Transient increase in plasma quinidine concentrations during ketoconazole-quinidine therapy. *Clin Pharmacol* 1989;8:222–225.

137. Kambam JR, Franks JJ, Naukam R, Sastry BV. Effect of quinidine on plasma cholinesterase activity and succinylcholine neuromuscular blockade. *Anesthesiology* 1987;67:858–860.

138. Data JL, Wilkinson GR, Nies AS. Interaction with quinidine and anticonvulsant drugs. *N Engl J Med* 1976;294:699–702.

139. Strayhorn VA, Self TH, Baciewicz AM. Update on rifampin drug interactions, III. *Arch Intern Med* 1997;157:2453–2458.

140. Schneider D, Gannon R, Sweeney K, Shore E. Theophylline and antiparasitic drug interactions: a case report and study of the influence of thiabendazole on theophylline pharmacokinetics in adults. *Chest* 1990;97:84–87.

141. Bittencourt PR, Garcia CM, Martins R, et al. Phenytoin and carbamazepine decrease oral bioavailability of praziquantel. *Neurology* 1992; 42:492–496.

142. Jung H, Sotelo J, Corona T, Castro N, Medina R. Pharmacokinetic study of praziquantel administered alone and in combination with cimetidine in a single-day therapeutic regimen. *Antimicrob Agents Chemother* 1997;41:1256–1259.

143. Na-Bangchang K, Karbwang J, Vanijanonta S. Plasma concentrations of praziquantel during the therapy of neurocysticerosis with praziquantel, in the presence of antiepileptics and dexamethasone. *Southeast Asian J Trop Med Public Health* 1995;26:120–123.

implications of recent clinical trials on prophylaxis and treatment. *AIDS Clin Rev* 1997;98:271–287.

CHAPTER 47

Antifungals

Janne T. Backman, Kari T. Kivistö, Jun-Sheng Wang, and Pertti J. Neuvonen

Because of increasing use of broad-spectrum antibiotics and immunosuppressive therapy, the significance of fungal infections has increased during the last decades. Fortunately, some important advances in antifungal therapy have also been achieved, especially after the introduction of the triazoles, itraconazole and fluconazole (1). However, because fungal cells are eukaryotic and thus resemble mammalian cells, it has been difficult to find specific cellular targets for antifungal agents. Consequently, many antifungal agents have been associated with problems, such as toxicity and drug interactions.

One of the most important problems has arisen from inhibition of mammalian cytochrome P450 (CYP) enzymes by the azole antifungal agents, that is, the azoles are not selective for their target, the fungal cytochrome P450 enzyme lanosterol 14-demethylase. By inhibiting drug-metabolizing CYPs, the systemically administered azoles—ketoconazole, itraconazole, and fluconazole—substantially increase the plasma concentrations of a large number of drugs. In many cases, the interactions can have harmful consequences as a result of potentiated adverse effects. Apart from azoles, no other antifungals have been clearly associated with inhibition of drug metabolism.

The three main classes of systemic antifungals include the azoles, the polyene macrolides, and the allylamines. Griseofulvin and flucytosine have also been used as systemic antifungals for a long time. The effects of antifungal agents on the oxidative metabolism and pharmacokinetics of drugs have been extensively studied in numerous studies *in vitro* and *in vivo*. This chapter systematically reviews each antifungal agent as an inhibitor of metabolic enzymes. First, the clinical pharmacokinetics of the antifungal agent are summarized to provide a view of the exposure of drug-metabolizing tissues to the antifungal. Thereafter, both the inhibitory effects of the antifungal on specific enzymes *in vitro* and its pharmacokinetic interactions are reviewed, including an assessment of the degree of *in vitro–in vivo* agreement.

AZOLES

Azoles are a broad class of antifungals, some of which (e.g., clotrimazole and econazole) are only used topically. Systemically administerd azoles include the imidazoles miconazole and ketoconazole and the triazoles itraconazole and fluconazole. The antifungal effect of the azoles is based on inhibition of ergosterol synthesis by binding to the fungal cytochrome P450 enzyme lanosterol 14-demethylase, which catalyzes the initial step in the conversion of lanosterol to ergosterol (2,3). In addition to inhibiting the fungal enzyme, virtually all clinically used azoles have been observed to inhibit human drug-metabolizing CYP enzymes, thereby being able to impair the metabolism of a large number of drugs.

Ketoconazole

After ketoconazole was synthesized in 1977, it became the first significant orally administered broad-spectrum azole antimycotic drug (2–4). In the past, ketoconazole was widely used for a variety of non–life-threatening fungal infections, such as dermatophytosis, onychomycosis, *Candida* infections, and pityriasis versicolor. However, disappointing cure rates (5), variable gastrointestinal absorption, and rare occurrence of hepatotoxicity limited the use of systemic ketoconazole, especially after terbinafine and the triazoles itraconazole and fluconazole were introduced. Topical ketoconazole is still in wide use.

Ketoconazole is well absorbed when administered with a meal (2,6,7). However, its absorption is reduced during fasting and with diminished gastric acidity. Its recom-

J. T. Backman, K. T. Kivistö, Jun-Sheng Wang, and P. J. Neuvonen: Department of Clinical Pharmacology, University of Helsinki, Haartmaninkatu 4, FIN-00290 Helsinki, Finland

mended dosing is 200 to 400 mg daily. Peak plasma concentration (C_{max}) of ketoconazole is reached in about 2 to 4 hours after ingestion and averages 2.5 to 4 mg/L (i.e., 4.7–7.5 μM) in healthy volunteers after a single oral 200-mg dose (2,4). Under steady-state conditions, the mean plasma concentrations of ketoconazole have ranged from 2.7 to 4.8 mg/L (i.e., 5.1–9.0 μM) in patients receiving 200 to 600 mg ketoconazole daily, but its C_{max} can be more than two times higher (4). Ketoconazole is highly protein bound with a free fraction of less than 1%, and its volume of distribution (V_d) is only about 0.4 L/kg (6). In animal studies, the concentrations of ketoconazole in liver have been 0.5 to 3 times its total concentrations in plasma (8,9).

Ketoconazole is significantly metabolized during first pass and is also eliminated largely by way of metabolism, which appears to be mediated by CYP3A4. For example, the CYP3A4 enzyme inducers rifampicin and phenytoin markedly reduce the plasma concentrations of ketoconazole (10,11). The identities and quantities of its major metabolites are not known, but the metabolites are thought not to have antifungal activity (2). The elimination half-life ($t_{1/2}$) of ketoconazole approximates 6.5 to 9.6 hours. The pharmacokinetics of ketoconazole are dose dependent, presumably as a result of autoinhibition of metabolism (4,6,7).

As an imidazole, ketoconazole was early suspected and also confirmed to potently inhibit human oxidative drug metabolism both *in vitro* and *in vivo* (12–14). Thereafter, it has been reported to impair the metabolism of numerous drugs, leading to potentially dangerous drug interactions. In addition, ketoconazole has been reported to block adrenal and testicular CYP-mediated steroid and testosterone synthesis, which has occasionally led to symptoms of androgen deficiency in patients (15–18).

Ketoconazole as an Inhibitor of Metabolic Enzymes
In Vitro

In vitro, ketoconazole is a highly potent and relatively selective inhibitor of CYP3A4. Because of its selectivity, ketoconazole has been widely used as a "diagnostic" inhibitor of CYP3A4 *in vitro*. In human liver microsomes, ketoconazole was shown to inhibit the CYP3A4-mediated biotransformation of midazolam (19), cyclosporine (20–25), nifedipine (26), erythromycin (24), testosterone (23,27,28), and cortisol (22) with an IC_{50} ranging from 0.04 to 2.1 μM. In contrast, the IC_{50} values of ketoconazole for CYP1A1, CYP1A2, CYP2A6, CYP2B6, CYP2C9, CYP2C19, CYP2D6, and CYP2E1 activities were at least an order of magnitude higher (21,23,24,26–29). However, in some cases the IC_{50} values were relatively low (12–28 μM) for CYP2C19 (23,24), CYP1A2, CYP2C9, and CYP2D6 (23).

In studies with several CYP3A4 substrates including alprazolam (30), midazolam (31), triazolam (8), terfena-dine (32–34), and cyclosporine (20,22,35), ketoconazole was reported to produce competitive inhibition. However, in some other reports, inhibition by ketoconazole was consistent with a noncompetitive mechanism when midazolam (36,37) or cyclosporine (25) was used as a substrate. In one study with nifedipine, ketoconazole was described to produce mixed inhibition (26). In most studies, ketoconazole was a very potent inhibitor of CYP3A4, with a K_i ranging from 0.0037 to 0.7 μM. However, in two studies with terfenadine (32) and tacrolimus (38), the K_i of ketoconazole was 3 and 11 μM, respectively. In addition to inhibiting CYP3A4, ketoconazole seems to potently inhibit P-glycoprotein; for example, in concentrations approximating normal therapeutic plasma levels, it effectively reversed the resistance of cells to vinblastine and doxorubicin in a study using a multidrug-resistant human cell line (39). Furthermore, ketoconazole reduced the basoapical secretion of digoxin across monolayers of cultured renal tubular cells originating from dogs (40).

Although ketoconazole slightly inhibits also other CYP enzymes, the K_i values are clearly higher than those for CYP3A4. For example, ketoconazole has inhibited the CYP2C9-mediated tolbutamide 4-hydroxylation with a K_i of 8.5 μM (29) and diclofenac 4-hydroxylation with a K_i of about 85 μM (36). In one study, ketoconazole was found to be a mixed inhibitor of the CYP2C19-mediated 4-hydroxylation of mephenytoin with a K_i of 31 μM (41). Furthermore, the K_i of ketoconazole for desipramine hydroxylation, a reaction primarily catalyzed by CYP2D6, was 10.3 μM (42). In addition, ketoconazole inhibited coumarin 7-hydroxylation (CYP2A6) with a K_i of 24 μM (43) and zidovudine glucuronidation with a K_i of 80 μM (44). Inhibition of CYP2E1 by ketoconazole was also weak even at 100 μM (45).

Effects of Ketoconazole on the Metabolism of Drugs
In Vivo

The effects of ketoconazole on the metabolism and pharmacokinetics of drugs have been assessed in numerous studies in healthy volunteers and patients. In two studies in normal subjects, ketoconazole 400 mg daily for 5 to 7 days had no significant effect on antipyrine clearance (46,47). However, in a crossover study in six healthy nonsmoking volunteers, administration of 400 mg ketoconazole daily for 7 days decreased antipyrine clearance by 25% when antipyrine was administered on day 5 of the ketoconazole treatment (13). Although the effect of ketoconazole on the disposition of antipyrine, which is metabolized by several CYPs (48), seems to be small, ketoconazole is a potent inhibitor of CYP3A4-mediated reactions *in vivo*. For example, 200 mg ketoconazole daily reduced the 24-hour urinary ratio of 6β-hydroxy-cortisol to 17-hydroxycorticosteroids by more than 50% in eight normal subjects (49), most likely reflecting inhibition of CYP3A4. In three recent studies in ovarian cancer patients and healthy volunteers, ketoconazole also markedly inhibited hepatic CYP3A4 activity as assessed by the erythromycin breath test (50–52).

In randomized, placebo-controlled crossover studies, ketoconazole has been shown to markedly increase the plasma concentrations and effects of orally administered midazolam and triazolam, both of which are specific substrates of CYP3A4 (Fig. 47-1) (8,53–55). After taking 400 mg ketoconazole daily for 4 days, the area under the plasma concentration versus time curve (AUC) of midazolam was increased 16-fold and the C_{max} about four-fold in a study with nine healthy volunteers (see Fig. 47-1) (54). In another study, 200 mg ketoconazole daily for 1 week increased the AUC of midazolam 12-fold in five healthy subjects (56).

Treatment with 400 mg ketoconazole daily for 4 days increased the AUC of oral triazolam 22-fold and its C_{max} about three-fold in nine healthy volunteers (see Fig. 47-1) (55). In a recent study in nine healthy volunteers, the AUC of triazolam was increased nine-fold by administering 200-mg doses of ketoconazole 1 and 17 hours before taking 0.125 mg triazolam (8,53). In all these studies, ketoconazole also prolonged the half-life and markedly increased the effects of midazolam and triazolam, indicating that ketoconazole can increase the deepness of sleep and prolong the hypnotic effect of orally administered midazolam and triazolam.

In a study with eight patients with epilepsy stabilized on carbamazepine, administration of 200 mg ketoconazole daily for 10 days was associated with a 29% increase in plasma carbamazepine concentrations, whereas concentrations of its active epoxymetabolite were unchanged (57). In an early study, the plasma clearance of intravenously given chlordiazepoxide was decreased by about 40% after taking 400 mg ketoconazole daily for 5 days in five normal subjects (12). In addition, the AUC of the N-

desmethyl metabolite of chlordiazepoxide was decreased, probably because of inhibition of its formation by ketoconazole. However, single 200- and 400-mg doses of ketoconazole only slightly reduced the clearance of chlordiazepoxide. In one study with six healthy male volunteers, 200 mg ketoconazole daily for 1 week decreased the clearance of alfentanil by 82% after an intravenous dose of alfentanil (52). In a study in two groups of six healthy subjects, 200 mg ketoconazole daily for 2 weeks slightly increased the AUC of imipramine by inhibiting its CYP3A4 mediated N-demethylation without affecting the CYP2D6-mediated 2-hydroxylation of imipramine or metabolically derived desipramine (58).

Two case reports have described elevated terfenadine levels, prolongation of the QT interval, and torsades de pointes arrhythmia in two patients during concomitant treatment with terfenadine and ketoconazole (59,60). In a study in six normal subjects, 60 mg terfenadine was administered twice daily for 1 week to achieve steady-state levels (61). After 200 mg ketoconazole twice daily was added to the regimen, markedly increased serum levels of unmetabolised terfenadine developed in all subjects within 4 to 7 days (Fig. 47-2), leading to a prolongation from 416 to 490 msec in the mean QT interval. In another study, 400 mg ketoconazole four times daily for 1 week increased the C_{max} of terfenadine from less than 10 μg/L (limit of detection) to 27 μg/L after a single 120-mg dose of terfenadine in 12 healthy subjects, and the C_{max} as well as the apparent clearance of the active metabolite of terfenadine were reduced (62). Because ketoconazole inhibits the metabolism of astemizole *in vitro* (63), it is likely that treatment with ketoconazole also increases the plasma concentrations of astemizole in patients. This

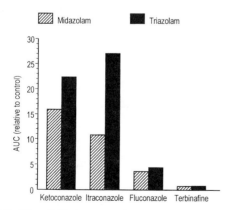

FIG. 47-1. The AUC (mean value relative to control phase mean) of midazolam and triazolam after a single oral dose following administration of 400 mg ketoconazole (54,55), 200 mg itraconazole (54,55), 200 mg fluconazole (148,218) or 250 mg terbinafine (150,217) once daily for 4 days (400 mg fluconazole on day 1).

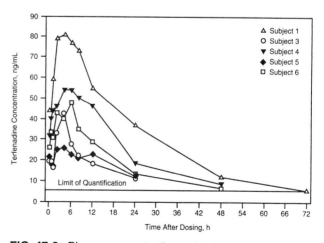

FIG. 47-2. Plasma concentrations of terfenadine in five subjects following coadministration of 60 mg terfenadine and 200 mg ketoconazole twice daily for 6 days. (From Honig PK, Wortham DC, Zamani K, Conner DP, Mullin JC, Cantilena LR. Terfenadine-ketoconazole interaction. Pharmacokinetic and electrocardiographic consequences. *JAMA* 1993;269: 1513–1518, with permission.)

probably explains the reported occurrence of QT prolongation and torsades de pointes ventricular tachycardia during combined use of astemizole and ketoconazole in one patient (64).

In contrast to terfenadine and astemizole, the other H_1 receptor antagonists have not been associated with cardiac arrhythmias. Ketoconazole 200 mg twice daily for 1 week simultaneously with azelastine 4.4 mg twice daily had no effect on electrocardiograms (ECGs) of 12 normal volunteers (65). However, in a placebo-controlled study in 12 normal volunteers, 200 mg ketoconazole twice daily for 8 days increased the C_{max} and the AUC of loratadine two- to three-fold after a single 20-mg dose of loratadine (66). In another study with 24 volunteers taking 10 mg loratadine daily, addition of 200 mg ketoconazole daily for 10 days increased serum loratadine levels four-fold, but no sedation, syncope, or any clinically relevant changes in ECG were reported (67). In one crossover study, addition of 400 mg ketoconazole for 8 days to volunteers taking 10 mg loratadine or 20 mg ebastine daily increased the AUCs of loratadine and ebastine 4.5-fold and 40-fold, respectively, but only slightly prolonged the QTc interval (68).

QT-prolongation and ventricular arrhythmias have developed in several patients during concomitant ketoconazole and cisapride administration (69,70). According to Stockley (71), the addition of 200 mg ketoconazole twice daily increased the AUC of cisapride four- to eight-fold when four to five consecutive 10-mg doses of cisapride were administered within a 24-hour period in a controlled study in 14 healthy volunteers.

Based on a case report, ketoconazole also seems to increase the plasma concentrations of quinidine (72). An elderly man had been given 300 mg quinidine four times daily with serum quinidine levels in a range of 1.4 to 2.7 mg/L. One week after starting 200 mg of ketoconazole daily for candidal esophagitis, his quinidine levels had increased to 6.9 mg/L and the half-life of quinidine had prolonged to 25 hours.

Ketoconazole has been documented to increase the concentrations of the immunosuppressants cyclosporine and tacrolimus that are substrates for both CYP3A4 and P-glycoprotein. In a recent study, the pharmacokinetics of single oral and intravenous doses (separated by 6 days) of tacrolimus were studied before and during 200 mg of ketoconazole given daily for 12 days in six healthy subjects (73). Ketoconazole treatment doubled the mean oral bioavailability of tacrolimus (30% versus 14%), but had no significant effect on its intravenous clearance and half-life. The calculated hepatic bioavailability was not changed by ketoconazole, and thus the interaction most likely resulted from an increase in the intestinal bioavailability of tacrolimus, suggesting inhibition of the intestinal CYP3A4 and P-glycoprotein by ketoconazole.

In several controlled studies and case reports, ketoconazole has been described to increase serum cyclospor-

ine concentrations, thereby increasing the risk of cyclosporine toxicity (74–79). In a study in five normal subjects, the pharmacokinetics of intravenous and oral cyclosporine were studied before and during treatment with 200 mg ketoconazole daily for 10 days (76). Ketoconazole increased the oral bioavailability of cyclosporine 2.6-fold and decreased its systemic clearance 1.8-fold, which would lead to an about five-fold increase in the AUC of oral cyclosporine. Because the calculated hepatic bioavailability of cyclosporine increased from 75% to 86% only, it was estimated that the observed increase in total bioavailability was mainly due to a 2.3-fold increase in the intestinal bioavailability, that is, fraction of the dose absorbed and bypassing intestinal metabolism.

In studies with transplant patients, administration of ketoconazole reduced cyclosporine dose requirements by almost 80%, leading to more than 50% savings in the cost of treatments during the first year after transplantation (75,78,80–83). Therefore, it has been suggested that ketoconazole should be routinely used in combination with cyclosporine for economical reasons. However, this approach has also been criticized, because the use of this combination may increase the risk of adverse effects of cyclosporine, impair treatment compliance, and increase the need for monitoring (84,85). However, in a recent randomized study in cardiac transplant patients, administration of 200 mg ketoconazole daily with cyclosporine not only reduced the dose of cyclosporine needed to maintain target levels but also reduced the rate of rejection in the first month after transplantation in 23 patients compared to 20 patients given cyclosporine alone (86). Thus, ketoconazole might even improve the clinical results of transplantations.

In two studies with six normal volunteers, treatment with 200 mg ketoconazole daily for 6 or 7 days decreased the systemic clearance of methylprednisolone by 46% to 60% and increased its AUC about 2.4-fold after a single 15- to 30-mg intravenous dose of methylprednisolone, leading to increased adrenal suppression (87,88). However, the effect of ketoconazole on prednisone and prednisolone pharmacokinetics seems to be smaller. In one study, treatment with 200 mg of ketoconazole daily for 7 days decreased the systemic clearance of prednisolone by almost 30% and reduced the urinary excretion of its 6-betahydroxy metabolite following a single intravenous dose of prednisolone in 10 normal subjects (49). In addition, ketoconazole increased the AUC of prednisone and prednisolone by almost 50% after a single dose of oral prednisone. However, in two small studies with four to six subjects, a similar course of ketoconazole only nonsignificantly reduced the clearance of prednisolone after a single dose of oral prednisone or intravenous prednisolone (89,90).

In unpublished studies (see Ref. 71), the coadministration of ketoconazole 200 mg daily with saquinavir (a protease inhibitor metabolized by CYP3A4) 600 mg three times daily resulted in a three-fold increase in saquinavir plasma concentrations compared to saquinavir alone, and a single 400-mg dose of ketoconazole increased the AUC of indinavir by 68%. In studies in 12 healthy subjects, ketoconazole 400 mg daily for 7 days also slightly (by 20%–30%) increased the plasma concentrations of nelfinavir when 500 mg nelfinavir was administered three times daily for 5 days (91) and those of ritonavir when 500 mg ritonavir was given twice daily for 10 days (92).

Ketoconazole has been shown to moderately increase the plasma concentrations of omeprazole, a proton pump inhibitor, and tirilazad mesylate, an inhibitor of membrane lipid peroxidation. In a study in ten healthy subjects including extensive and poor metabolizers of (S)-mephenytoin, 200 mg ketoconazole daily for 4 days increased the AUC (0–6 hours) of omeprazole 1.4- and 2.0-fold in extensive and poor metabolizers, respectively, and markedly decreased the concentrations of omeprazole sulfone (93). Thus, it was presumed that omeprazole sulfoxidation is catalyzed by CYP3A4. In a crossover study in 12 healthy volunteers, 200 mg ketoconazole daily for 1 week increased the oral bioavailability of tirilazad mesylate from 9% to 21% and decreased its systemic clearance, leading to a 4.1-fold increase in its AUC (94).

In a study in seven normal subjects, 200 mg ketoconazole daily for 7 days increased the half-life of tolbutamide, a CYP2C9 substrate, 3.3-fold and its AUC 1.8-fold (95). As a result, the hypoglycemic effects of tolbutamide were increased. However, ketoconazole has shown no unequivocal effects on the pharmacokinetics of other substrates of CYP2C9. According to a case report, administration of ketoconazole to two patients receiving warfarin was associated with potentiation of the anticoagulant effect (96). A positive dechallenge was also reported. However, in some other individuals, ketoconazole had no effect on response to warfarin (97).

In a randomized crossover study, ketoconazole 200 mg twice daily for 6 days had no effect on serum phenytoin concentrations after a single oral dose of phenytoin in nine healthy volunteers (98). In another crossover study, 400 mg ketoconazole daily for 6 days had no significant effect on the pharmacokinetics of intravenous losartan or its active metabolite E-3174 in 11 normal subjects (99). Moreover, a single 200-mg dose of ketoconazole had no effect on the 24-hour urinary recovery of sulfamethoxazole or its metabolites in a study with ten healthy male subjects, consistent with lack of significant effect on the CYP2C9-catalyzed oxidation of sulfamethoxazole (100). In a study in seven ovarian cancer patients, 200 mg ketoconazole given 3 hours before or 100 to 1600 mg ketoconazole given 3 hours after starting an intravenous 3-hour infusion of paclitaxel, an anticancer agent metabolized primarily by CYP2C8, had no effect on the pharmacokinetics of paclitaxel (50).

In 12 normal male subjects including two poor metabolizers of debrisoquine, 400 mg ketoconazole daily reduced the 0- to 8-hour urinary R/S ratio of mephenytoin to 43% of its baseline value after 28 days of treatment, suggesting that ketoconazole markedly inhibits the CYP2C19-catalyzed 4-hydroxylation of (S)-mephenytoin in vivo (101). In addition, the 0- to 8-hour urinary ratio of debrisoquine to 4-hydroxydebrisoquine, an index of CYP2D6 activity, was increased slightly (by 31%) on the 28th day of ketoconazole administration, suggesting slight inhibition of CYP2D6. However, in one study with limited documentation, 200 mg ketoconazole three times daily had no effect on CYP2D6 as assessed by using debrisoquine as a probe in a group of cancer patients (102). One male patient who had been taking propafenone, a CYP2D6 substrate, for 4 years was reported to have experienced convulsions 2 days after starting treatment with ketoconazole (103), but no other reports have described possible interactions between ketoconazole and substrates of CYP2D6.

A dosage of 400 or 200 mg ketoconazole daily for 5 to 7 days had no significant effect on the pharmacokinetics of intravenous aminophylline, a CYP1A2 substrate, in studies with six (12) and ten (104) nonsmoking healthy volunteers, respectively. However, in another study in six healthy volunteers, ketoconazole increased the half-life of theophylline by 22% (105). Correspondingly, a single 400-mg dose of ketoconazole had no apparent effect on the pharmacokinetics of intravenous caffeine in a study in eight normal volunteers (106). In a study in a group of cancer patients, 200 mg ketoconazole three times daily significantly decreased (by 60%) the acetylation ratio (N-acetyltransferase), but had no effect on CYP2E1 as assessed by using chlorzoxazone as a probe (102).

Ketoconazole as an Inhibitor of Metabolic Enzymes

Based on a large number of studies, ketoconazole is a potent inhibitor of CYP3A4 in vitro and in vivo (see Fig. 47-1). It has been estimated with some oral substrates of CYP3A4 that the in vivo inhibitory potency of ketoconazole is in good agreement with its in vitro potency against CYP3A4, if its active inhibitory concentrations in drug metabolizing tissues are assumed to be similar to its total concentrations in plasma (9). In addition to inhibiting CYP3A4, ketoconazole inhibits P-glycoprotein in vitro and the CYPs responsible for steroid and testosterone biosynthesis in vitro and in vivo. Because of inhibition of CYP3A4 (and P-glycoprotein), ketoconazole can markedly increase the plasma concentrations of drugs metabolized by CYP3A4.

In contrast, ketoconazole is a weak inhibitor of other drug-metabolizing CYPs in vitro. However, because the K_i of ketoconazole against CYP2A6, CYP2C9, CYP2C19, and CYP2D6 is close to its normal therapeutic maximum plasma concentrations, ketoconazole may slightly inhibit these enzymes also in vivo. In fact, ketoconazole seems to slightly impair (or have no effect on) drug metabolism mediated by CYP2C9, CYP2C19, and CYP2D6 *in vivo*. However, according to a limited number of studies, it appears to have no effect on CYP1A2, CYP2C8, and CYP2E1 *in vivo*.

Miconazole

Miconazole was introduced in 1969 (2). It is an imidazole derivative that is active against a broad spectrum of fungal pathogens including dermatophytes and *Candida* species. Miconazole is used orally in tablet and gel forms in treatment of candidiosis and fungal colonization of the gastrointestinal tract, and parenterally in treatment of deep fungal infections. In addition, several forms of miconazole nitrate are available for topical use. Because of the large number of side effects, parenteral miconazole is no longer a first line drug for most systemic mycoses, and miconazole is mainly used topically.

Although miconazole is relatively poorly absorbed after oral application, at least 20% of an oral dose is absorbed (107). Single oral doses of 500 to 1000 mg have been reported to produce mean C_{max} values of 0.37 and 1.16 mg/L (i.e., 0.9 and 2.8 μM) 2 to 4 hours after administration (108). The usual oral dose of miconazole is 250 mg at 6-hour intervals in treatment of oral and gastrointestinal tract candidiosis. After intravenous injection of 4 to 18 mg/kg of miconazole, peak serum levels of up to 2 mg/L were produced (109). In another study, an intravenous 522-mg dose of miconazole produced a mean C_{max} ranging from 2 to 33 mg/L (i.e., 4.8–79 μM) in 12 subjects including healthy volunteers and patients with mild renal impairment (110). Intravenous dosages ranging from 200 to 1200 mg three times daily are used clinically. About 90% of miconazole is protein bound in plasma (111). It is metabolized in the liver and eliminated in the urine and feces as inactive metabolites. The terminal elimination half-life of miconazole is about 24 hours (110).

Miconazole as an Inhibitor of Metabolic Enzymes *In Vitro*

In vitro, miconazole has been shown to be a strong but relatively nonspecific inhibitor of CYP-mediated reactions. In particular, miconazole potently inhibits CYP2C9-catalyzed reactions in human liver microsomes, including (S)-warfarin 6- and 7-hydroxylation (112) and tolbutamide 4-hydroxylation (29). The inhibition of the 7-hydroxylation of (S)-warfarin by miconazole was consistent with a mixed mechanism with a K_i of 0.5 μM (112). The IC_{50} of miconazole for tolbutamide hydroxylation was 0.85 μM, that is, approximately 20 times less than that of ketoconazole and one-third that of clotrimazole (29).

In studies with human hepatocytes and hepatic microsomes, miconazole was also a strong inhibitor of

CYP3A4, with a K_i of 0.9 to 1.3 μM for cyclosporine oxidation (24,35). In addition, miconazole inhibited the metabolism of tacrolimus, another CYP3A4 substrate, in human hepatic microsomes with an average K_i of 15 μM (38). In each study, miconazole was only slightly less potent as an inhibitor of CYP3A4 on a molar basis than ketoconazole.

In human hepatic microsomes, miconazole competitively inhibited the 6-hydroxylation of (R)-warfarin with a K_i of about 4 μM (212), suggesting inhibition of CYP1A2 (113). In addition, miconazole was a potent (K_i = 0.22 μM) competitive inhibitor of the CYP2A6-mediated coumarin 7-hydroxylation (43,114) and a noncompetitive inhibitor of the CYP2E1-mediated 4-nitrophenol hydroxylation with a K_i of 4 μM (45). However, it only weakly inhibited zidovudine glucuronidation with a K_i of 180 μM (44) in human liver microsomes.

Miconazole as an Inhibitor of Drug Metabolism *In Vivo*

Like ketoconazole, miconazole seems to impair testosterone biosynthesis (115). In addition, miconazole has been reported to impair the clearance of several substrates of CYP2C9. Miconazole given parenterally or as an oral gel has been associated with enhanced hypoprothrombinemia and bleeding in several patients receiving oral anticoagulants, including nicoumalone, tioclomarol, phenindione, and warfarin (116–123). In a study with six normal subjects, 125 mg miconazole administered orally once a day (a low dosage) for 3 days decreased the systemic clearance of (R)- and (S)-warfarin, leading to a three-fold increase in the AUC and a marked increase in the anticoagulant effect after a single oral dose of pseudoracemic warfarin (112). The oxidation of (S)-warfarin (catalyzed by CYP2C9) (124), in particular its 7-hydroxylation, was most strongly inhibited, with an about 80% decrease in its clearance. In human liver microsomes, miconazole also inhibited the oxidation of (S)-warfarin more than it affected the oxidation of (R)-warfarin (112). Thus, the interaction was mainly caused by inhibition of CYP2C9 by miconazole, with possible inhibition of other CYPs playing a minor role. (S)-warfarin is at least five times more potent as an anticoagulant than (R)-warfarin, thus explaining the documented increase in the anticoagulant effects of warfarin. In practice, careful monitoring of oral anticoagulant effects is needed whenever miconazole is used in patients on oral anticoagulants.

According to case reports, parenterally given miconazole also seems to inhibit the metabolism of other CYP2C9 substrates, including phenytoin and some sulfonylureas. Initiation of treatment with parenteral miconazole 500 mg three times daily to a patient, whose phenytoin dose had remained unchanged for 5 years, was soon followed by symptoms and signs of phenytoin toxicity and plasma phenytoin concentrations well above the recommended therapeutic range (125). A decrease in plasma phenytoin concentrations was seen when antifungal treatment was stopped with no change in phenytoin dosage or formulation. Another case of phenytoin intoxication was reported after starting 500 mg miconazole daily (120). In addition, several cases of hypoglycemia were reported in patients with diabetes receiving sulfonylureas (tolbutamide, glibenclamide [glyburide], gliclazide) within 2 to 10 days after beginning treatment with miconazole (120,126). Furthermore, intravenous miconazole substantially increased the plasma levels and decreased the systemic clearance of pentobarbital in five intensive care patients (127).

According to some case reports, miconazole may also inhibit CYP3A4 *in vivo*. In one study, a single intravenous 200-mg dose of miconazole reduced CYP3A4 activity (erythromycin breath test) in an ovarian cancer patient (50). In one report, administration of 1 g of miconazole intravenously three times daily to a patient receiving cyclosporine increased cyclosporine plasma concentrations by about 65% within 3 days after starting miconazole (77). This finding was also confirmed by a rechallenge with miconazole, suggesting inhibition of the CYP3A4-mediated metabolism of cyclosporine (35) *in vivo*. In another report, signs of carbamazepine toxicity developed in a patient on long-term treatment with carbamazepine during administration of intravenous miconazole (120).

Miconazole as an Inhibitor of Metabolic Enzymes

Miconazole is a potent inhibitor of CYP2C9 and CYP3A4 *in vitro*. Based on several case reports and one controlled study with warfarin, miconazole seems to be a potent inhibitor of CYP2C9 also *in vivo*. Moreover, based on the similar potency of *in vitro* inhibition of CYP3A4 and CYP2C9 by miconazole and two case reports, it seems reasonable to assume that, during intravenous or oral administration, the concentrations of miconazole are high enough to produce clinically significant inhibition of CYP3A4 also. In particular, oral miconazole may impair the gastrointestinal metabolism of orally administered CYP3A4 substrates. However, the magnitude of the *in vivo* inhibitory effect of miconazole on CYP3A4 is unclear. It is likely that even low doses of orally or parenterally administered miconazole can considerably impair the metabolism of drugs that are substrates for CYP2C9 or CYP3A4. Furthermore, there may also be a risk of interactions with substrates of CYP1A2, CYP2A6, and CYP2E1, which are potently inhibited by miconazole *in vitro*.

Topically Used Imidazoles

In addition to ketoconazole and miconazole, there are a number of other imidazole antimycotics that are in wide use as topical formulations, including clotrimazole, econazole, and tioconazole. Clotrimazole and econazole, for example, are relatively potent competitive inhibitors of CYP3A4-mediated reactions (19,24) and moderate or weak inhibitors of some other CYPs in human liver microsomes (29,43,45). Although the risk of metabolic drug interactions is very small when these drugs are administered topically, administration to the gastrointestinal tract can probably impair drug metabolism as seems to occur when clotrimazole troches are given orally.

Clotrimazole is a chlorinated imidazole derivative used to treat superficial dermatomycoses and oropharyngeal and vaginal candidiasis (2). It is useful only when administered locally, because even with low systemic doses, clotrimazole causes marked induction of hepatic oxidation, including its own metabolism (128). Clotrimazole is probably metabolized by CYP3A4, because clotrimazole was shown to relatively selectively induce the CYP3A4 isoenzyme in human hepatocytes (24). In addition, it was shown to induce CYP3A4, CYP3A5, and P-glycoprotein in human colon carcinoma cells (129).

In a clinical situation, clotrimazole has been suggested to behave as an inhibitor of CYP3A4, because inhibition of cyclosporine oxidation was observed to overtake induction of CYP3A4 in human hepatocyte cultures (24). In human liver microsomes, clotrimazole was a potent inhibitor of CYP3A4, with a K_i of 0.15 μM for cyclosporine oxidation (24) and an IC_{50} of less than 1 μM for midazolam α- and 4-hydroxylation (19). In addition, clotrimazole competitively inhibited the CYP2C9-mediated hydroxylation of tolbutamide with a K_i of 1.1 μM (29) and the CYP2A6-mediated 7-hydroxylation of coumarin with a K_i of 0.42 μM (43), and uncompetitively inhibited the CYP2E1-mediated hydroxylation of 4-nitrophenol with a K_i of 12 μM (45) in human liver microsomes.

In one case report, elevated serum tacrolimus and creatinine concentrations developed in a liver transplant patient receiving tacrolimus (15 mg/day) and prednisone during concomitant treatment with 10 mg clotrimazole troches four times daily (130). After a rechallenge with clotrimazole, the AUC of tacrolimus was almost doubled. Because clotrimazole from the troche eventually reaches the intestine and is at least partly absorbed, the interaction presumably resulted from inhibition of the intestinal and hepatic CYP3A4-mediated metabolism of tacrolimus.

Taken together, clotrimazole is a potent inhibitor of CYP2A6, CYP2C9, and CYP3A4 *in vitro*. According to one case report, oral administration of clotrimazole probably leads to clinically significant inhibition of CYP3A4 and increases the concentrations of CYP3A4 substrates, such as cyclosporine and tacrolimus. However, after cutaneous or vaginal therapy, inhibition of hepatic microsomal enzymes is probably not a problem, because only less than 0.5% or 3% to 10% of the dose is absorbed, respectively (131,132).

Itraconazole

Itraconazole is a triazole antifungal agent that has an even broader spectrum of activity than ketoconazole, with efficacy against infections caused by dermatophytes, yeasts, and some molds (1,133,134). In clinical use, it is superior to ketoconazole in the treatment of common dermatophyte infections and certain opportunistic fungal infections. Its pharmacokinetics allow effective short-term treatment of, for example, onychomycosis with high rates of cure, and it rarely causes serious side effects.

Itraconazole is currently available only as an oral capsule, but an intravenous formulation is already in clinical trials (7,133–135). Itraconazole is a highly lipohilic, weakly basic compound, and gastric acidity is needed for its dissolution and absorption. Like ketoconazole, itraconazole is well absorbed when administered with a meal, but its absorption is reduced during fasting and in diminished gastric acidity, for example, in patients with acquired immunodeficiency syndrome (AIDS). The recommended daily doses of itraconazole range from 100 to 400 mg. In normal volunteers its C_{max} averages 0.1 and 0.3 mg/L after single oral doses of 100 and 200 mg taken with a meal, respectively, and is reached within 1.5 to 4 hours after ingestion (136). After 2 weeks of treatment with 100 mg itraconazole daily (steady-state), the peak and trough plasma concentrations of itraconazole are about 0.4 to 0.6 and 0.2 mg/L, respectively (133,136). During treatment with 200 mg itraconazole once or twice daily, the C_{max} at steady-state averages 1.1 or 2.0 mg/L (i.e., 1.6 or 2.8 μM), respectively (136). It is noteworthy that, after a single oral dose of itraconazole as well as during continuous administration, the plasma levels of the active metabolite, hydroxyitraconazole, are approximately two-fold compared to those of the parent drug (135,137,138).

Itraconazole is highly protein bound with most of the drug bound to plasma proteins (95%) and blood cells (5%), and only 0.2% to 3% of the drug being free in plasma (133,135,139). The V_d of itraconazole is about 11 L/kg, that is, at least 20 times that of ketoconazole, indicating extensive tissue distribution. Because of the lipophilicity of itraconazole, its concentrations may be three to ten times higher in skin and ten to 20 times higher in liver than in plasma (135,140). Itraconazole has a significant first pass metabolism and is eliminated largely by way of metabolism. Its half-life ranges from 20 to 60 hours. The half-life and plasma concentrations increase more than proportionally with increasing doses and duration of therapy (136,141), suggesting saturable metabolism. Itraconazole seems to be metabolized by CYP3A4, in that CYP3A4 enzyme inducers, such as rifampicin, carbamazepine, and phenytoin, markedly reduce the plasma concentrations of itraconazole (11,142,143).

Itraconazole as an Inhibitor of Metabolic Enzymes
In Vitro

Itraconazole was earlier claimed to have a specific effect on fungal CYP enzymes and not to be able to inhibit human drug-metabolizing enzymes, because it had no effect on the pharmacokinetics of several drugs in experimental animals and antipyrine in humans (135,144, 145). Furthermore, unlike ketoconazole, itraconazole did not inhibit the synthesis of androgens and cortisol at doses up to 400 mg/day (134).

However, like ketoconazole, itraconazole turned out to be a relatively potent and selective inhibitor of the CYP3A4-mediated hydroxylations of midazolam, cyclosporine, terfenadine, and cortisol in vitro (19,20,22,36, 146). In human liver microsomes, itraconazole competitively inhibited the hydroxylation of cyclosporine with a K_i of 0.7 μM (20,22), the α-hydroxylation of midazolam with a K_i of 0.275 μM (31), and the oxidation of terfenadine to desalkyl- and hydroxyterfenadine with a K_i of 0.28 and 2.05 μM (34) or 4 and 11 μM (32), respectively. In one report, the inhibition of α-hydroxylation of midazolam by itraconazole was described as noncompetitive with a K_i of 6 μM (36). In addition, itraconazole seems to potently inhibit P-glycoprotein. In one study, 0.7 to 10 μM itraconazole reversed the resistance of P-glycoprotein–expressing human leukemia cells to adriamycin and etoposide in vitro (147). In more recent studies, itraconazole inhibited the secretion of digoxin across cultured dog renal tubular cell monolayers even more effectively than ketoconazole (40), and potently reduced the uptake of vincristine and vinblastine by cultured mouse brain capillary cells (140).

Notably, there are very few studies on the effects of itraconazole on other drug-metabolizing enzymes in human liver microsomes. In one study published as an abstract, itraconazole was more than ten times less potent as an inhibitor of dextromethorphan O-demethylation (CYP2D6) and tolbutamide hydroxylation (CYP2C9) than as an inhibitor of CYP3A4 (146). In addition, itraconazole at a 100- and 200-μM concentration had very little effect on 4-nitrophenol hydroxylation, a CYP2E1-catalyzed reaction (45), and diclofenac 4-hydroxylation, a CYP2C9-specific reaction (36), respectively. Similarly, the inhibition of coumarin 7-hydroxylation (CYP2A6) by itraconazole was weak with a K_i of more than 200 μM (43).

Itraconazole as an Inhibitor of Metabolic Enzymes
In Vivo

In humans, itraconazole markedly increases the plasma concentrations and half-lives of many drugs metabolized by CYP3A4. In several crossover studies, itraconazole has been shown to strongly inhibit the metabolism of midazolam and triazolam during both first pass and elimination phases (see Fig. 47-1), leading to increased and prolonged psychomotor effects after oral administration. In three separate studies in healthy volunteers, 200 mg itraconazole daily for 4 to 6 days increased the mean AUC of oral midazolam 7- to 11-fold and its half-life 3.1- to 3.6-fold (54,148,149). In addition, the systemic clearance of midazolam was decreased to 31% of its control value and the oral bioavailability increased from 39% to 96% by itraconazole (148). In one study, itraconazole also greatly decreased the ratio of α-hydroxymidazolam to midazolam in plasma (149), indicating that the interaction resulted from inhibition of CYP3A4 by itraconazole. Moreover, the AUC of oral midazolam was increased 3.4-fold already after a single 200-mg dose of itraconazole (148) and 2.6-fold still 4 days after stopping a 4-day treatment with 200 mg itraconazole daily (149), demonstrating potent enzyme inhibition at relatively low plasma levels of itraconazole. Furthermore, 100 mg itraconazole daily for 4 days significantly affected the pharmacokinetics of oral midazolam, increasing its AUC 5.8-fold in a placebo-controlled crossover study in 12 healthy volunteers (150).

In other studies, itraconazole has been shown to increase the plasma concentrations and effects of oral triazolam even more than those of midazolam (see Fig. 47-1) (55,151). Treatment with 200 mg itraconazole daily for 4 days increased the AUC of oral triazolam 27-fold, its C_{max} about three-fold, and its half-life more than six-fold in nine healthy volunteers (see Fig. 47-1) (55). In addition, a single 200-mg dose of itraconazole ingested simultaneously with triazolam or 3, 12, or 24 hours before increased the AUC of triazolam 3.1- to 4.8-fold and its half-life about three-fold in a study with ten healthy subjects (151).

In contrast to midazolam and triazolam, treatment with 200 mg itraconazole daily for 4 days only slightly increased (by 14%–70%) the plasma concentrations and half-life of zopiclone (152), temazepam (153), diazepam (154), and zolpidem (137) after single oral doses of the hypnotics in crossover studies with ten healthy subjects. These slight increases in plasma levels of the hypnotics are probably clinically insignificant, because no relevant changes in the psychomotor effects of the drugs were observed.

The concentrations of buspirone, a nonbenzodiazepine anxiolytic agent, are greatly increased by itraconazole (Fig. 47-3). In healthy volunteers, 100 mg itraconazole twice daily for 4 days increased the AUC of buspirone 19-fold and the C_{max} 13-fold without significantly affecting the half-life of buspirone (155). Increased buspirone effects and side effects were also noted during itraconazole administration. In contrast, 200 mg itraconazole daily for 4 days had no effect on the pharmacokinetics of intravenous fentanyl, a synthetic opioid, in a study in ten healthy volunteers (156), although it has been reported to be metabolized by CYP3A4 *in vitro*. Furthermore, itraconazole seems to have no effect on the disposition of

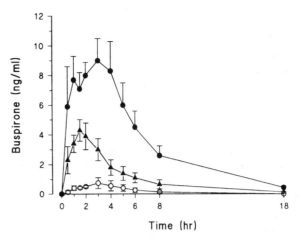

FIG. 47-3. Mean (± SEM) plasma concentrations of buspirone in eight subjects after a single oral dose following administration of 500 mg erythromycin three times daily (▲), 100 mg itraconazole twice daily (●) or placebo (○) for 4 days. (From Kivistö KT, Lamberg TS, Kantola T, Neuvonen PJ. Plasma buspirone concentrations are greatly increased by erythromycin and itraconazole. *Clin Pharmacol Ther* 1997;62:348–354, with permission.)

clozapine, an atypical neuroleptic partially metabolized by CYP3A4. In a placebo-controlled crossover trial in seven schizophrenic inpatients receiving clozapine, addition of 200 mg itraconazole daily for 7 days had no effect on serum clozapine and *N*-desmethylclozapine concentrations on days 3 and 7 after starting itraconazole (157).

Like ketoconazole, itraconazole also increases the serum concentrations of cyclosporine. An average 56% reduction in the dose of cyclosporine was required in seven lung and heart transplant patients after initiating itraconazole treatment (158). In three other patients, cyclosporine levels increased two- to three-fold after starting itraconazole (159–161). In a cross-sectional population pharmacokinetic study in 182 transplant patients receiving cyclosporine, the ratio of cyclosporine dose rate to its trough concentrations in patients receiving 200 mg itraconazole twice daily was about 50% of that in patients receiving no inhibitors of CYP3A4, suggesting that the dose of cyclosporine should be reduced by about 50% in patients receiving 400 mg/day itraconazole (83). However, in another study, 14 patients receiving 100 mg itraconazole twice daily for 4 to 7 weeks had cyclosporine levels similar to those in 20 patients on cyclosporine without itraconazole (162).

In one study in ten lung transplant patients receiving either cyclosporine or tacrolimus, 100 mg itraconazole twice daily reduced the dose requirement of the immunosuppressants at steady-state by an average of 50% to 66% (163). In addition, itraconazole has increased serum concentrations and side effects of tacrolimus in some patients (164,165). Itraconazole also markedly increased the ratio of the trough concentration to dose rate of tacrolimus in a retrospective analysis of 14 patients given either tacrolimus alone or tacrolimus combined with itraconazole (166).

Itraconazole can markedly increase the plasma concentrations and effects of methylprednisolone. In a placebo-controlled study in ten healthy volunteers, 200 mg itraconazole daily for 4 days increased the AUC of methylprednisolone 3.9-fold after a single 16-mg oral dose, resulting in considerably increased adrenal suppression (167). In a case report, corticosteroid side effects (myopathy and diabetes) were reported to have developed in an organ transplant patient receiving cyclosporine, azathioprine, and methylprednisolone after addition of itraconazole (168).

Treatment with itraconazole has also been associated with increased plasma concentrations and adverse effects of certain chemotherapeutic agents. In a study comparing busulfan pharmacokinetics in 13 bone marrow transplant patients receiving itraconazole to those in matched control patients who received either fluconazole or no antifungals, itraconazole treatment was accompanied by about a 20% reduction in the systemic clearance of busulfan (169). In six patients with acute lymphoblastic leukemia receiving chemotherapy containing vincristine, unusually severe vincristine-induced neurotoxicity was observed during simultaneous treatment with itraconazole, according to two case reports (170,171). In addition, itraconazole can increase the concentrations of oxybutynin, an anticholinergic drug used for symptomatic treatment of urinary incontinence. In a crossover study in ten healthy subjects, 200 mg itraconazole daily for 4 days almost doubled the AUC of oxybutynin (172). However, the concentrations of the active metabolite of oxybutynin were not significantly affected by itraconazole.

In patients receiving terfenadine, treatment with itraconazole has been attributed to cardiac toxicity including episodes of syncope, QT prolongation, and ventricular arrhythmias (173–175). In a study in six normal subjects, administration of 200 mg itraconazole once daily resulted in increased concentrations of terfenadine with its C_{max} at about 14 ng/mL and significant changes in cardiac repolarization (176). The elimination of the active metabolite of terfenadine was also delayed. In addition, there is a possibility for a dangerous interaction between itraconazole and astemizole, another antihistamine capable of prolonging QT interval. In a study in 12 healthy volunteers, 200 mg itraconazole twice daily for 2 weeks increased the AUC of astemizole 2.8-fold and the AUC of desmethylastemizole 2.0-fold when a single dose of astemizole was administered on day 11 of the treatment (177). Itraconazole also inhibited the metabolism of astemizole in vitro (63). According to Stockley (71), itraconazole inhibits the metabolism of cisapride in vitro and increases cisapride plasma concentrations and the risk of QT prolongation and ventricular arrhythmias in vivo. In fact, in some patients, QT prolongation and ventricular

arrhythmias have developed during concomitant administration of itraconazole and cisapride (69,70).

In case reports, coadministration of itraconazole has been associated with the occurrence of rhabdomyolysis in patients given the cholesterol-lowering agents lovastatin and simvastatin (178–180). This association most probably results from a drastic increase in the concentrations of these statins caused by itraconazole. Compared to placebo, 200 mg itraconazole daily for 4 days increased the AUC of lovastatin and lovastatin acid, the active metabolite, at least 20-fold after a single dose of lovastatin in a crossover study in 12 healthy volunteers (Fig. 47-4) (181). In one subject, plasma creatine kinase was increased ten-fold after lovastatin during the itraconazole treatment. In a similar study with a 100-mg daily dose of itraconazole, the AUC of lovastatin and its acid form were increased about 15-fold by itraconazole (182). In a crossover study in ten healthy volunteers, treatment with 200 mg itraconazole daily for 4 days increased the AUC of simvastatin and total simvastatin acid after a single oral dose of simvastatin 10-fold and 19-fold, respectively (138).

As opposed to lovastatin and simvastatin, the pharmacokinetics of other statins are less susceptible to the effects of itraconazole. In a crossover study in ten healthy volunteers, 200 mg itraconazole daily for 4 days increased the AUC of the acid and lactone forms of atorvastatin three- to four-fold and greatly decreased the C_{max} of their 2-hydroxy metabolites after a single oral dose of atorvastatin (183). However, the concentrations of fluvastatin and pravastatin were only nonsignificantly increased by 100 and 200 mg itraconazole daily for 4 days, respectively (138,182).

Itraconazole also seems to substantially increase the plasma concentrations and effects of dihydropyridine calcium channel blockers. Two patients on felodipine were reported to have experienced leg and ankle swelling soon after starting additional treatment with itraconazole; the edema disappeared within 4 days of stopping itraconazole and felodipine (184). Similarly, increased side effects were reported in patients on isradipine and nifedipine when given itraconazole (184–186). The interaction between itraconazole and felodipine was verified in a recent crossover study, which showed an almost eight-fold increase in the C_{max} of felodipine and a twofold prolongation in its half-life after a single oral dose of felodipine following treatment with 200 mg itraconazole daily for 4 days (Fig. 47-5) (187). Increased effects of felodipine on blood pressure and heart rate were also observed during itraconazole administration.

Itraconazole also increases the plasma concentrations of quinidine, which probably explains the reported quinidine-induced QT prolongation in one patient during concomitant treatment with itraconazole (188). In a study in nine healthy volunteers, 200 mg itraconazole daily for 4 days increased the AUC of quinidine 2.4-fold after a sin-

---

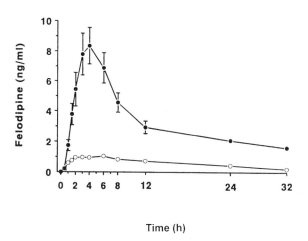

FIG. 47-5. Mean (± SEM) plasma concentrations of felodipine in 12 subjects after a single oral dose following administration of 200 mg itraconazole (●) or placebo (○) once daily for 4 days. (From Jalava KM, Olkkola KT, Neuvonen PJ. Effect of itraconazole on the pharmacokinetics and pharmacodynamics of zopiclone. *Eur J Clin Pharmacol* 1996;51: 331–334, with permission.)

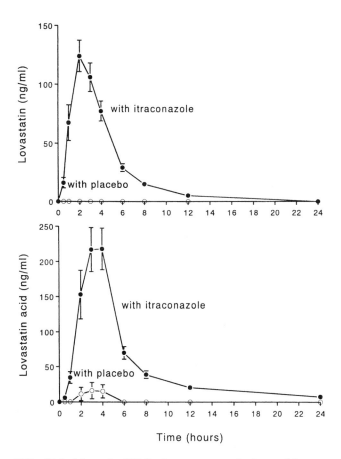

FIG. 47-4. Mean (± SEM) plasma concentrations of lovastatin and lovastatin acid in 12 subjects after a single oral dose of lovastatin following administration of 200 mg itraconazole (●) or placebo (○) once daily for 4 days. (From Neuvonen PJ, Jalava KM. Itraconazole drastically increases plasma concentrations of lovastatin and lovastatin acid. *Clin Pharmcol Ther* 1996;60:54–61, with permission.)

gle oral dose of quinidine sulfate (189). Both the C_{max} and the half-life of quinidine were increased 1.6-fold by itraconazole. In addition, the ratio of 3-hydroxyquinidine to unchanged quinidine in plasma was decreased to 20%, indicating that itraconazole inhibited the 3-hydroxylation of quinidine. However, the renal clearance of quinidine was also reduced by itraconazole, suggesting that itraconazole also inhibits the P-glycoprotein–mediated tubular secretion of quinidine.

Although lidocaine is thought to be metabolized by CYP3A4, 200 mg itraconazole daily for 4 days had no significant effect on the pharmacokinetics of intravenous lidocaine or monoethylglycinexylidide, one of its major metabolites, in a crossover study in nine healthy volunteers (190). In a similar study, 200 mg itraconazole daily for 5 days had no effect on the pharmacokinetics of oral levosimendan, a new calcium-sensitizing drug (191).

Only about 10% of the cardiac glycoside digoxin is eliminated by metabolism with most of the drug excreted directly in urine and bile (192) by active transport mediated by P-glycoprotein (193). In several case reports, treatment with itraconazole has been associated with digoxin toxicity and increased serum concentrations (194–198). In a crossover study in ten normal subjects, treatment with 200 mg itraconazole once daily increased serum digoxin levels almost two-fold after 10 days of concomitant treatment, compared to digoxin alone (199). Later, 200 mg itraconazole daily for 5 days was shown to increase the AUC of digoxin by about 50% and decrease its renal clearance by about 20% after a single oral dose in a crossover study in ten healthy volunteers (200), suggesting that the interaction is primarily caused by inhibition of P-glycoprotein by itraconazole.

There seem to be very few studies on the effects of itraconazole on CYPs other than CYP3A4 *in vivo*. In one report, initiation of 200 mg itraconazole twice daily was described to have increased the anticoagulant effects of warfarin, leading to bruising and bleeding in a woman stabilized on 5 mg warfarin daily and receiving concomitant treatment with other drugs including omeprazole and quinine sulphate (201). Because warfarin is also a substrate for CYP3A4, the interaction could have resulted from inhibition of CYP3A4 by itraconazole. Furthermore, 200 mg itraconazole daily for 4 days had no effect on the single-dose pharmacokinetics of losartan in a crossover study in 11 normal subjects (202), suggesting that itraconazole does not significantly inhibit CYP2C9. The lack of effect of 200 mg itraconazole daily on serum clozapine and *N*-desmethylclozapine concentrations (157) indicates that itraconazole is not an inhibitor of CYP1A2. Because 200 mg itraconazole daily for 4 days increased the AUC and half-life of diazepam only by 32% and 34%, respectively (154), it is likely that itraconazole does not inhibit CYP2C19 and that the interaction resulted from inhibition of CYP3A4.

Itraconazole as an Inhibitor of Metabolic Enzymes

According to studies in humans, itraconazole inhibits CYP3A4 with a potency similar to that of ketoconazole *in vivo,* being able to substantially increase the plasma concentrations of CYP3A4 substrates (see Fig. 47-1). However, the plasma concentrations of itraconazole are clearly lower and its *in vitro* K_i for CYP3A4 is clearly higher than those of ketoconazole. Therefore, it is likely that the active inhibitory concentrations of itraconazole in liver (and intestinal wall) are much higher than its total concentrations in plasma (9), as also suggested by the observed high levels of itraconazole in liver tissue in animal studies (135,140). On the other hand, its major metabolite, hydroxyitraconazole, is also a potent inhibitor of CYP3A4 *in vitro* (203) and could partly explain the potent *in vivo* inhibition of CYP3A4 caused by itraconazole. In addition to inhibiting CYP3A4, itraconazole potently inhibits P-glycoprotein *in vitro* and probably also *in vivo.*

Notably, there are only a few studies on the effects of itraconazole on enzymes other than CYP3A4. According to some *in vitro* studies, itraconazole is more than ten times less potent as an inhibitor of CYP2A6, CYP2C9, CYP2D6, and CYP2E1 than as an inhibitor of CYP3A4, suggesting lack of inhibition toward these enzymes *in vivo.* Based on two studies with clozapine and losartan in humans, itraconazole is unable to inhibit CYP1A2 and CYP2C9 *in vivo.* In addition, it seems to have no significant effect on CYP2C19 *in vivo.*

Fluconazole

Fluconazole is a broad-spectrum triazole antifungal agent, which was synthesized in 1982 (204). It is effective in *Candida* and dermatophyte infections (134,204,205). It is widely used in the treatment of mucocutaneous and disseminated candidiasis and, for example, cryptococcal meningitis (1). The pharmacokinetic properties of fluconazole differ markedly from those of the other systemic azoles, because it is water soluble and can be administered both orally and intravenously.

The oral bioavailability of fluconazole is more than 90% and practically unaltered by changes in intragastric pH or intake of food (204–206). Normal daily doses of fluconazole range from 50 to 400 mg/day, depending on the severity of the infection. Within this range, the pharmacokinetics of fluconazole exhibit dose linearity. The mean C_{max} of fluconazole averages 2 mg/L after a single 100-mg oral dose and 7 mg/L after a single 400-mg dose (205). Steady-state fluconazole levels are two to three times higher than the concentrations after a single dose,

and are reached within 10 days (206). The C_{max} of fluconazole at steady-state during treatment with 100, 200, and 400 mg fluconazole daily have been reported to approximate 6.3, 10, and 19 mg/L, respectively (i.e., about 21–62 µM).

Fluconazole is only 11% to 12% protein bound with most of the drug free in plasma (7,134,205). Its V_d is about 0.8 L/kg and its concentrations in most body fluids are similar to those in plasma. Even higher concentrations have been measured in cerebrospinal fluid. Unlike ketoconazole and itraconazole, fluconazole is not significantly metabolized during first pass and is primarily (80%) eliminated by renal excretion (134,205). Only about 10% of the drug is eliminated as metabolites. Its elimination half-life ranges from 20 to 40 hours in healthy volunteers, but is prolonged in patients with impaired renal function.

Fluconazole as an Inhibitor of Metabolic Enzymes *In Vitro*

Compared with ketoconazole and itraconazole, fluconazole is a fairly weak inhibitor of CYP3A4-mediated reactions *in vitro* (19,20,22,24,31,32,34,36). In studies with human liver microsomes, fluconazole inhibited cyclosporine oxidation according to a mixed mechanism with a K_i of 40 (20,22) or 63 µM (24), or a noncompetitive mechanism with a K_i of 25.1 µM (25). In three other reports, inhibition of midazolam α-hydroxylation by fluconazole was described as competitive or noncompetitive with a K_i ranging from 1.27 to greater than 80 µM (31,36,146). In addition, fluconazole inhibited the *N*-dealkylation and hydroxylation of terfenadine with a K_i of 6 and 11 µM, respectively (32), or greater than 15 µM (34). In one study, fluconazole was also found to competitively inhibit the CYP3A4-catalyzed 10-hydroxylation of (R)-warfarin with a K_i of 15 to 18 µM (113). However, unlike ketoconazole and itraconazole, fluconazole even at 100 µM had virtually no effect on the flux of digoxin across dog renal tubular cell monolayers (40), suggesting lack of significant effects on the function of P-glycoprotein.

Fluconazole has been demonstrated to be a relatively potent inhibitor of a number of CYP2C9-mediated reactions *in vitro,* including tolbutamide hydroxylation (29), diclofenac 4-hydroxylation (36), and (S)-warfarin 6- and 7-hydroxylation (113). In studies with human liver microsomes, the inhibition of the 7-hydroxylation of (S)-warfarin by fluconazole was consistent with a mixed mechanism with a K_i of 7 to 8 µM (113), whereas fluconazole competitively inhibited the 4-hydroxylation of diclofenac with a K_i of 17 µM (113).

In studies with human liver microsomes, fluconazole was also found to be a potent competitive inhibitor (K_i = 2.0 µM) of the CYP2C19-catalyzed 4-hydroxylation of (S)-mephenytoin and 8-hydroxylation of (R)-warfarin

(207). In contrast, the CYP1A2-dependent 6-hydroxyla-tion of (R)-warfarin was only very weakly inhibited by fluconazole with a K_i greater than 800 µM (113). Also, the inhibition of coumarin 7-hydroxylation (CYP2A6) by fluconazole was weak with a K_i of greater than 200 µM (43). In addition, the inhibition of 4-nitrophenol hydroxy-lation (CYP2E1) and zidovudine glucuronidation (K_i = 1400 µM) by fluconazole was weak (44,45). In one study, the IC_{50} of fluconazole for zidovudine glucuronidation was about 160 µM (208).

Fluconazole as an Inhibitor of Metabolic Enzymes *In Vivo*

The effects of fluconazole on drug metabolism have been studied in a large number of studies. Although 50 mg oral fluconazole daily for 7 or 10 days had no significant effect on antipyrine half-life in two early studies in healthy volunteers (209,210), the half-life of antipyrine was pro-longed by 15% and the 24-hour urinary excretion of 6-β-hydroxycortisol was decreased by 28% after 400 mg oral fluconazole daily for 1 week in a recent study in ten male patients with AIDS (211). In one study, 200 mg oral flu-conazole daily also decreased the urinary 6-β-hydroxy-cortisol to cortisol ratio by 50% (212), indicating inhibi-tion of CYP3A4 by fluconazole. In addition, fluconazole has been demonstrated to impair the CYP3A4- and CYP2C9-mediated metabolism of several drugs. How-ever, in contrast to ketoconazole, 400 mg oral fluconazole daily for 6 days slightly increased the levels of endoge-nous testosterone in a study in nine healthy males (98).

In a study in six healthy subjects, 200 mg oral flucona-zole daily for 7 days increased the AUC of the active metabolite of terfenadine by 34% when 60 mg terfena-dine had been given twice daily for 2 weeks (213). How-ever, the plasma concentrations of the parent drug remained undetectable (<5 ng/mL) and cardiac repolar-ization was not significantly affected by either of the study drugs. In another study, the AUC of terfenadine was increased by 52% and the QTc interval was prolonged after 800 mg fluconazole once daily for 1 week in six nor-mal subjects having detectable plasma levels of terfena-dine during treatment with terfenadine 60 mg twice daily (214). In addition, the concentrations of the active metabolite of terfenadine were elevated by fluconazole.

Fluconazole has been shown to increase the plasma concentrations and effects of midazolam and triazolam (see Fig. 47-1). The effects of 200 mg oral fluconazole daily for 6 days (400 mg on day 1) on the pharmacoki-netics of intravenous and oral midazolam were studied in a placebo-controlled crossover study in 12 healthy sub-jects (148). Fluconazole reduced the systemic clearance of midazolam by 51% as assessed by administering an intravenous dose of midazolam on day 4 of the treatment. When an oral dose of midazolam was given 1 hour after the first (400 mg) dose of fluconazole, the AUC of mida-

zolam was increased 3.5-fold with a 2.5-fold increase in its C_{max} and a 1.7-fold prolongation in its half-life. On the sixth day of fluconazole administration, the oral bioavail-ability of midazolam was increased from 39% to 67% and its AUC was increased 3.6-fold (see Fig. 47-1), that is, not more than on day 1, although the plasma levels of fluconazole were almost 50% higher. The lack of differ-ence between days 1 and 6 was probably due to a stronger inhibition of the intestinal metabolism of midazolam after the 400-mg oral dose of fluconazole on day 1 than after the 200-mg dose on day 6. This explanation is also supported by the results of a subsequent study in nine healthy volunteers, which showed that a single oral 400-mg dose of fluconazole increased the C_{max} and AUC (0–3 hours) of oral midazolam more than an intravenous 400-mg dose of fluconazole, although the concentrations of fluconazole in plasma during absorption of midazolam were even higher after the intravenous dose than after the oral dose (215). In a previous study focusing on midazo-lam pharmacodynamics, a single oral 150-mg dose of flu-conazole slightly increased the 0- to 90-minute post-dose concentrations and effects of midazolam in five healthy volunteers (216). Unfortunately, the concentrations of midazolam were not measured after 90 minutes.

In a randomized, placebo-controlled study in 12 healthy subjects, 100 mg oral fluconazole once daily for 4 days increased the AUC of oral triazolam 2.4-fold and almost doubled its half-life, considerably increasing its pharmacodynamic effects (217). In a study investigating the dependency of the interaction on the dose of flucona-zole in eight healthy volunteers, 50, 100, or 200 mg (400 mg on day 1) oral fluconazole once daily for 4 days increased the AUC of triazolam 1.6-, 2.1-, and 4.4-fold (see Fig. 47-1), respectively (218). Correspondingly, the mean half-life of triazolam was prolonged 1.3- to 2.3-fold by the different fluconazole dosages, clearly demonstrat-ing the dose-dependency of the interaction.

The effect of intravenous and oral fluconazole on the pharmacokinetics of intravenous alfentanil was studied in a placebo-controlled, randomized, crossover study in nine healthy volunteers (219). A single 400 mg dose of oral or intravenous fluconazole reduced the systemic clearance of alfentanil by 55% to 58%. As a result, the extent and duration of the pharmacologic effects of alfentanil were increased. The effect of oral fluconazole on the disposi-tion of methadone was studied in 25 patients on methadone maintenance therapy (220). The patients were randomized to receive either 200 mg fluconazole daily or placebo. After 14 days, the AUC, C_{max}, and trough con-centrations of methadone were increased by 35%, 27%, and 48%, respectively, in the fluconazole group but not in the placebo group. However, signs or symptoms of nar-cotic overdose were not observed in any of the patients.

Fluconazole administration seems to produce a small increase in plasma clarithromycin concentrations. When 500 mg clarithromycin was administered twice daily for

8 days to 20 healthy subjects, its minimum plasma concentration and AUC (0–12 hours) increased by 33% and 18%, respectively, after adding 200 mg oral fluconazole daily for 4 days (221). Furthermore, fluconazole was shown to increase the concentrations of rifabutin in a study in 12 patients with human immunodeficiency virus (HIV) receiving maintenance therapy with zidovudine (222). The AUC of rifabutin over a dosing interval was increased by 80% after 2 weeks of concomitant use of oral fluconazole 200 mg daily and rifabutin 300 mg daily, compared to rifabutin alone. In addition, the concentrations of the 25-desacetyl metabolite of rifabutin were increased. In one study, fluconazole was also shown to inhibit the metabolism of rifabutin in human liver microsomes (223). The increase in the plasma concentrations of rifabutin caused by fluconazole may lead to increased efficacy and toxicity of rifabutin (224,225).

Fluconazole has also been shown to cause a small and clinically insignificant increase in the plasma concentrations of the HIV protease inhibitor ritonavir. When eight healthy subjects were given 200 mg ritonavir four times daily for 4 days alone followed by concomitant oral fluconazole 200 mg daily for 5 days (400 mg on day 1), the AUC and C_{max} of ritonavir during the last four ritonavir dosing intervals were increased by less than 15% by fluconazole (226). However, 400 mg oral fluconazole daily for 8 days had no significant effect on the pharmacokinetics of concomitantly administered indinavir in a study in 13 HIV-infected patients (227).

In a crossover study in 12 HIV-positive men, the AUC of zidovudine was increased by 74% and its terminal half-life by 130% when 400 mg oral fluconazole was given once daily concomitantly with 200 mg zidovudine three times daily for 1 week, compared to zidovudine alone (228). In addition, the urinary excretion of zidovudine glucuronide was decreased by fluconazole, suggesting inhibition of the glucuronidation of zidovudine. However, in another study, 400 mg oral fluconazole once daily for 1 week only slightly (by 15%) prolonged the half-life of zidovudine and had no effect on the disposition of its glucuronide after a single 500-mg oral dose of zidovudine in ten HIV-positive patients (211). In addition, 400 mg oral fluconazole daily for 2 weeks increased the steady-state levels of oral atevirdine mesylate by 30% in a study in HIV-positive patients (229). In a similar study in parallel groups of eight and five HIV-infected patients, 400 mg oral fluconazole daily for 2 weeks had no significant effect on the steady-state pharmacokinetics of oral delavirdine (230). Furthermore, 200 mg oral fluconazole daily for 1 week (400 mg on day 1) had no effect on the pharmacokinetics of didanosine in 12 HIV-positive patients given oral didanosine twice daily (231).

According to several studies, at least high doses of fluconazole can increase the serum levels of cyclosporine. In one study, 16 renal transplant patients receiving a constant dose of cyclosporine were randomized to receive either placebo or 200 mg oral fluconazole once daily for 2 weeks (232,233). Fluconazole almost doubled trough serum levels of cyclosporine and increased its AUC over 24 hours from about 2200 to 4000 ng h/mL. In other reports, serum levels of cyclosporine increased two- to three-fold within 6 to 11 days of starting 100 to 200 mg fluconazole daily (234–236), sometimes even leading to nephrotoxicity (237). However, in studies in ten bone marrow transplant patients, 100 mg oral fluconazole daily for 14 days had no effect on serum cyclosporine levels at steady-state (209,238,239). This discrepancy may be explained by dose-dependent inhibition of the metabolism of cyclosporine by fluconazole (240). Moreover, the effect of intravenous fluconazole on the pharmacokinetics of cyclosporine seems to be smaller than that of oral fluconazole. A study in six bone marrow transplant patients found that the mean steady-state concentrations of cyclosporine were increased only by 21% after 2 weeks of 400 mg intravenous fluconazole daily (241).

In a diabetic liver transplant patient immunosuppressed with tacrolimus, treatment with fluconazole led to highly elevated plasma levels of tacrolimus and serum levels of creatinine (242). The increase in tacrolimus levels was later confirmed by a rechallenge with fluconazole. In addition, oral fluconazole 100 mg daily was successfully used to improve the oral bioavailability of tacrolimus in one pediatric patient (243). In 20 organ transplant patients on tacrolimus, addition of either 100 or 200 mg oral fluconazole daily increased the trough levels of tacrolimus 1.4- and 3.1-fold, respectively, after 1 day of therapy with fluconazole (244). Thereafter, a median reduction of 56% in the dosage of tacrolimus was required. In one patient, the AUC of tacrolimus decreased from 13 to 5.4 ng h/mL after 100 mg fluconazole daily was stopped. In contrast to the above reports concerning orally administered fluconazole, 400 mg fluconazole intravenously once daily for 2 weeks only statistically nonsignificantly increased the steady-state levels of tacrolimus in 15 bone marrow transplant patients (241).

In one study, 50 mg oral fluconazole daily for 10 days had no effect on the pharmacokinetics of ethinyl estradiol and norgestrel after a single dose of an oral contraceptive in ten healthy female volunteers (209). However, a single 150-mg oral dose of fluconazole slightly increased the plasma concentrations of ethinyl estradiol in a study in 20 women regularly taking oral contraceptives containing ethinyl estradiol (245). Moreover, in unpublished studies, 200 mg fluconazole daily increased the levels of ethinyl estradiol and levonorgestrel by 40% and 24%, respectively (71).

In addition to moderately inhibiting CYP3A4, fluconazole has been shown to considerably impair CYP2C9-mediated drug metabolism in humans. Several case reports have described increased phenytoin levels and toxic symptoms after starting treatment with fluconazole to patients on phenytoin (246–248). In a study comparing ten subjects given 200 mg oral fluconazole daily for 14 days with ten subjects not receiving fluconazole, fluconazole increased the AUC of phenytoin over 24 hours after an intravenous dose of phenytoin (following 200 mg phenytoin orally for 3 days) by 75% and the trough serum levels of phenytoin by 130% (209,249). In another study, 400 mg oral fluconazole daily for 6 days increased the AUC over 48 hours following a single oral dose of phenytoin by 33% and the phenytoin concentration at 48 hours by 133% in nine healthy male subjects (98). Because of the saturable metabolism of phenytoin and its long half-life, it is likely that the extent of this interaction is much greater in patients on continuous treatment with phenytoin.

In several case reports, treatment with fluconazole has been associated with an increased hypoprothrombinemic response to warfarin (250–254). In seven men stabilized on warfarin, 100 mg oral fluconazole daily for 1 week increased the prothrombin time by about 40% (255). In a crossover study in 13 volunteers, 200 mg oral fluconazole daily for 1 week increased the effects of warfarin on prothrombin time by about 10% after a single 15-mg dose of warfarin (209). In another crossover study in six subjects, 400 mg oral fluconazole daily for 1 week substantially increased the prothrombin time after a single oral 0.75-mg/kg dose of pseudoracemic warfarin (256). This was mainly due to a 2.8-fold increase in the AUC of the active S-enantiomer caused by inhibition of its CYP2C9 catalyzed 6- and 7-hydroxylation by fluconazole, as reflected in the formation clearances of the respective metabolites. The AUC of the less active R-enenatiomer was increased 2.1-fold as a result of reduced formation of its 6-, 7-, 8-, and 10-hydroxy metabolites, which can be explained by inhibition of CYP2C19, CYP3A4, and some undefined CYP isoforms. The mean half-life values of (R)- and (S)-warfarin were increased by about 110% and 180% as a result of 54% and 68% reductions in the systemic clearances (assuming 100% bioavailability), respectively. Based on the observed total plasma concentrations of fluconazole and formation clearances of (S)-7-hydroxy warfarin and (R)-8-hydroxy warfarin, an in vivo K_i of 22.5 μM and 76 μM was calculated for CYP2C9 and CYP3A4, respectively (257), suggesting that the active inhibitory concentration of fluconazole at the enzyme site is about one-third of its total plasma concentration.

In one study with limited documentation, 100 mg oral fluconazole daily for 1 week increased the AUC and prolonged the half-life of tolbutamide after a single 500-mg dose by 58% to 59% in 13 healthy volunteers (209), suggesting inhibition of the metabolism of tolbutamide by fluconazole. According to Stockley (71), 100 mg fluconazole daily for 6 to 7 days increased the AUCs of chlorpropamide, glipizide, glibenclamide, and tolbutamide by 30% to 50% after single oral doses of the antidiabetics in controlled studies in healthy subjects. In most of the studies, the proportion of subjects reporting

hypoglycemic symptoms was also increased during fluconazole administration. One published case report also describes a patient on glipizide in whom severe hypoglycemia developed during treatment with fluconazole (258).

The effect of 200 mg oral fluconazole daily for 4 days (400 mg on day 1) on the pharmacokinetics of a single oral dose of losartan, a CYP2C9 substrate, was studied in a randomized, double-blind, placebo-controlled trial in 11 healthy subjects (202). Fluconazole decreased the AUC and C_{max} of E-3174, the active metabolite of losartan, by 53% and 70%, respectively, and only nonsignificantly increased the AUC of unchanged losartan. In another study, 16 volunteers received 100 mg losartan once daily for 20 days and 200 mg oral fluconazole once daily from day 11 to 20 of the losartan administration (259). After administration of fluconazole, the AUC and C_{max} of losartan were increased by 66% and 30% and those of E-3174 decreased by 43% and 56%, respectively. In a similar study, 200 mg oral fluconazole daily had no effect on the disposition of eprosartan (259).

In six healthy volunteers, 200 mg oral fluconazole daily for 3 days (400 mg on day 1) decreased the apparent oral clearance of sulfamethoxazole by 26% when a single oral dose of sulfamethoxazole and trimethoprim was given 24 hours after the first dose of fluconazole (260). In particular, the formation of sulfamethoxazole hydroxylamine, the metabolite putatively responsible for sulfamethoxazole toxicity, was decreased by fluconazole as shown by the 93% decrease in its AUC. The formation of the hydroxylamine was inhibited by fluconazole also in vitro. In another study, a 150-mg oral dose of fluconazole reduced the urinary recovery of sulfamethoxazole hydroxylamine over 24 hours by 50% after a single oral dose of cotrimoxazole in ten healthy volunteers (100).

There are only a few reports on the effects of fluconazole on the pharmacokinetics of drugs metabolized by enzymes other than CYP3A4 or CYP2C9. A study with limited documentation in six young and five elderly subjects found that 200 mg or 400 mg oral fluconazole daily for 10 days reduced the systemic clearance of caffeine, a drug primarily metabolized by CYP1A2, by 17% or 32%, respectively (261). There was also a significant correlation between the AUC of fluconazole and the reduction in the clearance of caffeine. In a crossover study in five normal subjects, 100 mg oral fluconazole twice daily for 3 days had no significant effect on the pharmacokinetics of theophylline after a single oral 300-mg dose of aminophylline (262). However, an undetailed report describes a patient in whom an elevation in theophylline levels developed during treatment with fluconazole (254).

In a crossover study in six healthy volunteers, 200 mg oral fluconazole daily for 7 days had no effect on the pharmacokinetics of mexiletine, a CYP2D6 substrate (263). However, an isolated case report describes an elderly patient on nortriptyline, in whom a 70% increase in serum nortriptyline levels developed 13 days after starting 100 mg oral fluconazole daily (264). Furthermore, 100 to 400 mg oral fluconazole daily appeared to significantly increase serum amitriptyline concentrations in three male adults (265). These possible interactions can be explained by inhibition of the demethylation of nortriptyline and amitriptyline, which is probably mediated by CYP2C9, CYP2C19, or CYP3A4. In a crossover study in eight fast and eight slow acetylators of isoniazid, 400 mg oral fluconazole daily for 1 week had no significant effect on the pharmacokinetics of isoniazid (266).

Fluconazole as an Inhibitor of Metabolic Enzymes

Based on *in vivo* studies, fluconazole is a moderately potent inhibitor of CYP3A4, being able to increase the plasma concentrations of CYP3A4 substrates roughly as much as erythromycin, for example, but less than ketoconazole and itraconazole (see Fig. 47-1). This is also in good agreement with the *in vitro* potency of fluconazole against CYP3A4, because its plasma concentrations during administration of 100 to 400 mg daily range from 20 to 60 μM (206), exceeding or equaling its *in vitro* K_i values for CYP3A4. According to a number of studies, fluconazole is a fairly potent inhibitor of CYP2C9 both *in vitro* and *in vivo,* and may therefore cause harmful interactions with drugs metabolized by CYP2C9, such as warfarin, phenytoin, and tolbutamide. Furthermore, based on potent inhibition of CYP2C19 *in vitro,* it is likely that fluconazole also significantly impairs CYP2C19-mediated metabolism *in vivo.* In contrast, because fluconazole seems to have no effect on CYP1A2 *in vitro* or on the pharmacokinetics of theophylline *in vivo,* it is probably not an inhibitor of CYP1A2 *in vivo,* although it slightly reduced the clearance of caffeine in one study. Furthermore, because fluconazole seems to have virtually no effect on CYP2A6 and CYP2E1 *in vitro,* it is likely that it does not inhibit these enzymes *in vivo.*

New Azoles

In addition to itraconazole and fluconazole, several new azoles are under development (1). For example, the triazoles voriconazole (UK-109496) and ZD-0870 showed a promising antifungal spectrum in preclinical studies. However, no studies on their effects on drug-metabolizing enzymes have been reported so far.

ALLYLAMINES (TERBINAFINE)

Allylamines act by inhibiting a non-CYP enzyme, squalene epoxidase in the fungal ergosterol synthesis (134,267). Currently, terbinafine is the only systemic allylamine antimycotic agent in wide clinical use (1,268). Terbinafine is available as oral and topical formulations. It is active and clinically effective against dermatophytes

and molds, but its activity against yeasts is weaker and more variable. Therefore, its main indications are onychomycosis, tinea infections, and pityriasis versicolor. In addition, the topical form is used for treatment of cutaneous yeast infections.

After oral administration, approximately 70% to 80% of terbinafine is absorbed (3,134,268,269). Intake of food does not significantly affect its bioavailability. The recommended oral dose is 250 mg/day, and after a single 250-mg dose, the C_{max} approximates 0.8 mg/L and is reached about 2 hours after ingestion (3,269). After administration of terbinafine 250 mg/day for 10 to 14 days (steady-state), the C_{max} is approximately 1.3 mg/L (i.e., 4.5 μM). The plasma protein binding of terbinafine exceeds 99% (269). As a highly lipophilic agent, it is widely distributed within the body, with a V_d of about 14 L/kg at steady-state. High concentrations are found in skin, hair, and nails. Terbinafine undergoes extensive metabolism and at least 15 metabolites have been identified, none with significant antifungal activity (269). Its elimination is triphasic, with average half-life values of 1.2, 16, and 100 hours (268). The metabolism of terbinafine is influenced by agents affecting CYP enzyme activity, such as rifampicin, phenobarbital, and cimetidine (270).

Terbinafine as an Inhibitor of Metabolic Enzymes

Terbinafine seems to have a low potential for drug–drug interactions because of inhibition or induction of CYP2C9 and CYP3A4. In studies with human hepatic microsomes, terbinafine even at 100 μM did not significantly inhibit cyclosporine, cortisol, tolbutamide, or ethoxycoumarin metabolism (20–22,271), suggesting lack of inhibitory effects on CYP2C9 and CYP3A4. The reaction most affected by terbinafine was ethinyl estradiol 2-hydroxylation with a 35% reduction at 50 μM (21).

In a crossover study in eight healthy subjects, 125 mg terbinafine twice daily for 8 days had no effect on antipyrine clearance (272). Furthermore, a single 500-mg dose of terbinafine or 500 mg terbinafine daily for 8 days had no effect on serum testosterone levels in two crossover studies in healthy male subjects (273,274). In agreement with *in vitro* studies, 250 mg terbinafine once daily for 4 days also had no effect on the pharmacokinetics of the orally taken CYP3A4 substrates midazolam and triazolam in placebo-controlled crossover studies with 12 normal subjects (see Fig. 47-1) (150,217). In addition, 250 mg terbinafine daily for 18 days slightly reduced the trough plasma concentrations of the acid metabolite of terfenadine, and caused no accumulation of unchanged terfenadine in a crossover study in 26 healthy subjects (275).

In a study in 20 male volunteers, 250 mg terbinafine daily for 1 week did not increase, but decreased the peak blood concentration and AUC of cyclosporine by 13% to 14% (276). A similar slight decrease in blood trough levels of cyclosporine was observed during administration of 250 mg terbinafine daily for 12 weeks in a study in 11 transplant patients (277). In a recent case report based on four renal transplant patients, administration of 250 mg terbinafine daily was also reported to have slightly (by up to 35%) reduced blood cyclosporine levels (278). In a crossover study in 16 healthy volunteers, 250 mg terbinafine daily for 12 days had no effect on the pharmacokinetics of oral digoxin (279).

In a crossover study in eight healthy volunteers, a single 500-mg dose of terbinafine reduced the systemic clearance of caffeine by 21% and increased its AUC by 29% after an intravenous bolus dose (106). In another crossover study in 12 normal subjects, 250 mg terbinafine daily for 4 days increased the AUC and half-life of oral theophylline by 16% and 24%, respectively (280), which raises the question about the possible inhibition of CYP1A2 by terbinafine. However, in a recent crossover study in 12 healthy nonsmoking volunteers, 250 mg terbinafine daily for 3 days had no effect on CYP1A2, N-acetyltransferase or xanthine oxidase as assessed by using caffeine as a probe (281).

In two contrasting case reports, treatment with terbinafine was described to have either decreased (282) or increased (283) the anticoagulant effects of warfarin. However, in a crossover study in 16 healthy volunteers, 250 mg terbinafine once daily for 14 days had no significant effects on the pharmacokinetics of a single dose of warfarin (284) excluding the possibility of any major effects on the metabolism of warfarin by terbinafine.

One case report describes a patient on nortriptyline in whom nortriptyline intoxication developed within 2 weeks after starting treatment with 250 mg terbinafine daily (285). An increase in serum nortriptyline concentrations was also observed after a rechallenge with terbinafine. In one study, treatment with terbinafine was associated with a substantially elevated metabolic ratio of dextromethorphan in two genotypically extensive metabolizers, suggesting that terbinafine is an inhibitor of CYP2D6 (286). In subsequent studies, terbinafine was also found to be a strong inhibitor ($K_i = 0.028–0.044 \mu M$) of CYP2D6 in human liver microsomes (J.S. Leeder, personal communication).

Taken together, when terbinafine is used in normal therapeutic doses, it does not inhibit the CYP3A4-mediated metabolism of drugs such as triazolam, midazolam, terfenadine, or cyclosporine (see Fig. 47-1), and it seems to have no effect on the CYP2C9-mediated biotransformation of warfarin, for example. These results are also in excellent agreement with the lack of effect on CYP3A4 and CYP2C9 activity $in vitro$. However, based on slightly conflicting $in vivo$ studies, 250 or 500 mg terbinafine daily may slightly impair CYP1A2-mediated drug metabolism $in vivo$. Moreover, in view of some recent $in vitro$ and $in vivo$ observations, terbinafine seems to be a potent inhibitor of CYP2D6.

POLYENES

Since nystatin was discovered in 1951, almost 90 polyene antibiotics have been reported (2). However, most of them have caused problems that have prevented their widespread clinical use. Therefore, only nystatin, natamycin, and amphotericin B are clinically important. Nystatin and natamycin are used topically only and have not been associated with inhibition of drug metabolism.

Amphotericin B became the first commercially available systemic antifungal agent in 1960. It is presumed to act by binding to ergosterol in the fungal cell membrane, leading to disruption of the cell membrane (2,287). Amphotericin B is a first line agent in the treatment of certain systemic mycoses, such as fungal meningitis (1,288). For systemic mycoses, it is used parenterally, because it is not absorbed following oral administration. It is also available as topical forms, which can be used for treatment of cutaneous and mucocutaneous candidiasis, but have no significant activity against dermatophytes. The use of amphotericin B is limited by adverse effects, such as nephrotoxicity; therefore, less toxic liposomal amphotericin B formulations have been developed (289).

Amphotericin B is associated with certain clinically important pharmacodynamic drug interactions, such as increased nephrotoxicity with cyclosporine or gentamicin (290), and enhanced digitalis toxicity and prolonged muscle relaxation with succinylcholine resulting from amphotericin B–induced hypokalemia (291,292). However, amphotericin B has not been reported to cause drug interactions by enzyme inhibition. Moreover, in human liver microsomes and primary cultures of hepatocytes, 100 μM amphotericin B did not significantly inhibit the oxidation of cyclosporine (35). In another study, amphotericin B only weakly ($K_i = 130 \mu M$) inhibited zidovudine glucuronidation in human hepatic microsomes (44). Thus, although the C_{max} of amphotericin B at steady-state may average 90 μM during high-dose liposomal amphotericin B treatment (289), it seems unlikely that amphotericin B would significantly inhibit CYP3A4 or zidovudine glucuronidation $in vivo$.

GRISEOFULVIN

Griseofulvin was the first orally administered antifungal agent used for dermatophyte infections. It is presumed to act by inhibiting fungal cell mitosis, leading to interruption of fungal cell division (2,293). Its therapeutic indications include dermatophytic infections of the skin, nails, and hair caused by *Microsporum, Trichophyton,* and *Epidermophyton* species, but it is not effective against *Candida* species and certain molds (294). In humans, treatment with griseofulvin has been associated with decreased plasma concentrations of or therapeutic failure with some drugs (e.g., cyclosporine, oral contraceptives, warfarin, theophylline, and salicylate); therefore, it has been suggested that griseofulvin is an enzyme inducer (295–301). However, there seem to be no reports about possible enzyme inhibition by griseofulvin.

FLUCYTOSINE

Flucytosine is a fluorinated pyrimidine, which is used as oral and parenteral preparations in the management of deep seated candidosis and cryptococcosis. In fungi, the drug is converted to 5-fluorouracil, which disturbs RNA and DNA synthesis, leading to cell death (302). Therefore, flucytosine may interact with drugs that are cytotoxic or myelotoxic by increasing the risk of hematologic toxicity (303). However, there seem to be no reports about the effects of flucytosine on drug metabolism.

REFERENCES

1. Kauffman CA, Carver PL. Antifungal agents in the 1990s. Current status and future developments. *Drugs* 1997;53:539–549.
2. Gupta AK, Sauder DN, Shear NH. Antifungal agents: an overview. Part I. *J Am Acad Dermatol* 1994;30:677–698.
3. Meinhof W. Kinetics and spectrum of activity of oral antifungals: the therapeutic implications. *J Am Acad Dermatol* 1993;29[Suppl]:37–41.
4. Heel RC, Brogden RN, Carmine A, Morley PA, Speight TM, Avery GS. Ketoconazole: a review of its therapeutic efficacy in superficial and systemic fungal infections. *Drugs* 1982;23:1–36.
5. Svejgaard E. Oral ketoconazole as an alternative to griseofulvin in recalcitrant dermatophyte infections and onychomycosis. *Acta Derm Venereol* 1985;65:143–149.
6. Daneshmend TK, Warnock DW. Clinical pharmacokinetics of ketoconazole. *Clin Pharmacokinet* 1988;14:13–34.
7. Schäfer-Korting M. Pharmacokinetic optimisation of oral antifungal therapy. *Clin Pharmacokinet* 1993;25:329–341.
8. von Moltke LL, Greenblatt DJ, Harmatz JS, et al. Triazolam biotransformation by human liver microsomes in vitro: effects of metabolic inhibitors and clinical confirmation of a predicted interaction with ketoconazole. *J Pharmacol Exp Ther* 1996;276:370–379.
9. von Moltke LL, Greenblatt DJ, Schmider J, Wright CE, Harmatz JS, Shader RI. In vitro approaches to predicting drug interactions in vivo. *Biochem Pharmacol* 1998;55:113–122.
10. Doble N, Shaw R, Rowland-Hill C, Lush M, Warnock DW, Keal EE. Pharmacokinetic study of the interaction between rifampicin and ketoconazole. *J Antimicrob Chemother* 1988;21:633–635.
11. Tucker RM, Denning DW, Hanson LH, et al. Interaction of azoles with rifampin, phenytoin, and carbamazepine: in vitro and clinical observations. *Clin Infect Dis* 1992;14:165–174.
12. Brown MW, Maldonado AL, Meredith CG, Speeg KV Jr. Effect of ketoconazole on hepatic oxidative drug metabolism. *Clin Pharmacol Ther* 1985;37:290–297.
13. D'Mello AP, D'Souza MJ, Bates TR. Pharmacokinetics of ketoconazole-antipyrine interaction. *Lancet* 1985;2:209–210.
14. Pasanen M, Taskinen T, Iscan M, Sotaniemi EA, Kairaluoma M, Pelkonen O. Inhibition of human hepatic and placental xenobiotic monooxygenases by imidazole antimycotics. *Biochem Pharmacol* 1988;37:3861–3866.
15. Pont A, Williams PL, Loose DS, et al. Ketoconazole blocks adrenal steroid synthesis. *Ann Intern Med* 1982;97:370–372.
16. Pont A, Williams PL, Azhar S, et al. Ketoconazole blocks testosterone synthesis. *Arch Intern Med* 1982;142:2137–2140.
17. Pont A, Graybill JR, Craven PC. High-dose ketoconazole therapy and adrenal and testicular function in humans. *Arch Intern Med* 1984;144:2150–2153.
18. Sikka SC, Swerdloff RS, Rajfer J. In vitro inhibition of testosterone biosynthesis by ketoconazole. *Endocrinology* 1985;116:1920–1925.
19. Gascon MP, Dayer P. In vitro forecasting of drugs which may interfere with the biotransformation of midazolam. *Eur J Clin Pharmacol* 1991;41:573–578.
20. Back DJ, Tjia JF. Comparative effects of the antimycotic drugs ketoconazole, fluconazole, itraconazole and terbinafine on the metabolism of cyclosporin by human liver microsomes. *Br J Clin Pharmacol* 1991;32:624–626.
21. Back DJ, Stevenson P, Tjia JF. Comparative effects of two antimycotic agents, ketoconazole and terbinafine on the metabolism of tolbutamide, ethinyloestradiol, cyclosporin and ethoxycoumarine by human liver microsomes in vitro. *Br J Clin Pharmacol* 1989;28:166–170.
22. Back DJ, Tjia JF, Abel SM. Azoles, allylamines and drug metabolism. *Br J Dermatol* 1992;126[Suppl]:14–18.
23. Baldwin SJ, Bloomer JC, Smith GJ, Ayrton AD, Clarke SE, Chenery RJ. Ketoconazole and sulphaphenazole as the respective selective inhibitors of P4503A and 2C9. *Xenobiotica* 1995;25:261–270.
24. Maurice M, Pichard L, Daujat M, et al. Effect of imidazole derivatives on cytochromes P450 from human hepatocytes in primary culture. *FASEB J* 1992;6:752–758.
25. Omar G, Whiting PH, Hawksworth GM, Humphrey MJ, Burke MD. Ketoconazole and fluconazole inhibition of the metabolism of cyclosporin A by human liver in vitro. *Ther Drug Monit* 1997;19:436–445.
26. Bourrié M, Meunier V, Berger Y, Fabre G. Cytochrome P450 isoform inhibitors as a tool for the investigation of metabolic reactions catalyzed by human liver microsomes. *Pharmacol Exp Ther* 1996;277:321–332.
27. Eagling VA, Tjia JF, Back DJ. Differential selectivity of cytochrome P450 inhibitors against probe substrates in human and rat liver microsomes. *Br J Clin Pharmacol* 1998;45:107–114.
28. Newton DJ, Wang RW, Lu AY. Cytochrome P450 inhibitors. Evaluation of specificities in the in vitro metabolism of therapeutic agents by human liver microsomes. *Drug Metab Dispos* 1995;23:154–158.
29. Back DJ, Tjia JF, Karbwang J, Colbert J. In vitro inhibition studies of tolbutamide hydroxylase activity of human liver microsomes by azoles, sulphonamides and quinolines. *Br J Clin Pharmacol* 1988;26:23–29.
30. von Moltke LL, Greenblatt DJ, Cotreau-Bibbo MM, Harmatz JS, Shader RI. Inhibitors of alprazolam metabolism in vitro: effect of serotonin-reuptake-inhibitor antidepressants, ketoconazole and quinidine. *Br J Clin Pharmacol* 1994;38:23–31.
31. von Moltke LL, Greenblatt DJ, Schmider J, Duan SX, Wright CE, Harmatz JS, Shader RI. Midazolam hydroxylation by human liver microsomes in vitro: inhibition by fluoxetine, norfluoxetine, and by azole antifungal agents. *J Clin Pharmacol* 1996;36:783–791.
32. Jurima-Romet M, Crawford K, Cyr T, Inaba T. Terfenadine metabolism in human liver. In vitro inhibition by macrolide antibiotics and azole antifungals. *Drug Metab Dispos* 1994;22:849–857.
33. von Moltke LL, Greenblatt DJ, Duan SX, Harmatz JS, Shader RI. In vitro prediction of the terfenadine-ketoconazole pharmacokinetic interaction. *J Clin Pharmacol* 1994;34:1222–1227.
34. von Moltke LL, Greenblatt DJ, Duan SX, Harmatz JS, Wright CE, Shader RI. Inhibition of terfenadine metabolism in vitro by azole antifungal agents and by selective serotonin reuptake inhibitor antidepressants: relation to pharmacokinetic interactions in vivo. *J Clin Psychopharmacol* 1996;16:104–112.
35. Pichard L, Fabre I, Fabre G, et al. Cyclosporin A drug interactions. Screening for inducers and inhibitors of cytochrome P-450 (cyclosporin A oxidase) in primary cultures of human hepatocytes and in liver microsomes. *Drug Metab Dispos* 1990;18:595–606.
36. Hargreaves JA, Jezequel S, Houston JB. Effect of azole antifungals on human microsomal metabolism of diclofenac and midazolam. *Br J Clin Pharmacol* 1994;38:175P (abstr.).
37. Wrighton SA, Ring BJ. Inhibition of human CYP3A catalyzed 1'-hydroxy midazolam formation by ketoconazole, nifedipine, erythromycin, cimetidine and nizatidine. *Pharm Res* 1994;11:921–924.
38. Christians U, Schmidt G, Bader A, et al. Identification of drugs inhibiting the in vitro metabolism of tacrolimus by human liver microsomes. *Br J Clin Pharmacol* 1996;41:187–190.
39. Siegsmund MJ, Cardarelli C, Aksentijevich I, Sugimoto Y, Pastan I, Gottesman MM. Ketoconazole effectively reverses multidrug resistance in highly resistant KB cells. *J Urol* 1994;151:485–491.
40. Woodland C, Ito S, Koren G. A model for the prediction of digoxin-drug interactions at the renal tubular cell level. *Ther Drug Monit* 1998;20:134–138.
41. Hall SD, Guengerich FP, Branch RA, Wilkinson GR. Characterization and inhibition of mephenytoin 4-hydroxylase activity in human liver microsomes. *J Pharmacol Exp Ther* 1987;240:216–222.

42. von Moltke LL, Greenblatt DJ, Cotreau-Bibbo MM, Duan SX, Harmatz JS, Shader RI. Inhibition of desipramine hydroxylation in vitro by serotonin-reuptake-inhibitor antidepressants, and by quinidine and ketoconazole: a model system to predict drug interactions in vivo. *J Pharmacol Exp Ther* 1994;268:1278–1283.

43. Draper AJ, Madan A, Parkinson A. Inhibition of coumarin 7-hydroxylase activity in human liver microsomes. *Arch Biochem Biophys* 1997; 341:47–61.

44. Sampol E, Lacarelle B, Rajaonarison JF, Catalin J, Durand A. Comparative effects of antifungal agents on zidovudine glucuronidation by human liver microsomes. *Br J Clin Pharmacol* 1995;40:83–86.

45. Tassaneeyakul W, Birkett DJ, Miners JO. Inhibition of human hepatic cytochrome P4502E1 by azole antifungals, CNS-active drugs and nonsteroidal anti-inflammatory agents. *Xenobiotica* 1998;28:293–301.

46. Blyden GT, Abernethy DR, Greenblatt DJ. Ketoconazole does not impair antipyrine clearance in humans. *Int J Clin Pharmacol Ther Toxicol* 1986;24:225–226.

47. Daneshmend TK, Warnock DW, Ene MD, et al. Multiple dose pharmacokinetics of ketoconazole and their effects on antipyrine kinetics in man. *J Antimicrob Chemother* 1983;12:185–188.

48. Engel G, Hofmann U, Heidemann H, Cosme J, Eichelbaum M. Antipyrine as a probe for human oxidative drug metabolism: identification of the cytochrome P450 enzymes catalyzing 4-hydroxyantipyrine, 3-hydroxymethylantipyrine, and norantipyrine formation. *Clin Pharmacol Ther* 1996;59:613–623.

49. Zürcher RM, Frey BM, Frey FJ. Impact of ketoconazole on the metabolism of prednisolone. *Clin Pharmacol Ther* 1989;45:366–372.

50. Jamis-Dow CA, Pearl ML, Watkins PB, Blake DS, Klecker RW, Collins JM. Predicting drug interactions in vivo from experiments in vitro. Human studies with paclitaxel and ketoconazole. *Am J Clin Oncol* 1997;20:592–599.

51. Kinirons MT, Krivoruk Y, Wilkinson GR, Wood AJJ. Cytochrome P4503A and the dapsone recovery ratio: lack of inhibition by ketoconazole. *Clin Pharmacol Ther* 1995;57:186(abstr).

52. Krivoruk Y, Kinirons MT, Wood AJJ, Wood M. Alfentanil disposition in vivo is mediated by CYP3A4 in humans. *Anesthesiology* 1994;81: A380(abstr).

53. Greenblatt DJ, von Moltke LL, Harmatz JS, et al. Interaction of triazolam and ketoconazole. *Lancet* 1995;345:191.

54. Olkkola KT, Backman JT, Neuvonen PJ. Midazolam should be avoided in patients receiving the systemic antimycotics ketoconazole or itraconazole. *Clin Pharmacol Ther* 1994;55:481–485.

55. Varhe A, Olkkola KT, Neuvonen PJ. Oral triazolam is potentially hazardous to patients receiving systemic antimycotics ketoconazole or itraconazole. *Clin Pharmacol Ther* 1994;56:601–607.

56. Lam YWF, Alfaro CL, Ereshefsky L, Miller M. Effect of antidepressants (AD) and ketoconazole (K) on oral midazolam (M) pharmacokinetics (PK). *Clin Pharmacol Ther* 1998;63:229(abstr).

57. Spina E, Arena D, Scordo MG, Fazio A, Pisani F, Perucca E. Elevation of plasma carbamazepine concentrations by ketoconazole in patients with epilepsy. *Ther Drug Monit* 1997;19:535–538.

58. Spina E, Avenoso A, Campo GM, Scordo MG, Caputi AP, Perucca E. Effect of ketoconazole on the pharmacokinetics of imipramine and desipramine in healthy subjects. *Br J Clin Pharmacol* 1997;43: 315–318.

59. Monahan BP, Ferguson CL, Killeavy ES, Lloyd BK, Troy J, Cantilena LR Jr. Torsades de pointes occurring in association with terfenadine use. *JAMA* 1990;264:2788–2790.

60. Zimmermann M, Duruz H, Guinand O, et al. Torsades de pointes after treatment with terfenadine and ketoconazole. *Eur Heart J* 1992;13:1002–1003.

61. Honig PK, Wortham DC, Zamani K, Conner DP, Mullin JC, Cantilena LR. Terfenadine-ketoconazole interaction. Pharmacokinetic and electrocardiographic consequences. *JAMA* 1993;269:1513–1518.

62. Eller MG, Okerholm RA. Pharmacokinetic interaction between terfenadine and ketoconazole. *Clin Pharmacol Ther* 1991;49:130(abstr).

63. Lavrijsen K, Van Houdt J, Meuldermans W, Janssens M, Heykants J. The interaction of ketoconazole, itraconazole and erythromycin with the in vitro metabolism of antihistamines in human liver microsomes. *Allergy* 1993;48[Suppl]:34.

64. Tsai WC, Tsai LM, Chen JH. Combined use of astemizole and ketoconazole resulting in torsades de pointes. *J Formos Med Assoc* 1997; 96:144–146.

65. Morganroth J, Lyness WH, Perhach JL, et al. Lack of effect of aze-lastine and ketoconazole coadministration on electrocardiographic parameters in healthy volunteers. *J Clin Pharmacol* 1997;37: 1065–1072.

66. van Peer A, Crabbé R, Woestenborghs R, Heykants J, Janssens M. Ketoconazole inhibits loratadine metabolism in man. *Allergy* 1993;48 [Suppl 16]:34(abstr).

67. Brannan MD, Reidenberg P, Radwanski E, Shneyer L, Lin C, Affrime MB. Evaluation of pharmacokinetic and electrocardiographic parameters following 10 days of concomitant administration of loratadine with ketoconazole. *J Clin Pharmacol* 1994;34:1016(abstr).

68. Gillen M, Pentikis H, Rhodes G, et al. Pharmacokinetic (PK) and cardiac safety studies of ebastine (EBA) and loratadine (LOR) administered with ketoconazole (keto). *J Clin Pharmacol* 1998;38:842–886.

69. Chan-Tompkins NH, Babinchak TJ. Cardiac arrhythmias associated with coadministration of azole compounds and cisapride. *Clin Infect Dis* 1997;24:1285.

70. Wysowski DK, Bacsanyi J. Cisapride and fatal arrhythmia. *N Engl J Med* 1996;335:290–291.

71. Stockley IH. *Drug interactions,* 4th ed. London: The Pharmaceutical Press, 1996.

72. McNulty RM, Lazor JA, Sketch M. Transient increase in plasma quinidine concentrations during ketoconazole-quinidine therapy. *Clin Pharm* 1989;8:222–225.

73. Floren LC, Bekersky I, Benet LZ, et al. Tacrolimus oral bioavailability doubles with coadministration of ketoconazole. *Clin Pharmacol Ther* 1997;62:41–49.

74. Dieperink H, Møller J. Ketoconazole and cyclosporin. *Lancet* 1982; 2:1217.

75. First MR, Schroeder TJ, Alexander JW, Stephens GW, Weiskittel P, Myre SA, Pesce AJ. Cyclosporine dose reduction by ketoconazole administration in renal transplant recipients. *Transplantation* 1991; 51:365–370.

76. Gomez DY, Wacher VJ, Tomlanovich SJ, Hebert MF, Benet LZ. The effects of ketoconazole on the intestinal metabolism and bioavalibility of cyclosporine. *Clin Pharmacol Ther* 1995;58:15–19.

77. Horton CM, Freeman CD, Nolan PE Jr, Copeland JG 3d. Cyclosporine interactions with miconazole and other azole-antimycotics: a case report and review of the literature. *J Heart Lung Transplant* 1992;11:1127–1132.

78. Patton PR, Brunson ME, Pfaff WW, Howard RJ, Peterson JC, Ramos EL, Karlix JL. A preliminary report of diltiazem and ketoconazole. Their cyclosporine-sparing effect and impact on transplant outcome. *Transplantation* 1994;57:889–892.

79. Shepard JH, Canafax DM, Simmons RL, Najarian JS. Cyclosporine-ketoconazole: a potentially dangerous drug-drug interaction. *Clin Pharm* 1986;5:468.

80. Butman SM, Wild JC, Nolan PE, et al. Prospective study of the safety and financial benefit of ketoconazole as adjunctive therapy to cyclosporine after heart transplantation. *J Heart Lung Transplant* 1991;10:351–358.

81. First MR, Schroeder TJ, Michael A, Hariharan S, Weiskittel P, Alexander JW. Safety and efficacy of long-term cyclosporine-ketoconazole administration and preliminary results of a randomized trial. *Transplant Proc* 1993;25:591–594.

82. Foradori A, Mezzano S, Videla C, Pefaur J, Elberg A. Modification of the pharmacokinetics of cyclosporine A and metabolites by the concomitant use of Neoral and diltiazem or ketoconazol in stable adult kidney transplants. *Transplant Proc* 1998;30:1685–1687.

83. McLachlan AJ, Tett SE. Effect of metabolic inhibitors on cyclosporine pharmacokinetics using a population approach. *Ther Drug Monit* 1998;20:390–395.

84. Chapman SA, Lake KD, Solbrack DF, Milfred SK, Marshall PS, Kamps MA. Considerations for using ketoconazole in solid organ transplant recipients receiving cyclosporine immunosuppression. *J Transpl Coord* 1996;6:148–154.

85. Jones TE. The use of other drugs to allow a lower dosage of cyclosporin to be used. Therapeutic and pharmacoeconomic considerations. *Clin Pharmacokinet* 1997;32:357–367.

86. Keogh A, Spratt P, McCosker C, Macdonald P, Mundy J, Kaan A. Ketoconazole to reduce the need for cyclosporine after cardiac transplantation. *N Engl J Med* 1995;333:628–633.

87. Glynn AM, Slaughter RL, Brass C, D'Ambrosio R, Jusko WJ. Effects of ketoconazole on methylprednisolone pharmacokinetics and cortisol secretion. *Clin Pharmacol Ther* 1986;39:654–659.

88. Kandrotas RJ, Slaughter RL, Brass C, Jusko WJ. Ketoconazole effects on methylprednisolone disposition and their joint suppression of endogenous cortisol. *Clin Pharmacol Ther* 1987;42:465–470.

89. Ludwig EA, Slaughter RL, Savliwala M, Brass C, Jusko WJ. Steroid-specific effects of ketoconazole on corticosteroid disposition: unaltered prednisolone elimination. *DICP* 1989;23:858–861.

90. Yamashita SK, Ludwig EA, Middleton E Jr, Jusko WJ. Lack of pharmacokinetic and pharmacodynamic interactions between ketoconazole and prednisolone. *Clin Pharmacol Ther* 1991;49:558–570.

91. Kerr BM, Yuen GJ, Sandoval T, Wu E, Shetty BV, Anderson R. The pharmacokinetics of nelfinavir administered alone and with ketoconazole in healthy volunteers. *Clin Pharmacol Ther* 1997;61:147(abstr).

92. Bertz R, Wong C, Carothers L, Lauva I, Dennis S, Valdes J. Evaluation of the pharmacokinetics of multiple dose ritonavir and ketoconazole in combination. *Clin Pharmacol Ther* 1998;63:230(abstr).

93. Böttiger Y, Tybring G, Götharson E, Bertilsson L. Inhibition of the sulfoxidation of omeprazole by ketoconazole in poor and extensive metabolizer of S-mephenytoin. *Clin Pharmacol Ther* 1997;62:384–391.

94. Fleishaker JC, Pearson PG, Wienkers LC, Pearson LK, Peters GR. Biotransformation of tirilazad in humans: 2. Effect of ketoconazole on tirilazad clearance and oral bioavailability. *J Pharmacol Exp Ther* 1996;277:991–998.

95. Krishnaiah YS, Satyanarayana S, Visweswaram D. Interaction between tolbutamide and ketoconazole in healthy subjects. *Br J Clin Pharmacol* 1994;37:205–207.

96. Smith AG. Potentiation of oral anticoagulants by ketoconazole. *BMJ (Clin Res Ed)* 1984;288:188–189.

97. Stevens DA, Stiller RL, Williams PL, Sugar AM. Experience with ketoconazole in three major manifestations of progressive coccidioidomycosis. *Am J Med* 1983;74:58–63.

98. Touchette MA, Chandrasekar PH, Milad MA, Edwards DJ. Contrasting effects of fluconazole and ketoconazole on phenytoin and testosterone disposition in man. *Br J Clin Pharmacol* 1992;34:75–78.

99. McCrea JB, Lo MW, Furtek CI, et al. Ketoconazole does not effect the systemic conversion of losartan to E-3174. *Clin Pharmacol Ther* 1996;59:169(abstr).

100. Gill HJ, Maggs JL, Madden S, Pirmohamed M, Park BK. The effect of fluconazole and ketoconazole on the metabolism of sulphamethoxazole. *Br J Clin Pharmacol* 1996;42:347–353.

101. Atiba JO, Blaschke TF, Wilkinson GR. Effects of ketoconazole on the polymorphic 4-hydroxylations of S-mephenytoin and debrisoquine. *Br J Clin Pharmacol* 1989;28:161–165.

102. Adedoyin A, Trump DL, Brufsky A, Frye RF, Hofacker J, Branch RA. Selective alteration of specific metabolizing enzyme activities by disulfiram and ketoconazole. *Clin Pharmacol Ther* 1998;63:154(abstr).

103. Duvelleroy Hommet C, Jonville-Bera AP, Autret A, Saudeau D, Autret E, Fauchier JP. Convulsive seizures in a patient treated with propafenone and ketoconazole. *Therapie* 1995;50:164–165.

104. Heusner JJ, Dukes GE, Rollins DE, Tolman KG, Galinsky RE. Effect of chronically administered ketoconazole on the elimination of theophylline in man. *Drug Intell Clin Pharm* 1987;21:514–517.

105. Naline E, Sanceaume M, Pays M, Advenier C. Application of theophylline metabolite assays to the exploration of liver microsome oxidative function in man. *Fund Clin Pharmacol* 1988;2:341–351.

106. Wahlländer A, Paumgartner G. Effect of ketoconazole and terbinafine on the pharmacokinetics of caffeine in healthy volunteers. *Eur J Clin Pharmacol* 1989;37:279–283.

107. Brugmans J, Van Cutsem J, Heykants J, Schuermans V, Thienpont D. Systemic antifungal potential, safety, biotransport and transformation of miconazole nitrate. *Eur J Clin Pharmacol* 1972;51:93–99.

108. Boelaert J, Daneels R, Van Landuyt H, Symoens J. Miconazole plasma levels in healthy subjects and in patients with impaired renal function. *Chemotherapy* 1976;6:165–169.

109. Stevens DA. Miconazole in the treatment of coccidioidomycosis. *Drugs* 1983;26:347–354.

110. Lewi PJ, Boelaert J, Daneels R, et al. Pharmacokinetic profile of intravenous miconazole in man: comparison of normal subjects and patients with renal insufficiency. *Eur J Clin Pharmacol* 1976;10:49–54.

111. Stevens DA, Levine HB, Deresinski SC. Miconazole incoccidioidomycosis. II. Therapeutic and pharmacologic studies in man. *Am J Med* 1976;60:191–202.

112. O'Reilly RA, Goulart DA, Kunze KL, et al. Mechanisms of the stereoselective interaction between miconazole and racemic wafarin in human subjects. *Clin Pharmacol Ther* 1992;51:656–667.

113. Kunze KL, Wienkers LC, Thummel KE, Trager WF. Warfarin-fluconazole. I. Inhibition of the human cytochrome P450-dependent metabolism of warfarin by fluconazole: in vitro studies. *Drug Metab Dispos* 1996;24:414–421.

114. Mäenpää J, Sigusch H, Raunio H, et al. Differential inhibition of coumarin 7-hydroxylase activity in mouse and human liver microsomes. *Biochem Pharmacol* 1993;45:1035–1042.

115. Morita K, Ono T, Shimakawa H. Inhibition of testosterone biosynthesis in testicular microsomes by various imidazole drugs. Comparative study with ketoconazole. *J Pharmacobiodyn* 1990;13:336–343.

116. Ariyaratnam S, Thakker NS, Sloan P, Thornhill MH. Potentiation of warfarin anticoagulant activity by miconazole oral gel. *BMJ* 1997;314:349.

117. Colquhoun MC, Daly M, Stewart P, Beeley L. Interaction between warfarin and miconazole oral gel. *Lancet* 1987;1:695–696.

118. Goenen M, Reymert M, Jaumin P, Chalant CH, Tremouroux J. A case of *Candida albicans* endocarditis 3 years after an aortic valve replacement: successful combined medical and surgical therapy. *J Cardiovasc Surg* 1977;18:391–396.

119. Long E. Warfarin-miconazole interaction. *Arch Intern Med* 1983;143:2214–2215.

120. Loupi E, Descotes J, Lery N, Evreux JC. Interactions medicamenteuses et miconazole. *Therapie* 1982;37:437–441.

121. Pemberton MN, Sloan P, Ariyaratnam S, Thakker NS, Thornhill MH. Derangement of warfarin anticoagulation by miconazole oral gel. *Br Dent J* 1998;84:68–69.

122. Shenfield GM, Page M. Potentiation of warfarin action by miconazole oral gel. *Aust NZ J Med* 1991;21:928.

123. Watson PG, Lochan RG, Redding VJ. Drug interactions with coumarin derivative anticoagulants. *BMJ* 1982;285:1045–1046.

124. Rettie AE, Korzekwa KR, Kunze KL, et al. Hydroxylation of warfarin by human cDNA-expressed cytochrome, a role for P-4502C9 in the etiology of (S)-warfarin-drug interactions. *Chem Res Toxicol* 1992;5:54–59.

125. Rolan PE, Somogyi AA, Drew MJ, Cobain WG, South D, Bochner F. Phenytoin intoxication during treatment with parenteral miconazole. *BMJ (Clin Res Ed)* 1983;287:1760.

126. Meurice JC, Lecomte P, Renard JP, Girard JJ. Interaction miconazole et sulfamides hypoglycemiants. *Presse Med* 1983;12:1670.

127. Heinemeyer G, Roots I, Schultz H, Dennhardt R. Hemmung der Pentobarbital-Elimination bei Intensivtherapie des erhohten intracraniellen Druckes. *Intensivmed* 1988;22:164–167.

128. Burgess MA, Bodey GP. Clotrimazole (Bay b 5097): in vitro and clinical pharmacological studies. *Antimicrob Agents Chemother* 1972;2:423–426.

129. Schuetz EG, Beck WT, Schuetz JD. Modulators and substrates of P-glycoprotein and cytochrome P4503A coordinately up-regulate these proteins in human colon carcinoma cells. *Mol Pharmacol* 1996;49:311–318.

130. Mieles L, Venkataramanan R, Yokoyama I, Warty VJ, Starzl TE. Interaction between FK506 and clotrimazole in a liver transplant recipient. *Transplantation* 1991;52:1086–1087.

131. Duhm B, Medenwald H, Puetter J, Maul W, Patzschke K, Wegner LA. The pharmacokinetics of clotrimazole ^{14}C. *Postgrad Med J* 1974;50[Suppl 1]:13–16.

132. Ritter W. Pharmacokinetic fundamentals of vaginal treatment with clotrimazole. *Am J Obstet Gynecol* 1985;152:945–947.

133. Grant SM, Clissold SP. Itraconazole. A review of its pharmacodynamic and pharmacokinetic properties, and therapeutic use in superficial and systemic mycoses. *Drugs* 1989;37:310–344.

134. Gupta AK, Sauder DN, Shear NH. Antifungal agents: an overview. Part II. *J Am Acad Dermatol* 1994;30:911–933.

135. Heykants J, Van Peer A, Van de Velde V, et al. The clinical pharmacokinetics of itraconazole: an overview. *Mycoses* 1989;32[Suppl 1]:67–87.

136. Hardin TC, Graybill JR, Fetchick R, Woestenborghs R, Rinaldi MG, Kuhn JG. Pharmacokinetics of itraconazole following oral administration to normal volunteers. *Antimicrob Agents Chemother* 1988;32:1310–1313.

137. Luurila H, Kivistö KT, Neuvonen PJ. Effect of itraconazole on the pharmacokinetics and pharmacodynamics of zolpidem. *Eur J Clin Phamacol* 1998;54:163–166.

138. Neuvonen PJ, Kantola T, Kivistö KT. Simvastatin but not pravastatin is very susceptible to interaction with the CYP3A4 inhibitor itraconazole. *Clin Pharmacol Ther* 1998;63:332–341.

139. Arredondo G, Calvo R, Marcos F, Martinez-Jorda R, Suarez E. Protein binding of itraconazole and fluconazole in patients with cancer. *Int J Clin Pharmacol Ther* 1995;33:449–452.

140. Miyama T, Takanaga H, Matsuo H, et al. P-glycoprotein-mediated transport of itraconazole across the blood-brain barrier. *Antimicrob Agents Chemother* 1998;42:1738–1744.

141. van Peer A, Woestenborghs R, Heykants J, Gasparini R, Gauwenbergh G. The effects of food and dose on the oral systemic availability of itraconazole in healthy subjects. *Eur J Clin Pharmacol* 1989;36:423–426.

142. Ducharme MP, Slaughter RL, Warbasse LH, et al. Itraconazole and hydroxyitraconazole serum concentrations are reduced more than tenfold by phenytoin. *Clin Pharmacol Ther* 1995;58:617–624.

143. Jaruratanasirikul S, Sriwiriyajan S. Effect of rifampicin on the pharmacokinetics of itraconazole in normal volunteers and AIDS patients. *Eur J Clin Pharmacol* 1998;54:155–158.

144. Damanhouri Z, Gumbleton M, Nicholls PJ, Shaw MA. In-vivo effects of itraconazole on hepatic mixed-function oxidase. *J Antimicrob Chemother* 1988;21:187–194.

145. Heykants J, Van Peer A, Lavrijsen K, Meuldermans W, Woestenborghs R, Cauwenbergh G. Pharmacokinetics of oral antifungals and their clinical implications. *Br J Clin Pract Suppl* 1990;71:50–56.

146. Gascon MP, Oestreicher-Kondo M, Dayer P. Comparative effects of imidazole antifungals on liver monooxygenases. *Clin Pharmacol Ther* 1991;49:158(abstr).

147. Kurosawa M, Okabe M, Hara N, et al. Reversal effect of itraconazole on adriamycin and etoposide resistance in human leukemia cells. *Ann Hematol* 1996;72:17–21.

148. Olkkola KT, Ahonen J, Neuvonen PJ. The effects of the systemic antimycotics, itrconazole and fluconazole, on the pharmacokinetics and pharmacodynamics of intravenous and oral midazolam. *Anesth Analg* 1996;82:511–516.

149. Backman JT, Kivistö KT, Olkkola KT, Neuvonen PJ. The area under the plasma concentration-time curve for oral midazolam is 400-fold larger during treatment with itraconazole than with rifampicin. *Eur J Clin Pharmacol* 1998;54:53–58.

150. Ahonen J, Olkkola KT, Neuvonen PJ. Effect of itraconazole and terbinafine on the pharmacokinetics and pharmacodynamics of midazolam in healthy volunteers. *Br J Clin Pharmacol* 1995;40:270–272.

151. Neuvonen PJ, Varhe A, Olkkola KT. The effect of ingestion time interval on the interaction between itraconazole and triazolam. *Clin Pharmacol Ther* 1996;60:326–331.

152. Jalava KM, Olkkola KT, Neuvonen PJ. Effect of itraconazole on the pharmacokinetics and pharmacodynamics of zopiclone. *Eur J Clin Pharmacol* 1996;51:331–334.

153. Ahonen J, Olkkola KT, Neuvonen PJ. Lack of effect of antimycotic itraconazole on the pharmacokinetics or pharmacodynamics of temazepam. *Ther Drug Monit* 1996;18:124–127.

154. Ahonen J, Olkkola KT, Neuvonen PJ. The effect of the antimycotic itraconazole on the pharmacokinetics and pharmacodynamics of diazepam. *Fund Clin Pharmacol* 1996;10:314–318.

155. Kivistö KT, Lamberg TS, Kantola T, Neuvonen PJ. Plasma buspirone concentrations are greatly increased by erythromycin and itraconazole. *Clin Pharmacol Ther* 1997;62:348–354.

156. Palkama VJ, Neuvonen PJ, Olkkola KT. The CYP3A4 inhibitor itraconazole has no effect on the pharmacokinetics of i.v. fentanyl. *Br J Anaesth* 1998;81:598–600.

157. Raaska K, Neuvonen PJ. Serum concentrations of clozapine and N-desmethylclozapine are unaffected by the potent CYP3A4 inhibitor itraconazole. *Eur J Clin Pharmacol* 1998;54:167–170.

158. Kramer MR, Marshall SE, Denning DW, et al. Cyclosporine and itraconazole interaction in heart and lung transplant recipients. *Ann Intern Med* 1990;113:327–329.

159. Jones TE, Morris RG. Diltiazem does not always increase blood cyclosporin concentration. *Br J Clin Pharmacol* 1996;42:642–644.

160. Kwan JT, Foxall PJ, Davidson DG, Bending MR, Eisinger AJ. Interaction of cyclosporin and itraconazole. *Lancet* 1987;2:282.

161. Trenk D, Brett W, Jahnchen E, Birnbaum D. Time course of cyclosporin/itraconazole interaction. *Lancet* 1987;2:1335–1336.

162. Novakova I, Donnelly P, de Witte T, de Pauw B, Boezeman J, Veltman G. Itraconazole and cyclosporin nephrotoxicity. *Lancet* 1987;2:920–921.

163. Kramer MR, Merin G, Rudis E, Bar I, Nesher T, Bublil M, Milgalter E. Dose adjustment and cost of itraconazole prophylaxis in lung transplant recipients receiving cyclosporine and tacrolimus (FK 506). *Transplant Proc* 1997;29:2657–2659.

164. Furlan V, Parquin F, Penaud JF, et al. Interaction between tacrolimus and itraconazole in a heart-lung transplant recipient. *Transplant Proc* 1998;30:187–188.

165. Katari SR, Magnone M, Shapiro R, et al. Clinical features of acute reversible tacrolimus (FK 506) nephrotoxicity in kidney transplant recipients. *Clin Transplant* 1997;11:237–242.

166. Billaud EM, Guillemain R, Tacco F, Chevalier P. Evidence for a pharmacokinetic interaction between itraconazole and tacrolimus in organ transplant patients. *Br J Clin Pharmacol* 1998;46:271–272.

167. Varis T, Kaukonen KM, Kivistö KT, Neuvonen PJ. Plasma concentrations and effects of oral methylprednisolone are considerably increased by itraconazole. *Clin Pharmacol Ther* 1998;64:363–368.

168. Linthoudt H, Van Raemdonck D, Lerut T, Demedts M, Verleden G. The association of itraconazole and methylprednisolone may give rise to important steroid-related side effects. *J Heart Lung Transplant* 1996;15:1165.

169. Buggia I, Zecca M, Alessandrino EP, et al. Itraconazole can increase systemic exposure to busulfan in patients given bone marrow transplantation. GITMO (Gruppo Italiano Trapianto di Midollo Osseo). *Anticancer Res* 1996;16:2083–2088.

170. Bohme A, Ganser A, Hoelzer D. Aggravation of vincristine-induced neurotoxicity by itraconazole in the treatment of adult ALL. *Ann Hematol* 1995;71:311–312.

171. Gillies J, Hung KA, Fitzsimons E, Soutar R. Severe vincristine toxicity in combination with itraconazole. *Clin Lab Haematol* 1998;20:123–124.

172. Lukkari E, Juhakoski A, Aranko K, Neuvonen PJ. Itraconazole moderately increases serum concentrations of oxybutynin but does not affect those of the active metabolite. *Eur J Clin Pharmacol* 1997;52:403–406.

173. Crane JK, Shih HT. Syncope and cardiac arrhythmia due to an interaction between itraconazole and terfenadine. *Am J Med* 1993;95:445–446.

174. Pohjola-Sintonen S, Viitasalo M, Toivonen L, Neuvonen P. Itraconazole prevents terfenadine metabolism and increases risk of torsades de pointes ventricular tachycardia. *Eur J Clin Pharmacol* 1993;45:191–193.

175. Pohjola-Sintonen S, Viitasalo M, Toivonen L, Neuvonen P. Torsades de pointes after terfenadine-itraconazole interaction. *BMJ* 1993;306:186.

176. Honig PK, Wortham DC, Hull R, Zamani K, Smith JE, Cantilena LR. Itraconazole affects single-dose terfenadine pharmacokinetics and cardiac repolarization pharmacodynamics. *J Clin Pharmacol* 1993;33:1201–1206.

177. Lefebvre RA, Van Peer A, Woestenborghs R. Influence of itraconazole on the pharmacokinetics and electrocardiographic effects of astemizole. *Br J Clin Pharmacol* 1997;43:319–322.

178. Horn M. Coadministration of itraconazole with hypolipidemic agents may induce rhabdomyolysis in healthy individuals. *Arch Dermatol* 1996;132:1254.

179. Lees RS, Lees AM. Rhabdomyolysis from the coadministration of lovastatin and the antifungal agent itraconazole. *N Engl J Med* 1995;333:664–665.

180. Segaert MF, De Soete C, Vandewiele I, Verbanck J. Drug-interaction-induced rhabdomyolysis. *Nephrol Dial Transplant* 1996;11:1846–1847.

181. Neuvonen PJ, Jalava KM. Itraconazole drastically increases plasma concentrations of lovastatin and lovastatin acid. *Clin Pharmcol Ther* 1996;60:54–61.

182. Kivistö KT, Kantola T, Neuvonen PJ. Different effects of itraconazole on the pharmacokinetics of fluvastatin and lovastatin. *Br J Clin Pharmacol* 1998;46:49–53.

183. Kantola T, Kivistö KT, Neuvonen PJ. Effect of itraconazole on the pharmacokinetics of atorvastatin. *Clin Pharmacol Ther* 1998;64:58–65.

184. Neuvonen PJ, Suhonen R. Itraconazole interacts with felodipine. *J Am Acad Dermatol* 1995;33:134–135.

185. Rosen T. Debilitating edema associated with itraconazole therapy. *Arch Dermatol* 1994;130:260–261.

186. Tailor SA, Gupta AK, Walker SE, Shear NH. Peripheral edema due to

nifedipine-itraconazole interaction: a case report. *Arch Dermatol* 1996;132:350–352.

187. Jalava KM, Olkkola KT, Neuvonen PJ. Itraconazole greatly increases plasma concentrations and effects of felodipine. *Clin Pharmacol Ther* 1997;61:410–415.

188. Cruccu V, Pedretti D, Confalonieri F. A case of pulmonary aspergillosis effectively treated with itraconazole. Possible interaction of the antimycotic agent with hydroquinidine. *Clin Ter* 1995;146:383–839.

189. Kaukonen KM, Olkkola KT, Neuvonen PJ. Itraconazole increases plasma concentrations of quinidine. *Clin Pharmacol Ther* 1997;62: 510–517.

190. Isohanni MH, Neuvonen PJ, Palkama VJ, Olkkola KT. Effect of erythromycin and itraconazole on the pharmacokinetics of intravenous lignocaine. *Eur J Clin Pharmacol* 1998;54:561–565.

191. Antila S, Honkanen T, Lehtonen L, Neuvonen PJ. The CYP3A4 inhibitor itraconazole does not affect the pharmacokinetics of a new calcium-sensitizing drug levosimendan. *Int J Clin Pharmacol Ther* 1998;36:446–449.

192. Hinderling PH, Hartmann D. Pharmacokinetics of digoxin and main metabolites/derivatives in healthy humans. *Ther Drug Monit* 1991;13: 381–401.

193. de Lannoy IA, Silverman M. The MDR1 gene product, P-glycoprotein, mediates the transport of the cardiac glycoside, digoxin. *Biochem Biophys Res Commun* 1992;189:551–557.

194. Alderman CP, Allcroft PD. Digoxin–itraconazole interaction: possible mechanisms. *Ann Pharmacother* 1997;31:438–440.

195. Cone LA, Himelman RB, Hirschberg JN, Hutcheson JW. Itraconazole-related amaurosis and vomiting due to digoxin toxicity. *West J Med* 1996;165:322.

196. McClean KL, Sheehan GJ. Interaction between itraconazole and digoxin. *Clin Infect Dis* 1994;18:259–260.

197. Rex J. Itraconazole-digoxin interaction. *Ann Intern Med* 1992;116: 525.

198. Sachs MK, Blanchard LM, Green PJ. Interaction of itraconazole and digoxin. *Clin Infect Dis* 1993;16:400–403.

199. Partanen J, Jalava KM, Neuvonen PJ. Itraconazole increases serum digoxin concentration. *Pharmacol Toxicol* 1996;79:274–276.

200. Jalava KM, Partanen J, Neuvonen PJ. Itraconazole decreases renal clearance of digoxin. *Ther Drug Monit* 1997;19:609–613.

201. Yeh J, Soo SC, Summerton C, Richardson C. Potentiation of action of warfarin by itraconazole. *BMJ* 1990;301:669.

202. Kaukonen KM, Olkkola KT, Neuvonen PJ. Fluconazole but not itraconazole decreases the metabolism of losartan to E-3174. *Eur J Clin Pharmacol* 1998;53:445–449.

203. von Moltke LL, Greenblatt DJ, Duan SX, Harmatz JS, Shader RI. Inhibition of triazolam hydroxylation by ketoconazole, itraconazole, hydroxyitraconazole and fluconazole in-vitro. *Pharm Pharmacol Commun* 1998;4:443–445.

204. Debruyne D. Clinical pharmacokinetics of fluconazole in superficial and systemic mycoses. *Clin Pharmacokinet* 1997;33:52–77.

205. Grant SM, Clissold SP. Fluconazole. A review of its pharmacodynamic and pharmacokinetic properties, and therapeutic potential in superficial and systemic mycoses. *Drugs* 1990;39:877–916.

206. Brammer KW, Farrow PR, Faulkner JK. Pharmacokinetics and tissue penetration of fluconazole in humans. *Rev Infect Dis* 1990;12[Suppl 3]:S318–S326.

207. Wienkers LC, Wurden CJ, Storch E, Kunze KL, Rettie AE, Trager WF. Formation of (R)-8-hydroxywarfarin in human liver microsomes. A new metabolic marker for the (S)-mephenytoin hydroxylase, P4502C19. *Drug Metab Dispos* 1996;24:610–614.

208. Trapnell CB, Klecker RW, Jamis-Dow C, Collins JM. Glucuronidation of 3′-azido-3′-deoxythymidine (zidovudine) by human liver microsomes: relevance to clinical pharmacokinetic interactions with atovaquone, fluconazole, methadone, and valproic acid. *Antimicrob Agents Chemother* 1998;42:1592–1596.

209. Lazar JD, Wilner KD. Drug interactions with fluconazole. *Rev Infect Dis* 1990;12[Suppl 3]:327–333.

210. Purba HS, Back DJ. Effect of fluconazole (UK-49,858) on antipyrine metabolism. *Br J Clin Pharmacol* 1986;21:603(abstr).

211. Brockmeyer NH, Tillmann I, Mertins L, Barthel B, Goos M. Pharmacokinetic interaction of fluconazole and zidovudine in HIV-positive patients. *Eur J Med Res* 1997;2:377–383.

212. Morita K, Konishi H, Shimakawa H. Fluconazole: a potent inhibitor of cytochrome P450-dependent drug-metabolism in mice and humans

in vivo. Comparative study with ketoconazole. *Chem Pharm Bull (Tokyo)* 1992;40:1247–1251.

213. Honig PK, Worham DC, Zamani K, Mullin JC, Conner DP, Cantilena LR. The effect of fluconazole on the steady-state pharmacokinetics and electrocardiographic pharmacodynamics of terfenadine in humans. *Clin Pharmacol Ther* 1993;53:630–636.

214. Cantilena LR, Sorrels S, Wiley T, Wortham T. Fluconazole alters terfenadine pharmacokinetics and electrocardiographic pharmacodynamics. *Clin Pharmacol Ther* 1995;57:185(abstr).

215. Ahonen J, Olkkola KT, Neuvonen PJ. Effect of route of administration of fluconazole on the interaction between fluconazole and midazolam. *Eur J Clin Pharmacol* 1997;51:415–419.

216. Vanakoski J, Mattila MJ, Vainio P, Idänpään-Heikkilä JJ, Törnwall M. 150 mg fluconazole does not substantially increase the effects of 10 mg midazolam or the plasma midazolam concentrations in healthy subjects. *Int J Clin Pharmacol Ther* 1995;33:518–523.

217. Varhe A, Olkkola KT, Neuvonen PJ. Fluconazole, but not terbinafine, enhances the effects of triazolam by inhibiting its metabolism. *Br J Clin Pharmacol* 1996;41:319–323.

218. Varhe A, Olkkola KT, Neuvonen PJ. Effect of fluconazole dose on the extent of fluconazole-triazolam interaction. *Br J Clin Pharmacol* 1996;42:465–470.

219. Palkama VJ, Isohanni MH, Neuvonen PJ, Olkkola KT. The effect of intravenous and oral fluconazole on the pharmacokinetics and pharmacodynamics of intravenous alfentanil. *Anesth Analg* 1998;87: 190–194.

220. Cobb MN, Desai J, Brown LS Jr, Zannikos PN, Rainey PM. The effect of fluconazole on the clinical pharmacokinetics of methadone. *Clin Pharmacol Ther* 1998;63:655–662.

221. Gustavson LE, Shi H, Palmer RN, Siepman NC, Craft JC. Drug interaction between clarithromycin and fluconazole in healthy subjects. *Clin Pharmacol Ther* 1996;59:185(abstr).

222. Trapnell CB, Narang PK, Li R, Lavelle JP. Increased plasma rifabutin levels with concomitant fluconazole therapy in HIV-infected patients. *Ann Intern Med* 1996;124:573–576.

223. Iatsimirskaia E, Tulebaev S, Storozhuk E, et al. Metabolism of rifabutin in human enterocyte and liver microsomes: kinetic parameters, identification of enzyme systems, and drug interactions with macrolides and antifungal agents. *Clin Pharmacol Ther* 1997;61:554–562.

224. Narang PK, Trapnell CB, Schoenfelder JR, Lavelle JP, Bianchine JR. Fluconazole and enhanced effect of rifabutin prophylaxis. *N Engl J Med* 1994;330:1316–1317.

225. Tseng AL, Walmsley SL. Rifabutin-associated uveitis. *Ann Pharmacother* 1995;29:1149–1155.

226. Cato A 3rd, Cao G, Hsu A, Cavanaugh J, Leonard J, Granneman R. Evaluation of the effect of fluconazole on the pharmacokinetics of ritonavir. *Drug Metab Dispos* 1997;25:1104–1106.

227. De Wit S, Debier M, De Smet M, et al. Effect of fluconazole on indinavir pharmacokinetics in human immunodeficiency virus-infected patients. *Antimicrob Agents Chemother* 1998;42:223–227.

228. Sahai J, Gallicano K, Pakuts A, Cameron DW. Effect of fluconazole on zidovudine pharmacokinetics in patients infected with human immunodeficiency virus. *J Infect Dis* 1994;169:1103–1107.

229. Borin MT, Driver MR, Wajszczuk CP, Anderson RD. The effect of fluconazole (FLU) on the pharmacokinetics of atevirdine mesylate (ATV) in HIV+ patients. *Clin Pharmacol Ther* 1994;55:193(abstr).

230. Borin MT, Cox SR, Herman BD, Carel BJ, Anderson RD, Freimuth WW. Effect of fluconazole on the steady-state pharmacokinetics of delavirdine in human immunodeficiency virus-positive patients. *Antimicrob Agents Chemother* 1997;41:1892–1897.

231. Bruzzese VL, Gillum JG, Israel DS, Johnson GL, Kplowitz LG, Polk RE. Effect of fluconazole on pharmacokinetics of 2′,3′-dideoxyinosine in patients seropositive for human immunodeficency virus. *Antimicrob Agents Chemother* 1995;39:1050–1053.

232. Canafax DM, Graves NM, Hilligoss DM, Carleton BC, Gardner MJ, Matas AJ. Increased cyclosporine levels as a result of simultaneous fluconazole and cyclosporine therapy in renal transplant recipients: a double-blind, randomized pharmacokinetic and safety study. *Transplant Proc* 1991;23:1041–1042.

233. Canafax DM, Graves NM, Hilligoss DM, Carleton BC, Gardner MJ, Matas AJ. Interaction between cyclosporine and fluconazole in renal allograft recipients. *Transplantation* 1991;51:1014–1018.

234. Barbara JA, Clarkson AR, LaBrooy J, McNeil JD, Woodroffe AJ. *Candida albicans* arthritis in a renal allograft recipient with an interaction

between cyclosporin and fluconazole. *Nephrol Dial Transplant* 1993; 8:263–266.

235. Sugar AM, Saunders C, Idelson BA, Bernard DB. Interaction of fluconazole and cyclosporine. *Ann Intern Med* 1989;110:844.

236. Torregrosa V, De la Torre M, Campistol JM, Oppenheimer F, Ricart MJ, Vilardell J, Andreu J. Interaction of fluconazole with cyclosporin A. *Nephron* 1992;60:125–126.

237. Collignon P, Hurley B, Mitchell D. Interaction of fluconazole with cyclosporin. *Lancet* 1989;1:1262.

238. Ehninger G, Jaschonek K, Schuler U, Kruger HU. Interaction of fluconazole with cyclosporin. *Lancet* 1989;2:104–105.

239. Krüger HU, Schuler U, Zimmermann R, Ehninger G. Absence of significant interaction of fluconazole with cyclosporin. *J Antimicrob Chemother* 1989;24:781–786.

240. López-Gil JA. Fluconazole-cyclosporine interaction: a dose-dependent effect? *Ann Pharmacother* 1993;27:427–430.

241. Osowski CL, Dix SP, Lin LS, Mullins RE, Geller RB, Wingard JR. Evaluation of the drug interaction between intravenous high-dose fluconazole and cyclosporine or tacrolimus in bone marrow transplant patients. *Transplantation* 1996;61:1268–1272.

242. Assan R, Fredj G, Larger E, Feutren G, Bismuth H. FK 506/fluconazole interaction enhances FK 506 nephrotoxicity. *Diabetes Metab* 1994;20:49–52.

243. Dhawan A, Tredger JM, North-Lewis PJ, Gonde CE, Mowat AP, Heaton NJ. Tacrolimus (FK506) malabsorption: management with fluconazole coadministration. *Transpl Int* 1997;10:331–334.

244. Mañez R, Martin M, Raman D, et al. Fluconazole therapy in transplant recipients receiving FK506. *Transplantation* 1994;57:1521–1523.

245. Sinofsky FE, Pasquale SA. The effect of fluconazole on circulating ethinyl estradiol levels in women taking oral contraceptives. *Am J Obstet Gynecol* 1998;178:300–304.

246. Cadle RM, Zenon GJ 3rd, Rodriguez-Barradas MC, Hamill RJ. Fluconazole-induced symptomatic phenytoin toxicity. *Ann Pharmacother* 1994;28:191–195.

247. Howitt KM, Oziemski MA. Phenytoin toxicity induced by fluconazole. *Med J Aust* 1989;151:603–604.

248. Mitchell AS, Holland JT. Fluconazole and phenytoin: a predictable interaction. *BMJ* 1989;298:1315.

249. Blum RA, Wilton JH, Hilligoss DM, et al. Effect of fluconazole on the disposition of phenytoin. *Clin Pharmacol Ther* 1991;49:420–425.

250. Baciewicz AM, Menke JJ, Bokar JA, Baud EB. Fluconazole-warfarin interaction. *Ann Pharmacother* 1994;28:1111.

251. Gericke KR. Possible interaction between warfarin and fluconazole. *Pharmacotherapy* 1993;13:508–509.

252. Kerr HD. Case report: potentiation of warfarin by fluconazole. *Am J Med Sci* 1993;305:164–165.

253. Seaton TL, Celum CL, Black DJ. Possible potentiation of warfarin by fluconazole. *DICP* 1990;24:1177–1178.

254. Tett S, Carey D, Lee HS. Drug interactions with fluconazole. *Med J Aust* 1992;156:365.

255. Crussell-Porter LL, Rindone JP, Ford MA, Jaskar DW. Low-dose fluconazole therapy potentiates the hypoprothrombinemic response of warfarin sodium. *Arch Intern Med* 1993;153:102–104.

256. Black DJ, Kunze KL, Wienkers LC, et al. Warfarin-fluconazole. II. A metabolically based drug interaction: in vivo studies. *Drug Metab Dispos* 1996;24:422–428.

257. Kunze KL, Trager WF. Warfarin-fluconazole. III. A rational approach to management of a metabolically based drug interaction. *Drug Metab Dispos* 1996;24:429–435.

258. Fournier JP, Schneider S, Martinez P, et al. Hypoglycemic coma in a patient treated with glipizide and fluconazole: a possible interaction? *Therapie* 1992;47:446–447.

259. Kazierad DJ, Martin DE, Blum RA, et al. Effect of fluconazole on the pharmacokinetics of eprosartan and losartan in healthy male volunteers. *Clin Pharmacol Ther* 1997;62:417–425.

260. Mitra AK, Thummel KE, Kalhorn TF, Kharasch ED, Unadkat JD, Slattery JT. Inhibition of sulfamethoxazole hydroxylamine formation by fluconazole in human liver microsomes and healthy volunteers. *Clin Pharmacol Ther* 1996;59:332–340.

261. Nix DE, Zelenitsky SA, Symonds WT, Spivey JM, Norman A. The effect of fluconazole on the pharmacokinetics of caffeine in young and elderly subjects. *Clin Pharmacol Ther* 1992;51:183(abstr).

262. Konishi H, Morita K, Yamaji A. Effect of fluconazole on theophylline disposition in humans. *Eur J Clin Pharmacol* 1994;46:309–312.

263. Ueno K, Yamaguchi R, Tanaka K, et al. Lack of a kinetic interaction between fluconazole and mexiletine. *Eur J Clin Pharmacol* 1996;50: 129–131.

264. Gannon RH, Anderson ML. Fluconazole-nortriptyline drug interaction. *Ann Pharmacother* 1992;26:1456–1457.

265. Newberry DL, Bass SN, Mbanefo CO. A fluconazole/amitriptyline drug interaction in three male adults. *Clin Infect Dis* 1997;24: 270–271.

266. Buss DC, Routledge PA, Hutchings A, Brammer KW, Thorpe JE. The effect of fluconazole on the acetylation of isoniazid. *Hum Exp Toxicol* 1991;10:85–86.

267. Birnbaum JE. Pharmacology of the allylamines. *J Am Acad Dermatol* 1990;23:782–785.

268. Balfour JA, Faulds D. Terbinafine. A review of its pharmacodynamic and pharmacokinetic properties, and therapeutic potential in superficial mycoses. *Drugs* 1992;43:259–284.

269. Jensen JC. Clinical pharmacokinetics of terbinafine (Lamisil). *Clin Exp Dermatol* 1989;14:110–113.

270. Breckenridge A. Clinical significance of interactions with antifungal agents. *Br J Dermatol* 1992;126:19–22.

271. Shah IA, Whiting PH, Omar G, Ormerod AD, Burke MD. The effects of retinoids and terbinafine on the human hepatic microsomal metabolism of cyclosporin. *Br J Dermatol* 1993;129:395–398.

272. Seyffer R, Eichelbaum M, Jensen JC, Klotz U. Antipyrine metabolism is not affected by terbinafine, a new antifungal agent. *Eur J Clin Pharmacol* 1989;37:231–233.

273. Effendy I, Krause W. In vivo effects of terbinafine and ketoconazole on testosterone plasma levels in healthy males. *Dermatologica* 1989; 178:103–106.

274. Nashan D, Knuth UA, Weidinger G, Nieschlag E. The antimycotic drug terbinafine in contrast to ketoconazole lacks acute effects on the pituitary-testicular function of healthy men: a placebo-controlled double-blind trial. *Acta Endocrinol (Copenh)* 1989;120:677–681.

275. Robbins B, Chang CT, Cramer JA, et al. Safe coadministration of terbinafine and terfenadine: a placebo-controlled crossover study of pharmacokinetic and pharmacodynamic interactions in healthy volunteers. *Clin Pharmacol Ther* 1996;59:275–283.

276. Long CC, Hill SA, Thomas RC, Johnston A, Smith SG, Kendall F, Finlay AY. Effect of terbinafine on the pharmacokinetics of cyclosporin in humans. *J Invest Dermatol* 1994;102:740–743.

277. Jensen P, Lehne G, Fauchald P, Simonsen S. Effect of oral terbinafine treatment on cyclosporin pharmacokinetics in organ transplant recipients with dermatophyte nail infection. *Acta Derm Venereol* 1996;76: 280–281.

278. Lo AC, Lui SL, Lo WK, Chan DT, Cheng IK. The interaction of terbinafine and cyclosporine A in renal transplant patients. *Br J Clin Pharmacol* 1997;43:340–341.

279. Tarral A, Francheteau P, Guerret M. Effects of terbinafine on the pharmacokinetics of digoxin in healthy volunteers. *Pharmacotherapy* 1997;17:791–795.

280. Trépanier EF, Nafziger AN, Amsden GW. Effect of terbinafine on theophylline pharmacokinetics in healthy volunteers. *Antimicrob Agents Chemother* 1998;42:695–697.

281. Trépanier EF, Nafziger AN, Kearns GL, Kashuba AD, Amsden GW. Absence of effect of terbinafine on the activity of CYP1A2, NAT-2, and xanthine oxidase. *J Clin Pharmacol* 1998;38:424–428.

282. Warwick JA, Corrall RJ. Serious interaction between warfarin and oral terbinafine. *BMJ* 1998;316:440.

283. Gupta AK, Ross GS. Interaction between terbinafine and warfarin. *Dermatology* 1998;196:266–267.

284. Guerret M, Francheteau P, Hubert M. Evaluation of effects of terbinafine on single oral dose pharmacokinetics and anticoagulant actions of warfarin in healthy volunteers. *Pharmacotherapy* 1997;17: 767–773.

285. van der Kuy PH, Hooymans PM, Verkaaik AJB. Nortriptyline intoxication induced by terbinafine. *BMJ* 1998;316:441.

286. Leeder JS, Gotschall RR, Gaedigk A, Kearns GL. CYP2D6 phenotype-genotype discordance and potential new drug–drug interactions. *Clin Pharmacol Ther* 1998;63:216(abstr).

287. Medoff G. The mechanism of action of amphotericin B. In: van den Bosshe H, Mackenzie DWR, Cauwenbergh G, eds. *Aspergillus and aspergillosis.* New York: Plenum Press, 1988:161–164.

288. Gallis HA, Drew RH, Pickard WW. Amphotericin B: 30 years of clinical experience. *Rev Infect Dis* 1990;12:308–329.

289. Coukell AJ, Brogden RN. Liposomal amphotericin B. Therapeutic use in the management of fungal infections and visceral leishmaniasis. *Drugs* 1998;55:585–612.
290. Kennedy MS, Deeg HJ, Siegel M, Crowley JJ, Storb R, Thomas ED. Acute renal toxicity with combined use of amphotericin B and cyclosporine after marrow trasplantation. *Transplantation* 1983;35:211–215.
291. Cushard WG Jr, Kohanim M, Lantis LR. Blastomycosis of bone. Treatment with intramedullary amphotericin-B. *J Bone Joint Surg* 1969;51:704–712.
292. Miller RP, Bates JH. Amphotericin B toxicity. A follow-up report of 53 patients. *Ann Intern Med* 1969;71:1089–1095.
293. Roobol A, Gull K, Pogson CI. Griseofulvin-induced aggregation of microtubule protein. *Biochem J* 1977;167:39–43.
294. Davies RR. Griseofulvin. In: Spiller DCE, ed. *Antifungal chemotherapy.* John Wiley and Sons, 1980:149–182.
295. Abu-Romeh SH, Rashed A. Cyclosporin A and griseofulvin: another drug interaction. *Nephron* 1991;58:237.
296. Klintmalm G, Sawe J. High dose methylprednisolone increases plasma cyclosporin level in renal transplant recipients. *Lancet* 1984;1: 731.
297. McDaniel PA, Caldroner RD. Oral contraceptives and griseofulvin interaction. *Drug Intell Clin Pham* 1986;20:384.
298. Okino K, Weibert RT. Warfarin-griseofulvin interaction. *Drug Intell Clin Pharm* 1986;20:291–293.
299. Phillips KR, Wideman SD, Cochran EB, Becker JA. Griseofulvin significantly decreases serum salicylate concentrations. *Pediatr Infect Dis J* 1993;12:350–352.
300. Rasmussen BB, Jeppesen U, Gaist D, Brosen K. Griseofulvin and fluvoxamine interactions with the metabolism of theophylline. *Ther Drug Monit* 1997;19:56–62.
301. van Dijke CP, Weber JC. Interaction between oral contraceptives and griseofulvin. *BMJ* 1984;288:1125–1126.
302. Polak A, Scholer HJ. Mode of action of 5-fluorocytosine and mechanisms of resistance. *Chemotherapy* 1975;21:113–130.
303. Albengres E, Le Louet H, Tillement JP. Systemic antifungal agents. Drug interactions of clinical significance. *Drug Saf* 1998;18:83–97.

CHAPTER 48

Protease Inhibitors

Jashvant D. Unadkat and Yi Wang

In the life cycle of human immunodeficiency retrovirus type 1 (HIV-1), the virally encoded enzyme, HIV-1 protease, is critical for the assembly of new infectious virons in the host cells (1). Because this enzyme is viral specific, it constitutes a unique therapeutic target (2). To date, five HIV-1 protease inhibitors (PIs) have been developed and approved for the treatment of HIV-1 infection: amprenavir (Agenerase), indinavir sulfate (Crixivan), nelfinavir mesylate (Viracept), ritonavir (Norvir), and saquinavir mesylate (Invirase, hard-gel capsule, and Fortovase, soft-gel capsule). These drugs, when combined with anti-HIV nucleoside reverse transcriptase inhibitors, have been remarkably successful in the clinic in suppressing viremia (3–7). PIs are extensively metabolized *in vivo,* primarily by cytochrome P450 (CYP) 3A4/5 (see Chapter 31). Many of the PIs are also potent inhibitors of CYP3A4/5. In addition, the PIs are substrates and inhibitors of the efflux pump P-glycoprotein (8–11) (see Chapter 11). Consequently, the potential for *in vivo* interactions of PIs with other drugs metabolized by CYP3A4/5 or transported by P-glycoprotein is high. This potential for drug interactions is particularly high in people with acquired immunodeficiency syndrome (AIDS). They receive multiple drugs for treatment of HIV infection and prophylaxis for various opportunistic infections; many of these drugs are extensively metabolized by CYP3A4/5 or are substrates of P-glycoprotein (11,12). In this chapter, the inhibitory profiles and *in vivo* metabolic drug interactions of the PIs are discussed. Refer to Chapter 31 for the metabolic profiles of the PIs.

INHIBITORY PROFILES OF PROTEASE INHIBITORS

All PIs are substrates of CYP3A4/5—enzymes that by their strategic location in the liver and the intestine play an important role in the first pass metabolism of a wide range of drug molecules (13). Except for amprenavir, the pharmacokinetics of all PIs demonstrate a dose-dependent decrease in their oral clearance (see Chapter 31), indicating that their metabolism by CYP3A enzymes is saturable within the dose range used in the clinic. Therefore, it is not surprising that many of the PIs are potent inhibitors of CYP3A4/5.

The degree to which the PIs will inhibit the *in vivo* clearance of other CYP3A4/5 substrates in the clinic depends on many factors, including the contribution of CYP3A4/5 enzymes to the overall clearance of the substrates, the concentration of the inhibitor at the site of metabolism, and the *in vivo* inhibitory capacity of the inhibitor (*in vivo* K_i) (14). Because the latter two values are generally not available, the average concentration of the inhibitor in the plasma ([I]) is generally assumed to reflect the concentration of the drug at the site of metabolism (see Chapter 31 for discussion of unbound versus total plasma concentration), and the *in vitro* K_i value is assumed to reflect the *in vivo* K_i. In the presence of a competitive or a noncompetitive inhibition mechanism, assuming that the concentration of the substrate is less than the K_m, the degree of inhibition of the *in vivo* clearance of a drug by an inhibitor may be estimated from the formula $AUC_i/AUC = 1 + [I]/K_i$, where AUC_i and AUC are the area under the plasma concentration-time profile of a drug in the presence and absence of the inhibitor (15). Thus, a ratio of $[I]/K_i$ that is much greater than unity would predict a clinically significant drug interaction with the inhibitor.

As shown in Table 48-1, the *in vitro* potency of inhibition of all PIs is highest toward CYP3A4/5, regardless of the substrate used to measure CYP3A activity. Moreover, except for saquinavir, the reported CYP3A4/5 K_i (or IC_{50}) values relative to the average steady-state clinical plasma concentration of the inhibitor ([I]) predict that these PIs should be potent inhibitors of CYP3A4/5 *in vivo*. This potency of inhibition (I/K_i) decreases in the

J. D. Unadkat and Y. Wang: Department of Pharmaceutics, University of Washington, Box 357610, H272 Health Sciences Building, Seattle, Washington 98195 -7610

TABLE 48-1. In vitro *inhibitory potencies (K_i or IC_{50} values) of protease inhibitors toward P450 enzymes in human liver microsomes*

Protease inhibitor	$C_{ss,av}$ (μM)	CYP isoform	Protein concentration (μg/mL)	K_i (μM)	IC_{50} (μM)	Probe pathway	Mechanism	Reference
Amprenavir	3.0	3A4/5	0.5	0.5		Testosterone 6β-hydroxylation	—	25
Indinavir	3.8	3A4/5	0.5	0.17 ± 0.01		Testosterone 6β-hydroxylation	—	26
		3A4/5	4.0	0.5		Testosterone 6β-hydroxylation	—	27
		3A4/5	1.0	0.68		Testosterone 6β-hydroxylation	—	28
		3A4/5	1.0		0.51 ± 0.03	Triazolam hydroxylation	—	29
		3A4/5	0.25	0.86 ± 0.72		Dextromethorphan *N*-demethylation	Competitive	30
		3A4/5	0.05	0.2		Saquinavir oxidation	—	19
		2C9	1.0		230 ± 57	Tolbutamide hydroxylation	—	29
		2D6	1.0	15.6		Desipramine hydroxylation	Mixed type	31
		2D6	1.0		84 ± 1.2	Desipramine hydroxylation	—	29
		2D6	1.0		245 ± 26	Dextromethorphan *O*-demethylation	—	29
Nelfinavir	4.0	3A4/5	1.0	4.8		Testosterone 6β-hydroxylation	Competitive	28
		3A4/5	1.0		3.35 ± 0.14	Triazolam hydroxylation	—	29
		3A4/5	0.25	0.31 ± 0.16		Dextromethorphan *N*-demethylation	Competitive	30
		1A2	1.0	190		Phenacetin *O*-deethylation	Competitive	28
		2C9	1.0		87 ± 11	Tolbutamide hydroxylation	—	29
		2C19	1.0	68.0		S-mephenytoin hydroxylation	Competitive	28
		2D6	1.0	126		Dextromethorphan *O*-demethylation	Competitive	28
		2D6	1.0	51.9		Desipramine hydroxylation	Mixed-type	31
Ritonavir	5.0	3A4/5	0.5	0.019 ± 0.004		Testosterone 6β-hydroxylation	—	26
		3A4/5	1.0	0.11		Testosterone 6β-hydroxylation	Competitive	28
		3A4/5	1.0		0.07	Nifedipine oxidation	—	32
		3A4/5	1.0		0.14	Terfenadine hydroxylation	—	32
		3A4/5	1.0		0.38 ± 0.05	Triazolam hydroxylation	—	29
		3A4/5	0.25		0.46 ± 0.37	Dextromethorphan *N*-demethylation	Noncompetitive	30
		2C9	0.5	4.2 ± 1.3		Tolbutamide hydroxylation	—	26
		2C9	1.0		8.0	Tolbutamide hydroxylation	—	32
		2C9	1.0		6.2 ± 0.5	Tolbutamide hydroxylation	—	29
		2C19	1.0		23.5 ± 3.8	(S)-mephenytoin hydroxylation	—	29
		2D6	1.0	4.8		Desipramine hydroxylation	Mixed type	31
		2D6	1.0		2.5	Dextromethorpan *O*-demethylation	—	32
		2D6	1.0		17.3 ± 1.7	Dextromethorphan *O*-demethylation	—	29
		2D6	1.0		14.1 ± 0.7	Desipramine hydroxylation	—	29
Saquinavir	1.4	3A4/5	0.5	2.99 ± 0.87		Testosterone 6β-hydroxylation	—	26
		3A4/5	1.0	4.0		Testosterone 6β-hydroxylation	—	28
		3A4/5	1.0		11.5 ± 1.9	Triazolam hydroxylation	—	29
		3A4/5	0.25	4.36 ± 0.54		Dextromethorphan *N*-demethylation	Competitive	30
		3A4/5	0.05	0.7		Terfenadine hydroxylation	—	19
		2C9	0.5	53.9 ± 9.9		Tolbutamide hydroxylation	—	26
		2D6	1.0		130 ± 6	Desipramine hydroxylation	—	29
		2D6	1.0	24.0		Desipramine hydroxylation	Mixed type	31

$C_{ss,av}$, average steady-state plasma concentration.

following order: ritonavir > indinavir ≈ nelfinavir ≈ amprenavir > saquinavir. Therefore, except saquinavir, coadministration of PIs with drugs that are predominantly cleared by CYP3A4/5 enzymes should lead to clinically significant drug interactions. With respect to inhibition of other CYP isoforms *in vivo,* only ritonavir is predicted to achieve plasma concentration in the clinic comparable to the *in vitro* K_i (or IC_{50}) values for CYP2C9 and CYP2D6.

In Vivo Metabolic Drug Interactions with CYP3A4/5 Substrates

The *in vivo* capacities of PIs to inhibit the oral clearance of CYP3A4/5 substrates decreases in the order predicted from the *in vitro* inhibitory data (Table 48-2 and see Table 48-1). The potent PIs (e.g., ritonavir and indinavir) significantly increase the plasma AUC of other PIs (e.g., nelfinavir and saquinavir) and non–anti-HIV CYP3A4/5 substrates (e.g., clarithromycin and rifabutin), but not that of nonnucleoside reverse transcriptase

inhibitors. The less potent PIs (e.g., nelfinavir and amprenavir) affect the plasma AUC of other PIs to a lesser degree. As indicated in Chapter 31, the lack of clinically significant interaction of the PIs with the nonnucleoside reverse transcriptase inhibitors is most likely because CYP3A4/5 enzymes are not the predominant ones involved in the disposition of these drugs.

Although there is a general rank-order correlation of the *in vivo* data with the predicted potency of CYP3A4 inhibitors, this correlation is not perfect or quantitative. First, based on the $[I]/K_i$ ratio, amprenavir, indinavir, and nelfinavir are predicted to significantly and substantially decrease the *in vivo* clearance of other PIs. However, except for saquinavir (see later text), they either do not affect their clearance or only affect it marginally. There are several possible explanations for this lack of quantitative correlation with the *in vivo* data. The formula ($[I]/K_i$ ratio) assumes that the substrate is present at a concentration less than the K_m of the enzyme, CYP3A4. However, at the doses used in the clinic, the pharmacokinetics of the substrate may be nonlinear (e.g., most PIs, clar-

TABLE 48-2. *Effect of protease inhibitors (dose in parentheses) on the pharmacokinetics (% changes in AUC) of CYP3A4/5 substrates*

Protease inhibitor	Protease inhibitors					Nonnucleoside reverse transcriptase inhibitors			Other drugs				
	Amprenavir	Indinavir	Nelfinavir	Ritonavir	Saquinavir	Efavirenz	Delavirdine	Nevirapine	Clarithromycin	Ketoconazole	Rifabutin	Terfenadine	Sildenafil
Amprenavir	—	38↓[a] (800 mg[b])	15↑ (800 mg)	—	18↓ (800 mg)	16↑ (1200 mg)	—	—	17↓–11↑ (1200 mg b.i.d.)	44↑ (1200 mg b.i.d.)	193↑ (1200 mg b.i.d.)	—	—
Indinavir	33↑ (800 mg t.i.d.)	—	83↑ (1000 mg b.i.d.)	—	620↑[c] (800 mg t.i.d.)[33]	0↔ (800 mg t.i.d.)	0↔ (800 mg)[34]	0↔ (800 mg t.i.d.)	53↑ (800 mg t.i.d.)	—	50↑ (800 mg q.i.d.)	—	—
Nelfinavir	15↑ (750 mg t.i.d.)	51↑ (750 mg b.i.d.)	—	—	500↑ (750 mg b.i.d.[c])[35]	—	58↓ (750 mg t.i.d.)[36]	0↔ (750 mg b.i.d.)[37]	—	—	207↑ (750 mg t.i.d.)	—	—
Ritonavir	—	475↑ (400 mg q.i.d.)[38]	152↑ (500 mg b.i.d.)	—	>5000↑ (600 mg)[39]	21↑ (600 mg b.i.d.)[40]	0↔ (300 mg b.i.d.)[41]	0↔ (600 mg b.i.d.)	77↑ (200 mg q.i.d.)[42]	330↑ (500 mg b.i.d.)[43]	400↑ (500 mg b.i.d.)[44]	—	1000↑ (400 mg b.i.d.)
Saquinavir	32↓ (800 mg t.i.d.)	—	18↑ (1200 mg t.i.d.[c])	6.4↑ (600 mg)[39]	—	12↓ (1200 mg t.i.d.[c])	0↔ (600 mg t.i.d.)[45]	3↓ (600 mg t.i.d.)[46]	45↑ (1200 mg t.i.d.[c])[33]	0↔ (600 mg t.i.d.)	—	368↑ (1200 mg t.i.d.)[33]	140↑ (1200 mg t.i.d.)[c]

[a]Data without citation are from pharmaceutical companies' package inserts.
[b]Dose of the inhibitor used in the study.
[c]Soft-gel saquinavir (Fortovase) was used in the study.

TABLE 48-3. *Effect of protease inhibitors (dose in parentheses) on the pharmacokinetics (% changes in AUC) of drugs that are metabolized by enzymes other than CYP3A4/5*

Protease inhibitor	Atovaquone	Desipramine	Ethinylestradiol	Fluconazole	Isoniazid	Lamivudine	Methadone	Rifampin	Stavudine	Theophylline	Zidovudine
Amprenavir	—	—	—	—	—	3–17↑[a] (1200 mg b.i.d.)[b]	—	13↓–12↑ (1200 mg b.i.d.)	—	—	40↑ (1200 mg b.i.d.)
Indinavir	13↑ (800 mg t.i.d.)[47]	—	24↑ (800 mg t.i.d.)	0↔ (1000 mg t.i.d.)[48]	13↑ (800 mg t.i.d.)	—	—	—	25↑ (800 mg t.i.d.)	—	17↑ (1000 mg t.i.d.)
Nelfinavir	—	—	47↓ (750 mg t.i.d.)	—	—	10↑ (750 mg t.i.d.)	—	—	0↔ (750 mg t.i.d.)	—	35↓ (750 mg t.i.d.)
Ritonavir	—	145↑ (500 mg b.i.d.)	41↓ (500 mg b.i.d.)[22]	—	—	—	36↓ (500 mg b.i.d.)[49]	—	—	16↓ (500 mg b.i.d.)[24]	26↓ (500 mg b.i.d.)[23]
Saquinavir	—	—	—	—	—	—	—	—	—	—	0↔ (600 mg t.i.d.)[50]

[a]Data without citation are from pharmaceutical companies' package inserts.
[b]Dose of the inhibitor used in the study

ithromycin), indicating saturation of their metabolism, presumably by CYP3A4. Second, the assumption that metabolism by CYP3A4 is the predominant elimination pathway of the substrate may not be correct. Third, most of the aforementioned PIs are substrates or inhibitors of the P-glycoprotein efflux pump (16,17), which is expressed in the intestine and in the bile canalicular membrane (18). Thus, many of the interactions are likely to be taking place at the level of inhibition of both CYP3A4/5 and P-glycoprotein efflux. For example, the inhibition of CYP3A4/5-mediated metabolism of saquinavir in both the intestine and the liver and inhibition of P-glycoprotein efflux in the intestine are the most likely explanations for the observation that interaction of CYP3A4 inhibitors with saquinavir is quantitatively the largest among all the PIs (16,19). The role of P-glycoprotein efflux in the absorption of saquinavir is supported by the observation that cyclosporine, a poor inhibitor of CYP3A4 but a potent inhibitor of P-glycoprotein, increases the AUC of saquinavir by 430% (20).

In Vivo Metabolic Interactions with Substrates of Enzymes Other than CYP3A4/5

Except for ritonavir, amprenavir-zidovudine, and nelfinavir-ethinylestradiol, the remaining interactions of PIs with non-CYP3A4/5 substrates are clinically insignificant (Table 48-3). The interaction of amprenavir with zidovudine and that of nelfinavir with ethinylestradiol cannot be evaluated because they have not been published in peer-reviewed manuscripts.

The *in vitro* K_i of ritonavir toward CYP2D6 is comparable to the *in vivo* concentrations of the drug achieved in the clinic. Therefore, ritonavir significantly affects the oral clearance of desipramine, a CYP2D6 substrate (21). As indicated in Chapter 31, ritonavir is not only a potent inhibitor of CYP3A4/5, it may also be an inducer of other enzymes. The hypothesis that ritonavir may be an enzyme inducer appears to be supported by the observation that ritonavir moderately increases the oral clearance of ethinyl estradiol (22), zidovudine (23), and theophylline (24) (see Table 48-3).

CONCLUSION

Except for ritonavir, the PIs approved to date appear to be relatively specific inhibitors of CYP3A4/5. However, their potencies to inhibit these enzymes, both *in vitro* and *in vivo,* spans a wide range; ritonavir is the most potent and saquinavir is the least potent. Coadministration of ritonavir with drugs cleared predominantly by CYP2D6 is also likely to lead to clinically significant drug interactions. The hypothesis that ritonavir is an inducer of drug-metabolizing enzymes needs to be substantiated with detailed *in vivo* mechanistic pharmacokinetic studies.

REFERENCES

1. Kohl NE, Emini EA, Schleif WA, et al. Active human immunodeficiency virus protease is required for viral infectivity. *Proc Natl Acad Sci USA* 1988;85(13):4686–9460.
2. Dreyer GB, Metcalf BW, Tomaszek TA Jr. Inhibition of human immunodeficiency virus 1 protease in vitro: rational design of substrate analogue inhibitors. *Proc Natl Acad Sci USA* 1989;86(24):9752–9756.
3. Murphy RL, Gulick RM, DeGruttola V, et al. Treatment with amprenavir alone or amprenavir with zidovudine and lamivudine in adults with human immunodeficiency virus infection. AIDS Clinical Trials Group 347 Study Team. *J Infect Dis* 1999;179(4):808–816.
4. Notermans DW, Jurriaans S, de Wolf F, et al. Decrease of HIV-1 RNA levels in lymphoid tissue and peripheral blood during treatment with ritonavir, lamivudine and zidovudine. Ritonavir/3TC/ZDV Study Group. *AIDS* 1998;12(2):167–173.
5. Gulick RM, Mellors JW, Havlir D. Simultaneous vs sequential initiation of therapy with indinavir, zidovudine, and lamivudine for HIV-1 infection: 100-week follow-up. *JAMA* 1998;280(1):35–41.
6. Markowitz M, Conant M, Hurley A, et al. A preliminary evaluation of nelfinavir mesylate, an inhibitor of human immunodeficiency virus (HIV)-1 protease, to treat HIV infection. *J Infect Dis* 1998;177(6):1533–1540.
7. McDonald CK, Kuritzkes DR. Human immunodeficiency virus type 1 protease inhibitors. *Arch Intern Med* 1997;157(9):951–959.
8. Srinivas RV, Middlemas D, Flynn P, Fridland A. Human immunodeficiency virus protease inhibitors serve as substrates for multidrug transporter proteins MDR1 and MRP1 but retain antiviral efficacy in cell lines expressing these transporters. *Antimicrob Agents Chemother* 1998;42(12):3157–3162.
9. Lee CG, Gottesman MM, Cardarelli CO, et al. HIV-1 protease inhibitors are substrates for the MDR1 multidrug transporter. *Biochemistry* 1998;37(11):3594–3601.
10. Kim AE, Dintaman JM, Waddell DS, Silverman JA. Saquinavir, an HIV protease inhibitor, is transported by P-glycoprotein. *J Pharmacol Exp Ther* 1998;286(3):1439–1445.
11. Kim RB, Fromm MF, Wandel C, et al. The drug transporter P-glycoprotein limits oral absorption and brain entry of HIV-1 protease inhibitors. *J Clin Invest* 1998;101(2):289–294.
12. Iatsimirskaia E, Tulebaev S, Storozhuk E, et al. Metabolism of rifabutin in human enterocyte and liver microsomes: kinetic parameters, identification of enzyme systems, and drug interactions with macrolides and antifungal agents. *Clin Pharmacol Ther* 1997;61(5):554–562.
13. Thummel KE, Wilkinson GR. In vitro and in vivo drug interactions involving human CYP3A. *Annu Rev Pharmacol Toxicol* 1998;38:389–430.
14. Bertz RJ, Granneman GR. Use of in vitro and in vivo data to estimate the likelihood of metabolic pharmacokinetic interactions. *Clin Pharmacokinet* 1997;32(3):210–258.
15. Shaw PN, Houston JB. Kinetics of drug metabolism inhibition: use of metabolite concentration-time profiles. *J Pharmacokinet Biopharm* 1987;15(5):497–510.
16. Alsenz J, Steffen H, Alex R. Active apical secretory efflux of the HIV protease inhibitors saquinavir and ritonavir in Caco-2 cell monolayers [published erratum appears in *Pharm Res* 1998 Jun;15(6):958]. *Pharm Res* 1998;15(3):423–428.
17. Washington CB, Duran GE, Man MC, Sikic BI, Blaschke TF. Interaction of anti-HIV protease inhibitors with the multidrug transporter P-glycoprotein (P-gp) in human cultured cells. *J Acquir Immune Defic Syndr Hum Retrovirol* 1998;19(3):203–209.
18. Pavelic ZP, Reising J, Pavelic L, Kelley DJ, Stambrook PJ, Gluckman JL. Detection of P-glycoprotein with four monoclonal antibodies in normal and tumor tissues. *Arch Otolaryngol Head Neck Surg* 1993;119(7):753–757.
19. Fitzsimmons ME, Collins JM. Selective biotransformation of the human immunodeficiency virus protease inhibitor saquinavir by human small-intestinal cytochrome P4503A4: potential contribution to high first-pass metabolism. *Drug Metab Dispos* 1997;25(2):256–266.
20. Brinkman K, Huysmans F, Burger DM. Pharmacokinetic interaction between saquinavir and cyclosporine [letter]. *Ann Intern Med* 1998;129(11):914–915.
21. von Moltke L, Greenblatt D, Duan S, Daily J, Harmatz J, Shader R. Inhibition of desipramine hydroxylation (Cytochrome P450-2D6) in

vitro by quinidine and by viral protease inhibitors: relation to drug interactions in vivo. *J Pharm Sci* 1998;87(10):1184–1189.

22. Ouellet D, Hsu A, Qian J, et al. Effect of ritonavir on the pharmacokinetics of ethinyl oestradiol in healthy female volunteers. *Br J Clin Pharmacol* 1998;46(2):111–116.

23. Cato A 3rd, Qian J, Hsu A, Levy B, Leonard J, Granneman R. Multidose pharmacokinetics of ritonavir and zidovudine in human immunodeficiency virus-infected patients. *Antimicrob Agents Chemother* 1998;42(7):1788–1793.

24. Hsu A, Granneman G, Witt G, Cavanaugh J, Leonard J. Assessment of multiple doses of ritonavir on the pharmacokinetics of theophylline. *Int Conf AIDS* 1996;11:89.

25. Decker CJ, Laitinen LM, Bridson GW, Raybuck SA, Tung RD, Chaturvedi PR. Metabolism of amprenavir in liver microsomes: role of CYP3A4 inhibition for drug interactions. *J Pharm Sci* 1998;87(7): 803–807.

26. Eagling VA, Back DJ, Barry MG. Differential inhibition of cytochrome P450 isoforms by the protease inhibitors, ritonavir, saquinavir and indinavir. *Br J Clin Pharmacol* 1997;44(2):190–194.

27. Chiba M, Hensleigh M, Nishime JA, Balani SK, Lin JH. Role of cytochrome P450 3A4 in human metabolism of MK-639, a potent human immunodeficiency virus protease inhibitor. *Drug Metab Dispos* 1996;24(3):307–314.

28. Lillibridge JH, Liang BH, Kerr BM, et al. Characterization of the selectivity and mechanism of human cytochrome P450 inhibition by the human immunodeficiency virus-protease inhibitor nelfinavir mesylate. *Drug Metab Dispos* 1998;26(7):609–616.

29. von Moltke LL, Greenblatt DJ, Grassi JM, et al. Protease inhibitors as inhibitors of human cytochromes P450: high risk associated with ritonavir. *J Clin Pharmacol* 1998;38(2):106–111.

30. Wang Y, Unadkat J. Differential inhibitory capacities of indinavir (IND) and ritonavir (RIT) towards cytochrome P450 (CYP) enzymes 3A4 and 3A5. *Pharm Sci* 1998;1:1128.

31. von Moltke L, Greenblatt D, Duan S, Daily J, Harmatz J, Shader R. Inhibition of desipramine hydroxylation (Cytochrome P450-2D6) in vitro by quinidine and by viral protease inhibitors: relation to drug interactions in vivo. *J Pharm Sci* 1998;87(10):1184–1189.

32. Kumar G, Rodrigues A, Buko A, Denissen J. Cytochrome P450-mediated metabolism of the HIV-1 protease inhibitor ritonavir (ABT-538) in human liver microsomes. *J Pharmacol Exp Ther* 1996;277(1): 423–431.

33. Buss N. Saquinavir soft gel capsule (Fortovase): pharmacokinetics and drug interactions. 5th Conf Retrovir Oppor Infect 1998:145.

34. Ferry JJ, Herman BD, Carel BJ, Carlson GF, Batts DH. Pharmacokinetic drug-drug interaction study of delavirdine and indinavir in healthy volunteers. *J Acquir Immune Defic Syndr Hum Retrovirol* 1998;18(3): 252–259.

35. Merry C, Barry MG, Mulcahy F, Halifax KL, Back DJ. Saquinavir pharmacokinetics alone and in combination with nelfinavir in HIV-infected patients. *AIDS* 1997;11(15):F117–F120.

36. Cox S, Schneck D, Herman B, et al. Delavirdine (DLV) and nelfinavir (NFV): a pharmacokinetic (PK) drug-drug interaction study in healthy adult volunteers. 5th Conf Retrovir Oppor Infect 1998:144 (abstract no. 345).

37. Skowron G, Leoung G, Kerr B, et al. Lack of pharmacokinetic interaction between nelfinavir and nevirapine [editorial; comment]. *AIDS* 1998;12(10):1243–1244.

38. Hsu A, Granneman GR, Cao G, et al. Pharmacokinetic interaction between ritonavir and indinavir in healthy volunteers. *Antimicrob Agents Chemother* 1998;42(11):2784–2791.

39. Hsu A, Granneman GR, Cao G, et al. Pharmacokinetic interactions between two human immunodeficiency virus protease inhibitors, ritonavir and saquinavir. *Clin Pharmacol Ther* 1998;63(4):453–464.

40. Fiske W, Benedek I, Joseph J, et al. Pharmacokinetics of efavirenz (EFV) and ritonavir (RIT) after multiple oral doses in healthy volunteers. *Int Conf AIDS* 1998;12:827 (abstract no. 42269).

41. Ferry J, Schneck D, Carlson G, et al. Evaluation of the pharmacokinetic (PK) interaction between ritonavir (RIT) and delavirdine (DLV) in healthy volunteers. 4th Conf Retrovir Oppor Infect 1997.

42. Ouellet D, Hsu A, Granneman GR, et al. Pharmacokinetic interaction between ritonavir and clarithromycin. *Clin Pharmacol Ther* 1998; 64(4):355–362.

43. Bertz R, Wong C, Carother L, et al. Evaluation of the pharmacokinetics of multiple dose ritonavir and ketoconazole in combination. *Clin Pharmacol Ther* 1998;63:230.

44. Cato A 3rd, Cavanaugh J, Shi H, Hsu A, Leonard J, Granneman R. The effect of multiple doses of ritonavir on the pharmacokinetics of rifabutin. *Clin Pharmacol Ther* 1998;63(4):414–421.

45. Cox S, Batts D, Stewart F, et al. Evaluation of the pharmacokinetic (PK) interaction between saquinavir (SQV) and delavirdine (DLV) in healthy volunteers. 4th Conf Retrovir Oppor Infect 1997.

46. Sahai J, Cameron W, Salgo M, Stewart F, Myers M, Lamson M, Gagnier P. Drug interaction study between saquinavir (SQV) and nevirapine (NVP). 4th Conf Retrovir Oppor Infect 1997 (abstract no. 614).

47. Emmanuel A, Gillotin C, Farinotti R, Sadler BM. Atovaquone suspension and indinavir have minimal pharmacokinetic interactions. *Int Conf AIDS* 1998;12:90(abstract no. 12384).

48. De Wit S, Debier M, De Smet M, et al. Effect of fluconazole on indinavir pharmacokinetics in human immunodeficiency virus-infected patients. *Antimicrob Agents Chemother* 1998;42(2):223–227.

49. Hsu A, Granneman G, Carothers L, et al. Ritonavir does not increase methadone exposure in healthy volunteers. 5th Conf Retrovir Oppor Infect 1998:143(abstract no. 342).

50. Vanhove G, Kastrissios H, Gries J, et al. Pharmacokinetics of saquinavir, zidovudine, and zalcitabine in combination therapy. *Antimicrob Agents Chemother* 1997;41(11):2428–2432.

CHAPTER 49

H₂-Receptor Antagonists

Mary F. Paine

HISTORICAL PERSPECTIVES

Before the advent of the histamine₂ (H₂)-receptor antagonists, treatments for various acid-related gastrointestinal disorders were limited to antacids, anticholinergic agents, and even surgical intervention (1–3). Since the debut of cimetidine in the late 1970s, the H₂ antagonists revolutionized the management of such disorders, including peptic ulcer disease, reflux esophagitis, and Zollinger-Ellison syndrome. These drugs effectively reduce acid secretion by competitively inhibiting the binding of histamine to H₂-receptors located in gastric parietal cells. When taken alone, the H₂ antagonists have an extremely low propensity for causing adverse reactions (<1%–3%), in part because of their poor penetration across the blood–brain barrier and the limited physiologic function of H₂-receptors in organs other than the stomach (2). When coadministered with certain other drugs, however, the potential for such adverse reactions is greatly increased. The majority of these drug–drug interactions result from the inhibition of the metabolism of the "object" drug (i.e., the drug *affected* by the interaction) (4) by the H₂ antagonist. Other mechanisms, including an increase in the absorption and/or a decrease in the renal tubular secretion of the object drug (4–7) are beyond the scope of this review.

Throughout the 1980s, the H₂ antagonists were the drugs of choice for the management of acid peptic disorders. Since the advent of the proton pump inhibitors (omeprazole, lansoprazole and rabeprazole), the H₂ antagonists have been increasingly considered as secondary agents and detailed discussion of metabolically based drug–drug interactions involving the H₂ antagonists may seem unnecessary. However, because they have

recently become available over-the-counter (Table 49-1), and are heavily advertised as effective for the relief of "heartburn" and "indigestion," the indiscriminate use of these agents by patients may lead to an increased incidence of adverse reactions (3,8). This chapter describes the nature of these interactions, beginning with the first documented cimetidine–drug interaction, followed by the mechanisms deduced from *in vitro* studies that might explain the adverse effects observed *in vivo*.

Cimetidine–Warfarin Interaction

Of the four commercially available H₂ antagonists, cimetidine has been the most frequently implicated in potentially serious metabolic drug–drug interactions. One of the earliest cases, reported over 20 years ago, involved a 70-year-old woman stabilized on warfarin for 7 years following aortic and mitral valve replacement (9). Shortly after cimetidine was added to her therapy, she noticed an ache behind her left knee. Three days later, when she could no longer bear weight on this knee and had painless, gross hematuria, she was admitted to the hospital. Notable findings during her evaluation included a tender left popliteal fossa hematoma and a prothrombin time of 83 seconds, a tripling of the value reported 2

M. F. Paine: General Clinical Research Center, University of North Carolina Hospitals, Room 3005 Main Building, CB# 7600, Chapel Hill, North Carolina 27599-7600 and Division of Pharmacotherapy, School of Pharmacy, University of North Carolina, CB# 7360 Beard Hall, Chapel Hill, North Carolina 27599-7360

TABLE 49-1. *Commercially available H₂ antagonists*

Generic name	Trade name	Year approved by the FDA	Usual daily dose[a] (mg)
Cimetidine	Tagamet	1977	800–1200
Ranitidine	Zantac	1983	300
Famotidine	Pepcid	1986	20
Nizatidine	Axid	1988	300

[a]For active duodenal ulcer

weeks earlier before starting cimetidine. Both cimetidine and warfarin were discontinued, and a single dose of vitamin K was administered intravenously. Ten hours later, the patient's prothrombin time had decreased to 16 seconds. One day later warfarin was reinstituted, and the patient was discharged after 5 more days with a prothrombin time of 19 seconds.

The concomitant administration of cimetidine and warfarin was shown to prolong prothrombin time in several more case reports (10–13). Subsequent controlled studies in patients and healthy volunteers revealed that cimetidine significantly increased plasma concentrations of warfarin by decreasing its apparent oral clearance, with a mean percent decrease ranging from 22% to 36% (14–17). Further investigations revealed that cimetidine only interacts with the less pharmacologically active R-enantiomer of warfarin (18,19).

Studies and case reports showing that cimetidine decreases the systemic or apparent oral clearance of numerous additional drugs soon appeared in the literature (Table 49-2). Except for a few isolated reports involving ranitidine (15,20) or famotidine (21), the other H_2 antagonists do not significantly alter the clearance of other drugs (16,22–27). Thus the question arises: why is cimetidine, and not the remaining H_2 antagonists, so highly prone to such phenomena?

TABLE 49-2. *Drugs whose metabolism is significantly inhibited by cimetidine, classified according to the cytochrome P450 isoforms known to mediate part or all of their metabolism*

CYP1A2	
Caffeine	Theophylline[a]
Theobromine	
CYP2C9	
Phenytoin[a]	(S)-warfarin
CYP2C19	
Diazepam	
CYP2D6	
Amitriptyline[a]	Nortriptyline[a]
Desipramine[a]	Metoprolol
Flecainide	Propranolol
Imipramine[a]	
CYP2E1	
Caffeine	
CYP3A4	
Alprazolam	Nifedipine[a]
Diazepam	Quinidine[a]
Lidocaine	Triazolam[a]
Midazolam	(R)-warfarin[a]
Isoform selectivity unknown or unavailable	
Chlordiazepoxide	Meperidine
Chlormethiazole[a]	Metronidazole
Clobazam	Nitrazepam
Flurazepam	

[a]Potentially serious adverse effects reported. Compiled from references 7, 59, 61–63, 67–69, and 81.

MECHANISMS OF METABOLIC DRUG INTERACTIONS

Metabolic Pathways Involved

The majority of metabolic drug–drug interactions involving the H_2 antagonists are through the inhibition of oxidative reactions catalyzed by the cytochromes P450 (CYP), the possible mechanisms of which are described later. A few investigators have reported that the H_2 antagonists also inhibit another phase I enzyme, gastric alcohol dehydrogenase, resulting in a statistically significant increase in blood alcohol levels or area under the curve (AUC) (reviewed in 4,7,28). However, in a recent and thorough critique of this topic, Hansten states "these have all been small absolute value increases and have been observed only under experimental conditions (4)." Interactions between H_2 antagonists and alcohol are probably of little clinical importance (2,4,7,28).

As for phase II enzyme–mediated reactions, the H_2 antagonists appear not to affect glucuronidation, sulfation, or acetylation. For example, cimetidine does not impair the glucuronidation of morphine (29), phenprocoumon (30), oxazepam (31–33), lorazepam (32–34), or temazepam (35,36); the sulfation of acetaminophen (37,38); nor the acetylation of dapsone (39), isoniazid (40,41), or procainamide (42). In summary, the cytochromes P450 appear to be the only drug-metabolizing enzymes affected by the H_2 antagonists.

Cytochrome P450 Binding Studies

Several early *in vitro* studies with both rat and human liver microsomes revealed that cimetidine binds directly but reversibly to the cytochromes P450 (43–45). When cimetidine was added to a microsomal suspension, a "type II" optical difference spectrum resulted. Type II difference spectra, characterized by a trough at approximately 390 nm and an absorption peak at approximately 430 nm, are indicative of direct binding to the heme moiety (i.e., a ligand type interaction). Such compounds displace water from the distal heme pocket to form a stronger low-spin state, thus preventing the reduction of ferric iron and subsequent metabolism of the substrate (46,47). Pasanen and colleagues (47), using human liver microsomes, compared the spectral binding constants (K_s) for the four H_2 antagonists and found cimetidine to be the most potent with a K_s of 0.87 mM. Ranitidine exhibited a very weak type II spectral change with a K_s of 5.1 mM, whereas famotidine and nizatidine exhibited no spectral change at concentrations up to 4 mM. In support of these findings, Wang and co-workers (48) observed a pronounced type II spectral change for cimetidine but no change for famotidine at equimolar concentrations (0.3 mM).

As the different CYP isoforms became known, Knodell and associates (49) later conducted binding studies with cimetidine using human liver microsomes and purified human liver CYP2C and CYP3A4. In agreement with results from the prior study, these investigators found the K_s for cimetidine in whole microsomes to average 0.64 ± 0.21 mM (n = 2). This value was similar to that for purified CYP3A4 (0.70 mM), but approximately six-fold lower than that for purified CYP2C (4.42 mM). These findings suggested that cimetidine may inhibit CYP3A4-mediated reactions to a greater extent than CYP2C-mediated reactions.

The differences in CYP-binding potencies among the H₂ antagonists are likely to be caused by differences in their chemical structures (Fig. 49-1) rather than by differences in H₂-receptor blockade (5,6,50). Cimetidine contains an imidazole ring, whereas ranitidine contains a furan ring, and famotidine and nizatidine each contain a thiazole ring. For cimetidine, the imidazole and especially the cyano group on the side chain (i.e., the cyanoguanidine) appear to be important for the ligand interaction between the drug and heme moiety (51–55). Moreover, the cyanoguanidine side chain enhances the lipophilicity of the compound, which facilitates its penetration across lipid membranes and hydrophobic binding to the enzyme (51,55). This cimetidine-heme interaction prevents reduction of ferric iron, and thereby dioxygen binding, thus slowing the rate of metabolism of susceptible substrates. This, in turn, can lead to a reduction in overall clearance and a potential for adverse reactions or toxicity. As the binding studies indicate, the three other H₂ antagonists bind very weakly to the enzyme, explaining their virtual lack of metabolic drug interactions. Although famotidine contains a guanidine group, it is probably sterically hindered because of its close proxim-

ity to the thiazole ring, effectively preventing its interaction with the heme (1).

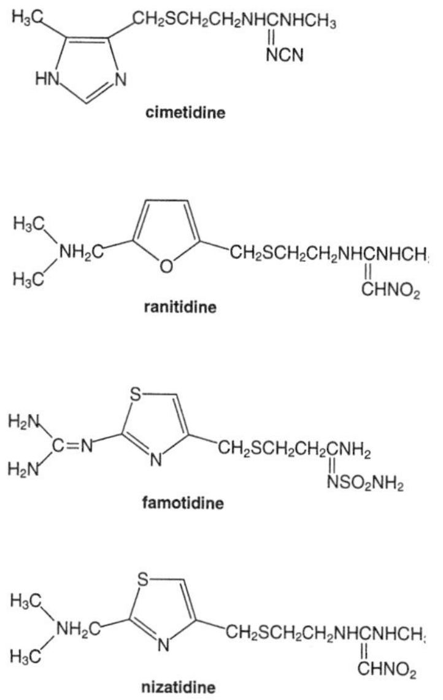

In Vitro Inhibition Studies

Similar to the *in vivo* observations and results from the binding studies, all *in vitro* metabolic studies have shown that, of the H₂ antagonists, cimetidine is the most potent inhibitor of cytochrome P450-mediated reactions. For example, an early investigation with rat liver microsomes revealed cimetidine to be nearly 30-fold more potent than ranitidine as a mixed inhibitor of the nonselective reaction, aminopyrine N-demethylation (56). The inhibition constant (K_i) estimated for each compound was 0.13 and 3.69 mM, respectively. In human liver microsomes, cimetidine inhibited meperidine demethylation and pentobarbital hydroxylation at a concentration of 3 mM, whereas ranitidine had no effect at the same concentration (44). Likewise, cimetidine was more potent than famotidine as an inhibitor of 7-ethoxycoumarin O-deethylation and benzphetamine N-demethylation in rat and human liver microsomes at concentrations ranging from 0.25 to 2 mM (48). Finally, as an inhibitor of aminopyrine N-demethylase, nizatidine was near control values at concentrations as high as 10 mM (57). Moreover, Wrighton and Ring (58) found cimetidine to be ten-fold more potent than nizatidine in inhibiting midazolam $1'$-hydroxylation, a selective CYP3A-mediated reaction, as evidenced by a K_i estimated for each compound of 0.27 and 2.9 mM, respectively.

Knodell and co-workers (49) have examined the inhibitory effect of cimetidine on the major human cytochromes P450 using substrates that are selective for the various isoforms. The following enzyme activities were measured in four to six different human liver microsomal preparations: tolbutamide and hexobarbital hydroxylation (CYP2C9), nifedipine oxidation and erythromycin N-demethylation (CYP3A4), bufuralol hydroxylation (CYP2D6), ethoxyresorufin O-deethylation (CYP1A), and aniline hydroxylation (CYP2E1).

In agreement with prior binding studies (47–49), nifedipine oxidase activity was inhibited to a greater extent (range 60%–93%) than either tolbutamide or hexobarbital hydroxylase activities (4%–50% and 32%–57%, respectively) at a cimetidine concentration of 3 mM. Moreover, nifedipine oxidase was sensitive to cimetidine concentrations as low as 50 µM (no K_i was reported). Unexpectedly, erythromycin demethylase activity was inhibited by a much lesser degree (range 1%–17%). This discrepancy may have been due to the 25-fold higher erythromycin concentration used compared to nifedipine (2.5 versus 0.1 mM). The authors also speculated that the two substrates may bind to different sites on the CYP3A4 molecule such that the erythromycin binding site is not impeded by the interaction of cimetidine with the heme moiety.

FIG. 49-1. Chemical structures of the commercially available H₂ antagonists.

Cimetidine inhibited bufuralol hydroxylase activity to a degree similar to that observed for nifedipine oxidase activity (range 69%–100%). A Dixon plot of bufuralol hydroxylation rates against increasing concentrations of cimetidine revealed a K_i of 50 μM. The K_i for ethoxyresorufin deethylase activity, however, was 12-fold higher (0.6 mM), corresponding to the modest inhibition observed with 3 mM cimetidine (range 14%–28%). Finally, the extent of inhibition of aniline hydroxylase was on a par with the CYP2C-mediated reactions and ranged from 11% to 55%.

Another important observation from this study is that there were large interindividual variations in the extent of inhibition of each CYP isoform-mediated reaction. It is well known that the different human CYP isoforms are highly variably expressed, from 20-fold for CYP3A4 and CYP2E1 to greater than 1000-fold for the polymorphically expressed CYP2D6 (59). This may explain in part why some individuals are more susceptible to the effects of an interaction between cimetidine and certain drugs. That is, a patient with low levels of a particular isoform may be more prone to experience the effects of a cimetidine–drug interaction compared to one who has high levels of the same enzyme.

Collectively, the inhibition studies with human liver microsomes suggest that CYP3A4 and CYP2D6 are most sensitive to the effects of cimetidine, followed by CYP2C9 and CYP2E1, followed by CYP1A. These results are consistent with many of the interactions listed in Table 49-2, even though the concentrations of cimetidine used in vitro are much higher than plasma concentrations typically observed (approximately 1–10 μM) (1,60). Although diazepam is metabolized by more than one isoform (CYP3A4 and CYP2C19), CYP3A4 is probably the major isoform that contributes to its overall metabolism (61–63).

Racemic warfarin is also metabolized by more than one isoform. As discussed earlier, cimetidine only interacts with the less active R-enantiomer. However, Choonara and colleagues (64) demonstrated that a dose of R-warfarin as small as 1 mg can cause a measurable increase in prothrombin time. Thus, a plausible explanation for the in vivo effect is that cimetidine inhibits the CYP3A-mediated metabolism of the R-enantiomer, causing an additive hypoprothrombinemic effect to that of the S-enantiomer.

Soon after the introduction of cimetidine, theophylline, like warfarin, was also frequently reported to cause potentially serious adverse reactions when coadministered with cimetidine. Grand mal seizures, sinus tachycardia, and severe nausea have been observed in patients receiving the two medications concurrently (65,66). In a review by Somogyi and Muirhead (7), the mean percent decrease in theophylline systemic or apparent oral clearance by cimetidine in patients with asthma, chronic obstructive pulmonary disease, and cirrhosis ranged from 20% to 44%. Theophylline is believed to be primarily a substrate for CYP1A2 (67–69). Because cimetidine was found to be a relatively weak inhibitor of this isoform in vitro (49), it is difficult to explain this in vivo effect. Likewise, in vitro–in vivo correlations with other CYP1A2 substrates, as well as CYP2C9 and CYP2E1 substrates, appear to be lacking. Thus, it is likely there are other mechanisms whereby cimetidine inhibits the cytochromes P450.

Metabolite–Intermediate Complex Formation

A major criticism of the cytochrome P450 binding and inhibition studies is that the concentrations of H_2 antagonists used are 100 to 1000 times higher than concentrations associated with inhibition of drug metabolism in vivo (1,60). Some investigators have shown that cimetidine inhibits the cytochromes P450 at much lower concentrations by forming a metabolite–intermediate (MI) complex. The antibiotic troleandomycin (70), the antidepressant nortriptyline (71), and the antiparkinsonian agent orphenadrine (72–74) have all been shown to inhibit some cytochrome P450 isoforms by this mechanism.

Jensen and Gugler (75), using rat liver microsomes, found cimetidine to inhibit 7-ethoxycoumarin O-deethylase activity in a mixed type manner when the reaction was initiated with an NADPH-generating system. A large K_i of 0.8 mM resulted. However, if the microsomes were preincubated with cimetidine and NADPH, and the reaction was initiated by the addition of substrate, then the degree of inhibition by cimetidine was enhanced. This enhancement of inhibition was also accompanied by a decrease in total CYP content as measured by the Fe(II)-carbon monoxide–binding difference spectrum. Moreover, the decrease in enzyme activity and CYP content were attenuated if potassium ferricyanide, a compound that destroys CYP complexes by oxidizing the ferrous heme to liberate the free enzyme (70), was added to the microsomal suspension. Similarly, 7-ethoxycoumarin O-deethylase activity and CYP content in liver microsomes prepared from cimetidine-treated rats were near the values obtained in control rats if the former microsomes were washed with potassium ferricyanide. From these findings, the authors proposed that a complex between a cimetidine intermediate and the CYP isoforms might be responsible for the inhibition of enzyme activity.

Chang and colleagues (76) conducted similar experiments with rat liver microsomes using testosterone as the substrate. As with the previous study, these investigators found that when incubations containing substrate and high concentrations of cimetidine (0.25–10 mM) were initiated with NADPH, the different metabolic pathways of testosterone (2α-, 2β-, 6β-, and 16α-hydroxylation) were inhibitable, with IC_{50} values ranging from 1.0 to 7.4 mM. However, when microsomes were preincubated with a lower concentration of cimetidine (0.05 mM) and NADPH, the inhibition potency increased, again suggesting the formation of an MI complex. Moreover, cimetidine only inhibited the reaction mediated by the male-specific CYP2C11 (2α-hydroxylase).

Further investigation of the CYP2C11 complex revealed that the spectral peak observed at 428 to 430 nm was dependent on the presence of NADPH and the concentration of cimetidine (77). That is, the amplitude of the peak increased with an increase in cimetidine concentration, from 0.01 to 0.5 mM. In addition, this peak was not dissociated by the addition of potassium ferricyanide, suggesting that the cimetidine intermediate forms a stable complex with this particular isoform in its ferric state.

Collectively, these studies indicate that cimetidine is capable of forming an MI complex at concentrations lower than those used in traditional (i.e., competitive or mixed-type) inhibition studies. The drug also appears to be isoform selective, at least in the rat. Although investigations involving human CYP isoforms are lacking, this mechanism could explain *in vivo* cimetidine–drug interactions that are inconsistent with the ligand-binding mechanism. Elucidation of the human CYP isoforms that form complexes with the metabolite intermediate, as well as the nature of the intermediate itself, would help fill a gap in modern understanding of the mechanisms behind these important drug interactions.

EFFECT OF DOSE AND LENGTH OF TREATMENT

As shown *in vitro*, the degree of inhibition of drug metabolism by the H$_2$ antagonists *in vivo* also appears to be dose dependent. Somogyi and Muirhead (7) concluded that a daily cimetidine dose of 300 to 400 mg generally inhibits metabolism of the object drug by 10% to 20%, a dose of 400 to 800 mg inhibits by 20% to 30%, and a dose of 800 to 1600 mg inhibits by 30% to 40%. Although rarely prescribed, a daily cimetidine dose greater than 2000 mg generally inhibits metabolism by 40% to 50%. In addition, the few reports of significant ranitidine or famotidine drug interactions usually involved higher-than-normal doses of the H$_2$ antagonist. For example, the prolongation of prothrombin time by the coadministration of ranitidine and warfarin only occurred at a ranitidine daily dose of 600 mg; no effect was observed at the usual daily dose of 300 mg (20). Moreover, the significant increase in mean theophylline AUC by famotidine occurred at a nightly famotidine dose of 40 mg (21).

The onset of inhibition of drug metabolism by cimetidine is generally rapid. Maximum inhibition can occur as early as 24 hours after starting the drug and is maintained for at least 30 days if continued (4,7,78). However, the time required for the object drug to reach a new steady-state concentration, whether cimetidine is contin-

ued or discontinued, depends on the half-life of the object drug (4). For example, a patient receiving theophylline will achieve a new steady-state concentration within 1 to 3 days after starting or stopping cimetidine. A patient receiving warfarin, however, will not achieve a new steady state for at least 1 week. This is due to warfarin having a much longer half-life compared to theophylline (approximately 35 hours and 6 to 10 hours for racemic warfarin and theophylline, respectively) (78,79). Thus it is important to monitor concentrations of the object drug regularly when cimetidine is added or discontinued, especially if the object drug has a narrow therapeutic index.

SUMMARY

The H$_2$ antagonists represent the first class of drugs to have a profound impact on the treatment of acid peptic conditions. These novel agents dramatically increased duodenal and gastric ulcer healing rates and greatly decreased the need for surgical intervention. Even though all of these drugs enjoy a remarkably low incidence of adverse reactions when given alone, cimetidine has been implicated in a long list of significant metabolically based drug–drug interactions. Such interactions appear to arise from the inhibition of the cytochrome P450 isoforms responsible for the metabolism of the object drug.

One proposed mechanism for the inhibitory effect of cimetidine is competitive (or mixed) inhibition of the CYP isoforms, of which CYP3A4 and CYP2D6 appear to be the most sensitive. Many of the drugs involved in clinically reported interactions are substrates for these isoforms (see Table 49-2). However, a disturbing fact common to all of the CYP-binding and competitive-type (i.e., NADPH-initiated) inhibition experiments is that the concentrations of cimetidine needed are in the millimolar range. This conflicts with the micromolar concentrations observed *in vivo*. The formation of a metabolite–intermediate complex at lower concentrations of cimetidine thus represents an attractive, alternative mechanism, although this has not been adequately investigated in humans.

In agreement with *in vitro* observations, the degree of inhibition of drug metabolism by cimetidine *in vivo* appears to increase with an increase in dose. The onset of effect is generally rapid, with no tolerance to the inhibitory effects. The time for the object drug to reach a new steady-state concentration, whether cimetidine is started or stopped, depends on its half-life.

In conclusion, despite 20 years of experience with cimetidine, there is still much that is not known about the nature of its metabolic drug interactions. In addition, the recent availability of the H$_2$ antagonists as over-the-counter medications emphasizes the need for clinicians to understand these interactions and to question their patients about nonprescription drug use.

REFERENCES

1. Mitchard M, McIsaac RL, Bell JA. H$_2$-receptor antagonists. In: Damani LA, ed. *Sulphur-containing drugs and related organic compounds: chemistry, biochemistry and toxicology,* Vol. 3, Part A. Chichester: Ellis Horwood, 1989:53–86.

2. Brunton LL. Agents for control of gastric acidity and treatment of peptic ulcers. In: Hardman JG, Limbird LL, Molinoff PB, Ruddon RW, Goodman LS, Gilman A, eds. *Goodman and Gilman's the pharmacological basis of therapeutics,* 9th ed. New York: McGraw-Hill, 1996:901–915.

3. Sanders SW. Pathogenesis and treatment of acid peptic disorders: comparison of proton pump inhibitors with other antiulcer drugs. *Clin Ther* 1996;18:2–34.

4. Hansten PD. Drug interactions of gastrointestinal drugs. In: Lewis JH, ed. *A pharmacological approach to gastrointestinal disorders.* Baltimore: Williams & Wilkins, 1994:535–563.

5. Sedman AJ. Cimetidine-drug interactions. *Am J Med* 1984;76:109–114.

6. Nazario M. The hepatic and renal mechanisms of drug interactions with cimetidine. *Drug Intell Clin Pharm* 1986;20:342–348.

7. Somogyi A, Muirhead M. Pharmacokinetic interactions of cimetidine 1987. *Clin Pharmacokinet* 1987;12:321–366.

8. Honig PK, Gillespie BK. Drug interactions between prescribed and over-the-counter medications. *Drug Saf* 1995;13:296–303.

9. Silver BA, Bell WR. Cimetidine potentiation of the hypoprothrombinemic effect of warfarin. *Ann Intern Med* 1979;90:348–349.

10. Wallin BA, Jacknowitz A, Raich P. Cimetidine and effect of warfarin. *Ann Intern Med* 1979;90:993.

11. Hetzel D, Birkett D, Miners J. Cimetidine interaction with warfarin. *Lancet* 1979;2:639.

12. Ovedoff DL. Cimetidine and warfarin. *Med J Aust* 1979;1:96.

13. Kerley B, Ali M. Cimetidine potentiation of warfarin action. *Can Med Assoc J* 1982;126:116.

14. Serlin MJ, Sibeon RG, Mossman S, Breckenridge AM. Cimetidine: interaction with oral anticoagulants in man. *Lancet* 1979;2:317–319.

15. Desmond PV, Mashford ML, Harman PJ, Morphett BJ, Breen KJ, Wang YM. Decreased oral warfarin clearance after ranitidine and cimetidine. *Clin Pharmacol Ther* 1984;35:338–341.

16. O'Reilly RA. Comparative interaction of cimetidine and ranitidine with racemic warfarin in man. *Arch Intern Med* 1984;144:989–991.

17. Sax MJ, Randolph WC, Peace KE, et al. Effect of two cimetidine regimens on prothrombin time and warfarin pharmacokinetics during long-term warfarin therapy. *Clin Pharm* 1987;6:492–495.

18. Choonara IA, Cholerton S, Haynes BP, Breckenridge AM, Park BK. Stereoselective interaction between the R enantiomer of warfarin and cimetidine. *Br J Clin Pharmacol* 1986;21:271–277.

19. Toon S, Hopkins KJ, Garstang FM, Rowland M. Comparative effects of ranitidine and cimetidine on the pharmacokinetics and pharmacodynamics of warfarin in man. *Eur J Clin Pharmacol* 1987;32:165–172.

20. Baciewicz AM, Morgan PJ. Ranitidine-warfarin interaction. *Ann Intern Med* 1990;112:76–77.

21. Dal Negro R, Pomari C, Turco P. Famotidine and theophylline pharmacokinetics. An unexpected cimetidine-like interaction in patients with chronic obstructive pulmonary disease. *Clin Pharmacokinet* 1993;24:255–258.

22. Kirch W, Hoensch H, Janisch HD. Interactions and non-interactions with ranitidine. *Clin Pharmacokinet* 1984;9:493–510.

23. Secor JW, Speeg KV, Meredith CG, Johnson RF, Snowdy P, Schenker S. Lack of effect of nizatidine on hepatic drug metabolism in man. *Br J Clin Pharmacol* 1985;20:710–713.

24. Somerville KW, Kitchingman GA, Langman MJS. Effect of famotidine on oxidative drug metabolism. *Eur J Clin Pharmacol* 1986;30:279–281.

25. Krishna DR, Klotz U. Newer H$_2$-receptor antagonists. Clinical pharmacokinetics and drug interaction potential. *Clin Pharmacokinet* 1988;15:205–215.

26. Smith RS, Kendall MJ. Ranitidine versus cimetidine. A comparison of their potential to cause clinically important drug interactions. *Clin Pharmacokinet* 1988;15:44–56.

27. Klotz U, Kroemer HK. The drug interaction potential of ranitidine:an update. *Pharmacol Ther* 1991;50:233–244.

28. Fraser A. Pharmacokinetic interactions between alcohol and other drugs. *Clin Pharmacokinet* 1997;33:79–90.

29. Mojaverian P, Fedder IL, Vlasses PH, et al. Cimetidine does not alter morphine disposition in man. *Br J Clin Pharmacol* 1982;14:809–813.

30. Harenberg J, Zimmermann R, Staiger C, de Vries JX, Walter E, Weber E. Lack of effect of cimetidine on action of phenprocoumon. *Eur J Clin Pharmacol* 1982;23:365–367.

31. Klotz U, Reimann I. Influence of cimetidine on the pharmacokinetics of desmethyldiazepam and oxazepam. *Eur J Clin Pharmacol* 1980;18:517–520.

32. Patwardhan RV, Yarborough GW, Desmond PV, Johnson RF, Schenker S, Speeg KV. Cimetidine spares the glucuronidation of lorazepam and oxazepam. *Gastroenterology* 1980;79:912–916.

33. Greenblatt DJ, Abernethy DR, Keopke HH, Shader RI. Interaction of cimetidine with oxazepam, lorazepam, and flurazepam. *J Clin Pharmacol* 1984;24:187–193.

34. Abernethy DR, Greenblatt DJ, Divoll M, Ameer B, Shader RI. Differential effect of cimetidine on drug oxidation (antipyrine and diazepam) vs. conjugation (acetaminophen and lorazepam): prevention of acetaminophen toxicity by cimetidine. *J Pharmacol Exper Ther* 1983;224:508–513.

35. Greenblatt DJ, Abernethy DR, Divoll M, Locniskar A, Harmatz JS, Shader RI. Noninteraction of temazepam and cimetidine. *J Pharm Sci* 1984;73:399–401.

36. Elliot P, Dundee JW, Elwood RJ, Collier PS. The influence of H$_2$ receptor antagonists on the plasma concentrations of midazolam and temazepam. *Eur J Anaesth* 1984;1:245–251.

37. Miners JO, Attwood JA, Birkett DJ. Determinants of acetaminophen metabolism: effect of inducers and inhibitors of drug metabolism on acetaminophen's metabolic pathways. *Clin Pharmacol Ther* 1984;35:480–486.

38. Mitchell MC, Schenker S, Speeg KV. Selective inhibition of acetaminophen oxidation and toxicity by cimetidine and other histamine H$_2$-receptor antagonists in vivo and in vitro in the rat and man. *J Clin Invest* 1984;73:383–391.

39. Wright JT, Goodman RP, Bethel AMM, Lambert CM. Cimetidine and dapsone acetylation. *Drug Metab Dispos* 1984;12:782–783.

40. Lauterberg BH, Todd EL, Smith CV, Mitchell JR. Cimetidine inhibits the formation of the reactive, toxic metabolite of isoniazid in rats but not in man. *Hepatology* 1985;5:607–609.

41. Paulsen O, Höglund P, Nilsson L-G, Gredeby H. No interaction between H$_2$ blockers and isoniazid. *Eur J Respir Dis* 1986;68:286–290.

42. Somogyi A, Heinzow B. Cimetidine reduces procainamide elimination. *N Engl J Med* 1982;307:1080.

43. Rendic S, Sunjic V, Toso R, Kajfez F. Interaction of cimetidine with liver microsomes. *Xenobiotica* 1979;9:555–564.

44. Knodell RG, Holtzman JL, Crankshaw DL, Steele NM, Stanley LN. Drug metabolism by rat and human hepatic microsomes in response to interaction with H$_2$-receptor antagonists. *Gastroenterology* 1982;82:84–88.

45. Bast A, Savenije-Chapel EM, Droes BH. Inhibition of mono-oxygenase and oxidase activity of rat-hepatic cytochrome P-450 by H$_2$-receptor blockers. *Xenobiotica* 1984;14:399–408.

46. Trager WF. Oxidative functionalization reactions. In: Jenner P, Testa B, eds. *Concepts in drug metabolism, Part A.* New York: Marcel Dekker, 1980;177–209.

47. Pasanen M, Arvela P, Pelkonen O, Sotaniemi E, Klotz U. Effect of five structurally diverse H$_2$-receptor antagonists on drug metabolism. *Biochem Pharmacol* 1986;35:4457–4461.

48. Wang RW, Miwa GT, Argenbright LS, Lu AYH. *In vitro* studies on the interaction of famotidine with liver microsomal cytochrome P-450. *Biochem Pharmacol* 1988;37:3049–3053.

49. Knodell RG, Browne DG, Gwozdz GP, Brian WR, Guengerich FP. Differential inhibition of individual human liver cytochrome P-450 by cimetidine. *Gastroenterology* 1991;101:1680–1691.

50. Breen KJ, Bury R, Desmond PV, et al. Effects of cimetidine and ranitidine on hepatic drug metabolism. *Clin Pharmacol Ther* 1982;31:297–300.

51. Wilkinson CF, Hetnarski K, Yellin TO. Imidazole derivatives—a new class of microsomal enzyme inhibitors. *Biochem Pharmacol* 1972;21:3187–3192.

52. Bell JA, Gower AJ, Martin LE, Mills ENC, Smith WP. Interaction of H$_2$-receptor antagonists with drug-metabolizing enzymes. *Biochem Soc Trans* 1981;9:113–114.

53. Mihaly GW, Smallwood RA, Anderson JD, Jones DB, Webster LK, Vajda FJ. H$_2$-receptor antagonists and hepatic drug disposition. *Hepatology* 1982;2:828–831.

54. Rendic S, Kajfez F, Ruf H-H. Characterization of cimetidine, raniti-

dine, and related structures' interaction with cytochrome P-450. *Drug Metab Dispos* 1983;11:137–142.

55. Rekka E, Sterk GJ, Timmerman H, Bast A. Identification of structural characteristics of some potential H$_2$-receptor antagonists that determine the interaction with rat hepatic P-450. *Chem Biol Interact* 1988;67: 117–127.

56. Speeg KV, Patwardhan RV, Avant GR, Mitchell MC, Schenker S. Inhibition of microsomal drug metabolism by histamine H$_2$-receptor antagonists studied in vivo and in vitro in rodents. *Gastroenterology* 1982; 82:89–96.

57. Meredith CG, Speeg KV, Schenker S. Nizatidine, a new histamine H$_2$-receptor antagonist, and hepatic oxidative drug metabolism in the rat: a comparison with structurally related compounds. *Toxicol Appl Pharmacol* 1985;77:315–324.

58. Wrighton SA, Ring BJ. Inhibition of human CYP3A catalyzed 1′-hydroxy midazolam formation by ketoconazole, nifedipine, erythromycin, cimetidine, and nizatidine. *Pharm Res* 1994;11:921–924.

59. Guengerich FP. Human cytochrome P450 enzymes. In: Ortiz de Montellano, ed. *Cytochrome P450: structure, mechanism, and biochemistry*, 2nd ed. New York: Plenum Press, 1995:473–535.

60. Lauritsen K, Laursen LS, Rask-Madsen J. Clinical pharmacokinetics of drugs used in the treatment of gastrointestinal diseases (part 1). *Clin Pharmacokinet* 1990;19:11–31.

61. Andersson T, Miners JO, Veronese ME, Birkett DJ. Diazepam metabolism by human liver microsomes is mediated by both S-mephenytoin hydroxylase and CYP3A isoforms. *Br J Clin Pharmacol* 1994;38: 131–137.

62. Flockhart DA. Drug interactions and the cytochrome P450 system. The role of cytochrome P450 2C19. *Clin Pharmacokinet* 1995;29[Suppl 1]: 45–52.

63. Ono S, Hatanaka T, Miyazawa S, et al. Human liver microsomal diazepam metabolism using cDNA-expressed cytochrome P450s: role of CYP2B6, 2C19 and the 3A subfamily. *Xenobiotica* 1996;26: 1155–1166.

64. Choonara IA, Haynes BP, Cholerton S, Breckenridge AM, Park BK. Enantiomers of warfarin and vitamin K$_1$ metabolism. *Br J Clin Pharmacol* 1986;22:729–732.

65. Bauman JH, Kimelblatt BJ, Caraccio TR, Silverman HM, Simon GI, Beck GJ. Cimetidine-theophylline interaction: report of four patients. *Ann Allergy* 1982;48:100–102.

66. Lofgren RP, Gilbertson RA. Cimetidine and theophylline. *Ann Intern Med* 1982;96:378.

67. Gu L, Gonzalez FJ, Kalow W, Tang BK. Biotransformation of caffeine, paraxanthine, theobromine and theophylline by cDNA-expressed human CYP1A2 and CYP2E1. *Pharmacogenetics* 1992;2:73–77.

68. Tassaneeyakul W, Birkett DJ, McManus ME, et al. Caffeine metabolism by human hepatic cytochromes P450: contributions of 1A2, 2E1 and 3A isoforms. *Biochem Pharmacol* 1994;47:1767–1776.

69. Brosen K. Drug interactions and the cytochrome P450 system. The role of cytochrome P450 1A2. *Clin Pharmacokinet* 1995;29[Suppl1]: 20–25.

70. Pessayre D, Larrey D, Vitaux J, Breil P, Belghiti J, Benhamou J-P. Formation of an inactive cytochrome P-450 Fe(II)-metabolite complex after administration of troleandomycin in humans. *Biochem Pharmacol* 1982;31:1699–1704.

71. Murray M. Metabolite intermediate complexation of microsomal cytochrome P450 2C11 in male rat liver by nortriptyline. *Mol Pharmacol* 1992;42:931–938.

72. Bast A, van Kemenade FAA, Savenije-Chapel EM, Noordhoek J. Product inhibition in orphenadrine metabolism as a result of a stable cytochrome P-450-metabolic intermediate complex formed during the disposition of mono-N-desmethylorphenadrine (tofenacine) in the rat. *Res Commun Chem Pathol Pharmacol* 1983;40:391–403.

73. Reidy GF, Mehta I, Murray M. Inhibition of oxidative drug metabolism by orphenadrine: *in vitro* and *in vivo* evidence for isozyme-specific complexation of cytochrome P-450 and inhibition kinetics. *Mol Pharmacol* 1989;35:736–743.

74. Roos PH, Mahnke A. Metabolite complex formation of orphenadrine with cytochrome P450. *Biochem Pharmacol* 1996;52:73–84.

75. Jensen JC, Gugler R. Cimetidine interaction with liver microsomes *in vitro* and *in vivo*. Involvement of an activated complex with cytochrome P-450. *Biochem Pharmacol* 1985;34:2141–2146.

76. Chang T, Levine M, Bellward GD. Selective inhibition of rat hepatic microsomal cytochrome P-450. II. Effect of the *in vitro* administration of cimetidine. *J Pharmacol Exper Ther* 1992;260:1450–1455.

77. Levine M, Bellward GD. Effect of cimetidine on hepatic cytochrome P450: evidence for formation of a metabolite-intermediate complex. *Drug Metab Dispos* 1995;23:1407–1411.

78. Holford NHG. Clinical pharmacokinetics and pharmacodynamics of warfarin. Understanding the dose-effect relationship. *Clin Pharmacokinet* 1986;11:483–504.

79. Hendeles L, Weinberger M. Theophylline. A "state of the art" review. *Pharmacotherapy* 1983;3:2–44.

80. von Moltke LL, Greenblatt DJ, Cotreau-Bibbo MM, Harmatz JS, Shader RI. Inhibitors of alprazolam metabolism *in vitro*: effect of serotonin-reuptake-inhibitor antidepressants, ketoconazole and quinidine. *Br J Clin Pharmacol* 1994;38:23–31.

81. Lauritsen K, Laursen LS, Rask-Madsen J. Clinical pharmacokinetics of drugs used in the treatment of gastrointestinal diseases (part II). *Clin Pharmacokinet* 1990;19:94–125.

CHAPTER 50

Inhibitors in the Diet: Grapefruit Juice–Drug Interactions

David G. Bailey, J. Malcolm O. Arnold, and J. David Spence

In 1991, we reported the original observation that grapefruit juice can markedly increase the oral bioavailability and augment the effect of two dihydropyridine calcium channel blockers—felodipine and nifedipine (1). Subsequently, grapefruit juice was shown to interact with a number of drugs in diverse therapeutic categories. The topic of grapefruit juice–drug interactions has been the subject of several recent reviews (2–5).

Grapefruit juice is classified as a food product and is considered inherently safe for human consumption. Therefore, it does not come under the same scrutiny as therapeutic agents. Historically, the potential for food–drug interactions has not been fully appreciated. Since the early 1990s, however, research has shown that grapefruit juice can cause clinically relevant changes in plasma drug concentrations and that this type of interaction is probably more common than was once thought. Prescribing information has been changed or is being changed for some medications cautioning against consumption of grapefruit juice during therapy. A warning label for application to drug prescription vials is currently available at pharmacies. Some hospitals have taken the initiative to exclude grapefruit juice from patients' meals to prevent the possibility of a drug interaction. Thus, the initial observation and subsequent research has gone "from bench top to bedside."

D.G. Bailey, J. M.O. Arnold: Departments of Medicine and Pharmacology and Toxicology, University of Western Ontario and Department of Medicine, London Health Sciences Centre, 375 South Street, London, Ontario N6A 4G5 Canada

J.D. Spence: Departments of Clinical Neurological Sciences, Internal Medicine, and Pharmacology and Toxicology, University of Western Ontario and Stroke Prevention and Atherosclerosis Research Centre, Robarts Research Institute, 1400 Western Road, London, Ontario N6C 2V2 Canada

This chapter retraces discovery of this novel interaction, reviews the mechanism of action, summarizes studied medications, and discusses potentially active ingredients in grapefruit juice.

DISCOVERY

Originally, we set out to assess the possibility of an interaction between ethanol and felodipine (6). Because ethanol and felodipine both cause vasodilatation and diuresis and because ethanol might inhibit felodipine metabolism, enhanced cardiovascular effects seemed probable with the combination. The choice of grapefruit juice to mask the taste of the ethanol was based on an assessment of ethanol with every juice in a home refrigerator one Saturday evening. White grapefruit juice, particularly double-strength juice (single dilution of frozen concentrate), most effectively blinded the participants to the taste of ethanol. The results of the study showed that the combination of a nonintoxicating dose of ethanol and felodipine regular-release tablet resulted in lower standing blood pressure and a high frequency of orthostatic hypotension compared to felodipine alone in patients with untreated borderline hypertension (6). Plasma felodipine concentrations were not different between treatments supporting an additive or synergistic interaction between the vasodilatation/diuretic properties of the two components. However, the relevant observation for discussion was that felodipine concentrations were several-fold higher than observed in other pharmacokinetic investigations using the same dose of drug. A systematic examination of obvious possible causes, such as incorrect tablet strength or drug assay problems, did not resolve this discrepancy. Because previous studies had administered felodipine with water and not grapefruit juice, a pilot project was undertaken in one of the authors (DGB) to judge the potential role of the juice. In this individual, plasma felodipine concentrations with 350 mL double-strength grapefruit juice were five-fold greater than with water.

MECHANISM OF THE INTERACTION

Felodipine Disposition and Metabolism

Felodipine has been the most extensively studied probe for grapefruit juice–drug interactions. Following oral administration, felodipine is completely absorbed from the gastrointestinal tract (7). However, it undergoes high presystemic (first pass) metabolism, resulting in low absolute bioavailability averaging 15% (7) but ranging from 4% to 36% among individuals (8). Both the gut wall and the liver appear responsible for presystemic felodipine elimination (9).

Felodipine is biotransformed to a single primary inactive metabolite, dehydrofelodipine, which is subsequently oxidized by two secondary pathways (10). Cytochrome P450 3A4 (CYP3A4) catalyzes the formation of both dehydrofelodipine (11) and the major secondary metabolite, M3 (12). Apical enterocytes of the small bowel and hepatocytes of the liver both contain CYP3A4 (13,14). The content of CYP3A4 in both tissues ranges at least ten-fold among individuals and appears to be regulated independently of the other (15).

Grapefruit Juice Effects

The first report of this interaction revealed that grapefruit juice, but not orange juice, tripled mean plasma felodipine area under the curve (AUC) compared to water in borderline hypertensive patients (1). Blood pressure reduction, heart rate increase, and frequency of vasodilatation-related adverse events were also greater. Grapefruit juice markedly elevated plasma peak felodipine concentration (C_{max}) but did not alter systemic felodipine elimination half-life ($t_{1/2}$). Because grapefruit juice did not change intravenous felodipine pharmacokinetics (9), it indicates that the interaction with grapefruit juice resulted from inhibition of presystemic drug metabolism.

Grapefruit juice reduced dehydrofelodipine to felodipine AUC ratio and increased absolute dehydrofelodipine AUC (1). The decrease in the AUC ratio was compatible with inhibition of the primary metabolic pathway. The absolute increase in dehydrofelodipine AUC indicated that a subsequent metabolic pathway might also be inhibited, and this was supported by measurements showing that the M3 metabolite AUC was reduced (12). Thus, grapefruit juice appeared to inhibit CYP3A4, an important isozyme of cytochrome P450, because it oxidizes a broad range of drugs and xenobiotics (16).

Recently, the effect of a normal amount of grapefruit juice (250 mL three times daily) on drug-metabolizing enzymes of the small bowel and liver was reported in an *in vivo* investigation in humans (17). Grapefruit juice consumption for 5 days caused a mean 62% reduction of small bowel enterocyte CYP3A4 and CYP3A5 protein content associated with a greater than three- and five-fold increase in felodipine AUC and C_{max}, respectively. In contrast, liver CYP3A4 activity, as measured by the erythromycin breath test, and colon CYP3A5 protein content were not altered. Also, intestinal CYP2D6 and CYP1A1 protein content were not affected. Although these changes were measured after 5 days of grapefruit juice, preliminary data also showed that small bowel CYP3A4 can be markedly reduced 4 hours after a single glass of juice. Consequently, it was concluded that grapefruit juice acted by selectively inhibiting CYP3A isozymes of the small bowel to cause greater felodipine oral bioavailability.

Decreased expression of CYP3A isoforms by grapefruit juice implied that the interaction was not simple competition for substrate metabolism. Because small bowel CYP3A4 mRNA was not changed (17), grapefruit juice likely decreased CYP3A4 protein content by a post-transcriptional mechanism, possibly involving accelerated CYP3A4 degradation through mechanism-based (suicide) enzyme inactivation. Thus, the return of CYP3A4 activity would require de novo enzyme synthesis.

The duration of activity of grapefruit juice has been studied. In one study, consumption of a single glass (200 mL) of juice at various time intervals before felodipine showed that the extent of increase in felodipine AUC and C_{max} was maximal between simultaneous and 4-hour previous juice administration with drug (18). Then, the magnitude of the interaction declined slowly with increasing time interval between grapefruit juice and felodipine administration. The half-life of effect of grapefruit juice was estimated at 12 hours. Higher felodipine C_{max} was still evident when grapefruit juice was consumed 24 hours before felodipine. In another investigation, the effect of routine grapefruit juice consumption was evaluated (17). One glass (250 mL) of grapefruit juice augmented mean felodipine AUC and C_{max} to 267% and 345%, respectively, in comparison to water. Grapefruit juice three times daily with meals for 5 days further increased felodipine AUC and C_{max} to 345% and 538% in comparison to water, showing a cumulative effect of the juice.

The magnitude of the interaction was highly variable among individuals, ranging from no change to six-fold greater plasma felodipine AUC and C_{max} with grapefruit juice compared to water under single dose conditions (2,5,17,19). However, results were reproducible within individuals following repeat testing and, thus, were dependent on factors inherent to the individual (19). Grapefruit juice reduced small bowel CYP3A4 content contingent upon pretreatment levels (17). Individuals with the highest small bowel CYP3A4 content before grapefruit juice had the largest reduction in CYP3A4 and highest increase in felodipine C_{max} with grapefruit juice. Consequently, individual disparity in the magnitude of interaction with grapefruit juice appears at least partially explained by innate differences in baseline small bowel CYP3A4 protein content.

MEDICATIONS ASSESSED FOR INTERACTION WITH GRAPEFRUIT JUICE

Drugs Interacting with Grapefruit Juice

Medications that produce a pharmacokinetic interaction with grapefruit juice are listed in Table 50-1 and all are substrates for CYP3A4. The most extensively studied are the dihydropyridine calcium channel antagonists, that is, felodipine (1,9,12,17–21), amlodipine (22,23), nicardipine (24), nifedipine (1,25–27), nitrendipine (28,29), nisoldipine (30), and nimodipine (31), which vary markedly in their extent of presystemic drug metabolism and oral bioavailability (32). Based on the mechanism of interaction, it would be expected that the inherent oral bioavailability of a dihydropyridine would influence the magnitude of the interaction with grapefruit juice. This appears to be partially true. For example, nisoldipine and amlodipine have very low and very high innate oral bioavailability, respectively. The mean

TABLE 50-1. *Drugs interacting with grapefruit juice*

Cardiovascular agents
  Felodipine (1,9,12,17–21)
  Nicardipine (24)
  Nifedipine (1,25–27)
  Nimodipine (31)
  Nisoldipine (30)
  Nitrendipine (28,29)
  Verapamil (38)
Histamine H_1 antagonists
  Astemizole (65)
  Terfenadine (57–60)
Gastrointestinal agents
  Cisapride (66)
Antilipemic agents
  Atorvastatin (74)
  Lovastatin (72)
  Simvastatin (73)
Central nervous system agents
  Buspirone (75)
  Carbamazepine (76)
  Diazepam (83)
  Midazolam (81)
  Triazolam (82)
Immunosuppressive agents
  Cyclosporine (85–91)
  Tacrolimus (93)
Antiinfective agents
  Saquinavir (94)
Estrogens
  Ethinylestradiol (96)

(range) magnitude of increase of plasma drug C_{max} concentrations of nisoldipine (30) and amlodipine (22) with grapefruit juice were four-fold greater (no change to 8.5-fold higher) and no change (no change to 1.6-fold higher), respectively. Thus, nisoldipine had a greater proportional increase in both mean and individual variability of plasma drug concentrations compared to amlodipine. This larger and more unpredictable effect with nisoldipine should alert health professionals to the potential consequences of the interaction between grapefruit juice and a dihydropyridine possessing low innate oral bioavailability.

All dihydropyridines, apart from nifedipine, have a chiral center with the activity primarily residing with a particular enantiomer (10). Therefore, the relevance of an interaction with grapefruit juice would depend mostly on the magnitude of increase of the more active enantiomer. For nitrendipine, the S-enantiomer appears to possess all the activity (33,34). Grapefruit juice produced proportional enhancement of both enantiomers, indicating that the increase in plasma total nitrendipine concentration was predictive of the pharmacodynamic extent of interaction (28). For nicardipine, the S-enantiomer has one third the activity of the R-enantiomer (35). Grapefruit juice augmented S-nicardipine AUC and C_{max} by 1.5- and 1.2-fold more, respectively, than R-nicardipine, demonstrating that the increase in plasma total nicardipine concentration may slightly overestimate associated clinical consequences (24).

The opposite situation may exist for the nondihydropyridine calcium channel antagonist, verapamil. The S-enantiomer of verapamil has at least ten times the dromotropic activity compared to the R-enantiomer (36). Although grapefruit juice did not change verapamil pharmacokinetics under single-dose conditions (37), it produced mean plasma total verapamil and norverapamil AUCs that were 143% and 128%, respectively, of that of water, following repeated drug and juice administration (38). Despite these relatively small changes in pharmacokinetics, first degree heart block (PR interval > 240 msec) was observed in only subjects (4 of 24) who received verapamil with grapefruit juice. Although the intersubject variation of the interaction was not reported, it is possible that grapefruit juice preferentially augmented S-verapamil and thus the increase in plasma total verapamil concentrations would underestimate the importance of the interaction.

The nonsedating antihistamines, terfenadine (39–48) and astemizole (49), and the gastrointestinal prokinetic agent, cisapride (50), can cause a life threatening ventricular arrhythmia, torsades de pointes. Conditions in which there is electrocardiographic QT interval prolongation increase the risk of development of this arrhythmia. Terfenadine and likely astemizole and cisapride appear to act in a concentration-dependent manner to block the potassium rectifier current in cardiac conduction pathways, which is the basis for QT interval prolongation (51–60). Thus, conditions in which plasma concentrations of these drugs are markedly elevated are associated with increased risk of development of torsades de pointes. Terfenadine has almost complete presystemic elimination (61,62), whereas astemizole undergoes very high presystemic metabolism, resulting in an estimated 3% oral bioavailability (63). Cisapride normally has intermediate presystemic metabolism by CYP3A4 and a 40% to 50% absolute oral bioavailability (64). Because grapefruit juice can increase the oral bioavailability of terfenadine (57–60), astemizole (65), and cisapride (66), it is prudent to avoid consumption of this juice with these medications. Alternative pharmacotherapy could include the nonsedating antihistamines, cetirizine, fexofenadine (active metabolite of terfenadine), or loratidine, which do not appear to prolong QT interval. Metoclopramide or domperidone are possible alternatives for cisapride.

The HMG-CoA reductase inhibitors, lovastatin (67–69) and simvastatin (70,71), belong to an important class of cholesterol-lowering medications, but their use can be associated with diffuse myalgia and marked elevation of creatine phosphokinase. There have been reports of severe rhabdomyolysis that precipitated acute renal failure. The mechanism of this adverse drug effect has not been clearly defined. However, it appears to occur in conditions in which plasma concentrations of the parent drug and metabolite are profoundly elevated, suggesting that this adverse effect has a pharmacokinetic basis. Both lovastatin and simvastatin have very low oral bioavailability from high presystemic metabolism by CYP3A4. Grapefruit juice produced more than ten-fold higher plasma concentrations of lovastatin (72) and simvastatin (73), indicating that a clinically important interaction may occur between this juice and these two medications. Grapefruit juice doubled atorvastatin AUC (74). The effect on cerivastatin and fluvastatin has not been reported to our knowledge. However, pravastatin is not metabolized by CYP3A4 to any significant extent and pravastatin did not interact with grapefruit juice (74).

Buspirone is an anxiolytic agent that produces less sedation and impairment of psychomotor function than benzodiazepines. It has only about 5% oral bioavailability because of extensive first pass metabolism. Concomitant grapefruit juice administration substantially increased plasma buspirone concentrations (75). Buspirone AUC and C_{max} were 920% and 430% higher, respectively, with grapefruit juice compared to water. A visual analogue scale used to measure overall drug activity showed that the effect of buspirone was increased when it was administered with grapefruit juice.

Carbamazepine is an effective anticonvulsant with a narrow therapeutic index, but it is still considered a drug of first choice for the management of partial and tonic-clonic seizures. Carbamazepine is metabolized to an active metabolite, 10,11-epoxide, by CYP3A4. Hospital-

ized epileptic patients who routinely received carbamazepine, 200 mg three times daily, were given their morning dose of carbamazepine with grapefruit juice (76). Single-dose administration of grapefruit juice increased carbamazepine AUC, C_{max}, and C_{min} to 140% compared to water. It was concluded that improved carbamazepine bioavailability by grapefruit juice warrants clinicians to instruct patients to avoid consumption of grapefruit juice with this drug because of the possibility of adverse effects.

Midazolam is an ultra-short–acting benzodiazepine hypnotic with low oral bioavailability because of high presystemic drug metabolism. Substantial presystemic metabolism appears to occur in both the small bowel and liver (77,78). The major primary metabolite, 1'-hydroxy-midazolam, is generated by CYP3A4 (79,80). Grapefruit juice did not alter midazolam intravenous pharmacokinetics (81). However, it produced mean oral midazolam AUC and C_{max} that were 152% and 156%, respectively, those of water (81). This was caused by an estimated 41% decrease of small bowel midazolam metabolism. The time to midazolam C_{max} (t_{max}) was increased to 179% that of water. Psychometric tests (reaction times, Digit Symbol Substitution Test) showed greater patient impairment when oral midazolam was administered with grapefruit juice compared to water. Grapefruit juice augmented triazolam AUC, C_{max}, and t_{max} to 148%, 130%, and 156%, respectively, of that of water (82). Triazolam $t_{1/2}$ was not changed. Drowsiness was significantly enhanced. Diazepam AUC and C_{max} were increased to 320% and 150% by grapefruit juice compared to water (83).

Cyclosporine is the cornerstone for immunosuppression therapy following transplantation. Plasma cyclosporine concentrations must be maintained within a narrow range to achieve adequate immunosuppression without nephrotoxicity. However, cyclosporine possesses low and variable oral bioavailability. Although this has been attributed to poor drug solubility and diffusion characteristics, more recent work has supported presystemic cyclosporine metabolism as a factor (84). In two studies of healthy volunteers, grapefruit juice produced mean oral cyclosporine AUCs that were 162% and 143% those with water (85,86). Intravenous cyclosporine pharmacokinetics were not altered (85). Orange juice did not augment cyclosporine AUC (86). Several studies were conducted in medically stable renal transplant patients (87–91). Grapefruit juice was given with the patient's usual oral dose of cyclosporine to achieve steady-state effects. The effect of grapefruit juice on cyclosporine pharmacokinetics varied among studies. Plasma cyclosporine AUC (88,90,91) and trough concentration (87,90), which is commonly used during therapeutic drug monitoring, were augmented in some investigations. The largest mean interaction was a cyclosporine AUC and trough concentration with grapefruit juice that were 134% and 177%, respectively, of that compared to water

(90). There was more than a tripling in plasma trough cyclosporine concentration in at least one patient, which undoubtedly is clinically important (91). Because cyclosporine is very expensive, administration with grapefruit juice has been suggested as a technique to decrease drug costs (86). However, the magnitude of the effect was variable among individuals, and the constancy of the interaction with repeat dosing among brands or batches of grapefruit juice has not been documented. Thus, concurrent administration of grapefruit juice cannot be recommended as a therapeutic strategy for such patients (92). Another immunosuppressant, tacrolimus, is extensively metabolized by CYP3A4 and it is indicated that grapefruit juice should be avoided with this drug as well (93).

Saquinavir, a drug used in patients with acquired immunodeficiency syndrome (AIDS), belongs to a new class of agents known as protease inhibitors. Its very low bioavailability is, in part, due to presystemic metabolism by CYP3A4. A glass of grapefruit juice (400 mL) increased the absolute oral bioavailability of saquinavir by a factor of two, from 0.7% to 1.4% (94). Grapefruit juice did not alter intravenous saquinavir pharmacokinetics. Although most grapefruit juice–drug interactions have the potential for increased drug toxicity, this does not appear to be the case for saquinavir. Thus, concomitant administration of grapefruit juice has been suggested as a strategy to increase saquinavir bioavailability. Although the magnitude of the interaction may be variable among patients, it appears to have only the potential to enhance therapeutic benefit. However, it would still be appropriate to confirm sustained elevated plasma saquinavir concentrations with chronic drug and grapefruit juice administration and lack of adverse interaction with other medications in the AIDS patient's regimen.

Ethinylestradiol has an oral bioavailability of 42% as a result of extensive first pass biotransformation (95). In contrast to herbal tea, single-dose grapefruit juice increased ethinylestradiol AUC and C_{max} to 128% and 137% in healthy volunteers (96). Whether the extent of this effect is clinically important requires investigation in long-term studies.

Drugs Not Interacting with Grapefruit Juice

Medications that were not affected by grapefruit juice are listed in Table 50-2. Based on the proposed mechanism of action of grapefruit juice, it might be expected that plasma concentrations of amlodipine (22,23), clomipramine (97), haloperidol (98), acenocoumarol (99), warfarin (100), theophylline (101), and prednisone (89) would not be increased by grapefruit juice. These drugs inherently have high or nearly complete oral bioavailability. Thus, selective inhibition of small bowel drug metabolism by grapefruit juice would not be anticipated to increase plasma drug concentrations. Also, theophylline and prednisone are not substrates for CYP3A4.

TABLE 50-2. *Drugs not affected by grapefruit juice*

Cardiovascular agents
  Amlodipine (22,23)
  Diltiazem (104)
  Propafenone (106)
  Quinidine (105)
Central nervous system agents
  Clomipramine (97)
  Haloperidol (98)
Anticoagulants
  Acenocoumarol (99)
  Warfarin (100)
Antiinfective agents
  Clarithromycin (102)
  Itraconazole (103)
Antiasthmatic agents
  Theophylline (101)
Antiinflammatory agents
  Prednisone (89)
Estrogens
  17β-Estradiol (107)
Antilepmic agents
  Pravastatin (74)

On the other hand, the CYP3A4 substrates, clarithromycin (102) and itraconazole (103), have incomplete oral bioavailability but this appears mainly to be the result of inferior drug absorption rather than presystemic drug metabolism.

Other medications showing little interaction with grapefruit juice include diltiazem (104), quinidine (105), propafenone (106), and 17β-estradiol (107). Although these drugs are substrates for CYP3A4 and have at least some presystemic elimination, the lack of interaction with grapefruit juice may be explained by alternative major pathways of presystemic biotransformation. Therefore, inactivation of CYP3A4 by grapefruit juice might be expected merely to shift metabolism to other pathways.

ACTIVE INGREDIENTS IN GRAPEFRUIT JUICE

Identification of the active ingredients in grapefruit juice would permit prediction and evaluation of similar effects with other foods. In addition, grapefruit juice or the active ingredients it contains might be used to improve the therapeutic benefit of orally administered drugs (2,5), which is the preferred route of dosing because of better tolerability and suitability for long-term treatment. This strategy could be applied to drugs that undergo complete presystemic metabolism involving small bowel CYP3A4 and therefore are currently active and available only by the intravenous route. This approach could also be clinically useful for drugs with higher but incomplete presystemic elimination to produce greater and more dependable drug bioavailability and clinical response. Also, grapefruit juice did not alter hepatic CYP3A4 activity (17), indicating that addition of the active ingredients may not jeopardize a major mechanism for the inactivation of numerous medications and environmental substances. However, the persistence of hepatic CYP3A4 activity means that grapefruit juice would not be expected to produce complete oral drug bioavailability.

Because flavonoids have long been known to inhibit *in vitro* drug oxidative metabolism (108), they were initially considered as possible active constituents in grapefruit juice. Flavonoids are widely distributed in fruits and vegetables (109). Naringin is the most prevalent flavonoid in grapefruit juice, attaining relatively high concentrations (1 mmol/L). It is absent from orange juice, which did not increase plasma concentrations of felodipine (1) or cyclosporine (86). The effects of naringin and other flavonoids on the oxidation of felodipine and nifedipine by human liver microsomes have been studied (110,111). Although naringin inhibited the metabolism of these dihydropyridines, it was much less potent than its aglycone, naringenin (110). Naringenin is not normally present in grapefruit juice (109), but oral administration of the juice resulted in renal excretion of naringenin conjugates demonstrating *in vivo* formation of this potentially active species (112). Because naringenin was not detected in plasma and the total amount recovered in urine represented only a small percentage of the oral naringin dose in the juice (112), naringenin appears to have low systemic availability, which is consistent with the hypothesis of inhibition of felodipine metabolism localized to the small bowel. Nevertheless, commercially available naringin, in the same amount as found in grapefruit juice and administered as an aqueous solution with felodipine (21) or in a capsule with nisoldipine (30), produced little or no increase in plasma drug concentrations. The reasons for lack of *in vivo* activity of commercially available pure naringin have not been elucidated. Possible explanations include (a) loss of activity of naringin during purification from grapefruit juice, such as change in optical isomer composition (113), (b) lack of conversion to the more biologically active species, such as naringenin (2), (c) the requirement for several components in grapefruit juice to interact in order to produce inhibition of felodipine metabolism, or (d) naringin is not involved in the interaction (2).

Recently, furanocoumarins have been proposed as active ingredients in grapefruit juice. Initially, 6',7'-dihydroxybergamottin was suggested as a potentially active substance (114). It is present in grapefruit juice, but not orange juice, and produced inhibition of CYP3A-mediated testosterone oxidation by rat liver microsomes. In a Caco-2 cell culture model of human intestinal epithelium, 6',7'-dihydroxybergamottin was subsequently demonstrated to cause a dose-dependent decrease in CYP3A4 catalytic activity and immunoreactive CYP3A4 protein concentration (115). The concentration of 6',7'-dihydroxybergamottin in grapefruit juice was shown to exceed the IC_{50} for loss of CYP3A4 activity. CYP1A1

and CYP2D6 protein content was not affected. Recombinant CYP3A4 was initially competitively inhibited followed by mechanism-based inactivation. Thus, *in vitro* results initially suggested that 6',7'-dihydroxybergamottin may be a major active ingredient in grapefruit juice.

Subsequently, a study was conducted in humans to evaluate the role of naringin and 6',7'-dihydroxybergamottin in grapefruit juice–drug interactions (116). The approach was to separate grapefruit juice by centrifugation into two fractions (supernatant and particulate), which contained different amounts of these two substances. The effect of these fractions, grapefruit juice containing a comparable amount of both fractions, and water on the pharmacokinetics of oral felodipine were compared. Because the supernatant fraction had nearly all of the naringin and three-fold higher 6',7'-dihydroxybergamottin content than the particulate fraction, it was postulated that the activity of the supernatant fraction would range from being greater than that of the particulate fraction and equivalent to that of the grapefruit juice. However, this was not the case. Although the supernatant fraction was active compared to water, it produced a felodipine AUC that was less than that obtained with the particulate fraction. Thus, the hypothesis that naringin and/or 6',7'-dihydroxybergamottin were the main active substances in grapefruit juice was not supported. However, they may possess some *in vivo* activity. The findings of this study also underline the necessity of *in vivo* human testing when attempting to identify the active inhibitors of intestinal CYP3A4 in grapefruit juice and possibly other foodstuffs.

Recently, a more lipophilic analogue and metabolic precursor of 6',7'-dihydroxybergamottin, bergamottin, was shown to be the major furanocoumarin in juice from fresh pink grapefruit sections and to act as a potent *in vitro* mechanism-based inhibitor of CYP3A4 (117). Preliminary data from our laboratory also indicated that bergamottin is found in high concentrations in commercial white grapefruit juice and was measurable only in the particulate fraction (116). Other furanocoumarin dimers isolated from grapefruit juice also have been reported to inhibit the *in vitro* activity of human CYP3A4 (115, 118). However, a final decision on their importance in grapefruit juice–drug interactions must await results from testing in human subjects.

CONCLUSION

A single normal amount of grapefruit juice has the potential to augment the oral bioavailability and to enhance the beneficial or adverse effects of a broad range of medications, even when juice is consumed hours beforehand. Grapefruit juice acts by reducing presystemic drug metabolism through inactivation of CYP3A isoforms in the small bowel. Isolation of the active ingredients may lead to identification of other foods producing this interaction or to its incorporation into pharmaceutical formulations. The serendipitous observation of increased plasma felodipine concentrations by grapefruit juice has provided fundamental new knowledge to improve pharmacotherapy and to stimulate research.

REFERENCES

1. Bailey DG, Spence JD, Munoz C, Arnold JMO. Interaction of citrus juices with felodipine and nifedipine. *Lancet* 1991;337:268–269.
2. Bailey DG, Arnold JMO, Spence JD. Grapefruit juice and drugs: how significant is the interaction? *Clin Pharmacokinet* 1994;26:91–98.
3. Ameer B, Weintraub RA. Drug interactions with grapefruit juice. *Clin Pharmacokinet* 1997;33:103–121.
4. Fuhr U. Drug interactions with grapefruit juice. Extent, probable mechanism and clinical relevance. *Drug Saf* 1998;18:251–272.
5. Bailey DG, Arnold JMO, Spence JD. Grapefruit juice-drug interactions. *Br J Clin Pharmacol* 1998;46:101–110.
6. Bailey DG, Spence JD, Edgar B, Bayliff CD, Arnold JMO. Ethanol enhances the hemodynamic effects of felodipine. *Clin Invest Med* 1989;12:357–362.
7. Edgar B, Regardh CG, Johnsson G, et al. Felodipine kinetics in healthy man. *Clin Pharmacol Ther* 1985;38:205–211.
8. Blychert E, Edgar B, Elmfeldt D, Hedner T. A population study of the pharmaco-kinetics of felodipine. *Br J Clin Pharmacol* 1991;31:15–24.
9. Lundahl J, Regardh CG, Edgar B, Johnsson G. Effects of grapefruit juice ingestion—pharmacokinetics and haemodynamics of intravenously and orally administered felodipine in healthy men. *Eur J Clin Pharmacol* 1997;52:139–145.
10. Regardh CG, Baarnhielm C, Edgar B, Hoffman KJ. Pharmacokinetics and biotransformation of 1,4-dihydropyridine calcium antagonists. *Prog Drug Metab* 1990;12:41–86.
11. Guengerich FP, Brian WR, Iwasaki M, Sari MA, Baarnhielm C, Berntsson P. Oxidation of dihydropyridine calcium channel blockers and analogues by human liver cytochrome P450IIIA4. *J Med Chem* 1991;34:1834–1844.
12. Bailey DG, Bend JR, Arnold JMO, Tran LT, Spence JD. Erythromycin-felodipine interaction:magnitude, mechanism, and comparison with grapefruit juice. *Clin Pharmacol Ther* 1996;60:25–33.
13. Kolars JC, Schmiedlin-Rem P, Schuetz JD, Fang C, Watkins PB. Identification of rifampicin-inducible P450IIIA4 (CYP3A4) in human small bowel enterocytes. *J Clin Invest* 1992;90:1871–1878.
14. De Waziers I, Cugnenc PH, Yan CS, Leroux JP, Beaune PH. Cytochrome P450 isoenzymes, epoxide hydrolase and glutathione transferases in rat and human hepatic and extrahepatic tissues. *J Pharmacol Exp Ther* 1990;253:287–294.
15. Lown KS, Kolars JC, Thummel KE, et al. Interpatient heterogeneity in expression of CYP3A4 and CYP3A5 in small bowel—lack of prediction by the erythromycin breath test. *Drug Metab Dispos* 1994;22:947–955.
16. Guengerich FP. Catalytic selectivity of human cytochrome P450 enzymes: relevance to drug metabolism and toxicity. *Toxicol Let* 1994;70:133–138.
17. Lown KS, Bailey DG, Fontana RJ, et al. Grapefruit juice increases felodipine oral availability in humans by decreasing intestinal CYP3A protein expression. *J Clin Invest* 1997;99:2545–2553.
18. Lundahl J, Regardh CG, Edgar B, Johnsson G. Relationship between time of intake of grapefruit juice and its effect on pharmacokinetics and pharmacodynamics of felodipine in healthy subjects. *Eur J Clin Pharmacol* 1995;49:61–67.
19. Bailey DG, Arnold JMO, Bend JR, Tran LT, Spence JD. Grapefruit juice-felodipine interaction:reproducibility and characterization with the extended release drug formulation. *Br J Clin Pharmacol* 1995;40:135–140.
20. Edgar B, Bailey DG, Bergstrand R, Johnsson G, Regardh CG. Acute effects of drinking grapefruit juice on the pharmacokinetics and pharmacodyanmics of felodipine—and its potential clinical relevance. *Eur J Clin Pharmacol* 1992;42:313–317.
21. Bailey DG, Arnold JMO, Munoz C, Spence JD. Grapefruit juice-felodipine interaction: mechanism, predictability and effect of naringin. *Clin Pharmacol Ther* 1993;53:637–642.
22. Josefsson M, Zackrisson AL, Ahlner J. Effect of grapefruit juice on the pharmacokinetics of amlodipine in healthy volunteers. *Eur J Clin Pharmacol* 1996;51:189–193.
23. Vincent J, Foulds G, Dogolo LC, Willavize SA, Friedman HL. Grapefruit juice does not alter the pharmacokinetics of amlodipine in man (abstr). *Clin Pharmacol Ther* 1997;61:233.
24. Uno T, Ohkubo T, Sugawara K, Higashiyama A, Motomura S. Effect of grapefruit juice on the disposition of nicardipine after administration of intravenous and oral doses (abstr). *Clin Pharmacol Ther* 1997;61:209.
25. Rashid J, McKinstry C, Renwick AG, Dirnhuber M, Waller DG, George CF. Quercetin, an in vitro inhibitor of CYP3A, does not contribute to the interaction between nifedipine and grapefruit juice. *Br J Clin Pharmacol* 1993;36:460–463.
26. Rashid TJ, Martin U, Clarke H, Waller DG, Renwick AG, George CF. Factors affecting the absolute bioavailability of nifedipine. *Br J Clin Pharmacol* 1995;40:51–58.
27. Sigush H, Hippius M, Henschel L, Kaufmann K, Hoffmann A. Influence of grapefruit juice on the pharmacokinetics of a slow release nifedipine formulation. *Pharmazie* 1994;49:522–524.
28. Soons PA, Vogels BAPM, Roosemalen MCM, et al. Grapefruit juice and cimetidine inhibit stereoselective metabolism of nitrendipine in man. *Clin Pharmacol Ther* 1991;50:394–403.
29. Bailey DG, Munoz C, Arnold JMO, Strong HA, Spence JD. Grapefruit juice and naringin interaction with nitrendipine (abstr). *Clin Pharmacol Ther* 1992;51:156.
30. Bailey DG, Arnold JMO, Strong HA, Munoz C, Spence JD. Effect of grapefruit juice and naringin on nisoldipine pharmacokinetics. *Clin Pharmacol Ther* 1993;54:589–594.
31. Fuhr U, Maier-Bruggemann A, Blume H, et al. Grapefruit juice increases oral nimodipine bioavailability. *In J Clin Pharmacol Ther* 1998;36:126–132.
32. Abernethy DR, Schwartz JB. Pharmacokinetics of calcium antagonists under development. *Clin Pharmacokinet* 1988;15:1–14.
33. Mikus G, Mast V, Ratge D, Wisser H, Eichelbaum M. Pharmacokinetics, hemodynamics and biochemical effects of the nitrendipine enantiomers (abstr). *Eur J Clin Pharmacol* 1989;36[Suppl]:A19.
34. Eltze M, Boer R, Sanders KH, Boss H, Ulrich WR, Flockerzi D. Stereoselective inhibition of thromboxane-induced coronary vasoconstriction by 1,4-dihydropyridine calcium channel antagonists. *Chirality* 1990;2:233–240.
35. Takenaka T, Miyazaki I, Asano M, Higuchi S, Maeno H. Vasodilator and hypotensive effects of the optical isomers of nicardipine (YC-93), a new Ca^{2+} antagonist. *Jpn J Pharmacol* 1982;32:665–670.
36. Echizen H, Manz M, Eichelbaum M. Electrophysiological effects of dextro- and levo-verapamil on sinus node and AV node function in humans. *J Cardiovasc Pharmacol* 1988;12:543–546.
37. Zaidenstein R, Dishi V, Gips M, et al. The effect of grapefruit juice on the pharmacokinetics of orally administered verapamil. *Eur J Clin Pharmacol* 1998;54:337–340.
38. Fuhr U, Harder S, Lopez-Rojas P, Muller-Peltzer H, Kern R, Staib AH. Increase of verapamil concentrations in steady state by coadministration of grapefruit juice (abstr). *Naunyn Schmiedebergs Arch Pharmacol* 1994;349[suppl]:R134.
39. Monahan BP, Ferguson CL, Killeavy ES, Lloyd BK, Troy J, Cantilena LR. Torsades de pointes occurring in association with terfenadine use. *JAMA* 1990;264:2788–2790.
40. Matthews DR, McNutt B, Okerholm R, Flicker M, McBride G. Torsades de pointes occurring in association with terfenadine use. *JAMA* 1991;266:2375–2376.
41. Zimmermann M, Duruz H, Guinand O, et al. Torsades de pointes after treatment with terfenadine and ketoconazole. *Eur Heart J* 1992;13:1002–1003.
42. Pratt CM, Hertz RP, Ellis BE, Cromwell SP, Louv W, Moye L. Risk of developing life-threatening ventricular arrhythmia associated with terfenadine in comparison with over-the-counter antihistamines, ibuprofen and clemastine. *Am J Cardiol* 1994;73:346–352.
43. Crane JK, Shih H-T. Syncope and cardiac arrhythmia due to an interaction between itraconazole and terfenadine. *Am J Med* 1993;95:445–446.
44. Pohjola-Sintonen S, Viitasalo L, Toivonen L, Neuvonen P. Torsades de pointes after terfenadine-itraconazole interaction. *BMJ* 1993;306:186.
45. Paris DG, Parente TF, Bruschetta HR, Guzman E, Niarchos AP. Torsades de pointes induced by erythromycin and terfenadine. *Am J Emerg Med* 1994;12:636–638.

46. Koh KK, Rim MS, Yoon J, Kim SS. Torsades de pointes induced by terfenadine in a patient with long QT syndrome. *J Electrocardiol* 1994; 27:343–346.

47. Kamisako T, Adachi Y, Nakagawa H, Yamamoto T. Torsades de pointes associated with terfenadine in a case of liver cirrhosis and hepatocellular carcinoma. *Intern Med* 1995;34:92–95.

48. Spence JD. Drug interactions with grapefruit: whose responsibility is to warn the public? *Clin Pharmacol Ther* 1997;61:395–400.

49. Tsai WC, Tasi LM, Chen JH. Combined use of astemizole and ketoconazole resulting in torsades de pointes. *J Formos Med Assoc* 1997; 96:144–146.

50. Wysowsk DK, Bacsanyi J. Cisapride and fatal arrhythmia. *N Engl J Med* 1996;335:290–291.

51. Woosley RL, Chen Y, Freiman JP, Gillis RA. Mechanism of the cardiotoxic actions of terfenadine. *JAMA* 1993;269:1532–1536.

52. Yang T, Prakash C, Roden DM, Snyders DJ. Mechanism of block of a human cardiac potassium channel by terfenadine racemate and enantiomers. *Br J Pharmacol* 1995;115:267–274.

53. Rampe D, Wible B, Brown AM, Dage RC. Effects of terfenadine and its metabolites on a delayed rectifier K+ channel cloned from human heart. *Mol Pharmacol* 1993;44:1240–1245.

54. Honig PK, Wortham DC, Zamani K, Conner DP, Mullin JC, Cantilena LR. Terfenadine-ketoconazole interaction: pharmacokinetic and electrocardiographic consequences. *JAMA* 1993;269:1513–1518.

55. Honig PK, Worthman DC, Hull R, Zamani K, Smith JE, Cantilena LR. Itraconazole affects single-dose terfenadine pharmacokinetics and cardiac repolarization pharmacodynamics. *J Clin Pharmacol* 1993;33: 1201–1206.

56. Honig PK, Woosley RL, Samani K, Conner DP, Cantilena LR. Changes in the pharmacokinetics and electrocardiographic pharmacodynamics of terfenadine with concomitant administration of erythromycin. *Clin Pharmacol Ther* 1992;52:231–238.

57. Benton RE, Honig PK, Zamani K, Cantilena LR, Woosley RL. Grapefruit juice alters terfenadine pharmacokinetics, resulting in prolongation of repolarization on the electrocardiogram. *Clin Pharmacol Ther* 1996; 59:383–388.

58. Honig PK, Wortham DC, Lazarev A, Cantilena LR. Grapefruit juice alters the systemic bioavailability and cardiac repolarization of terfenadine in poor metabolizers of terfenadine. *J Clin Pharmacol* 1996;36: 345–351.

59. Rau SE, Bend JR, Arnold JMO, Tran LT, Spence JD, Bailey DG. Grapefruit juice-terfenadine single-dose interaction: magnitude, mechanism, and relevance. *Clin Pharmacol Ther* 1997;61:401–409.

60. Clifford CP, Adams DA, Murray S, et al. The cardiac effect of terfenadine after inhibition of its metabolism by grapefruit juice. *Eur J Clin Pharmacol* 1997;52:311–315.

61. Garteiz DA, Hook RH, Walker BJ, Okerholm RA. Pharmacokinetics and biotransformation studies of terfenadine in man. *Arzneim Forsch Drug Res* 1982;32:1185–1190.

62. Yun C-H, Okerholm RA, Guengerich FP. Oxidation of the antihistamine drug terfenadine in human liver microsomes. Role of cytochrome P-4503A(4) in N-dealkylation and C-hydroxylation. *Drug Metab Dispos* 1993;21:403–409.

63. Krstenansky PM, Cluxton RJ. Astemizole: a long-acting, nonsedating antihistamine. *Drug Intell Clin Pharm* 1987;21:947–953.

64. Bedford TA, Rowbotham DJ. Cisapride: drug interactions of clinical significance. *Drug Saf* 1996;15:167–175.

65. Johnson & Johnson—Merck Consumer Pharmaceuticals of Canada. *Hismanal Product Monograph.* Guelph, Ontario, 1999.

66. Gross AS, Goh YD, Addison RS, Shenfield GM. Influence of grapefruit juice on cisapride pharmacokinetics. *Clin Pharmacol Ther* 1999; 65:395–401.

67. Lees RS, Lees AM. Rhabdomyolysis from the coadministration of lovastatin and the antifungal agent itraconazole. *N Engl J Med* 1995; 333:664–665.

68. Spach DH, Bauwens JE, Clark CD, Burke WG. Rhabdomyolysis associated with lovastatin and erythromycin use. *West J Med* 1991;154: 213–215.

69. Norman DJ, Illingworth DR, Murson J, Hosenpud J. Myolysis and acute renal failure in a heart-transplant patient receiving lovastatin. *N Engl J Med* 1988;318:46–47.

70. Meier C, Stey C, Brack T, Maggiorini M, Risti B, Krahenbuhl S. Rhabdomyolysis in patients treated with simvastatin and cyclosporin: role of the hepatic cytochrome P450 enzyme system activity. *Schweiz Med Wochenschr* 1995;125:1342–1346.

71. Deslypere JP, Vermeulen A. Rhabdomyolysis and simvastatin. *Ann Intern Med* 1991;114:342.

72. Kantola T, Kivisto KT, Neuvonen PJ. Grapefruit juice greatly increases serum concentrations of lovastatin and lovastatin acid. *Clin Pharmacol Ther* 1998;63:397–402.

73. Lilja JJ, Kivisto KT, Neuvonen PJ. Grapefruit juice-simvastatin interaction: effect on serum concentrations of simvastatin, simvastatin acid, and HMG-CoA reductase inhibitors. *Clin Pharmacol Ther* 1998;64: 477–483.

74. Neuvonen PJ, Lilja J, Kivisto KT. Grapefruit juice increases serum simvastatin and atorvastatin but not pravastatin (abstr). *Clin Pharmacol Ther* 1999;65:180.

75. Lilja JJ, Kivisto KT, Backman JT, Lamberg TS, Neuvonen PJ. Grapefruit juice substantially increases plasma concentrations of buspirone. *Clin Pharmacol Ther* 1998;64:655–660.

76. Garg SJ, Kumar N, Bhargava VK, Prabhakar SK. Effect of grapefruit juice on carbamazepine bioavailability in patients with epilepsy. *Clin Pharmacol Ther* 1998;64:286–288.

77. Thummel KE, O'Shea D, Paine MF, et al. Oral first-pass elimination of midazolam involves both gastrointestinal and hepatic CYP3A-mediated metabolism. *Clin Pharmacol Ther* 1996;59:491–502.

78. Paine MF, Shen DD, Kunze KL, et al. First-pass metabolism of midazolam by the human intestine. *Clin Pharmacol Ther* 1996;60: 14–24.

79. Kronbach T, Mathys D, Umeno M, Gonzalez FJ, Meyer UA. Oxidation of midazolam and triazolam by human liver cytochrome P450IIIA4. *Mol Pharmacol* 1989;36:89–96.

80. Gorski JC, Hall SD, Jones DR, VandenBranden M, Wrighton SA. Regioselective biotransformation of midazolam by members of the human cytochrome P450 3A (CYP3A) subfamily. *Biochem Pharmacol* 1994;47:1643–1653.

81. Kupferschmidt HHT, Ha HR, Ziegler WH, Meir PJ, Krahenbuhl S. Interaction between grapefruit juice and midazolam in humans. *Clin Pharmacol Ther* 1995;58:20–28.

82. Hukkinen SK, Varhe A, Olkkola KT, Neuvonen PJ. Plasma concentrations of triazolam are increased by concomitant ingestion of grapefruit juice. *Clin Pharmacol Ther* 1995;58:127–131.

83. Ozedemir M, Aktan Y, Boydag BS, Cingi MI, Musmul A. Interaction between grapefruit juice and diazepam in humans. *Eur J Drug Metab Pharmacokinet* 1998;1:55–59.

84. Kolars JC, Awni WM, Merion RM, Watkins PB. First-pass metabolism of cyclosporin by the gut. *Lancet* 1991;338:1488–1490.

85. Ducharme MP, Warbasse LH, Edwards DJ. Disposition of intravenous and oral cyclosporine after administration with grapefruit juice. *Clin Pharmacol Ther* 1995;57:485–491.

86. Yee GC, Stanley DL, Pessa JL, et al. Effect of grapefruit juice on blood cyclosporin concentration. *Lancet* 1995;345:955–956.

87. Ducharme MP, Provenzano R, Dehoorne-Smith M, Edwards DJ. Trough concentrations of cyclosporine following administration with grapefruit juice. *Br J Clin Pharmacol* 1993;36:457–459.

88. Herlitz H, Edgar B, Hedner T, Lidman K, Karlberg I. Grapefruit juice: a possible source of variability in blood concentration of cyclosporin A (letter). *Nephrol Dial Transplant* 1993;8:375.

89. Hollander AAMJ, van Rooij J, Lentjes EGWM, et al. The effect of grapefruit juice on cyclosporin and prednisone metabolism in transplant patients. *Clin Pharmacol Ther* 1995;57:318–324.

90. Proppe DG, Hoch OD, McLean AJ, Visser KE. Influence of chronic ingestion of grapefruit juice on steady state blood concentrations of cyclosporine A in renal transplant patients with stable graft function. *Br J Clin Pharmacol* 1995;39:337.

91. Min DI, Ku Y-M, Perry PJ, et al. Effect of grapefruit juice on cyclosporine pharmacokinetics in renal transplant patients. *Transplantation* 1996;62:123–125.

92. Johnston A, Holt DW. Effect of grapefruit juice on blood cyclosporin concentration. *Lancet* 1995;346:122–123.

93. Fujisawa Canada Inc. Prograf Product Monograph. Markham, Ontario, 1999.

94. Kupferschmidt HH, Fattinger KE, Ha HR, Follath F, Krahenbuhl S. Grapefruit juice enhances the bioavailability of the HIV protease inhibitor saquinavir in man. *Br J Clin Pharmacol* 1998;45:355–359.

95. Back DJ, Breckenridge AM, Crawford FE. An investigation of the phar-

macokinetics of ethinylestradiol in women using radioimmunoassay. *Contraception* 1979;20:263–273.

96. Weber A, Jager R, Borner A, et al. Can grapefruit juice influence ethinylestradiol bioavailability? *Contraception* 1996;53:41–47.

97. Oesterheld J, Kallepalli BR. Grapefruit juice and clomipramine: shifting metabolic ratios (letter). *J Clin Psychopharmacol* 1997;1:62–63.

98. Yasui N, Kondo T, Suzuki A, et al. Lack of significant pharmacokinetic interaction between haloperidol and grapefruit juice. *Int Clin Psychopharmacol* 1999;14:113–118.

99. van Rooij J, van der Meer FJM, Schoemaker HC, Cohen AF. Comparison of the effect of grapefruit juice and cimetidine on pharmacokinetics and anticoagulant effect of a single dose of acenocoumarol (abstr). *Br J Clin Pharmacol* 1993;35:548P.

100. Sullivan DM, Ford MA, Boyden TW. Grapefruit juice and the response to warfarin. *Am J Health Syst Pharm* 1998;55:1581–1583.

101. Fuhr U, Maier A, Keller A, Steinijans VW, Sauter R, Staib AH. Lacking effect of grapefruit juice on theophylline pharmacokinetics. *Int J Clin Pharmacol Ther* 1995;33:311–314.

102. Cheng KL, Nafziger AN, Peloquin CA, Amsden GW. Effect of grapefruit juice on clarithromycin pharmacokinetics. *Antimicrob Agents Chemother* 1998;42:927–929.

103. Kawakami M, Suzuki K, Ishizuka T, Hidaka T, Matsuki Y, Nakamura H. Effect of grapefruit juice on pharmacokinetics of itraconazole in healthy subjects. *Int J Clin Pharmacol Ther* 1998;36:306–308.

104. Sigusch H, Henschel L, Kraul H, Merkel U, Hoffmann A. Lack of effect of grapefruit juice on diltiazem bioavailability in normal subjects. *Pharmazie* 1994;49:675–679.

105. Min DI, Ku Y-M, Geraets DR, Lee H-C. Effect of grapefruit juice on the pharmacokinetics and pharmacodynamics of quinidine in healthy volunteers. *J Clin Pharmacol*;36:469–476.

106. Munoz CE, Ito S, Bend JR, et al. Propafenone interaction with CYP3A4 inhibitors in man (abstract). *Clin Pharmacol Ther* 1997;61:154.

107. Schubert W, Cullberg G, Edgar B, Hedner T. Inhibition of 17β-estradiol metabolism by grapefruit juice in ovariectomized women. *Maturitas* 1994;20:155–163.

108. Buening MK, Change RL, Huang MT, Fortner JG, Wood AW, Conney AH. Activation and inhibition of benzo(a)pyrene and aflatoxin B_1 metabolism in human liver microsomes by naturally occurring flavonoids. *Cancer Res* 1981;41:67–72.

109. Kuhnau J. The flavonoids: a class of semi-essential food components; their role in human nutrition. *World Rev Nutr Diet* 1976;24:117–191.

110. Guengerich FP, Kim DH. In vitro inhibition of dihydropyridine oxidation and aflatoxin B_1 activation in human liver microsomes by naringenin and other flavonoids. *Carcinogenesis* 1990;11:2275–2279.

111. Miniscalco A, Lundahl J, Regardh CG, Edgar B, Eriksson UG. Inhibition of dihydropyridine metabolism in rat and human liver microsomes by flavonoids found in grapefruit juice. *J Pharmacol Exp Therap* 1992;261:1196–1199.

112. Fuhr U, Kummert AL. The fate of naringin in humans: a key to grapefruit juice-drug interactions? *Clin Pharmacol Ther* 1995;58:365–373.

113. Gaffield W, Lundin RE, Gentilli B, Horowitz RM. C-2 stereochemistry of naringin and its relation to taste and biosynthesis in maturing grapefruit. *Bioorg Chem* 1975;4:259–269.

114. Edwards DJ, Bellevue FH, Woster PM. Identification of 6′,7′-dihydroxybergamottin, a cytochrome P450, in grapefruit juice. *Drug Metab Dispos* 1996;24:1287–1290.

115. Schmiedlin-Ren P, Edwards DJ, Fitzsimmons ME, et al. Mechanisms of enhanced oral availability of CYP3A4 substrates by grapefruit juice constituents: decreased enterocyte CYP3A4 concentration and mechanism-based inactivation by furanocoumarins. *Drug Metab Dispos* 1997;25:1228–1233.

116. Bailey DG, Kreeft JH, Munoz C, Freeman DJ, Bend JR. Grapefruit juice-felodipine interaction: effect of naringin and 6′,7′-dihydroxybergamottin in humans. *Clin Pharmacol Ther* 1998;64:248–256.

117. He K, Iyer KR, Hayes RN, Sinz MW, Woolf TF, Hollenberg PF. Inactivation of cytochrome P450 3A4 by bergamottin, a component in grapefruit juice. *Chem Res Toxicol* 1998;11:252–259.

118. Fukuda K, Ohta T, Oshima Y, Ohashi N, Yoshikawa M, Yamazoe Y. Specific CYP3A4 inhibitors in grapefruit juice: furocoumarin dimers as components of drug interaction. *Pharmacogenetics* 1997;5:391–396.

Drugs as Inducers
of Metabolic Enzymes

CHAPTER 51

Phenobarbital, Phenytoin, and Carbamazepine

Susan M. Abdel-Rahman and J. Steven Leeder

PHENOBARBITAL

Pharmacology

Phenobarbital is among the oldest of the currently used anticonvulsant agents, approved for use by the Food and Drug Administration (FDA) in 1939. As with all barbiturates, phenobarbital exerts its activity by elevating seizure threshold in the motor cortex and limiting the spread of discharges from a seizure focus in the cortex, thalamus, and limbic systems. Thus, both presynaptic and postsynaptic excitability are diminished. Although the exact mechanism of action has not been fully elucidated, phenobarbital may modulate the activity of γ-aminobutyric acid.

Effects on Drug-Metabolizing Enzymes *In Vitro*

Phenobarbital is a pleiotropic agent that, among other effects, causes proliferation of hepatic smooth endoplasmic reticulum and induction of several drug-metabolizing enzymes, including cytochromes P450 and glucuronosyl transferases. Its inductive effects have been known for more than 40 years; indeed, phenobarbital is recognized as the prototypical inducer of a class of compounds with diverse chemical structures (1). Extensively studied in rodents and rodent-based systems, induction of members of the CYP2A, CYP2B, CYP2C, and CYP3A subfamilies by phenobarbital is well characterized (2).

Early *in vitro* investigations of phenobarbital induction in humans were limited to studies with panels of human

S. M. Abdel-Rahman: Departments of Pharmacy and Pediatrics, University of Missouri, Kansas City and Department of Clinical Pharmacology and Experimental Therapeutics, Children's Mercy Hospital, 2401 Gillham Road, Kansas City, Missouri 64108-4698

J. S. Leeder: Department of Pediatrics, University of Missouri, Kansas City and Department of Clinical Pharmacology and Toxicology, Children's Mercy Hospital, 2401 Gillham Road, Kansas City, Missouri 64108-4698

liver microsomes. In one study of eight individual samples, the concentration of a cytochrome P450 designated HLp (currently known as CYP3A4) was significantly increased in two patients having received dexamethasone, phenytoin (PHT), and phenobarbital (3). While the authors attributed the observed induction primarily to dexamethasone, studies with human-based systems in which all requisite regulatory elements are present and functional clearly indicate that phenobarbital is also capable of inducing cytochromes P450 (CYPs) and glucuronosyl transferases *in vitro*. For example, when primary cultures of human hepatocytes were incubated with 3.2 mM phenobarbital for 7 days, total P450 content increased 1.7- to 2-fold (4). A similar increase in pentoxyresorufin *O*-dealkylase activity was observed following 72 hours of culture with 2 mM phenobarbital (5). Donato and colleagues observed that optimal induction of ethoxycoumarin *O*-deethylation, a nonselective P450 substrate, was achieved with a 48-hour exposure to 1.5 mM phenobarbital and, furthermore, that this increased activity was accompanied by a two-fold increase in total P450 content (6). However, even though the results of these studies document the ability of phenobarbital to induce P450s in primary human hepatocytes, the specific isoforms induced were not identified.

More recent studies have been able to overcome this apparent deficiency through improvements in culture techniques and the development of isoform-specific reagents. In cultured hepatocytes from seven different donors, exposure to 2 mM phenobarbital for 48 to 72 hours produced 4.0- to 33-fold increases in microsomal immunoreactive CYP3A protein relative to the vehicle (DMSO) alone. The increased CYP3A content was accompanied by a 140% to 637% increase in cyclosporin A metabolism, a prototypic CYP3A substrate (7). In contrast, 48-hour exposure to 3.2 mM phenobarbital produced a modest (1.4- to 1.8-fold) increase in CYP2C8/9 immunoreactive protein and no change in CYP3A4 protein by another group (8,9). Donato and colleagues (10) reported 2.0- to 2.5-fold increases in testosterone hydroxylation in the 16α- and 16β-positions with smaller increases in 2β- and 6β-hydroxylated metabolites, suggesting moderated induction of the human CYP3A and CYP2C subfamilies. Chang and associates observed increases in immunoreactive CYP2B6, CYP2C8, CYP2C9, and CYP3A4 proteins following phenobarbital treatment (2 mM, 96 hours), whereas CYP1A1 and CYP1A2 expression was not affected (11). In this study, induction was accompanied by 1.9- to 6.8-fold increases in cyclophosphamide activation and 2.0- to 8.2-fold increases in ifosfamide activation, catalytic reactions that have been attributed to these CYP isoforms in humans (11). Approximately two-fold increases in CYP3A4-specific mRNA have also been observed (12,13). Studies with replicating human hepatoma cell lines (HepG2, TONG/HCC) indicate that phenobarbital also induces CYP3A7, but not CYP3A5, mRNA, or immunoreactive protein (12).

Cumulatively, the data indicate that phenobarbital produces moderate induction of CYP2C subfamily members and induces both CYP3A4 protein and catalytic activities, but is less potent as an inducer than dexamethasone or rifampin. The degree of induction observed in the various studies cited is highly variable, most likely as a consequence of the range of culture conditions (i.e., attachment surface, culture medium, and confluency of cultures) employed in different laboratories. With more standardized conditions, induction by phenobarbital and other inducers has been found to be highly reproducible in multiple laboratories, and phenobarbital is often used as a prototype inducer for *in vitro* induction studies (14). A more important issue is the fact that there is considerable intersubject variability in the extent of induction observed *in vitro*, consistent with the variability observed *in vivo*. Induction of phase II enzyme activities by phenobarbital has not been extensively studied, however. Induction of glucuronosyl transferases (UGTs) (15,16), glutathione S-transferase α (17), and epoxide hydrolase (18) activities by phenobarbital has been reported. However, almost all clinically significant drug–drug interactions involving phenobarbital induction involve the cytochromes P450.

Effects on Specific Drug-Metabolizing Enzymes *In Vivo*

Early studies of oxidative drug biotransformation in humans often used antipyrine as a general probe of cytochrome P450 activity. Chronic administration of phenobarbital, PHT, or carbamazepine (CBZ) is consistently associated with increased antipyrine clearance and, thus, microsomal drug oxidation capacity (19,20). More recent detailed studies of the P450s responsible for antipyrine

biotransformation indicate that CYPs 1A2, 2A6, 2C8, 2C9, 2C19, 2E1, and 3A4 all participate to some extent, but implicate CYPs 1A2 and 2C9 in the formation of 3-hydroxyantipyrine, CYPs 1A2 and 3A4 in the formation of 4-hydroxyantipyrine, and predominantly CYPs 2C9 and 1A2 in norantipyrine formation (21,22). However, no consistent patterns in antipyrine metabolite profiles have been observed in studies with healthy volunteers (23), and, therefore, no conclusions concerning induction of individual P450 isoforms can be made.

The urinary ratio of 6β-hydroxycortisol to cortisol has been proposed as a marker of CYP3A activity. Although correlations with other markers of CYP3A activity such as erythromycin *N*-demethylase activity have generated mixed results (24), the 6β-hydroxycortisol to cortisol ratio does appear to be a reasonable measure of CYP3A induction in humans (25). In children with epilepsy treated with phenobarbital and PHT, four- to seven-fold greater urinary 6β-hydroxycortisol to cortisol ratio has been observed compared to age-matched control subjects (26,27). Similar results have also been reported in healthy adult volunteers, although significant increases in the ratio were not attained until day 13 of a 100 mg/day regimen (28). In contrast, a regimen of phenobarbital, 100 mg/day for 7 days, resulted in a moderate increase in urinary ratio that did not reach statistical significance (29). In an additional study, however, phenobarbital, 100 mg/day for 14 days, resulted in a 2.4- to 3.0-fold increase in urinary ratio ($p < 0.05$) that was independent of CYP2D6 phenotype (23). Thus, the cumulative *in vivo* data support induction of CYP3A activity by phenobarbital in humans. Because of the long half-life of the drug, however, maximum effect may not be observed until after 10 to 14 days of therapy.

Studies or Reports of Interactions *In Vivo*

Interactions with Other Antiepileptic Drugs

Carbamazepine

Phenobarbital significantly increases CBZ clearance in patients receiving concurrent therapy. In one study, patients with epilepsy who received both agents displayed lower steady-state CBZ concentrations and higher CBZ-epoxide concentrations compared to patients on CBZ monotherapy (30). Similar findings of lower CBZ concentrations and higher concentrations of the epoxide and dihydrodiol metabolites have been noted by others, although these differences (10%–15% changes) were modest (31). Riva and colleagues reported data indicating that children concurrently given phenobarbital had 15% lower CBZ concentrations (25.2 ± 5.9 μM versus 29.8 ± 8.8 μM) despite receiving higher CBZ doses (21.1 ± 8.1 versus 18.4 ± 7.2 mg/kg/day) than children given CBZ alone (32). CBZ concentrations were similarly decreased in adults. In neither age group was any change in CBZ-epoxide observed. More extensive reviews of the phenobarbital–CBZ interaction indicate that steady-state CBZ concentrations may decrease as much as 50%, whereas CBZ-epoxide concentrations remain unchanged during combination therapy with phenobarbital (33). Clinically, higher doses of CBZ are required in the presence of coadministered phenobarbital (34).

Phenytoin

Because PHT and phenobarbital have similar induction profiles and are subject to biotransformation by human CYP2C enzymes, the possibility of reciprocal induction and competitive inhibition exists. The net outcome of an interaction between the two drugs in a given individual will therefore reflect which, if either, mechanism predominates. Browne and colleagues (35) observed that, compared to pretreatment values, PHT clearance, half-life, or volume of distribution was not significantly altered at 4 and 12 weeks following the initiation of phenobarbital. In addition, there were no significant differences in the urinary recovery of unchanged PHT, its major *p*-hydroxylated metabolite, or the dihydrodiol metabolite in the presence or absence of phenobarbital. Using single point determinations of PHT concentration, Diamond and colleagues also determined that the addition of phenobarbital to, or the removal of phenobarbital from, a stable regimen of PHT produced no change in PHT concentrations (36). Because PHT is subject to saturable metabolism, inhibition by phenobarbital may be expected under conditions in which maximum induction has been achieved and PHT concentrations are in the high therapeutic range (33).

Lamotrigine

N-glucuronidation accounts for approximately 80% of lamotrigine clearance in humans (37). Several pharmacokinetic studies indicate that the lamotrigine half-life is shorter (approximately 14 hours) in the presence of a P450-inducing anticonvulsant (CBZ, PHT, or phenobarbital) relative to lamotrigine and valproic acid (VPA) (40–45 hours) or lamotrigine plus an inducing anticonvulsant and VPA (approximately 30 hours) (38–40). Data from a therapeutic drug monitoring service demonstrate that the lamotrigine serum concentration to dose ratio is lower in patients receiving the drug in combination with phenobarbital (ratio = 0.52), PHT (0.32), or CBZ (0.57) compared to monotherapy (0.98; $p < 0.05$). These results provide further indirect evidence for enzyme induction (41). In the absence of metabolite data, however, alternative mechanisms for lower lamotrigine concentrations may also be operative.

Interactions with Other Concomitantly Administered Drugs

Phenobarbital, PHT, and CBZ have been reported to increase the clearance or decrease the therapeutic efficacy of many different compounds as described in detail in the following sections. Additional drugs not specifically addressed are listed in Table 51-1.

Calcium Channel Blockers

The influence of phenobarbital has been evaluated on select agents in the dihydropyridine class including nimodipine and felodipine. Tartara and colleagues compared the pharmacokinetics of nimodipine in control subjects and individuals receiving enzyme-inducing antiepileptics, alone or in combination, and observed significantly lower C_{max} and AUC values (90% and 86%, respectively) and a 57% shorter half-life in the anticonvulsant-treated group (42). A similar evaluation of felodipine suggested a comparable reduction in C_{max} and AUC by 82% and 94%, respectively (43).

Corticosteroids

Implications of induced corticosteroid metabolism involve several disease states, including asthma, autoimmune disorders, and transplantation. In a study comparing the pharmacokinetics of prednisolone in subjects receiving phenobarbital and PHT, alone or in combina-

TABLE 51-1. *Drugs of clinical interest for which coadministration of phenobarbital (PB), phenytoin (PHT), and carbamazepine (CBZ) is associated with increased clearance or decreased pharmacologic effect*

Drug	Inducer	References
Antidepressants	PB, PHT, CBZ	137
Amitriptyline		
Clomipramine		
Desipramine		168
Doxepin		
Imipramine		
Nortriptyline		
Clozapine	CBZ	170
Disopyramide	PB, PHT	171–173
Ethosuximide	PB, PHT, CBZ	33, 174, 175
Fentanyl	PB, PHT, CBZ	176
Haloperidol	PB, PHT	177
Methadone	PHT	178, 179
Mexiletine	PHT	180
Neuromuscular blockers		
Atracurium	CBZ	181
Doxacurium	CBZ	182
Pipecuronium	CBZ	183
Paroxetine	PHT	169
Quinidine	PB, PHT	184
Thioridazine	PB, PHT	177

tion, versus control subjects receiving no concurrent medications, there was a significantly shorter half-life (32%) and a significantly greater total body clearance (44%) of prednisolone with no significant change in volume of distribution or protein binding in the anticonvulsant-treated group (44). Additionally, patients receiving anticonvulsants had more than a two-fold mean elevation in their early morning hydrocortisone peak concentrations, suggesting that the concurrent administration of anticonvulsant enzyme inducer with an exogenously administered corticosteroid resulted in less suppression of the hypothalamic–pituitary axis and a more normal circadian rhythm of endogenous steroid production (44). Brooks and associates suggested that the half-life of prednisolone was shortened (25%) in rheumatoid arthritis patients, and the signs and symptoms of disease significantly worsened (e.g., articular index worsened by 31%, pain score doubled, duration of morning stiffness increased 117%) with the addition of phenobarbital (45).

In 16 asthmatic subjects before and 3 weeks after the initiation of phenobarbital, the half-life of intravenously administered dexamethasone decreased significantly (45%) and clearance increased significantly (87%) over pre-phenobarbital values (46). The authors further described three subjects for whom changes (i.e., worsening) in forced expiratory volume (FEV), maximal midexpiratory flow rate (MMEF), eosinophilia, and clinical degree of bronchospasm were observed while receiving phenobarbital, with subsequent improvement in these measurements upon discontinuation. Similar changes in pharmacokinetic parameters have been reported for intravenously administered methylprednisolone, although changes in the pharmacokinetics of the more water-soluble methylprednisolone-sodium hemisuccinate were less dramatic (47). The clinical significance of enzyme induction is most evident in transplant patients. Wassner and colleagues provide evidence of decreased graft survival and increased risk of graft failure in patients receiving anticonvulsant enzyme inducers compared with control transplant recipients receiving no such agents (48).

Cyclosporin A

Several case reports detail the clinical significance of an interaction between phenobarbital and cyclosporin A in patients receiving the two medications concurrently. Carstensen and associates report subtherapeutic cyclosporine concentrations in a child receiving phenobarbital followed by an increase in cyclosporine concentrations as the dose of phenobarbital was reduced (49). Similarly, Burckart and co-workers described a 70% reduction in the clearance of cyclosporine (from 12.6 mL/min/kg to 3.8 mL/min/kg) when phenobarbital was discontinued from the regimen of a young child following renal transplantation (50).

Metronidazole

Several authors have reported failure of metronidazole treatment in cases of vaginal trichomoniasis and giardiasis when phenobarbital is prescribed concurrently. Consequently, an increase in dose is necessary to effect a microbiologic cure (51,52). In a crossover study of six patients with chronic disease, metronidazole AUC and half-life were significantly decreased by 30% and 23%, respectively. No significant difference in apparent volume of distribution was observed, although the AUC of the hydroxy metabolite was increased by 29% (53).

Oral Contraceptives

The potential for decreased efficacy of oral contraceptive therapy secondary to the use of enzyme-inducing anticonvulsants has been recognized for several years (54). This interaction has frequently been attributed to enhanced metabolism of both estrogenic and progestin components, but alterations in protein binding, specifically serum hormone binding globulin (SHBG), appear also to be involved. In a prospective evaluation of plasma ethynyl estradiol concentrations in the presence and absence of phenobarbital, two of four subjects demonstrated 64% and 72% reductions from baseline values. However, the overall change for all subjects was not statistically significant given only a moderate decrease in the third subject and an increase in ethynyl estradiol concentrations in the fourth. In contrast, SHBG capacity increased 15% to 49% in all subjects following the administration of phenobarbital. Of clinical interest, breakthrough bleeding developed in the women who demonstrated reductions in plasma ethynyl estradiol concentrations (55). Thus, a pharmacodynamic interaction can be expected with the concurrent administration of oral contraceptives and phenobarbital; however, whether this is a result of alterations in metabolism or a consequence of altered protein binding remains to be elucidated.

Theophylline

Although scant, there is evidence to suggest that phenobarbital induces the metabolism of theophylline in older children and adults. In one crossover study with six subjects, theophylline clearance increased 34% after phenobarbital coadministration (56). In seven children with asthma, theophylline clearance increased by 42% and average steady-state concentrations decreased by 30% (57). In contrast, Kandrotas and colleagues found no change in the clearance and dose requirements of aminophylline in premature neonates receiving the agent alone or in combination with phenobarbital (58).

Warfarin

The plasma half-life and apparent total body clearance of (R)-warfarin and (S)-warfarin were evaluated in three subjects administered each enantiomer separately before and concurrently with phenobarbital. For all subjects, the mean (R)- and (S)-enantiomer half-lives decreased by 40% and 38%, respectively. Similarly, (R)- and (S)-warfarin clearance increased by 65% and 50%, respectively (59). The increased warfarin clearance translated into an approximately 25% decrease in prothrombin time over a 3-week period (60). CYP2C9 appears to be the principal form of human hepatic P450 modulating levels of the pharmacologically more active S-enantiomer with a minor contribution from CYP3A4, whereas CYP3A4 and CYP1A2 are involved in (R)-warfarin biotransformation (61). The lack of stereospecificity suggests that multiple P450 pathways are induced while the decreased pharmacologic effects likely reflect CYP2C9 induction. Regardless of P450 isoforms induced, studies with phenobarbital and other barbiturates indicate that induction may persist for 3 or 4 weeks after drug discontinuation (62).

PHENYTOIN

Pharmacology

PHT is a hydantoin anticonvulsant first synthesized in 1908 and approved for use by the FDA in 1939. This agent is primarily used in the treatment of generalized tonic-clonic seizures and complex partial seizures. Unlike other anticonvulsants, which elevate seizure threshold, PHT exerts its action by limiting the spread of seizure activity, essentially stabilizing the neuronal membrane against hyperexcitability (possibly by way of promoting sodium efflux from neurons). Because the stabilizing effect of PHT is evident on all neuronal membranes, including peripheral nerves, the agent has also been used in the management of peripheral neuropathies and arrhythmias. PHT is available for administration both orally and parenterally and has most recently been approved for intravenous administration in a prodrug form as fosphenytoin.

Effects on Drug Metabolizing Enzymes *In Vitro*

PHT is often referred to as a "phenobarbital-like" inducer (15,63), but its ability to induce CYP isoforms *in vitro* has not been extensively characterized relative to phenobarbital. As cited earlier, expression of CYP3A proteins is reported to be higher in human liver microsomal samples obtained from individuals exposed to PHT and phenobarbital (3,63). When primary cultures of human hepatocytes were maintained in the presence of 50 µM PHT for 48 to 72 hours, cyclosporin A oxidase activity was increased 1.4- to 5.9-fold relative to

untreated cultures, equivalent to the increase in activity observed with phenobarbital. Under these same conditions, the amount of immunoreactive CYP3A protein increased 5.2- to 8.2-fold (7). The ability of PHT to induce other CYP isoforms in cultured human hepatocytes has not been addressed.

Induction of hepatic CYP3A4 by PHT and its reversibility upon drug discontinuation has been studied immunohistochemically in posttransplant liver biopsies (64). In biopsy samples obtained from patients receiving long-term PHT treatment for suspected cyclosporine neurotoxicity, there was strong staining of CYP3A4 protein in all hepatocytes, whereas acute PHT treatment was associated with CYP3A4-positive staining in pericentral and midzonal, but not periportal, hepatocytes. Cumulatively, the data suggested that induction of CYP3A4 occurs rapidly (2–5 days) in the pericentral and midzonal areas, whereas more prolonged exposure to PHT is required for increased expression in the periportal region. Reversion to a pericentral distribution pattern for CYP3A4 occurs approximately 2 weeks after drug discontinuation (64).

Effects on Specific Drug-Metabolizing Enzymes *In Vivo*

As with phenobarbital, studies with antipyrine have indicated that PHT is a potent inducer of oxidative drug biotransformation in humans. In patients with epilepsy treated primarily with PHT monotherapy for at least 2 years, antipyrine total body clearance in patients without evidence of hepatic dysfunction was almost two-fold greater (50.4 ± 17.5 mL/min/kg) than that of control subjects (26.6 ± 7.0 mL/min/kg). Patients with hepatic abnormalities ranging from mild fat infiltration to cirrhosis with moderate hepatitis also had significantly greater antipyrine clearance ($p < 0.01$). Total P450 content in biopsy specimens was increased in the healthy epileptic group only (16.6 ± 4.4 nmol/g versus 11.3 ± 2.2 nmol/g; $p < 0.001$). This study also evaluated liver blood flow using a technetium-based imaging technique but found no significant differences among the three treatment groups when values were corrected for body weight (65).

Several studies have consistently demonstrated a two- to three-fold increase in urinary 6β-hydroxycortisol to cortisol ratio with PHT (66–68), consistent with induction of CYP3A activity. When the relative effects of anticonvulsants have been compared, PHT has been less potent than CBZ with respect to CYP3A4, but is associated with a greater increase in acetaminophen glucuronidation (68). The ability of PHT to induce its own metabolism (as discussed later) indicates that CYP2C9 activity is also induced.

Studies or Reports of Interactions *In Vivo*

Autoinduction

PHT is a prochiral compound that is principally hydroxylated to (S)- and (R)-5-(4-hydroxyphenyl)-5-phenylhydantoin (*p*-HPPH) in a ratio of 19:1 (69). The formation of *p*-HPPH has been attributed to members of the CYP2C subfamily (70) and it has previously been observed that (S)-*p*-HPPH/(R)-*p*-HPPH ratios greater than 40 were likely to occur in poor metabolizers of PHT (69). Recent work has confirmed that CYP2C9 and CYP2C19 catalyze the formation of both enantiomers but that CYP2C9 is highly (S)-enantiospecific, whereas CYP2C19 is not. Because the CYP2C9 K_m (5 μM) is ten-fold lower than the CYP2C19 K_m (70 μM), CYP2C9 predominates at lower PHT concentrations but is readily saturated as the therapeutic range of 40 to 80 μM is approached (71). Although several authors provide data suggesting that PHT may induce its own metabolism, confirming this finding remains complicated because of the nonlinear pharmacokinetics of PHT and the difficulty in estimating rate constants after a single dose.

Miller and colleagues report two cases in which steady-state PHT plasma concentrations demonstrated a marked decline and the calculated V_{max} values increased by approximately 11% over the course of therapy (72). In a more controlled setting, Chetty and co-workers evaluated the single-dose pharmacokinetics of PHT in three capsule formulations in a randomized crossover study. An equivalent dose of PHT was administered in each arm of the study with a 6-day washout between doses. In evaluating total exposure between study phases, the mean $AUC_{0-\infty}$ for phase 2 declined modestly to 94.7% (90% CI 83.8% to 105.7%) of that observed in phase 1. However, by phase 3, $AUC_{0-\infty}$ declined significantly to 76.25% (90% CI 65.3% to 87.2%) of that observed in phase 1 and was formulation independent (73). Examination of the plasma concentration versus time plot demonstrates a decrease in C_{max} and AUC with no apparent change in PHT half-life and, thus, an interaction at the level of the intestine (e.g., increased presystemic metabolism, diminished absorption) cannot be excluded. In a similar study of two formulations, Dickinson and associates reported a slight but significant increase in the urinary excretion of conjugated and unconjugated *p*-HPPH between the first and second dose (74). The relatively small drug challenge in the latter studies (i.e., a single dose) resulted in an apparent decrease in total body exposure of parent drug and an apparent increase in the excretion of metabolite, despite a washout of approximately 1 week between doses. Thus, if autoinduction is a real and consistent phenomenon, it may require only relatively small doses and persist for an extended period of time.

Interactions with Other Antiepileptic Drugs

Carbamazepine

The main pathway of CBZ biotransformation is oxidation to CBZ 10,11 epoxide and subsequent hydration to the corresponding *trans*-dihydrodiol. Minor oxidative metabolites include 2-hydroxy-carbamazepine, 3-hydroxy-carbamazepine, and 9-hydroxymethyl-10-carbamoylacridan. Most of the products of oxidative biotransformation are found in the urine as glucuronide conjugates (75). CYP3A4 is the primary human cytochrome P450 isoform catalyzing the 10,11-epoxidation reaction, whereas CYP2C8 is a minor contributor (76); formation of the *trans*-dihydrodiol has been attributed to microsomal epoxide hydrolase activity. CBZ displays a relatively narrow therapeutic index such that concomitant medications that induce drug metabolism may result in subtherapeutic CBZ concentrations and inadequate seizure control.

The evaluation of CBZ steady-state levels in the presence and absence of PHT suggests that the combination regimen can result in CBZ levels that, on average, are approximately 34% lower than those observed in patients on monotherapy (34). This change is not reflective of maximal induction in that the addition of a third inducer (e.g., phenobarbital) to the regimen of CBZ and PHT resulted in steady-state levels that were 45% lower than those of subjects on the monotherapy regimen (34). Alternatively, when chronic PHT therapy was withdrawn, total CBZ concentrations increased by 48% and free CBZ concentrations increased by 30% without any change in CBZ-epoxide levels (77).

Although these data are suggestive of induction of CBZ metabolism by PHT, single point determinations alone do not allow one to rule out changes in other pharmacokinetic processes, including absorption or distribution. PHT does appear to decrease exposure to CBZ but does not appear to influence the levels of the epoxide and *trans*-dihydrodiol metabolites (31). PHT induction of epoxide hydrolase and glucuronosyl transferase may also be involved, but has not been addressed in detail.

Primidone/Phenobarbital

An initial study evaluating the steady-state levels of primidone and its metabolite phenobarbital in patients receiving equivalent doses of primidone alone or in combination with PHT demonstrated that mean serum primidone levels were lower (8.2 ± 0.7 mg/L versus 12.2 ± 1.6 mg/L) and mean phenobarbital levels were higher (30.6 ± 2.9 mg/L versus 14.4 ± 3.3 mg/L) in individuals receiving primidone concurrently with PHT. Although the decrease in serum primidone concentrations could be influenced by decreased intestinal absorption, this would not be consistent with the greater than two-fold increase in serum phenobarbital concentrations (78). These results were corroborated in an individual who experienced an 18% decrease in primidone concentrations and a corresponding 74% increase in phenobarbital plasma concentration when PHT was added to existing primidone therapy. Likewise, urinary recovery of phenobarbital was increased and urinary levels of primidone were decreased. Further oxidation of phenobarbital to p-hydroxyphenobarbital apparently was decreased during PHT therapy, but 1 month after PHT was discontinued, levels of all three compounds returned to their baseline values (79).

Although the above findings are consistent with induction of primidone metabolism by PHT and possible inhibition of phenobarbital metabolism, several studies report that the combination of PHT and primidone resulted in no change in primidone levels when compared with patients on monotherapy, yet resulted in up to a 2.5-fold increase in phenobarbital levels. In fact, when a third agent (CBZ) was added to the regimen of primidone and phenobarbital, primidone levels remained unchanged yet phenobarbital levels increased approximately four-fold (80,81). In subjects receiving phenobarbital, PHT has been observed to have no effect in one study and to significantly increase plasma phenobarbital concentrations in another (80,82). It appears that the coadministration of PHT and primidone can be expected to ultimately increase phenobarbital levels, but whether this represents increased conversion of primidone to phenobarbital or inhibition of phenobarbital biotransformation has not been resolved.

Valproic Acid

Even though glucuronide conjugation and subsequent renal excretion account for 70% to 80% of VPA elimination, this agent does undergo CYP-mediated oxidative biotransformation. In subjects receiving VPA and PHT alone or in combination with other enzyme-inducing anticonvulsants, mean VPA plasma concentrations were lower compared to VPA monotherapy (75.3 ± 13.8 mg/L versus 90.3 ± 8.7 mg/L) despite larger mean VPA doses (41.6 ± 12.3 mg/kg versus 25.4 ± 4.9 mg/kg) (83). Similarly, May and Rambeck (84) reported that serum concentrations of VPA in patients with epilepsy concurrently receiving PHT were approximately 50% those of patients on VPA monotherapy. The further addition of either phenobarbital or CBZ, or both, to a regimen of VPA and PHT did not appear to further magnify the induction of VPA metabolism, but when PHT was withdrawn after long-term coadministration, VPA concentrations increased by approximately 19% (77). Although these findings are consistent with enzyme induction, single point determinations do not allow one to rule out alternative factors, including changes in absorption or volume of distribution.

Interactions with Other Concomitantly Administered Drugs

Antineoplastics

High-dose busulfan is used in combination with cyclophosphamide as a myeloablative regimen before bone marrow transplantation. Given that the dose-dependent neurotoxicity observed with busulfan typically manifests as seizures, seizure prophylaxis is recommended with this regimen and typically includes PHT. Data from a study evaluating busulfan pharmacokinetics before and after 15 days of PHT therapy revealed no change in C_{max} and volume of distribution. However, AUC and half-life were significantly decreased and clearance was increased in the presence of PHT (85).

Similarly, clearance of the epipodophyllotoxin teniposide was studied over multiple courses in pediatric control subjects and in children on anticonvulsant therapy (PHT n = 4, phenobarbital n = 2) and was found to be 2.5 times higher in the anticonvulsant group. Even though teniposide is a highly protein-bound drug with a high unbound clearance, no significant change in the volume of distribution was observed in this study (86). The clinical consequences of induction of antineoplastic metabolism are significant given the direct impact these agents have on patient mortality rates. Enhanced metabolism of antineoplastic drugs decreases efficacy and therefore, dosage increases are necessary to achieve the same level of exposure.

Benzodiazepines

Clonazepam undergoes extensive hepatic metabolism to a number of inactive metabolites, with the major pathway thought to be mediated by CYP3A4 (87). In the presence of PHT, clonazepam clearance increased by greater than 50%, elimination rate constant increased by 45%, and half-life decreased by 31%, with no change in volume of distribution or protein binding (88). In a separate evaluation of five subjects, initiation of PHT resulted in 31% to 70% reductions in plasma clonazepam concentrations. Concentrations of 7-amino-clonazepam were also decreased in three patients in whom measurements were made (range 45%–81%), suggesting that either induction occurred by way of a pathway other than that involved in formation of this metabolite, absorption was decreased, or there was increased presystemic biotransformation of the parent compound (89). Given the wide therapeutic index of clonazepam, the clinical significance of this interaction is limited.

Oxazepam is almost exclusively eliminated by glucuronide conjugation and subsequent renal elimination. Administration of PHT and other anticonvulsant inducers appears to significantly accelerate clearance, presumably through induction of glucuronyl transferase activity. In a study evaluating the influence of PHT (n = 6) or the combination of PHT and phenobarbital (n = 3) on the metabolism of oxazepam, coadministration of enzyme inducer decreased oxazepam AUC by 45% and half-life by 53%, with an 81% increase in systemic clearance. The lack of any appreciable changes in C_{max} and protein binding argue against alterations in absorption and volume of distribution contributing to the findings (90).

Cyclosporin A

Original reports evaluating the influence of PHT on cyclosporine attempted to suggest a role for the induction of cyclosporine metabolism based on the findings of decreased serum concentrations and half-life of cyclosporine in blood (91). In contrast, when concentrations in serum were analyzed, the cyclosporine half-life was not affected by PHT and concentrations of the metabolites M-17 and M-18 were significantly decreased (91). The data were analyzed by a second group who attributed the observed interaction to a change in absorption, possibly by way of a mechanism analogous to that of the formulation-dependent griseofulvin–phenobarbital interaction (92). An alternative explanation is a PHT-induced increase in presystemic metabolism analogous to that reported with rifampin (93). Although the mechanism cannot be clearly elucidated from these data, concurrent administration of these two agents can result in a clinically significant decrease in cyclosporine levels, necessitating an increase in dose.

Itraconazole

Although most antiinfectives demonstrate a relatively wide therapeutic index, enzyme induction can pose a specific concern of subtherapeutic plasma and tissue concentrations with the risk of treatment failure. The azole antifungals are used frequently in the management of fungal infections, and central nervous system infections in particular may require coadministration of an anticonvulsant agent in case of seizures. Ducharme and co-workers (94) evaluated the pharmacokinetics of itraconazole and its hydroxy metabolite alone and after 15 days of PHT administration. PHT markedly decreased itraconazole C_{max}, AUC, and half-life by 83%, 93%, and 83%, respectively. Total body clearance was increased nearly 15-fold. Hydroxyitraconazole C_{max}, AUC, and half-life were also decreased by 95%, 84%, and 74%, respectively, suggesting that the principal interaction occurred at the intestinal level. Unlike most of the other agents discussed earlier, the magnitude of the effect of itraconazole concentrations is so large that one may not be able to compensate by increasing the dose, and alternative antifungal agents may need to be considered.

Meperidine

Meperidine, a synthetic narcotic analgesic used acutely for the management of pain, undergoes N-demethylation to an active metabolite, normeperidine, in a CYP-dependent process. A crossover study evaluating the pharmacokinetic parameters of meperidine in the presence and absence of PHT demonstrated that the coadministration of PHT with this analgesic resulted in a shortened half-life (33%) and a 26% increase in total body clearance. Concurrently, both the C_{max} and AUC of normeperidine were increased by 44% and 53%, respectively, consistent with enzyme induction as the primary mechanism for this interaction (95). Clinical consequences of this interaction include hypoalgesia secondary to subtherapeutic meperidine plasma concentrations and increased normeperidine concentrations leading to sedation in the general population and potentially resulting in seizures in specific high-risk conditions (e.g., porphyria) (96).

Oral Contraceptives

Odlind and colleagues (97) reported significantly higher free and total norethisterone concentrations in five healthy subjects receiving hormone therapy compared with a single patient with epilepsy receiving hormone therapy concurrently with PHT. Free and total norethisterone concentrations increased over the 21-day course of therapy in all subjects, although concentrations at 1, 2, and 3 weeks of therapy were approximately three-fold higher in the subjects receiving no concurrent therapy. However, SHBG levels were approximately two- to threefold lower in these same individuals during this time frame. Although the authors suggested that the terminal elimination half-life of norethisterone after 21 days was higher in the patients with epilepsy, the data were derived from a limited sampling scheme and may not be truly reflective of total body clearance (97). An additional case report by the same authors (98) and data reported by Victor and associates (99) appear to corroborate these findings, suggesting that, in a large majority of women receiving PHT, SHBG levels are greater than 2 standard deviations above the mean values for women on no concurrent therapy. Although the interaction between PHT and the steroid sex hormones may be multifactorial, regardless of the mechanism, the clinical consequences remain the same. These include symptomatic changes in menstrual cycle (98), unplanned pregnancies (98,100), and increased signs and symptoms of menopause (101) when PHT is added to therapy comprised of oral or implantable hormone therapy.

Theophylline

Theophylline has been associated with several drug interactions because of its narrow therapeutic index and the number of metabolic pathways involved in its bio-transformation. Marquis and associates (102) evaluated the pharmacokinetic profile of theophylline, administered parenterally as aminophylline, before and after 10 days of oral PHT therapy. No change in C_{max} and volume of distribution were observed. However, there was a significant decrease in half-life and AUC (48% and 47%, respectively) with a concurrent increase in total body clearance of 73%. Several reports have evaluated PHT-dependent induction of theophylline metabolism, taking into consideration both age and smoking status. The coadministration of both agents resulted in an increase in both clearance and elimination rate constant ranging from 36% to 45% and 36% to 42%, respectively, with no change in volume of distribution (103,104). Even though smoking is reported to induce theophylline metabolism, a similar increase in clearance and elimination rate constant (39% and 43%, respectively) was observed in a "preinduced" smoking population with, again, no change in volume of distribution. Thus, the magnitude of induction appears to be independent of smoking status (103).

The disposition of theophylline was further evaluated with respect to its predominant metabolites: 3-methyl-xanthine, 1-methyluric acid, and 1,3-dimethyluric acid. In both smokers and nonsmokers, induction of the formation of all three metabolites by PHT increased by the same magnitude approximately 60% and 40%, respectively (66). Miller and colleagues reported 55%, 43%, 62%, and 57% increases 24-hour urinary recovery of 1-methyluric acid, 3-methylxanthine, 1,3-dimethyluric acid, and theophylline, respectively (104). Even though hepatic enzyme induction may account for the increased formation of theophylline metabolites, other mechanisms clearly must be involved in the observed increase in urinary excretion of theophylline itself. Studies with human liver microsomes (105) and heterologously expressed enzymes (106) support a major role for CYP1A2 and, to a lesser extent, CYP2E1 in formation of all three major theophylline metabolites with minor, if any at all, involvement by CYP3A4. Thus, although the nonselective induction of all three metabolites would be consistent with induction of the CYP1A2 pathway, this conclusion is speculative. However, the inducing effect of CBZ on theophylline metabolism is similar to that of PHT (107), and recent data suggest that CBZ may induce CYP1A2 activity (108).

Warfarin

Based on the effects of phenobarbital and other barbiturates on warfarin metabolism described earlier, one would expect PHT also to be associated with an enhanced hypoprothrombinemic response and increased warfarin dosage requirements. In fact, the PHT–warfarin interaction appears to be complex, possibly involving displace-ment from plasma protein-binding sites, PHT effects on vitamin K-dependent clotting factor synthesis, and inhibition of warfarin biotransformation as well as induction (62). Most information concerning this interaction is derived from case reports with conflicting results. One study characterizing the interaction between PHT and dicoumarol reported that dicoumarol concentrations decreased after a few days of concomitant therapy and recovered two to three weeks after PHT discontinuation. Decreased dicoumarol concentrations were accompanied by an increase in the prothrombin–convertin concentration. Only limited patient data are presented; therefore, it is difficult to determine the extent of the interaction (109). Despite the limited information available, it seems likely that addition of PHT to a stable regimen of warfarin initially will be accompanied by increased warfarin response either by displacement of warfarin from its plasma protein binding sites, inhibition of its biotransformation, or a combination of both potential mechanisms. Longer term PHT administration may result in decreased warfarin effect resulting from P450 induction. Regardless, close monitoring is necessary to maintain the desired anticoagulant response.

CARBAMAZEPINE

Pharmacology

CBZ was approved by the FDA for use as an anticonvulsant in adults in 1974 and in children older than 6 years of age in 1978. In 1987, the age restriction was lifted. An iminostilbene derivative, CBZ is structurally related to the tricyclic antidepressant imipramine and is effective in the treatment of simple partial, complex partial, and generalized tonic-clonic seizures. It is also widely used in the treatment of bipolar depression and trigeminal neuralgia. Although there is evidence supporting actions on synaptic transmission and receptors for neurotransmitters such as acetylcholine and N-methyl-D-aspartate, the main mechanism of CBZ anticonvulsant activity appears related to enhancement of sodium channel inactivation and a reduced ability of neurons to fire at high frequency (110).

Effects on Drug-Metabolizing Enzymes In Vitro

Although there are numerous clinical investigations describing the inductive properties of CBZ, there is a paucity of data characterizing this phenomenon in vitro. In primary cultures of human hepatocytes, CBZ treatment produced a 16-fold increase in immunoreactive CYP3A protein. In contrast, CYP3A catalytic activity as measured by cyclosporine oxidase activity was 56% of that observed in control cultures. Because studies with human hepatic microsomes failed to confirm CBZ as a

CYP3A inhibitor, the authors attributed the decreased cyclosporine activity observed in intact cells to possible cytotoxicity (7). In preliminary studies with a reporter gene assay system based on approximately 1 kb of the CYP3A4 regulatory region, CBZ (100 µM) produced a 2.8-fold increase in reporter gene activity. In comparison, the same concentration of rifampin, a well-documented inducer of CYP3A4, was associated with a four-fold induction of reporter gene activity (111). Thus, available *in vitro* activity support the role of CBZ as an inducer of CYP3A4 activity.

Effects on Specific Drug Metabolizing Enzymes
In Vivo

Antipyrine clearance is reported to be increased by approximately 50% after treatment of healthy volunteers with 200 mg CBZ daily for 25 days. Although CBZ induction of biotransformation pathways is the most likely explanation for these results, the absence of metabolite data precludes any definitive conclusions concerning the individual P450 isoforms induced from being drawn (112). Measurement of urinary 6β-hydroxycortisol excretion in this study, however, revealed a two-fold increase upon completion of the CBZ treatment, consistent with induction of CYP3A4 activity. A three-fold induction of urinary 6β-hydroxycortisol excretion (expressed as the ratio to urinary free cortisol) has also been reported in Chinese patients with epilepsy on long-term CBZ therapy relative to healthy control subjects (68).

Human hepatic CYP1A2 activity can be conveniently estimated using an orally administered dose of caffeine and measuring the urinary production of its 3-*N*-demethylated metabolite (113). Alternatively, caffeine can be labeled with a stable isotope ($[^{13}C]$) in the 3-*N*-position, and enrichment of $[^{13}C]$ carbon dioxide in expired air used to measure caffeine 3-demethylation, and thus, CYP1A2 activity. Using this latter method, CYP1A2 activity was determined in five children aged 6 to 17 years before and after 2 to 3 weeks of CBZ treatment. The percentage recovery of $[^{13}C]$-labeled carbon dioxide in the 2-hour collection period increased from 3.47% to 7.65% over the CBZ treatment period (108). Closer examination of the data indicates that the increase in $[^{13}C]$-labeled carbon dioxide was less than 2.5-fold in four of the patients (1.2- to 2.4-fold increases) and 6.7-fold in the fifth patient. In contrast, an earlier study concluded that CBZ had no effect on caffeine clearance but did not measure metabolite levels, relying instead on estimations of caffeine clearance derived from two data points. This same study demonstrated that PHT increased caffeine clearance approximately 2.4-fold (114). Thus, it appears that CBZ therapy may be associated with moderate induction of CYP1A2 activity, although considerable intersubject variability exists.

Studies or Reports of Interactions *In Vivo*
Autoinduction

The possibility that CBZ induces its own metabolism (autoinduction) first became apparent when steady-state concentrations predicted from single-dose pharmacokinetic studies overestimated those actually observed in patients treated long term. More detailed study in four patients undergoing treatment for recalcitrant headaches indicated that the CBZ half-life declined from a mean value of 36 hours after a single dose to approximately 21 hours at steady-state, and that CBZ concentrations decreased continually during the first few days of multiple dosing (115). Studies using deuterium-labeled CBZ in children provided direct evidence for autoinduction. In three children aged 10 to 13 years, CBZ clearance increased from a mean of 0.028 L/hr/kg on the first day of treatment to 0.036 L/hr/kg and had doubled to 0.056 L/hr/kg after 17 to 32 days of therapy. No further increase in clearance was observed over the following 4 months, indicating that the autoinduction process was completed within the first 4 weeks of treatment (116). Similar results have also been observed in adults (117).

Autoinduction of CBZ clearance is accompanied by increased urinary excretion of metabolites from the epoxide-diol pathway, apparently without any appreciable change in excretion of 2-hydroxy and 3-hydroxy metabolites (118). Whereas *trans*-dihydrodiol formation from the 10,11-epoxide is also induced (albeit to a lesser extent than the formation of CBZ 10,11-epoxide formation from CBZ), the increased formation of these two metabolites is consistent with the documented role of CBZ as an inducer of CYP3A4 activity.

Interactions with Other Antiepileptic Drugs
Phenytoin

PHT concentrations are reported to be decreased (119), increased (120,121), or unaffected (119,120) by concurrent CBZ therapy. Treatment with 600 mg CBZ daily for 9 days in five patients with epilepsy reduced the half-life of intravenously administered PHT to 6.4 hours from a pretreatment level of 10.6 hours (119). When the same CBZ dose was added after steady PHT concentrations had been achieved, PHT concentrations were markedly decreased in three patients and were unchanged in four others. The lack of an effect on PHT plasma protein binding and decreased PHT half-life after intravenous PHT administration argues strongly for induced hepatic biotransformation to be the mechanism of the interaction with CBZ in this study (119). In contrast, addition of CBZ to steady-state concentrations of PHT was associated with an almost two-fold increase in PHT levels in 12 of 24 patients studied (120). Using a stable isotope technique, addition of CBZ to monotherapy with PHT resulted in decreased PHT clearance, which was accompanied by decreased *p*-HPPH and PHT dihydrodiol production and increased dose-related toxicity (121).

As discussed earlier, the ten-fold difference in CYP2C9 and CYP2C19 K_m values indicates that CYP2C9 will predominate at lower PHT concentrations but would be readily saturated as the therapeutic range of 40 to 80 μM is approached (71). Thus it is possible that CBZ induces one P450 isoform (CYP2C9) and inhibits another (CYP2C19) with the clinical consequences of concomitant CBZ therapy dependent upon the relative contributions of the two CYP2C isoforms in a given individual, among other considerations. However, none of the studies cited have addressed the effects of CBZ on (S)- and (R)-*p*HPPH formation, nor is there any direct experimental evidence for CBZ induction of CYP2C9 activity. As is discussed in more detail in this section, a CBZ interaction with warfarin is suggestive of CYP2C9 induction. However, because addition of CBZ to a patient stably maintained on PHT may have unpredictable consequences, close monitoring is warranted. Likewise, due caution should be exercised whenever withdrawal of CBZ is contemplated.

Primidone and Phenobarbital

Addition of CBZ to patients given primidone resulted in increased concentrations of the active primidone metabolite, phenobarbital (80). Because concurrent CBZ apparently does not affect phenobarbital clearance (122), the increased phenobarbital concentrations can be attributed to formation from primidone rather than reduced phenobarbital clearance per se. The enzymes responsible for primidone biotransformation have not been identified whereas preliminary data suggest that CYPs 2C9 and 2C19 are primarily responsible for the *p*-hydroxylation of phenobarbital (123).

Valproic Acid

In healthy volunteers, CBZ administration (200 mg daily) was associated with a 21% decrease in trough steady-state VPA concentration but no change in the elimination rate constant during the dosing interval (124). A second study in healthy volunteers (125) demonstrated that the same dose of CBZ increased plasma VPA clearance 40% compared to pretreatment values (1.26 ± 0.24 L/hr versus 0.90 ± 0.18 L/hr; $p < 0.05$) with a corresponding 40% decrease in trough steady-state VPA concentrations. A decrease in serum half-life from 14.0 ± 10.6 hours to 10.6 ± 1.4 hours ($p < 0.05$) in the absence of a significant change in distribution volume is consistent with enzyme induction. However, the increase in VPA clearance was not accompanied by an increase in the urinary recovery of VPA conjugates, suggesting that there may also be a component of reduced absorption. Levy and colleagues conducted a detailed analysis of the

changes in the formation and excretion of 15 VPA metabolites in patients undergoing treatment with VPA monotherapy, VPA and CBZ, and VPA in combination with PHT. They observed 50% and 90% increases in VPA clearance in the CBZ and PHT groups relative to the VPA monotherapy group (126). The urinary recovery of VPA metabolites tended to be lower in the VPA/CBZ and VPA/PHT groups compared to the patients receiving VPA alone, although the differences did not reach statistical significance. CBZ was not associated with a change in the formation clearance of conjugation (mostly glucuronidation) and beta oxidation pathways, but did produce a two-fold increase in the formation of cytochrome P450–dependent metabolites 4-hydroxy-VPA, 5-hydroxy VPA, and the potentially hepatotoxic metabolite 4-ene-VPA. Recent data indicate that induction of CYP2C9 and CYP2A6 is more likely to be responsible for increased 4-ene-VPA production than induction of CYP3A4 (127). Based on the data summarized earlier, it appears that CBZ can produce clinically significant reductions in VPA concentrations, probably through enzyme induction and decreased absorption. From a toxicologic perspective, induction of pathways leading to the formation of potentially hepatotoxic metabolites may account for the increased incidence of VPA-related toxicity in patients given concurrent treatment with P450 inducers (128).

Lamotrigine

Because CBZ data are usually included with those of other "enzyme-inducing" anticonvulsants, CBZ effects on lamotrigine plasma concentrations and clearance are discussed in the phenobarbital section.

Newer Anticonvulsants

The clearance of several new anticonvulsants is also accelerated in the presence of CBZ therapy. Whereas only about 20% of a felbamate dose appears to be metabolized by CYP3A4- or CYP2E1-dependent pathways (129), two population studies indicate that CBZ can increase felbamate apparent clearance by 32% (130) to 49% (131) compared to felbamate monotherapy. In a zonisamide add-on study, the mean plasma half-life of the drug was 36.4 hours in the presence of CBZ (132), 40% to 50% shorter than that observed in healthy volunteers (133). Zonisamide biotransformation is complex but *in vitro* data indicate that CYP3A4 is responsible for reductive cleavage of the isoxazole ring (134), a pathway that accounts for approximately 20% of human biotransformation (133). CBZ is also reported to decrease the half-lives of topiramate and tiagabine, presumably through induction of CYP3A4 activity (33,133,135). One topiramate add-on study reported two- to three-fold higher apparent clearance when CBZ was coadministered (136) but, in general, studies of these newer antiepileptic agents have not specifically investigated CYP3A4 induction by

CBZ as the mechanism of decreased drug concentrations and, therefore, decreased bioavailability cannot be excluded as a possible mechanism.

Interactions with Other Concomitantly Administered Drugs

Benzodiazepines

Several benzodiazepines and structurally related compounds are substrates for CYP3A4, although the actual contribution of CYP3A4 to overall metabolic disposition varies for a given compound, depending on the relative contributions of alternative pathways (137). The results of prospective (138) and retrospective (139) therapeutic drug monitoring studies have indicated that concurrent CBZ or PHT therapy was associated with decreased clobazam serum concentrations, whereas the concentration of its major metabolite, N-desmethylclobazam, was increased. A detailed pharmacokinetic study in healthy volunteers demonstrated that CBZ, 200 mg twice daily for 2 weeks, increased clobazam apparent clearance 2.6-fold over pre-CBZ values (6.7 ± 2.0 L/hr versus 2.6 ± 0.9 L/hr), and the observed 61% decrease in steady-state clobazam concentrations was accompanied by a 44% increase in N-desmethylclobazam concentrations. N-desmethylclobazam half-life was also reduced by CBZ (81.5 ± 34.0 hours versus 48 ± 19 hours), but the increase in metabolite formation was greater than the increase in its clearance, leading to accumulation (140).

CBZ 200 mg daily also decreased clonazepam steady concentrations by 17% to 37% over a 5- to 15-day period, accompanied by a 30% decrease in clonazepam half-life relative to the control period (141). Although metabolite concentrations were not measured in this study, the CBZ effect is consistent with induction of CYP3A4, the major CYP isoform involved in clonazepam nitroreduction (87).

Following an intravenous dose, diazepam clearance was increased in patients receiving chronic anticonvulsant therapy compared to a group of healthy control subjects (142). This increased diazepam clearance was accompanied by higher concentrations of the pharmacologically active N-desmethyl metabolite that accounts for approximately 60% of diazepam biotransformation in humans (143). Diazepam N-demethylase activity segregates with CYP2C19 phenotype in vivo (143), and data from several in vitro studies confirm that CYP2C19 is a high-affinity diazepam N-demethylase with an apparent K_m value of 20 μM (144,145). CYP3A4 is largely responsible for 3-hydroxylation of both diazepam and N-desmethyldiazepam (146), and has been identified as a low-affinity diazepam N-demethylase (K_m approximately 320 μM) in both CYP2C19 rapid and poor metabolizers (144). As discussed by Levy and colleagues (140), there are several scenarios that could account for the observa-

tions of Dhillon and colleagues summarized earlier. This most certainly is a complex process in that the ratio of N-desmethyldiazepam to 3-hydroxydiazepam formation in vitro has been reported to increase as diazepam concentration decreases (147), and under in vivo conditions, the ratio would be affected by the relative changes in CYP3A4 and possibly CYP2C19 activities under inducing conditions. Thus, it is difficult to ascertain the relative roles that CYP3A4 and CYP2C19 induction would play in this process. Even so, because the N-demethylated metabolites of diazepam and clobazam are pharmacologically active, enzyme induction by CBZ and PHT may not affect the therapeutic efficacy of these compounds to an appreciable extent.

CYP3A4 is also an important determinant of alprazolam biotransformation in vitro (148) and in vivo (149). When compared in healthy volunteers receiving a 10-day course of CBZ 300 mg/day or matched placebo, alprazolam half-life was decreased (7.7 ± 1.7 hours versus 17.1 ± 4.9 hours, $p < 0.001$) and apparent oral clearance increased (2.13 ± 0.54 mL/min/kg versus 0.90 ± 0.21 mL/min/kg; $p < 0.001$) during CBZ treatment. Peak plasma concentrations and measures of psychomotor functions were not significantly different in the two treatment periods. The authors attributed the latter to the sedative effects of CBZ itself (150).

Midazolam is a validated probe for CYP3A activity that is used widely to characterize the effects of various disease states and exogenous factors on this particular CYP activity in humans (24,151). Midazolam clearance in vivo correlates better with in vitro hepatic CYP3A content after intravenous administration of the drug ($r = 0.84$, $p < 0.01$) (64) compared to after oral administration ($r = 0.54$, $p < 0.05$) (152) as a result of substantial CYP3A-mediated metabolism on transit through the intestinal mucosa (153). In patients with epilepsy treated with CBZ or PHT, peak midazolam concentrations and AUC following a 15-mg oral dose are only 7.4% and 5.7% of those observed in control subjects. Similarly, the elimination half-life was reduced from a mean of 3.1 hours in controls to 1.3 hours in patients, and was accompanied by reduced pharmacodynamic effects (154). Thus, using midazolam as a substrate, it appears that treatment with CBZ or PHT is associated with profound induction of CYP3A activity, and for drugs that are subject to extensive first pass metabolism, it is likely that this induction occurs at both the hepatic and intestinal levels.

Bupropion

Bupropion is an aminoketone antidepressant agent chemically unrelated to antidepressants with tricyclic and tetracyclic structures as well as serotonin selective reuptake inhibitors. It undergoes extensive biotransformation to metabolites that are pharmacologically active and have slower clearances than the parent compound (155). The major pathway involves hydroxylation of the *tert*-butyl moiety to form hydroxybupropion, which accumulates to a level 40-fold greater than that of bupropion at steady-state. The enzymes involved in bupropion biotransformation have not been characterized, although available data suggest that CYP2D6 (156) and CYP1A2 (157) are unlikely to play significant roles. In patients meeting Diagnostic and Statistical Manual of Mental Disorders, 3rd Edition, Revised (DSM-III-R) criteria for major affective disorders, concurrent CBZ therapy (minimum of 3 weeks of treatment) decreased bupropion AUC by 84% and increased the AUC of hydroxybupropion by 50%, consistent with induction of bupropion biotransformation; examination of the hydroxybupropion data presented in this chapter suggests that clearance of the metabolite is also increased by CBZ therapy (158). Because hydroxybupropion and other metabolites may contribute to therapeutic or adverse events, the clinical consequences of induction have not been definitively established.

Cyclosporin A

Like PHT and phenobarbital, CBZ is thought to induce cyclosporin A biotransformation but the data consist largely of anecdotal reports of increased dosage requirements for cyclosporine when CBZ was added to existing therapy or of increased cyclosporine concentrations when CBZ was discontinued (159). One exception is a study in which cyclosporine pharmacokinetics were determined in three pediatric renal transplant patients aged 3 years, 7 years, and 14 years receiving CBZ doses of 16.4 to 20.8 mg/kg/day. Compared to control patients matched for age, body weight, and surface area, steady-state trough concentrations of cyclosporine were significantly lower in the CBZ group (57 ± 14 ng/mL versus 162 ± 22 ng/mL) despite receiving a higher dose of cyclosporine (16.2 ± 8.8 mg/kg/day versus 10.8 ± 5.2 mg/kg/day). Average steady-state cyclosporine concentrations expressed as a function of the administered dose were approximately 40% lower in the CBZ group, whereas the elimination half-life was not different (160). Although decreased cyclosporine bioavailability cannot be completely ruled out, data in adults (93,161) and children (162) indicate that cyclosporine is subject to presystemic biotransformation by intestinal CYP3A4. Given that all children studied by Cooney and colleagues received the same formulation of cyclosporine, the most likely explanation for the decreased steady-state concentrations of cyclosporine during CBZ treatment is induction of intestinal and hepatic CYP3A4.

Oral Contraceptives

Both breakthrough bleeding and contraceptive failure have been reported in women taking oral contraceptives concurrently with CBZ (163). In a pharmacokinetic study conducted in four women, 8 to 12 weeks of CBZ therapy was associated with a 40% decrease in the area under the plasma concentration-time curves for both 17α-ethinylestradiol and levonorgestrel relative to pretreatment levels (164). Given the role of CYP3A4, and possibly human CYP2C isoforms, in the formation of 2-hydroxy-17α-ethinylestradiol (165,166), it is likely that induction of at least CYP3A4 is responsible for this clinically significant interaction.

Warfarin

Several published case reports imply that CBZ may induce warfarin biotransformation (62), but no studies have yet addressed this directly. In two of three patients in whom CBZ was added to a stable warfarin regimen, warfarin serum concentrations and half-life decreased by approximately 50% (119). In this study, pharmacokinetic estimates were obtained following intravenous administration of warfarin and, therefore, reduced absorption and increased presystemic clearance cannot account for the observed effects of concurrent CBZ administration. Likewise, two-fold reductions in warfarin dose have been necessary when chronic CBZ therapy has been discontinued (62). Although the effect of CBZ enzyme induction on (S)- and (R)-warfarin biotransformation has not been studied as it has for rifampin (167), it seems unlikely that CBZ induction solely at the CYP3A4 level [affecting primarily the pharmacologically less active (R)-warfarin] could account for the observed 50% increase in warfarin clearance and hypoprothrombinemic activity. Therefore, some induction of CYP2C9-mediated S-7-hydroxylation must also occur.

SUMMARY

A large number of the interactions presented in this chapter can be attributed to induction of CYP3A4 activity. Although most pharmacokinetic studies are not able to differentiate between interactions occurring at the level of the intestine or liver, both are theoretically possible. Evidence for induction of other pathways, such as CYP2C9 and UGTs, is largely inferred from pharmacokinetic studies of drugs known to be dependent upon those particular biotransformation pathways as determined by *in vitro* investigations. As a general rule, phenobarbital, PHT, and CBZ will increase the clearance of any drug that is primarily dependent upon CYP3A4 activity (and possibly CYP2C9 activity) for the majority of its elimination from the body. However, there are also cases in which these anticonvulsants have been reported to induce the metabolism of drugs primarily metabolized by CYP isoforms other than CYP3A4. For example, CYP2D6 plays a predominant role in the disposition of desipramine and paroxetine *in vivo*. Even though 30% to 40% increases in clearance have been reported in the presence of phenobarbital or PHT (168,169), no convincing evidence of CYP2D6 induction by "enzyme-inducing" anticonvulsants is available to attribute induction to CYP2D6.

It is important to recognize that all individuals have a unique complement of CYP isoforms expressed in their liver and other tissues and this will impact upon the potential for induction with a given inducer. It is also conceivable that new discoveries in gene regulation will reveal new determinants of interindividual variability in response to inducing agents. Nevertheless, the clinical significance of enzyme induction is dependent on additional factors, including the therapeutic index of the drug in question, the presence and contribution of numerous competing drug biotransformation pathways, and the pharmacologic or toxicologic potential of the metabolites produced. Recognition of these factors will help minimize unexpected adverse responses in patients when enzyme-inducing anticonvulsants are added to existing treatment regimens.

REFERENCES

1. Conney AH. Pharmacological implications of microsomal enzyme induction. *Pharmacol Rev* 1967;19:317–366.
2. Waxman DJ, Azaroff L. Phenobarbital induction of cytochrome P-450 gene expression. *Biochem J* 1992;281:577–592.
3. Watkins PB, Wrighton SA, Maurel P, et al. Identification of an inducible form of cytochrome P-450 in human liver. *Proc Natl Acad Sci USA* 1985;82:6310–6314.
4. Guillouzo A, Beaune P, Gascoin M-N, et al. Maintenance of cytochrome P-450 in cultured adult human hepatocytes. *Biochem Pharmacol* 1985;34:2991–2995.
5. Grant MH, Burke MD, Hawksworth GM, Duthie SJ, Engeset J, Petri JC. Human adult hepatocytes in primary monolayer culture. Maintenance of mixed function oxidase and conjugation pathways of drug metabolism. *Biochem Pharmacol* 1987;36:2311–2316.
6. Donato MT, Gómez-Lechón MJ, Castell JV. Effect of xenobiotics on monooxygenase activities in cultured human hepatocytes. *Biochem Pharmacol* 1990;39:1321–1326.
7. Pichard L, Fabre I, Fabre G, et al. Screening for inducers and inhibitors of cytochrome P-450 (cyclosporin A oxidase) in primary cultures of human hepatocytes and in liver microsomes. *Drug Metab Dispos* 1990;18:595–606.
8. Morel F, Beaune P, Ratanasavanh D, Flinois JP, Guengerich FP, Guillouzo A. Effects of various inducers on the expression of cytochromes P-450 IIC8, 9, 10 and IIIA in cultured adult human hepatocytes. *Toxicol In Vitro* 1990;4:458–460.
9. Morel F, Beaune PH, Ratanasavanh D, et al. Expression of cytochrome P-450 enzymes in cultured human hepatocytes. *Eur J Biochem* 1990;191:437–444.
10. Donato MT, Gómez-Lechón MJ, Castell JV. Effect of model inducers on cytochrome P450 activities of human hepatocytes in primary culture. *Drug Metab Dispos* 1995;23:553–558.
11. Chang TKH, Yu L, Maurel P, Waxman DJ. Enhanced cyclophosphamide and ifosfamide activation in primary human hepatocyte cultures: response to cytochrome P-450 inducers and autoinduction by oxazaphosphorines. *Cancer Res* 1997;57:1946–1954.
12. Schuetz EG, Schuetz JD, Strom SC, et al. Regulation of human liver cytochromes P-450 in family 3A in primary and continuous culture of human hepatocytes. *Hepatology* 1993;18:1254–1262.
13. Kocarek TA, Schuetz EG, Strom SC, Fisher RA, Guzelian PS. Comparative analysis of cytochrome P4503A induction in primary cultures of rat, rabbit, and human hepatocytes. *Drug Metab Dispos* 1995;23:415–421.
14. Li AP, Maurel P, Gomez-Lechon MJ, Cheng LC, Jurima-Romet M. Preclinical evaluation of drug-drug interaction potential: present status of the application of primary human hepatocytes in the evaluation of cytochrome P450 induction. *Chem Biol Interact* 1997;107:5–16.
15. Bock KW, Bock-Hennig BS. Differential induction of human liver UDP-glucuronosyltransferase activities by phenobarbital-type inducers. *Biochem Pharmacol* 1987;36:4137–4143.
16. Doostdar H, Grant MH, Melvin WT, Wolf CR, Burke MD. The effects of inducing agents on cytochrome P450 and UDP-glucuronsyltransferase activities in human HepG2 hepatoma cells. *Biochem Pharmacol* 1993;46:629–635.
17. Morel F, Fardel O, Meyer DJ, et al. Preferential increase of glutathione S-transferase class a transcripts in cultured human hepatocytes by phenobarbital, 3-methylcholanthrene, and dithiolethiones. *Cancer Res* 1993;53:231–234.
18. Hassett C, Laurenzana EM, Sidhu JS, Omiecinski CJ. Effects of chemical inducers on human microsomal epoxide hydrolase in primary hepatocyte cultures. *Biochem Pharmacol* 1998;55:1059–1069.
19. Byrne E, Harman AW, Frewin DB, Hallpike JF. Antipyrine half-life as a measure of hepatic enzyme induction: clinical applications in a chronic epileptic population. *Clin Exp Neurol* 1979;16:183–189.
20. Perucca E, Hedges A, Makki KA, Ruprah M, Wilson JF, Richens A. A comparative study of the relative enzyme inducing properties of anticonvulsant drugs in epileptic patients. *Br J Clin Pharmacol* 1984;18:401–410.
21. Sharer JE, Wrighton SA. Identification of the human hepatic cytochromes P450 involved in the *in vitro* oxidation of antipyrine. *Drug Metab Dispos* 1996;24:487–494.
22. Engel G, Hofmann U, Heidemann H, Cosme J, Eichelbaum M. Antipyrine as a probe for human oxidative drug metabolism: identification of the cytochrome P450 enzymes catalyzing 4-hydroxyantipyrine, 3-hydroxymethylantipyrine, and norantipyrine formation. *Clin Pharmacol Ther* 1996;59:613–623.
23. Leclercq V, Desager JP, Horsmans Y, van Nieuwenhuyze Y, Harvengt C. Influence of rifampicin, phenobarbital and cimetidine on mixed function monooxygenase in extensive and poor metabolizers of debrisoquine. *Int J Clin Pharmacol Ther Toxicol* 1989;27:593–598.
24. Watkins PB. Noninvasive tests of CYP3A enzymes. *Pharmacogenetics* 1994;4:171–184.
25. Ged C, Rouillon JM, Pichard L, et al. The increase in urinary excretion of 6 beta-hydroxycortisol as a marker of human hepatic cytochrome P450IIA induction. *Br J Clin Pharmacol* 1989;28:373–387.
26. Saenger P, Forster E, Kream J. 6β-Hydroxycortisol: a noninvasive indicator of enzyme induction. *J Clin Endocrinol Metab* 1981;52:381–384.
27. Saenger P. 6β–Hydroxycortisol in random urine samples as an indicator of enzyme induction. *Clin Pharmacol Ther* 1983;34:818–821.
28. Ohnhaus EE, Breckenridge AM, Park BK. Urinary excretion of 6β-hydroxycortisol and the time course measurement of induction of man. *Eur J Clin Pharmacol* 1989;36:39–46.
29. Eichelbaum M, Mineshita S, Ohnhaus EE, Zekorn C. The influence of enzyme induction of polymorphic sparteine oxidation. *Br J Clin Pharmcol* 1986;22:49–53.
30. Ramsay R, McManus D, Guterman A, et al. Carbamazepine metabolism in humans: effect of concurrent anticonvulsant therapy. *Ther Drug Monit* 1990;12:235–241.
31. Liu H, Delgado MR. Interactions of phenobarbital and phenytoin with carbamazepine and its metabolites' concentrations, concentration ratios, and level/dose ratios in epileptic children. *Epilepsia* 1995;36:249–254.
32. Riva R, Contin M, Albani F, Perucca E, Procaccianti G, Baruzzi A. Free concentration of carbamazepine and carbamazepine-10,11-epoxide in children and adults. Influence of age and phenobarbitone co-medication. *Clin Pharmacokinet* 1985;10:524–531.
33. Riva R, Albani F, Contin M, Baruzzi A. Pharmacokinetic interactions between antiepileptic drugs. Clinical considerations. *Clin Pharmacokinet* 1996;31:470–493.
34. Christiansen J, Dam M. Influence of phenobarbital and diphenylhydantoin on plasma carbamazepine levels in patients with epilepsy. *Acta Neurol Scand* 1973;49:543–546.
35. Browne T, Szabo G, Evans J, Greenblatt D, Mikati M. Phenobarbital does not alter phenytoin steady-state serum concentration or pharmacokinetics. *Neurology* 1988;38:639–642.

36. Diamond W, Buchanan R. A clinical study of the effect of phenobarbital on diphenylhydantoin plasma levels. *J Clin Pharmacol* 1970;10: 306–311.

37. Rambeck B, Wolf P. Lamotrigine clinical pharmacokinetics. *Clin Pharmacokin* 1993;25:433–443.

38. Binnie CD, van Emde Boas W, Kasteleijn-Nolste-Trenite DG, et al. Acute effects of lamotrigine (BW430C) in persons with epilepsy. *Epilepsia* 1986;27:248–254.

39. Jawad S, Yuen WC, Peck AW, Hamilton MJ, Oxley JR, Richens A. Lamotrigine: single-dose pharmacokinetics and initial 1 week experience in refractory epilepsy. *Epilepsy Res* 1987;1:194–201.

40. Eriksson AS, Hoppu K, Nergårdh A, Boreus L. Pharmacokinetic interactions between lamotrigine and other antiepileptic drugs in children with intractable epilepsy. *Epilepsia* 1996;37:769–773.

41. May TW, Rambeck B, Jurgens U. Serum concentrations of lamotrigine in epileptic patients: the influence of dose and comedication. *Ther Drug Monitor* 1996;18:523–531.

42. Tartara A, Galimberti C, Manni R, et al. Differential effects of valproic acid and enzyme-inducing anticonvulsants on nimodipine pharmacokinetics in epileptic patients. *Br J Clin Pharmacol* 1991;32: 335–340.

43. Capewell S, Freestone S, Critchley J, Pottage A, Prescott L. Reduced felodipine bioavailability in patients taking anticonvulsants. *Lancet* 1988:480–482.

44. Gambertoglio J, Holford N, Kapusnik J, et al. Disposition of total and unbound prednisolone in renal transplant patients receiving anticonvulsants. *Kidney Int* 1984;25:119–123.

45. Brooks P, Buchanan W, Grove M, Downie W. Effects of enzyme induction on metabolism of prednisolone. Clinical and laboratory study. *Ann Rheum Dis* 1976;35:339–343.

46. Brooks S, Werk E, Ackerman S, Sullivan I, Thrasher K. Adverse effects of phenobarbital on corticosteroid metabolism in patients with bronchial asthma. *N Engl J Med* 1972;286:1125–1128.

47. Stjernholm M, Katz F. Effects of diphenylhydantoin, phenobarbital, and diazepam on the metabolism of methylprednisolone and its sodium succinate. *J Clin Endocrinol Metab* 1975;41:887–893.

48. Wassner S, Pennisi A, Malekzadeh M, Fine R. The adverse effect of anticonvulsant therapy on renal allograft survival. A preliminary report. *J Pediatr* 1976;88:134–137.

49. Carstensen H, Jacobsen N, Dieperink H. Interaction between cyclosporin A and phenobarbitone. *Br J Clin Pharmacol* 1986;21:550–551.

50. Burckart G, Venkataramanan R, Starzl T, Ptachcinski J, Gartner J, Rosenthal T. Cyclosporin clearance in children following organ transplantation (abstr). *J Clin Pharmacol* 1984;24:412.

51. Mead P, Gibson M, Schentag J, Ziemniak J. Possible alteration of metronidazole metabolism by phenobarbital. *N Engl J Med* 1982;306: 1409.

52. Gupte S. Phenobarbital and metabolism of metronidazole. *N Engl J Med* 1983;308:529.

53. Eradiri O, Jamali F, Thomson A. Interaction of metronidazole with phenobarbital, cimetidine, prednisone, and sulfasalazine in Crohn's disease. *Biopharm Drug Dispos* 1988;9:219–227.

54. Shane–McWorter L, Cerveny JD, MacFarlane LL, Osborn C. Enhanced metabolism of levonorgestrel during phenobarbital treatment and resultant pregnancy. *Pharmacotherapy* 1998;18:1360–1364.

55. Back D, Bates M, Bowden A, et al. The interaction of phenobarbital and other anticonvulsants with oral contraceptives. *Contraception* 1980;22:495–503.

56. Landay R, Gonzalez M, Taylor J. Effect of phenobarbital on theophylline disposition. *J Allergy Clin Immunol* 1978;62:27–29.

57. Saccar C, Danish M, Ragni M, et al. The effect of phenobarbital on theophylline disposition in children with asthma. *J Allergy Clin Immunol* 1985;75:716–719.

58. Kandrotas R, Cranfield T, Gal P, Ransom J, Weaver R. Effect of phenobarbital administration on theophylline clearance in premature neonates. *Ther Drug Monit* 1990;12:139–143.

59. Orme M, Breckenridge A. Enantiomers of warfarin and phenobarbital. *N Engl J Med* 1976;295:1482.

60. Udall J. Clinical implications of warfarin interactions with five sedatives. *Am J Cardiol* 1975;35:67–71.

61. Rettie AE, Korzekwa KR, Kunze KL, et al. Hydroxylation of warfarin by human cDNA-expressed cytochrome P-450: A role for P-4502C9 in the etiology of (*S*)-warfarin-drug interactions. *Chem Res Toxicol* 1992; 5:54–59.

62. Cropp JS, Bussey HI. A review of enzyme induction of warfarin metabolism with recommendations for patient management. *Pharmacotherapy* 1997;17:917–928.

63. Wrighton SA, Ring BJ, Watkins PB, Vandenbranden M. Identification of a polymorphically expressed member of the human cytochrome P-450III family. *Mol Pharmacol* 1989;36:97–105.

64. Thummel KE, Shen DD, Podoll TD, et al. Use of midazolam as a human cytochrome P450 3A probe: II. Characterization of inter- and intraindividual hepatic CYP3A variability after liver transplantation. *J Pharmacol Exp Ther* 1994;271:557–566.

65. Pirttiaho HI, Sotaniemi EA, Pelkonen RO, Pitkänen U. Hepatic blood flow and drug metabolism in patients on enzyme-inducing anticonvulsants. *Eur J Clin Pharmacol* 1982;22:441–445.

66. Crowley JJ, Cusack BJ, Jue SG, Koup JR, Park BK, Vestal RE. Aging and drug interactions. II. Effect of phenytoin and smoking on the oxidation of theophylline and cortisol in healthy men. *J Pharmacol Exp Ther* 1988;245:513–523.

67. Fleishaker JC, Pearson LK, Peters GR. Phenytoin causes a rapid increase in 6β-hydroxycortisol urinary excretion in humans—a putative measure of CYP3A induction. *J Pharm Sci* 1995;84:292–294.

68. Tomlinson B, Young RP, Ng MC, Anderson PJ, Kay R, Critchley JA. Selective liver enzyme induction by carbamazepine and phenytoin in Chinese epileptics. *Eur J Clin Pharmacol* 1996;50:411–415.

69. Fritz S, Lindner W, Roots I, Frey BM, Küpfer A. Stereochemistry of aromatic phenytoin hydroxylation in various drug hydroxylation phenotypes in humans. *J Pharmacol Exp Ther* 1987;241:615–622.

70. Veronese ME, Mackenzie PI, Doecke CJ, McManus ME, Miners JO, Birkett DJ. Tolbutamide and phenytoin hydroxylations by cDNA-expressed human liver cytochrome P4502C9. *Biochem Biophys Res Commun* 1991;175:1112–1118.

71. Bajpai M, Roskos LK, Shen DD, Levy RH. Roles of cytochrome P4502C9 and cytochrome P4502C19 in the stereoselective metabolism of phenytoin to its major metabolite. *Drug Metab Dispos* 1996;24: 1401–1403.

72. Miller R, Bill P, DuToit J. Phenytoin auto-induction? *S Afr Med J* 1989;75:332–333.

73. Chetty M, Miller R, Seymour M. Phenytoin auto-induction. *Ther Drug Monit* 1998;20:60–62.

74. Dickinson R, Hooper W, Patterson M, Eadie M, Maguire B. Extent of urinary excretion of p-hydroxyphenytoin in healthy subjects given phenytoin. *Ther Drug Monit* 1985;7:283–289.

75. Lertratanangkoon K, Horning MG. Metabolism of carbamazepine. *Drug Metab Dispos* 1982;10:1–10.

76. Kerr BM, Thummel KE, Wurden CJ, et al. Human liver carbamazepine metabolism. Role of CYP3A4 and CYP2C8 in 10,11-epoxide formation. *Biochem Pharmacol* 1994;47:1969–1979.

77. Duncan J, Patsalos P, Shorvon S. Effects of discontinuation of phenytoin, carbamazepine, and valproate of concomitant antiepileptic medication. *Epilepsia* 1991;32:101–115.

78. Fincham R, Schottelius D, Sahs A. The influence of diphenylhydantoin on primidone metabolism. *Arch Neurol* 1974;30:259–262.

79. Porro M, Kupferberg H, Porter R, Theodore W, Newmark M. Phenytoin: an inhibitor and inducer of primidone metabolism in an epileptic patient. *Br J Clin Pharmacol* 1982;14:294–297.

80. Callaghan N, Feely M, Duggan F, O'Callaghan M, Seldrup J. The effect of anticonvulsant drugs which induce liver microsomal enzymes on derived and ingested phenobarbitone levels. *Acta Neurol Scand* 1977; 56:1–6.

81. Reynolds E, Fenton G, Fenwick P, Johnson A, Laundy M. Interaction of phenytoin and primidone. *BMJ* 1975;2:594–595.

82. Gambie D, Johnson R. The effects of phenytoin on phenobarbitone and primidone metabolism. *J Neurol Neurosurg Psychiatr* 1981;44: 148–151.

83. Mihlay G, Vajda F, Miles J, Louis W. Single and chronic dose pharmacokinetic studies of sodium valproate in epileptic patients. *Eur J Clin Pharmacol* 1979;16:23–29.

84. May T, Rambeck B. Serum concentration of valproic acid: influence of dose and comedication. *Ther Drug Monit* 1985;7:387–390.

85. Hassan M, Oberg G, Bjorkholm M, Wallin I, Lindgren M. Influence of prophylactic anticonvulsant therapy on high-dose busulphan kinetics. *Cancer Chemother Pharmacol* 1993;33:181–186.

86. Baker DK, Relling MV, Pui C-H, Christensen ML, Evans WE, Rodman JH. Increased teniposide clearance with concomitant anticonvulsant therapy. *J Clin Oncol* 1992;10:311–315.

87. Seree EJ, Pisano PJ, Placidi M, Rahmani R, Barra YA. Identification of the human and animal hepatic cytochromes P450 involved in clonazepam metabolism. *Fund Clin Pharmacol* 1995;7:69–75.

88. Khoo K. Influence of phenytoin and phenobarbital on the disposition of a single dose of clonazepam. *Clin Pharmacol Ther* 1980;28:368.

89. Sjo O, Hvidberg E, Naestoft J, Lund M. Pharmacokinetics and side-effects of clonazepam and its 7-amino-metabolite in man. *Eur J Clin Pharmacol* 1975;8:249–254.

90. Scott A, Khir A, Steele W, Hawksworth G, Petrie J. Oxazepam pharmacokinetics in patients with epilepsy treated long-term with phenytoin alone or in combination with phenobarbitone. *Br J Clin Pharmacol* 1983;16:441–444.

91. Freeman D, Laupacis A, Keown P, Stiller C, Carruthers S. Evaluation of cyclosporin–phenytoin interaction with observations on cyclosporin metabolites. *Br J Clin Pharmacol* 1984;18:887–893.

92. Rowland M, Gupta S. Cyclosporin-phenytoin interaction: re-evaluation using metabolite data. *Br J Clin Pharmacol* 1987;24:329–334.

93. Hebert MF, Roberts JP, Prueksaritanont T, Benet LZ. Bioavailability of cyclosporine with concomitant rifampin administration is markedly less than predicted by hepatic enzyme induction. *Clin Pharmacol Ther* 1993;52:453–457.

94. Ducharme MP, Slaughter RL, Warbasse LH, et al. Itraconazole and hydroxyitraconazole serum concentrations are reduced more than tenfold by phenytoin. *Clin Pharmacol Ther* 1995;58:617–624.

95. Pond S, Kretschzmar K. Effect of phenytoin on meperidine clearance and normeperidine formation. *Clin Pharmacol Ther* 1981;30:680–686.

96. Deeg M, Rajamani K. Normeperidine-induced seizures in hereditary coproporphyria. *South Med J* 1990;83:1307–1308.

97. Odlind V, Johansson E. Free norethisterone as reflected by saliva concentrations of norethisterone during oral contraceptive use. *Acta Endocrinol* 1981;98:470–476.

98. Odlind V, Olsson S. Enhanced metabolism of levonorgestrel during phenytoin treatment in a woman with Norplant implants. *Contraception* 1986;33:257–261.

99. Victor A, Lundberg P, Johansson E. Induction of sex hormone binding globulin by phenytoin. *BMJ* 1977;2:934–935.

100. Kenyon I. Unplanned pregnancy in an epileptic. *BMJ* 1972;1:686–687.

101. Notelovitz M, Tjapkes J, Ware M. Interaction between estrogen and dilantin in a menopausal woman. *N Engl J Med* 1981;304:788–789.

102. Marquis J, Carruthers S, Spence J, Brownstone Y, Toogood J. Phenytoin-theophylline interaction. *N Engl J Med* 1982;307:1189–1190.

103. Crowley JJ, Cusack BJ, Jue SG, Koup JR, Vestal RE. Cigarette smoking and theophylline metabolism: effects of phenytoin. *Clin Pharmacol Ther* 1987;42:334–340.

104. Miller M, Cosgriff J, Kwong T, Morken DA. Influence of phenytoin on theophylline clearance. *Clin Pharmacol Ther* 1984;35:666–669.

105. Tjia JF, Colbert J, Back DJ. Theophylline metabolism in human liver microsomes: inhibition studies. *J Pharmacol Exp Ther* 1996;276:912–917.

106. Ha HR, Chen J, Freiburghaus AU, Follath F. Metabolism of theophylline by cDNA-expressed human cytochromes P-450. *Br J Clin Pharmacol* 1995;39:321–326.

107. Jonkman JH, Upton RA. Pharmacokinetic drug interactions with theophylline. *Clin Pharmacokinet* 1984;9:309–334.

108. Parker AC, Pritchard P, Preston T, Choonara I. Induction of CYP1A2 activity by carbamazepine in children using the caffeine breath test. *Br J Clin Pharmacol* 1998;45:176–178.

109. Hansen JM, Siersback-Nielsen K, Kristensen M, Skovsted L, Christensen LK. Effect of diphenylhydantoin on the metabolism of dicoumarol in man. *Acta Med Scand* 1971;189:15–19.

110. Macdonald RL. Carbamazepine. Mechanisms of Action. In: Levy RH, Mattson RH, Meldrum BS, eds. *Antiepileptic drugs,* 4th ed. New York: Raven Press, 1995:491–498.

111. Ogg MS, Gray TJB, Gibson GG. Development of an in vitro reporter gene assay to assess xenobiotic induction of the human CYP3A4 gene. *Eur J Drug Metab Pharmacokinet* 1997;22:311–313.

112. Macphee GJA, Thompson GG, Scobie G, et al. Effects of cimetidine on carbamazepine auto- and hetero-induction in man. *Br J Clin Pharmacol* 1984;18:411–419.

113. Butler MA, Lang NP, Young JF, et al. Determination of CYP1A2 and NAT2 phenotypes in human populations by analysis of caffeine urinary metabolites. *Pharmacogenetics* 1992;2:116–127.

114. Wietholtz H, Zysset TH, Kreiten K, Dohl D, Büchsel R, Matern S. Effect of phenytoin, carbamazepine and valproic acid on caffeine metabolism. *Eur J Clin Pharmacol* 1989;36:401–406.

115. Eichelbaum M, Ekbom K, Bertilsson L, Ringberger VA, Rane A. Plasma kinetics of carbamazepine and its epoxide metabolite in man after single and multiple doses. *Eur J Clin Pharmacol* 1975;8:337–341.

116. Bertilsson L, Hojer B, Tybring G, Osterloh J, Rane A. Autoinduction of carbamazepine metabolism in children examined by a stable isotope technique. *Clin Pharmacol Ther* 1980;27:83–88.

117. McNamara PJ, Colburn WA, Gibaldi M. Time course of carbamazepine self-induction. *J Pharmacokin Biopharm* 1979;7:63–68.

118. Eichelbaum M, Köthe KW, Hoffman F, von Unruh GE. Use of stable labelled carbamazepine to study its kinetics during chronic carbamazepine treatment. *Eur J Clin Pharmacol* 1982;23:241–244.

119. Hansen JM, Siersback-Nielsen K, Skovsted L. Carbamazepine-induced acceleration of diphenylhydantoin and warfarin metabolism in man. *Clin Pharmacol Ther* 1971;12:539–543.

120. Zielinski JJ, Haidukewych D, Leheta BJ. Carbamazepine-phenytoin interaction: elevation of plasma phenytoin concentrations due to carbamazepine comedication. *Ther Drug Monit* 1985;7:51–53.

121. Browne TR, Szabo GK, Evans JH, Evans BA, Greenblatt DJ, Mikati MA. Carbamazepine increases phenytoin serum concentration and reduces phenytoin clearance. *Neurology* 1988;38:1146–1150.

122. Eadie MJ, Lander CM, Hooper WD, Tyrer JH. Factors influencing plasma phenobarbitone levels in epileptic patients. *Br J Clin Pharmacol* 1977;4:541–547.

123. Hargreaves JA, Howald WN, Racha JK, Levy RH. Identification of enzymes responsible for the metabolism of phenobarbital. *ISSX Proceedings* 1996;10:259.

124. Bowdle TA, Levy RH, Cutler RE. Effects of carbamazepine on valproic acid kinetics in normal subjects. *Clin Pharmacol Ther* 1979;26:629–634.

125. Panesar SK, Orr JM, Farrell K, Burton RW, Kassahun K, Abbott FS. The effect of carbamazepine on valproic disposition in adult volunteers. *Br J Clin Pharmacol* 1989;27:323–328.

126. Levy RH, Rettenmeier AW, Anderson GD, et al. Effects of polytherapy with phenytoin, carbamazepine, and stiripentol on formation of 4-ene-valproate, a hepatotoxic metabolite of valproic acid. *Clin Pharmacol Ther* 1990;48:225–235.

127. Sadeque AJM, Fisher MB, Korzekwa KR, Gonzalez FJ, Rettie AE. Human CYP2C9 and CYP2A6 mediate formation of the hepatotoxin 4-ene-valproic acid. *J Pharmacol Exp Ther* 1997;283:698–703.

128. Dreifuss FE, Santilli N, Langer DH, Sweeney KP, Moline KA, Menander KB. Valproic acid hepatic fatalities: a retrospective review. *Neurology* 1987;37:379–385.

129. Glue P, Banfield CR, Perhach JL, Mather GG, Racha JK, Levy RH. Pharmacokinetic interactions with felbamate. *In vitro-in vivo* correlation. *Clin Pharmacokinet* 1997;33:214–224.

130. Banfield CR, Zhu GR, Jen JF, et al. The effect of age on the apparent clearance of felbamate: a retrospective analysis using nonlinear mixed-effects modeling. *Ther Drug Monitor* 1996;18:19–29.

131. Kelley MT, Walson PD, Cox S, Dusci LJ. Population pharmacokinetics of felbamate in children. *Ther Drug Monitor* 1997;19:29–36.

132. Ojemann LM, Shastri RA, Wilensky AJ, et al. Comparative pharmacokinetics of zonisamide (CI-912) in epileptic patients. *Ther Drug Monitor* 1986;8:293–296.

133. Perucca E, Bialer M. The clinical pharmacokinetics of the newer antiepileptic drugs. Focus on topiramate, zonisamide and tiagabine. *Clin Pharmacokinet* 1996;31:29–46.

134. Nakasa H, Nakamura H, Ono S, et al. Prediction of drug-drug interactions of zonisamide metabolism in humans from in vitro data. *Eur J Clin Pharmacol* 1998;54:177–183.

135. Rambeck B, Specht U, Wolf P. Pharmacokinetic interactions of the new antiepileptic drugs. *Clin Pharmacokinet* 1996;31:309–324.

136. Sachdeo RC, Sachdeo SK, Walker SA, Kramer LD, Nayak RK, Doose DR. Steady-state pharmacokinetics of topiramate and carbamazepine in patients with epilepsy during monotherapy and concomitant therapy. *Epilepsia* 1996;37:774–780.

137. Ketter TA, Flockhart DA, Post RM, et al. The emerging role of P450 3A in psychopharmacology. *J Clin Psychopharmacol* 1995;15:387–398.

138. Theis JG, Koren G, Daneman R, et al. Interactions of clobazam with conventional antiepileptics in children. *J Child Neurol* 1997;12:208–213.

139. Sennoune S, Mesdjian E, Bonneton J, Genton P, Dravet C, Roger J. Interactions between clobazam and standard antiepileptic drugs in patients with epilepsy. *Ther Drug Monitor* 1992;14:269–274.

140. Levy RH, Lane EA, Guyot M, Brachet-Liermain A, Cenraud B, Loiseau P. Analysis of parent drug-metabolite relationship in the presence of an inducer. Application to the carbamazepine-clobazam interaction in normal man. *Drug Metab Dispos* 1983;11:286–292.

141. Lai AA, Levy RH, Cutler RE. Time-course of interaction between carbamazepine and clonazepam in normal man. *Clin Pharmacol Ther* 1978;24:316–323.

142. Dhillon S, Richens A. Pharmacokinetics of diazepam in epileptic patients and normal volunteers following intravenous administration. *Br J Clin Pharmacol* 1981;12:841–844.

143. Bertilsson L, Henthorn TK, Sanz E, Tybring G, Säwe J, Villén T. Importance of genetic factors in the regulation of diazepam metabolism: relationship to S-mephenytoin, but not debrisoquin, hydroxylation phenotype. *Clin Pharmacol Ther* 1989;45:348–355.

144. Yasumori T, Qing-Hua L, Yamazoe Y, Ueda M, Tsuzuki T, Kato R. Lack of low Km diazepam N-demethylase in livers of poor metabolizers for S-mephenytoin 4′-hydroxylation. *Pharmacogenetics* 1994;4:323–331.

145. Jung F, Richardson TH, Raucy JL, Johnson EF. Diazepam metabolism by cDNA-expressed human 2C P450s: identification of P4502C18 and P4502C19 as low K_M diazepam N-demethylases. *Drug Metab Dispos* 1997;25:133–139.

146. Ono S, Hatanaka T, Miyazaki S, et al. Human liver microsomal diazepam metabolism using cDNA-expressed cytochrome P450s: role of CYP2B6, 2C19 and the 4A subfamily. *Xenobiotica* 1996;26:1155–1166.

147. Andersson T, Miners JO, Veronese ME, Birkett DJ. Diazepam metabolism by human microsomes is mediated by both S-mephenytoin hydroxylase and CYP3A isoforms. *Br J Clin Pharmacol* 1994;38:131–137.

148. von Moltke LL, Greenblatt DJ, Cotreau-Bibbo MM, Harmatz JS, Shader RI. Inhibitors of alprazolam metabolism in vitro: effect of serotonin-reuptake-inhibitor antidepressants, ketoconazole and quinidine. *Br J Clin Pharmacol* 1994;38:23–31.

149. Yasui N, Otani K, Kaneko S, et al. A kinetic and dynamic study of oral alprazolam with and without erythromycin in humans: in vivo evidence for the involvement of CYP3A4 in alprazolam metabolism. *Clin Pharmacol Ther* 1996;59:514–519.

150. Furukori H, Otani K, Yasui N, et al. Effect of carbamazepine on the single oral dose pharmacokinetics of alprazolam. *Neuropsychopharmacology* 1998;18:364–369.

151. Thummel KE, Shen DD, Podoll TD, et al. Use of midazolam as a human cytochrome P450 3A probe: I. In vitro-in vivo correlations in liver transplant patients. *J Pharmacol Exp Ther* 1994;271:549–556.

152. Wandel C, Böcker RH, Böhrer H, et al. Relationship between hepatic cytochrome P450 3A content and activity and the disposition of midazolam administered orally. *Drug Metab Dispos* 1998;26:110–114.

153. Paine MF, Shen DD, Kunze KL, et al. First-pass metabolism of midazolam by the human intestine. *Clin Pharmacol Ther* 1996;60:14–24.

154. Backman JT, Olkkola KT, Ojala M, Laaksovirta H, Neuvonen PJ. Concentrations and effects of oral midazolam are greatly reduced in patients treated with carbamazepine or phenytoin. *Epilepsia* 1996;37:253–257.

155. Laizure SC, DeVane CL, Stewart JT, Dommisse CS, Lai AA. Pharmacokinetics of bupropion and its major basic metabolites in normal subjects after a single dose. *Clin Pharmacol Ther* 1985;38:586–589.

156. Pollock BG, Sweet RA, Kirshner M, Reynolds CFI. Bupropion plasma levels and CYP2D6 phenotype. *Ther Drug Monitor* 1995;18:581–585.

157. Hsyu PH, Singh A, Giargiari TD, Dunn JA, Ascher JA, Johnston JA. Pharmacokinetics of bupropion and its metabolites in cigarette smokers versus nonsmokers. *J Clin Pharmacol* 1997;37:737–743.

158. Ketter TA, Jenkins JB, Schroeder DH, et al. Carbamazepine but not valproate induces bupropion metabolism. *J Clin Psychopharmacol* 1995;15:327–333.

159. Campana C, Regazzi MB, Buggia I, Molinaro M. Clinically significant drug interactions with cyclosporin. An update. *Clin Pharmacokinet* 1996;30:141–179.

160. Cooney GF, Mochon M, Kaiser B, Dunn SP, Goldsmith B. Effects of carbamazepine on cyclosporine metabolism in pediatric renal transplant recipients. *Pharmacotherapy* 1995;15:353–356.

161. Kolars JC, Awni WM, Merion RM, Watkins PB. First-pass metabolism of cyclosproine by the gut. *Lancet* 1990;338:1488–1490.

162. Hoppu K, Koskimies O, Holmberg C, Hirvisalo E. Evidence for pre-hepatic metabolism of oral cyclosporine in children. *Br J Clin Pharmacol* 1991;32:477–481.

163. Back DJ, Orme ML. Pharmacokinetic drug interactions with oral contraceptives. *Clin Pharmacokinet* 1990;18:472–484.

164. Crawford P, Chadwick DJ, Martin C, Tjia J, Back DJ, Orme M. The interaction of phenytoin and carbamazepine with combined oral contraceptive steroids. *Br J Clin Pharmacol* 1990;30:892–896.

165. Guengerich FP. Oxidation of 17α–ethynylestradiol by human liver cytochrome P-450. *Mol Pharmacol* 1988;33:500–508.

166. Ball SE, Forrester LM, Wolf CR, Back DJ. Differences in the cytochrome P-450 isoenzymes involved in the 2-hydroxylation of oestradiol and 17 alpha-ethinyloestradiol. Relative activities of rat and human liver enzymes. *Biochem J* 1990;267:221–226.

167. Heimark LD, Gibaldi M, Trager WF, O'Reilly RA, Goulart DA. The mechanism of the warfarin-rifampin drug interaction in humans. *Clin Pharmacol Ther* 1987;42:388–394.

168. Spina E, Avenoso A, Campo G, Caputi A, Perucca E. Phenobarbital induces the 2-hydroxylation of desipramine. *Ther Drug Monit* 1996;18:60–64.

169. Kaye C, Haddock R, Langley P, et al. A review of the metabolism and pharmacokinetics of paroxetine in man. *Acta Psychiatr Scand Suppl* 1989;350:60–75.

170. Jerling M, Linström L, Bondesson U, Bertilsson L. Fluvoxamine inhibition and carbamazepine induction of the metabolism of clozapine: evidence from a therapeutic drug monitoring service. *Ther Drug Monitor* 11994;16:368–374.

170. Kapil R, Axelson J, Mansfield I, et al. Disopyramide pharmacokinetics and metabolism: effect of inducers. *Br J Clin Pharmacol* 1987;24:781–791.

171. Aitio M, Mansury L, Tala E, Haataja M, Aitio A. The effect of enzyme induction on the metabolism of disopyramide in man. *Br J Clin Pharmacol* 1981;11:279–285.

172. Nightingale J, Nappi J. Effect of phenytoin on serum disopyramide concentrations. *Clin Pharm* 1987;6:46–50.

173. Giaccone M, Bartoli A, Gatti G, et al. Effect of enzyme inducing anticonvulsants on ethosuximide pharmacokinetics in epileptic patients. *Br J Clin Pharmacol* 1996;41:575–579.

174. Bachmann KA, Jauregi L. Use of single sample clearance estimates of cytochrome P450 substrates to characterize human hepatic CYP status in vivo. *Xenobiotica* 1993;23:307–315.

175. Tempelhoff R, Modica PA, Spitnagel EL. Anticonvulsant therapy increases fentanyl requirements during anesthesia for craniotomy. *Can J Anaesth* 1990;37:327–332.

176. Linnoila M, Viukari M, Vaisanen K, Auvinen J. Effect of anticonvulsants on plasma haloperidol and thioridazine levels. *Am J Psychiatry* 1980;137:819–821.

177. Finelli P. Phenytoin and methadone tolerance. *N Engl J Med* 1976;294:227.

178. Tong T, Pond S, Kreek M, Jaffery N, Benowitz N. Phenytoin-induced methadone withdrawal. *Ann Intern Med* 1981;94:349–351.

179. Begg E, Chinwah P, Webb C, Day R, Wade D. Enhanced metabolism of mexiletine after phenytoin administration. *Br J Clin Pharmacol* 1982;14:219–223.

180. Spacek A, Neiger FX, Spiss CK, Kress HG. Atracurium-induced neuromuscular block is not affected by chronic anticonvulsant therapy with carbamazepine. *Acta Anaesthesiol Scand* 1997;41:1308–1311.

181. Ornstein E, Matteo RS, Weinstein JA, Halevy JD, Young WL, Abou-Donia MM. Accelerated recovery from doxacurium-induced neuromuscular blockade in patients receiving chronic anticonvulsant therapy. *J Clin Anesth* 1991;3:108–111.

182. Jellish WS, Modica PA, Tempelhoff R. Accelerated recovery from pipecuronium in patients treated with chronic anticonvulsant therapy. *J Clin Anesth* 1993;5:105–108.

183. Data JL, Wilkinson GR, Nies AS. Interaction of quinidine with anticonvulsant drugs. *N Engl J Med* 1976;294:699–702.

CHAPTER 52

Rifampin, Dexamethasone, and Omeprazole

Graham R. Jang and Patrick J. P. Maurel

RIFAMPIN

Pharmacology

Rifampin (RIF) was developed in the 1960s as the first orally active derivative of rifamycin [isolated from *Nocardia (Streptomyces) mediteranae*] (1) and is bactericidal for *Mycobacterium tuberculosis*, *M. leprae*, gram-positive bacteria (especially staphylococci), and certain gram-negative forms (e.g., *Neisseria meningitidis, N. gonorrhoeae, Haemophilus influenzae,* and *Legionella*). It acts by complexing and thus inhibiting bacterial DNA-dependent RNA polymerase (2). This antibiotic is a mainstay in the treatments of tuberculosis and leprosy (frequently administered with other agents to prevent the development of resistance) and also is used in prophylaxis for numerous types of infections. Quite clearly, these clinical characteristics (widespread and long-term use, potential combination therapy) contribute to making the drug particularly prone to provoking significant drug–drug interactions.

For nearly all indications, RIF is administered in daily oral doses of 450 to 600 mg. As previously reviewed (3), peak plasma concentrations of 7 to 9 μg/mL (9–11 μM) are attained in 2 to 4 hours (after a 600-mg dose) and reported elimination half-lives ($t_{1/2}$) range from 2 to 5 hours. Roughly 80% of the drug is bound to plasma proteins (primarily α_1-acid glycoprotein), and it is metabolized in the liver to active 25-desacetylrifampin. The enzyme(s) mediating RIF oxidation have not been elucidated, although on continued administration, the drug induces its own metabolism (assuming no change in its apparent volume of distribution, V_d), as evidenced by a decrease in its $t_{1/2}$ after 1 week of daily use (4).

Effects on Drug-Metabolizing Enzyme Expression

Nearly 25 years ago, it was recognized that RIF altered (augmented) the metabolism of several coadministered agents (5–7). Early work in our laboratory with rabbit hepatocytes in primary culture demonstrated that RIF induces cytochromes P450 (CYPs) of the 2B and 3A subfamilies at the mRNA, protein, and activity levels (8). Further studies in the rabbit demonstrated that RIF activates CYP3A6 transcription and has no effect on messenger half-life in cultured hepatocytes and *in vivo* (9–11). We further demonstrated that RIF principally induces cyclosporin A oxidase and cortisol 6β-hydroxylase in human liver *in vivo*, and that this enzyme is indeed CYP3A4 (12,13). Additionally, by using human hepatocytes in primary culture, we and others have demonstrated that RIF induces CYP3A4 mRNA (14–17), immunodetectable protein (15–19), and specific monooxygenase activities (16–21). RIF also induces CYPs 2A6 (22), 2B6, 2C8, 2C9, and 2C19 in cell culture (15,19) (S. Gerbal, unpublished data), although generally to lesser extents than its induction of CYP3A4. RIF has been demonstrated to increase the 0- to 8-hour urinary R-/S-mephenytoin ratio and urinary excretion of 4'-hydroxy-S-mephenytoin in extensive (but not poor) metabolizers of the anticonvulsant (23), consistent with induction of CYP2C19 *in vivo* (see Chapter 7 for details of this polymorphism). Indeed, other reported interactions further suggest that RIF induces CYP2C enzymes *in vivo* (and are discussed later).

RIF is now considered a prototypical CYP3A4 inducer in human liver, but also activates *CYP3A4* transcription in the intestine. The presence of CYP3A4 mRNA and protein in jejunal enterocytes was first demonstrated by Watkins et al. (24). de Waziers et al. (25) reported the expression of CYP3A4, CYP2D6, and CYP2C isoforms in the small intestine, and that the level of CYP3A4 protein decreases gradually in the proximal-to-distal direction (duodenum $\rightarrow$ jejunum $\rightarrow$ ileum $\rightarrow$ colon), a trend

G. R. Jang: Department of Metabolism and Pharmacokinetics, Bristol-Myers Squibb, Pharmaceutical Research Institute, P.O. Box 4000, Princeton, New Jersey 08548-4000

P. J. P. Maurel: INSERM U128, IFR24, 1919 Route de Mende, 34293 Montpellier, France

recently confirmed by Paine et al. (26) at both the protein and activity levels in 20 donor organs. Kolars et al. (27,28) demonstrated that mRNA for CYPs 3A4 and 3A5 (but not 3A7) are found throughout the digestive tract and that intestinal CYP3A4 mRNA and protein are induced by RIF in vivo (27).

The expression of CYP3A enzymes in other extrahepatic sites suggests additional tissues in which RIF may act as an inducer. In 25 human kidneys, CYP3A5 was found to be uniformly and CYP3A4 polymorphically (40%) expressed (29), although the contribution of renal CYP3A forms to drug elimination and the effects of RIF on their expression are not known. In lung tissues, the O-deethylation of 7-ethoxycoumarin was significantly higher in biopsies from patients receiving RIF (as part of multidrug tuberculosis therapy) relative to mean activity in control tissues (from patients with nonmalignant lung disease) (30). The major CYPs expressed in human lung are 1A1, 2A6, 2C9, 2E1, and 3A4 (31,32), suggesting that RIF induces CYPs 2A6, 2C9, and/or 3A4 in the lung in vivo [recombinant forms of these three enzymes have been shown to catalyze this oxidation effectively (33)].

The effects of RIF on the expression of other phase I and on phase II enzymes have not been clearly characterized. In the previously mentioned lung study, RIF did not induce epoxide hydrolase or glutathione-S-transferase activities in this tissue (30). In primary human hepatocytes, RIF induced sulfotransferase activity two-fold (34) and 1-naphthol uridine diphosphate (UDP)-glucuronosyltransferase (UGT) (35), whereas in HepG2 cells, it increased the rate of bilirubin (but not 1-naphthol, morphine, or testosterone) glucuronidation (36). Studies in other hepatocarcinoma cell lines further indicate that RIF likely induces UGTs in an isoform-specific manner (35,37). Several reported drug interactions involving RIF suggest that it induces UGTs in vivo (discussed later). Because numerous non-CYP phase I and phase II enzymes (particularly UGTs and sulfotransferases) are expressed in the gastrointestinal tract and could play important roles in oral drug bioavailability, further studies characterizing the effects of RIF on their expression in this tissue and in the liver may identify additional loci of potential RIF-induced drug interactions.

The mechanism by which RIF induces CYP3A and other gene expression has not yet been elucidated at the molecular level. However, we recently demonstrated that this molecule is able to bind and activate the human glucocorticoid receptor (38), making this ligand-activated transcription factor a potential candidate as mediator of the inductive effects.

Studies or Reports of Interaction In Vivo

Because of the clinical characteristics of RIF use, its now well-documented ability to induce CYP3A4 potently and the important role of this enzyme in xenobiotic metabolism, it is far from surprising that the literature describing drug interactions involving the antibiotic is extensive. At present, more than 65 drugs have been reported to interact with RIF coadministration in vivo (Table 52-1). The majority are substrates of CYP3A4, for which this isoform is their primary metabolizing enzyme (e.g., midazolam and verapamil). Many literature reports, particularly those of single-case studies, describe a decrease or abolition of efficacy, and others describe observations of lowered plasma or serum drug concentrations necessitating dosage adjustment. For these reports, limited data preclude mechanistic evaluation, but they are clearly consistent with RIF (a) causing a decrease in oral bioavailability (F_{oral}) through induction of CYP3A4 in the intestine and/or liver, and/or (b) causing an increase in the drugs systemic clearance (CL) via induction of liver CYP3A4. In other instances, it also is reported that the $t_{1/2}$ of the coadministered drug is decreased, confirming a pronounced effect on its systemic (presumably hepatic) clearance (assuming no change in V_d). Reports that are of particular interest demonstrate differential effects of RIF-mediated enzyme induction in the intestine versus liver or interactions with RIF despite (normally) minor contribution of CYP3A4 to the metabolism of those drugs. Furthermore, the likely importance of RIF coadministration with drugs used to treat human immunodeficiency virus (HIV)-positive patients is presented.

Studies Illustrating Differential Effects of Intestinal versus Liver Enzyme Induction

The identification of inducible CYP3A4 in the human small intestine indicated that its activity in the enterocyte, in addition to that in the hepatocyte, likely contributes to observed drug interactions and the often limited or highly variable F_{oral} of CYP3A4 substrates (27). As recently described by Thummel et al. (39), it is likely that the relative contributions of intestinal and hepatic CYP3A4 to F_{oral} depend principally on the metabolic capacity of the intestine for the considered CYP3A4 substrate. In brief, the investigators calculated intestinal intrinsic clearances (CL_{int}) for numerous CYP3A4 substrates (possessing relatively low F_{oral}) from in vitro, liver microsome-derived Michaelis–Menten parameters, adjusting V_{max} for relative intestinal CYP3A content. These CL_{int} values were then used to calculate intestinal extraction ratios (ERs), thus allowing estimation of intestinal metabolic capacities for the substrates (taking into account intestinal transit times based on mean times to peak concentrations). Their results suggest that the contribution of intestinal (vs. liver) CYP3A4 to first pass extraction is predominant for nifedipine, saquinavir, and tacrolimus, equivalent for midazolam, but very minor for quinidine, cyclosporine, and terfenadine (suggested to be due to enzyme saturation in the case of quinidine and to low intestinal metabolic capaci-

TABLE 52-1. *Drugs for which a significant interaction with RIF coadministration has been reported during clinical use or in* in vivo *studies*

	Increased		Decreased		
	CL/F_{oral}	CL_{iv}	$t_{1/2}$	Levels and/or effect	Ref(s).
Antipyrine	✓		✓		(58,113–116)
Azole antifungals					
Fluconazole	✓	✓	✓		(163–165)
Itraconazole				✓	(166–168)
Ketoconazole	✓				(169,170)
β-Adrenergic receptor blockers					
Alprenolol	✓				(171)
Bisoprolol	✓		✓		(172)
Metoprolol	✓				(171)
Propranolol	✓		No		(90,91,171)
Benzodiazepines					
Midazolam	✓		✓	✓	(47,173)
Triazolam	✓		✓	✓	(174)
Caffeine		✓	✓		(65)
Calcium channel blockers					
Barnidipine				✓	(175)
Manidipine				✓	(175)
Nifedipine	✓	n.s.	n.s.	✓	(41–43,175,176)
Nisoldipine				✓	(175)
Chloramphenicol				✓	(177)
Clarithromycin				✓	(123)
Clofibrate				[a]	(178)
Corticosteroids					
Cortisol		✓	✓		(179,180)
Dexamethasone		✓	✓		(180)
Hydrocortisone		✓		✓	(181)
Prednisolone		✓	✓		(180,182)
Coumarin derivatives					
Phenprocoumon				✓	(183)
Warfarin	✓		✓	✓	(5,108,184–187)
Cyclosporine	✓	✓	✓	✓	(48,50,188–191)
Dapsone				✓	(121)
Debrisoquine				[b]	(58)
Delavirdine mesylate	✓		✓		(120)
Dextromethorphan				[c]	(61)
Diazepam		✓			(109)
Digitoxin				✓	(192,193)
Digoxin				✓	(194,195)
Disopyramide				✓	(196,197)
Doxycycline	✓		✓	✓	(198)
FK 506				✓	(199)
Fluoroquinolones					
Fleroxacin	✓		✓		(200)
Perfloxacin		✓	✓		(201)
Haloperidol		✓	✓		(202–204)
Hexobarbitone	✓	✓	✓		(7,83,205)
HIV protease inhibitors (indinavir, nelfinavir, saquinavir, ritonavir)	✓			✓	(119)
Lorcainide				✓	(206)
Mephenytoin				[d]	(23)
Mexiletine	✓		✓		(113)
Nortriptyline				✓	(207,208)
Opioid analgesics					
Alfentanil		✓	✓		(209)
Codeine	✓			✓	(100)
Methadone			✓	✓	(116,210,211)
Morphine	✓			✓	(92)
Oral contraceptives				✓	(6,212–214)
Phenytoin		✓		✓	(81,215)
Propafenone				✓	(64)
Quinidine				✓	(194)
Quinine				✓	(216)
Sulfonylurea hypoglycemic agents					
Chlorpropamide				✓	(217)
Glibenclamide				✓	(218,219)
Tolbutamide		✓	✓		(7,82,83)
Sulfasalazine				[e]	(220)
Theophylline	✓	✓	✓		(68–72)
Thyroid hormone				✓	(221)
Tocainide	✓		✓		(222)
Verapamil	✓	✓		✓	(44,223,224)
Zidovudine	✓			✓	(118,225)
Zopiclone			✓	✓	(226)

n.s., change not statistically significant.

[a] Decreased steady-state levels of its primary metabolite (due to lower F_{oral}?).
[b] RIF decreases its urinary metabolic ratio in PMs.
[c] RIF decreases its urinary metabolic ratio in EMs and PMs.
[d] Increased 0- to 8-hr urinary R/S mephenytoin ratio and excretion of 4′-hydroxy-S-mephenytoin RIF in extensive metabolizers.
[e] RIF alters subsequent disposition of sulfapyridine formed by sulfasalazine acetylation.

ties relative to the doses commonly administered of the latter two drugs).

With these analyses in mind, it is clear that the effects of RIF-mediated CYP3A4 induction in the intestine and/or liver on the disposition of coadministered CYP3A4 substrates will vary significantly. These effects will depend on the route (usually p.o.), dose, duration, and timing of RIF administration, the resulting extents of intestinal and liver CYP3A4 induction, and the relative ERs of the two organs for the concomitantly administered agent. Recent *in vivo* reports or studies of drug interactions between RIF and nifedipine, midazolam, and cyclosporine illustrate the effects of the antibiotic on the disposition of drugs for which intestinal CYP3A4 appears to contribute to varying degrees to F_{oral}.

Nifedipine has an F_{oral} of roughly 50% (40), and the estimates made by Thummel et al. (39) predict that much of its first pass extraction is attributable to intestinal CYP3A4 metabolism (the calculated intestinal blood and plasma extraction ratios were 0.36 and 0.52, respectively). Two early case reports demonstrated that concomitant RIF administration abolished the therapeutic efficacy of nifedipine by apparently increasing its oral clearance (CL/F_{oral}) (41,42). Holtbecker et al. (43) recently assessed the pharmacokinetics of oral and i.v. nifedipine before and after RIF administration (600 mg/day for 1 week). RIF tended to decrease i.v. nifedipine area under the curve (AUC; hence increase systemic clearance) and $t_{1/2}$, but the changes were not significant. The mean oral nifedipine AUC decreased roughly 12-fold (CL/F_{oral} increased 14-fold) after RIF treatment (both changes highly significant). Pre- and post-RIF F_{oral} were 41% and 5%, respectively. RIF administration increased estimated ERs for the liver and intestine from 0.47 to 0.67 and 0.22 to 0.76, respectively, with only the change in intestinal ER being statistically significant. This study suggests that for a drug whose F_{oral} is governed largely by intestinal CYP3A4 (high intestinal metabolic capacity) and whose systemic clearance is primarily hepatic and less affected by changes in metabolic CL_{int} (i.e., an intermediate- to high-hepatic ER drug), RIF administration will decrease F_{oral} but affect less its $t_{1/2}$. Although the changes in i.v. nifedipine pharmacokinetics were not significant, their trend suggests that RIF (at these doses) does alter slightly the systemic clearance of drugs with intermediate liver ER. Similar results were recently reported for verapamil, wherein RIF treatment affected its CL/F_{oral} much more significantly than its systemic clearance (44).

In addition to the earlier noted estimates of intestinal metabolic capacity by Thummel et al. (39), these investigators have demonstrated that the intestine and liver share roughly equivalent roles in the first pass oral extraction of midazolam. Mean intestinal and hepatic ERs of 0.43 and 0.44, respectively, were estimated from pharmacokinetic data obtained after i.v. and oral midazolam administration (45). Furthermore, administering the benzodiazepine to 10 liver transplant recipients during the anhepatic phase of surgery directly demonstrated that the mean intestinal extraction of an intraduodenal dose (in five subjects) was 0.43 and that intestinal extraction of an i.v. dose (in the remaining five patients) through the splanchnic vascular bed was 0.08 (46). The latter result indicates that intestinal CYP3A4 contributes little to the systemic clearance of midazolam (this likely applies to most CYP3A4 substrates). Backman et al. (47) recently reported a clinical study in which the effects of RIF (600 mg/day for 5 days) on the pharmacokinetics and pharmacodynamics of oral midazolam were assessed. The mean AUC and peak concentration decreased from 10.2 to 0.42 µg/min/mL and 55 to 3.5 ng/mL, respectively (both, $p < 0.001$). Moreover, the mean $t_{1/2}$ decreased from 3.1 to 1.3 hours, and there were decreases in its effects as assessed by numerous psychomotor tests (both decreases, $p < 0.001$). Thus for midazolam, RIF-induced CYP3A4 in both the intestine and liver contribute to decreased F_{oral}, resulting in a greater decrease in its oral AUC than that for nifedipine (24-fold vs. 12-fold) and more significant alteration of its $t_{1/2}$.

An interaction between cyclosporine and RIF was first reported in 1983 in a patient who had undergone renal transplantation and was receiving antituberculosis therapy (48). This and numerous other reports were, at the time, logically attributed to the RIF-mediated induction of hepatic CYP3A4. With the subsequent characterization of intestinal CYP3A forms, Kolars et al. (49) demonstrated that metabolites of cyclosporine were formed in the intestine *in vivo*. Hebert et al. (50) administered oral and i.v. cyclosporine to six subjects before and after treatment with RIF and reported an increase in systemic cyclosporine clearance and a decrease in F_{oral} only partly accounted for by the increase in hepatic clearance, suggesting a significant effect of intestinal CYP3A4 induction. The characterization of P-glycoprotein [the *mdr1* gene product, an adenosine triphosphate (ATP)-dependent drug efflux pump] expression in the apical, brush-border membranes of the human small intestine (51,52), and its ability to transport cyclosporine (53,54) indicated that this transporter may also be an important factor in the low and highly variable F_{oral} of the drug. Recently the groups of Watkins and Benet performed stepwise forward regression analyses with cyclosporine CL/F_{oral} (measured in 25 kidney transplant patients) as the dependent variable and duodenal CYP3A4 and P-glycoprotein levels (from pinch biopsies), hepatic CYP3A4 activity (assessed by the i.v. erythromycin breath test), and other measures as potential independent variables (55). The results indicate that 56% and 17% of the variability in the CL/F_{oral} of cyclosporine is accounted for by hepatic CYP3A4 activity ($p < 0.0001$) and duodenal P-glycoprotein concentration ($p < 0.0059$), respectively, with none of the other measures, most notably intestinal CYP3A4 content, contributing significantly to the predictiveness of the model. These findings confirm the previously noted estimate of

Thummel et al. (45) that intestinal CYP3A4 plays a very limited role in governing the F_{oral} of this immunosuppressant. However, RIF induction of CYP3A4 in the intestine may increase its metabolic capacity for cyclosporine (increased V_{max} and thus CL_{int}), leading to increased contribution of the intestinal enzyme pool in induced subjects. Additionally, RIF may also decrease cyclosporine F_{oral} by induction of intestinal P-glycoprotein. To our knowledge, this possibility has not yet been explored, although it has been shown that RIF induces P-glycoprotein expression in a human colon carcinoma–derived cell line (56).

Interactions with Drugs for Which CYP3A4 Is Not the Principal Metabolizing Enzyme

CYP3A4 does not catalyze the principal oxidations of numerous drugs reported to interact with RIF in vivo (see Table 52-1). In fact, some are considered prototypical substrates of CYPs 1A2 (caffeine, theophylline), 2C9 (warfarin), or 2D6 (debrisoquine, propranolol), or to be chiefly metabolized by glucuronidation (morphine). These interactions are very likely explained by (a) a relatively minor role of CYP3A4 in the oxidation of the drug in the noninduced state, but a more significant contribution to its metabolism after induction, and/or (b) the induction of an enzyme other than CYP3A4 in the intestine and/or liver. These examples illustrate that the consideration of metabolic drug interactions involving RIF should not be limited to compounds principally metabolized by CYP3A4, but extended to drugs for which a relatively minor CYP3A4-catalyzed metabolic pathway may gain importance and, moreover, to certain substrates of CYP2C9, CYP2C19, and UGTs.

Reports Indicating an Increased Metabolic Role of CYP3A4 on Its Induction

Debrisoquine was one of the first drugs for which a polymorphism in its metabolism (4-hydroxylation) was reported (57), leading to the characterization of CYP2D6 and the existence of several mutant alleles that result in the absence of functional protein (see Chapter 8). RIF has been reported to decrease the debrisoquine/4-hydroxydebrisoquine urinary metabolic ratio in poor (PM) but not extensive (EM) metabolizers of the drug (58), consistent with RIF augmenting 4-hydroxylase activity in those for whom CYP3A4 or other enzymes catalyze the reaction, while having very little effect in EM for whom CYP2D6 activity predominates. Dextromethorphan is O-demethylated by CYP2D6 (59) and N-demethylated (to 3-methoxymorphinan) by CYP3A4 (60). RIF treatment decreased the dextromethorphan/3-methoxymorphinan urinary metabolic ratio (in both PMs and EMs) in a manner consistent with eight-fold induction of liver CYP3A4 activity (61). Finally, another CYP2D6 substrate, propafenone (through 5-hydroxylation) (62), is N-dealkylated

by CYPs 1A2 and 3A4 (63). RIF was reported to reduce plasma concentrations and therapeutic effects of this antiarrhythmic (64), likely through increased first pass and/or systemic metabolism through N-dealkylation. Thus RIF can potentially interact with substrates of the polymorphically expressed CYP2D6 if CYP3A4 also contributes to their metabolism. However, the clinical significance of this will likely vary, depending on the patient phenotype (PM vs. EM) and the relative metabolic contribution of CYP3A4 in the noninduced state.

It was reported that RIF administration caused an increase in the clearance of caffeine and a decrease in its $t_{1/2}$, which was attributed to induction of hepatic CYP1A2 (65). In human liver microsomes, caffeine N-demethylations are catalyzed principally by CYP1A2 (and by CYP2E1 with low affinity), but its 8-hydroxylation is catalyzed by CYP3A4 (66,67). Because RIF does not induce CYPs 1A2 or 2E1, it seems more plausible that induction of CYP3A4 leads to greater metabolism by the 8-hydroxylation pathway. The N7-demethylation of caffeine gives rise to theophylline, for which numerous cases of interaction with RIF coadministration have been reported (68–72). In humans, theophylline is metabolized by N-demethylations and 8-hydroxylation (the major route), reactions in which CYP1A2 activity predominates, but to which CYPs 2E1, 2D6, and 3A4 also may contribute (73–77). The reported interactions with RIF suggest that significant induction of CYP3A4 may increase its role in intestinal and hepatic extraction of theophylline. Because the hepatic ER for theophylline is low, its systemic (hepatic) clearance is more significantly altered by changes in its metabolic CL_{int}.

Cases Suggesting the Induction of Other Enzymes

Phenytoin is eliminated primarily by oxidation to (R)- and (S)-enantiomers of 5-(4-hydroxyphenyl)-5-phenylhydantoin by CYPs 2C9 and 2C19 (78–80). In six subjects, RIF administration caused a two-fold increase in the mean systemic clearance of i.v. phenytoin (81), likely because of the induction of both CYP2C isoforms. Consistent with these observations are reports that RIF increased the systemic clearance (by roughly two-fold) and shortened the $t_{1/2}$ of tolbutamide (7,82,83), a drug also predominantly metabolized by CYP2C enzymes (78,79,84).

Propranolol is principally metabolized by N-deisopropylation and aromatic (4- and 5-) hydroxylations (85,86), reactions that are catalyzed predominantly by CYPs 1A2 and 2D6, respectively (87–89). This β-blocker also is eliminated by glucuronidation (accounting for roughly 10% to 20% of its clearance) (85,86). In six subjects, concomitant RIF treatment caused a roughly three-fold increase in the CL/F_{oral} of propranolol, but no changes in its $t_{1/2}$ or plasma protein–binding characteristics (90). This report suggests a significant effect of RIF on oral first pass propranolol extraction and few effects on its systemic clearance. In a subsequent study, RIF caused a four-fold increase in the CL/F_{oral} of propranolol in both EMs and PMs of debrisoquine, a similar increase in urinary glucuronide excretion in both phenotypes, but an increase in 4-hydroxylation that was 15-fold greater in EMs relative to the increase in PMs (91). Although glucuronidation represents a relatively minor contribution to systemic clearance, it seems possible that RIF-mediated induction of UGTs in the intestine (in addition to liver) could contribute to decreased F_{oral}. Interestingly, the increase in 4-hydroxylation activity by RIF (which was much more pronounced in EMs) suggests induction of CYP2D6. However, at present, no known inducers of this enzyme have been reported in the literature (RIF does not induce CYP2D6 mRNA or protein in human hepatocytes in primary culture). This could perhaps indicate RIF-mediated induction of an enzyme expressed or functional only in EMs (other than CYP2D6) that also has significant propranolol 4-hydroxylase activity.

Concomitant RIF administration increased the CL/F_{oral} of morphine and abolished its analgesic effects (92). Importantly, there were also decreases in the AUCs and urinary excretion of the 3- and 6-glucuronides, indicating that the effects of RIF were likely not the result of induction of liver UGTs. The mean rate of morphine glucuronidation in human intestinal homogenates was found to be roughly half that observed in liver homogenates (93), suggesting that the intestine may contribute significantly to the first pass extraction of the opioid (which has an F_{oral} of 24% ± 12%) (40). In anesthetized rabbits, the intestinal, liver, and pulmonary ERs of morphine were found to be 0.65, 0.52, and 0.33, respectively (94). In human liver, morphine 3- and 6-glucuronidation are catalyzed primarily by UGT2B7 (95), but the levels of expression and activity of this isozyme in the intestine are unknown. The decreases in parent drug, in 3- and 6-glucuronide AUCs, and in urinary glucuronide excretion are best explained by RIF increasing intestinal extraction, perhaps by induction of UGT2B7 or another isoform in this tissue. The increased intestinal activity may not have been detected through analysis of urinary glucuronide excretion (depending on intestinal absorption of the glucuronides). Additionally, morphine has been demonstrated to be a substrate of P-glycoprotein in multidrug-resistant cells (96) and in mice in vivo (97), suggesting that induction of intestinal P-glycoprotein by RIF may also contribute to decreased morphine F_{oral}.

Interactions in Which Induction of CYP3A4 and Other Enzymes May Both Contribute

Codeine is O-demethylated (to form morphine) by CYP2D6 (98), N-demethylated by CYP3A4 (99), and glucuronidated by UGT2B7 (95). Caraco et al. (100) reported that RIF administration increased the CL/F_{oral} of

codeine in both PMs and EMs of debrisoquine through increased N-demethylation and glucuronidation, consistent with induction of CYP3A4 and UGT2B7. Interestingly, codeine O-demethylation also was induced, but only in EMs (similar to the results noted earlier for propranolol 4-hydroxylation).

(S)-warfarin is hydroxylated predominantly by CYP2C9 (101,102), but the (R)-enantiomer is metabolized by numerous enzymes including CYPs 1A2, 2C19, and 3A4 (102–107). It appears that the induction of CYPs 2C9, 2C19, and 3A4 by RIF all likely contribute to the numerous reported interactions between RIF and warfarin. Indeed, one report described increases in the clearances of (S)- and (R)-warfarin by two- and three-fold, respectively (108), indicating that induction of enzymes metabolizing both enantiomers had occurred. Similarly, RIF was reported to increase the systemic clearance of diazepam roughly three-fold through induction of its principal metabolic pathways, N-demethylation and 3-hydroxylation (109), reactions catalyzed primarily by CYPs 2C19 and 3A4 (110–112). These reports, as well as the previously described effects of RIF on phenytoin, tolbutamide, and S-mephenytoin disposition, indicate that the observations of CYP2C9 and CYP2C19 induction in human hepatocytes in primary culture can indeed be extrapolated to the in vivo administration of therapeutic doses of RIF.

Finally, the clearance of antipyrine has often been used as a general measure of liver CYP activity, and numerous interactions with antipyrine and RIF coadministration have been reported (58,113–116). RIF appears to induce antipyrine elimination predominantly through increased N-demethylation to norantipyrine (115), a reaction that CYPs 1A2, 2A6, 2C9, 2C19, 2D6, 2E1, and 3A4 have been shown to catalyze in vitro (117). It is therefore likely that RIF-mediated induction of CYPs 2A6, 2C9, 2C19, and 3A4 in the intestine and/or liver accounts for the observed interactions.

Use of Rifampin and a Newer Derivative, Rifabutin, in Patients with HIV

The high incidence of RIF administration for antituberculosis therapy in patients with HIV disease makes interactions with other therapeutic agents in this population (often receiving multidrug regimens) particularly likely. RIF was reported to increase the CL/F_{oral} of the nucleoside analogue zidovudine (AZT) (118) and to increase the metabolism of the HIV protease inhibitors saquinavir, ritonavir, indinavir, and nelfinavir, resulting in subtherapeutic levels of these agents (119). In HIV patients receiving delavirdine mesylate (a nonnucleoside HIV reverse transcriptase inhibitor), concomitant RIF therapy caused a 27-fold increase in its CL/F_{oral}, negligible plasma trough levels, and a significant decrease in its $t_{1/2}$ (120). Additionally, an interaction with RIF appeared to prevent effective dapsone use as prophylaxis for *Pneumocystis carinii* pneumonia (121). Finally, significant interactions with methadone were reported in HIV-positive, former i.v. narcotics abusers (116).

A newer rifamycin derivative, rifabutin, is similar in structure and activity to RIF, equally effective in the treatment of pulmonary tuberculosis, but more active against *M. avium-intracellulare* complex, and thus increasingly used in the prophylaxis and treatment of this common infection in HIV patients (122). Numerous reports suggest that it induces CYP3A4 (and perhaps other enzymes) *in vivo*, but to a lesser extent than RIF (72,115,123–125). Thus rifabutin represents a first step toward finding newer rifamycin derivatives that are equally or more bactericidal than RIF but do not induce metabolic enzymes, therefore diminishing therapeutic complications associated with the numerous and significant drug interactions involving RIF.

DEXAMETHASONE

Pharmacology

Dexamethasone (DEX) is a potent synthetic glucocorticoid that lacks mineralocorticoid activity. Its principal indications are the treatment of cerebral edema in malignancy, diagnosis of Cushing's syndrome (by suppression of corticotropin secretion), prevention of nausea and vomiting subsequent to cancer chemotherapy, and in bacterial meningitis, to reduce inflammation and hearing loss. For most uses, doses of 0.5 to 10 mg are administered intravenously or orally every 2 to 24 hours. DEX is well absorbed in the intestine, and the F_{oral} ranges from 50% to 80% (126). Its major metabolite is formed by 6β-hydroxylation catalyzed by liver CYP3A4 (127).

Effects on Drug-Metabolizing Enzyme Expression

Members of the CYP3A subfamily were originally isolated, characterized, and cloned as antiglucocorticoid or glucocorticoid-inducible CYPs in several experimental species and in humans (see Chapter 10). DEX is thus a well-established inducer of CYP3A4 in human hepatocytes in primary culture (11,16,18,128) and in the liver *in vivo* (129–131). To our knowledge, induction of human intestinal CYP3A forms by DEX has not been thoroughly investigated, although the drug induces CYP3A enzymes in rat intestine (24). In addition, we and others have demonstrated that DEX induces CYPs 2B6, 2C8, 2C9, and 2C19 in human hepatocytes in primary culture, as evidenced by mRNA and/or protein accumulation (19; S. Gerbal, unpublished data). DEX also induces bilirubin UGT in HepG2 cells (36) and (class I) alcohol dehydrogenase mRNA in a rat hepatoma cell line (132), suggesting that it may have the same effects in human intestine and/or liver.

Studies or Reports of Interaction *In Vivo*

In comparison to RIF, relatively few significant drug interactions involving DEX have been reported (Table 52-2), which may be largely attributable to the previously mentioned clinical characteristics of its use (i.e., relatively low doses and frequency of use, short-term courses of therapy). We have previously described an induction protocol for CYP3A enzymes *in vivo* in the rat or rabbit by using a dose of 150 mg/kg/day for 4 days (11). In contrast, the largest dose of DEX administered to patients (for cerebral edema with inoperable brain tumors) is roughly 2 to 3 mg/kg/day, gradually decreased over a period of several days. Furthermore, we have generally noted that its potency and extent of CYP3A4 induction in human hepatocytes in primary culture are significantly lower than those of RIF (11,16,18). Thus its potency as a glucocorticoid necessitates low therapeutic doses, which are perhaps insufficient for significant CYP induction in many patients. Shorter-term therapy (relative to RIF use) and limited concomitant administration of other agents also likely contribute to the paucity of reported interactions. Nevertheless, the limited reports suggest that drug interactions can indeed occur because of DEX-mediated induction of CYPs.

An evaluation of the population pharmacokinetics of caffeine in neonates and infants revealed an increased clearance with concomitant DEX administration (133). The mechanism may be that indicated earlier for observed RIF–caffeine interactions, wherein CYP3A4 induction results in increased elimination through 8-hydroxylation.

In nine patients awaiting bone marrow transplantation, a single high dose of the anticancer prodrug cyclophosphamide (in combination with DEX) resulted in increased systemic clearance of both drugs (on their readministration 24 hours later) and increased 4-hydroxycyclophosphamide formation (the principal cytotoxic metabolite) (134). Repeated cyclophosphamide administration had previously been reported to decrease its $t_{1/2}$ (135,136). CYP2A6, CYP2B6, all members of the CYP2C subfamily, and CYP3A4 can all catalyze cyclophosphamide 4-hydroxylation *in vitro* (137,138). In human hepatocytes in primary culture, cyclophosphamide and DEX induce CYPs 2C8, 2C9, and 3A4 (DEX also induces CYP2B6), and both drugs increase rates of cyclophosphamide 4-hydroxylation *in cellulo* (19). Thus the earlier interaction likely results from the combined

TABLE 52-2. *Drugs whose disposition was altered by the* in vivo *enzyme inductive effects of dexamethasone or omeprazole*

DEX	Ref(s).	OM	Ref(s).
Caffeine	(133)	Caffeine	(159–161,227)
Cyclophosphamide	(134,139)	Cyclosporine	(162)
Misonidazole	(140)		
Phenytoin	(144)		
Praziquantel	(145)		

inductive effects of cyclophosphamide and DEX on the indicated liver CYP forms that are capable of catalyzing the 4-hydroxylation. Prior treatment with DEX alone was also reported to increase the clearance of cyclophosphamide significantly (139).

In five patients, DEX administration (8 mg/day for 3 weeks) caused significant reductions in the AUC and $t_{1/2}$ of orally administered misonidazole (a radiosensitizer) and an increase in its 24-hour urinary excretion (but no change in glomerular filtration rate in the one subject evaluated) (140). However, the AUC and urinary excretion of the major demethylated metabolite were unaltered. A role of CYP3A4 in misonidazole demethylation has not been demonstrated, but similar changes in its disposition were reported for other CYP inducers (phenobarbital and phenytoin), but accompanied by increased metabolite AUCs (141,142). In this case, the data are most consistent with a primary role of increased renal elimination (perhaps through induction of a transporter). Increased intestinal metabolite formation and absorption, resulting in similar metabolite AUCs, also may have contributed.

An early report of increased mean (24-hour) phenytoin serum concentrations with simultaneous DEX administration is consistent with enzyme inhibition and suggests that the two drugs may be partly metabolized by the same enzyme(s) (143). In contrast, a later single-case report described an increase in i.v. phenytoin clearance with concurrent DEX administration (requiring an increase in the phenytoin maintenance dose), with a subsequent increase in serum levels on DEX discontinuation (144). This interaction may perhaps be attributed to DEX-mediated induction of CYPs 2C9 and 2C19 in the liver.

Simultaneous administration of the antiparasitic drug praziquantel and DEX resulted in decreased plasma levels of the former (145). As for misonidazole, a rigorous examination of the CYP forms responsible for praziquantel metabolism has not been reported to date. However, phenytoin and carbamazepine increase its CL/F_{oral} in humans (146), and ketoconazole and miconazole have the opposite effects in the rat (147), suggesting that intestinal and/or hepatic CYP3A enzymes largely contribute to first pass praziquantel extraction. The interaction therefore appears to be a manifestation of DEX-mediated induction of these enzymes.

OMEPRAZOLE

Pharmacology

The substituted benzimidazole omeprazole (OM) is a potent irreversible inhibitor of H^+,K^+-ATPase (or the "proton pump") and therefore blocks gastric acid secretion from parietal cells. It is commonly used in the treatments of gastroesophageal reflux, peptic ulcer, and Zollinger–Ellison syndrome (a disease characterized by hypersecretion of gastric acid). For most uses, daily oral doses of 20 to 40 mg are administered, although doses up to 120 mg/day may be used for the latter indication. OM is rapidly absorbed, and F_{oral} ranges from 40% to 58%. It is extensively metabolized in the liver through 5-hydroxylation and sulfoxidation, reactions catalyzed predominantly by CYPs 2C19 and 3A4, respectively (148). Principal involvement of CYP2C19 in its metabolism results in polymorphic metabolism in humans, with PMs displaying roughly five- to ten-fold greater AUCs and significantly longer $t_{1/2}$ values than do EMs (149).

Effects on Drug-Metabolizing Enzyme Expression

Nearly a decade ago, we reported that OM is an inducer of CYP1A1 and CYP1A2 mRNA and CYP1A-specific activities in human hepatocytes in primary culture, and of liver CYP1A2 immunoreactive protein and CYP1A-specific activities in five patients in vivo (150). This generated significant controversy regarding the clinical relevance of the cell-culture results, the validity of the in vivo data, and the suggested implications for CYP1A-mediated activation of potential carcinogens. Subsequently, both OM and lansoprazole were shown to induce CYPs 1A1, 1A2, and 3A4 at the mRNA, protein, and activity levels in hepatocytes, with the induction of CYP3A4 displaying apparent polymorphism (observed in five of ten cultures) (17).

Induction of CYP1A enzymes by aryl hydrocarbons is mediated by the dioxin (Ah) receptor, for which OM and its sulfone are not ligands (151). However, we and others have shown that OM activates this receptor, as evidenced by gel mobility shift assays or transcriptional activation from a heterologous promoter containing the xenobiotic-response element (to which the activated Ah receptor binds) (152,153). OM does not activate the Ah receptor in mouse primary hepatocytes or hepatoma cells, and appears to be a precursor to a true Ah receptor ligand and activator that is produced in a species-specific manner (154,155). Regarding the apparent polymorphism of OM-mediated CYP3A4 induction, this could potentially involve the polymorphic expression of a transcription (or other protein) factor or an enzyme that converts OM to a CYP3A4-inducing species distinct from that inducing CYP1A forms.

McDonnell et al. (156) demonstrated the constitutive presence of CYP1A1 mRNA and 7-ethoxyresorufin O-deethylation (EROD) activity in the duodenum of six healthy subjects, as well as the inducibility of both by therapeutic doses of OM (20 mg/day for 1 week) in five of the six. The nonresponsive subject later displayed increased CYP1A1 mRNA and EROD activity after receiving 60 mg/day for 1 week, and two of the six subjects also demonstrated induction of CYP1A2 mRNA. Another work using duodenal biopsies reported increased CYP1A immunoreactive protein and EROD activities in patients taking OM (20–60 mg/day for at least 1 week) relative to a control group of other nonsmokers (157). In a further study, duodenal biopsies from six subjects before and after OM ingestion (20 mg/day, for 10 days) indicated increased EROD and nonspecific UGT activities, whereas total glutathione-S-transferase activity was unchanged (158). Clinical doses of OM therefore appear to induce CYP1A1 in the small intestine nearly uniformly, although the clinical relevance of this in terms of altered xenobiotic disposition or cancer risk remains to be determined. At present, we are unaware of studies evaluating potential induction of CYP3A enzymes by OM in gastrointestinal tissues.

Studies or Reports of Interaction *In Vivo* or Lack Thereof

A vital question after the initial report of CYP1A induction by OM in primary human hepatocytes and in the livers of five subjects *in vivo* was whether therapeutic use of the drug truly results in increased liver CYP1A2 levels and activity. Along with the subsequent characterization of OM metabolism (involvement of CYP2C19 and resulting polymorphism), numerous clinical studies have been reported that now allow this question to be addressed quite thoroughly.

Only two drugs (see Table 52-2) have been reported to demonstrate an interaction with concomitant OM use (in a manner consistent with enzyme induction) in clinical studies (caffeine) or in a single case report (cyclosporine). Rost et al. (159) demonstrated that the predominantly CYP1A2-catalyzed N3-demethylation of caffeine (assessed by $^{13}CO_2$ release in the breath) was increased by OM (40 mg/day for 7 days) in PMs but not in EMs of S-mephenytoin, but that an increased dose (120 mg/day for 1 week) significantly increased $^{13}CO_2$ release and caffeine plasma clearance in EMs (160). Interestingly, the latter study also demonstrated that urinary 6β-hydroxy-

cortisol excretion was unchanged in all subjects, consistent with a lack of liver CYP3A4 induction. These investigators also demonstrated that the polymorphism and dose-dependency of response was equally well detected by estimates of $^{13}CO_2$ release, plasma clearance, or urinary metabolite ratios (N-demethylated products/8-hydroxylated) (161). In the case of the CYP3A4 substrate cyclosporine, a bone marrow transplant patient maintained on the immunosuppressant (1.5 mg/kg b.i.d., i.v.) was given concomitant OM at 40 mg/day, i.v., for 11 days, during which time the serum cyclosporine levels decreased precipitately (by 70%), increasing again to previous levels 4 days after cessation of OM use (162). A possible scenario is that this patient represents a cosegregation of the CYP2C19-deficient and CYP3A4-inducible (by OM) phenotypes, which resulted in greater systemic benzimidazole exposure (from the relatively large intravenous dose) and hence significant induction of liver CYP3A4 (and presumably CYP1A2). We have previously reported that OM at concentrations up to 100 μM did not inhibit the metabolism of 5 μM cyclosporine in primary human hepatocytes (18), suggesting that OM should not inhibit induced cyclosporine metabolism *in vivo*.

Far more numerous are the reported clinical studies in which substrates of CYPs 1A2 and/or 3A4 were shown not to interact with multiple-dose OM therapy (see Table 52-3).It is important to note that virtually all of these studies were performed by using subjects who were healthy (except for the cyclosporine and second warfarin reports) and uncharacterized for CYP2C19 phenotype (except the diazepam work). In this collective study population (very likely comprised predominantly of EMs), OM when used at common therapeutic doses did not significantly induce *mean* CYP1A2 or CYP3A4 activities in the liver. Because the frequency of the PM phenotype for S-mephenytoin 4'-hydroxylation in whites and Asians is

TABLE 52-3. *Drugs partly or principally metabolized by CYP1A2 and/or CYP3A4 whose* in vivo *metabolism in healthy volunteers (unless otherwise noted) was not increased by concomitant, multiple-dose OM treatment*

Drug	Active CYP(s)	OM dose/day (mg × days)	Result	Ref(s).
Caffeine, p.o.	1A2/2E1/3A4	20 × 7	No change in urinary (sum-N-demethylated)/	(228)
		20 × 14	hydroxylated metabolite ratio	(229)
Cyclosporine, p.o.	3A4	20 × 14	Unchanged steady-state trough levels[a]	(230)
Diazepam, i.v.	2C19/3A4	20 × 14	Increased AUC, longer $t_{1/2}$ in extensive metabolizers	(231)
Lidocaine, i.v.	3A4	40 × 7	Unchanged AUC and $t_{1/2}$	(232)
Nifedipine, p.o.	3A4	20 × 8	Increased AUC	(233)
Phenacetin, p.o.	1A2	20 × 8	Unchanged AUC and $t_{1/2}$	(234)
Prednisone, p.o.	3A4	40 × 7	Unchanged AUC and $t_{1/2}$	(235)
Propranolol, p.o.	1A2/2D6	20 × 8	Unchanged steady-state AUC	(236)
Quinidine, p.o.	3A4	40 × 7	Unaltered AUC, effects	(237)
Theophylline, p.o.	1A2/3A4	20 × 7	Unchanged steady-state AUC	(238)
R-warfarin, p.o.	1A2/3A4/2C19	20 × 14	Slight *increases* in mean plasma concentration[b]	(239,240)
		20 × 21		

[a]In renal transplant patients.
[b]Three-week study conducted in patients receiving anticoagulation therapy.

roughly 2% to 3% and 15% to 20%, respectively, this result can be extrapolated to the vast majority of prospective OM users.

In summary, current evidence indicates that the induction of liver CYP1A2 by therapeutic doses of OM is not likely except in patients known to be PMs of S-mephenytoin or those requiring larger doses of the benzimidazole (e.g., patients with Zollinger–Ellison syndrome). The inductive effects may not be clinically important unless the coadministered CYP1A2 substrate displays a low hepatic ER (hepatic CL thus being more dependent on CL_{int}) and a narrow therapeutic range. Similarly, OM therapy does not seem to induce liver (or intestinal) CYP3A4 significantly, although this may have occurred in an isolated case.

REFERENCES

1. Sensi P. History of the development of rifampin. *Rev Infect Dis* 1983; 5(suppl 3):S402–S406.
2. Wehrli W. Rifampin: mechanisms of action and resistance. *Rev Infect Dis* 1983;5(suppl 3):S407–S411.
3. Holdiness MR. Clinical pharmacokinetics of the antituberculosis drugs. *Clin Pharmacokinet* 1984;9:511–544.
4. Immanuel C, Jayasankar K, Narayana AS, Santha T, Sundaram V, Sarma GR. Induction of rifampicin metabolism during treatment of tuberculous patients with daily and fully intermittent regimens containing the drug. *Indian J Chest Dis Allied Sci* 1989;31:251–257.
5. O'Reilly RA. Interaction of sodium warfarin and rifampin: studies in man. *Ann Intern Med* 1974;81:337–340.
6. Bolt HM, Bolt M. [Interaction between the effect of rifampicin and oral contraceptives]. *Internist (Berl)* 1974;15:571–572.
7. Zilly W, Breimer DD, Richter E. Induction of drug metabolism in man after rifampicin treatment measured by increased hexobarbital and tolbutamide clearance. *Eur J Clin Pharmacol* 1975;9:219–227.
8. Daujat M, Pichard L, Dalet C, et al. Expression of five forms of microsomal cytochrome P-450 in primary cultures of rabbit hepatocytes treated with various classes of inducers. *Biochem Pharmacol* 1987;36: 3597–3606.
9. Potenza CL, Pendurthi UR, Strom DK, et al. Regulation of the rabbit cytochrome P-450 3c gene: age-dependent expression and transcriptional activation by rifampicin. *J Biol Chem* 1989;264:16222–16228.
10. Daujat M, Clair P, Astier C, et al. Induction, regulation and messenger half-life of cytochromes P450 IA1, IA2 and IIIA6 in primary cultures of rabbit hepatocytes: CYP 1A1, 1A2 and 3A6 chromosome location in the rabbit and evidence that post-transcriptional control of gene IA2 does not involve mRNA stabilization. *Eur J Biochem* 1991;200: 501–510.
11. Daujat M, Pichard L, Fabre I, et al. Induction protocols for cytochromes P450IIIA in vivo and in primary cultures of animal and human hepatocytes. *Methods Enzymol* 1991;206:345–353.
12. Combalbert J, Fabre I, Fabre G, et al. Metabolism of cyclosporin A. IV: purification and identification of the rifampicin-inducible human liver cytochrome P-450 (cyclosporin A oxidase) as a product of P450IIIA gene subfamily. *Drug Metab Dispos* 1989;17:197–207.
13. Ged C, Rouillon JM, Pichard L, et al. The increase in urinary excretion of 6 beta-hydroxycortisol as a marker of human hepatic cytochrome P450IIIA induction. *Br J Clin Pharmacol* 1989;28:373–387.
14. Daujat M, Fabre I, Diaz D, et al. Inducibility and expression of class 1A and 3A cytochromes P450 in primary cultures of adult human hepatocytes. *Biochem Pharmacol* 1990;9:315–326.
15. Morel F, Beaune PH, Ratanasavanh D, et al. Expression of cytochrome P-450 enzymes in cultured human hepatocytes. *Eur J Biochem* 1990; 191:437–444.
16. Pichard L, Fabre I, Daujat M, Domergue J, Joyeux H, Maurel P. Effect of corticosteroids on the expression of cytochromes P450 and on cyclosporin A oxidase activity in primary cultures of human hepatocytes. *Mol Pharmacol* 1992;41:1047–1055.
17. Curi-Pedrosa R, Daujat M, Pichard L, et al. Omeprazole and lansoprazole are mixed inducers of CYP1A and CYP3A in human hepatocytes in primary culture. *J Pharmacol Exp Ther* 1994;269:384–392.
18. Pichard L, Fabre I, Fabre G, et al. Cyclosporin A drug interactions: screening for inducers and inhibitors of cytochrome P-450 (cyclosporin A oxidase) in primary cultures of human hepatocytes and in liver microsomes. *Drug Metab Dispos* 1990;18:595–606.
19. Chang TK, Yu L, Maurel P, Waxman DJ. Enhanced cyclophosphamide and ifosfamide activation in primary human hepatocyte cultures: response to cytochrome P-450 inducers and autoinduction by oxazaphosphorines. *Cancer Res* 1997;57:1946–1954.
20. Lemoine A, Gautier JC, Azoulay D, et al. Major pathway of imipramine metabolism is catalyzed by cytochromes P-450 1A2 and P-450 3A4 in human liver. *Mol Pharmacol* 1993;43:827–832.
21. Li AP, Rasmussen A, Xu L, Kaminski DL. Rifampicin induction of lidocaine metabolism in cultured human hepatocytes. *J Pharmacol Exp Ther* 1995;274:673–677.
22. Dalet-Beluche I, Boulenc X, Fabre G, Maurel P, Bonfils C. Purification of two cytochrome P450 isozymes related to CYP2A and CYP3A gene families from monkey (baboon, *Papio papio*) liver microsomes. *Eur J Biochem* 1992;204:641–648.
23. Zhou HH, Anthony LB, Wood AJ, Wilkinson GR. Induction of polymorphic 4'-hydroxylation of S-mephenytoin by rifampicin. *Br J Clin Pharmacol* 1990;30:471–475.
24. Watkins PB, Wrighton SA, Schuetz EG, Molowa DT, Guzelian PS. Identification of glucocorticoid-inducible cytochromes P-450 in the intestinal mucosa of rats and man. *J Clin Invest* 1987;80:1029–1036.
25. de Waziers I, Cugnenc PH, Yang CS, Leroux JP, Beaune PH. Cytochrome P 450 isoenzymes, epoxide hydrolase and glutathione transferases in rat and human hepatic and extrahepatic tissues. *J Pharmacol Exp Ther* 1990;253:387–394.
26. Paine MF, Khalighi M, Fisher JM, et al. Characterization of interintestinal and intraintestinal variations in human CYP3A-dependent metabolism. *J Pharmacol Exp Ther* 1997;283:1552–1562.
27. Kolars JC, Schmiedlin-Ren P, Schuetz JD, Fang C, Watkins PB. Identification of rifampin-inducible P450IIIA4 (CYP3A4) in human small bowel enterocytes. *J Clin Invest* 1992;90:1871–1878.
28. Kolars JC, Lown KS, Schmiedlin-Ren P, et al. CYP3A gene expression in human gut epithelium. *Pharmacogenetics* 1994;4:247–259.
29. Haehner BD, Gorski JC, Vandenbranden M, et al. Bimodal distribution of renal cytochrome P450 3A activity in humans. *Mol Pharmacol* 1996; 50:52–59.
30. Ohnhaus EE, Bluhm RC. Induction of the monooxygenase enzyme system in human lung. *Eur J Clin Invest* 1987;17:488–492.
31. Murray GI, Burke MD. Immunohistochemistry of drug metabolizing enzymes. *Biochem Pharmacol* 1995;50:895–903.
32. Shimada T, Yamazaki H, Mimura M, et al. Characterization of microsomal cytochrome P450 enzymes involved in the oxidation of xenobiotic chemicals in human fetal livers and adult lungs. *Drug Metab Dispos* 1996;24:515–522.
33. Waxman DJ, Lapenson DP, Aoyama T, Gelboin HV, Gonzalez FJ, Korzekwa K. Steroid hormone hydroxylase specificities of eleven cDNA-expressed human cytochrome P450s. *Arch Biochem Biophys* 1991; 290:160–166.
34. Kern A, Bader A, Pichlmayr R, Sewing KF. Drug metabolism in hepatocyte sandwich cultures of rats and humans. *Biochem Pharmacol* 1997;54:761–772.
35. Abid A, Sabolovic N, Magdalou J. Expression and inducibility of UDP-glucuronosyltransferases 1-naphthol in human cultured hepatocytes and hepatocarcinoma cell lines. *Life Sci* 1997;60:1943–1951.
36. Doostdar H, Grant MH, Melvin WT, Wolf CR, Burke MD. The effects of inducing agents on cytochrome P450 and UDP-glucuronyltransferase activities in human HEPG2 hepatoma cells. *Biochem Pharmacol* 1993;46:629–635.
37. Abid A, Sabolovic N, Magdalou J. Inducibility of ethoxyresorufin deethylase and UDP-glucuronosyltransferase activities in two human hepatocarcinoma cell lines KYN-2 and Mz-Hep-1. *Cell Biol Toxicol* 1996;12:115–123.
38. Calleja C, Pascussi JM, Mani JC, Maurel P, Vilarem MJ. The antibiotic rifampicin is a nonsteroidal ligand and activator of the human glucocorticoid receptor. *Nat Med* 1998;4:92–96.
39. Thummel KE, Kunze KL, Shen DD. Enzyme-catalyzed processes of first-pass hepatic and intestinal drug extraction. *Adv Drug Deliv Rev* 1997;27:99–128.

40. Benet LZ, Oie S, Schwartz JB. Design and optimization of dosage regimens: pharmacokinetic data. In: Hardman JG, Limbard LE, Molinoff PB, Ruddon RW, Gilman AG, eds. *The pharmacological basis of therapeutics.* New York: McGraw-Hill, 1996:1707–1792.

41. Tsuchihashi K, Fukami K, Kishimoto H, et al. A case of variant angina exacerbated by administration of rifampicin. *Heart Vessels* 1987;3: 214–217.

42. Tada Y, Tsuda Y, Otsuka T, et al. Case report: nifedipine-rifampicin interaction attenuates the effect on blood pressure in a patient with essential hypertension. *Am J Med Sci* 1992;303:25–27.

43. Holtbecker N, Fromm MF, Kroemer HK, Ohnhaus EE, Heidemann H. The nifedipine-rifampin interaction: evidence for induction of gut wall metabolism. *Drug Metab Dispos* 1996;24:1121–1123.

44. Fromm MF, Busse D, Kroemer HK, Eichelbaum M. Differential induction of prehepatic and hepatic metabolism of verapamil by rifampin. *Hepatology* 1996;24:796–801.

45. Thummel KE, O'Shea D, Paine MF, et al. Oral first-pass elimination of midazolam involves both gastrointestinal and hepatic CYP3A-mediated metabolism. *Clin Pharmacol Ther* 1996;59:491–502.

46. Paine MF, Shen DD, Kunze KL, et al. First-pass metabolism of midazolam by the human intestine. *Clin Pharmacol Ther* 1996;60:14–24.

47. Backman JT, Olkkola KT, Neuvonen PJ. Rifampin drastically reduces plasma concentrations and effects of oral midazolam. *Clin Pharmacol Ther* 1996;59:7–13.

48. Langhoff E, Madsen S. Rapid metabolism of cyclosporin and prednisone in kidney transplant patient receiving tuberculostatic treatment [Letter]. *Lancet* 1983;2:1031.

49. Kolars JC, Awni WM, Merion RM, Watkins PB. First-pass metabolism of cyclosporin by the gut. *Lancet* 1991;338:1488–1490.

50. Hebert MF, Roberts JP, Prueksaritanont T, Benet LZ. Bioavailability of cyclosporine with concomitant rifampin administration is markedly less than predicted by hepatic enzyme induction. *Clin Pharmacol Ther* 1992;52:453–457.

51. Thiebaut F, Tsuruo T, Hamada H, Gottesman MM, Pastan I, Willingham MC. Cellular localization of the multi-drug resistance gene product P-glycoprotein in normal human tissues. *Proc Natl Acad Sci USA* 1987;84:7735–7738.

52. Penny JI, Campbell FC. Active transport of benzo-(a)pyrene in apical membrane vesicles from normal human intestinal epithelium. *Biochim Biophys Acta* 1994;1226:232–236.

53. Tsuji A, Tamai I, Sakata A, Tenda Y, Terasaki T. Restricted transport of cyclosporin A across the blood-brain barrier by a multi-drug transporter, P-glycoprotein. *Biochem Pharmacol* 1993;46:1096–1099.

54. Saeki T, Ueda K, Tanigawara Y, Hori R, Komano T. Human P-glycoprotein transports cyclosporin A and FK506. *J Biol Chem* 1993;268: 6077–6080.

55. Lown KS, Mayo RR, Leichtman AB, et al. Role of intestinal P-glycoprotein (mdr1) in interpatient variation in the oral bioavailability of cyclosporine. *Clin Pharmacol Ther* 1997;62:248–260.

56. Schuetz EG, Beck WT, Schuetz JD. Modulators and substrates of P-glycoprotein and cytochrome P4503A coordinately up-regulate these proteins in human colon carcinoma cells. *Mol Pharmacol* 1996;49: 311–318.

57. Mahgoub A, Idle JR, Dring LG, Lancaster R, Smith RL. Polymorphic hydroxylation of debrisoquin in man. *Lancet* 1977;2:584–586.

58. Leclercq V, Desager JP, Horsmans Y, Van Nieuwenhuyze Y, Harvengt C. Influence of rifampicin, phenobarbital and cimetidine on mixed function monooxygenase in extensive and poor metabolizers of debrisoquine. *Int J Clin Pharmacol Ther Toxicol* 1989;27:593–598.

59. Schmid B, Bircher J, Preisig R, Kupfer A. Polymorphic dextromethorphan metabolism: co-segregation of oxidative O-demethylation with debrisoquin hydroxylation. *Clin Pharmacol Ther* 1985;38: 618–624.

60. Gorski JC, Jones DR, Wrighton SA, Hall SD. Characterization of dextromethorphan N-demethylation by human liver microsomes: contribution of the cytochrome P450 3A (CYP3A) subfamily. *Biochem Pharmacol* 1994;48:173–182.

61. Jones DR, Gorski JC, Haehner BD, O'Mara EM Jr, Hall SD. Determination of cytochrome P450 3A4/5 activity in vivo with dextromethorphan N-demethylation. *Clin Pharmacol Ther* 1996;60:374–384.

62. Kroemer HK, Mikus G, Kronbach T, Meyer UA, Eichelbaum M. In vitro characterization of the human cytochrome P-450 involved in polymorphic oxidation of propafenone. *Clin Pharmacol Ther* 1989;45: 28–33.

63. Botsch S, Gautier JC, Beaune P, Eichelbaum M, Kroemer HK. Identification and characterization of the cytochrome P450 enzymes involved in N-dealkylation of propafenone: molecular base for interaction potential and variable disposition of active metabolites. *Mol Pharmacol* 1993; 43:120–126.

64. Castel JM, Cappiello E, Leopaldi D, Latini R. Rifampicin lowers plasma concentrations of propafenone and its antiarrhythmic effect. *Br J Clin Pharmacol* 1990;30:155–156.

65. Wietholtz H, Zysset T, Marschall HU, Generet K, Matern S. The influence of rifampin treatment on caffeine clearance in healthy man. *J Hepatol* 1995;22:78–81.

66. Tassaneeyakul W, Mohamed Z, Birkett DJ, et al. Caffeine as a probe for human cytochromes P450: validation using cDNA-expression, immunoinhibition and microsomal kinetic and inhibitor techniques. *Pharmacogenetics* 1992;2:173–183.

67. Tassaneeyakul W, Birkett DJ, McManus ME, et al. Caffeine metabolism by human hepatic cytochromes P450: contributions of 1A2, 2E1 and 3A isoforms. *Biochem Pharmacol* 1994;47:1767–1776.

68. Straughn AB, Henderson RP, Lieberman PL, Self TH. Effect of rifampin on theophylline disposition. *Ther Drug Monit* 1984;6:153–156.

69. Robson RA, Miners JO, Wing LM, Birkett DJ. Theophylline-rifampicin interaction: non-selective induction of theophylline metabolic pathways. *Br J Clin Pharmacol* 1984;18:445–448.

70. Powell-Jackson PR, Jamieson AP, Gray BJ, Moxham J, Williams R. Effect of rifampicin administration on theophylline pharmacokinetics in humans. *Am Rev Respir Dis* 1985;131:939–940.

71. Boyce EG, Dukes GE, Rollins DE, Sudds TW. The effect of rifampin on theophylline kinetics. *J Clin Pharmacol* 1986;26:696–699.

72. Gillum JG, Sesler JM, Bruzzese VL, Israel DS, Polk RE. Induction of theophylline clearance by rifampin and rifabutin in healthy male volunteers. *Antimicrob Agents Chemother* 1996;40:1866–1869.

73. McManus ME, Miners JO, Gregor D, Stupans I, Birkett DJ. Theophylline metabolism by human, rabbit and rat liver microsomes and by purified forms of cytochrome P450. *J Pharm Pharmacol* 1988;40:388–391.

74. Sarkar MA, Jackson BJ. Theophylline N-demethylations as probes for P4501A1 and P4501A2. *Drug Metab Dispos* 1994;22:827–834.

75. Zhang ZY, Kaminsky LS. Characterization of human cytochromes P450 involved in theophylline 8-hydroxylation. *Biochem Pharmacol* 1995;50:205–211.

76. Ha HR, Chen J, Freiburghaus AU, Follath F. Metabolism of theophylline by cDNA-expressed human cytochromes P-450. *Br J Clin Pharmacol* 1995;39:321–326.

77. Tjia JF, Colbert J, Back DJ. Theophylline metabolism in human liver microsomes: inhibition studies. *J Pharmacol Exp Ther* 1996;276: 912–917.

78. Doecke CJ, Veronese ME, Pond SM, et al. Relationship between phenytoin and tolbutamide hydroxylations in human liver microsomes. *Br J Clin Pharmacol* 1991;31:125–130.

79. Veronese ME, Mackenzie PI, Doecke CJ, McManus ME, Miners JO, Birkett DJ. Tolbutamide and phenytoin hydroxylations by cDNA-expressed human liver cytochrome P4502C9. *Biochem Biophys Res Commun* 1991;175:1112–1118.

80. Bajpai M, Roskos LK, Shen DD, Levy RH. Roles of cytochrome P4502C9 and cytochrome P4502C19 in the stereoselective metabolism of phenytoin to its major metabolite. *Drug Metab Dispos* 1996;24: 1401–1403.

81. Kay L, Kampmann JP, Svendsen TL, et al. Influence of rifampicin and isoniazid on the kinetics of phenytoin. *Br J Clin Pharmacol* 1985;20: 323–326.

82. Syvalahti E, Pihlajamaki K, Iisalo E. Effect of tuberculostatic agents on the response of serum growth hormone and immunoreactive insulin to intravenous tolbutamide, and on the half-life of tolbutamide. *Int J Clin Pharmacol Biopharm* 1976;13:83–89.

83. Zilly W, Breimer DD, Richter E. Stimulation of drug metabolism by rifampicin in patients with cirrhosis or cholestasis measured by increased hexobarbital and tolbutamide clearance. *Eur J Clin Pharmacol* 1977;11:287–293.

84. Relling MV, Aoyama T, Gonzalez FJ, Meyer UA. Tolbutamide and mephenytoin hydroxylation by human cytochrome P450s in the CYP2C subfamily. *J Pharmacol Exp Ther* 1990;252:442–447.

85. Walle T, Walle UK, Olanoff LS. Quantitative account of propranolol metabolism in urine of normal man. *Drug Metab Dispos* 1985;13: 204–209.

86. Walle T, Walle UK, Olanoff LS, Conradi EC. Partial metabolic clear-

ances as determinants of the oral bioavailability of propranolol. *Br J Clin Pharmacol* 1986;22:317–323.

87. Marathe PH, Shen DD, Nelson WL. Metabolic kinetics of pseudo-racemic propranolol in human liver microsomes: enantioselectivity and quinidine inhibition. *Drug Metab Dispos* 1994;22:237–247.

88. Masubuchi Y, Hosokawa S, Horie T, et al. Cytochrome P450 isozymes involved in propranolol metabolism in human liver microsomes: the role of CYP2D6 as ring-hydroxylase and CYP1A2 as *N*-desisopropylase. *Drug Metab Dispos* 1994;22:909–915.

89. Yoshimoto K, Echizen H, Chiba K, Tani M, Ishizaki T. Identification of human CYP isoforms involved in the metabolism of propranolol enantiomers: *N*-desisopropylation is mediated mainly by CYP1A2. *Br J Clin Pharmacol* 1995;39:421–431.

90. Herman RJ, Nakamura K, Wilkinson GR, Wood AJ. Induction of propranolol metabolism by rifampicin. *Br J Clin Pharmacol* 1983;16:565–569.

91. Shaheen O, Biollaz J, Koshakji RP, Wilkinson GR, Wood AJ. Influence of debrisoquin phenotype on the inducibility of propranolol metabolism. *Clin Pharmacol Ther* 1989;45:439–443.

92. Fromm MF, Eckhardt K, Li S, et al. Loss of analgesic effect of morphine due to coadministration of rifampin. *Pain* 1997;72:261–267.

93. Pacifici GM, Bencini C, Rane A. Presystemic glucuronidation of morphine in humans and rhesus monkeys: subcellular distribution of the UDP-glucuronyltransferase in the liver and intestine. *Xenobiotica* 1986;16:123–128.

94. Abdallah C, Besner JG, du Souich P. Presystemic elimination of morphine in anesthetized rabbits: contribution of the intestine, liver, and lungs. *Drug Metab Dispos* 1995;23:584–589.

95. Coffman BL, Rios GR, King CD, Tephly TR. Human UGT2B7 catalyzes morphine glucuronidation. *Drug Metab Dispos* 1997;25:1–4.

96. Callaghan R, Riordan JR. Synthetic and natural opiates interact with P-glycoprotein in multidrug-resistant cells. *J Biol Chem* 1993;268:16059–16064.

97. Schinkel AH, Wagenaar E, van-Deemter L, Mol CA, Borst P. Absence of the mdr1a P-glycoprotein in mice affects tissue distribution and pharmacokinetics of dexamethasone, digoxin, and cyclosporin A. *J Clin Invest* 1995;96:698–705.

98. Mortimer O, Persson K, Ladona MG, et al. Polymorphic formation of morphine from codeine in poor and extensive metabolizers of dextromethorphan: relationship to the presence of immunoidentified cytochrome P-450IID1. *Clin Pharmacol Ther* 1990;47:27–35.

99. Caraco Y, Tateishi T, Guengerich FP, Wood AJ. Microsomal codeine *N*-demethylation: cosegregation with cytochrome P4503A4 activity. *Drug Metab Dispos* 1996;24:761–764.

100. Caraco Y, Sheller J, Wood AJ. Pharmacogenetic determinants of codeine induction by rifampin: the impact on codeine's respiratory, psychomotor and miotic effects. *J Pharmacol Exp Ther* 1997;281:330–336.

101. Rettie AE, Eddy AC, Heimark LD, Gibaldi M, Trager WF. Characteristics of warfarin hydroxylation catalyzed by human liver microsomes. *Drug Metab Dispos* 1989;17:265–270.

102. Rettie AE, Korzekwa KR, Kunze KL, et al. Hydroxylation of warfarin by human cDNA expressed cytochrome P450: a role for CYP2C9 in the etiology of (S)-warfarin drug interactions. *Chem Res Toxicol* 1992;5:54–59.

103. Brian WB, Sari MA, Iwasaki M, Shimada T, Kaminsky LS, Guengerich FP. Catalytic activities of human liver cytochrome P450 3A4 expressed in *Saccharomyces cerevisiae*. *Biochemistry* 1990;29:11280–11292.

104. Kunze KL, Trager WF. Isoform-selective mechanism-based inhibition of human cytochrome P450 1A2 by furafylline. *Chem Res Toxicol* 1993;6:649–656.

105. Kaminsky LS, de Morais SM, Faletto MB, Dunbar DA, Goldstein JA. Correlation of human cytochrome P450 2C substrate specificities with primary structure: warfarin as a probe. *Mol Pharmacol* 1993;43:234–239.

106. Gallagher EP, Wienkers LC, Stapleton PL, Kunze KL, Eaton DL. Role of human microsomal and human complementary DNA-expressed cytochromes P450 1A2 and P450 3A4 in the bioactivation of aflatoxin B1. *Cancer Res* 1994;54:101–108.

107. Wienkers LC, Wurden CJ, Storch E, Kunze KL, Rettie AE, Trager WF. Formation of (R)-8-hydroxywarfarin in human liver microsomes: a new metabolic marker for the (S)-mephenytoin hydroxylase, P4502C19. *Drug Metab Dispos* 1996;24:610–614.

108. Heimark LD, Gibaldi M, Trager WF, O'Reilly RA, Goulart DA. The mechanism of the warfarin-rifampin drug interaction in humans. *Clin Pharmacol Ther* 1987;42:388–394.

109. Ohnhaus EE, Brockmeyer N, Dylewicz P, Habicht H. The effect of antipyrine and rifampin on the metabolism of diazepam. *Clin Pharmacol Ther* 1987;42:148–156.

110. Andersson T, Miners J, Veronese M, Birkett D. Diazepam metabolism by human liver microsomes is mediated by both S-mephenytoin hydroxylase and CYP3A isoforms. *Br J Clin Pharmacol* 1994;38:131–137.

111. Ono S, Hatanaka T, Miyazawa S, et al. Human liver microsomal diazepam metabolism using cDNA-expressed cytochrome P450s: role of CYP2B6, 2C19 and the 3A subfamily. *Xenobiotica* 1996;26:1155–1166.

112. Jung F, Richardson T, Raucy J, Johnson E. Diazepam metabolism by cDNA-expressed human 2C P450s: identification of P4502C18 and P4502C19 as low K(M) diazepam *N*-demethylases. *Drug Metab Dispos* 1997;25:133–139.

113. Pentikainen PJ, Koivula IH, Hiltunen HA. Effect of rifampicin treatment on the kinetics of mexiletine. *Eur J Clin Pharmacol* 1982;23:261–266.

114. Schulte HM, Monig H, Benker G, Pagel H, Reinwein D, Ohnhaus EE. Pharmacokinetics of aldosterone in patients with Addison's disease: effect of rifampicin treatment on glucocorticoid and mineralocorticoid metabolism. *Clin Endocrinol (Oxf)* 1987;27:655–662.

115. Perucca E, Grimaldi R, Frigo GM, Sardi A, Monig H, Ohnhaus EE. Comparative effects of rifabutin and rifampicin on hepatic microsomal enzyme activity in normal subjects. *Eur J Clin Pharmacol* 1988;34:595–599.

116. Brockmeyer NH, Mertins L, Goos M. Pharmacokinetic interaction of antimicrobial agents with levomethadon in drug-addicted AIDS patients. *Klin Wochenschr* 1991;69:16–18.

117. Sharer JE, Wrighton SA. Identification of the human hepatic cytochromes P450 involved in the *in vitro* oxidation of antipyrine. *Drug Metab Dispos* 1996;24:487–494.

118. Burger DM, Meenhorst PL, ten Napel CH, et al. Pharmacokinetic variability of zidovudine in HIV-infected individuals: subgroup analysis and drug interactions. *AIDS* 1994;8:1683–1689.

119. Clinical update: impact of HIV protease inhibitors on the treatment of HIV-infected tuberculosis patients with rifampin. *Morb Mortal Wkly Rep* 1996;45:921–925.

120. Borin MT, Chambers JH, Carel BJ, Gagnon S, Freimuth WW. Pharmacokinetic study of the interaction between rifampin and delavirdine mesylate. *Clin Pharmacol Ther* 1997;61:544–553.

121. Huengsberg M, Castelino S, Sherrard J, O'Farrell N, Bingham J. Does drug interaction cause failure of PCP prophylaxis with dapsone? [Letter]. *Lancet* 1993;341:48.

122. Brogden RN, Fitton A. Rifabutin. A review of its antimicrobial activity, pharmacokinetic properties and therapeutic efficacy. *Drugs* 1994;47:983–1009.

123. Wallace RJ Jr, Brown BA, Griffith DE, Girard W, Tanaka K. Reduced serum levels of clarithromycin in patients treated with multidrug regimens including rifampin or rifabutin for *Mycobacterium avium-M. intracellulare* infection. *J Infect Dis* 1995;171:747–750.

124. Brown LS, Sawyer RC, Li R, Cobb MN, Colborn DC, Narang PK. Lack of a pharmacologic interaction between rifabutin and methadone in HIV-infected former injecting drug users. *Drug Alcohol Depend* 1996;43:71–77.

125. Borin MT, Chambers JH, Carel BJ, Freimuth WW, Aksentijevich S, Piergies AA. Pharmacokinetic study of the interaction between rifabutin and delavirdine mesylate in HIV-1 infected patients. *Antiviral Res* 1997;35:53–63.

126. Brophy T, McCafferty J, Tyrer J, Eadie M. Bioavailability of oral dexamethasone during high dose steroid therapy in neurological patients. *Eur J Clin Pharmacol* 1983;24:103–108.

127. Gentile DM, Tomlinson ES, Maggs JL, Park BK, Back DJ. Dexamethasone metabolism by human liver in vitro: metabolite identification and inhibition of 6-hydroxylation. *J Pharmacol Exp Ther* 1996;277:105–112.

128. Kocarek TA, Schuetz EG, Strom SC, Fisher RA, Guzelian PS. Comparative analysis of cytochrome P4503A induction in primary cultures of rat, rabbit, and human hepatocytes. *Drug Metab Dispos* 1995;23:415–421.

129. Watkins PB, Wrighton SA, Maurel P, et al. Identification of an inducible form of cytochrome P-450 in human liver. *Proc Natl Acad Sci USA* 1985;82:6310–6314.

130. Molowa DT, Schuetz EG, Wrighton SA, et al. Complete cDNA sequence of a cytochrome P-450 inducible by glucocorticoids in human liver. *Proc Natl Acad Sci USA* 1986;83:5311–5315.

131. Watkins PB, Murray SA, Winkelman LG, Heuman DM, Wrighton SA, Guzelian PS. Erythromycin breath test as an assay of glucocorticoid-inducible liver cytochromes P-450: studies in rats and patients. *J Clin Invest* 1989;83:688–697.

132. Dong Y, Poellinger L, Okret S, et al. Regulation of gene expression of class I alcohol dehydrogenase by glucocorticoids. *Proc Natl Acad Sci USA* 1988;85:767–771.

133. Thomson AH, Kerr S, Wright S. Population pharmacokinetics of caffeine in neonates and young infants. *Ther Drug Monit* 1996;18: 245–253.

134. Moore MJ, Hardy RW, Thiessen JJ, Soldin SJ, Erlichman C. Rapid development of enhanced clearance after high-dose cyclophosphamide. *Clin Pharmacol Ther* 1988;44:622–628.

135. Graham MI, Shaw IC, Souhami RL, Sidau B, Harper PG, McLean AE. Decreased plasma half-life of cyclophosphamide during repeated high-dose administration. *Cancer Chemother Pharmacol* 1983;10: 192–193.

136. Sladek NE, Doeden D, Powers JF, Krivit W. Plasma concentrations of 4-hydroxycyclophosphamide and phosphoramide mustard in patients repeatedly given high doses of cyclophosphamide in preparation for bone marrrow transplantation. *Cancer Treat Rep* 1984;68:1247–1254.

137. Chang TK, Weber GF, Crespi CL, Waxman DJ. Differential activation of cyclophosphamide and ifosphamide by cytochromes P-450 2B and 3A in human liver microsomes. *Cancer Res* 1993;53:5629–5637.

138. Chang TK, Yu L, Goldstein JA, Waxman DJ. Identification of the polymorphically expressed CYP2C19 and the wild-type CYP2C9-ILE359 allele as low-K_m catalysts of cyclophosphamide and ifosfamide activation. *Pharmacogenetics* 1997;7:211–221.

139. Yule SM, Boddy AV, Cole M, et al. Cyclophosphamide pharmacokinetics in children. *Br J Clin Pharmacol* 1996;41:13–19.

140. Jones DH, Bleehen NM, Workman P, Walton MI. The role of dexamethasone in the modification of misonidazole pharmacokinetics. *Br J Cancer* 1983;48:553–557.

141. Jones D, Bleehen N, Workman P, Smith N. The role of microsomal enzyme inducers in the reduction of misonidazole neurotoxicity. *Br J Radiol* 1983;56:865–870.

142. Williams K, Begg E, Wade D, O'Shea K. Effects of phenytoin, phenobarbital, and ascorbic acid on misonidazole elimination. *Clin Pharmacol Ther* 1983;33:314–321.

143. Lawson LA, Blouin RA, Smith RB, Rapp RP, Young AB. Phenytoin-dexamethasone interaction: a previously unreported observation. *Surg Neurol* 1981;16:23–24.

144. Lackner TE. Interaction of dexamethasone with phenytoin. *Pharmacotherapy* 1991;11:344–347.

145. Vazquez ML, Jung H, Sotelo J. Plasma levels of praziquantel decrease when dexamethasone is given simultaneously. *Neurology* 1987;37: 1561–1562.

146. Bittencourt P, Gracia C, Martins R, Fernandes A, Diekmann H, Jung W. Phenytoin and carbamazepine decreased oral bioavailability of praziquantel. *Neurology* 1992;42:492–496.

147. Diekmann H, Schneidereit M, Overbosch D. Inhibitory effects of cimetidine ketoconazole and miconazole on the metabolism of praziquantel. *Acta Leiden* 1989;57:217–228.

148. Karam WG, Goldstein JA, Lasker JM, Ghanayem BI. Human CYP2C19 is a major omeprazole 5-hydroxylase, as demonstrated with recombinant cytochrome P450 enzymes. *Drug Metab Dispos* 1996;24: 1081–1087.

149. Andersson T, Regardh CG, Lou YC, Zhang Y, Dahl ML, Bertilsson L. Polymorphic hydroxylation of S-mephenytoin and omeprazole metabolism in Caucasian and Chinese subjects. *Pharmacogenetics* 1992;2: 25–31.

150. Diaz D, Fabre I, Daujat M, et al. Omeprazole is an aryl hydrocarbon-like inducer of human hepatic cytochrome P450. *Gastroenterology* 1990;99:737–747.

151. Daujat M, Peryt B, Lesca P, et al. Omeprazole, an inducer of human CYP1A1 and 1A2, is not a ligand for the Ah receptor. *Biochem Biophys Res Commun* 1992;188:820–825.

152. Quattrochi LC, Tukey RH. Nuclear uptake of the Ah (dioxin) receptor in response to omeprazole: transcriptional activation of the human CYP1A1 gene. *Mol Pharmacol* 1993;43:504–508.

153. Daujat M, Charrasse S, Fabre I, et al. Induction of CYP1A1 gene by benzimidazole derivatives during Caco-2 cell differentiation: evidence for an aryl-hydrocarbon receptor-mediated mechanism. *Eur J Biochem* 1996;237:642–652.

154. Lesca P, Peryt B, Larrieu G, et al. Evidence for the ligand-independent activation of the AH receptor. *Biochem Biophys Res Commun* 1995; 209:474–482.

155. Dzeletovic N, McGuire J, Daujat M, et al. Regulation of dioxin receptor function by omeprazole. *J Biol Chem* 1997;272:12705–12713.

156. McDonnell WM, Scheiman JM, Traber PG. Induction of cytochrome P450IA genes (CYP1A) by omeprazole in the human alimentary tract. *Gastroenterology* 1992;103:1509–1516.

157. Buchthal J, Grund KE, Buchmann A, Schrenk D, Beaune P, Bock KW. Induction of cytochrome P4501A by smoking or omeprazole in comparison with UDP-glucuronosyltransferase in biopsies of human duodenal mucosa. *Eur J Clin Pharmacol* 1995;47:431–435.

158. Kashfi K, McDougall CJ, Dannenberg MD. Comparative effects of omeprazole on xenobiotic metabolizing enzymes in the rat and human. *Clin Pharmacol Ther* 1995;58:625–630.

159. Rost KL, Brosicke H, Brockmoller J, Scheffler M, Helge H, Roots I. Increase of cytochrome P450IA2 activity by omeprazole: evidence by the ^{13}C-[*N*-3-methyl]-caffeine breath test in poor and extensive metabolizers of S-mephenytoin. *Clin Pharmacol Ther* 1992;52:170–180.

160. Rost KL, Brosicke H, Heinemeyer G, Roots I. Specific and dose-dependent enzyme induction by omeprazole in human beings. *Hepatology* 1994;20:1204–1212.

161. Rost KL, Roots I. Accelerated caffeine metabolism after omeprazole treatment is indicated by urinary metabolite ratios: coincidence with plasma clearance and breath test. *Clin Pharmacol Ther* 1994;55: 402–411.

162. Arranz R, Yanez E, Franceschi JL, Fernandez-Ranada JM. More about omeprazole-cyclosporine interaction [Letter; comment]. *Am J Gastroenterol* 1993;88:154–155.

163. Coker RJ, Tomlinson DR, Parkin J, Harris JR, Pinching AJ. Interaction between fluconazole and rifampicin. *BMJ* 1990;301:818.

164. Apseloff G, Hilligoss DM, Gardner MJ, et al. Induction of fluconazole metabolism by rifampin: in vivo study in humans. *J Clin Pharmacol* 1991;31:358–361.

165. Nicolau DP, Crowe HM, Nightingale CH, Quintiliani R. Rifampin-fluconazole interaction in critically ill patients. *Ann Pharmacother* 1995; 29:994–996.

166. Tucker RM, Denning DW, Hanson LH, et al. Interaction of azoles with rifampin, phenytoin, and carbamazepine: in vitro and clinical observations. *Clin Infect Dis* 1992;14:165–174.

167. Drayton J, Dickinson G, Rinaldi MG. Coadministration of rifampin and itraconazole leads to undetectable levels of serum itraconazole [Letter]. *Clin Infect Dis* 1994;18:266.

168. Hecht FM, Wheat J, Korzun AH, et al. Itraconazole maintenance treatment for histoplasmosis in AIDS: a prospective, multicenter trial. *J AIDS Hum Retrovirol* 1997;16:100–107.

169. Doble N, Shaw R, Rowland-Hill C, Lush M, Warnock DW, Keal EE. Pharmacokinetic study of the interaction between rifampicin and ketoconazole. *J Antimicrob Chemother* 1988;21:633–635.

170. Pilheu JA, Galati MR, Yunis AS, et al. [Pharmacokinetic interaction of ketoconazole, isoniazid and rifampicin]. *Medicina (B Aires)* 1989;49: 43–47.

171. Branch RA, Herman RJ. Enzyme induction and beta-adrenergic receptor blocking drugs. *Br J Clin Pharmacol* 1984;17(suppl 1):77S–84S.

172. Kirch W, Rose I, Klingmann I, Pabst J, Ohnhaus EE. Interaction of bisoprolol with cimetidine and rifampicin. *Eur J Clin Pharmacol* 1986; 31:59–62.

173. Abernethy DR, Greenblatt DJ, Ochs HR, Shader RI. Benzodiazepine drug-drug interactions commonly occurring in clinical practice. *Curr Med Res Opin* 1984;8(suppl 4):80–93.

174. Villikka K, Kivisto KT, Backman JT, Olkkola KT, Neuvonen PJ. Triazolam is ineffective in patients taking rifampin. *Clin Pharmacol Ther* 1997;61:8–14.

175. Yoshimoto H, Takahashi M, Saima S. [Influence of rifampicin on antihypertensive effects of dihydropyridine calcium-channel blockers in four elderly patients]. *Nippon Ronen Igakkai Zasshi* 1996;33:692–696.

176. Ndanusa BU, Mustapha A, Abdu-Aguye I. The effect of single does of rifampicin on the pharmacokinetics of oral nifedipine. *J Pharm Biomed Anal* 1997;15:1571–1575.

177. Kelly HW, Couch RC, Davis RL, Cushing AH, Knott R. Interaction of chloramphenicol and rifampin. *J Pediatr* 1988;112:817–820.

178. Houin G, Tillement JP. Clofibrate and enzymatic induction in man. *Int J Clin Pharmacol Biopharm* 1978;16:150–154.

179. Kyriazopoulou V, Parparousi O, Vagenakis AG. Rifampicin-induced adrenal crisis in addisonian patients receiving corticosteroid replacement therapy. *J Clin Endocrinol Metab* 1984;59:1204–1206.

180. Kawai S. [A comparative study of the accelerated metabolism of cortisol, prednisolone and dexamethasone in patients under rifampicin therapy]. *Nippon Naibunpi Gakkai Zasshi* 1985;61:145–161.

181. Kitao T, Kondo K, Nakao S, Asakura H, Arai Y. [Interaction of rifampicin and hydrocortisone-succinate.] *Kekkaku* 1986;61:71–74.

182. Lee KH, Shin JG, Chong WS, et al. Time course of the changes in prednisolone pharmacokinetics after co-administration or discontinuation of rifampin. *Eur J Clin Pharmacol* 1993;45:287–289.

183. Held H. [Interaction of rifampicin with phenprocoumon (author's transl).] *Dtsch Med Wochenschr* 1979;104:1311–1314.

184. O'Reilly RA. Interaction of chronic daily warfarin therapy and rifampin. *Ann Intern Med* 1975;83:506–508.

185. Self TH, Mann RB. Interaction of rifampin and warfarin. *Chest* 1975;67:490–491.

186. Romankiewicz JA, Ehrman M. Rifampin and warfarin: a drug interaction. *Ann Intern Med* 1975;82:224–225.

187. Fox P. Warfarin-rifampicin interaction [Letter]. *Med J Aust* 1982;1:60.

188. Daniels NJ, Dover JS, Schachter RK. Interaction between cyclosporin and rifampicin [Letter]. *Lancet* 1984;2:639.

189. Cassidy MJ, Van Zyl-Smit R, Pascoe MD, Swanepoel CR, Jacobson JE. Effect of rifampicin on cyclosporin A blood levels in a renal transplant recipient [Letter]. *Nephron* 1985;41:207–208.

190. Offermann G, Keller F, Molzahn M. Low cyclosporin A blood levels and acute graft rejection in a renal transplant recipient during rifampin treatment. *Am J Nephrol* 1985;5:385–387.

191. Allen RD, Hunnisett AG, Morris PJ. Cyclosporin and rifampicin in renal transplantation [Letter]. *Lancet* 1985;1:980.

192. Boman G, Eliasson K, Odar-Cederlof I. Acute cardiac failure during treatment with digitoxin: an interaction with rifampicin. *Br J Clin Pharmacol* 1980;10:89–90.

193. Poor DM, Self TH, Davis HL. Interaction of rifampin and digitoxin. *Arch Intern Med* 1983;143:599.

194. Bussey HI, Merritt GJ, Hill EG. The influence of rifampin on quinidine and digoxin. *Arch Intern Med* 1984;144:1021–1023.

195. Gault H, Longerich L, Dawe M, Fine A. Digoxin-rifampin interaction. *Clin Pharmacol Ther* 1984;35:750–754.

196. Aitio ML, Mansury L, Tala E, Haataja M, Aitio A. The effect of enzyme induction on the metabolism of disopyramide in man. *Br J Clin Pharmacol* 1981;11:279–285.

197. Staum JM. Enzyme induction: rifampin-disopyramide interaction. *DICP* 1990;24:701–703.

198. Colmenero JD, Fernandez-Gallardo LC, Agundez JA, Sedeno J, Benitez J, Valverde E. Possible implications of doxycycline-rifampin interaction for treatment of brucellosis. *Antimicrob Agents Chemother* 1994;38:2798–2802.

199. Furlan V, Perello L, Jacquemin E, Debray D, Taburet AM. Interactions between FK506 and rifampicin or erythromycin in pediatric liver recipients. *Transplantation* 1995;59:1217–1218.

200. Schrenzel J, Dayer P, Leemann T, Weidekamm E, Portmann R, Lew DP. Influence of rifampin on fleroxacin pharmacokinetics. *Antimicrob Agents Chemother* 1993;37:2132–2138.

201. Humbert G, Brumpt I, Montay G, et al. Influence of rifampin on the pharmacokinetics of pefloxacin. *Clin Pharmacol Ther* 1991;50:682–687.

202. Takeda M, Nishinuma K, Yamashita S, Matsubayashi T, Tanino S, Nishimura T. Serum haloperidol levels of schizophrenics receiving treatment for tuberculosis. *Clin Neuropharmacol* 1986;9:386–397.

203. Kim YH, Cha IJ, Shim JC, et al. Effect of rifampin on the plasma concentration and the clinical effect of haloperidol concomitantly administered to schizophrenic patients. *J Clin Psychopharmacol* 1996;16:247–252.

204. Decocq G, Compagnon M, Andrejak M, Guedj B, Doutrellot C. [Adverse effects related to the use of antitubercular drugs in psychiatric centers: retrospective study at the Philippe Pinel CH in Amiens 1994.] *Therapie* 1996;51:543–549.

205. Smith DA, Chandler MH, Shedlofsky SI, Wedlund PJ, Blouin RA. Age-dependent stereoselective increase in the oral clearance of hexobarbitone isomers caused by rifampicin. *Br J Clin Pharmacol* 1991;32:735–739.

206. Mauro VF, Somani P, Temesy-Armos PN. Drug interaction between lorcainide and rifampicin [Letter]. *Eur J Clin Pharmacol* 1987;31:737–738.

207. Self T, Corley CR, Nabhan S, Abell T. Case report: interaction of rifampin and nortriptyline. *Am J Med Sci* 1996;311:80–81.

208. Bebchuk JM, Stewart DE. Drug interaction between rifampin and nortriptyline: a case report. *Int J Psychiatry Med* 1991;21:183–187.

209. Kharasch ED, Russell M, Mautz D, et al. The role of cytochrome P450 3A4 in alfentanil clearance: implications for interindividual variability in disposition and perioperative drug interactions. *Anesthesiology* 1997;87:36–50.

210. Kreek MJ, Garfield JW, Gutjahr CL, Giusti LM. Rifampin-induced methadone withdrawal. *N Engl J Med* 1976;294:1104–1106.

211. Holmes VF. Rifampin-induced methadone withdrawal in AIDS [Letter]. *J Clin Psychopharmacol* 1990;10:443–444.

212. Dommisse J. Letter: oral contraceptive failure due to drug interaction. *S Afr Med J* 1976;50:796.

213. Burley DM. Rifampicin, enzyme induction, oestrogens and the "pill." In: Grahame-Smith DG, ed. *Drug interactions.* Baltimore: University Park Press, 1977:293–299.

214. Gupta KC, Ali MY. Failure of oral contraceptive with rifampicin. *Med J Zambia* 1980;15:23.

215. Abajo FJ. Phenytoin interaction with rifampicin. *BMJ* 1988;297:1048.

216. Wanwimolruk S, Wong SM, Zhang H, Coville PF, Walker RJ. Metabolism of quinine in man: identification of a major metabolite, and effects of smoking and rifampicin pretreatment. *J Pharm Pharmacol* 1995;47:957–963.

217. Self TH, Morris T. Interaction of rifampin and chlorpropamide. *Chest* 1980;77:800–801.

218. Surekha V, Peter JV, Jeyaseelan L, Cherian AM. Drug interaction: rifampicin and glibenclamide. *Natl Med J India* 1997;10:11–12.

219. Self TH, Tsiu SJ, Fowler JW Jr. Interaction of rifampin and glyburide [Letter]. *Chest* 1989;96:1443–1444.

220. Shaffer JL, Houston JB. The effect of rifampicin on sulphapyridine plasma concentrations following sulphasalazine administration. *Br J Clin Pharmacol* 1985;19:526–528.

221. Ohnhaus EE, Studer H. A link between liver microsomal enzyme activity and thyroid hormone metabolism in man. *Br J Clin Pharmacol* 1983;15:71–76.

222. Rice TL, Patterson JH, Celestin C, Foster JR, Powell JR. Influence of rifampin on tocainide pharmacokinetics in humans. *Clin Pharm* 1989;8:200–205.

223. Rahn KH, Mooy J, Bohm R, v.d. Vet A. Reduction of bioavailability of verapamil by rifampin [Letter]. *N Engl J Med* 1985;312:920–921.

224. Barbarash RA. Verapamil-rifampin interaction. *DICP* 1985;19:559–560.

225. Burger DM, Meenhorst PL, Koks CH, Beijnen JH. Pharmacokinetic interaction between rifampin and zidovudine. *Antimicrob Agents Chemother* 1993;37:1426–1431.

226. Villikka K, Kivisto KT, Lamberg TS, Kantola T, Neuvonen PJ. Concentrations and effects of zopiclone are greatly reduced by rifampicin. *Br J Clin Pharmacol* 1997;43:471–474.

227. Nousbaum JB, Berthou F, Carlhant D, Riche C, Robaszkiewicz M, Gouerou H. Four-week treatment with omeprazole increases the metabolism of caffeine [published erratum appears in *Am J Gastroenterol* 1994;89:1135] [see comments]. *Am J Gastroenterol* 1994;89:371–375.

228. Andersson T, Bergstrand R, Cederberg C, Eriksson S, Lagerstrom PO, Skanberg I. Omeprazole treatment does not affect the metabolism of caffeine. *Gastroenterology* 1991;101:943–947.

229. Rizzo N, Padoin C, Palombo S, Scherrmann JM, Girre C. Omeprazole and lansoprazole are not inducers of cytochrome P4501A2 under conventional therapeutic conditions. *Eur J Clin Pharmacol* 1996;49:491–495.

230. Blohme I, Idstrom J, Andersson T. A study of the interaction between omeprazole and cyclosporine in renal transplant patients. *Br J Clin Pharmacol* 1993;35:156–160.

231. Andersson T, Cederberg C, Edvardsson G, Heggelund A, Lundborg P. Effect of omeprazole treatment on diazepam plasma levels in slow versus normal rapid metabolizers of omeprazole. *Clin Pharmacol Ther* 1990;47:79–85.

232. Noble D, Bannister J, Lamont M, Andersson T, Scott D. The effect of oral omeprazole on the disposition of lignocaine. *Anaesthesia* 1994;49:497–500.

233. Soons PA, van den Berg G, Danhof M, et al. Influence of single- and

multiple-dose omeprazole treatment on nifedipine pharmacokinetics and effects in healthy subjects. *Eur J Clin Pharmacol* 1992;42:319–324.

234. Xiaodong S, Gatti G, Bartoli A, Cipolla G, Crema F, Perucca E. Omeprazole does not enhance the metabolism of phenacetin, a marker of CYP1A2 activity, in healthy volunteers. *Ther Drug Monit* 1994;16: 248–250.

235. Cavanaugh JH, Karol MD. Lack of pharmacokinetic interaction after administration of lansoprazole or omeprazole with prednisone. *J Clin Pharmacol* 1996;36:1064–1071.

236. Henry D, Brent P, Whyte I, Mihaly G, Devenish-Meares S. Propranolol steady-state pharmacokinetics are unaltered by omeprazole. *Eur J Clin Pharmacol* 1987;33:369–373.

237. Ching MS, Elliott SL, Stead CK, et al. Quinidine single dose pharmacokinetics and pharmacodynamics are unaltered by omeprazole. *Aliment Pharmacol Ther* 1991;5:523–531.

238. Taburet AM, Geneve J, Bocquentin M, Simoneau G, Caulin C, Singlas E. Theophylline steady state pharmacokinetics is not altered by omeprazole. *Eur J Clin Pharmacol* 1992;42:343–345.

239. Sutfin T, Balmer K, Bostrom H, Eriksson S, Hoglund P, Paulsen O. Stereoselective interaction of omeprazole with warfarin in healthy men. *Ther Drug Monit* 1989;11:176–184.

240. Unge P, Svedberg LE, Nordgren A, et al. A study of the interaction of omeprazole and warfarin in anticoagulated patients. *Br J Clin Pharmacol* 1992;34:509–512.

CHAPTER 53

Isoniazid and Ethanol

John T. Slattery

Ethanol and isoniazid are both inhibitors and inducers of CYP2E1. Ethanol and isopentanol (present in alcoholic beverages) also induce CYP3A in primary cultures of human hepatocytes (1), although there are no clinical reports of drug interactions attributable to induction of CYP3A. As discussed in Chapter 9, the regulatory mechanisms for CYP2E1 are diverse. With regard to drug interactions, the most interesting regulatory mechanism is stabilization of the enzyme by the binding of a ligand to the active site. This phenomenon simultaneously inhibits the catalytic activity of the enzyme and causes the amount of enzyme to increase because of a decreased rate of degradation. Thus when one considers the pharmacokinetic result of a drug interaction occurring through such a mechanism, it quickly becomes clear that the clearance of the substrate could either increase through the induction of the enzyme, decrease through competitive inhibition, or perhaps, if these two effects balance, not be altered at all.

The clinically most important substrates of CYP2E1 are ethanol, chlorzoxazone acetaminophen, and halogenated anesthetics. The ligand stabilizers that have been most studied are isoniazid and ethanol. This chapter focuses on the influence of isoniazid and ethanol on the clearance of substrates of CYP2E1 with particular attention to studies that address the dual nature of interactions that occur through ligand stabilization: those with isoniazid and ethanol as the CYP2E1 ligand.

ISONIAZID

Pharmacology

Isoniazid is a mainstay in the treatment and prophylaxis of tuberculosis. Interestingly, its mechanism of action is

J. T. Slattery: Department of Pharmaceutics, University of Washington, Box 357610, H272J Health Sciences Building, Seattle, Washington 98195-7610

not known, although effects on lipids, nucleic acid biosynthesis, and glycolysis have been suggested (2).

Effects as an Inducer of CYP2E1

The mechanism by which isoniazid induces CYP2E1 is somewhat controversial. Park et al. (3) suggested that isoniazid induces CYP2E1 by translational activation, based on the observations that enhanced CYP2E1 levels required protein synthesis and did not involve enhanced levels of specific mRNA. However, their data showed that isoniazid prevented the loss of CYP2E1 in rat liver over an 18-hour period when synthesis of protein was inhibited by administration of cyclohexamide. Eighteen hours is sufficiently long that loss of enzyme should have been observed based on its reported degradation kinetics (4); the absence of loss of CYP2E1 suggests that its degradation was inhibited, most likely by stabilization of the enzyme. This interpretation of the results presented by Park et al. (3) are supported by recent studies in which the effect of isoniazid administration on the degradation of radiolabeled CYP2E1 in the liver of rats was studied (5). Direct examination of the effects of isoniazid administration on the synthesis and degradation of CYP2E1 has shown that synthesis is unchanged, whereas the rapid phase of CYP2E1 degradation is slowed. It has also been reported that isoniazid competitively inhibits CYP2E1 activity with a K_i of 40 μM, suggesting that isoniazid binds to the active site of CYP2E1 (6). Thus the available evidence strongly supports the conclusion that isoniazid induces CYP2E1 through ligand stabilization.

A series of studies of the influence of isoniazid administration on the clearance of chlorzoxazone, eliminated to a large extent through the formation of 4-hydroxychlorzoxazone by CYP2E1 (7), and the formation clearance of the acetaminophen reactive metabolite, N-acetyl-p-aminobenzoquinone imine (NAPQI), in human subjects has been reported. NAPQI formation is catalyzed by

707

CYP2E1, CYP1A2, and CYP3A4 in human liver microsomes and by the same cDNA-expressed human enzymes (8,9). However, more recent pharmacokinetic studies in humans with inducers of CYP1A2 and CYP3A4 have failed to demonstrate enhanced formation of NAPQI (10,11), whereas its formation is strongly inhibited by administration of single-dose disulfiram (11). Thus in humans *in vivo*, NAPQI appears to be formed almost exclusively by CYP2E1.

In the first two of these studies (13–17), NAPQI formation kinetics were determined on three occasions in healthy subjects who received isoniazid daily for several days: before isoniazid administration was initiated, together with isoniazid, and 48 hours after the last dose of isoniazid (14). When acetaminophen was ingested together with isoniazid, a 66% inhibition was observed in the oxidation of acetaminophen to NAPQI. At 48 hours after the discontinuation of isoniazid, NAPQI formation had returned to the preisoniazid value. In the second study (17), NAPQI formation was inhibited by 66% when acetaminophen was taken together with isoniazid. At 24 hours after the last dose of isoniazid, a 56% increase in the formation of NAPQI was observed, which returned to the preinduced level 72 hours after the discontinuation of isoniazid. When chlorzoxazone was taken together with isoniazid, chlorzoxazone clearance was inhibited by 58% in comparison with the preisoniazid control. At 48 hours after the last dose of isoniazid, a 50% increase in chlorzoxazone clearance was observed, which had returned to the preisoniazid level 96 hours after the last isoniazid dose.

The influence of isoniazid acetylation status on the interaction between isoniazid and acetaminophen was studied in patients receiving a morning dose of isoniazid for a period of at least 6 months for prophylaxis of tuberculosis, and was found to be consistent with the studies in healthy volunteers (13). Acetaminophen was administered on separate occasions, either with the morning dose of isoniazid or in the evening 12 hours after the morning dose of isoniazid. At the conclusion of isoniazid therapy, a time-matched control phase (morning vs. evening) of acetaminophen administration was performed. When acetaminophen and isoniazid were coadministered, the mean NAPQI formation clearance was inhibited by 64% in slow acetylators, and by 52% in fast acetylators. When acetaminophen was given 12 hours after isoniazid, the mean NAPQI formation clearance in fast acetylators was increased 37% from the value observed in the absence of isoniazid therapy, but remained inhibited by 32% in slow acetylators, as expected if isoniazid was still present in those individuals in whom it would be eliminated more slowly.

A similar study was conducted in which chlorzoxazone was used as a probe of CYP2E1 activity (15). Coadministration of chlorzoxazone with isoniazid resulted in 80% inhibition of chlorzoxazone clearance in slow acetylators

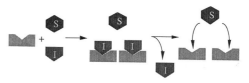

FIG. 53-1. Stabilization of CYP2E1 by active site occupation. Inhibitor/inducer and substrate are I and S, respectively, and CYP2E1 is represented by the shaded block. Competitive inhibition of CYP2E1 occurs as the inhibitor/inducer binds to the active site, blocking the substrate access. As a consequence of binding, CYP2E1 accumulates because of stabilization. As the inhibitor/inducer is removed, substrate regains access to the active site, and the metabolism of substrate is enhanced. From Chien JY, Thummel KE, Slattery JT. Pharmacokinetic consequences of induction of CYP2E1 by ligand stabilization. *Drug Metab Dispos* 1997;25:1165–1174.

and 60% in fast acetylators. At 48 hours after the last dose of isoniazid, 6-hydroxy chlorzoxazone formation in slow acetylators was still increased by 60%, and had returned to the preisoniazid value in fast acetylators.

This biphasic interaction between two CYP2E1 substrates and isoniazid, an inhibitor and inducer of the enzyme, illustrates that the clearance of CYP2E1 substrates is inhibited while isoniazid is present, increases above the preisoniazid value as isoniazid is removed, and then returns to its preisoniazid value. The time course of the interactions is consistent with the stabilization of CYP2E1 by binding of isoniazid to the active site. This mechanism is illustrated in Fig. 53-1. When isoniazid is present and bound to the active site, CYP2E1-mediated clearance is inhibited, but the amount of enzyme present increases because of a stabilization rendering it less susceptible to degradation. When administration of isoniazid is stopped, isoniazid concentration declines, and if this happens faster than the CYP2E1 is degraded, substrate clearance increases as long as CYP2E1 levels remain elevated.

Perhaps the most interesting feature of this mechanism of interaction is that it does not result simply in inhibition or induction, but in both. In fact, the isoniazid–acetaminophen and isoniazid–chlorzoxazone studies demonstrate that this interaction can endlessly cycle between inhibited and enhanced CYP2E1-mediated clearance, depending on the time between administration of isoniazid and the CYP2E1 substrate.

ETHANOL

Pharmacology

The central nervous system (CNS) depressant and sedative/ataxic effects by ethanol were once thought to be caused by increasing the fluidity of lipid membranes. More recently, however, evidence has accumulated implicating receptor-mediated actions on glutamate and γ-aminobutyric acid (GABA)-mediated ion channels. In addition to its effects on the CNS, ethanol also has direct effects on the cardiovascular system, plasma lipoproteins, skeletal muscle, and body temperature. Effects on the liver include fatty changes, thought to be mediated by depletion of hepatic reduced nicotinamide adenine dinucleotide (NADH) stores through the oxidation of ethanol to acetaldehyde by alcohol dehydrogenase. Acetaldehyde oxidizes lipids, damages mitochondria, depletes glutathione, certain vitamins, and trace metals, and decreases transport of certain proteins. These effects result in hepatocyte engorgement with fat, protein, and water, and the progression to the necrosis and fibrosis found in cirrhotic livers (18).

Effects as an Inducer of CYP2E1

The ethanol–acetaminophen interaction has been a topic of investigation for at least 20 years. Early reports noted that short-term ethanol administration resulted in a protection from acetaminophen hepatotoxicity, whereas prolonged administration enhanced toxicity in laboratory animals. For many years, it was thought that ethanol was simply both an inhibitor and inducer of CYP2E1, acting in the respective roles by separate mechanisms.

More recent studies have demonstrated that ethanol induces CYP2E1 in rats by ligand stabilization (19), but also appears to induce by enhanced transcription at high urinary (and presumably plasma) levels (20–22). In alcoholic patients, apoenzyme is found abundantly in periportal and pericentral regions of the hepatic acinus, whereas it is relatively restricted to the pericentral regions in healthy individuals (23). Enhanced specific mRNA levels have also been reported in the liver of alcoholics (23). Because starvation enhances CYP2E1 gene transcription (24), it is difficult to conclude that enhanced CYP2E1 mRNA in alcoholic patients is due to ethanol and is not influenced by malnutrition associated with alcoholism. Nevertheless, it appears that ethanol may induce CYP2E1 by two mechanisms, ligand stabilization and enhanced transcription. Enhanced transcription has been demonstrated or suggested only when plasma levels of ethanol are relatively high.

Simultaneous ingestion of ethanol and acetaminophen results in inhibition of NAPQI formation (25,26). However, it has recently been shown that even short-term ethanol administration enhances NAPQI formation in humans (27). In this study, ethanol was administered intravenously for 6 hours, achieving a steady-state concentration of approximately 100 mg/dL. Acetaminophen was administered 8 hours after the infusion of ethanol was stopped, at a time when ethanol concentration in plasma had declined to less than 10 mg/dL, and the formation clearance of NAPQI was seen to be enhanced by 22%. Thus the pharmacokinetic aspects of the effect of ethanol on NAPQI formation are similar to those of isoniazid: diminished NAPQI formation while ethanol is present, followed by enhanced formation as ethanol is eliminated.

Only the pharmacokinetic aspects of the interaction between ethanol and acetaminophen have been discussed here. There are other mechanisms by which ethanol might modulate the toxicity of NAPQI once formed, such as selective modulation of hepatocyte mitochondrial glutathione stores (28). Moreover, alcoholism introduces a constellation of effects that might further influence NAPQI toxicity (16).

PREDICTABILITY OF DRUG INTERACTIONS BY LIGAND STABILIZATION OF CYP2E1

The binding of ligand to the active site of CYP2E1 slows the degradation of the enzyme, resulting in its accumulation. However, clearance of substrate is competitively inhibited as long as the ligand is present. At least one key question arises from a consideration of this mechanism: Can clearance of substrate increase above the value observed in the absence of the ligand while the ligand is still present?

This question is very difficult to address experimentally, but it can be approached theoretically because the key features of the system are known and can easily be represented mathematically. A kinetic model that relates the inhibition/induction of CYP2E1-dependent clearance to substrate concentration (S) and the substrate Michaelis constant (K_m), and the concentration of the inhibitor/inducer (I) and its enzyme dissociation constant (K_i) has recently been described (12). Based on experimental data (14,17), the model includes two physical pools of CYP2E1, one subject to both rapid and slow degradation, and the second, in which only the slow process operates (Fig. 53-2). Rat studies have shown that ligand stabilizes the enzyme from degradation by the rapid process without affecting the slower one (4,19). The model treats CYP2E1 inhibition as competitive and provides for enzyme to accumulate as a consequence of its stabilization through occupation of the active site by ligand.

The agreement between predictions of this model and the results of the isoniazid interactions with chlorzoxazone and acetaminophen in humans is shown in Fig. 53-3. The simulations in Fig. 53-3 take a value of S/K_m of 0.1. In humans, the dose of acetaminophen administered produces a maximal concentration in plasma of approximately 56 μM (13), and the dose of chlorzoxazone, a maximal unbound concentration of 3 μM (29). The K_m of acetaminophen for CYP2E1 is approximately 1 mM (30,31), and that of chlorzoxazone is 45 μM in human liver microsomes (7,31). The half-lives of CYP2E1 have been established in the rat, but not in humans. In addition to conducting simulations with CYP2E1 half-lives of 7 and 37 hours, as observed in the rat, we also performed

Pool 1   Pool 2

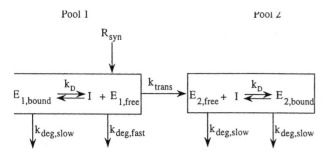

FIG. 53-2. Two-compartment model consisting of two physically distinct pools of CYP2E1. R_{syn} is the rate of synthesis, a constant zero-order input into pool 1. The rapid degradation rate constant of the unbound enzyme in pool 1 (E1, free) is kdeg, fast. The degradation rate constant of the stabilized enzyme E1, bound and the bound and unbound enzyme in pool 2 (E2, bound and E2, free) is kdeg, slow. The transfer rate constant of enzyme from pool 1 to pool 2 is ktrans. From Chien JY, Thummel KE, Slattery JT. Pharmacokinetic consequences of induction of CYP2E1 by ligand stabilization. *Drug Metab Dispos* 1997;25:1165–1174.

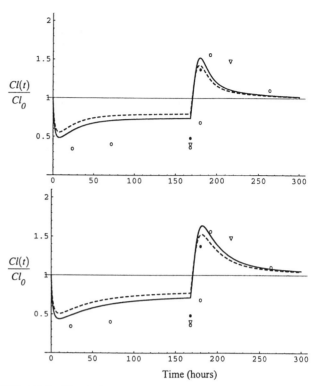

Time (hours)

FIG. 53-3. Simulation of the time course of the interaction between isoniazid and acetaminophen assuming I/K_i of 1.5, (stippled line) and 2.0 (solid line). S/K_m = 0.1 in all simulations. Top, CYP2E1 half-lives of 7 and 37 hours; bottom, 15 and 79 hours. Circles represent data from studies of the formation of NAPQI from acetaminophen (13,14,17), and triangles, the formation of 6-hydroxychlorzoxazone from chlorzoxazone (17). Open symbols represent slow acetylators of isoniazid, and closed symbols, rapid acetylators. In each study, isoniazid was administered as 300 mg once daily in the morning for several days. Acetaminophen (500 mg) and chlorzoxazone (750 mg) were administered before isoniazid was begun (14,17) or well after CYP2E1 induction had reversed after isoniazid (13), during the period of administration of isoniazid, and shortly after isoniazid was stopped. Acetaminophen (14,17) and chlorzoxazone (17) were given together with isoniazid during the period of isoniazid administration, except in one case in which acetaminophen was given either together with isoniazid or 12 hours after the dose of isoniazid (13). From Chien JY, Thummel KE, Slattery JT. Pharmacokinetic consequences of induction of CYP2E1 by ligand stabilization. *Drug Metab Dispos* 1997;25:1165–1174.

simulations with values of 15 and 79 hours, as the half-life in humans is expected to be longer than that of the rat. The time for alcoholics to return to an uninduced CYP2E1 activity has been estimated to be 60 hours (32). The longer half-life values used provide the same distribution of enzyme between the two pools we estimated in the rat. Peak isoniazid concentration in plasma is reported to vary between 36 and 73 μM at a dose of 300 mg (33,34), and a K_i of 40 μM for human CYP2E1 has been reported (6).

Figure 53-3 shows data from the human studies and simulations with the literature parameters for I/K_i of 1.5 and 2, and CYP2E1 half-lives of 3 and 37 hours and 15 and 79 hours. The simulation with the longer half-lives and larger I/K_i best fit the data, although both agree qualitatively well with the time course of the interaction, inhibited clearance giving way to enhanced clearance.

This model also was used to address the question posed earlier: Can clearance of substrate increase above the value observed in the absence of the ligand while the ligand is still present? The result of model-based computer simulations addressing this issue is shown in Fig. 53-4. The simulation considers the case of both ligand and substrate being infused to steady state, at which the ratio of S/K_m and I/K_i can be known. At low S/K_m, the usual clinical condition with substrate concentration low relative K_m, increasing I relative to K_i results in inhibition of clearance. The question posed earlier is answered by considering the effect of increasing S relative to K_m at any given value of I/K_i. As the figure shows, this results in a *decrease* in the clearance of the substrate under all conditions. At first glance, this result may seem counterintuitive. However, for the substrate to compete successfully for enzyme, substrate concentration must increase such that S becomes appreciable relative to K_m. This condition results in a decrease in clearance due to saturation of enzyme with substrate. Thus although access of the substrate to the active site of the enzyme is increased, clearance is less than the value observed at low substrate concentration in the absence of ligand because of saturation of the enzyme with substrate, just as would be observed with simple Michaelis–Menten kinetics.

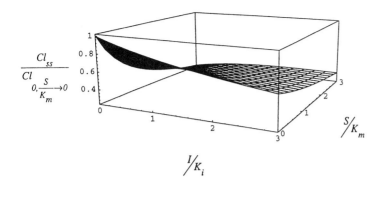

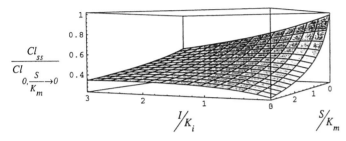

FIG. 53-4. The effect of the administration of inhibitor/inducer on the clearance of substrate expressed relative to clearance at vanishingly low substrate concentration. By clearance declines relative to the value observed at low substrate, concentration in the absence of inhibitor as either I/K_i or S/K_m increases. The lower panel is a 180-degree rotation of the upper panel. From Chien JY, Thummel KE, Slattery JT. Pharmacokinetic consequences of induction of CYP2E1 by ligand stabilization. *Drug Metab Dispos* 1997;25:1165–1174.

Conclusions

The class of drug interactions that accrues through ligand stabilization of CYP2E1 may be unique to this enzyme. Induction of CYP3A isoforms by *N*-substituted imidazoles and macrolides may represent variants of this mechanism (see 35–37). They represent an unusual case in which the effect of one drug on the other is not inhibition or induction, but both. The result of the effect of the inhibitor/inducer on the clearance of the substrate is predictable from the synthesis and degradation kinetics of the enzyme and the affinities and concentrations of the inhibitor/inducer and substrate. The unusual feature of this interaction is that although induction of CYP2E1 begins as soon as the inhibitor/inducer is administered, enhanced clearance of substrate in relation to the preinhibitor/inducer condition is observed only after the inducer is removed. The isoniazid–acetaminophen interaction illustrates that it is possible for the interaction to cycle between inhibited and enhanced clearance within a dosing interval of the inhibitor/inducer. The ethanol–acetaminophen interaction shows a similar biphasic effect.

REFERENCES

1. Kostrubsky VE, Strom SC, Wood SG, Wrighton SA, Sinclair PR, Sinclair JF. Ethanol and isopentanol increase CYP3A and CYP2E in primary cultures of human hepatocytes. *Arch Biochem Biophys* 1995;322:516–520.
2. Manell GL, Petri WA. Antimicrobial agents: drugs used in the chemotherapy of tuberculosis and leprosy. In: Hardman JG, Limbird LE, Molinoff PB, Ruddon RW, Gilman AG, eds. *Goodman and Gilman's the pharmacological basis of therapeutics.* 9th ed. New York: McGraw-Hill, 1996:1156–1158.
3. Park KS, Sohn DH, Veech RL, Song BJ. Translational activation of ethanol-inducible cytochrome P450 (CYP2E1) by isoniazid. *Eur J Pharmacol* 1993;248:7–14.
4. Song BJ, Veech RL, Park SS, Gelboin HV, Gonzelez FJ. Induction of rat hepatic *N*-nitrosodimethylamine demethylase by acetone is due to protein stabilization. *J Biol Chem* 1988;264:3568–3572.
5. Manyike PT. CYP2E1: mechanisms of induction by isoniazid and role in acetaminophen oxidation. PhD dissertation, University of Washington, 1999.
6. Peter RM, Chen W, Darbyshire JF, Kunze KT, Nelson SD. Inhibition of human CYP2E1 and metabolic intermediate complex formation by isoniazid. *ISSX Proc* 1996;10:245.
7. Peter R, Bocker R, Beaune PH, Iwasaki M, Guengerich FP, Yang CS. Hydroxylation of chlorzoxazone as a specific probe for human liver cytochrome P-450IIEI. *Chem Res Toxicol* 1990;3:566–573.
8. Raucy JL, Lasker JM, Lieber CS, Black M. Acetaminophen activation by human liver microsomes P450IIE1 and P450IA2. *Arch Biochem Biophys* 1989;271:270–283.
9. Thummel KE, Lee CA, Kunze KL, Nelson SD, Slattery JT. Oxidation of acetaminophen to *N*-acetyl-*p*-benzoquinone imine by human CYP3A4. *Biochem Pharmacol* 1993;45:1563–1569.
10. Sarich T, Kalhorn TF, Magee S, et al. The effect of omeprazole pretreatment on acetaminophen metabolism in rapid and slow metabolizers of S-mephenytoin. *Clin Pharmacol Ther* 1997;62:21–28.
11. Manyike PT, Kharasch ED, Kalhorn TF, Slattery JT. Contribution of CYP2E1 and CYP3A4 to acetaminophen reactive metabolite formation. *Clin Pharmacol Ther* 2000 (*in press*).
12. Chien JY, Thummel KE, Slattery JT. Pharmacokinetic consequences of induction of CYP2E1 by ligand stabilization. *Drug Metab Dispos* 1997;25:1165–1174.
13. Chien JY, Peter RM, Nolan CM, et al. Influence of polymorphic N-acetyltransferase phenotype on the inhibition and induction of acetaminophen bioactivation with long-term isoniazid. *Clin Pharmacol Ther* 1997;61:24–34.
14. Epstein MM, Nelson SD, Slattery JT, Kalhorn TF, Wall RA, Wright JM. Inhibition of the metabolism of paracetamol by isoniazid. *Br J Clin Pharmacol* 1991;31:139–142.
15. O'Shea D, Rim RB, Wilkinson GR. Modulation of CYP2E1 activity by isoniazid in rapid and slow N-acetylators. *Br J Clin Pharmacol* 1997;43:99–103.
16. Slattery JT, Nelson SD, Thummel KE. The complex interaction between ethanol and acetaminophen. *Clin Pharmacol Ther* 1996;60:241–246.
17. Zand R, Nelson SD, Slattery JT, et al. Inhibition and induction of

cytochrome P4502E1-catalyzed oxidation by isoniazid in humans. *Clin Pharmacol Ther* 1993;54:142–149.

18. Hobbs WR, Rall TW, Verdoorn TA. Hypnotics and sedatives: ethanol. In: Hardman JG, Limdird KO, Molinoff PB, Ruddon RW, Gilman AG, eds. *Goodman and Gilman's the pharmacological basis of therapeutics*. 9th ed. New York: McGraw-Hill, 1996:388–389.

19. Roberts BJ, Song BJ, Soh Y, Park SS, Shoaf SE. Ethanol induces CYP2E1 by protein stabilization: role of ubiquitin conjugation in the rapid degradation of CYP2E1. *J Biol Chem* 1995;270: 29632–29635.

20. Badger TM, Huang J, Ronis M, Lumpkin CK. Induction of cytochrome P450 2E1 during chronic ethanol exposure occurs via transcription of the CYP 2E1 gene when blood alcohol concentrations are high. *Biochem Biophys Res Commun* 1993;190:780–785.

21. Ronis MJJ, Huang J, Crouch J, et al. Cytochrome P450 CYP 2E1 induction during chronic alcohol exposure occurs by a two-step mechanism associated with blood alcohol concentrations in rats. *J Pharmacol Exp Ther* 1993;264:944–950.

22. Tsutsumi M, Lasker JM, Takahashi T, Lieber CS. In vivo induction of hepatic P4502E1 by ethanol: role of increased enzyme synthesis. *Arch Biochem Biophys* 1993;304:209–218.

23. Takahashi T, Lasker JM, Rosman AS, Lieber CS. Induction of cytochrome P-4502E1 in the human liver by ethanol is caused by a corresponding increase in encoding messenger RNA. *Hepatology* 1993; 17:236–245.

24. Johansson I, Lindros KO, Eriksson H, Ingleman-Sundberg M. Transcriptional control of CYP2E1 in the perivenous liver region and during starvation. *Biochem Biophys Res Commun* 1990;173:331–338.

25. Banda PW, Quart BD. The effect of mild alcohol consumption on the metabolism of acetaminophen in man. *Res Commun Chem Pathol Pharmacol* 1982;38:57–70.

26. Forrest JAH, Clements JA, Prescott LF. Clinical pharmacokinetics of paracetamol. *Clin Pharmacokinet* 1982;7:93–107.

27. Thummel KE, Slattery JT, Ro H, et al. Ethanol and production of the hepatoxic metabolite of acetaminophen in healthy adults. *Clin Pharmacol Ther* 2000 (*in press*).

28. Fernandez-Checa JC, Ookhtens M, Kaplowitz N. Effects of chronic ethanol feeding on rat hepatocytic gluthathione: relationship of cytosolic glutathione to efflux and mitochondrial sequestration. *J Clin Invest* 1989;83:1274–1252.

29. De Vries JD, Salphati L, Horie S, Becker CE, Hoener BA. Variability in the disposition of chlorzoxazone. *Biopharm Drug Dispos* 1994;15: 587–597.

30. Chen W, Peter RM, McArdle S, Thummel KE, Sigle RO, Nelson SD. Baculovirus expression and purification of human and rat cytochrome P450 2E1. *Arch Biochem Biophys* 1996;331:123–130.

31. Patten CJ, Thomas PE, Guy RL, et al. Cytochrome P450 enzymes involved in acetaminophen activation by rat and human liver microsomes and their kinetics. *Chem Res Toxicol* 1993;6:511–518.

32. Lucas D, Ménez C, Girre C, Bodénez P, Hispard E, Ménez JF. Decrease in cytochrome P4502E1 as assessed by the rate of chlorzoxazone hydroxylation in alcoholics during the withdrawal phase. *Alcohol Clin Exp Res* 1995;19:362–366.

33. Breda M, Pianezzola E, Benedetti MS, et al. A study of the effects of rifabutin on isoniazid pharmacokinetics and metabolism in healthy volunteers. *Drug Metab Drug Interact* 1992;10:323–341.

34. Weber WW, Hein DW. Clinical pharmacokinetics of isoniazid. *Clin Pharmacokinet* 1979;4:401–422.

35. Danan G, Descatoire V, Pessayre D. Self-induction by erythromycin of its own transformation into a metabolite forming an inactive complex with reduced cytochrome P450. *J Pharmacol Exp Ther* 1981;218: 509–514.

36. Pappas JB, Franklin MR. Hepatic clotrimazole concentrations and hepatic drug metabolizing enzyme activities in adult male Sprague-Dawley rats. *Toxicology* 1993;80:27–35.

37. Ritter JK, Franklin MR. Induction and inhibition of rat hepatic drug metabolism by *N*-substituted imidazole drugs. *Drug Metab Dispos* 1987;15:335–343.

SECTION VI

Clinical Considerations

CHAPTER 54

Clinical and Pharmacoeconomic Significance of Metabolic Drug Interactions

Philip D. Hansten

Most published reports on drug–drug interactions are designed to study the changes in pharmacokinetics resulting from the interaction and the mechanisms by which these changes occur. Pharmacokinetic and mechanistic investigations are vital to our understanding of how two or more drugs interact, and may allow us to predict the interactive properties of new drugs. Nonetheless, it is rarely possible to determine with any degree of assurance how often patients receiving a given drug combination will actually manifest an adverse outcome. Historically most epidemiologic studies of drug interactions have addressed patient *exposures* to potentially interacting drug combinations rather than patient outcomes (1,2). Even when epidemiologic data on adverse outcomes from a drug interaction are available—which is rarely the case—it is often difficult to determine whether a given patient is actually at risk. For example, suppose a particular interacting drug combination is found to produce adverse consequences in approximately 10% of patients. How does the clinician know whether the patient in question will be in the 10% of patients with an adverse outcome, or in the 90% of patients who are not adversely affected? For some drug interactions, factors that increase the risk of an adverse outcome have been identified, and one can determine whether a patient is at higher than average risk based on the presence of one or more risk factors. But unfortunately, for most drug interactions, only some of the factors that predispose the patient to adverse consequences from the interaction are known, and the assessment of risk is only a rough guide.

TYPES OF ADVERSE OUTCOMES

When a metabolic drug interaction occurs, the drug that causes the interaction is called the "precipitant drug," and the drug whose effect is altered by the interaction is termed the "object drug." Metabolic drug interactions tend to result in an increase or decrease in the serum concentrations of the object drug, which in turn enhances or reduces the pharmacodynamic response to the object drug. If the magnitude of the alteration in pharmacodynamic response is sufficient, the patient can develop object drug toxicity or an inadequate therapeutic response to the object drug.

Toxicity of Object Drug

Object drug toxicity can occur when an enzyme-inhibiting precipitant drug is added to the patient's therapy. For example, a patient receiving prolonged theophylline therapy is at risk of developing theophylline toxicity if a CYP1A2 inhibitor such as ciprofloxacin is added to the therapy (3,4). Toxicity can also occur with the reverse order of administration—that is, when object drug is started in the presence of therapy with an enzyme-inhibiting precipitant drug. This is particularly true if the prescriber is unaware of the interaction. For example, beginning theophylline therapy in a patient receiving long-term fluvoxamine—a potent CYP1A2 inhibitor—may result in theophylline toxicity if appropriate precautions are not taken (i.e., conservative doses of theophylline and close monitoring of theophylline response).

Although perhaps not so well appreciated by clinicians, object drug toxicity can also occur when an enzyme-inducing precipitant drug is discontinued. For example, a patient receiving long-term therapy with an

P. D. Hansten: Department of Pharmacy, University of Washington, 1959 NE Pacific Street, Seattle, Washington 98195-7630

enzyme-inducing precipitant drug such as phenytoin who is then started with theophylline is likely to require larger than expected doses of theophylline to achieve therapeutic theophylline concentrations (5). If, however, the enzyme-inducing agent is subsequently discontinued in the presence of continued theophylline therapy, the enzyme induction will gradually dissipate, and the theophylline serum concentration is likely to increase.

Reduced Therapeutic Response to Object Drug

When an enzyme-inducing precipitant drug is added to a susceptible object drug, the pharmacodynamic effect of the object drug tends to decrease. If the magnitude of the interaction is large enough, the therapeutic response to the object drug may be reduced or in some cases abolished. For example, in a hypertensive patient receiving long-term oral therapy with the calcium channel blocker, verapamil, the addition of an enzyme inducer such as rifampin is likely to reduce verapamil serum concentrations markedly and decrease the antihypertensive response (6). Unfortunately, drug interactions resulting in reduced response tend to be more difficult to detect than drug toxicity, at least in the short term. In our hypertensive patient taking verapamil, the increased blood pressure may not be detected until the patient's next office visit. Moreover, even when the decreased therapeutic effect is recognized, there is a tendency to attribute the lack of response to factors other than a drug interaction. In our example, the increased blood pressure may result in the prescription of additional antihypertensive medications and/or an increase in verapamil dosage, actions that may result in excessive hypotension if the enzyme inducer (rifampin) is discontinued.

Reduced object drug response also can occur when an enzyme-inhibiting precipitant drug is discontinued. For example, a patient stabilized on long-term therapy with both fluconazole (a CYP2C9 inhibitor) and warfarin (a CYP2C9 substrate) is likely to manifest a reduced anticoagulant response to warfarin if the fluconazole is discontinued (7–9). Reduced object drug response also may occur when the desired pharmacologic effect resides not with the object drug but with a primary metabolite, and the precipitant drug inhibits the enzyme converting the object prodrug to active metabolite. Although unreported, such an interaction might be expected between an inhibitor of CYP2C19 (i.e., fluconazole) and the antimalarial prodrug, chlorquanide. As with the other types of metabolic drug interactions described earlier, knowledge of the interactive properties of drugs enables one to anticipate the interaction and take appropriate precautions to avoid an adverse outcome.

Other Adverse Outcomes

Although the vast majority of metabolic drug interactions result in an increase or decrease in the effect of the object drug, occasionally other types of adverse reactions occur. For example, some drugs—such as acetaminophen—have minor metabolic pathways in the liver that produce toxic metabolites. Prior administration of drugs that induce the enzymes involved can increase the proportion of acetaminophen converted to these reactive metabolites. This appears to be the mechanism by which prolonged alcohol abuse can increase the hepatotoxicity of acetaminophen (10).

ESTIMATING CLINICAL IMPORTANCE OF DRUG INTERACTIONS

The process of estimating the clinical importance of specific drug interactions has proved to be a difficult task. Few epidemiologic data are available on the risk of specific drug interactions; thus estimates must generally be made indirectly, based on a variety of factors.

Adequacy of Documentation

The amount and quality of published information on a given drug interaction is obviously an important consideration in estimating its clinical importance. Unfortunately, failure to assess the primary literature critically has resulted in the circulation of a great deal of misleading information on drug interactions. This, in turn, has generated skepticism on the part of many clinicians when they attempt to use this information in their practices.

Pharmacokinetic studies of drug interactions must be carefully designed to provide valid results. Important study details include:

- How many subjects or patients were involved? Because the magnitude of drug interactions tends to be highly variable from person to person, it is important to use enough subjects to avoid type II errors.
- Were pertinent pharmacogenetic factors controlled for? When the cytochrome P450 isozyme involved in the drug interaction exhibits genetic polymorphism, it is important to assess the isoenzyme activity of the subjects.
- Were potentially interfering habits of subjects addressed? Because the activity of cytochrome P450 isozymes can be affected by alcohol (11,12), smoking (13,14), birth control pills (13), caffeine, drugs of abuse (14), and dietary factors, it is important to consider such intake in selecting subjects. Unfortunately, some studies of metabolic drug interactions fail to control carefully for intake of these substances.
- Were other drugs taken by the subjects accounted for? This is generally more a problem when the study

involves the use of patients instead of healthy subjects. Because it is usually not possible to find patients who are taking no drugs other than the study drugs, it is important to list all of the drugs that each patient is taking—including over-the-counter (OTC) products. It is not useful simply to state, "None of the patients took drugs known to interact with the object drug." This presumes that the authors are aware of all interactions of the object drug, which may or may not be the case.

- Was the study design appropriate? Pharmacokinetic studies of metabolic drug interactions tend to be performed in a randomized, crossover manner, which allows one to compare—in the same subject—the pharmacokinetics of the object drug alone with the object drug given with the precipitant drug. Parallel designs, in which one group of subjects receives the object drug alone and another group receives the object drug plus the precipitant drug, can be especially problematic for studies of metabolic drug interactions, because drug metabolism is influenced by so many factors. As a result, large numbers of subjects are generally needed to obtain valid results.

- Were the doses of the drugs appropriate? Because most metabolic drug interactions are dose related, it is important to assure that reasonable doses were used. Unrealistic doses are sometimes used in error, and sometimes because the authors would like to achieve a certain outcome from the study.

- Was the duration of drug administration suitable? If the object drug is normally given for a prolonged period, one can usually obtain more clinically useful information by studying its drug interactions after multiple doses. Nonetheless, valuable information on mechanisms, magnitude, and other characteristics can often be gained from studies by using a single dose of the object drug. On the other hand, single doses of the *precipitant* drug are often insufficient to result in an adequate test of metabolic drug interactions. It usually takes multiple doses of the precipitant drug for it to achieve serum concentrations typical of the clinical situation. In addition, some drugs will precipitate an enzyme primarily as the result of the formation of inhibitory metabolite. Prolonged dosing of such drugs (e.g., erythromycin) is necessary for the maximal accumulation of the inhibitory species. Moreover, for enzyme-inducing precipitant drugs, multiple doses over days or, in some cases, weeks are necessary to test fully the ability of the drug to cause enzyme induction.

- What was the timing of administration of the interacting drugs? The timing of administration of the two drugs relative to each other can be critical to achieving valid results when studying metabolic drug interactions. One must consider the individual pharmacokinetics of the two drugs and the likely mechanism of interaction to design the timing of administration appropriately.

Although they are usually the initial basis for detailed interaction studies to elucidate the phenomenon, case reports of drug interactions must also be carefully assessed to determine the strength of the proposed causal relationship. It is rare to find case reports of drug interactions that contain all of the information needed to establish conclusively a causal relationship between the drug interaction and the observed reaction. Accordingly, there has been a tendency to place more credence on case reports than is warranted. Moreover, in those rare instances in which the details of the case report have been checked for accuracy after publication of the case, it has not been unusual to find that the original published report contained factual errors. Nonetheless, as long as these limitations are recognized, much can be learned from case reports of drug interactions. Patterns among case reports can emerge, for example, that shed light on characteristics of the interaction, such as risk factors, time course, and typical symptoms. Case reports are also particularly useful if well-controlled pharmacokinetic studies of the interaction in question involve only single doses of the object drug in healthy subjects. In this situation, case reports can provide important information on the time course of the interaction.

A number of questions should be addressed when evaluating a case report of a possible metabolic drug interaction:

- Is the time course of the onset and offset of the interaction reasonable? To assess what is "reasonable," one must consider the pharmacokinetic properties of the drugs involved, the proposed mechanism of the interaction, and the time course from previous case reports, if any. If the time course of the interaction in the case in question is clearly inconsistent with the expected findings, one should consider alternative explanations.

- Did the interaction remit on dechallenge of the precipitant drug and/or reappear with rechallenge of the precipitant drug? A positive dechallenge (especially if accompanied by a positive rechallenge) strongly suggests that the observed effect was caused by the interaction. Rechallenge is not regularly performed in practice, however, because most patients and clinicians are understandably reluctant to reenact the process that caused the adverse outcome in the first place.

- Were there alternative reasonable causes for the event (e.g., diseases, other interacting drugs, changes in compliance)? In most case reports, it is not possible to investigate thoroughly all possible alternative causes for the adverse outcome. This is especially true for seriously ill patients with fluctuating disease processes and receiving multiple and changing drug therapy.

- Was the drug interaction confirmed by any objective evidence (e.g., drug serum concentrations, laboratory tests, physical examination)? In many case reports of possible metabolic drug interactions, objective evidence is presented. Some types of drug-interaction case reports, however, are more difficult to assess. Purported drug interactions that produce adverse psychiatric effects, for example, are particularly difficult to assess, because little objective evidence is available.

Magnitude of Interaction

For most metabolic drug interactions, we have a general idea of the magnitude of the interaction. This is useful information, because for a given object drug, the greater the magnitude of precipitant drug effect, the higher the likelihood of adverse outcomes. Nonetheless, it is important to realize that estimates of drug-interaction magnitude are based on less than perfect pharmacokinetic studies and case reports. Pharmacokinetic studies typically use healthy subjects, and the magnitude may differ in patients receiving the two interacting drugs therapeutically. Moreover, other aspects of pharmacokinetic study design may not typify the clinical situation, resulting in overestimation or underestimation of the magnitude. Case reports of drug interactions are even more likely to be misleading with regard to magnitude, because they are likely to have reporting bias. That is, patients in whom the interaction is larger (due to the presence of predisposing factors) are the most likely to be reported in the literature.

When considering the magnitude of drug interactions, it is best to keep in mind that most interactions are remarkably variable from one person to another. Differences in type and severity of disease do not appear to play a large role in this variability; even pharmacokinetic studies of drug interactions in healthy subjects typically yield a wide range of values. Thus *mean* changes in object drug serum concentrations or pharmacodynamic effect are useful only as a general guide, because your patient may be at either end of the bell-shaped curve.

Theoretical Considerations

Judicious application of theoretical principles can be a useful adjunct to the "hard" data discussed earlier in the estimation of the clinical importance of drug interactions.

- Is the drug interaction consistent with the known interactive properties of precipitant and object drugs? Given that metabolic drug interactions tend to be predictable, it is important to consider if the two drugs *ought* to interact based on their respective interactive properties. If, on the other hand, the observed effects are inconsistent with the interactive properties of the two drugs, one should look carefully for alternative explanations.
- What are the potential toxicities of the object drug? Even when a particular drug interaction is based only on pharmacokinetic data in healthy subjects, one can estimate the clinical importance of the interaction by

considering the toxicity of the object drug. For example, adding even a moderately potent CYP2C9-inhibiting precipitant drug, such as fluconazole, to warfarin therapy can result in life-threatening bleeding episodes.
- What is the potential adverse outcome of reduced object drug effect? When the interaction results in reduced pharmacodynamic effect of the object drug, one must consider the clinical implications of impaired *therapeutic* response to the object drug. In some cases, the effect can be serious (e.g., thrombosis from inadequate anticoagulant response to warfarin, caused by concurrent administration of a CYP2C9 inducer).
- What is the likelihood that the adverse outcome will be detected early with no special monitoring? Some drug interactions produce effects that are likely to be detected with the usual monitoring for object drug effects. For example, a hospitalized patient taking warfarin may have international normalized ratios (INRs) done frequently enough so that any drug interactions will be detected early and counteracted through adjustments in warfarin dose.
- What is the likelihood that the drugs will be used together in practice? Some combinations appear to be rather unlikely (e.g., a pediatric drug plus a drug used to treat Alzheimer's disease). One must be careful in making such assumptions, however, because drugs are often used for indications not included in the product labeling.

PREDICTING RISK IN SPECIFIC PATIENTS

Some drug interactions result in adverse outcomes in virtually every patient who receives the combination. These "predictable" interactions are rare, however, and the vast majority of reported drug interactions result in adverse outcomes in a minority of patients who receive the interacting combination (see Fig. 54-1). Thus for most drug interactions, it is necessary to assess each patient situation individually.

Patient-Related Risk Factors

Some of the factors affecting the risk of adverse drug interactions are related to the patient behaviors.

- Pharmacogenetics. As discussed elsewhere in this book, some of the cytochrome P450 isozymes are

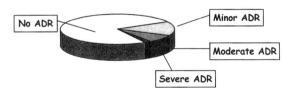

FIG. 54-1. Typical findings in patients receiving interacting drug combinations.

under genetic control—most notably CYP2D6, CYP2C9, and CYP2C19. The activity of *N*-acetyl transferases (1 and 2) and glucuronosyltransferases are also genetically determined. Unfortunately, in most clinical situations, the genotype and phenotypic activity of the patient's drug-metabolizing enzymes is not known to the clinicians caring for the patient.

- Disease states. Diseases of the kidney can slow the renal elimination of some drugs, thus potentially increasing the serum concentrations and pharmacodynamic response of drugs eliminated primarily unchanged in the urine. This would theoretically increase the risk of adverse drug interactions involving such drugs. There are relatively few examples of this phenomenon, however, at least partly because the majority of drugs are inactivated in the intestinal mucosa and liver before elimination by the kidneys. Hepatic disease would theoretically impair drug metabolism and increase the risk of adverse drug interactions, but impaired drug metabolism does not usually occur until the liver is severely damaged.
- In some cases, the disease states of the patient affect the risk of an adverse drug interaction indirectly. Drugs may be given in different doses or duration, depending on the disease being treated. For example, some antibiotics and antifungal agents that affect the activity of cytochrome P450 isozymes can be used for only a day or two in the prevention or treatment of certain infections. In general, this type of short-term use of a precipitant drug would be much less likely to result in an adverse drug interaction than would administration for a more prolonged period.
- Habits. Cigarette smoking is a potent inducer of CYP1A2, and patients who smoke tend to have very low serum concentrations of CYP1A2 substrates such as theophylline and olanzapine. Smoking does not appear to affect cytochrome P450 isozymes other than CYP1A2 to nearly the same extent. Prolonged alcohol abuse results in enzyme induction of CYP2E1 as well as other cytochrome P450 isozymes, but this inducing effect is observed only when the person is sober. Acute alcohol intoxication tends to inhibit hepatic drug metabolism (see Chapter 53). Eventually, long-term alcohol abuse can lead to enough liver damage to impair drug metabolism, but this is usually observed only in the late stages of the disease. These changes in drug metabolism due to cigarettes or alcohol should be considered when evaluating the risk of metabolic drug interactions in patients.
- Age. Elderly patients appear to be at greater risk of manifesting adverse drug interactions, based on epidemiologic studies, case reports, and the clinical experience of those who care for older patients. The elderly are clearly *exposed* to more interacting drug combinations than are younger patients (2), but the extent to which aging *per se* increases the risk of

adverse drug interactions is not established. Indeed, it may well be that older patients are at greater risk primarily because they take more medications and have more diseases that impair their ability to withstand the physiologic insult of a drug interaction (15,16) (see Chapter 56).

Drug Administration–Related Factors

Dose

Most metabolic drug interactions are dose related. That is, as the dose of the precipitant drug is increased over its usual dosage range, the magnitude of its effect on the object drug tends to increase. Thus the dose of the precipitant drug is often an important determinant of risk to the patient. In some cases, the precipitant drug is such a potent inhibitor of a drug-metabolizing enzyme that its dose is of little importance. Quinidine, for example, is a potent inhibitor of CYP2D6, so that even when low quinidine doses are used, it is capable of substantially inhibiting the metabolism of drugs metabolized by CYP2D6 (17).

The properties of the object drug also can be important. If an object drug is highly susceptible to inhibition of metabolism, the interaction may be so large with moderate doses of the precipitant drug that most patients become toxic. Thus the risk of an adverse drug interaction is only marginally increased if large doses of the precipitant drug are used.

The dose of the object drug also may affect the risk of an adverse drug interaction. For example, a patient taking small doses of an object drug with serum concentrations at the low end of the target range is, on average, at lower risk from the addition of an enzyme-inhibiting precipitant drug than would be a patient taking large doses of the same object drug.

Route of Administration

Route of administration is an important risk factor for some nonmetabolic drug interactions (for example, when one drug binds with another in the gastrointestinal tract). But route can be important for metabolic drug interactions as well, particularly when the object drug undergoes extensive first pass metabolism in the gut wall and liver by CYP3A4. For example, the calcium channel blocker, verapamil, undergoes first pass CYP3A4 metabolism. When verapamil is given orally in the presence of therapy with rifampin (a potent CYP3A4 inducer), the first pass metabolism of verapamil is dramatically increased, and the verapamil serum concentrations may decrease to undetectable levels. Parenteral verapamil, on the other hand, is only minimally affected by the concurrent administration of rifampin (6).

Duration of Administration of Precipitant Drug

Most drug interactions have a characteristic time course over which the effects of the interaction develop. In some cases, the interaction is slow to develop, taking days to weeks, and short-term administration of the precipitant drug may be of little clinical importance. For example, the addition of cimetidine to a patient receiving long-term warfarin therapy results in a new steady-state hypoprothrombinemic response in about 7 to 10 days (18). This is because warfarin has a long half-life, and it takes approximately 5 half-lives (now prolonged by the cimetidine) to see a new steady-state warfarin serum concentration. Thus giving cimetidine for 1 or 2 days is unlikely to have much effect on the anticoagulant response to warfarin.

Sequence of Administration of the Interacting Drugs

Most adverse metabolic drug interactions occur when a precipitant drug is started in a patient stabilized with an object drug. Depending on whether the precipitant drug is an enzyme inhibitor or inducer, the pharmacodynamic response of the object drug will increase or decrease, with the accompanying risk of drug toxicity or therapeutic failure. On the other hand, when the object drug is started in the presence of long-term therapy with the precipitant drug, the risk is at least theoretically less. This is because most drugs with significant dose-related toxicity are titrated to effect at the beginning of therapy. The titration process for the object drug should thus reduce the risk of an adverse outcome. The danger with this sequence of administration (object drug added to precipitant drug) occurs when the precipitant drug is later discontinued in the presence of continued therapy with the object drug. For example, a patient starting warfarin in the presence of long-term therapy with an enzyme inducer such as carbamazepine is likely to require relatively large doses of warfarin (19). If the carbamazepine is subsequently discontinued, warfarin serum concentrations will increase, and the patient is likely to become overanticoagulated and at increased risk of a bleeding episode.

The sequence of administration of the object drug and precipitant drug can also affect the time course of metabolic drug interactions. For example, if an enzyme inducer such as rifampin is started in a patient stabilized with a calcium channel blocker such as nifedipine, the increase in enzyme activity will occur gradually. Accordingly, the reduction in nifedipine pharmacodynamic response will generally take place gradually over a week or more. On the other hand, if nifedipine therapy is started in a patient receiving long-term rifampin therapy, the lack of nifedipine response will occur immediately.

PHARMACOECONOMIC SIGNIFICANCE OF DRUG INTERACTIONS

When a patient develops a clinically apparent adverse drug interaction, the cost of medical care is likely to increase. Although some data have been presented on the cost of adverse drug interactions in individual patients, little is known about larger patient groups. What is the aggregate cost of adverse drug interactions in a population of patients? There is virtually no information available on this point.

In a retrospective study, charts of all outpatients receiving theophylline ($n = 913$) were reviewed for concomitant use of cimetidine ($n = 124$), erythromycin ($n = 66$), or ciprofloxacin ($n = 39$). Two patients were identified as being hospitalized for drug interactions: one after cimetidine, and one after ciprofloxacin. The cost of a hospital stay for the patient admitted because of cimetidine-induced theophylline toxicity was $7,372, and for the patient admitted with ciprofloxacin-induced theophylline toxicity, hospital costs were $5,492 (20). The results of this study are consistent with the impressions of many clinicians, that most patients who receive interacting drugs do not manifest severe adverse consequences. It also suggests that the few severe adverse drug interactions that do occur can be costly. Moreover, this study was not designed to detect adverse drug interactions of insufficient severity to result in hospitalization. Hence, any additional costs resulting from outpatient physician visits due to adverse drug interactions would not have been considered.

A retrospective study in two community teaching hospitals looked at all inpatients who received warfarin or theophylline over a 1-year period (21). The patients were divided into two groups: those who received concomitant interacting drugs, and those who did not. The total number of drugs received by each patient was also considered as a rough indicator of illness severity. Outcome measures included length of stay, number of laboratory tests, and laboratory test results. In those patients receiving theophylline, there was no difference in these outcomes, whether or not the patient was receiving interacting drugs. With warfarin, however, patients receiving concurrent therapy with interacting drugs incurred on average almost $1,000 more in hospital expenses (early 1990s dollars) because of increased length of stay and more laboratory tests, compared with patients receiving warfarin in the absence of interacting drugs. Although these results are not definitive, they do suggest that drug interactions with warfarin may increase substantially the cost of hospitalization.

The pharmacoeconomics of drug interactions may also be an important consideration for health care organizations in the selection of a preferred drug within a class of drugs. Unfortunately, for most drug classes, little is known about the pharmacoeconomic implications of potential drug interactions. The H_2-receptor antagonists are a good example. Cimetidine is known to inhibit the metabolism of numerous drugs that are metabolized by cytochrome P450 isozymes, whereas famotidine, nizatidine, and ranitidine appear to have little effect on these enzymes. Before the H_2-receptor antagonists were available without prescription, health care organizations had to make a difficult pharmacoeconomic decision: which H_2-receptor antagonist should be their "preferred" agent? Whereas cimetidine was more likely than other H_2-receptor antagonists to interact with other drugs, the clinical evidence suggested that most patients receiving cimetidine with interacting object drugs did not manifest significant adverse outcomes. Moreover, at that time, cimetidine was considerably less expensive than the other H_2-receptor antagonists. Thus some health care organizations chose to switch as many patients as possible to cimetidine. Did this save money? Probably, but we may never know. There were (and still are) no reliable data on the incidence of severe (and hence expensive) adverse drug interactions with cimetidine. Severe adverse drug interactions due to cimetidine appear to be rare, but can cause significant morbidity when they do occur (20,22–24). Given the large number of patients in these health care organizations, there were almost certainly some severe adverse consequences from cimetidine drug interactions. But the hundreds of thousands of dollars saved by using cimetidine could easily have been greater than the cost of treating the adverse drug interactions from cimetidine.

Herein lies an ethical dilemma. Is it appropriate to save money for the organization, knowing that in doing so, many patients will be placed at increased risk, and a few patients are likely to have adverse consequences? Does the decision depend on how much money is saved, or on how severe the adverse drug interactions are likely to be? How is this different from an automobile manufacturer continuing to produce a car with, say, a defective gas tank, knowing that some small number of people will be killed in explosions, but also knowing that settling the ensuing lawsuits will be cheaper than correcting the problem? As we learn more about drug interactions, such dilemmas are likely to increase rather than decrease.

CONCLUSIONS

Drug–drug interactions can produce a wide variety of adverse outcomes, depending on the interactive properties of the interacting drugs. Although it is possible to estimate the clinical importance of drug interactions in a general way, individual patients vary widely in their response to interacting drugs. Thus it is often difficult to predict the magnitude of a given drug interaction in a specific patient, even when risk factors for the interaction are considered. Little is known regarding the pharmacoeconomics of

adverse drug interactions, but it is clear that they increase the costs of medical care in individual patients.

REFERENCES

1. Pashko S, Somons WR, Sena MM, Stoddard ML. Rate of exposure to theophylline-drug interactions. *Clin Ther* 1994;16:1068–1077.
2. Sipilä J, Klaukka T, Martikainen J, Himberg J-J. Occurrence of potentially harmful drug combinations among Finnish primary care patients. *Int Pharm J* 1995;9:104–107.
3. Loi C-M, Perker BM, Cusack BJ, Vestal RE. Aging and drug interactions. III: individual and combined effects of cimetidine and ciprofloxacin on theophylline metabolism in healthy male and female nonsmokers. *J Pharmacol Exp Ther* 1997;280:627–637.
4. Andrews PA. Interactions with ciprofloxacin and erythromycin leading to aminophylline toxicity. *Nephrol Dial Transplant* 1998;13:1006–1008.
5. Miller M, Cosgriff J, Kwong T, Morken DA. Influence of phenytoin on theophylline clearance. *Clin Pharmacol Ther* 1984:35:666–669.
6. Fromm MF, Busse D, Kroemer HK, Eichelbaum M. Differential induction of prehepatic and hepatic metabolism of verapamil by rifampin. *Hepatology* 1996;24:796–801.
7. Black DJ, Kunze KL, Wienkers LC, et al. Warfarin-fluconazole. II. A metabolically based drug interaction: in vivo studies. *Drug Metab Dispos* 1996;24:422–428.
8. Kunze KL, Wienkers LC, Thummel KE, Trager WF. Warfarin-fluconazole. I: Inhibition of the human cytochrome P450-dependent metabolism of warfarin by fluconazole: in vitro studies. *Drug Metab Dispos* 1996;24:414–421.
9. Kunze KL, Trager WF. Warfarin-fluconazole. III: A rational approach to management of a metabolically based drug interaction. *Drug Metab Dispos* 1996;24:429–435.
10. Slattery JT, Nelson SD, Thummel KE. The complex interaction between ethanol and acetaminophen. *Clin Pharmacol Ther* 1996;60:241–246.
11. Fraser AG. Pharmacokinetic interactions between alcohol and other drugs. *Clin Pharmacokinet* 1997;33:79–90.
12. Adams WL. Interactions between alcohol and other drugs. *Int J Addict* 1995;30:1903–1923.
13. Scavone JM, Greenblatt DJ, Abernethy DR, Luna BG, Harmatz JS, Shader RI. Influence of oral contraceptive use and cigarette smoking, alone and together, on antipyrine pharmacokinetics. *J Clin Pharmacol* 1997;37:437–441.
14. Wiseman EJ, McMillan DE. Combined use of cocaine with alcohol or cigarettes. *Am J Drug Alcohol Abuse* 1996;22:577–587.
15. Vestal RE, Cusack BJ, Crowley JJ, Loi C-M. Aging and the response to inhibition and induction of theophylline metabolism. *Exp Gerontol* 1993;28:421–433.
16. Tanaka E. In vivo age-related changes in hepatic drug-oxidizing capacity in humans. *J Clin Pharm Ther* 1998;23:247–255.
17. von Moltke LL, Greenblatt DJ, Duan SX, Daily JP, Harmatz JS, Shader RI. Inhibition of desipramine hydroxylation (cytochrome P450-2D6) in vitro by quinidine and by viral protease inhibitors: relation to drug interactions in vivo. *J Pharm Sci* 1998;87:1184–1189.
18. Serlin MJ, Sibeon RG, Mossman S, et al. Cimetidine: interaction with oral anticoagulants in man. *Lancet* 1979;2:317–319.
19. Massey EW. Effect of carbamazepine on coumadin metabolism. *Ann Neurol* 1983;13:691–692.
20. Hamilton RA, Gordon T. Incidence and cost of hospital admissions secondary to drug interactions involving theophylline. *Ann Pharmacother* 1992;26:1507–1511.
21. Jankel CA, McMillan JA, Martin BC. Effect of drug interactions on outcomes of patients receiving warfarin or theophylline. *Am J Hosp Pharm* 1994;51:661–666.
22. Derby LE, Jick SS, Langlois JC, Johnson LE, Jick H. Hospital admission for xanthine toxicity. *Pharmacotherapy* 1990;10:112–114.
23. Andersen M, Schou JS. Adverse reactions to H_2-receptor antagonists in Denmark before and after transfer of cimetidine and ranitidine to over-the-counter status. *Pharmacol Toxicol* 1991;69:253–258.
24. Ben-Joseph R, Segal R, Russell WL. Risk for adverse events among patients receiving intravenous histamine2-receptor antagonists. *Ann Pharmacother* 1993;27:1532–1537.

Pharmacist Management of Drug Interactions

Philip D. Hansten

Pharmacists are in a particularly advantageous position to prevent adverse drug interactions, because patients often go to the same pharmacy to have their prescriptions filled (1). Management of drug interactions by pharmacists involves three steps: identification of patients receiving—or about to receive—potentially interacting drugs; determining which of these patients is at significant risk of an adverse outcome from the interaction; and selection of a course of action to minimize the likelihood of an adverse outcome.

IDENTIFICATION OF PATIENTS RECEIVING INTERACTING DRUGS

When adverse drug–drug interactions were first generally recognized as a potential problem in the late 1960s, there were no tools for systematic drug-interaction detection. Pharmacists and physicians typically relied on the "hit and miss" method wherein the only drug interactions identified were those that the health professional happened to notice during normal activities. As one might guess, this "method" was not optimal in identifying potential drug-interaction problems. Unfortunately, this method is still popular today, despite all of the efforts made to computerize and summarize and codify drug interactions.

Over the years, several manual systems of drug-interaction detection have been proposed, involving wall charts and the like. These have generally not proved useful, at least partly because the yield of clinically useful information does not appear to justify the time spent in using them.

Computerized drug-interaction screening has dramatically increased the number of potential drug interactions detected by pharmacists. This has been both a blessing and a curse. Although the computer is ideally suited for rapid checking of new prescriptions for potential interactions with current medications, the resulting alerts, for a variety of reasons, have not been uniformly successful in preventing patients from receiving interacting drug combinations (see Computerized Prevention of Adverse Drug Interactions, below).

No matter what system is used for detecting drug interactions in patients, there are several impediments to the process. First, many patients receive prescriptions from more than one prescriber and/or receive their drugs from more than one pharmacy. This may result in the pharmacist and physician having less than complete information on all of the drugs the patient is taking. Second, patients taking prescribed medications often take over-the-counter (OTC) medications concurrently. Such nonprescription medications often remain undetected by drug-interaction screening systems. Third, the concurrent use of herbal medications represents a variety of problems for drug-interactions detection. Like OTC drugs, they rarely appear on a patient's medication profile, and there is also a lack of clinical information on how they might interact with prescribed drugs. Moreover, given the lack of standardization of herbals, their actual composition is often not known with certainty.

ASSESSING RISK OF DRUG INTERACTIONS IN SPECIFIC PATIENTS

Because very few drug interactions cause adverse outcomes in everyone who receives the interacting combination, it is necessary to estimate the risk for each patient to avoid unnecessary preventive action for those at minimal risk. Risk factors include *patient* risk factors such as diseases, renal function, genetics, gender, age, and habits such as smoking and drinking alcohol. Drug-administration factors can also be important and include

P. D. Hansten: School of Pharmacy, University of Washington, 1959 NE Pacific Street, Seattle, Washington 98195-7630 dose of both precipitant and object drugs, duration of therapy, timing of doses of each drug, and route of administration.

The most common method of assessing the risk of an adverse drug interaction in specific patients is to use the tools immediately available to health-care practitioners: clinical experience, intuition, and common sense. All of these can be useful, but they often fall short in determining the risk of drug interactions. Most drug–drug interactions, even serious ones, cause adverse consequences in only a small percentage of patients who receive the combination. Thus there is a tendency for clinicians to discount the clinical importance of many drug interactions because most patients taking interacting combinations seem to do well. Conversely, a physician or pharmacist whose patient manifests a serious adverse drug interaction may tend to overestimate the clinical importance of that interaction in subsequent patients.

Standard textbooks on drug interactions can also be used to assess the risk of drug interactions in specific patients. The better drug-interaction texts provide, when possible, information on risk factors for specific drug interactions. Nonetheless, accessing and applying such information takes more time than many busy health-care practitioners are able or willing to spend. Decision-support systems for drug interactions may prove useful, but are currently not widely used (2).

ACTIONS TO REDUCE RISK OF ADVERSE DRUG INTERACTIONS

Use of Alternative Noninteracting Medications

For a few drug–drug interactions, the risk of a serious adverse consequence substantially outweighs the benefit of using the combination. Such combinations are therefore considered contraindicated, and the use of a noninteracting alternative is clearly necessary. An example of such an interaction would be that between cisapride and CYP3A4 inhibitors such as erythromycin or clarithromycin (3,4). In this case, an alternative must be found for either the object drug (cisapride) or the precipitant drug (erythromycin or clarithromycin). Accordingly, because azithromycin does not appear to inhibit CYP3A4, it might be considered as an alternative antibiotic to erythromycin or clarithromycin (5,6).

Even when an interacting drug pair is not absolutely contraindicated, it may still be possible to increase the benefit-to-risk ratio by using a noninteracting alternative for one of the drugs. For virtually all drug classes, there are differences in the interactive properties of at least some members of the class (Table 55-1). Thus it is almost always possible to select an alternative to the object drug or precipitant drug that would pose less risk to the patient.

Adjust Dose of Object Drug

If the decision is made to use the interacting drug pair, it may be possible to reduce the risk to the patient by adjusting the dose of the object drug. When possible, it is generally better to adjust the object-drug dose based on changes in the response rather than prophylactically. When the dose of the object drug is adjusted prophylactically at the same time as the precipitant drug is started, it is difficult to know precisely how much to adjust the object-drug dose. The magnitude of drug interactions varies dramatically from patient to patient, and it is quite unlikely that the selected dosage adjustment will exactly offset the effect of the precipitant drug. Thus the patient often is at risk of developing a subtherapeutic or toxic serum concentration of the object drug. O'Connor and Fris (7) demonstrated the difficulty of achieving accurate prophylactic dosage adjustments in five patients taking carbamazepine who were then given clarithromycin. Even though the carbamazepine dose was decreased by 30% to 40%, three of the patients still developed toxic carbamazepine serum concentrations. If one were to prophylactically to decrease carbamazepine dose enough to prevent *any* patients from developing toxic carbamazepine serum concentrations due to clarithromycin, it might be difficult to avoid the risk of subtherapeutic carbamazepine serum concentrations in some patients.

Adjust Dosing Times

For interactions involving binding in the gastrointestinal tract, it may be possible to minimize binding by separating the doses of the binding agent from the object drug. It was formerly thought that a 1- to 2-hour separation of doses was sufficient to minimize the binding, but it is now clear that to minimize the interaction, the object drug should be taken at least 2 hours before or 6 hours after the binding agent (8). Even this amount of separation may not be sufficient to avoid the interaction completely if the object drug undergoes enterohepatic circulation. Drugs undergoing enterohepatic circulation include warfarin, thyroid hormones, and several of the nonsteroidal antiinflammatory drugs.

Monitor for Altered Response

In some cases it is desirable to monitor object drug serum concentrations or increase the frequency of other laboratory tests that measure object-drug response such as an international normalized ratio (INR) or blood glucose concentration. Before doing so, however, one should rule out the use of an alternative noninteracting drug to replace the precipitant drug. Even if the alternative drug is more expensive, it may well cost less than the increased laboratory monitoring. In addition to increased laboratory monitoring, one may wish to increase the frequency

TABLE 55-1. *Drug classes: Differences in interactive properties*

Drug class	Interactive property	Members with interactive property	Members lacking interactive property
Benzodiazepines	Susceptible to CYP3A4 inhibitors	Alprazolam Diazepam[a] Midazolam (oral) Triazolam	Lorazepam[b] Oxazepam[b] Temazepan
Calcium channel blockers	Inhibition of CYP3A4	Diltiazem Verapamil	Dihydropyridine calcium channel blockers[c]
Comarin anticoagulants	Susceptible to CYP2C9 inhibitors	Acenocoumarol Warfarin	Phenprocoumon[d]
HMG-CoA reductase inhibitors	Highly susceptible to inhibition by CYP3A4 inhibitors	Lovastatin Simvastatin	Atorvastatin[e] Cerivastatin[f] Fluvastatin[g] Pravastatin[h]
H₂-receptor antagonists	Inhibition of various CYP450 isozymes	Cimetidine	Famotidine Nizatidine Ranitidine
Macrolide antibiotics	Inhibition of CYP3A4	Clarithromycin Erthromycin	Azithromycin Dirithromycin
Quinolone antibiotics	Inhibition of CYP1A2	Ciprofloxacin Enoxacin Grepafloxacin	Levofloxacin Lovafloxacin Ofloxacin Sparfloxacin Trovafloxacin
Selective serotonin reuptake inhibitors	Inhibition of CYP2D6	Fluoxetine Paroxetine	Citalopram Fluvoxamine[i] Sertraline[j]

[a]Diazepam also is metabolized by CYP2C19 and is only modestly affected by CYP3A4 inhibitors.
[b]Metabolized primarily by glucuronidation.
[c]Dihydropyridines appear unlikely to inhibit CYP3A4, but not all of them have been studied.
[d]Phenprocoumon is metabolized primarily by glucuronide conjugation.
[e]Atorvastatin is metabolized by CYP3A4 but is only moderately affected by CYP3A4 inhibitors.
[f]Cerivastatin is metabolized by CYP3A4 but is only minimally affected by CYP3A4 inhibitors.
[g]Fluvastatin is metabolized by CYP2C9, so it is not affected by CYP3A4 inhibitors.
[h]Pravastatin is not metabolized by cytochrome P450 isozymes.
[i]Fluvoxamine inhibits several other CYP450 enzymes (e.g., CYP1A2, CYP2C19, CYP3A4).
[j]7Sertraline is only a weak inhibitor of CYP2D6.

of physical assessments for altered object-drug response. An example would be increased frequency of blood pressure monitoring if a nonsteroidal antiinflammatory drug is added to antihypertensive drug therapy (9). Finally, if the precipitant drug is expected to increase the effect of the object drug, one should monitor for evidence of object-drug toxicity. For example, a patient taking lovastatin or simvastatin who subsequently takes a CYP3A4 inhibitor such as itraconazole should be alert for evidence of myopathy (e.g., muscle pain and weakness, darkened urine) (10).

COMPUTERIZED PREVENTION OF ADVERSE DRUG INTERACTIONS

Although computers initially seemed to be the ideal tool to detect potential adverse drug interactions, early enthusiasm has given way to recognition of the limitations of computerized drug-interaction screening. Indeed, evidence from studies suggests that, despite computers, physicians regularly prescribe and pharmacists regularly dispense interacting drugs with potentially serious outcomes (1,11–13). The popular media, including *US News and World Report* and the television program, *Dateline*, have also presented evidence to suggest that important drug interactions are not handled appropriately in US pharmacies. There are numerous possible reasons for the suboptimal performance, as described later.

Problems Not Amenable to Rapid Correction

- The sheer volume of the available information. More than 2,000 drug interactions have been described in the medical and pharmaceutical literature, and new interactions are described with every passing month. Clearly most pharmacists and physicians feel overwhelmed by this onslaught and are unable to keep abreast of recent developments in drug interactions.
- Lack of rapid dissemination of data on drug interactions. Many drug interactions are published in medical specialty journals or clinical pharmacology journals that are not read by many practicing pharmacists or

primary care physicians. Thus most health-care practitioners must wait for the interaction to appear in textbooks and computer systems, a process that can take 1 to 2 years or more.

- Lack of epidemiologic information. Even when well-controlled pharmacokinetic studies show that one drug substantially affects the serum concentrations of another, we seldom know how often this produces adverse effects. More epidemiologic studies are needed to put the pharmacokinetic studies and case reports in clinical perspective.
- Complex patients taking many drugs. Patients taking eight to ten drugs or more have an enormous number of possible combinations of drugs to interact with each other. This has been a problem for many years, and is not likely to change soon, given the aging of the population.

Systemic Flaws

- Inadequacy of computer screening systems. This is a major problem. Computer systems have tended to overwhelm pharmacists with excessive drug-interaction alerts. Pharmacists thus become inured to the incessant warnings, and pressing the "override" key often becomes a conditioned response. Pharmacy computer systems may also fail to give alerts when an alert is warranted. Thus computer systems tend to generate too many "overcalls" and too many "undercalls."
- Health professionals with too little time. Some pharmacists, physicians, and other prescribers are simply not afforded enough time, or feel that they do not have enough time, to perform their professional duties adequately regarding drug interactions.

Patient-Induced Problems

- Patient has multiple prescribers and/or multiple pharmacies. Sometimes multiple prescribers or pharmacies are necessary, but the patient should make sure *someone* has a complete record of the medications. Ideally, this would be the primary care physician as well as the primary pharmacy. Unfortunately, this is often not the case.
- Adherence (compliance) problems. Failing to follow directions on how much to take, when to take doses, or what other drugs to avoid can increase the risk of adverse drug interactions. This is a particular problem for drug interactions, because patients taking numerous medications are more likely to have problems adhering to prescribed dosing schedules and are also at greater risk of taking interacting drugs.

Improving the Impact of Computerized Drug-Interaction Screening

Because so much time and money are being expended on drug-interaction research and on computerized drug-interaction screening systems, efforts should be made to improve their impact on patient care. Suggestions for improvement follow.

- Improve the data on computerized drug-interaction screening systems. Most of the available computer systems leave much to be desired. They have both too many drug interactions of questionable clinical importance and too many important drug interactions missing. If one is inundated with drug-interaction alerts, it is only human nature to ignore them. Most pharmacists state that they would use a computerized drug-interaction system if it were accurate and credible.
- Do more epidemiologic studies. Epidemiologic studies are needed to help determine which drug interactions are the most important from a public health standpoint. Drug interactions supported by valid epidemiologic data are more credible than those based on case reports or pharmacokinetic data alone.
- Address the causes of poor performance by some pharmacists. Assuming that pharmacists are like other health-care professionals, lack of knowledge may not be the biggest obstacle. To protect the public health, we need to address the root causes of the observed failure to perform. It may be that attitudes, working conditions, and inadequate systems, are at least as important as lack of knowledge.

SUMMARY

Monitoring for drug interactions involves three steps: identification of patients receiving (or about to receive) potentially interacting drugs; determination of which of these patients is at significant risk of an adverse outcome from the interaction; and selection of a course of action to minimize the likelihood of an adverse outcome. To perform these three steps effectively and efficiently, several questions must be addressed.

What system will be used to identify patients receiving interacting drugs? Most pharmacists use computers for this purpose, but computerized drug-interaction screening has not proved uniformly successful.

How many drug interactions will be included in the system? Too many interactions (the most common mistake) can result in sensory overload; too few bring the risk of adverse outcomes.

How will the clinical significance of drug interactions in specific patients be determined? Decision support systems are needed to aid the pharmacist in this task.

How will the prescriber be notified? Immediate contact by telephone is rarely needed.

How will pharmacist recommendations to prescribers be recorded? The record can document pharmacist's professional activities, as well as provide medicolegal protection.

Are there alternatives to notifying the prescriber? Patient education may be the best way to handle some drug interactions.

Will there be follow-up to determine whether the pharmacist's recommendations were instituted, and whether an adverse outcome occurred?

All of these questions must be addressed appropriately if the incidence of adverse drug interactions is to be reduced.

REFERENCES

1. Zechnich AD, Hedges JR, Eiselt-Proteau D, Haxby D. Possible interactions with terfenadine or astemizole. *West J Med* 1994;160:321–325.
2. Hansten PD. *Drug interactions decision support tables.* Spokane: Applied Therapeutics, 1987.
3. Gray VS. Syncopal episodes associated with cisapride and concurrent drugs. *Ann Pharmacother* 1998;32:648–651.
4. van Haarst AD, van't Klooster GA, van Gerven JM, et al. The influence of cisapride and clarithromycin on QT intervals in healthy volunteers. *Clin Pharmacol Ther* 1998;64:542–546.
5. Harris S, Hilligoss DM, Colangelo PM, Eller M, Okerholm R. Azithromycin and terfenadine: lack of drug interaction. *Clin Pharmacol Ther* 1995;58:310–315.
6. Nahata MJ. Drug interactions with azithromycin and the macrolides: an overview. *Antimicrob Chemother* 1996;37(suppl C):133–142.
7. O'Connor NK, Fris J. Clarithromycin-carbamazepine interaction in a clinical setting. *J Am Board Fam Pract* 1994;7:489–492.
8. Nix DE, Watson WA, Lener ME, et al. Effects of aluminum and magnesium antacids and ranitidine on the absorption of ciprofloxacin. *Clin Pharmacol Ther* 1989;46:700–705.
9. Polonia J. Interaction of antihypertensive drugs with anti-inflammatory drugs. *Cardiology* 1997;88(suppl 3):47–51.
10. Neuvonen PJ, Kantola T, Kivisto KT. Simvastatin but not pravastatin is very susceptible to interaction with the CYP3A4 inhibitor itraconazole. *Clin Pharmacol Ther* 1998;63:332–341.
11. Thompson D, Oster G. Use of terfenadine and contraindicated drugs. *JAMA* 1961;275:1339–1341.
12. Cavuto NJ, Woosley RL, Sale M. Pharmacies and prevention of potentially fatal drug interactions [Letter]. *JAMA* 1996;275:1086–1087.
13. Burkhart GA, Sevka MJ, Temple R, Honig PK. Temporal decline in filling prescriptions for terfenadine closely in time with those for either ketoconazole or erythromycin. *Clin Pharmacol Ther* 1997;61:93–96.

CHAPTER 56

Interactions in the Elderly

Robert E. Vestal and Barry J. Cusack

Elderly patients often present unique challenges to the clinician. Frequently they have multiple chronic illnesses, and as a result, they require treatment with a greater number and variety of medications than do younger patients. The combined effects of drugs and the acute or chronic diseases for which they are prescribed may stress the already diminished physiologic reserves of patients in this age group. Age-related changes in physiology may influence the disposition and response to drug therapy. Thus prescribing for the elderly is complicated by polypharmacy and by altered pharmacokinetics and pharmacodynamics. Although metabolic drug–drug interactions are the main focus of this chapter, a review of drug use, pharmacokinetics, and pharmacodynamics in the elderly will provide the context.

DRUG USE AND POLYPHARMACY

It is self-evident that the use of medications in elderly patients is extensive (1–4). This only adds to the difficulties of prescribing in this age group. Although they compose only 12.5% of the population, older ambulatory patients use three-fold more medications than do younger patients. They account for approximately 25% of physician visits, approximately 30% of medication mentions in surveys, and approximately 35% of drug expenditures. Surveys indicate that 80% to 90% of older patients use at least one medication, with an average of at least four prescription drugs. Two thirds of elderly persons take at least one over-the-counter preparation, and these account for

about 40% of total drug expenditures by this age group. Based on the 1987 National Medical Expenditure sample, it is concerning that an estimated 24% of community-dwelling persons aged 65 years or older (6.64 million Americans) received at least one of 20 inappropriate prescription drugs, and 20% of these persons received two or more (5).

The type of medication used most often varies with the setting. Analgesics, diuretics, cardiovascular drugs, and sedatives are the most frequently prescribed agents in this setting, whereas for nursing home residents, antipsychotics and sedative–hypnotics are most commonly prescribed, followed by diuretics, antihypertensives, analgesics, cardiac drugs, and antibiotics (1–4).

In spite of the known risks of polypharmacy and psychoactive drugs in particular, data clearly show that drug use in elderly nursing home patients is very high. For example, a study in 12 Massachusetts intermediate-care facilities, involving 850 patients with a mean age of 85 years, 84% of whom were female patients, found that the average number of different medications was 8.1 per patient (6). Only 35 (4%) patients had no medication orders. Nearly two thirds of the residents were prescribed one or more psychoactive medications. In another study, based on explicit criteria developed by experts through a consensus process, 40% of 1,106 California nursing home residents received at least one inappropriate medication order, and 10% received two or more inappropriate medication orders (7).

It is important to recognize that self-medication with nonprescription drugs includes the use of herbal (botanical) medications. According to one survey, 3% of the general population use herbal medications (8), but use by the elderly may be considerably greater. A preliminary report of a study conducted in a New Mexico senior health center revealed that 70% to 80% of Hispanic and 35% to 50% of non-Hispanic geriatric patients use herbal medicines (9). Very little is known about the basic and

R. E. Vestal: Early Clinical Development, Covance Incorporated, 2121 North California Boulevard, Suite 500, Walnut Creek, California 94596 and Department of Medicine, University of Washington School of Medicine, Seattle, Washington 98195

B. J. Cusack: Clinical Pharmacology and Gerontology Research Unit, Department of Veterans Affairs Medical Center and Mountain States Medical Research Institute, 500 West Fort Street, Boise, Idaho, 83702

clinical pharmacology of these botanicals and how they may interact with other drugs, either favorably or unfavorably. Unfortunately, the manufacturing processes are not standardized, and they are not regulated as drugs by the Food and Drug Administration. These concerns are being addressed the US Pharmacopeia (USP), which is responsible for establishing manufacturing standards for drug products in this country.

Studies evaluating the appropriateness of prescribing are few. In one study, doses of cimetidine, flurazepam, and digoxin were analyzed on a milligram-per-kilogram basis. It was found that patients weighing 50 kg or less received doses that were 31% to 46% higher than the group mean, and 70% to 80% higher than for patients weighing more than 90 kg (10). Although body weight declined with age, doses in older patients were not decreased proportionately. Because low body weight and advanced age are both risk factors for adverse drug reactions, commonly used drug doses may be excessive in some elderly patients and must be reduced to achieve the desired therapeutic outcome without adverse effects. Evaluation of the appropriateness of prescribing is difficult, and in one study of patients admitted to the hospital, the number of drugs prescribed was not considered to be inappropriate (11). Nevertheless, the prescriber is obliged to reevaluate the need for multiple medications and to be alert to the increased risk of drug interactions in patients taking multiple drugs.

PHARMACOKINETICS

The effects of age on pharmacokinetics are best understood in the context of age-related changes in physiologic function (Table 56-1) (2–4,12–18). Although a number of interesting and important changes in physiology may influence drug absorption, they do not appear to have clinically important effects. For example, in our studies with theophylline, there were no significant age differences in bioavailability or absorption (19–21), and this is true for a variety of other drugs. A delay averaging 60 min. in the time to peak concentration of digoxin has been observed in elderly patients, but the total area under the plasma concentration–time curve was not significantly different, indicating complete absorption (22). The potential exists for drug interactions that might slow absorption or interfere with absorption because of binding in the gastrointestinal tract, but it is unlikely that such an effect would differ significantly with age.

Several important physiological factors may influence drug distribution (2–4,12–18). These include an age-related increase in the proportion of body fat in men (two-fold, from 18% to 36%) and in women (from 33% to 45%), which may account in part for the increase in volume of distribution that has been shown for lipid-soluble drugs such as benzodiazepines (23). For a hydrophilic drug, such as alcohol, the volume of distribution declines,

and at equivalent doses, this will lead to a higher peak plasma concentration (24). This can be explained by the decrease in lean body mass, which includes a 10% to 15% decrease in total body water.

Plasma albumin concentration has been shown to be either decreased or unchanged, and α_1-acid glycoprotein concentration is either increased or unchanged (2–4, 12–18). Usually the effect of plasma binding of drugs is not clinically important. Furthermore, an age-related increase in the unbound fraction by more than 50% occurs with only a few drugs, such as acetazolamide, valproate, diflusinal, salicylate, and naproxen (25). In malnourished patients, however, such as those with advanced cancer, serum albumin can be quite low. This may result in increased unbound concentrations of low-clearance, highly bound drugs, which in turn may lead to unexpected toxicity (26).

Biochemical studies in hepatic tissue from primates and liver biopsy specimens from humans have shown that phase I or phase II (conjugation) enzyme activity does not differ with age (27). Much more important is the age-related decrease in liver mass. Absolute liver weight declines 20% to 50% across the age span up to age 80 years, and ultrasound studies show that liver volume decreases by about 25%. Galactose clearance, a nondrug marker of hepatic functional mass, is decreased by 25%. Associated with the age-related decrease in liver mass is a 35% decrease in hepatic blood flow between the third and seventh decades. Adjusted for liver volume, this corresponds to a decrease in liver perfusion of 10% to 15%. The decrease in liver mass will influence the clearance of drugs that are oxidized by the liver, and in some cases, this affects drugs that are eliminated by conjugation. For example, this reported decrease in liver mass probably accounts for the 20% to 25% decrease in the clearance of theophylline, a substrate for cytochrome P450 (CYP) 1A2 in the liver with a low extraction ratio and only 40% to 50% protein binding, in healthy elderly men and women compared with that in young subjects (19–21). Similarly, Wynne et al. (28) sought to explain the decrease in warfarin dose requirement with advancing age. Pharmacokinetic studies have not provided a definitive explanation. A decline in liver volume was confirmed by ultrasound in 39 patients older than 50 years. In these patients with stable international normalized ratio (INR) values, there was an age-related decline in the mean weekly dose of warfarin. Multivariate analysis revealed significant relations between and warfarin dose and liver volume. A small (36%) additive effect on the total variance was explained when age was included, but liver volume was the most critical variable for predicting warfarin dose requirement.

The age-related decrease in liver blood flow results in decreased first pass metabolism, systemic bioavailability, and plasma concentrations of drugs that are highly excreted by the liver, such as labetalol, propranolol, ver-

TABLE 56-1. *Factors affecting drug disposition in the geriatric patient*

Pharmacokinetic parameter	Age-related physiological change	Pharmacokinetic effect	Examples of affected drugs	Pathologic condition	Therapeutic and environmental factors
Absorption	↑ Gastric pH ↓ Absorptive surface ↓ Splanchnic blood flow ↓ GI motility	NC		Achlorhydria Diarrhea Postgastrectomy Malabsorption syndromes Pancreatitis	Antacids Anticholinergics Cholestyramine Drug–drug interactions Food or meals
First pass metabolism	↓ Hepatic blood flow	↑ Bioavailability for high-extraction drugs	Labetolol Metoprolol Nifedipine Propranolol Verapamil	Congestive heart failure Hepatic failure	Drug–drug interactions
Distribution Volume	↓ Lean body mass ↓ Total body water ↑ Total body fat	↑ $t_{1/2}$ of some fat-soluble drugs ↑ Plasma levels of some water-soluble drugs	Diazepam Midazolam Alcohol Antipyrine	Congestive heart failure Dehydration Edema or ascites Hepatic failure Malnutrition Renal failure	Drug–drug interactions Protein-binding displacement
Protein-binding	↓ (or NC) serum albumin concentration ↑ (or NC) α_1-AGP concentration	↑ (or NC) unbound drug concentration ↓ (or NC) unbound drug concentration	Phenytoin Warfarin Imipramine		
Metabolism	↓ Hepatic mass ↓ Hepatic blood flow	↓ (or NC) plasma CL ↑ (or NC) $t_{1/2}$	Fosinopril Imipramine Levodopa Lidocaine Morphine Propranolol Nortriptyline Theophylline	Congestive heart failure Fever Frailty Hepatic insufficiency Malignancy Malnutrition Thyroid disease Viral infection	Dietary composition Drug–drug interactions Insecticides Tobacco (smoke)
Excretion	↓ Renal blood flow ↓ GFR ↓ Tubular secretion	↓ Plasma CL ↑ $t_{1/2}$	ACE inhibitors Amantidine Chlorpropamide Cimetidine Furosemide Gentamicin Metformin Procainamide Ranitidine	Hypovolemia Renal insufficiency	Drug–drug interactions

α_1-AGP, α_1-acid glycoprotein; $t_{1/2}$, half-life; CL, clearance; GFR, glomerular filtration rate; ACE, angiotensin-converting enzyme; ↑, increase; ↓, decrease; NC, no change.

Adapted from Vestal RE, Dawson GW. Pharmacology and aging. In: Finch CE, Schneider EL, eds. *Handbook of the biology of aging*. 2nd ed. New York: Van Nostrand Reinhold, 1985:744–819, and Vestal RE. Aging and pharmacology. *Cancer* 1997;80:1302–1310.

apamil, and morphine (14,15,27). In addition, enzyme activity in the intestine may influence first pass metabolism and systemic bioavailability. Cytochrome CYP3A4, the predominant P450 isoform in the liver, is present in the intestinal mucosa, where it also may influence first pass metabolism and systemic bioavailability (29). The effect of age on the *in vivo* clearance of various substrates for specific cytochrome P450 isoforms is summarized in Table 56-2. Recognizing that age differences probably reflect factors other than intrinsic enzyme activity, it is apparent that information is available for only half of the P450 isoforms.

Some evidence suggests that the response to environmental factors may differ with age. For example, the inducibility of the metabolism of antipyrine, a substrate for several hepatic cytochromes P450, in older cigarette smokers is less than that in younger smokers (39). This may represent a cohort effect related to survival of older

TABLE 56-2. *Effect of age on* in vivo *clearance of typical substrates by cytochrome P450 isoforms*

CYP	Typical substrate	Clinical relevance	Inducers	Effect of age in vivo	References
1A1	Polycyclic hydrocarbons	?Cancer risk linked with mutations	?Dietary and smokers	Not known	NA
1A2	Caffeine, theophylline, paracetamol (acetaminophen)	Bioactivation of carcinogens	Smoking and omeprazole	Reduction	19–21
2A	Warfarin	Polymorphic	Polymorphic	Probably no reduction	30
2B	NA	NA	?Phenobarbital	Not known	NA
2C8	?Retinoic acid	NA	NA	Not known	NA
2C9 and 10	Tolbutamide, hexobarbital	Autoimmune hepatitis	Phenobarbital	Reduction	31,32
2C18 and 19	Mephenytoin, diazepam, omeprazole	Drug toxicity and lack of efficacy	Phenobarbital and rifampin	Reduction	33
2D6	Debrisoquine, sparteine, β-blockers, tricyclic antidepressants, codeine	Drug toxicity and the lack of efficacy, lung cancer, Parkinson's disease	Rifampin	No reduction	34
2E1	Chloroxazone	Cancer and drug toxicity	Alcohol, starvation, and diabetes	Possible reduction	35,36
3A3/4	Nifedipine, erythromycin		Rifampin	Reduction	37
3A5	Nifedipine[a]			Reduction	38
3A7	Steroids			NA	NA

[a]CYP3A5 does not metabolize erythromycin or quinidine, indicating a difference in metabolic profile between CYP3A4 and CYP3A5. The reduction in clearance reflects changes in physiological factors such as organ blood flow and organ volume.

NA, not available.

From Kinirons MT, Crome P. Clinical pharmacokinetics considerations in the elderly: an update. *Clin Pharmacokinet* 1997;33:302–312.

smokers with reduced inducibility and selective mortality of smokers with more inducible P450-mediated hepatic metabolism. In smaller studies with theophylline, however, a similar age difference in the effect of smoking has not been shown (19,20).

Because virtually no research has been performed related to the effect of age and diet on drug metabolism, the potential importance is largely speculative. Reviews of this topic reflect this lack of specific information (40). From studies in young individuals, we know that alterations in diet can have a profound effect on drug metabolism (26). A high-protein, low-carbohydrate diet is associated with an increase in clearance of a marker substrate such as antipyrine. The converse is true when diets are switched to a low-protein, high-carbohydrate content. Individuals with malnutrition have markedly impaired drug metabolism. This becomes an important consideration when treating patients who may be malnourished because of anorexia associated with chronic illness.

Although genetic polymorphisms are another potentially important consideration in the use of drug therapy in the elderly, there are very few studies of possible age differences in the frequency distribution of genetic polymorphisms or their phenotypic expression. The available studies have not identified significant age effects. Variants of CYP2D6, which is responsible for oxidizing many therapeutic drugs, are found in 7% to 10% of the white

population who have a "poor metabolizer" phenotype. Data from Sweden, Germany, and France indicate that there is no age difference in the frequency distribution of poor and extensive metabolizers (41–43). A study of acetylator phenotype in 512 subjects in the Baltimore Longitudinal Study of Aging did not show an age difference in the nearly equal distribution of rapid and slow acetylator phenotypes (44). These results are consistent with the majority of smaller studies.

Stereoselective drug metabolism is yet another consideration (17), but again, the available data are very limited. A 58% decrease in the clearance of L-hexobarbital compared with D-hexobarbital was found in older compared with younger subjects (32). However, studies with enantiomers of ibuprofen and propranolol do not show age differences in metabolism (17). The results of additional research will be of interest.

Frailty is a another variable that has received scant attention, but a study from Newcastle indicates that it may be quite important (45). Although a significant 28% decrease in the clearance of acetaminophen was found in fit elderly compared with the young, this age difference disappeared when the data were normalized by an estimate of liver volume obtained with ultrasound. The 42% decrease in the clearance of acetaminophen in frail elderly also diminished, but remained significant, even when adjusted for liver volume.

Changes in renal function have profound effects on the excretion of drugs and their metabolites (46). Renal mass decreases 25% to 30% across the age span, renal blood flow decreases about 1% per year after age 50, and glomerular filtration rate decreases approximately 35% in healthy individuals between age 20 and 90 years. There also are decreases in tubular function, impairment of *para*-aminohippurate (PAH) secretion, and reduced ability to concentrate and dilute the urine. However, careful longitudinal studies in some individuals show maintenance of normal renal function into later life. In fact, a few individuals actually have small increases in creatinine clearance. In general, however, because renal function declines with aging, the clearance of drugs that are secreted or filtered by the kidney is decreased in a predictable manner. All studies that have investigated the effect of age on the clearance of renally excreted drugs have found age-related decreases.

PHARMACODYNAMICS

The effects of age on pharmacodynamic responses have been studied less extensively than pharmacokinetics (2–4,12–16,18,47). Cardiovascular and central nervous system (CNS) effects have received the most attention. Several studies have found that the chronotropic response to intravenous isoproterenol is diminished with aging (48). The dose required to achieve the 25-beat increase in heart rate in older compared with younger subjects is larger (49). Based largely on studies with cardiac tissue from animals, the explanation for this age difference in response has been thought to reside at the level of receptor–effector coupling (48). Radioligand-binding experiments with antagonists do not show an age-related decrease in total β-adrenergic receptor density. Studies with agonists, however, indicate that the ability to form the high-affinity receptor is diminished with an associated decrease in cyclic adenosine monophosphate (AMP) production and adenylyl cyclase activation. In addition to these biochemical changes, it is also quite possible that structural differences in the sinus node with fibrosis and loss of pacemaker cells may be important mechanisms for the altered response to isoproterenol. In the presence of autonomic blockade, the cardiac chronotropic sensitivity to isoproterenol in elderly subjects was similar to that found in young subjects (50). This indicates that the age-associated reduction in cardiac chronotropic responses to bolus isoproterenol is primarily due to an age-related reduction in the influence of reflex cardiovascular responses on heart rate and not to an age-related reduction in cardiac β-adrenergic sensitivity. In addition, because theophylline eliminated the age difference in chronotropic response in another study, it has been suggested that excessive production or an increased effect of adenosine is partly responsible for the cardiac chronotropic resistance to isoproterenol (51). Altered

adrenergic receptor sensitivity may have practical clinical significance. For example, airway β2-adrenergic receptor responsiveness is diminished in old age, resulting in an increased dose requirement for albuterol to achieve bronchial relaxation after methacholine challenge (52).

Although there are concerns related to the design of some of the studies, it is generally accepted that the sensitivity to psychoactive drugs, such as anxiolytics and hypnotics in the benzodiazepine drug class, is greater in older persons (23). There is also an increased frequency of adverse effects, particularly falls and hip fractures, from benzodiazepines and other psychotropic drugs that have long half-lives of parent drug or active metabolite (53–55). The use of these agents must be avoided in the elderly. Although treatment with tricyclic antidepressants (TCAs) may be effective, adverse effects are more frequent than in younger patients. Most data indicate that plasma concentrations of many tricyclic and newer antidepressants are increased with age (56). This probably is due to decreased clearance, but this may vary with the specific metabolic pathway or pathways involved in biotransformation. For example, one study showed a decrease with age in the clearance of imipramine, but not desipramine (57). Care is needed to avoid pharmacodynamic interactions resulting from polypharmacy. TCAs antagonize α1-adrenoceptor activation and can potentiate the effects of diuretics or β-adrenergic blockers, resulting in profound hypotension. They also increase the depressant effects of alcohol and benzodiazepines, and they may potentiate the effects of some antiarrhythmics (58).

The selective serotonin reuptake inhibitors (SSRIs), such as fluoxetine, sertraline, and paroxetine, are being used increasingly in frail elderly patients because of their favorable safety profile and apparent clinical efficacy (58). Because SSRIs are inhibitors of several cytochromes P450, particularly CYP2D6, CYP1A2, CYP3A, and CYP2C19 (59), reduced clearance of a number of commonly used drugs, including TCAs, phenothiazines, anticoagulants, and class IC antiarrhythmics, can result when these drugs are coadministered. Care is needed to avoid unexpected reactions in elderly patients, who are more likely to be receiving one or more of these drugs.

The effect of age on the response to drugs used for pain management is noteworthy. It has been known for many years that the elderly have a greater response to the analgesics morphine and pentazocine (60). Subsequently it was reported that the maximal degree of pain relief after intramuscular morphine (8 or 16 mg) was similar, or even somewhat greater in the oldest patients (aged 70–89 years), but the duration of pain relief was markedly prolonged with increasing age (61). This effect probably is due in part to pharmacokinetic differences. Peak serum concentrations of morphine at 2 minutes after intravenous injection increase with age, but by 10 minutes, this difference no longer is present (62). Paradoxically, detailed pharmacokinetic studies subsequently showed a decreased, rather than increased, half-life in the older individuals, indicating faster elimination by that parameter (63,64). However, a 50% decrease in the volume of distribution of morphine results in an overall decrease of about 20% in total plasma clearance. Thus the pharmacokinetic characteristics of narcotic analgesics in the elderly are complex.

Pharmacokinetic age differences provide only a partial explanation for age differences in response. For example, brain sensitivity to intravenous fentanyl and alfentanil is increased in elderly patients undergoing general anesthesia compared with younger patients (65). Before surgery, intravenous fentanyl or alfentanil was infused into individuals ranging in age from 20 to 89 years. During the infusions, subjects were monitored with electroencephalogram (EEG) recordings. The infusions were discontinued when delta waves (less than 4 Hz) were observed. Fourier transformations were used to convert the raw EEG data into spectral edge tracings. From this information, median inhibitory concentration (IC_{50}) values were determined to quantify brain sensitivity. They were 22% and 35% lower in the elderly for fentanyl and alfentanil, respectively. This occurred despite comparable plasma levels, which facilitates the interpretation of pharmacodynamic responses. These results are consistent with other data for CNS-active drugs, such as benzodiazepines, showing that the elderly are more sensitive to the pharmacodynamic responses (23).

ADVERSE DRUG EVENTS

The elderly experience more adverse drug events (ADEs) than do younger patients (2–4,12,16,66,67). For example, in outpatient elderly populations, the prevalence is approximately 30%. Up to 20% of hospital admissions in elderly patients are caused by ADEs. In older hospitalized patients, the incidence of ADEs ranges from 10% to 25%. Approximately half of deaths are related to ADEs in patients older than 60 years. It is important to recognize that age itself is a less important factor than the number of diseases that are typical of this age group and the number of drugs that older patients take (66–68). In one study of patients older than 50 years who were admitted to the hospital through the emergency department, there was no relation between age and the number of ADEs, but there were positive correlations between ADEs and the number of diagnoses and the number of drugs taken (68). Predicable ADEs are common in high-risk older outpatients, and they result in considerable medication modification and substantial health-care use. A study of 167 high-risk (taking at least five scheduled medications) ambulatory older veterans participating in a year-long health-service intervention trial revealed 80 self-reported ADEs (69). These 80 ADEs involved 72 medications taken by 58 (35%) of the patients, as determined by close-out interviews. Seventy-six (95%) were classified as predictable.

Sixty-three percent of patients with ADEs required physician contacts; 10%, emergency department visits; and 11%, hospitalizations. Twenty percent of medications implicated in ADEs required dosage changes, and 48% of ADE-related medications were discontinued. In addition to multiple diseases and polypharmacy, impairment of the homeostatic mechanisms that regulate blood pressure (decreased baroreceptor and autonomic function), body temperature, and intravascular volume (decreased thirst, antidiuretic hormone response, maximum urine osmolality, and excretion of a water load) all influence the ability of patients to adapt to the effects of various drugs (16). They are particularly vulnerable to the side effects of anticancer drugs (70).

DRUG INTERACTIONS

Drug interactions as a broad category include drug–disease interactions (Table 56-3), drug–food interactions (related to malnutrition, altered drug absorption, and induction or inhibition of biotransformation), drug–laboratory test interactions (related to methodologic interference or biologic alteration), drug–alcohol (related to the combined effects of alcohol and a drug), and drug–drug interactions (mainly impaired drug absorption and induction or inhibition of biotransformation) (71). When two or more drugs are administered concurrently or within temporal proximity, a drug interaction may result in synergistic, potentiated, or antagonistic effects. Synergism is rare, but occurs when the combined action of two drugs exceeds the summation of their independent actions. Potentiation occurs when two active drugs produce a greater effect than would be expected on the basis of their dose–response curves. Antagonism results from the reduction or blockade of the clinical effect of one drug by another.

Rates of prevalence of drug interactions vary among studies because of the lack of consensus on what constitutes a significant interaction, the lack of adequately standardized criteria and methodology, and the use of multiple reference materials from different sources and databases to perform drug-interaction identification (72). Potential interactions are reported to range from as low as 2.7% to as high as 68.9% of patients, depending on the criteria and specific patient population (73–79). It is important to note, however, that these reports do not document actual clinical events, only potential events. A chart review revealed no serious actual interaction among 1,052 potential interactions (310 drug–food, 316 drug–alcohol, and 426 drug–drug), even though the potential interactions were categorized as highly significant for 27% of the drug–drug, 11% of the drug–alcohol, and 3% of the drug–food interactions (76). Thus many or perhaps even most of the potential drug–drug interactions that are identified by computerized and other screening methods may have no real clinical significance. Nevertheless, such systems can help increase the health-care provider's awareness

TABLE 56-3. *Selected drug–disease interactions in older persons*

Disease	Drugs	Adverse effect
Benign prostatic hypertrophy	Anticholinergics, decongestants	Decreased bladder emptying, urinary retention
Cardiac conduction abnormalities	Verapamil, TCAs, β-blockers	Heart block
Chronic obstructive pulmonary disease	β-Blockers, narcotic analgesics	Bronchoconstriction Respiratory depression
Chronic renal insufficiency	NSAIDs, contrast agents, aminoglycosides	Acute renal failure
Congestive heart failure (systolic)	β-Blockers, verapamil	Acute renal failure
Dementia	Anticholinergics, benzodiazepines, levodopa, opiates, antidepressants	Delirium
Diabetes mellitus	Diuretics, corticosteroids	Hyperglycemia
Angle-closure glaucoma	Anticholinergics	Acute exacerbation of glaucoma
Hypertension	NSAIDs	Increased blood pressure
Hypokalemia	Digoxin	Cardiac arrhythmias
Hyponatremia	Oral hypoglycemics, diuretics, carbamazepine	Decreased sodium concentration
Peptic ulcer disease	Anticoagulants, NSAIDs	Upper gastrointestinal bleeding
Postural hypotension	Diuretics, TCAs, levodopa, vasodilators	Syncope, falls, hip fracture

TCAs, tricyclic antidepressants; NSAIDs, nonsteroidal antiinflammatory drugs. From Parker BM, Cusack BJ. Pharmacology and appropriate prescribing. In: Reuben DB, Yoshikawa TT, Besdine RW, eds. *Geriatrics review syllabus: a core curriculum in geriatric medicine.* Dubuque: Kendall/Hunt Publishing, 1996:29–36.

of possibly interacting drug combinations, which in turn may lead to prevention of unintended ADEs (74,77,80).

Studies of the effects of age on drug interactions are few (81) (Table 56-4). In addition, most of the earlier studies failed to include measurements of the plasma concentrations of the interacting drugs. Without this information, it is not possible to be certain that young and old subjects were exposed to similar concentrations of the inducer or inhibitor drug. Research in our laboratory using an inducer (phenytoin) and inhibitors (cimetidine, ciprofloxacin) of

theophylline metabolism by hepatic CYP1A2 have not shown the older subjects to differ significantly from the young in the proportionate effects of concomitant drug administration (Figs. 56-1 to 56-3) (19–21). This means that this age group is at least equally vulnerable to the potential untoward effects of reduced or increased plasma levels (undertreatment or toxicity, respectively). In our studies, plasma levels of substrate as well as inducer or inhibitor(s) were measured to assure that comparable levels were achieved, or in the case of cimetidine, that the

TABLE 56-4. *Effect of age on induction and inhibition of drug metabolism by the liver in humans*

Interacting drug	Marker drug substrate	Effects in old versus young subjects	Reference
Inducer			
Dichloralphenazone	Antipyrine	Decreased	82
	Quinine	Decreased	82
Glutethimide	Antipyrine	Same or increased	83
Phenytoin	Theophylline	Same	20
	Cortisol	Same[a]	20
Rifampin	Antipyrine	Decreased	84
	Propranolol	Same or decreased	85
Inhibitor			
Cimetidine	Antipyrine	Same	86
	Desmethyldiazepam	Same	86
	Theophylline	Same	87
			88
			21
			19
	Cortisol	Same[a]	19
Ciprofloxacin	Theophylline	Same	21
Ciprofloxacin plus cimetidine	Theophylline	Same	21

[a]Urinary excretion of 6β-hydroxycortisol.
Adapted from Vestal RE, Cusack BJ. Pharmacology and aging. In: Schneider EL, Rowe JW, eds. *Handbook of the biology of aging.* 3rd ed. San Diego: Academic Press, 1990:349–383, and Vestal RE, Cusack BJ, Crowley, Loi CM. Aging and the response to inhibition and induction of theophylline metabolism. *Exp Gerontol* 1993;28:421–433.

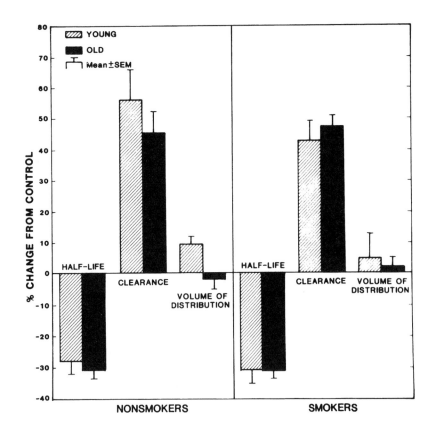

FIG. 56-1. Effect of age and smoking on the proportionate change in half-life, clearance, and volume of distribution of theophylline in young and old subjects after treatment with phenytoin. From Crowley JJ, Cusack BJ, Jue SG, Koup JR, Park BK, Vestal RE. Aging and drug interactions. II: Effect of phenytoin and smoking on the oxidation of theophylline and cortisol in healthy men. *J Pharmacol Exp Ther* 1988;245:513–523, with permission.

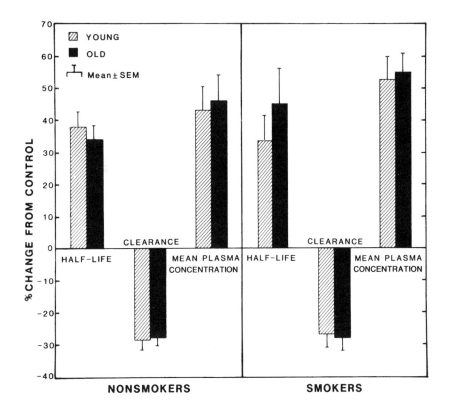

FIG. 56-2. The effect of age and smoking on the proportionate change in half-life, clearance, and mean plasma concentration in young and old subjects after treatment with cimetidine. From Vestal RE, Cusack BJ, Mercer GD, Dawson GW, Park BK. Aging and drug interactions. I: Effect of cimetidine and smoking on the oxidation of theophylline and cortisol in healthy men. *J Pharmacol Exp Ther* 1987;241:488–500, with permission.

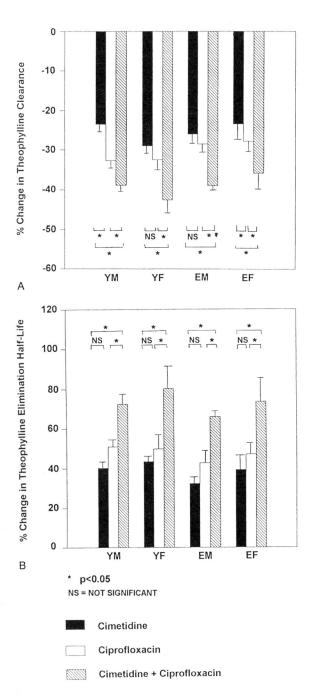

A

B

* p<0.05
NS = NOT SIGNIFICANT

- ■ Cimetidine
- □ Ciprofloxacin
- ▨ Cimetidine + Ciprofloxacin

FIG. 56-3. Proportionate change in plasma theophylline elimination: **(A)** clearance, and **(B)** half-life after treatment with cimetidine and ciprofloxacin. YM, young males; YF, young females; EM, elderly males; EF, elderly females. From Loi CM, Parker BM, Cusack BJ, Vestal RE. Aging and drug interactions. III: Individual and combined effects of cimetidine and ciprofloxacin on theophylline metabolism in healthy male and female nonsmokers. *J Pharmacol Exp Ther* 1997;280: 627–637, with permission.

decrease in theophylline clearance could not be explained by differences in values of area under the curve (AUC) (19). With phenytoin, the study was complicated by the nonlinear kinetics and the possibility of autoinduction. Therefore the study design included an initial assessment of phenytoin disposition followed by dose administration and mid-study adjustments based on the plasma levels of phenytoin that were achieved (90; Fig. 56-4). From our own work and that of others (see Table 56-4), it is reasonable to conclude that the response to induction is variable without clear age differences, and that age appears to have no effect of the response to the inhibitory effects of cimetidine and ciprofloxacin. However, similar elevations in plasma levels induced by inhibitors may result in greater toxicity in the elderly. For example, chronic theophylline toxicity in the elderly often is more serious because of increased vulnerability to the cardiac electrophysiologic and neurophysiologic effects (91). Studies are needed with substrates that are specific for individual isozymes of cytochrome P450. The important caveat, however, is that the few available studies, including our own, have been performed in healthy older persons who may not be representative of the frail elderly patients who are likely to be more susceptible to the adverse effects of complex drug regimens.

Examples of drug–drug interactions of potential clinical importance in the elderly are listed in Table 56-5. They include both pharmacokinetic and pharmacodynamic interactions. Drugs most commonly implicated are those that are used to treat chronic illness in the elderly, and agents with a low therapeutic index (small difference between therapeutic and toxic dose) require the most careful monitoring to recognize signs of toxicity early in dose titration (92). Such agents include digoxin, diuretics, calcium channel blockers, oral hypoglycemic agents, tricyclic antidepressants, antiarrhythmic drugs, warfarin, nonsteroidal antiinflammatory drugs (NSAIDS; including aspirin), phenytoin, centrally acting analgesics, antacids, theophylline, and antipsychotics. Drug combinations that pose the greatest risk for untoward effects include inhibitors and inducers of the hepatic microsomal drug-metabolizing enzymes, any drug combination that causes a decrease in blood pressure, any combination of drugs with additive sedative effects, combinations of drugs with anticholinergic effects, and any drug combination with coumarin anticoagulants, most commonly warfarin (92). Inhibition of renal organic cationic drug excretion appears not to be age related (93).

More than 60% of patients with cancer are older than 65 years. Important drug–drug interactions include methotrexate and salicylates, cisplatin and aminoglycosides, mercaptopurine and allopurinol, procarbazine and tricyclic antidepressants, and vincristine and opioid analgesics (70). CYP3A isoforms are involved in the biotransformation of a number of anticancer drugs including cyclophosphamide and ifosfamide, epipodophyllotoxins

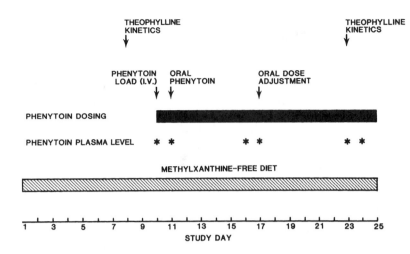

FIG. 56-4. Protocol to study the effect of age and smoking on the induction of theophylline metabolism by phenytoin. From Crowley JJ, Cusack BJ, Jue SG, Koup JR, Vestal RE. Cigarette smoking and theophylline metabolism: effects of phenytoin. *Clin Pharmacol Ther* 1987;42:334–340, with permission.

(etoposide, teniposide), paclitaxel, tamoxifen, and *Vinca* alkaloids (vinblastine, vincristine, and navelbine). These drugs are also substrates for P-glycoprotein. Appropriate caution should be exercised when combining P-glycoprotein inhibitors and potential CYP3A inhibitors such as cyclosporine, calcium channel blockers (verapamil, nifedipine), macrolide antibiotics (erythromycin), and imidazole antifungals (ketoconazole, miconazole, itraconazole) with cancer chemotherapy (94).

There is little available information on drug–food, drug–laboratory test, and drug–alcohol interactions in the elderly. However, alcohol abuse remains a public health concern in the elderly (95). Among those aged 65 to 75 years, it is estimated that 42% use alcohol. This figure declines to 30% in those older than 75 years. Furthermore, about 6% of the elderly are considered to be heavy drinkers (more than two drinks per day), and about 5% to 12% of men and 1% to 2% women in their sixties are considered to be problem drinkers. Alcohol use can impair the effectiveness of drug therapy, or it can create new medical problems requiring additional therapy. Thus the possibility of drug–alcohol interactions must be an important consideration in elderly as well as in young and middle-aged patients (95,96). Community surveys have shown that between 25% and 38% of elderly respondents used alcohol together with one or more drugs with the potential to act adversely when combined (97,98). Elderly patients are particularly susceptible to the additional sedation resulting from the synergism between alcohol and psychotropic drugs (antipsychotics, antidepressants, anxiolytics, and sedative–hypnotics) and to gastrointestinal bleeding that results from the interaction of alcohol with aspirin and other NSAIDs (95,96). The risk of upper gastrointestinal bleeding is increased nearly 13-fold in older patients taking NSAIDs and warfarin compared with age-matched controls (99).

STRATEGIES TO AVOID DRUG INTERACTIONS

Because elderly patients may have multiple disease states and may require a wide variety of drugs, the potential for drug interactions and associated ADEs is increased. It is helpful to be aware of the numerous other factors that may lead to polypharmacy (Table 56-6). Although computerized alerting mechanisms may be helpful (74,80,92), they are not a substitute for thoughtful and appropriate prescribing (Table 56-7). A clear understanding of the risks and benefits of drug treatment for each patient is essential. Each treatment regimen should be adjusted for the individual patient to maximize the benefits and minimize the risks.

A careful drug history should be obtained in every elderly patient, with attention to all prescription and nonprescription drugs, a directed history of previous drug reactions, and information about the patient's use of tobacco, alcohol, caffeine, and illicit drugs. The possibility of additional medications prescribed by other providers should be explored. A comprehensive list of medications should be maintained and reviewed at each patient visit. Drugs that are no longer needed or appropriate should be discontinued, and nondrug therapy always should be considered. It often is helpful to ask patients to bring their medications to the office so that they can be reviewed, and discarded if necessary, by the health-care provider. When a new drug is added to the regimen, new or unusual symptoms, or nonspecific complaints such as confusion, unsteady gait, lethargy, weakness, dizzy spells, incontinence, urinary retention, depression, and falling should prompt a careful look at the patient's medication list for a possible drug–drug interaction. Not all drug–drug interactions require discontinuation of the interacting medication. Instead, the suspected mechanism may indicate a change in dosage or

TABLE 56-5. *Important drug–drug interactions*

Mechanism	Drug	Interacting drug	Effect
Pharmacokinetic interactions			
Decreased absorption	Digoxin	Antacids, cholestyramine, colestipol	Decreased digoxin effect
	Ciprofloxacin	Sucralfate	Decreased antibiotic response
Altered rate of gastric emptying	Most drugs	Metoclopramide	Increased rate of drug absorption
	Most drugs	Anticholinergic drugs	Decreased rate of drug absorption
Displacement of plasma protein binding	Warfarin	Aspirin, furosemide	Possible increased anticoagulation effect
Inhibition of drug metabolism	Warfarin	Cimetidine, omeprazole, trimethoprim–sulfamethoxazole, metronidazole, amiodarone	Increased anticoagulation, bleeding
	Theophylline	Cimetidine, erythromycin, ciprofloxacin, enoxacin	Theophylline toxicity
Induction of drug metabolism	Warfarin	Barbiturates, rifampin, carbamazepine	Decreased anticoagulation
	Phenytoin	Barbiturates, rifampin	Loss of seizure control
	Theophylline	Phenytoin, rifampin, carbamazepine, smoking	Increased dyspnea
Decreased active renal tubular secretion	Methotrexate	Salicylate, penicillins, probenecid, other organic acids	Methotrexate toxicity
Decreased renal or nonrenal clearance	Digoxin	Quinidine, verapamil, amiodarone, diltiazem	Digitalis toxicity
	Lithium	NSAIDs, thiazide diuretics	Lithium toxicity
Pharmacodynamic interactions			
Specific receptor-mediated interactions			
Additive effect on cholinergic receptors	Benztropine	Other anticholinergics (e.g. tricyclic antidepressants, thioridazine, antihistamines)	Confusion, urinary retention
Competitive blockade of β-adrenergic receptors	Albuterol	β-Blockers	Decreased bronchodilator response
Nonspecific pharmacodynamic interactions			
Effects on cardiac conduction	β-Blockers	Verapamil, diltiazem, digoxin	Bradycardia, heart block
Hypokalemia	Digoxin	Diuretics	Digitalis toxicity
Orthostatic hypotension	Diuretics	ACE inhibitors, tricyclic antidepressants, α-blockers, phenothiazines, vasodilators, levodopa	Falls, weakness, syncope
Reduced renal function	ACE inhibitors	NSAIDs	Hyperkalemia, renal impairment
Reduced renal perfusion	Diuretics	NSAIDs	Renal impairment
Effects on platelet function, coagulation, and mucosal integrity	Aspirin	Warfarin	Gastrointestinal bleeding

ACE, angiotensin-converting enzyme; NSAIDs, nonsteroidal antiinflammatory drugs. Adapted from Cusack BJ, Vestal RE. Clinical pharmacology. In: Abrams WB, Beers MH, Berkow R, eds *The Merck manual of geriatrics.* 2nd ed. Whitehouse Station: Merck Research Laboratories, 1995:255–276.

TABLE 55-6. *Predisposing factors to polypharmacy*

Multiple prescribing physicians
Multiple filling pharmacies
Propensity of physicians to prescribe
Expectations of patients
Use of medications for symptoms rather than diagnoses
Reluctance of physicians and patients to discontinue old
  medications
Automatic refills
Multiple over-the-counter medications
Borrowing medications from family and friends

From Vestal RE. Aging and pharmacology. *Cancer* 1997;
80:1302–1310.

timing of administration, which might obviate interference with drug absorption. Understanding what happened may allow the use of approaches for future prevention. Consultation with a clinical pharmacologist or a clinical pharmacist may help improve older patients' drug regimens and minimize drug interactions.

CONCLUSIONS

The complexity of disease and medication use in elderly patients, combined with age-related alterations in pharmacokinetics and pharmacodynamics, places this patient population at particularly high risk for drug interactions. Surprisingly, there are few studies that carefully evaluated drug–drug interactions or other types of drug interactions in this age group. The available data indicate that the age-dependent effects of inducers are inconsistent, whereas uniformly, the effects of inhibitors are similar in young and old age groups. Although simultaneous use of potentially interacting drugs is inevitable and often unavoidable in clinical practice, an awareness of the most important interactions and their adverse effects will help diminish the morbidity experienced by elderly patients.

TABLE 56-7. *Principles of appropriate prescribing*

Obtain a complete history of medications, habits, and diet
Evaluate the need for drug therapy
Know the pharmacology of drugs prescribed
Titrate from smaller initial doses to therapeutic response
Simplify the therapeutic regimen
Encourage treatment adherence and use of home health
  services
Review treatment plan regularly and discontinue drugs no
  longer needed
Use new drugs with caution
Monitor for adverse drug events

From Vestal RE. Aging and pharmacology. *Cancer* 1997;
80:1302–1310.

REFERENCES

1. Chrischilles EA, Foley DJ, Wallace RB, et al. Use of medications by persons 65 and over: data from the established populations for epidemiologic studies of the elderly. *J Gerontol* 1992;47:M137–M144.
2. Vestal RE, Gurwitz JH. Geriatric clinical pharmacology. In: Carruthers GS, Hoffman BB, Nierenberg DW, Melmon KL, eds. *Melmon and Morrelli's clinical pharmacology: basic principles in therapeutics.* 4th ed. New York: McGraw-Hill, 2000.
3. Cusack BJ, Vestal RE. Clinical pharmacology. In: Abrams WB, Beers MH, Berkow R, eds. *The Merck manual of geriatrics.* 2nd ed. Whitehouse Station: Merck Research Laboratories, 1995:255–276.
4. Cusack BJ, Nielson CP, Vestal RE. Geriatric clinical pharmacology and therapeutics. In: Speight TM, Holford NHG, eds. *Avery's drug treatment.* 4th ed. Auckland: Adis International, 1996:173–223.
5. Wilcox SM, Himmelstein DU, Woolhandler S. Inappropriate drug prescribing for the community-dwelling elderly. *JAMA* 1994;272:292–296.
6. Beers M, Avorn J, Soumerai SB, Everitt DE, Sherman DS, Salem S. Psychoactive medication use in intermediate-care facility residents. *JAMA* 1988;260:3016–3020.
7. Beers MH, Ouslander JG, Fingold SF, et al. Inappropriate medication prescribing in skilled-nursing facilities. *Ann Intern Med* 1992;117:684–689.
8. Eisenberg DM, Kessler RC, Foster C, Norlock FE, Calkins DR, Delbanco TL. Unconventional medicine in the United States: prevalence, costs, and patterns of use. *N Engl J Med* 1993;328:246–252.
9. Zeilmann C. The utilization of herbal remedies by ambulatory Hispanic and non-Hispanic white elderly in New Mexico: presented at the USP Open Conference on Botanicals for Medical and Dietary Uses: Standards and Information Issues, Washington: 1996.
10. Campion EW, Avorn J, Reder VA, Olins NJ. Overmedication of the low-weight elderly. *Arch Intern Med* 1987;147:945–947.
11. Gosney M, Tallis R. Prescription of contraindicated and interacting drugs in elderly patients admitted to hospital. *Lancet* 1984;2:564–567.
12. Vestal RE, Dawson GW. Pharmacology and aging. In: Finch CE, Schneider EL, eds. *Handbook of the biology of aging.* 2nd ed. New York: Van Nostrand Reinhold, 1985:744–819.
13. Montamat SC, Cusack BJ, Vestal RE. Management of drug therapy in the elderly. *N Engl J Med* 1989;321:303–309.
14. Dawling S, Crome P. Clinical pharmacokinetic considerations in the elderly: an update. *Clin Pharmacokinet* 1989;17:236–263.
15. Durnas C, Loi CM, Cusack BJ. Hepatic drug metabolism and aging. *Clin Pharmacokinet* 1990;19:359–389.
16. Parker BM, Cusack BJ. Pharmacology and appropriate prescribing. In: Reuben DB, Yoshikawa TT, Besdine RW, eds. *Geriatrics review syllabus: a core curriculum in geriatric medicine.* Dubuque: Kendall/Hunt Publishing, 1996:29–36.
17. Kinirons MT, Crome P. Clinical pharmacokinetics considerations in the elderly: an update. *Clin Pharmacokinet* 1997;33:302–312.
18. Vestal RE. Aging and pharmacology. *Cancer* 1997;80:1302–1310.
19. Vestal RE, Cusack BJ, Mercer GD, Dawson GW, Park BK. Aging and drug interactions. I: Effect of cimetidine and smoking on the oxidation of theophylline and cortisol in healthy men. *J Pharmacol Exp Ther* 1987;241:488–500.
20. Crowley JJ, Cusack BJ, Jue SG, Koup JR, Park BK, Vestal RE. Aging and drug interactions. II: Effect of phenytoin and smoking on the oxidation of theophylline and cortisol in healthy men. *J Pharmacol Exp Ther* 1988;245:513–523.
21. Loi CM, Parker BM, Cusack BJ, Vestal RE. Aging and drug interactions. III: Individual and combined effects of cimetidine and ciprofloxacin on theophylline metabolism in healthy male and female nonsmokers. *J Pharmacol Exp Ther* 1997;280:627–637.
22. Cusack B, Kelly J, O'Mally K, Noel J, Lavan J, Hogan J. Digoxin in the elderly: pharmacokinetic consequences of old age. *Clin Pharmacol Ther* 1979;25:772–776.
23. Greenblatt DJ, Harmatz JS, Shader RI. Clinical pharmacokinetics of anxiolytics and hypnotics in the elderly: therapeutic considerations. *Clin Pharmacokinet* 1991;21:165–177, 262–273.
24. Vestal RE, McGuire EA, Tobin JD, Andres R, Norris AH, Mezey E. Aging and ethanol metabolism in man. *Clin Pharmacol Ther* 1977;21:343–354.
25. Verbeeck RK, Cardinal J-A, Wallace SM. Effect of age and sex on the

plasma binding of acidic and basic drugs. *Eur J Clin Pharmacol* 1984; 27:91–97.

26. Walter-Sack I, Klotz U. Influence of diet and nutritional status on drug metabolism. *Clin Pharmacokinet* 1996;31:47–64.

27. Woodhouse K, Wynne HA. Age-related changes in hepatic function: implications for drug therapy. *Drugs Aging* 1992;2:243–255.

28. Wynne H, Cope L, Kelly P, Whittingham T, Edwards, Kamali F. The influence of age, liver size and enantiomer concentrations on warfarin requirements. *Br J Clin Pharmacol* 1995;40:203–207.

29. Kolars JC, Lown KS, Schmiedlin-Ren P, et al. CYP3A4 gene expression in human gut epithelium. *Pharmacogenetics* 1994;4:247–259.

30. Wynne HA, Kamali F, Edwards C, Long A, Kelly P. Effect of ageing upon warfarin dose requirements: a longitudinal study. *Age Ageing* 1991;25:429–431.

31. Knodell RG, Dubey RK, Wildinson GR, Guengerich FP. Oxidative metabolism of hexobarbital in human liver: relationship to polymorphic S-mephenytoin 4-hydroxylation. *J Pharmacol Exp Ther* 1988:245:845–849.

32. Chandler MHH, Scott SR, Blouin RA. Age-associated stereoselective alterations in hexobarbital metabolism. *Clin Pharmacol Ther* 1988;43:436–441.

33. Klotz U, Avant GR, Hoyumpa A, Schenker S, Wilkinson GR. The effects of age and liver disease on the disposition and elimination of diazepam in adult man. *J Clin Invest* 1975;55:347–359.

34. May DG, Porter J, Wilkinson GR, Branch RA. Frequency distribution of dapsone *N*-hydroxylase: a putative probe for P4503A4 activity in a Caucasian population. *Clin Pharmacol Ther* 1994;55:492–500.

35. O'Shea D, Davis SN, Kim RB, Wilkinson GR. Effect of fasting and obesity in humans on the 6-hydroxylation of chlorzoxazone: a putative probe for CYP2E1 activity. *Clin Pharmacol Ther* 1996;56:359–367.

36. Kim R, O'Shea D, Wilkinson GR. Relationship in healthy subjects between CYP2E1 genetic polymorphism and the 6-hydroxylation of chlorzoxazone: a putative measure of CYP2E1. *Pharmacogenetics* 1994;4:162–165.

37. Miglioli PA, Pivetta P, Strazzabosco M, Orlando R, Okolicsanyi L, Palatini P. Effect of age on single and multiple dose pharmacokinetics of erythromycin. *Eur J Clin Pharmacol* 1990;39:161–164.

38. Robertson DR, Waller DG, Renwick AG, George CF. Age related changes in the pharmacokinetics and pharmacodynamics of nifedipine. *Br J Clin Pharmacol* 1988;25:297–305.

39. Vestal RE, Norris AH, Tobin JD, Cohen BH, Shock NW, Andres R. Antipyrine metabolism in man: influence of age, alcohol, caffeine and smoking. *Clin Pharmacol Ther* 1975;18:425–432.

40. Thomas JA. Drug-nutrient interactions. *Nutr Rev* 1995;53:271–282.

41. Steiner E, Bertilsson L, Säwe J, Ingegärd B, Sjöqvist F. Polymorphic debrisoquin hydroxylation in 757 Swedish subjects. *Clin Pharmacol Ther* 1988;44:431–435.

42. Siegmund W, Hanke W, Zschiesche M, Franke G, Biebler KE, Wilke A. *N*-acetylation and debrisoquine type oxidation polymorphism in Caucasians—with reference to age and sex. *Int J Clin Pharmacol Ther Toxicol* 1990;28:504–509.

43. Laurent-Kenesi MA, Jacqz-Aigrain E, Lejonc JL, Jaillon P, Funck-Brentano C. Assessment of CYP2D6 activity in very elderly healthy subjects. *Fund Clin Pharmacol* 1996;10:158–159.

44. Korrapati MR, Sorkin JD, Andres R, et al. Acetylator phenotype in relation to age and gender in the Baltimore Longitudinal Study of Aging. *J Clin Pharmacol* 1997;37:83–91.

45. Wynne HA, Cope LH, James OFW, Rawlins MD, Woodhouse KW. The effect of age and frailty upon acetanilide clearance in man. *Age Ageing* 1989;18:415–418.

46. Lindeman RD. Changes in renal function with aging: implications for treatment. *Drugs Aging* 1992;2:423–431.

47. Lamy P. Physiological changes due to age: pharmacodynamic changes of drug action and implications for therapy. *Drugs Aging* 1991;1:385–404.

48. Scarpace PJ, Tumer N, Mader SL. β-Adrenergic function in aging: basic mechanisms and clinical implications. *Drugs Aging* 1991;1:116–129.

49. Vestal RE, Wood AJJ, Shand DG. Reduced β-adrenoceptor sensitivity in the elderly. *Clin Pharmacol Ther* 1979;26:181–186.

50. Ford GA, James OFW. Effect of "autonomic blockade" on cardiac β-adrenergic chronotropic responsiveness in healthy young, healthy elderly and endurance-trained elderly subjects. *Clin Sci* 1994;87:297–302.

51. Suteparuk S, Nies AS, Andros E, Gerber JG. The role of adenosine in promoting cardiac β-adrenergic subsensitivity in aging humans. *J Gerontol* 1995;50A:B128–B134.

52. Connolly MJ, Crowley JJ, Charan NB, Nielson CP, Vestal RE. Impaired bronchodilator response to albuterol in healthy elderly men and women. *Chest* 1995;108:401–406.

53. Greenblatt DJ, Allen MD, Shader RI. Toxicity of high-dose flurazepam in the elderly. *Clin Pharmacol Ther* 1977;21:355–361.

54. MacDonald JB, MacDonald ET. Nocturnal femoral fractures and continued widespread use of barbiturate hypnotics. *Br Med J* 1977;2:483–485.

55. Ray W. Psychotropic drugs and injuries in the elderly: a review. *J Clin Pharmacol* 1992;12:386–396.

56. von Moltke LL, Greenblatt DJ, Shader RI. Clinical pharmacokinetics of antidepressants in the elderly: therapeutic implications. *Clin Pharmacokinet* 1993;24:141–160.

57. Abernethy DR, Greenblatt DJ, Shader DJ. Imipramine and desipramine disposition in the elderly. *J Pharmacol Exp Ther* 1985;232:183–188.

58. Skerritt U, Evans R, Montgomery SA. Selective serotonin reuptake inhibitors in older patients: a tolerability perspective. *Drugs Aging* 1997;10:209–218.

59. Sproule BA, Naranjo CA, Brenner Ke, Hassan PC. Selective serotonin reuptake inhibitors and CNS drug interactions: a critical review of the evidence. *Clin Pharmacokinet* 1997;33:454–471.

60. Bellville JW, Forrest WH, Miller E, Brown BW. Influence of age on pain relief from analgesics: a study of postoperative patients. *JAMA* 1971;217:1835–1841.

61. Kaiko RF. Age and morphine analgesia in cancer patients with postoperative pain. *Clin Pharmacol Ther* 1980;28:823–826.

62. Berkowitz BA, Ngai SH, Yang JC, Hempstead J, Spector S. The disposition of morphine in surgical patients. *Clin Pharmacol Ther* 1975;17:629–635.

63. Stanski DR, Greenblatt DJ, Lowenstein E. Kinetics of intravenous and intramuscular morphine. *Clin Pharmacol Ther* 1978;24:52–59.

64. Owen JA, Sitar DS, Berger L, Brownell L, Duke PC, Mitenko PA. Age-related morphine kinetics. *Clin Pharmacol Ther* 1983;34:364–368.

65. Scott JC, Stanski DR. Decreased fentanyl and alfentanil dose requirements with age: a simultaneous pharmacokinetic and pharmacodynamic evaluation. *J Pharmacol Exp Ther* 1987;240:159–166.

66. Nolan L, O'Malley K. Prescribing for the elderly. I: Sensitivity of the elderly to adverse drug reactions. *J Am Geriatr Soc* 1988;36:142–149.

67. Gurwitz JH, Avorn J. The ambiguous relation between aging and adverse drug reactions. *Ann Intern Med* 1991;114:956–966.

68. Grymonpre RE, Mitenko PA, Sitar DS, Aoki FY, Montgomery PR. Drug-associated hospital admissions in older medical patients. *J Am Geriatr Soc* 1988;36:1092–1098.

69. Hanlon JT, Schmader KE, Koronkowski MJ, et al. Adverse drug events in high risk older outpatients. *J Am Geriatr Soc* 1997;45:945–948.

70. Phister JE, Jue SG, Cusack BJ. Problems in the use of anticancer drugs in the elderly. *Drugs* 1989;37:551–565.

71. Lamy PP. The elderly and drug interactions. *J Am Geriatr Soc* 1986;34:586–592.

72. Simonson W, Pratt CC. Pharmacist's perceptions of geriatric pharmacy practice. *Drug Intell Clin Pharm* 1983;17:134–138.

73. Armstrong WA Jr, Driever CW, Hays RL. Analysis of drug-drug interactions in geriatric population. *Am J Hosp Pharm* 1980;37:385–387.

74. Blaschke TF, Cohen SN, Tatro DS, Rubin PC. Drug-drug interactions and aging. In: Jarvik LF, Greenblatt DJ, Harman D, eds. *Clinical pharmacology and the aged patient (Aging, Vol 16)*. New York: Raven Press, 1981:11–26.

75. Lamy P. Drug interactions and the elderly. *J Gerontol Nurs* 1986;12:36–37.

76. Kurfess JF, Dotson RL. Drug interactions in the elderly. *J Fam Pract* 1987;25:477–488.

77. Davidson KW, Kahn A, Price RD. Reduction of adverse drug reactions by computerized drug interaction screening. *J Fam Pract* 1987;4:371–375.

78. Tamai IY, Strome S, Marshall CE, Mooradian AD. Analysis of drug-drug interactions among nursing home residents. *Am J Hosp Pharm* 1989;46:1567–1569.

79. Bergendal L, Friberg A, Schaffrath AM. Potential drug-drug interactions in 5,125 mostly elderly out-patients in Gothenburg, Sweden. *Pharm World Sci* 1995;17:152–157.

80. Haumschild MJ, Ward ES, Bishop JM, Haumschild MS. Pharmacy-

based computer system for monitoring and reporting drug interactions. *Am J Hosp Pharm* 1987;44:345–348.

81. Vestal RE, Cusack BJ, Crowley, Loi CM. Aging and the response to inhibition and induction of theophylline metabolism. *Exp Gerontol* 1993;28:421–433.

82. Salem SAM, Rajjayabun P, Shepherd AMM, Stevenson IH. Reduced induction of drug metabolism in the elderly. *Age Ageing* 1978;7:68–73.

83. Pearson MW, Roberts CJC. Drug induction of hepatic enzymes in the elderly. *Age Ageing* 1984;13:313–316.

84. Twum-Barima Y, Finnigan T, Habsh AI, Cape RDT, Carruthers SG. Impaired enzyme induction by rifampicin in the elderly. *Br J Clin Pharmacol* 1984;17:595–597.

85. Herman RJ, Biolliaz J, Shaheen O, Wood AJJ, Wilkinson GR. Induction of propranolol metabolism by rifampin in the elderly. *Acta Pharmacol Toxicol* 1986;59(suppl V):102.

86. Divoll M, Greenblatt DJ, Abernethy DR, Shader RI. Cimetidine impairs clearance of antipyrine and desmethyldiazepam in the elderly. *J Am Geriatr Soc* 1982;30:684–689.

87. Adebayo GI, Coker AHB. Cimetidine inhibition of theophylline elimination: the influence of adult age and the time course. *Biopharm Drug Dispos* 1987;8:149–158.

88. Feely J, Pereira L, Guy E, Hockings N. Factors affecting the response to inhibition of drug metabolism by cimetidine—dose response and sensitivity of elderly and induced subjects. *Br J Clin Pharmacol* 1984;17:77–81.

89. Vestal RE, Cusack BJ. Pharmacology and aging. In: Schneider EL, Rowe JW, eds. *Handbook of the biology of aging*. 3rd ed. San Diego: Academic Press, 1990:349–383.

90. Crowley JJ, Cusack BJ, Jue SG, Koup JR, Vestal RE. Cigarette smoking and theophylline metabolism: effects of phenytoin. *Clin Pharmacol Ther* 1987;42:334–340.

91. Shannon M, Lovejoy FH Jr. The influence of age vs peak serum concentration on life-threatening events after chronic theophylline intoxication. *Arch Intern Med* 1990;150:2045–2048.

92. Seymour RM, Routledge PA. Important drug-drug interactions in the elderly. *Drugs Aging* 1998;12:485–494.

93. Gaudry SE, Sitar DS, Smyth DD, McKenzie JK, Aoki FY. Gender and age as factors in the inhibition of renal clearance of amantadine by quinine and quinidine. *Clin Pharmacol Ther* 1993;54:23–27.

94. Kivistö KT, Droemer HK, Eichelbaum M. The role of human cytochrome P450 enzymes in the metabolism of anticancer agents: implications for drug interactions. *Br J Clin Pharmacol* 1995;40:523–530.

95. Korrapati MR, Vestal RE. Alcohol and medications in the elderly: complex interactions. In: Beresford T, Gomberg E, eds. *Alcohol and aging*. New York: Oxford University Press, 1995:42–55.

96. Fraser AG. Pharmacokinetic interactions between alcohol and other drugs. *Clin Pharmacokinet* 1997;33:79–90.

97. Adams WL. Potential for adverse drug-alcohol interactions among retirement community residents. *J Am Geriatr Soc* 1995;43:1021–1025.

98. Forster LE, Pollow R, Stoller EP. Alcohol use and potential risk for alcohol-related adverse drug reactions among community based elderly. *J Community Health* 1993;18:225–239.

99. Shorr RI, Ray WA, Daugherty JR, Griffin MR. Concurrent use of nonsteroidal anti-inflammatory drugs and oral anticoagulants places elderly persons at high risk for hemorrhagic peptic ulcer disease. *Arch Intern Med* 1993;153:1665–1670.

SECTION VII

Appendix

Other Drugs

Kenneth E. Thummel and René H. Levy

There are numerous drugs for which the potential to cause or be susceptible to a metabolically based drug interaction has not been addressed in preceding chapters. Except for specific compounds discussed in a later section of this chapter, their absence indicates either no known mechanistic basis for an interaction, or insufficient availability of data for comment.

DRUGS FOR WHICH P450S DO NOT CONTRIBUTE SIGNIFICANTLY TO THEIR ELIMINATION

For many drugs, metabolism is not a significant mode of elimination; this includes a number of the antibiotics (e.g., aminoglycosides, penicillins, and cephalosporins), bisphosphonates (e.g., alendronate, residronate, and telidronate), anticholinesterases (e.g., pyridostigmine and neostigmine), the uricosuric agents probenecid and sulfinpyrazone, renal loop diuretics (e.g., furosemide, bumetanide, torsemide, and ethacrynic acid) and angiotensin-converting enzyme (ACE) inhibitors (captopril and lisinopril). Thus they are not the objects of enzyme inhibition or induction. However, some, such as fluconazole and some of the fluoroquinolone antibiotics, are eliminated primarily by the kidney but inhibit hepatic CYP2C9/3A4 and CYP1A2, respectively. These precipitants of drug interactions have been presented within the relevant drug classes. Some renally cleared drugs also may alter the function of drug transporters or be susceptible to the effects of transporter inhibitors/inducers. Except for substrates or modifiers of P-glycoprotein (see Chapter 11), discussions of this type of drug–drug inter-

action have not been included in the scope of this edition of this textbook.

Other drugs, such as substrates for plasma or hepatic/intestinal esterases (e.g., the neuromuscular blockers succinylcholine, pancuronium, and tubocurarine), the antiplatelet drugs clopidogrel and aspirin, and miscellaneous drugs such as reserpine, procaine, carbimazole, methylphenidate, and misoprostil, are all metabolized predominantly by an enzyme family that does not appear to be susceptible to significant modification of enzyme expression or activity.

Substrates for the phase II enzymes are potential objects and precipitants of drug–drug interactions, either through direct competition for the enzyme active site or by indirect competition for a limited cofactor pool (see Chapters 13–15). This includes the N-acetyltransferases, its cofactor acetyl coenzyme A (CoA), and representative substrates (isoniazid, ethionamide, aminosalicylic acid, and dapsone) that are used in the treatment of tuberculosis, *Mycobacterium-avium* complex (MAC), or leprosy, and some of the sympathomimetic agents (e.g., dopamine, dobutamine, and isoproterenol) that are substrates for catechol O-methyl transferase, with its cofactor S-adenosyl methionine. Similarly, substrates for the sulfotransferases (e.g., ethinyl estradiol, acetaminophen, lamotrigine, metoclopramide, terbutaline, and other sympathomimetic catecholamines), as well as substrates for the family of glucuronosyl transferases (e.g., mycophenolic acid, acetaminophen, zidovudine, minoxidil, metoclopramide, lorazepam, diflunisal, valproic acid, propofol, morphine and other structurally related opioid analgesic agents), may be the object of interactions with other drugs that compete for binding to the enzyme or use of cofactor (PAPS and UDPGA, respectively). However, metabolic interactions involving phase II enzymes are generally less frequent compared with those involving P450 enzymes and not so well understood in terms of kinetic mechanisms and predictability.

K. E. Thummel and R. H. Levy: Department of Pharmaceutics, University of Washington, Box 357610, H272 Health Sciences Building, Seattle, Washington 98195-7610

DRUGS WITH LIMITED INFORMATION ON P450 MODULATION AND RECENTLY APPROVED DRUGS

Clarithromycin and Erythromycin As a class, the macrolide antibiotics are noted for the inhibitory effects they exert on the clearance of substrates for cytochrome P450 3A4 (see Chapter 46). Less importance is given to their own susceptibility to modulators of drug clearance processes. However, some clinically significant interactions by this mechanism have been described, the best characterized of which involves clarithromycin. Clarithromycin is eliminated by both renal and non-renal routes. Approximately 20-40% of an oral dose is excreted unchanged into urine (1). The rest of the dose is converted primarily into an active metabolite, 14-hydroxy clarithromycin, and an inactive metabolite, *N*-demethyl clarithromycin (1). The metabolites are excreted into bile, accounting for up to 50% of the clarithromycin dose (2). Formation of the hydroxy and desmethyl metabolites appears to be catalyzed exclusively by the CYP3A subfamily (3). These reactions appear to be saturable *in vivo*, as evidenced by marked dose-dependent elimination kinetics (2). Because of the role of CYP3A in the elimination of clarithromycin, one can expect significant pharmacokinetic and clinically meaningful interactions with CYP3A modulators. For example, both rifampin and rifabutin induce the clearance of clarithromycin (4), whereas the potent CYP3A inhibitor ritonavir markedly increases and decreases plasma concentrations of clarithromycin and 14-hydroxy clarithromycin, respectively (5). However, in both cases a clinical interpretation of the interaction is complicated by the pharmacological activity of the metabolite.

Erythromycin also undergoes significant hepatic CYP3A-dependent metabolism, yielding an *N*-demethyl metabolite. Indeed, the demethylation of erythromycin forms the biochemical basis for the Erythromycin Breath Test, an *in vivo* probe for hepatic CYP3A activity (6). The desmethyl metabolite of erythromycin is excreted into bile and fecal elimination accounts for a significant fraction of the dose. Numerous studies with the Erythromycin Breath Test have demonstrated the anticipated effects of CYP3A inducers [e.g., rifampin, dexamethasone (6)] and inhibitors [e.g., troleandomycin (6), ketoconazole (7), delavirdine (8)] on the *N*-demethylation pathway. However, little has been written on the consequences of these interactions in clinical practice.

Rifampin and Rifabutin The macrocyclic antibiotics agents, rifampin and rifabutin, are eliminated from the body to varying degrees by both metabolic and excretory routes. Rifampin is deacetylated by esterases to an active metabolite and both parent drug and metabolite are excreted into bile (9). The drug undergoes enterohepatic recycling such that most of the dose is eventually recovered as metabolite in feces and urine. Rifampin clearance is increased with multiple dose administration, suggest-

ing auto-induction of the esterase or transport pathways. Rifabutin also undergoes *O*-deacetylation at the 25-position but, in addition, it is metabolized by CYP3A to several metabolites: 27-*O*-demethylrifabutin and 20-, 31-, 32-hydroxyrifabutin (10). CYP3A pathways of elimination appear to be significant, since known inhibitors of the enzyme (i.e., clarithromycin and fluconazole) elevate rifabutin levels *in vivo* (11-13). These changes are reportedly sufficient to warrant dose adjustment. It should also be remembered that both rifampin and rifabutin will alter the metabolic clearance of numerous drugs through induction of hepatic and intestinal biotransformation enzymes. These interactions are discussed in Chapter 52.

A number of drugs marketed recently provide new modalities for the treatment of human disease. As such, there are relatively few members in the drug class, and there is generally only limited peer-reviewed information available. The following is a brief overview of some of these new drugs that have been identified as substrates/inhibitors of cytochrome P450.

Zafirlukast (Accolate; Zeneca) is an orally active selective cysteinyl leukotriene-1 receptor antagonist that blocks the contraction of bronchial smooth muscle triggered by the release of endogenous leukotrienes (e.g., LTD$_4$) during asthmatic attacks. In animals, zafirlukast undergoes hydrolysis of the amide linkage at the 5-aminoindole position and various aromatic and aliphatic hydroxylations (14). According to the Physician's Desk Reference (15), zafirlukast undergoes undefined CYP2C9-mediated hydroxylation(s) in humans, and metabolism is the predominant route of its elimination. Although no *in vivo* studies have been reported, inhibition of zafirlukast metabolic clearance by fluconazole and induction by rifampin may occur. The clinical consequences of such interactions are unknown.

Zafirlukast reportedly is also a potent inhibitor of CYP2C9 and CYP3A4, based on results from interaction experiments with human liver microsomes and pharmacokinetic studies in healthy volunteers (15). After multiple-dose administration, it inhibited the metabolic clearance of the CYP2C9 substrate warfarin but, surprisingly, not the CYP3A4 substrate terfenadine. Interestingly, a significant inhibitory interaction between zafirlukast and theophylline was recently reported (16). This finding suggests that zafirlukast might also be an inhibitor of CYP1A2, although it showed lower inhibitory potency for this enzyme *in vitro* compared with its effect on CYP2C9 and CYP3A4.

Montelukast (Singulair; Merck) is also a cysteinyl leukotriene-1 receptor antagonist used for the treatment of asthma. It undergoes diastereomeric *S*-oxidation, benzylic hydroxylation at position-21, and methyl hydroxylation at position-36 of the molecule (17,18). Additional metabolites have been reported, including an acyl glucuronide, a 25-hydroxy alcohol, and a dicarboxylic acid derived from secondary oxidation of the primary 36-

hydroxymethyl metabolite (18). Formation of the major, primary metabolite (36-hydroxymontelukast) is catalyzed by CYP2C9, whereas the sulfoxide and 21-hydroxymontelukast are formed by CYP3A4 (17). *In vivo* interaction studies reveal induction of montelukast clearance by phenobarbital (an inducer of CYP3A4 and CYP2C9 in human hepatocytes). Although undocumented, inhibition of montelukast clearance by the potent CYP3A4 inhibitors ketoconazole and erythromycin, as well as the CYP2C9 inhibitor fluconazole, is predicted.

Zileuton (Zyflo; Abbott) is a potent inhibitor of 5-lipoxygenase, a mediator of leukotriene biosynthesis and smooth muscle contraction in asthma. It is eliminated from the body by both conjugative and oxidative metabolic processes. *O*-glucuronidation is the dominant metabolic pathway *in vivo* (19), and the metabolites are formed stereoselectively from zileuton isomers (20). An unusual minor pathway for zileuton elimination involves formation of an inactive *N*-dehydroxy metabolite. Additional zileuton metabolites include a sulfoxide formed primarily by CYP3A4 and a ring-hydroxylated metabolite formed primarily by CYP1A2 (21). Zileuton appears to be an inhibitor of CYP3A4 and CYP1A2 *in vivo*, based on a respective weak to moderate inhibition of terfenadine and theophylline clearance (22,23). Interestingly, zileuton was also reported to have reduced by half the metabolic clearance of propranolol (22), a drug whose clearance is mediated largely through glucuronidation, CYP2D6-catalyzed 4-hydroxylation, and CYP1A2-catalyzed *N*-deisopropylation. Although the interaction may be mediated through the P450 isozymes, it is also possible that the interaction involves competition for a glucuronosyl transferase.

Cisapride (Propulsid; Janssen) stimulates gastric motility presumably by enhancing the release of acetylcholine at the myenteric plexus or acting as an agonist at the 5HT$_4$ (serotonin) receptor. Because of its favorable efficacy/toxicity profile in comparison to metoclopramide, it is considered the drug of choice for treatment of various small bowel–motility disorders. It is cleared from the body primarily by *N*-demethylation to norcisapride (24). Other metabolic pathways include *O*-dealkylation, aromatic hydroxylation, and formation of an N^4-glucuronide. There is little peer-reviewed information available on the enzyme(s) catalyzing cisapride demethylation, but the manufacturer states that it is a CYP3A4-mediated process (25). This information is consistent with a list of notable pharmacokinetic interactions with concomitantly administered drugs, including ketoconazole, itraconazole, fluconazole, miconazole, erythromycin, troleandomycin, and clarithromycin (26), and with grapefruit juice (27). Elevation of cisapride blood levels with most of these CYP3A4 inhibitors has been associated with prolongation of the cardiac QT interval and, in some cases, development of a potentially fatal arrhythmia (28–31). These findings have led to a black-box warning by the manufacturer against the concomitant administration of cisapride with recognized CYP3A4 inhibitors (25).

Finasteride (Proscar and Propecia; Merck) is a potent inhibitor of type II 5α-reductase that is used in the treatment of benign prostatic hyperplasia and male-pattern baldness. It is eliminated from the body almost exclusively through CYP3A4-mediated oxidation of the *t*-butyl side chain (19,20). A minor metabolic pathway involves 6α-hydroxylation. The primary ω-hydroxy metabolite is oxidized further to a monocarboxylic acid that is excreted in urine and feces. Given the role of CYP3A4 in the clearance of finasteride, pharmacokinetic interactions with ketoconazole, erythromycin, and other CYP3A4 inhibitors are expected. However, such interactions might not be clinically significant because the drug appears to be relatively safe under aggressive dosing conditions (34).

Flutamide (Eulexin; Schering Corp.) is a nonsteroidal antiandrogen used in the management of prostatic carcinoma. It is extensively metabolized and yields a number of urinary products. Formation of the major circulating and active metabolite, 2-hydroxyflutamide (35,36), is catalyzed principally by CYP1A2 (37). Flutamide can cause anomalous adverse reactions in cancer patients, including hepatic toxicity and methemoglobinemia. It has been suggested that some of these events may be related to increased or decreased metabolic activity through the CYP1A2 pathway (37). Thus inhibitors or inducers of CYP1A2, such as the fluoroquinolone antibiotics and cigarette smoking, respectively, may influence the frequency of events, although there are no clinical data in support of this position.

Sildenafil (Viagra; Pfizer) is a cyclic guanosine monophosphate (cGMP)-specific phosphodiesterase type 5 inhibitor approved for the treatment of male erectile dysfunction. It undergoes extensive biotransformation to a number of metabolites, including an active, circulating piperazine desmethyl metabolite that contributes to the overall pharmacologic effect, and an inactive piperazine *N,N'*-desethyl metabolite (38). CYP3A4 (major) and CYP2C9 (minor) are reported to be the principal catalysts of sildenafil metabolism (39). Not surprisingly, CYP3A4 inhibitors (e.g., erythromycin and cimetidine) reduce the oral clearance of sildenafil when coadministered with the drug (40). Interestingly, an analysis of phase II/III clinical data suggests no relation between the use of CYP3A4 inhibitors and the frequency of adverse events (40,41). Nonetheless, a low starting dose is recommended in patients taking known CYP3A4 inhibitors (40). Given the nature of sildenafil clearance, coadministration of a standard dose with known CYP3A4 inducers such as rifampin might be expected to result in reduced efficacy.

Sibutramine (Meridia; Knoll Pharmaceuticals) is an inhibitor of monoamine reuptake used in the treatment of obesity. It undergoes extensive CYP3A4-dependent first pass metabolism after oral administration, yielding a primary and secondary amine, each possessing pharmacologic activity (42). These molecules undergo further hydroxylation to pharmacologically inactive metabolites. The manufacturer reports that concomitant ketoconazole and erythromycin administration increased the area under the curve (AUC) of sibutramine *in vivo*, but only modestly (58% and 14%, respectively) in comparison to the effect of these inhibitors on other highly extracted CYP3A substrates (e.g., terfenadine and midazolam). Thus although there is the potential for an inhibitory drug–drug interaction, the clinical significance appears to be minimal. Because the pharmacologic activity of sibutramine resides primarily with its metabolites, coadministration with a CYP3A4 inducer may have no significant clinical effect, unless alternative pathways for the clearance of the active metabolites are preferentially induced.

REFERENCES

1. Ferrero JL, Bopp BA, Marsh KC, et al. Metabolism and disposition of clarithromycin in man. *Drug Metab Dispos* 1990;18:441–446.
2. Fraschini F, Scaglione F, Demartini G. Clarithromycin clinical pharmacokinetics. *Clin Pharmacokinet* 1993;25:189–204.
3. Rodrigues AD, Roberts EM, Mulford DJ, Yao Y, Ouellet D. Oxidative metabolism of clarithromycin in the presence of human liver microsomes. Major role for the cytochrome P4503A (CYP3A) subfamily. *Drug Metab Dispos* 1997;25:623–630.
4. Wallace RJ Jr, Brown BA, Griffith DE, Girard W, Tanaka K. Reduced serum levels of clarithromycin in patients treated with multidrug regimens including rifampin or rifabutin for Mycobacterium avium-M. intracellulare infection. *J Infect Dis* 1995;171:747–750.
5. Ouellet D, Hsu A, Granneman GR, et al. Pharmacokinetic interaction between ritonavir and clarithromycin. *Clin Pharmacol Ther* 1998;64: 355–362.
6. Watkins PB, Murray SA, Winkelman LG, Heuman DM, Wrighton SA, Guzelian PS. Erythromycin breath test as an assay of glucocoricoid-inducible liver cytochromes P-450. Studies in rats and patients. *J Clin Invest* 1989;83:688–697.
7. Jamis-Dow CA, Pearl ML, Watkins PB, Blake DS, Klecker RW, Collins JM. Predicting drug interactions in vivo from experiments in vitro. Human studies with paclitaxel and ketoconazole. *Am J Clin Oncol* 1997;20:592–599.
8. Cheng C-L, Smith DE, Carver PL, et al. Steady-state pharmacokinetics of delavirdine in HIV-positive patients: effect on erythromycin breath test. *Clin Pharmacol Ther* 1997;61:531–543.
9. Mandell GL, Petri WA. Antimicrobial agents: drugs used in the chemotherapy of tuberculosis, mycobacterium avium complex disease, and leprosy. In: *Goodman and Gilman's the pharmacological basis of therapeutics.* New York: McGraw-Hill, 1996, pp. 1155–1174.
10. Iatsimirskaia E, Tulebaev S, Storozhuk E, et al. Metabolism of rifabutin in human enterocyte and liver microsomes: kinetic paramters, identification of enzyme systems, and drug interactions with macrolides and antifungal agents. *Clin Pharmacol Ther* 1997;61:554–562.
11. Apseloff G, Foulds G, LaBoy-Goral L, Willavize S, Vincent J. Comparison of azithromycin and clarithromycin in their interactions with rifabutin in healthy volunteers. *J Clin Pharmacol* 1998;38:830–835.
12. Hafner R, Bethel J, Power M, et al. Tolerance and pharmacokinetic interactions of rifabutin and clarithromycin in human immunodeficiency virus-infected volunteers. *Antimicrob Agents Chemother* 1998; 42:631–639.
13. Trapnell CB, Narang PK, Li R, Lavelle JP. Increased plasma rifabutin levels with concomitant fluconazole therapy in HIV-infected patients. *Ann Intern Med* 1996;124:573–576.
14. Savidge RD, Bui KH, Birmingham BK, Morse JL, Spreen RC. Metabolism and excretion of zafirlukast in dogs, rats, and mice. *Drug Metab Dispos* 1998;26:1069–1076.
15. *Physicians' desk reference.* 53rd ed. Montvale, NJ: Medical Economics Company, 1999:3402–3204.
16. Katial RH, Stelzle RC, Bonner MW, Marino M, Cantilena LR, Smith LJ. A drug interaction between zafirlukast and theophylline. *Arch Intern Med* 1998;158:1713–1715.
17. Chiba M, Xu X, Nishime JA, Balani SK, Lin JH. Hepatic microsomal metabolism of montelukast, a potent leukotriene D_4 receptor antagonist, in humans. *Drug Metab Dispos* 1997;25:1022–1031.
18. Balani SK, Xu X, Pratha V, et al. Metabolic profiles of montelukast sodium (Singulair), a potent cysteinyl leukotriene1 receptor antagonist, in human plasma and bile. *Drug Metab Dispos* 1997;25:1282–1287.
19. Wong SL, Awni WM, Cavenaugh J, El-Shourbagy T, Locke CS, Dubé LM. The pharmacokinetics of single oral doses of zileuton 200 to 800 mg, its enantiomers, and its metabolites, in normal volunteers. *Clin Pharmacokinet* 1995;29(suppl 2):9–21.
20. Sweeny DJ, Nellans HN. Stereoselective glucuronidation of zileuton isomers by human hepatic microsomes. *Drug Metab Dispos* 1995;23: 149–153.
21. Machinist JM, Mayer MD, Shet MS, Ferrero JL, Rodrigues AD. Identification of the human liver cytochrome P450 enzymes involved in the metabolism of zileuton (ABT-077) and its N-dehydroxylated metabolite, Abbott-66193. *Drug Metab Dispos* 1995;23:1163–1174.
22. *Physicians' desk reference.* 53rd ed. Montvale, NJ: Medical Economics Company, 1999:481–483.
23. Granneman GR, Braekman RA, Locke CS, Cavanaugh JH, Dubé LM, Awni WM. Effect of zileuton on theophylline pharmacokinetics. *Clin Pharmacokinet* 1995;29(suppl 2):77–83.
24. Meuldermans W, Peer AV, Hendrickx J, et al. Excretion and biotransformation of cisapride in dogs and humans after oral administration. *Drug Metab Dispos* 1988;16:403–409.
25. *Physicians' desk reference.* 53rd ed. Montvale, NJ: Medical Economics Company, 1999:1430–1432.
26. Bedford TA, Rowbotham DJ. Cisapride: drug interactions of clinical significance. *Drug Safety* 1996;15:167–175.
27. Gross AS, Goh YD, Addison RS, Shenfield GM. Influence of grapefruit juice on cisapride pharmacokinetics. *Clin Pharmacol Ther* 1999;65: 395–401.
28. Wysowski DK, Bacsanyi J. Cisapride and fatal arrhythmia. *N Engl J Med* 1996;335:290–291.
29. Haarst ADV, Klooster GAEVT, Gerven JMAV, et al. The influence of cisapride and clarithromycin on QT intervals in volunteers. *Clin Pharmacol Ther* 1998;64:542–546.
30. Piquette RK. Torsades de pointes induced by cisapride/clarithromycin interaction. *Ann Pharmacother* 1999;33:22–26.
31. Thomas AR, Chan LN, Bauman JL, Olopade CO. Prolongation of the QT interval related to cisapride-diltiazem interaction. *Pharmacotherapy* 1998;18:381–385.
32. Huskey SW, Dean DC, Miller RR, Rasmusson GH, Chiu S-HL. Identification of human cytochrome P450 isozymes responsible for the in vitro oxidative metabolism of finasteride. *Drug Metab Dispos* 1995;23: 1126–1135.
33. Steiner JF. Clinical pharmacokinetics and pharmacodynamics of finasteride. *Clin Pharmacokinet* 1996;30:16–27.
34. *Physicians' desk reference.* 53rd ed. Montvale, NJ: Medical Economics Company, 1999:1877–1883.
35. Radwanski E, Perentesis G, Symchowicz S, Zampaglione N. Single and multiple dose pharmacokinetic evaluation of flutamide in normal geriatric volunteers. *J Clin Pharmacol* 1989;29:554–558.
36. Anjum S, Swan SK, Lambrecht LJ, et al. Pharmacokinetics of flutamide in patients with renal insufficiency. *Br J Clin Pharmacol* 1999; 47:43–47.
37. Shet MS, McPhaul M, Fisher CW, Stallings NR, Estabrook RW. Metabolism of the antiandrogenic drug (flutamide) by human CYP1A2. *Drug Metab Dispos* 1997;25:1298–1303.
38. Walker DK, Ackland MJ, James GC, et al. Pharmacokinetics and metabolism of sildenafil in mouse, rat, rabbit, dog and man. *Xenobiotica* 1999;29:297–310.
39. *Physicians' desk reference.* 53rd ed. Montvale, NJ: Medical Economics Company, 1999:2424–2427.
40. Zusman RM, Morales A, Glasser DB, Osterloh IH. Overall cardiovascular profile of sildenafil citrate. *Am J Cardiol* 1999;83:35C–44C.
41. Goldenberg MM. Safety and efficacy of sildenafil citrate in the treatment of male erectile dysfunction. *Clin Ther* 1998;20:1033–1048.
42. *Physicians' desk reference.* 53rd ed. Montvale, NJ: Medical Economics Company, 1999:1494–1498.

Drug Interaction Index

General Index

CYP2A6 inhibition, 150
CYP2B6 induction, 153
Skin cancer, 182
Smoking. *See* Cigarette smoking
Soluble epoxide hydrolases, 207–208
Somatostatin
codeine and, 305–306
Sorivudine
5-fluorouracil and, 547
Sotalol
fluoxetine and, 351–352l
Sparteine
codeine and, 306
CYP2D6 reactivity, 88
polymorphism, 87
dextromethorphan and, 300
metabolism, 397
paroxetine and, 570
quinidine and, 603, 605–606
Spiramycin
carbamazepine and, 223
Spironolactone
antipyrine and, 374
digoxin and, 385
metabolism, 372–374
SSRIs.*See* Selective serotonin reuptake
inhibitors
Stavudine
metabolism, 425
zidovudine and, 426, 429
Steady-state blood concentration, 14–16
Stereoisomer interaction, 44–45
Stereospecific metabolism, 44
in elderly, 732
Steroids, 277
cytochrome P450 enzyme induction, 53
drug interactions, 503–504
metabolism, 502–503
therapeutic development, 511
UGT1A7 reactivity, 166
See also specific steroid
tranS-Stilbene oxide
glutathione *S*-transferase reactivity, 179, 180
soluble epoxide hydrolase reactivity, 207
Stomach cancer, 182
Styrene
CYP2B6 interaction, 152
microsomal epoxide hydrolase reactivity, 210
Substrate characteristics, 21–22
cholesterol oxide hydrolase, 206
CYP1A, 66–70
CYP2A6, 147–149
CYP2B6, 151–152
CYP2C, 76–79
CYP2D6, 89
CYP2E1, 102–103, 110
CYP3A, 118
CYP3A5, 117
CYP4A11, 154–155
CYP450 form-selective catalytic activity,
32–33, 53
enzyme interactions predicting inhibitor
interaction, 26
glutathione *S*-transferases, 179
hepoxilin A3 hydrolase, 206
inhibitory profile, 26
leukotriene A4 hydrolase, 207
methyltransferases, 191, 197
microsomal epoxide hydrolase, 210
soluble epoxide hydrolase, 208

sulfotransferases, 191, 192, 195
UDPGTs, 161
UGT1A1, 162–163
UGT1A3,4,5, 164–165
UGT2B, 167
UGT2B7, 168
UGT2B17, 170–171
Substrate concentration
clinical significance, 29
determinants of, 29
enzyme induction modeling, 14–16
major *vs.* minor drug interactions, 4
mathematical modeling, 4–5
Substrate elimination
in enzyme induction, 14–16
identification of enzyme catalysts, 23, 24
in reversible enzyme inhibition, 4–5
Succinylcholine, amphoteracin B and, 639
Sucralfate, digoxin and, 385
Sudden infant death syndrome, 81
Sufentanil
erythromycin and, 312, 619
gestodene and, 312
metabolism, 312
midazolam and, 312
pharmacology, 312
propofol and, 277
troleandomycin and, 312
Suicide inhibitors, 5–7
CYP2E1, 103–104
CYP3A subfamily, 126–127
pharmacokinetic consequences, 12
Sulfadiazine
phenytoin and, 225
Sulfahydryls, 198–200
Sulfamethazine
chlorpropamide and, 532
Sulfamethizole
phenytoin and, 225
tolbutamide and, 534
Sulfamethoxazole
fluconazole and, 637
ketoconazole and, 627
phenytoin and, 225
Sulfaphenazole
CYP2C9 inhibition, 82
dextromethorphan and, 300, 301
losartan and, 361
phenytoin and, 225
theophylline and, 472
tolbutamide and, 9, 534
torsemide and, 372
warfarin and, 24
Sulfaslazine
digoxin and, 385
Sulfinpyrazone, 82
acenocoumarol and, 411
acetaminophen and, 450
phenprocoumon and, 410
theobromine and, 475
theophylline and, 474
torsemide and, 372
warfarin and, 409
Sulfisoxazole
chlorpropamide and, 532
tolbutamide and, 534
Sulfonamide antibiotics, 532
tolbutamide and, 534
Sulfonylurea drugs, 530–531
drug interactions, 540

first generation, 531–536
metformin and, 539
second generation, 536–538
See also specific drug
Sulfonylureas
miconazole and, 629
Sulfotransferases
acetaminophen, 447
biochemistry, 195–196
classification, 191–193
clinical significance, 191, 192, 196, 201
cytosolic catalysis, 192, 195
estrogen, 195, 196
future research prospects, 201
hydroxysteroid, 195, 196
inhibitors, 196
interindividual variation, 194–195
isoform properties, 195–196
phenol, 193–194, 195, 196
structure, 192, 193–194
substrates, 191, 192, 195
Sulindac, 462–463
lithium and, 465
tolbutamide and, 536
Sulpiride
bufuralol and, 586
metabolism, 582
pharmacokinetics, 581
Sumatriptan
drug interactions, 325
furazolidone and, 325
metabolism, 324–325
monoamine oxidase and, 325
monoamine oxidase inhibitors and, 325
pharmacokinetics, 324
procarbazine and, 325
propranolol and, 325
tranylcypromine and, 325

T
Tacrine, 70
cimetidine and, 322–323
CYP1A2 interaction, 322
diazepam and, 323
digoxin and, 323
enoxacin and, 322, 616
fluvoxamine and, 322
furafylline and, 322
haloperidol and, 322
ibuprofen and, 322
metabolism, 321–322
pharmacokinetics, 321
quinidine and, 323
theophylline and, 323
Tacrolimus, 505
clarithromycin and, 617
clotrimazole and, 629
fluconazole and, 636
fluoroquinolones and, 616
itraconazole and, 631–632
ketoconazole and, 624, 626
miconazole and, 628
nifedipine and, 597
verapamil and, 592
Tamoxifen, 103, 126
aminoglutethimide and, 551
bromocriptine and, 551
CYP2B6 interaction, 152
drug interactions, 551
metabolism, 515–517, 551